Basic & Clinical Pharmacology

ninth edition

Edited by

Bertram G. Katzung, MD, PhD
Professor Emeritus
Department of Cellular & Molecular Pharmacology
University of California, San Francisco

Lange Medical Books/McGraw-Hill
Medical Publishing Division

New York   Chicago   San Francisco   Lisbon   London   Madrid   Mexico City
Milan   New Delhi   San Juan   Singapore   Sydney   Toronto

Basic & Clinical Pharmacology, Ninth Edition

34567890 DOC/DOC 098765

Set ISBN: 0-07-141092-9

Book ISBN: 0-07-144097-6

Student Online Resource Center Card: 0-07-144098-4

ISSN: 0891-2033

Notice

Medicine is an ever-changing science. As new research and clinical experience broaden our knowledge, changes in treatment and drug therapy are required. The authors and the publisher of this work have checked with sources believed to be reliable in their efforts to provide information that is complete and generally in accord with the standards accepted at the time of publication. However, in view of the possibility of human error or changes in medical sciences, neither the authors nor the publisher nor any other party who has been involved in the preparation or publication of this work warrants that the information contained herein is in every respect accurate or complete, and they disclaim all responsibility for any errors or omissions or for the results obtained from use of the information contained in this work. Readers are encouraged to confirm the information contained herein with other sources. For example and in particular, readers are advised to check the product information sheet included in the package of each drug they plan to administer to be certain that the information contained in this work is accurate and that changes have not been made in the recommended dose or in the contraindications for administration. This recommendation is of particular importance in connection with new or infrequently used drugs.

This book was set in Garamond by Rainbow Graphics.
The editors were Jennifer Bernstein, Jim Ransom, Janet Foltin, and Barbara Holton.
The production supervisor was Phil Galea.
The index was prepared by Alexandra Nickerson.
RR Donnelley was printer and binder.

This book is printed on acid-free paper.

Contents

iii

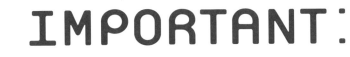

IMPORTANT:

HERE IS YOUR REGISTRATION CODE TO ACCESS YOUR PREMIUM STUDENT ONLINE RESOURCE CENTER.

For key premium online resources you need THIS CODE to gain access. Once the code is entered, you will be able to use the Web resources for the length of your course.

Access is provided if you have purchased a new book. If the registration code is missing from this book, the registration screen on our Website will tell you how to obtain your new code.

Registering for the STUDENT ONLINE RESOURCE CENTER

TO gain access to the STUDENT ONLINE RESOURCE CENTER, simply follow the steps below:

1. USE YOUR WEB BROWSER TO GO TO: http://www.KatzungOnline.com
2. CLICK ON **FIRST TIME USER**.
3. ENTER THE REGISTRATION CODE* PRINTED ON THE RIGHT.
4. AFTER YOU HAVE ENTERED YOUR REGISTRATION CODE, CLICK **REGISTER**.
5. FOLLOW THE INSTRUCTIONS TO SET-UP YOUR PERSONAL UserID AND PASSWORD.
6. WRITE YOUR UserID AND PASSWORD DOWN FOR FUTURE REFERENCE. KEEP IT IN A SAFE PLACE.

Thank you, and welcome to the STUDENT ONLINE RESOURCE CENTER!

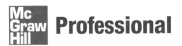

* YOUR REGISTRATION CODE CAN BE USED ONLY ONCE TO ESTABLISH ACCESS. IT IS NOT TRANSFERABLE.

P/N 144098-4 PART OF 0-07-141092-9
KATZUNG: BASIC & CLINICAL PHARMACOLOGY, 9/E.

MCGRAW-HILL
STUDENT ONLINE RESOURCE CENTER

REGISTRATION CODE

BYIA-SSQT-QEJN-LHJU-OORA

 Professional

Preface

This book is designed to provide a complete, authoritative, current, and readable pharmacology textbook for medical, pharmacy, and other health science students. It also offers special features that make it useful to house officers and practicing clinicians.

Information is organized according to the sequence used in many pharmacology courses: basic principles; autonomic drugs; cardiovascular-renal drugs; drugs with important actions on smooth muscle; central nervous system drugs; drugs used to treat inflammation, gout, and diseases of the blood; endocrine drugs; chemotherapeutic drugs; toxicology; and special topics. This sequence builds new information on a foundation of information already assimilated. For example, early presentation of autonomic pharmacology allows students to integrate the physiology and neuroscience they know with the pharmacology they are learning and prepares them to understand the autonomic effects of other drugs. This is especially important for the cardiovascular and central nervous system drug groups. However, chapters can be used equally well in courses that present these topics in a different sequence.

Within each chapter, emphasis is placed on discussion of drug groups and prototypes rather than offering repetitive detail about individual drugs. Selection of the subject matter and the order of its presentation are based on the accumulated experience of teaching this material to thousands of medical, pharmacy, dental, podiatry, nursing, and other health science students.

Major features that make this book especially useful to professional students include sections that specifically address the clinical choice and use of drugs in patients and the monitoring of their effects—in other words, *clinical pharmacology* is an integral part of this text. Lists of the commercial preparations available, including trade and generic names and dosage formulations, are provided at the end of each chapter for easy reference by the house officer or practitioner writing a chart order or prescription.

Significant revisions in this edition include the following:

- Major revisions of the chapters on antiarrhythmic drugs, antidiabetic drugs, anthelmintics, antiviral drugs, and drugs used for gastrointestinal conditions
- New figures, most in color, that help to clarify important concepts in pharmacology
- Many descriptions of important developments based on genetically modified mice ("knockout" and "knockin" mice), a research tool of great importance in pharmacology
- Continuing expansion of the coverage of general concepts relating to receptors and listings of newly discovered receptors
- Descriptions of important new drugs released through August 2003
- Extensively revised bibliographies with many new references through August 2003
- Free access to the Student Online Resource Center, which features chapter learning objectives, chapter questions and answers with rationales, and a 50-question practice exam

An important related source of information is *Katzung & Trevor's Pharmacology: Examination & Board Review,* 6th ed. (Trevor AJ, Katzung BG, & Masters SB: McGraw-Hill, 2002). This book provides a succinct review of pharmacology with one of the largest available collections of sample examination questions and answers. It is especially helpful to students preparing for board-type examinations. A more highly condensed source of information suitable for review purposes is *USMLE Road Map: Pharmacology* (Katzung BG, Trevor AJ: McGraw-Hill, 2003).

The widespread acceptance of the first eight editions of *Basic & Clinical Pharmacology* over more than 20 years suggests that this book fills an important need. We believe that the ninth edition will satisfy this need even more successfully. Spanish, Portuguese, Italian, French, Czech, Indonesian, Japanese, and Chinese translations are available. Translations into other languages are under way; the publisher may be contacted for further information.

I wish to acknowledge the ongoing efforts of my contributing authors and the major contributions of the staff at Appleton & Lange and more recently at McGraw-Hill, and of our editors, Jennifer Bernstein and James Ransom. I also wish to thank my wife, Alice, for her expert proofreading contributions since the first edition.

Suggestions and comments about *Basic & Clinical Pharmacology* are always welcome. They may be sent to me at the Department of Cellular & Molecular Pharmacology, Box 0450, University of California, San Francisco, CA 94143-0450.

Bertram G. Katzung, MD, PhD
San Francisco
December 2003

Authors

Emmanuel T. Akporiaye, PhD
Professor, Department of Microbiology and Immunology, University of Arizona Health Sciences Center, Tucson

Michael J. Aminoff, MD, DSc, FRCP
Professor, Department of Neurology, University of California, San Francisco

Allan I. Basbaum, PhD
Professor and Chair, Department of Anatomy and W.M. Keck Foundation Center for Integrative Neuroscience, University of California, San Francisco

Neal L. Benowitz, MD
Professor of Medicine, Psychiatry, and Biopharmaceutical Sciences, University of California, San Francisco

Barry A. Berkowitz, PhD
Corporate Vice President, Albany Molecular Research, Inc., Albany, New York

Daniel D. Bikle, MD, PhD
Professor of Medicine, Department of Medicine, and Co-Director, Special Diagnostic and Treatment Unit, University of California, San Francisco, and Veterans Affairs Medical Center, San Francisco

Henry R. Bourne, MD
Professor, Department of Cellular & Molecular Pharmacology, University of California, San Francisco

Homer A. Boushey, MD
Chief, Asthma Clinical Research Center and Division of Allergy & Immunology; Professor of Medicine, Department of Medicine, University of California, San Francisco

Adrienne D. Briggs, MD
Clinical Director, Blood & Marrow Transplant Program, Assistant Professor of Clinical Medicine, University of Arizona; Arizona Cancer Center, Tucson

Henry F. Chambers, MD
Professor of Medicine, University of California, San Francisco; Chief of Infectious Diseases, San Francisco General Hospital

Kanu Chatterjee, FRCP, FCCP, FACC, MACP
Ernest Gallo Distinguished Professor of Medicine, University of California, San Francisco

George P. Chrousos, MD
Chief, Section on Pediatric Endocrinology; Chief, Pediatric and Reproductive Endocrinology Branch; National Institute of Child Health and Human Development, National Institutes of Health, Bethesda

Edward Chu, MD
Professor of Medicine and Pharmacology; Director, VACT Cancer Center; Associate Director, Yale Cancer Center; Yale University School of Medicine, New Haven

Robin L. Corelli, PharmD
Associate Clinical Professor, Department of Clinical Pharmacy, School of Pharmacy, University of California, San Francisco

Maria Almira Correia, PhD
Professor of Pharmacology, Pharmaceutical Chemistry and Biopharmaceutical Sciences, Department of Cellular & Molecular Pharmacology, University of California, San Francisco

Cathi E. Dennehy, PharmD
Associate Clinical Professor, Department of Clinical Pharmacy, School of Pharmacy, University of California, San Francisco

Betty J. Dong, PharmD
Professor of Clinical Pharmacy and Clinical Professor of Family and Community Medicine, Department of Clinical Pharmacy and Department of Family and Community Medicine, Schools of Pharmacy and Medicine, University of California, San Francisco

Paul A. Fitzgerald, MD
Clinical Professor of Medicine and Attending Physician, Department of Medicine, Division of Endocrinology, University of California, San Francisco

Marie L. Foegh, MD, DSc
Professor, Department of Surgery, Georgetown University Medical Center, Washington

Daniel E. Furst, MD
Carl M. Pearson Professor of Rheumatology, Director, Rheumatology Clinical Research Center, Department of Rheumatology, University of California, Los Angeles

Robert S. Goldsmith, MD, DTM&H
Professor Emeritus of Tropical Medicine and Epidemiology, Department of Epidemiology and Biostatistics, University of California, San Francisco

Augustus O. Grant, MD, PhD
Professor of Medicine, Cardiovascular Division, Duke University Medical Center, Durham

Francis S. Greenspan, MD
Clinical Professor of Medicine and Radiology and Chief, Thyroid Clinic, Division of Endocrinology, Department of Medicine, University of California, San Francisco

Julie Hambleton, MD
Associate Clinical Professor, Department of Medicine, University of California, San Francisco

Philip D. Hansten, PharmD
Professor of Pharmacy, School of Pharmacy, University of Washington, Seattle

Brian B. Hoffman, MD
Visiting Professor of Medicine, Harvard Medical School, Boston; Co-Chief of Medicine, Veterans Administration Boston Health Care System, West Roxbury, Massachusetts

Nicholas H.G. Holford, MBChB, MSc, MRCP(UK), FRACP
Associate Professor, Department of Pharmacology and Clinical Pharmacology, University of Auckland Medical School, Auckland

Leo E. Hollister, MD[†]
Professor Emeritus of Psychiatry, University of Texas Medical School, Houston; Life Fellow, Emeritus, Clinical Psychopharmacology

Joseph R. Hume, PhD
Professor and Chairman, Department of Pharmacology; Adjunct Professor, Department of Physiology and Cell Biology, University of Nevada School of Medicine, Reno

Harlan E. Ives, MD, PhD
Professor of Medicine, Department of Medicine, University of California, San Francisco

John P. Kane, MD, PhD
Professor of Medicine, Department of Medicine; Professor of Biochemistry and Biophysics; Associate Director, Cardiovascular Research Institute, University of California, San Francisco

John H. Karam, MD[†]
Professor Emeritus, Department of Medicine, University of California, San Francisco

Bertram G. Katzung, MD, PhD
Professor Emeritus, Department of Cellular & Molecular Pharmacology, University of California, San Francisco

Puja Khanna, MD, MPH
Division of Rheumatology, University of California, Los Angeles

Gideon Koren, MD, FABMT, FRCPC
Director, The Motherisk Program, Professor of Pediatrics, Pharmacology, Pharmacy, Medicine, and Medical Genetics, The University of Toronto; Senior Scientist, The Research Institute, The Hospital for Sick Children, Toronto

Michael J. Kosnett, MD, MPH
Associate Clinical Professor of Medicine, Division of Clinical Pharmacology and Toxicology, University of Colorado Health Sciences Center, Denver

Thomas R. Kosten, MD
Professor of Psychiatry, Department of Psychiatry, Yale University School of Medicine, New Haven; Deputy Chief of Psychiatry, Veterans Affairs, Connecticut

Douglas F. Lake, PhD
Assistant Professor, Department of Microbiology & Immunology and Arizona Cancer Center, University of Arizona Health Services Center, Tucson

†Deceased

Harry W. Lampiris, MD
Assistant Professor of Medicine, School of
Medicine, University of California, San Francisco

Paul W. Lofholm, PharmD
Clinical Professor of Pharmacy, School of
Pharmacy, University of California, San Francisco

Daniel S. Maddix, PharmD
Assistant Clinical Professor of Pharmacy,
University of California, San Francisco

Howard I. Maibach, MD
Professor of Dermatology, Department of
Dermatology, University of California, San
Francisco

Mary J. Malloy, MD
Clinical Professor of Pediatrics and Medicine,
Departments of Pediatrics and Medicine,
Cardiovascular Research Institute, University of
California, San Francisco

Susan B. Masters, PhD
Adjunct Professor of Pharmacology, Department of
Cellular & Molecular Pharmacology, University of
California, San Francisco

Kenneth R. McQuaid, MD
Professor of Clinical Medicine, Department of
Medicine, University of California, San Francisco;
Director of Gastrointestinal Endoscopy, San
Francisco Veterans Affairs Medical Center, San
Francisco

Brian S. Meldrum, MB, PhD
Professor Emeritus, GKT School of Medicine,
Guy's Campus, London

Roger A. Nicoll, MD
Professor of Pharmacology and Physiology,
Departments of Cellular & Molecular
Pharmacology and Physiology, University of
California, San Francisco

Martha S. Nolte, MD
Associate Clinical Professor, Department of
Medicine, University of California, San Francisco

Kent R. Olson, MD
Clinical Professor, Departments of Medicine,
and Pharmacy, University of California,
San Francisco; Medical Director, San Francisco
Division, California Poison Control System

Achilles J. Pappano, PhD
Professor, Department of Pharmacology, University
of Connecticut Health Center, Farmington

William W. Parmley, MD, MACC
Emeritus Professor of Medicine, University of
California, San Francisco

Gabriel L. Plaa, PhD
Professeur Émérite de Pharmacologie, Départment
de Pharmacologie, Faculté de Médecine, Université
de Montréal

Roger J. Porter, MD
Adjunct Professor of Neurology, University of
Pennsylvania, Philadelphia; Adjunct Professor of
Pharmacology, Uniformed Services University of
the Health Sciences, Bethesda

William Z. Potter, MD, PhD
Executive Director, Medical, Neuroscience
Therapeutic Area, Lilly Research Laboratories, A
Division of Eli Lilly and Company, Indianapolis

Peter W. Ramwell, PhD
Professor Emeritus, Department of Surgery and
Department of Physiology, Georgetown University
Medical Center, Washington

Ian A. Reid, PhD
Professor Emeritus, Department of Physiology,
University of California, San Francisco

Dirk B. Robertson, MD
Professor of Clinical Dermatology, Department of
Dermatology, Emory University School of
Medicine, Atlanta

Philip J. Rosenthal, MD
Professor, Department of Medicine, San Francisco
General Hospital, University of California, San
Francisco

Sharon Safrin, MD
Associate Clinical Professor, Department of
Medicine, University of California, San Francisco

Alan C. Sartorelli, PhD
Alfred Gilman Professor of Pharmacology,
Department of Pharmacology, Yale University
School of Medicine, New Haven

Mark A. Schumacher, PhD, MD
Associate Professor, Department of Anesthesia and
Perioperative Care, University of California, San
Francisco

Don Sheppard, MD
Visiting Scientist, Harbor-UCLA Research and
Education Institute, Division of Infectious
Diseases, Torrance

George Thomas, PhD
Associate Director, Icos Corporation, Bothell,
Washington

Anthony J. Trevor, PhD
Professor Emeritus, Department of Cellular &
Molecular Pharmacology, University of California,
San Francisco

Candy Tsourounis, PharmD
Associate Professor of Clinical Pharmacy,
Department of Clinical Pharmacy, School of
Pharmacy, University of California, San Francisco

Mark von Zastrow, MD, PhD
Associate Professor, Departments of Psychiatry and
Cellular & Molecular Pharmacology, University of
California, San Francisco

William Wagner, MD
Clinical Research Coordinator, David Geffen
School of Medicine at the University of California,
Los Angeles

Alice Lee Wang, PhD
Associate Research Chemist, Department of
Pharmaceutical Chemistry, University of
California, San Francisco

Ching Chung Wang, PhD
Professor of Chemistry and Pharmaceutical
Chemistry, Department of Pharmaceutical
Chemistry, University of California, San Francisco

Walter L. Way, MD
Professor Emeritus, Departments of Anesthesia and
Cellular & Molecular Pharmacology, University of
California, San Francisco

Paul F. White, PhD, MD
Professor and Holder of the Margaret Milam
McDermott Distinguished Chair of
Anesthesiology, Department of Anesthesiology and
Pain Management, University of Texas
Southwestern Medical Center at Dallas
Southwestern Medical School, Dallas

SECTION I
Basic Principles

Introduction

Bertram G. Katzung, MD, PhD

Pharmacology can be defined as the study of substances that interact with living systems through chemical processes, especially by binding to regulatory molecules and activating or inhibiting normal body processes. These substances may be chemicals administered to achieve a beneficial therapeutic effect on some process within the patient or for their toxic effects on regulatory processes in parasites infecting the patient. Such deliberate therapeutic applications may be considered the proper role of **medical pharmacology**, which is often defined as the science of substances used to prevent, diagnose, and treat disease. **Toxicology** is that branch of pharmacology which deals with the undesirable effects of chemicals on living systems, from individual cells to complex ecosystems.

History of Pharmacology

Prehistoric people undoubtedly recognized the beneficial or toxic effects of many plant and animal materials. The earliest written records from China and from Egypt list remedies of many types, including a few still recognized today as useful drugs. Most, however, were worthless or actually harmful. In the 2500 years or so preceding the modern era there were sporadic attempts to introduce rational methods into medicine, but none were successful owing to the dominance of systems of thought that purported to explain all of biology and disease without the need for experimentation and observation. These schools promulgated bizarre notions such as the idea that disease was caused by excesses of bile or blood in the body, that wounds could be healed by applying a salve to the weapon that caused the wound, and so on.

Around the end of the 17th century, reliance on observation and experimentation began to replace theorizing in medicine, following the example of the physical sciences. As the value of these methods in the study of disease became clear, physicians in Great Britain and on the Continent began to apply them to the effects of traditional drugs used in their own practices. Thus, materia medica—the science of drug preparation and the medical use of drugs—began to develop as the precursor to pharmacology. However, any understanding of the mechanisms of action of drugs was prevented by the absence of methods for purifying active agents from the crude materials that were available and—even more—by the lack of methods for testing hypotheses about the nature of drug actions.

In the late 18th and early 19th centuries, François Magendie and later his student Claude Bernard began to develop the methods of experimental animal physiology and pharmacology. Advances in chemistry and the further development of physiology in the 18th, 19th, and early 20th centuries laid the foundation needed for understanding how drugs work at the organ and tissue levels. Paradoxically, real advances in basic pharmacology during this time were accompanied by an outburst of unscientific promotion by manufacturers and marketers of worthless "patent medicines." It was not until the concepts of rational therapeutics, especially that of the controlled clinical trial, were reintroduced into medicine—about 50 years ago—that it became possible to accurately evaluate therapeutic claims.

About 50 years ago, there also began a major expansion of research efforts in all areas of biology. As new concepts and new techniques were introduced, information accumulated about drug action and the biologic substrate of that action, the receptor. During the last half-century, many fundamentally new drug groups and new members of old groups were introduced. The last 3 decades have seen an even more rapid growth of information and understanding of the molecular basis for drug action. The molecular mechanisms of action of many drugs have now been identified, and numerous receptors have been isolated, structurally characterized, and cloned. In fact, the use of receptor identification methods (described in Chapter 2) has led to the discovery of many orphan receptors—receptors for which no ligand has been discovered and whose function can only be surmised. Studies of the local molecular environment of receptors have shown that receptors and effectors do not function in isolation—they are strongly influenced by companion regulatory proteins. Decoding of the genomes of many species—from bacteria to humans—has led to the recognition of unsuspected relationships between receptor families. Pharmacogenomics—the relation of the individual's genetic makeup to his or her response to specific drugs—is close to becoming a practical area of therapy (see Box: Pharmacology & Genetics). Much of that progress is summarized in this book.

The extension of scientific principles into everyday therapeutics is still going on, though the medication consuming public, unfortunately, is still exposed to vast amounts of inaccurate, incomplete, or unscientific information regarding the pharmacologic effects of chemicals. This has resulted in the faddish use of innumerable expensive, ineffective, and sometimes harmful remedies and the growth of a huge "alternative health care" industry. Conversely, lack of understanding of basic scientific principles in biology and statistics and the absence of critical thinking about public health issues has led to rejection of medical science by a segment of the public and a common tendency to assume that all adverse drug effects are the result of malpractice. Two general principles that the student should always remember are, first, that all substances can under certain circumstances be toxic; and second, that all therapies promoted as health-enhancing should meet the same standards of evidence of efficacy and safety, ie, there should be no artificial separation between scientific medicine and "alternative" or "complementary" medicine.

PHARMACOLOGY & GENETICS

During the last 5 years, the genomes of humans, mice, and many other organisms have been decoded in considerable detail. This has opened the door to a remarkable range of new approaches to research and treatment. It has been known for centuries that certain diseases are inherited, and we now understand that individuals with such diseases have a heritable abnormality in their DNA. It is now possible in the case of some inherited diseases to define exactly which DNA base pairs are anomalous and in which chromosome they appear. In a small number of animal models of such diseases, it has been possible to correct the abnormality by **"gene therapy,"** ie, insertion of an appropriate "healthy" gene into somatic cells. Human somatic cell gene therapy has been attempted, but the technical difficulties are great.

Studies of a newly discovered receptor or endogenous ligand are often confounded by incomplete knowledge of the exact role of that receptor or ligand. One of the most powerful of the new genetic techniques is the ability to breed animals (usually mice) in which the gene for the receptor or its endogenous ligand has been "knocked out," ie, mutated so that the gene product is absent or non-functional. Homozygous **"knockout"** mice will usually have complete suppression of that function, while heterozygous animals will usually have partial suppression. Observation of the behavior, biochemistry, and physiology of the knockout mice will often define the role of the missing gene product very clearly. When the products of a particular gene are so essential that even heterozygotes do not survive to birth, it is sometimes possible to breed "knockdown" versions with only limited suppression of function. Conversely, "knockin" mice have been bred that overexpress certain receptors of interest.

Some patients respond to certain drugs with greater than usual sensitivity. (Such variations are discussed in Chapter 4.) It is now clear that such increased sensitivity is often due to a very small genetic modification that results in decreased activity of a particular enzyme responsible for eliminating that drug. **Pharmacogenomics** (or pharmacogenetics) is the study of the genetic variations that cause individual differences in drug response. Future clinicians may screen every patient for a variety of such differences before prescribing a drug.

The Nature of Drugs

In the most general sense, a drug may be defined as any substance that brings about a change in biologic function through its chemical actions. In the great majority of cases, the drug molecule interacts with a specific molecule in the biologic system that plays a regulatory role. This molecule is called a **receptor.** The nature of receptors is discussed more fully in Chapter 2. In a very small number of cases, drugs known as chemical antagonists may interact directly with other drugs, while a few other drugs (eg, osmotic agents) interact almost exclusively with water molecules. Drugs may be synthesized within the body (eg, **hormones**) or may be chemicals *not* synthesized in the body, ie, **xenobiotics** (from Gr *xenos* "stranger"). **Poisons** are drugs. **Toxins** are usually defined as poisons of biologic origin, ie, synthesized by plants or animals, in contrast to inorganic poisons such as lead and arsenic.

In order to interact chemically with its receptor, a drug molecule must have the appropriate size, electrical charge, shape, and atomic composition. Furthermore, a drug is often administered at a location distant from its intended site of action, eg, a pill given orally to relieve a headache. Therefore, a useful drug must have the necessary properties to be transported from its site of administration to its site of action. Finally, a practical drug should be inactivated or excreted from the body at a reasonable rate so that its actions will be of appropriate duration.

A. THE PHYSICAL NATURE OF DRUGS

Drugs may be solid at room temperature (eg, aspirin, atropine), liquid (eg, nicotine, ethanol), or gaseous (eg, nitrous oxide). These factors often determine the best route of administration. For example, some liquid drugs are easily vaporized and can be inhaled in that form, eg, halothane, amyl nitrite. The most common routes of administration are listed in Table 3–3. The various classes of organic compounds—carbohydrates, proteins, lipids, and their constituents—are all represented in pharmacology. Many drugs are weak acids or bases. This fact has important implications for the way they are handled by the body, because pH differences in the various compartments of the body may alter the degree of ionization of such drugs (see below).

B. DRUG SIZE

The molecular size of drugs varies from very small (lithium ion, MW 7) to very large (eg, alteplase [t-PA], a protein of MW 59,050). However, the vast majority of drugs have molecular weights between 100 and 1000. The lower limit of this narrow range is probably set by the requirements for specificity of action. In order to have a good "fit" to only one type of receptor, a drug molecule must be sufficiently unique in shape, charge, etc, to prevent its binding to other receptors. To achieve such selective binding, it appears that a molecule should in most cases be at least 100 MW units in size. The upper limit in molecular weight is determined primarily by the requirement that drugs be able to move within the body (eg, from site of administration to site of action). Drugs much larger than MW 1000 will not diffuse readily between compartments of the body (see Permeation, below). Therefore, very large drugs (usually proteins) must be administered directly into the compartment where they have their effect. In the case of alteplase, a clot-dissolving enzyme, the drug is administered directly into the vascular compartment by intravenous infusion.

C. DRUG REACTIVITY AND DRUG-RECEPTOR BONDS

Drugs interact with receptors by means of chemical forces or bonds. These are of three major types: covalent, electrostatic, and hydrophobic. Covalent bonds are very strong and in many cases not reversible under biologic conditions. Thus, the covalent bond formed between the activated form of phenoxybenzamine and the α receptor for norepinephrine (which results in blockade of the receptor) is not readily broken. The blocking effect of phenoxybenzamine lasts long after the free drug has disappeared from the bloodstream and is reversed only by the synthesis of new α receptors, a process that takes about 48 hours. Other examples of highly reactive, covalent bond-forming drugs are the DNA-alkylating agents used in cancer chemotherapy to disrupt cell division in the neoplastic tissue.

Electrostatic bonding is much more common than covalent bonding in drug-receptor interactions. Electrostatic bonds vary from relatively strong linkages between permanently charged ionic molecules to weaker hydrogen bonds and very weak induced dipole interactions such as van der Waals forces and similar phenomena. Electrostatic bonds are weaker than covalent bonds.

Hydrophobic bonds are usually quite weak and are probably important in the interactions of highly lipid-soluble drugs with the lipids of cell membranes and perhaps in the interaction of drugs with the internal walls of receptor "pockets."

The specific nature of a particular drug-receptor bond is of less practical importance than the fact that drugs which bind through weak bonds to their receptors are generally more selective than drugs which bind through very strong bonds. This is because weak bonds require a very precise fit of the drug to its receptor if an interaction is to occur. Only a few receptor types are likely to provide such a precise fit for a particular drug structure. Thus, if we wished to design a highly selective short-acting drug for a particular receptor, we would avoid highly reactive molecules that form covalent bonds and instead choose molecules that form weaker bonds.

A few substances that are almost completely inert in the chemical sense nevertheless have significant pharmacologic effects. For example, xenon, an "inert gas," has anesthetic effects at elevated pressures.

D. DRUG SHAPE

The shape of a drug molecule must be such as to permit binding to its receptor site. Optimally, the drug's shape is complementary to that of the receptor site in the same way that a key is complementary to a lock. Furthermore, the phenomenon of **chirality** (**stereoisomerism**) is so common in biology that more than half of all useful drugs are chiral molecules, ie, they exist as enantiomeric pairs. Drugs with two asymmetric centers have four diastereomers, eg, ephedrine, a sympathomimetic drug. In the great majority of cases, one of these enantiomers will be much more potent than its mirror image enantiomer, reflecting a better fit to the receptor molecule. For example, the (S)(+) enantiomer of methacholine, a parasympathomimetic drug, is over 250 times more potent than the (R)(−) enantiomer. If one imagines the receptor site to be like a glove into which the drug molecule must fit to bring about its effect, it is clear why a "left-oriented" drug will be more effective in binding to a left-hand receptor than will its "right-oriented" enantiomer.

The more active enantiomer at one type of receptor site may not be more active at another type, eg, a receptor type that may be responsible for some unwanted effect. For example, carvedilol, a drug that interacts with adrenoceptors, has a single chiral center and thus two enantiomers (Table 1–1). One of these enantiomers, the

(S)(−) isomer, is a potent β-receptor blocker. The (R)(+) isomer is 100-fold weaker at the β receptor. However, the isomers are approximately equipotent as α-receptor blockers. Ketamine is an intravenous anesthetic. The (+) enantiomer is a more potent anesthetic and is less toxic than the (−) enantiomer. Unfortunately, the drug is still used as the racemic mixture.

Finally, because enzymes are usually stereoselective, one drug enantiomer is often more susceptible than the other to drug-metabolizing enzymes. As a result, the duration of action of one enantiomer may be quite different from that of the other.

Unfortunately, most studies of clinical efficacy and drug elimination in humans have been carried out with racemic mixtures of drugs rather than with the separate enantiomers. At present, only about 45% of the chiral drugs used clinically are marketed as the active isomer—the rest are available only as racemic mixtures. As a result, many patients are receiving drug doses of which 50% or more is either inactive or actively toxic. However, there is increasing interest—at both the scientific and the regulatory levels—in making more chiral drugs available as their active enantiomers.

E. RATIONAL DRUG DESIGN

Rational design of drugs implies the ability to predict the appropriate molecular structure of a drug on the basis of information about its biologic receptor. Until recently, no receptor was known in sufficient detail to permit such drug design. Instead, drugs were developed through random testing of chemicals or modification of drugs already known to have some effect (see Chapter 5). However, during the past 3 decades, many receptors have been isolated and characterized. A few drugs now in use were developed through molecular design based on a knowledge of the three-dimensional structure of the receptor site. Computer programs are now available that can iteratively optimize drug structures to fit known receptors. As more becomes known about receptor structure, rational drug design will become more feasible.

F. RECEPTOR NOMENCLATURE

The spectacular success of newer, more efficient ways to identify and characterize receptors (see Chapter 2, Box, How Are New Receptors Discovered?) has resulted in a variety of differing systems for naming them. This in turn has led to a number of suggestions regarding more rational methods of naming them. The interested reader is referred for details to the efforts of the International Union of Pharmacology (IUPHAR) *Committee on Receptor Nomenclature and Drug Classification* (reported in various issues of *Pharmacological Reviews*) and to the annual *Receptor and Ion Channel Nomenclature Supplements* published as special issues by the journal *Trends in*

Table 1–1. Dissociation constants (K_d) of the enantiomers and racemate of carvedilol. The K_d is the concentration for 50% saturation of the receptors and is inversely proportionate to the affinity of the drug for the receptors.[1]

Form of Carvedilol	Inverse of Affinity for α Receptors (K_d, nmol/L)	Inverse of Affinity for β Receptors (K_d, nmol/L)
R(+) enantiomer	14	45
S(−) enantiomer	16	0.4
R,S(+/−) enantiomers	11	0.9

[1]Data from Ruffolo RR et al: The pharmacology of carvedilol. Eur J Pharmacol 1990;38:S82.

Pharmacological Sciences (TIPS). The chapters in this book mainly use these sources for naming receptors.

Drug-Body Interactions

The interactions between a drug and the body are conveniently divided into two classes. The actions of the drug on the body are termed **pharmacodynamic** processes; the principles of pharmacodynamics are presented in greater detail in Chapter 2. These properties determine the group in which the drug is classified and often play the major role in deciding whether that group is appropriate therapy for a particular symptom or disease. The actions of the body on the drug are called **pharmacokinetic** processes and are described in Chapters 3 and 4. Pharmacokinetic processes govern the absorption, distribution, and elimination of drugs and are of great practical importance in the choice and administration of a particular drug for a particular patient, eg, one with impaired renal function. The following paragraphs provide a brief introduction to pharmacodynamics and pharmacokinetics.

Pharmacodynamic Principles

As noted above, most drugs must bind to a receptor to bring about an effect. However, at the molecular level, drug binding is only the first in what is often a complex sequence of steps.

A. TYPES OF DRUG-RECEPTOR INTERACTIONS

Agonist drugs bind to and *activate* the receptor in some fashion, which directly or indirectly brings about the effect. Some receptors incorporate effector machinery in the same molecule, so that drug binding brings about the effect directly, eg, opening of an ion channel or activation of enzyme activity. Other receptors are linked through one or more intervening coupling molecules to a separate effector molecule. The several types of drug-receptor-effector coupling systems are discussed in Chapter 2. Pharmacologic antagonist drugs, by binding to a receptor, *prevent* binding by other molecules. For example, acetylcholine receptor blockers such as atropine are antagonists because they prevent access of acetylcholine and similar agonist drugs to the acetylcholine receptor and they stabilize the receptor in its inactive state. These agents reduce the effects of acetylcholine and similar drugs in the body.

B. "AGONISTS" THAT *INHIBIT* THEIR BINDING MOLECULES AND PARTIAL AGONISTS

Some drugs mimic agonist drugs by inhibiting the molecules responsible for terminating the action of an endogenous agonist. For example, acetylcholinesterase inhibitors, by slowing the destruction of endogenous acetylcholine, cause cholinomimetic effects that closely resemble the actions of cholinoceptor agonist molecules even though cholinesterase inhibitors do not—or only incidentally do—bind to cholinoceptors (see Chapter 7, Cholinoceptor-Activating & Cholinesterase-Inhibiting Drugs). Other drugs bind to receptors and activate them but do not evoke as great a response as so-called full agonists. Thus, pindolol, a β adrenoceptor "partial agonist," may act as either an agonist (if no full agonist is present) or as an antagonist (if a full agonist such as isoproterenol is present). (See Chapter 2.)

C. DURATION OF DRUG ACTION

Termination of drug action at the receptor level results from one of several processes. In some cases, the effect lasts only as long as the drug occupies the receptor, so that dissociation of drug from the receptor automatically terminates the effect. In many cases, however, the action may persist after the drug has dissociated, because, for example, some coupling molecule is still present in activated form. In the case of drugs that bind covalently to the receptor, the effect may persist until the drug-receptor complex is destroyed and new receptors are synthesized, as described previously for phenoxybenzamine. Finally, many receptor-effector systems incorporate desensitization mechanisms for preventing excessive activation when agonist molecules continue to be present for long periods. See Chapter 2 for additional details.

D. RECEPTORS AND INERT BINDING SITES

To function as a receptor, an endogenous molecule must first be selective in choosing ligands (drug molecules) to bind; and second, it must change its function upon binding in such a way that the function of the biologic system (cell, tissue, etc) is altered. The first characteristic is required to avoid constant activation of the receptor by promiscuous binding of many different ligands. The second characteristic is clearly necessary if the ligand is to cause a pharmacologic effect. The body contains many molecules that are capable of binding drugs, however, and not all of these endogenous molecules are regulatory molecules. Binding of a drug to a nonregulatory molecule such as plasma albumin will result in no detectable change in the function of the biologic system, so this endogenous molecule can be called an inert binding site. Such binding is not completely without significance, however, since it affects the distribution of drug within the body and will determine the amount of free drug in the circulation. Both of these factors are of pharmacokinetic importance (see below and Chapter 3).

Pharmacokinetic Principles

In practical therapeutics, a drug should be able to reach its intended site of action after administration by some convenient route. In some cases, a chemical that is readily absorbed and distributed is administered and then converted to the active drug by biologic processes—inside the body. Such a chemical is called a **prodrug**. In only a few situations is it possible to directly apply a drug to its target tissue, eg, by topical application of an anti-inflammatory agent to inflamed skin or mucous membrane. Most often, a drug is administered into one body compartment, eg, the gut, and must move to its site of action in another compartment, eg, the brain. This requires that the drug be **absorbed** into the blood from its site of administration and **distributed** to its site of action, **permeating** through the various barriers that separate these compartments. For a drug given orally to produce an effect in the central nervous system, these barriers include the tissues that comprise the wall of the intestine, the walls of the capillaries that perfuse the gut, and the "blood-brain barrier," the walls of the capillaries that perfuse the brain. Finally, after bringing about its effect, a drug should be **eliminated** at a reasonable rate by metabolic inactivation, by excretion from the body, or by a combination of these processes.

A. Permeation

Drug permeation proceeds by four primary mechanisms. Passive diffusion in an aqueous or lipid medium is common, but active processes play a role in the movement of many drugs, especially those whose molecules are too large to diffuse readily.

1. Aqueous diffusion—Aqueous diffusion occurs within the larger aqueous compartments of the body (interstitial space, cytosol, etc) and across epithelial membrane tight junctions and the endothelial lining of blood vessels through aqueous pores that—in some tissues—permit the passage of molecules as large as MW 20,000–30,000.*

Aqueous diffusion of drug molecules is usually driven by the concentration gradient of the permeating drug, a downhill movement described by Fick's law (see below). Drug molecules that are bound to large plasma proteins (eg, albumin) will not permeate these aqueous pores. If the drug is charged, its flux is also influenced by electrical fields (eg, the membrane potential and—in parts of the nephron—the transtubular potential).

2. Lipid diffusion—Lipid diffusion is the most important limiting factor for drug permeation because of the large number of lipid barriers that separate the compartments of the body. Because these lipid barriers separate aqueous compartments, the lipid:aqueous partition coefficient of a drug determines how readily the molecule moves between aqueous and lipid media. In the case of weak acids and weak bases (which gain or lose electrical charge-bearing protons, depending on the pH), the ability to move from aqueous to lipid or vice versa varies with the pH of the medium, because charged molecules attract water molecules. The ratio of lipid-soluble form to water-soluble form for a weak acid or weak base is expressed by the Henderson-Hasselbalch equation (see below).

3. Special carriers—Special carrier molecules exist for certain substances that are important for cell function and too large or too insoluble in lipid to diffuse passively through membranes, eg, peptides, amino acids, glucose. These carriers bring about movement by active transport or facilitated diffusion and, unlike passive diffusion, are saturable and inhibitable. Because many drugs are or resemble such naturally occurring peptides, amino acids, or sugars, they can use these carriers to cross membranes.

Many cells also contain less selective membrane carriers that are specialized for expelling foreign molecules, eg, the **P-glycoprotein** or **multidrug-resistance type 1 (MDR1) transporter** found in the brain, testes, and other tissues, and in some drug-resistant neoplastic cells. A similar transport molecule, the **multidrug resistance-associated protein-type 2 (MRP2) transporter**, plays an important role in excretion of some drugs or their metabolites into urine and bile.

4. Endocytosis and exocytosis—A few substances are so large or impermeant that they can enter cells only by endocytosis, the process by which the substance is engulfed by the cell membrane and carried into the cell by pinching off of the newly formed vesicle inside the membrane. The substance can then be released inside the cytosol by breakdown of the vesicle membrane. This process is responsible for the transport of vitamin B_{12}, complexed with a binding protein (intrinsic factor), across the wall of the gut into the blood. Similarly, iron is transported into hemoglobin-synthesizing red blood cell precursors in association with the protein transferrin. Specific receptors for the transport proteins must be present for this process to work. The reverse process (exocytosis) is responsible for the secretion of many substances from cells. For example, many neurotransmitter substances are stored in membrane-bound vesicles in nerve endings to protect them from metabolic destruction in the cytoplasm. Appropriate activation of the nerve ending causes fusion of the storage vesicle with the cell membrane and expulsion of its contents into the extracellular space (see Chapter 6).

---

* The capillaries of the brain, the testes, and some other tissues are characterized by absence of the pores that permit aqueous diffusion of many drug molecules into the tissue. They may also contain high concentrations of drug export pumps (MDR pumps; see text). These tissues are therefore "protected" or "sanctuary" sites from many circulating drugs.

B. Fick's Law of Diffusion

The passive flux of molecules down a concentration gradient is given by Fick's law:

Flux (molecules per unit time) =

$$(C_1 - C_2) \times \frac{\text{Area} \times \text{Permeability coefficient}}{\text{Thickness}}$$

where C_1 is the higher concentration, C_2 is the lower concentration, area is the area across which diffusion is occurring, permeability coefficient is a measure of the mobility of the drug molecules in the medium of the diffusion path, and thickness is the thickness (length) of the diffusion path. In the case of lipid diffusion, the lipid:aqueous partition coefficient is a major determinant of mobility of the drug, since it determines how readily the drug enters the lipid membrane from the aqueous medium.

C. Ionization of Weak Acids and Weak Bases; the Henderson-Hasselbalch Equation

The electrostatic charge of an ionized molecule attracts water dipoles and results in a polar, relatively water-soluble and lipid-insoluble complex. Since lipid diffusion depends on relatively high lipid solubility, ionization of drugs may markedly reduce their ability to permeate membranes. A very large fraction of the drugs in use are weak acids or weak bases (Table 1–2). For drugs, a weak acid is best defined as a neutral molecule that can reversibly dissociate into an anion (a negatively charged molecule) and a proton (a hydrogen ion). For example, aspirin dissociates as follows:

$$C_8H_7O_2COOH \rightleftharpoons C_8H_7O_2COO^- + H^+$$

| Neutral aspirin | Aspirin anion | Proton |

A drug that is a weak base can be defined as a neutral molecule that can form a cation (a positively charged molecule) by combining with a proton. For example, pyrimethamine, an antimalarial drug, undergoes the following association-dissociation process:

$$C_{12}H_{11}ClN_3NH_3^+ \rightleftharpoons C_{12}H_{11}ClN_3NH_2 + H^+$$

| Pyrimethamine cation | Neutral pyrimethamine | Proton |

Note that the protonated form of a weak acid is the neutral, more lipid-soluble form, whereas the unprotonated form of a weak base is the neutral form. The law of mass action requires that these reactions move to the left in an acid environment (low pH, excess protons available) and to the right in an alkaline environment. The Henderson-Hasselbalch equation relates the ratio of protonated to unprotonated weak acid or weak base to the molecule's pK_a and the pH of the medium as follows:

$$\log \frac{\text{(Protonated)}}{\text{(Unprotonated)}} = pK_a - pH$$

This equation applies to both acidic and basic drugs. Inspection confirms that the lower the pH relative to the pK_a, the greater will be the fraction of drug in the protonated form. Because the uncharged form is the more lipid-soluble, more of a weak acid will be in the lipid-soluble form at acid pH, while more of a basic drug will be in the lipid-soluble form at alkaline pH.

An application of this principle is in the manipulation of drug excretion by the kidney. Almost all drugs are filtered at the glomerulus. If a drug is in a lipid-soluble form during its passage down the renal tubule, a significant fraction will be reabsorbed by simple passive diffusion. If the goal is to accelerate excretion of the drug, it is important to prevent its reabsorption from the tubule. This can often be accomplished by adjusting urine pH to make certain that most of the drug is in the ionized state, as shown in Figure 1–1 on page 9. As a result of this pH partitioning effect, the drug will be "trapped" in the urine. Thus, weak acids are usually excreted faster in alkaline urine; weak bases are usually excreted faster in acidic urine. Other body fluids in which pH differences from blood pH may cause trapping or reabsorption are the contents of the stomach and small intestine; breast milk; aqueous humor; and vaginal and prostatic secretions (Table 1–3).

As suggested by Table 1–2, a large number of drugs are weak bases. Most of these bases are amine-containing molecules. The nitrogen of a neutral amine has three atoms associated with it plus a pair of unshared electrons—see the display below. The three atoms may consist of one carbon (designated "R") and two hydrogens (a *primary* amine), two carbons and one hydrogen (a *secondary* amine), or three carbon atoms (a *tertiary* amine). Each of these three forms may reversibly bind a proton with the unshared electrons. Some drugs have a fourth carbon-nitrogen bond; these are *quaternary* amines. However, the quaternary amine is permanently charged and has no unshared electrons with which to reversibly bind a proton. Therefore, primary, secondary, and tertiary amines may undergo reversible protonation and vary their lipid solubility with pH, but quaternary amines are always in the poorly lipid-soluble charged form.

Primary	Secondary	Tertiary	Quaternary
H	R	R	R
R:N:	R:N:	R:N:	R:N:R
H	H	R	R

Table 1-2. Ionization constants of some common drugs.

Drug	pK$_a$[1]	Drug	pK$_a$[1]	Drug	pK$_a$[1]
Weak acids		**Weak bases (cont'd)**		**Weak bases (cont'd)**	
Acetaminophen	9.5	Amiloride	8.7	Methamphetamine	10.0
Acetazolamide	7.2	Amiodarone	6.56	Methyldopa	10.6
Ampicillin	2.5	Amphetamine	9.8	Metoprolol	9.8
Aspirin	3.5	Atropine	9.7	Morphine	7.9
Chlorothiazide	6.8, 9.4[2]	Bupivacaine	8.1	Nicotine	7.9, 3.1[2]
Chlorpropamide	5.0	Chlordiazepoxide	4.6	Norepinephrine	8.6
Ciprofloxacin	6.09, 8.74[2]	Chloroquine	10.8, 8.4[2]	Pentazocine	7.9
Cromolyn	2.0	Chlorpheniramine	9.2	Phenylephrine	9.8
Ethacrynic acid	2.5	Chlorpromazine	9.3	Physostigmine	7.9, 1.8[2]
Furosemide	3.9	Clonidine	8.3	Pilocarpine	6.9, 1.4[2]
Ibuprofen	4.4, 5.2[2]	Cocaine	8.5	Pindolol	8.6
Levodopa	2.3	Codeine	8.2	Procainamide	9.2
Methotrexate	4.8	Cyclizine	8.2	Procaine	9.0
Methyldopa	2.2, 9.2[2]	Desipramine	10.2	Promazine	9.4
Penicillamine	1.8	Diazepam	3	Promethazine	9.1
Pentobarbital	8.1	Dihydrocodeine	3	Propranolol	9.4
Phenobarbital	7.4	Diphenhydramine	8.8	Pseudoephedrine	9.8
Phenytoin	8.3	Diphenoxylate	7.1	Pyrimethamine	7.0
Propylthiouracil	8.3	Ephedrine	9.6	Quinidine	8.5, 4.4[2]
Salicylic acid	3.0	Epinephrine	8.7	Scopolamine	8.1
Sulfadiazine	6.5	Ergotamine	6.3	Strychnine	8.0, 2.3[2]
Sulfapyridine	8.4	Fluphenazine	8.0, 3.9[2]	Terbutaline	10.1
Theophylline	8.8	Guanethidine	11.4, 8.3[2]	Thioridazine	9.5
Tolbutamide	5.3	Hydralazine	7.1	Tolazoline	10.6
Warfarin	5.0	Imipramine	9.5		
Weak bases		Isoproterenol	8.6		
Albuterol	9.3	Kanamycin	7.2		
(salbutamol)		Lidocaine	7.9		
Allopurinol	9.4, 12.3	Metaraminol	8.6		
Alprenolol	9.6	Methadone	8.4		

[1]The pK$_a$ is that pH at which the concentrations of the ionized and un-ionized forms are equal.
[2]More than one ionizable group.

Drug Groups

To learn each pertinent fact about each of the many hundreds of drugs mentioned in this book would be an impractical goal and, fortunately, is in any case unnecessary. Almost all of the several thousand drugs currently available can be arranged in about 70 groups. Many of the drugs within each group are very similar in pharmacodynamic actions and often in their pharmacokinetic properties as well. For most groups, one or more **prototype drugs** can be identified that typify the most important characteristics of the group. This permits classification of other important drugs in the group as variants of the prototype, so that only the prototype must be learned in detail and, for the remaining drugs, only the differences from the prototype.

Sources of Information

Students who wish to review the field of pharmacology in preparation for an examination are referred to *Pharmacology: Examination and Board Review,* by Trevor, Katzung, and Masters (McGraw-Hill, 2002) or *USMLE Road Map: Pharmacology,* by Katzung and Trevor (McGraw-Hill, 2003).

The references at the end of each chapter in this book were selected to provide information specific to those chapters.

Specific questions relating to basic or clinical research are best answered by resort to the general pharmacology and clinical specialty serials. For the student and the physician, three periodicals can be recommended as especially useful sources of current informa-

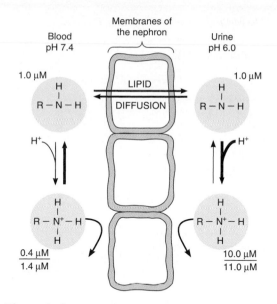

Figure 1–1. Trapping of a weak base (pyrimethamine) in the urine when the urine is more acidic than the blood. In the hypothetical case illustrated, the diffusible uncharged form of the drug has equilibrated across the membrane but the total concentration (charged plus uncharged) in the urine is almost eight times higher than in the blood.

tion about drugs: *The New England Journal of Medicine,* which publishes much original drug-related clinical research as well as frequent reviews of topics in pharmacology; *The Medical Letter on Drugs and Therapeutics,* which publishes brief critical reviews of new and old therapies, mostly pharmacologic; and *Drugs,* which publishes extensive reviews of drugs and drug groups.

Other sources of information pertinent to the USA should be mentioned as well. The "package insert" is a summary of information the manufacturer is required to place in the prescription sales package; *Physicians' Desk Reference (PDR)* is a compendium of package inserts published annually with supplements twice a year; *Facts and Comparisons* is a more complete looseleaf drug information service with monthly updates; and the *USP DI* (vol 1, *Drug Information for the Health Care Professional*) is a large drug compendium with monthly updates that is now published on the Internet by the Micromedex Corporation. The package insert consists of a brief description of the pharmacology of the product. While this brochure contains much practical information, it is also used as a means of shifting liability for untoward drug reactions from the manufacturer onto the practitioner. Therefore, the manufacturer typically lists every toxic effect ever reported, no matter how rare. A useful and objective handbook that presents information on drug toxicity and interactions is *Drug Interactions.* Finally, the FDA has an Internet World Wide Web site that carries news regarding recent drug

Table 1–3. Body fluids with potential for drug "trapping" through the pH-partitioning phenomenon.

Body Fluid	Range of pH	Total Fluid: Blood Concentration Ratios for Sulfadiazine (acid, pK$_a$ 6.5)[1]	Total Fluid: Blood Concentration Ratios for Pyrimethamine (base, pK$_a$ 7.0)[1]
Urine	5.0–8.0	0.12–4.65	72.24–0.79
Breast milk	6.4–7.6[2]	0.2–1.77	3.56–0.89
Jejunum, ileum contents	7.5–8.0[3]	1.23–3.54	0.94–0.79
Stomach contents	1.92–2.59[2]	0.11[4]	85,993–18,386
Prostatic secretions	6.45–7.4[2]	0.21	3.25–1.0
Vaginal secretions	3.4–4.2[3]	0.11[4]	2848–452

[1]Body fluid protonated-to-unprotonated drug ratios were calculated using each of the pH extremes cited; a blood pH of 7.4 was used for blood:drug ratio. For example, the steady-state urine:blood ratio for sulfadiazine is 0.12 at a urine pH of 5.0; this ratio is 4.65 at a urine pH of 8.0. Thus, sulfadiazine is much more effectively trapped and excreted in alkaline urine.

[2]Lentner C (editor): *Geigy Scientific Tables,* vol 1, 8th ed. Ciba Geigy, 1981.

[3]Bowman WC, Rand MJ: *Textbook of Pharmacology,* 2nd ed. Blackwell, 1980.

[4]Insignificant change in ratios over the physiologic pH range.

approvals, withdrawals, warnings, etc. It can be reached using a personal computer equipped with Internet browser software at http://wwwfda.gov.

The following addresses are provided for the convenience of readers wishing to obtain any of the publications mentioned above:

Drug Interactions
Lea & Febiger
600 Washington Square
Philadelphia, PA 19106

Facts and Comparisons
111 West Port Plaza, Suite 300
St. Louis, MO 63146

Pharmacology: Examination & Board Review, 6th ed
McGraw-Hill Companies, Inc
2 Penn Plaza 12th Floor
New York, NY 10121-2298

USMLE Road Map: Pharmacology
McGraw-Hill Companies, Inc
2 Penn Plaza 12th Floor
New York, NY 10121-2298

The Medical Letter on Drugs and Therapeutics
56 Harrison Street
New Rochelle, NY 10801

The New England Journal of Medicine
10 Shattuck Street
Boston, MA 02115

Physicians' Desk Reference
Box 2017
Mahopac, NY 10541

United States Pharmacopeia Dispensing Information
Micromedex, Inc.
6200 S. Syracuse Way, Suite 300
Englewood, CO 80111

Drug Receptors & Pharmacodynamics

2

Henry R. Bourne, MD, & Mark von Zastrow, MD, PhD

Therapeutic and toxic effects of drugs result from their interactions with molecules in the patient. Most drugs act by associating with specific macromolecules in ways that alter the macromolecules' biochemical or biophysical activities. This idea, more than a century old, is embodied in the term **receptor:** the component of a cell or organism that interacts with a drug and initiates the chain of biochemical events leading to the drug's observed effects.

Receptors have become the central focus of investigation of drug effects and their mechanisms of action (pharmacodynamics). The receptor concept, extended to endocrinology, immunology, and molecular biology, has proved essential for explaining many aspects of biologic regulation. Many drug receptors have been isolated and characterized in detail, thus opening the way to precise understanding of the molecular basis of drug action.

The receptor concept has important practical consequences for the development of drugs and for arriving at therapeutic decisions in clinical practice. These consequences form the basis for understanding the actions and clinical uses of drugs described in almost every chapter of this book. They may be briefly summarized as follows:

(1) **Receptors largely determine the quantitative relations between dose or concentration of drug and pharmacologic effects.** The receptor's affinity for binding a drug determines the concentration of drug required to form a significant number of drug-receptor complexes, and the total number of receptors may limit the maximal effect a drug may produce.

(2) **Receptors are responsible for selectivity of drug action.** The molecular size, shape, and electrical charge of a drug determine whether—and with what affinity—it will bind to a particular receptor among the vast array of chemically different binding sites available in a cell, tissue, or patient. Accordingly, changes in the chemical structure of a drug can dramatically increase or decrease a new drug's affinities for different classes of receptors, with resulting alterations in therapeutic and toxic effects.

(3) **Receptors mediate the actions of both pharmacologic agonists and antagonists.** Some drugs and many natural ligands, such as hormones and neurotransmitters, regulate the function of receptor macromolecules as agonists; ie, they activate the receptor to signal as a direct result of binding to it. Other drugs function as pharmacologic antagonists; ie, they bind to receptors but do not activate generation of a signal; consequently, they interfere with the ability of an agonist to activate the receptor. Thus, the effect of a so-called "pure" antagonist on a cell or in a patient depends entirely on its preventing the binding of agonist molecules and blocking their biologic actions. Some of the most useful drugs in clinical medicine are pharmacologic antagonists.

MACROMOLECULAR NATURE OF DRUG RECEPTORS

Most receptors are proteins, presumably because the structures of polypeptides provide both the necessary diversity and the necessary specificity of shape and electrical charge. The Box, How Are New Receptors Discovered? describes some of the methods by which receptors are discovered and defined (see page 12).

The best-characterized drug receptors are **regulatory proteins,** which mediate the actions of endogenous chemical signals such as neurotransmitters, autacoids, and hormones. This class of receptors mediates the effects of many of the most useful therapeutic agents. The molecular structures and biochemical mechanisms of these regulatory receptors are described in a later section entitled Signaling Mechanisms & Drug Action.

Other classes of proteins that have been clearly identified as drug receptors include **enzymes,** which may be inhibited (or, less commonly, activated) by binding a drug (eg, dihydrofolate reductase, the receptor for the antineoplastic drug methotrexate); **transport proteins** (eg, Na^+/K^+ ATPase, the membrane receptor for cardioactive digitalis glycosides); and **structural proteins** (eg, tubulin, the receptor for colchicine, an anti-inflammatory agent).

HOW ARE NEW RECEPTORS DISCOVERED?

Because today's new receptor sets the stage for tomorrow's new drug, it is important to know how new receptors are discovered. Receptor discovery often begins by studying the relations between structures and activities of a group of drugs on some conveniently measured response. Binding of radioactive ligands defines the molar abundance and binding affinities of the putative receptor and provides an assay to aid in its biochemical purification.

Analysis of the pure receptor protein identifies the number of its subunits, its size, and (sometimes) provides a clue to how it works (eg, agonist-stimulated autophosphorylation on tyrosine residues, seen with receptors for insulin and many growth factors). These classic steps in receptor identification serve as a warming-up exercise for molecular cloning of the segment of DNA that encodes the receptor. Receptors within a specific class or subclass generally contain highly conserved regions of similar or identi-

cal amino acid (and therefore DNA) sequence. This has led to an entirely different approach toward identifying receptors by sequence homology to already known (cloned) receptors.

Cloning of new receptors by sequence homology has identified a number of subtypes of known receptor classes, such as α-adrenoceptors and serotonin receptors, the diversity of which was only partially anticipated from pharmacologic studies. This approach has also led to the identification of receptors whose existence was not anticipated from pharmacologic studies. These putative receptors, identified only by their similarity to other known receptors, are termed **orphan** receptors until their native ligands are identified. Identifying such receptors and their ligands is of great interest because this process may elucidate entirely new signaling pathways and therapeutic targets.

This chapter deals with three aspects of drug receptor function, presented in increasing order of complexity: (1) Receptors as determinants of the quantitative relation between the concentration of a drug and the pharmacologic response. (2) Receptors as regulatory proteins and components of chemical signaling mechanisms that provide targets for important drugs. (3) Receptors as key determinants of the therapeutic and toxic effects of drugs in patients.

RELATION BETWEEN DRUG CONCENTRATION & RESPONSE

The relation between dose of a drug and the clinically observed response may be complex. In carefully controlled in vitro systems, however, the relation between concentration of a drug and its effect is often simple and can be described with mathematical precision. This idealized relation underlies the more complex relations between dose and effect that occur when drugs are given to patients.

Concentration-Effect Curves & Receptor Binding of Agonists

Even in intact animals or patients, responses to low doses of a drug usually increase in direct proportion to dose. As doses increase, however, the response increment diminishes; finally, doses may be reached at which no further increase in response can be achieved. In idealized or in vitro systems, the relation between drug con-

centration and effect is described by a hyperbolic curve (Figure 2–1A) according to the following equation:

$$E = \frac{E_{max} \times C}{C + EC_{50}}$$

where E is the effect observed at concentration C, E_{max} is the maximal response that can be produced by the drug, and EC_{50} is the concentration of drug that produces 50% of maximal effect.

This hyperbolic relation resembles the mass action law, which predicts association between two molecules of a given affinity. This resemblance suggests that drug agonists act by binding to ("occupying") a distinct class of biologic molecules with a characteristic affinity for the drug receptor. Radioactive receptor ligands have been used to confirm this occupancy assumption in many drug-receptor systems. In these systems, drug bound to receptors (B) relates to the concentration of free (unbound) drug (C) as depicted in Figure 2–1B and as described by an analogous equation:

$$B = \frac{B_{max} \times C}{C + K_D}$$

in which B_{max} indicates the total concentration of receptor sites (ie, sites bound to the drug at infinitely high concentrations of free drug). K_D (the equilibrium dissociation constant) represents the concentration of free drug at which half-maximal binding is observed. This constant characterizes the receptor's affinity for binding

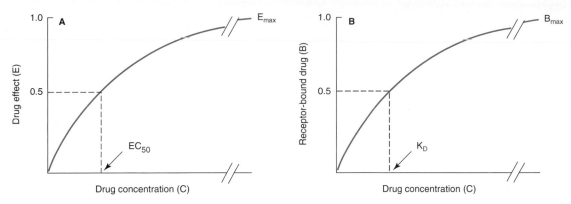

Figure 2–1. Relations between drug concentration and drug effect (panel **A**) or receptor-bound drug (panel **B**). The drug concentrations at which effect or receptor occupancy is half-maximal are denoted EC_{50} and K_D, respectively.

the drug in a reciprocal fashion: If the K_D is low, binding affinity is high, and vice versa. The EC_{50} and K_D may be identical, but need not be, as discussed below. Dose-response data is often presented as a plot of the drug effect (ordinate) against the *logarithm* of the dose or concentration (abscissa). This mathematical maneuver transforms the hyperbolic curve of Figure 2–1 into a sigmoid curve with a linear midportion (eg, Figure 2–2). This expands the scale of the concentration axis at low concentrations (where the effect is changing rapidly) and compresses it at high concentrations (where the effect is changing slowly), but has no special biologic or pharmacologic significance.

Receptor-Effector Coupling & Spare Receptors

When a receptor is occupied by an agonist, the resulting conformational change is only the first of many steps usually required to produce a pharmacologic response. The transduction process between occupancy of receptors and drug response is often termed **coupling**. The relative efficiency of occupancy-response coupling is partially determined by the initial conformational change in the receptor—thus, the effects of full agonists can be considered more efficiently coupled to receptor occupancy than can the effects of partial agonists, as described below. Coupling efficiency is also determined by the biochemical events that transduce receptor occupancy into cellular response.

High efficiency of receptor-effector interaction may also be envisioned as the result of spare receptors. Receptors are said to be "spare" for a given pharmacologic response when the maximal response can be elicited by an agonist at a concentration that does not result in occupancy of the full complement of available receptors. Spare receptors are not qualitatively different from nonspare receptors. They are not hidden or unavailable, and when they are occupied they can be coupled to response. Experimentally, spare receptors may be demonstrated by using irreversible antagonists to prevent binding of agonist to a proportion of available receptors and showing that high concentrations of agonist can still produce an undiminished maximal response (Figure 2–2). Thus, a maximal inotropic response of heart muscle to catecholamines can be elicited even under conditions where 90% of the β-adrenoceptors are occupied by a quasi-irreversible antagonist. Accordingly, myocardial cells are said to contain a large proportion of spare β-adrenoceptors.

How can we account for the phenomenon of spare receptors? In a few cases, the biochemical mechanism is understood, such as for drugs that act on some regulatory receptors. In this situation, the effect of receptor activation—eg, binding of guanosine triphosphate (GTP) by an intermediate—may greatly outlast the agonist-receptor interaction (see the following section on G Proteins & Second Messengers). In such a case, the "spareness" of receptors is *temporal* in that the response initiated by an individual ligand-receptor binding event persists longer than the binding event itself.

In other cases, where the biochemical mechanism is not understood, we imagine that the receptors might be *spare in number*. If the concentration or amount of a cellular component other than the receptor limits the coupling of receptor occupancy to response, then a maximal response can occur without occupancy of all receptors. This concept helps explain how the sensitivity of a cell or tissue to a particular concentration of agonist depends not only on the *affinity* of the receptor for binding the agonist (characterized by the K_D) but also on the *degree of spareness*—the total number of receptors

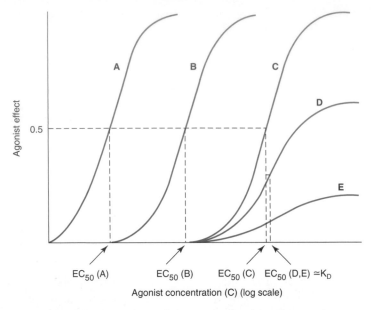

Figure 2–2. Logarithmic transformation of the dose axis and experimental demonstration of spare receptors, using different concentrations of an irreversible antagonist. Curve **A** shows agonist response in the absence of antagonist. After treatment with a low concentration of antagonist (curve **B**), the curve is shifted to the right; maximal responsiveness is preserved, however, because the remaining available receptors are still in excess of the number required. In curve **C,** produced after treatment with a larger concentration of antagonist, the available receptors are no longer "spare"; instead, they are just sufficient to mediate an undiminished maximal response. Still higher concentrations of antagonist (curves **D** and **E**) reduce the number of available receptors to the point that maximal response is diminished. The apparent EC_{50} of the agonist in curves **D** and **E** may approximate the K_D that characterizes the binding affinity of the agonist for the receptor.

present compared to the number actually needed to elicit a maximal biologic response. The K_D of the agonist-receptor interaction determines what fraction (B/B_{max}) of total receptors will be occupied at a given free concentration (C) of agonist regardless of the receptor concentration:

$$\frac{B}{B_{max}} = \frac{C}{C + K_D}$$

Imagine a responding cell with four receptors and four effectors. Here the number of effectors does not limit the maximal response, and the receptors are *not* spare in number. Consequently, an agonist present at a concentration equal to the K_D will occupy 50% of the receptors, and half of the effectors will be activated, producing a half-maximal response (ie, two receptors stimulate two effectors). Now imagine that the number of receptors increases 10-fold to 40 receptors but that the total number of effectors remains constant. Most of the receptors are now spare in number. As a result, a much lower concentration of agonist suffices to occupy two of

the 40 receptors (5% of the receptors), and this same low concentration of agonist is able to elicit a half-maximal response (two of four effectors activated). Thus, it is possible to change the sensitivity of tissues with spare receptors by changing the receptor concentration.

Competitive & Irreversible Antagonists

Receptor antagonists bind to receptors but do not activate them. In general, the effects of these antagonists result from preventing agonists (other drugs or endogenous regulatory molecules) from binding to and activating receptors. Such antagonists are divided into two classes depending on whether or not they *reversibly* compete with agonists for binding to receptors.

In the presence of a fixed concentration of agonist, increasing concentrations of a **competitive antagonist** progressively inhibit the agonist response; high antagonist concentrations prevent response completely. Conversely, sufficiently high concentrations of agonist can completely surmount the effect of a given concentration of the antagonist; ie, the E_{max} for the agonist remains the same for any fixed concentration of antagonist (Figure 2–3A). Because the antagonism is competitive, the presence of antagonist increases the agonist concentration required for a given degree of response, and so the agonist concentration-effect curve is shifted to the right.

The concentration (C') of an agonist required to produce a given effect in the presence of a fixed concentration ([I]) of competitive antagonist is greater than the agonist concentration (C) required to produce the same effect in the absence of the antagonist. The ratio of these two agonist concentrations (the "dose ratio") is related to the dissociation constant (K_I) of the antagonist by the Schild equation:

$$\frac{C'}{C} = 1 + \frac{[I]}{K_I}$$

Pharmacologists often use this relation to determine the K_I of a competitive antagonist. Even without knowledge of the relationship between agonist occupancy of the receptor and response, the K_I can be determined simply and accurately. As shown in Figure 2–3, concentration response curves are obtained in the presence and in the absence of a fixed concentration of competitive antagonist; comparison of the agonist concentrations required to produce identical degrees of pharmacologic effect in the two situations reveals the antagonist's K_I. If C' is twice C, for example, then [I] = K_I.

For the clinician, this mathematical relation has two important therapeutic implications:

(1) The degree of inhibition produced by a competitive antagonist depends on the concentration of antagonist. Different patients receiving a fixed dose of propranolol, for example, exhibit a wide range of plasma concentrations, owing to differences in clearance of the drug. As a result, the effects of a fixed dose of this competitive antagonist of norepinephrine may vary widely in patients, and the dose must be adjusted accordingly.

(2) Clinical response to a competitive antagonist depends on the concentration of agonist that is competing for binding to receptors. Here also propranolol provides a useful example: When this competitive β-adrenoceptor antagonist is administered in doses sufficient to block the effect of basal levels of the neurotransmitter norepinephrine, resting heart rate is decreased. However, the increase in release of norepinephrine and epinephrine that occurs with exercise, postural changes, or emotional stress may suffice to overcome competitive antagonism by propranolol and increase heart rate, and thereby can influence therapeutic response.

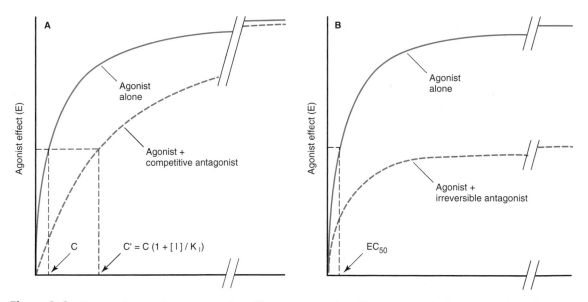

Figure 2–3. Changes in agonist concentration-effect curves produced by a competitive antagonist (panel **A**) or by an irreversible antagonist (panel **B**). In the presence of a competitive antagonist, higher concentrations of agonist are required to produce a given effect; thus the agonist concentration (C') required for a given effect in the presence of concentration [I] of an antagonist is shifted to the right, as shown. High agonist concentrations can overcome inhibition by a competitive antagonist. This is not the case with an irreversible antagonist, which reduces the maximal effect the agonist can achieve, although it may not change its EC_{50}.

Some receptor antagonists bind to the receptor in an **irreversible** or nearly irreversible fashion, ie, not competitive. The antagonist's affinity for the receptor may be so high that for practical purposes, the receptor is unavailable for binding of agonist. Other antagonists in this class produce irreversible effects because after binding to the receptor they form covalent bonds with it. After occupancy of some proportion of receptors by such an antagonist, the number of remaining unoccupied receptors may be too low for the agonist (even at high concentrations) to elicit a response comparable to the previous maximal response (Figure 2–3B). If spare receptors are present, however, a lower dose of an irreversible antagonist may leave enough receptors unoccupied to allow achievement of maximum response to agonist, although a higher agonist concentration will be required (Figures 2–2B and C; see Receptor-Effector Coupling and Spare Receptors, above).

Therapeutically, irreversible antagonists present distinctive advantages and disadvantages. Once the irreversible antagonist has occupied the receptor, it need not be present in unbound form to inhibit agonist responses. Consequently, the duration of action of such an irreversible antagonist is relatively independent of its own rate of elimination and more dependent on the rate of turnover of receptor molecules.

Phenoxybenzamine, an irreversible α-adrenoceptor antagonist, is used to control the hypertension caused by catecholamines released from pheochromocytoma, a tumor of the adrenal medulla. If administration of phenoxybenzamine lowers blood pressure, blockade will be maintained even when the tumor episodically releases very large amounts of catecholamine. In this case, the ability to prevent responses to varying and high concentrations of agonist is a therapeutic advantage. If overdose occurs, however, a real problem may arise. If the α-adrenoceptor blockade cannot be overcome, excess effects of the drug must be antagonized "physiologically," ie, by using a pressor agent that does not act via α receptors.

Partial Agonists

Based on the maximal pharmacologic response that occurs when all receptors are occupied, agonists can be divided into two classes: **partial agonists** produce a lower response, at full receptor occupancy, than do **full agonists.** Partial agonists produce concentration-effect curves that resemble those observed with full agonists in the presence of an antagonist that irreversibly blocks some of the receptor sites (compare Figures 2–2 [curve D] and 2–4B). It is important to emphasize that the failure of partial agonists to produce a maximal response is not due to decreased affinity for binding to receptors. Indeed, a partial agonist's inability to cause a maximal

pharmacologic response, even when present at high concentrations that saturate binding to all receptors, is indicated by the fact that partial agonists competitively inhibit the responses produced by full agonists (Figure 2–4C). Many drugs used clinically as antagonists are in fact weak partial agonists.

Other Mechanisms of Drug Antagonism

Not all of the mechanisms of antagonism involve interactions of drugs or endogenous ligands at a single type of receptor. Indeed, **chemical antagonists** need not involve a receptor at all. Thus, one drug may antagonize the actions of a second drug by binding to and inactivating the second drug. For example, protamine, a protein that is positively charged at physiologic pH, can be used clinically to counteract the effects of heparin, an anticoagulant that is negatively charged; in this case, one drug antagonizes the other simply by binding it and making it unavailable for interactions with proteins involved in formation of a blood clot.

The clinician often uses drugs that take advantage of **physiologic antagonism** between endogenous regulatory pathways. For example, several catabolic actions of the glucocorticoid hormones lead to increased blood sugar, an effect that is physiologically opposed by insulin. Although glucocorticoids and insulin act on quite distinct receptor-effector systems, the clinician must sometimes administer insulin to oppose the hyperglycemic effects of glucocorticoid hormone, whether the latter is elevated by endogenous synthesis (eg, a tumor of the adrenal cortex) or as a result of glucocorticoid therapy.

In general, use of a drug as a physiologic antagonist produces effects that are less specific and less easy to control than are the effects of a receptor-specific antagonist. Thus, for example, to treat bradycardia caused by increased release of acetylcholine from vagus nerve endings, the physician could use isoproterenol, a β-adrenoceptor agonist that increases heart rate by mimicking sympathetic stimulation of the heart. However, use of this physiologic antagonist would be less rational—and potentially more dangerous—than would use of a receptor-specific antagonist such as atropine (a competitive antagonist at the receptors at which acetylcholine slows heart rate).

SIGNALING MECHANISMS & DRUG ACTION

Until now we have considered receptor interactions and drug effects in terms of equations and concentration-effect curves. We must also understand the molecular mechanisms by which a drug acts. Such understanding allows us to ask basic questions with important clinical implications:

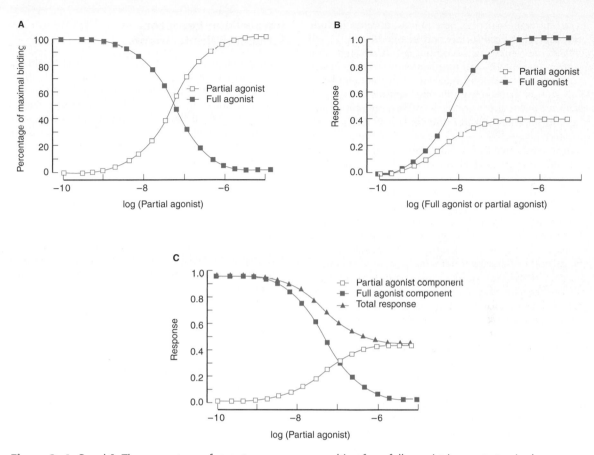

Figure 2–4. Panel **A:** The percentage of receptor occupancy resulting from full agonist (present at a single concentration) binding to receptors in the presence of increasing concentrations of a partial agonist. Because the full agonist (filled squares) and the partial agonist (open squares) compete to bind to the same receptor sites, when occupancy by the partial agonist increases, binding of the full agonist decreases. Panel **B:** When each of the two drugs is used alone and response is measured, occupancy of all the receptors by the partial agonist produces a lower maximal response than does similar occupancy by the full agonist. Panel **C:** Simultaneous treatment with a single concentration of full agonist and increasing concentrations of the partial agonist produces the response patterns shown in the bottom panel. The fractional response caused by a single concentration of the full agonist (filled squares) decreases as increasing concentrations of the partial agonist compete to bind to the receptor with increasing success; at the same time the portion of the response caused by the partial agonist (open squares) increases, while the total response—ie, the sum of responses to the two drugs (filled triangles)—gradually decreases, eventually reaching the value produced by partial agonist alone (compare panel **B**).

- Why do some drugs produce effects that persist for minutes, hours, or even days after the drug is no longer present?
- Why do responses to other drugs diminish rapidly with prolonged or repeated administration?
- How do cellular mechanisms for amplifying external chemical signals explain the phenomenon of spare receptors?

- Why do chemically similar drugs often exhibit extraordinary selectivity in their actions?
- Do these mechanisms provide targets for developing new drugs?

Most transmembrane signaling is accomplished by a small number of different molecular mechanisms. Each type of mechanism has been adapted, through the evolution of distinctive protein families, to transduce many different signals. These protein families include receptors on the cell surface and within the cell, as well as enzymes and other components that generate, amplify, coordinate, and terminate postreceptor signaling by chemical second messengers in the cytoplasm. This section first discusses the mechanisms for carrying chemical information across the plasma membrane and then outlines key features of cytoplasmic second messengers.

Five basic mechanisms of transmembrane signaling are well understood (Figure 2–5). Each uses a different strategy to circumvent the barrier posed by the lipid bilayer of the plasma membrane. These strategies use (1) a lipid-soluble ligand that crosses the membrane and acts on an intracellular receptor; (2) a transmembrane receptor protein whose intracellular enzymatic activity is allosterically regulated by a ligand that binds to a site on the protein's extracellular domain; (3) a transmembrane receptor that binds and stimulates a protein tyrosine kinase; (4) a ligand-gated transmembrane ion channel that can be induced to open or close by the binding of a ligand; or (5) a transmembrane receptor protein that stimulates a GTP-binding signal transducer protein (G protein), which in turn modulates production of an intracellular second messenger.

While the five established mechanisms do not account for all the chemical signals conveyed across cell membranes, they do transduce many of the most important signals exploited in pharmacotherapy.

Intracellular Receptors for Lipid-Soluble Agents

Several biologic signals are sufficiently lipid-soluble to cross the plasma membrane and act on intracellular receptors. One of these is a gas, nitric oxide (NO), that acts by stimulating an intracellular enzyme, guanylyl cyclase, which produces cyclic guanosine monophosphate (cGMP). Signaling via cGMP is described in more detail later in this chapter. Receptors for another class of ligands—including corticosteroids, mineralocorticoids, sex steroids, vitamin D, and thyroid hormone—stimulate the transcription of genes in the nucleus by binding to specific DNA sequences near the gene whose expression is to be regulated. Many of the target DNA sequences (called **response elements**) have been identified.

These "gene-active" receptors belong to a protein family that evolved from a common precursor. Dissection of the receptors by recombinant DNA techniques has provided insights into their molecular mechanism. For example, binding of glucocorticoid hormone to its normal receptor protein relieves an inhibitory constraint on the transcription-stimulating activity of the protein. Figure 2–6 schematically depicts the molecular mechanism of glucocorticoid action: In the absence of hormone, the receptor is bound to hsp90, a protein that appears to prevent normal folding of several structural domains of the receptor. Binding of hormone to the ligand-binding domain triggers release of hsp90. This allows the DNA-binding and transcription-activating

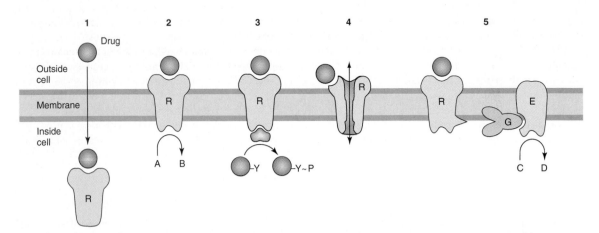

Figure 2–5. Known transmembrane signaling mechanisms: **1:** A lipid-soluble chemical signal crosses the plasma membrane and acts on an intracellular receptor (which may be an enzyme or a regulator of gene transcription); **2:** the signal binds to the extracellular domain of a transmembrane protein, thereby activating an enzymatic activity of its cytoplasmic domain; **3:** the signal binds to the extracellular domain of a transmembrane receptor bound to a protein tyrosine kinase, which it activates; **4:** the signal binds to and directly regulates the opening of an ion channel; **5:** the signal binds to a cell-surface receptor linked to an effector enzyme by a G protein. (A, C, substrates; B, D, products; R, receptor; G, G protein; E, effector [enzyme or ion channel]; Y, tyrosine; P, phosphate.)

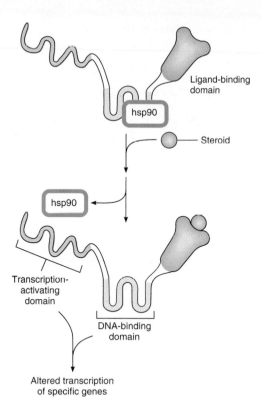

Figure 2–6. Mechanism of glucocorticoid action. The glucocorticoid receptor polypeptide is schematically depicted as a protein with three distinct domains. A heat-shock protein, hsp90, binds to the receptor in the absence of hormone and prevents folding into the active conformation of the receptor. Binding of a hormone ligand (steroid) causes dissociation of the hsp90 stabilizer and permits conversion to the active configuration.

domains of the receptor to fold into their functionally active conformations, so that the activated receptor can initiate transcription of target genes.

The mechanism used by hormones that act by regulating gene expression has two therapeutically important consequences:

(1) All of these hormones produce their effects after a characteristic lag period of 30 minutes to several hours—the time required for the synthesis of new proteins. This means that the gene-active hormones cannot be expected to alter a pathologic state within minutes (eg, glucocorticoids will not immediately relieve the symptoms of acute bronchial asthma).

(2) The effects of these agents can persist for hours or days after the agonist concentration has been reduced to zero. The persistence of effect is primarily due to the relatively slow turnover of most enzymes and proteins, which can remain active in cells for hours or days after they have been synthesized. Consequently, it means that the beneficial (or toxic) effects of a gene-active hormone will usually decrease slowly when administration of the hormone is stopped.

Ligand-Regulated Transmembrane Enzymes Including Receptor Tyrosine Kinases

This class of receptor molecules mediates the first steps in signaling by insulin, epidermal growth factor (EGF), platelet derived growth factor (PDGF), atrial natriuretic peptide (ANP), transforming growth factor-β (TGF-β), and many other trophic hormones. These receptors are polypeptides consisting of an extracellular hormone-binding domain and a cytoplasmic enzyme domain, which may be a protein tyrosine kinase, a serine kinase, or a guanylyl cyclase (Figure 2–7). In all these receptors, the two domains are connected by a hydrophobic segment of the polypeptide that crosses the lipid bilayer of the plasma membrane.

The receptor tyrosine kinase signaling pathway begins with ligand binding to the receptor's extracellular domain. The resulting change in receptor conformation causes receptor molecules to bind to one another, which in turn brings together the tyrosine kinase domains, which become enzymatically active, and phosphorylate one another as well as additional downstream signaling proteins. Activated receptors catalyze phosphorylation of tyrosine residues on different target signaling proteins, thereby allowing a single type of activated receptor to modulate a number of biochemical processes. Insulin, for example, uses a single class of receptors to trigger increased uptake of glucose and amino acids and to regulate metabolism of glycogen and triglycerides in the cell. Similarly, each of the growth factors initiates in its specific target cells a complex program of cellular events ranging from altered membrane transport of ions and metabolites to changes in the expression of many genes. At present, a few compounds have been found to produce effects that may be due to inhibition of tyrosine kinase activities. It is easy to imagine therapeutic uses for specific inhibitors of growth factor receptors, especially in neoplastic disorders where excessive growth factor signaling is often observed. For example, a monoclonal antibody (trastuzumab) that acts as an antagonist of the HER2/neu receptor tyrosine kinase is effective in therapy of human breast cancers associated with overexpression of this growth factor receptor.

The intensity and duration of action of EGF, PDGF, and other agents that act via receptor tyrosine kinases are

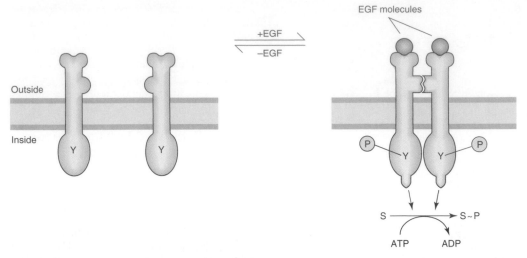

Figure 2–7. Mechanism of activation of the epidermal growth factor (EGF) receptor, a representative receptor tyrosine kinase. The receptor polypeptide has extracellular and cytoplasmic domains, depicted above and below the plasma membrane. Upon binding of EGF (circle), the receptor converts from its inactive monomeric state (left) to an active dimeric state (right), in which two receptor polypeptides bind noncovalently in the plane of the membrane. The cytoplasmic domains become phosphorylated (*P*) on specific tyrosine residues (*Y*) and their enzymatic activities are activated, catalyzing phosphorylation of substrate proteins (*S*).

limited by receptor down-regulation. Ligand binding induces accelerated endocytosis of receptors from the cell surface, followed by the degradation of those receptors (and their bound ligands). When this process occurs at a rate faster than de novo synthesis of receptors, the total number of cell-surface receptors is reduced (down-regulated) and the cell's responsiveness to ligand is correspondingly diminished. A well-understood process by which many tyrosine kinases are down-regulated is via ligand-induced internalization of receptors followed by trafficking to lysosomes, where receptors are proteolyzed. EGF causes internalization and subsequent proteolytic down-regulation after binding to the EGF receptor protein tyrosine kinase; genetic mutations that interfere with this process of down-regulation cause excessive growth factor–induced cell proliferation and are associated with an increased susceptibility to certain types of cancer. Internalization of certain receptor tyrosine kinases, most notably receptors for nerve growth factor, serves a very different function. Internalized nerve growth factor receptors are not rapidly degraded. Instead, receptors remain intact and are translocated in endocytic vesicles from the distal axon (where receptors are activated by nerve growth factor released from the innervated tissue) to the cell body (where the signal is transduced to transcription factors regulating the expression of genes controlling cell survival). This process effectively transports a critical survival signal released from the target tissue over a remarkably long distance—more than 1 meter in certain sensory neurons. A number of regulators of growth and differentiation, including TGF-β, act on another class of transmembrane receptor enzymes that phosphorylate serine and threonine residues. ANP, an important regulator of blood volume and vascular tone, acts on a transmembrane receptor whose intracellular domain, a guanylyl cyclase, generates cGMP (see below). Receptors in both groups, like the receptor tyrosine kinases, are active in their dimeric forms.

Cytokine Receptors

Cytokine receptors respond to a heterogeneous group of peptide ligands that includes growth hormone, erythropoietin, several kinds of interferon, and other regulators of growth and differentiation. These receptors use a mechanism (Figure 2–8) closely resembling that of receptor tyrosine kinases, except that in this case, the protein tyrosine kinase activity is not intrinsic to the receptor molecule. Instead, a separate protein tyrosine kinase, from the Janus-kinase (JAK) family, binds noncovalently to the receptor. As in the case of the EGF-receptor, cytokine receptors dimerize after they bind the activating ligand, allowing the bound JAKs to become activated and to phosphorylate tyrosine residues on the receptor. Tyrosine phosphates on the receptor then set in motion a complex signaling dance by binding

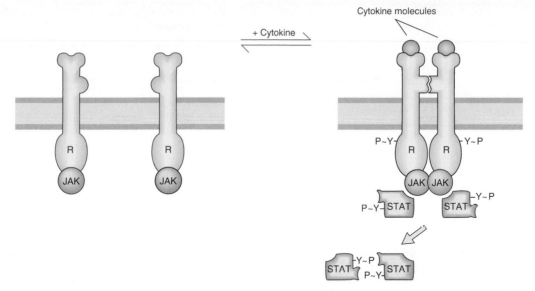

Figure 2–8. Cytokine receptors, like receptor tyrosine kinases, have extracellular and intracellular domains and form dimers. However, after activation by an appropriate ligand, separate mobile protein tyrosine kinase molecules (JAK) are activated, resulting in phosphorylation of signal transducers and activation of transcription (STAT) molecules. STAT dimers then travel to the nucleus, where they regulate transcription.

another set of proteins, called STATs (signal transducers and activators of transcription). The bound STATs are themselves phosphorylated by the JAKs, two STAT molecules dimerize (attaching to one another's tyrosine phosphates), and finally the STAT/STAT dimer dissociates from the receptor and travels to the nucleus, where it regulates transcription of specific genes.

Ligand-Gated Channels

Many of the most useful drugs in clinical medicine act by mimicking or blocking the actions of endogenous ligands that regulate the flow of ions through plasma membrane channels. The natural ligands include acetylcholine, serotonin, γ-aminobutyric acid (GABA), and the excitatory amino acids (eg, glycine, aspartate, and glutamate). All of these agents are synaptic transmitters.

Each of their receptors transmits its signal across the plasma membrane by increasing transmembrane conductance of the relevant ion and thereby altering the electrical potential across the membrane. For example, acetylcholine causes the opening of the ion channel in the nicotinic acetylcholine receptor (AChR), which allows Na^+ to flow down its concentration gradient into cells, producing a localized excitatory postsynaptic potential—a depolarization.

The AChR (Figure 2–9) is one of the best-characterized of all cell-surface receptors for hormones or neuro-

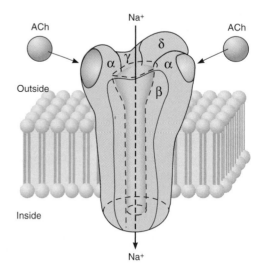

Figure 2–9. The nicotinic acetylcholine receptor, a ligand-gated ion channel. The receptor molecule is depicted as embedded in a rectangular piece of plasma membrane, with extracellular fluid above and cytoplasm below. Composed of five subunits (two α, one β, one γ, and one δ), the receptor opens a central transmembrane ion channel when acetylcholine (ACh) binds to sites on the extracellular domain of its α subunits.

transmitters. One form of this receptor is a pentamer made up of five polypeptide subunits (eg, two α chains plus one β, one γ, and one δ chain, all with molecular weights ranging from 43,000 to 50,000). These polypeptides, each of which crosses the lipid bilayer four times, form a cylindric structure 8 nm in diameter. When acetylcholine binds to sites on the α subunits, a conformational change occurs that results in the transient opening of a central aqueous channel through which sodium ions penetrate from the extracellular fluid into the cell.

The time elapsed between the binding of the agonist to a ligand-gated channel and the cellular response can often be measured in milliseconds. The rapidity of this signaling mechanism is crucially important for moment-to-moment transfer of information across synapses. Ligand-gated ion channels can be regulated by multiple mechanisms, including phosphorylation and internalization. In the central nervous system, these mechanisms contribute to synaptic plasticity involved in learning and memory.

G Proteins & Second Messengers

Many extracellular ligands act by increasing the intracellular concentrations of second messengers such as cyclic adenosine-3′,5′-monophosphate (cAMP), calcium ion, or the phosphoinositides (described below). In most cases they use a transmembrane signaling system with three separate components. First, the extracellular ligand is specifically detected by a cell-surface receptor. The receptor in turn triggers the activation of a G protein located on the cytoplasmic face of the plasma membrane. The activated G protein then changes the activity of an effector element, usually an enzyme or ion channel. This element then changes the concentration of the intracellular second messenger. For cAMP, the effector enzyme is adenylyl cyclase, a transmembrane protein that converts intracellular adenosine triphosphate (ATP) to cAMP. The corresponding G protein, G_s, stimulates adenylyl cyclase after being activated by hormones and neurotransmitters that act via a specific receptor (Table 2–1).

G_s and other G proteins use a molecular mechanism that involves binding and hydrolysis of GTP (Figure 2–10). This mechanism allows the transduced signal to be amplified. For example, a neurotransmitter such as norepinephrine may encounter its membrane receptor for only a few milliseconds. When the encounter generates a GTP-bound G_s molecule, however, the duration of activation of adenylyl cyclase depends on the longevity of GTP binding to G_s rather than on the receptor's affinity for norepinephrine. Indeed, like other G proteins, GTP-bound G_s may remain active for tens of seconds, enormously amplifying the original signal.

Table 2–1. A partial list of endogenous ligands and their associated second messengers.

Ligand	Second Messenger
Adrenocorticotropic hormone	cAMP
Acetylcholine (muscarinic receptors)	Ca^{2+}, phosphoinositides
Angiotensin	Ca^{2+}, phosphoinositides
Catecholamines (α_1-adrenoceptors)	Ca^{2+}, phosphoinositides
Catecholamines (β-adrenoceptors)	cAMP
Chorionic gonadotropin	cAMP
Follicle-stimulating hormone	cAMP
Glucagon	cAMP
Histamine (H_2 receptors)	cAMP
Luteinizing hormone	cAMP
Melanocyte-stimulating hormone	cAMP
Parathyroid hormone	cAMP
Platelet-activating factor	Ca^{2+}, phosphoinositides
Prostacyclin, prostaglandin E_2	cAMP
Serotonin ($5\text{-}HT_4$ receptors)	cAMP
Serotonin ($5\text{-}HT_{1C}$ and $5\text{-}HT_2$ receptors)	Ca^{2+}, phosphoinositides
Thyrotropin	cAMP
Thyrotropin-releasing hormone	Ca^{2+}, phosphoinositides
Vasopressin (V_1 receptors)	Ca^{2+}, phosphoinositides
Vasopressin (V_2 receptors)	cAMP

Key: cAMP = cyclic adenosine monophosphate.

This mechanism explains how signaling by G proteins produces the phenomenon of spare receptors (described above). At low concentrations of agonist the proportion of agonist-bound receptors may be much less than the proportion of G proteins in the active (GTP-bound) state; if the proportion of active G proteins correlates with pharmacologic response, receptors will appear to be spare (ie, a small fraction of receptors occupied by agonist at any given time will appear to produce a proportionately larger response).

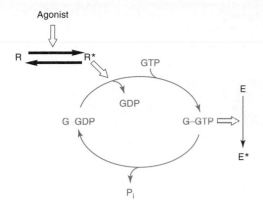

Figure 2–10. The guanine nucleotide-dependent activation-inactivation cycle of G proteins. The agonist activates the receptor (R), which promotes release of GDP from the G protein (G), allowing entry of GTP into the nucleotide binding site. In its GTP-bound state (G-GTP), the G protein regulates activity of an effector enzyme or ion channel (E). The signal is terminated by hydrolysis of GTP, followed by return of the system to the basal unstimulated state. Open arrows denote regulatory effects. (P_i, inorganic phosphate.)

The family of G proteins contains several functionally diverse subfamilies (Table 2–2), each of which mediates effects of a particular set of receptors to a distinctive group of effectors. Receptors coupled to G proteins comprise a family of "seven-transmembrane" or "serpentine" receptors, so called because the receptor polypeptide chain "snakes" across the plasma membrane seven times (Figure 2–11). Receptors for adrenergic amines, serotonin, acetylcholine (muscarinic but not nicotinic), many peptide hormones, odorants, and even visual receptors (in retinal rod and cone cells) all belong to the serpentine family. All were derived from a common evolutionary precursor. Some serpentine receptors exist as dimers, but it is thought that dimerization is not usually required for activation.

Serpentine receptors transduce signals across the plasma membrane in essentially the same way. Often the agonist ligand—eg, a catecholamine, acetylcholine, or the photon-activated chromophore of retinal photoreceptors—is bound in a pocket enclosed by the transmembrane regions of the receptor (as in Figure 2–11). The resulting change in conformation of these regions is transmitted to cytoplasmic loops of the receptor, which in turn activate the appropriate G protein by promoting replacement of GDP by GTP, as described above. Considerable biochemical evidence indicates that G proteins interact with amino acids in the third cytoplasmic loop of the serpentine receptor polypeptide (shown by arrows in Figure 2–11). The carboxyl terminal tails of these receptors, also located in the cytoplasm, can regulate the receptors' ability to interact with G proteins, as described below.

Receptor Regulation

Receptor-mediated responses to drugs and hormonal agonists often desensitize with time (Figure 2–12, top). After reaching an initial high level, the response (eg, cellular cAMP accumulation, Na^+ influx, contractility, etc) gradu-

Table 2–2. G proteins and their receptors and effectors.

G Protein	Receptors for:	Effector/Signaling Pathway
G_s	β-Adrenergic amines, glucagon, histamine, serotonin, and many other hormones	↑ Adenylyl cyclase → ↑ cAMP
G_{i1}, G_{i2}, G_{i3}	α_2-Adrenergic amines, acetylcholine (muscarinic), opioids, serotonin, and many others	Several, including: ↓Adenylyl cyclase → ↓ cAMP Open cardiac K^+ channels → ↓heart rate
G_{olf}	Odorants (olfactory epithelium)	↑Adenylyl cyclase → ↑ cAMP
G_o	Neurotransmitters in brain (not yet specifically identified)	Not yet clear
G_q	Acetylcholine (eg, muscarinic), bombesin, serotonin (5-HT$_{1C}$), and many others	↑Phospholipase C → ↑ IP$_3$, diacylglycerol, cytoplasmic Ca^{2+}
G_{t1}, G_{t2}	Photons (rhodopsin and color opsins in retinal rod and cone cells)	↑cGMP phosphodiesterase → ↓ cGMP (phototransduction)

Key: cAMP = cyclic adenosine monophosphate; cGMP = cyclic guanosine monophosphate.

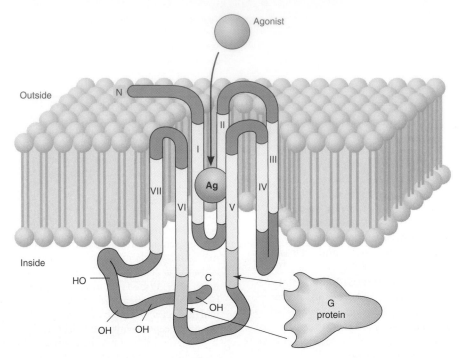

Figure 2–11. Transmembrane topology of a typical serpentine receptor. The receptor's amino (N) terminal is extracellular (above the plane of the membrane), and its carboxyl (C) terminal intracellular. The terminals are connected by a polypeptide chain that traverses the plane of the membrane seven times. The hydrophobic transmembrane segments (light color) are designated by roman numerals (I–VII). The agonist (Ag) approaches the receptor from the extracellular fluid and binds to a site surrounded by the transmembrane regions of the receptor protein. G proteins (G) interact with cytoplasmic regions of the receptor, especially with portions of the third cytoplasmic loop between transmembrane regions V and VI. The receptor's cytoplasmic terminal tail contains numerous serine and threonine residues whose hydroxyl (–OH) groups can be phosphorylated. This phosphorylation may be associated with diminished receptor-G protein interaction.

ally diminishes over seconds or minutes, even in the continued presence of the agonist. This desensitization is usually reversible; a second exposure to agonist, if provided a few minutes after termination of the first exposure, results in a response similar to the initial response.

Although many kinds of receptors undergo desensitization, the mechanism is in many cases obscure. A molecular mechanism of desensitization has been worked out in some detail, however, in the case of the β-adrenoceptor (Figure 2–12, bottom). The agonist-induced change in conformation of the receptor causes it to bind, activate, and serve as a substrate for a specific kinase, β-adrenoceptor kinase (also called βARK). βARK then phosphorylates serine or threonine residues in the receptor's carboxyl terminal tail. The presence of phosphoserines increases the receptor's affinity for binding a third protein, β-arrestin. Binding of β-arrestin to cytoplasmic loops of the receptor diminishes the receptor's ability to

interact with G_s, thereby reducing the agonist response (ie, stimulation of adenylyl cyclase). Upon removal of agonist, however, cellular phosphatases remove phosphates from the receptor and βARK stops putting them back on, so that the receptor—and consequently the agonist response—return to normal. This mechanism of desensitization, which rapidly and reversibly modulates the ability of the receptor to signal to G protein, turns out to regulate many G protein–coupled receptors. Another important regulatory process is down-regulation. Down-regulation, which decreases the actual number of receptors present in the cell or tissue, occurs more slowly than rapid desensitization and is less readily reversible. This is because down-regulation involves a net degradation of receptors present in the cell, requiring new receptor biosynthesis for recovery, in contrast to rapid desensitization which involves reversible phosphorylation of existing receptors. Many G protein–coupled

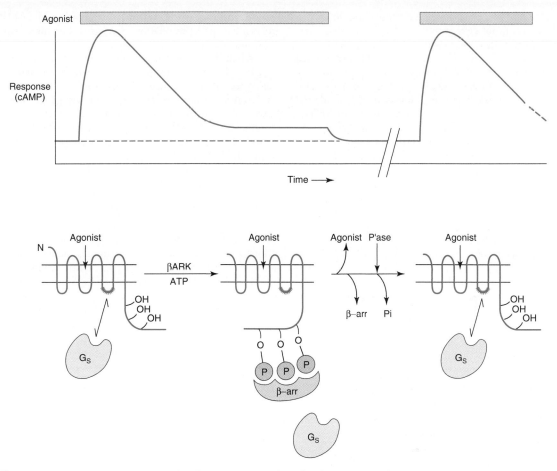

Figure 2–12. Possible mechanism for desensitization of the β-adrenoceptor. The upper part of the figure depicts the response to a β-adrenoceptor agonist (ordinate) versus time (abscissa). The break in the time axis indicates passage of time in the absence of agonist. Temporal duration of exposure to agonist is indicated by the light-colored bar. The lower part of the figure schematically depicts agonist-induced phosphorylation (P) by β-adrenoceptor kinase (β-adrenergic receptor kinase, βARK) of carboxyl terminal hydroxyl groups (–OH) of the β-adrenoceptor. This phosphorylation induces binding of a protein, β-arrestin (β-arr), which prevents the receptor from interacting with G_s. Removal of agonist for a short period of time allows dissociation of β-arr, removal of phosphate (Pi) from the receptor by phosphatases (P'ase), and restoration of the receptor's normal responsiveness to agonist.

receptors are down-regulated by undergoing ligand-induced endocytosis and delivery to lysosomes, similar to down-regulation of protein tyrosine kinases such as the EGF receptor. Down-regulation generally occurs only after prolonged or repeated exposure of cells to agonist (over hours to days). Brief periods of agonist exposure (several minutes) can also induce internalization of receptors. In this case, many receptors, including the β-adrenoceptor, do not down-regulate but instead recycle intact to the plasma membrane. This rapid cycling through endocytic vesicles promotes dephosphorylation

of receptors, increasing the rate at which fully functional receptors are replenished in the plasma membrane. Thus, depending on the particular receptor and duration of activation, internalization can mediate quite different effects on receptor signaling and regulation.

Well-Established Second Messengers

A. CYCLIC ADENOSINE MONOPHOSPHATE (cAMP)

Acting as an intracellular second messenger, cAMP mediates such hormonal responses as the mobilization of stored energy (the breakdown of carbohydrates in liver or triglycerides in fat cells stimulated by β-adrenomimetic catecholamines), conservation of water by the kidney (mediated by vasopressin), Ca^{2+} homeostasis (regulated by parathyroid hormone), and increased rate and contraction force of heart muscle (β-adrenomimetic catecholamines). It also regulates the production of adrenal and sex steroids (in response to corticotropin or follicle-stimulating hormone), relaxation of smooth muscle, and many other endocrine and neural processes.

cAMP exerts most of its effects by stimulating cAMP-dependent protein kinases (Figure 2–13). These kinases are composed of a cAMP-binding regulatory (R) dimer and two catalytic (C) chains. When cAMP binds to the R dimer, active C chains are released to diffuse through the cytoplasm and nucleus, where they transfer phosphate from ATP to appropriate substrate proteins, often enzymes. The specificity of cAMP's regulatory effects resides in the distinct protein substrates of the kinases that are expressed in different cells. For example, liver is rich in phosphorylase kinase and glycogen syn-

thase, enzymes whose reciprocal regulation by cAMP-dependent phosphorylation governs carbohydrate storage and release.

When the hormonal stimulus stops, the intracellular actions of cAMP are terminated by an elaborate series of enzymes. cAMP-stimulated phosphorylation of enzyme substrates is rapidly reversed by a diverse group of specific and nonspecific phosphatases. cAMP itself is degraded to 5′-AMP by several cyclic nucleotide phosphodiesterases (PDE, Figure 2–13). Competitive inhibition of cAMP degradation is one way caffeine, theophylline, and other methylxanthines produce their effects (see Chapter 20).

B. CALCIUM AND PHOSPHOINOSITIDES

Another well-studied second messenger system involves hormonal stimulation of phosphoinositide hydrolysis (Figure 2–14). Some of the hormones, neurotransmitters, and growth factors that trigger this pathway (see Table 2–1) bind to receptors linked to G proteins, while others bind to receptor tyrosine kinases. In all cases, the crucial step is stimulation of a membrane enzyme, phospholipase C (PLC), which splits a minor phospholipid component of the plasma membrane, phosphatidylinositol-4,5-bisphosphate (PIP_2), into two second messengers, diacylglycerol and inositol-1,4,5-trisphosphate

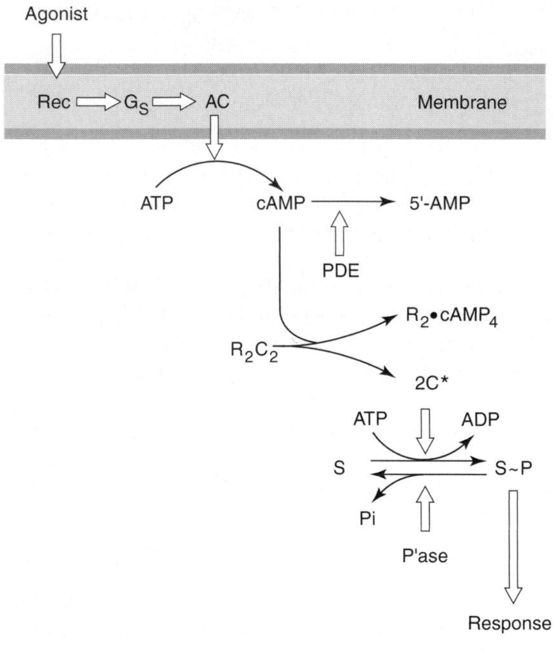

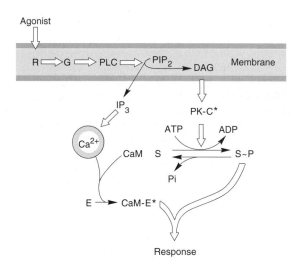

Figure 2–13. The cAMP second messenger pathway. Key proteins include hormone receptors (Rec), a stimulatory G protein (G_s), catalytic adenylyl cyclase (AC), phosphodiesterases (PDE) that hydrolyze cAMP, cAMP-dependent kinases, with regulatory (R) and catalytic (C) subunits, protein substrates (S) of the kinases, and phosphatases (P′ase), which remove phosphates from substrate proteins. Open arrows denote regulatory effects.

Figure 2–14. The Ca^{2+}-phosphoinositide signaling pathway. Key proteins include hormone receptors (R), a G protein (G), a phosphoinositide-specific phospholipase C (PLC), protein kinase C substrates of the kinase (S), calmodulin (CaM), and calmodulin-binding enzymes (E), including kinases, phosphodiesterases, etc. (PIP_2, phosphatidylinositol-4,5-bisphosphate; DAG, diacylglycerol. Asterisk denotes activated state. Open arrows denote regulatory effects.)

(IP$_3$ or InsP$_3$). Diacylglycerol is confined to the membrane where it activates a phospholipid- and calcium-sensitive protein kinase called protein kinase C. IP$_3$ is water-soluble and diffuses through the cytoplasm to trigger release of Ca^{2+} from internal storage vesicles. Elevated cytoplasmic Ca^{2+} concentration promotes the binding of Ca^{2+} to the calcium-binding protein calmodulin, which regulates activities of other enzymes, including calcium-dependent protein kinases.

With its multiple second messengers and protein kinases, the phosphoinositide signaling pathway is much more complex than the cAMP pathway. For example, different cell types may contain one or more specialized calcium- and calmodulin-dependent kinases with limited substrate specificity (eg, myosin light chain kinase) in addition to a general calcium- and calmodulin-dependent kinase that can phosphorylate a wide variety of protein substrates. Furthermore, at least nine structurally distinct types of protein kinase C have been identified.

As in the cAMP system, multiple mechanisms damp or terminate signaling by this pathway. IP$_3$ is inactivated by dephosphorylation; diacylglycerol is either phosphorylated to yield phosphatidic acid, which is then converted back into phospholipids, or it is deacylated to yield arachidonic acid; Ca^{2+} is actively removed from the cytoplasm by Ca^{2+} pumps.

These and other nonreceptor elements of the calcium-phosphoinositide signaling pathway are now becoming targets for drug development. For example, the therapeutic effects of lithium ion, an established agent for treating manic-depressive illness, may be mediated by effects on the metabolism of phosphoinositides (see Chapter 29).

C. Cyclic Guanosine Monophosphate (cGMP)

Unlike cAMP, the ubiquitous and versatile carrier of diverse messages, cGMP has established signaling roles in only a few cell types. In intestinal mucosa and vascular smooth muscle, the cGMP-based signal transduction mechanism closely parallels the cAMP-mediated signaling mechanism. Ligands detected by cell surface receptors stimulate membrane-bound guanylyl cyclase to produce cGMP, and cGMP acts by stimulating a cGMP-dependent protein kinase. The actions of cGMP in these cells are terminated by enzymatic degradation of the cyclic nucleotide and by dephosphorylation of kinase substrates.

Increased cGMP concentration causes relaxation of vascular smooth muscle by a kinase-mediated mechanism that results in dephosphorylation of myosin light chains (see Figure 12–2). In these smooth muscle cells, cGMP synthesis can be elevated by two different transmembrane signaling mechanisms utilizing two different guanylyl cyclases. ANP, a blood-borne peptide hormone, stimulates a transmembrane receptor by binding to its extracellular domain, thereby activating the guanylyl cyclase activity that resides in the receptor's intracellular domain. The other mechanism mediates responses to NO (see Chapter 19), which is generated in vascular endothelial cells in response to natural vasodilator agents such as acetylcholine and histamine (NO is also called endothelium-derived relaxing factor [EDRF]). After entering the target cell, NO binds to and activates a cytoplasmic guanylyl cyclase. A number of useful vasodilating drugs act by generating or mimicking NO, or by interfering with the metabolic breakdown of cGMP by phosphodiesterase (see Chapters 11 and 12).

Interplay Among Signaling Mechanisms

The calcium-phosphoinositide and cAMP signaling pathways oppose one another in some cells and are complementary in others. For example, vasopressor agents that contract smooth muscle act by IP$_3$-mediated mobilization of Ca^{2+}, whereas agents that relax smooth muscle often act by elevation of cAMP. In contrast, cAMP and phosphoinositide second messengers act together to stimulate glucose release from the liver.

Phosphorylation: A Common Theme

Almost all second messenger signaling involves reversible phosphorylation, which performs two principal functions in signaling: amplification and flexible regulation. In **amplification,** rather like GTP bound to a G protein, the attachment of a phosphoryl group to a serine, threonine, or tyrosine residue powerfully amplifies the initial regulatory signal by recording a molecular memory that the pathway has been activated; dephosphorylation erases the memory, taking a longer time to do so than is required for dissociation of an allosteric ligand. In **flexible regulation,** differing substrate specificities of the multiple protein kinases regulated by second messengers provide branch points in signaling pathways that may be independently regulated. In this way, cAMP, Ca^{2+}, or other second messengers can use the presence or absence of particular kinases or kinase substrates to produce quite different effects in different cell types. Inhibitors of protein kinases have great potential as therapeutic agents, particularly in neoplastic diseases. Trastuzumab, an antibody that antagonizes growth factor receptor signaling, was discussed earlier as a therapeutic agent for breast cancer. Another example of this general approach is imatinib (Gleevec, STI571), a small molecule inhibitor of the cytoplasmic tyrosine kinase Bcr/Abl, which is activated by growth factor signaling pathways and is overexpressed in chronic myelogenous leukemia (CML). This compound, a promising agent for treating CML, was recently approved by the US Food and Drug Administration (FDA) for clinical use.

RECEPTOR CLASSES & DRUG DEVELOPMENT

The existence of a specific drug receptor is usually inferred from studying the **structure-activity relationship** of a group of structurally similar congeners of the drug that mimic or antagonize its effects. Thus, if a series of related agonists exhibits identical relative potencies in producing two distinct effects, it is likely that the two effects are mediated by similar or identical receptor molecules. In addition, if identical receptors mediate both effects, a competitive antagonist will inhibit both responses with the same K_I; a second competitive antagonist will inhibit both responses with its own characteristic K_I. Thus, studies of the relation between structure and activity of a series of agonists and antagonists can identify a species of receptor that mediates a set of pharmacologic responses.

Exactly the same experimental procedure can show that observed effects of a drug are mediated by *different* receptors. In this case, effects mediated by different receptors may exhibit different orders of potency among agonists and different K_I values for each competitive antagonist.

Wherever we look, evolution has created many different receptors that function to mediate responses to any individual chemical signal. In some cases, the same chemical acts on completely different structural receptor classes. For example, acetylcholine uses ligand-gated ion channels (nicotinic AChRs) to initiate a fast excitatory postsynaptic potential (EPSP) in postganglionic neurons. Acetylcholine also activates a separate class of G protein–coupled receptors (muscarinic AChRs), which modulate responsiveness of the same neurons to the fast EPSP. In addition, each structural class usually includes multiple subtypes of receptor, often with significantly different signaling or regulatory properties. For example, norepinephrine activates many structurally related receptors, including β-adrenergic (stimulation of G_s, increased heart rate), α_1-adrenergic (stimulation of G_q, vasoconstriction), and α_2-adrenergic (stimulation of G_i, opening of K^+ channels) (see Table 2–2). The existence of multiple receptor classes and subtypes for the same endogenous ligand has created important opportunities for drug development. For example, propranolol, a selective antagonist of β-adrenergic receptors, can reduce an accelerated heart rate without preventing the sympathetic nervous system from causing vasoconstriction, an effect mediated by α_1 receptors.

The principle of drug selectivity may even apply to structurally identical receptors expressed in different cells, eg, receptors for steroids such as estrogen (Figure 2–6). Different cell types express different accessory proteins, which interact with steroid receptors and change the functional effects of drug-receptor interaction. For example, tamoxifen acts as an *antagonist* on estrogen receptors expressed in mammary tissue but as an *agonist* on estrogen receptors in bone. Consequently, tamoxifen may be useful not only in the treatment and prophylaxis of breast cancer but also in the prevention of osteoporosis by increasing bone density (see Chapters 40 and 42). Tamoxifen may also create complications in postmenopausal women, however, by exerting an agonist action in the uterus, stimulating endometrial cell proliferation.

New drug development is not confined to agents that act on receptors for extracellular chemical signals. Pharmaceutical chemists are now determining whether elements of signaling pathways distal to the receptors may also serve as targets of selective and useful drugs. For example, clinically useful agents might be developed that act selectively on specific G proteins, kinases, phosphatases, or the enzymes that degrade second messengers.

RELATION BETWEEN DRUG DOSE & CLINICAL RESPONSE

We have dealt with receptors as molecules and shown how receptors can quantitatively account for the relation between dose or concentration of a drug and pharmacologic responses, at least in an idealized system. When faced with a patient who needs treatment, the prescriber must make a choice among a variety of possible drugs and devise a dosage regimen that is likely to produce maximal benefit and minimal toxicity. In order to make rational therapeutic decisions, the prescriber must understand how drug-receptor interactions underlie the relations between dose and response in patients, the nature and causes of variation in pharmacologic responsiveness, and the clinical implications of selectivity of drug action.

Dose & Response in Patients

A. Graded Dose-Response Relations

To choose among drugs and to determine appropriate doses of a drug, the prescriber must know the relative **pharmacologic potency** and **maximal efficacy** of the drugs in relation to the desired therapeutic effect. These two important terms, often confusing to students and clinicians, can be explained by refering to Figure 2–15, which depicts graded dose-response curves that relate dose of four different drugs to the magnitude of a particular therapeutic effect.

1. **Potency**—Drugs A and B are said to be more potent than drugs C and D because of the relative positions of

their dose-response curves along the dose axis of Figure 2–15. Potency refers to the concentration (EC_{50}) or dose (ED_{50}) of a drug required to produce 50% of that drug's maximal effect. Thus, the pharmacologic potency of drug A in Figure 2–15 is less than that of drug B, a partial agonist, because the EC_{50} of A is greater than the EC_{50} of B. Potency of a drug depends in part on the affinity (K_D) of receptors for binding the drug and in part on the efficiency with which drug-receptor interaction is coupled to response. Note that some doses of drug A can produce larger effects than any dose of drug B, despite the fact that we describe drug B as pharmacologically more potent. The reason for this is that drug A has a larger maximal efficacy, as described below.

For clinical use, it is important to distinguish between a drug's potency and its efficacy. The clinical effectiveness of a drug depends not on its potency (EC_{50}), but on its maximal efficacy (see below) and its ability to reach the relevant receptors. This ability can depend on its route of administration, absorption, distribution through the body, and clearance from the blood or site of action. In deciding which of two drugs to administer to a patient, the prescriber must usually consider their relative effectiveness rather than their relative potency. Pharmacologic potency can largely determine the administered dose of the chosen drug.

For therapeutic purposes, the potency of a drug should be stated in dosage units, usually in terms of a particular therapeutic end point (eg, 50 mg for mild sedation, 1 μg/kg/min for an increase in heart rate of 25 beats/min). Relative potency, the ratio of equi-effective doses (0.2, 10, etc), may be used in comparing one drug with another.

2. Maximal efficacy—This parameter reflects the limit of the dose-response relation on the **response axis**. Drugs A, C, and D in Figure 2–15 have equal maximal efficacy, while all have greater maximal efficacy than drug B. The maximal efficacy (sometimes referred to simply as efficacy) of a drug is obviously crucial for making clinical decisions when a large response is needed. It may be determined by the drug's mode of interactions with receptors (as with partial agonists, described above)* or by characteristics of the receptor-effector system involved.

---

* Note that "maximal efficacy," used in a therapeutic context, does not have exactly the same meaning the term denotes in the more specialized context of drug-receptor interactions described earlier in this chapter. In an idealized in vitro system, efficacy denotes the relative maximal efficacy of agonists and partial agonists that act via the same receptor. In therapeutics, efficacy denotes the extent or degree of an effect that can be achieved in the intact patient. Thus, therapeutic efficacy may be affected by the characteristics of a particular drug-receptor interaction, but it also depends on a host of other factors as noted in the text.

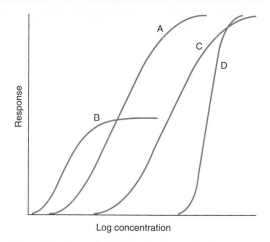

Figure 2–15. Graded dose-response curves for four drugs, illustrating different pharmacologic potencies and different maximal efficacies. (See text.)

Thus, diuretics that act on one portion of the nephron may produce much greater excretion of fluid and electrolytes than diuretics that act elsewhere. In addition, the practical efficacy of a drug for achieving a therapeutic end point (eg, increased cardiac contractility) may be limited by the drug's propensity to cause a toxic effect (eg, fatal cardiac arrhythmia) even if the drug could otherwise produce a greater therapeutic effect.

B. SHAPE OF DOSE-RESPONSE CURVES

While the responses depicted in curves A, B, and C of Figure 2–15 approximate the shape of a simple Michaelis-Menten relation (transformed to a logarithmic plot), some clinical responses do not. Extremely steep dose-response curves (eg, curve D) may have important clinical consequences if the upper portion of the curve represents an undesirable extent of response (eg, coma caused by a sedative-hypnotic). Steep dose-response curves in patients could result from cooperative interactions of several different actions of a drug (eg, effects on brain, heart, and peripheral vessels, all contributing to lowering of blood pressure).

C. QUANTAL DOSE-EFFECT CURVES

Graded dose-response curves of the sort described above have certain limitations in their application to clinical decision making. For example, such curves may be impossible to construct if the pharmacologic response is an either-or (quantal) event, such as prevention of convulsions, arrhythmia, or death. Furthermore, the clinical relevance of a quantitative dose-response relationship in a single patient, no matter how precisely defined, may be limited in application to other patients, owing to the great potential variability among patients in severity of disease and responsiveness to drugs.

Some of these difficulties may be avoided by determining the dose of drug required to produce a specified magnitude of effect in a large number of individual patients or experimental animals and plotting the cumulative frequency distribution of responders versus the log dose (Figure 2–16). The specified quantal effect may be chosen on the basis of clinical relevance (eg, relief of headache) or for preservation of safety of experimental subjects (eg, using low doses of a cardiac stimulant and specifying an increase in heart rate of 20 beats/min as the quantal effect), or it may be an inherently quantal event (eg, death of an experimental animal). For most drugs, the doses required to produce a specified quantal effect in individuals are lognormally distributed; ie, a frequency distribution of such responses plotted against the log of the dose produces a gaussian normal curve of variation (colored area, Figure 2–16). When these responses are summated, the resulting cumulative frequency distribution constitutes a quantal dose-effect curve (or dose-percent curve) of the proportion or percentage of individuals who exhibit the effect plotted as a function of log dose (Figure 2–16).

The quantal dose-effect curve is often characterized by stating the **median effective dose (ED$_{50}$),** the dose at which 50% of individuals exhibit the specified quantal effect. (Note that the abbreviation ED$_{50}$ has a different meaning in this context from its meaning in relation to graded dose-effect curves, described above.) Similarly, the dose required to produce a particular toxic effect in 50% of animals is called the **median toxic dose (TD$_{50}$)** If the toxic effect is death of the animal, a **median lethal dose (LD$_{50}$)** may be experimentally defined. Such values provide a convenient way of comparing the potencies of drugs in experimental and clinical settings: Thus, if the ED$_{50}$s of two drugs for producing a specified quantal effect are 5 and 500 mg, respectively, then the first drug can be said to be 100 times more potent than the second for that particular effect. Similarly, one can obtain a valuable index of the selectivity of a drug's action by comparing its ED$_{50}$s for two different quantal effects in a population (eg, cough suppression versus sedation for opioid drugs).

Quantal dose-effect curves may also be used to generate information regarding the margin of safety to be expected from a particular drug used to produce a specified effect. One measure, which relates the dose of a drug required to produce a desired effect to that which produces an undesired effect, is the **therapeutic index.** In animal studies, the therapeutic index is usually defined as the ratio of the TD$_{50}$ to the ED$_{50}$ for some therapeutically relevant effect. The precision possible in animal experiments may make it useful to use such a therapeutic index to estimate the potential benefit of a drug in humans. Of course, the therapeutic index of a drug in humans is almost never known with real precision; instead, drug trials and accumulated clinical experience often reveal a range of usually effective doses and a different (but sometimes overlapping) range of possibly toxic doses. The clinically acceptable risk of toxicity depends critically on the severity of the disease being treated. For example, the dose range that provides relief from an ordinary headache in the great majority of patients should be very much lower than the dose range that produces serious toxicity, even if the toxicity occurs in a small minority of patients. However, for treatment of a lethal disease such as Hodgkin's lymphoma, the acceptable difference between therapeutic and toxic doses may be smaller.

Finally, note that the quantal dose-effect curve and the graded dose-response curve summarize somewhat different sets of information, although both appear sigmoid in shape on a semilogarithmic plot (compare Figures 2–15 and 2–16). Critical information required for making rational therapeutic decisions can be obtained from each type of curve. Both curves provide information regarding the **potency** and **selectivity** of drugs; the

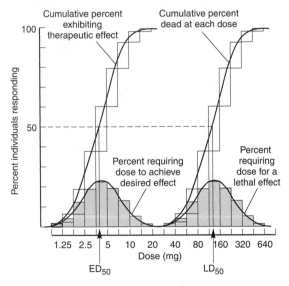

Figure 2–16. Quantal dose-effect plots. Shaded boxes (and the accompanying curves) indicate the frequency distribution of doses of drug required to produce a specified effect; ie, the percentage of animals that required a particular dose to exhibit the effect. The open boxes (and the corresponding curves) indicate the cumulative frequency distribution of responses, which are lognormally distributed.

graded dose-response curve indicates the **maximal efficacy** of a drug, and the quantal dose-effect curve indicates the potential **variability** of responsiveness among individuals.

Variation in Drug Responsiveness

Individuals may vary considerably in their responsiveness to a drug; indeed, a single individual may respond differently to the same drug at different times during the course of treatment. Occasionally, individuals exhibit an unusual or **idiosyncratic** drug response, one that is infrequently observed in most patients. The idiosyncratic responses are usually caused by genetic differences in metabolism of the drug or by immunologic mechanisms, including allergic reactions.

Quantitative variations in drug response are in general more common and more clinically important. An individual patient is **hyporeactive** or **hyperreactive** to a drug in that the intensity of effect of a given dose of drug is diminished or increased in comparison to the effect seen in most individuals. (*Note:* The term **hypersensitivity** usually refers to allergic or other immunologic responses to drugs.) With some drugs, the intensity of response to a given dose may change during the course of therapy; in these cases, responsiveness usually decreases as a consequence of continued drug administration, producing a state of relative **tolerance** to the drug's effects. When responsiveness diminishes rapidly after administration of a drug, the response is said to be subject to **tachyphylaxis.**

Even before administering the first dose of a drug, the prescriber should consider factors that may help in predicting the direction and extent of possible variations in responsiveness. These include the propensity of a particular drug to produce tolerance or tachyphylaxis as well as the effects of age, sex, body size, disease state, genetic factors, and simultaneous administration of other drugs.

Four general mechanisms may contribute to variation in drug responsiveness among patients or within an individual patient at different times.

A. Alteration in Concentration of Drug That Reaches the Receptor

Patients may differ in the rate of absorption of a drug, in distributing it through body compartments, or in clearing the drug from the blood (see Chapter 3). By altering the concentration of drug that reaches relevant receptors, such pharmacokinetic differences may alter the clinical response. Some differences can be predicted on the basis of age, weight, sex, disease state, liver and kidney function, and by testing specifically for genetic differences that may result from inheritance of a functionally distinctive complement of drug-metabolizing enzymes (see Chapters 3 and 4).

B. Variation in Concentration of an Endogenous Receptor Ligand

This mechanism contributes greatly to variability in responses to pharmacologic antagonists. Thus, propranolol, a β-adrenoceptor antagonist, will markedly slow the heart rate of a patient whose endogenous catecholamines are elevated (as in pheochromocytoma) but will not affect the resting heart rate of a well-trained marathon runner. A partial agonist may exhibit even more dramatically different responses: Saralasin, a weak partial agonist at angiotensin II receptors, lowers blood pressure in patients with hypertension caused by increased angiotensin II production and raises blood pressure in patients who produce small amounts of angiotensin.

C. Alterations in Number or Function of Receptors

Experimental studies have documented changes in drug responsiveness caused by increases or decreases in the number of receptor sites or by alterations in the efficiency of coupling of receptors to distal effector mechanisms. In some cases, the change in receptor number is caused by other hormones; for example, thyroid hormones increase both the number of β receptors in rat heart muscle and cardiac sensitivity to catecholamines. Similar changes probably contribute to the tachycardia of thyrotoxicosis in patients and may account for the usefulness of propranolol, a β-adrenoceptor antagonist, in ameliorating symptoms of this disease.

In other cases, the agonist ligand itself induces a decrease in the number (eg, down-regulation) or coupling efficiency (eg, desensitization) of its receptors. These mechanisms (discussed above, under Signaling Mechanisms & Drug Actions) may contribute to two clinically important phenomena: first, tachyphylaxis or tolerance to the effects of some drugs (eg, biogenic amines and their congeners), and second, the "overshoot" phenomena that follow withdrawal of certain drugs. These phenomena can occur with either agonists or antagonists. An antagonist may increase the number of receptors in a critical cell or tissue by preventing down-regulation caused by an endogenous agonist. When the antagonist is withdrawn, the elevated number of receptors can produce an exaggerated response to physiologic concentrations of agonist. Potentially disastrous withdrawal symptoms can result for the opposite reason when administration of an agonist drug is discontinued. In this situation, the number of receptors, which has been decreased by drug-induced down-regulation, is too low for endogenous agonist to produce effective stimulation. For example, the withdrawal of clonidine (a drug whose α_2-adrenoceptor agonist activity reduces blood pressure) can produce hypertensive crisis, probably because the drug down-regulates α_2-adrenoceptors (see Chapter 11).

Genetic factors also can play an important role in altering the number or function of specific receptors. For example, a specific genetic variant of the α_{2C}-adrenoceptor—when inherited together with a specific variant of the β_1-adrenoceptor—confers a greatly increased risk for developing congestive heart failure which may be reduced by early intervention using antagonist drugs. The identification of such genetic factors, part of the rapidly developing field of **pharmacogenetics,** holds exciting promise for clinical diagnosis and may help physicians design the most appropriate pharmacologic therapy for individual patients.

D. CHANGES IN COMPONENTS OF RESPONSE DISTAL TO THE RECEPTOR

Although a drug initiates its actions by binding to receptors, the response observed in a patient depends on the functional integrity of biochemical processes in the responding cell and physiologic regulation by interacting organ systems. Clinically, changes in these postreceptor processes represent the largest and most important class of mechanisms that cause variation in responsiveness to drug therapy.

Before initiating therapy with a drug, the prescriber should be aware of patient characteristics that may limit the clinical response. These characteristics include the age and general health of the patient and—most importantly—the severity and pathophysiologic mechanism of the disease. The most important potential cause of failure to achieve a satisfactory response is that the diagnosis is wrong or physiologically incomplete. Drug therapy will always be most successful when it is accurately directed at the pathophysiologic mechanism responsible for the disease.

When the diagnosis is correct and the drug is appropriate, an unsatisfactory therapeutic response can often be traced to compensatory mechanisms in the patient that respond to and oppose the beneficial effects of the drug. Compensatory increases in sympathetic nervous tone and fluid retention by the kidney, for example, can contribute to tolerance to antihypertensive effects of a vasodilator drug. In such cases, additional drugs may be required to achieve a useful therapeutic response.

Clinical Selectivity: Beneficial Versus Toxic Effects of Drugs

Although we classify drugs according to their principal actions, it is clear that *no drug causes only a single, specific effect.* Why is this so? It is exceedingly unlikely that any kind of drug molecule will bind to only a single type of receptor molecule, if only because the number of potential receptors in every patient is astronomically large.

Even if the chemical structure of a drug allowed it to bind to only one kind of receptor, the biochemical processes controlled by such receptors would take place in multiple cell types and would be coupled to many other biochemical functions; as a result, the patient and the prescriber would probably perceive more than one drug effect. Accordingly, drugs are only *selective*—rather than specific—in their actions, because they bind to one or a few types of receptor more tightly than to others and because these receptors control discrete processes that result in distinct effects.

It is only because of their selectivity that drugs are useful in clinical medicine. Selectivity can be measured by comparing binding affinities of a drug to different receptors or by comparing $ED_{50}s$ for different effects of a drug in vivo. In drug development and in clinical medicine, selectivity is usually considered by separating effects into two categories: **beneficial** or **therapeutic effects** versus **toxic effects.** Pharmaceutical advertisements and prescribers occasionally use the term **side effect,** implying that the effect in question is insignificant or occurs via a pathway that is to one side of the principal action of the drug; such implications are frequently erroneous.

A. BENEFICIAL AND TOXIC EFFECTS MEDIATED BY THE SAME RECEPTOR-EFFECTOR MECHANISM

Much of the serious drug toxicity in clinical practice represents a direct pharmacologic extension of the therapeutic actions of the drug. In some of these cases (bleeding caused by anticoagulant therapy; hypoglycemic coma due to insulin), toxicity may be avoided by judicious management of the dose of drug administered, guided by careful monitoring of effect (measurements of blood coagulation or serum glucose) and aided by ancillary measures (avoiding tissue trauma that may lead to hemorrhage; regulation of carbohydrate intake). In still other cases, the toxicity may be avoided by not administering the drug at all, if the therapeutic indication is weak or if other therapy is available.

In certain situations, a drug is clearly necessary and beneficial but produces unacceptable toxicity when given in doses that produce optimal benefit. In such situations, it may be necessary to add another drug to the treatment regimen. In treating hypertension, for example, administration of a second drug often allows the prescriber to reduce the dose and toxicity of the first drug (see Chapter 11).

B. BENEFICIAL AND TOXIC EFFECTS MEDIATED BY IDENTICAL RECEPTORS BUT IN DIFFERENT TISSUES OR BY DIFFERENT EFFECTOR PATHWAYS

Many drugs produce both their desired effects and adverse effects by acting on a single receptor type in different tissues. Examples discussed in this book include:

digitalis glycosides, which act by inhibiting Na^+/K^+ ATPase in cell membranes; methotrexate, which inhibits the enzyme dihydrofolate reductase; and glucocorticoid hormones.

Three therapeutic strategies are used to avoid or mitigate this sort of toxicity. First, the drug should always be administered at the lowest dose that produces acceptable benefit. Second, adjunctive drugs that act through different receptor mechanisms and produce different toxicities may allow lowering the dose of the first drug, thus limiting its toxicity (eg, use of other immunosuppressive agents added to glucocorticoids in treating inflammatory disorders). Third, selectivity of the drug's actions may be increased by manipulating the concentrations of drug available to receptors in different parts of the body, for example, by aerosol administration of a glucocorticoid to the bronchi in asthma.

C. BENEFICIAL AND TOXIC EFFECTS MEDIATED BY DIFFERENT TYPES OF RECEPTORS

Therapeutic advantages resulting from new chemical entities with improved receptor selectivity were mentioned earlier in this chapter and are described in detail in later chapters. Such drugs include the α- and β-selective adrenoceptor agonists and antagonists, the H_1 and H_2 antihistamines, nicotinic and muscarinic blocking agents, and receptor-selective steroid hormones. All of these receptors are grouped in functional families, each responsive to a small class of endogenous agonists. The receptors and their associated therapeutic uses were discovered by analyzing effects of the physiologic chemical signals—catecholamines, histamine, acetylcholine, and corticosteroids.

A number of other drugs were discovered by exploiting therapeutic or toxic effects of chemically similar agents observed in a clinical context. Examples include quinidine, the sulfonylureas, thiazide diuretics, tricyclic antidepressants, opioid drugs, and phenothiazine antipsychotics. Often the new agents turn out to interact with receptors for endogenous substances (eg, opioids and phenothiazines for endogenous opioid and dopamine receptors, respectively). It is likely that other new drugs will be found to do so in the future, perhaps leading to the discovery of new classes of receptors and endogenous ligands for future drug development.

Thus, the propensity of drugs to bind to different classes of receptor sites is not only a potentially vexing problem in treating patients, it also presents a continuing challenge to pharmacology and an opportunity for developing new and more useful drugs.

REFERENCES

Aaronson DS, Horvath CM: A road map for those who know JAK-STAT. Science 2002;296:1653.

Arteaga CL, Moulder SL, Yakes FM: HER (erbB) tyrosine kinase inhibitors in the treatment of breast cancer. Semin Oncol 2002;29:4.

Bootman MD et al: Calcium signalling–an overview. Semin Cell Dev Biol 2001;12:3.

Bourne HR: How receptors talk to trimeric G proteins. Curr Opin Cell Biol 1997;9:134.

Catterall WA: From ionic currents to molecular mechanisms: the structure and function of voltage-gated sodium channels. Neuron 2000;26:13.

Civelli O et al: Novel neurotransmitters as natural ligands of orphan G-protein-coupled receptors. Trends Neurosci 2001;24:230.

Derynck R, Akhurst RJ, Balmain A: TGF-beta signaling in tumor suppression and cancer progression. Nat Genet 2001;29:117.

Farfel Z, Bourne HR, Iiri T: The expanding spectrum of G protein diseases. N Engl J Med 1999;340:1012.

Ginty DD, Segal RA: Retrograde neurotrophin signaling: Trk-ing along the axon. Curr Opin Neurobiol 2002;12:268.

Hermiston ML et al: Reciprocal regulation of lymphocyte activation by tyrosine kinases and phosphatases. J Clin Invest 2002;109:9.

Jan LY, Stevens CF: Signalling mechanisms: a decade of signalling. Curr Opin Neurobiol 2000;10:625.

Kenakin T: Efficacy at G-protein-coupled receptors. Nat Rev Drug Discov 2002;1:103.

Pierce KL, Premont RT, Lefkowitz RJ: Seven-transmembrane receptors. Nature Rev Mol Cell Biol 2002;3:639.

Mitlak BH, Cohen FJ: Selective estrogen receptor modulators: A look ahead. Drugs 1999;57:653.

Moghal N, Sternberg PW: Multiple positive and negative regulators of signaling by the EGF-receptor. Curr Opin Cell Biol 1999;11:190.

Roden DM, George AL Jr: The genetic basis of variability in drug responses. Nat Rev Drug Discov 2002;1:37.

Rotella DP: Phosphodiesterase 5 inhibitors: current status and potential applications. Nat Rev Drug Discov 2002;1:674.

Schlessinger J: Cell signaling by receptor tyrosine kinases. Cell 2000;103:193.

Small KM et al: Synergistic Polymorphisms of β_1- and α_{2C}-Adrenergic Receptors and the Risk of Congestive Heart Failure. N Engl J Med 2002;347:1135.

Tsao P, von Zastrow M: Downregulation of G protein-coupled receptors. Curr Opin Neurobiol 2000;10:365.

Williams D, Mitchell T: Latest developments in crystallography and structure-based design of protein kinase inhibitors as drug candidates. Curr Opin Pharmacol 2002;2:567.

Pharmacokinetics & Pharmacodynamics: Rational Dosing & the Time Course of Drug Action

3

Nicholas H.G. Holford, MB, ChB, FRACP

The goal of therapeutics is to achieve a desired beneficial effect with minimal adverse effects. When a medicine has been selected for a patient, the clinician must determine the dose that most closely achieves this goal. A rational approach to this objective combines the principles of pharmacokinetics with pharmacodynamics to clarify the dose-effect relationship (Figure 3–1). Pharmacodynamics governs the concentration-effect part of the interaction, whereas pharmacokinetics deals with the dose-concentration part (Holford & Sheiner, 1981). The pharmacokinetic processes of absorption, distribution, and elimination determine how rapidly and for how long the drug will appear at the target organ. The pharmacodynamic concepts of maximum response and sensitivity determine the magnitude of the effect at a particular concentration (see E_{max} and EC_{50}, Chapter 2).

Figure 3–1 illustrates a fundamental hypothesis of pharmacology, namely, that a relationship exists between a beneficial or toxic effect of a drug and the concentration of the drug. This hypothesis has been documented for many drugs, as indicated by the Target Concentrations and Toxic Concentrations columns in Table 3–1. The apparent lack of such a relationship for some drugs does not weaken the basic hypothesis but points to the need to consider the time course of concentration at the actual site of pharmacologic effect (see below).

Knowing the relationship between dose, drug concentration and effects allows the clinician to take into account the various pathologic and physiologic features of a particular patient that make him or her different from the average individual in responding to a drug. The importance of pharmacokinetics and pharmacodynamics in patient care thus rests upon the improvement in therapeutic benefit and reduction in toxicity that can be achieved by application of these principles.

PHARMACOKINETICS

The "standard" dose of a drug is based on trials in healthy volunteers and patients with average ability to absorb, distribute, and eliminate the drug (see Clinical Trials: The IND and NDA in Chapter 5). This dose will not be suitable for every patient. Several physiologic processes (eg, maturation of organ function in infants) and pathologic processes (eg, heart failure, renal failure) dictate dosage adjustment in individual patients. These processes modify specific pharmacokinetic parameters. The two basic parameters are **clearance,** the measure of the ability of the body to eliminate the drug; and **volume of distribution,** the measure of the apparent space in the body available to contain the drug. These parameters are illustrated schematically in Figure 3–2 (page 39), where the volume of the compartments into which the drugs diffuse represents the volume of distribution and the size of the outflow "drain" in Figures 3–2B and 3–2D represents the clearance.

Volume of Distribution

Volume of distribution (V_d) relates the amount of drug in the body to the concentration of drug (C) in blood or plasma:

$$V_d = \frac{\text{Amount of drug in body}}{C} \qquad (1)$$

The volume of distribution may be defined with respect to blood, plasma, or water (unbound drug), depending on the concentration used in equation (1) ($C = C_b$, C_p, or C_u).

That the V_d calculated from equation (1) is an *apparent* volume may be appreciated by comparing the volumes of distribution of drugs such as digoxin or

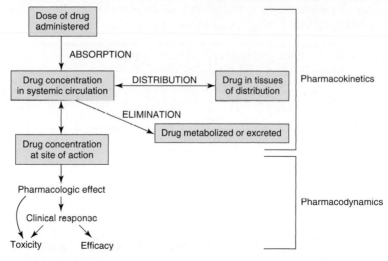

Figure 3–1. The relationship between dose and effect can be separated into pharmacokinetic (dose-concentration) and pharmacodynamic (concentration-effect) components. Concentration provides the link between pharmacokinetics and pharmacodynamics and is the focus of the target concentration approach to rational dosing. The three primary processes of pharmacokinetics are absorption, distribution, and elimination.

chloroquine (Table 3–1) with some of the physical volumes of the body (Table 3–2). Volume of distribution can vastly exceed any physical volume in the body because it is the volume apparently necessary to contain the amount of drug *homogeneously* at the concentration found in the blood, plasma, or water. Drugs with very high volumes of distribution have much higher concentrations in extravascular tissue than in the vascular compartment, ie, they are *not* homogeneously distributed. Drugs that are completely retained within the vascular compartment, on the other hand, have a minimum possible volume of distribution equal to the blood component in which they are distributed, eg, 0.04 L/kg body weight or 2.8 L/70 kg (Table 3–2) for a drug that is restricted to the plasma compartment.

Clearance

Drug clearance principles are similar to the clearance concepts of renal physiology. Clearance of a drug is the factor that predicts the rate of elimination in relation to the drug concentration:

$$CL = \frac{\text{Rate of elimination}}{C} \qquad (2)$$

Clearance, like volume of distribution, may be defined with respect to blood (CL_b), plasma (CL_p), or unbound in water (CL_u), depending on the concentration measured.

It is important to note the additive character of clearance. Elimination of drug from the body may involve processes occurring in the kidney, the lung, the liver, and other organs. Dividing the rate of elimination at each organ by the concentration of drug presented to it yields the respective clearance at that organ. Added together, these separate clearances equal total systemic clearance:

$$CL_{renal} = \frac{\text{Rate of elimination}_{kidney}}{C} \qquad (3a)$$

$$CL_{liver} = \frac{\text{Rate of elimination}_{liver}}{C} \qquad (3b)$$

$$CL_{other} = \frac{\text{Rate of elimination}_{other}}{C} \qquad (3c)$$

$$CL_{systemic} = CL_{renal} + CL_{liver} + CL_{other} \qquad (3d)$$

"Other" tissues of elimination could include the lungs and additional sites of metabolism, eg, blood or muscle.

The two major sites of drug elimination are the kidneys and the liver. Clearance of unchanged drug in the urine represents renal clearance. Within the liver, drug elimination occurs via biotransformation of parent drug to one or more metabolites, or excretion of unchanged drug into the bile, or both. The pathways of biotransfor-

Table 3–1. Pharmacokinetic and pharmacodynamic parameters for selected drugs.
(See Speight & Holford, 1997, for a more comprehensive listing.)

Drug	Oral Availability (F) (%)	Urinary Excretion (%)	Bound in Plasma (%)	Clearance (L/h/70 kg)[1]	Volume of Distribution (L/70 kg)	Half-Life (h)	Target Concentrations	Toxic Concentrations
Acetaminophen	88	3	0	21	67	2	15 mg/L	>300 mg/L
Acyclovir	23	75	15	19.8	48	2.4	...	...
Amikacin	...	98	4	5.46	19	2.3	...	...
Amoxicillin	93	86	18	10.8	15	1.7	...	...
Amphotericin	...	4	90	1.92	53	18	...	...
Ampicillin	62	82	18	16.2	20	1.3	...	...
Aspirin	68	1	49	39	11	0.25	...	...
Atenolol	56	94	5	10.2	67	6.1	1 mg/L	...
Atropine	50	57	18	24.6	120	4.3	...	...
Captopril	65	38	30	50.4	57	2.2	50 ng/mL	...
Carbamazepine	70	1	74	5.34	98	15	6 mg/L	>9 mg/L
Cephalexin	90	91	14	18	18	0.9	...	...
Cephalothin	...	52	71	28.2	18	0.57	...	...
Chloramphenicol	80	25	53	10.2	66	2.7	...	...
Chlordiazepoxide	100	1	97	2.28	21	10	1 mg/L	...
Chloroquine	89	61	61	45	13000	214	20 ng/mL	250 ng/mL
Chlorpropamide	90	20	96	0.126	6.8	33	...	...
Cimetidine	62	62	19	32.4	70	1.9	0.8 mg/L	...
Ciprofloxacin	60	65	40	25.2	130	4.1	...	...
Clonidine	95	62	20	12.6	150	12	1 ng/mL	...
Cyclosporine	23	1	93	24.6	85	5.6	200 ng/mL	>400 ng/mL
Diazepam	100	1	99	1.62	77	43	300 ng/mL	...
Digitoxin	90	32	97	0.234	38	161	10 ng/mL	>35 ng/mL
Digoxin	70	60	25	7	500	50	1 ng/mL	>2 ng/mL
Diltiazem	44	4	78	50.4	220	3.7	...	...
Disopyramide	83	55	[2]	5.04	41	6	3 mg/L	>8 mg/L
Enalapril	95	90	55	9	40	3	> 0.5 ng/mL	...
Erythromycin	35	12	84	38.4	55	1.6	...	...

(continued)

Table 3–1. Pharmacokinetic and pharmacodynamic parameters for selected drugs *(continued)*.

Drug	Oral Availability (F) (%)	Urinary Excretion (%)	Bound in Plasma (%)	Clearance (L/h/70 kg)[1]	Volume of Distribution (L/70 kg)	Half-Life (h)	Target Concentrations	Toxic Concentrations
Ethambutol	77	79	5	36	110	3.1	...	>10 mg/L
Fluoxetine	60	3	94	40.2	2500	53	...	...
Furosemide	61	66	99	8.4	7.7	1.5	...	>25 mg/L
Gentamicin	...	90	10	5.4	18	2.5	...	...
Hydralazine	40	10	87	234	105	1	100 ng/mL	...
Imipramine	40	2	90	63	1600	18	200 ng/mL	>1 mg/L
Indomethacin	98	15	90	8.4	18	2.4	1 mg/L	>5 mg/L
Labetalol	18	5	50	105	660	4.9	0.1 mg/L	...
Lidocaine	35	2	70	38.4	77	1.8	3 mg/L	>6 mg/L
Lithium	100	95	0	1.5	55	22	0.7 mEq/L	>2 mEq/L
Meperidine	52	12	58	72	310	3.2	0.5 mg/L	...
Methotrexate	70	48	34	9	39	7.2	750 μM-h[3]	>950 μM-h
Metoprolol	38	10	11	63	290	3.2	25 ng/mL	...
Metronidazole	99	10	10	5.4	52	8.5	4 mg/L	...
Midazolam	44	56	95	27.6	77	1.9	...	...
Morphine	24	8	35	60	230	1.9	60 ng/mL	...
Nifedipine	50	0	96	29.4	55	1.8	50 ng/mL	...
Nortriptyline	51	2	92	30	1300	31	100 ng/mL	>500 ng/mL
Phenobarbital	100	24	51	0.258	38	98	15 mg/L	>30 mg/L
Phenytoin	90	2	89	Conc-dependent[4]	45	Conc-dependent[5]	10 mg/L	>20 mg/L
Prazosin	68	1	95	12.6	42	2.9	...	...
Procainamide	83	67	16	36	130	3	5 mg/L	>14 mg/L
Propranolol	26	1	87	50.4	270	3.9	20 ng/mL	...
Pyridostigmine	14	85	...	36	77	1.9	75 ng/mL	...
Quinidine	80	18	87	19.8	190	6.2	3 mg/L	>8 mg/L
Ranitidine	52	69	15	43.8	91	2.1	100 ng/mL	...
Rifampin	?	7	89	14.4	68	3.5	...	...
Salicylic acid	100	15	85	0.84	12	13	200 mg/L	>200 mg/L

(continued)

Table 3–1. Pharmacokinetic and pharmacodynamic parameters for selected drugs *(continued)*.

Drug	Oral Availability (F) (%)	Urinary Excretion (%)	Bound in Plasma (%)	Clearance (L/h/70 kg)[1]	Volume of Distribution (L/70 kg)	Half-Life (h)	Target Concentrations	Toxic Concentrations
Sulfamethoxazole	100	14	62	1.32	15	10	...	...
Terbutaline	14	56	20	14.4	125	14	2 ng/mL	...
Tetracycline	77	58	65	7.2	105	11	...	...
Theophylline	96	18	56	2.8	35	8.1	10 mg/L	>20 mg/L
Tobramycin	...	90	10	4.62	18	2.2	...	...
Tocainide	89	38	10	10.8	210	14	10 mg/L	...
Tolbutamide	93	0	96	1.02	7	5.9	100 mg/L	...
Trimethoprim	100	69	44	9	130	11	...	...
Tubocurarine	...	63	50	8.1	27	2	0.6 mg/L	...
Valproic acid	100	2	93	0.462	9.1	14	75 mg/L	>150 mg/L
Vancomycin	...	79	30	5.88	27	5.6	...	...
Verapamil	22	3	90	63	350	4	...	...
Warfarin	93	3	99	0.192	9.8	37	...	...
Zidovudine	63	18	25	61.8	98	1.1	...	...

[1]Convert to mL/min by multiplying the number given by 16.6.
[2]Varies with concentration.
[3]Target area under the concentration time curve after a single dose.
[4]Can be estimated from measured C_p using $CL = V_{max}/(K_m + C_p)$; $V_{max} = 415$ mg/d, $K_m = 5$ mg/L. See text.
[5]Varies because of concentration-dependent clearance.

mation are discussed in Chapter 4. For most drugs, clearance is constant over the concentration range encountered in clinical settings, ie, elimination is not saturable, and the rate of drug elimination is directly proportional to concentration (rearranging equation [2]):

$$\text{Rate of elimination} = CL \times C \qquad (4)$$

This is usually referred to as first-order elimination. When clearance is first-order, it can be estimated by calculating the **area under the curve** (AUC) of the time-concentration profile after a dose. Clearance is calculated from the dose divided by the AUC.

A. Capacity-Limited Elimination

For drugs that exhibit capacity-limited elimination (eg, phenytoin, ethanol), clearance will vary depending on the concentration of drug that is achieved (Table 3–1). Capacity-limited elimination is also known as saturable, dose- or concentration-dependent, nonlinear, and Michaelis-Menten elimination.

Most drug elimination pathways will become saturated if the dose is high enough. When blood flow to an organ does not limit elimination (see below), the relation between elimination rate and concentration (C) is expressed mathematically in equation (5):

$$\text{Rate of elimination} = \frac{V_{max} \times C}{K_m + C} \qquad (5)$$

The maximum elimination capacity is V_{max}, and K_m is the drug concentration at which the rate of elimination is 50% of V_{max}. At concentrations that are high relative to the K_m, the elimination rate is almost independent of concentration—a state of "pseudo-zero order" elimination. If dosing rate exceeds elimination capacity, steady state cannot be achieved: The concentration will keep on rising as long as dosing continues. This pattern of capacity-limited elimination is important for three drugs in common use: ethanol, phenytoin, and aspirin. Clearance has no real meaning for drugs with capacity-

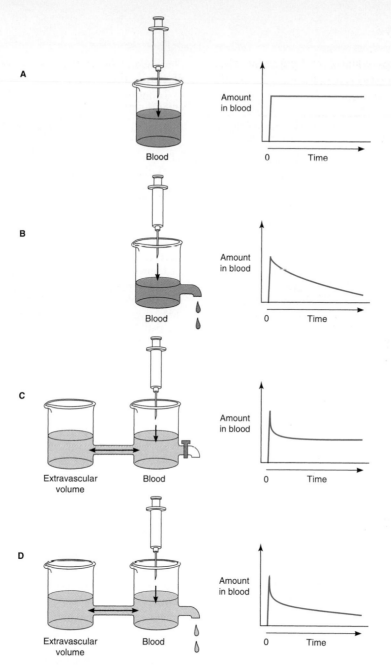

Figure 3–2. Models of drug distribution and elimination. The effect of adding drug to the blood by rapid intravenous injection is represented by expelling a known amount of the agent into a beaker. The time course of the amount of drug in the beaker is shown in the graphs at the right. In the first example (**A**), there is no movement of drug out of the beaker, so the graph shows only a steep rise to maximum followed by a plateau. In the second example (**B**), a route of elimination is present, and the graph shows a slow decay after a sharp rise to a maximum. Because the level of material in the beaker falls, the "pressure" driving the elimination process also falls, and the slope of the curve decreases. This is an exponential decay curve. In the third model (**C**), drug placed in the first compartment ("blood") equilibrates rapidly with the second compartment ("extravascular volume") and the amount of drug in "blood" declines exponentially to a new steady state. The fourth model (**D**) illustrates a more realistic combination of elimination mechanism and extravascular equilibration. The resulting graph shows an early distribution phase followed by the slower elimination phase.

Table 3–2. Physical volumes (in L/kg body weight) of some body compartments into which drugs may be distributed.

Compartment and Volume	Examples of Drugs
Water	
Total body water (0.6 L/kg[1])	Small water-soluble molecules: eg, ethanol.
Extracellular water (0.2 L/kg)	Larger water-soluble molecules: eg, gentamicin.
Blood (0.08 L/kg); plasma (0.04 L/kg)	Strongly plasma protein-bound molecules and very large molecules: eg, heparin.
Fat (0.2–0.35 L/kg)	Highly lipid-soluble molecules: eg, DDT.
Bone (0.07 L/kg)	Certain ions: eg, lead, fluoride.

[1]An average figure. Total body water in a young lean man might be 0.7 L/kg; in an obese woman, 0.5 L/kg.

limited elimination, and AUC cannot be used to describe the elimination of such drugs.

B. Flow-Dependent Elimination

In contrast to capacity-limited drug elimination, some drugs are cleared very readily by the organ of elimination, so that at any clinically realistic concentration of the drug, most of the drug in the blood perfusing the organ is eliminated on the first pass of the drug through it. The elimination of these drugs will thus depend primarily on the rate of drug delivery to the organ of elimination. Such drugs (see Table 4–7) can be called "high-extraction" drugs since they are almost completely extracted from the blood by the organ. Blood flow to the organ is the main determinant of drug delivery, but plasma protein binding and blood cell partitioning may also be important for extensively bound drugs that are highly extracted.

Half-Life

Half-life ($t_{1/2}$) is the time required to change the amount of drug in the body by one-half during elimination (or during a constant infusion). In the simplest case—and the most useful in designing drug dosage regimens—the body may be considered as a single compartment (as

illustrated in Figure 3–2B) of a size equal to the volume of distribution (V_d). The time course of drug in the body will depend on both the volume of distribution and the clearance:

$$t_{1/2} = \frac{0.7^* \times V_d}{CL} \qquad (6)$$

Half-life is useful because it indicates the time required to attain 50% of steady state—or to decay 50% from steady-state conditions—after a change in the rate of drug administration. Figure 3–3 shows the time course of drug accumulation during a constant-rate drug infusion and the time course of drug elimination after stopping an infusion that has reached steady state.

Disease states can affect both of the physiologically related primary pharmacokinetic parameters: volume of distribution and clearance. A change in half-life will not necessarily reflect a change in drug elimination. For example, patients with chronic renal failure have decreased renal clearance of digoxin but also a decreased volume of distri-

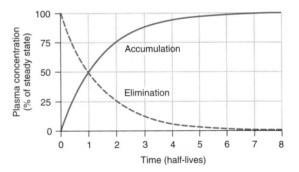

Figure 3–3. The time course of drug accumulation and elimination. **Solid line:** Plasma concentrations reflecting drug accumulation during a constant rate infusion of a drug. Fifty percent of the steady-state concentration is reached after one half-life, 75% after two half-lives, and over 90% after four half-lives. **Dashed line:** Plasma concentrations reflecting drug elimination after a constant rate infusion of a drug had reached steady state. Fifty percent of the drug is lost after one half-life, 75% after two half-lives, etc. The "rule of thumb" that four half-lives must elapse after starting a drug-dosing regimen before full effects will be seen is based on the approach of the accumulation curve to over 90% of the final steady-state concentration.

---

* The constant 0.7 in equation (6) is an approximation to the natural logarithm of 2. Because drug elimination can be described by an exponential process, the time taken for a twofold decrease can be shown to be proportional to ln(2).

bution; the increase in digoxin half-life is not as great as might be expected based on the change in renal function. The decrease in volume of distribution is due to the decreased renal and skeletal muscle mass and consequent decreased tissue binding of digoxin to Na^+/K^+ ATPase.

Many drugs will exhibit multicompartment pharmacokinetics (as illustrated in Figures 3–2C and 3–2D). Under these conditions, the "true" terminal half-life, as given in Table 3–1, will be greater than that calculated from equation (6).

Drug Accumulation

Whenever drug doses are repeated, the drug will accumulate in the body until dosing stops. This is because it takes an infinite time (in theory) to eliminate all of a given dose. In practical terms, this means that if the dosing interval is shorter than four half-lives, accumulation will be detectable.

Accumulation is inversely proportional to the fraction of the dose lost in each dosing interval. The fraction lost is 1 minus the fraction remaining just before the next dose. The fraction remaining can be predicted from the dosing interval and the half-life. A convenient index of accumulation is the **accumulation factor.**

$$\text{Accumulation factor} = \frac{1}{\text{Fraction lost in one dosing interval}}$$

$$= \frac{1}{1 - \text{Fraction remaining}}$$

(7)

For a drug given once every half-life, the accumulation factor is 1/0.5, or 2. The accumulation factor predicts the ratio of the steady-state concentration to that seen at the same time following the first dose. Thus, the peak concentrations after intermittent doses at steady state will be equal to the peak concentration after the first dose multiplied by the accumulation factor.

Bioavailability

Bioavailability is defined as the fraction of unchanged drug reaching the systemic circulation following administration by any route (Table 3–3). The area under the blood concentration-time curve (area under the curve, AUC) is a common measure of the extent of bioavailability for a drug given by a particular route (Figure 3–4). For an intravenous dose of the drug, bioavailability is assumed to be equal to unity. For a drug administered orally, bioavailability may be less than 100% for two main reasons—incomplete extent of absorption and first-pass elimination.

Table 3–3. Routes of administration, bioavailability, and general characteristics.

Route	Bioavailability (%)	Characteristics
Intravenous (IV)	100 (by definition)	Most rapid onset
Intramuscular (IM)	75 to ≤100	Large volumes often feasible; may be painful
Subcutaneous (SC)	75 to ≤100	Smaller volumes than IM; may be painful
Oral (PO)	5 to <100	Most convenient; first-pass effect may be significant
Rectal (PR)	30 to <100	Less first-pass effect than oral
Inhalation	5 to <100	Often very rapid onset
Transdermal	80 to ≤100	Usually very slow absorption; used for lack of first-pass effect; prolonged duration of action

A. EXTENT OF ABSORPTION

After oral administration, a drug may be incompletely absorbed, eg, only 70% of a dose of digoxin reaches the systemic circulation. This is mainly due to lack of absorption from the gut. Other drugs are either too hydrophilic (eg, atenolol) or too lipophilic (eg, acyclovir) to be absorbed easily, and their low bioavailability is also due to incomplete absorption. If too hydrophilic, the drug cannot cross the lipid cell membrane; if too lipophilic, the drug is not soluble enough to cross the water layer adjacent to the cell. Drugs may not be absorbed because of a reverse transporter associated with P-glycoprotein. This process actively pumps drug out of gut wall cells back into the gut lumen. Inhibition of P-glycoprotein and gut wall metabolism, eg, by grapefruit juice, may be associated with substantially increased drug absorption.

B. FIRST-PASS ELIMINATION

Following absorption across the gut wall, the portal blood delivers the drug to the liver prior to entry into the systemic circulation. A drug can be metabolized in the gut wall (eg, by the CYP3A4 enzyme system) or even in the portal blood, but most commonly it is the liver that is responsible for metabolism before the drug reaches the systemic circulation. In addition, the liver can excrete the drug into the bile. Any of these sites can contribute to this reduction in bioavailability, and the overall process is known as first-pass elimination. The effect of first-pass hepatic elimination on bioavailability is expressed as the extraction ratio (ER):

$$ER = \frac{CL_{liver}}{Q} \qquad (8a)$$

where Q is hepatic blood flow, normally about 90 L/h in a person weighing 70 kg.

The systemic bioavailability of the drug (F) can be predicted from the extent of absorption (f) and the extraction ratio (ER):

$$F = f \times (1 - ER) \qquad (8b)$$

A drug such as morphine is almost completely absorbed (f = 1), so that loss in the gut is negligible. However, the hepatic extraction ratio for morphine is 0.67, so (1 − ER) is 0.33. The bioavailability of morphine is therefore expected to be about 33%, which is close to the observed value (Table 3–1).

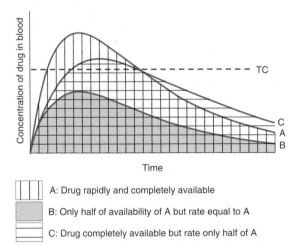

Figure 3–4. Blood concentration-time curves, illustrating how changes in the rate of absorption and extent of bioavailability can influence both the duration of action and the effectiveness of the same total dose of a drug administered in three different formulations. The dashed line indicates the target concentration (TC) of the drug in the blood.

C. RATE OF ABSORPTION

The distinction between rate and extent of absorption is shown in Figure 3–4. The rate of absorption is determined by the site of administration and the drug formulation. Both the rate of absorption and the extent of input can influence the clinical effectiveness of a drug. For the three different dosage forms depicted in Figure 3–4, there would be significant differences in the intensity of clinical effect. Dosage form B would require twice the dose to attain blood concentrations equivalent to those of dosage form A. Differences in rate of availability may become important for drugs given as a single dose, such as a hypnotic used to induce sleep. In this case, drug from dosage form A would reach its target concentration earlier than drug from dosage form C; concentrations from A would also reach a higher level and remain above the target concentration for a longer period. In a multiple dosing regimen, dosage forms A and C would yield the same average blood level concentrations, although dosage form A would show somewhat greater maximum and lower minimum concentrations.

The mechanism of drug absorption is said to be zero-order when the rate is independent of the amount of drug remaining in the gut, eg, when it is determined by the rate of gastric emptying or by a controlled-release drug formulation. In contrast, when the full dose is dissolved in gastrointestinal fluids, the rate of absorption is usually proportional to the gastrointestinal concentration and is said to be first-order.

Extraction Ratio & the First-Pass Effect

Systemic clearance is not affected by bioavailability. However, clearance can markedly affect the extent of availability because it determines the extraction ratio (equation [8a]). Of course, therapeutic blood concentrations may still be reached by the oral route of administration if larger doses are given. However, in this case, the concentrations of the drug *metabolites* will be increased significantly over those that would occur following intravenous administration. Lidocaine and verapamil are both used to treat cardiac arrhythmias and have bioavailability less than 40%, but lidocaine is never given orally because its metabolites are believed to contribute to central nervous system toxicity. Other drugs that are highly extracted by the liver include isoniazid, morphine, propranolol, verapamil, and several tricyclic antidepressants (Table 3–1).

Drugs with high extraction ratios will show marked variations in bioavailability between subjects because of differences in hepatic function and blood flow. These differences can explain the marked variation in drug concentrations that occurs among individuals given similar doses of highly extracted drugs. For drugs that are highly extracted by the liver, shunting of blood past hepatic sites of elimination will result in substantial increases in drug availability, whereas for drugs that are poorly extracted by the liver (for which the difference between entering and exiting drug concentration is small), shunting of blood past the liver will cause little change in availability. Drugs in Table 3–1 that are poorly extracted by the liver include chlorpropamide, diazepam, phenytoin, theophylline, tolbutamide, and warfarin.

Alternative Routes of Administration & the First-Pass Effect

There are several reasons for different routes of administration used in clinical medicine (Table 3–3)—for convenience (eg, oral), to maximize concentration at the site of action and minimize it elsewhere (eg, topical), to prolong the duration of drug absorption (eg, transdermal), or to avoid the first-pass effect.

The hepatic first-pass effect can be avoided to a great extent by use of sublingual tablets and transdermal preparations and to a lesser extent by use of rectal suppositories. Sublingual absorption provides direct access to systemic—not portal—veins. The transdermal route offers the same advantage. Drugs absorbed from suppositories in the lower rectum enter vessels that drain into the inferior vena cava, thus bypassing the liver. However, suppositories tend to move upward in the rectum into a region where veins that lead to the liver predominate. Thus, only about 50% of a rectal dose can be assumed to bypass the liver.

Although drugs administered by inhalation bypass the hepatic first-pass effect, the lung may also serve as a site of first-pass loss by excretion and possibly metabolism for drugs administered by nongastrointestinal ("parenteral") routes.

THE TIME COURSE OF DRUG EFFECT

The principles of pharmacokinetics (discussed in this chapter) and those of pharmacodynamics (discussed in Chapter 2; Holford & Sheiner, 1981) provide a framework for understanding the time course of drug effect.

Immediate Effects

In the simplest case, drug effects are directly related to plasma concentrations, but this does not necessarily mean that effects simply parallel the time course of concentrations. Because the relationship between drug concentration and effect is not linear (recall the E_{max} model described in Chapter 2), the effect will not usually be linearly proportional to the concentration.

Consider the effect of an angiotensin-converting enzyme (ACE) inhibitor, such as enalapril, on plasma ACE. The half-life of enalapril is about 3 hours. After an oral dose of 10 mg, the peak plasma concentration at 3 hours is about 64 ng/mL. Enalapril is usually given once a day, so seven half-lives will elapse from the time of peak concentration to the end of the dosing interval. The concentration of enalapril after each half-life and the corresponding extent of ACE inhibition are shown in Figure 3–5. The extent of inhibition of ACE is calculated using the E_{max} model, where E_{max}, the maximum extent of inhibition, is 100% and the EC_{50} is about 1 ng/mL.

Note that plasma concentrations of enalapril change by a factor of 16 over the first 12 hours (four half-lives) after the peak, but ACE inhibition has only decreased by 20%. Because the concentrations over this time are so high in relation to the EC_{50}, the effect on ACE is almost constant. After 24 hours, ACE is still 33% inhibited. This explains why a drug with a short half-life can be given once a day and still maintain its effect throughout the day. The key factor is a high initial concentration in relation to the EC_{50}. Even though the plasma concentration at 24 hours is less than 1% of its peak, this low concentration is still half the EC_{50}. This is very common for drugs that act on enzymes (eg, ACE inhibitors) or compete at receptors (eg, propranolol).

When concentrations are in the range between one fourth and four times the EC_{50}, the time course of effect is essentially a linear function of time—13% of the effect is lost every half-life over this concentration range. At concentrations below one fourth the EC_{50}, the effect becomes almost directly proportional to concentration and the time course of drug effect will follow the exponential decline of concentration. It is only when the

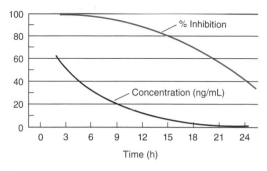

Figure 3–5. Time course of angiotensin-converting enzyme (ACE) inhibitor concentrations and effects. The black line shows the plasma enalapril concentrations in nanograms per milliliter after a single oral dose. The colored line indicates the percentage inhibition of its target, ACE. Note the different shapes of the concentration-time course (exponentially decreasing) and the effect-time course (linearly decreasing in its central portion).

concentration is low in relation to the EC_{50} that the concept of a "half-life of drug effect" has any meaning.

Delayed Effects

Changes in drug effects are often delayed in relation to changes in plasma concentration. This delay may reflect the time required for the drug to distribute from plasma to the site of action. This will be the case for almost all drugs. The delay due to distribution is a pharmacokinetic phenomenon that can account for delays of a few minutes. This distributional delay can account for the lag of effects after rapid intravenous injection of central nervous system (CNS)–active agents such as thiopental.

A common reason for more delayed drug effects—especially those that take many hours or even days to occur—is the slow turnover of a physiologic substance that is involved in the expression of the drug effect (Jusko & Ko, 1994). For example, warfarin works as an anticoagulant by inhibiting vitamin K epoxidase in the liver. This action of warfarin occurs rapidly, and inhibition of the enzyme is closely related to plasma concentrations of warfarin. The clinical effect of warfarin, eg, on the prothrombin time, reflects a decrease in the concentration of the prothrombin complex of clotting factors (see Figure 34–7). Inhibition of vitamin K epoxidase decreases the synthesis of these clotting factors, but the complex has a long half-life (about 14 hours), and it is this half-life that determines how long it takes for the concentration of clotting factors to reach a new steady state and for a drug effect to become manifest that reflects the warfarin plasma concentration.

Cumulative Effects

Some drug effects are more obviously related to a cumulative action than to a rapidly reversible one. The renal toxicity of aminoglycoside antibiotics (eg, gentamicin) is greater when administered as a constant infusion than with intermittent dosing. It is the accumulation of aminoglycoside in the renal cortex that is thought to cause renal damage. Even though both dosing schemes produce the same average steady-state concentration, the intermittent dosing scheme produces much higher peak concentrations, which saturate an uptake mechanism into the cortex; thus, total aminoglycoside accumulation is less. The difference in toxicity is a predictable consequence of the different patterns of concentration and the saturable uptake mechanism.

The effect of many drugs used to treat cancer also reflects a cumulative action—eg, the extent of binding of a drug to DNA is proportional to drug concentration and is usually irreversible. The effect on tumor growth is therefore a consequence of cumulative exposure to the drug. Measures of cumulative exposure, such as AUC, provide a means to individualize treatment (Evans et al, 1998).

THE TARGET CONCENTRATION APPROACH TO DESIGNING A RATIONAL DOSAGE REGIMEN

A rational dosage regimen is based on the assumption that there is a **target concentration** that will produce the desired therapeutic effect. By considering the pharmacokinetic factors that determine the dose-concentration relationship, it is possible to individualize the dose regimen to achieve the target concentration. The effective concentration ranges shown in Table 3–1 are a guide to the concentrations measured when patients are being effectively treated. The initial target concentration should usually be chosen from the lower end of this range. In some cases, the target concentration will also depend on the specific therapeutic objective—eg, the control of atrial fibrillation by digoxin often requires a target concentration of 2 ng/mL, while heart failure is usually adequately managed with a target concentration of 1 ng/mL.

Maintenance Dose

In most clinical situations, drugs are administered in such a way as to maintain a steady state of drug in the body, ie, just enough drug is given in each dose to replace the drug eliminated since the preceding dose. Thus, calculation of the appropriate maintenance dose is a primary goal. Clearance is the most important pharmacokinetic term to be considered in defining a rational steady state drug dosage regimen. At steady state, the dosing rate ("rate in") must equal the rate of elimination ("rate out"). Substitution of the target concentration (TC) for concentration (C) in equation (4) predicts the maintenance dosing rate:

$$\text{Dosing rate}_{ss} = \text{Rate of elimination}_{ss}$$

$$= \text{CL} \times \text{TC} \qquad (9)$$

Thus, if the desired target concentration is known, the clearance in that patient will determine the dosing rate. If the drug is given by a route that has a bioavailability less than 100%, then the dosing rate predicted by equation (9) must be modified. For oral dosing:

$$\text{Dosing rate}_{oral} = \frac{\text{Dosing rate}}{F_{oral}} \qquad (10)$$

If intermittent doses are given, the maintenance dose is calculated from:

Maintenance dose =

$$\text{Dosing rate} \times \text{Dosing interval} \qquad (11)$$

(See Box, Example: Maintenance Dose Calculation.)

EXAMPLE: MAINTENANCE DOSE CALCULATION

A target plasma theophylline concentration of 10 mg/L is desired to relieve acute bronchial asthma in a patient. If the patient is a nonsmoker and otherwise normal except for asthma, we may use the mean clearance given in Table 3–1, ie, 2.8 L/h/70 kg. Since the drug will be given as an intravenous infusion, F = 1.

$$\text{Dosing rate} = CL \times TC$$
$$= 2.8\ L/h/70\ kg \times 10\ mg/L$$
$$= 28\ mg/h/70\ kg$$

Therefore, in this patient, the proper infusion rate would be 28 mg/h/70 kg.

If the asthma attack is relieved, the clinician might want to maintain this plasma level using oral theophylline, which might be given every 12 hours using an extended-release formulation to approximate a continuous intravenous infusion. According to Table 3–1, F_{oral} is 0.96. When the dosing interval is 12 hours, the size of each maintenance dose would be:

$$\text{Maintenance dose} = \frac{\text{Dosing rate}}{F} \times \text{Dosing interval}$$
$$= \frac{28\ mg/h}{0.96} \times 12\ hours$$
$$= 350\ mg$$

A tablet or capsule size close to the ideal dose of 350 mg would then be prescribed at 12-hourly intervals. If an 8-hour dosing interval was used, the ideal dose would be 233 mg; and if the drug was given once a day, the dose would be 700 mg. In practice, F could be omitted from the calculation since it is so close to 1.

Note that the steady-state concentration achieved by continuous infusion or the *average* concentration following intermittent dosing depends only on clearance. The volume of distribution and the half-life need not be known in order to determine the average plasma concentration expected from a given dosing rate or to predict the dosing rate for a desired target concentration.

Figure 3–6 shows that at different dosing intervals, the concentration time curves will have different maximum and minimum values even though the average level will always be 10 mg/L.

Estimates of dosing rate and average steady-state concentrations, which may be calculated using clearance, are independent of any specific pharmacokinetic

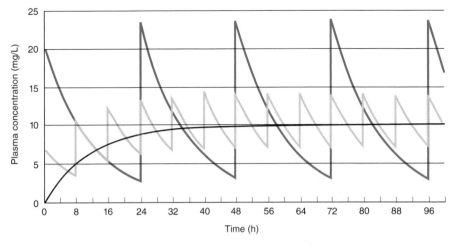

Figure 3–6. Relationship between frequency of dosing and maximum and minimum plasma concentrations when a steady-state theophylline plasma level of 10 mg/L is desired. The smoothly rising line (solid black) shows the plasma concentration achieved with an intravenous infusion of 28 mg/h. The doses for 8-hourly administration (light color) are 224 mg; for 24-hourly administration (dark color), 672 mg. In each of the 3 cases, the mean steady-state plasma concentration is 10 mg/L.

model. In contrast, the determination of maximum and minimum steady-state concentrations requires further assumptions about the pharmacokinetic model. The accumulation factor (equation [7]) assumes that the drug follows a one-compartment body model (Figure 3–2B), and the peak concentration prediction assumes that the absorption rate is much faster than the elimination rate. For the calculation of estimated maximum and minimum concentrations in a clinical situation, these assumptions are usually reasonable.

Loading Dose

When the time to reach steady state is appreciable, as it is for drugs with long half-lives, it may be desirable to administer a loading dose that promptly raises the concentration of drug in plasma to the target concentration. In theory, only the amount of the loading dose need be computed—not the rate of its administration—and, to a first approximation, this is so. The volume of distribution is the proportionality factor that relates the total amount of drug in the body to the concentration in the plasma (C_p); if a loading dose is to achieve the target concentration, then from equation (1):

$$\text{Loading dose} = \begin{array}{c}\text{Amount in the body}\\ \text{immediately following}\\ \text{the loading dose}\end{array}$$
$$= V_d \times TC \qquad (12)$$

For the theophylline example given in the Box, Example: Maintenance Dose Calculation, the loading dose would be 350 mg (35 L × 10 mg/L) for a 70 kg person. For most drugs, the loading dose can be given as a single dose by the chosen route of administration.

Up to this point, we have ignored the fact that some drugs follow more complex multicompartment pharmacokinetics, eg, the distribution process illustrated by the two-compartment model in Figure 3–2. This is justified in the great majority of cases. However, in some cases the distribution phase may not be ignored, particularly in connection with the calculation of loading doses. If the rate of absorption is rapid relative to distribution (this is always true for intravenous bolus administration), the concentration of drug in plasma that results from an appropriate loading dose—calculated using the apparent volume of distribution—can initially be considerably higher than desired. Severe toxicity may occur, albeit transiently. This may be particularly important, for example, in the administration of antiarrhythmic drugs such as lidocaine, where an almost immediate toxic response may occur. Thus, while the estimation of the *amount* of a loading dose may be quite correct, the *rate of administration* can sometimes be crucial in preventing excessive drug concentrations, and slow administration

of an intravenous drug (over minutes rather than seconds) is almost always prudent practice. For intravenous doses of theophylline, initial injections should be given over a 20-minute period to reduce the possibility of high plasma concentrations during the distribution phase.

When intermittent doses are given, the loading dose calculated from equation (12) will only reach the average steady-state concentration and will not match the peak steady-state concentration (see Figure 3–6). To match the peak steady-state concentration, the loading dose can be calculated from equation (13):

$$\text{Loading dose} = \text{Maintenance dose} \times$$
$$\text{Accumulation factor} \qquad (13)$$

THERAPEUTIC DRUG MONITORING: RELATING PHARMACOKINETICS & PHARMACODYNAMICS

The basic principles outlined above can be applied to the interpretation of clinical drug concentration measurements on the basis of three major pharmacokinetic variables: absorption, clearance, and volume of distribution (and the derived variable, half-life); and two pharmacodynamic variables: maximum effect attainable in the target tissue and the sensitivity of the tissue to the drug. Diseases may modify all of these parameters, and the ability to predict the effect of disease states on pharmacokinetic parameters is important in properly adjusting dosage in such cases. (See Box, The Target Concentration Strategy.)

Pharmacokinetic Variables

A. Absorption

The amount of drug that enters the body depends on the patient's compliance with the prescribed regimen and on the rate and extent of transfer from the site of administration to the blood.

Overdosage and underdosage relative to the prescribed dosage—both aspects of failure of compliance—can frequently be detected by concentration measurements when gross deviations from expected values are obtained. If compliance is found to be adequate, absorption abnormalities in the small bowel may be the cause of abnormally low concentrations. Variations in the extent of bioavailability are rarely caused by irregularities in the manufacture of the particular drug formulation. More commonly, variations in bioavailability are due to metabolism during absorption.

B. Clearance

Abnormal clearance may be anticipated when there is major impairment of the function of the kidney, liver, or

THE TARGET CONCENTRATION STRATEGY

Recognition of the essential role of concentration in linking pharmacokinetics and pharmacodynamics leads naturally to the target concentration strategy. Pharmacodynamic principles can be used to predict the concentration required to achieve a particular degree of therapeutic effect. This target concentration can then be achieved by using pharmacokinetic principles to arrive at a suitable dosing regimen (Holford, 1999). The target concentration strategy is a process for optimizing the dose in an individual on the basis of a measured surrogate response such as drug concentration:

1. Choose the target concentration, TC.

2. Predict volume of distribution (V_d) and clearance (CL) based on standard population values (eg, Table 3–1) with adjustments for factors such as weight and renal function.
3. Give a loading dose or maintenance dose calculated from TC, V_d, and CL.
4. Measure the patient's response and drug concentration.
5. Revise V_d and/or CL based on the measured concentration.
6. Repeat steps 3–5, adjusting the predicted dose to achieve TC.

---

heart. Creatinine clearance is a useful quantitative indicator of renal function. Conversely, drug clearance may be a useful indicator of the functional consequences of heart, kidney, or liver failure, often with greater precision than clinical findings or other laboratory tests. For example, when renal function is changing rapidly, estimation of the clearance of aminoglycoside antibiotics may be a more accurate indicator of glomerular filtration than serum creatinine.

Hepatic disease has been shown to reduce the clearance and prolong the half-life of many drugs. However, for many other drugs known to be eliminated by hepatic processes, no changes in clearance or half-life have been noted with similar hepatic disease. This reflects the fact that hepatic disease does not always affect the hepatic intrinsic clearance. At present, there is no reliable marker of hepatic drug-metabolizing function that can be used to predict changes in liver clearance in a manner analogous to the use of creatinine clearance as a marker of renal drug clearance.

C. VOLUME OF DISTRIBUTION

The apparent volume of distribution reflects a balance between binding to tissues, which decreases plasma concentration and makes the apparent volume larger, and binding to plasma proteins, which increases plasma concentration and makes the apparent volume smaller. Changes in either tissue or plasma binding can change the apparent volume of distribution determined from plasma concentration measurements. Older people have a relative decrease in skeletal muscle mass and tend to have a smaller apparent volume of distribution of digoxin (which binds to muscle proteins). The volume of distribution may be overestimated in obese patients if based on body weight and the drug does not enter fatty

tissues well, as is the case with digoxin. In contrast, theophylline has a volume of distribution similar to that of total body water. Adipose tissue has almost as much water in it as other tissues, so that the apparent total volume of distribution of theophylline is proportional to body weight even in obese patients.

Abnormal accumulation of fluid—edema, ascites, pleural effusion—can markedly increase the volume of distribution of drugs such as gentamicin that are hydrophilic and have small volumes of distribution.

D. HALF-LIFE

The differences between clearance and half-life are important in defining the underlying mechanisms for the effect of a disease state on drug disposition. For example, the half-life of diazepam increases with age. When clearance is related to age, it is found that clearance of this drug does not change with age. The increasing half-life for diazepam actually results from changes in the volume of distribution with age; the metabolic processes responsible for eliminating the drug are fairly constant.

Pharmacodynamic Variables

A. MAXIMUM EFFECT

All pharmacologic responses must have a maximum effect (E_{max}). No matter how high the drug concentration goes, a point will be reached beyond which no further increment in response is achieved.

If increasing the dose in a particular patient does not lead to a further clinical response, it is possible that the maximum effect has been reached. Recognition of maximum effect is helpful in avoiding ineffectual increases of dose with the attendant risk of toxicity.

B. SENSITIVITY

The sensitivity of the target organ to drug concentration is reflected by the concentration required to produce 50% of maximum effect, the EC_{50}. Failure of response due to diminished sensitivity to the drug can be detected by measuring—in a patient who is not getting better—drug concentrations that are usually associated with therapeutic response. This may be a result of abnormal physiology—eg, hyperkalemia diminishes responsiveness to digoxin—or drug antagonism—eg, calcium channel blockers impair the inotropic response to digoxin.

Increased sensitivity to a drug is usually signaled by exaggerated responses to small or moderate doses. The pharmacodynamic nature of this sensitivity can be confirmed by measuring drug concentrations that are low in relation to the observed effect.

INTERPRETATION OF DRUG CONCENTRATION MEASUREMENTS

Clearance

Clearance is the single most important factor determining drug concentrations. The interpretation of measurements of drug concentrations depends on a clear understanding of three factors that may influence clearance: the dose, the organ blood flow, and the intrinsic func-

tion of the liver or kidneys. Each of these factors should be considered when interpreting clearance estimated from a drug concentration measurement. It must also be recognized that changes in protein binding may lead the unwary to believe there is a change in clearance when in fact drug elimination is not altered (see Box, Plasma Protein Binding: Is It Important?). Factors affecting protein binding include the following:

1. Albumin concentration: Drugs such as phenytoin, salicylates, and disopyramide are extensively bound to plasma albumin. Albumin levels are low in many disease states, resulting in lower total drug concentrations.

2. Alpha$_1$-acid glycoprotein concentration: α_1-Acid glycoprotein is an important binding protein with binding sites for drugs such as quinidine, lidocaine, and propranolol. It is increased in acute inflammatory disorders and causes major changes in total plasma concentration of these drugs even though drug elimination is unchanged.

3. Capacity-limited protein binding: The binding of drugs to plasma proteins is capacity-limited. Therapeutic concentrations of salicylates and prednisolone show concentration-dependent protein binding. Because unbound drug concentration is determined by dosing rate and clearance—which is not altered, in the case of these low-extraction-ratio drugs, by protein binding—increases in dosing rate will cause corre-

---

PLASMA PROTEIN BINDING: IS IT IMPORTANT?

Plasma protein binding is often mentioned as a factor playing a role in pharmacokinetics, pharmacodynamics, and drug interactions. However, there are no clinically relevant examples of changes in drug disposition or effects that can be clearly ascribed to changes in plasma protein binding (Benet & Hoener 2002). The idea that if a drug is displaced from plasma proteins it would increase the unbound drug concentration and increase the drug effect and, perhaps, produce toxicity seems a simple and obvious mechanism. Unfortunately, this simple theory, which is appropriate for a test tube, does not work in the body, which is an open system capable of eliminating unbound drug.

First, a seemingly dramatic change in the unbound fraction from 1% to 10% releases less than 5% of the total amount of drug in the body into the unbound pool because less than one third of the drug in the body is bound to plasma proteins even in the most extreme cases, eg, warfarin. Drug displaced from plasma protein will of course distribute

throughout the volume of distribution, so that a 5% increase in the amount of unbound drug in the body produces at most a 5% increase in pharmacologically active unbound drug at the site of action.

Second, when the amount of unbound drug in plasma increases, the rate of elimination will increase (if unbound clearance is unchanged), and after four half-lives the unbound concentration will return to its previous steady state value. When drug interactions associated with protein binding displacement and clinically important effects have been studied, it has been found that the displacing drug is also an inhibitor of clearance, and it is the change in *clearance* of the *unbound* drug that is the relevant mechanism explaining the interaction.

The clinical importance of plasma protein binding is only to help interpretation of measured drug concentrations. When plasma proteins are lower than normal, then total drug concentrations will be lower but unbound concentrations will not be affected.

sponding changes in the pharmacodynamically important unbound concentration. Total drug concentration will increase less rapidly than the dosing rate would suggest as protein binding approaches saturation at higher concentrations.

Dosing History

An accurate dosing history is essential if one is to obtain maximum value from a drug concentration measurement. In fact, if the dosing history is unknown or incomplete, a drug concentration measurement loses all predictive value.

Timing of Samples for Concentration Measurement

Information about the rate and extent of drug absorption in a particular patient is rarely of great clinical importance. However, absorption usually occurs during the first 2 hours after a drug dose and varies according to food intake, posture, and activity. Therefore, it is important to avoid drawing blood until absorption is complete (about 2 hours after an oral dose). Attempts to measure peak concentrations early after oral dosing are usually unsuccessful and compromise the validity of the measurement, because one cannot be certain that absorption is complete.

Some drugs such as digoxin and lithium take several hours to distribute to tissues. Digoxin samples should be taken at least 6 hours after the last dose and lithium just before the next dose (usually 24 hours after the last dose). Aminoglycosides distribute quite rapidly, but it is still prudent to wait 1 hour after giving the dose before taking a sample.

Clearance is readily estimated from the dosing rate and mean steady-state concentration. Blood samples should be appropriately timed to estimate steady-state concentration. Provided steady state has been approached (at least three half-lives of constant dosing), a sample obtained near the midpoint of the dosing interval will usually be close to the mean steady-state concentration.

Initial Predictions of Volume of Distribution & Clearance

A. Volume of Distribution

Volume of distribution is commonly calculated for a particular patient using body weight (70 kg body weight is assumed for the values in Table 3–1). If a patient is obese, drugs that do not readily penetrate fat (eg, gentamicin and digoxin) should have their volumes calculated from ideal body weight as shown below:

$$\text{Ideal body wt (kg)} = 52 + 1.9 \text{ kg/in height}$$
$$\text{over 5 ft (men)} \qquad (14)$$
$$= 49 + 1.7 \text{ kg/in height}$$
$$\text{over 5 ft (women)}$$

Patients with edema, ascites, or pleural effusions offer a larger volume of distribution to the aminoglycoside antibiotics (eg, gentamicin) than is predicted by body weight. In such patients, the weight should be corrected as follows: Subtract an estimate of the weight of the excess fluid accumulation from the measured weight. Use the resultant "normal" body weight to calculate the normal volume of distribution. Finally, this normal volume should be increased by 1 L for each estimated kilogram of excess fluid. This correction is important because of the relatively small volumes of distribution of these water-soluble drugs.

B. Clearance

Drugs cleared by the renal route often require adjustment of clearance in proportion to renal function. This can be conveniently estimated from the creatinine clearance, calculated from a single serum creatinine measurement and the predicted creatinine production rate.

The predicted creatinine production rate in women is 85% of the calculated value, because they have a smaller muscle mass per kilogram and it is muscle mass that determines creatinine production. Muscle mass as a fraction of body weight decreases with age, which is why age appears in the Cockcroft-Gault equation.[*]

The decrease of renal function with age is independent of the decrease in creatinine production. Because of the difficulty of obtaining complete urine collections, creatinine clearance calculated in this way is at least as reliable as estimates based on urine collections. Ideal body weight should be used for obese patients, and correction should be made for muscle wasting in severely ill patients.

Revising Individual Estimates of Volume of Distribution & Clearance

The commonsense approach to the interpretation of drug concentrations compares predictions of pharmacokinetic parameters and expected concentrations to measured values. If measured concentrations differ by more than 20% from predicted values, revised estimates of V_d or CL for that patient should be calculated using equation (1) or equation (2). If the change calculated is more than a 100% increase or 50% decrease in either V_d or

---

[*] The Cockcroft-Gault equation is given in Chapter 61.

CL, the assumptions made about the timing of the sample and the dosing history should be critically examined.

For example, if a patient is taking 0.25 mg of digoxin a day, a clinician may expect the digoxin concentration to be about 1 ng/mL. This is based on typical values for bioavailability of 70% and total clearance of about 7 L/h (CL_{renal} 4 L/h, $CL_{nonrenal}$ 3 L/h). If the patient has heart failure, the nonrenal (hepatic) clearance might be halved because of hepatic congestion and hypoxia, so the expected clearance would become 5.5 L/h. The concentration is then expected to be about 1.3 ng/mL. Suppose that the concentration actually measured is 2 ng/mL. Common sense would suggest halving the daily dose to achieve a target concentration of 1 ng/mL. This approach implies a revised clearance of 3.5 L/h. The smaller clearance compared with the expected value of 5.5 L/h may reflect additional renal functional impairment due to heart failure.

This technique will often be misleading if steady state has not been reached. At least a week of regular dosing (three to four half-lives) must elapse before the implicit method will be reliable.

REFERENCES

Benet LZ, Hoener B: Changes in plasma protein binding have little clinical relevance. Clin Pharmacol Ther 2002;71:115.

Evans WE et al: Conventional compared with individualized chemotherapy for childhood acute lymphoblastic leukemia. N Engl J Med 1998;338:499.

Holford NHG: Pharmacokinetic and pharmacodynamic principles. 2003; http://www.health.auckland.ac.nz/courses/Humanbio251/.

Holford NHG, Sheiner LB: Understanding the dose-effect relationship. Clin Pharmacokinet 1981;6:429.

Holford NHG: Target concentration intervention: Beyond Y2K. Br J Clin Pharmacol 1999;48:9.

Jusko WJ, Ko HC: Physiologic indirect response models characterize diverse types of pharmacodynamic effects. Clin Pharmacol Ther 1994;56:406.

Speight T, Holford NHG: *Avery's Drug Treatment,* 4th ed. Adis International, 1997.

Drug Biotransformation

Maria Almira Correia, PhD

Humans are exposed daily to a wide variety of foreign compounds called **xenobiotics**—substances absorbed across the lungs or skin or, more commonly, ingested either unintentionally as compounds present in food and drink or deliberately as drugs for therapeutic or "recreational" purposes. Exposure to environmental xenobiotics may be inadvertent and accidental or—when they are present as components of air, water, and food—inescapable. Some xenobiotics are innocuous, but many can provoke biologic responses. Such biologic responses often depend on conversion of the absorbed substance into an active metabolite. The discussion that follows is applicable to xenobiotics in general (including drugs) and to some extent to endogenous compounds.

WHY IS DRUG BIOTRANSFORMATION NECESSARY?

Renal excretion plays a pivotal role in terminating the biologic activity of some drugs, particularly those that have small molecular volumes or possess polar characteristics such as functional groups that are fully ionized at physiologic pH. However, many drugs do not possess such physicochemical properties. Pharmacologically active organic molecules tend to be lipophilic and remain un-ionized or only partially ionized at physiologic pH. They are often strongly bound to plasma proteins. Such substances are not readily filtered at the glomerulus. The lipophilic nature of renal tubular membranes also facilitates the reabsorption of hydrophobic compounds following their glomerular filtration. Consequently, most drugs would have a prolonged duration of action if termination of their action depended solely on renal excretion.

An alternative process that may lead to the termination or alteration of biologic activity is metabolism. In general, lipophilic xenobiotics are transformed to more polar and hence more readily excretable products. The role metabolism may play in the inactivation of lipid-soluble drugs can be quite dramatic. For example, lipophilic barbiturates such as thiopental and pentobarbital would have extremely long half-lives if it were not for their metabolic conversion to more water-soluble compounds.

Metabolic products are often less pharmacodynamically active than the parent drug and may even be inactive. However, some biotransformation products have *enhanced* activity or toxic properties. It is noteworthy that the synthesis of endogenous substrates such as steroid hormones, cholesterol, active vitamin D congeners and bile acids involves many pathways catalyzed by enzymes associated with the metabolism of xenobiotics. Finally, drug-metabolizing enzymes have been exploited in the design of pharmacologically inactive prodrugs that are converted to active molecules in the body.

THE ROLE OF BIOTRANSFORMATION IN DRUG DISPOSITION

Most metabolic biotransformations occur at some point between absorption of the drug into the general circulation and its renal elimination. A few transformations occur in the intestinal lumen or intestinal wall. In general, all of these reactions can be assigned to one of two major categories called **phase I** and **phase II reactions** (Figure 4–1).

Phase I reactions usually convert the parent drug to a more polar metabolite by introducing or unmasking a functional group ($-OH$, $-NH_2$, $-SH$). Often these metabolites are inactive, although in some instances activity is only modified.

If phase I metabolites are sufficiently polar, they may be readily excreted. However, many phase I products are not eliminated rapidly and undergo a subsequent reaction in which an endogenous substrate such as glucuronic acid, sulfuric acid, acetic acid, or an amino acid combines with the newly incorporated functional group to form a highly polar conjugate. Such conjugation or synthetic reactions are the hallmarks of phase II metabolism. A great variety of drugs undergo these sequential biotransformation reactions, although in some instances the parent drug may already possess a functional group that may form a conjugate directly. For example, the hydrazide moiety of isoniazid is known to form an *N*-acetyl conjugate in a phase II reaction. This conjugate is then a substrate for a phase I type reaction, namely, hydrolysis to isonicotinic acid (Figure 4–2). Thus, phase II reactions may actually precede phase I reactions.

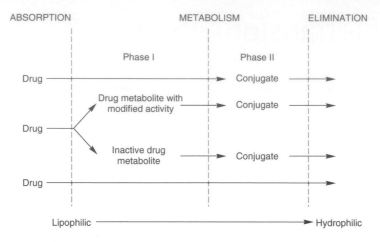

Figure 4–1. Phase I and phase II reactions in drug biodisposition. Phase II reactions may also precede phase I reactions.

WHERE DO DRUG BIOTRANSFORMATIONS OCCUR?

Although every tissue has some ability to metabolize drugs, the liver is the principal organ of drug metabolism. Other tissues that display considerable activity include the gastrointestinal tract, the lungs, the skin, and the kidneys. Following oral administration, many drugs (eg, isoproterenol, meperidine, pentazocine, morphine) are absorbed intact from the small intestine and transported first via the portal system to the liver, where they undergo extensive metabolism. This process has

been called a **first-pass effect** (see Chapter 3). Some orally administered drugs (eg, clonazepam, chlorpromazine) are more extensively metabolized in the intestine than in the liver. Thus, intestinal metabolism may contribute to the overall first-pass effect. First-pass effects may so greatly limit the bioavailability of orally administered drugs that alternative routes of administration must be used to achieve therapeutically effective blood levels. The lower gut harbors intestinal microorganisms that are capable of many biotransformation reactions. In addition, drugs may be metabolized by gastric acid (eg, penicillin), by digestive enzymes (eg, polypeptides such as insulin), or by enzymes in the wall of the intestine (eg, sympathomimetic catecholamines).

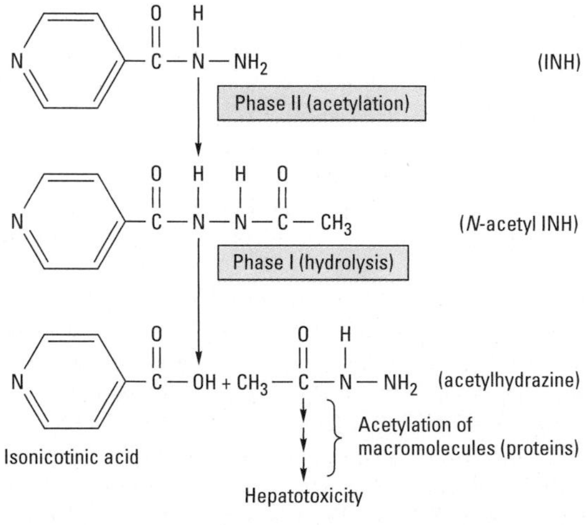

Although drug biotransformation in vivo can occur by spontaneous, noncatalyzed chemical reactions, the vast majority of transformations are catalyzed by specific cellular enzymes. At the subcellular level, these enzymes may be located in the endoplasmic reticulum, mitochondria, cytosol, lysosomes, or even the nuclear envelope or plasma membrane.

MICROSOMAL MIXED FUNCTION OXIDASE SYSTEM & PHASE I REACTIONS

Many drug-metabolizing enzymes are located in the lipophilic membranes of the endoplasmic reticulum of the liver and other tissues. When these lamellar membranes are isolated by homogenization and fractionation of the cell, they re-form into vesicles called **microsomes.** Microsomes retain most of the morphologic and functional characteristics of the intact membranes, including the rough and smooth surface features of the rough

Figure 4–2. Phase II activation of isoniazid (INH) to a hepatotoxic metabolite.

(ribosome-studded) and smooth (no ribosomes) endoplasmic reticulum. Whereas the rough microsomes tend to be dedicated to protein synthesis, the smooth microsomes are relatively rich in enzymes responsible for oxidative drug metabolism. In particular, they contain the important class of enzymes known as the **mixed function oxidases** (MFOs), or monooxygenases. The activity of these enzymes requires both a reducing agent (NADPH) and molecular oxygen; in a typical reaction, one molecule of oxygen is consumed (reduced) per substrate molecule, with one oxygen atom appearing in the product and the other in the form of water.

In this oxidation-reduction process, two microsomal enzymes play a key role. The first of these is a flavoprotein, **NADPH-cytochrome P450 reductase.** One mole of this enzyme contains 1 mol each of flavin mononucleotide (FMN) and flavin adenine dinucleotide (FAD). The second microsomal enzyme is a hemoprotein called **cytochrome P450** that serves as the terminal oxidase. In fact, the microsomal membrane harbors multiple forms of this hemoprotein, and this multiplicity is increased by repeated administration of exogenous chemicals (see below). The name cytochrome P450 (abbreviated as CYP or P450) is derived from the spectral properties of this hemoprotein. In its reduced (ferrous) form, it binds carbon monoxide to give a complex that absorbs light maximally at 450 nm. The relative abundance of P450, compared with that of the reductase in the liver, contributes to making P450 heme reduction a rate-limiting step in hepatic drug oxidations.

Microsomal drug oxidations require P450, P450 reductase, NADPH, and molecular oxygen. A simplified scheme of the oxidative cycle is presented in Figure 4–3. Briefly, oxidized (Fe^{3+}) P450 combines with a drug substrate to form a binary complex (step ①). NADPH donates an electron to the flavoprotein reductase, which in turn reduces the oxidized P450-drug complex (step ②). A second electron is introduced from NADPH via the same flavoprotein reductase, which serves to reduce molecular oxygen and to form an "activated oxygen"-P450-substrate complex (step ③). This complex in turn transfers activated oxygen to the drug substrate to form the oxidized product (step ④).

The potent oxidizing properties of this activated oxygen permit oxidation of a large number of substrates. Substrate specificity is very low for this enzyme complex. High solubility in lipids is the only common structural feature of the wide variety of structurally unrelated drugs and chemicals that serve as substrates in this system (Table 4–1).

Enzyme Induction

Some of these chemically dissimilar drug substrates, on repeated administration, "induce" P450 by enhancing

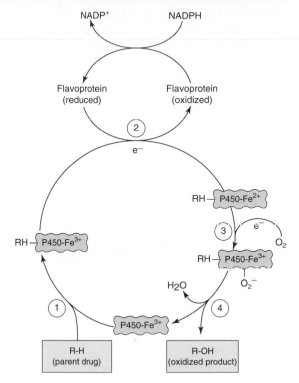

Figure 4–3. Cytochrome P450 cycle in drug oxidations. (R-H, parent drug; R-OH, oxidized metabolite; e⁻, electron.)

the rate of its synthesis or reducing its rate of degradation. Induction results in an acceleration of substrate metabolism and usually in a decrease in the pharmacologic action of the inducer and also of coadministered drugs. However, in the case of drugs metabolically transformed to reactive metabolites, enzyme induction may exacerbate metabolite-mediated toxicity.

Various substrates appear to induce P450 isoforms having different molecular masses and exhibiting different substrate specificities and immunochemical and spectral characteristics. The isoforms that have been most extensively studied include CYP2B1 (formerly P450b), induced by phenobarbital treatment; CYP1A1 ($P_1$450 or P448), induced by polycyclic aromatic hydrocarbons ("PAHs" such as benzo[a]pyrene and 3-methylcholanthrene); CYPs3A (including CYPs 3A4 and 3A5, the major human liver isoforms) induced by glucocorticoids, macrolide antibiotics, anticonvulsants, and some steroids. Chronic administration of isoniazid or ethanol induces a different isoform, CYP2E1, that oxidizes ethanol and activates carcinogenic nitrosamines. The VLDL-lowering drug clofibrate induces other distinct

Table 4–1. Phase I reactions.

Reaction Class	Structural Change	Drug Substrates
Oxidations		
Cytochrome P450-dependent oxidations: Aromatic hydroxylations		Acetanilide, propranolol, phenobarbital, phenytoin, phenylbutazone, amphetamine, warfarin, 17α-ethinyl estradiol, naphthalene, benzpyrene
Aliphatic hydroxylations	$RCH_2CH_3 \rightarrow RCH_2CH_2OH$ $RCH_2CH_3 \rightarrow RCHCH_3$ $\qquad\qquad\qquad\ \ |$ $\qquad\qquad\qquad OH$	Amobarbital, pentobarbital, secobarbital, chlorpropamide, ibuprofen, meprobamate, glutethimide, phenylbutazone, digitoxin
Epoxidation	$RCH{=}CHR \rightarrow R{-}\overset{\displaystyle H}{\underset{\displaystyle}{C}}\overset{\displaystyle O}{\diagdown\diagup}\overset{\displaystyle H}{\underset{\displaystyle}{C}}{-}R$	Aldrin
Oxidative dealkylation N-Dealkylation	$RNHCH_3 \rightarrow RNH_2 + CH_2O$	Morphine, ethylmorphine, benzphetamine, aminopyrine, caffeine, theophylline
O-Dealkylation	$ROCH_3 \rightarrow ROH + CH_2O$	Codeine, *p*-nitroanisole
S-Dealkylation	$RSCH_3 \rightarrow RSH + CH_2O$	6-Methylthiopurine, methitural
N-Oxidation Primary amines	$RNH_2 \rightarrow RNHOH$	Aniline, chlorphentermine
Secondary amines	R_1 $\quad\diagdown$ $\quad\ NH \rightarrow \quad N{-}OH$ $\quad\diagup$ R_2	2-Acetylaminofluorene, acetaminophen
Tertiary amines	R_1 $\quad\diagdown$ $R_2{-}N \rightarrow R_2{-}N{\rightarrow}O$ $\quad\diagup$ R_3	Nicotine, methaqualone
S-Oxidation	R_1 $\quad\diagdown$ $\quad\ S \rightarrow \quad S{=}O$ $\quad\diagup$ R_2	Thioridazine, cimetidine, chlorpromazine
Deamination	$\qquad\qquad\qquad OH$ $\qquad\qquad\qquad |$ $RCHCH_3 \rightarrow R{-}C{-}CH_3 \rightarrow R{-}CCH_3 + NH_3$ $\quad |\qquad\qquad\ \ |\qquad\qquad\ \ \|$ $\ NH_2\qquad\quad NH_2\qquad\qquad O$	Amphetamine, diazepam
Desulfuration	R_1 $\quad\diagdown$ $\quad\ C{=}S \rightarrow \quad C{=}O$ $\quad\diagup$ R_2	Thiopental

Table 4–1. Phase I reactions (cont'd).

Reaction Class	Structural Change	Drug Substrates
Cytochrome P450-dependent oxidations: (cont'd)	$$\begin{array}{c}R_1\\ \backslash\\ P{=}S \to\\ /\\ R_2\end{array}\quad \begin{array}{c}R_1\\ \backslash\\ P{=}O\\ /\\ R_2\end{array}$$	Parathion
Dechlorination	$CCl_4 \to [CCl_3{}^{\cdot}] \to CHCl_3$	Carbon tetrachloride
Cytochrome P450-independent oxidations:		
Flavin monooxygenase (Ziegler's enzyme)	$R_3N \longrightarrow R_3N^+ {\to} O^- \xrightarrow{H^+} R_3N^+OH$	Chlorpromazine, amitriptyline, benzphetamine
	$RCH_2N{-}CH_2R \to RCH_2{-}\underset{OH}{N}{-}CH_2R \to$ $RCH{=}N{-}CH_2R$	Desipramine, nortriptyline
	$\begin{array}{c}-N\\ \quad\\ C{-}SH \to\\ \quad\\ -N\end{array}\; \begin{array}{c}-N\\ \quad\\ C{-}SOH \to\\ \quad\\ -N\end{array}\; \begin{array}{c}-N\\ \quad\\ C{-}SO_2H\\ \quad\\ -N\end{array}$	Methimazole, propylthiouracil
Amine oxidases	$RCH_2NH_2 \to RCHO + NH_3$	Phenylethylamine, epinephrine
Dehydrogenations	$RCH_2OH \to RCHO$	Ethanol
Reductions Azo reductions	$RN{=}NR_1 \to RNH{-}NHR_1 \to RNH_2 + R_1NH_2$	Prontosil, tartrazine
Nitro reductions	$RNO_2 \to RNO \to RNHOH \to RNH_2$	Nitrobenzene, chloramphenicol, clonazepam, dantrolene
Carbonyl reductions	$R\underset{O}{\overset{||}{C}}R' \to R\underset{OH}{\overset{|}{C}}HR'$	Metyrapone, methadone, naloxone
Hydrolyses Esters	$R_1COOR_2 \to R_1COOH + R_2OH$	Procaine, succinylcholine, aspirin, clofibrate, methylphenidate
Amides	$RCONHR_1 \to RCOOH + R_1NH_2$	Procainamide, lidocaine, indomethacin

enzymes of the CYP4A class that are responsible for ω-hydroxylation of several fatty acids, leukotrienes, and prostaglandins.

Environmental pollutants are also capable of inducing P450 enzymes. As noted above, exposure to benzo[*a*]pyrene and other polycyclic aromatic hydrocarbons, which are present in tobacco smoke, charcoal-broiled meat, and other organic pyrolysis products, is known to induce CYP1A enzymes and to alter the rates of drug metabolism. Other environmental chemicals known to induce specific P450s include the polychlorinated biphenyls (PCBs), which were used widely in industry as insulating materials and plasticizers, and 2,3,7,8-tetrachlorodibenzo-*p*-dioxin (dioxin, TCDD), a trace byproduct of the chemical synthesis of the defoliant 2,4,5-T (see Chapter 57).

Increased P450 synthesis requires enhanced transcription and translation. A cytoplasmic receptor (termed AhR) for polycyclic aromatic hydrocarbons (eg, benzo[*a*]pyrene, dioxin) has been identified, and the translocation of the inducer-receptor complex into the nucleus and subsequent activation of regulatory elements of genes have been documented. A pregnane X receptor (PXR), a member of the steroid-retinoid-thyroid hormone receptor family, has recently been shown to mediate CYP3A induction by various chemicals (dexamethasone, rifampin) in the liver and intestinal mucosa. A similar receptor, the constitutive androstane receptor (CAR) has been identified for the phenobarbital class of inducers (Sueyoshi, 2001; Willson, 2002).

P450 enzymes may also be induced by "substrate stabilization," ie, decreased degradation, as is the case with troleandomycin- or clotrimazole-mediated induction of CYP3A enzymes and the ethanol-mediated induction of CYP2E1.

Enzyme Inhibition

Certain drug substrates may inhibit cytochrome P450 enzyme activity. Imidazole-containing drugs such as cimetidine and ketoconazole bind tightly to the P450 heme iron and effectively reduce the metabolism of endogenous substrates (testosterone) or other coadministered drugs through competitive inhibition. However, macrolide antibiotics such as troleandomycin, erythromycin, and other erythromycin derivatives are metabolized, apparently by CYP3A, to metabolites that complex the cytochrome heme-iron and render it catalytically inactive. Another compound that acts through this mechanism is the well-known inhibitor proadifen (SKF-525-A), which binds tightly to the heme-iron and quasi-irreversibly inactivates the enzyme, thereby inhibiting the metabolism of potential substrates.

Some substrates irreversibly inhibit P450s via covalent interaction of a metabolically generated reactive intermediate that may react with the P450 apoprotein or heme moiety or even cause the heme to fragment and irreversibly modify the apoprotein. The antibiotic chloramphenicol is metabolized by CYP2B1 to a species that modifies its protein and thus also inactivates the enzyme. A growing list of "**suicide inhibitors**"—inactivators that attack the heme or the protein moiety—includes the steroids ethinyl estradiol, norethindrone, and spironolactone; the anesthetic agent fluroxene; the barbiturate allobarbital; the analgesic sedatives allylisopropylacetylurea, diethylpentenamide, and ethchlorvynol; the solvent carbon disulfide; and propylthiouracil. On the other hand, the barbiturate secobarbital is found to inactivate CYP2B1 by modification of both its heme and protein moieties.

Human Liver P450 Enzymes

Immunoblotting analyses—coupled with the use of relatively selective functional markers and selective P450 inhibitors—have identified numerous P450 isoforms (CYPs 1A2, 2A6, 2B6, 2C9, 2C19, 2D6, 2E1, 3A4, 3A5, 4A11 and 7) in human liver microsomal preparations. Of these, CYPs 1A2, 2A6, 2C9, 2D6, 2E1, and 3A4 appear

to be the major forms, accounting for approximately, 12, 4, 20, 4, 6, and 28 percent, respectively, of the total human liver P450 content. Together they are responsible for catalyzing the bulk of the hepatic drug and xenobiotic metabolism (Table 4–2). It is noteworthy that CYP3A4 alone is responsible for metabolism of more than 50% of the clinically prescribed drugs metabolized by the liver. The involvement of individual P450s in the metabolism of a given drug may be screened in vitro by means of selective functional markers, selective chemical P450 inhibitors, and anti-P450 antibodies. In vivo, such screening may be accomplished by means of relatively selective noninvasive markers, which include breath tests or urinary analyses of specific metabolites after administration of a P450-selective substrate probe.

PHASE II REACTIONS

Parent drugs or their phase I metabolites that contain suitable chemical groups often undergo coupling or conjugation reactions with an endogenous substance to yield drug conjugates (Table 4–3). In general, conjugates are polar molecules that are readily excreted and often inactive. Conjugate formation involves high-energy intermediates and specific transfer enzymes. Such enzymes (transferases) may be located in microsomes or in the cytosol. They catalyze the coupling of an activated endogenous substance (such as the uridine 5′-diphosphate [UDP] derivative of glucuronic acid) with a drug (or endogenous compound), or of an activated drug (such as the S-CoA derivative of benzoic acid) with an endogenous substrate. Because the endogenous substrates originate in the diet, nutrition plays a critical role in the regulation of drug conjugations.

Drug conjugations were once believed to represent terminal inactivation events and as such have been viewed as "true detoxification" reactions. However, this concept must be modified, since it is now known that certain conjugation reactions (acyl glucuronidation of nonsteroidal anti-inflammatory drugs, O-sulfation of N-hydroxyacetylaminofluorene, and N-acetylation of isoniazid) may lead to the formation of reactive species responsible for the hepatotoxicity of the drugs. Furthermore, sulfation is known to activate the orally active prodrug minoxidil into a very efficacious vasodilator.

METABOLISM OF DRUGS TO TOXIC PRODUCTS

It has become evident that metabolism of drugs and other foreign chemicals may not always be an innocuous biochemical event leading to detoxification and elimination of the compound. Indeed, several compounds have been shown to be metabolically transformed to reactive intermediates that are toxic to various organs. Such toxic

Table 4–2. Human liver P450s (CYPs), and some of the drugs metabolized (substrates), inducers, and drugs used for screening (noninvasive markers).

CYP	Substrates	Inducers	Noninvasive Markers
1A2	Acetaminophen, antipyrine, caffeine, clomipramine, phenacetin, tamoxifen, theophylline, warfarin	Smoking, charcoal-broiled foods, cruciferous vegetables, omeprazole	Caffeine
2A6	Coumarin		Coumarin
2B6	Artemisinin, bupropion, cyclophosphamide, S-mephobarbital, S-mephenytoin (N-demethylation to nirvanol), propofol, selegiline, sertraline	Phenobarbital, cyclophosphamide	S-Mephenytoin
2C9	Hexobarbital, ibuprofen, phenytoin, tolbutamide, trimethadione, sulfaphenazole, S-warfarin, ticrynafen	Barbiturates, rifampin	Tolbutamide, warfarin
2C19	Diazepam, S-mephenytoin, naproxen, nirvanol, omeprazole, propranolol	Barbiturates, rifampin	S-Mephenytoin
2D6	Bufuralol, bupranolol, clomipramine, clozapine, codeine, debrisoquin, dextromethorphan, encainide, flecainide, fluoxetine, guanoxan, haloperidol, hydrocodone, 4-methoxy-amphetamine, metoprolol, mexiletine, oxycodone, paroxetine, phenformin, propafenone, propoxyphene, risperidone, selegiline (deprenyl), sparteine, thioridazine, timolol, tricyclic antidepressants	None known	Debrisoquin, dextromethorphan
2E1	Acetaminophen, chlorzoxazone, enflurane, halothane, ethanol (a minor pathway)	Ethanol, isoniazid	Chlorzoxazone
3A4	Acetaminophen, alfentanil, amiodarone, astemizole, cocaine, cortisol, cyclosporine, dapsone, diazepam, dihydroergot-amine, dihydropyridines, diltiazem, ethinyl estradiol, gestodene, indinavir, lidocaine, lovastatin, macrolides, methadone, miconazole, midazolam, mifepristone (RU 486), paclitaxel, progesterone, quinidine, rapamycin, ritonavir, saquinavir, spironolactone, sulfamethoxazole, sufentanil, tacrolimus, tamoxifen, terfenadine, testosterone, tetrahydro-cannabinol, triazolam, troleandomycin, verapamil	Barbiturates, carbamazepine, macrolides, glucocorticoids, pioglitazone, phenytoin, rifampin	Erythromycin, 6β-hydroxycortisol

reactions may not be apparent at low levels of exposure to parent compounds when alternative detoxification mechanisms are not yet overwhelmed or compromised and the availability of endogenous detoxifying cosubstrates (glutathione [GSH], glucuronic acid, sulfate) is not limited. However, when these resources are exhausted, the toxic pathway may prevail, resulting in overt organ toxicity or carcinogenesis. The number of specific examples of such drug-induced toxicity is expanding rapidly. An example is acetaminophen (paracetamol)-induced hepatotoxicity (Figure 4–4). This analgesic antipyretic drug is quite safe in therapeutic doses (1.2 g/d for an adult). It normally undergoes glucuronidation and sulfation to the corresponding conjugates, which together comprise 95% of the total excreted metabolites. The alternative P450-dependent

glutathione conjugation pathway accounts for the remaining 5%. When acetaminophen intake far exceeds therapeutic doses, the glucuronidation and sulfation pathways are saturated, and the P450-dependent pathway becomes increasingly important. Little or no hepatotoxicity results as long as glutathione is available for conjugation. However, with time, hepatic glutathione is depleted faster than it can be regenerated, and a reactive and toxic metabolite accumulates. In the absence of intracellular nucleophiles such as glutathione, this reactive metabolite (*N*-acetylbenzoiminoquinone) reacts with nucleophilic groups of cellular proteins, resulting in hepatotoxicity (Figure 4–4).

The chemical and toxicologic characterization of the electrophilic nature of the reactive acetaminophen metabolite has led to the development of effective anti-

Table 4–3. Phase II reactions.

Type of Conjugation	Endogenous Reactant	Transferase (Location)	Types of Substrates	Examples
Glucuronidation	UDP glucuronic acid	UDP glucuronosyl-transferase (microsomes)	Phenols, alcohols, carboxylic acids, hydroxylamines, sulfonamides	Nitrophenol, morphine, acetaminophen, diazepam, *N*-hydroxydapsone, sulfathiazole, meprobamate, digitoxin, digoxin
Acetylation	Acetyl-CoA	*N*-Acetyltransferase (cytosol)	Amines	Sulfonamides, isoniazid, clonazepam, dapsone, mescaline
Glutathione conjugation	Glutathione	GSH-*S*-transferase (cytosol, microsomes)	Epoxides, arene oxides, nitro groups, hydroxylamines	Ethacrynic acid, bromobenzene
Glycine conjugation	Glycine	Acyl-CoA glycinetransferase (mitochondria)	Acyl-CoA derivatives of carboxylic acids	Salicylic acid, benzoic acid, nicotinic acid, cinnamic acid, cholic acid, deoxycholic acid
Sulfate conjugation	Phosphoadenosyl phosphosulfate	Sulfotransferase (cytosol)	Phenols, alcohols, aromatic amines	Estrone, aniline, phenol, 3-hydroxycoumarin, acetaminophen, methyldopa
Methylation	*S*-adenosyl-methionine	Transmethylases (cytosol)	Catecholamines, phenols, amines	Dopamine, epinephrine, pyridine, histamine, thiouracil
Water conjugation	Water	Epoxide hydrolase (microsomes)	Arene oxides, *cis*-disubstituted and monosubstituted oxiranes	Benzopyrene 7,8-epoxide, styrene 1,2-oxide, carbamazepine epoxide
		(cytosol)	Alkene oxides, fatty acid epoxides	Leukotriene A_4

dotes—cysteamine and *N*-acetylcysteine. Administration of *N*-acetylcysteine (the safer of the two) within 8–16 hours following acetaminophen overdosage has been shown to protect victims from fulminant hepatotoxicity and death (see Chapter 59).

CLINICAL RELEVANCE OF DRUG METABOLISM

The dose and the frequency of administration required to achieve effective therapeutic blood and tissue levels vary in different patients because of individual differences in drug distribution and rates of drug metabolism and elimination. These differences are determined by genetic factors and nongenetic variables such as age, sex, liver size, liver function, circadian rhythm, body temperature, and nutritional and environmental factors such as concomitant exposure to inducers or inhibitors of drug metabolism. The discussion that follows summarizes the most important of these variables.

Individual Differences

Individual differences in metabolic rate depend on the nature of the drug itself. Thus, within the same popula-

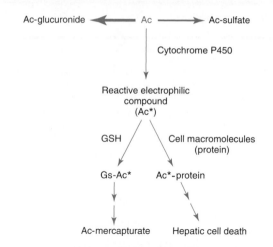

Figure 4–4. Metabolism of acetaminophen (Ac) to hepatotoxic metabolites. (GSH, glutathione; GS, glutathione moiety; Ac*, reactive intermediate.)

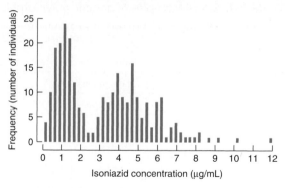

Figure 4–5. Genetic polymorphism in drug metabolism. The graph shows the distribution of plasma concentrations of isoniazid in 267 individuals 6 hours after an oral dose of 9.8 mg/kg. This distribution is clearly bimodal. Individuals with a plasma concentration greater than 2.5 mg/mL at 6 hours are considered slow acetylators. (Redrawn, with permission, from Evans DAP, Manley KA, McKusick VA: Genetic control of isoniazid metabolism in man. Br Med J 1960;2:485.)

tion, steady-state plasma levels may reflect a 30-fold variation in the metabolism of one drug and only a twofold variation in the metabolism of another.

Genetic Factors

Genetic factors that influence enzyme levels account for some of these differences. Succinylcholine, for example, is metabolized only half as rapidly in persons with genetically determined defects in pseudocholinesterase as in persons with normally functioning pseudocholinesterase. Analogous pharmacogenetic differences are seen in the acetylation of isoniazid (Figure 4–5) and the hydroxylation of warfarin. The defect in slow acetylators (of isoniazid and similar amines) appears to be caused by the synthesis of less of the enzyme rather than of an abnormal form of it. Inherited as an autosomal recessive trait, the slow acetylator phenotype occurs in about 50% of blacks and whites in the USA, more frequently in Europeans living in high northern latitudes, and much less commonly in Asians and Inuits (Eskimos). Similarly, genetically determined defects in the oxidative metabolism of debrisoquin, phenacetin, guanoxan, sparteine, phenformin, warfarin and others have been reported (Table 4–4). The defects are apparently transmitted as autosomal recessive traits and may be expressed at any one of the multiple metabolic transformations that a chemical might undergo.

Of the several recognized genetic variations of drug metabolism polymorphisms, three have been particularly well characterized and afford some insight into possible underlying mechanisms. First is the debrisoquin-sparteine oxidation type of polymorphism, which apparently occurs in 3–10% of whites and is inherited

as an autosomal recessive trait. In affected individuals, the CYP2D6-dependent oxidations of debrisoquin and other drugs (see Table 4–2) are impaired. These defects in oxidative drug metabolism are probably coinherited. The precise molecular basis for the defect appears to be faulty expression of the P450 protein, resulting in little or no isoform-catalyzed drug metabolism. More recently, however, another polymorphic genotype has been reported that results in ultrarapid metabolism of relevant drugs due to the presence of 2D6 allelic variants with up to 13 gene copies in tandem. This genotype is most common in Ethiopians and Saudi Arabians, populations that display it in up to one third of individuals. As a result, these subjects require twofold to threefold higher daily doses of nortriptyline (a 2D6 substrate) to achieve therapeutic plasma levels. Conversely, in these ultrarapidly metabolizing populations, the prodrug codeine (another 2D6 substrate) is metabolized much faster to morphine, often resulting in undesirable side effects of morphine such as severe abdominal pain.

A second well-studied genetic drug polymorphism involves the stereoselective aromatic (4)-hydroxylation of the anticonvulsant mephenytoin, catalyzed by CYP2C19. This polymorphism, which is also inherited as an autosomal recessive trait, occurs in 3–5% of Caucasians and 18–23% of Japanese populations. It is genetically independent of the debrisoquin-sparteine polymorphism. In normal "extensive metabolizers," (S)-mephenytoin is extensively hydroxylated by CYP2C19 at the 4 position of the phenyl ring before its glucuronidation and rapid excretion in the urine, whereas

Table 4–4. Some examples of genetic polymorphisms in drug metabolism.

Defect	Drug and Therapeutic Use	Clinical Consequences[1]
Oxidation	Bufuralol (β-adrenoceptor blocker)	Exacerbation of β-blockade, nausea
Oxidation	Codeine (analgesic)[2]	Reduced analgesia
Oxidation	Debrisoquin (antihypertensive)	Orthostatic hypotension
N-Demethylation	Ethanol	Facial flushing, cardiovascular symptoms
Oxidation	Ethanol	Facial flushing, cardiovascular symptoms
N-Acetylation	Hydralazine (antihypertensive)	Lupus erythematosus-like syndrome
N-Acetylation	Isoniazid (antitubercular)	Peripheral neuropathy
Oxidation	Mephenytoin (antiepileptic)	Overdose toxicity
Thiopurine methyl-transferase	Mercaptopurines (antileukemic)	Myelotoxicity
Oxidation	Nicotine (stimulant)	Lesser addiction
Oxidation	Nortriptyline (antidepressant)	Toxicity
O-Demethylation	Omeprazole (antiulcer)	Increased therapeutic efficacy
Oxidation	Sparteine	Oxytocic symptoms
Ester hydrolysis	Succinylcholine (neuromuscular blocker)	Prolonged apnea
Oxidation	S-warfarin (anticoagulant)	Bleeding
Oxidation	Tolbutamide (hypoglycemic)	Cardiotoxicity

[1]Observed or predictable.
[2]Prodrug

(R)-mephenytoin is slowly N-demethylated to nirvanol, an active metabolite. "Poor metabolizers," however, appear to totally lack the stereospecific (S)-mephenytoin hydroxylase activity, so both (S)- and (R)-mephenytoin enantiomers are N-demethylated to nirvanol, which accumulates in much higher concentrations. Thus, poor metabolizers of mephenytoin show signs of profound sedation and ataxia after doses of the drug that are well tolerated by normal metabolizers. The molecular basis for this defect is a single base pair mutation in exon 5 of the CYP2C19 gene that creates an aberrant splice site, a correspondingly altered reading frame of the mRNA, and, finally, a truncated nonfunctional protein. It is clinically important to recognize that the safety of a drug may be severely reduced in individuals who are poor metabolizers.

The third genetic polymorphism recently characterized is that of CYP2C9. Two well-characterized variants of this enzyme exist, each with amino acid mutations that result in altered metabolism: CYP2C9*2 allele encodes an Arg144Cys mutation, exhibiting impaired functional interactions with P450 reductase. The other allelic variant, CYP2C9*3, encodes an enzyme with an Ile359Leu mutation that has lowered affinity for many substrates. Consequently, individuals displaying the CYP2C9*3 phenotype have greatly reduced tolerance for the anticoagulant warfarin. The warfarin clearance in CYP2C9*3-homozygous individuals is only 10% of normal values, and these people can tolerate much smaller daily doses of the drug than those who are homozygous for the normal wild type allele. These individuals also have a much higher risk of adverse effects with warfarin (eg, bleeding) and with other CYP2C9 substrates such as phenytoin, losartan, tolbutamide, and some NSAIDs.

Allelic variants of CYP3A4 have also been reported but their contribution to its well-known interindividual variability in drug metabolism apparently is limited. On the other hand, the expression of CYP3A5, another human liver isoform, is markedly polymorphic, ranging from 0% to 100% of the total hepatic CYP3A content. This CYP3A5 protein polymorphism is now known to result from a single nucleotide polymorphism (SNIP) within intron 3 which enables normally spliced

CYP3A5 transcripts in 5% of Caucasians, 29% of Japanese, 27% of Chinese, 30% of Koreans, and 73% of African Americans. Thus, it can significantly contribute to interindividual differences in the metabolism of preferential CYP3A5 substrates such as midazolam.

Additional genetic polymorphisms in drug metabolism that are inherited independently from those already described are being discovered. Studies of theophylline metabolism in monozygotic and dizygotic twins that included pedigree analysis of various families have revealed that a distinct polymorphism may exist for this drug and may be inherited as a recessive genetic trait. Genetic drug metabolism polymorphisms also appear to occur for aminopyrine and carbocysteine oxidations. Regularly updated information on human P450-polymorphisms is available at www.imm.ki.se/CYPalleles/.

Although genetic polymorphisms in drug oxidations often involve specific P450 enzymes, such genetic variations can occur at other sites. The recent descriptions of a polymorphism in the oxidation of trimethylamine, believed to be metabolized largely by the flavin monooxygenase (Ziegler's enzyme), suggest that genetic variants of other non-P450-dependent oxidative enzymes may also contribute to such polymorphisms.

Diet & Environmental Factors

Diet and environmental factors also contribute to individual variations in drug metabolism. Charcoal-broiled foods and cruciferous vegetables are known to induce CYP1A enzymes, whereas grapefruit juice is known to inhibit the CYP3A metabolism of coadministered drug substrates. Cigarette smokers metabolize some drugs more rapidly than nonsmokers because of enzyme induction (see above). Industrial workers exposed to some pesticides metabolize certain drugs more rapidly than nonexposed individuals. Such differences make it difficult to determine effective and safe doses of drugs that have narrow therapeutic indices.

Age & Sex

Increased susceptibility to the pharmacologic or toxic activity of drugs has been reported in very young and old patients compared with young adults (see Chapters 60 and 61). Although this may reflect differences in absorption, distribution, and elimination, differences in drug metabolism also plays a role. Slower metabolism could be due to reduced activity of metabolic enzymes or reduced availability of essential endogenous cofactors.

Sex-dependent variations in drug metabolism have been well documented in rats but not in other rodents. Young adult male rats metabolize drugs much faster than mature female rats or prepubertal male rats. These differences in drug metabolism have been clearly associated with androgenic hormones. Clinical reports suggest that similar sex-dependent differences in drug metabolism also exist in humans for ethanol, propranolol, some benzodiazepines, estrogens, and salicylates.

Drug-Drug Interactions During Metabolism

Many substrates, by virtue of their relatively high lipophilicity, are retained not only at the active site of the enzyme but remain nonspecifically bound to the lipid membrane of the endoplasmic reticulum. In this state, they may induce microsomal enzymes; depending on the residual drug levels at the active site, they also may competitively inhibit metabolism of a simultaneously administered drug.

Enzyme-inducing drugs include various sedative-hypnotics, tranquilizers, anticonvulsants, and insecticides (Table 4–5). Patients who routinely ingest barbiturates, other sedative-hypnotics, or tranquilizers may require considerably higher doses of warfarin (an oral anticoagulant) to maintain a prolonged prothrombin

Table 4–5. Partial list of drugs that enhance drug metabolism in humans.

Inducer	Drug Whose Metabolism Is Enhanced
Benzo[a]pyrene	Theophylline
Chlorcyclizine	Steroid hormones
Ethchlorvynol	Warfarin
Glutethimide	Antipyrine, glutethimide, warfarin
Griseofulvin	Warfarin
Phenobarbital and other barbiturates[1]	Barbiturates, chloramphenicol, chlorpromazine, cortisol, coumarin anticoagulants, desmethylimipramine, digitoxin, doxorubicin, estradiol, phenylbutazone, phenytoin, quinine, testosterone
Phenylbutazone	Aminopyrine, cortisol, digitoxin
Phenytoin	Cortisol, dexamethasone, digitoxin, theophylline
Rifampin	Coumarin anticoagulants, digitoxin, glucocorticoids, methadone, metoprolol, oral contraceptives, prednisone, propranolol, quinidine

[1]Secobarbital is an exception. See Table 4–6 and text.

time. On the other hand, discontinuance of the sedative may result in reduced metabolism of the anticoagulant and bleeding—a toxic effect of the ensuing enhanced plasma levels of the anticoagulant. Similar interactions have been observed in individuals receiving various combination drug regimens such as antipsychotics or sedatives with contraceptive agents, sedatives with anticonvulsant drugs, and even alcohol with hypoglycemic drugs (tolbutamide).

It must also be noted that an inducer may enhance not only the metabolism of other drugs but also its own metabolism. Thus, continued use of some drugs may result in a pharmacokinetic type of tolerance—progressively reduced effectiveness due to enhancement of their own metabolism.

Conversely, simultaneous administration of two or more drugs may result in impaired elimination of the more slowly metabolized drug and prolongation or potentiation of its pharmacologic effects (Table 4–6). Both competitive substrate inhibition and irreversible substrate-mediated enzyme inactivation may augment plasma drug levels and lead to toxic effects from drugs with narrow therapeutic indices. Similarly, allopurinol both prolongs the duration and enhances the chemotherapeutic action of mercaptopurine by competitive inhibition of xanthine oxidase. Consequently, to avoid bone marrow toxicity, the dose of mercaptopurine is usually reduced in patients receiving allopurinol. Cimetidine, a drug used in the treatment of peptic ulcer, has been shown to potentiate the pharmacologic actions of anticoagulants and sedatives. The metabolism of the sedative chlordiazepoxide has been shown to be inhibited by 63% after a single dose of cimetidine; such effects are reversed within 48 hours after withdrawal of cimetidine.

Impaired metabolism may also result if a simultaneously administered drug irreversibly inactivates a common metabolizing enzyme. These inhibitors, in the course of their metabolism by cytochrome P450, inactivate the enzyme and result in impairment of their own metabolism and that of other cosubstrates.

Interactions Between Drugs & Endogenous Compounds

Various drugs require conjugation with endogenous substrates such as glutathione, glucuronic acid, and sulfate for their inactivation. Consequently, different drugs may compete for the same endogenous substrates, and the faster-reacting drug may effectively deplete endogenous substrate levels and impair the metabolism of the slower-reacting drug. If the latter has a steep dose-response curve or a narrow margin of safety, potentiation of its pharmacologic and toxic effects may result.

Table 4–6. Partial list of drugs that inhibit drug metabolism in humans.

Inhibitor	Drug Whose Metabolism Is Inhibited
Allopurinol, chloramphenicol, isoniazid	Antipyrine, dicumarol, probenecid, tolbutamide
Cimetidine	Chlordiazepoxide, diazepam, warfarin, others
Dicumarol	Phenytoin
Diethylpentenamide	Diethylpentenamide
Disulfiram	Antipyrine, ethanol, phenytoin, warfarin
Ethanol	Chlordiazepoxide (?), diazepam (?), methanol
Grapefruit juice[1]	Alprazolam, atorvastatin, cisapride, cyclosporine, midazolam, triazolam
Ketoconazole	Cyclosporine, astemizole, terfenadine
Nortriptyline	Antipyrine
Oral contraceptives	Antipyrine
Phenylbutazone	Phenytoin, tolbutamide
Secobarbital	Secobarbital
Troleandomycin	Theophylline, methylprednisolone

[1]Active components in grapefruit juice include furanocoumarins such as 6′,7′-dihydroxybergamottin (which is known to inactivate both intestinal and liver CYP3A4) as well as other unknown components that inhibit P-glycoprotein-mediated intestinal drug efflux and consequently further enhance the bioavailability of certain drugs such as cyclosporine.

Diseases Affecting Drug Metabolism

Acute or chronic diseases that affect liver architecture or function markedly affect hepatic metabolism of some drugs. Such conditions include alcoholic hepatitis, active or inactive alcoholic cirrhosis, hemochromatosis, chronic active hepatitis, biliary cirrhosis, and acute viral or drug-induced hepatitis. Depending on their severity, these conditions may significantly impair hepatic drug-metabolizing enzymes, particularly microsomal oxidases, and thereby markedly affect drug elimination. For example, the half-lives of chlordiazepoxide and diazepam in patients with liver cirrhosis or acute viral hepatitis are greatly increased, with a corresponding prolongation of their

Table 4–7. Rapidly metabolized drugs whose hepatic clearance is blood flow-limited.

Alprenolol	Lidocaine
Amitriptyline	Meperidine
Clomethiazole	Morphine
Desipramine	Pentazocine
Imipramine	Propoxyphene
Isoniazid	Propranolol
Labetalol	Verapamil

effects. Consequently, these drugs may cause coma in patients with liver disease when given in ordinary doses.

Some drugs are metabolized so readily that even marked reduction in liver function does not significantly prolong their action. However, cardiac disease, by limiting blood flow to the liver, may impair disposition of those drugs whose metabolism is flow-limited (Table 4–7). These drugs are so readily metabolized by the liver that hepatic clearance is essentially equal to liver blood flow. Pulmonary disease may also affect drug metabolism as indicated by the impaired hydrolysis of procainamide and procaine in patients with chronic respiratory insufficiency and the increased half-life of antipyrine in patients with lung cancer. Impairment of enzyme activity or defective formation of enzymes associated with heavy metal poisoning or porphyria also results in reduction of hepatic drug metabolism.

Although the effects of endocrine dysfunction on drug metabolism have been well-explored in experimental animal models, corresponding data for humans with endocrine disorders are scanty. Thyroid dysfunction has been associated with altered metabolism of some drugs and of some endogenous compounds as well. Hypothyroidism increases the half-life of antipyrine, digoxin, methimazole, and practolol, whereas hyperthyroidism has the opposite effect. A few clinical studies in diabetic patients indicate no apparent impairment of drug metabolism although impairment has been noted in diabetic rats. Malfunctions of the pituitary, adrenal cortex, and gonads markedly impair hepatic drug metabolism in rats. On the basis of these findings, it may be supposed that such disorders could significantly affect drug metabolism in humans. However, until sufficient evidence is obtained from clinical studies in patients, such extrapolations must be considered tentative.

REFERENCES

Correia MA, Ortiz de Montellano P: Inhibitors of cytochrome P-450 and possibilities for their therapeutic application. In: Ruckpaul K (editor). *Frontiers in Biotransformation,* vol 8. Taylor & Francis, 1993.

Correia MA: Rat and human liver cytochromes P450: Substrate and inhibitor specificities and functional markers. In: Ortiz de Montellano P (editor). *Cytochrome P450: Structure, Mechanism and Biochemistry,* 2nd ed. Plenum Press, 1995.

Desmond PV et al: Cimetidine impairs elimination of chlordiazepoxide (Librium) in man. Ann Intern Med 1980;93:266.

Hustert E et al: The genetic determinants of the CYP3A5 polymorphism. Pharmacogenetics 2001;11:773.

Gilmore DA et al: Age and gender influence the stereoselective pharmacokinetics of propranolol. J Pharmacol Exp Ther 1992;261:1181.

Gonzalez F: The molecular biology of cytochrome P450s. Pharmacol Rev 1989;40:243.

Guengerich FP: Human cytochrome P450 enzymes. In: Ortiz de Montellano P (editor). *Cytochrome P450: Structure, Mechanism and Biochemistry,* 2nd ed. Plenum Press, 1995.

Guengerich FP: Role of cytochrome P450 enzymes in drug-drug interactions. Adv Pharmacol 1997;43:7.

Guengerich FP: Cytochrome P-450 3A4: Regulation and role in drug metabolism. Annu Rev Pharmacol Toxicol 1999;39:1.

Ingelman-Sundberg M: Pharmacogenetics: an opportunity for a safer and more efficient pharmacotherapy. J Intern Med 2001;250:186.

Jenner P, Testa B (editors): *Concepts in Drug Metabolism.* Part B of: *Drugs and the Pharmaceutical Science Series,* vol 10. Marcel Dekker, 1981.

Kroemer HK, Klotz U: Glucuronidation of drugs: A reevaluation of the pharmacological significance of the conjugates and modulating factors. Clin Pharmacokinet 1992;23:292.

Meyer UA: Pharmacogenetics and adverse drug reactions. Lancet 2000;356:1667.

Miller LG: Recent developments in the study of the effects of cigarette smoking on clinical pharmacokinetics and clinical pharmacodynamics. Clin Pharmacokinet 1989;17:90.

Murray M: P450 enzymes: Inhibition mechanisms, genetic regulation, and effects of liver disease. Clin Pharmacokinet 1992;23:132.

Nelson DR et al: The P450 superfamily: Update on new sequences, gene mapping, accession numbers, and nomenclature. Pharmacogenetics 1996;6:1.

Nelson DR et al: Updated human P450 sequences available at http://drnelson.utmem.edu/human.P450.seqs.html.

Ortiz de Montellano PR, Correia MA: Inhibition of cytochrome P450 enzymes. In: Ortiz de Montellano P (editor). *Cytochrome P450: Structure, Mechanism and Biochemistry,* 2nd ed. Plenum Press, 1995.

Sueyoshi T, Negishi M: Phenobarbital response elements of cytochrome P450 genes and nuclear receptors. Annu Rev Pharmacol Toxicol 2001;41:123.

Thummel KE, Wilkinson GR: In vitro and in vivo drug interactions involving human CYP3A. Annu Rev Pharmacol Toxicol 1998;38:389.

Willson TM, Kliewer SA: PXR, CAR and drug metabolism. Nat Rev Drug Discov 2002;1:259.

Xu C et al: CYP2A6 genetic variation and potential consequences Adv Drug Delivery Rev 2002;54:1245.

Basic & Clinical Evaluation of New Drugs

5

*Barry A. Berkowitz, PhD**

New drug developments have revolutionized the practice of medicine, converting many once fatal or debilitating diseases into almost routine therapeutic exercises. For example, deaths from cardiovascular disease and stroke have decreased by more than 50% in the USA over the past 30 years. This decline is due—in part—to the discovery and increased use of antihypertensives, cholesterol synthesis inhibitors, and drugs that prevent or dissolve blood clots. The process of drug discovery and development has been greatly affected by investment in new technology and by governmental support of medical research.

In most countries, the testing of therapeutic agents is now regulated by legislation and closely monitored by governmental agencies. This chapter summarizes the process by which new drugs are discovered, developed, and regulated. While the examples used reflect the experience in the USA, the pathway of new drug development is generally the same worldwide.

One of the first steps in the development of a new drug is the discovery or synthesis of a potential new drug molecule and correlating this molecule with an appropriate biologic target. Repeated application of this approach leads to compounds with increased potency and selectivity (Figure 5–1). By law, the safety and efficacy of drugs must be defined before they can be marketed. In addition to in vitro studies, most of the biologic effects of the molecule must be characterized in animals before human drug trials can be started. Human testing must then go forward in three conventional phases before the drug can be considered for approval for general use. A fourth phase of data gathering and safety monitoring follows after approval for general use.

Enormous costs, from $150 million to over $800 million, are involved in the research and development of a single successful new drug. Thousands of compounds may be synthesized and hundreds of thousands tested from existing libraries of compounds for each successful new drug that reaches the market. It is primarily because of the economic investment and risks involved as well as the need for multiple interdisciplinary technologies that most new drugs are developed in pharmaceutical companies. At the same time, the incentives to succeed in drug development are equally enormous. The worldwide market for ethical (prescription) pharmaceuticals in 2001 was $364 billion. Moreover, it has been estimated that during the second half of the 20th century, medications produced by the pharmaceutical industry saved more than 1.5 million lives and $140 billion in the costs of treatment for tuberculosis, poliomyelitis, coronary artery disease, and cerebrovascular disease alone. In the USA, approximately 10% of the health care dollar is presently spent on prescription drugs.

DRUG DISCOVERY

Most new drug candidates are launched through one or more of five approaches:

1. Identification or elucidation of a new drug target

2. Rational drug design based on an understanding of biologic mechanisms, drug receptor structure, and drug structure

3. Chemical modification of a known molecule

4. Screening for biologic activity of large numbers of natural products; banks of previously discovered chemical entities; and large libraries of peptides, nucleic acids, and other organic molecules

5. Biotechnology and cloning using genes to produce larger peptides and proteins. Moreover, automation, miniaturization and informatics have facilitated the process known as "high through-put screening," which permits millions of assays per month.

Major attention is now being given to the discovery of entirely new targets for drug therapy. These targets are emerging from studies with genomics, proteomics,

* Acknowledgment: I thank Wallace Dairman for comments and Kevin Abbey and Sema Ashkouri for their research and administrative efforts.

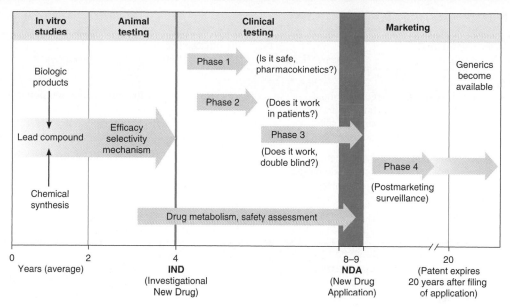

Figure 5–1. The development and testing process required to bring a drug to market in the USA. Some of the requirements may be different for drugs used in life-threatening diseases.

and molecular pharmacology and are expected to increase the number of useful biologic or disease targets ten-fold and thus be a positive driver for new and improved drugs.

Drug Screening

Regardless of the source or the key idea leading to a drug candidate molecule, testing it involves a sequence of experimentation and characterization called **drug screening.** A variety of biologic assays at the molecular, cellular, organ system, and whole animal levels are used to define the activity and selectivity of the drug. The type and number of initial screening tests depend on the pharmacologic goal. Anti-infective drugs will generally be tested first against a variety of infectious organisms, hypoglycemic drugs for their ability to lower blood sugar, etc. In addition, the molecule will also be studied for a broad array of other actions to establish the mechanism of action and selectivity of the drug. This has the advantage of demonstrating unsuspected toxic effects and occasionally discloses a previously unsuspected therapeutic action. The selection of molecules for further study is most efficiently conducted in animal models of human disease. Where good predictive models exist (eg, hypertension or thrombotic disease), we generally have adequate drugs. Good drugs are conspicuously lacking for diseases for which models are poor or not yet available, eg, Alzheimer's disease.

Some of the studies performed during drug screening are listed in Table 5–1 and define the **pharmacologic profile** of the drug. For example, a broad range of tests would be performed on a drug designed to act as an antagonist at vascular α-adrenoceptors for the treatment of hypertension. At the molecular level, the compound would be screened for receptor binding affinity to cell membranes containing α receptors, possibly cloned human receptors, other receptors, and binding sites on enzymes. Early studies would be done on liver cytochrome P450 enzymes to determine whether the molecule of interest is likely to be a substrate or inhibitor of these enzymes.

Effects on cell function would be studied to determine the efficacy of the compound. Evidence would be obtained about whether the drug is an agonist, partial agonist, or antagonist at α receptors. Isolated tissues would be utilized to characterize the pharmacologic activity and selectivity of the new compound in comparison with reference compounds. Comparison with other drugs would also be undertaken in other in vitro preparations such as gastrointestinal and bronchial smooth muscle. At each step in this process, the compound would have to meet specific performance criteria to be carried further.

Whole animal studies are generally necessary to determine the effect of the drug on organ systems and disease models. Cardiovascular and renal function studies of all new drugs are first performed in normal animals. For the

Table 5–1. Pharmacologic profile tests.

Experimental Method or Target Organ	Species or Tissue	Route of Administration	Measurement
Molecular			
Receptor binding (example: β-adrenoceptors)	Cell membrane fractions from organs or cultured cells; cloned receptors	In vitro	Receptor affinity and selectivity
Enzyme activity (examples: tyrosine hydroxylase, dopamine-3-hydroxylase, monoamine oxidase)	Sympathetic nerves; adrenal glands; purified enzymes	In vitro	Enzyme inhibition and selectivity
Cytochrome P450	Liver	In vitro	Enzyme inhibition; effects on drug metabolism
Cellular			
Cell function	Cultured cells	In vitro	Evidence for receptor activity— agonism or antagonism (example: effects on cyclic nucleotides)
Isolated tissue	Blood vessels, heart, lung, ileum (rat or guinea pig)	In vitro	Effects on vascular contraction and relaxation; selectivity for vascular receptors; effects on other smooth muscles
Systems/disease models			
Blood pressure	Dog, cat (anesthetized)	Parenteral	Systolic-diastolic changes
	Rat, hypertensive (conscious)	Oral	Antihypertensive effects
Cardiac effects	Dog (conscious)	Oral	Electrocardiography
	Dog (anesthetized)	Parenteral	Inotropic, chronotropic effects, cardiac output, total peripheral resistance
Peripheral autonomic nervous system	Dog (anesthetized)	Parenteral	Effects on response to known drugs and electrical stimulation of central and peripheral autonomic nerves
Respiratory effects	Dog, guinea pig	Parenteral	Effects on respiratory rate and amplitude, bronchial tone
Diuretic activity	Dog	Oral, parenteral	Natriuresis, kaliuresis, water diuresis, renal blood flow, glomerular filtration rate
Gastrointestinal effects	Rat	Oral	Gastrointestinal motility and secretions
Circulating hormones, cholesterol, blood sugar	Rat, dog	Parenteral, oral	Serum concentration
Blood coagulation	Rabbit	Oral	Coagulation time, clot retraction, prothrombin time
Central nervous system	Mouse, rat	Parenteral, oral	Degree of sedation, muscle relaxation, locomotor activity, stimulation

hypothetical antihypertensive drug, animals with hypertension would then be treated to see if blood pressure was lowered and to characterize other effects of the compound. Evidence would be collected on duration of action and efficacy following oral and parenteral administration. If the agent possessed useful activity, it would be further studied for possible adverse effects on other major organ systems, including the respiratory, gastrointestinal, endocrine, and central nervous systems.

These studies might suggest the need for further chemical modification to achieve more desirable pharmacokinetic or pharmacodynamic properties. For example, oral administration studies might show that the drug was poorly absorbed or rapidly metabolized in the liver; modification to improve bioavailability might be indicated. If the drug was to be administered long-term, an assessment of tolerance development would be made. For drugs related to those known to cause physical dependence, abuse potential would also be studied. Finally, for each major action, a pharmacologic mechanism would be sought.

The result of this procedure (which may have to be repeated several times with variants of the original molecules) is called a **lead compound,** ie, a leading candidate for a successful new drug. A patent application may then be filed for a novel compound (composition of matter patent) that is efficacious, or for a new and nonobvious therapeutic use (use patent) for a previously known chemical entity.

Advances in molecular biology and biotechnology have introduced new approaches and new problems into the drug development process. New information about the structure of drug targets such as receptors is making possible more rational drug design. A better understanding of second messenger processes is revealing second messenger receptors as a new class of drug targets. Insertion of the genes for active peptides or proteins into bacteria, yeast, or mammalian cells makes it possible to prepare large quantities of molecules that are impractical to synthesize in the test tube. Human insulin, human growth hormone, interferon, hepatitis vaccines, tissue plasminogen activator, erythropoietin, antihemophilic factor, and bone marrow growth factors produced by these biotechnology approaches are now available for general clinical use. Antibodies used as drugs are increasingly successful.

PRECLINICAL SAFETY & TOXICITY TESTING

Candidate drugs that survive the initial screening and profiling procedures must be carefully evaluated for potential risks before and during clinical testing. Depending on the proposed use of the drug, preclinical toxicity testing includes most or all of the procedures shown in Table 5–2. While no chemical can be certified as completely "safe" (free of risk), since every chemical is toxic at some dosage, it is usually possible to estimate the risk associated with exposure to the chemical under specified conditions if appropriate tests are performed.

The goals of preclinical toxicity studies include: identifying all potential human toxicities; designing tests to further define the toxic mechanisms; and predicting the specific and the most relevant toxicities to be monitored in clinical trials. The major kinds of information needed from preclinical toxicity studies are (1) acute toxicity—effects of large single doses up to the lethal level; (2) subacute and chronic toxicity—effects of multiple doses, which are especially important if the drug is intended for prolonged use in humans; (3) effects on reproductive functions, including teratogenicity and postnatal development; (4) carcinogenicity; (5) mutagenicity; and (6) investigative toxicology. In addition to the studies shown in Table 5–2, several quantitative estimates are desirable. These include the "no-effect" dose—the maximum dose at which a specified toxic effect is not seen; the **minimum lethal dose**—the smallest dose that is observed to kill any animal; and, if necessary, the **median lethal dose** (LD_{50})—the dose that kills approximately 50% of the animals. Historically, the LD_{50} was determined with a high degree of precision and was used to compare toxicities of compounds relative to their therapeutic doses. Presently, the LD_{50} is now estimated from the smallest number of animals possible. These doses are used to calculate the initial dose to be tried in humans, usually taken as one hundredth to one tenth of the no-effect dose in animals.

It is important to recognize the limitations of preclinical testing. These include the following:

1. Toxicity testing is time-consuming and expensive. During the last decade, the total cost of preclinical pharmacology and toxicology studies was estimated to be at least 41 million *per successful drug.* Two to 5 years may be required to collect and analyze data before the drug can be considered ready for testing in humans.

2. Large numbers of animals are needed to obtain valid preclinical data. Scientists are properly concerned about this situation, and progress has been made toward reducing the numbers required while still obtaining valid data. Cell and tissue culture in vitro methods are increasingly being used, but their predictive value is still severely limited. Nevertheless, some segments of the public attempt to halt all animal testing in the unfounded belief that it has become unnecessary.

3. Extrapolation of toxicity data from animals to humans is not completely reliable. For any given compound, the total toxicity data from all species

Table 5–2. Safety tests.

Type of Test	Approach	Comment
Acute toxicity	Acute dose that is lethal in approximately 50% of animals and the maximum tolerated dose. Usually two species, two routes, single dose.	Compare with therapeutic dose.
Subacute toxicity	Three doses, two species. 4 weeks to 3 months may be necessary prior to clinical trial. The longer the duration of expected clinical use, the longer the subacute test.	Clinical chemistry, physiologic signs, autopsy studies, hematology, histology, electron microscopy studies. Identify target organs of toxicity.
Chronic toxicity	Rodent and non-rodent species. 6 months or longer. Required when drug is intended to be used in humans for prolonged periods. Usually run concurrently with clinical trial.	Goals of subacute and chronic tests are to show which organs are susceptible to drug toxicity. Tests as noted above for subacute. 3 dose levels plus controls.
Effect on reproductive performance	Effects on animal mating behavior, reproduction, parturition, progeny, birth defects, postnatal development.	Examines fertility, teratology, perinatal and postnatal effects, lactation.
Carcinogenic potential	Two years, two species. Required when drug is intended to be used in humans for prolonged periods.	Hematology, histology, autopsy studies. Tests in transgenic mice for shorter periods may be permitted as one species.
Mutagenic potential	Effects on genetic stability and mutations in bacteria (Ames test) or mammalian cells in culture; dominant lethal test and clastogenicity in mice.	Increasing interest in this potential problem.
Investigative toxicology	Determine sequence and mechanisms of toxic action. Discover the genes, proteins, pathways involved. Develop new methods for assessing toxicity.	May allow rational and earlier design and identification of safer drugs. Possibly run at higher compound throughput.

have a very high predictive value for its toxicity in humans. However, there are limitations on the amount of information it is practical to obtain.

4. For statistical reasons, rare adverse effects are unlikely to be detected.

EVALUATION IN HUMANS

Less than one third of the drugs tested in clinical trials reach the marketplace. Federal law in the USA requires that the study of new drugs in humans be conducted in accordance with stringent guidelines. Scientifically valid results are not guaranteed simply by conforming to government regulations, however, and the design and execution of a good clinical trial requires the efforts of clinician-scientists or clinical pharmacologists, statisticians, and frequently other professionals as well. The need for careful design and execution is based on three major confounding factors inherent in the study of any thera-

peutic measure—pharmacologic or nonpharmacologic—in humans.

Confounding Factors in Clinical Trials

A. THE VARIABLE NATURAL HISTORY OF MOST DISEASES

Many diseases tend to wax and wane in severity; some disappear spontaneously with time; even malignant neoplasms may, on occasion, undergo spontaneous remissions. A good experimental design must take into account the natural history of the disease under study by evaluating a large enough population of subjects over a sufficient period of time. Further protection against errors of interpretation caused by fluctuations in severity of the manifestations of disease is provided by using a crossover design, which consists of alternating periods of administration of test drug, placebo preparation (the control), and the standard treatment (positive control), if any, in each subject. These sequences are systematically varied, so that different subsets of patients receive each of the possible sequences of treatment. An example of such a design is shown in Table 5–3.

B. THE PRESENCE OF OTHER DISEASES AND RISK FACTORS

Known and unknown diseases and risk factors (including lifestyles of subjects) may influence the results of a clinical study. For example, some diseases alter the pharmacokinetics of drugs (see Chapters 3 and 4). Concentrations of a blood component being monitored as a measure of the effect of the new agent may be influenced by other diseases or other drugs. Attempts to avoid this hazard usually involve the crossover technique (when feasible) and proper selection and assignment of patients to each of the study groups. This requires that careful medical and pharmacologic histories (including use of recreational drugs) be obtained and that statistically valid methods of randomization be used in assigning subjects to particular study groups.

C. SUBJECT AND OBSERVER BIAS

Most patients tend to respond in a positive way to any therapeutic intervention by interested, caring, and enthusiastic medical personnel. The manifestation of this phenomenon in the subject is the placebo response (Latin "I shall please") and may involve objective physiologic and biochemical changes as well as changes in subjective complaints associated with the disease. The placebo response is usually quantitated by administration of an inert material, with exactly the same physical appearance, odor, consistency, etc, as the active dosage form. The magnitude of the response varies considerably from patient to patient. However, the incidence of the placebo response is fairly constant, being observed

Table 5–3. Typical crossover design for comparing a mythical new analgesic, "Novent," with placebo and a known active drug, aspirin, in the management of chronic pain. Each therapeutic period lasts 7 days, with 1 week between each treatment period for washout of the preceding medication.

Patient Group	Medication Given		
	Week 1	Week 3	Week 5
I	Aspirin	Placebo	"Novent"
II	Placebo	"Novent"	Aspirin
III	"Novent"	Aspirin	Placebo

in 20–40% of patients in almost all studies. Placebo "toxicity" also occurs but usually involves subjective effects: stomach upset, insomnia, sedation, etc.

Subject bias effects can be quantitated—and discounted from the response measured during active therapy—by the **single-blind design**. This involves use of a placebo or dummy medication, as described above, which is administered to the same subjects in a crossover design, if possible, or to a separate control group of subjects. Observer bias can be taken into account by disguising the identity of the medication being used—placebo or active form—from both the subjects and the personnel evaluating the subjects' responses (**double-blind design**). In this design, a third party holds the code identifying each medication packet, and the code is not broken until all of the clinical data have been collected.

The Food & Drug Administration

The FDA is the administrative body that oversees the drug evaluation process in the USA and grants approval for marketing of new drug products. The FDA's authority to regulate drug marketing derives from several pieces of legislation (Table 5–4). If a drug has not been shown through adequately controlled testing to be "safe and effective" for a specific use, it cannot be marketed in interstate commerce for this use.* Unfortunately, "safe" means different things to the patient, the physician, and society. As noted above, complete absence of risk is impossible to demonstrate (and probably never occurs), but this fact is not well understood by the average member of the public, who assumes that any medication sold with the approval of the FDA must indeed be free of serious "side effects." This confusion continues to be a major cause of litigation and dissatisfaction with medical care.

The history of drug regulation reflects several medical and public health events that precipitated major shifts in public opinion. The Pure Food and Drug Act of 1906 (Table 5–4) became law mostly in response to revelations of unsanitary and unethical practices in the meat-packing industry. The Federal Food, Drug, and Cosmetic Act of 1938 was largely a reaction to a series of deaths associated with the use of a preparation of sulfanilamide that was marketed before it and its vehicle were adequately tested. Thalidomide is another example of a drug that altered drug testing methods and stimulated drug regulating legislation. This agent was introduced in Europe in 1957 and 1958 and, based on animal tests then commonly used, was promoted as a "nontoxic" hypnotic. In 1961, the first reports were published suggesting that thalidomide was responsible

---

* Although the FDA does not directly control drug commerce within states, a variety of state and federal laws control interstate production and marketing of drugs.

Table 5–4. Major legislation pertaining to drugs in the United States.

Law	Purpose and Effect
Pure Food and Drug Act of 1906	Prohibited mislabeling and adulteration of drugs.
Opium Exclusion Act of 1909	Prohibited importation of opium.
Amendment (1912) to the Pure Food and Drug Act	Prohibited false or fraudulent advertising claims.
Harrison Narcotic Act of 1914	Established regulations for use of opium, opiates, and cocaine (marijuana added in 1937).
Food, Drug, and Cosmetic Act of 1938	Required that new drugs be safe as well as pure (but did not require proof of efficacy). Enforcement by FDA.
Durham-Humphrey Act of 1952	Vested in the FDA the power to determine which products could be sold without prescription.
Kefauver-Harris Amendments (1962) to the Food, Drug, and Cosmetic Act	Required proof of efficacy as well as safety for new drugs and for drugs released since 1938; established guidelines for reporting of information about adverse reactions, clinical testing, and advertising of new drugs.
Comprehensive Drug Abuse Prevention and Control Act (1970)	Outlined strict controls in the manufacture, distribution, and prescribing of habit-forming drugs; established programs to prevent and treat drug addiction.
Orphan Drug Amendments of 1983	Amended Food, Drug, and Cosmetic Act of 1938, providing incentives for development of drugs that treat diseases with less than 200,000 patients in USA.
Drug Price Competition and Patent Restoration Act of 1984	Abbreviated new drug applications for generic drugs. Required bioequivalence data. Patent life extended by amount of time drug delayed by FDA review process. Cannot exceed 5 extra years or extend to more than 14 years post-NDA approval.
Expedited Drug Approval Act (1992)	Allowed accelerated FDA approval for drugs of high medical need. Required detailed postmarketing patient surveillance.
Prescription Drug User Fee Act (1992) Reauthorized 1997 and 2002.	Manufacturers pay user fees for certain new drug applications. FDA claims review time for new chemical entities dropped from 30 months in 1992 to 20 months in 1994.
Dietary Supplement Health and Education Act (1994)	Amended the Federal Food, Drug, and Cosmetic Act of 1938 to establish standards with respect to dietary supplements. Required the establishment of specific ingredient and nutrition information labeling that defines dietary supplements and classifies them as part of the food supply.
Bioterrorism Act of 2002	Enhanced controls on dangerous biologic agents and toxins. Seeks to protect safety of food, water, and drug supply.

for a dramatic increase in the incidence of a rare birth defect called **phocomelia,** a condition involving shortening or complete absence of the limbs. Epidemiologic studies soon provided strong evidence for the association of this defect with thalidomide use by women during the first trimester of pregnancy, and the drug was withdrawn from sale worldwide. An estimated 10,000 children were born with birth defects because of maternal exposure to this one agent. The tragedy led to the requirement for more extensive testing of new drugs for teratogenic effects and played an important role in stimulating passage of the Kefauver-Harris Amendments of

1962, even though the drug was not then approved for use in the USA. In spite of its disastrous fetal toxicity, thalidomide is a relatively safe drug for humans after birth. Even the most serious risk of toxicities may be avoided or managed if understood, and despite its toxicity thalidomide is now available in the USA for limited use as a potent immunoregulatory agent and to treat leprosy.

Of course it is impossible, as noted above, to certify that a drug is absolutely safe, ie, free of all risk. It is possible, however, to identify most of the hazards likely to be associated with use of a new drug and to place some statistical limits on frequency of occurrence of such events in the population under study. As a result, an operational and pragmatic definition of "safety" can usually be reached that is based on the nature and incidence of drug-associated hazards compared with the hazard of nontherapy of the target disease.

Clinical Trials: The IND & NDA

The new drug approval process involves a systematic series of events (Guarino, 2000). Once a drug is judged ready to be studied in humans, a Notice of Claimed Investigational Exemption for a New Drug (IND) must be filed with the FDA (Figure 5–1). The IND includes (1) information on the composition and source of the drug, (2) manufacturing information, (3) all data from animal studies, (4) clinical plans and protocols, and (5) the names and credentials of physicians who will conduct the clinical trials.

It often requires 4–6 years of clinical testing to accumulate all required data. Testing in humans is begun after sufficient acute and subacute animal toxicity studies have been completed. Chronic safety testing in animals is usually done concurrently with clinical trials. In each of the three formal phases of clinical trials, volunteers or patients must be informed of the investigational status of the drug as well as possible risks and must be allowed to decline or to consent to participate and receive the drug. These regulations are based on the ethical principles set forth in the Declaration of Helsinki (Editor's Page, 1966). In addition to the approval of the sponsoring organization and the FDA, an interdisciplinary institutional review board at the facility where the clinical drug trial will be conducted must review and approve the plans for testing in humans.

In **phase 1,** the effects of the drug as a function of dosage are established in a small number (25–50) of healthy volunteers. (If the drug is expected to have significant toxicity, as is often the case in cancer and AIDS therapy, volunteer patients with the disease are used in phase 1 rather than normal volunteers.) Phase 1 trials are done to determine whether humans and animals show significantly different responses to the drug and to establish the probable limits of the safe clinical dosage range. These trials are nonblind or "open," ie, both the investigators and the subjects know what is being given. Many predictable toxicities are detected in this phase. Pharmacokinetic measurements of absorption, half-life, and metabolism are often done in phase 1. Phase 1 studies are usually performed in research centers by specially trained clinical pharmacologists.

In **phase 2,** the drug is studied for the first time in patients with the target disease to determine its efficacy. A small number of patients (100–200) are studied in great detail. A single-blind design is often used, with an inert placebo medication and an older active drug (positive control) in addition to the investigational agent. Phase 2 trials are usually done in special clinical centers (eg, university hospitals). A broader range of toxicities may be detected in this phase.

In **phase 3,** the drug is evaluated in much larger numbers of patients—sometimes thousands—to further establish safety and efficacy. Using information gathered in phases 1 and 2, phase 3 trials are designed to minimize errors caused by placebo effects, variable course of the disease, etc. Therefore, double-blind and crossover techniques (like that set out in Table 5–3) are frequently used. Phase 3 trials are usually performed in settings similar to those anticipated for the ultimate use of the drug. Phase 3 studies can be difficult to design and execute and are usually expensive because of the large numbers of patients involved and the masses of data that must be collected and analyzed. The investigators are usually specialists in the disease being treated. Certain toxic effects—especially those caused by immunologic processes—may first become apparent in phase 3.

If phase 3 results meet expectations, application will be made for permission to market the new agent. The process of applying for marketing approval requires submission of a **New Drug Application** (NDA) to the FDA. The application contains, often in hundreds of volumes, full reports of all preclinical and clinical data pertaining to the drug under review. The FDA review of this material and a decision on approval may take 3 years or longer. In cases where an urgent need is perceived (eg, cancer chemotherapy), the process of preclinical and clinical testing and FDA review may be greatly accelerated. For serious diseases, the FDA may permit extensive but controlled marketing of a new drug before phase 3 studies are completed; for life-threatening diseases, it may permit controlled marketing even before phase 2 studies have been completed.

Once approval to market a drug has been obtained, **phase 4** begins. This constitutes monitoring the safety of the new drug under actual conditions of use in large numbers of patients. The importance of careful and complete reporting of toxicity by physicians after marketing begins can be appreciated by noting that many important drug-induced effects have an incidence of 1 in 10,000 or less. The sample size required to disclose drug-induced events or toxicities is very large for such rare events. For example, several hundred thousand patients may have to be exposed before the first case is observed of a toxicity that occurs with an average incidence of 1 in 10,000. Therefore low-incidence drug effects will not generally be detected before phase 4 no matter how carefully the studies are executed. Phase 4 has no fixed duration.

The time from the filing of a patent application to approval for marketing of a new drug may be 5 years or considerably longer. Since the lifetime of a patent is 20 years in the USA, the owner of the patent (usually a pharmaceutical company) has exclusive rights for marketing the product for only a limited time after approval of the NDA. Because the FDA review process can be lengthy, the time consumed by the review process is sometimes added to the patent life. However, the extension (up to 5 years) cannot increase the total life of the patent to more than 14 years post NDA approval. After expiration of the patent, any company may produce and market the drug as a **generic** product without paying license fees to the original patent owner. However, a trademark (the drug's proprietary trade name) may be legally protected indefinitely. Therefore, pharmaceutical companies are strongly motivated to give their new drugs easily remembered trade names. For example, "Prilosec" is the trade name for the antiulcer and heartburn drug "omeprazole" (see Box, Case Study: Discovery & Development of a Blockbuster Drug—Omeprazole). For the same reason, the company's advertising material will emphasize the trade name. Generic prescribing is described in Chapter 66.

The FDA drug approval process is one of the rate-limiting factors in the time it takes for a drug to be marketed and reach patients. The Prescription Drug User Fee Act (PDUFA) of 1992, reauthorized in 1997 and 2002, attempts to make the drug approval process more

---

CASE STUDY: DISCOVERY & DEVELOPMENT OF A BLOCKBUSTER DRUG—OMEPRAZOLE

Background

Considerable clinical success in the treatment of gastritis, heartburn, and duodenal ulcers was achieved with the introduction of the H_2-receptor antagonist cimetidine and follow-up drugs such as ranitidine. Dr George Sachs hypothesized that control of acid secretion was accomplished via several pathways (including histamine H_2 receptors) that converged on a common target—the acid (proton) pump. He speculated that pharmacologic control of the proton pump was possible and offered a new drug target (Berkowitz and Sachs, 2002). However, because of the success of cimetidine, its producer lowered the priority for research into the direct control of the proton pump. Sachs continued his basic research on the molecular biology of this potential drug target and later began collaborating on this project with scientists at a small pharmaceutical company in Sweden.

The success of the H_2-receptor antagonist drugs significantly improved therapy, provided better regulation of gastric acid, and increased the diagnosis of acid-related disorders. However, H_2 blockers required dosing several times per day, were associated with undesirable fluctuations in gastric acid levels, and failed to optimally treat more severe disorders such as gastroesophageal reflux disease (GERD) and Zollinger-Ellison syndrome.

Sachs and his colleagues had begun work that would show that H^+/K^+-ATPase, as the proton pump, moves acid across the membranes of gastric parietal cells (Blum et al, 1971). Scientists at the Swedish firm had focused on imidazoles and specifically, benzimidazoles, apparently in part because cimetidine (like histamine) is an imidazole. By adding a benzimidazole moiety to pyridine-2-thioacetamide, a known antisecretory agent, a new class of substituted benzimidazoles, which would later yield omeprazole was created (Fellenius, 1981). These congeners were sufficiently novel so that patent approval, a necessary component of the project, was likely if the compounds proved useful.

Research, Development, & Marketing

Initial results yielded drugs that were found to suppress acid secretion but were too unstable, too toxic, or insufficiently selective. However, application of the drug development process described above eventually led to better molecules and omeprazole (Prilosec) was discovered in 1978. Human testing began in 1983 and 1984 (Lind et al, 1983 and Lambers et al, 1984) and marketing approval occurred in 1989. Thus, 12 years had passed between project launch and approval for use in patients).

In 1999, worldwide sales of omeprazole were $5.9 billion. By 2001, sales were $5.7 billion, and the worldwide market for ulcer drugs exceeded 14 billion. There are now five benzimidazole compounds available from a number of companies. Omeprazole went off patent in 2001 and is now available as generic drug.

efficient by collecting fees from the drug companies that produce certain human drugs and biologic products.

Orphan Drugs

Drugs for rare diseases—so-called orphan drugs—can be difficult to research, develop, and market. Proof of drug safety and efficacy in small populations must be established, but doing so effectively is a complex process. For example, clinical testing of drugs in children is severely restricted, even for common diseases, and a number of rare diseases affect the very young. Furthermore, because basic research in the pathophysiology and mechanisms of rare diseases tends to receive little attention or funding in both academic and industrial settings, recognized rational targets for drug action may be relatively few. In addition, the cost of developing a drug can greatly influence priorities when the target population is relatively small.

The Orphan Drug Act of 1983, which amended the 1938 Federal Food, Drug, and Cosmetic Act, provides incentives for the development of drugs for treatment of diseases affecting fewer than 200,000 patients in the USA. The FDA maintains an office of Orphan Product Development to provide special assistance and grants to scientists with an interest in these products. Information on orphan drugs is also available from The National Organization for Rare Disorders.

As of 1999, more than 500 biologic or drug products were registered with the FDA as orphan drugs, most of which were products currently in development. Since 1983, the FDA has approved marketing applications for 120 orphan drugs to treat more than 82 rare diseases.

Adverse Reactions to Drugs

Severe adverse reactions to marketed drugs are uncommon, although less dangerous toxic effects, as noted elsewhere in this book, are frequent for some drug groups. Life-threatening reactions probably occur in less than 2% of patients admitted to medical wards. The mechanisms of these reactions fall into two main categories. Those in the first group are often extensions of known pharmacologic effects and thus are predictable. These toxicities are generally discovered by pharmacologists, toxicologists, and clinicians involved in phase 1–3 testing. Those in the second group, which may be immunologic or of unknown mechanism (Rawlins, 1981), are generally unexpected and may not be recognized until a drug has been marketed for many years. These toxicities are therefore usually discovered by clinicians. It is thus important that practitioners be aware of the various types of allergic reactions to drugs. These include IgE-mediated reactions such as anaphylaxis, urticaria, and angioedema; IgG- or IgM-mediated reactions of the lupus erythematosus type; IgG-mediated responses of the serum sickness type, which involve vasculitis; and cell-mediated allergies involved in contact dermatitis. They are discussed in Chapter 56.

Evaluating a Clinical Drug Study

The periodical literature should be the chief source of clinical information about new drugs, especially those very recently released for general use. Such information may include new indications or major new toxicities and contraindications. Therefore, health practitioners should be familiar with the sources of such information (noted in Chapter 1) and should be prepared to evaluate it. Certain general principles can be applied to such evaluations and are discussed in detail in the Cohen (1994) and Nowak (1994) references listed below.

REFERENCES

Berkowitz BA, Sachs G: Life Cycle of a Block Buster: Discovery and Development of Omeprazole (Prilosec™). Molecular Interventions 2002;2:6.

Beyer KH: *Discovery, Development, and Delivery of New Drugs.* SP Medical & Scientific Books, 1978.

Billstein SA: How the pharmaceutical industry brings an antibiotic drug to market in the United Sates. Antimicrob Agents Chemother 1994;38:2679.

Black J: Drugs from emasculated hormones: The principle of syntopic antagonism. Science 1989;245:486.

Blum AL et al: Properties of soluble ATPase of gastric mucosa. Biochim Biophys Acta 1971;249:101.

Chappell WR, Mordenti J: Extrapolation of toxicological and pharmacological data from animals to humans. Adv Drug Res 1991;20:1.

Cohen J: Clinical trial monitoring: Hit or miss? Science 1994;264:1534.

Collins JM, Grieshaber CK, Chabner BA: Pharmacologically guided phase I clinical trials based upon preclinical drug development. J Natl Cancer Inst 1990;82:1321.

DiMasi JA: Success rates for new drugs entering clinical testing in the United States. Clin Pharmacol Ther 1995;58:1.

Dimasi JA: Risks in new drug development: approval success rates for investigational drugs. Clin Pharmacol Ther 2001;69:297.

Editor's Page: Code of ethics of the World Medical Association: Declaration of Helsinki. Clin Res 1966;14:193.

Fellenius E et al: Substituted benzimidazoles inhibit gastric acid secretion by blocking H^+,K^+-ATPase. Nature 1981;290:159.

Guarino RA: New Drug Approval Process. *Drugs and Pharmaceutical Sciences,* Volume 100. Marcel Decker, 2000.

Jelovsek FR, Mattison DR, Chen JJ: Prediction of risk for human developmental toxicity: How important are animal studies? Obstet Gynecol 1989;74:624.

Janzen WP: *High Throughput Screening, Methods and Protocols.* Humana Press, 2002.

Kessler DA: The regulation of investigational drugs. N Engl J Med 1989;320:281.

Laughren TP: The review of clinical safety data in a new drug application. Psychopharmacol Bull 1989;25:5.

Lambers CB et al: Omeprazole in Zollinger-Ellison syndrome. N Engl J Med 1984;310:758.

Lind T et al: Effect of omeprazole—a gastric proton pump inhibitor. Gut 1983;24:270.

Mattison N, Trimble AG, Lasagna L: New drug development in the United States, 1963 through 1984. Clin Pharmacol 1988;43:290.

McKhann GM: The trials of clinical trials. Arch Neurol 1989;46:611.

Moscucci M et al: Blinding, unblinding, and the placebo effect: An analysis of patients' guesses of treatment assignment in a double-blind clinical trial. Clin Pharmacol Ther 1987;41:259.

The Nordic GORD Study Group: The cost of long term therapy for gastro-oesophageal reflux disease. Gut 2001;49:488.

Nowak R: Problems in clinical trials go far beyond misconduct. Science 1994;264:1538.

Rawlins MD: Clinical pharmacology: Adverse reactions to drugs. Br Med J 1981;282:974.

Sibille M et al: Adverse events in phase one studies: A study in 430 healthy volunteers. Eur J Clin Pharmacol 1992;42:389.

Spilker B: The development of orphan drugs: An industry perspective. In: Scheinberg JH, Walshe JM (editors). *Orphan Diseases and Orphan Drugs*. Manchester Univ Press, 1986.

Waller PC: Measuring the frequency of adverse drug reactions. Br J Clin Pharmacol 1992;33:249.

Young FE, Nightingale SL: FDA's newly designated treatment INDs. JAMA 1988;260:224.

SECTION II
Autonomic Drugs

Introduction to Autonomic Pharmacology

6

Bertram G. Katzung, MD, PhD

The motor (efferent) portion of the nervous system can be divided into two major subdivisions: **autonomic** and **somatic.** The **autonomic nervous system (ANS)** is largely autonomous (independent) in that its activities are not under direct conscious control. It is concerned primarily with visceral functions—cardiac output, blood flow to various organs, digestion, etc—that are necessary for life. The somatic division is largely concerned with consciously controlled functions such as movement, respiration, and posture. Both systems have important afferent (sensory) inputs that provide sensation and modify motor output through reflex arcs of varying size and complexity.

The nervous system has several properties in common with the endocrine system, which is the other major system for control of body function. These include high-level integration in the brain, the ability to influence processes in distant regions of the body, and extensive use of negative feedback. Both systems use chemicals for the transmission of information. In the nervous system, chemical transmission occurs between nerve cells and between nerve cells and their effector cells. Chemical transmission takes place through the release of small amounts of transmitter substances from the nerve terminals into the synaptic cleft. The transmitter crosses the cleft by diffusion and activates or inhibits the postsynaptic cell by binding to a specialized receptor molecule.

By using drugs that mimic or block the actions of chemical transmitters, we can selectively modify many autonomic functions. These functions involve a variety of effector tissues, including cardiac muscle, smooth muscle, vascular endothelium, exocrine glands, and presynaptic nerve terminals. Autonomic drugs are useful in many clinical conditions. Conversely, a very large number of drugs used for other purposes have unwanted effects on autonomic function.

ANATOMY OF THE AUTONOMIC NERVOUS SYSTEM

The autonomic nervous system lends itself to division on anatomic grounds into two major portions: the **sympathetic (thoracolumbar)** division and the **parasympathetic (craniosacral)** division (Figure 6–1). Both divisions originate in nuclei within the central nervous system and give rise to preganglionic efferent fibers that exit from the brain stem or spinal cord and terminate in motor ganglia. The sympathetic preganglionic fibers leave the central nervous system through the thoracic and lumbar spinal nerves. The parasympathetic preganglionic fibers leave the central nervous system through the cranial nerves (especially the third, seventh, ninth, and tenth) and the third and fourth sacral spinal roots.

Most of the sympathetic preganglionic fibers terminate in ganglia located in the paravertebral chains that lie on either side of the spinal column. The remaining sympathetic preganglionic fibers terminate in prevertebral ganglia, which lie in front of the vertebrae. From the ganglia, postganglionic sympathetic fibers run to the

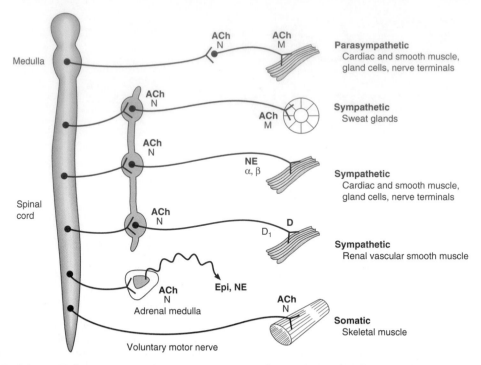

Figure 6–1. Schematic diagram comparing some anatomic and neurotransmitter features of autonomic and somatic motor nerves. Only the primary transmitter substances are shown. Parasympathetic ganglia are not shown because most are in or near the wall of the organ innervated. Note that some sympathetic postganglionic fibers release acetylcholine or dopamine rather than norepinephrine. The adrenal medulla, a modified sympathetic ganglion, receives sympathetic preganglionic fibers and releases epinephrine and norepinephrine into the blood. (ACh, acetylcholine; D, dopamine; Epi, epinephrine; NE, norepinephrine; N, nicotinic receptors; M, muscarinic receptors.)

tissues innervated. Some preganglionic parasympathetic fibers terminate in parasympathetic ganglia located outside the organs innervated: the ciliary, pterygopalatine, submandibular, otic, and several pelvic ganglia. The majority of parasympathetic preganglionic fibers terminate on ganglion cells distributed diffusely or in networks in the walls of the innervated organs. Note that the terms "sympathetic" and "parasympathetic" are anatomic ones and do not depend on the type of transmitter chemical released from the nerve endings nor on the kind of effect—excitatory or inhibitory—evoked by nerve activity.

In addition to these clearly defined peripheral motor portions of the autonomic nervous system, there are large numbers of afferent fibers that run from the periphery to integrating centers, including the enteric plexuses in the gut, the autonomic ganglia, and the central nervous system. Many of the sensory neurons that end in the central nervous system terminate in the integrating centers of the hypothalamus and medulla and evoke reflex motor activity that is carried to the effector

cells by the efferent fibers described above. There is increasing evidence that some of these sensory fibers also have important peripheral motor functions (see Nonadrenergic, Noncholinergic Systems, below).

The **enteric nervous system** (**ENS**) is a large and highly organized collection of neurons located in the walls of the gastrointestinal system (Figure 6–2). It is sometimes considered a third division of the ANS. The enteric nervous system includes the myenteric plexus (the plexus of Auerbach) and the submucous plexus (the plexus of Meissner). These neuronal networks receive preganglionic fibers from the parasympathetic system as well as postganglionic sympathetic axons. They also receive sensory input from within the wall of the gut. Fibers from the cell bodies in these plexuses travel to the smooth muscle of the gut to control motility. Other motor fibers go to the secretory cells. Sensory fibers transmit information from the mucosa and from stretch receptors to motor neurons in the plexuses and to postganglionic neurons in the sympathetic ganglia. The parasympathetic and sympathetic fibers that synapse on

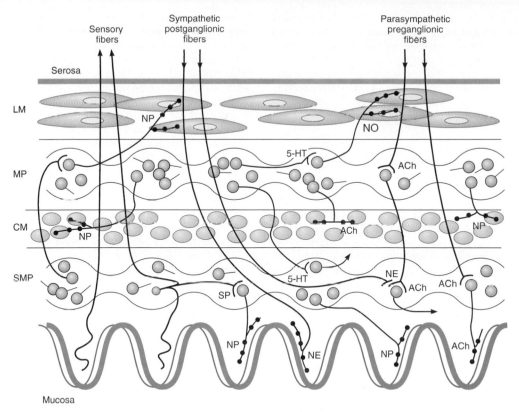

Figure 6–2. A highly simplified diagram of the intestinal wall and some of the circuitry of the enteric nervous system (ENS). The ENS receives input from both the sympathetic and the parasympathetic systems and sends afferent impulses to sympathetic ganglia and to the central nervous system. Many transmitter or neuromodulator substances have been identified in the ENS; see Table 6–1. (LM, longitudinal muscle layer; MP, myenteric plexus; CM, circular muscle layer; SMP, submucosal plexus; ACh, acetylcholine; NE, norepinephrine; NO, nitric oxide; NP, neuropeptides; SP, substance P; 5-HT, serotonin.)

enteric plexus neurons appear to play a modulatory role, as indicated by the observation that deprivation of input from both ANS divisions does not completely halt activity in the plexuses nor in the smooth muscle and glands innervated by them.

NEUROTRANSMITTER CHEMISTRY OF THE AUTONOMIC NERVOUS SYSTEM

An important traditional classification of autonomic nerves is based on the primary transmitter molecules—acetylcholine or norepinephrine—released from their terminal boutons and varicosities. A large number of peripheral autonomic nervous system fibers synthesize and release acetylcholine; they are **cholinergic** fibers, ie, they act by releasing acetylcholine. As shown in Figure 6–1, these include all preganglionic efferent autonomic fibers and the somatic (nonautonomic) motor fibers to skeletal muscle as well. Thus, almost all efferent fibers leaving the central nervous system are cholinergic. In addition, most parasympathetic postganglionic and a few sympathetic postganglionic fibers are cholinergic. A significant number of parasympathetic postganglionic neurons utilize nitric oxide or peptides for transmission. Most postganglionic sympathetic fibers release norepinephrine (noradrenaline); they are **noradrenergic** (often called simply "adrenergic") fibers—ie, they act by releasing norepinephrine. These transmitter characteristics are presented schematically in Figure 6–1. As noted above, a few sympathetic fibers release acetylcholine. Dopamine is a very important transmitter in the central nervous system, and there is evidence that it is released by some peripheral sympathetic fibers. Adrenal medullary cells, which are embryologically analogous to postganglionic sympathetic neurons, release a mixture of epinephrine and norepinephrine. Finally, most autonomic nerves also release several transmitter substances, or *cotransmitters,* in addition to the primary transmitter.

Five key features of neurotransmitter function represent potential targets of pharmacologic therapy: synthesis, storage, release, activation of receptors, and termination of action. These processes are discussed in detail below.

Cholinergic Transmission

The terminals of cholinergic neurons contain large numbers of small membrane-bound vesicles concentrated near the synaptic portion of the cell membrane (Figure 6–3) as well as a smaller number of large dense-cored vesicles located farther from the synaptic membrane. The large vesicles contain a high concentration of peptide cotransmitters (Table 6–1), while the smaller clear vesicles contain most of the acetylcholine. Vesicles are initially synthesized in the neuron soma and transported to the terminal. They may also be recycled several times within the terminal.

Acetylcholine is synthesized in the cytoplasm from acetyl-CoA and choline through the catalytic action of the enzyme choline acetyltransferase (ChAT). Acetyl-CoA is synthesized in mitochondria, which are present in large numbers in the nerve ending. Choline is transported from the extracellular fluid into the neuron terminal by a sodium-dependent membrane carrier (Figure 6–3, carrier A). This carrier can be blocked by a group of drugs called **hemicholiniums.** Once synthesized, acetylcholine is transported from the cytoplasm into the vesicles by an antiporter that removes protons (Figure 6–3, carrier B). This transporter can be blocked by **vesamicol.** Acetylcholine synthesis is a rapid process capable of supporting a very high rate of transmitter release. Storage of acetylcholine is accomplished by the packaging of "quanta" of acetylcholine molecules (usually 1000–50,000 molecules in each vesicle).

Release of transmitter is dependent on extracellular calcium and occurs when an action potential reaches the terminal and triggers sufficient influx of calcium ions. The increased Ca^{2+} concentration "destabilizes" the storage vesicles by interacting with special proteins associated with the vesicular membrane. Fusion of the vesicular membranes with the terminal membrane occurs through the interaction of vesicular proteins (vesicle-associated membrane proteins, **VAMPs**), eg, synaptotagmin and synaptobrevin, with several proteins of the terminal membrane (synaptosome-associated proteins, **SNAPs**), eg, SNAP-25 and syntaxin. Fusion of the membranes results in exocytotic expulsion of—in the case of somatic motor nerves—several hundred quanta of acetylcholine into the synaptic cleft. The amount of

transmitter released by one depolarization of an autonomic postganglionic nerve terminal is probably smaller. In addition to acetylcholine, several cotransmitters will be released at the same time (Table 6–1). The ACh vesicle release process is blocked by botulinum toxin through the enzymatic removal of two amino acids from one or more of the fusion proteins.

After release from the presynaptic terminal, acetylcholine molecules may bind to and activate an acetylcholine receptor (**cholinoceptor**). Eventually (and usually very rapidly), all of the acetylcholine released will diffuse within range of an **acetylcholinesterase** (AChE) molecule. AChE very efficiently splits acetylcholine into choline and acetate, neither of which has significant transmitter effect, and thereby terminates the action of the transmitter (Figure 6–3). Most cholinergic synapses are richly supplied with acetylcholinesterase; the half-life of acetylcholine in the synapse is therefore very short. Acetylcholinesterase is also found in other tissues, eg, red blood cells. (Another cholinesterase with a lower specificity for acetylcholine, butyrylcholinesterase [pseudocholinesterase], is found in blood plasma, liver, glia, and many other tissues.)

Adrenergic Transmission

Adrenergic neurons (Figure 6–4, page 81) also transport a precursor molecule into the nerve ending, then synthesize the catecholamine transmitter, and finally store it in membrane-bound vesicles, but—as indicated in Figure 6–5—the synthesis of the catecholamine transmitters is more complex than that of acetylcholine. In most sympathetic postganglionic neurons, norepinephrine is the final product. In the adrenal medulla and certain areas of the brain, norepinephrine is further converted to epinephrine. Conversely, synthesis terminates with dopamine in the dopaminergic neurons of the central nervous system. Several important processes in these nerve terminals are potential sites of drug action. One of these, the conversion of tyrosine to dopa, is the rate-limiting step in catecholamine transmitter synthesis. It can be inhibited by the tyrosine analog **metyrosine** (Figure 6–4). A high-affinity carrier for catecholamines located in the wall of the storage vesicle can be inhibited by the **reserpine** alkaloids (Figure 6–4, carrier B). Depletion of transmitter stores results. Another carrier transports norepinephrine and similar molecules into the cell cytoplasm (Figure 6–4, carrier 1, commonly called uptake 1 or reuptake 1). It can be inhibited by **cocaine** and **tricyclic antidepressant** drugs, resulting in an increase of transmitter activity in the synaptic cleft.

Release of the vesicular transmitter store from noradrenergic nerve endings is similar to the calcium-dependent process described above for cholinergic terminals. In addition to the primary transmitter (norepinephrine),

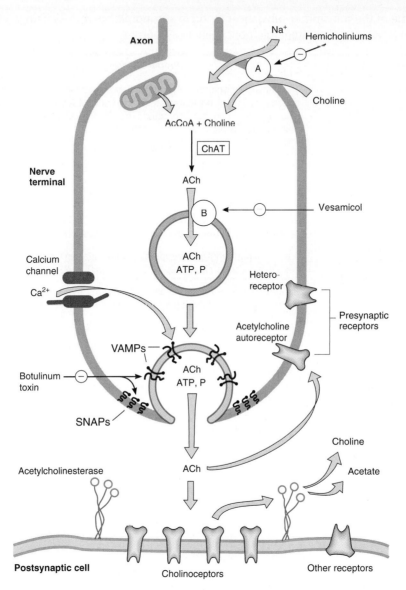

Figure 6–3. Schematic illustration of a generalized cholinergic junction (not to scale). Choline is transported into the presynaptic nerve terminal by a sodium-dependent carrier *(A).* This transport can be inhibited by hemicholinium drugs. ACh is transported into the storage vesicle by a second carrier *(B)* that can be inhibited by vesamicol. Peptides *(P),* ATP, and proteoglycan are also stored in the vesicle. Release of transmitter occurs when voltage-sensitive calcium channels in the terminal membrane are opened, allowing an influx of calcium. The resulting increase in intracellular calcium causes fusion of vesicles with the surface membrane and exocytotic expulsion of ACh and cotransmitters into the junctional cleft. This step is blocked by botulinum toxin. Acetylcholine's action is terminated by metabolism by the enzyme acetylcholinesterase. Receptors on the presynaptic nerve ending regulate transmitter release. (SNAPs, synaptosome-associated proteins; VAMPs, vesicle-associated membrane proteins.)

Table 6–1. Some of the transmitter substances found in autonomic nervous system (ANS), enteric nervous system (ENS), and nonadrenergic, noncholinergic neurons.

Substance	Probable Roles
Acetylcholine (ACh)	The primary transmitter at ANS ganglia, at the somatic neuromuscular junction, and at parasympathetic postganglionic nerve endings. A primary excitatory transmitter to smooth muscle and secretory cells in the ENS. Probably also the major neuron-to-neuron ("ganglionic") transmitter in the ENS.
Adenosine triphosphate (ATP)	May act as a cotransmitter at inhibitory ENS neuromuscular junctions. Inhibits release of ACh and norepinephrine from ANS nerve endings. An excitatory transmitter in sympathetic–smooth muscle synapses.
Calcitonin gene-related peptide (CGRP)	Found with substance P in cardiovascular sensory nerve fibers. Present in some secretomotor ENS neurons and interneurons. A cardiac stimulant.
Cholecystokinin (CCK)	May act as a cotransmitter in some excitatory neuromuscular ENS neurons.
Dopamine	A possible postganglionic sympathetic transmitter in renal blood vessels. Probably a modulatory transmitter in some ganglia and the ENS.
Enkephalin and related opioid peptides	Present in some secretomotor and interneurons in the ENS. Appear to inhibit ACh release and thereby inhibit peristalsis. May *stimulate* secretion.
Galanin	Present in secretomotor neurons; may play a role in appetite-satiety mechanisms.
GABA (γ-aminobutyric acid)	May have presynaptic effects on excitatory ENS nerve terminals. Has some relaxant effect on the gut. Probably not a major transmitter in the ENS.
Gastrin-releasing peptide (GRP)	Extremely potent excitatory transmitter to gastrin cells. Also known as mammalian bombesin.
Neuropeptide Y (NPY)	Present in some secretomotor neurons in the ENS and may inhibit secretion of water and electrolytes by the gut. Causes long-lasting vasoconstriction. It is also a cotransmitter in many parasympathetic postganglionic neurons and sympathetic postganglionic noradrenergic vascular neurons.
Nitric oxide (NO)	A cotransmitter at inhibitory ENS neuromuscular junctions; especially important at sphincters. Probable transmitter for parasympathetic vasodilation.
Norepinephrine (NE)	The primary transmitter at most sympathetic postganglionic nerve endings.
Serotonin (5-HT)	A major transmitter at excitatory neuron-to-neuron junctions in the ENS.
Substance P (and related "tachykinins")	Substance P is an important sensory neuron transmitter in the ENS and elsewhere. Tachykinins appear to be excitatory cotransmitters with ACh at ENS neuromuscular junctions. Found with CGRP in cardiovascular sensory neurons. Substance P is a vasodilator (probably via release of nitric oxide).
Vasoactive intestinal peptide (VIP)	Excitatory secretomotor transmitter in the ENS; may also be an inhibitory ENS neuromuscular cotransmitter. A probable cotransmitter in many cholinergic neurons. A vasodilator (found in many perivascular neurons) and cardiac stimulant.

ATP, dopamine-β-hydroxylase, and peptide cotransmitters are also released into the synaptic cleft. Indirectly acting sympathomimetics—eg, **tyramine** and **amphetamines**—are capable of releasing stored transmitter from noradrenergic nerve endings. These drugs are poor agonists (some are inactive) at adrenoceptors but are taken up into noradrenergic nerve endings by uptake 1. In the nerve ending, they may displace norepinephrine from storage vesicles, inhibit monoamine oxidase, and have other effects that result in increased norepinephrine activity in the synapse. Their action does not require vesicle exocytosis and is not calcium-dependent.

Norepinephrine and epinephrine can be metabolized by several enzymes, as shown in Figure 6–6. Because of

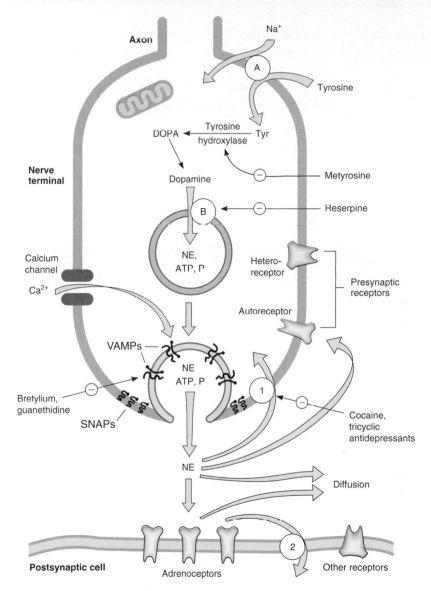

Figure 6–4. Schematic diagram of a generalized noradrenergic junction (not to scale). Tyrosine is transported into the noradrenergic ending or varicosity by a sodium-dependent carrier *(A)*. Tyrosine is converted to dopamine (see Figure 6–5 for details), which is transported into the vesicle by a carrier *(B)* that can be blocked by reserpine. The same carrier transports norepinephrine *(NE)* and several other amines into these granules. Dopamine is converted to NE in the vesicle by dopamine-β-hydroxylase. Release of transmitter occurs when an action potential opens voltage-sensitive calcium channels and increases intracellular calcium. Fusion of vesicles with the surface membrane results in expulsion of norepinephrine, cotransmitters, and dopamine-β-hydroxylase. Release can be blocked by drugs such as guanethidine and bretylium. After release, norepinephrine diffuses out of the cleft or is transported into the cytoplasm of the terminal (uptake 1 *[1],* blocked by cocaine, tricyclic antidepressants) or into the postjunctional cell (uptake 2 *[2]*). Regulatory receptors are present on the presynaptic terminal. (SNAPs, synaptosome-associated proteins; VAMPs, vesicle-associated membrane proteins.)

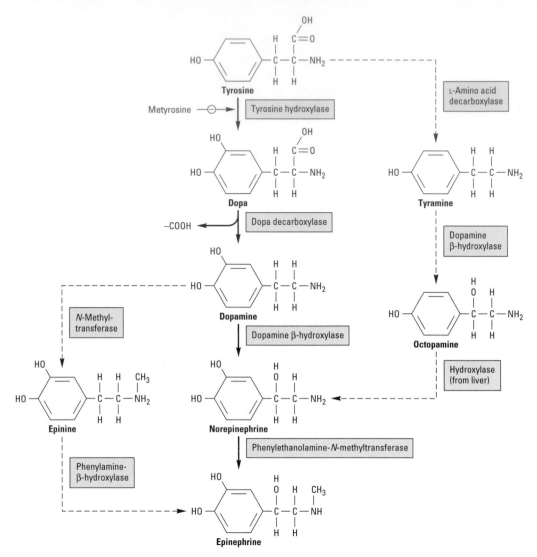

Figure 6–5. Biosynthesis of catecholamines. The rate-limiting step, conversion of tyrosine to dopa, can be inhibited by metyrosine (α-methyltyrosine). The alternative pathways shown by the dashed arrows have not been found to be of physiologic significance in humans. However, tyramine and octopamine may accumulate in patients treated with monoamine oxidase inhibitors. (Reproduced, with permission, from Greenspan FS, Gardner DG (editors): *Basic and Clinical Endocrinology*, 7th ed. McGraw-Hill, 2003.)

the high activity of monoamine oxidase in the mitochondria of the nerve terminal, there is a significant turnover of norepinephrine even in the resting terminal. Since the metabolic products are excreted in the urine, an estimate of catecholamine turnover can be obtained from laboratory analysis of total metabolites (sometimes referred to as "VMA and metanephrines") in a 24-hour urine sample. However, metabolism is not the primary

mechanism for termination of action of norepinephrine physiologically released from noradrenergic nerves. Termination of noradrenergic transmission results from several processes, including simple diffusion away from the receptor site (with eventual metabolism in the plasma or liver) and reuptake into the nerve terminal (**uptake 1**) or into perisynaptic glia or smooth muscle cells (**uptake 2**) (Figure 6–4).

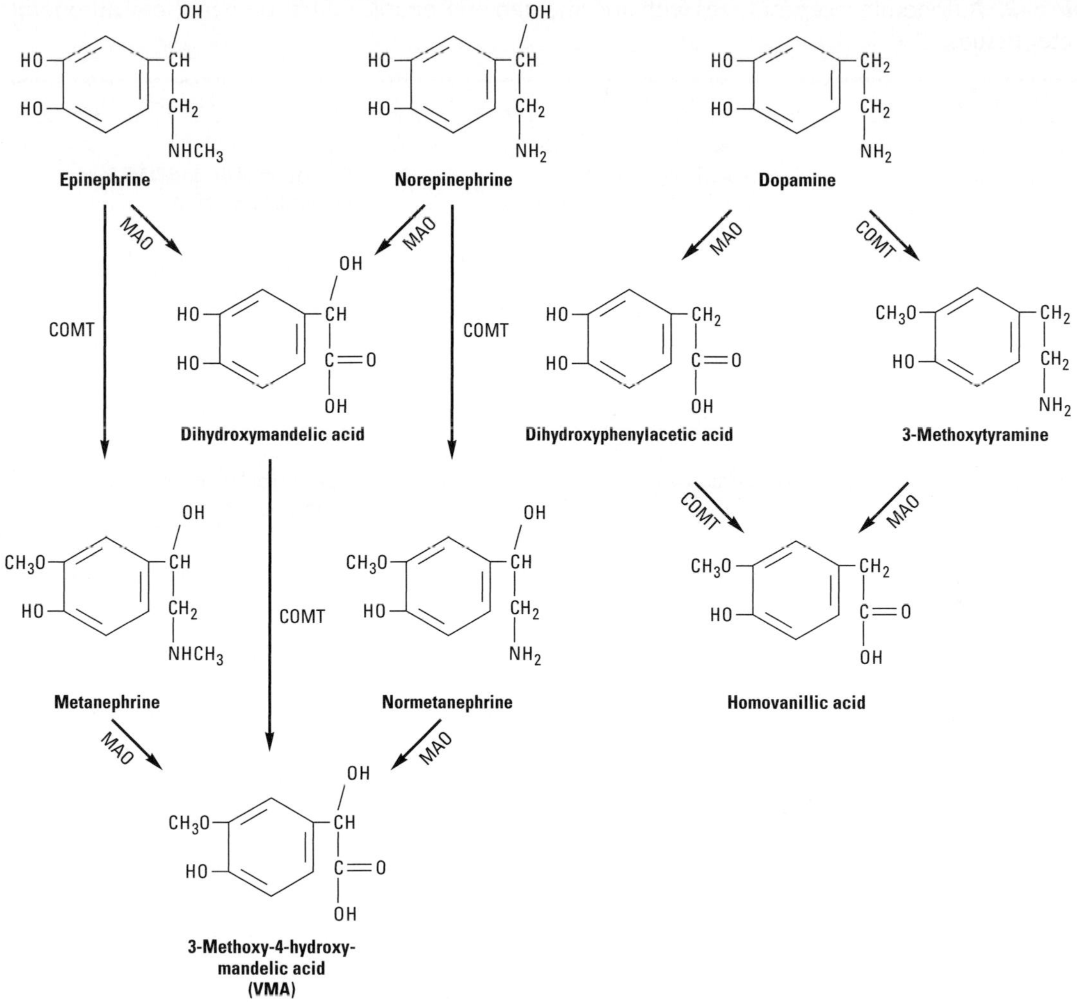

Figure 6–6. Metabolism of catecholamines by catechol-*O*-methyltransferase (*COMT*) and monoamine oxidase (*MAO*). (Modified and reproduced, with permission, from Greenspan FS, Gardner DG (editors): *Basic and Clinical Endocrinology,* 7th ed. McGraw-Hill, 2003.)

Cotransmitters in Cholinergic & Adrenergic Nerves

As previously noted, the vesicles of both cholinergic and adrenergic nerves contain other substances in addition to the primary transmitter. Some of the substances identified to date are listed in Table 6–1. Many of these substances are also *primary* transmitters in the nonadrenergic, noncholinergic nerves described below. Their roles in the function of nerves that release acetylcholine or norepinephrine are not yet fully understood. In some cases, they provide a faster or slower action to supplement or modulate the effects of the primary transmitter.

They also participate in feedback inhibition of the same and nearby nerve terminals.

AUTONOMIC RECEPTORS

Historically, structure-activity analyses, with careful comparisons of the potency of series of autonomic agonist and antagonist analogs, led to the definition of different autonomic receptor subtypes, including muscarinic and nicotinic cholinoceptors, and α, β, and dopamine adrenoceptors (Table 6–2). Molecular biology now provides techniques for the discovery and

Table 6–2. Autonomic receptor types with documented or probable effects on peripheral autonomic effector tissues.

Receptor Name	Typical Locations	Result of Ligand Binding
Cholinoceptors		
Muscarinic M_1	CNS neurons, sympathetic postganglionic neurons, some presynaptic sites	Formation of IP_3 and DAG, increased intracellular calcium
Muscarinic M_2	Myocardium, smooth muscle, some presynaptic sites	Opening of potassium channels, inhibition of adenylyl cyclase
Muscarinic M_3	Exocrine glands, vessels (smooth muscle and endothelium)	Formation of IP_3 and DAG, increased intracellular calcium
Nicotinic N_N	Postganglionic neurons, some presynaptic cholinergic terminals	Opening of Na^+, K^+ channels, depolarization
Nicotinic N_M	Skeletal muscle neuromuscular end plates	Opening of Na^+, K^+ channels, depolarization
Adrenoceptors		
Alpha$_1$	Postsynaptic effector cells, especially smooth muscle	Formation of IP_3 and DAG, increased intracellular calcium
Alpha$_2$	Presynaptic adrenergic nerve terminals, platelets, lipocytes, smooth muscle	Inhibition of adenylyl cyclase, decreased cAMP
Beta$_1$	Postsynaptic effector cells, especially heart, lipocytes, brain; presynaptic adrenergic and cholinergic nerve terminals	Stimulation of adenylyl cyclase, increased cAMP
Beta$_2$	Postsynaptic effector cells, especially smooth muscle and cardiac muscle	Stimulation of adenylyl cyclase and increased cAMP. Activates cardiac G_i under some conditions.
Beta$_3$	Postsynaptic effector cells, especially lipocytes	Stimulation of adenylyl cyclase and increased cAMP
Dopamine receptors		
D_1 (DA_1), D_5	Brain; effector tissues, especially smooth muscle of the renal vascular bed	Stimulation of adenylyl cyclase and increased cAMP
D_2 (DA_2)	Brain; effector tissues especially smooth muscle; presynaptic nerve terminals	Inhibition of adenylyl cyclase; increased potassium conductance
D_3	Brain	Inhibition of adenylyl cyclase
D_4	Brain, cardiovascular system	Inhibition of adenylyl cyclase

expression of genes that code for related receptors within these groups. (See Chapter 2 Box, How Are New Receptors Discovered?)

The primary acetylcholine receptor subtypes were named after the alkaloids originally used in their identification: muscarine and nicotine. These nouns are read-ily converted into adjectives—thus, **muscarinic** and **nicotinic receptors.** In the case of receptors associated with noradrenergic nerves, the coining of simple adjectives from the names of the agonists (noradrenaline, phenylephrine, isoproterenol, etc) was not practicable. Therefore, the term **adrenoceptor** is widely used to describe receptors that respond to catecholamines such as norepinephrine. By analogy, the term **cholinoceptor** denotes receptors (both muscarinic and nicotinic) that respond to acetylcholine. In North America, receptors were colloquially named after the nerves that usually innervate them; thus, **adrenergic** (or noradrenergic) **receptors** and **cholinergic receptors.** The adrenoceptors can be subdivided into α-**adrenoceptor** and β-**adrenoceptor** types on the basis of both agonist and antagonist selectivity. Development of more selective blocking drugs has led to the naming of subclasses within these major types; eg, within the α-adrenoceptor class, α_1 and α_2 receptors differ in both agonist and antagonist selectivity. Specific examples of such selective drugs are given in the chapters that follow.

NONADRENERGIC, NONCHOLINERGIC NEURONS

It has been known for many years that autonomic effector tissues (eg, gut, airways, bladder) contain nerve fibers that do not show the histochemical characteristics of either cholinergic or adrenergic fibers. Both motor and sensory nonadrenergic, noncholinergic fibers are present. Although peptides are the most common transmitter substances found in these nerve endings, other substances, eg, nitric oxide synthase and purines, are also present in many nerve terminals (Table 6–1). Improved immunologic assay methods now permit accurate identification and quantitation of peptides stored in and released from the fiber terminals. Capsaicin, a neurotoxin derived from chili peppers, can cause the release of transmitter (especially substance P) from such neurons and, if given in high doses, destruction of the neuron.

The enteric system in the gut wall (Figure 6–2) is the most extensively studied system containing nonadrenergic, noncholinergic neurons in addition to cholinergic and adrenergic fibers. In the small intestine, for example, these neurons contain one or more of the following: nitric oxide synthase, calcitonin gene-related peptide, cholecystokinin, dynorphin, enkephalins, gastrin-releasing peptide, 5-hydroxytryptamine (serotonin), neuropeptide Y, somatostatin, substance P, and vasoactive intestinal peptide. Some neurons contain as many as five different transmitters. The ENS functions in a semiautonomous manner, utilizing input from the motor outflow of the ANS for modulation of gastrointestinal activity and sending sensory information back to the central nervous system. The ENS provides the necessary synchronization of impulses that, for example, ensures forward, not backward, propulsion of gut contents and relaxation of sphincters when the gut wall contracts.

The sensory fibers in the nonadrenergic, noncholinergic systems are probably better termed "sensory-efferent" or "sensory-local effector" fibers because, when activated by a sensory input, they are capable of releasing transmitter peptides from the sensory ending itself, from local axon branches, and from collaterals that terminate in the autonomic ganglia. These peptides are potent agonists at many autonomic effector tissues.

FUNCTIONAL ORGANIZATION OF AUTONOMIC ACTIVITY

A basic understanding of the interactions of autonomic nerves with each other and with their effector organs is essential for an appreciation of the actions of autonomic drugs, especially because of the significant reflex (compensatory) effects that may be evoked by these agents.

Central Integration

At the highest level—midbrain and medulla—the two divisions of the autonomic nervous system and the endocrine system are integrated with each other, with sensory input, and with information from higher central nervous system centers. These interactions are such that early investigators called the parasympathetic system a **trophotropic** one (ie, leading to growth) used to "rest and digest" and the sympathetic system an **ergotropic** one (ie, leading to energy expenditure) that is activated for "fight or flight." While such terms offer little insight into the mechanisms involved, they do provide simple descriptions applicable to many of the actions of the systems (Table 6–3). For example, slowing of the heart and stimulation of digestive activity are typical energy-conserving actions of the parasympathetic system. In contrast, cardiac stimulation, increased blood sugar, and cutaneous vasoconstriction are responses produced by sympathetic discharge that are suited to fighting or surviving attack.

At a more subtle level of interactions in the brain stem, medulla, and spinal cord, there are important cooperative interactions between the parasympathetic and sympathetic systems. For some organs, sensory fibers associated with the parasympathetic system exert reflex control over motor outflow in the sympathetic system. Thus, the sensory carotid sinus baroreceptor fibers in the glossopharyngeal nerve have a major influence on sympathetic outflow from the vasomotor center. This example is described in greater detail below. Similarly, parasympathetic sensory fibers in the wall of the urinary bladder significantly influence sympathetic inhibitory outflow to that organ. Within the enteric nervous system, sensory fibers from the wall of the gut synapse on both preganglionic and postganglionic motor cells that control intestinal smooth muscle and secretory cells (Figure 6–2).

Table 6–3. Direct effects of autonomic nerve activity on some organ systems.

| | Effect of | | | |
| | Sympathetic Activity | | Parasympathetic Activity | |
Organ	Action[1]	Receptor[2]	Action	Receptor[2]
Eye				
Iris				
Radial muscle	Contracts	α_1	...	...
Circular muscle	...	...	Contracts	M_3
Ciliary muscle	[Relaxes]	β	Contracts	M_3
Heart				
Sinoatrial node	Accelerates	β_1, β_2	Decelerates	M_2
Ectopic pacemakers	Accelerates	β_1, β_2	...	...
Contractility	Increases	β_1, β_2	Decreases (atria)	M_2
Blood vessels				
Skin, splanchnic vessels	Contracts	α	...	...
Skeletal muscle vessels	Relaxes	β_2	...	...
	[Contracts]	α	...	...
	Relaxes	M^3	...	...
Endothelium			Releases EDRF	$M_3{}^4$
Bronchiolar smooth muscle	Relaxes	β_2	Contracts	M_3
Gastrointestinal tract				
Smooth muscle				
Walls	Relaxes	$\alpha_2,{}^5 \beta_2$	Contracts	M_3
Sphincters	Contracts	α_1	Relaxes	M_3
Secretion	...	...	Increases	M_3
Myenteric plexus			Activates	M_1
Genitourinary smooth muscle				
Bladder wall	Relaxes	β_2	Contracts	M_3
Sphincter	Contracts	α_1	Relaxes	M_3
Uterus, pregnant	Relaxes	β_2	...	...
	Contracts	α	Contracts	M_3
Penis, seminal vesicles	Ejaculation	α	Erection	M
Skin				
Pilomotor smooth muscle	Contracts	α	...	...
Sweat glands			...	...
Thermoregulatory	Increases	M	...	...
Apocrine (stress)	Increases	α	...	...
Metabolic functions				
Liver	Gluconeogenesis	β_2, α	...	...
Liver	Glycogenolysis	β_2, α	...	...
Fat cells	Lipolysis	β_3	...	...
Kidney	Renin release	β_1	...	...
Autonomic nerve endings				
Sympathetic	...	...	Decreases NE release	M^6
Parasympathetic	Decreases ACh release	α	...	...

[1]Less important actions are shown in brackets.

[2]Specific receptor type: α = alpha, β = beta, M = muscarinic.

[3]Vascular smooth muscle in skeletal muscle has sympathetic cholinergic dilator fibers.

[4]The endothelium of most blood vessels releases EDRF (endothelium-derived relaxing factor), which causes marked vasodilation, in response to muscarinic stimuli. However, unlike the receptors innervated by sympathetic cholinergic fibers in skeletal muscle blood vessels, these muscarinic receptors are not innervated and respond only to circulating muscarinic agonists.

[5]Probably through presynaptic inhibition of parasympathetic activity.

[6]Probably M_1 but M_2 may participate in some locations.

Integration of Cardiovascular Function

Autonomic reflexes are particularly important in understanding cardiovascular responses to autonomic drugs. As indicated in Figure 6–7, the primary controlled variable in cardiovascular function is **mean arterial pressure.** Changes in any variable contributing to mean arterial pressure (eg, a drug-induced increase in peripheral vascular resistance) will evoke powerful **homeostatic** secondary responses that tend to compensate for the directly evoked change. The homeostatic response may be sufficient to reduce the change in mean arterial pressure and to reverse the drug's effects on heart rate. A slow infusion of norepinephrine provides a useful example. This agent produces direct effects on both vascular and cardiac muscle. It is a powerful vasoconstrictor and, by increasing peripheral vascular resistance, increases mean arterial pressure. In the absence of reflex control—in a patient who has had a heart transplant, for example—the drug's effect on the heart is also stimulatory; ie, it increases heart rate and contractile force. However, in a subject with intact reflexes, the negative feedback baroreceptor response to increased mean arterial pressure causes decreased sympathetic outflow to the heart and a powerful increase in parasympathetic (vagus nerve) discharge at the cardiac pacemaker. As a result, the *net* effect of ordinary pressor doses of norepinephrine is to produce a marked increase in peripheral vascular resistance, an increase in mean arterial pressure, and a consistent *slowing* of heart rate. Bradycardia, the reflex compensatory response elicited by this agent, is the *exact opposite* of the drug's direct action; yet it is completely predictable if the integration of cardiovascular function by the autonomic nervous system is understood.

Presynaptic Regulation

The principle of negative feedback control is also found at the presynaptic level of autonomic function. Impor-

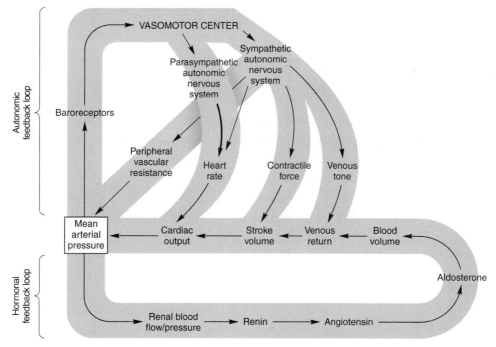

Figure 6–7. Autonomic and hormonal control of cardiovascular function. Note that two feedback loops are present: the autonomic nervous system loop and the hormonal loop. The sympathetic nervous system directly influences four major variables: peripheral vascular resistance, heart rate, force, and venous tone. It also directly modulates renin production (not shown). The parasympathetic nervous system directly influences heart rate. Angiotensin II directly increases peripheral vascular resistance and facilitates sympathetic effects (not shown). The net feedback effect of each loop is to compensate for changes in arterial blood pressure. Thus, decreased blood pressure due to blood loss would evoke increased sympathetic outflow and renin release. Conversely, elevated pressure due to the administration of a vasoconstrictor drug would cause reduced sympathetic outflow and renin release and increased parasympathetic (vagal) outflow.

tant presynaptic feedback inhibitory control mechanisms have been shown to exist at most nerve endings. A well-documented mechanism involves an α_2 receptor located on noradrenergic nerve terminals. This receptor is activated by norepinephrine and similar molecules; activation diminishes further release of norepinephrine from these nerve endings (Table 6–4). Conversely, a presynaptic β receptor appears to facilitate the release of norepinephrine. Presynaptic receptors that respond to the transmitter substances released by the nerve ending are called **autoreceptors.** Autoreceptors are usually inhibitory, but many cholinergic fibers, especially somatic motor fibers, have excitatory nicotinic autoreceptors.

Control of transmitter release is not limited to modulation by the transmitter itself. Nerve terminals also carry regulatory receptors that respond to many other substances. Such **heteroreceptors** may be activated by substances released from other nerve terminals that synapse with the nerve ending. For example, some vagal fibers in the myocardium synapse on sympathetic noradrenergic nerve terminals and inhibit norepinephrine release. Alternatively, the ligands for these receptors may diffuse to the receptors from the blood or from nearby tissues. Some of the transmitters and receptors identified to date are listed in Table 6–4. Presynaptic regula-

tion by a variety of endogenous chemicals probably occurs in all nerve fibers.

Postsynaptic Regulation

Postsynaptic regulation can be considered from two perspectives: modulation by the prior history of activity at the primary receptor (which may up- or down-regulate receptor number or desensitize receptors; see Chapter 2) and modulation by other temporally associated events.

The first mechanism has been well documented in several receptor-effector systems. Up- and down-regulation are known to occur in response to decreased or increased activation, respectively, of the receptors. An extreme form of up-regulation occurs after denervation of some tissues, resulting in **denervation supersensitivity** of the tissue to activators of that receptor type. In skeletal muscle, for example, nicotinic receptors are normally restricted to the end plate regions underlying somatic motor nerve terminals. Surgical denervation results in marked proliferation of nicotinic cholinoceptors over all parts of the fiber, including areas not previously associated with any motor nerve junctions. A pharmacologic supersensitivity related to denervation supersensitivity occurs in autonomic effector tissues after administration of drugs that deplete transmitter

Table 6–4. Autoreceptor, heteroreceptor, and modulatory effects in peripheral synapses.[1]

Transmitter/Modulator	Receptor Type	Neuron Terminals Where Found
Inhibitory effects		
Acetylcholine	M_2	Adrenergic, enteric nervous system
Norepinephrine	Alpha$_2$	Adrenergic
Dopamine	D_2; less evidence for D_1	Adrenergic
Serotonin (5-HT)	5-HT$_1$, 5-HT$_2$, 5-HT$_3$	Cholinergic preganglionic
ATP and adenosine	P_2 (ATP), P_1 (adenosine)	Adrenergic autonomic and ENS cholinergic neurons
Histamine	H_3, possibly H_2	H_3 type identified on CNS adrenergic and serotonergic neurons
Enkephalin	Delta (also mu, kappa)	Adrenergic, ENS cholinergic
Neuropeptide Y	NPY	Adrenergic, some cholinergic
Prostaglandin E_1, E_2	EP$_3$	Adrenergic
Excitatory effects		
Epinephrine	Beta$_2$	Adrenergic, somatic motor cholinergic
Acetylcholine	N_M	Somatic motor cholinergic, ANS cholinergic
Angiotensin II	AT$_1$	Adrenergic

[1]A provisional list. The number of transmitters and locations will undoubtedly increase with additional research.

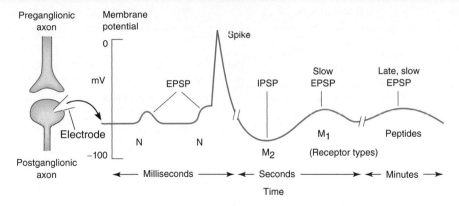

Figure 6–8. Excitatory and inhibitory postsynaptic potentials *(EPSP* and *IPSP)* in an autonomic ganglion cell. The postganglionic neuron shown at the left with a recording electrode might undergo the membrane potential changes shown schematically in the recording. The response begins with two EPSP responses to nicotinic *(N)* receptor activation, the first not achieving threshold. The action potential is followed by an IPSP, probably evoked by M_2 receptor activation (with possible participation from dopamine receptor activation). The IPSP is, in turn, followed by a slower M_1-dependent EPSP, and this is sometimes followed by a still slower peptide-induced excitatory postsynaptic potential.

stores and prevent activation of the postsynaptic receptors for a sufficient period of time. For example, administration of large doses of reserpine, a norepinephrine depleter, can cause increased sensitivity of the smooth muscle and cardiac muscle effector cells served by the depleted sympathetic fibers.

The second mechanism involves modulation of the primary transmitter-receptor event by events evoked by the same or other transmitters acting on different postsynaptic receptors. Ganglionic transmission is a good example of this phenomenon (Figure 6–8). The postganglionic cells are activated (depolarized) as a result of binding of an appropriate ligand to a nicotinic (N_N) acetylcholine receptor. The resulting fast excitatory postsynaptic potential (EPSP) evokes a propagated action potential if threshold is reached. This event is often followed by a small and slowly developing but longer-lasting hyperpolarizing afterpotential—a slow inhibitory postsynaptic potential (IPSP). The hyperpolarization involves opening of potassium channels by M_2 cholinoceptors. The IPSP is followed by a small, slow excitatory postsynaptic potential caused by closure of potassium channels linked to M_1 cholinoceptors. Finally, a late, very slow EPSP may be evoked by peptides released from other fibers. These slow potentials serve to modulate the responsiveness of the postsynaptic cell to subsequent primary excitatory presynaptic nerve activity. (See Chapter 21 for additional examples.)

PHARMACOLOGIC MODIFICATION OF AUTONOMIC FUNCTION

Because transmission involves different mechanisms in different segments of the autonomic nervous system, some drugs produce highly specific effects while others are much less selective in their actions. A summary of the steps in transmission of impulses, from the central nervous system to the autonomic effector cells, is presented in Table 6–5. Drugs that block action potential propagation (local anesthetics) are very nonselective in their action, since they act on a process that is common to all neurons. On the other hand, drugs that act on the biochemical processes involved in transmitter synthesis and storage are more selective, since the biochemistry of adrenergic transmission is very different from that of cholinergic transmission. Activation or blockade of effector cell receptors offers maximum flexibility and selectivity of effect: adrenoceptors are easily distinguished from cholinoceptors. Furthermore, individual subgroups can often be selectively activated or blocked within each major type. Some examples are given in the Box, Pharmacology of the Eye.

The next four chapters provide many more examples of this useful diversity of autonomic control processes.

Table 6–5. Steps in autonomic transmission: Effects of drugs.

Process	Drug Example	Site	Action
Action potential propagation	Local anesthetics, tetrodotoxin,[1] saxitoxin[2]	Nerve axons	Block sodium channels; block conduction
Transmitter synthesis	Hemicholinium	Cholinergic nerve terminals: membrane	Blocks uptake of choline and slows synthesis
	α-Methyltyrosine (metyrosine)	Adrenergic nerve terminals and adrenal medulla: cytoplasm	Blocks synthesis
Transmitter storage	Vesamicol	Cholinergic terminals: vesicles	Prevents storage, depletes
	Reserpine	Adrenergic terminals: vesicles	Prevents storage, depletes
Transmitter release	Many[3]	Nerve terminal membrane receptors	Modulate release
	ω-Conotoxin GVIA[4]	Nerve terminal calcium channels	Blocks calcium channels, reduces transmitter release
	Botulinum toxin	Cholinergic vesicles	Prevents release
	Alpha-latrotoxin[5]	Cholinergic and adrenergic vesicles	Causes explosive release
	Tyramine, amphetamine	Adrenergic nerve terminals	Promote transmitter release
Transmitter uptake after release	Cocaine, tricyclic antidepressants	Adrenergic nerve terminals	Inhibit uptake; increase transmitter effect on postsynaptic receptors
	6-Hydroxydopamine	Adrenergic nerve terminals	Destroys the terminals
Receptor activation or blockade	Norepinephrine	Receptors at adrenergic junctions	Binds α receptors; causes activation
	Phentolamine	Receptors at adrenergic junctions	Binds α receptors; prevents activation
	Isoproterenol	Receptors at adrenergic junctions	Binds β receptors; activates adenylyl cyclase
	Propranolol	Receptors at adrenergic junctions	Binds β receptors; prevents activation
	Nicotine	Receptors at nicotinic cholinergic junctions (autonomic ganglia, neuromuscular end plates)	Binds nicotinic receptors; opens ion channel in postsynaptic membrane
	Tubocurarine	Neuromuscular end plates	Prevents activation
	Bethanechol	Receptors, parasympathetic effector cells (smooth muscle, glands)	Binds and activates muscarinic receptors
	Atropine	Receptors, parasympathetic effector cells	Binds muscarinic receptors; prevents activation
Enzymatic inactivation of transmitter	Neostigmine	Cholinergic synapses (acetylcholinesterase)	Inhibits enzyme; prolongs and intensifies transmitter action
	Tranylcypromine	Adrenergic nerve terminals (monoamine oxidase)	Inhibits enzyme; increases stored transmitter pool

[1]Toxin of puffer fish, California newt.

[2]Toxin of *Gonyaulax* (red tide organism).

[3]Norepinephrine, dopamine, acetylcholine, peptides, various prostaglandins, etc.

[4]Toxin of marine snails of the genus *Conus*.

[5]Black widow spider venom.

PHARMACOLOGY OF THE EYE

The eye is a good example of an organ with multiple ANS functions, controlled by several different autonomic receptors. As shown in Figure 6–9, the anterior chamber is the site of several tissues controlled by the ANS. These tissues include three different muscles (pupillary dilator and constrictor muscles in the iris and the ciliary muscle) and the secretory epithelium of the ciliary body.

Muscarinic cholinomimetics mediate contraction of the circular pupillary constrictor muscle and of the ciliary muscle. Contraction of the pupillary constrictor muscle causes miosis, a reduction in pupil size. Miosis is usually present in patients exposed to large systemic or small topical doses of cholinomimetics, especially organophosphate cholinesterase inhibitors. Ciliary muscle contraction causes accommodation of focus for near vision. Marked contraction of the ciliary muscle, which often occurs with cholinesterase inhibitor intoxication, is called *cyclospasm*. Ciliary muscle contraction also puts tension on the trabecular meshwork, opening its pores and facilitating outflow of the aqueous humor into the canal of Schlemm. Increased outflow reduces intraocular pressure, a very useful result in patients with glaucoma. All of these effects are prevented or reversed by muscarinic blocking drugs such as atropine.

Alpha adrenoceptors mediate contraction of the radially oriented pupillary dilator muscle fibers in the iris and result in mydriasis. This occurs during sympathetic discharge and when alpha agonist drugs such as phenylephrine are placed in the conjunctival sac. Beta-adrenoceptors on the ciliary epithelium facilitate the secretion of aqueous humor. Blocking these receptors (with β-blocking drugs) reduces the secretory activity and reduces intraocular pressure, providing another therapy for glaucoma.

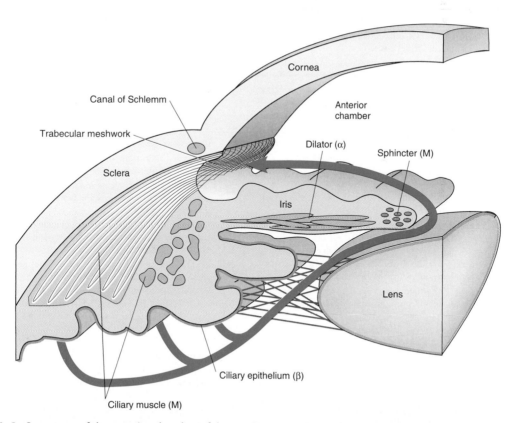

Figure 6–9. Structures of the anterior chamber of the eye. Tissues with significant autonomic functions and the associated ANS receptors are shown in this schematic diagram. Aqueous humor is secreted by the epithelium of the ciliary body, flows through the anterior chamber, and exits via the canal of Schlemm (arrow). Blockade of the β adrenoceptors associated with the ciliary epithelium causes decreased secretion of aqueous. Blood vessels (not shown) in the sclera are also under autonomic control and influence aqueous drainage.

REFERENCES

Altman JD et al: Abnormal regulation of the sympathetic nervous system in alpha$_{2A}$-adrenergic receptor knockout mice. Mol Pharmacol 1999;56:154.

Anderson K-E: Pharmacology of lower urinary tract smooth muscles and penile erectile tissues. Pharmacol Rev 1993;45:253.

Bernardi L et al: Demonstrable cardiac reinnervation after human heart transplantation by carotid baroreflex modulation of RR interval. Circulation 1995;92:2895.

Bernstein D: Cardiovascular and metabolic alterations in mice lacking beta$_1$- and beta$_2$-adrenergic receptors. Trends Cardiovasc Med 2002;12:287.

Boehm S, Kubista H: Fine tuning of sympathetic transmitter release via ionotropic and metabotropic presynaptic receptors. Pharmacol Rev 2002;54:43.

Burnstock G, Hoyle CHV: *Autonomic Neuroeffector Mechanisms.* Harwood Academic Publishers, 1992.

Burnstock G: Noradrenaline and ATP: Cotransmitters and neuromodulators. J Physiol Pharmacol 1995;46:365.

Chang HY, Mashimo H, Goyal RK: Musings on the wanderer: What's new in our understanding of the vago-vagal reflex? IV. Current concepts of vagal efferent projections to the gut. Am J Physiol Gastrointest Liver Physiol 2003;284:G357.

Chen D et al: Rat stomach ECL cells up-date of biology and physiology. Gen Pharmacol 1999;32:413.

deGroat WC, Yoshimura N: Pharmacology of the lower urinary tract. Annu Rev Pharmacol Toxicol 2001;41:691.

Docherty JR: Age-related changes in adrenergic neuroeffector transmission. Auton Neurosci 2002;96:8.

Eglen RM, Hegde SS, Watson N: Muscarinic receptor subtypes and smooth muscle function. Pharmacol Rev 1996;48:531.

Fetscher C et al: M$_3$ muscarinic receptors mediate contraction of human urinary bladder. Br J Pharmacol 2002;136:641.

Furchgott RF: Role of endothelium in responses of vascular smooth muscle to drugs. Annu Rev Pharmacol Toxicol 1984;24:175.

Furness JB et al: Roles of peptides in transmission in the enteric nervous system. Trends Neurosci 1992;15:66.

Galligan JJ: Ligand-gated ion channels in the enteric nervous system. Neurogastroenterol Motil 2002;14:611.

Gershon MD, Kirchgessner AL, Wade PR: Functional anatomy of the enteric nervous system. In: *Physiology of the Gastrointestinal Tract,* 3rd ed. Johnson LR (editor). Raven Press, 1994.

Goldstein DS et al: Dysautonomias: clinical disorders of the autonomic nervous system. Ann Intern Med 2002;137:753.

Goyal RK, Hirano I: The enteric nervous system. N Engl J Med 1996;334:1106.

Hallett M: One man's poison—Clinical applications of botulinum toxin. (Editorial.) N Engl J Med 1999;341:118.

Hansen G et al: Absence of muscarinic cholinergic airway responses in mice deficient in the cyclic nucleotide phosphodiesterase PDE4D. Proc Natl Acad Sci U S A 2000;97:6751.

Huikuri HV, Makikallio TH: Heart rate variability in ischemic heart disease. Auton Neurosci 2001;90:95.

Jarvis SE, Zamponi GW: Interactions between presynaptic Ca^{2+} channels, cytoplasmic messengers and proteins of the synaptic vesicle complex. Trends Pharmacol Sci 2001;22:519.

Kellogg DL Jr et al: Cutaneous active vasodilation in humans is mediated by cholinergic nerve cotransmission. Circ Res 1995; 77:1222.

Kumada M, Terui N, Kuwaki T: Arterial baroreceptor reflex: Its central and peripheral neural mechanisms. Prog Neurobiol 1990; 35:331.

Lee TJF, Liu J, Evans S: Cholinergic-nitrergic transmitter mechanisms in the cerebral circulation. Microsc Res Tech 2001; 53:119.

Lepori L et al: Interaction between cholinergic and nitrergic vasodilation: a novel mechanism of blood pressure control. Cardiovasc Res 2001;51:767.

Lundberg JM: Pharmacology of cotransmission in the autonomic nervous system: Integrative aspects on amines, neuropeptides, adenosine triphosphate, amino acids and nitric oxide. Pharmacol Rev 1996;48:113.

MacDermott AB, Role LW, Siegelbaum SA: Presynaptic ionotropic receptors and the control of neurotransmitter release. Annu Rev Neurosci 1999;22:443.

MacDonald A et al: Contributions of α_1-adrenoceptors, α_2-adrenoceptors, and P$_{2x}$-purinoceptors to neurotransmission in several rabbit isolated blood vessels: Role of neuronal uptake and autofeedback. Br J Pharmacol 1992;105:347.

Miller RJ: Presynaptic receptors. Annu Rev Pharmacol Toxicol 1998;38:201.

Montecucco C, Schiavo G: Structure and function of tetanus and botulinum neurotoxins. Q Rev Biophys 1995;28:423.

1999 Receptor and ion channel nomenclature supplement. Trends Pharmacol Sci 1999(Suppl):1.

Ralevic V, Burnstock G: Receptors for purines and pyrimidines. Pharmacol Rev 1998;50:413.

Rohrer DK et al: Cardiovascular and metabolic alterations in mice lacking both β_1- and β_2-adrenergic receptors. J Biol Chem 1999;274:16701.

Südhof TC: The synaptic vesicle cycle: A cascade of protein-protein interactions. Nature 1995;375:645.

Sang Q et al: Innervation of the esophagus in mice that lack MASH1. J Comp Neurol 1999;408:1.

Santicioli P, Maggi CA: Myogenic and neurogenic factors in the control of pyeloureteral motility and ureteral peristalsis. Pharmacol Rev 1998;50:683.

Schiavo G et al: Tetanus and botulinum-B neurotoxins block neurotransmitter release by proteolytic cleavage of synaptobrevin. Nature 1992;359:832.

Schlicker E, Gothert M: Interactions between the presynaptic alpha$_2$-autoreceptor and the presynaptic inhibitory heteroreceptors on noradrenergic neurons. Brain Res Bull 1998; 47:129.

Serone AP, Wright CE, Angus JA: Heterogeneity of prejunctional NPY receptor-mediated inhibition of cardiac neurotransmission. Br J Pharmacol 1999;127:99.

Skok VI: Nicotinic acetylcholine receptors in autonomic ganglia. Auton Neurosci 2002;97:1.

Slutsky I, Parnas H, Parnas I: Presynaptic effects of muscarine on ACh release at the frog neuromuscular junction. J Physiol (Lond) 1999;514:769.

Tetrodotoxin poisoning associated with eating puffer fish transported from Japan—California, 1996. MMWR Morbid Mortal Wkly Rep 1996;45:389.

Thiel G: Recent breakthroughs in neurotransmitter release: Paradigm for regulated exocytosis. News Physiol Sci 1995;10:42.

Toda N, Okamura T: The pharmacology of nitric oxide in the peripheral nervous system of blood vessels. Pharmacol Rev 2003;55:271.

Todorov LD et al: Differential cotransmission in sympathetic nerves: Role of frequency of stimulation and prejunctional autoreceptors. J Pharmacol Exp Ther 1999;290:241.

Westfall DP, Todorov LD, Mihaylova-Todorova ST: ATP as a cotransmitter in sympathetic nerves and its inactivation by releasable enzymes. J Pharmacol Exp Ther 2002;303:439.

Wilson RF et al: Regional differences in sympathetic reinnervation after human orthotopic cardiac transplantation. Circulation 1993;88:165.

Zanzinger J: Role of nitric oxide in the neural control of cardiovascular function. Cardiovasc Res 1999;43:639.

Zhou X, Galligan JJ: Synaptic activation and properties of 5-hydroxytryptamine(3) receptors in myenteric neurons of guinea pig intestine. J Pharmacol Exp Ther 1999;290:803.

Cholinoceptor-Activating & Cholinesterase-Inhibiting Drugs

Achilles J. Pappano, PhD

Acetylcholine receptor stimulants and cholinesterase inhibitors together comprise a large group of drugs that mimic acetylcholine (cholinomimetic agents) (Figure 7–1). Cholinoceptor stimulants are classified pharmacologically by their spectrum of action depending on the type of receptor—muscarinic or nicotinic—that is activated. They are also classified by their mechanism of action because some cholinomimetic drugs bind directly to (and activate) cholinoceptors while others act indirectly by inhibiting the hydrolysis of endogenous acetylcholine.

SPECTRUM OF ACTION OF CHOLINOMIMETIC DRUGS

Early studies of the parasympathetic nervous system showed that the alkaloid **muscarine** mimicked the effects of parasympathetic nerve discharge, ie, the effects were **parasympathomimetic.** Application of muscarine to ganglia and to autonomic effector tissues (smooth muscle, heart, exocrine glands) showed that the parasympathomimetic action of the alkaloid occurred

through an action on receptors at effector cells, not those in ganglia. The effects of acetylcholine itself and of other cholinomimetic drugs at autonomic neuroeffector junctions are called parasympathomimetic effects, and are mediated by muscarinic receptors. In contrast, low concentrations of the alkaloid **nicotine** stimulated autonomic ganglia and skeletal muscle neuromuscular junctions but not autonomic effector cells. The ganglion and skeletal muscle receptors were therefore labeled nicotinic. When acetylcholine was later identified as the physiologic transmitter at both muscarinic and nicotinic receptors, both receptors were recognized as cholinoceptor subtypes.

Cholinoceptors are members of either G protein-linked (muscarinic) or ion channel (nicotinic) families on the basis of their transmembrane signaling mechanisms. Muscarinic receptors contain seven transmembrane domains whose third cytoplasmic loop is coupled to G proteins that function as intramembrane transducers (see Figure 2–11). In general, these receptors regulate the production of intracellular second messengers. Agonist selectivity is determined by the subtypes of muscarinic receptors and G proteins that are present in a

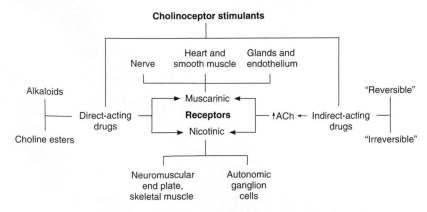

Fi... major groups of cholinoceptor-activating drugs, receptors, and target tissues.

Table 7–1. Subtypes and characteristics of cholinoceptors.

Receptor Type	Other Names	Location	Structural Features	Postreceptor Mechanism
M_1	M_{1a}	Nerves	Seven transmembrane segments, G protein-linked	IP_3, DAG cascade
M_2	M_{2a}, cardiac M_2	Heart, nerves, smooth muscle	Seven transmembrane segments, G protein-linked	Inhibition of cAMP production, activation of K^+ channels
M_3	M_{2b}, glandular M_2	Glands, smooth muscle, endothelium	Seven transmembrane segments, G protein-linked	IP_3, DAG cascade
m_4[1]		?CNS	Seven transmembrane segments, G protein-linked	Inhibition of cAMP production
m_5[1]		?CNS	Seven transmembrane segments, G protein-linked	IP_3, DAG cascade
N_M	Muscle type, end plate receptor	Skeletal muscle neuromuscular junction	Pentamer $(\alpha_2\beta\delta\gamma)$[2]	Na^+, K^+ depolarizing ion channel
N_N	Neuronal type, ganglion receptor	Postganglionic cell body, dendrites	α and β subunits only as $\alpha_2\beta_2$ or $\alpha_3\beta_3$	Na^+, K^+ depolarizing ion channel

[1]Genes have been cloned, but functional receptors have not been incontrovertibly identified.

[2]Structure in *Torpedo* electric organ and fetal mammalian muscle. In adult muscle, the γ subunit is replaced by an ε subunit. Several different α and β subunits have been identified in different mammalian tissues (Lukas et al, 1999).

given cell (Table 7–1). Muscarinic receptors are located on plasma membranes of cells in the central nervous system, in organs innervated by parasympathetic nerves as well as on some tissues that are not innervated by these nerves, eg, endothelial cells (Table 7–1), and on those tissues innervated by postganglionic sympathetic cholinergic nerves.

Nicotinic receptors are part of a transmembrane polypeptide whose subunits form cation-selective ion channels (see Figure 2–9). These receptors are located on plasma membranes of postganglionic cells in all autonomic ganglia, of muscles innervated by somatic motor fibers, and of some central nervous system neurons (see Figure 6–1).

Unselective cholinoceptor stimulants in sufficient dosage can produce very diffuse and marked alterations in organ system function because acetylcholine has multiple sites of action where it initiates both excitatory and inhibitory effects. Fortunately, drugs are available that have a degree of selectivity, so that desired effects can often be achieved while avoiding or minimizing adverse effects. Selectivity of action is based on several factors. Some drugs stimulate either muscarinic receptors or nicotinic receptors selectively. Some agents stimulate

nicotinic receptors at neuromuscular junctions preferentially and have less effect on nicotinic receptors in ganglia. Organ selectivity can also be achieved by using appropriate routes of administration ("pharmacokinetic selectivity"). For example, muscarinic stimulants can be administered topically to the surface of the eye to modify ocular function while minimizing systemic effects.

MODE OF ACTION OF CHOLINOMIMETIC DRUGS

Direct-acting cholinomimetic agents directly bind to and activate muscarinic or nicotinic receptors (Figure 7–1). Indirect-acting agents produce their primary effects by inhibiting acetylcholinesterase, which hydrolyzes acetylcholine to choline and acetic acid (see Figure 6–3). By inhibiting acetylcholinesterase, the indirect-acting drugs increase the endogenous acetylcholine concentration in synaptic clefts and neuroeffector junctions, and the excess acetylcholine in turn stimulates cholinoceptors to evoke increased responses. These drugs act primarily where acetylcholine is physiologically released and are *amplifiers* of endogenous acetylcholine.

Some cholinesterase inhibitors also inhibit butyrylcholinesterase (pseudocholinesterase). However, inhibition of butyrylcholinesterase plays little role in the action of indirect-acting cholinomimetic drugs because this enzyme is not important in the physiologic termination of synaptic acetylcholine action. Some quaternary cholinesterase inhibitors also have a modest direct action as well, eg, neostigmine, which activates neuromuscular nicotinic cholinoceptors directly in addition to blocking cholinesterase.

I. BASIC PHARMACOLOGY OF THE DIRECT-ACTING CHOLINOCEPTOR STIMULANTS

The direct-acting cholinomimetic drugs can be divided on the basis of chemical structure into esters of choline (including acetylcholine) and alkaloids (such as muscarine and nicotine). A few of these drugs are highly selective for the muscarinic or for the nicotinic receptor. Many have effects on both receptors; acetylcholine is typical.

Chemistry & Pharmacokinetics

A. Structure

Four important choline esters that have been studied extensively are shown in Figure 7–2. Their permanently charged quaternary ammonium group renders them relatively insoluble in lipids. Many naturally occurring and synthetic cholinomimetic drugs that are not choline esters have been identified; a few of these are shown in Figure 7–3. The muscarinic receptor is strongly stereoselective: *(S)*-bethanechol is almost 1000 times more potent than *(R)*-bethanechol.

B. Absorption, Distribution, and Metabolism

Choline esters are poorly absorbed and poorly distributed into the central nervous system because they are hydrophilic. Although all are hydrolyzed in the gastrointestinal tract (and less active by the oral route), they differ markedly in their susceptibility to hydrolysis by cholinesterase in the body. Acetylcholine is very rapidly hydrolyzed (see Chapter 6); large amounts must be infused intravenously to achieve concentrations high enough to produce detectable effects. A large intravenous bolus injection has a brief effect, typically 5–20 seconds, whereas intramuscular and subcutaneous injections produce only local effects. Methacholine is more resistant to hydrolysis, and the carbamic acid esters carbachol and bethanechol are still more resistant to hydrolysis by cholinesterase and have correspondingly

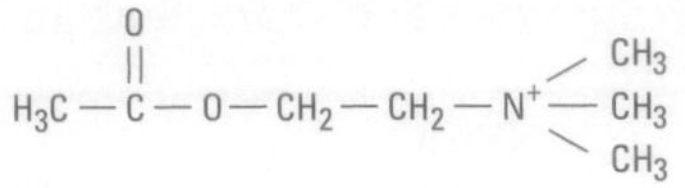

Acetylcholine

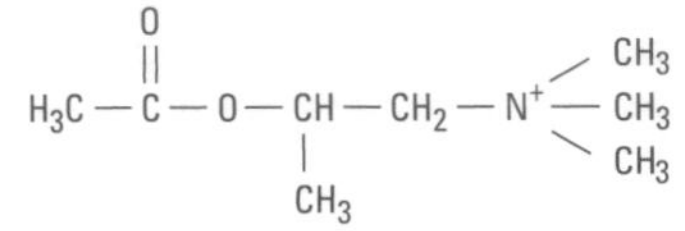

Methacholine (acetyl-β-methylcholine)

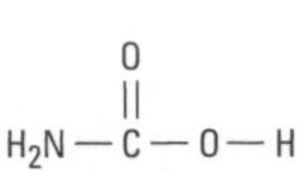

Carbamic acid

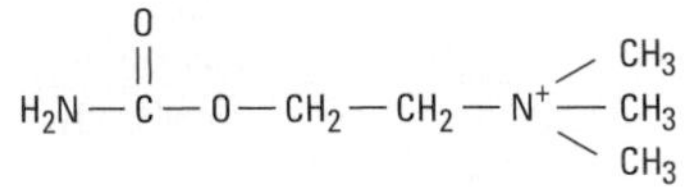

Carbachol (carbamoylcholine)

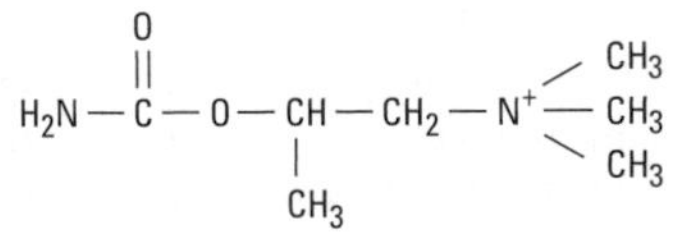

Bethanechol (carbamoyl-β-methylcholine)

Figure 7–2. Molecular structures of four choline esters and carbamic acid. Acetylcholine and methacholine are acetic acid esters of choline and β-methylcholine, respectively. Carbachol and bethanechol are carbamic acid esters of the same alcohols.

longer durations of action. The β-methyl group (methacholine, bethanechol) reduces the potency of these drugs at nicotinic receptors (Table 7–2).

The tertiary natural cholinomimetic alkaloids (pilocarpine, nicotine, lobeline; Figure 7–3) are well absorbed from most sites of administration. Nicotine, a liquid, is sufficiently lipid-soluble to be absorbed across the skin. Muscarine, a quaternary amine, is less completely absorbed from the gastrointestinal tract than the tertiary amines but is nevertheless toxic when ingested,

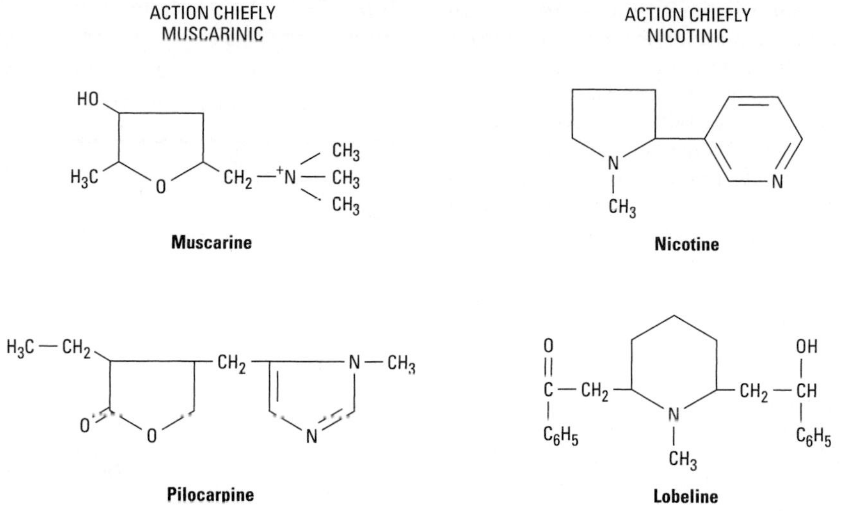

ACTION CHIEFLY
MUSCARINIC

ACTION CHIEFLY
NICOTINIC

Muscarine

Nicotine

Pilocarpine

Lobeline

Figure 7–3. Structures of some cholinomimetic alkaloids.

eg, in certain mushrooms, and even enters the brain. Lobeline is a plant derivative similar to nicotine. These amines are excreted chiefly by the kidneys. Acidification of the urine accelerates clearance of the tertiary amines.

Pharmacodynamics

A. MECHANISM OF ACTION

Activation of the parasympathetic nervous system modifies organ function by two major mechanisms. First, acetylcholine released from parasympathetic nerves activates muscarinic receptors on effector cells to alter organ function directly. Second, acetylcholine released from parasympathetic nerves interacts with muscarinic receptors on nerve terminals to inhibit the release of their

Table 7–2. Properties of choline esters.

Choline Ester	Susceptibility to Cholinesterase	Muscarinic Action	Nicotinic Action
Acetylcholine chloride	++++	+++	+++
Methacholine chloride	+	++++	None
Carbachol chloride	Negligible	++	+++
Bethanechol chloride	Negligible	++	None

neurotransmitter. By this mechanism, acetylcholine release and circulating muscarinic agonists indirectly alter organ function by modulating the effects of the parasympathetic and sympathetic nervous systems and perhaps nonadrenergic, noncholinergic systems.

The mechanisms by which muscarinic stimulants alter cellular function continue to be investigated. As indicated in Chapter 6, muscarinic receptor subtypes have been characterized by binding studies and cloned. Several cellular events occur when muscarinic receptors are activated, one or more of which might serve as second messengers for muscarinic activation. All muscarinic receptors appear to be of the G-protein coupled type (see Chapter 2 and Table 7–1). Muscarinic agonist binding activates the IP_3, DAG cascade. Some evidence implicates DAG in the opening of smooth muscle calcium channels; IP_3 releases calcium from endoplasmic and sarcoplasmic reticulum. Muscarinic agonists also increase cellular cGMP concentrations. Activation of muscarinic receptors also increases potassium flux across cardiac cell membranes and decreases it in ganglion and smooth muscle cells. This effect is mediated by the binding of an activated G protein directly to the channel. Finally, muscarinic receptor activation in some tissues (eg, heart, intestine) inhibits adenylyl cyclase activity. Moreover, muscarinic agonists can attenuate the activation of adenylyl cyclase and modulate the increase in cAMP levels induced by hormones such as catecholamines. These muscarinic effects on cAMP generation cause a reduction of the physiologic response of the organ to stimulatory hormones.

The mechanism of nicotinic receptor activation has been studied in great detail, taking advantage of three factors: (1) the receptor is present in extremely high concentration in the membranes of the electric organs of electric fish; (2) α-bungarotoxin, a component of certain snake venoms, is tightly bound to the receptors and readily labeled as a marker for isolation procedures; and (3) receptor activation results in easily measured electrical and ionic changes in the cells involved. The nicotinic receptor in muscle tissues is a pentamer of four types of glycoprotein subunits (one monomer occurs twice) with a total molecular weight of about 250,000 (see Figure 2–9). The neuronal nicotinic receptor consists of α and β subunits only (Table 7–1). Each subunit has four transmembrane segments. Each α subunit has a receptor site that, when occupied by a nicotinic agonist, causes a conformational change in the protein (channel opening) that allows sodium and potassium ions to diffuse rapidly down their concentration gradients. While binding of an agonist molecule by one of the two α subunit receptor sites only modestly increases the probability of channel opening, simultaneous binding of agonist by both of the receptor sites greatly enhances opening probability. The primary effect of nicotinic receptor activation is depolarization of the nerve cell or neuromuscular end plate membrane.

Prolonged agonist occupancy of the nicotinic receptor abolishes the effector response; ie, the postganglionic neuron stops firing (ganglionic effect), and the skeletal muscle cell relaxes (neuromuscular end plate effect). Furthermore, the continued presence of the nicotinic agonist prevents electrical recovery of the postjunctional membrane. Thus, a state of "depolarizing blockade" is induced that is refractory to reversal by other agonists. As noted below, this effect can be exploited for producing muscle paralysis.

B. ORGAN SYSTEM EFFECTS

Most of the direct organ system effects of muscarinic cholinoceptor stimulants are readily predicted from a knowledge of the effects of parasympathetic nerve stimulation (see Table 6–3) and the distribution of muscarinic receptors. Effects of a typical agent such as acetylcholine are listed in Table 7–3. The effects of nicotinic agonists are similarly predictable from a knowledge of the physiology of the autonomic ganglia and skeletal muscle motor end plate.

1. Eye—Muscarinic agonists instilled into the conjunctival sac cause contraction of the smooth muscle of the iris sphincter (resulting in miosis) and of the ciliary muscle (resulting in accommodation). As a result, the iris is pulled away from the angle of the anterior chamber, and the trabecular meshwork at the base of the ciliary muscle is opened. Both effects facilitate aqueous humor outflow into the canal of Schlemm, which drains the anterior chamber.

Table 7–3. Effects of direct-acting cholinoceptor stimulants. Only the direct effects are indicated; homeostatic responses to these direct actions may be important (see text).

Organ	Response
Eye	
Sphincter muscle of iris	Contraction (miosis)
Ciliary muscle	Contraction for near vision
Heart	
Sinoatrial node	Decrease in rate (negative chronotropy)
Atria	Decrease in contractile strength (negative inotropy). Decrease in refractory period
Atrioventricular node	Decrease in conduction velocity (negative dromotropy). Increase in refractory period
Ventricles	Small decrease in contractile strength
Blood vessels	
Arteries	Dilation (via EDRF). Constriction (high-dose direct effect)
Veins	Dilation (via EDRF). Constriction (high-dose direct effect)
Lung	
Bronchial muscle	Contraction (bronchoconstriction)
Bronchial glands	Stimulation
Gastrointestinal tract	
Motility	Increase
Sphincters	Relaxation
Secretion	Stimulation
Urinary bladder	
Detrusor	Contraction
Trigone and sphincter	Relaxation
Glands	
Sweat, salivary, lacrimal, nasopharyngeal	Secretion

2. Cardiovascular system—The primary cardiovascular effects of muscarinic agonists are reduction in peripheral vascular resistance and changes in heart rate. The direct effects listed in Table 7–3 are modified by important homeostatic reflexes, as described in Chapter 6 and depicted in Figure 6–7. Intravenous infusions of minimal effective doses of acetylcholine in humans (eg, 20–50 µg/min) cause vasodilation, resulting in a reduction in blood pressure, often accompanied by a reflex increase in heart rate. Larger doses of acetylcholine produce bradycardia and decrease atrioventricular node conduction velocity in addition to the hypotensive effect.

The direct cardiac actions of muscarinic stimulants include the following: (1) an increase in a potassium current ($I_{K(ACh)}$) in atrial muscle cells and in the cells of the sinoatrial and atrioventricular nodes as well; (2) a decrease in the slow inward calcium current (I_{Ca}) in heart cells; and (3) a reduction in the hyperpolarization-activated current (I_f) that underlies diastolic depolarization. All of these actions are mediated by M_2 receptors and contribute to slowing the pacemaker rate. Effects (1) and (2) cause hyperpolarization and decrease the contractility of atrial cells.

The direct slowing of sinoatrial rate and atrioventricular conduction that is produced by muscarinic agonists is often opposed by reflex sympathetic discharge, elicited by the decrease in blood pressure. The resultant sympathetic-parasympathetic interaction is complex because of the muscarinic modulation of sympathetic influences that occurs by inhibition of norepinephrine release and by postjunctional cellular effects. Muscarinic receptors that are present on postganglionic parasympathetic nerve terminals allow neurally released acetylcholine to inhibit its own secretion. The neuronal muscarinic receptors need not be the same subtype as found on effector cells. Therefore, the net effect on heart rate depends on local concentrations of the agonist in the heart and in the vessels and on the level of reflex responsiveness.

Parasympathetic innervation of the ventricles is much less extensive than that of the atria and activation of ventricular muscarinic receptors results in much less physiologic effect than that seen in atria. However, during sympathetic stimulation, the effects of muscarinic agonists on ventricular function are clearly evident because of muscarinic modulation of sympathetic effects ("accentuated antagonism"; Levy et al, 1994).

In the intact organism, muscarinic agonists produce marked vasodilation. However, in earlier studies, isolated blood vessels often showed a contractile response to these agents. It is now known that acetylcholine-induced vasodilation requires the presence of intact endothelium (Figure 7–4). Muscarinic agonists release a substance (endothelium-derived relaxing factor, or EDRF) from the endothelial cells that relaxes smooth muscle. Isolated vessels prepared with the endothelium preserved consistently reproduce the vasodilation seen in the intact organism. EDRF appears to be largely nitric oxide (NO). This substance activates guanylyl cyclase and increases cGMP in smooth muscle, resulting in relaxation (see Figure 12–2).

The cardiovascular effects of all of the choline esters are similar to those of acetylcholine, the main difference being in their potency and duration of action. Because of the resistance of methacholine, carbachol, and bethanechol to acetylcholinesterase, lower doses given intravenously are sufficient to produce effects similar to those of acetylcholine, and the duration of action of these synthetic choline esters is longer. The cardiovascular effects of most of the cholinomimetic natural alkaloids and the synthetic analogs are also generally similar to those of acetylcholine.

Pilocarpine is an interesting exception to the above statement. If given intravenously (an experimental exercise), it may produce hypertension after a brief initial hypotensive response. The longer-lasting hypertensive effect can be traced to sympathetic ganglionic discharge caused by activation of postganglionic cell membrane

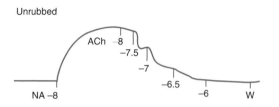
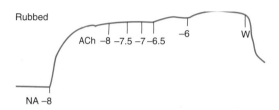

Figure 7–4. Activation of endothelial cell muscarinic receptors by acetylcholine releases endothelium-derived relaxing factor (nitric oxide) (EDRF [NO]), which causes relaxation of vascular smooth muscle precontracted with norepinephrine. Removal of the endothelium by rubbing eliminates the relaxant effect and reveals contraction caused by direct action of acetylcholine on vascular smooth muscle. (Modified and reproduced, with permission, from Furchgott RF, Zawadzki JV: The obligatory role of endothelial cells in the relaxation of arterial smooth muscle by acetylcholine. Nature 1980;288:373.)

M_1 receptors, which close K^+ channels and elicit slow excitatory (depolarizing) postsynaptic potentials. This effect, like the hypotensive effect, can be blocked by atropine, an antimuscarinic drug.

3. Respiratory system—Muscarinic stimulants contract the smooth muscle of the bronchial tree. In addition, the glands of the tracheobronchial mucosa are stimulated to secrete. This combination of effects can occasionally cause symptoms, especially in individuals with asthma.

4. Gastrointestinal tract—Administration of muscarinic agonists, like parasympathetic nervous system stimulation, increases the secretory and motor activity of the gut. The salivary and gastric glands are strongly stimulated; the pancreas and small intestinal glands less so. Peristaltic activity is increased throughout the gut, and most sphincters are relaxed. Stimulation of contraction in this organ system involves depolarization of the smooth muscle cell membrane and increased calcium influx.

5. Genitourinary tract—Muscarinic agonists stimulate the detrusor muscle and relax the trigone and sphincter muscles of the bladder, thus promoting voiding. The human uterus is not notably sensitive to muscarinic agonists.

6. Miscellaneous secretory glands—Muscarinic agonists stimulate secretion by thermoregulatory sweat, lacrimal, and nasopharyngeal glands.

7. Central nervous system—The central nervous system contains both muscarinic and nicotinic receptors, the brain being relatively richer in muscarinic sites and the spinal cord containing a preponderance of nicotinic sites. The physiologic roles of these receptors are discussed in Chapter 21.

The role of muscarinic receptors in the central nervous system has been confirmed by experiments in knockout mice (see Chapter 1). Predictably, carbachol did not inhibit atrial rate in animals with mutated M_2 receptors. The central nervous system effects of the synthetic muscarinic agonist oxotremorine (tremor, hypothermia, and antinociception) were also lacking in mice with homozygously mutated M_2 receptors. Knockout of M_1 receptors is associated with different changes in the peripheral and central nervous systems. Oxotremorine did not suppress M current in sympathetic ganglia, and pilocarpine did not induce epileptic seizures in M_1 mutant mice.

In spite of the smaller ratio of nicotinic to muscarinic receptors in the brain, nicotine and lobeline (Figure 7–3) have important effects on the brainstem and cortex. The mild alerting action of nicotine absorbed from inhaled tobacco smoke is the best-known of these effects. In larger concentrations, nicotine induces tremor, emesis, and stimulation of the respiratory center. At still higher levels, nicotine causes convulsions, which may terminate in fatal coma. The lethal effects on the central nervous system and the fact that nicotine is readily absorbed form the basis for the use of nicotine as an insecticide. Dimethylphenylpiperazinium (DMPP), a synthetic nicotinic stimulant used in research is relatively free of these central effects because it does not cross the blood-brain barrier.

8. Peripheral nervous system—The autonomic ganglia are important sites of nicotinic synaptic action. The nicotinic agents shown in Figure 7–3 cause marked activation of these nicotinic receptors and initiate action potentials in postganglionic neurons. Nicotine itself has a somewhat greater affinity for neuronal than for skeletal muscle nicotinic receptors. The action is the same on both parasympathetic and sympathetic ganglia. The initial response therefore often resembles simultaneous discharge of both the parasympathetic and the sympathetic nervous systems. In the case of the cardiovascular system, the effects of nicotine are chiefly sympathomimetic. Dramatic hypertension is produced by parenteral injection of nicotine; sympathetic tachycardia may alternate with a vagally mediated bradycardia. In the gastrointestinal and urinary tracts, the effects are largely parasympathomimetic: nausea, vomiting, diarrhea, and voiding of urine are commonly observed. Prolonged exposure may result in depolarizing blockade of the ganglia.

Neuronal nicotinic receptors are present on sensory nerve endings—especially afferent nerves in coronary arteries and the carotid and aortic bodies as well as on the glomus cells of the latter. Activation of these receptors by nicotinic stimulants and of muscarinic receptors on glomus cells by muscarinic stimulants elicits complex medullary responses, including respiratory alterations and vagal discharge.

9. Neuromuscular junction—The nicotinic receptors on the neuromuscular end plate apparatus are similar but not identical to the receptors in the autonomic ganglia (see Table 7–1). Both types respond to acetylcholine and nicotine. (However, as discussed in Chapter 8, the receptors differ in their structural requirements for nicotinic blocking drugs.) When a nicotinic agonist is applied directly (by iontophoresis or by intra-arterial injection), an immediate depolarization of the end plate results, caused by an increase in permeability to sodium and potassium ions. Depending on the synchronization of depolarization of end plates throughout the muscle, the contractile response will vary from disorganized fasciculations of independent motor units to a strong contraction of the entire muscle. Depolarizing nicotinic agents that are not rapidly hydrolyzed (like nicotine itself) cause rapid development of depolarization blockade; transmission blockade persists even when the membrane has repolarized (discussed further in Chapters 8 and 27). In the case of skeletal muscle, this block is manifested as flaccid paralysis.

II. BASIC PHARMACOLOGY OF THE INDIRECT-ACTING CHOLINOMIMETICS

The actions of acetylcholine released from autonomic and somatic motor nerves are terminated by enzymatic destruction of the molecule. Hydrolysis is accomplished by the action of acetylcholinesterase, which is present in high concentrations in cholinergic synapses. The indirect-acting cholinomimetics have their primary effect at the active site of this enzyme, although some also have direct actions at nicotinic receptors. The chief differences between members of the group are chemical and pharmacokinetic—their pharmacodynamic properties are almost identical.

Chemistry & Pharmacokinetics

A. STRUCTURE

The commonly used cholinesterase inhibitors fall into three chemical groups: (1) simple alcohols bearing a quaternary ammonium group, eg, edrophonium; (2) carbamic acid esters of alcohols bearing quaternary or tertiary ammonium groups (carbamates, eg, neostigmine); and (3) organic derivatives of phosphoric acid (organophosphates, eg, echothiophate). Examples of the first two groups are shown in Figure 7–5. Edrophonium, neostigmine, and ambenonium are synthetic quaternary ammonium agents used in medicine. Physostigmine (eserine) is a naturally occurring tertiary amine of greater lipid solubility that is also used in therapeutics. Carbaryl (carbaril) is typical of a large group of carbamate insecticides designed for very high lipid solubility, so that absorption into the insect and distribution to its central nervous system are very rapid.

A few of the estimated 50,000 organophosphates are shown in Figure 7–6. Many of the organophosphates (echothiophate is an exception) are highly lipid-soluble liquids. Echothiophate, a thiocholine derivative, is of clinical value because it retains the very long duration of action of other organophosphates but is more stable in aqueous solution. Soman is an extremely potent "nerve gas." Parathion and malathion are thiophosphate insecticides that are inactive as such; they are converted to the phosphate derivatives in animals and plants and are used as insecticides.

B. ABSORPTION, DISTRIBUTION, AND METABOLISM

Absorption of the quaternary carbamates from the conjunctiva, skin, and lungs is predictably poor, since their permanent charge renders them relatively insoluble in

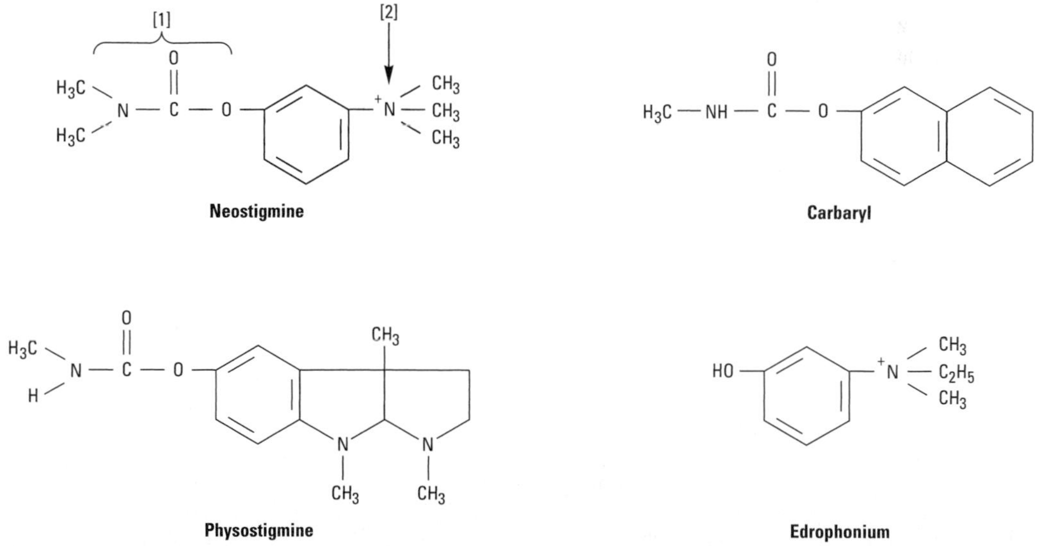

Figure 7–5. Cholinesterase inhibitors. Neostigmine exemplifies the typical compound that is an ester of carbamic acid ([1]) and a phenol bearing a quaternary ammonium group ([2]). Physostigmine, a naturally occurring carbamate, is a tertiary amine. Edrophonium is not an ester but binds to the active site of the enzyme.

lipids. Similarly, much larger doses are required for oral administration than for parenteral injection. Distribution into the central nervous system is negligible. Physostigmine, in contrast, is well absorbed from all sites and can be used topically in the eye (Table 7–4). It is distributed into the central nervous system and is more toxic than the more polar quaternary carbamates. The carbamates are relatively stable in aqueous solution but can be metabolized by nonspecific esterases in the body as well as by cholinesterase. However, the duration of their effect is determined chiefly by the stability of the inhibitor-enzyme complex (see Mechanism of Action, below), not by metabolism or excretion.

The organophosphate cholinesterase inhibitors (except for echothiophate) are well absorbed from the skin, lung, gut, and conjunctiva—thereby making them dangerous to humans and highly effective as insecticides. They are relatively less stable than the carbamates when dissolved in water and thus have a limited half-life in the environment (compared with the other major class of insecticides, the halogenated hydrocarbons, eg, DDT). Echothiophate is highly polar and more stable than most other organophosphates. It can be made up in aqueous solution for ophthalmic use and retains its activity for weeks.

The thiophosphate insecticides (parathion, malathion, and related compounds) are quite lipid-soluble and are rapidly absorbed by all routes. They must be activated in the body by conversion to the oxygen analogs (Figure 7–6), a process that occurs rapidly in both insects and vertebrates. Malathion and certain other organophosphate insecticides are also rapidly metabolized by other pathways to inactive products in birds and mammals but not in insects; these agents are therefore considered safe enough for sale to the general public. Unfortunately, fish cannot detoxify malathion, and significant numbers of fish have died from the heavy use of this agent on and near waterways. Parathion is not detoxified effectively in vertebrates; thus, it is considerably more dangerous than malathion to humans and livestock and is not available for general public use.

All of the organophosphates except echothiophate are distributed to all parts of the body, including the central nervous system. Poisoning with these agents therefore includes an important component of central nervous system toxicity.

Pharmacodynamics

A. MECHANISM OF ACTION

Acetylcholinesterase is the primary target of these drugs, but butyrylcholinesterase is also inhibited. Acetylcholinesterase is an extremely active enzyme. In the initial step, acetylcholine binds to the enzyme's active site and is hydrolyzed, yielding free choline and the acetylated enzyme. In the second step, the covalent acetylenzyme bond is split, with the addition of water (hydra-

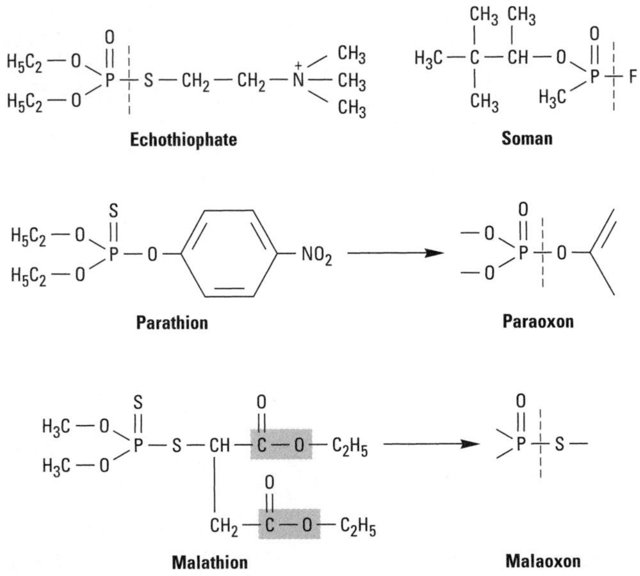

Figure 7–6. Structures of some organophosphate cholinesterase inhibitors. The dashed lines indicate the bond that is hydrolyzed in binding to the enzyme. The shaded ester bonds in malathion represent the points of detoxification of the molecule in mammals and birds.

tion). The entire process takes place in approximately 150 microseconds.

All of the cholinesterase inhibitors increase the concentration of endogenous acetylcholine at cholinoceptors by inhibiting acetylcholinesterase. However, the molecular details of their interaction with the enzyme vary according to the three chemical subgroups mentioned above.

The first group, of which edrophonium is the major example, consists of quaternary alcohols. These agents reversibly bind electrostatically and by hydrogen bonds to the active site, thus preventing access of acetylcholine. The enzyme-inhibitor complex does not involve a covalent bond and is correspondingly short-lived (on the order of 2–10 minutes). The second group consists of carbamate esters, eg, neostigmine and physostigmine. These agents undergo a two-step hydrolysis sequence analogous to that described for acetylcholine. However, the covalent bond of the *carbamoylated* enzyme is considerably more resistant to the second (hydration) process, and this step is correspondingly prolonged (on the order of 30 minutes to 6 hours). The third group consists of the organophosphates. These agents also undergo initial binding and hydrolysis by the enzyme, resulting in a *phosphorylated* active site. The covalent phosphorus-enzyme bond is extremely stable and hydrolyzes in water at a very slow rate (hundreds of hours). After the initial binding-hydrolysis step, the phosphorylated enzyme complex may undergo a process called **aging.** This process apparently involves the breaking of one of the oxygen-phosphorus bonds of the inhibitor and further strengthens the phosphorus-enzyme bond. The rate of aging varies with the particular organophosphate compound. If given before aging has occurred, strong nucleophiles like pralidoxime are able to split the phosphorus-enzyme bond and can be used as "cholinesterase regenerator" drugs for organophosphate insecticide poisoning (see Chapter 8). Once aging has occurred, the enzyme-inhibitor complex is even more stable and is more difficult to split, even with oxime regenerator compounds.

Because of the marked differences in duration of action, the organophosphate inhibitors are sometimes referred to as "irreversible" cholinesterase inhibitors, and edrophonium and the carbamates are considered "reversible" inhibitors. However, the molecular mechanisms of action of the three groups do not support this simplistic description.

B. Organ System Effects

The most prominent pharmacologic effects of cholinesterase inhibitors are on the cardiovascular and gastrointestinal systems, the eye, and the skeletal muscle neuromuscular junction. Because the primary action is to amplify the actions of endogenous acetylcholine, the effects are similar (but not always identical) to the effects of the direct-acting cholinomimetic agonists.

1. Central nervous system—In low concentrations, the lipid-soluble cholinesterase inhibitors cause diffuse activation on the electroencephalogram and a subjective alerting response. In higher concentrations, they cause generalized convulsions, which may be followed by coma and respiratory arrest.

2. Eye, respiratory tract, gastrointestinal tract, urinary tract—The effects of the cholinesterase inhibitors on these organ systems, all of which are well innervated by the parasympathetic nervous system, are qualitatively quite similar to the effects of the direct-acting cholinomimetics.

3. Cardiovascular system—The cholinesterase inhibitors can increase activation in both sympathetic and parasympathetic ganglia supplying the heart and at the acetylcholine receptors on neuroeffector cells (cardiac and vascular smooth muscles) that receive cholinergic innervation.

In the heart, the effects on the parasympathetic limb predominate. Thus, cholinesterase inhibitors such as edrophonium, physostigmine, or neostigmine mimic the effects of vagal nerve activation on the heart. Negative chronotropic, dromotropic, and inotropic effects are produced, and cardiac output falls. The fall in cardiac output is attributable to bradycardia, decreased atrial contractility, and some reduction in ventricular contractility. The latter effect occurs as a result of prejunctional inhibition of norepinephrine release as well as inhibition of postjunctional cellular sympathetic effects.

Cholinesterase inhibitors have less marked effects on vascular smooth muscle and on blood pressure than direct-acting muscarinic agonists. This is because indirect-acting drugs can modify the tone of only those vessels that are innervated by cholinergic nerves and because the net effects on vascular tone may reflect activation of both the parasympathetic and sympathetic nervous systems. The cholinomimetic effect at the smooth muscle effector tissue is minimal since few vascular beds receive cholinergic innervation. Activation of sympathetic ganglia may increase vascular resistance.

The *net* cardiovascular effects of moderate doses of cholinesterase inhibitors therefore consist of modest bradycardia, a fall in cardiac output, and no change or a modest fall in blood pressure. Large (toxic) doses of these drugs cause more marked bradycardia (occasionally tachycardia) and hypotension.

4. Neuromuscular junction—The cholinesterase inhibitors have important therapeutic and toxic effects at the skeletal muscle neuromuscular junction. Low (therapeutic) concentrations moderately prolong and intensify the actions of physiologically released acetylcholine. This increases strength of contraction, especially in muscles weakened by curare-like neuromuscular blocking agents or by myasthenia gravis. At higher concentrations, the accumulation of acetylcholine may result in fibrillation of muscle fibers. Antidromic firing of the motor neuron may also occur, resulting in fasciculations that involve an entire motor unit. With marked inhibition of acetylcholinesterase, depolarizing neuromuscular blockade occurs and that may be followed by a phase of nondepolarizing blockade as seen with succinylcholine (see Table 27–2 and Figure 27–6).

Some quaternary carbamate cholinesterase inhibitors, eg, neostigmine, have an additional *direct* nicotinic agonist effect at the neuromuscular junction. This may contribute to the effectiveness of these agents as therapy for myasthenia.

III. CLINICAL PHARMACOLOGY OF THE CHOLINOMIMETICS

The major therapeutic uses of the cholinomimetics are for diseases of the eye (glaucoma, accommodative esotropia), the gastrointestinal and urinary tracts (postoperative atony, neurogenic bladder), the neuromuscular junction (myasthenia gravis, curare-induced neuromuscular paralysis), and rarely, the heart (certain atrial arrhythmias). Cholinesterase inhibitors are occasionally used in the treatment of atropine overdosage. Several newer cholinesterase inhibitors are being used to treat patients with Alzheimer's disease.

Clinical Uses

A. THE EYE

Glaucoma is a disease characterized by increased intraocular pressure. Muscarinic stimulants and cholinesterase inhibitors reduce intraocular pressure by causing contraction of the ciliary body so as to facilitate outflow of aqueous humor and perhaps also by diminishing the rate of its secretion (see Figure 6–9). In the past, glaucoma was treated with either direct agonists (pilocarpine, methacholine, carbachol) or cholinesterase inhibitors (physostigmine, demecarium, echothiophate, isoflurophate). For chronic glaucoma, these drugs have been largely replaced by topical β-blockers and prostaglandin derivatives.

Acute angle-closure glaucoma is a medical emergency that is frequently treated initially with drugs but usually requires surgery for permanent correction. Initial therapy often consists of a combination of a direct muscarinic agonist and a cholinesterase inhibitor (eg, pilocarpine plus physostigmine) as well as other drugs. Once the intraocular pressure is controlled and the danger of vision loss is diminished, the patient can be prepared for corrective surgery (iridectomy). Open-angle glaucoma and some cases of secondary glaucoma are chronic diseases that are not amenable to traditional surgical correction although newer laser techniques appear to be useful. Other treatments for glaucoma are described in the Box, Treatment of Glaucoma in Chapter 10.

Accommodative esotropia (strabismus caused by hypermetropic accommodative error) in young children is sometimes diagnosed and treated with cholinomimetic agonists. Dosage is similar to or higher than that used for glaucoma.

B. GASTROINTESTINAL AND URINARY TRACTS

In clinical disorders that involve depression of smooth muscle activity *without obstruction,* cholinomimetic drugs with direct or indirect muscarinic effects may be helpful. These disorders include postoperative ileus (atony or paralysis of the stomach or bowel following surgical manipulation) and congenital megacolon. Urinary retention may occur postoperatively or postpartum or may be secondary to spinal cord injury or disease (neurogenic bladder). Cholinomimetics are also sometimes used to increase the tone of the lower esophageal sphincter in patients with reflux esophagitis. Of the choline esters, bethanechol is the most widely used for these disorders. For gastrointestinal problems, it is usually administered orally in a dose of 10–25 mg three or four times daily. In patients with urinary retention, bethanechol can be given subcutaneously in a dose of 5 mg and repeated in 30 minutes if necessary. Of the cholinesterase inhibitors, neostigmine is the most widely used for these applications. For paralytic ileus or atony of the urinary bladder, neostigmine can be given subcutaneously in a dose of 0.5–1 mg. If patients are able to take the drug by mouth, neostigmine can be given orally in a dose of 15 mg. In all of these situations, the clinician must be certain that there is no mechanical obstruction to outflow prior to using the cholinomimetic. Otherwise, the drug may exacerbate the problem and may even cause perforation as a result of increased pressure.

Pilocarpine has long been used to increase salivary secretion. Cevimeline is a new direct-acting muscarinic agonist used for the treatment of dry mouth associated with Sjögren's syndrome.

C. NEUROMUSCULAR JUNCTION

Myasthenia gravis is a disease affecting skeletal muscle neuromuscular junctions. An autoimmune process causes production of antibodies that decrease the number of functional nicotinic receptors on the postjunctional end plates. Frequent findings are ptosis, diplopia, difficulty in speaking and swallowing, and extremity weakness. Severe disease may affect all the muscles, including those necessary for respiration. The disease resembles the neuromuscular paralysis produced by *d*-tubocurarine and similar nondepolarizing neuromuscular blocking drugs (see Chapter 27). Patients with myasthenia are exquisitely sensitive to the action of curariform drugs and other drugs that interfere with neuromuscular transmission, eg, aminoglycoside antibiotics.

Cholinesterase inhibitors—but not direct-acting acetylcholine receptor agonists—are extremely valuable as therapy for myasthenia. Almost all patients are also treated with immunosuppressant drugs and some with thymectomy.

Edrophonium is sometimes used as a diagnostic test for myasthenia. A 2 mg dose is injected intravenously after baseline measurements of muscle strength have been obtained. If no reaction occurs after 45 seconds, an additional 8 mg may be injected. Some clinicians divide the 8 mg dose into two doses of 3 and 5 mg given at 45-second intervals. If the patient has myasthenia gravis, an improvement in muscle strength that lasts about 5 minutes will usually be observed.

Edrophonium is also used to assess the adequacy of treatment with the longer-acting cholinesterase inhibitors in patients with myasthenia gravis. If excessive amounts of cholinesterase inhibitor have been used, patients may become paradoxically weak because of nicotinic depolarizing blockade of the motor end plate. These patients may also exhibit symptoms of excessive stimulation of muscarinic receptors (abdominal cramps, diarrhea, increased salivation, excessive bronchial secretions, miosis, bradycardia). Small doses of edrophonium (1–2 mg intravenously) will produce no relief or even worsen weakness if the patient is receiving excessive cholinesterase inhibitor therapy. On the other hand, if the patient improves with edrophonium, an increase in cholinesterase inhibitor dosage may be indicated. Clinical situations in which severe myasthenia (myasthenic crisis) must be distinguished from excessive drug therapy (cholinergic crisis) usually occur in very ill myasthenic patients and must be managed in hospital with adequate emergency support systems (eg, mechanical ventilators) available.

Long-term therapy for myasthenia gravis is usually accomplished with neostigmine, pyridostigmine, or ambenonium. The doses are titrated to optimum levels based on changes in muscle strength. These agents are relatively short-acting and therefore require frequent dosing (every 4 hours for neostigmine and every 6 hours for pyridostigmine and ambenonium; Table 7–4). Sustained-release preparations are available but should be used only at night and if needed. Longer-acting cholinesterase inhibitors such as the organophosphate agents are not used, because the dose requirement in this disease changes too rapidly to permit smooth control with long-acting drugs.

Table 7–4. Therapeutic uses and durations of action of cholinesterase inhibitors.

	Uses	Approximate Duration of Action
Alcohols		
Edrophonium	Myasthenia gravis, ileus, arrhythmias	5–15 minutes
Carbamates and related agents		
Neostigmine	Myasthenia gravis, ileus	0.5–2 hours
Pyridostigmine	Myasthenia gravis	3–6 hours
Physostigmine	Glaucoma	0.5–2 hours
Ambenonium	Myasthenia gravis	4–8 hours
Demecarium	Glaucoma	4–6 hours
Organophosphates		
Echothiophate	Glaucoma	100 hours

If muscarinic effects of such therapy are prominent, they can be controlled by the administration of antimuscarinic drugs such as atropine. Frequently, tolerance to the muscarinic effects of the cholinesterase inhibitors develops, so atropine treatment is not required.

Neuromuscular blockade is frequently produced as an adjunct to surgical anesthesia, using nondepolarizing neuromuscular relaxants such as pancuronium and newer agents (see Chapter 27). Following surgery, it is usually desirable to reverse this pharmacologic paralysis promptly. This can be easily accomplished with cholinesterase inhibitors; neostigmine and edrophonium are the drugs of choice. They are given intravenously or intramuscularly for prompt effect.

D. HEART

The short-acting cholinesterase inhibitor edrophonium had been used to treat supraventricular tachyarrhythmias, particularly paroxysmal supraventricular tachycardia. In this application, edrophonium has been replaced by newer drugs (adenosine and the calcium channel blockers verapamil and diltiazem).

E. ANTIMUSCARINIC DRUG INTOXICATION

Atropine intoxication is potentially lethal in children (see Chapter 8) and may cause prolonged severe behavioral disturbances and arrhythmias in adults. The tricyclic antidepressants, when taken in overdosage (often with suicidal intent), also cause severe muscarinic blockade (see Chapter 30). The muscarinic receptor blockade produced by all these agents is competitive in nature and can be overcome by increasing the amount of endogenous acetylcholine present at the neuroeffector junctions. Theoretically, a cholinesterase inhibitor could be used to reverse these effects. Physostigmine has been used for this application, because it enters the central nervous system and reverses the central as well as the peripheral signs of muscarinic blockade. However, as noted previously, physostigmine itself can produce dangerous central nervous system effects, and such therapy is therefore used only in patients with dangerous elevation of body temperature or very rapid supraventricular tachycardia.

F. Central Nervous System

Tacrine is a drug with anticholinesterase and other cholinomimetic actions that has been used for the treatment of mild to moderate Alzheimer's disease. Evidence for tacrine's efficacy is modest and hepatic toxicity is significant. Donepezil, galantamine, and rivastigmine are newer, more selective acetylcholinesterase inhibitors that appear to have the same modest clinical benefit as tacrine in treatment of cognitive dysfunction in Alzheimer's patients. Donepezil may be given once daily because of its long half-life, and it lacks the hepatotoxic effect of tacrine. However, no comparative trials of these newer drugs and tacrine have been reported. These drugs are discussed in Chapter 61.

Toxicity

The toxic potential of the cholinoceptor stimulants varies markedly depending on their absorption, access to the central nervous system, and metabolism.

A. Direct-Acting Muscarinic Stimulants

Drugs such as pilocarpine and the choline esters cause predictable signs of muscarinic excess when given in overdosage. These effects include nausea, vomiting, diarrhea, salivation, sweating, cutaneous vasodilation, and bronchial constriction. The effects are all blocked competitively by atropine and its congeners.

Certain mushrooms, especially those of the genus *Inocybe,* contain muscarinic alkaloids. Ingestion of these mushrooms causes typical signs of muscarinic excess within 15–30 minutes. Treatment is with atropine, 1–2 mg parenterally. (*Amanita muscaria,* the first source of muscarine, contains very low concentrations of the alkaloid.)

B. Direct-Acting Nicotinic Stimulants

Nicotine itself is the only common cause of this type of poisoning. The acute toxicity of the alkaloid is well-defined but much less important than the chronic effects associated with smoking. In addition to tobacco products, nicotine is also used in insecticides.

1. Acute toxicity—The fatal dose of nicotine is approximately 40 mg, or 1 drop of the pure liquid. This is the amount of nicotine in two regular cigarettes. Fortunately, most of the nicotine in cigarettes is destroyed by burning or escapes via the "sidestream" smoke. Ingestion of nicotine insecticides or of tobacco by infants and children is usually followed by vomiting, limiting the amount of the alkaloid absorbed.

The toxic effects of a large dose of nicotine are simple extensions of the effects described previously. The most dangerous are (1) central stimulant actions, which cause convulsions and may progress to coma and respiratory arrest; (2) skeletal muscle end plate depolarization, which may lead to depolarization blockade and respiratory paralysis; and (3) hypertension and cardiac arrhythmias.

Treatment of acute nicotine poisoning is largely symptom-directed. Muscarinic excess resulting from parasympathetic ganglion stimulation can be controlled with atropine. Central stimulation is usually treated with parenteral anticonvulsants such as diazepam. Neuromuscular blockade is not responsive to pharmacologic treatment and may require mechanical respiration.

Fortunately, nicotine is metabolized and excreted relatively rapidly. Patients who survive the first 4 hours usually recover completely if hypoxia and brain damage have not occurred.

2. Chronic nicotine toxicity—The health costs of tobacco smoking to the smoker and its socioeconomic costs to the general public are still incompletely understood. However, the 1979 *Surgeon General's Report on Health Promotion and Disease Prevention* stated that "cigarette smoking is clearly the largest single preventable cause of illness and premature death in the United States." This statement has been supported by numerous studies. Unfortunately, the fact that the most important of the tobacco-associated diseases are delayed in onset reduces the health incentive to stop smoking.

It is clear that the addictive power of cigarettes is directly related to their nicotine content. It is not known to what extent nicotine per se contributes to the other well-documented adverse effects of chronic tobacco use. It appears highly probable that nicotine contributes to the increased risk of vascular disease and sudden coronary death associated with smoking. It is also probable that nicotine contributes to the high incidence of ulcer recurrences in smokers with peptic ulcer.

C. Cholinesterase Inhibitors

The acute toxic effects of the cholinesterase inhibitors, like those of the direct-acting agents, are direct extensions of their pharmacologic actions. The major source of such intoxications is pesticide use in agriculture and in the home. Approximately 100 organophosphate and 20 carbamate cholinesterase inhibitors are available in pesticides and veterinary vermifuges used in the USA.

Acute intoxication must be recognized and treated

promptly in patients with heavy exposure. The dominant inirial signs are those of muscarinic excess: miosis, salivation, sweating, bronchial constriction, vomiting, and diarrhea. Central nervous system involvement usually follows rapidly, accompanied by peripheral nicotinic effects, especially depolarizing neuromuscular blockade. Therapy always includes (1) maintenance of vital signs—respiration in particular may be impaired; (2) decontamination to prevent further absorption—this may require removal of all clothing and washing of the skin in cases of expo-

sure to dusts and sprays; and (3) atropine parenterally in large doses, given as often as required to control signs of muscarinic excess. Therapy often also includes treatment with pralidoxime as described in Chapter 8.

Chronic exposure to certain organophosphate compounds, including some organophosphate cholinesterase inhibitors, causes neuropathy associated with demyelination of axons. **Triorthocresylphosphate,** an additive in lubricating oils, is the prototype agent of this class. The effects are not caused by cholinesterase inhibition.

PREPARATIONS AVAILABLE

DIRECT-ACTING CHOLINOMIMETICS
Acetylcholine (Miochol-E)
Ophthalmic: 1:100 (10 mg/mL) intraocular solution
Bethanechol (generic, Urecholine)
Oral: 5, 10, 25, 50 mg tablets
Parenteral: 5 mg/mL for SC injection
Carbachol
Ophthalmic (topical, Isopto Carbachol, Carboptic): 0.75, 1.5, 2.25, 3% drops
Ophthalmic (intraocular, Miostat, Carbastat): 0.01% solution
Cevimeline (Evoxac)
Oral: 30 mg capsules
Pilocarpine (generic, Isopto Carpine)
Ophthalmic (topical): 0.25, 0.5, 1, 2, 3, 4, 6, 8, 10% solutions, 4% gel
Ophthalmic sustained-release inserts (Ocusert Pilo-20, Ocusert Pilo-40): release 20 and 40 μg pilocarpine per hour for 1 week, respectively
Oral (Salagen): 5 mg tablets

CHOLINESTERASE INHIBITORS
Ambenonium (Mytelase)
Oral: 10 mg tablets

Demecarium (Humorsol)
Ophthalmic: 0.125, 0.25% drops
Donepezil (Aricept)
Oral: 5, 10 mg tablets
Echothiophate (Phospholine)
Ophthalmic: Powder to reconstitute for 0.03, 0.06, 0.125, 0.25% drops
Edrophonium (generic, Tensilon)
Parenteral: 10 mg/mL for IM or IV injection
Galantamine (Reminyl)
Oral: 4, 8, 12 mg capsules; 4 mg/mL solution
Neostigmine (generic, Prostigmin)
Oral: 15 mg tablets
Parenteral: 1:1000 in 10 mL; 1:2000, 1:4000 in 1 mL
Physostigmine, eserine (generic)
Parenteral: 1 mg/mL for IM or slow IV injection
Pyridostigmine (Mestinon, Regonol)
Oral: 60 mg tablets; 180 mg sustained-release tablets; 15 mg/mL syrup
Parenteral: 5 mg/mL for IM or slow IV injection
Rivastigmine (Exelon)
Oral: 1.5, 3, 4.5, 6 mg tablets; 2 mg/mL solution
Tacrine (Cognex)
Oral: 10, 20, 30, 40 mg tablets

REFERENCES

Abou-Donia MB, Lapadula DM: Mechanisms of organophosphorus ester-induced delayed neurotoxicity: Type I and type II. Annu Rev Pharmacol 1990;30:405.

Accili EA, Redaelli G, DiFrancesco D: Two distinct pathways of muscarinic current responses in rabbit sino-atrial node myocytes. Pflugers Arch 1998;437:164.

Aquilonius S-M, Hartvig P: Clinical pharmacology of cholinesterase inhibitors. Clin Pharmacokinet 1986;11:236.

Benowitz NL: Pharmacology of nicotine: Addiction and therapeutics. Annu Rev Pharmacol Toxicol 1996;36:597.

Boehm S, Kubista H: Fine tuning of sympathetic transmitter release via ionotropic and metabotropic presynaptic receptors. Pharmacol Rev 2002;54:43.

Brodde O-E, Michel MC: Adrenergic and muscarinic receptors in the human heart. Pharmacol Rev 1999;51:651.

Caulfield MP, Birdsall NJM: International Union of Pharmacology. XVII. Classification of muscarinic acetylcholine receptors. Pharmacol Rev 1998;50:279.

Costello RW et al: Localization of eosinophils to airway nerves and effect on neuronal M_2 muscarinic receptor function. Am J Physiol 1997;273:L93.

Devillers-Thiéry A et al: Functional architecture of the nicotinic acetylcholine receptor: A prototype of ligand-gated ion channels. J Membrane Biol 1993;136:97.

Eglen RM, Hedge SS, Watson N: Muscarinic receptor subtypes and smooth muscle function. Pharmacol Rev 1996;48:531.

Furchgott RF, Zawadzki JV: The obligatory role of endothelial cells in the relaxation of arterial smooth muscle by acetylcholine. Nature 1980;288:373.

Gomeza J et al: Pronounced pharmacologic deficits in M_2 muscarinic acetylcholine receptor knockout mice. Proc Natl Acad Sci U S A 1999;96:1692.

González C (editor): *The Carotid Body Chemoreceptors.* Chapman & Hall, 1997.

Hamilton SE et al: Disruption of the M_1 receptor gene ablates muscarinic receptor-dependent M current regulation and seizure activity in mice. Proc Natl Acad Sci U S A 1997;94:13311.

Hobbiger F: Pharmacology of anticholinesterase drugs. In: Zaimis E (editor): *Handbook of Experimental Pharmacology. Vol 42: Neuromuscular Junction.* Springer, 1976.

Irvine RF, Schell MJ: Back in the water: the return of the inositol phosphates. Nat Rev Mol Cell Biol 2001;2:327.

Levine RR, Birdsall NJM, Nathanson NM (editors): Subtypes of muscarinic receptors. Life Sci 1999;64:355.

Levy MN, Schwartz PJ (editors): *Vagal Control of the Heart.* Futura, 1994.

Lindstrom J et al: Structural and functional heterogeneity of nicotinic receptors. In: Bock G, Marsh J (editors): *The Biology of Nicotine Dependence.* Ciba Symposium 152. Wiley, 1990.

Lucas RJ et al: International Union of Pharmacology. XX. Current status of the nomenclature for nicotinic acetylcholine receptors and their subunits. Pharmacol Rev 1999;51:397.

Méry P-F et al: Muscarinic regulation of the L-type calcium current in isolated cardiac myocytes. Life Sci 1997;60:1113.

Molitor H: A comparative study of the effects of five choline compounds used in therapeutics: Acetylcholine chloride, acetyl-beta-methylcholine chloride, carbaminoyl choline, ethyl ether beta-methylcholine chloride, carbaminoyl beta-methylcholine chloride. J Pharmacol Exp Ther 1936;58:337.

Moncada S et al: Nitric oxide: Physiology, pathophysiology, and pharmacology. Pharmacol Rev 1991;43:109.

Newton GE et al: Muscarinic receptor modulation of basal and beta-adrenergic stimulated function of the failing human left ventricle. J Clin Invest 1996;98:2756.

Noronha-Blob L et al: Muscarinic receptors: Relationships among phosphoinositide breakdown, adenylate cyclase inhibition, in vitro detrusor muscle contraction, and in vivo cystometrogram studies in guinea pig bladder. J Pharmacol Exp Ther 1989;249:843.

Okamoto H et al: Muscarinic agonist potencies at three different effector systems linked to the M(2) or M(3) receptor in longitudinal smooth muscle of guinea-pig small intestine. Br J Pharmacol 2002;135:1765.

Pappano AJ: Modulation of the heartbeat by the vagus nerve. In: Zipes DP, Jalife J (editors): *Cardiac Electrophysiology: From Cell to Bedside.* Saunders, 1995.

Pfeiffer A et al: Muscarinic receptors mediating acid secretion in isolated rat gastric mucosa cells are of M3 type. Gastroenterology 1990;98:218.

Rand MJ: Neuropharmacological effects of nicotine in relation to cholinergic mechanisms. Prog Brain Res 1989;79:3.

Smoking and cardiovascular disease. MMWR Morb Mortal Wkly Rep 1984;32:677.

The Surgeon General: *Smoking and Health.* US Department of Health and Human Services, 1964.

Sussman JL et al: Atomic structure of acetylcholinesterase from *Torpedo californica:* A prototypic acetylcholine-binding protein. Science 1991;253:872.

Taylor P, Radic Z: The cholinesterases: From genes to proteins. Annu Rev Pharmacol Toxicol 1994;34:281.

Vincent A, Drachman DB: Myasthenia gravis. Adv Neurol 2002;88:159.

Wickman KD, Clapham DE: Ion channel regulation by G proteins. Physiol Rev 1995;75:865.

Cholinoceptor-Blocking Drugs

8

Achilles J. Pappano, PhD, & Bertram G. Katzung, MD, PhD

Cholinoceptor antagonists, like agonists, are divided into muscarinic and nicotinic subgroups on the basis of their specific receptor affinities. The antinicotinic drugs consist of ganglion-blockers and neuromuscular junction blockers. The ganglion-blocking drugs have little clinical use and are discussed at the end of this chapter. The neuromuscular blockers are discussed in Chapter 27. This chapter emphasizes drugs that block muscarinic cholinoceptors.

As noted in Chapters 6 and 7, five subtypes of muscarinic receptors have been described, primarily on the basis of data from ligand-binding and cDNA-cloning experiments. A standard terminology (M_1 through M_5) for these subtypes is now in common use, and evidence, based mostly on selective agonists and antagonists, indicates that functional differences exist between several of these subtypes.

As suggested in Chapter 6, the M_1 receptor subtype appears to be located on central nervous system neurons, sympathetic postganglionic cell bodies, and many presynaptic sites. M_2 receptors are located in the myocardium, smooth muscle organs, and some neuronal sites. M_3 receptors are most common on effector cell membranes, especially glandular and smooth muscle cells.

I. BASIC PHARMACOLOGY OF THE MUSCARINIC RECEPTOR-BLOCKING DRUGS

Muscarinic antagonists are often called parasympatholytic because they block the effects of parasympathetic autonomic discharge. However, they do not "lyse" parasympathetic nerves, and they have some effects that are not predictable from block of the parasympathetic nervous system. For these reasons, the term "antimuscarinic" is preferable.

Naturally occurring compounds with antimuscarinic effects have been known and used for millennia as medicines, poisons, and cosmetics. Atropine is the prototype of these drugs. Many similar plant alkaloids are known,

and hundreds of synthetic antimuscarinic compounds have been prepared.

Chemistry & Pharmacokinetics

A. SOURCE AND CHEMISTRY

Atropine and its naturally occurring congeners are tertiary amine alkaloid esters of tropic acid (Figure 8–1). Atropine (hyoscyamine) is found in the plant *Atropa belladonna,* or deadly nightshade, and in *Datura stramonium,* also known as jimsonweed (Jamestown weed) or thorn apple. Scopolamine (hyoscine) occurs in *Hyoscyamus niger,* or henbane, as the *l*(–) stereoisomer. Naturally occurring atropine is *l*(–)-hyoscyamine, but the compound readily racemizes, so the commercial material is racemic *d,l*-hyoscyamine. The *l*(–) isomers of both alkaloids are at least 100 times more potent than the *d*(+) isomers.

A variety of semisynthetic and fully synthetic molecules have antimuscarinic effects.

The tertiary members of these classes (Figure 8–2) are often used for their effects on the eye or the central nervous system. Many antihistaminic (see Chapter 16), antipsychotic (see Chapter 29), and antidepressant (see Chapter 30) drugs have similar structures and, predictably, significant antimuscarinic effects.

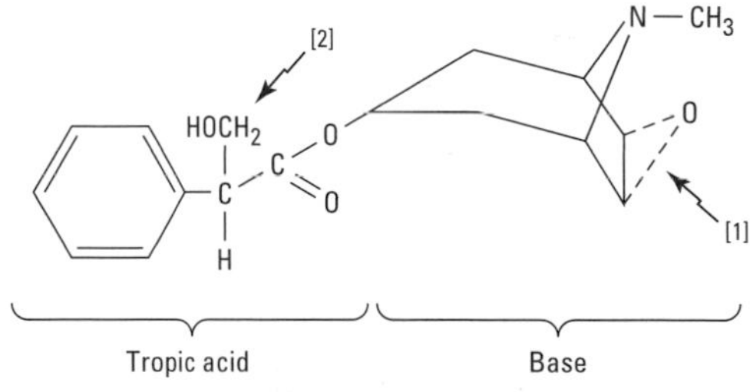

Figure 8–1. The structure of atropine (oxygen at *[1]* is missing) or scopolamine (oxygen present). In homatropine, the hydroxymethyl at *[2]* is replaced by a hydroxyl group, and the oxygen at *[1]* is absent.

Quaternary amines for gastrointestinal applications (peptic disease, hypermotility):

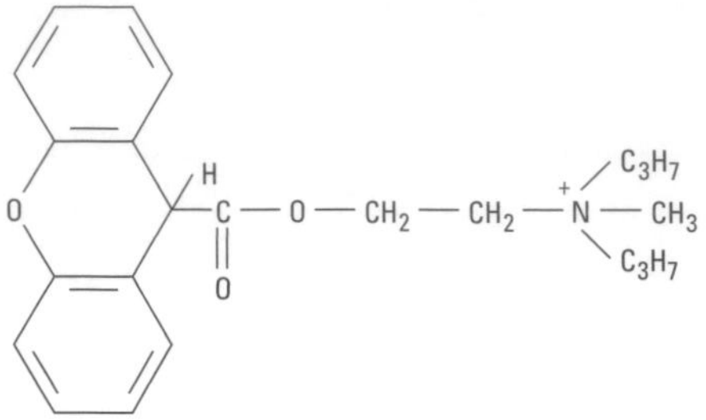

Propantheline

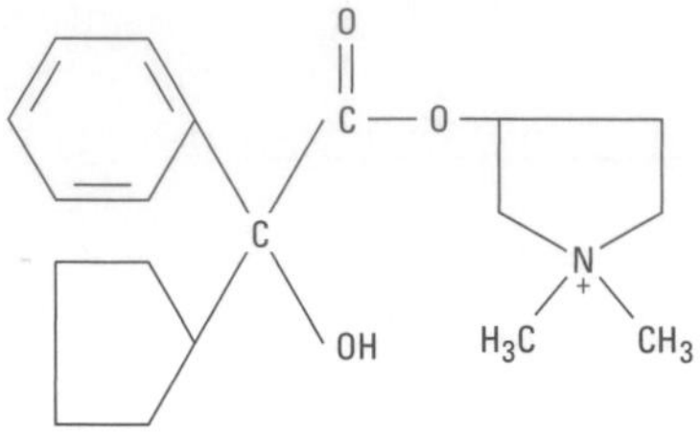

Glycopyrrolate

Tertiary amines for peripheral applications:

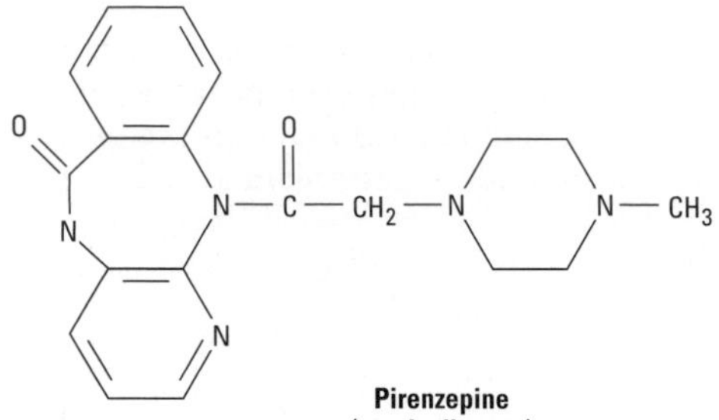

Pirenzepine
(peptic disease)

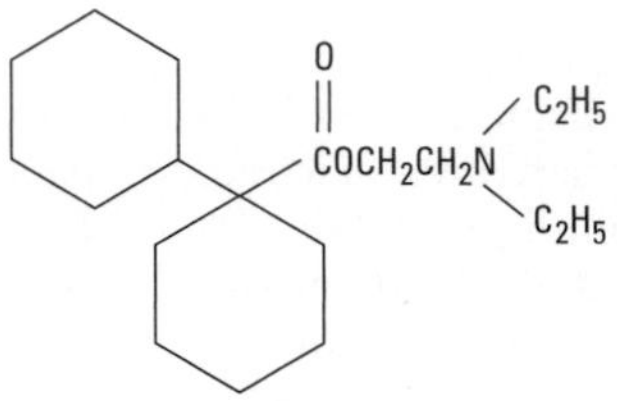

Dicyclomine
(peptic disease, hypermotility)

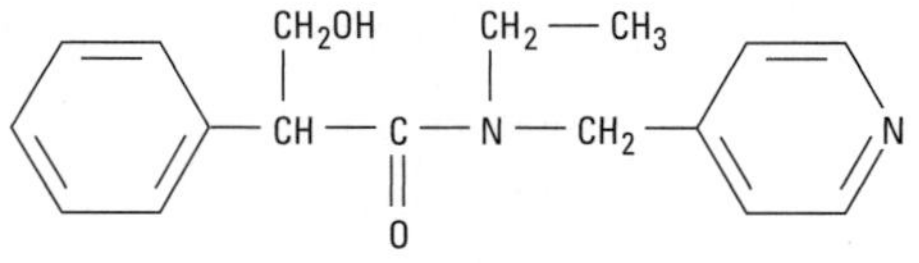

Tropicamide
(mydriatric, cycloplegic)

Quaternary amine for use in asthma:

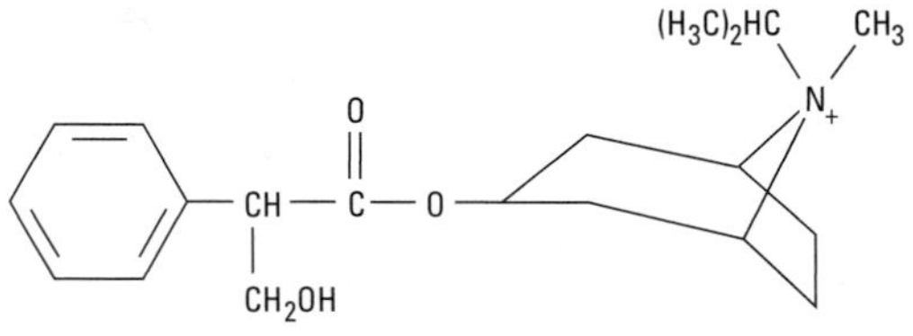

Tertiary amine for Parkinson's disease:

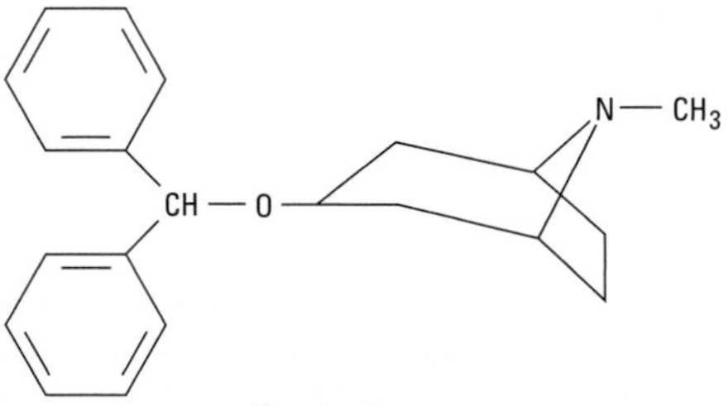

Ipratropium

Benztropine

Figure 8–2. Structures of some semisynthetic and synthetic antimuscarinic drugs.

Quaternary amine antimuscarinic agents (Figure 8–2) have been developed to produce more peripheral effects with reduced central nervous system effects.

B. ABSORPTION

The natural alkaloids and most tertiary antimuscarinic drugs are well absorbed from the gut and conjunctival membranes. When applied in a suitable vehicle, some (eg, scopolamine) are even absorbed across the skin (transdermal route). In contrast, only 10–30% of a dose of a quaternary antimuscarinic drug is absorbed after oral administration, reflecting the decreased lipid solubility of the charged molecule.

C. DISTRIBUTION

Atropine and the other tertiary agents are widely distributed in the body. Significant levels are achieved in the central nervous system within 30 minutes to 1 hour, and this may limit the dose tolerated when the drug is taken for its peripheral effects. Scopolamine is rapidly and fully distributed into the central nervous system where it has greater effects than most other antimuscarinic drugs. In contrast, the quaternary derivatives are poorly taken up by the brain and therefore are relatively free—at low doses—of central nervous system effects.

D. METABOLISM AND EXCRETION

Atropine disappears rapidly from the blood after administration, with a half-life of 2 hours. About 60% of the dose is excreted unchanged in the urine. Most of the rest appears in the urine as hydrolysis and conjugation products. The drug's effect on parasympathetic function declines rapidly in all organs except the eye. Effects on the iris and ciliary muscle persist for ≥ 72 hours.

Pharmacodynamics

A. MECHANISM OF ACTION

Atropine causes reversible (surmountable) blockade of cholinomimetic actions at muscarinic receptors—ie, blockade by a small dose of atropine can be overcome by a larger concentration of acetylcholine or equivalent muscarinic agonist. Mutation experiments suggest that a specific amino acid is required in the receptor to form the characteristic bond with the nitrogen atom of acetylcholine; this amino acid is also required for binding of antimuscarinic drugs. When atropine binds to the muscarinic receptor, it prevents the actions described in Chapter 7 such as the release of inositol trisphosphate (IP_3) and the inhibition of adenylyl cyclase that are caused by muscarinic agonists.

The effectiveness of antimuscarinic drugs varies with the tissue under study and with the source of agonist. Tissues most sensitive to atropine are the salivary, bronchial, and sweat glands. Secretion of acid by the

gastric parietal cells is the least sensitive. In most tissues, antimuscarinic agents block exogenously administered cholinoceptor agonists more effectively than endogenously released acetylcholine.

Atropine is highly selective for muscarinic receptors. Its potency at nicotinic receptors is much lower, and actions at nonmuscarinic receptors are generally undetectable clinically.

Atropine does not distinguish between the M_1, M_2, and M_3 subgroups of muscarinic receptors. In contrast, other antimuscarinic drugs have moderate selectivity for one or another of these subgroups (Table 8–1). Most synthetic antimuscarinic drugs are considerably less selective than atropine in interactions with nonmuscarinic receptors. For example, some quaternary amine antimuscarinic agents have significant ganglion-blocking actions, and others are potent histamine receptor blockers. The antimuscarinic effects of other groups, eg, antipsychotic and antidepressant drugs, have been mentioned. Their relative selectivity for muscarinic receptor subtypes has not been defined.

B. ORGAN SYSTEM EFFECTS

1. Central nervous system—In the doses usually used, atropine has minimal stimulant effects on the central nervous system, especially the parasympathetic medullary centers, and a slower, longer-lasting sedative effect on the brain. Scopolamine has more marked central effects, producing drowsiness when given in recommended dosages and amnesia in sensitive individuals. In toxic doses, scopolamine and to a lesser degree atropine can cause excitement, agitation, hallucinations, and coma.

The tremor of Parkinson's disease is reduced by centrally acting antimuscarinic drugs, and atropine—in the form of belladonna extract—was one of the first drugs used in the therapy of this disease. As discussed in Chapter 28, parkinsonian tremor and rigidity seem to result from a *relative* excess of cholinergic activity because of a deficiency of dopaminergic activity in the basal ganglia-striatum system. The combination of an antimuscarinic agent with a dopamine precursor drug (levodopa) may provide more effective therapy than either drug alone.

Vestibular disturbances, especially motion sickness, appear to involve muscarinic cholinergic transmission. Scopolamine is often effective in preventing or reversing these disturbances.

2. Eye—The pupillary constrictor muscle (see Figure 6–9) depends on muscarinic cholinoceptor activation. This activation is blocked by topical atropine and other tertiary antimuscarinic drugs and results in unopposed sympathetic dilator activity and mydriasis (Figure 8–3). Dilated pupils were considered cosmetically desirable during the Renaissance and account for the name bel-

Table 8–1. Muscarinic receptor subgroups and their antagonists. (Acronyms identify selective antagonists used in research studies only.)

Property	Subgroup		
	M$_1$	M$_2$	M$_3$
Primary locations	Nerves	Heart, nerves, smooth muscle	Glands, smooth muscle, endothelium
Dominant effector system	↑ IP$_3$, ↑ DAG	↓ cAMP, ↑ K$^+$ channel current	↑ IP$_3$, ↑ DAG
Antagonists	Pirenzepine, telenzepine dicyclomine,[2] trihexyphenidyl[3]	Gallamine,[1] methoctramine, AF-DX 116	4-DAMP, HHSD, darifenacin
Approximate dissociation constant[4]			
Atropine	1	1	1
Pirenzepine	10	50	200
AF-DX 116	800	100	3000
HHSD	40	200	2

[1]In clinical use as a neuromuscular blocking agent.

[2]In clinical use as an intestinal antispasmodic agent.

[3]In clinical use in the treatment of Parkinson's disease.

[4]Relative to atropine. Smaller numbers indicate higher affinity.

AF-DX 116, 11-({2-[(Diethylamino)methyl]-1-piperidinyl}acetyl)-5,11-dihydro-6H-pyrido-[2,3-b](1,4)benzodiaz-epin-6-one; DAG, Diacylglycerol; IP$_3$, Inositol trisphosphate; 4-DAMP, 4-Diphenylacetoxy-N-methylpiperidine; HHSD, Hexahydrosiladifenidol

ladonna (Italian, "beautiful lady") applied to the plant and its active extract because of the use of the extract as eye drops during that time.

The second important ocular effect of antimuscarinic drugs is weakening of contraction of the ciliary muscle, or **cycloplegia.** The result of cycloplegia is loss of the ability to accommodate; the fully atropinized eye cannot focus for near vision (Figure 8–3).

Both mydriasis and cycloplegia are useful in ophthalmology. They are also potentially hazardous, since acute glaucoma may be precipitated in patients with a narrow anterior chamber angle.

A third ocular effect of antimuscarinic drugs is reduction of lacrimal secretion. Patients occasionally complain of dry or "sandy" eyes when receiving large doses of antimuscarinic drugs.

3. Cardiovascular system—The sinoatrial node is very sensitive to muscarinic receptor blockade. The effect of moderate to high therapeutic doses of atropine in the innervated and spontaneously beating heart is a block-

ade of vagal slowing and a relative tachycardia. However, lower doses often result in initial bradycardia before the effects of peripheral vagal block become manifest (Figure 8–4). This slowing may be due to block of presynaptic muscarinic receptors on vagal postganglionic fibers that normally limit acetylcholine release in the sinus node and other tissues. The same mechanisms operate in the control of atrioventricular node function; in the presence of high vagal tone, atropine can significantly reduce the PR interval of the ECG by blocking muscarinic receptors in the atrioventricular node. Muscarinic effects on atrial muscle are similarly blocked, but these effects are of no clinical significance except in atrial flutter and fibrillation. Because of a lesser degree of muscarinic control, the ventricles are less affected by antimuscarinic drugs at therapeutic levels. In toxic concentrations, the drugs can cause intraventricular conduction block by an unknown mechanism.

Blood vessels receive no direct innervation from the parasympathetic nervous system. However, parasympathetic nerve stimulation dilates coronary arteries, and

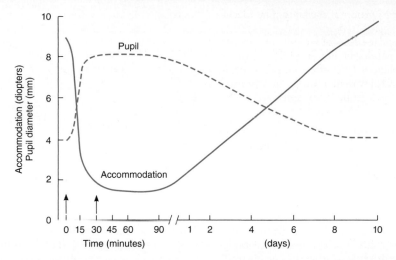

Figure 8–3. Effects of topical scopolamine drops on pupil diameter (mm) and accommodation (diopters) in the normal human eye. One drop of 0.5% solution of drug was applied at zero time, and a second drop was administered at 30 minutes (*arrows*). The responses of 42 eyes were averaged. Note the extremely slow recovery. (Redrawn from Marron J: Cycloplegia and mydriasis by use of atropine, scopolamine, and homatropine-paredrine. Arch Ophthalmol 1940;23:340.)

sympathetic cholinergic nerves cause vasodilation in the skeletal muscle vascular bed (see Chapter 6). Atropine can block this vasodilation. Furthermore, almost all vessels contain endothelial muscarinic recep-tors that mediate vasodilation (see Chapter 7). These receptors are readily blocked by antimuscarinic drugs. At toxic doses, and in some individuals at normal doses, antimuscarinic agents cause cutaneous vasodilation,

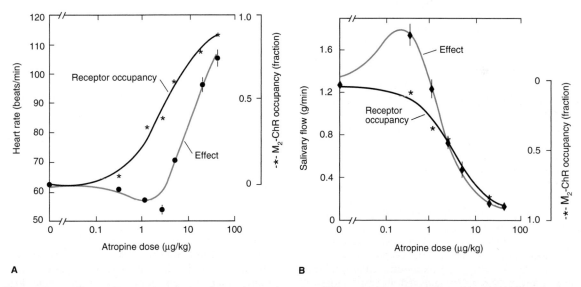

Figure 8–4. Effects of increasing doses of atropine on heart rate (**A**) and salivary flow (**B**) compared with muscarinic receptor occupancy in humans. The parasympathomimetic effect of low-dose atropine is attributed to blockade of prejunctional muscarinic receptors that suppress acetylcholine release. (Modified and reproduced, with permission, from Wellstein A, Pitschner HF: Complex dose-response curves of atropine in man explained by different functions of M_1 and M_2 cholinoceptors. Naunyn Schmiedebergs Arch Pharmacol 1988;338:19.)

especially in the upper portion of the body. The mechanism is unknown.

The net cardiovascular effects of atropine in patients with normal hemodynamics are not dramatic: tachycardia may occur, but there is little effect on blood pressure. However, the cardiovascular effects of administered direct-acting muscarinic stimulants are easily prevented.

4. Respiratory system—Both smooth muscle and secretory glands of the airway receive vagal innervation and contain muscarinic receptors. Even in normal individuals, some bronchodilation and reduction of secretion can be measured after administration of atropine. The effect is more significant in patients with airway disease, although the antimuscarinic drugs are not as useful as the β-adrenoceptor stimulants in the treatment of asthma (see Chapter 20). The effectiveness of unselective antimuscarinic drugs in treating chronic obstructive pulmonary disease (COPD) is limited because block of autoinhibitory M_2 receptors on postganglionic parasympathetic nerves can oppose the bronchodilation caused by block of M_3 receptors on airway smooth muscle. Nevertheless, antimuscarinic agents are valuable in some patients with asthma or COPD.

Antimuscarinic drugs are frequently used prior to administration of inhalant anesthetics to reduce the accumulation of secretions in the trachea and the possibility of laryngospasm.

5. Gastrointestinal tract—Blockade of muscarinic receptors has dramatic effects on motility and some of the secretory functions of the gut. However, even complete muscarinic block cannot totally abolish activity in this organ system since local hormones and noncholinergic neurons in the enteric nervous system (see Chapters 6 and 63) also modulate gastrointestinal function. As in other tissues, exogenously administered muscarinic stimulants are more effectively blocked than the effects of parasympathetic (vagal) nerve activity. The removal of autoinhibition, a negative feedback mechanism by which neural acetylcholine suppresses its own release, might explain the greater efficacy of antimuscarinic drugs against exogenous muscarinic stimulants.

Antimuscarinic drugs have marked effects on salivary secretion; dry mouth occurs frequently in patients taking antimuscarinic drugs for Parkinson's disease or urinary conditions (Figure 8–5). Gastric secretion is blocked less effectively: the volume and amount of acid, pepsin, and mucin are all reduced, but large doses of atropine may be required. Basal secretion is blocked more effectively than that stimulated by food, nicotine, or alcohol. Pirenzepine and a more potent analog, telenzepine, reduce gastric acid secretion with fewer adverse effects than atropine and other less selective agents. This

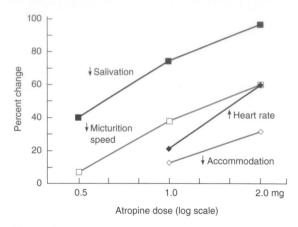

Figure 8–5. Effects of subcutaneous injection of atropine on salivation, speed of micturition (voiding), heart rate, and accommodation in normal adults. Note that salivation is the most sensitive of these variables, accommodation the least. (Data from Herxheimer A: Br J Pharmacol 1958;13:184.)

results from a selective blockade of presynaptic excitatory muscarinic receptors on vagal nerve endings as suggested by their high ratio of M_1 to M_3 affinity (Table 8–1). Pirenzepine and telenzepine are investigational in the USA. Pancreatic and intestinal secretion are little affected by atropine; these processes are primarily under hormonal rather than vagal control.

Gastrointestinal smooth muscle motility is affected from the stomach to the colon. In general, the walls of the viscera are relaxed, and both tone and propulsive movements are diminished. Therefore, gastric emptying time is prolonged, and intestinal transit time is lengthened. Diarrhea due to overdosage with parasympathomimetic agents is readily stopped, and even that caused by nonautonomic agents can usually be temporarily controlled. However, intestinal "paralysis" induced by antimuscarinic drugs is temporary; local mechanisms within the enteric nervous system will usually reestablish at least some peristalsis after 1–3 days of antimuscarinic drug therapy.

6. Genitourinary tract—The antimuscarinic action of atropine and its analogs relaxes smooth muscle of the ureters and bladder wall and slows voiding (Figure 8–5). This action is useful in the treatment of spasm induced by mild inflammation, surgery, and certain neurologic conditions, but it can precipitate urinary retention in elderly men, who may have prostatic hyperplasia (see following section, Clinical Pharmacology of the Muscarinic Receptor-Blocking Drugs). The antimuscarinic drugs have no significant effect on the uterus.

7. Sweat glands—Atropine suppresses thermoregulatory sweating. Sympathetic cholinergic fibers innervate eccrine sweat glands, and their muscarinic receptors are readily accessible to antimuscarinic drugs. In adults, body temperature is elevated by this effect only if large doses are administered, but in infants and children even ordinary doses may cause "atropine fever."

II. CLINICAL PHARMACOLOGY OF THE MUSCARINIC RECEPTOR-BLOCKING DRUGS

Therapeutic Applications

A. CENTRAL NERVOUS SYSTEM DISORDERS

1. Parkinson's disease—As described in Chapter 28, the treatment of Parkinson's disease is often an exercise in polypharmacy, since no single agent is fully effective over the course of the disease. Most antimuscarinic drugs promoted for this application (see Table 28–1) were developed before levodopa became available. Their use is accompanied by all of the adverse effects described below, but the drugs remain useful as adjunctive therapy in some patients.

2. Motion sickness—Certain vestibular disorders respond to antimuscarinic drugs (and to antihistaminic agents with antimuscarinic effects). Scopolamine is one of the oldest remedies for seasickness and is as effective as any more recently introduced agent. It can be given by injection, by mouth, or as a transdermal patch. The patch formulation produces significant blood levels over 48–72 hours. Unfortunately, useful doses by any route usually cause significant sedation and dry mouth.

B. OPHTHALMOLOGIC DISORDERS

Accurate measurement of refractive error in uncooperative patients, eg, young children, requires ciliary paralysis. Also, ophthalmoscopic examination of the retina is greatly facilitated by mydriasis. Therefore, antimuscarinic agents, administered topically as eye drops or ointment, are extremely helpful in doing a complete examination. For adults and older children, the shorter-acting drugs are preferred (Table 8–2). For younger children, the greater efficacy of atropine is sometimes necessary, but the possibility of antimuscarinic poisoning is correspondingly increased. Drug loss from the conjunctival sac via the nasolacrimal duct into the nasopharynx can be diminished by the use of the ointment form instead of drops. In the past, ophthalmic antimuscarinic drugs have been selected from the tertiary amine subgroup to ensure good penetration after conjunctival application. Recent experiments in animals, however, suggest that glycopyrrolate, a quaternary agent, is as rapid in onset and as long-lasting as atropine.

Antimuscarinic drugs should never be used for mydriasis unless cycloplegia or prolonged action is required. Alpha-adrenoceptor stimulant drugs, eg, phenylephrine, produce a short-lasting mydriasis that is usually sufficient for funduscopic examination (see Chapter 9).

A second ophthalmologic use is to prevent synechia (adhesion) formation in uveitis and iritis. The longer-lasting preparations, especially homatropine, are valuable for this indication.

C. RESPIRATORY DISORDERS

The use of atropine became part of routine preoperative medication when anesthetics such as ether were used, because these irritant anesthetics markedly increased airway secretions and were associated with frequent episodes of laryngospasm. Preanesthetic injection of atropine or scopolamine could prevent these hazardous effects. Scopolamine also produces significant amnesia for the events associated with surgery and obstetric delivery, a side effect that was considered desirable. On the other hand, urinary retention and intestinal hypomotility following surgery were often exacerbated by antimuscarinic drugs. Newer inhalational anesthetics are far less irritating to the airways.

As described in Chapter 20, the hyperactive neural bronchoconstrictor reflex present in most individuals with asthma is mediated by the vagus, acting on muscarinic receptors on bronchial smooth muscle cells. **Ipratropium** (Figure 8–2), a synthetic analog of atropine, is used as an inhalational drug in asthma. The aerosol route of administration provides the advantages of maximal concentration at the bronchial target tissue with reduced systemic effects. This application is discussed in greater detail in Chapter 20. Ipratropium has also proved useful in COPD, a condition that occurs with higher frequency in older patients, particularly chronic smokers. Patients with COPD benefit from bronchodilators, especially

Table 8–2. Antimuscarinic drugs used in ophthalmology.

Drug	Duration of Effect (days)	Usual Concentration (%)
Atropine	7–10	0.5–1
Scopolamine	3–7	0.25
Homatropine	1–3	2–5
Cyclopentolate	1	0.5–2
Tropicamide	0.25	0.5–1

antimuscarinic agents such as ipratropium. Investigational agents in this category include **tiotropium**, a long-acting quaternary aerosol antimuscarinic drug.

D. CARDIOVASCULAR DISORDERS

Marked reflex vagal discharge sometimes accompanies the pain of myocardial infarction and may result in sufficient depression of sinoatrial or atrioventricular node function to impair cardiac output. Parenteral atropine or a similar antimuscarinic drug is appropriate therapy in this situation. Rare individuals without other detectable cardiac disease have hyperactive carotid sinus reflexes and may experience faintness or even syncope as a result of vagal discharge in response to pressure on the neck, eg, from a tight collar. Such individuals may benefit from the judicious use of atropine or a related antimuscarinic agent.

Pathophysiology can influence muscarinic activity in other ways as well. Circulating autoantibodies against the second extracellular loop of cardiac muscarinic receptors have been detected in some patients with idiopathic dilated cardiomyopathy. These antibodies exert parasympathomimetic actions on the heart that are prevented by atropine. Although their role in the pathology of heart failure is unknown, they should provide clues to the molecular basis of receptor activation.

E. GASTROINTESTINAL DISORDERS

Antimuscarinic agents are now rarely used for peptic ulcer disease in the USA (see Chapter 63). Antimuscarinic agents can provide some relief in the treatment of common traveler's diarrhea and other mild or self-limited conditions of hypermotility. They are often combined with an opioid antidiarrheal drug, an extremely effective therapy. In this combination, however, the very low dosage of the antimuscarinic drug functions primarily to discourage abuse of the opioid agent. The classic combination of atropine with diphenoxylate, a nonanalgesic congener of meperidine, is available under many names (eg, Lomotil) in both tablet and liquid form (see Chapter 63).

F. URINARY DISORDERS

Atropine and other antimuscarinic drugs have been used to provide symptomatic relief in the treatment of urinary urgency caused by minor inflammatory bladder disorders (Table 8–3). However, specific antimicrobial therapy is essential in bacterial cystitis.

Oxybutynin is often used to relieve bladder spasm after urologic surgery, eg, prostatectomy. It is also valuable in reducing involuntary voiding in patients with neurologic disease, eg, children with meningomyelocele. Oral oxybutynin or instillation of the drug by catheter into the bladder in such patients appears to improve bladder capacity and continence and to reduce infection

Table 8–3. Antimuscarinic drugs used in gastrointestinal and genitourinary conditions.

Drug	Usual Dosage
Quaternary amines	
Anisotropine	50 mg tid
Clidinium	2.5 mg tid–qid
Glycopyrrolate	1 mg bid–tid
Isopropamide	5 mg bid
Mepenzolate	25–50 mg qid
Methantheline	50–100 mg qid
Methscopolamine	2.5 mg qid
Oxyphenonium	5–10 mg qid
Propantheline	15 mg qid
Tertiary amines	
Atropine	0.4 mg tid–qid
Dicyclomine	10–20 mg qid
Oxybutynin	5 mg tid
Oxyphencyclimine	10 mg bid
Propiverine	15 mg bid–tid
Scopolamine	0.4 mg tid
Tolterodine	2 mg bid
Tridihexethyl	25–50 mg tid–qid

and renal damage. **Tolterodine,** an M_3-selective antimuscarinic, is available for use in adults with urinary incontinence.

Imipramine, a tricyclic antidepressant drug with strong antimuscarinic actions, has long been used to reduce incontinence in institutionalized elderly patients. It is moderately effective but causes significant central nervous system toxicity. **Propiverine,** a newer antimuscarinic agent, has been approved for this purpose.

The antimuscarinic agents have also been used in urolithiasis to relieve the ureteral smooth muscle spasm caused by passage of the stone. However, their usefulness in this condition is debatable.

G. CHOLINERGIC POISONING

Severe cholinergic excess is a medical emergency, especially in rural communities where the use of cholinesterase inhibitor insecticides is common and in cultures where wild mushrooms are commonly eaten. The potential use of cholinesterase inhibitors as chemical warfare "nerve gases" also requires an awareness of the methods for treating acute poisoning (see Chapter 59).

1. Antimuscarinic therapy—As noted in Chapter 7, both the nicotinic and the muscarinic effects of the cholinesterase inhibitors can be life-threatening. Unfortunately, there is no effective method for directly blocking the nicotinic effects of cholinesterase inhibition, because nicotinic agonists *and* blockers cause blockade of transmission (see Chapter 27). To reverse the muscarinic effects, a tertiary (not quaternary) amine drug must be used (preferably atropine), since the central nervous system effects as well as the peripheral effects of the organophosphate inhibitors must be treated. Large doses of atropine may be needed to combat the muscarinic effects of extremely potent agents like parathion and chemical warfare nerve gases: 1–2 mg of atropine sulfate may be given intravenously every 5–15 minutes until signs of effect (dry mouth, reversal of miosis) appear. The drug may have to be repeated many times, since the acute effects of the anticholinesterase agent may last for 24–48 hours or longer. In this life-threatening situation, as much as 1 g of atropine per day may be required for as long as 1 month for full control of muscarinic excess.

2. Cholinesterase regenerator compounds—A second class of compounds, capable of regenerating active enzyme from the organophosphorus-cholinesterase complex, is also available to treat organophosphorus poisoning. These oxime agents include pralidoxime (PAM), diacetylmonoxime (DAM), and others.

Pralidoxime   **Diacetylmonoxime**

The oxime group (=NOH) has a very high affinity for the phosphorus atom, and these drugs are able to hydrolyze the phosphorylated enzyme if the complex has not "aged" (see Chapter 7). Pralidoxime is the most extensively studied—in humans—of the agents shown and the only one available for clinical use in the USA. It is most effective in regenerating the cholinesterase associated with skeletal muscle neuromuscular junctions. Because of its positive charge, it does not enter the central nervous system and is ineffective in reversing the central effects of organophosphate poisoning. Diacetylmonoxime, on the other hand, does cross the blood-brain barrier and, in experimental animals, can regenerate some of the central nervous system cholinesterase.

Pralidoxime is administered by intravenous infusion, 1–2 g given over 15–30 minutes. In spite of the likeli-

hood of aging of the phosphate-enzyme complex, recent reports suggest that administration of multiple doses of pralidoxime over several days may be useful in severe poisoning. In excessive doses, pralidoxime can induce neuromuscular weakness and other adverse effects. Pralidoxime is *not* recommended for the reversal of inhibition of acetylcholinesterase by carbamate inhibitors. Further details of treatment of anticholinesterase toxicity are given in Chapter 59.

A third approach to protection against excessive AChE inhibition lies in *pretreatment* with reversible inhibitors of the enzyme to prevent binding of the irreversible organophosphate inhibitor. This prophylaxis can be achieved with pyridostigmine or physostigmine but is reserved for situations in which possibly lethal poisoning is anticipated, eg, chemical warfare. Simultaneous use of atropine is required to control muscarinic excess.

Mushroom poisoning has traditionally been divided into rapid-onset and delayed-onset types. The rapid-onset type is usually apparent within 15–30 minutes following ingestion of the mushrooms. It is often characterized entirely by signs of muscarinic excess: nausea, vomiting, diarrhea, vasodilation, reflex tachycardia (occasionally bradycardia), sweating, salivation, and sometimes bronchoconstriction. Although *Amanita muscaria* contains muscarine (the alkaloid was named after the mushroom), numerous other alkaloids, including antimuscarinic agents, are found in this fungus. In fact, ingestion of *A muscaria* may produce signs of atropine poisoning, not muscarine excess. Other mushrooms, especially those of the *Inocybe* genus, cause rapid-onset poisoning of the muscarinic excess type. Parenteral atropine, 1–2 mg, is effective treatment in such intoxications.

Delayed-onset mushroom poisoning, usually caused by *Amanita phalloides, A virosa, Galerina autumnalis,* or *G marginata,* manifests its first symptoms 6–12 hours after ingestion. Although the initial symptoms usually include nausea and vomiting, the major toxicity involves hepatic and renal cellular injury by amatoxins that inhibit RNA polymerase. Atropine is of no value in this form of mushroom poisoning (see Chapter 59).

H. Other Applications

Hyperhidrosis is sometimes reduced by antimuscarinic agents. However, relief is incomplete at best, probably because apocrine rather than eccrine glands are usually involved.

Adverse Effects

Treatment with atropine or its congeners directed at one organ system almost always induces undesirable effects in other organ systems. Thus, mydriasis and cycloplegia are adverse effects when an antimuscarinic agent is being used to reduce gastrointestinal secretion or motility, even though they are therapeutic effects when the drug is used in ophthalmology.

At higher concentrations, atropine causes block of all parasympathetic functions. However, atropine is a remarkably safe drug *in adults*. Atropine poisoning has occurred as a result of attempted suicide, but most cases are due to attempts to induce hallucinations. Poisoned individuals manifest dry mouth, mydriasis, tachycardia, hot and flushed skin, agitation, and delirium for as long as a week. Body temperature is frequently elevated. These effects are memorialized in the adage, "dry as a bone, blind as a bat, red as a beet, mad as a hatter."

Unfortunately, children, especially infants, are very sensitive to the hyperthermic effects of atropine. Although accidental administration of over 400 mg has been followed by recovery, deaths have followed doses as small as 2 mg. Therefore, atropine should be considered a highly dangerous drug when overdose occurs in infants or children.

Overdoses of atropine or its congeners are generally treated symptomatically (see Chapter 59). In the past, physostigmine or another cholinesterase inhibitor was recommended, but most poison control experts now consider physostigmine more dangerous and no more effective in most patients than symptomatic management. When physostigmine is deemed necessary, *small* doses are given *slowly* intravenously (1–4 mg in adults, 0.5–1 mg in children). Symptomatic treatment may require temperature control with cooling blankets and seizure control with diazepam.

Poisoning caused by high doses of the quaternary antimuscarinic drugs is associated with all of the peripheral signs of parasympathetic blockade but few or none of the central nervous system effects of atropine. These more polar drugs may cause significant ganglionic blockade, however, with marked orthostatic hypotension (see below). Treatment of the antimuscarinic effects, if required, can be carried out with a quaternary cholinesterase inhibitor such as neostigmine. Control of hypotension may require the administration of a sympathomimetic drug such as phenylephrine.

Contraindications

Contraindications to the use of antimuscarinic drugs are relative, not absolute. *Obvious muscarinic excess, especially that caused by cholinesterase inhibitors, can always be treated with atropine.*

Antimuscarinic drugs are contraindicated in patients with glaucoma, especially angle-closure glaucoma. Even systemic use of moderate doses may precipitate angle closure (and acute glaucoma) in patients with shallow anterior chambers.

In elderly men, antimuscarinic drugs should always be used with caution and should be avoided in those with a history of prostatic hyperplasia.

Because the antimuscarinic drugs slow gastric emptying, they may *increase* symptoms in patients with gastric ulcer. Nonselective antimuscarinic agents should never be used to treat acid-peptic disease (see Chapter 63).

III. BASIC & CLINICAL PHARMACOLOGY OF THE GANGLION-BLOCKING DRUGS

These agents block the action of acetylcholine and similar agonists at the nicotinic receptors of both parasympathetic and sympathetic autonomic ganglia. Some members of the group also block the ion channel that is gated by the nicotinic cholinoceptor. The ganglion-blocking drugs are still important and useful in pharmacologic and physiologic research because of their ability to block all autonomic outflow. However, their lack of selectivity confers such a broad range of undesirable effects that they have been abandoned for clinical use.

Chemistry & Pharmacokinetics

All ganglion-blocking drugs of interest are synthetic amines. The first to be recognized as having this action was **tetraethylammonium (TEA)**. Because of the very short duration of action of TEA, **hexamethonium** ("C6") was developed and was soon introduced into clinical medicine as the first effective drug for management of hypertension. As shown in Figure 8–6, there is an obvious relationship between the structures of the agonist acetylcholine and the nicotinic antagonists tetraethylammonium and hexamethonium. Decamethonium, the "C10" analog of hexamethonium, is an effective neuromuscular depolarizing blocking agent.

Because the quaternary amine ganglion-blocking compounds were poorly and erratically absorbed after oral administration, **mecamylamine,** a secondary amine, was developed to improve the degree and extent of absorption from the gastrointestinal tract. **Trimethaphan,** a short-acting ganglion blocker, is inactive orally and is given by intravenous infusion.

Pharmacodynamics

A. MECHANISM OF ACTION

Ganglionic nicotinic receptors, like those of the skeletal muscle neuromuscular junction, are subject to both

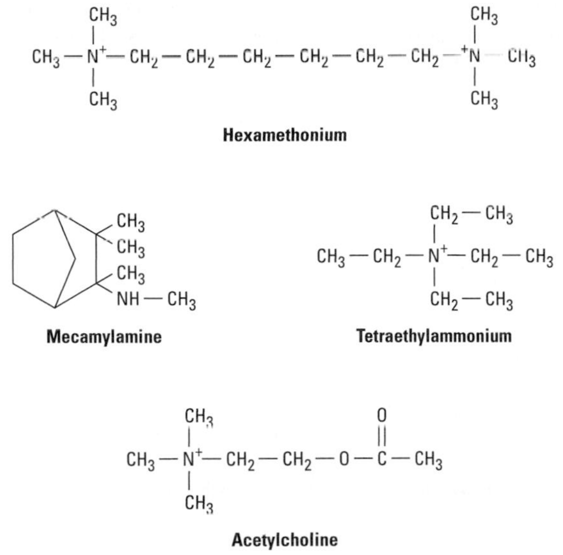

Figure 8–6. Some ganglion-blocking drugs. Acetylcholine is shown for reference.

depolarizing and nondepolarizing blockade (see Chapters 7 and 27). Nicotine itself, carbamoylcholine, and even acetylcholine (if amplified with a cholinesterase inhibitor) can produce depolarizing ganglion block.

The drugs presently used as ganglion blockers are classified as nondepolarizing competitive antagonists. However, evidence suggests that hexamethonium actually produces most of its blockade by occupying sites in or on the ion channel that is controlled by the acetylcholine receptor, not by occupying the cholinoceptor itself. In contrast, trimethaphan appears to block the nicotinic receptor, not the channel. Blockade can be at least partially overcome by increasing the concentration of normal agonists, eg, acetylcholine.

B. ORGAN SYSTEM EFFECTS

1. Central nervous system—The quaternary amine agents and trimethaphan lack central effects because they do not cross the blood-brain barrier. Mecamylamine, however, readily enters the central nervous system. Sedation, tremor, choreiform movements, and mental aberrations have all been reported as effects of the latter drug.

2. Eye—Because the ciliary muscle receives innervation primarily from the parasympathetic nervous system, the ganglion-blocking drugs cause a predictable cycloplegia with loss of accommodation. The effect on the pupil is not so easily predicted, since the iris receives both sym-

pathetic innervation (mediating pupillary dilation) and parasympathetic innervation (mediating pupillary constriction). Because parasympathetic tone is usually dominant in this tissue, ganglionic blockade usually causes moderate dilation of the pupil.

3. Cardiovascular system—The blood vessels receive chiefly vasoconstrictor fibers from the sympathetic nervous system; therefore, ganglionic blockade causes a very important decrease in arteriolar and venomotor tone. The blood pressure may drop precipitously, because both peripheral vascular resistance and venous return are decreased (see Figure 6–7). Hypotension is especially marked in the upright position (orthostatic or postural hypotension), because postural reflexes that normally prevent venous pooling are blocked.

Cardiac effects include diminished contractility and, because the sinoatrial node is usually dominated by the parasympathetic nervous system, a moderate tachycardia.

4. Gastrointestinal tract—Secretion is reduced, although not enough to effectively treat peptic disease. Motility is profoundly inhibited, and constipation may be marked.

5. Other systems—Genitourinary smooth muscle is partially dependent on autonomic innervation for normal function. Ganglionic blockade therefore causes hesitancy in urination and may precipitate urinary retention in men with prostatic hyperplasia. Sexual function is impaired in that both erection and ejaculation may be prevented by moderate doses.

Thermoregulatory sweating is blocked by the ganglion-blocking drugs. However, hyperthermia is not a problem except in very warm environments, because cutaneous vasodilation is usually sufficient to maintain a normal body temperature.

6. Response to autonomic drugs—Because the effector cell receptors (muscarinic, α, and β) are not blocked, patients receiving ganglion-blocking drugs are fully responsive to autonomic drugs acting on these receptors. In fact, responses may be exaggerated or even reversed (eg, norepinephrine may cause tachycardia rather than bradycardia), because homeostatic reflexes, which normally moderate autonomic responses, are absent.

Clinical Applications & Toxicity

Because of the availability of more selective autonomic blocking agents, the applications of the ganglion blockers have almost disappeared. Mecamylamine is being studied for possible use in reducing nicotine craving in patients attempting to quit smoking and for some other central indications. Trimethaphan is occasionally used in the treatment of hypertensive emergencies and dissecting aortic aneurysm, to produce controlled hypotension, which can be of value in neurosurgery to reduce bleeding in the operative field, and in patients undergoing electroconvulsive therapy. The toxicity of the gan-glion-blocking drugs is limited to the autonomic effects already described. For most patients, these effects are intolerable except for acute use.

PREPARATIONS AVAILABLE

Antimuscarinic Anticholinergic Drugs*

Atropine (generic)
Oral: 0.4 mg tablets
Parenteral: 0.05, 0.1, 0.3, 0.4, 0.5, 0.8, 1 mg/mL for injection
Ophthalmic (generic, Isopto Atropine): 0.5, 1, 2% drops; 1% ointments

Belladonna alkaloids, extract or tincture (generic)
Oral: 0.27–0.33 mg/mL liquid

Clidinium (Quarzan)
Oral: 2.5, 5 mg capsules

Cyclopentolate (generic, Cyclogyl, others)
Ophthalmic: 0.5, 1, 2% drops

Dicyclomine (generic, Bentyl, others)
Oral: 10, 20 mg capsules; 20 mg tablets; 10 mg/5 mL syrup
Parenteral: 10 mg/mL for injection

Flavoxate (Urispas)
Oral: 100 mg tablets

Glycopyrrolate (generic, Robinul)
Oral: 1, 2 mg tablets
Parenteral: 0.2 mg/mL for injection

Homatropine (generic, Isopto Homatropine)
Ophthalmic: 2, 5% drops

l-Hyoscyamine (Anaspaz, Cystospaz-M, Levsinex)
Oral: 0.125, 0.15 mg tablets; 0.375 mg timed-release capsules; 0.125 mg/5 mL oral elixir and solution
Parenteral: 0.5 mg/mL for injection

Ipratropium (generic, Atrovent)
Aerosol: 200 dose metered-dose inhaler
Solution for nebulizer: 0.02%
Nasal spray: 0.03, 0.06%

Mepenzolate (Cantil)
Oral: 25 mg tablets

Methantheline (Banthine)
Oral: 50 mg tablets

Methscopolamine (Pamine)
Oral: 2.5 mg tablets

Oxybutynin (generic, Ditropan)
Oral: 5 mg tablets; 5, 10, 15 mg extended-release tablets; 5 mg/5 mL syrup

Propantheline (generic, Pro-Banthine)
Oral: 7.5, 15 mg tablets

Scopolamine (generic)
Oral: 0.4 mg tablets
Parenteral: 0.3, 0.4, 0.65, 0.86, 1 mg/mL for injection
Ophthalmic (Isopto Hyoscine): 0.25% solution
Transdermal (Transderm Scop): 1.5 mg (delivers 0.5 mg) patch

Tolterodine (Detrol)
Oral: 1, 2 mg tablets; 2, 4 mg extended-release capsules

Tridihexethyl (Pathilon)
Oral: 25 mg tablets

Tropicamide (generic, Mydriacyl Ophthalmic, others)
Ophthalmic: 0.5, 1% drops

Ganglion Blockers

Mecamylamine (Inversine)
Oral: 2.5 mg tablets

Trimethaphan (Arfonad)
Parenteral: 50 mg/mL

Cholinesterase Regenerator

Pralidoxime (generic, Protopam)
Parenteral: 1 g vial with 20 mL diluent for IV administration; 600 mg in 2 mL autoinjector

---

* Antimuscarinic drugs used in parkinsonism are listed in Chapter 28.

REFERENCES

Amitai Y et al: Atropine poisoning in children during the Persian Gulf crisis. JAMA 1992;268:630.

Andersson KE, Hedlund P: Pharmacologic perspective on the pathophysiology of the lower urinary tract. Urology 2002;60(5 Suppl 1):13.

Berdie GJ et al: Angle closure glaucoma precipitated by aerosolized atropine. Arch Intern Med 1991;151:1658.

Brodde O-E, Michel MC: Adrenergic and muscarinic receptors in the human heart. Pharmacol Rev 1999;51:651.

Campbell SC: Clinical aspects of inhaled anticholinergic therapy. Respir Care 2001;46:275.

Chapple CR, Yamanishi T, Chess-Williams R: Muscarinic receptor types and management of the overactive bladder. Urology 2002;60(5 Suppl 1):82.

Christofi FL, Palmer JM, Wood JD: Neuropharmacology of the muscarinic antagonist telenzepine in myenteric ganglia of the guinea-pig small intestine. Eur J Pharmacol 1991;195:333.

Doods HN et al: Selectivity of muscarinic antagonists in radioligand and *in vivo* experiments for the putative M_1, M_2, and M_3 receptors. J Pharmacol Exp Ther 1987;242:257.

Fukusaki M et al: Effects of controlled hypotension with sevoflurane anesthesia on hepatic function of surgical patients. Eur J Anaesthesiol 1999;16:111.

Gurney AM, Rang HP: The channel-blocking action of methonium compounds on rat submandibular ganglion cells. Br J Pharmacol 1984;82:623.

Holtmann G, Küppers U, Singer MV: Telenzepine, a new M_1-receptor antagonist, is a more potent inhibitor of pentagastrin-stimulated gastric acid output than pirenzepine in dogs. Scand J Gastroenterol 1990;25:293.

Jimson weed poisoning-Texas, New York, and California, 1994. MMWR Morbid Mortal Wkly Rep 1995;44:41.

Kranke P et al: The efficacy and safety of transdermal scopolamine for the prevention of postoperative nausea and vomiting: a quantitative systematic review. Anesth Analg 2002;95:133.

Lee AM, Jacoby DB, Fryer AD: Selective muscarinic receptor antagonists for airway diseases. Curr Opin Pharmacol 2001;1:223.

Maesen FP et al: Tiotropium bromide, a new long-acting antimuscarinic bronchodilator: A pharmacodynamic study in patients with chronic obstructive pulmonary disease (COPD). Eur Respir J 1995;8:1506.

Matsui S et al: Beneficial effect of muscarinic-2 antagonist on dilated cardiomyopathy induced by autoimmune mechanism against muscarinic-2 receptor. J Cardiovasc Pharmacol 2001;38(Suppl 1):S43.

Mazur D et al: Clinical and urodynamic effects of propiverine in patients suffering from urgency and urge incontinence: A multicentre dose-optimizing study. Scand J Urol Nephrol 1995;29:289.

Olson K: Mushrooms. In: Olson K (editor). *Poisoning & Drug Overdose,* 3rd ed. McGraw-Hill, 1998.

Petrides G et al: Trimethaphan (Arfonad) control of hypertension and tachycardia during electroconvulsive therapy: a double-blind study. J Clin Anesth 1996;8:104.

Rascol O et al: Antivertigo medications and drug-induced vertigo: A pharmacological review. Drugs 1995;50:777.

Schneider F et al: Plasma and urine concentrations of atropine after the ingestion of cooked deadly nightshade berries. J Toxicol 1996;34:113.

Simpson JI et al: Trimethaphan versus sodium nitroprusside for the control of proximal hypertension during aortic cross-clamping: the effects on spinal cord ischemia. Anest Analg 1996;82:68.

Smellie JM et al: Nocturnal enuresis: A placebo-controlled trial of two antidepressant drugs. Arch Dis Child 1996;75:62.

Varssano D et al: The mydriatic effect of topical glycopyrrolate. Graefes Arch Clin Exp Ophthalmol 1996;234:205.

Wellstein A, Pitschner HF: Complex dose-response curves of atropine in man explained by different functions of M_1- and M_2-cholinoceptors. Naunyn Schmiedebergs Arch Pharmacol 1988;338:19.

Young JM et al: Mecamylamine: new therapeutic uses and toxicity/risk profile. Clin Ther 2001;23:532.

Treatment of Anticholinesterase Poisoning

Cannon JG et al: Structure-activity studies on a potent antagonist to organophosphate-induced toxicity. J Med Chem 1991;34:1582.

deKort WLAM, Kiestra SH, Sangster B: The use of atropine and oximes in organophosphate intoxications: A modified approach. Clin Toxicol 1988;26:199.

Farrar HC, Wells TG, Kearns GL: Use of continuous infusion of pralidoxime for treatment of organophosphate poisoning in children. J Pediatr 1990;116:658.

Loke WK, Simm MK, Go ML: O-substituted derivatives of pralidoxime: muscarinic properties and protection against soman effects in rats. Eur J Pharmacol 2002;442:279.

Solana RP et al: Evaluation of a two-drug combination pretreatment against organophosphorus exposure. Toxicol Appl Pharmacol 1990;102:421.

Adrenoceptor-Activating & Other Sympathomimetic Drugs

9

Brian B. Hoffman, MD

The sympathetic nervous system is an important regulator of the activities of organs such as the heart and peripheral vasculature, especially in responses to stress (see Chapter 6). The ultimate effects of sympathetic stimulation are mediated by release of norepinephrine from nerve terminals that serve to activate the adrenoceptors on postsynaptic sites. Also, in response to a variety of stimuli, such as stress, the adrenal medulla releases epinephrine, which is transported in the blood to target tissues—in other words, epinephrine acts as a hormone. Drugs that mimic the actions of epinephrine or norepinephrine—**sympathomimetic drugs**—would be expected to have a wide range of effects. An understanding of the pharmacology of these agents is thus a logical extension of what we know about the physiologic role of the catecholamines.

The Mode & Spectrum of Action of Sympathomimetic Drugs

Like the cholinomimetic drugs, the sympathomimetics can be grouped by mode of action and by the spectrum of receptors that they activate. Some of these drugs (eg, norepinephrine, epinephrine) act by a *direct* mode, ie, they directly interact with and activate adrenoceptors. Others act *indirectly;* their actions are dependent on the release of endogenous catecholamines. These indirect agents may have either of two different mechanisms: (1) displacement of stored catecholamines from the adrenergic nerve ending (eg, amphetamine and tyramine) or (2) inhibition of reuptake of catecholamines already released (eg, cocaine and tricyclic antidepressants). Some drugs have both direct and indirect actions. Both types of sympathomimetics, direct and indirect, ultimately cause activation of adrenoceptors, leading to some or all of the characteristic effects of catecholamines. The selectivity of different sympathomimetics for various types of adrenoceptors is discussed below.

I. BASIC PHARMACOLOGY OF SYMPATHOMIMETIC DRUGS

IDENTIFICATION OF ADRENOCEPTORS

The effort to understand the molecular mechanisms by which catecholamines act has a long and rich history. A great conceptual debt is owed to the work done by John Langley and Paul Ehrlich 100 years ago in developing the hypothesis that drugs have their effects by interacting with specific "receptive" substances. Raymond Ahlquist in 1948 rationalized a large body of observations by his conjecture that catecholamines acted via two principal receptors. He termed these receptors α and β. Alpha receptors are those that have the comparative potencies epinephrine $\geq$ norepinephrine $>>$ isoproterenol. Beta receptors have the comparative potencies isoproterenol $>$ epinephrine $\geq$ norepinephrine. Ahlquist's hypothesis was dramatically confirmed by the development of drugs that selectively antagonize β receptors but not α receptors (see Chapter 10). More recent evidence suggests that α receptors comprise two major families. At present, therefore, it appears appropriate to classify adrenoceptors into three major groups, namely, β, α_1, and α_2 receptors. Each of these major groups of receptors has also three subtypes.

A. Beta Adrenoceptors

Soon after the demonstration of separate α and β receptors, it was found that there were at least two *subtypes* of β receptors, designated β_1 and β_2. Beta$_1$ and β_2 Receptors are operationally defined by their affinities for epinephrine and norepinephrine: β_1 receptors have approximately equal affinity for epinephrine and norepinephrine, whereas β_2 receptors have a higher affinity for epinephrine than for norepinephrine. Subsequently, β_3 receptors were identified as a novel and distinct third β adrenoceptor subtype. Some of the properties of each of these receptor types are listed in Table 9–1.

B. Alpha Adrenoceptors

Following the demonstration of the β subtypes, it was found that there are two major groups of α receptors: α_1 and α_2. These receptors were originally identified with antagonist drugs that distinguished between α_1 and α_2 receptors. For example, α adrenoceptors were identified in a variety of tissues by measuring the binding of radiolabeled antagonist compounds that are considered to have a high affinity for these receptors, eg, dihydroergocryptine (α_1 and α_2), prazosin (α_1), and yohimbine (α_2). These radioligands were used to measure the num-

Table 9–1. Adrenoceptor types and subtypes.

Receptor	Agonist	Antagonist	Effects	Gene on Chromosome
α_1 **type**	Phenylephrine, methoxamine	Prazosin, corynanthine	$\uparrow IP_3$, DAG common to all	
α_{1A}		WB4101, prazosin		C5
α_{1B}		CEC (irreversible)		C8
α_{1D}		WB4101		
α_2 **type**		Rauwolscine, yohimbine	$\downarrow$ cAMP common to all	C20
α_{2A}	Clonidine, BHT920 Oxymetazoline		$\downarrow$ cAMP; $\uparrow K^+$ channels; $\downarrow Ca^{2+}$ channels	C10
α_{2B}		Prazosin	$\downarrow$ cAMP; $\downarrow Ca^{2+}$ channels	C2
α_{2C}		Prazosin	$\downarrow$ cAMP	C4
β **type**	Isoproterenol	Propranolol	$\uparrow$ cAMP common to all	
β_1	Dobutamine	Betaxolol	$\uparrow$ cAMP	C10
β_2	Procaterol, terbutaline	Butoxamine	$\uparrow$ cAMP	C5
β_3	BRL37344		$\uparrow$ cAMP	C8
Dopamine type	Dopamine			
D_1	Fenoldopam		$\uparrow$ cAMP	C5
D_2	Bromocriptine		$\downarrow$ cAMP; $\uparrow K^+$ channels; $\downarrow Ca^{2+}$ channels	C11
D_3	Quinpirol	AJ76	$\downarrow$ cAMP; $\uparrow K^+$ channels; $\uparrow Ca^{2+}$ channels	C3
D_4		Clozapine	$\downarrow$ cAMP	C11
D_5			$\uparrow$ cAMP	C4

Key: BRL37344 = Sodium-4-(2-[2-hydroxy-{3-chlorophenyl}ethylamino]propyl)phenoxyacetate
BHT920 = 6-Allyl-2-amino-5,6,7,8-tetrahydro-4*H*-thiazolo-[4,5-*d*]-azepine
CEC = Chloroethylclonidine
DAG = Diacylglycerol
IP_3 = Inositol trisphosphate
WB4101 = *N*-[2-(2,6-dimethoxyphenoxy)ethyl]-2,3-dihydro-1,4-benzodioxan-2-methanamine

ber of receptors in tissues and to determine the affinity (by displacement of the radiolabeled ligand) of other drugs that interact with the receptors.

The concept of subtypes *within* the α_1 group emerged out of pharmacologic experiments that demonstrated complex shapes of agonist dose-response curves of smooth muscle contraction as well as differences in antagonist affinities in inhibiting contractile responses in various tissues. These experiments demonstrated the existence of two subtypes of α_1 receptor that could be distinguished on the basis of their reversible affinities for a variety of drugs and experimental compounds. A third α_1 receptor subtype was subsequently identified by molecular cloning techniques. These α_1 receptors are termed α_{1A}, α_{1B}, and α_{1D} receptors. There is evidence that the α_{1A} receptor has splice variants. A major current area of investigation is determining the importance of each of these various subtypes in mediating α_1 receptor responses in a variety of organs.

The hypothesis that there are subtypes of α_2 receptors emerged from pharmacologic experiments and molecular cloning. It is now known that there are three subtypes of α_2 receptors, termed α_{2A}, α_{2B}, and α_{2C}, that are products of distinct genes.

C. DOPAMINE RECEPTORS

The endogenous catecholamine dopamine produces a variety of biologic effects that are mediated by interactions with specific dopamine receptors (Table 9–1). These receptors are distinct from α and β receptors and are particularly important in the brain (see Chapters 21 and 29) and in the splanchnic and renal vasculature. There is now considerable evidence for the existence of at least five subtypes of dopamine receptors. Pharmacologically distinct dopamine receptor subtypes, termed D_1 and D_2, have been known for some time. Molecular cloning has identified several distinct genes encoding each of these subtypes. Further complexity occurs because of the presence of introns within the coding region of the D_2-like receptor genes, which allows for alternative splicing of the exons in this major subtype. There is extensive polymorphic variation in the D_4 human receptor gene. The terminology of the various subtypes is D_1, D_2, D_3, D_4, and D_5. They comprise two D_1-like receptors (D_1 and D_5) and three D_2-like (D_2, D_3, and D_4). These subtypes may have importance for understanding the efficacy and adverse effects of novel antipsychotic drugs (see Chapter 29).

Receptor Selectivity

Examples of clinically useful sympathomimetic agonists that are relatively selective for α_1-, α_2-, and β-adrenoceptor subgroups are compared with some nonselective agents in Table 9–2. Selectivity means that a drug may

Table 9–2. Relative selectivity of adrenoceptor agonists.

	Relative Receptor Affinities
Alpha agonists	
Phenylephrine, methoxamine	$\alpha_1 > \alpha_2 >>>>> \beta$
Clonidine, methylnorepinephrine	$\alpha_2 > \alpha_1 >>>>> \beta$
Mixed alpha and beta agonists	
Norepinephrine	$\alpha_1 = \alpha_2; \beta_1 >> \beta_2$
Epinephrine	$\alpha_1 = \alpha_2; \beta_1 = \beta_2$
Beta agonists	
Dobutamine[1]	$\beta_1 > \beta_2 >>>> \alpha$
Isoproterenol	$\beta_1 = \beta_2 >>>> \alpha$
Terbutaline, metaproterenol, albuterol, ritodrine	$\beta_2 >> \beta_1 >>>> \alpha$
Dopamine agonists	
Dopamine	$D_1 = D_2 >> \beta >> \alpha$
Fenoldopam	$D_1 >> D_2$

[1]See text.

preferentially bind to one subgroup of receptors at concentrations too low to interact extensively with another subgroup. For example, norepinephrine preferentially activates β_1 receptors as compared with β_2 receptors. However, selectivity is not usually absolute (nearly absolute selectivity has been termed "specificity"), and at higher concentrations related classes of receptor may also interact with the drug. As a result, the "numeric" subclassification of adrenoceptors is clinically important mainly for drugs that have relatively marked selectivity. Given interpatient variations in drug kinetics and dynamics, the extent of a drug's selectivity should be kept in mind if this property is viewed as clinically important in the treatment of an individual patient.

The exact number of adrenoceptor subtypes that are actually expressed in human tissues is uncertain, but expression of subtypes has been demonstrated in tissues where the physiologic or pharmacologic importance of the subtype is not yet known. These results suggest the possibility of designing novel drugs to exploit the expression of a particular receptor subtype in a single target tissue. For example, determining which blood vessels express which subtypes of α_1 and α_2 receptors could lead to design of drugs having selectivity for certain vascular beds such as the splanchnic or coronary vessels. Similarly, there has been extensive investigation into the α_1 receptor subtypes mediating pharmacologic responses in the human prostate.

MOLECULAR MECHANISMS OF SYMPATHOMIMETIC ACTION

The effects of catecholamines are mediated by cell surface receptors. As described in Chapter 2, these receptors are coupled by G proteins to the various effector proteins whose activities are regulated by those receptors. Each G protein is a heterotrimer consisting of α, β, and γ subunits. G proteins are classified on the basis of their distinctive α subunits. G proteins of particular importance for adrenoceptor function include G_s, the stimulatory G protein of adenylyl cyclase; G_i, the inhibitory G protein of adenylyl cyclase; and G_q, the protein coupling α receptors to phospholipase C. The activation of G protein-coupled receptors by catecholamines promotes the dissociation of GDP from the α subunit of the appropriate G protein. GTP then binds to this G protein, and the α subunit dissociates from the β-γ unit. The activated GTP-bound α subunit then regulates the activity of its effector. Effectors of adrenoceptor-activated α subunits include adenylyl cyclase, cGMP phosphodiesterase, phospholipase C, and ion channels. The α subunit is inactivated by hydrolysis of the bound GTP to GDP and P_i, and the subsequent reassociation of the α subunit with the β-γ subunit. The β-γ subunits have additional independent effects, acting on a variety of effectors such as ion channels and enzymes.

Receptor Types

A. ALPHA RECEPTORS

Alpha$_1$ receptors stimulate polyphosphoinositide hydrolysis, leading to the formation of inositol 1,4,5-trisphosphate (IP_3) and diacylglycerol (DAG) (Figure 9–1). G proteins in the G_q family couple α_1 receptors to phospholipase C. IP_3 promotes the release of sequestered Ca^{2+} from intracellular stores, which increases the cytoplasmic concentration of free Ca^{2+} and the activation of various calcium-dependent protein kinases. Activation of these receptors may also increase influx of calcium across the cell's plasma membrane. Inositol 1,4,5-trisphosphate is sequentially dephosphorylated, which ultimately leads to the formation of free inositol. DAG activates protein kinase C that modulates activity of many signaling pathways. In addition, α_1 receptors activate signal transduction pathways that were originally described for peptide growth factor receptors which activate tyrosine kinases. For example, α_1 receptors have been found to activate mitogen-activated kinases (MAP kinases) and polyphosphoinositol-3-kinase (PI-3 kinase). These pathways may have importance for the α_1 receptor-mediated stimulation of cell growth and proliferation through the regulation of gene expression. The physiologic significance of this "cross talk" between major signaling pathways remains to be determined.

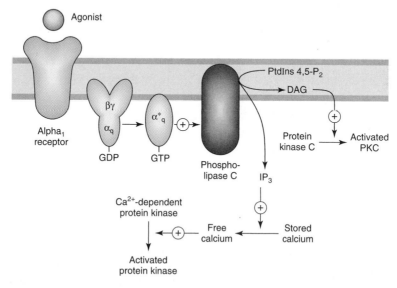

Figure 9–1. Activation of α_1 responses. Stimulation of α_1 receptors by catecholamines leads to the activation of a G_q coupling protein. The α subunit of this G protein activates the effector, phospholipase C, which leads to the release of IP_3 (inositol 1,4,5-trisphosphate) and DAG (diacylglycerol) from phosphatidylinositol 4,5-bisphosphate (PtdIns 4,5-P_2). IP_3 stimulates the release of sequestered stores of calcium, leading to an increased concentration of cytoplasmic Ca^{2+}. Ca^{2+} may then activate Ca^{2+}-dependent protein kinases, which in turn phosphorylate their substrates. DAG activates protein kinase C. See text for additional effects of α_1 receptor activation.

Alpha$_2$ receptors inhibit adenylyl cyclase activity and cause intracellular cAMP levels to decrease. In addition to this well-documented effect, activation of α_2-receptors utilize additional signaling pathways, including regulation of ion channel activities and the activities of important enzymes involved in signal transduction. Alpha$_2$-receptor–mediated inhibition of adenylyl cyclase activity is transduced by the inhibitory regulatory protein, G$_i$, which couples α_2 receptors to the inhibition of adenylyl cyclase (Figure 9–2). How the activation of G$_i$ leads to the inhibition of adenylyl cyclase is unclear, but it is likely that both α and the β-γ subunits of G$_i$ contribute to this response. In addition, some of the effects of α_2 adrenoceptors are independent of their ability to inhibit adenylyl cyclase; for example, α_2-receptor agonists cause platelet aggregation and a decrease in platelet cAMP levels, but it is not clear that aggregation is the result of the decrease in cAMP or other mechanisms involving G$_i$-regulated effectors.

B. Beta Receptors

The mechanism of action of β agonists has been studied in considerable detail. Activation of all three receptor subtypes (β_1, β_2, and β_3) results in activation of adenylyl cyclase and increased conversion of ATP to cAMP (Figure 9–2). Activation of the cyclase enzyme is mediated by the stimulatory coupling protein G$_s$. cAMP is the major second messenger of β-receptor activation. For example, in the liver of many species, β-receptor activation increases cAMP synthesis, which leads to a cascade of events culminating in the activation of glycogen phosphorylase. In the heart, β-receptor activation increases the influx of calcium across the cell membrane and its sequestration inside the cell. Beta-receptor activation also promotes the relaxation of smooth muscle. While the mechanism is uncertain, it may involve the phosphorylation of myosin light chain kinase to an inactive form (see Figure 12–1). Beta adrenoceptors may activate voltage-

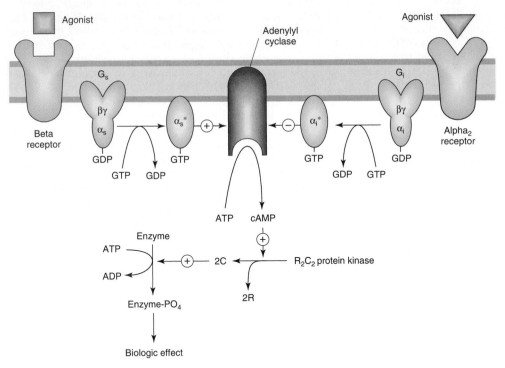

Figure 9–2. Activation and inhibition of adenylyl cyclase by agonists that bind to catecholamine receptors. Binding to β adrenoceptors stimulates adenylyl cyclase by activating the stimulatory G protein, G$_s$, which leads to the dissociation of its α subunit charged with GTP. This α_s subunit directly activates adenylyl cyclase, resulting in an increased rate of synthesis of cAMP. Alpha$_2$ adrenoceptor ligands inhibit adenylyl cyclase by causing dissociation of the inhibitory G protein, G$_i$, into its subunits; ie, an α_i subunit charged with GTP and a β-γ unit. The mechanism by which these subunits inhibit adenylyl cyclase is uncertain. cAMP binds to the regulatory subunit (R) of cAMP-dependent protein kinase, leading to the liberation of active catalytic subunits (C) that phosphorylate specific protein substrates and modify their activity. These catalytic units also phosphorylate the cAMP response element binding protein (CREB), which modifies gene expression. See text for other actions of β and α_2 adrenoceptors.

sensitive calcium channels in the heart via G_s-mediated enhancement independently of changes in cAMP concentration. Under certain circumstances, β_2 receptors may couple to G_i proteins. These receptors have been demonstrated to activate additional kinases, such as MAP kinases, by forming multi-subunit complexes, found within cells, containing multiple signaling molecules. In addition, recent evidence suggests that formation of dimers of β receptors themselves (both homodimers and heterodimers of β_1 and β_2 receptors) is importantly involved in their signaling mechanisms.

C. DOPAMINE RECEPTORS

The D_1 receptor is typically associated with the stimulation of adenylyl cyclase (Table 9–1); for example, D_1-receptor-induced smooth muscle relaxation is presumably due to cAMP accumulation in the smooth muscle of those vascular beds where dopamine is a vasodilator. D_2 receptors have been found to inhibit adenylyl cyclase activity, open potassium channels, and decrease calcium influx.

Receptor Regulation

Responses mediated by adrenoceptors are not fixed and static. The number and function of adrenoceptors on the cell surface and their responses may be regulated by catecholamines themselves, other hormones and drugs, age, and a number of disease states. These changes may modify the magnitude of a tissue's physiologic response to catecholamines and can be important clinically during the course of treatment. One of the best-studied examples of receptor regulation is the **desensitization** of adrenoceptors that may occur after exposure to catecholamines and other sympathomimetic drugs. After a cell or tissue has been exposed for a period of time to an agonist, that tissue often becomes less responsive to further stimulation by that agent. Other terms such as tolerance, refractoriness, and tachyphylaxis have also been used to denote desensitization. This process has potential clinical significance because it may limit the therapeutic response to sympathomimetic agents.

Many mechanisms have been found to contribute to desensitization. Operating at transcriptional, translational, and protein levels, some mechanisms function relatively slowly—over the course of hours or days. Other mechanisms of desensitization occur quickly, within minutes. Rapid modulation of receptor function in desensitized cells may involve critical covalent modification of the receptor, especially by phosphorylation on specific amino acid residues, association of these receptors with other proteins, or changes in their subcellular location.

There are two major categories of desensitization of responses mediated by G protein coupled receptors.

Homologous desensitization refers to loss of responsiveness exclusively of the receptors that have been exposed to repeated or sustained activation by a drug. *Heterologous* desensitization refers to loss of responsiveness of some cell surface receptors that have not been directly activated by the drug in question.

A major mechanism of desensitization that occurs rapidly involves phosphorylation of receptors by members of the G protein-coupled receptor kinase (GRK) family, of which there are at least seven members. Specific adrenoreceptors are substrates for these kinases only when they are bound to an agonist. This mechanism is an example of homologous desensitization since it specifically involves only agonist-occupied receptors.

Phosphorylation of these receptors enhances their affinity for β-arrestins; upon binding of a β-arrestin molecule, the capacity of the receptor to activate G proteins is blunted, presumably due to steric hindrance (see Figure 2–12). Arrestins constitute another large family of widely expressed proteins. Receptor phosphorylation followed by β-arrestin binding has been linked to subsequent endocytosis of the receptor. This response may be facilitated by the capacity of β-arrestins to bind to the structural protein clathrin. In addition to blunting responses requiring the presence of the receptor on the cell surface, these regulatory processes may also contribute to novel mechanisms of receptor signaling via intracellular pathways.

Receptor desensitization may also be mediated by second-messenger feedback. For example, β adrenoceptors stimulate cAMP accumulation, which leads to activation of protein kinase A; protein kinase A can phosphorylate residues on β receptors, resulting in inhibition of receptor function. For example, for the β_2 receptor, phosphorylation occurs on serine residues both in the third cytoplasmic loop and carboxyl terminal tail of the receptor. Similarly, activation of protein kinase C by G_q-coupled receptors may lead to phosphorylation of this class of G protein-coupled receptors. This second-messenger feedback mechanism has been termed *heterologous* desensitization because activated protein kinase A or protein kinase C may phosphorylate any structurally similar receptor with the appropriate consensus sites for phosphorylation by these enzymes.

ADRENORECEPTOR POLYMORPHISMS

Since elucidation of the sequences of the genes encoding the α_1, α_2, and β subtypes of adrenoceptors, it has become clear that there are relatively common genetic polymorphisms for many of these receptor subtypes in humans. Some of these may lead to changes in critical amino acid sequences that have pharmacologic importance. There is evidence that some of these polymorphisms may change the susceptibility to diseases such as heart failure, alter the propensity of a receptor to desensitize, and alter therapeutic responses to drugs in diseases such as asthma.

CHEMISTRY & PHARMACOKINETICS OF SYMPATHOMIMETIC DRUGS

Phenylethylamine may be considered the parent compound from which sympathomimetic drugs are derived (Figure 9–3). This compound consists of a benzene ring with an ethylamine side chain. Substitutions may be made (1) on the terminal amino group, (2) on the benzene ring, and (3) on the α or β carbons. Substitution by –OH groups at the 3 and 4 positions yields sympathomimetic drugs collectively known as catecholamines. The effects of modification of phenylethylamine are to change the affinity of the drugs for α and β receptors as well as to influence the intrinsic ability to activate the receptors. In addition, chemical structure determines the pharmacokinetic properties of these molecules. Sympathomimetic drugs may activate both α and β receptors; however, the relative α-receptor versus β-receptor activity spans the range from almost pure α activity (methoxamine) to almost pure β activity (isoproterenol).

A. SUBSTITUTION ON THE AMINO GROUP

Increasing the size of alkyl substituents on the amino group tends to increase β-receptor activity. For example, methyl substitution on norepinephrine, yielding epi-

nephrine, enhances activity at β_2 receptors. Beta activity is further enhanced with isopropyl substitution at the amino nitrogen (isoproterenol). Beta$_2$-selective agonists generally require a large amino substituent group. The larger the substituent on the amino group, the lower the activity at α receptors; eg, isoproterenol is very weak at α receptors.

B. SUBSTITUTION ON THE BENZENE RING

Maximal α and β activity are found with catecholamines (drugs having –OH groups at the 3 and 4 positions). The absence of one or the other of these groups, particularly the hydroxyl at C_3, without other substitutions on the ring may dramatically reduce the potency of the drugs. For example, phenylephrine (Figure 9–4) is much less potent than epinephrine; indeed, α receptor affinity is decreased about 100-fold and β activity is almost negligible except at very high concentrations. However, catecholamines are subject to inactivation by catechol-*O*-methyltransferase (COMT), an enzyme found in gut and liver (see Chapter 6). Therefore, absence of one or both –OH groups on the phenyl ring increases the bioavailability after oral administration and prolongs the duration of action. Furthermore, absence of ring –OH groups tends to increase the distribution of the molecule to the central nervous system. For example, ephedrine and amphetamine (Figure 9–4) are orally active, have a prolonged duration of action, and produce central nervous system effects not typically observed with the catecholamines.

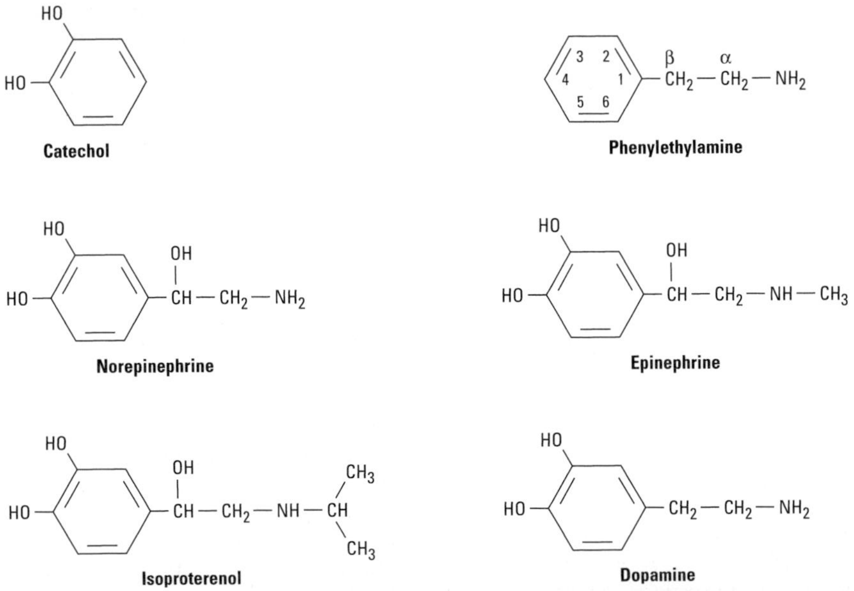

Figure 9–3. Phenylethylamine and some important catecholamines. Catechol is shown for reference.

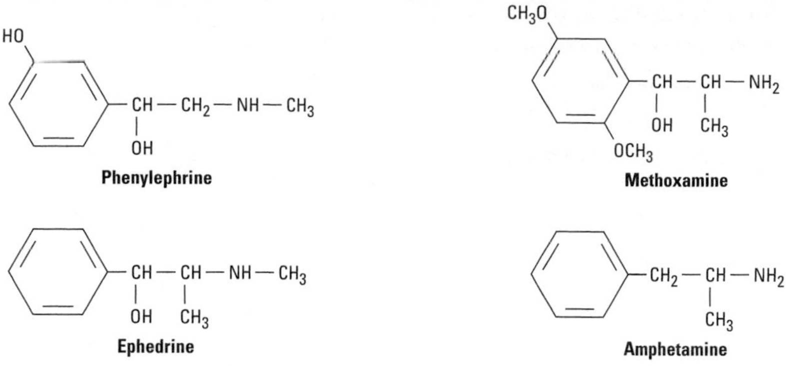

Figure 9–4. Some examples of noncatecholamine sympathomimetic drugs.

C. Substitution on the Alpha Carbon

Substitutions at the α carbon block oxidation by monoamine oxidase (MAO) and prolong the action of such drugs, particularly the noncatecholamines. Ephedrine and amphetamine are examples of α-substituted compounds (Figure 9–4). Alpha-methyl compounds are also called phenylisopropylamines. In addition to their resistance to oxidation by MAO, some phenylisopropylamines have an enhanced ability to displace catecholamines from storage sites in noradrenergic nerves. Therefore, a portion of their activity is dependent upon the presence of normal norepinephrine stores in the body; they are indirectly acting sympathomimetics.

D. Substitution on the Beta Carbon

Direct-acting agonists typically have a β-hydroxyl group, though dopamine does not. In addition to activating adrenoceptors, this hydroxyl group may be important for storage of sympathomimetic amines in neural vesicles.

ORGAN SYSTEM EFFECTS OF SYMPATHOMIMETIC DRUGS

General outlines of the cellular actions of sympathomimetics are presented in Tables 6–3 and 9–3. The net effect of a given drug in the intact organism depends on its relative receptor affinity (α or β), intrinsic activity, and the compensatory reflexes evoked by its direct actions.

Cardiovascular System

A. Blood Vessels

Vascular smooth muscle tone is regulated by adrenoceptors; consequently, catecholamines are important in controlling peripheral vascular resistance and venous capacitance. Alpha receptors increase arterial resistance, whereas β_2 receptors promote smooth muscle relaxation. There are major differences in receptor types in the various vascular beds (Table 9–4). The skin vessels have predominantly α receptors and constrict in the presence of epinephrine and norepinephrine, as do the splanchnic vessels. Vessels in skeletal muscle may constrict or dilate depending on whether α or β receptors are activated. Consequently, the overall effects of a sympathomimetic drug on blood vessels depend on the relative activities of that drug at α and β receptors and the anatomic sites of the vessels affected. In addition, D_1 receptors promote vasodilation of renal, splanchnic, coronary, cerebral, and perhaps other resistance vessels. Activation of the D_1 receptors in the renal vasculature may play a major role in the natriuresis induced by pharmacologic administration of dopamine.

B. Heart

Direct effects on the heart are determined largely by β_1 receptors, although β_2 and to a lesser extent α receptors are also involved. Beta-receptor activation results in increased calcium influx in cardiac cells. This has both electrical (Figure 9–5) and mechanical consequences. Pacemaker activity, both normal (sinoatrial node) and abnormal (eg, Purkinje fibers), is increased (positive chronotropic effect). Conduction velocity in the atrioventricular node is increased, and the refractory period is decreased. Intrinsic contractility is increased (positive inotropic effect), and relaxation is accelerated. As a result, the twitch response of isolated cardiac muscle is increased in tension but abbreviated in duration. In the intact heart, intraventricular pressure rises and falls more rapidly, and ejection time is decreased. These direct effects are easily demonstrated in the absence of reflexes evoked by changes in blood pressure, eg, in isolated myocardial preparations and in patients with ganglionic blockade. In the presence of normal reflex activ-

Table 9–3. Distribution of adrenoceptor subtypes.

Type	Tissue	Actions
α_1	Most vascular smooth muscle (innervated)	Contraction
	Pupillary dilator muscle	Contraction (dilates pupil)
	Pilomotor smooth muscle	Erects hair
	Prostate	Contraction
	Heart	Increases force of contraction
α_2	Postsynaptic CNS adrenoceptors	Probably multiple
	Platelets	Aggregation
	Adrenergic and cholinergic nerve terminals	Inhibition of transmitter release
	Some vascular smooth muscle	Contraction
	Fat cells	Inhibition of lipolysis
β_1	Heart	Increases force and rate of contraction
β_2	Respiratory, uterine, and vascular smooth muscle	Promotes smooth muscle relaxation
	Skeletal muscle	Promotes potassium uptake
	Human liver	Activates glycogenolysis
β_3	Fat cells	Activates lipolysis
D_1	Smooth muscle	Dilates renal blood vessels
D_2	Nerve endings	Modulates transmitter release

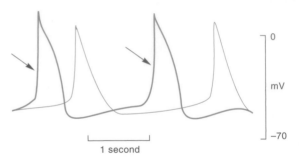

Figure 9–5. Effect of epinephrine on the transmembrane potential of a pacemaker cell in the frog heart. The arrowed trace was recorded after the addition of epinephrine. Note the increased slope of diastolic depolarization and decreased interval between action potentials. This pacemaker acceleration is typical of β_1-stimulant drugs. (Modified and reproduced, with permission, from Brown H, Giles W, Noble S: Membrane currents underlying rhythmic activity in frog sinus venosus. In: *The Sinus Node: Structure, Function, and Clinical Relevance.* Bonke FIM [editor]. Martinus Nijhoff, 1978.)

ity, the direct effects on heart rate may be dominated by a reflex response to blood pressure changes. Physiologic stimulation of the heart by catecholamines tends to increase coronary blood flow.

C. BLOOD PRESSURE

The effects of sympathomimetic drugs on blood pressure can be explained on the basis of their effects on the heart, the peripheral vascular resistance, and the venous return (see Figure 6–7 and Table 9–4). A relatively pure α agonist such as phenylephrine increases peripheral arterial resistance and decreases venous capacitance. The enhanced arterial resistance usually leads to a dose-dependent rise in blood pressure (Figure 9–6). In the presence of normal cardiovascular reflexes, the rise in blood pressure elicits a baroreceptor-mediated increase in vagal tone with slowing of the heart rate, which may be quite marked. However, cardiac output may not diminish in proportion to this reduction in rate, since increased venous return may increase stroke volume; furthermore, direct α-adrenoceptor stimulation of the heart may have a modest positive inotropic action. While these are the expected effects of pure α agonists in normal subjects, their use in hypotensive patients usually does not lead to brisk reflex responses because in this situation blood pressure is returning to normal, not exceeding normal.

The blood pressure response to a pure β-adrenoceptor agonist is quite different. Stimulation of β receptors in the heart increases cardiac output. A relatively pure β agonist such as isoproterenol also decreases peripheral resistance by activating β_2 receptors, leading to vasodilation in certain vascular beds (Table 9–4). The net effect is to maintain or slightly increase systolic pressure while permitting a fall in diastolic pressure owing to enhanced diastolic runoff (Figure 9–6). The actions of drugs with both α and β effects (eg, epinephrine and norepinephrine) are discussed below.

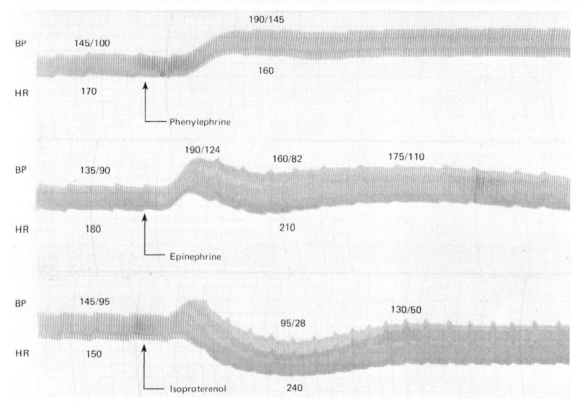

Figure 9–6. Effects of an α-selective (phenylephrine), β-selective (isoproterenol), and nonselective (epinephrine) sympathomimetic, given as an intravenous bolus injection to a dog. (BP, blood pressure; HR, heart rate.) Reflexes are blunted but not eliminated in this anesthetized animal.

Eye

The radial pupillary dilator muscle of the iris contains α receptors; activation by drugs such as phenylephrine causes mydriasis (Figure 6–9). Alpha and β stimulants also have important effects on intraocular pressure. Present evidence suggests that α agonists increase the outflow of aqueous humor from the eye, while β antagonists decrease the production of aqueous humor. These effects are important in the treatment of glaucoma (see Chapter 10), a leading cause of blindness. Beta stimulants relax the ciliary muscle to a minor degree, causing an insignificant decrease in accommodation. In addition, adrenergic drugs may directly protect neuronal cells in the retina.

Respiratory Tract

Bronchial smooth muscle contains β_2 receptors that cause relaxation. Activation of these receptors results in bronchodilation (see Chapter 20 and Table 9–3). The

blood vessels of the upper respiratory tract mucosa contain α receptors; the decongestant action of adrenoceptor stimulants is clinically useful (see Clinical Pharmacology).

Gastrointestinal Tract

Relaxation of gastrointestinal smooth muscle can be brought about by both α- and β-stimulant agents. Beta receptors appear to be located directly on the smooth muscle cells and mediate relaxation via hyperpolarization and decreased spike activity in these cells. Alpha stimulants, especially α_2-selective agonists, decrease muscle activity *indirectly* by presynaptically reducing the release of acetylcholine and possibly other stimulants within the enteric nervous system (see Chapter 6). The α-receptor-mediated response is probably of greater pharmacologic significance than the β-stimulant response. Alpha$_2$ receptors may also decrease salt and water flux into the lumen of the intestine.

Table 9–4. Cardiovascular responses to sympathomimetic amines.[1]

	Phenyl-ephrine	Epi-nephrine	Isopro-terenol
Vascular resistance (tone)			
Cutaneous, mucous membranes (α)	↑↑	↑↑	0
Skeletal muscle (β_2, α)	↑	↓ or ↑	↓↓
Renal (α, β)	↑	↑	↓
Splanchnic (α)	↑↑	↓ or ↑[2]	↓
Total peripheral resistance	↑↑↑	↓ or ↑[2]	↓↓
Venous tone (α, β)	↑	↑	↓
Cardiac			
Contractility (β_1)	0 or ↑	↑↑↑	↑↑↑
Heart rate (predominantly β_1)	↓↓ (vagal reflex)	↑ or ↓	↑↑↑
Stroke volume	0, ↓, ↑	↑	↑
Cardiac output	↓	↑	↑↑
Blood pressure			
Mean	↑↑	↑	↓
Diastolic	↑↑	↓ or ↑[2]	↓↓
Systolic	↑↑	↑↑	0 or ↓
Pulse pressure	0	↑↑	↑↑

[1]↑ = increase; ↓ = decrease; 0 = no change.

[2]Small doses decrease, large doses increase.

Genitourinary Tract

The human uterus contains α and β_2 receptors. The fact that the β receptors mediate relaxation may be clinically useful in pregnancy (see Clinical Pharmacology). The bladder base, urethral sphincter, and prostate contain α receptors that mediate contraction and therefore promote urinary continence. The specific subtype of α_1 receptor involved in mediating constriction of the bladder base and prostate is uncertain, but α_{1A} receptors probably play an important role. The β_2 receptors of the bladder wall mediate relaxation. Ejaculation depends upon normal α-receptor (and possibly purinergic receptor) activation in the ductus deferens, seminal vesicles, and prostate. The detumescence of erectile tissue that normally follows ejaculation is also brought about by norepinephrine (and possibly neuropeptide Y) released from sympathetic nerves. Alpha activation appears to have a similar detumescent effect on erectile tissue in female animals.

Exocrine Glands

The salivary glands contain adrenoceptors that regulate the secretion of amylase and water. However, certain sympathomimetic drugs, eg, clonidine, produce symptoms of dry mouth. The mechanism of this effect is uncertain; it is likely that central nervous system effects are responsible, though peripheral effects may contribute.

The apocrine sweat glands, located on the palms of the hands and a few other areas, respond to adrenoceptor stimulants with increased sweat production. These are the apocrine nonthermoregulatory glands usually associated with psychologic stress. (The diffusely distributed thermoregulatory eccrine sweat glands are regulated by *sympathetic cholinergic* postganglionic nerves that activate muscarinic cholinoceptors; see Chapter 6.)

Metabolic Effects

Sympathomimetic drugs have important effects on intermediary metabolism. Activation of β adrenoceptors in fat cells leads to increased lipolysis with enhanced release of free fatty acids and glycerol into the blood. Beta$_3$ adrenoceptors play a role in mediating this response. There is considerable interest in developing β_3 receptor-selective agonists, which could be useful in some metabolic disorders. Human lipocytes also contain α_2 receptors that inhibit lipolysis by decreasing intracellular cAMP. Sympathomimetic drugs enhance glycogenolysis in the liver, which leads to increased glucose release into the circulation. In the human liver, the effects of catecholamines are probably mediated mainly by β receptors, though α_1 receptors may also play a role. Catecholamines in high concentration may also cause metabolic acidosis. Activation of β_2 adrenoceptors by endogenous epinephrine or by sympathomimetic drugs promotes the uptake of potassium into cells, leading to a fall in extracellular potassium. This may lead to a fall in the plasma potassium concentration during stress or protect against a rise in plasma potassium during exercise. Blockade of these receptors may accentuate the rise in plasma potassium that occurs during exercise. Beta receptors and α_2 receptors that are expressed in pancreatic islets tend to increase and decrease, respectively, insulin secretion, although the major regulator of insulin release is the plasma concentration of glucose.

Effects on Endocrine Function & Leukocytosis

Catecholamines are important endogenous regulators of hormone secretion from a number of glands. As mentioned above, insulin secretion is stimulated by β receptors and inhibited by α_2 receptors. Similarly, renin secretion is stimulated by β_1 and inhibited by α_2 receptors; indeed, β-receptor antagonist drugs may lower plasma renin and blood pressure in patients with hypertension at least in part by this mechanism. Adrenoceptors also modulate the secretion of parathyroid hormone, calcitonin, thyroxine, and gastrin; however, the physiologic significance of these control mechanisms is probably limited. In high concentrations, epinephrine and related agents cause leukocytosis, in part by promoting demargination of white blood cells sequestered away from the general circulation.

Effects on the Central Nervous System

The action of sympathomimetics on the central nervous system varies dramatically, depending on their ability to cross the blood-brain barrier. The catecholamines are almost completely excluded by this barrier, and subjective central nervous system effects are noted only at the highest rates of infusion. These effects have been described as ranging from "nervousness" to "a feeling of impending disaster," sensations that are undesirable. Furthermore, peripheral effects of β adrenoceptor agonists such as tachycardia and tremor are similar to the somatic manifestations of anxiety. In contrast, noncatecholamines with indirect actions, such as amphetamines, which readily enter the central nervous system from the circulation, produce qualitatively very different central nervous system effects. These actions vary from mild alerting, with improved attention to boring tasks; through elevation of mood, insomnia, euphoria, and anorexia; to full-blown psychotic behavior. These effects are not readily assigned to either α- or β-mediated actions and may represent enhancement of dopamine-mediated processes or other effects of these drugs in the central nervous system.

SPECIFIC SYMPATHOMIMETIC DRUGS

Catecholamines

Epinephrine (adrenaline) is a very potent vasoconstrictor and cardiac stimulant. The rise in systolic blood pressure that occurs after epinephrine release or administration is caused by its positive inotropic and chronotropic actions on the heart (predominantly β_1 receptors) and the vasoconstriction induced in many vascular beds (α receptors). Epinephrine also activates β_2 receptors in some vessels (eg, skeletal muscle blood vessels), leading to their dilation. Consequently, total peripheral resistance may actually fall, explaining the fall in diastolic pressure that is sometimes seen with epinephrine injection (Figure 9–6; Table 9–4). Activation of these β_2 receptors in skeletal muscle contributes to increased blood flow during exercise. Under physiologic conditions, epinephrine functions largely as a hormone; after release from the adrenal medulla into the blood, it acts on distant cells.

Norepinephrine (levarterenol, noradrenaline) and epinephrine have similar effects on β_1 receptors in the heart and similar potency at α receptors. Norepinephrine has relatively little effect on β_2 receptors. Consequently, norepinephrine increases peripheral resistance and both diastolic and systolic blood pressure. Compensatory vagal reflexes tend to overcome the direct positive chronotropic effects of norepinephrine; however, the positive inotropic effects on the heart are maintained (Table 9–4).

Isoproterenol (isoprenaline) is a very potent β-receptor agonist and has little effect on α receptors. The drug has positive chronotropic and inotropic actions; because isoproterenol activates β receptors almost exclusively, it is a potent vasodilator. These actions lead to a marked increase in cardiac output associated with a fall in diastolic and mean arterial pressure and a lesser decrease or a slight increase in systolic pressure (Table 9–4; Figure 9–6).

Dopamine, the immediate metabolic precursor of norepinephrine, activates D_1 receptors in several vascular beds, which leads to vasodilation. The effect this has on renal blood flow may be of clinical value, though this is uncertain. The activation of presynaptic D_2 receptors, which suppress norepinephrine release, contributes to these effects to an unknown extent. In addition, dopamine activates β_1 receptors in the heart. At low doses, peripheral resistance may decrease. At higher rates of infusion, dopamine activates vascular α receptors, leading to vasoconstriction, including in the renal vascular bed. Consequently, high rates of infusion of dopamine may mimic the actions of epinephrine.

Fenoldopam is a D_1 receptor agonist that selectively leads to peripheral vasodilation in some vascular beds. The primary indication for fenoldopam is as an intravenously administered drug for the treatment of severe hypertension (Chapter 11). Continuous infusions of the drug have prompt effects on blood pressure.

Dopamine agonists with central actions are of considerable value for the treatment of Parkinson's disease and prolactinemia. These agents are discussed in Chapters 28 and 37.

Dobutamine is a relatively β_1-selective synthetic catecholamine. As discussed below, dobutamine also activates α_1 receptors.

Other Sympathomimetics

These agents are of interest because of pharmacokinetic features (oral activity, distribution to the central nervous system) or because of relative selectivity for specific receptor subclasses.

Phenylephrine was previously described as an example of a relatively pure α agonist (Table 9–2). It acts directly on the receptors. Because it is not a catechol derivative (Figure 9–4), it is not inactivated by COMT and has a much longer duration of action than the catecholamines. It is an effective mydriatic and decongestant and can be used to raise the blood pressure (Figure 9–6).

Methoxamine acts pharmacologically like phenylephrine, since it is predominantly a direct-acting α_1-receptor agonist. It may cause a prolonged increase in blood pressure due to vasoconstriction; it also causes a vagally mediated bradycardia. Methoxamine is available for parenteral use, but clinical applications are rare and limited to hypotensive states.

Midodrine is a prodrug that is enzymatically hydrolyzed to desglymidodrine, an α_1 receptor-selective agonist. The peak concentration of desglymidodrine is achieved about 1 hour after midodrine is administered. The primary indication for midodrine is the treatment of postural hypotension, typically due to impaired autonomic nervous system function. While the drug has efficacy in diminishing the fall of blood pressure when the patient is standing, it may cause hypertension when the subject is supine.

Ephedrine occurs in various plants and has been used in China for over 2000 years; it was introduced into Western medicine in 1924 as the first orally active sympathomimetic drug. It is found in Ma-huang, a popular herbal medication (see Chapter 65). Ma-huang contains multiple ephedrine-like alkaloids in addition to ephedrine. Because ephedrine is a noncatechol phenylisopropylamine (Figure 9–4), it has high bioavailability and a relatively long duration of action—hours rather than minutes. As is the case with many other phenylisopropylamines, a significant fraction of the drug is excreted unchanged in the urine. Since it is a weak base, its excretion can be accelerated by acidification of the urine.

Ephedrine has not been extensively studied in humans in spite of its long history of use. Its ability to activate β receptors probably accounted for its earlier use in asthma. Because it gains access to the central nervous system, it is a mild stimulant. Ingestion of ephedrine alkaloids contained in Ma-huang has raised important safety concerns. Pseudoephedrine, one of four ephedrine enantiomers, is available over the counter as a component of many decongestant mixtures.

Xylometazoline and **oxymetazoline** are direct-acting α agonists. These drugs have been used as topical decongestants because of their ability to promote constriction of the nasal mucosa. When taken in large doses, oxymetazoline may cause hypotension, presumably because of a central clonidine-like effect (Chapter 11). (As noted in Table 9–1, oxymetazoline has significant affinity for α_{2A} receptors.)

Amphetamine is a phenylisopropylamine (Figure 9–4) that is important chiefly because of its use and misuse as a central nervous system stimulant (see Chapter 32). Its pharmacokinetics are similar to those of ephedrine; however, amphetamine very readily enters the central nervous system, where it has marked stimulant effects on mood and alertness and a depressant effect on appetite. Its peripheral actions are mediated primarily through the release of catecholamines. **Methamphetamine** (N-methylamphetamine) is very similar to amphetamine with an even higher ratio of central to peripheral actions. **Phenmetrazine** (see Figure 32–1) is a variant phenylisopropylamine with amphetamine-like effects. It has been promoted as an anorexiant and is also a popular drug of abuse. **Methylphenidate** and **pemoline** are amphetamine variants whose major pharmacologic effects and abuse potential are similar to those of amphetamine. These two drugs appear to have efficacy in some children with attention deficit hyperactivity disorder (see Clinical Pharmacology). Pemoline must be used with great caution because of an association with life-threatening hepatic failure. **Modafinil** is a new drug with both similarities to and differences from amphetamine. It has significant effects on central α_{1B} receptors but in addition appears to affect GABAergic, glutaminergic, and serotonergic synapses (see Clinical Pharmacology). **Phenylpropanolamine** (PPA) is a sympathomimetic drug that for many years was used as an over-the-counter agent in numerous weight reduction and cold medications. It has been withdrawn from over-the-counter use in the USA because of concerns regarding an association with hemorrhagic stroke.

Receptor-Selective Sympathomimetic Drugs

Alpha$_2$-selective agonists have an important ability to decrease blood pressure through actions in the central nervous system even though direct application to a blood vessel may cause vasoconstriction. Such drugs (eg, clonidine, methyldopa, guanfacine, guanabenz) are useful in the treatment of hypertension (and some other conditions) and are discussed in Chapter 11. **Dexmedetomidine** is a centrally acting α_2-selective agonist that is indicated for sedation of initially intubated and mechanically ventilated patients during treatment in an intensive care setting.

Beta-selective agonists are very important because of the separation of β_1 and β_2 effects that has been achieved (Table 9–2). Although this separation is incomplete, it is sufficient to reduce adverse effects in several clinical applications.

Beta$_1$-selective agents include dobutamine and a partial agonist, prenalterol (Figure 9–7). Because they are less effective in activating vasodilator β_2 receptors, they may increase cardiac output with less reflex tachycardia

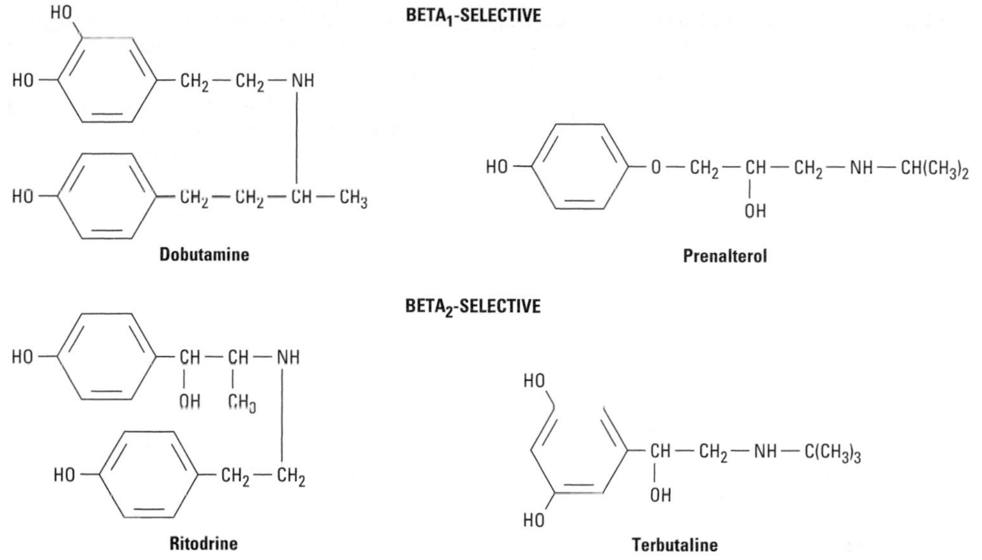

BETA₁-SELECTIVE

Dobutamine

Prenalterol

BETA₂-SELECTIVE

Ritodrine

Terbutaline

Figure 9–7. Examples of β_1- and β_2-selective agonists.

than occurs with nonselective β agonists such as isoproterenol. Dobutamine consists of two isomers, administered as a racemic mixture. The (+) isomer is a potent β_1 agonist and an α_1 receptor antagonist. The (–) isomer is a potent α_1 agonist, capable of causing significant vasoconstriction when given alone. This action tends to reduce vasodilation and may also contribute to the positive inotropic action caused by the isomer with predominantly β-receptor activity. A major limitation with these drugs—as with other direct-acting sympathomimetic agents—is that tolerance to their effects may develop with prolonged use and the likelihood that chronic cardiac stimulation in patients with heart failure may worsen long-term outcome.

Beta₂-selective agents have achieved an important place in the treatment of asthma and are discussed in Chapter 20. An additional application is to achieve uterine relaxation in premature labor (ritodrine; see below). Some examples of β_2-selective drugs currently in use are shown in Figures 9–7 and 20–4; many more are available or under investigation.

Special Sympathomimetics

Cocaine is a local anesthetic with a peripheral sympathomimetic action that results from inhibition of transmitter reuptake at noradrenergic synapses (see Chapter 6). It readily enters the central nervous system and produces an amphetamine-like effect that is shorter lasting and more intense. The major action of cocaine in the central

nervous system is to inhibit dopamine reuptake into neurons in the "pleasure centers" of the brain. These properties and the fact that it can be smoked, "snorted" into the nose, or injected for rapid onset of effect have made it a heavily abused drug (see Chapter 32). Interestingly, dopamine-transporter knockout mice still self-administer cocaine, suggesting that cocaine may have additional pharmacologic targets.

Tyramine (see Figure 6–5) is a normal by-product of tyrosine metabolism in the body and is also found in high concentrations in fermented foods such as cheese (Table 9–5). It is readily metabolized by MAO in the liver and is normally inactive when taken orally because of a very high first-pass effect, ie, low bioavailability. If administered parenterally, it has an indirect sympathomimetic action caused by the release of stored catecholamines. Consequently, its spectrum of action is similar to that of norepinephrine. In patients treated with MAO inhibitors—particularly inhibitors of the MAO-A isoform—this effect of tyramine may be greatly intensified, leading to marked increases in blood pressure. This occurs on account of increased bioavailability of tyramine and increased neuronal stores of catecholamines. Patients taking MAO inhibitors must be very careful to avoid tyramine-containing foods. There are differences in the effects of various MAO inhibitors on tyramine bioavailability, and isoform-specific or reversible enzyme antagonists may be safer (see Chapters 28 and 30).

Table 9–5. Foods reputed to have a high content of tyramine or other sympathomimetic agents. In a patient taking an irreversible MAO inhibitor drug, 20–50 mg of tyramine in a meal may increase the blood pressure significantly (see also Chapter 30). Note that only cheese, sausage, pickled fish, and yeast supplements contain sufficient tyramine to be consistently dangerous. This does not rule out the possibility that some preparations of other foods might contain significantly greater than average amounts of tyramine.

Food	Tyramine Content of an Average Serving
Beer	(No data)
Broad beans, fava beans	Negligible (but contains dopamine)
Cheese, natural or aged	Nil to 130 mg (Cheddar, Gruyère, and Stilton especially high)
Chicken liver	Nil to 9 mg
Chocolate	Negligible (but contains phenylethylamine)
Sausage, fermented (eg, salami, pepperoni, summer sausage)	Nil to 74 mg
Smoked or pickled fish (eg, pickled herring)	Nil to 198 mg
Snails	(No data)
Wine (red)	Nil to 3 mg
Yeast (eg, dietary brewer's yeast supplements)	2–68 mg

II. CLINICAL PHARMACOLOGY OF SYMPATHOMIMETIC DRUGS

The rationale for the use of sympathomimetic drugs in therapy rests on a knowledge of the physiologic effects of catecholamines on tissues. Selection of a particular sympathomimetic drug from the host of compounds available depends upon such factors as whether activation of α, β_1, or β_2 receptors is desired; the duration of action desired; and the preferred route of administration. Sympathomimetic drugs are very potent and can have profound effects on a variety of organ systems, particularly the heart and peripheral circulation. Therefore, great caution is indicated when these agents are used parenterally. In most cases, rather than using fixed doses of the drugs, careful monitoring of pharmacologic response is required to determine the appropriate dosage, especially if the drug is being infused. Generally, it is desirable to use the minimum dose required to achieve the desired response. The adverse effects of these drugs are generally understandable in terms of their known physiologic effects.

Cardiovascular Applications

A. CONDITIONS IN WHICH BLOOD FLOW OR PRESSURE IS TO BE ENHANCED

Hypotension may occur in a variety of settings such as decreased blood volume, cardiac arrhythmias, neurologic disease, adverse reactions to medications such as antihypertensive drugs, and infection. If cerebral, renal, and cardiac perfusion is maintained, hypotension itself does not usually require vigorous direct treatment. Rather, placing the patient in the recumbent position and ensuring adequate fluid volume—while the primary problem is determined and treated—is usually the correct course of action. The use of sympathomimetic drugs merely to elevate a blood pressure that is not an immediate threat to the patient may increase morbidity (see Toxicity of Sympathomimetic Drugs, below). Sympathomimetic drugs may be used in a hypotensive emergency to preserve cerebral and coronary blood flow. Such situations might arise in severe hemorrhage, spinal cord injury, or overdoses of antihypertensive or central nervous system depressant medications. The treatment is usually of short duration while the appropriate intravenous fluid or blood is being administered. Direct-acting α agonists such as norepinephrine, phenylephrine, or methoxamine have been utilized in this setting if vasoconstriction is desired. For the treatment of chronic orthostatic hypotension, oral ephedrine has been the traditional therapy. Midodrine, an orally active α agonist, may be the preferred sympathomimetic in this application if further studies confirm its long-term safety and efficacy.

Shock is a complex acute cardiovascular syndrome that results in a critical reduction in perfusion of vital tissues and a wide range of systemic effects. Shock is usually associated with hypotension, an altered mental state, oliguria, and metabolic acidosis. If untreated, shock usually progresses to a refractory deteriorating state and death. The three major mechanisms responsible for shock are hypovolemia, cardiac insufficiency, and altered vascular resistance. Volume replacement and treatment of the underlying disease are the mainstays of the treatment of shock. While sympathomimetic drugs have been used in the treatment of virtually all forms of shock, their efficacy is unclear. In most forms of shock, vasoconstriction mediated by the sympathetic nervous system is already intense. Indeed, efforts aimed at reducing rather than increasing peripheral resistance may be more fruitful if cerebral, coronary, and renal perfusion are improved. A decision to use vasoconstrictors or vasodilators is best made on the basis of information about the underlying cause, which may require invasive monitoring.

Cardiogenic shock, usually due to massive myocardial infarction, has a poor prognosis. Mechanically assisted perfusion and emergency cardiac surgery have been utilized in some settings. Optimal fluid replacement requires monitoring of pulmonary capillary wedge pressure and other parameters of cardiac function. Positive inotropic agents such as dopamine or dobutamine may have a role in this situation. In low to moderate doses, these drugs may increase cardiac output and, compared with norepinephrine, cause relatively little peripheral vasoconstriction. Isoproterenol increases heart rate and work more than either dopamine or dobutamine. See Chapter 13 and Table 13–6 for a discussion of shock associated with myocardial infarction.

Unfortunately, the patient with shock may not respond to any of these therapeutic maneuvers; the temptation is then great to use vasoconstrictors to maintain adequate blood pressure. While coronary perfusion may be improved, this gain may be offset by increased myocardial oxygen demands as well as more severe vasoconstriction in blood vessels to the abdominal viscera. Therefore, the goal of therapy in shock should be to optimize tissue perfusion, not blood pressure.

B. Conditions in Which Blood Flow Is to Be Reduced

Reduction of regional blood flow is desirable for achieving hemostasis in surgery, for reducing diffusion of local anesthetics away from the site of administration, and for reducing mucous membrane congestion. In each instance, α-receptor activation is desired, and the choice of agent depends upon the maximal efficacy required, the desired duration of action, and the route of administration.

Effective pharmacologic hemostasis, often necessary for facial, oral, and nasopharyngeal surgery, requires drugs of high efficacy that can be administered in high concentration by local application. Epinephrine is usually applied topically in nasal packs (for epistaxis) or in a gingival string (for gingivectomy). **Cocaine** is still sometimes used for nasopharyngeal surgery, because it combines a hemostatic effect with local anesthesia. Occasionally, cocaine is mixed with epinephrine for maximum hemostasis and local anesthesia.

Combining α agonists with some local anesthetics greatly prolongs the duration of infiltration nerve block; the total dose of local anesthetic (and the probability of toxicity) can therefore be reduced. **Epinephrine,** 1:200,000, is the favored agent for this application, but norepinephrine, phenylephrine, and other α agonists have also been used. Systemic effects on the heart and peripheral vasculature may occur even with local drug administration.

Mucous membrane decongestants are α agonists that reduce the discomfort of hay fever and, to a lesser extent, the common cold by decreasing the volume of the nasal mucosa. These effects are probably mediated by α_1 receptors. Unfortunately, rebound hyperemia may follow the use of these agents, and repeated topical use of high drug concentrations may result in ischemic changes in the mucous membranes, probably as a result of vasoconstriction of nutrient arteries. Constriction of these vessels may involve activation of α_2 receptors. For example, phenylephrine is often used in nasal decongestant sprays. A longer duration of action—at the cost of much lower local concentrations and greater potential for cardiac and central nervous system effects—can be achieved by the oral administration of agents such as ephedrine or one of its isomers, pseudoephedrine. Long-acting topical decongestants include xylometazoline and oxymetazoline. All of these mucous membrane decongestants are available as over-the-counter products.

C. Cardiac Applications

Catecholamines such as isoproterenol and epinephrine have been utilized in the temporary emergency management of complete heart block and cardiac arrest. Epinephrine may be useful in cardiac arrest in part by redistributing blood flow during cardiopulmonary resuscitation to coronaries and to the brain. However, electronic pacemakers are both safer and more effective in heart block and should be inserted as soon as possible if there is any indication of continued high-degree block.

Heart failure may respond to the positive inotropic effects of drugs such as dobutamine. These applications are discussed in Chapter 13. The development of tolerance or desensitization is a major limitation to the use of catecholamines in heart failure.

Pulmonary Applications

One of the most important uses of sympathomimetic drugs is in the therapy of bronchial asthma. This use is discussed in Chapter 20. Nonselective drugs (epinephrine), β-selective agents (isoproterenol), and β_2-selective agents (metaproterenol, terbutaline, albuterol) are all available for this indication. Sympathomimetics other than the β_2-selective drugs are now rarely used because they are likely to have more adverse effects than the selective drugs.

Anaphylaxis

Anaphylactic shock and related immediate (type I) IgE-mediated reactions affect both the respiratory and the cardiovascular systems. The syndrome of bronchospasm, mucous membrane congestion, angioedema, and severe hypotension usually responds rapidly to the parenteral administration of **epinephrine**, 0.3–0.5 mg (0.3–0.5 mL of 1:1000 epinephrine solution). Intramuscular injection may be the preferred route of administration, since skin blood flow (and hence systemic drug absorption from subcutaneous injection) may be unpredictable in hypotensive patients. In some patients with impaired cardiovascular function, very cautious intravenous injection of epinephrine may be required. Epinephrine is the agent of choice because of extensive experimental and clinical experience with the drug in anaphylaxis and because epinephrine activates α, β_1, and β_2 receptors, all of which may be important in reversing the pathophysiologic processes underlying anaphylaxis. Glucocorticoids and antihistamines (both H_1 and H_2 receptor antagonists) may be useful as secondary therapy in anaphylaxis; however, epinephrine is the initial treatment.

Ophthalmic Applications

Phenylephrine is an effective mydriatic agent frequently used to facilitate examination of the retina. It is also a useful decongestant for minor allergic hyperemia and itching of the conjunctival membranes. Sympatho-mimetics administered as ophthalmic drops are also useful in localizing the lesion in Horner's syndrome. (See Box, An Application of Basic Pharmacology to a Clinical Problem.)

Glaucoma responds to a variety of sympathomimetic and sympathoplegic drugs. (See box in Chapter 10: The Treatment of Glaucoma.) Epinephrine and its prodrug dipivefrin are now rarely used, but β-blocking agents are among the most important therapies. **Apraclonidine** and **brimonidine** are α_2-selective agonists that also lower intraocular pressure and are approved for use in glaucoma. The mechanism of action of these drugs in treating glaucoma is still uncertain; direct neuroprotective effects may be involved in addition to the benefits of lowering intraocular pressure.

Genitourinary Applications

As noted above, β_2-selective agents relax the pregnant uterus. **Ritodrine, terbutaline,** and similar drugs have been used to suppress premature labor. The goal is to defer labor long enough to ensure adequate maturation of the fetus. These drugs may delay labor for several days. This may afford time to administer corticosteroid drugs, which decrease the incidence of neonatal respiratory distress syndrome. However, meta-analysis of older trials and a randomized study suggest that β-agonist therapy may have no significant benefit on perinatal infant mortality and may increase maternal morbidity.

AN APPLICATION OF BASIC PHARMACOLOGY TO A CLINICAL PROBLEM

Horner's syndrome is a condition—usually unilateral—that results from interruption of the sympathetic nerves to the face. The effects include vasodilation, ptosis, miosis, and loss of sweating on the side affected. The syndrome can be caused by either a preganglionic or a postganglionic lesion, such as a tumor. Knowledge of the location of the lesion (preganglionic or postganglionic) helps determine the optimal therapy.

An understanding of the effects of denervation on neurotransmitter metabolism permits the clinician to use drugs to localize the lesion. In most situations, a localized lesion in a nerve will cause degeneration of the distal portion of that fiber and loss of transmitter contents from the degenerated nerve ending—without affecting neurons innervated by the fiber. Therefore, a preganglionic lesion will leave the postganglionic adrenergic neuron intact, whereas a postganglionic lesion results in degeneration of the adrenergic nerve endings and loss of stored catecholamines from them. Because indirectly acting sympathomimetics require normal stores of catecholamines, such drugs can be used to test for the presence of normal adrenergic nerve endings. The iris, because it is easily visible and responsive to topical sympathomimetics, is a convenient assay tissue in the patient.

If the lesion of Horner's syndrome is postganglionic, indirectly acting sympathomimetics (eg, cocaine, hydroxyamphetamine) will not dilate the abnormally constricted pupil—because catecholamines have been lost from the nerve endings in the iris. In contrast, the pupil will dilate in response to phenylephrine, which acts directly on the α receptors on the smooth muscle of the iris. A patient with a preganglionic lesion, on the other hand, will show a normal response to both drugs, since the postganglionic fibers and their catecholamine stores remain intact in this situation.

Oral sympathomimetic therapy is occasionally useful in the treatment of stress incontinence. Ephedrine or pseudoephedrine may be tried.

Central Nervous System Applications

As noted above, the amphetamines have a mood-elevating (euphoriant) effect; this effect is the basis for the widespread abuse of this drug and some of its analogs (see Chapter 32). The amphetamines also have an alerting, sleep-deferring action that is manifested by improved attention to repetitive tasks and by acceleration and desynchronization of the EEG. A therapeutic application of this effect is in the treatment of narcolepsy. **Modafinil,** a new amphetamine substitute, is approved for use in narcolepsy and is claimed to have fewer disadvantages (excessive mood changes, insomnia, abuse potential) than amphetamine in this condition. The appetite-suppressing effect of these agents is easily demonstrated in experimental animals. In obese humans, an encouraging initial response may be observed, but there is no evidence that long-term improvement in weight control can be achieved with amphetamines alone, especially when administered for a relatively short course. A final application of the CNS-active sympathomimetics is in the attention-deficit hyperactivity disorder (ADHD) of children, a poorly defined and overdiagnosed behavioral syndrome consisting of short attention span, hyperkinetic physical behavior, and learning problems. Some patients with this syndrome respond well to low doses of methylphenidate and related agents or to clonidine. Extended-release formulations of methylphenidate may simplify dosing regimens and increase adherence to therapy, especially in school-age children. Evidence from several clinical trials suggests that modafinil may also be useful in ADHD.

Additional Therapeutic Uses

While the primary use of the α_2 agonist clonidine is in the treatment of hypertension (Chapter 11), the drug has been found to have efficacy in the treatment of diarrhea in diabetics with autonomic neuropathy, perhaps due to its ability to enhance salt and water absorption from the intestines. In addition, clonidine has efficacy in diminishing craving for narcotics and alcohol during withdrawal and may facilitate cessation of cigarette smoking. Clonidine has also been used to diminish menopausal hot flushes and is being used experimentally to reduce hemodynamic instability during general anesthesia. Dexmedetomidine is indicated for sedation under intensive care circumstances.

TOXICITY OF SYMPATHOMIMETIC DRUGS

The adverse effects of adrenoceptor agonists are primarily extensions of their pharmacologic effects in the cardiovascular and central nervous systems.

Adverse cardiovascular effects seen with intravenously infused pressor agents include marked elevations in blood pressure that cause increased cardiac work, which may precipitate cardiac ischemia and failure. Systemically administered β receptor-stimulant drugs may cause sinus tachycardia and may even provoke serious ventricular arrhythmias. Sympathomimetic drugs may lead to myocardial damage, particularly after prolonged infusion. Special caution is indicated in elderly patients or those with hypertension or coronary artery disease. To avoid excessive pharmacologic responses, it is essential to monitor the blood pressure when administering sympathomimetic drugs parenterally.

If an adverse sympathomimetic effect requires urgent reversal, a specific adrenoceptor antagonist can be used (see Chapter 10).

Central nervous system toxicity is rarely observed with catecholamines or drugs such as phenylephrine. In moderate doses, amphetamines commonly cause restlessness, tremor, insomnia, and anxiety; in high doses, a paranoid state may be induced. Cocaine may precipitate convulsions, cerebral hemorrhage, arrhythmias, or myocardial infarction. Therapy is discussed in Chapter 59.

PREPARATIONS AVAILABLE[1]

Amphetamine, racemic mixture (generic)
Oral: 5, 10 mg tablets
Oral (Adderall): 1:1:1:1 mixtures of amphetamine sulfate, amphetamine aspartate, dextroamphetamine sulfate, and dextroamphetamine saccharate, formulated to contain a total of 5, 7.5, 10, 12.5, 15, 20, or 30 mg in tablets; or 10, 20, or 30 mg in capsules

Apraclonidine (Iopidine)
Topical: 0.5, 1% solutions

Brimonidine (Alphagan)
Topical: 0.15, 0.2% solution

Dexmedetomidine (Precedex)
Parenteral: 100 μg/mL

Dexmethylphenidate (Focalin)
Oral: 2.5, 5, 10 mg tablets

Dextroamphetamine (generic, Dexedrine)
Oral: 5, 10 mg tablets
Oral sustained-release: 5, 10, 15 mg capsules
Oral mixtures with amphetamine: see Amphetamine (Adderall)

Dipivefrin (generic, Propine)
Topical: 0.1% ophthalmic solution

Dobutamine (generic, Dobutrex)
Parenteral: 12.5 mg/mL in 20 mL vials for injection

Dopamine (generic, Intropin)
Parenteral: 40, 80, 160 mg/mL for injection; 80, 160, 320 mg/100 mL in 5% D/W for injection

Ephedrine (generic)
Oral: 25 mg capsules
Parenteral: 50 mg/mL for injection
Nasal: 0.25% spray

Epinephrine (generic, Adrenalin Chloride, others)
Parenteral: 1:1000 (1 mg/mL), 1:2000 (0.5 mg/mL), 1:10,000 (0.1 mg/mL), 1:100,000 (0.01 mg/mL) for injection
Parenteral autoinjector (Epipen): 1:2000 (0.5 mg/mL)
Ophthalmic: 0.1, 0.5, 1, 2% drops
Nasal: 0.1% drops and spray
Aerosol for bronchospasm (Primatene Mist, Bronkaid Mist): 0.16, 0.2 mg/spray
Solution for aerosol: 1:100

Fenoldopam (Corlopam)
Parenteral: 10 mg/mL for IV infusion

Hydroxyamphetamine (Paredrine)
Ophthalmic: 1% drops

Isoproterenol (generic, Isuprel)
Parenteral: 1:5000 (0.2 mg/mL), 1:50,000 (0.02 mg/mL) for injection

Mephentermine (Wyamine Sulfate)
Parenteral: 15, 30 mg/mL for injection

Metaraminol (Aramine)
Parenteral: 10 mg/mL for injection

Methamphetamine (Desoxyn)
Oral: 5 mg tablets

Methoxamine (Vasoxyl)
Parenteral: 20 mg/mL for injection

Methylphenidate (generic, Ritalin, Ritalin-SR)
Oral: 5, 10, 20 mg tablets
Oral sustained-release: 10, 18, 20, 27, 36, 54 mg tablets; 20, 30, 40 mg capsules

Midodrine (ProAmatine)
Oral: 2.5, 5 mg tablets

Modafinil (Provigil)
Oral: 100, 200 mg tablets

Naphazoline (Privine)
Nasal: 0.05% drops and spray
Ophthalmic: 0.012, 0.02, 0.03% drops

Norepinephrine (generic, Levophed)
Parenteral: 1 mg/mL for injection

Oxymetazoline (generic, Afrin, Neo-Synephrine 12 Hour, others)
Nasal: 0.025, 0.05% sprays
Ophthalmic: 0.025% drops

Pemoline (generic, Cylert)
Oral: 18.75, 37.5, 75 mg tables; 37.5 mg chewable tablets

Phendimetrazine (generic)
Oral: 35 mg tablets, capsules; 105 mg sustained-release capsules

Phenylephrine (generic, Neo-Synephrine)
Oral: 10 mg chewable tablets
Parenteral: 10 mg/mL for injection
Nasal: 0.125, 0.16, 0.25, 0.5, 1% drops and spray; 0.5% jelly

Pseudoephedrine (generic, Sudafed, others)
Oral: 30, 60 mg tablets; 60 mg capsules; 15, 30 mg/5 mL syrups; 7.5 mg/0.8 mL drops
Oral extended-release: 120, 240 mg tablets, capsules

Tetrahydrozoline (generic, Tyzine)
Nasal: 0.05, 0.1% drops
Ophthalmic: 0.05% drops

Xylometazoline (generic, Otrivin, Neo-Synephrine Long-Acting, Chlorohist LA)
Nasal: 0.05 drops, 0.1% drops and spray

---

[1] α_2-Agonists used in hypertension are listed in Chapter 11. β_2-Agonists used in asthma are listed in Chapter 20.

REFERENCES

Angers S et al: Detection of beta$_2$-adrenergic receptor dimerization in living cells using bioluminescence resonance energy transfer (BRET). Proc Natl Acad Sci U S A 2000;97:3684.

Bray GA: Use and abuse of appetite-suppressant drugs in the treatment of obesity. Ann Intern Med 1993;119(7 Part 2):707.

Brogden RN, Markham A: Fenoldopam: A review of its pharmacodynamic and pharmacokinetic properties and intravenous clinical potential in the management of hypertensive urgencies and emergencies. Drugs 1997;54:634.

Brodde O-E et al: Presence, distribution and physiological function of adrenergic and muscarinic receptor subtypes in the human heart. Basic Res Cardiol 2001;96:528.

Bylund DB et al: International Union of Pharmacology nomenclature of adrenoceptors. Pharmacol Rev 1994;46:121.

Evans WE, McLeod HL: Pharmacogenomics—drug disposition, drug targets, and side effects. N Engl J Med 2003;348:538.

Ewan PW: Anaphylaxis. BMJ 1998;316:1442.

Glassman AH et al: Heavy smokers, smoking cessation, and clonidine: Results of a double-blind, randomized trial. JAMA 1988;259:2863.

Goldenberg RL, Rouse DJ: Prevention of premature birth. N Engl J Med 1998;339:313.

Graham RM et al: Alpha$_1$-adrenergic receptor subtypes. Molecular structure, function, and signaling. Circ Res 1996;78:737.

Hieble JP et al: International Union of Pharmacology. X. Recommendation for nomenclature of alpha$_1$-adrenoceptors: Consensus update. Pharmacol Rev 1995;47:267.

Jordan J: New trends in the treatment of orthostatic hypotension. Curr Hypertens Rep 2001;3:216.

Koshimizu T et al: Recent progress in alpha$_1$-adrenoceptor pharmacology. Biol Pharm Bull 2002;25:401.

Lin JS et al: Role of catecholamines in the modafinil and amphetamine induced wakefulness, a comparative pharmacological study in the cat. Brain Res 1992;591:319.

McCabe BJ: Dietary tyramine and other pressor amines in MAOI regimens: A review. J Am Diet Assoc 1986;86:1059.

McClellan KJ, Wiseman LR, Wilde MI: Midodrine. A review of its therapeutic use in the management of orthostatic hypotension. Drugs Aging 1998;12:7.

Mitler MM, Hayduk R: Benefits and risks of pharmacotherapy for narcolepsy. Drug Saf 2002;25:791.

Missale C et al: Dopamine receptors: From structure to function. Physiol Rev 1998;78:189.

1999 Receptor and Ion Channel Nomenclature Supplement. Trends Pharmacol Sci 1999.

Perry SJ, Lefkowitz RJ: Arresting developments in heptahelical receptor signaling and regulation. Trends Cell Biol 2002;12:130.

Philipp M, Brede M, Hein L: Physiological significance of alpha$_2$-adrenergic receptor subtype diversity: one receptor is not enough. Am J Physiol Integrative Comp Physiol 2002;283:R287.

Pierce KL, Lefkowitz RJ: Classical and new roles of beta-arrestins in the regulation of G-protein-coupled receptors. Nat Rev Neurosci 2001;2:727.

Post SR, Hammond HK, Insel PA: Beta-adrenergic receptors and receptor signaling in heart failure. Annu Rev Pharmacol Toxicol 1999;39:343.

Rocha BA et al: Cocaine self-administration in dopamine-transporter knockout mice. Nat Neurosci 1998;2:132.

Rockman HA, Koch WJ, Lefkowitz RJ: Seven-transmembrane-spanning receptors and heart function. Nature 2002;415:206.

Rohrer DK, Kobilka BK: Insights from in vivo modification of adrenergic receptor gene expression. Annu Rev Pharmacol Toxicol 1998;38:351.

Ruffolo RR Jr, Hieble JP: Adrenoceptor pharmacology: Urogenital applications. Eur Urol 1999;36(Suppl 1):17.

Ruffolo RR Jr: Fundamentals of receptor theory: Basics for shock research. Circ Shock 1992;37:176.

Small KM, McGraw DW, Liggett SB: Pharmacology and physiology of human adrenergic receptor polymorphisms. Ann Rev Pharmacol Toxicol 2003;43:381.

Soltau JB, Zimmerman TJ: Changing paradigms in the medical treatment of glaucoma. Surv Ophthalmol 2002;47(Suppl 1):S2.

Spitzer WO et al: The use of β-agonists and the risk of death and near death from asthma. N Engl J Med 1992;326:501.

Sunahara RK, Dessauer CW, Gilman AG: Complexity and diversity of mammalian adenylyl cyclases. Annu Rev Pharmacol Toxicol 1996;36:461.

Treatment of preterm labor with the beta-adrenergic agonist ritodrine. The Canada Preterm Labor Investigators Group. N Engl J Med 1992;327:308.

Trendelenburg A-U et al: A study of presynaptic alpha$_2$-autoreceptors in alpha$_{2A/D}$-, alpha$_{2B}$-, and alpha$_{2C}$- adrenoceptor-deficient mice. Naunyn Schmiedebergs Arch Pharmacol 2001;364:117.

Tsao P, von Zastrow M: Downregulation of G protein-coupled receptors. Curr Opin Neurobiol 2000;10:365.

Weyer C, Gautier JF, Danforth E Jr: Development of β$_3$-adrenoceptor agonists for the treatment of obesity and diabetes—an update. Diabetes Metab 1999;25:11.

Wheeler LA, Gil DW, WoldeMussie E: Role of alpha-2 adrenergic receptors in neuroprotection and glaucoma. Surv Ophthalmol 2001;45(Suppl 3):S290.

Zhong H, Minneman KP: Alpha$_1$-adrenoceptor subtypes. Eur J Pharmacol 1999;375:26.

Adrenoceptor Antagonist Drugs

Brian B. Hoffman, MD

Since catecholamines play a role in a variety of physiologic and pathophysiologic responses, drugs that block adrenoceptors have important effects, some of which are of great clinical value. These effects vary dramatically according to the drug's selectivity for α and β receptors. The classification of adrenoceptors into α_1, α_2, and β subtypes and the effects of activating these receptors are discussed in Chapters 6 and 9. Blockade of peripheral dopamine receptors is of no recognized clinical importance at present. In contrast, blockade of central nervous system dopamine receptors is very important; drugs that act on these receptors are discussed in Chapters 21 and 29. This chapter deals with pharmacologic antagonist drugs whose major effect is to occupy either α_1, α_2, or β receptors outside the central nervous system and prevent their activation by catecholamines and related agonists.

For pharmacologic research, α_1- and α_2-adrenoceptor antagonist drugs have been very useful in the experimental exploration of autonomic nervous system function. In clinical therapeutics, nonselective α antagonists have been used in the treatment of pheochromocytoma (tumors that secrete catecholamines), and α_1-selective antagonists are used in primary hypertension and benign prostatic hyperplasia. Beta-receptor antagonist drugs have been found useful in a much wider variety of clinical conditions and are firmly established in the treatment of hypertension, ischemic heart disease, arrhythmias, endocrinologic and neurologic disorders, and other conditions.

I. BASIC PHARMACOLOGY OF THE ALPHA-RECEPTOR ANTAGONIST DRUGS

Mechanism of Action

Alpha-receptor antagonists may be reversible or irreversible in their interaction with these receptors. Reversible antagonists dissociate from receptors; irreversible drugs do not. Phentolamine (Figure 10–1) and tolazoline are examples of reversible antagonists. Pra-

zosin (and analogs) and labetalol—drugs used primarily for their antihypertensive effects—as well as several ergot derivatives (see Chapter 16) are also reversible α-adrenoceptor antagonists. Phenoxybenzamine, an agent related to the nitrogen mustards, forms a reactive ethyleneimonium intermediate (Figure 10–1) that covalently binds to α receptors, resulting in irreversible blockade. Figure 10–2 illustrates the effects of a reversible drug in comparison with those of an irreversible agent.

The duration of action of a reversible antagonist is largely dependent on the half-life of the drug in the body and the rate at which it dissociates from its receptor: The shorter the half-life of the drug in the body or of binding to its receptor, the less time it takes for the effects of the drug to dissipate. However, the effects of an irreversible antagonist may persist long after the drug has been cleared from the plasma. In the case of phenoxybenzamine, the restoration of tissue responsiveness after extensive α-receptor blockade is dependent on synthesis of new receptors, which may take several days. The rate of return of α_1 adrenoceptor drug effect may be particularly important in patients having a sudden cardiovascular event or who become candidates for urgent surgery.

Pharmacologic Effects

A. CARDIOVASCULAR EFFECTS

Because arteriolar and venous tone are determined to a large extent by α receptors on vascular smooth muscle, α-receptor antagonist drugs cause a lowering of peripheral vascular resistance and blood pressure (Figure 10–3). These drugs can prevent the pressor effects of usual doses of α agonists; indeed, in the case of agonists with both α and β_2 effects (eg, epinephrine), selective α_1 receptor antagonism may convert a pressor to a depressor response (Figure 10–3). This change in response is called **epinephrine reversal**; it illustrates how the activation of both α and β receptors in the same tissue may lead to opposite responses. Alpha-receptor antagonists may cause postural hypotension and reflex tachycardia. Postural hypotension is due to antagonism of sympathetic nervous system stimulation of α_1 receptors in venous smooth muscle; contraction of veins is an

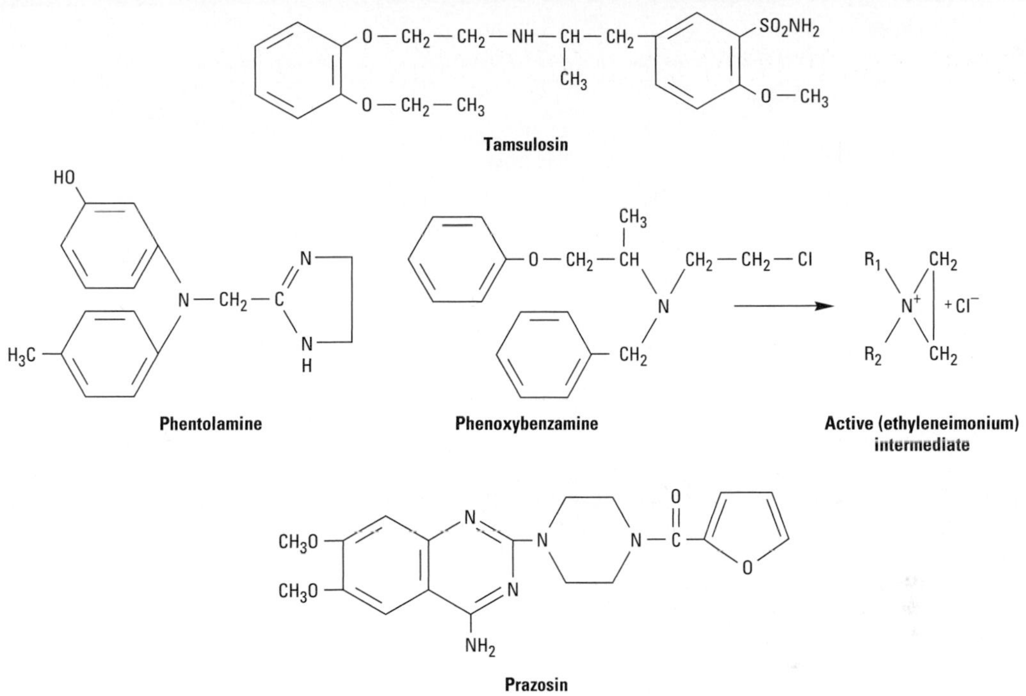

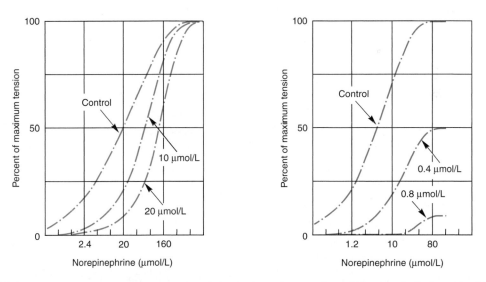

Figure 10–1. Structure of several α-receptor-blocking drugs.

Figure 10–2. Dose-response curves to norepinephrine in the presence of two different α-adrenoceptor-blocking drugs. The tension produced in isolated strips of cat spleen, a tissue rich in α receptors, was measured in response to graded doses of norepinephrine. **Left:** Tolazoline, a reversible blocker, shifted the curve to the right without decreasing the maximum response when present at concentrations of 10 and 20 μmol/L. **Right:** Dibenamine, an analog of phenoxybenzamine and irreversible in its action, reduced the maximum response attainable at both concentrations tested. (Modified and reproduced, with permission, from Bickerton RK: The response of isolated strips of cat spleen to sympathomimetic drugs and their antagonists. J Pharmacol Exp Ther 1963;142:99.)

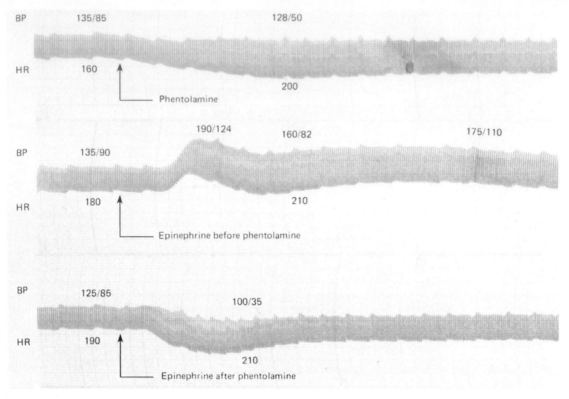

Figure 10–3. **Top:** Effects of phentolamine, an α receptor-blocking drug, on blood pressure in an anesthetized dog. Epinephrine reversal is demonstrated by tracings showing the response to epinephrine before (**middle**) and after (**bottom**) phentolamine. All drugs given intravenously. (BP, blood pressure; HR, heart rate.)

important component of the capacity to maintain blood pressure in the upright position since it decreases venous pooling in the periphery. Constriction of arterioles in the legs may also contribute to the postural response. Tachycardia may be more marked with agents that block α_2-presynaptic receptors in the heart (Table 10–1), since the augmented release of norepinephrine will further stimulate β receptors in the heart.

B. OTHER EFFECTS

Minor effects that signal the blockade of α receptors in other tissues include miosis and nasal stuffiness. $Alpha_1$-receptor blockade of the base of the bladder and the prostate is associated with decreased resistance to the flow of urine. Individual agents may have other important effects in addition to α-receptor antagonism (see below).

SPECIFIC AGENTS

Phentolamine, an imidazoline derivative, is a potent competitive antagonist at both α_1 and α_2 receptors

Table 10–1. Relative selectivity of antagonists for adrenoceptors.

	Receptor Affinity
α Antagonists	
Prazosin, terazosin, doxazosin	$\alpha_1 >>>> \alpha_2$
Phenoxybenzamine	$\alpha_1 > \alpha_2$
Phentolamine	$\alpha_1 = \alpha_2$
Rauwolscine, yohimbine, tolazoline	$\alpha_2 >> \alpha_1$
Mixed antagonists	
Labetalol, carvedilol	$\beta_1 = \beta_2 \geq \alpha_1 > \alpha_2$
β Antagonists	
Metoprololol, acebutolol, alprenolol, atenolol, betaxolol, celiprolol, esmolol	$\beta_1 >>> \beta_2$
Propranolol, carteolol, penbutolol, pindolol, timolol	$\beta_1 = \beta_2$
Butoxamine	$\beta_2 >>> \beta_1$

(Table 10–1). Phentolamine causes a reduction in peripheral resistance through blockade of α_1 receptors and possibly α_2 receptors on vascular smooth muscle. The cardiac stimulation induced by phentolamine is due to sympathetic stimulation of the heart resulting from baroreflex mechanisms. Furthermore, since phentolamine potently blocks α_2 receptors, antagonism of presynaptic α_2 receptors may lead to enhanced release of norepinephrine from sympathetic nerves. Enhanced norepinephrine release may contribute to cardiac stimulation via unblocked β adrenoceptors, especially after intravenous injection. In addition to being an α_1- and α_2-receptor antagonist, phentolamine also inhibits responses to serotonin and may be an agonist at muscarinic and H_1 and H_2 histamine receptors. Consequently, phentolamine has multiple potential actions, though it is not clear which if any of these are clinically significant.

Phentolamine has limited absorption after oral administration. Its pharmacokinetic properties are not well known; it may reach peak concentrations within an hour after oral administration and has a half-life of about 5–7 hours. The principal adverse effects are related to cardiac stimulation, which may cause severe tachycardia, arrhythmias, and myocardial ischemia, especially after intravenous administration. With oral administration, adverse effects include tachycardia, nasal congestion, and headache.

Phentolamine has been used in the treatment of pheochromocytoma—especially intraoperatively—as well as for male erectile dysfunction by injection intracavernosally and when taken orally (see below).

Tolazoline is similar to phentolamine. Tolazoline has very limited clinical application in the treatment of pulmonary hypertension in newborn infants with respiratory distress syndrome. Its efficacy in this condition is doubtful, and the drug is rarely used.

Ergot derivatives—eg, ergotamine, dihydroergotamine—cause reversible α-receptor blockade. However, most of the clinically significant effects of these drugs are the result of other actions; eg, ergotamine probably acts at serotonin receptors in the treatment of migraine (Chapter 16).

Phenoxybenzamine binds covalently to α receptors, causing irreversible blockade of long duration (14–48 hours or longer). It is somewhat selective for α_1 receptors but less so than prazosin (Table 10–1). The drug also inhibits reuptake of released norepinephrine by presynaptic adrenergic nerve terminals. Phenoxybenzamine blocks histamine (H_1), acetylcholine, and serotonin receptors as well as α receptors (see Chapter 16).

The pharmacologic actions of phenoxybenzamine are primarily related to antagonism of α-receptor-mediated events. Most importantly, phenoxybenzamine attenuates catecholamine-induced vasoconstriction.

While phenoxybenzamine causes relatively little fall in blood pressure in normal supine individuals, it reduces blood pressure when sympathetic tone is high, eg, as a result of upright posture or because of reduced blood volume. Cardiac output may be increased because of reflex effects and because of some blockade of presynaptic α_2 receptors in cardiac sympathetic nerves.

Phenoxybenzamine is absorbed after oral administration, although bioavailability is low and its kinetic properties are not well known. The drug is usually given orally, starting with low doses of 10–20 mg/d and progressively increasing the dose until the desired effect is achieved. Less than 100 mg/d is usually sufficient to achieve adequate α-receptor blockade. The major use of phenoxybenzamine is in the treatment of pheochromocytoma (see below).

Many of the adverse effects of phenoxybenzamine derive from its α-receptor-blocking action; the most important are postural hypotension and tachycardia. Nasal stuffiness and inhibition of ejaculation also occur. Since phenoxybenzamine enters the central nervous system, it may cause less specific effects, including fatigue, sedation, and nausea. Since phenoxybenzamine is an alkylating agent, it may have other adverse effects that have not yet been characterized. Phenoxybenzamine causes tumors in animals, but the clinical implications of this observation are unknown.

Prazosin is a piperazinyl quinazoline effective in the management of hypertension (see Chapter 11). It is highly selective for α_1 receptors, having relatively low affinity for α_2 receptors (typically 1000-fold less potent). This may partially explain the relative absence of tachycardia seen with prazosin as compared to what is reported with phentolamine and phenoxybenzamine. Prazosin leads to relaxation of both arterial and venous smooth muscle due to blockade of α_1 receptors. Prazosin is extensively metabolized in humans; because of metabolic degradation by the liver, only about 50% of the drug is available after oral administration. The half-life is normally about 3 hours.

Terazosin is another reversible α_1-selective antagonist that is effective in hypertension (Chapter 11); it has also been approved for use in men with urinary symptoms due to benign prostatic hyperplasia (BPH). Terazosin has high bioavailability but is extensively metabolized in the liver, with only a small fraction of unchanged drug excreted in the urine. The half-life of terazosin is 9–12 hours.

Doxazosin is efficacious in the treatment of hypertension and BPH. It differs from prazosin and terazosin in having a longer half-life of about 22 hours. It has moderate bioavailability and is extensively metabolized, with very little parent drug excreted in urine or feces. Doxazosin has active metabolites, although their contribution to the drug's effects is probably small.

Tamsulosin is a competitive α_1 antagonist with a structure quite different from that of most other α_1-receptor blockers. It has high bioavailability and a long half-life of 9–15 hours. It is metabolized extensively in the liver. Tamsulosin has higher affinity for α_{1A} and α_{1D} receptors than for the α_{1B} subtype. The drug's efficacy in BPH suggests that the α_{1A} subtype may be the most important α subtype mediating prostate smooth muscle contraction. Evidence suggests that tamsulosin has relatively greater potency in inhibiting contraction in *prostate* smooth muscle versus *vascular* smooth muscle, compared with other α_1-selective antagonists, which have equal or greater effects in vascular smooth muscle. This finding suggests that α_{1A} receptors are less important in mediating contraction in human arteries and veins. Furthermore, compared with other antagonists, tamsulosin has less effect on standing blood pressure in patients. Nonetheless, caution is appropriate in using any α antagonist in patients with diminished sympathetic nervous system function.

OTHER ALPHA-ADRENOCEPTOR ANTAGONISTS

Alfuzosin is an α_1-selective quinazoline derivative that has also been shown to be efficacious in BPH. It has a bioavailability of about 60%, is extensively metabolized, and has an elimination half-life of about 5 hours. This drug is not currently available in the USA. **Indoramin** is another α_1-selective antagonist that also has efficacy as an antihypertensive. **Urapidil** is an α_1 antagonist (its primary effect) that also has weak α_2-agonist and 5-HT$_{1A}$-agonist actions and weak antagonist action at β_1 receptors. It is used in Europe as an antihypertensive agent and for benign prostatic hyperplasia. **Labetalol** has both α_1-selective and β-antagonistic effects; it is discussed below. Neuroleptic drugs such as chlorpromazine and haloperidol are potent dopamine receptor antagonists but may also be antagonists at α receptors. Their antagonism of α receptors probably contributes to some of their adverse effects, particularly hypotension. Similarly, the antidepressant trazodone has the capacity to block α_1 receptors.

Yohimbine, an indole alkaloid, is an α_2-selective antagonist. It has no established clinical role. Theoretically, it could be useful in autonomic insufficiency by promoting neurotransmitter release through blockade of presynaptic α_2 receptors. It has been suggested that yohimbine improves male sexual function; however, evidence for this effect in humans is limited. Yohimbine can abruptly reverse the antihypertensive effects of an α_2-adrenoceptor agonist such as clonidine—a potentially serious adverse drug interaction.

II. CLINICAL PHARMACOLOGY OF THE ALPHA-RECEPTOR-BLOCKING DRUGS

Pheochromocytoma

The major clinical use of both phenoxybenzamine and phentolamine is in the management of pheochromocytoma. Pheochromocytoma is a tumor usually found in the adrenal medulla that releases a mixture of epinephrine and norepinephrine. Patients have many symptoms and signs of catecholamine excess, including intermittent or sustained hypertension, headaches, palpitations, and increased sweating.

The diagnosis of pheochromocytoma is usually made on the basis of chemical assay of circulating catecholamines and urinary excretion of catecholamine metabolites, especially 3-hydroxy-4-methoxymandelic acid, metanephrine, and normetanephrine. Measurement of plasma metanephrines has shown promise as an effective diagnostic tool. A variety of diagnostic techniques are available to localize a pheochromocytoma diagnosed biochemically, including CT and MRI scans as well as scanning with various radioisotopes.

Infusion of phentolamine was advocated in the past as a diagnostic test when pheochromocytoma was suspected, since patients with this tumor often manifest a greater drop in blood pressure in response to α-blocking drugs than do patients with primary hypertension. Provocative testing by infusion of histamine was occasionally used because this vasodilator drug may elicit a marked reflex rise in pressure in patients with pheochromocytoma. These tests are obsolete because measurement of circulating catecholamines and urinary catecholamines and their metabolites is a safer and far more reliable diagnostic approach.

Unavoidable release of stored catecholamines sometimes occurs during operative manipulation of pheochromocytoma; the resulting hypertension may be controlled with phentolamine or nitroprusside. Nitroprusside has many advantages, particularly since its effects can be more readily titrated and it has a shorter duration of action.

Alpha-receptor antagonists are most useful in the preoperative management of patients with pheochromocytoma (Figure 10–4). Administration of phenoxybenzamine in the preoperative period will help control hypertension and will tend to reverse chronic changes resulting from excessive catecholamine secretion such as plasma volume contraction, if present. Furthermore, the patient's operative course may be simplified. Oral doses of 10–20 mg/d may be increased at intervals of several days until hypertension is controlled. Some physicians

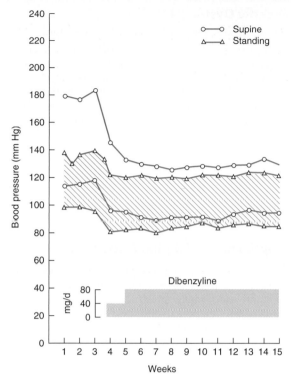

Figure 10–4. Effects of phenoxybenzamine (Dibenzyline) on blood pressure in a patient with pheochromocytoma. Dosage of the drug was begun in the third week as shown by the shaded bar. Supine systolic and diastolic pressures are indicated by the circles, the standing pressures by triangles and the hatched area. Note that the α-blocking drug dramatically reduced blood pressure. The reduction in orthostatic hypotension, which was marked before treatment, is probably due to normalization of blood volume, a variable that is sometimes markedly reduced in patients with longstanding pheochromocytoma-induced hypertension. (Redrawn and reproduced, with permission, from Engelman E, Sjoerdsma A: Chronic medical therapy for pheochromocytoma. Ann Intern Med 1961;61:229.)

give phenoxybenzamine to patients with pheochromocytoma for 1–3 weeks before surgery. Other surgeons prefer to operate on patients in the absence of treatment with phenoxybenzamine, counting on modern anesthetic techniques to control blood pressure and heart rate during surgery. Phenoxybenzamine may be very useful in the chronic treatment of inoperable or metastatic pheochromocytoma. Although there is less experience with alternative drugs, hypertension in patients with pheochromocytoma may also respond to reversible α₁-selective antagonists or to conventional calcium channel antagonists. Beta-receptor antagonists may be required after α-receptor blockade has been instituted to reverse the cardiac effects of excessive catecholamines. Beta antagonists should not be employed prior to establishing effective α-receptor blockade, since unopposed β-receptor blockade could theoretically cause blood pressure elevation from increased vasoconstriction.

Pheochromocytoma is rarely treated with **metyrosine** (α-methyltyrosine), the α-methyl analog of tyrosine. This agent is a competitive inhibitor of tyrosine hydroxylase and, in oral doses of 1–4 g/d, interferes with synthesis of dopamine (see Figure 6–5), thereby decreasing the amounts of norepinephrine and epinephrine secreted by the tumor. Metyrosine, while not an α-adrenoceptor antagonist, may act additively with phenoxybenzamine and a β-adrenoceptor antagonist in the treatment of pheochromocytoma. Metyrosine is especially useful in symptomatic patients with inoperable or metastatic pheochromocytoma.

Hypertensive Emergencies

The α-adrenoceptor antagonist drugs have limited application in the management of hypertensive emergencies, although labetalol has been used in this setting. In theory, α-adrenoceptor antagonists are most useful when increased blood pressure reflects excess circulating concentrations of α agonists. In this circumstance, which may result from pheochromocytoma, overdosage of sympathomimetic drugs, or clonidine withdrawal, phentolamine can be used to control high blood pressure. However, other drugs are generally preferable (see Chapter 11), since considerable experience is necessary to use phentolamine safely in these settings and few physicians have such experience.

Chronic Hypertension

Members of the prazosin family of α₁-selective antagonists are efficacious drugs in the treatment of mild to moderate systemic hypertension. They are generally well tolerated by most patients. However, their efficacy in preventing heart failure when used as monotherapy for hypertension has been questioned. Their major adverse effect is postural hypotension, which may be severe after the first dose but is otherwise uncommon (see Chapter 11). Nonselective α antagonists are not used in primary systemic hypertension. Prazosin and related drugs may also be associated with feelings of dizziness. This symptom may not be due to a fall in blood pressure, but postural changes in blood pressure should be checked routinely in any patient being treated for hypertension.

Interestingly, the use of α-adrenoceptor antagonists such as prazosin has been found to be associated with either no changes in plasma lipids or increased concentrations of HDL, which could be a favorable alteration. The mechanism for this effect is not known.

Peripheral Vascular Disease

Although α-receptor-blocking drugs have been tried in the treatment of peripheral vascular occlusive disease, there is no evidence that the effects are significant when morphologic changes limit flow in the vessels. Occasionally, individuals with Raynaud's phenomenon and other conditions involving excessive reversible vasospasm in the peripheral circulation do benefit from phentolamine, prazosin, or phenoxybenzamine, although calcium channel blockers may be preferable for many patients.

Local Vasoconstrictor Excess

Phentolamine has been used to reverse the intense local vasoconstriction caused by inadvertent infiltration of α agonists (eg, norepinephrine) into subcutaneous tissue during intended intravenous administration. The α antagonist is administered by local infiltration into the ischemic tissue.

Urinary Obstruction

Benign prostatic hyperplasia is a prevalent disorder in elderly men. A variety of surgical treatments are effective in relieving the urinary symptoms of BPH; however, drug therapy is efficacious in many patients. Alpha-receptor blockade was first found to be helpful in BPH using phenoxybenzamine in selected patients who were poor operative risks. The mechanism of action in improving urine flow involves partial reversal of smooth muscle contraction in the enlarged prostate and in the bladder base. It has been suggested that some α_1-receptor antagonists may have additional effects on cells in the prostate that help improve symptoms.

A number of well-controlled studies have demonstrated reproducible efficacy of several α_1-receptor antagonists in patients with BPH—lasting for several years in many cases. Prazosin, doxazocin, and terazosin are efficacious. These drugs are particularly useful in patients who also have hypertension. Considerable interest has focused on which α_1-receptor subtype is most important for smooth muscle contraction in the prostate: *subtype-selective* α_{1A}-receptor antagonists might lead to improved efficacy and safety in treating this disease. As indicated above, tamsulosin is also efficacious in BPH and has little if any effect on blood pressure. This drug may be preferred in patients who have experienced postural hypotension with other α_1-receptor antagonists. Some evidence suggests that the efficacy of α_1-receptor antagonists exceeds that of finasteride, the 5α-reductase inhibitor (see Chapter 40).

Erectile Dysfunction

A combination of the α-adrenoceptor antagonist phentolamine with the nonspecific vasodilator papaverine, when injected directly into the penis, may cause erections in men with sexual dysfunction. Fibrotic reactions may occur, especially with long-term administration. Systemic absorption may lead to orthostatic hypotension; priapism may require direct treatment with an α-adrenoceptor agonist such as phenylephrine. Orally administered phentolamine is being investigated in patients with erectile dysfunction (and in women with disorders of arousal.) Alternative therapies include prostaglandins (see Chapter 18), sildenafil, a cGMP phosphodiesterase inhibitor (see Chapter 12), and apomorphine.

Applications of Alpha₂ Antagonists

Alpha₂ antagonists have relatively little clinical usefulness. There has been experimental interest in the development of highly selective antagonists for use in Raynaud's phenomenon to inhibit smooth muscle contraction and in the treatment of type 2 diabetes (α_2 receptors inhibit insulin secretion) and psychiatric depression. It is not known to what extent the recognition of multiple subtypes of α_2 receptors will lead to development of clinically useful subtype-selective new drugs.

III. BASIC PHARMACOLOGY OF THE BETA-RECEPTOR-ANTAGONIST DRUGS

Drugs in this category share the common feature of antagonizing the effects of catecholamines at β adrenoceptors. Beta-blocking drugs occupy β receptors and competitively reduce receptor occupancy by catecholamines and other β agonists. (A few members of this group, used only for experimental purposes, bind irreversibly to β receptors.) Most β-blocking drugs in clinical use are pure antagonists; ie, the occupancy of a β receptor by such a drug causes no activation of the receptor. However, some are partial agonists; ie, they cause partial activation of the receptor, albeit less than that caused by the full agonists epinephrine and isoproterenol. As described in Chapter 2, partial agonists inhibit the activation of β receptors in the presence of high catecholamine concentrations but moderately activate the receptors in the absence of endogenous agonists. Another major difference among the many β-receptor-blocking drugs concerns their relative affinities for β_1 and β_2 receptors (Table 10–1). Some of these antagonists have a higher affinity for β_1 than for β_2 receptors, and this selectivity may have important clinical implications. Since none of the clinically available β receptor antagonists are absolutely specific for β_1 receptors, the selectivity is dose-related, ie, it tends to diminish at higher drug concentrations. Other major differences among β antagonists relate to their pharmacokinetic characteristics and local anesthetic membrane-stabilizing effects.

Chemically, the β-receptor-antagonist drugs (Figure 10–5) resemble isoproterenol (see Figure 9–3), a potent β receptor agonist.

Pharmacokinetic Properties of the Beta-Receptor Antagonists

A. ABSORPTION

Most of the drugs in this class are well absorbed after oral administration; peak concentrations occur 1–3 hours after ingestion. Sustained-release preparations of propranolol and metoprolol are available.

B. BIOAVAILABILITY

Propranolol undergoes extensive hepatic (first-pass) metabolism; its bioavailability is relatively low (Table 10–2). The proportion of drug reaching the systemic circulation increases as the dose is increased, suggesting that hepatic extraction mechanisms may become satu-

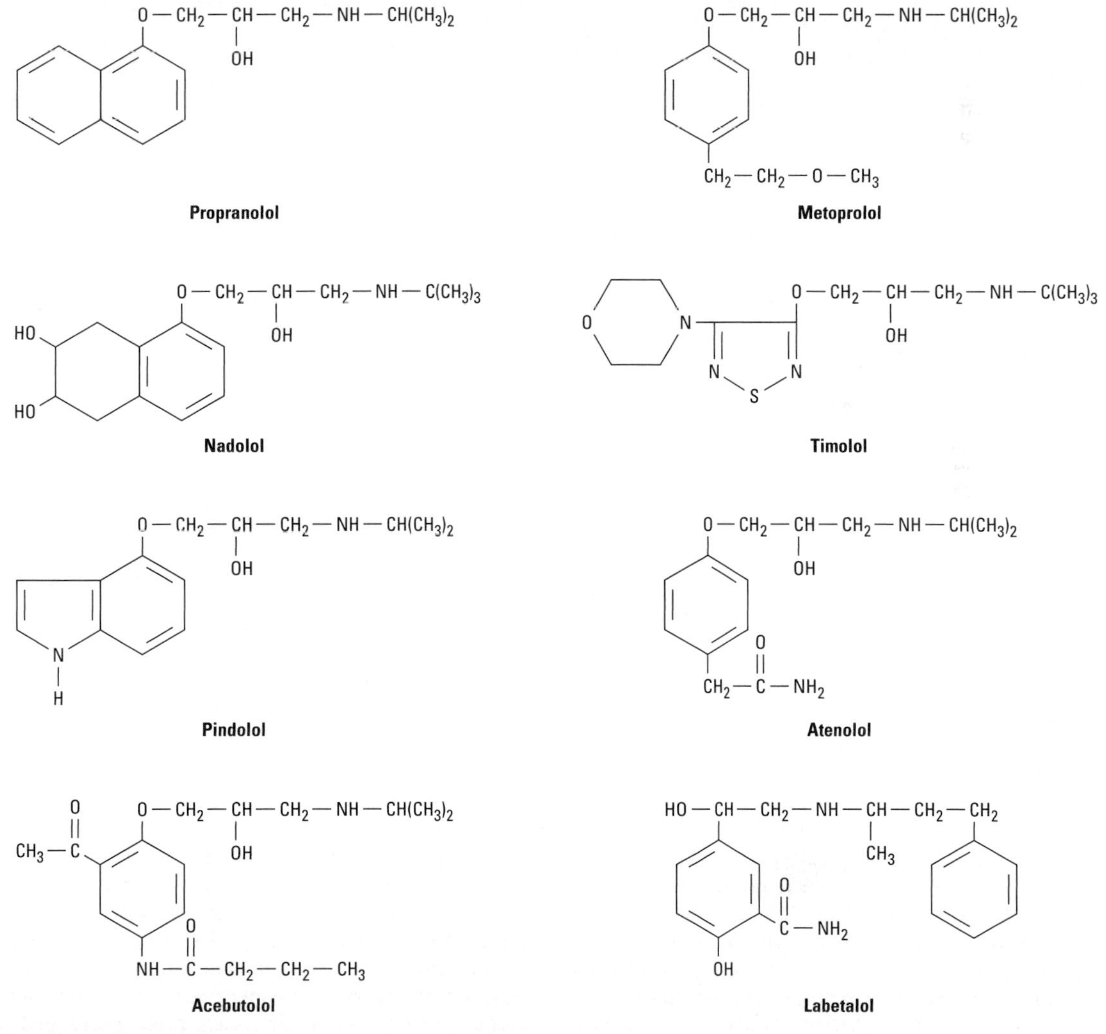

Figure 10–5. Structures of some β-receptor antagonists.

Table 10–2. Properties of several beta-receptor-blocking drugs.

	Selectivity	Partial Agonist Activity	Local Anesthetic Action	Lipid Solubility	Elimination Half-Life	Approximate Bioavailability
Acebutolol	β_1	Yes	Yes	Low	3–4 hours	50
Atenolol	β_1	No	No	Low	6–9 hours	40
Betaxolol	β_1	No	Slight	Low	14–22 hours	90
Bisoprolol	β_1	No	No	Low	9–12 hours	80
Carteolol	None	Yes	No	Low	6 hours	85
Carvedilol[1]	None	No	No	No data	6–8 hours	25–35
Celiprolol	β_1	Yes[2]	No	No data	4–5 hours	70
Esmolol	β_1	No	No	Low	10 minutes	–0
Labetalol[1]	None	Yes[1]	Yes	Moderate	5 hours	30
Metoprolol	β_1	No	Yes	Moderate	3–4 hours	50
Nadolol	None	No	No	Low	14–24 hours	33
Penbutolol	None	Yes	No	High	5 hours	>90
Pindolol	None	Yes	Yes	Moderate	3–4 hours	90
Propranolol	None	No	Yes	High	3.5–6 hours	30[3]
Sotalol	None	No	No	Low	12 hours	90
Timolol	None	No	No	Moderate	4–5 hours	50

[1]Carvedilol and labetalol also cause α_1 adrenoceptor blockade.
[2]Partial agonist effects at β_2 receptors.
[3]Bioavailability is dose-dependent.

rated. A major consequence of the low bioavailability of propranolol is that oral administration of the drug leads to much lower drug concentrations than are achieved after intravenous injection of the same dose. Because the first-pass effect varies among individuals, there is great individual variability in the plasma concentrations achieved after oral propranolol. Bioavailability is limited to varying degrees for most β antagonists with the exception of betaxolol, penbutolol, pindolol, and sotalol.

C. DISTRIBUTION AND CLEARANCE

The β antagonists are rapidly distributed and have large volumes of distribution. Propranolol and penbutolol are quite lipophilic and readily cross the blood-brain barrier (Table 10–2). Most β antagonists have half-lives in the range of 3–10 hours. A major exception is esmolol, which is rapidly hydrolyzed and has a half-life of approximately 10 minutes. Propranolol and metoprolol are extensively metabolized in the liver, with little unchanged drug appearing in the urine. The cytochrome P450 2D6 (CYP2D6) genotype is a major determinant of interindividual differences in metoprolol plasma clearance (Chapter 4). Poor metabolizers exhibit threefold to tenfold higher plasma concentrations after administration of metoprolol than extensive metabolizers. Atenolol, celiprolol, and pindolol are less completely metabolized. Nadolol is excreted unchanged in the urine and has the longest half-life of any available β antagonist (up to 24 hours). The half-life of nadolol is prolonged in renal failure. The elimination of drugs such as propranolol may be prolonged in the presence of liver disease, diminished hepatic blood flow, or hepatic enzyme inhibition. It is notable that the pharmacodynamic effects of these drugs are often prolonged well beyond the time predicted from half-life data.

Pharmacodynamics of the β-receptor-Antagonist Drugs

Most of the effects of these drugs are due to occupancy and blockade of β receptors. However, some actions may be due to other effects, including partial agonist activity at β receptors and local anesthetic action, which differ among the β-blockers (Table 10–2).

A. EFFECTS ON THE CARDIOVASCULAR SYSTEM

Beta-blocking drugs given chronically lower blood pressure in patients with hypertension. The mechanisms involved may include effects on the heart and blood vessels, suppression of the renin-angiotensin system, and perhaps effects in the central nervous system or elsewhere. Beta-adrenoceptor-blocking drugs are of major clinical importance in the treatment of hypertension (see Chapter 11). In contrast, conventional doses of these drugs do *not* usually cause hypotension in healthy individuals with normal blood pressure.

Beta-receptor antagonists have prominent effects on the heart (Figure 10–6). The negative inotropic and chronotropic effects are predictable from the role of adrenoceptors in regulating these functions. Slowed atrioventricular conduction with an increased PR interval is a related result of adrenoceptor blockade in the atrioventricular node. These effects may be clinically valuable in some patients but are potentially hazardous in others. In the vascular system, β-receptor blockade opposes β₂-mediated vasodilation. This may acutely lead to a rise in peripheral resistance from unopposed α-receptor-mediated effects as the sympathetic nervous system discharges in response to lowered blood pressure due to the fall in cardiac output. Beta-blocking drugs antagonize the release of renin caused by the sympathetic nervous system. As noted in Chapter 11, the relation between the effects on renin release and those on blood pressure is unclear. In any event, while the acute effects of these drugs may include a rise in peripheral resistance, chronic drug administration leads to a fall in peripheral resistance in patients with hypertension. How this adjustment occurs is not yet clear.

B. EFFECTS ON THE RESPIRATORY TRACT

Blockade of the β₂ receptors in bronchial smooth muscle may lead to an increase in airway resistance, particularly in patients with asthma. Beta₁-receptor antagonists such as metoprolol or atenolol may have some advantage over nonselective β antagonists when blockade of β₁ receptors in the heart is desired and β₂-receptor blockade is undesirable. However, no currently available β₁-selective antagonist is sufficiently specific to *completely* avoid interactions with β₂ adrenoceptors. Consequently, these drugs should generally be avoided in patients with asthma. On the other hand, some patients with chronic obstructive pulmonary disease (COPD) may tolerate these drugs quite well.

C. EFFECTS ON THE EYE

Several β-blocking agents reduce intraocular pressure, especially in glaucomatous eyes. The mechanism usually reported is decreased aqueous humor production. (See Clinical Pharmacology and Box, The Treatment of Glaucoma.)

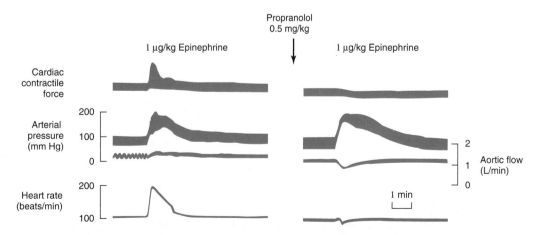

Figure 10–6. The effect in an anesthetized dog of the injection of epinephrine before and after propranolol. In the presence of a β-receptor-blocking agent, epinephrine no longer augments the force of contraction (measured by a strain gauge attached to the ventricular wall) nor increases cardiac rate. Blood pressure is still elevated by epinephrine because vasoconstriction is not blocked. (Reproduced, with permission, from Shanks RG: The pharmacology of b sympathetic blockade. Am J Cardiol 1966;18:312.)

THE TREATMENT OF GLAUCOMA

Glaucoma is a major cause of blindness and of great pharmacologic interest because the chronic form often responds to drug therapy. The primary manifestation is increased intraocular pressure not initially associated with symptoms. Without treatment, increased intraocular pressure results in damage to the retina and optic nerve, with restriction of visual fields and, eventually, blindness. Intraocular pressure is easily measured as part of the routine ophthalmologic examination. Two major types of glaucoma are recognized: open-angle and closed-angle (or narrow-angle). The closed-angle form is associated with a shallow anterior chamber, in which a dilated iris can occlude the outflow drainage pathway at the angle between the cornea and the ciliary body (Figure 6–9). This form is associated with acute and painful increases of pressure, which must be controlled on an emergency basis with drugs or prevented by surgical removal of part of the iris (iridectomy). The open-angle form of glaucoma is a chronic condition, and treatment is largely pharmacologic. Because intraocular pressure is a function of the balance between fluid input and drainage out of the globe, the strategies for the treatment of closed-angle glaucoma fall into two classes: reduction of aqueous humor secretion and enhancement of aqueous outflow. Five general groups of drugs—cholinomimetics, α agonists, β-blockers, prostaglandin $F_{2\alpha}$ analogs, and diuretics—have been found to be useful in reducing intraocular pressure and can be related to these strategies as shown in Table 10–3. Of the five drug groups listed in Table 10–3, the prostaglandin analogs and the β-blockers are the most popular. This popularity results from convenience (once- or twice-daily dosing) and relative lack of adverse effects (except, in the case of β-blockers, in patients with asthma or cardiac pacemaker or conduction pathway disease). Other drugs that have been reported to reduce intraocular pressure include prostaglandin E_2 and marijuana. The use of drugs in acute closed-angle glaucoma is limited to cholinomimetics, acetazolamide, and osmotic agents preceding surgery. The onset of action of the other agents is too slow in this situation.

Table 10–3. Drugs used in open-angle glaucoma.

	Mechanism	Methods of Administration
Cholinomimetics		
Pilocarpine, carbachol, physostigmine, echothiophate, demecarium	Ciliary muscle contraction, opening of trabecular meshwork; increased outflow	Topical drops or gel; plastic film slow-release insert
Alpha agonists		
Unselective	Increased outflow	Topical drops
Epinephrine, dipivefrin		
Alpha$_2$-selective	Decreased aqueous secretion	
Apraclonidine		Topical, postlaser only
Brimonidine		Topical
Beta-blockers		
Timolol, betaxolol, carteolol, levobunolol, metipranolol	Decreased aqueous secretion from the ciliary epithelium	Topical drops
Diuretics		
Dorzolamide, brinzolamide	Decreased secretion due to lack of HCO_3^-	Topical
Acetazolamide, dichlorphenamide, methazolamide		Oral
Prostaglandins		
Latanoprost, unoprostone	Increased outflow	Topical

D. Metabolic and Endocrine Effects

Beta-receptor antagonists such as propranolol inhibit sympathetic nervous system stimulation of lipolysis. The effects on carbohydrate metabolism are less clear, though glycogenolysis in the human liver is at least partially inhibited after β_2-receptor blockade. However, glucagon is the primary hormone employed to combat hypoglycemia. It is unclear to what extent β antagonists impair recovery from hypoglycemia, but they should be used with caution in insulin-dependent diabetic patients. This may be particularly important in diabetic patients with inadequate glucagon reserve and in pancreatectomized patients since catecholamines may be the major factors in stimulating glucose release from the liver in response to hypoglycemia. Beta$_1$-receptor-selective drugs may be less prone to inhibit recovery from hypoglycemia. Beta-receptor antagonists are much safer in those type 2 diabetic patients who do not have hypoglycemic episodes.

The chronic use of β-adrenoceptor antagonists has been associated with increased plasma concentrations of VLDL and decreased concentrations of HDL cholesterol. Both of these changes are potentially unfavorable in terms of risk of cardiovascular disease. Although LDL concentrations generally do not change, there is a variable decline in the HDL cholesterol/ LDL cholesterol ratio that may increase the risk of coronary artery disease. These changes tend to occur with both selective and nonselective β-blockers, though they are perhaps less likely to occur with β-blockers possessing intrinsic sympathomimetic activity (partial agonists). The mechanisms by which β-receptor antagonists cause these changes are not understood, though changes in sensitivity to insulin action may contribute.

E. Effects Not Related to Beta-Blockade

Partial β-agonist activity was significant in the first β-blocking drug synthesized, dichloroisoproterenol. It has been suggested that retention of some intrinsic sympathomimetic activity is desirable to prevent untoward effects such as precipitation of asthma or excessive bradycardia. Pindolol and other partial agonists are noted in Table 10–2. It is not yet clear to what extent partial agonism is clinically valuable. Furthermore, these drugs may not be as effective as the pure antagonists in secondary prevention of myocardial infarction. However, they may be useful in patients who develop symptomatic bradycardia or bronchoconstriction in response to pure antagonist β-adrenoceptor drugs, but only if they are strongly indicated for a particular clinical indication.

Local anesthetic action, also known as "membrane-stabilizing" action, is a prominent effect of several β-blockers (Table 10–2). This action is the result of typical local anesthetic blockade of sodium channels and can be demonstrated experimentally in isolated neurons, heart muscle, and skeletal muscle membrane. However, it is unlikely that this effect is important after systemic administration of these drugs, since the concentration in plasma usually achieved by these routes is too low for the anesthetic effects to be evident. These drugs are not used topically on the eye, where local anesthesia of the cornea would be highly undesirable. Sotalol is a nonselective β-receptor antagonist that lacks local anesthetic action but has marked class III antiarrhythmic effects, reflecting potassium channel blockade (see Chapter 14).

SPECIFIC AGENTS
(See Table 10–2.)

Propranolol is the prototypical β-blocking drug. It has low and dose-dependent bioavailability, the result of extensive first-pass metabolism in the liver. A long-acting form of propranolol is available; prolonged absorption of the drug may occur over a 24-hour period. The drug has negligible effects at α and muscarinic receptors; however, it may block some serotonin receptors in the brain, though the clinical significance is unclear. It has no detectable partial agonist action at β receptors.

Metoprolol, atenolol, and several other drugs (see Table 10–2) are members of the β_1-selective group. These agents may be safer in patients who experience bronchoconstriction in response to propranolol. Since their β_1 selectivity is rather modest, they should be used with great caution, if at all, in patients with a history of asthma. However, in selected patients with chronic obstructive lung disease the benefits may exceed the risks, eg, in patients with myocardial infarction. Beta$_1$-selective antagonists may be preferable in patients with diabetes or peripheral vascular disease when therapy with a β-blocker is required since β_2 receptors are probably important in liver (recovery from hypoglycemia) and blood vessels (vasodilation).

Nadolol is noteworthy for its very long duration of action; its spectrum of action is similar to that of timolol. **Timolol** is a nonselective agent with no local anesthetic activity. It has excellent ocular hypotensive effects when administered topically in the eye. **Levobunonol** (nonselective) and **betaxolol** (β_1-selective) are used for topical ophthalmic application in glaucoma; the latter drug may be less likely to induce bronchoconstriction than nonselective antagonists. **Carteolol** is a nonselective β-receptor antagonist.

Pindolol, acebutolol, carteolol, bopindolol,* oxprenolol,* celiprolol, and **penbutolol** are of interest because they have partial β-agonist activity. They are effective in the major cardiovascular applications of the β-blocking group (hypertension and

---

* Not Available in the USA.

angina). Although these partial agonists may be less likely to cause bradycardia and abnormalities in plasma lipids than are antagonists, the overall clinical significance of intrinsic sympathomimetic activity remains uncertain. Pindolol, perhaps as a result of actions on serotonin signaling, may potentiate the action of traditional antidepressant medications. Celiprolol* is a β_1-selective antagonist with a modest capacity to activate β_2 receptors.

There is limited evidence suggesting that celiprolol may have less adverse bronchoconstrictor effects in asthma and may even promote bronchodilation. Acebutolol is also a β_1-selective antagonist.

Labetalol is a reversible adrenoceptor antagonist available as a racemic mixture of two pairs of chiral isomers (the molecule has two centers of asymmetry). The (S,S)- and (R,S)-isomers are inactive, (S,R)- is a potent α-blocker, and the (R,R)-isomer is a potent β-blocker. Labetalol's affinity for α receptors is less than that of phentolamine, but labetalol is α_1-selective. Its β-blocking potency is somewhat lower than that of propranolol. Hypotension induced by labetalol is accompanied by less tachycardia than occurs with phentolamine and similar α-blockers.

Carvedilol, medroxalol, * and **bucindolol** * are nonselective β-receptor antagonists with some capacity to block α_1-adrenergic receptors.

Carvedilol antagonizes the actions of catecholamines more potently at β receptors than at α receptors. The drug has a half-life of 6–8 hours. It is extensively metabolized in the liver, and stereoselective metabolism of its two isomers is observed. Since metabolism of *(R)*-carvedilol is influenced by polymorphisms in cytochrome P450 2D6 activity and by drugs that inhibit this enzyme's activity (such as quinidine and fluoxetine), drug interactions may occur. Carvedilol also appears to attenuate oxygen free radical-initiated lipid peroxidation and to inhibit vascular smooth muscle mitogenesis independently of adrenoceptor blockade. These effects may contribute to the clinical benefits of the drug in chronic heart failure (see Chapter 13).

Esmolol is an ultra-short–acting β_1-selective adrenoceptor antagonist. The structure of esmolol contains an ester linkage; esterases in red blood cells rapidly metabolize esmolol to a metabolite that has a low affinity for β receptors. Consequently, esmolol has a short half-life (about 10 minutes). Therefore, during continuous infusions of esmolol, steady state concentrations are achieved quickly, and the therapeutic actions of the drug are terminated rapidly when its infusion is discontinued. Esmolol is potentially safer to use than longer-acting antagonists in critically ill patients who require a β-

adrenoceptor antagonist. Esmolol is useful in controlling supraventricular arrhythmias, arrhythmias associated with thyrotoxicosis, perioperative hypertension, and myocardial ischemia in acutely ill patients.

Butoxamine is selective for β_2 receptors. Selective β_2-blocking drugs have not been actively sought because there is no obvious clinical application for them and none are availale for clinical use.

IV. CLINICAL PHARMACOLOGY OF THE BETA-RECEPTOR-BLOCKING DRUGS

Hypertension

The β-adrenoceptor-blocking drugs have proved to be effective and well tolerated in hypertension. While many hypertensive patients will respond to a β-blocker used alone, the drug is often used with either a diuretic or a vasodilator. In spite of the short half-life of many β antagonists, these drugs may be administered once or twice daily and still have an adequate therapeutic effect. Labetalol, a competitive α and β antagonist, is effective in hypertension, though its ultimate role is yet to be determined. Use of these agents is discussed in detail in Chapter 11. There is some evidence that drugs in this class may be less effective in blacks and the elderly. However, these differences are relatively small and may not apply to an individual patient. Indeed, since effects on blood pressure are easily measured, the therapeutic outcome for this indication can be readily detected in any patient.

Ischemic Heart Disease

Beta-adrenoceptor blockers reduce the frequency of anginal episodes and improve exercise tolerance in many patients with angina (see Chapter 12). These actions relate to the blockade of cardiac β receptors, resulting in decreased cardiac work and reduction in oxygen demand. Slowing and regularization of the heart rate may contribute to clinical benefits (Figure 10–7). Multiple large-scale prospective studies indicate that the long-term use of timolol, propranolol, or metoprolol in patients who have had a myocardial infarction prolongs survival (Figure 10–8). At the present time, data are less compelling for the use of other than the three mentioned β-adrenoceptor antagonists for this indication. Importantly, surveys in many populations have indicated that the β-receptor antagonists are underused, leading to unnecessary morbidity and mortality. Studies in experimental animals suggest that use of β-receptor

---

* Not Available in the USA.

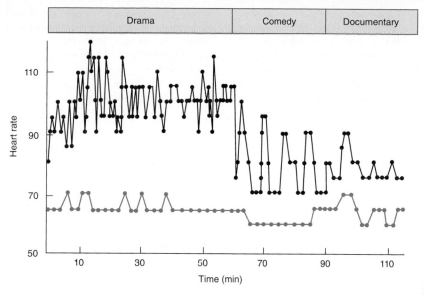

Figure 10–7. Heart rate in a patient with ischemic heart disease measured by telemetry while watching television. Measurements were begun 1 hour after receiving placebo (upper line, black) or 40 mg of oxprenolol (color), a nonselective β-antagonist with partial agonist activity. Not only was the heart rate decreased by the drug under the conditions of this experiment; it also varied much less in response to stimuli. (Modified and reproduced, with permission, from Taylor SH: Oxprenolol in clinical practice. Am J Cardiol 1983;52:34D.)

antagonists during the acute phase of a myocardial infarction may limit infarct size. However, this use is still controversial.

Cardiac Arrhythmias

Beta antagonists are effective in the treatment of both supraventricular and ventricular arrhythmias (see Chapter 14). It has been suggested that the improved survival following myocardial infarction in patients using β-antagonists (Figure 10–8; see above) is due to suppression of arrhythmias, but this has not been proved. By increasing the atrioventricular nodal refractory period, β antagonists slow ventricular response rates in atrial flutter and fibrillation. These drugs can also reduce ventricular ectopic beats, particularly if the ectopic activity has been precipitated by catecholamines. Sotalol has additional antiarrhythmic effects involving ion channel blockade in addition to its β-blocking action; these are discussed in Chapter 14.

Other Cardiovascular Disorders

Beta-receptor antagonists have been found to increase stroke volume in some patients with obstructive cardiomyopathy. This beneficial effect is thought to result from the slowing of ventricular ejection and decreased

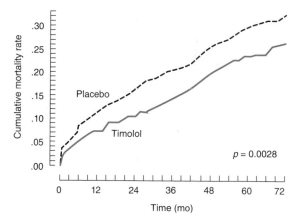

Figure 10–8. Effects of β-blocker therapy on life-table cumulated rates of mortality from all causes over 6 years among 1884 patients surviving myocardial infarctions. Patients were randomly assigned to treatment with placebo (dashed line) or timolol (color). (Reproduced, with permission, from Pederson TR: Six-year follow-up of the Norwegian multicenter study on timolol after acute myocardial infarction. N Engl J Med 1985;313:1055.)

outflow resistance. Beta-antagonists are useful in dissecting aortic aneurysm to decrease the rate of development of systolic pressure. Clinical trials have demonstrated that at least three β antagonists—metoprolol, bisoprolol, and carvedilol—are effective in treating chronic heart failure in selected patients. While administration of these drugs may acutely worsen congestive heart failure, cautious long-term use with gradual dose increments in patients who tolerate them may prolong life. While mechanisms are uncertain, there appear to be beneficial effects on myocardial remodeling and in decreasing the risk of sudden death (see Chapter 13).

Glaucoma
(See Box, p. 152, The Treatment of Glaucoma)

Systemic administration of β-blocking drugs for other indications was found serendipitously to reduce intraocular pressure in patients with glaucoma. Subsequently, it was found that topical administration also reduces intraocular pressure. The mechanism appears to involve reduced production of aqueous humor by the ciliary body, which is physiologically activated by cAMP. Timolol and related β antagonists are suitable for local use in the eye because they lack local anesthetic properties. Beta antagonists appear to have an efficacy comparable to that of epinephrine or pilocarpine in open-angle glaucoma and are far better tolerated by most patients. While the maximal daily dose applied locally (1 mg) is small compared with the systemic doses commonly used in the treatment of hypertension or angina (10–60 mg), sufficient timolol may be absorbed from the eye to cause serious adverse effects on the heart and airways in susceptible individuals. Topical timolol may interact with orally administered verapamil and increase the risk of heart block.

Betaxolol, carteolol, levobunolol, and metipranolol are newer β-receptor antagonists approved for the treatment of glaucoma. Betaxolol has the potential advantage of being β_1-selective; to what extent this potential advantage might diminish systemic adverse effects remains to be determined. The drug apparently has caused worsening of pulmonary symptoms in some patients.

Hyperthyroidism

Excessive catecholamine action is an important aspect of the pathophysiology of hyperthyroidism, especially in relation to the heart (see Chapter 38). The β antagonists have salutary effects in this condition. These beneficial effects presumably relate to blockade of adrenoceptors and perhaps in part to the inhibition of peripheral conversion of thyroxine to triiodothyronine. The latter action may vary from one β antagonist to another. Pro-

pranolol has been used extensively in patients with thyroid storm (severe hyperthyroidism); it is used cautiously in patients with this condition to control supraventricular tachycardias that often precipitate heart failure.

Neurologic Diseases

Several studies show a beneficial effect of propranolol in reducing the frequency and intensity of migraine headache. Other β-receptor antagonists with preventive efficacy include metoprolol and probably also atenolol, timolol, and nadolol. The mechanism is not known. Since sympathetic activity may enhance skeletal muscle tremor, it is not surprising that β antagonists have been found to reduce certain tremors (see Chapter 28). The somatic manifestations of anxiety may respond dramatically to low doses of propranolol, particularly when taken prophylactically. For example, benefit has been found in musicians with performance anxiety ("stage fright"). Propranolol may contribute to the symptomatic treatment of alcohol withdrawal in some patients.

Miscellaneous

Beta-receptor antagonists have been found to diminish portal vein pressure in patients with cirrhosis. There is evidence that both propranolol and nadolol decrease the incidence of the first episode of bleeding from esophageal varices and decrease the mortality rate associated with bleeding in patients with cirrhosis. Nadolol in combination with isosorbide mononitrate appears to be more efficacious than sclerotherapy in preventing rebleeding in patients who have previously bled from esophageal varices.

CHOICE OF A BETA-ADRENOCEPTOR ANTAGONIST DRUG

Propranolol is the standard against which newer β antagonists developed for systemic use have been compared. In many years of very wide use, it has been found to be a safe and effective drug for many indications. Since it is possible that some actions of a β-receptor antagonist may relate to some other effect of the drug, these drugs should not be considered interchangeable for all applications. For example, only β antagonists known to be effective in hyperthyroidism or in prophylactic therapy after myocardial infarction should be used for those indications. It is possible that the beneficial effects of one drug in these settings might not be shared by another drug in the same class. The possible advantages and disadvantages of β receptor antagonists that are partial agonists have not been clearly defined in clinical settings, although current evidence suggests that they are probably less efficacious in secondary prevention after a myocardial infarction compared to pure antagonists.

CLINICAL TOXICITY OF THE BETA-RECEPTOR ANTAGONIST DRUGS

A variety of minor toxic effects have been reported for propranolol. Rash, fever, and other manifestations of drug allergy are rare. Central nervous system effects include sedation, sleep disturbances, and depression. Rarely, psychotic reactions may occur. Discontinuing the use of β-blockers in any patient who develops a depression should be seriously considered if clinically feasible. It has been claimed that β-receptor antagonist drugs with low lipid solubility are associated with a lower incidence of central nervous system adverse effects than compounds with higher lipid solubility (Table 10–2). Further studies designed to compare the central nervous system adverse effects of various drugs are required before specific recommendations can be made, though it seems reasonable to try the hydrophilic drugs nadolol or atenolol in a patient who experiences unpleasant central nervous system effects with other β-blockers.

The major adverse effects of β-receptor antagonist drugs relate to the predictable consequences of β blockade. Beta$_2$-receptor blockade associated with the use of nonselective agents commonly causes worsening of pre-existing asthma and other forms of airway obstruction without having these consequences in normal individuals. Indeed, relatively trivial asthma may become severe after β blockade. However, because of their life-saving possibilities in cardiovascular disease, strong consideration should be given to individualized therapeutic trials in some classes of patients, eg, those with chronic obstructive pulmonary disease who have appropriate indications for β-blockers. While β$_1$-selective drugs may have less effect on airways than nonselective β antagonists, they must be used very cautiously, if at all, in patients with reactive airways. While β$_1$-selective antagonists are generally well tolerated in patients with mild to moderate peripheral vascular disease, caution is required in patients with severe peripheral vascular disease or vasospastic disorders.

Beta-receptor blockade depresses myocardial contractility and excitability. In patients with abnormal myocardial function, cardiac output may be dependent on sympathetic drive. If this stimulus is removed by β blockade, cardiac decompensation may ensue. Thus, caution must be exercised in using β-receptor antagonists in patients with compensated heart failure even though long-term use of these drugs in these patients may prolong life. A life-threatening adverse cardiac effect of a β antagonist may be overcome directly with isoproterenol or with glucagon (glucagon stimulates the heart via glucagon receptors, which are not blocked by β antagonists), but neither of these methods is without hazard. A very small dose of a β antagonist (eg, 10 mg of propranolol) may provoke severe cardiac failure in a susceptible individual. Beta-blockers may interact with the calcium antagonist verapamil; severe hypotension, bradycardia, heart failure, and cardiac conduction abnormalities have all been described. These adverse effects may even arise in susceptible patients taking a topical (ophthalmic) β-blocker and oral verapamil.

Some hazards are associated with abruptly discontinuing β antagonist therapy after chronic use. Evidence suggests that patients with ischemic heart disease may be at increased risk if β blockade is suddenly interrupted. The mechanism of this effect is uncertain but might involve up-regulation of the number of β receptors. Until better evidence is available regarding the magnitude of the risk, prudence dictates the gradual tapering rather than abrupt cessation of dosage when these drugs are discontinued, especially drugs with short half-lives, such as propranolol and metoprolol.

The incidence of hypoglycemic episodes in diabetics that are exacerbated by β-blocking agents is unknown. Nevertheless, it is inadvisable to use β antagonists in insulin-dependent diabetic patients who are subject to frequent hypoglycemic reactions if alternative therapies are available. Beta$_1$-selective antagonists offer some advantage in these patients, since the rate of recovery from hypoglycemia may be faster compared with diabetics receiving nonselective β adrenoceptor antagonists. There is considerable potential benefit from these drugs in diabetics after a myocardial infarction, so the balance of risk versus benefit must be evaluated in individual patients.

PREPARATIONS AVAILABLE

ALPHA BLOCKERS
Doxazosin (generic, Cardura)
 Oral: 1, 2, 4, 8 mg tablets
Phenoxybenzamine (Dibenzyline)
 Oral: 10 mg capsules
Phentolamine (generic, Regitine)
 Parenteral: 5 mg/vial for injection
Prazosin (generic, Minipress)
 Oral: 1, 2, 5 mg capsules
Tamsulosin (Flomax)
 Oral: 0.4 mg capsule
Terazosin (generic, Hytrin)
 Oral: 1, 2, 5, 10 mg tablets, capsules
Tolazoline (Priscoline)
 Parenteral: 25 mg/mL for injection

BETA BLOCKERS
Acebutolol (generic, Sectral)
 Oral: 200, 400 mg capsules
Atenolol (generic, Tenormin)
 Oral: 25, 50, 100 mg tablets
 Parenteral: 0.5 mg/mL for IV injection
Betaxolol
 Oral: 10, 20 mg tablets (Kerlone)
 Ophthalmic: 0.25%, 0.5% drops (generic, Betoptic)
Bisoprolol (Zebeta)
 Oral: 5, 10 mg tablets
Carteolol
 Oral: 2.5, 5 mg tablets (Cartrol)
 Ophthalmic: 1% drops (generic, Ocupress)
Carvedilol (Coreg)
 Oral: 3.125, 6.25, 12.5, 25 mg tablets
Esmolol (Brevibloc)
 Parenteral: 10 mg/mL for IV injection; 250 mg/mL for IV infusion

Labetalol (generic, Normodyne, Trandate)
 Oral: 100, 200, 300 mg tablets
 Parenteral: 5 mg/mL for injection
Levobunolol (Betagan Liquifilm, others)
 Ophthalmic: 0.25, 0.5% drops
Metipranolol (Optipranolol)
 Ophthalmic: 0.3% drops
Metoprolol (generic, Lopressor, Toprol)
 Oral: 50, 100 mg tablets
 Oral sustained-release: 25, 50, 100, 200 mg tablets
 Parenteral: 1 mg/mL for injection
Nadolol (generic, Corgard)
 Oral: 20, 40, 80, 120, 160 mg tablets
Penbutolol (Levatol)
 Oral: 20 mg tablets
Pindolol (generic, Visken)
 Oral: 5, 10 mg tablets
Propranolol (generic, Inderal)
 Oral: 10, 20, 40, 60, 80, 90 mg tablets; 4, 8, 80 mg/mL solutions
 Oral sustained release: 60, 80, 120, 160 mg capsules
 Parenteral: 1 mg/mL for injection
Sotalol (generic, Betapace)
 Oral: 80, 120, 160, 240 mg tablets
Timolol
 Oral: 5, 10, 20 mg tablets (generic, Blocadren)
 Ophthalmic: 0.25, 0.5% drops, gel (generic, Timoptic)

SYNTHESIS INHIBITOR
Metyrosine (Demser)
 Oral: 250 mg capsules

REFERENCES

Alward WLM: Medical management of glaucoma. N Engl J Med 1998;339:1298.

Becker AJ et al: Oral phentolamine as treatment for erectile dysfunction. J Urol 1998;159:1214.

Blaufarb I, Pfeifer TM, Frishman WH: Beta-blockers: Drug interactions of clinical significance. Drug Saf 1995;13:359.

Brantigan CO, Brantigan TA, Joseph N: Effect of beta blockade and beta stimulation on stage fright. Am J Med 1982;72:88.

Bristow M: Antiadrenergic therapy of chronic heart failure: surprises and new opportunities. Circulation 2003;107:1100.

Cheng J, Kamiya K, Kodama I: Carvedilol: molecular and cellular basis for its multifaceted therapeutic potential. Cardiovasc Drug Rev 2001;19:152.

Cleland JG: Beta-blockers for heart failure: why, which, when, and where. Med Clin North Am 2003;87:339.

Cooper KL, McKiernan JM, Kaplan SA: Alpha-adrenoceptor antagonists in the treatment of benign prostatic hyperplasia. Drugs 1999;57:9.

Fallon B: Intracavernous injection therapy for male erectile dysfunction. Urol Clin North Am 1995;22:833.

Fitzgerald JD: Do partial agonist beta-blockers have improved clinical utility? Cardiovasc Drugs Ther 1993; 7:303.

Freemantle N et al: Beta blockade after myocardial infarction: Systematic review and meta regression analysis. BMJ 1999;318: 1730.

Frishman WH: Carvedilol. N Engl J Med 1998;339:1759.

Gold EH et al: Synthesis and comparison of some cardiovascular properties of the stereoisomers of labetalol. J Med Chem 1982;25:1363.

Harada K, Ohmori M, Fujimura A: Comparison of the antagonistic activity of tamsulosin and doxazosin at vascular α_1-adrenoceptors in humans. Naunyn Schmiedebergs Arch Pharmacol 1996;354:557.

Kaplan SA et al: Combination therapy using oral α-blockers and intracavernosal injection in men with erectile dysfunction. Urology 1998;52:739.

Kyprianou N: Doxazosin and terazosin suppress prostate growth by inducing apoptosis: clinical significance. J Urol 2003;169:1520.

Lepor H et al: The efficacy of terazosin, finasteride, or both in benign prostate hyperplasia. N Engl J Med 1996; 335:533.

Nickerson M: The pharmacology of adrenergic blockade. Pharmacol Rev 1949;1:27.

Padma-Nathan H et al: Long-term safety and efficacy of oral phentolamine mesylate (Vasomax) in men with mild to moderate erectile dysfunction. Int J Impot Res 2002;14:266.

Rosen RC et al: Oral phentolamine and female sexual arousal disorder: A pilot study. J Sex Marital Ther 1999;25:137.

Ruffolo RR Jr et al: Pharmacologic and therapeutic applications of alpha$_2$-adrenoceptor subtypes. Annu Rev Pharmacol Toxicol 1993;32:243.

Ruffolo RR Jr, Hieble JP: Alpha-adrenoceptors. Pharmacol Ther 1994;61:1.

Teerlink JR, Massie BM: Beta-adrenergic blocker mortality trials in congestive heart failure. Am J Cardiol 1999;84(Suppl 9A):94R.

van Zwieten PA: An overview of the pharmacodynamic properties and therapeutic potential of combined alpha- and beta-adrenoceptor antagonists. Drugs 1993;45:509.

Villanueva C et al: Nadolol plus isosorbide mononitrate compared with sclerotherapy for prevention of variceal bleeding. N Engl J Med 1996;334:1624.

Wespes E: Intracavernous injection as an option for aging men with erectile dysfunction. Aging Male 2002;5:177.

Wilde MI, Fitton A, McTavish D: Alfuzosin. A review of its pharmacodynamic and pharmacokinetic properties, and therapeutic potential in benign prostatic hyperplasia. Drugs 1993;45:410.

Wilde MI, Fitton A, Sorkin EM: Terazosin. A review of its pharmacodynamic and pharmacokinetic properties, and therapeutic potential in benign prostatic hyperplasia. Drugs Aging 1993;3:258.

Wilde MI, McTavish D: Tamsulosin. A review of its pharmacological properties and therapeutic potential in the management of symptomatic benign prostatic hyperplasia. Drugs 1996;52:883.

Wilt TJ, MacDonald R, Rutks I: Tamsulosin for benign prostatic hyperplasia. Cochrane Database Syst Rev 2003;(1):CD002081.

Wuttke H et al: Increased frequency of cytochrome P450 2D6 poor metabolizers among patients with metoprolol-associated adverse effects. Clin Pharmacol Ther 2002;72:429.

Yedinak KC: Formulary considerations in selection of beta-blockers. Pharmacoeconomics 1993;4:104.

SECTION III
Cardiovascular-Renal Drugs

Antihypertensive Agents

Neal L. Benowitz, MD

Hypertension is the most common cardiovascular disease. Thus, the third National Health and Nutrition Examination Survey (NHANES III), conducted from 1992 to 1994, found that 27% of the USA adult population had hypertension. The prevalence varies with age, race, education, and many other variables. Sustained arterial hypertension damages blood vessels in kidney, heart, and brain and leads to an increased incidence of renal failure, coronary disease, cardiac failure, and stroke. Effective pharmacologic lowering of blood pressure has been shown to prevent damage to blood vessels and to substantially reduce morbidity and mortality rates. Many effective drugs are available. Knowledge of their antihypertensive mechanisms and sites of action allows accurate prediction of efficacy and toxicity. As a result, rational use of these agents, alone or in combination, can lower blood pressure with minimal risk of serious toxicity in most patients.

HYPERTENSION & REGULATION OF BLOOD PRESSURE

Diagnosis

The diagnosis of hypertension is based on repeated, reproducible measurements of elevated blood pressure. The diagnosis serves primarily as a prediction of consequences for the patient; it seldom includes a statement about the cause of hypertension.

Epidemiologic studies indicate that the risks of damage to kidney, heart, and brain are directly related to the extent of blood pressure elevation. Even mild hypertension (blood pressure ≥ 140/90 mm Hg) in young or middle-aged adults increases the risk of eventual end organ damage. The risks—and therefore the urgency of instituting therapy—increase in proportion to the magnitude of blood pressure elevation. The risk of end organ damage at any level of blood pressure or age is greater in black people and relatively less in premenopausal women than in men. Other positive risk factors include smoking, hyperlipidemia, diabetes, manifestations of end organ damage at the time of diagnosis, and a family history of cardiovascular disease.

It should be noted that the diagnosis of hypertension depends on measurement of blood pressure and not on symptoms reported by the patient. In fact, hypertension is usually asymptomatic until overt end organ damage is imminent or has already occurred.

Etiology of Hypertension

A specific cause of hypertension can be established in only 10–15% of patients. It is important to consider specific causes in each case, however, because some of them are amenable to definitive surgical treatment: renal artery constriction, coarctation of the aorta, pheochromocytoma, Cushing's disease, and primary aldosteronism.

Patients in whom no specific cause of hypertension can be found are said to have **essential hypertension.**[*]

---

[*] The adjective originally was intended to convey the now abandoned idea that blood pressure elevation was essential for adequate perfusion of diseased tissues.

In most cases, elevated blood pressure is associated with an overall increase in resistance to flow of blood through arterioles, while cardiac output is usually normal. Meticulous investigation of autonomic nervous system function, baroreceptor reflexes, the renin-angiotensin-aldosterone system, and the kidney has failed to identify a primary abnormality as the cause of increased peripheral vascular resistance in essential hypertension.

Elevated blood pressure is usually caused by a combination of several abnormalities (multifactorial). Epidemiologic evidence points to genetic inheritance, psychological stress, and environmental and dietary factors (increased salt and decreased potassium or calcium intake) as perhaps contributing to the development of hypertension. Increase in blood pressure with aging does not occur in populations with low daily sodium intake. Patients with labile hypertension appear more likely than normal controls to have blood pressure elevations after salt loading.

The heritability of essential hypertension is estimated to be about 30%. Mutations in several genes have been linked to various rare causes of hypertension. Functional variations of the genes for angiotensinogen, angiotensin-converting enzyme (ACE), and the β_2 adrenoceptor appear to contribute to some cases of essential hypertension.

Normal Regulation of Blood Pressure

According to the hydraulic equation, arterial blood pressure (BP) is directly proportionate to the product of the blood flow (cardiac output, CO) and the resistance to passage of blood through precapillary arterioles (peripheral vascular resistance, PVR):

$$BP = CO \times PVR$$

Physiologically, in both normal and hypertensive individuals, blood pressure is maintained by moment-to-moment regulation of cardiac output and peripheral vascular resistance, exerted at three anatomic sites (Figure 11–1): arterioles, postcapillary venules (capacitance vessels), and heart. A fourth anatomic control site, the kidney, contributes to maintenance of blood pressure by regulating the volume of intravascular fluid. Baroreflexes, mediated by autonomic nerves, act in combination with humoral mechanisms, including the renin-angiotensin-aldosterone system, to coordinate function at these four control sites and to maintain normal blood pressure. Finally, local release of hormones from vascular endothelium may also be involved in the regulation of vascular resistance. For example, nitric oxide (see Chapter 19) dilates and endothelin-1 (see Chapter 17) constricts blood vessels.

Blood pressure in a hypertensive patient is controlled by the same mechanisms that are operative in nor-

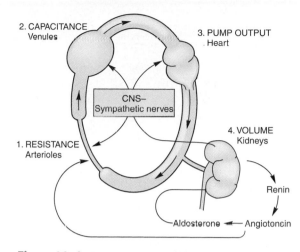

Figure 11–1. Anatomic sites of blood pressure control.

motensive subjects. Regulation of blood pressure in hypertensive patients differs from healthy patients in that the baroreceptors and the renal blood volume-pressure control systems appear to be "set" at a higher level of blood pressure. All antihypertensive drugs act by interfering with these normal mechanisms, which are reviewed below.

A. Postural Baroreflex (Figure 11–2)

Baroreflexes are responsible for rapid, moment-to-moment adjustments in blood pressure, such as in transition from a reclining to an upright posture. Central sympathetic neurons arising from the vasomotor area of the medulla are tonically active. Carotid baroreceptors are stimulated by the stretch of the vessel walls brought about by the internal pressure (blood pressure). Baroreceptor activation inhibits central sympathetic discharge. Conversely, reduction in stretch results in a reduction in baroreceptor activity. Thus, in the case of a transition to upright posture, baroreceptors sense the reduction in arterial pressure that results from pooling of blood in the veins below the level of the heart as reduced wall stretch, and sympathetic discharge is disinhibited. The reflex increase in sympathetic outflow acts through nerve endings to increase peripheral vascular resistance (constriction of arterioles) and cardiac output (direct stimulation of the heart and constriction of capacitance vessels, which increases venous return to the heart), thereby restoring normal blood pressure. The same baroreflex acts in response to any event that lowers arterial pressure, including a primary reduction in peripheral vascular resistance (eg, caused by a vasodilating agent) or a reduction in intravascular volume (eg, due to hemorrhage or to loss of salt and water via the kidney).

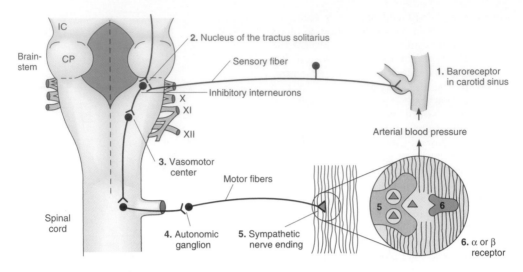

Figure 11–2. Baroreceptor reflex arc.

B. RENAL RESPONSE TO DECREASED BLOOD PRESSURE

By controlling blood volume, the kidney is primarily responsible for long-term blood pressure control. A reduction in renal perfusion pressure causes intrarenal redistribution of blood flow and increased reabsorption of salt and water. In addition, decreased pressure in renal arterioles as well as sympathetic neural activity (via β-adrenoceptors) stimulates production of renin, which increases production of angiotensin II (see Figure 11–1 and Chapter 17). Angiotensin II causes (1) direct constriction of resistance vessels and (2) stimulation of aldosterone synthesis in the adrenal cortex, which increases renal sodium absorption and intravascular blood volume. Vasopressin released from the posterior pituitary gland also plays a role in maintenance of blood pressure through its ability to regulate water reabsorption by the kidney (see Chapter 17).

I. BASIC PHARMACOLOGY OF ANTIHYPERTENSIVE AGENTS

All antihypertensive agents act at one or more of the four anatomic control sites depicted in Figure 11–1 and produce their effects by interfering with normal mechanisms of blood pressure regulation. A useful classification of these agents categorizes them according to the principal regulatory site or mechanism on which they act (Figure 11–3). Because of their common mechanisms of action, drugs within each category tend to pro-

duce a similar spectrum of toxicities. The categories include the following:

(1) **Diuretics,** which lower blood pressure by depleting the body of sodium and reducing blood volume and perhaps by other mechanisms.

(2) **Sympatholegic agents,** which lower blood pressure by reducing peripheral vascular resistance, inhibiting cardiac function, and increasing venous pooling in capacitance vessels. (The latter two effects reduce cardiac output.) These agents are further subdivided according to their putative sites of action in the sympathetic reflex arc (see below).

(3) **Direct vasodilators,** which reduce pressure by relaxing vascular smooth muscle, thus dilating resistance vessels and—to varying degrees—increasing capacitance as well.

(4) **Agents that block production or action of angiotensin** and thereby reduce peripheral vascular resistance and (potentially) blood volume.

The fact that these drug groups act by different mechanisms permits the combination of drugs from two or more groups with increased efficacy and, in some cases, decreased toxicity. (See Box, Monotherapy Versus Polypharmacy in Hypertension, p.174.)

DRUGS THAT ALTER SODIUM & WATER BALANCE

Dietary sodium restriction has been known for many years to decrease blood pressure in hypertensive

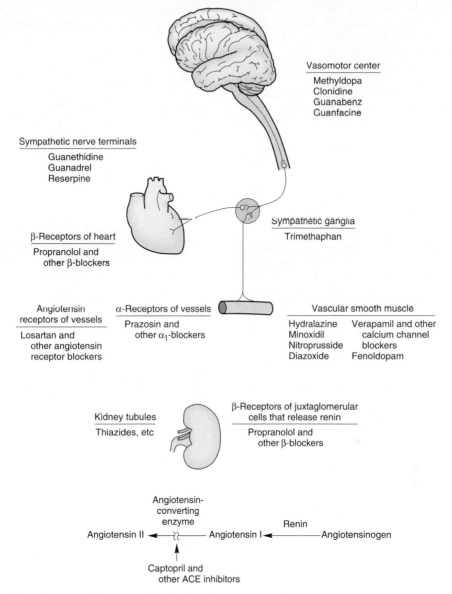

Vasomotor center

Methyldopa
Clonidine
Guanabenz
Guanfacine

Sympathetic nerve terminals

Guanethidine
Guanadrel
Reserpine

Sympathetic ganglia

Trimethaphan

β-Receptors of heart

Propranolol and
    other β-blockers

Angiotensin
receptors of vessels

Losartan and
    other angiotensin
    receptor blockers

α-Receptors of vessels

Prazosin and
    other α₁-blockers

Vascular smooth muscle

Hydralazine   Verapamil and other
Minoxidil   calcium channel
Nitroprusside   blockers
Diazoxide   Fenoldopam

Kidney tubules

Thiazides, etc

β-Receptors of juxtaglomerular
cells that release renin

Propranolol and
    other β-blockers

Angiotensin-
converting
enzyme

Renin

Angiotensin II ◄———⟨⟨——— Angiotensin I ◄——————— Angiotensinogen

Captopril and
other ACE inhibitors

Figure 11–3. Sites of action of the major classes of antihypertensive drugs.

patients. With the advent of diuretics, sodium restriction was thought to be less important. However, there is now general agreement that dietary control of blood pressure is a relatively nontoxic therapeutic measure and may even be preventive. Several studies have shown that even modest dietary sodium restriction lowers blood pressure (although to varying extents) in many hypertensive individuals.

Mechanisms of Action & Hemodynamic Effects of Diuretics

Diuretics lower blood pressure primarily by depleting body sodium stores. Initially, diuretics reduce blood pressure by reducing blood volume and cardiac output; peripheral vascular resistance may increase. After 6–8 weeks, cardiac output returns toward normal while peripheral vascular resistance declines. Sodium is believed to contribute to vascular resistance by increasing vessel stiffness and neural reactivity, possibly related to increased sodium-calcium exchange with a resultant increase in intracellular calcium. These effects are reversed by diuretics or sodium restriction.

Some diuretics have direct vasodilating effects in addition to their diuretic action. Indapamide is a nonthiazide sulfonamide diuretic with both diuretic and vasodilator activity. As a consequence of vasodilation, cardiac output remains unchanged or increases slightly. Amiloride inhibits smooth muscle responses to contractile stimuli, probably through effects on transmembrane and intracellular calcium movement that are independent of its action on sodium excretion.

Diuretics are effective in lowering blood pressure by 10–15 mm Hg in most patients, and diuretics alone often provide adequate treatment for mild or moderate essential hypertension. In more severe hypertension, diuretics are used in combination with sympathoplegic and vasodilator drugs to control the tendency toward sodium retention caused by these agents. Vascular responsiveness—ie, the ability to either constrict or dilate—is diminished by sympathoplegic and vasodilator drugs, so that the vasculature behaves like an inflexible tube. As a consequence, blood pressure becomes exquisitely sensitive to blood volume. Thus, in severe hypertension, when multiple drugs are used, blood pressure may be well controlled when blood volume is 95% of normal but much too high when blood volume is 105% of normal.

Use of Diuretics

The sites of action within the kidney and the pharmacokinetics of various diuretic drugs are discussed in Chapter 15. Thiazide diuretics are appropriate for most patients with mild or moderate hypertension and normal renal and cardiac function. More powerful diuretics (eg, those acting on the loop of Henle) are necessary in severe hypertension, when multiple drugs with sodium-retaining properties are used; in renal insufficiency, when glomerular filtration rate is less than 30 or 40 mL/min; and in cardiac failure or cirrhosis, where sodium retention is marked.

Potassium-sparing diuretics are useful both to avoid excessive potassium depletion, particularly in patients taking digitalis, and to enhance the natriuretic effects of other diuretics.

Some pharmacokinetic characteristics and the initial and usual maintenance dosages of hydrochlorothiazide are listed in Table 11–1. Although thiazide diuretics are more natriuretic at higher doses (up to 100–200 mg of hydrochlorothiazide), when used as a single agent, lower doses (25–50 mg) exert as much antihypertensive effect

as do higher doses. In contrast to thiazides, the blood pressure response to loop diuretics continues to increase at doses many times greater than the usual therapeutic dose.

Toxicity of Diuretics

In the treatment of hypertension, the most common adverse effect of diuretics (except for potassium-sparing diuretics) is potassium depletion. Although mild degrees of hypokalemia are tolerated well by many patients, hypokalemia may be hazardous in persons taking digitalis, those who have chronic arrhythmias, or those with acute myocardial infarction or left ventricular dysfunction. Potassium loss is coupled to reabsorption of sodium, and restriction of dietary sodium intake will therefore minimize potassium loss. Diuretics may also cause magnesium depletion, impair glucose tolerance, and increase serum lipid concentrations. Diuretics increase uric acid concentrations and may precipitate gout. The use of low doses minimizes these adverse metabolic effects without impairing the antihypertensive action. Several case-control studies have reported a small but significant excess risk of renal cell carcinoma associated with diuretic use.

DRUGS THAT ALTER SYMPATHETIC NERVOUS SYSTEM FUNCTION

In patients with moderate to severe hypertension, most effective drug regimens include an agent that inhibits function of the sympathetic nervous system. Drugs in this group are classified according to the site at which they impair the sympathetic reflex arc (Figure 11–2). This neuroanatomic classification explains prominent differences in cardiovascular effects of drugs and allows the clinician to predict interactions of these drugs with one another and with other drugs.

Most importantly, the subclasses of drugs exhibit different patterns of potential toxicity. Drugs that lower blood pressure by actions on the central nervous system tend to cause sedation and mental depression and may produce disturbances of sleep, including nightmares. Drugs that act by inhibiting transmission through autonomic ganglia produce toxicity from inhibition of parasympathetic regulation, in addition to profound sympathetic blockade. Drugs that act chiefly by reducing release of norepinephrine from sympathetic nerve endings cause effects that are similar to those of surgical sympathectomy, including inhibition of ejaculation, and hypotension that is increased by upright posture and after exercise. Drugs that block postsynaptic adrenoceptors produce a more selective spectrum of

Table 11–1. Pharmacokinetic characteristics and dosage of selected oral antihypertensive drugs.

Drug	Half-life (h)	Bioavailability (percent)	Suggested Initial Dose	Usual Maintenance Dose Range	Reduction of Dosage Required in Moderate Renal Insufficiency[1]
Atenolol	6	60	50 mg/d	50–100 mg/d	Yes
Captopril	2.2	65	50–75 mg/d	75–150 mg/d	Yes
Clonidine	8–12	95	0.2 mg/d	0.2–1.2 mg/d	Yes
Guanethidine	5 d	3–50	10 mg/d	25–50 mg/d	Yes
Hydralazine	1	25	100 mg/d	40–200 mg/d	No
Hydrochlorothiazide	12	70	25 mg/d	25–50 mg/d	No
Lisinopril	12	25	10 mg/d	10–80 mg/d	Yes
Losartan	1–2[2]	36	50 mg/d	2.5–100 mg/d	No
Methyldopa	2	25	1 g/d	1–2 g/d	No
Minoxidil	4	90	5–10 mg/d	40 mg/d	No
Nifedipine	2	50	30 mg/d	30–90 mg/d	No
Prazosin	3–4	70	3 mg/d	10–30 mg/d	No
Propranolol	3–6	25	80 mg/d	80–480 mg/d	No
Reserpine	24–48	NA	0.25 mg/d	0.25 mg/d	No
Verapamil	4–6	22	180 mg/d	240–480 mg/d	No

[1]Creatinine clearance $\geq$ 30 mL/min. Many of these drugs do require dosage adjustment if creatinine clearance falls below 30 mL/min.

[2]The active metabolite of losartan has a half-life of 3–4 hours.

effects depending on the class of receptor to which they bind.

Finally, one should note that *all* of the agents that lower blood pressure by altering sympathetic function can elicit compensatory effects through mechanisms that are not dependent on adrenergic nerves. Thus, the antihypertensive effect of any of these agents used alone may be limited by retention of sodium by the kidney and expansion of blood volume. For these reasons, sympathoplegic antihypertensive drugs are most effective when used concomitantly with a diuretic.

CENTRALLY ACTING SYMPATHOPLEGIC DRUGS

Mechanisms & Sites of Action

These agents reduce sympathetic outflow from vasopressor centers in the brainstem but allow these centers to retain or even increase their sensitivity to baroreceptor control. Accordingly, the antihypertensive and toxic actions of these drugs are generally less dependent on posture than are the effects of drugs that act directly on peripheral sympathetic neurons.

Methyldopa (L-α-methyl-3,4-dihydroxyphenylalanine) is an analog of L-dopa and is converted to α-methyldopamine and α-methylnorepinephrine; this pathway directly parallels the synthesis of norepinephrine from dopa illustrated in Figure 6–5. Alpha-methylnorepinephrine is stored in adrenergic nerve vesicles, where it stoichiometrically replaces norepinephrine, and is released by nerve stimulation to interact with postsynaptic adrenoceptors. However, this replacement of norepinephrine by a false transmitter in peripheral neurons is *not* responsible for methyldopa's antihypertensive effect, because the α-methylnorepinephrine released is an effective agonist at the α-adrenoceptors that mediate peripheral sympathetic constriction of arterioles and venules. Direct electrical stimulation of sympathetic nerves in methyldopa-treated animals produces sympathetic responses similar to those observed in untreated animals.

Indeed, methyldopa's antihypertensive action appears to be due to stimulation of central α-adrenoceptors by α-methylnorepinephrine or α-methyldopamine, based on the following evidence: (1) Much lower doses of methyldopa are required to lower blood pressure in animals when the drug is administered centrally by cerebral intraventricular injection rather than intravenously. (2) α-Receptor antagonists, especially α₂-selective antagonists, administered centrally, block the antihypertensive effect of methyldopa, whether the latter is given centrally or intravenously. (3) Potent inhibitors of dopa decarboxylase, administered centrally, block methyldopa's antihypertensive effect, thus showing that metabolism of the parent drug in the central nervous system is necessary for its action.

The antihypertensive action of **clonidine**, a 2-imidazoline derivative, was discovered in the course of testing the drug for use as a topically applied nasal decongestant.

After intravenous injection, clonidine produces a brief rise in blood pressure followed by more prolonged hypotension. The pressor response is due to direct stimulation of α-adrenoceptors in arterioles. The drug is classified as a partial agonist at α-receptors because it also inhibits pressor effects of other α-agonists.

Considerable evidence indicates that the hypotensive effect of clonidine is exerted at α-adrenoceptors in the medulla of the brain. In animals, the hypotensive effect of clonidine is prevented by central administration of α-antagonists. Clonidine reduces sympathetic and increases parasympathetic tone, resulting in blood pressure lowering and bradycardia. The reduction in pressure is accompanied by a decrease in circulating catecholamine levels. These observations suggest that clonidine sensitizes brainstem pressor centers to inhibition by baroreflexes.

Thus, studies of clonidine and methyldopa suggest that normal regulation of blood pressure involves central adrenergic neurons that modulate baroreceptor reflexes. Clonidine and α-methylnorepinephrine bind more tightly to α₂- than to α₁-adrenoceptors. As noted in Chapter 6, α₂-receptors are located on presynaptic adrenergic neurons as well as some postsynaptic sites. It is possible that clonidine and α-methylnorepinephrine act in the brain to reduce norepinephrine release onto relevant receptor sites. Alternatively, these drugs may act on postsynaptic α₂-adrenoceptors to inhibit activity of appropriate neurons. Finally, clonidine also binds to a nonadrenoceptor site, the **imidazoline receptor,** which may also mediate antihypertensive effects.

Methyldopa and clonidine produce slightly different hemodynamic effects: clonidine lowers heart rate and cardiac output more than does methyldopa. This difference suggests that these two drugs do not have identical sites of action. They may act primarily on different populations of neurons in the vasomotor centers of the brainstem.

Guanabenz and **guanfacine** are centrally active antihypertensive drugs that share the central α-adrenoceptor-stimulating effects of clonidine. They do not appear to offer any advantages over clonidine.

METHYLDOPA

Methyldopa is useful in the treatment of mild to moderately severe hypertension. It lowers blood pressure chiefly by reducing peripheral vascular resistance, with a variable reduction in heart rate and cardiac output.

Most cardiovascular reflexes remain intact after administration of methyldopa, and blood pressure reduction is not markedly dependent on maintenance of upright posture. Postural (orthostatic) hypotension sometimes occurs, particularly in volume-depleted patients. One potential advantage of methyldopa is that it causes reduction in renal vascular resistance.

α-Methyldopa
(α-methyl group in color)

Pharmacokinetics & Dosage

Pharmacokinetic characteristics of methyldopa are listed in Table 11–1. Methyldopa enters the brain via an aromatic amino acid transporter. An oral dose of methyldopa produces its maximal antihypertensive effect in 4–6 hours, and the effect can persist for up to 24 hours. Because the effect depends on accumulation and storage of a metabolite (α-methylnorepinephrine) in the vesicles of nerve endings, the action persists after the parent drug has disappeared from the circulation.

Toxicity

The most frequent undesirable effect of methyldopa is overt sedation, particularly at the onset of treatment. With long-term therapy, patients may complain of persistent mental lassitude and impaired mental concentration. Nightmares, mental depression, vertigo, and extrapyramidal signs may occur but are relatively infrequent. Lactation, associated with increased prolactin secretion, can occur both in men and in women treated with methyldopa. This toxicity is probably mediated by inhibition of dopaminergic mechanisms in the hypothalamus.

Other important adverse effects of methyldopa are development of a positive Coombs test (occurring in 10–20% of patients undergoing therapy for longer than

12 months), which sometimes makes cross-matching blood for transfusion difficult and rarely is associated with hemolytic anemia, as well as hepatitis and drug fever. Discontinuation of the drug usually results in prompt reversal of these abnormalities.

CLONIDINE

Hemodynamic studies indicate that blood pressure lowering by clonidine results from reduction of cardiac output due to decreased heart rate and relaxation of capacitance vessels, with a reduction in peripheral vascular resistance, particularly when patients are upright (when sympathetic tone is normally increased).

Reduction in arterial blood pressure by clonidine is accompanied by decreased renal vascular resistance and maintenance of renal blood flow. As with methyldopa, clonidine reduces blood pressure in the supine position and only rarely causes postural hypotension. Pressor effects of clonidine are not observed after ingestion of therapeutic doses of clonidine, but severe hypertension can complicate overdosage.

Clonidine

Pharmacokinetics & Dosage

Typical pharmacokinetic characteristics are listed in Table 11–1.

Clonidine is lipid-soluble and rapidly enters the brain from the circulation. Because of its relatively short half-life and the fact that its antihypertensive effect is directly related to blood concentration, oral clonidine must be given twice a day to maintain smooth blood pressure control. However, as is not the case with methyldopa, the dose-response curve of clonidine is such that increasing doses are more effective (but also more toxic).

A transdermal preparation of clonidine that reduces blood pressure for 7 days after a single application is also available. This preparation appears to produce less sedation than clonidine tablets but is often associated with local skin reactions.

Toxicity

Dry mouth and sedation are frequent and may be severe. Both effects are centrally mediated and dose-dependent and coincide temporally with the drug's antihypertensive effect.

The drug should not be given to patients who are at risk for mental depression and should be withdrawn if depression occurs during therapy. Concomitant treatment with tricyclic antidepressants may block the antihypertensive effect of clonidine. The interaction is believed to be due to α-adrenoceptor-blocking actions of the tricyclics.

Withdrawal of clonidine after protracted use, particularly with high dosages (greater than 1 mg/d), can result in life-threatening hypertensive crisis mediated by increased sympathetic nervous activity. Patients exhibit nervousness, tachycardia, headache, and sweating after omitting one or two doses of the drug. Although the incidence of severe hypertensive crisis is unknown, it is high enough to require that all patients who take clonidine be carefully warned of the possibility. If the drug must be stopped, this should be done gradually while other antihypertensive agents are being substituted. Treatment of the hypertensive crisis consists of reinstitution of clonidine therapy or administration of α- and β-adrenoceptor-blocking agents.

GANGLION-BLOCKING AGENTS

Historically, drugs that block stimulation of postganglionic autonomic neurons by acetylcholine were among the first agents used in the treatment of hypertension. Most such drugs are no longer available clinically because of intolerable toxicities related to their primary action (see below).

Ganglion blockers competitively block nicotinic cholinoceptors on postganglionic neurons in both sympathetic and parasympathetic ganglia. In addition, these drugs may directly block the nicotinic acetylcholine channel, in the same fashion as neuromuscular nicotinic blockers (see Figure 27–5).

The adverse effects of ganglion blockers are direct extensions of their pharmacologic effects. These effects include both sympathoplegia (excessive orthostatic hypotension and sexual dysfunction) and parasympathoplegia (constipation, urinary retention, precipitation of glaucoma, blurred vision, dry mouth, etc). These severe toxicities are the major reason for the abandonment of ganglion blockers for the therapy of hypertension.

ADRENERGIC NEURON-BLOCKING AGENTS

These drugs lower blood pressure by preventing normal physiologic release of norepinephrine from postganglionic sympathetic neurons.

GUANETHIDINE

In high enough doses, guanethidine can produce profound sympathoplegia. The resulting high maximal efficacy of this agent made it the mainstay of outpatient therapy of severe hypertension for many years. For the same reason, guanethidine can produce all of the toxicities expected from "pharmacologic sympathectomy," including marked postural hypotension, diarrhea, and impaired ejaculation. Because of these adverse effects, guanethidine is now rarely used.

Guanethidine

Guanethidine is too polar to enter the central nervous system. As a result, this drug has none of the central effects seen with many of the other antihypertensive agents described in this chapter.

Guanadrel is a guanethidine-like drug that is also available in the USA. **Bethanidine** and **debrisoquin**, antihypertensive agents not available for clinical use in the USA, are similar to guanethidine in mechanism of antihypertensive action.

Mechanism & Sites of Action

Guanethidine inhibits the release of norepinephrine from sympathetic nerve endings (Figure 11–4). This effect is probably responsible for most of the sympathoplegia that occurs in patients. Guanethidine is transported across the sympathetic nerve membrane by the same mechanism that transports norepinephrine itself (uptake 1), and uptake is essential for the drug's action. Once guanethidine has entered the nerve, it is concentrated in transmitter vesicles, where it replaces norepinephrine. Because it replaces norepinephrine, the drug causes a gradual depletion of norepinephrine stores in the nerve ending.

Inhibition of norepinephrine release is probably caused by guanethidine's local anesthetic properties on sympathetic nerve terminals. Although the drug does

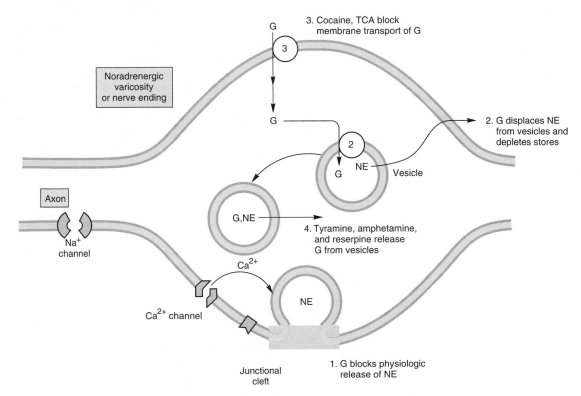

Figure 11–4. Guanethidine actions and drug interactions involving the adrenergic neuron. (G, guanethidine; NE, norepinephrine; TCA, tricyclic antidepressants.)

not impair axonal conduction in sympathetic fibers, local blockade of membrane electrical activity may occur in nerve endings because the nerve endings specifically take up and concentrate the drug.

Because neuronal uptake is necessary for the hypotensive activity of guanethidine, drugs that block the catecholamine uptake process or displace amines from the nerve terminal (see Chapter 6) block its effects. These include cocaine, amphetamine, tricyclic antidepressants, phenothiazines, and phenoxybenzamine.

Guanethidine increases sensitivity to the hypertensive effects of exogenously administered sympathomimetic amines. This results from inhibition of neuronal uptake of such amines and, after long-term therapy with guanethidine, supersensitivity of effector smooth muscle cells, in a fashion analogous to the process that follows surgical sympathectomy (see Chapter 6).

The hypotensive action of guanethidine early in the course of therapy is associated with reduced cardiac output, due to bradycardia and relaxation of capacitance vessels. With long-term therapy, peripheral vascular resistance decreases. Compensatory sodium and water retention may be marked during guanethidine therapy.

Pharmacokinetics & Dosage

Because of its long half-life (5 days) the onset of sympathoplegia is gradual (maximal effect in 1–2 weeks), and sympathoplegia persists for a comparable period after cessation of therapy. The dose should not ordinarily be increased at intervals shorter than 2 weeks.

Toxicity

Therapeutic use of guanethidine is often associated with symptomatic postural hypotension and hypotension following exercise, particularly when the drug is given in high doses, and may produce dangerously decreased blood flow to heart and brain or even overt shock.

Guanethidine-induced sympathoplegia in men may be associated with delayed or retrograde ejaculation (into the bladder). Guanethidine commonly causes diarrhea, which results from increased gastrointestinal motility due to parasympathetic predominance in controlling the activity of intestinal smooth muscle.

Interactions with other drugs may complicate guanethidine therapy. Sympathomimetic agents, at doses available in over-the-counter cold preparations, can produce hypertension in patients taking guanethidine. Similarly, guanethidine can produce hypertensive crisis by releasing catecholamines in patients with pheochromocytoma. When tricyclic antidepressants are administered to patients taking guanethidine, the drug's antihypertensive effect is attenuated, and severe hypertension may follow.

RESERPINE

Reserpine, an alkaloid extracted from the roots of an Indian plant, *Rauwolfia serpentina,* was one of the first effective drugs used on a large scale in the treatment of hypertension. At present, it is considered an effective and relatively safe drug for treating mild to moderate hypertension.

Mechanism & Sites of Action

Reserpine blocks the ability of aminergic transmitter vesicles to take up and store biogenic amines, probably by interfering with an uptake mechanism that depends on Mg^{2+} and ATP (Figure 6–4, carrier *B*). This effect occurs throughout the body, resulting in depletion of norepinephrine, dopamine, and serotonin in both central and peripheral neurons. Chromaffin granules of the adrenal medulla are also depleted of catecholamines, although to a lesser extent than are the vesicles of neurons. Reserpine's effects on adrenergic vesicles appear irreversible; trace amounts of the drug remain bound to vesicular membranes for many days. Although suffi-

Reserpine

ciently high doses of reserpine in animals can reduce catecholamine stores to zero, lower doses cause inhibition of neurotransmission that is roughly proportionate to the degree of amine depletion.

Depletion of peripheral amines probably accounts for much of the beneficial antihypertensive effect of reserpine, but a central component cannot be ruled out. The effects of low but clinically effective doses resemble those of centrally acting agents (eg, methyldopa) in that sympathetic reflexes remain largely intact, blood pressure is reduced in supine as well as in standing patients, and postural hypotension is mild. Reserpine readily enters the brain, and depletion of cerebral amine stores causes sedation, mental depression, and parkinsonism symptoms.

At lower doses used for treatment of mild hypertension, reserpine lowers blood pressure by a combination of decreased cardiac output and decreased peripheral vascular resistance.

Pharmacokinetics & Dosage

See Table 11–1.

Toxicity

At the low doses usually administered, reserpine produces little postural hypotension. Most of the unwanted effects of reserpine result from actions on the brain or gastrointestinal tract.

High doses of reserpine characteristically produce sedation, lassitude, nightmares, and severe mental depression; occasionally, these occur even in patients receiving low doses (0.25 mg/d). Much less frequently, ordinary low doses of reserpine produce extrapyramidal effects resembling Parkinson's disease, probably as a result of dopamine depletion in the corpus striatum. Although these central effects are uncommon, it should be stressed that they may occur at any time, even after months of uneventful treatment. Patients with a history of mental depression should not receive reserpine, and the drug should be stopped if depression appears.

Reserpine rather often produces mild diarrhea and gastrointestinal cramps and increases gastric acid secretion. The drug should probably not be given to patients with a history of peptic ulcer.

ADRENOCEPTOR ANTAGONISTS

The pharmacology of drugs that antagonize catecholamines at α- and β-adrenoceptors is presented in Chapter 10. This chapter will concentrate on two prototypical drugs, propranolol and prazosin, primarily in relation to their use in treatment of hypertension. Other adrenoceptor antagonists will be considered only briefly.

PROPRANOLOL

Propranolol was the first β-blocker shown to be effective in hypertension and ischemic heart disease. It is now clear that all β-adrenoceptor-blocking agents are very useful for lowering blood pressure in mild to moderate hypertension. In severe hypertension, β-blockers are especially useful in preventing the reflex tachycardia that often results from treatment with direct vasodilators. Beta blockers have been shown to reduce mortality in patients with heart failure, and they are particularly advantageous for treating hypertension in that population (see Chapter 13).

Mechanism & Sites of Action

Propranolol's efficacy in treating hypertension as well as most of its toxic effects result from nonselective β-blockade. Propranolol decreases blood pressure primarily as a result of a decrease in cardiac output. Other β-blockers may decrease cardiac output or decrease peripheral vascular resistance to various degrees, depending on cardioselectivity and partial agonist activities.

Beta-blockade in brain, kidney, and peripheral adrenergic neurons has been proposed as contributing to the antihypertensive effect observed with β-receptor blockers. In spite of conflicting evidence, the brain appears unlikely to be the primary site of the hypotensive action of these drugs, because some β-blockers that do not readily cross the blood-brain barrier (eg, nadolol, described below) are nonetheless effective antihypertensive agents.

Propranolol inhibits the stimulation of renin production by catecholamines (mediated by Beta$_1$-receptors). It is likely that propranolol's effect is due in part to depression of the renin-angiotensin-aldosterone system. Although most effective in patients with high plasma renin activity, propranolol also reduces blood pressure in hypertensive patients with normal or even low renin activity. Beta blockers might also act on peripheral presynaptic β-adrenoceptors to reduce sympathetic vasoconstrictor nerve activity.

In mild to moderate hypertension, propranolol produces a significant reduction in blood pressure without prominent postural hypotension.

Pharmacokinetics & Dosage

See Table 11–1. Resting bradycardia and a reduction in the heart rate during exercise are indicators of propranolol's β-blocking effect. Measures of these responses may be used as guides in regulating dosage. Propranolol can be administered once or twice daily.

Toxicity

The principal toxicities of propranolol result from blockade of cardiac, vascular, or bronchial β-receptors and are described in more detail in Chapter 10. The most important of these predictable extensions of the β-blocking action occur in patients with bradycardia or cardiac conduction disease, asthma, peripheral vascular insufficiency, and diabetes.

When propranolol is discontinued after prolonged regular use, some patients experience a withdrawal syndrome, manifested by nervousness, tachycardia, increased intensity of angina, or increase of blood pressure. Myocardial infarction has been reported in a few patients. Although the incidence of these complications is probably low, propranolol should not be discontinued abruptly. The withdrawal syndrome may involve up-regulation or supersensitivity of β-adrenoceptors.

OTHER BETA-ADRENOCEPTOR-BLOCKING AGENTS

Of the large number of β-blockers tested, most have been shown to be effective in lowering blood pressure. The pharmacologic properties of several of these agents differ from those of propranolol in ways that may confer therapeutic benefits in certain clinical situations.

1. Metoprolol

Metoprolol is approximately equipotent to propranolol in inhibiting stimulation of β_1-adrenoceptors such as those in the heart but 50- to 100-fold less potent than propranolol in blocking β_2-receptors. Although metoprolol is in other respects very similar to propranolol, its relative cardioselectivity may be advantageous in treating hypertensive patients who also suffer from asthma, diabetes, or peripheral vascular disease. Studies of small numbers of asthmatic patients have shown that metoprolol causes less bronchial constriction than propranolol at doses that produce equal inhibition of β_1-adrenoceptor responses. The cardioselectivity is not complete, however, and asthmatic symptoms have been exacerbated by metoprolol. Usual antihypertensive doses of metoprolol range from 100 to 450 mg/d.

2. Nadolol, Carteolol, Atenolol, Betaxolol, & Bisoprolol

Nadolol and carteolol, nonselective β-receptor antagonists, and atenolol, a β_1-selective blocker, are not appreciably metabolized and are excreted to a considerable extent in the urine. Betaxolol and bisoprolol are β_1-selective blockers that are primarily metabolized in the liver but have long half-lives. Because of these relatively long half-lives, these drugs can be administered once daily. Nadolol is usually begun at a dosage of 40 mg/d, atenolol at 50 mg/d, carteolol at 2.5 mg/d, betaxolol at 10 mg/d, and bisoprolol at 5 mg/d. Increases in dosage

to obtain a satisfactory therapeutic effect should take place no more often than every 4 or 5 days. Patients with reduced renal function should receive correspondingly reduced doses of nadolol, carteolol, and atenolol. It is claimed that atenolol produces fewer central nervous system-related effects than other more lipid-soluble β-antagonists.

3. Pindolol, Acebutolol, & Penbutolol

Pindolol, acebutolol, and penbutolol are partial agonists, ie, β-blockers with intrinsic sympathomimetic activity. They lower blood pressure by decreasing vascular resistance and appear to depress cardiac output or heart rate less than other β-blockers, perhaps because of significantly greater agonist than antagonist effects at β_2-receptors. This may be particularly beneficial for patients with bradyarrhythmias or peripheral vascular disease. Daily doses of pindolol start at 10 mg; of acebutolol, at 400 mg; and of penbutolol, at 20 mg.

4. Labetalol & Carvedilol

Labetalol is formulated as a racemic mixture of four isomers (it has two centers of asymmetry). Two of these isomers—the (S,S)- and (R,S)-isomers—are inactive, a third (S,R)- is a potent α-blocker, and the last (R,R)- is a potent β-blocker. The β-blocking isomer is thought to have selective β_2-agonist and nonselective β-antagonist action. Labetalol has a 3:1 ratio of β:α antagonism after oral dosing. Blood pressure is lowered by reduction of systemic vascular resistance without significant alteration in heart rate or cardiac output. Because of its combined α- and β-blocking activity, labetalol is useful in treating the hypertension of pheochromocytoma and hypertensive emergencies. Oral daily doses of labetalol range from 200 to 2400 mg/d. Labetalol is given as repeated intravenous bolus injections of 20–80 mg to treat hypertensive emergencies.

Carvedilol, like labetalol, is administered as a racemic mixture. The $S(-)$ isomer is a nonselective β-adrenoceptor blocker, but both $S(-)$ and $R(+)$ isomers have approximately equal α-blocking potency. The isomers are stereoselectively metabolized in the liver, which means that their elimination half-lives may differ. The average half-life is 7–10 hours. The usual starting dosage of carvedilol for ordinary hypertension is 6.25 mg twice daily.

5. Esmolol

Esmolol is a β_1-selective blocker that is rapidly metabolized via hydrolysis by red blood cell esterases. It has a short half-life (9 minutes) and is administered by constant intravenous infusion. Esmolol is generally administered as a loading dose (0.5–1 mg/kg), followed by a constant infusion. The infusion is typically started at 50–150 μg/kg/min, and the dose increased every 5 minutes, up to 300 μg/kg/min, as needed to achieve the desired therapeutic effect. Esmolol is used for management of intraoperative and postoperative hypertension, and sometimes for hypertensive emergencies, particularly when hypertension is associated with tachycardia.

PRAZOSIN & OTHER ALPHA₁ BLOCKERS

Mechanism & Sites of Action

Prazosin, terazosin, and doxazosin produce most of their antihypertensive effect by blocking α_1-receptors in arterioles and venules. Selectivity for α_1-receptors may explain why these agents produce less reflex tachycardia than do nonselective α-antagonists such as phentolamine. This receptor selectivity allows norepinephrine to exert unopposed negative feedback (mediated by presynaptic α_2-receptors) on its own release (see Chapter 6); in contrast, phentolamine blocks both presynaptic and postsynaptic α-receptors, with the result that reflex stimulation of sympathetic neurons produces greater release of transmitter onto β-receptors and correspondingly greater cardioacceleration.

Alpha blockers reduce arterial pressure by dilating both resistance and capacitance vessels. As expected, blood pressure is reduced more in the upright than in the supine position. Retention of salt and water occurs when these drugs are administered without a diuretic. The drugs are more effective when used in combination with other agents, such as a β-blocker and a diuretic, than when used alone.

Pharmacokinetics & Dosage

Pharmacokinetic characteristics of prazosin are listed in Table 11–1. Terazosin is also extensively metabolized but undergoes very little first-pass metabolism and has a half-life of 12 hours. Doxazosin has an intermediate bioavailability and a half-life of 22 hours.

Terazosin can often be given once daily, with doses of 5–20 mg/d. Doxazosin is usually given once daily starting at 1 mg/d and progressing to 4 mg/d or more as needed. Although long-term treatment with these α-blockers causes relatively little postural hypotension, precipitous drop in standing blood pressure develops in a number of patients shortly after the first dose is absorbed. For this reason, the first dose should be small and should be administered at bedtime. While the mechanism of this first-dose phenomenon is not clear, it occurs more commonly in patients who are salt- and volume-depleted.

Aside from the first-dose phenomenon, the reported toxicities of the α_1-blockers are relatively infrequent and mild. These include dizziness, palpitations, headache, and lassitude. Some patients develop a positive test for antinuclear factor in serum while on prazosin therapy, but this has not been associated with rheumatic symptoms. The α_1-blockers do not adversely and may even beneficially affect plasma lipid profiles but this action has not been shown to confer any benefit on clinical outcomes.

OTHER ALPHA ADRENOCEPTOR-BLOCKING AGENTS

Investigational α_1-selective blockers include pinacidil, urapidil, and cromakalim. The nonselective agents, **phentolamine** and **phenoxybenzamine,** are useful in diagnosis and treatment of pheochromocytoma and in other clinical situations associated with exaggerated release of catecholamines (eg, phentolamine may be combined with propranolol to treat the clonidine withdrawal syndrome, described above). Their pharmacology is described in Chapter 10.

VASODILATORS

Mechanism & Sites of Action

Within this class of drugs are the oral vasodilators, hydralazine and minoxidil, which are used for long-term outpatient therapy of hypertension; the parenteral vasodilators, nitroprusside, diazoxide, and fenoldopam, which are used to treat hypertensive emergencies; and the calcium channel blockers, which are used in both circumstances.

Chapter 12 contains a general discussion of vasodilators. All of the vasodilators useful in hypertension relax smooth muscle of arterioles, thereby decreasing systemic vascular resistance. Sodium nitroprusside also relaxes veins. Decreased arterial resistance and decreased mean arterial blood pressure elicit compensatory responses, mediated by baroreceptors and the sympathetic nervous system (Figure 11–5), as well as renin, angiotensin, and aldosterone. Because sympathetic reflexes are intact, vasodilator therapy does not cause orthostatic hypotension or sexual dysfunction.

Vasodilators work best in combination with other antihypertensive drugs that oppose the compensatory cardiovascular responses. (See Box, Monotherapy Versus Polypharmacy in Hypertension, p.174.)

HYDRALAZINE

Hydralazine, a hydrazine derivative, dilates arterioles but not veins. It has been available for many years,

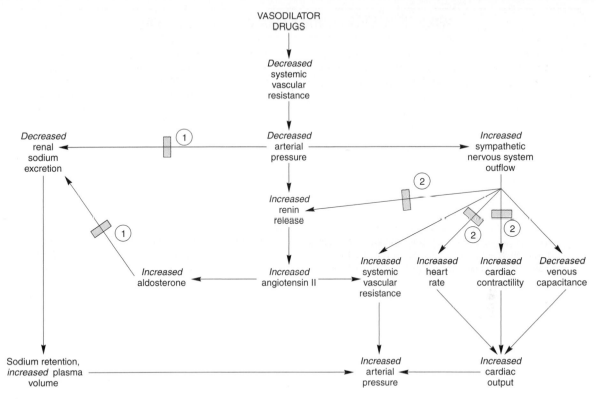

Figure 11–5. Compensatory responses to vasodilators; basis for combination therapy with β-blockers and diuretics. ① Effect blocked by diuretics. ② Effect blocked by β-blockers.

although it was initially thought not to be particularly effective because tachyphylaxis to hypertensive effects developed rapidly. The benefits of combination therapy are now recognized, and hydralazine may be used more effectively, particularly in severe hypertension.

Hydralazine

Pharmacokinetics & Dosage

Hydralazine is well absorbed and rapidly metabolized by the liver during the first pass, so that bioavailability is low (averaging 25%) and variable among individuals. It is metabolized in part by acetylation at a rate that appears to be bimodally distributed in the population (see Chapter 4). As a consequence, rapid acetylators have greater first-pass metabolism, lower bioavailability, and less antihypertensive benefit from a given dose than do slow acetylators. The half-life of hydralazine ranges from 2 to 4 hours, but vascular effects appear to persist longer than do blood concentrations, possibly due to avid binding to vascular tissue.

Usual dosage ranges from 40 mg/d to 200 mg/d. The higher dosage was selected as the dose at which there is a small possibility of developing the lupus erythematosus-like syndrome described in the next section. However, higher dosages result in greater vasodilation and may be used if necessary. Dosing two or three times daily provides smooth control of blood pressure.

Toxicity

The most common adverse effects of hydralazine are headache, nausea, anorexia, palpitations, sweating, and

---

MONOTHERAPY VERSUS POLYPHARMACY IN HYPERTENSION

Monotherapy of hypertension (treatment with a single drug) has become more popular because compliance is likely to be better and because in some cases adverse effects are fewer. However, moderate to severe hypertension is still commonly treated by a combination of two or more drugs, each acting by a different mechanism (polypharmacy). The rationale for polypharmacy is that each of the drugs acts on one of a set of interacting, mutually compensatory regulatory mechanisms for maintaining blood pressure (see Figures 6–7 and 11–1).

For example, because an adequate dose of hydralazine causes a significant decrease in peripheral vascular resistance, there will initially be a drop in mean arterial blood pressure, evoking a strong response in the form of compensatory tachycardia and salt and water retention (Figure 11–5). The result is an increase in cardiac output that is capable of almost completely reversing the effect of hydralazine. The addition of a β-blocker prevents the tachycardia; addition of a diuretic (eg, hydrochlorothiazide) prevents the salt and water retention. In effect, all three drugs increase the sensitivity of the cardiovascular system to each other's actions. Thus, partial impairment of one regulatory mechanism (sympathetic discharge to the heart) increases the antihypertensive effect of impairing regulation by another mechanism (peripheral vascular resistance). Finally, in some circumstances, a normal compensatory response accounts for the toxicity of an antihypertensive agent, and the toxic effect can be prevented by administering a second type of drug. In the case of hydralazine, compensatory tachycardia and increased cardiac output may precipitate angina in patients with coronary atherosclerosis. Addition of the β-blocker and diuretic can prevent this toxicity in many patients.

In practice, when hypertension does not respond adequately to a regimen of one drug, a second drug from a different class with a different mechanism of action and different pattern of toxicity is added. If the response is still inadequate and compliance is known to be good, a third drug may be added. The drugs least likely to be successful as monotherapy are the vasodilators hydralazine and minoxidil. It is not completely clear why other vasodilators such as calcium channel blockers cause less marked compensatory responses for the same amount of blood pressure lowering.

---

flushing. In patients with ischemic heart disease, reflex tachycardia and sympathetic stimulation may provoke angina or ischemic arrhythmias. With dosages of 400 mg/d or more, there is a 10–20% incidence—chiefly in persons who slowly acetylate the drug—of a syndrome characterized by arthralgia, myalgia, skin rashes, and fever that resembles lupus erythematosus. The syndrome is not associated with renal damage and is reversed by discontinuance of hydralazine. Peripheral neuropathy and drug fever are other serious but uncommon adverse effects.

MINOXIDIL

Minoxidil is a very efficacious orally active vasodilator. The effect appears to result from the opening of potassium channels in smooth muscle membranes by minoxidil sulfate, the active metabolite. This action stabilizes the membrane at its resting potential and makes contraction less likely. Like hydralazine, minoxidil dilates arterioles but not veins. Because of its greater potential antihypertensive effect, minoxidil should replace hydralazine when maximal doses of the latter are not effective or in patients with renal failure and severe hypertension, who do not respond well to hydralazine.

Minoxidil

Pharmacokinetics & Dosage

Pharmacokinetic parameters of minoxidil are listed in Table 11–1.

Even more than with hydralazine, the use of minoxidil is associated with reflex sympathetic stimulation and sodium and fluid retention. Minoxidil must be used in combination with a β-blocker and a loop diuretic.

Toxicity

Tachycardia, palpitations, angina, and edema are observed when doses of β-blockers and diuretics are inadequate. Headache, sweating, and hirsutism, which is particularly bothersome in women, are relatively common. Minoxidil illustrates how one person's toxicity may become another person's therapy. Topical minoxidil (as Rogaine) is now used as a stimulant to hair growth for correction of baldness.

SODIUM NITROPRUSSIDE

Sodium nitroprusside is a powerful parenterally administered vasodilator that is used in treating hypertensive emergencies as well as severe heart failure. Nitroprusside dilates both arterial and venous vessels, resulting in reduced peripheral vascular resistance and venous return. The action occurs as a result of activation of guanylyl cyclase, either via release of nitric oxide or by direct stimulation of the enzyme. The result is increased intracellular cGMP, which relaxes vascular smooth muscle.

In the absence of heart failure, blood pressure decreases, owing to decreased vascular resistance, while cardiac output does not change or decreases slightly. In patients with heart failure and low cardiac output, output often increases owing to afterload reduction.

Nitroprusside

Pharmacokinetics & Dosage

Nitroprusside is a complex of iron, cyanide groups, and a nitroso moiety. It is rapidly metabolized by uptake into red blood cells with liberation of cyanide. Cyanide in turn is metabolized by the mitochondrial enzyme rhodanase, in the presence of a sulfur donor, to the less toxic thiocyanate. Thiocyanate is distributed in extracellular fluid and slowly eliminated by the kidney.

Nitroprusside rapidly lowers blood pressure, and its effects disappear within 1–10 minutes after discontinuation. The drug is given by intravenous infusion. Sodium nitroprusside in aqueous solution is sensitive to light and must therefore be made up fresh before each administration and covered with opaque foil. Infusion solutions should be changed after several hours. Dosage typically begins at 0.5 μg/kg/min and may be increased up to 10 μg/kg/min as necessary to control blood pressure. Higher rates of infusion, if continued for more than an hour, may result in toxicity. Because of its efficacy and rapid onset of effect, the drug should be administered by infusion pump and arterial blood pressure continuously monitored via intra-arterial recording.

Toxicity

Other than excessive blood pressure lowering, the most serious toxicity is related to accumulation of cyanide; metabolic acidosis, arrhythmias, excessive hypotension, and death have resulted. In a few cases, toxicity after relatively low doses of nitroprusside suggested a defect in cyanide metabolism. Administration of sodium thiosulfate as a sulfur donor facilitates metabolism of cyanide. Hydroxocobalamin combines with cyanide to form the nontoxic cyanocobalamin. Both have been advocated for prophylaxis or treatment of cyanide poisoning during nitroprusside infusion. Thiocyanate may accumulate over the course of prolonged administration, usually a week or more, particularly in patients with renal insufficiency who do not excrete thiocyanate at a normal rate. Thiocyanate toxicity is manifested as weakness, disorientation, psychosis, muscle spasms, and convulsions, and the diagnosis is confirmed by finding serum concentrations greater than 10 mg/dL. Rarely, delayed hypothyroidism occurs, owing to thiocyanate inhibition of iodide uptake by the thyroid. Methemoglobinemia during infusion of nitroprusside has also been reported.

DIAZOXIDE

Diazoxide is an effective and relatively long-acting parenterally administered arteriolar dilator that is occasionally used to treat hypertensive emergencies. Injection of diazoxide results in a rapid fall in systemic vascular resistance and mean arterial blood pressure associated with substantial tachycardia and increase in cardiac output. Studies of its mechanism suggest that it prevents vascular smooth muscle contraction by opening potassium channels and stabilizing the membrane potential at the resting level.

Diazoxide

Pharmacokinetics & Dosage

Diazoxide is similar chemically to the thiazide diuretics but has no diuretic activity. It is bound extensively to serum albumin and to vascular tissue. Diazoxide is both metabolized and excreted unchanged; its metabolic pathways are not well characterized. Its half-life is approximately 24 hours, but the relationship between blood concentration and hypotensive action is not well established. The blood pressure-lowering effect after a rapid injection is established within 5 minutes and lasts for 4–12 hours.

When diazoxide was first marketed, a dose of 300 mg by rapid injection was recommended. It appears, however, that excessive hypotension can be avoided by beginning with smaller doses (50–150 mg). If necessary, doses of 150 mg may be repeated every 5 minutes until blood pressure is lowered satisfactorily. Nearly all patients respond to a maximum of three or four doses. Alternatively, diazoxide may be administered by intravenous infusion at rates of 15–30 mg/min. Because of reduced protein binding, hypotension occurs after smaller doses in persons with chronic renal failure, and smaller doses should be administered to these patients. The hypotensive effects of diazoxide are also greater if patients are pretreated with β-blockers to prevent the reflex tachycardia and associated increase in cardiac output.

Toxicity

The most significant toxicity from diazoxide has been excessive hypotension, resulting from the recommendation to use a fixed dose of 300 mg in all patients. Such hypotension has resulted in stroke and myocardial infarction. The reflex sympathetic response can provoke angina, electrocardiographic evidence of ischemia, and cardiac failure in patients with ischemic heart disease, and diazoxide should be avoided in this situation.

Diazoxide inhibits insulin release from the pancreas (probably by opening potassium channels in the β cell membrane) and is used to treat hypoglycemia secondary to insulinoma. Occasionally, hyperglycemia complicates diazoxide use, particularly in persons with renal insufficiency.

In contrast to the structurally related thiazide diuretics, diazoxide causes renal salt and water *retention*. However, because the drug is used for short periods only, this is rarely a problem.

FENOLDOPAM

Fenoldopam is a newer peripheral arteriolar dilator used for hypertensive emergencies and postoperative hypertension. It acts primarily as an agonist of dopamine D_1 receptors, resulting in dilation of peripheral arteries and natriuresis. The commercial product is a racemic mixture with the (R)-isomer mediating the pharmacologic activity.

Fenoldopam is rapidly metabolized, primarily by conjugation. Its half-life is 10 minutes. The drug is administered by continuous intravenous infusion. Fenoldopam is initiated at a low dosage (0.1 μg/kg/min), and the dose is then titrated upward every 15 or 20 minutes up to a maximum dose of 1.6 μg/kg/min or until the desired blood pressure reduction is achieved.

As with other direct vasodilators, the major toxicities are reflex tachycardia, headache, and flushing. Fenoldopam also increases intraocular pressure and should be avoided in patients with glaucoma.

CALCIUM CHANNEL BLOCKERS

In addition to their antianginal (see Chapter 12) and antiarrhythmic effects (see Chapter 14), calcium channel blockers also dilate peripheral arterioles and reduce blood pressure. The mechanism of action in hypertension (and, in part, in angina) is inhibition of calcium influx into arterial smooth muscle cells.

Verapamil, diltiazem, and the **dihydropyridine** family (**amlodipine, felodipine, isradipine, nicardipine, nifedipine,** and **nisoldipine**) are all equally effective in lowering blood pressure, and various formulations are currently approved for this use in the USA. Several others are under study. Hemodynamic differences among calcium channel blockers may influence the choice of a particular agent. Nifedipine and the other dihydropyridine agents are more selective as vasodilators and have less cardiac depressant effect than verapamil and diltiazem. Reflex sympathetic activation with slight tachycardia maintains or increases cardiac output in most patients given dihydropyridines. Verapamil has the greatest depressant effect on the heart and may decrease heart rate and cardiac output. Diltiazem has intermediate actions. The pharmacology and toxicity of these drugs is discussed in more detail in Chapter 12. Doses of calcium channel blockers used in treating hypertension are similar to those used in treating angina. Some epidemiologic studies reported an increased risk of myocardial infarction or mortality in patients receiving short-acting nifedipine for hypertension. While there is still debate about causation, it is recommended that short-acting dihydropyridines not be used for hypertension. Sustained-release calcium blockers or calcium blockers with long half-lives provide smoother blood pressure control and are more appropriate for treatment of chronic hypertension. Intravenous nicardipine is available for the treatment of hypertension when oral therapy is not feasible, although parenteral verapamil and diltiazem could be used for the same indication. Nicardipine is typically infused at rates of 2–15 mg/h. Oral short-acting nifedipine has been used in emergency management of severe hypertension.

INHIBITORS OF ANGIOTENSIN

Although the causative roles of renin, angiotensin, and aldosterone in essential hypertension are still controversial, there do appear to be differences in the activity of this system among individuals. Approximately 20% of patients with essential hypertension have inappropriately low and 20% have inappropriately high plasma renin activity. Blood pressure of patients with high-renin hypertension responds well to β-adrenoceptor blockers, which lower plasma renin activity, and to angiotensin inhibitors—supporting a role for excess renin and angiotensin in this population.

Mechanism & Sites of Action

Renin release from the kidney cortex is stimulated by reduced renal arterial pressure, sympathetic neural stimulation, and reduced sodium delivery or increased sodium concentration at the distal renal tubule (see Chapter 17). Renin acts upon angiotensinogen to split off the inactive precursor decapeptide angiotensin I. Angiotensin I is then converted, primarily by endothelial ACE, to the arterial vasoconstrictor octapeptide angiotensin II (Figure 11–6), which is in turn converted in the adrenal gland to angiotensin III. Angiotensin II has vasoconstrictor and sodium-retaining activity. Angiotensin II and III both stimulate aldosterone release. Angiotensin may contribute to maintaining high vascular resistance in hypertensive states associated with high plasma renin activity, such as renal arterial stenosis, some types of intrinsic renal disease, and malignant hypertension, as well as in essential hypertension after treatment with sodium restriction, diuretics, or vasodilators. However, even in low-renin hypertensive states, these drugs can lower blood pressure (see below).

A parallel system for angiotensin generation exists in several other tissues (eg, heart) and may be responsible for trophic changes such as cardiac hypertrophy. The converting enzyme involved in tissue angiotensin II synthesis is also inhibited by the ACE inhibitors.

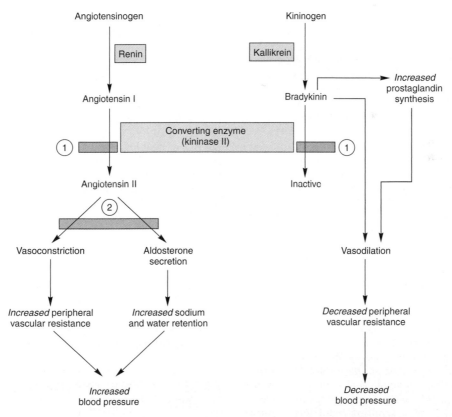

Figure 11–6. Sites of action of ACE inhibitors and angiotensin II receptor blockers. ① Site of ACE blockade. ② Site of receptor blockade.

Two classes of drugs act specifically on the renin-angiotensin system: the ACE inhibitors and the competitive inhibitors of angiotensin at its receptors, including losartan and other nonpeptide antagonists, and the peptide saralasin. (Saralasin is no longer in clinical use.)

ANGIOTENSIN-CONVERTING ENZYME (ACE) INHIBITORS

Captopril (see Figure 17–2) and other drugs in this class inhibit the converting enzyme peptidyl dipeptidase that hydrolyzes angiotensin I to angiotensin II and (under the name plasma kininase) inactivates bradykinin, a potent vasodilator, which works at least in part by stimulating release of nitric oxide and prostacyclin. The hypotensive activity of captopril results both from an inhibitory action on the renin-angiotensin system and a stimulating action on the kallikrein-kinin system (Figure 11–6). The latter mechanism has been demonstrated by showing that an experimental bradykinin receptor antagonist, icatibant, blunts the blood pressure-lowering effect of captopril.

Enalapril (see Figure 17–2) is a prodrug that is converted by deesterification to a converting enzyme inhibitor, enalaprilat, with effects similar to those of captopril. Enalaprilat itself is available only for intravenous use, primarily for hypertensive emergencies. **Lisinopril** is a lysine derivative of enalaprilat. **Benazepril, fosinopril, moexipril, perindopril, quinapril, ramipril,** and **trandolapril** are other long-acting members of the class. All are prodrugs, like enalapril, and are converted to the active agents by hydrolysis, primarily in the liver.

Angiotensin II inhibitors lower blood pressure principally by decreasing peripheral vascular resistance. Cardiac output and heart rate are not significantly changed. Unlike direct vasodilators, these agents do not result in reflex sympathetic activation and can be used safely in persons with ischemic heart disease. The absence of reflex tachycardia may be due to downward resetting of the baroreceptors or to enhanced parasympathetic activity.

Although converting enzyme inhibitors are most effective in conditions associated with high plasma renin activity, there is no good correlation among subjects between plasma renin activity and antihypertensive response. Accordingly, renin profiling is unnecessary.

ACE inhibitors have a particularly useful role in treating patients with diabetic nephropathy because they diminish proteinuria and stabilize renal function (even in the absence of lowering of blood pressure). These benefits probably result from improved intrarenal hemodynamics, with decreased glomerular efferent arteriolar resistance and a resulting reduction of intraglomerular capillary pressure. ACE inhibitors have also proved to be extremely useful in the treatment of heart failure, and after myocardial infarction (see Chapter 13).

Pharmacokinetics & Dosage

Captopril's pharmacokinetic parameters and dosing recommendations are set forth in Table 11–1.

Peak concentrations of enalaprilat, the active metabolite, occur 3–4 hours after dosing with enalapril. The half-life of enalaprilat is about 11 hours. Typical doses of enalapril are 10–20 mg once or twice daily.

Lisinopril has a half-life of 12 hours. Doses of 10–80 mg once daily are effective in most patients.

All of the ACE inhibitors except fosinopril and moexipril are eliminated primarily by the kidneys; doses of these drugs should be reduced in patients with renal insufficiency.

Toxicity

Severe hypotension can occur after initial doses of any ACE inhibitor in patients who are hypovolemic due to diuretics, salt restriction, or gastrointestinal fluid loss. Other adverse effects common to all ACE inhibitors include acute renal failure (particularly in patients with bilateral renal artery stenosis or stenosis of the renal artery of a solitary kidney), hyperkalemia, dry cough sometimes accompanied by wheezing, and angioedema. Hyperkalemia is more likely to occur in patients with renal insufficiency or diabetes. Bradykinin and substance P seem to be responsible for the cough and angioedema seen with ACE inhibition.

The use of ACE inhibitors is contraindicated during the second and third trimesters of pregnancy because of the risk of fetal hypotension, anuria, and renal failure, sometimes associated with fetal malformations or death. Captopril, particularly when given in high doses to patients with renal insufficiency, may cause neutropenia or proteinuria. Minor toxic effects seen more typically include altered sense of taste, allergic skin rashes, and drug fever, which may occur in as many as 10% of patients. The incidence of these adverse effects may be lower with the long-acting ACE inhibitors.

Important drug interactions include those with potassium supplements or potassium-sparing diuretics, which can result in hyperkalemia. Nonsteroidal anti-inflammatory drugs may impair the hypotensive effects of ACE inhibitors by blocking bradykinin-mediated vasodilation, which is at least in part, prostaglandin mediated.

ANGIOTENSIN RECEPTOR-BLOCKING AGENTS

Losartan and **valsartan** were the first marketed blockers of the angiotensin II type 1 (AT_1) receptor. More recently, candesartan, eprosartan, irbesartan, and telmisartan have been released. They have no effect on bradykinin metabolism and are therefore more selective blockers of angiotensin effects than ACE inhibitors. They also have the potential for more complete inhibition of angiotensin action compared with ACE inhibitors because there are enzymes other than ACE that are capable of generating angiotensin II. Losartan's pharmacokinetic parameters are listed in Table 11–1. The adverse effects are similar to those described for ACE inhibitors, including the hazard of use during pregnancy. Cough and angioedema can occur but are less common with angiotensin receptor blockers than with ACE inhibitors.

II. CLINICAL PHARMACOLOGY OF ANTIHYPERTENSIVE AGENTS

Hypertension presents a unique problem in therapeutics. It is usually a lifelong disease that causes few symptoms until the advanced stage. For effective treatment, medicines that may be expensive and often produce adverse effects must be consumed daily. Thus, the physician must establish with certainty that hypertension is persistent and requires treatment and must exclude secondary causes of hypertension that might be treated by definitive surgical procedures. Persistence of hypertension, particularly in persons with mild elevation of blood pressure, should be established by finding an elevated blood pressure on at least three different office visits. Ambulatory blood pressure monitoring may be the best predictor of risk and therefore of need for therapy in mild hypertension. Isolated systolic hypertension and hypertension in the elderly also benefit from therapy.

Once the presence of hypertension is established, the question of whether or not to treat and which drugs to use must be considered. The level of blood pressure, the age and sex of the patient, the severity of organ damage (if any) due to high blood pressure, and the presence of cardiovascular risk factors must all be considered. At this stage, the patient must be educated about the nature of hypertension and the importance of treatment so that he or she can make an informed decision regarding therapy.

Once the decision is made to treat, a therapeutic regimen must be developed. Selection of drugs is dictated by the level of blood pressure, the presence and severity of end-organ damage, and the presence of other diseases. Severe high blood pressure with life-threatening complications requires more rapid treatment with more potent drugs. Most patients with essential hypertension, however, have had elevated blood pressure for months or years, and therapy is best initiated in a gradual fashion.

Education about the natural history of hypertension and the importance of treatment compliance as well as potential side effects of drugs is essential. Follow-up visits should be frequent enough to convince the patient that the physician thinks the illness is serious. With each follow-up visit, the importance of treatment should be reinforced and questions particularly concerning dosing or side effects of medication encouraged. Other factors that may improve compliance are simplifying dosing regimens and having the patient monitor blood pressure at home.

OUTPATIENT THERAPY OF HYPERTENSION

The initial step in treating hypertension may be nonpharmacologic. As discussed previously, sodium restriction may be effective treatment for many patients with mild hypertension. The average American diet contains about 200 mEq of sodium per day. A reasonable dietary goal in treating hypertension is 70–100 mEq of sodium per day, which can be achieved by not salting food during or after cooking and by avoiding processed foods that contain large amounts of sodium.

Weight reduction even without sodium restriction has been shown to normalize blood pressure in up to 75% of overweight patients with mild to moderate hypertension. Regular exercise has been shown in some but not all studies to lower blood pressure in hypertensive patients.

For pharmacologic management of mild hypertension, blood pressure can be normalized in most patients with a single drug. Such "monotherapy" is also sufficient for some patients with moderate hypertension. Thiazide diuretics, β-blockers, and ACE inhibitors have been shown to reduce morbidity and mortality and are recommended for initial drug therapy in such patients. There has been concern that diuretics, by adversely affecting the serum lipid profile or impairing glucose tolerance, may add to the risk of coronary disease, thereby offsetting the benefit of blood pressure reduction. However a recent large clinical trial comparing different classes of antihypertensive mediations for initial therapy found that chlorthalidone (a thiazide diuretic) was as effective as other agents in reducing coronary heart disease death and nonfatal myocardial infarction, and was superior to amlodipine in preventing heart failure and superior to lisinopril in preventing stroke (ALLHAT Collaborative Research Group, 2002).

Alternative choices for initial monotherapy include angiotensin receptor blockers, calcium channel blockers, combination α- and β-blockers (labetalol or carvedilol), and central sympathoplegic agents (eg, clonidine). Alpha blockers should not be considered first-line therapy (ALLHAT, 2000). The presence of concomitant disease should influence selection of antihypertensive drugs because two diseases may benefit from a single drug. For example, ACE inhibitors are particularly useful in diabetic patients with evidence of renal disease. Beta blockers or calcium channel blockers are useful in patients who also have angina; diuretics, ACE inhibitors, or β-blockers in patients who also have heart failure; and α_1 blockers in men who have benign prostatic hyperplasia. Race may also affect drug selection: blacks respond better to diuretics and calcium channel blockers than to β-blockers and ACE inhibitors. Chinese are more sensitive to the effects of β-blockers and may require lower doses.

If a single drug does not adequately control blood pressure, drugs with different sites of action can be combined to effectively lower blood pressure while minimizing toxicity ("stepped care"). If a diuretic is not used initially, it is often selected as the second drug. If three drugs are required, combining a diuretic, a sympathoplegic agent or an ACE inhibitor, and a direct vasodilator (eg, hydralazine or a calcium channel blocker) is often effective. In the USA, fixed-dose drug combinations containing a β-blocker plus a thiazide, an ACE inhibitor plus a thiazide, an angiotensin receptor blocker plus a diuretic, and a calcium channel blocker plus an ACE inhibitor are available. Fixed-dose combinations have the drawback of not allowing for titration of individual drug doses but have the advantage of allowing fewer pills to be taken, potentially enhancing compliance.

Assessment of blood pressure during office visits should include measurement of recumbent, sitting, and standing pressures. An attempt should be made to normalize blood pressure in the posture or activity level that is customary for the patient. The recent large Hypertension Optimal Treatment study suggests that the optimal blood pressure end point is 138/83 mm Hg. Lowering blood pressure below this level produces no further benefit (Hansson et al, 1998). In diabetic patients, however, there is a continued reduction of event rates with progressively lower blood pressures. In addition to noncompliance with medication, causes of failure to respond to drug therapy include excessive sodium intake and inadequate diuretic therapy with excessive blood volume (this can be measured directly), and drugs such as tricyclic antidepressants, nonsteroidal anti-inflammatory drugs, over-the-counter sympathomimetics, abuse of stimulants (amphetamine or cocaine), or excessive doses of caffeine and oral contraceptives that can interfere with actions of some antihypertensive drugs or directly raise blood pressure.

MANAGEMENT OF HYPERTENSIVE EMERGENCIES

Despite the large number of patients with chronic hypertension, hypertensive emergencies are relatively rare. Marked or sudden elevation of blood pressure may be a serious threat to life, however, and prompt control of blood pressure is indicated. Most commonly, hypertensive emergencies occur in patients whose hypertension is severe and poorly controlled and in those who suddenly discontinue antihypertensive medications.

Clinical Presentation & Pathophysiology

Hypertensive emergencies include hypertension associated with vascular damage (termed malignant hypertension) and hypertension associated with hemodynamic complications such as heart failure, stroke, or dissecting aneurysm. The underlying pathologic process in malignant hypertension is a progressive arteriopathy with inflammation and necrosis of arterioles. Vascular lesions occur in the kidney, which releases renin, which in turn stimulates production of angiotensin and aldosterone, which further increase blood pressure.

Hypertensive encephalopathy is a classic feature of malignant hypertension. Its clinical presentation consists of severe headache, mental confusion, and apprehension. Blurred vision, nausea and vomiting, and focal neurologic deficits are common. If untreated, the syndrome may progress over a period of 12–48 hours to convulsions, stupor, coma, and even death.

Treatment of Hypertensive Emergencies

The general management of hypertensive emergencies requires monitoring the patient in an intensive care unit with continuous recording of arterial blood pressure. Fluid intake and output must be monitored carefully and body weight measured daily as an indicator of total body fluid volume during the course of therapy.

Parenteral antihypertensive medications are used to lower blood pressure rapidly (within a few hours); as soon as reasonable blood pressure control is achieved, oral antihypertensive therapy should be substituted, because this allows smoother long-term management of hypertension. The goal of treatment in the first few hours or days is not complete normalization of blood pressure because chronic hypertension is associated with autoregulatory changes in cerebral blood flow. Thus, rapid normalization of blood pressure may lead to cerebral hypoperfusion and brain injury. Rather, blood pressure should be lowered by about 25%, maintaining diastolic blood pressure at no less than 100–110 mm Hg. Subsequently, blood pressure can be reduced to normal levels using oral medications over several weeks. The drug most commonly used to treat hypertensive emergencies is the vasodilator sodium nitroprusside. Other parenteral drugs that may be effective include fenoldopam, nitroglycerin, labetalol, calcium channel blockers, diazoxide, and hydralazine. Esmolol is often used to manage intraoperative and postoperative hypertension. Diuretics such as furosemide are administered to prevent the volume expansion that typically occurs during administration of powerful vasodilators.

PREPARATIONS AVAILABLE

Beta Adrenoceptor Blockers
Acebutolol (generic, Sectral)
Oral: 200, 400 mg capsules
Atenolol (generic, Tenormin)
Oral: 25, 50, 100 mg tablets
Parenteral: 0.5 mg/mL for injection
Betaxolol (Kerlone)
Oral: 10, 20 mg tablets
Bisoprolol (Zebeta)
Oral: 5, 10 mg tablets
Carteolol (Cartrol)
Oral: 2.5, 5 mg tablets
Carvedilol (Coreg)
Oral: 3.125, 6.25, 12.5, 25 mg tablets
Esmolol (BreviBloc)
Parenteral: 10, 250 mg/mL for injection
Labetalol (generic, Normodyne, Trandate)
Oral: 100, 200, 300 mg tablets
Parenteral: 5 mg/mL for injection
Metoprolol (generic, Lopressor)
Oral: 50, 100 mg tablets
Oral extended-release (Toprol-XL): 25, 50, 100, 200 mg tablets
Parenteral: 1 mg/mL for injection
Nadolol (generic, Corgard)
Oral: 20, 40, 80, 120, 160 mg tablets
Penbutolol (Levatol)
Oral: 20 mg tablets
Pindolol (generic, Visken)
Oral: 5, 10 mg tablets
Propranolol (generic, Inderal)
Oral: 10, 20, 40, 60, 80, 90 mg tablets; 4, 8 mg/mL oral solution; Intensol, 80 mg/mL solution
Oral sustained-release (generic, Inderal LA): 60, 80, 120, 160 mg capsules
Parenteral: 1 mg/mL for injection
Timolol (generic, Blocadren)
Oral: 5, 10, 20 mg tablets

Centrally Acting Sympathoplegic Drugs
Clonidine (generic, Catapres)
Oral: 0.1, 0.2, 0.3 mg tablets
Transdermal (Catapres-TTS): patches that release 0.1, 0.2, 0.3 mg/24 h
Guanabenz (generic, Wytensin)
Oral: 4, 8 mg tablets
Guanfacine (Tenex)
Oral: 1, 2 mg tablets
Methyldopa (generic)
Oral: 250, 500 mg tablets
Parenteral: 50 mg/mL for injection

Postganglionic Sympathetic Nerve Terminal Blockers
Guanadrel (Hylorel)
Oral: 10, 25 mg tablets
Guanethidine (Ismelin)
Oral: 10, 25 mg tablets
Reserpine (generic)
Oral: 0.1, 0.25 mg tablets

Alpha$_1$ Selective Adrenoceptor Blockers
Doxazosin (generic, Cardura)
Oral: 1, 2, 4, 8 mg tablets
Prazosin (generic, Minipress)
Oral: 1, 2, 5 mg capsules
Terazosin (generic, Hytrin)
Oral: 1, 2, 5, 10 mg capsules and tablets

Ganglion-Blocking Agents
Mecamylamine (Inversine)
Oral: 2.5 mg tablets

Vasodilators Used in Hypertension
Diazoxide (Hyperstat IV)
Parenteral: 15 mg/mL ampule
Oral (Proglycem): 50 mg capsule; 50 mg/mL oral suspension
Fenoldopam (Corlopam)
Parenteral: 10 mg/mL for IV infusion
Hydralazine (generic, Apresoline)
Oral: 10, 25, 50, 100 mg tablets
Parenteral: 20 mg/mL for injection
Minoxidil (generic, Loniten)
Oral: 2.5, 10 mg tablets
Topical (Rogaine, etc): 2% lotion
Nitroprusside (generic, Nitropress)
Parenteral: 50 mg/vial

Calcium Channel Blockers
Amlodipine (Norvasc)
Oral 2.5, 5, 10 mg tablets
Diltiazem (generic, Cardizem)
Oral: 30, 60, 90, 120 mg tablets (unlabeled in hypertension)
Oral sustained-release (Cardizem CD, Cardizem SR, Dilacor XL): 60, 90, 120, 180, 240, 300, 360, 420 mg capsules
Parenteral: 5 mg/mL for injection
Felodipine (Plendil)
Oral extended-release: 2.5, 5, 10 mg tablets
Isradipine (DynaCirc)
Oral: 2.5, 5 mg capsules; 5, 10 mg controlled-release tablets

Nicardipine (generic, Cardene)
Oral: 20, 30 mg capsules
Oral sustained-release (Cardene SR): 30, 45, 60 mg capsules
Parenteral (Cardene I.V.): 2.5 mg/mL for injection
Nisoldipine (Sular)
Oral: 10, 20, 30, 40 mg extended-release tablets
Nifedipine (generic, Adalat, Procardia)
Oral: 10, 20 mg capsules (unlabeled in hypertension)
Oral extended-release (Adalat CC, Procardia-XL): 30, 60, 90 mg tablets
Verapamil (generic, Calan, Isoptin)
Oral: 40, 80, 120 mg tablets
Oral sustained-release (generic, Calan SR, Verelan): 120, 180, 240 mg tablets; 100, 120, 180, 200, 240, 300 mg capsules
Parenteral: 2.5 mg/mL for injection

ANGIOTENSIN-CONVERTING ENZYME INHIBITORS
Benazepril (Lotensin)
Oral: 5, 10, 20, 40, mg tablets
Captopril (generic, Capoten)
Oral: 12.5, 25, 50, 100 mg tablets
Enalapril (Vasotec)
Oral: 2.5, 5, 10, 20 mg tablets
Parenteral (Enalaprilat): 1.25 mg/mL for injection
Fosinopril (Monopril)
Oral: 10, 20, 40 mg tablets

Lisinopril (Prinivil, Zestril)
Oral: 2.5, 5, 10, 20, 40 mg tablets
Moexipril (Univasc)
Oral: 7.5, 15 mg tablets
Perindopril (Aceon)
Oral: 2, 4, 8 mg tablets
Quinapril (Accupril)
Oral: 5, 10, 20, 40 mg tablets
Ramipril (Altace)
Oral: 1.25, 2.5, 5, 10 mg capsules
Trandolapril (Mavik)
Oral: 1, 2, 4 mg tablets

ANGIOTENSIN RECEPTOR BLOCKERS
Candesartan (Atacand)
Oral: 4, 8, 16, 32 mg tablets
Eprosartan (Teveten)
Oral: 400, 600 mg tablets
Irbesartan (Avapro)
Oral; 75, 150, 300 mg tablets
Losartan (Cozaar)
Oral: 25, 50, 100 mg tablets
Olmisartan (Benicar)
Oral: 5, 20, 40 mg tablets
Telmisartan (Micardis)
Oral: 20, 40, 80 mg tablets
Valsartan (Diovan)
Oral: 40, 80, 160, 320 mg tablet

REFERENCES

ACE Inhibitors in Diabetic Nephropathy Trialist Group: Should all patients with type 1 diabetes mellitus and microalbuminuria receive angiotensin-converting enzyme inhibitors? A meta-analysis of individual patient data. Ann Intern Med 2001;134:370.

ALLHAT Officers and Coordinators for the ALLHAT Collaborative Research Group: Major cardiovascular events in hypertensive patients randomized to Doxazosin vs Chlorthalidone: The antihypertensive and lipid-lowering treatment to prevent heart attack trial. JAMA 2000;283:1967.

ALLHAT Officers and Coordinators for the ALLHAT Collaborative Research Group: Major outcomes of high-risk hypertensive patients randomized to angiotensin-converting enzyme inhibitor or calcium channel blockers vs diuretic: The antihypertensive and lipid-lowering treatment to prevent heart attack trial. JAMA 2002;288:2981.

August P: Initial treatment of hypertension. N Engl J Med 2003;348:610.

Bakris GL et al: Preserving renal function in adults with hypertension and diabetes: A consensus approach. Am J Kidney Dis 2000;363:646.

Brown NJ, Vaughan DE: Angiotensin-converting enzyme inhibitors. Circulation 1998;97:1411.

Burnier M: Cardiovascular Drugs: Angiotensin II type 1 receptor blockers. Circulation 2001;103:904.

Carretero OA, Oparil S: Clinical Cardiology: New Frontiers: Essential hypertension, Part I: definition and etiology. Circulation 2000;101:329.

Cooper H et al: Diuretics and risk of arrhythmic death in patients with left ventricular dysfunction. Circulation 1999;100:1311.

Cooper ME, Johnston CI: Optimizing treatment of hypertension in patients with diabetes. JAMA 2000;283:3177.

Corvol P et al: Seven lessons from two candidate genes in human essential hypertension: Angiotensinogen and epithelial sodium channel. Hypertension 1999;33:1324.

Garg J, Messerli AW, Bakris GL: Evaluation and treatment of patients with systemic hypertension. Circulation 2002;105:2458.

Hansson L et al: Effects of intensive blood-pressure lowering and low-dose aspirin in patients with hypertension: Principal results of the Hypertension Optimal Treatment (HOT) randomised trial. Lancet 1998;351:1755.

He J, Ogden L, Vupputuri S: Dietary sodium intake and subsequent risk of cardiovascular disease in overweight adults. JAMA 1999;282:2027.

Hyman DJ, Pavlik VN: Characteristics of patients with uncontrolled hypertension in the United States. N Engl J Med 2001;345:479.

Kaplan NM: Management of hypertension in patients with type 2 diabetes mellitus: guidelines based on current evidence. Ann Intern Med 2001;135:1079.

Ko DT et al: β-Blocker therapy and symptoms of depression, fatigue, and sexual dysfunction. JAMA 2002;288:351.

Mosterd A et al: Trends in the prevalence of hypertension, antihypertensive therapy, and left ventricular hypertrophy from 1950 to 1989. N Engl J Med 1999;340:1221.

Murphy MB, Murray C, Shorten GD: Fenoldopam—a selective peripheral dopamine-receptor agonist for the treatment of severe hypertension. N Engl J Med 2001;345:1548.

Palmer BF: Renal dysfunction complicating the treatment of hypertension. N Engl J Med 2002;347:1256.

Remuzzi G, Ruggenenti P, Perico N: Chronic renal diseases: renoprotective benefits of renin-angiotensin-system inhibition. Ann Intern Med 2002;136:604.

Sacks FM et al: Effects on blood pressure of reduced dietary sodium and the dietary approaches to stop hypertension (DASH) diet. N Engl J Med 2001;344:3.

Safian RD, Textor SC: Renal-artery stenosis. N Engl J Med 2001;344:431.

Sheffield JVL, Larson EB: Update in general internal medicine. Ann Intern Med 2001;135:269.

Sixth report of the Joint National Committee on prevention, detection, evaluation, and treatment of high blood pressure: Arch Intern Med 1997;157:2413.

Stevens VJ et al: Long-term weight loss and changes in blood pressure: results of the trials of hypertension prevention, phase II. Ann Intern Med 2001;134:1.

Vollmer WM et al: Effects of diet and sodium intake on blood pressure: Subgroup analysis of the DASH-Sodium trial. Ann Intern Med 2001;135:1019.

Wing LMH et al: A comparison of outcomes with angiotensin-converting-enzyme inhibitors and diuretics for hypertension in the elderly. N Engl J Med 2003;348:583.

Wright JT Jr et al: Effect of blood pressure lowering and antihypertensive drug class on progression of hypertensive kidney disease. Results from AASK Trial. JAMA 2002;288:2421.

Vasodilators & the Treatment of Angina Pectoris

Bertram G. Katzung, MD, PhD, & Kanu Chatterjee, MB, FRCP

Angina pectoris is the most common condition involving tissue ischemia in which vasodilator drugs are used. Angina (pain) is caused by the accumulation of metabolites in striated muscle; angina pectoris is the severe chest pain that occurs when coronary blood flow is inadequate to supply the oxygen required by the heart. The organic nitrates, eg, **nitroglycerin**, are the mainstay of therapy for the immediate relief of angina. Another group of vasodilators, the **calcium channel blockers,** is also important, especially for prophylaxis, and the β-**blockers,** which are *not* vasodilators, are also useful in prophylaxis. A new group of drugs (fatty acid oxidation inhibitors) that are not vasodilators but alter myocardial metabolism are under intense investigation.

Ischemic heart disease is the most common serious health problem in many Western societies. By far the most frequent cause of angina is atheromatous obstruction of the large coronary vessels (**atherosclerotic angina, classic angina**). However, transient spasm of localized portions of these vessels, which is usually associated with underlying atheromas, can also cause significant myocardial ischemia and pain (**angiospastic or variant angina**).

The primary cause of angina pectoris is an imbalance between the oxygen requirement of the heart and the oxygen supplied to it via the coronary vessels. In classic angina, the imbalance occurs when the myocardial oxygen requirement increases, as during exercise, and coronary blood flow does not increase proportionately. The resulting ischemia usually leads to pain. Classic angina is therefore "angina of effort." (In some individuals, the ischemia is not always accompanied by pain, resulting in "silent" or "ambulatory" ischemia.) In variant angina, oxygen delivery decreases as a result of reversible coronary vasospasm. Variant angina is also called vasospastic or Prinzmetal's angina.

In theory, the imbalance between oxygen delivery and myocardial oxygen demand can be corrected by **decreasing oxygen demand** or by **increasing delivery** (by increasing coronary flow). Oxygen demand can be reduced by decreasing cardiac work or, according to recent studies, by shifting myocardial metabolism to substrates that require less oxygen per unit of ATP produced. In effort angina, acute reduction of demand has traditionally been achieved by means of organic nitrates—potent vasodilators—and several other classes of drugs, which decrease cardiac work. Increased delivery via increased coronary flow is difficult to achieve rapidly by pharmacologic means when flow is limited by fixed atheromatous plaques. In this situation, invasive measures (coronary bypass grafts or angioplasty) may be needed if reduction of oxygen demand does not control symptoms. In variant angina, on the other hand, spasm of coronary vessels can be reversed by nitrates or calcium channel blockers. It should be emphasized that not all vasodilators are effective in angina and, conversely, that some agents useful in angina (eg, propranolol) are not vasodilators. Lipid-lowering drugs, especially the "statins," have become extremely important in the long-term treatment of atherosclerotic disease (see Chapter 35).

Unstable angina, an acute coronary syndrome, is said to be present when there are episodes of angina at rest and when there is a change in the character, frequency, and duration of chest pain as well as precipitating factors in patients with previously stable angina. Unstable angina is caused by episodes of increased epicardial coronary artery tone or small platelet clots occurring in the vicinity of an atherosclerotic plaque. In most cases, formation of labile nonocclusive thrombi at the site of a fissured or ulcerated plaque is the mechanism for reduction in flow. The course and the prognosis of unstable angina are variable, but this subset of acute coronary syndrome is associated with a high risk of myocardial infarction and death.

PATHOPHYSIOLOGY OF ANGINA

Determinants of Myocardial Oxygen Demand

The major and minor determinants of myocardial oxygen requirement are set forth in Table 12–1. Unlike

Table 12–1. Determinants of myocardial oxygen consumption.

Major
  Wall stress
    Intraventricular pressure
    Ventricular radius (volume)
    Wall thickness
  Heart rate
  Contractility

Minor
  Activation energy
  Resting metabolism

skeletal muscle, human cardiac muscle cannot develop an appreciable oxygen debt during stress and repay it later. As a consequence of its continuous activity, the heart's oxygen needs are relatively high, and it extracts approximately 75% of the available oxygen even under conditions of no stress. The myocardial oxygen requirement increases when there is an increase in heart rate, contractility, arterial pressure, or ventricular volume. These hemodynamic alterations frequently occur during physical exercise and sympathetic discharge, which often precipitate angina in patients with obstructive coronary artery disease. The relative contributions of basal metabolism and activation of contraction to the overall myocardial oxygen consumption appear to be small, but under pathologic conditions these apparently minor determinants of myocardial oxygen consumption may become relevant.

The heart favors fatty acids as a substrate for energy production. However, oxidation of fatty acids requires more oxygen per unit of ATP generated than oxidation of carbohydrates. Therefore, drugs that shift myocardial metabolism toward greater use of glucose (fatty acid oxidation inhibitors) have the potential of reducing the oxygen demand without altering hemodynamics. Experimental models suggest that ranolazine and trimetazidine may have this effect. Preliminary clinical trials have shown favorable results.

Determinants of Coronary Blood Flow & Myocardial Oxygen Supply

Increased myocardial demands for oxygen in the normal heart are met by augmenting coronary blood flow. Coronary blood flow is directly related to the perfusion pressure (aortic diastolic pressure) and the duration of diastole. Because coronary flow drops to negligible values during systole, the duration of diastole becomes a limiting factor for myocardial perfusion during tachycardia. Coronary blood flow is inversely proportional to coronary vascular bed resistance. Resistance is deter-

mined mainly by intrinsic factors, including metabolic products and autonomic activity; and by various pharmacologic agents. Damage to the endothelium of coronary vessels has been shown to alter their ability to dilate and to increase coronary vascular resistance.

Determinants of Vascular Tone

Arteriolar and venous tone (smooth muscle tension) both play a role in determining myocardial wall stress (Table 12–1). Arteriolar tone directly controls peripheral vascular resistance and thus arterial blood pressure. In systole, intraventricular pressure must exceed aortic pressure to eject blood; arterial blood pressure thus determines the *systolic* wall stress in an important way. Venous tone determines the capacity of the venous circulation and controls the amount of blood sequestered in the venous system versus the amount returned to the heart. Venous tone thereby determines the *diastolic* wall stress.

The regulation of smooth muscle contraction and relaxation is shown schematically in Figure 12–1. As

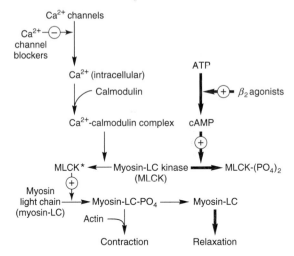

Figure 12–1. Control of smooth muscle contraction and site of action of calcium channel-blocking drugs. Contraction is triggered by influx of calcium (which can be blocked by calcium channel blockers) through transmembrane calcium channels. The calcium combines with calmodulin to form a complex that converts the enzyme myosin light chain kinase to its active form (*MLCK**). The latter phosphorylates the myosin light chains, thereby initiating the interaction of myosin with actin. Beta$_2$ agonists (and other substances that increase cAMP) may cause relaxation in smooth muscle by accelerating the inactivation of MLCK (heavy arrows) and by facilitating the expulsion of calcium from the cell (not shown).

shown in Figures 12–1 and 12–2, drugs may relax vascular smooth muscle in several ways:

1. Increasing cGMP—As indicated in Figure 12–2, cGMP facilitates the dephosphorylation of myosin light chains, preventing the interaction of myosin with actin. Nitric oxide is an effective activator of soluble guanylyl cyclase and acts mainly through this mechanism. Important molecular donors of nitric oxide include nitroprusside (see Chapter 11) and the organic nitrates used in angina.

2. Decreasing intracellular Ca^{2+}—Calcium channel blockers predictably cause vasodilation because they reduce intracellular Ca^{2+}, a major modulator of the activation of myosin light chain kinase. (Beta blockers and calcium channel blockers reduce Ca^{2+} *influx* in *cardiac* muscle, thereby reducing rate, contractility, and oxygen requirement unless reversed by compensatory responses.)

3. Stabilizing or preventing depolarization of the vascular smooth muscle cell membrane—The membrane potential of excitable cells is stabilized near the resting potential by increasing potassium permeability. Potassium channel openers, such as minoxidil sulfate, (see Chapter 11) increase the permeability of K^+ channels, probably ATP-dependent K^+ channels. Certain newer agents under investigation for use in angina (eg, nicorandil) may act, in part, by this mechanism.

4. Increasing cAMP in the vascular cells—As shown in Figure 12–1, an increase in cAMP increases

the rate of inactivation of myosin light chain kinase, the enzyme responsible for triggering the interaction of actin with myosin in these cells. This appears to be the mechanism of vasodilation caused by β_2-agonists, drugs that are *not* used in angina.

I. BASIC PHARMACOLOGY OF DRUGS USED TO TREAT ANGINA

Drug Action in Angina

All three of the drug groups currently approved for use in angina (organic nitrates, calcium channel blockers, and β-blockers) *decrease myocardial oxygen requirement* by decreasing the determinants of oxygen demand (heart rate, ventricular volume, blood pressure, and contractility). In some patients, a redistribution of coronary flow may increase oxygen delivery to ischemic tissue. In variant angina, the nitrates and the calcium channel blockers may also *increase myocardial oxygen delivery* by reversing coronary arterial spasm.

NITRATES & NITRITES

Chemistry

These agents are simple nitric and nitrous acid esters of polyalcohols. Nitroglycerin may be considered the prototype of the group. Although it is used in the manufacture of dynamite, the formulations of nitroglycerin used in medicine are not explosive. The conventional sublingual tablet form of nitroglycerin may lose potency when stored as a result of volatilization and adsorption to plastic surfaces. Therefore, it should be kept in tightly closed glass containers. It is not sensitive to light.

$$H_2C-O-NO_2$$
$$HC-O-NO_2$$
$$H_2C-O-NO_2$$

Nitroglycerin
(glyceryl trinitrate)

All therapeutically active agents in the nitrate group have identical mechanisms of action and similar toxicities. Therefore, pharmacokinetic factors govern the choice of agent and mode of therapy when using the nitrates.

Pharmacokinetics

The liver contains a high-capacity organic nitrate reductase that removes nitrate groups in a stepwise fashion

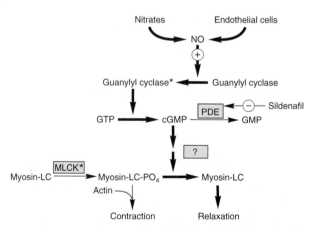

Figure 12–2. Mechanism of action of nitrates, nitrites, and other substances that increase the concentration of nitric oxide (NO) in smooth muscle cells. (MLCK*, activated myosin light chain kinase [see Figure 12–1]; guanylyl cyclase*, activated guanylyl cyclase; ?, unknown intermediate steps. Steps leading to relaxation are shown with heavy arrows.)

from the parent molecule and ultimately inactivates the drug. Therefore, oral bioavailability of the traditional organic nitrates (eg, nitroglycerin and isosorbide dinitrate) is very low (typically < 10–20%). The sublingual route, which avoids the first-pass effect, is therefore preferred for achieving a therapeutic blood level rapidly. Nitroglycerin and isosorbide dinitrate are both absorbed efficiently by this route and reach therapeutic blood levels within a few minutes. However, the total dose administered by this route must be limited to avoid excessive effect; therefore, the total duration of effect is brief (15–30 minutes). When much longer duration of action is needed, oral preparations can be given that contain an amount of drug sufficient to result in sustained systemic blood levels of the parent drug plus active metabolites. Other routes of administration available for nitroglycerin include transdermal and buccal absorption from slow-release preparations; these are described below.

Amyl nitrite and related nitrites are highly volatile liquids. Amyl nitrite is available in fragile glass ampules packaged in a protective cloth covering. The ampule can be crushed with the fingers, resulting in rapid release of inhalable vapors through the cloth covering. The inhalation route provides very rapid absorption and, like the sublingual route, avoids the hepatic first-pass effect. Because of its unpleasant odor and short duration of action, amyl nitrite is now obsolete for angina.

Once absorbed, the unchanged nitrate compounds have half-lives of only 2–8 minutes. The partially denitrated metabolites have much longer half-lives (up to 3 hours). Of the nitroglycerin metabolites (two dinitroglycerins and two mononitro forms), the dinitro derivatives have significant vasodilator efficacy; they probably provide most of the therapeutic effect of orally administered nitroglycerin. The 5-mononitrate metabolite of isosorbide dinitrate is an active metabolite of the latter drug and is available for clinical use as isosorbide mononitrate. It has a bioavailability of 100%.

Excretion, primarily in the form of glucuronide derivatives of the denitrated metabolites, is largely by way of the kidney.

Pharmacodynamics

A. MECHANISM OF ACTION IN SMOOTH MUSCLE

Nitroglycerin is denitrated by glutathione S-transferase. Free nitrite ion is released, which is then converted to nitric oxide (see Chapter 19). A different unknown enzymatic reaction releases nitric oxide directly from the parent drug molecule. As shown in Figure 12–2, nitric oxide (or an S-nitrosothiol derivative) causes activation of guanylyl cyclase and an increase in cGMP, which are the first steps toward smooth muscle relaxation. The production of prostaglandin E or prostacyclin (PGI_2) and membrane hyperpolarization may also be involved.

There is no evidence that autonomic receptors are involved in the primary nitrate response (although autonomic *reflex* responses are evoked when hypotensive doses are given).

As described below, tolerance is an important consideration in the use of nitrates. While tolerance may be caused in part by a decrease in tissue sulfhydryl groups, it can be only partially prevented or reversed with a sulfhydryl-regenerating agent. The site of this cellular tolerance may be in the unknown reaction responsible for the release of nitric oxide from the nitrate, since other agents, eg, acetylcholine, that cause vasodilation via release of nitric oxide from *endogenous* substrates do not show cross tolerance with the nitrates.

Nicorandil and several other investigational antianginal agents appear to combine the activity of nitric oxide release with potassium channel-opening action, thus providing an additional mechanism for causing vasodilation.

B. ORGAN SYSTEM EFFECTS

Nitroglycerin relaxes all types of smooth muscle irrespective of the cause of the preexisting muscle tone (Figure 12–3). It has practically no direct effect on cardiac or skeletal muscle.

1. Vascular smooth muscle—All segments of the vascular system from large arteries through large veins relax in response to nitroglycerin. Veins respond at the lowest concentrations, arteries at slightly higher ones. Arterioles and precapillary sphincters are dilated less than the large arteries and the veins, partly because of reflex responses and partly because different vessels vary in their ability to release nitric oxide (see Box, The Coronary Steal Phenomenon). The primary direct result of an effective dose of nitroglycerin is marked relaxation of veins with increased venous capacitance and decreased ventricular preload. Pulmonary vascular pressures and heart size are significantly reduced. In the absence of heart failure, cardiac output is reduced. Because venous capacitance is increased, orthostatic hypotension may be marked and syncope can result. Dilation of some large arteries (including the aorta) may be significant because of their large increase in compliance. Temporal artery pulsations and a throbbing headache associated with meningeal artery pulsations are frequent effects of nitroglycerin and amyl nitrite. In heart failure, preload is often abnormally high; the nitrates and other vasodilators, by reducing preload, may have a beneficial effect on cardiac output in this condition (see Chapter 13).

The indirect effects of nitroglycerin consist of those compensatory responses evoked by baroreceptors and hormonal mechanisms responding to decreased arterial pressure (see Figure 6–7); this consistently results in tachycardia and increased cardiac contractility. Retention of salt and water may also be significant, especially

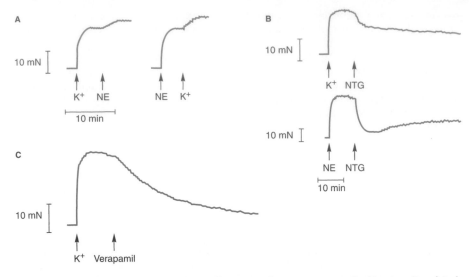

Figure 12–3. Effects of vasodilators on contractions of human vein segments studied in vitro. Panel A shows contractions induced by two vasoconstrictor agents, norepinephrine (NE) and potassium (K+). Panel B shows the relaxation induced by nitroglycerin (NTG), 4 µmol/L. The relaxation is prompt. Panel C shows the relaxation induced by verapamil, 2.2 µmol/L. The relaxation is slower but more sustained. (Modified and reproduced, with permission, from Mikkelsen E, Andersson KE, Bengtsson B: Effects of verapamil and nitroglycerin on contractile responses to potassium and noradrenaline in isolated human peripheral veins. Acta Pharmacol Toxicol 1978;42:14.)

THE CORONARY STEAL PHENOMENON

The development of useful vasodilators for management of angina has been marked by frustrating episodes when pharmacologists found that new drugs that were extremely effective vasodilators in normal animals were ineffective or even caused increased anginal symptoms in patients. It is now clear that potent arteriolar dilators (eg, hydralazine, dipyridamole) are generally ineffective in angina and may reduce perfusion of ischemic areas. In fact, dipyridamole is often used in imaging studies of the coronary circulation to demonstrate regions of poor perfusion. On the other hand, drugs that are more effective dilators of veins and large arteries and relatively ineffective dilators of resistance vessels (eg, nitrates) are very useful in angina. The reason for this apparent anomaly has been called the coronary steal phenomenon.

Coronary steal occurs when two branches from a main coronary vessel have differing degrees of obstruction. For example, one branch may be relatively normal and capable of dilating and constrict-

ing in response to changes in oxygen demand, while the other branch is significantly obstructed and has significant arteriolar dilation even when cardiac oxygen demand is low, because of the accumulation of metabolites in the ischemic tissue. Perfusion in the obstructed region may be adequate at rest, because perfusion pressure is well maintained in the main coronary artery. If a powerful arteriolar dilator drug is administered, the arterioles in the unobstructed vessel will be forced to dilate, reducing the resistance in this area and greatly increasing flow through the already adequately perfused tissue. As a result of the reduction in resistance in the normal branch, perfusion pressure in the main coronary will diminish, flow through the obstructed branch will *decrease,* and angina may worsen.

It has been suggested that the lesser potency of the nitrates in dilating arterioles is the result of a reduced ability of these vessels to release nitric oxide from the parent nitrate molecule.

with intermediate- and long-acting nitrates. These compensatory responses contribute to the development of tolerance.

In normal subjects without coronary disease, nitroglycerin can induce a significant, if transient, increase in total coronary blood flow. In contrast, there is no evidence that total coronary flow is increased in patients with angina due to atherosclerotic obstructive coronary artery disease. However, some studies suggest that *redistribution* of coronary flow from normal to ischemic regions may play a role in nitroglycerin's therapeutic effect. Nitroglycerin also exerts a weak negative inotropic effect via nitric oxide.

2. Other smooth muscle organs—Relaxation of smooth muscle of the bronchi, gastrointestinal tract (including biliary system), and genitourinary tract has been demonstrated experimentally. Because of their brief duration, these actions of the nitrates are rarely of any clinical value. During recent years, the use of amyl nitrite and isobutyl nitrite by inhalation as purported

recreational (sex-enhancing) drugs has become popular with some segments of the population. Nitrites release nitric oxide in erectile tissue as well as vascular smooth muscle and activate guanylyl cyclase. The resulting increase in cGMP causes dephosphorylation of myosin light chains and relaxation (Figure 12–2), which enhances erection. Drugs used in the treatment of erectile dysfunction are discussed in the Box, Drugs Used in the Treatment of Erectile Dysfunction.

3. Action on platelets—Nitric oxide released from nitroglycerin stimulates guanylyl cyclase in platelets as in smooth muscle. The increase in cGMP that results is responsible for a decrease in platelet aggregation. Unfortunately, recent prospective trials have established no survival benefit when nitroglycerin is used in acute myocardial infarction.

4. Other effects—*Nitrite* ion reacts with hemoglobin (which contains ferrous iron) to produce methemoglobin (which contains ferric iron). Because methemoglobin has a very low affinity for oxygen, large doses of

---

DRUGS USED IN THE TREATMENT OF ERECTILE DYSFUNCTION

Erectile dysfunction in men has long been the subject of research (by both amateur and professional scientists). Among the substances used in the past and generally discredited are "Spanish Fly" (a bladder and urethral irritant), yohimbine (an α_2-antagonist; see Chapter 10), nutmeg, and mixtures containing lead, arsenic, or strychnine. Substances currently favored by practitioners of herbal medicine include ginseng and kava (see Chapter 65).

Scientific studies of the process have shown that erection requires *relaxation* of the nonvascular smooth muscle of the corpora cavernosa. This relaxation permits inflow of blood at nearly arterial pressure into the sinuses of the cavernosa, and it is the pressure of the blood that causes erection. Physiologic erection occurs in response to the release of nitric oxide from nonadrenergic-noncholinergic nerves (see Chapter 6) associated with parasympathetic discharge. Thus, parasympathetic innervation must be intact and nitric oxide synthesis must be active. (It appears that a similar process occurs in female erectile tissues.) Certain other smooth muscle relaxants—eg, PGE$_1$ analogs, α-antagonists—if present in high enough concentration, can independently cause sufficient cavernosal relaxation to result in erection. As noted in the text, NO activates guanylyl cyclase, increases the concentration of cGMP, and the latter messenger stimulates the dephosphorylation of myosin light chains (see Figure 12–2) and

relaxation of the smooth muscle. Thus, any drug that increases cGMP might be of value in erectile dysfunction if normal innervation is present. **Sildenafil** (Viagra) acts to increase cGMP by inhibiting its breakdown by phosphodiesterase isoform 5. The drug has been very successful in the marketplace because it can be taken orally. However, sildenafil is of little or no value in men with loss of potency due to cord injury or other damage to innervation and in men lacking libido. Furthermore, sildenafil potentiates the action of nitrates used for angina, and severe hypotension and a few myocardial infarctions have been reported in men taking both drugs. It is recommended that at least 6 hours pass between use of a nitrate and the ingestion of sildenafil. Sildenafil also has effects on color vision, causing difficulty in blue-green discrimination. Two similar PDE-5 inhibitors **tadalafil** and **vardenafil,** were released in 2003.

The drug most commonly used in patients who do not respond to sildenafil is **alprostadil,** a PGE$_1$ analog (see Chapter 18) that can be injected directly into the cavernosa or placed in the urethra as a mini-suppository, from which it diffuses into the cavernosal tissue. Phentolamine can be used by injection into the cavernosa. These drugs will cause erection in most men who do not respond to sildenafil.

Another oral drug, apomorphine, acts by releasing dopamine in the central nervous system and is under investigation for erectile dysfunction.

nitrites can result in pseudocyanosis, tissue hypoxia, and death. Fortunately, the plasma level of *nitrite* resulting from even large doses of organic and inorganic *nitrates* is too low to cause significant methemoglobinemia in adults. However, sodium nitrite is used as a curing agent for meats. In nursing infants, the intestinal flora is capable of converting significant amounts of inorganic nitrate, eg, from well water, to nitrite ion. Thus, inadvertent exposure to large amounts of nitrite ion can occur and may produce serious toxicity.

One therapeutic application of this otherwise toxic effect of nitrite has been discovered. Cyanide poisoning results from complexing of cytochrome iron by the CN^- ion. Methemoglobin iron has a very high affinity for CN^-; thus, administration of sodium nitrite ($NaNO_2$) soon after cyanide exposure will regenerate active cytochrome. The cyanmethemoglobin produced can be further detoxified by the intravenous administration of sodium thiosulfate ($Na_2S_2O_3$); this results in formation of thiocyanate ion (SCN^-), a less toxic ion that is readily excreted. Methemoglobinemia, if excessive, can be treated by giving methylene blue intravenously.

Toxicity & Tolerance

A. Acute Adverse Effects

The major acute toxicities of organic nitrates are direct extensions of therapeutic vasodilation: orthostatic hypotension, tachycardia, and throbbing headache. Glaucoma, once thought to be a contraindication, does not worsen, and nitrates can be used safely in the presence of increased intraocular pressure. Nitrates are contraindicated, however, if intracranial pressure is elevated.

B. Tolerance

With continuous exposure to nitrates, isolated smooth muscle may develop complete tolerance (tachyphylaxis), and the intact human becomes progressively more tolerant when long-acting preparations (oral, transdermal) or continuous intravenous infusions are used for more than a few hours without interruption.

Continuous exposure to high levels of nitrates can occur in the chemical industry, especially where explosives are manufactured. When contamination of the workplace with volatile organic nitrate compounds is severe, workers find that upon starting their work week (Monday), they suffer headache and transient dizziness. After a day or so, these symptoms disappear owing to the development of tolerance. Over the weekend, when exposure to the chemicals is reduced, tolerance disappears, so symptoms recur each Monday. Other hazards of industrial exposure, including dependence, have been reported. There is no evidence that physical dependence develops as a result of the therapeutic use of short-acting nitrates for angina, even in large doses.

The mechanisms by which tolerance develops are not completely understood. As noted above, diminished release of nitric oxide may be partly responsible for tolerance to nitroglycerin. Systemic compensation also plays a role in tolerance in the intact human. Initially, significant sympathetic discharge occurs and after one or more days of therapy with long-acting nitrates, retention of salt and water may reverse the favorable hemodynamic changes normally caused by nitroglycerin.

C. Carcinogenicity of Nitrate and Nitrate Derivatives

Nitrosamines are small molecules with the structure R_2–N–NO formed from the combination of nitrates and nitrites with amines. Some nitrosamines are powerful carcinogens in animals, apparently through conversion to reactive derivatives. While there is no direct proof that these agents cause cancer in humans, there is a strong epidemiologic correlation between the incidence of esophageal and gastric carcinoma and the nitrate content of food in different cultures. Nitrosamines are also found in tobacco and in cigarette smoke. There is no evidence that the small doses of nitrates used in the treatment of angina result in significant body levels of nitrosamines.

Mechanisms of Clinical Effect

The beneficial and deleterious effects of nitrate-induced vasodilation are summarized in Table 12–2.

A. Nitrate Effects in Angina of Effort

Decreased venous return to the heart and the resulting reduction of intracardiac volume are the principal hemodynamic effects. Arterial pressure also decreases. Decreased intraventricular pressure and left ventricular volume are associated with decreased wall tension (Laplace relation) and decreased myocardial oxygen requirement. In rare instances, a paradoxical increase in myocardial oxygen demand may occur as a result of excessive reflex tachycardia and increased contractility.

Intracoronary, intravenous, or sublingual nitrate administration consistently increases the caliber of the large epicardial coronary arteries. Coronary arteriolar resistance tends to decrease, although to a lesser extent. However, nitrates administered by the usual systemic routes also consistently *decrease* overall coronary blood flow and myocardial oxygen consumption. The reduction in oxygen consumption is the major mechanism for the relief of angina.

B. Nitrate Effects in Variant Angina

Nitrates benefit patients with variant angina by relaxing the smooth muscle of the epicardial coronary arteries and relieving coronary artery spasm.

Table 12–2. Beneficial and deleterious effects of nitrates in the treatment of angina.

Effect	Result
Potential beneficial effects	
Decreased ventricular volume	Decreased myocardial oxygen requirement
Decreased arterial pressure	
Decreased ejection time	
Vasodilation of epicardial coronary arteries	Relief of coronary artery spasm
Increased collateral flow	Improved perfusion to ischemic myocardium
Decreased left ventricular diastolic pressure	Improved subendocardial perfusion
Potential deleterious effects	
Reflex tachycardia	Increased myocardial oxygen requirement
Reflex increase in contractility	
Decreased diastolic perfusion time due to tachycardia	Decreased myocardial perfusion

C. Nitrate Effects in Unstable Angina

Nitrates are also useful in the treatment of this acute coronary syndrome, but the precise mechanism for their beneficial effects is not clear. Because both increased coronary vascular tone and increased myocardial oxygen demand can precipitate rest angina in these patients, nitrates may exert their beneficial effects both by dilating the epicardial coronary arteries and by simultaneously reducing myocardial oxygen demand. As noted above, nitroglycerin also decreases platelet aggregation, and this effect may be of importance in unstable angina.

Clinical Use of Nitrates

Some of the forms of nitroglycerin and its congeners are listed in Table 12–3. Because of its rapid onset of action (1–3 minutes), sublingual nitroglycerin is the most frequently used agent for the immediate treatment of angina. Because its duration of action is short (not exceeding 20–30 minutes), it is not suitable for maintenance therapy. The onset of action of intravenous nitroglycerin is also rapid (minutes), but its hemodynamic effects are quickly reversed by stopping its infusion. Clinical application of intravenous nitroglycerin, therefore, is restricted to the treatment of severe, recurrent rest angina. Slowly absorbed preparations of nitroglycerin include a buccal form, oral preparations, and several transdermal forms. These formulations have been shown to provide blood concentrations for long periods but, as noted above, this leads to the development of tolerance.

Table 12–3. Nitrate and nitrite drugs used in the treatment of angina.

Drug	Dose	Duration of Action
"Short-acting"		
Nitroglycerin, sublingual	0.15–1.2 mg	10–30 minutes
Isosorbide dinitrate, sublingual	2.5–5 mg	10–60 minutes
Amyl nitrite, inhalant	0.18–0.3 mL	3–5 minutes
"Long-acting"		
Nitroglycerin, oral sustained-action	6.5–13 mg per 6–8 hours	6–8 hours
Nitroglycerin, 2% ointment, transdermal	1–1.5 inches per 4 hours	3–6 hours
Nitroglycerin, slow-release, buccal	1–2 mg per 4 hours	3–6 hours
Nitroglycerin, slow-release patch, transdermal	10–25 mg per 24 hours (one patch per day)	8–10 hours
Isosorbide dinitrate, sublingual	2.5–10 mg per 2 hours	1.5–2 hours
Isosorbide dinitrate, oral	10–60 mg per 4–6 hours	4–6 hours
Isosorbide dinitrate, chewable oral	5–10 mg per 2–4 hours	2–3 hours
Isosorbide mononitrate oral	20 mg per 12 hours	6–10 hours

The hemodynamic effects of sublingual or chewable isosorbide dinitrate and other organic nitrates are similar to those of nitroglycerin. The recommended dosage schedules for commonly used long-acting nitrate preparations, along with their durations of action, are listed in Table 12–3. Although transdermal administration may provide blood levels of nitroglycerin for 24 hours or longer, the full hemodynamic effects usually do not persist for more than 6–8 hours. The clinical efficacy of slow-release forms of nitroglycerin in maintenance therapy of angina is thus limited by the development of significant tolerance. Therefore, a nitrate-free period of at least 8 hours between doses should be observed to reduce or prevent tolerance.

CALCIUM CHANNEL-BLOCKING DRUGS

It has been known since the late 1800s that calcium influx was necessary for the contraction of smooth and cardiac muscle. The discovery of a calcium channel in cardiac muscle was followed by the finding of several different types of calcium channels in different tissues (Table 12–4). The discovery of these channels made possible the development of clinically useful blocking drugs. Although the successful therapeutic blockers developed to date have been exclusively L-type channel blockers, selective blockers of other types of calcium channels are under intensive investigation.

Chemistry & Pharmacokinetics

Verapamil, the first clinically useful member of this group, was the result of attempts to synthesize more active analogs of papaverine, a vasodilator alkaloid found in the opium poppy. Since then, dozens of agents of varying structure have been found to have the same fundamental pharmacologic action (Table 12–5). Three

chemically dissimilar calcium channel blockers are shown in Figure 12–4. Nifedipine is the prototype of the dihydropyridine family of calcium channel blockers; dozens of molecules in this family have been investigated, and eight are currently approved in the USA for angina and other indications. Nifedipine is the most extensively studied of this group, but the properties of the other dihydropyridines can be assumed to be similar to it unless otherwise noted.

The calcium channel blockers are orally active agents and are characterized by high first-pass effect, high plasma protein binding, and extensive metabolism. Verapamil and diltiazem are also used by the intravenous route.

Pharmacodynamics

A. MECHANISM OF ACTION

The L-type calcium channel is the dominant type in cardiac and smooth muscle and is known to contain several drug receptors. It has been demonstrated that nifedipine and other dihydropyridines bind to one site, while verapamil and diltiazem appear to bind to closely related but not identical receptors in another region. Binding of a drug to the verapamil or diltiazem receptors also affects dihydropyridine binding. These receptor regions are stereoselective, since marked differences in both stereoisomer-binding affinity and pharmacologic potency are observed for enantiomers of verapamil, diltiazem, and optically active nifedipine congeners.

Blockade by these drugs resembles that of sodium channel blockade by local anesthetics (see Chapters 14 and 26). The drugs act from the inner side of the membrane and bind more effectively to channels in depolarized membranes. Binding of the drug reduces the frequency of opening in response to depolarization. The

Table 12–4. Properties of several recognized voltage-activated calcium channels.

Type	Where Found	Properties of the Calcium Current	Blocked By
L	Muscle, neurons	Long, large, high threshold	Verapamil, DHPs, Cd^{2+}
T	Heart, neurons	Short, small, low threshold	sFTX, flunarizine[1], Ni^{2+}
N	Neurons	Short, high threshold	ω-CTX-GVIA, Cd^{2+}
P	Cerebellar Purkinje neurons	Long, high threshold	ω-CTX-MVIIC, ω-Aga-IVA

DHPs, dihydropyridines (eg, nifedipine); sFTX, synthetic funnel web spider toxin; ω-CTX, conotoxins extracted from several marine snails of the genus *Conus;* ω-Aga-IVA, a toxin of the funnel web spider, *Agelenopsis aperta.*
[1]An organic calcium channel blocker.

Table 12–5. Pharmacokinetics of some calcium channel-blocking drugs.

Drug	Oral Bioavailability	Onset of Action (route)	Plasma Half-Life (hours)	Disposition
Dihydropyridines				
Amlodipine	65–90%	No data available	30–50	> 90% bound to plasma proteins; extensively metabolized.
Felodipine	15–20%	2–5 hours (oral)	11–16	> 99% bound to plasma proteins; extensively metabolized.
Isradipine	15–25%	2 hours (oral)	8	95% bound to plasma protein; extensively metabolized.
Nicardipine	35%	20 minutes (oral)	2–4	95% bound; extensively metabolized in the liver.
Nifedipine	45–70%	< 1 minute (IV), 5–20 minutes (sublingual or oral)	4	About 90% bound to plasma protein; metabolized to an acid lactate. 80% of the drug and metabolites excreted in urine.
Nimodipine	13%	No data available	1–2	Extensively metabolized.
Nisoldipine	< 10%	No data available	6–12	Extensively metabolized.
Nitrendipine	10–30%	4 hours (oral)	5–12	98% bound; extensively metabolized.
Miscellaneous				
Bepridil	60%	60 minutes (oral)	24–40	> 99% bound to plasma proteins; extensively metabolized.
Diltiazem	40–65%	< 3 minutes (IV), > 30 minutes (oral)	3–4	70–80% bound to plasma protein; extensively deacylated. Drug and metabolites excreted in feces.
Verapamil	20–35%	< 1.5 minutes (IV), 30 minutes (oral)	6	About 90% bound to plasma protein. 70% eliminated by kidney; 15% by gastrointestinal tract.

result is a marked decrease in transmembrane calcium current associated in smooth muscle with a long-lasting relaxation (Figure 12–3) and in cardiac muscle with a reduction in contractility throughout the heart and decreases in sinus node pacemaker rate and in atrioventricular node conduction velocity.[*]

Smooth muscle responses to calcium influx through *receptor*-operated calcium channels are also reduced by these drugs but not as markedly. The block can be partially reversed by elevating the concentration of calcium, although the levels of calcium required are not easily attainable. Block can also be partially reversed by the use of drugs that increase the transmembrane flux of calcium, such as sympathomimetics.

Other types of calcium channels are less sensitive to blockade by these calcium channel blockers (Table 12–4). Therefore, tissues in which these channel types

---

[*] At very low doses and under certain circumstances, some dihydropyridines *increase* calcium influx. Some special dihydropyridines, eg, Bay K 8644, actually increase calcium influx over most of their dose range.

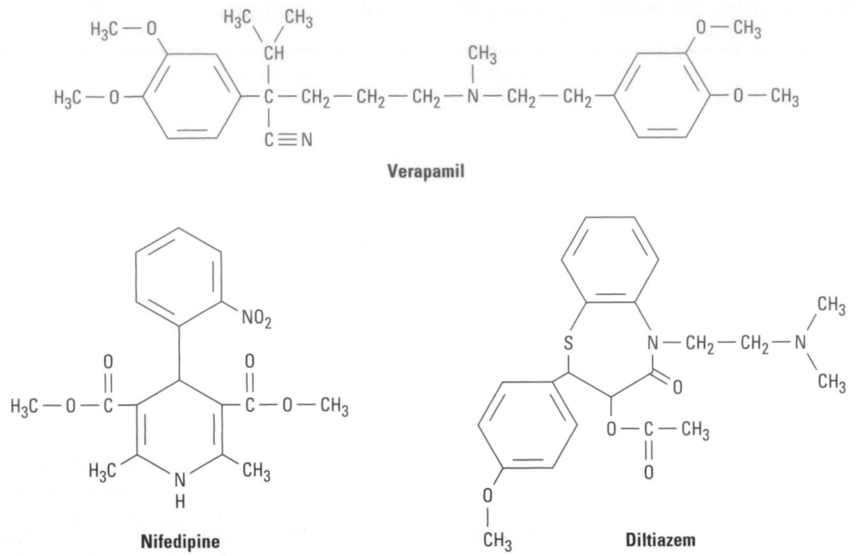

Figure 12–4. Chemical structures of several calcium channel-blocking drugs.

play a major role—neurons and most secretory glands—are much less affected by these drugs than are cardiac and smooth muscle.

B. ORGAN SYSTEM EFFECTS

1. Smooth muscle—Most types of smooth muscle are dependent on transmembrane calcium influx for normal resting tone and contractile responses. These cells are relaxed by the calcium channel blockers (Figure 12–3). Vascular smooth muscle appears to be the most sensitive, but similar relaxation can be shown for bronchiolar, gastrointestinal, and uterine smooth muscle. In the vascular system, arterioles appear to be more sensitive than veins; orthostatic hypotension is not a common adverse effect. Blood pressure is reduced with all calcium channel blockers. Women may be more sensitive than men to the hypotensive action of diltiazem. The reduction in peripheral vascular resistance is one mechanism by which these agents may benefit the patient with angina of effort. Reduction of coronary arterial tone has been demonstrated in patients with variant angina.

Important differences in vascular selectivity exist among the calcium channel blockers. In general, the dihydropyridines have a greater ratio of vascular smooth muscle effects relative to cardiac effects than do bepridil, diltiazem, and verapamil (Table 12–6). Furthermore, the dihydropyridines may differ in their potency in different vascular beds. For example, nimodipine is claimed to be particularly selective for cerebral blood vessels.

2. Cardiac muscle—Cardiac muscle is highly dependent upon calcium influx for normal function. Impulse generation in the sinoatrial node and conduction in the atrioventricular node—so-called slow response, or calcium-dependent, action potentials—may be reduced or blocked by all of the calcium channel blockers. Excitation-contraction coupling in all cardiac cells requires calcium influx, so these drugs reduce cardiac contractility in a dose-dependent fashion. In some cases, cardiac output may also decrease. This reduction in cardiac mechanical function is another mechanism by which the calcium channel blockers may reduce the oxygen requirement in patients with angina.

Important differences between the available calcium channel blockers arise from the details of their interactions with cardiac ion channels and, as noted above, differences in their relative smooth muscle versus cardiac effects. Cardiac *sodium* channels are blocked by bepridil but somewhat less effectively than are calcium channels. Sodium channel block is modest with verapamil and still less marked with diltiazem. It is negligible with nifedipine and other dihydropyridines. Verapamil and diltiazem interact kinetically with the calcium channel receptor in a different manner than the dihydropyridines; they block tachycardias in calcium-dependent cells, eg, the atrioventricular node, more selectively than do the dihydropyridines. (See Chapter 14 for additional details.) On the other hand, the dihydropyridines appear to block smooth muscle calcium channels at concentrations below those required for significant cardiac effects; they

Table 12–6. Vascular selectivity and clinical properties of some calcium channel-blocking drugs.

Drug	Vascular Selectivity[1]	Indications	Usual Dosage	Toxicity
Dihydropyridines				
Amlodipine	++	Angina, hypertension	5–10 mg orally once daily	Headache, peripheral edema
Felodipine	5.4	Hypertension, Raynaud's phenomenon, congestive heart failure	5–10 mg orally once daily	Dizziness, headache
Isradipine	7.4	Hypertension	2.5–10 mg orally every 12 hours	Headache, fatigue
Nicardipine	17.0	Angina, hypertension, congestive heart failure	20–40 mg orally every 8 hours	Peripheral edema, dizziness, headache, flushing
Nifedipine	3.1	Angina, hypertension, migraine, cardiomyopathy, Raynaud's phenomenon	3–10 µg/kg IV; 20–40 mg orally every 8 hours	Hypotension, dizziness, flushing, nausea, constipation, dependent edema
Nimodipine	++	Subarachnoid hemorrhage, migraine	60 mg orally every 4 hours	Headache, diarrhea
Nisoldipine	++	Hypertension	20–40 mg orally once daily	Probably similar to nifedipine
Nitrendipine	14.4	Investigational for angina, hypertension	20 mg orally once or twice daily	Probably similar to nifedipine
Miscellaneous				
Bepridil	–	Angina	200–400 mg orally once daily	Arrhythmias, dizziness, nausea
Diltiazem	0.3	Angina, hypertension, Raynaud's phenomenon	75–150 µg/kg IV; 30–80 mg orally every 6 hours	Hypotension, dizziness, flushing, bradycardia
Verapamil	1.3	Angina, hypertension, arrhythmias, migraine, cardiomyopathy	75–150 µg/kg IV; 80–160 mg orally every 8 hours	Hypotension, myocardial depression, constipation, dependent edema

[1]Numerical data (Spedding, 1990) give the ratio of vascular potency to cardiac potency; higher numbers mean greater vascular, less cardiac potency. Plus and minus signs reflect estimated ratio of vascular to cardiac potency: – = myocardial depression greater than vasodilation; ++ = significant degree of vasodilation greater than myocardial depression.

are therefore less depressant on the heart than verapamil or diltiazem. Bepridil also has a significant potassium channel blocking effect in the heart. This results in prolongation of cardiac repolarization (see Chapter 14) and a distinct risk of induction of arrhythmias.

3. Skeletal muscle—Skeletal muscle is not depressed by the calcium channel blockers because it uses intracellular pools of calcium to support excitation-contraction coupling and does not require as much transmembrane calcium influx.

4. Cerebral vasospasm and infarct following subarachnoid hemorrhage—Nimodipine, a member of the dihydropyridine group of calcium channel blockers, has a high affinity for cerebral blood vessels and appears to reduce morbidity following a subarachnoid hemorrhage. Nimodipine is therefore labeled for use in patients who have had a hemorrhagic stroke. Although evidence suggests that calcium channel blockers may also reduce cerebral damage following thromboembolic stroke in experimental animals, there is no evidence that this occurs in humans.

5. Other effects—Calcium channel blockers minimally interfere with stimulus-secretion coupling in glands and nerve endings because of differences between calcium channels in different tissues, as noted above. Verapamil has been shown to inhibit insulin release in humans, but the dosages required are greater than those used in management of angina.

A significant body of evidence suggests that the calcium channel blockers may interfere with platelet aggregation in vitro and prevent or attenuate the development of atheromatous lesions in animals. Clinical studies have not established their role in human blood clotting and atherosclerosis.

Verapamil has been shown to block the P170 glycoprotein responsible for the transport of many foreign drugs out of cancer (and other) cells; other calcium channel blockers appear to have a similar effect. This action is not stereospecific. Verapamil has been shown to partially reverse the resistance of cancer cells to many chemotherapeutic drugs in vitro. Some clinical results suggest similar effects in patients (see Chapter 55).

Toxicity

The most important toxic effects reported for the calcium channel blockers are direct extensions of their therapeutic action. Excessive inhibition of calcium influx can cause serious cardiac depression, including cardiac arrest, bradycardia, atrioventricular block, and heart failure. These effects have been rare in clinical use.

Retrospective case control studies reported that immediate-acting nifedipine increased the risk of myocardial infarction in patients with hypertension (Psaty, 1995). Slow-release and long-acting vasoselective calcium channel blockers are usually well tolerated. However, dihydropyridines, compared with angiotensin-converting enzyme inhibitors, have been reported to increase the risk of adverse cardiac events in patients with hypertension with or without diabetes (ABCD Trial, FACET Trial). These results suggest that relatively short-acting calcium channel blockers have the potential to enhance the risk of adverse cardiac events and should be avoided. Bepridil consistently prolongs the cardiac action potential and may cause a dangerous torsade de pointes arrhythmia in susceptible patients. It is contraindicated in patients with a history of serious arrhythmias or prolonged QT syndrome. Patients receiving β-adrenoceptor-blocking drugs are more sensitive to the cardiodepressant effects of calcium channel blockers. Minor toxicity (troublesome but not usually requiring discontinuance of therapy) includes flushing, dizziness, nausea, constipation, and peripheral edema (Table 12–6).

Mechanisms of Clinical Effects

Calcium channel blockers decrease myocardial contractile force, which reduces myocardial oxygen require-

ments. Inhibition of calcium entry into arterial smooth muscle is associated with decreased arteriolar tone and systemic vascular resistance, resulting in decreased arterial and intraventricular pressure. Some of these drugs (eg, verapamil) also possess a nonspecific antiadrenergic effect, which may contribute to peripheral vasodilation. As a result of all of these effects, left ventricular wall stress declines, which reduces myocardial oxygen requirements. Decreased heart rate with the use of verapamil, diltiazem, or bepridil causes a further decrease in myocardial oxygen demand. Calcium channel-blocking agents also relieve and prevent the primary cause of variant angina—focal coronary artery spasm. Use of these agents has thus emerged as the most effective prophylactic treatment for this form of angina pectoris.

Sinoatrial and atrioventricular nodal tissues, which are mainly composed of slow response cells, are affected markedly by verapamil, moderately by diltiazem, and much less by dihydropyridines. Thus, verapamil and diltiazem decrease atrioventricular nodal conduction and are effective in the management of supraventricular reentry tachycardia and in decreasing ventricular responses in atrial fibrillation or flutter. Nifedipine does not affect atrioventricular conduction. Nonspecific sympathetic antagonism is most marked with diltiazem and much less with verapamil. Nifedipine does not appear to have this effect. Thus, significant reflex tachycardia in response to hypotension occurs most frequently with nifedipine and less so with verapamil. These differences in pharmacologic effects should be considered in selecting calcium channel-blocking agents for the management of angina.

Clinical Uses of Calcium Channel-Blocking Drugs

In addition to angina, calcium channel blockers have well-documented efficacy in hypertension (see Chapter 11) and supraventricular tachyarrhythmias (see Chapter 14). They also show promise in a wide variety of other conditions, including hypertrophic cardiomyopathy, migraine, and Raynaud's phenomenon.

Approved and unlabeled indications and dosages for these drugs are set forth in Table 12–6. The choice of a particular calcium channel-blocking agent should be made with knowledge of its specific potential adverse effects as well as its pharmacologic properties. Nifedipine does not decrease atrioventricular conduction and therefore can be used more safely in the presence of atrioventricular conduction abnormalities. A combination of verapamil or diltiazem with β-blockers may produce atrioventricular block and depression of ventricular function. In the presence of overt heart failure, all calcium channel blockers can cause further worsening of heart failure as a result of their negative inotropic effect.

Amlodipine, however, does not increase the mortality of patients with heart failure due to left ventricular systolic dysfunction and can be used safely in these patients. In the presence of relatively low blood pressure, dihydropyridines can cause further deleterious lowering of pressure. Verapamil and diltiazem appear to produce less hypotension and may be better tolerated in these circumstances. In patients with a history of atrial tachycardia, flutter, and fibrillation, verapamil and diltiazem provide a distinct advantage because of their antiarrhythmic effects. In the patient receiving digitalis, verapamil should be used with caution, because it may increase digoxin blood levels through a pharmacokinetic interaction. Although increases in digoxin blood level have also been demonstrated with diltiazem and nifedipine, such interactions are less consistent than with verapamil.

In patients with unstable angina, immediate-release short-acting calcium channel blockers can increase the risk of adverse cardiac events and therefore are contraindicated (see Toxicity, above). However, in patients with non-Q-wave myocardial infarction, diltiazem can decrease the frequency of postinfarction angina and may be used.

BETA-ADRENOCEPTOR-BLOCKING DRUGS

Although they are not vasodilators, β-blocking drugs (see Chapter 10) are extremely useful in the management of angina pectoris associated with effort. The beneficial effects of β-blocking agents are related primarily to their hemodynamic effects—decreased heart rate, blood pressure, and contractility—which decrease myocardial oxygen requirements at rest and during exercise. Lower heart rate is also associated with an increase in diastolic perfusion time that may increase myocardial perfusion. However, reduction of heart rate and blood pressure and consequently decreased myocardial oxygen consumption appear to be the most important mechanisms for relief of angina and improved exercise tolerance. Beta blockers may also be valuable in treating silent or ambulatory ischemia. Because this condition causes no pain, it is usually detected by the appearance of typical electrocardiographic signs of ischemia. The total amount of "ischemic time" per day is reduced by long-term therapy with a β-blocker. Beta-blocking agents decrease mortality of patients with recent myocardial infarction and improve survival and prevent stroke in patients with hypertension. Randomized trials in patients with stable angina have shown better outcome and symptomatic improvement with β-blockers compared with calcium channel blockers (Gibbons, 1999).

Undesirable effects of β-blocking agents in angina include an increase in end-diastolic volume and an increase in ejection time. Increased myocardial oxygen requirements associated with increased diastolic volume partially offset the beneficial effects of β-blocking agents. These potentially deleterious effects of β-blocking agents can be balanced by the concomitant use of nitrates as described below.

The contraindications to the use of β-blockers are asthma and other bronchospastic conditions, severe bradycardia, atrioventricular blockade, bradycardia-tachycardia syndrome, and severe unstable left ventricular failure. Potential complications include fatigue, impaired exercise tolerance, insomnia, unpleasant dreams, worsening of claudication, and erectile dysfunction.

II. CLINICAL PHARMACOLOGY OF DRUGS USED TO TREAT ANGINA

Principles of Therapy for Angina

In addition to modification of the risk factors for coronary atherosclerosis (smoking, hypertension, hyperlipidemia), the treatment of angina and other manifestations of myocardial ischemia is based on reduction of myocardial oxygen demand and increase of coronary blood flow to the potentially ischemic myocardium to restore the balance between myocardial oxygen supply and demand. Pharmacologic therapy to prevent myocardial infarction and death is with antiplatelet agents (aspirin, clopidogrel) and lipid-lowering agents. Recently, angiotensin-converting enzyme inhibitors have also been reported to reduce the risk of adverse cardiac events in patients with high risk for coronary artery disease (Yusuf et al, 2000). In unstable angina and non-ST-segment elevation myocardial infarction, aggressive therapy with coronary stenting, antilipid drugs, heparin, and antiplatelet agents is recommended (Braunwald et al, 2000, 2002).

Angina of Effort

Many studies have demonstrated that nitrates, calcium channel blockers, and β-blockers increase time to onset of angina and ST depression during treadmill tests in patients with angina of effort (Figure 12–5). Although exercise tolerance increases, there is usually no change in the angina threshold, ie, the rate-pressure product at which symptoms occur.

For maintenance therapy of chronic stable angina, long-acting nitrates, calcium channel-blocking agents, or β-blockers may be chosen; the best choice of drug will depend on the individual patient's response. In hypertensive patients, monotherapy with either slow-release or long-acting calcium channel blockers or β-

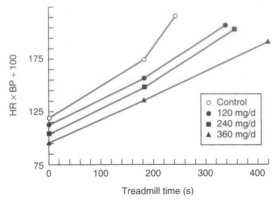

Figure 12–5. Effects of diltiazem on the double product (heart rate times systolic blood pressure) in a group of 20 patients with angina of effort. In a double-blind study using a standard protocol, patients were tested on a treadmill during treatment with placebo and three doses of the drug. Heart rate (HR) and systolic blood pressure (BP) were recorded at 180 seconds of exercise (midpoints of lines) and at the time of onset of anginal symptoms (rightmost points). Note that the drug treatment decreased the double product at all times during exercise and prolonged the time to appearance of symptoms. (Data from Lindenberg BS et al: Efficacy and safety of incremental doses of diltiazem for the treatment of angina. J Am Coll Cardiol 1983;2:1129. Used with permission of the American College of Cardiology.)

blockers may be adequate. In normotensive patients, long-acting nitrates may be suitable. The combination of a β-blocker with a calcium channel blocker (eg, propranolol with nifedipine) or two different calcium chan-

nel blockers (eg, nifedipine and verapamil) has been shown to be more effective than individual drugs used alone. If response to a single drug is inadequate, a drug from a different class should be added to maximize the beneficial reduction of cardiac work while minimizing undesirable effects (Table 12–7). Some patients may require therapy with all three drug groups.

Surgical revascularization (ie, coronary artery bypass grafting [CABG]) and catheter-based revascularization (ie, percutaneous coronary intervention [PCI]) are the primary methods for promptly restoring coronary blood flow and increasing oxygen supply to the myocardium. Major clinical trials suggest that coronary obstruction can also be decreased by vigorous antilipidemic therapy.

Vasospastic Angina

Nitrates and the calcium channel blockers are effective drugs for relieving and preventing ischemic episodes in patients with variant angina. In approximately 70% of patients treated with nitrates plus calcium channel blockers, angina attacks are completely abolished; in another 20%, marked reduction of frequency of anginal episodes is observed. Prevention of coronary artery spasm (in the presence or absence of fixed atherosclerotic coronary artery lesions) is the principal mechanism for this beneficial response. All presently available calcium channel blockers appear to be equally effective, and the choice of a particular drug should depend on the patient, as indicated above. Surgical revascularization and angioplasty are not indicated in patients with variant angina.

Unstable Angina & Acute Coronary Syndromes

In patients with unstable angina with recurrent ischemic episodes at rest, recurrent thrombotic occlusions of the

Table 12–7. Effects of nitrates alone and with β-blockers or calcium channel blockers in angina pectoris. (Undesirable effects are shown in italics.)

	Nitrates Alone	Beta Blockers or Calcium Channel Blockers	Combined Nitrates With Beta Blockers or Calcium Channel Blockers
Heart rate	*Reflex increase*	Decrease[1]	Decrease
Arterial pressure	Decrease	Decrease	Decrease
End-diastolic volume	Decrease	*Increase*	None or decrease
Contractility	*Reflex increase*	Decrease	None
Ejection time	Decrease	*Increase*	None

[1]Nifedipine may cause a *reflex increase* in heart rate and cardiac contractility.

offending coronary artery occur as the result of fissuring of atherosclerotic plaques and platelet aggregation. Anticoagulant and antiplatelet drugs play a major role in therapy (see Chapter 34). Aspirin has been shown to reduce the incidence of cardiac events in such patients. Intravenous heparin or subcutaneous low-molecular-weight heparin is indicated in most patients. Antiplatelet agents (ticlopidine, clopidogrel, and GPIIb/IIIa antagonists) have been found to be effective in decreasing risk in unstable angina (Braunwald et al 2000, 2002). In addition, therapy with nitroglycerin and β-blockers should be considered; calcium channel blockers should be added in refractory cases. Catheter-based or surgical myocardial revascularization is indicated in high-risk patients.

PREPARATIONS AVAILABLE

NITRATES & NITRITES

Amyl nitrite (generic, Aspirols, Vaporole)
Inhalant: 0.3 mL capsules
Isosorbide dinitrate (generic, Isordil, Sorbitrate)
Oral: 5, 10, 20, 30, 40 mg tablets; 5, 10 mg chewable tablets
Oral sustained-release (generic, Sorbitrate SA, Iso-Bid): 40 mg tablets and capsules
Sublingual: 2.5, 5, 10 mg sublingual tablets
Isosorbide mononitrate (Ismo, others)
Oral: 10, 20 mg tablets; extended-release 30, 60, 120 mg tablets
Nitroglycerin
Sublingual: 0.3, 0.4, 0.6 mg tablets; 0.4 mg/metered dose aerosol
Oral sustained-release (generic, Nitrong): 2.6, 6.5, 9 mg tablets; 2.5, 6.5, 9, 13 mg capsules
Buccal (Nitrogard): 2, 3 mg buccal tablets
Parenteral (Nitro-Bid IV, Tridil, generic): 0.5, 5 mg/mL for IV administration
Transdermal patches (Minitran, Nitro-Dur, Transderm-Nitro): to release at rates of 0.1, 0.2, 0.3, 0.4, 0.6, or 0.8 mg/h.
Topical ointment (generic, Nitrol): 20 mg/mL ointment (1 inch, or 25 mm, of ointment contains about 15 mg nitroglycerin)

CALCIUM CHANNEL BLOCKERS

Amlodipine (Norvasc)
Oral: 2.5, 5, 10 mg tablets
Bepridil (Vascor)
Oral: 200, 300 mg tablets

Diltiazem (Cardizem, generic)
Oral: 30, 60, 90, 120 mg tablets
Oral sustained-release (Cardizem SR, Dilacor XL, others): 60, 90, 120, 180, 240, 300, 360, 420 mg capsules
Parenteral: 5 mg/mL for injection
Felodipine (Plendil)
Oral extended-release: 2.5, 5, 10 mg tablets
Isradipine (DynaCirc)
Oral: 2.5, 5 mg capsules
Oral controlled release: 5, 10 mg tablets
Nicardipine (Cardene, others)
Oral: 20, 30 mg capsules
Oral sustained-release (Cardene SR): 30, 45, 60 mg capsules
Parenteral (Cardene I.V.): 2.5 mg/mL
Nifedipine (Adalat, Procardia, others)
Oral: 10, 20 mg capsules
Oral extended-release (Procardia XL, Adalat CC): 30, 60, 90 mg tablets
Nimodipine (Nimotop)
Oral: 30 mg capsules. (Labeled for use in subarachnoid hemorrhage, not angina.)
Nisoldipine (Sular)
Oral extended-release: 10, 20, 30, 40 mg tablets
Verapamil (generic, Calan, Isoptin)
Oral: 40, 80, 120 mg tablets
Oral sustained-release: 100, 120, 180, 240 mg tablets or capsules
Parenteral: 2.5 mg/mL for injection

BETA BLOCKERS

See Chapter 10.

REFERENCES

Bassenge E, Zanzinger J: Nitrates in different vascular beds, nitrate tolerance, and interactions with endothelial function. Am J Cardiol 1992;70(Suppl B):23B.

Boesgaard S et al: Nitrate tolerance in vivo is not associated with depletion of arterial or venous thiol levels. Circ Res 1994;74:115.

Braunwald E et al: ACC/AHA Guidelines for the management of patients with unstable angina and non-ST-segment elevation myocardial infarction: Executive summary and recommendations. A Report of the American College of Cardiology/American Heart Association Task Force on Practice Guidelines (Committee on the Management of Patients with Unstable Angina). Circulation 2000;102:1193.

Braunwald E et al: ACC/AHA Guideline update for the management of patients with unstable angina and non-ST-segment elevation myocardial infarction—2002. Circulation 2002;106:1893.

Carmichael P, Lieben J: Sudden death in explosives workers. Arch Environ Health 1963;7:50.

Chatterjee K: Ischemic heart disease. In: Stein JH (editor). *Internal Medicine,* 5th ed. Little, Brown, 1998.

Fung H-L, Bauer JA: Mechanisms of nitrate tolerance. Cardiovasc Drugs Ther 1994;8:489.

Furberg CD, Psaty BM, Meyer JV: Nifedipine. Dose-related increase in mortality in patients with coronary heart disease. Circulation 1995;92:1326.

Gibbons RJ et al: ACC/AHA/ACP-ASIM guidelines for the management of patients with chronic stable angina: executive summary and recommendations. A Report of the American College of Cardiology/American Heart Association Task Force on Practice Guidelines (Committee on Management of Patients with Chronic Stable Angina). J Am Coll Cardiol 1999;33:2829.

Gibbons RJ et al: ACC/AHA 2002 guideline update for the management of patients with chronic stable angina—summary article. J Am Coll Cardiol 2003;41:159.

Hartman PE: Review: Putative mutagens and carcinogens in foods. 1. Nitrate/nitrite ingestion and gastric cancer mortality. Environ Mutagen 1983;5:111.

Ho M, Belch JJ: Raynaud's phenomenon: State of the art 1998. Scand J Rheumatol 1998;27:319.

Hockerman GH et al: Molecular determinants of drug binding and action on L-type calcium channels. Annu Rev Pharmacol Toxicol 1997;37:361.

Ignarro LJ et al: Mechanism of vascular smooth muscle relaxation by organic nitrates, nitrites, nitroprusside, and nitric oxide: evidence for the involvement of S-nitrosothiols as active intermediates. J Pharmacol Exp Ther 1981;218:739.

Karlberg K-E et al: Dose-dependent effect of intravenous nitroglycerin on platelet aggregation, and correlation with plasma glyceryl dinitrate concentration in healthy men. Am J Cardiol 1992;69:802.

Kawanishi DT et al: Response of angina and ischemia to long-term treatment in patients with chronic stable angina: A double blind randomized individualized dosing trial of nifedipine, propranolol, and their combination. J Am Coll Cardiol 1992;19:409.

Lindenberg BS et al: Efficacy and safety of incremental doses of diltiazem for the treatment of stable angina pectoris. J Am Coll Cardiol 1983;2:1129.

McCormack JG, Stanley WC, Wolff AA: Ranolazine: a novel metabolic modulator for the treatment of angina. Gen Pharmac 1998;30:639.

Miljanich GP, Ramachandran J: Antagonists of neuronal calcium channels: Structure, function, and therapeutic implications. Annu Rev Pharmacol Toxicol 1995;35:707.

Packer M et al: Effect of amlodipine on morbidity and mortality in severe chronic heart failure. Prospective Randomized Amlodipine Survival Evaluation Study Group. N Engl J Med 1996;335:1107.

Pepine CJ, Wolff AA: A controlled trial with a novel anti-ischemic agent, ranolazine, in chronic stable angina pectoris that is responsive to conventional antianginal agents. Am J Cardiol 1999;84:46.

Psaty BM et al: The risk of myocardial infarction associated with antihypertensive drug therapies. JAMA 1995;274:620.

Schmidt HHHW et al: The nitric oxide and cGMP signal transduction system: regulation and mechanism of action. Biochim Biophys Acta 1993;1178:153.

Spedding M et al: Factors modifying the tissue selectivity of calcium-antagonists. J Neural Transm 1990;31(Suppl):5.

Spedding M, Kenny B, Chatelain P: New drug binding sites in Ca^{2+} channels. Trends Pharmacol Sci 1995;16:139.

Steering Committee, Transdermal Nitroglycerin Cooperative Study: Acute and chronic antianginal efficacy of continuous twenty-four hour application of transdermal nitroglycerin. Am J Cardiol 1991;68:1263.

Sturgill MG, Seibold JR: Rational use of calcium-channel antagonists in Raynaud's phenomenon. Curr Opin Rheumatol 1998;10:584.

Yusuf S et al: Effects of an angiotensin-converting enzyme inhibitor, ramipril, on cardiovascular events in high-risk patients. The Heart Outcomes Prevention Evaluation Study Investigators. N Engl J Med 2000;342:145.

Drugs Used in Heart Failure

13

Bertram G. Katzung, MD, PhD, & William W. Parmley, MD

Heart failure occurs when the cardiac output is inadequate to provide the oxygen needed by the body. It is a highly lethal condition, with a 5-year mortality rate conventionally said to be about 50%. The most common cause of heart failure in the USA is coronary artery disease. In systolic failure, the mechanical pumping action (contractility) and the ejection fraction of the heart are reduced. In diastolic failure, stiffening and loss of adequate relaxation plays a major role in reducing cardiac output and ejection fraction may be normal. Because other cardiovascular conditions are now being treated more effectively (especially myocardial infarction), more patients are surviving long enough for heart failure to develop, making this one of the cardiovascular conditions that is actually increasing in prevalence.

Although it is believed that the primary defect in early heart failure resides in the excitation-contraction coupling machinery of the heart, the clinical condition also involves many other processes and organs, including the baroreceptor reflex, the sympathetic nervous system, the kidneys, angiotensin II and other peptides, and death of cardiac cells. Recognition of these factors has resulted in evolution of a variety of treatment strategies (Table 13–1).

Clinical research has shown that therapy directed at noncardiac targets may be more valuable in the long-term treatment of heart failure than traditional positive inotropic agents (cardiac glycosides [digitalis]). Thus, drugs acting on the kidneys (diuretics) have long been considered at least as valuable as digitalis. Careful clinical trials have shown that angiotensin-converting enzyme (ACE) inhibitors, β-blockers, and spironolactone (a potassium-sparing diuretic) are the only agents in current use that actually prolong life in patients with chronic heart failure. Positive inotropic drugs, on the other hand, can be very helpful in acute failure. They also reduce symptoms in chronic failure.

Control of Normal Cardiac Contractility

The vigor of contraction of heart muscle is determined by several processes that lead to the movement of actin and myosin filaments in the cardiac sarcomere (Figure 13–1). Ultimately, contraction results from the interaction of calcium (during systole) with the actin-troponin-tropomyosin system, thereby releasing the actin-myosin interaction. This *activator* calcium is released from the sarcoplasmic reticulum (SR). The amount released depends on the amount stored in the SR and on the amount of *trigger* calcium that enters the cell during the plateau of the action potential.

A. SENSITIVITY OF THE CONTRACTILE PROTEINS TO CALCIUM

The determinants of calcium sensitivity, ie, the curve relating the shortening of cardiac myofibrils to the cytoplasmic calcium concentration, are incompletely understood, but several types of drugs can be shown to affect it in vitro. Levosimendan is the most recent example of a drug that increases calcium sensitivity (it may also inhibit phosphodiesterase) and reduces symptoms in models of heart failure.

B. THE AMOUNT OF CALCIUM RELEASED FROM THE SARCOPLASMIC RETICULUM

A small rise in free cytoplasmic calcium, brought about by calcium influx during the action potential, triggers the opening of calcium channels in the membrane of the SR and the rapid release of a large amount of the ion into the cytoplasm in the vicinity of the actin-troponin-tropomyosin complex. The amount released is proportional to the amount stored in the SR and the amount of trigger calcium that enters the cell through the cell membrane. Ryanodine is a potent *negative* inotropic plant alkaloid that *interferes* with the release of calcium through the SR channels. No drugs are available that increase the release of calcium through these channels.

C. THE AMOUNT OF CALCIUM STORED IN THE SARCOPLASMIC RETICULUM

The SR membrane contains a very efficient calcium uptake transporter, which maintains free cytoplasmic calcium at very low levels during diastole by pumping calcium into the SR. The amount of calcium sequestered in the SR is thus determined, in part, by the amount accessible to this transporter. This in turn is dependent on the balance of calcium influx (primarily through the voltage-gated membrane calcium channels)

201

Table 13–1. Drug groups commonly used in heart failure.

ACE inhibitors
Beta blockers
Angiotensin receptor blockers
Cardiac glycosides
Vasodilators
Beta agonists, dopamine
Bipyridines

ACE, angiotensin-converting enzyme.

and calcium efflux, the amount removed from the cell (primarily via the sodium-calcium exchanger, a transporter in the cell membrane).

D. THE AMOUNT OF TRIGGER CALCIUM

The amount of trigger calcium that enters the cell depends on the availability of calcium channels (primarily the L type) and the duration of their opening. As described in Chapters 6 and 9, sympathomimetics cause an increase in calcium influx through an action on these channels. Conversely, the calcium channel blockers (see Chapter 12) reduce this influx and depress contractility.

E. ACTIVITY OF THE SODIUM-CALCIUM EXCHANGER

This antiporter uses the sodium gradient to move calcium against its concentration gradient from the cytoplasm to the extracellular space. Extracellular concentrations of these ions are much less labile than intracellular concentrations under physiologic conditions. The sodium-calcium exchanger's ability to carry out this transport is thus strongly dependent on the intracellular concentrations of both ions, especially sodium.

F. INTRACELLULAR SODIUM CONCENTRATION AND ACTIVITY OF NA+/K+ ATPase

Na^+/K^+ ATPase, by removing intracellular sodium, is the major determinant of sodium concentration in the cell. The sodium influx through voltage-gated channels, which occurs as a normal part of almost all cardiac

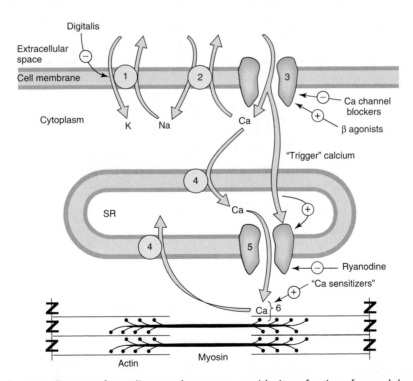

Figure 13–1. Schematic diagram of a cardiac muscle sarcomere, with sites of action of several drugs that alter contractility (numbered structures). Site *1* is Na^+/K^+ ATPase, the sodium pump. Site *2* is the sodium/calcium exchanger. Site *3* is the voltage-gated calcium channel. Site *4* is a calcium transporter that pumps calcium into the sarcoplasmic reticulum (SR). Site *5* is a calcium channel in the membrane of the SR that is triggered to release stored calcium by activator calcium. Site *6* is the actin-troponin-tropomyosin complex at which activator calcium brings about the contractile interaction of actin and myosin.

action potentials, is another determinant. As described below, Na+/K+ ATPase appears to be the primary target of cardiac glycosides.

Pathophysiology of Heart Failure

Heart failure is a syndrome with multiple causes that may involve the right ventricle, the left ventricle, or both. Cardiac output in heart failure is usually below the normal range. Systolic dysfunction, with reduced cardiac output and significantly reduced ejection fraction (less than 45%), is typical of acute failure, especially that resulting from myocardial infarction. Diastolic dysfunction often occurs as a result of hypertrophy and stiffening of the myocardium, and although cardiac output is reduced, ejection fraction may be normal. Heart failure due to diastolic dysfunction does not usually respond optimally to positive inotropic drugs.

Rarely, "high-output" failure may occur. In this condition, the demands of the body are so great that even increased cardiac output is insufficient. High-output failure can result from hyperthyroidism, beriberi, anemia, and arteriovenous shunts. This form of failure responds poorly to the drugs discussed in this chapter and should be treated by correcting the underlying cause.

The primary signs and symptoms of all types of heart failure include tachycardia, decreased exercise tolerance and shortness of breath, peripheral and pulmonary edema, and cardiomegaly. Decreased exercise tolerance with rapid muscular fatigue is the major direct consequence of diminished cardiac output. The other manifestations result from the attempts by the body to compensate for the intrinsic cardiac defect.

Neurohumoral (extrinsic) compensation involves two major mechanisms previously presented in Figure 6–7: the sympathetic nervous system and the renin-angiotensin-aldosterone hormonal response. Some of the pathologic as well as beneficial features of these compensatory responses are illustrated in Figure 13–2. The baroreceptor reflex appears to be reset, with a lower sensitivity to arterial pressure, in patients with heart failure. As a result, baroreceptor sensory input to the vasomotor center is reduced even at normal pressures; sympathetic outflow is increased, and parasympathetic outflow is decreased. Increased sympathetic outflow causes tachycardia, increased cardiac contractility, and increased vascular tone. While the increased preload, force, and heart rate initially increase cardiac output, increased arterial tone results in increased afterload and decreased ejection fraction, cardiac output, and renal perfusion. After a relatively short time, complex down-regulatory changes in the β_1-adrenoceptor-G protein-effector system take place that result in diminished stimulatory effects. Beta$_2$ receptors are *not* down-regulated and may develop increased

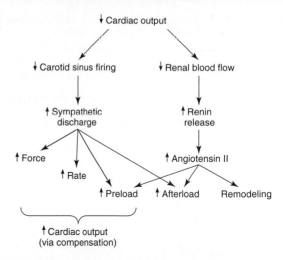

Figure 13–2. Some compensatory responses that occur during congestive heart failure. In addition to the effects shown, angiotensin II increases sympathetic effects by facilitating norepinephrine release.

coupling to the IP$_3$-DAG cascade. It has also been suggested that cardiac β_3 receptors (which do not appear to be down-regulated in failure) may mediate negative inotropic effects. Increased angiotensin II production leads to increased aldosterone secretion (with sodium and water retention), to increased afterload, and to remodeling of both heart and vessels (discussed below). Other hormones may also be released, including natriuretic peptide and endothelin (see Chapter 17).

The most important intrinsic compensatory mechanism is **myocardial hypertrophy**. This increase in muscle mass helps maintain cardiac performance. However, after an initial beneficial effect, hypertrophy can lead to ischemic changes, impairment of diastolic filling, and alterations in ventricular geometry. **Remodeling** is the term applied to dilation (other than that due to passive stretch) and slow structural changes that occur in the stressed myocardium. It may include proliferation of connective tissue cells as well as abnormal myocardial cells with some biochemical characteristics of fetal myocytes. Ultimately, myocytes in the failing heart die at an accelerated rate through apoptosis, leaving the remaining myocytes subject to even greater overload.

The severity of heart failure is usually described according to a scale devised by the New York Heart Association. Class I failure is associated with no limitations on ordinary activities and symptoms that occur only with greater than ordinary exercise. Class II is characterized by slight limitation of ordinary activities, which result in fatigue and palpitations. Class III results in no symptoms at rest, but fatigue, etc, with less than ordinary physical activity. Class IV is associated with symptoms even when the patient is at rest.

Pathophysiology of Cardiac Performance

Cardiac performance is a function of four primary factors:

1. Preload: When some measure of left ventricular performance such as stroke volume or stroke work is plotted as a function of left ventricular filling pressure, the resulting curve is termed the left ventricular function curve (Figure 13–3). The ascending limb (< 15 mm Hg filling pressure) represents the classic Frank-Starling relation. Beyond approximately 15 mm Hg, there is a plateau of performance. Preloads greater than 20–25 mm Hg result in pulmonary congestion. As noted above, preload is usually increased in heart failure because of increased blood volume and venous tone. Reduction of high filling pressure is the goal of salt restriction and diuretic therapy in heart failure. Venodilator drugs (eg, nitroglycerin) also reduce pre-load by redistributing blood away from the chest into peripheral veins.

2. Afterload: Afterload is the resistance against which the heart must pump blood and is represented by aortic impedance and systemic vascular resistance. As cardiac output falls in chronic failure, there is a reflex increase in systemic vascular resistance, mediated in part by increased sympathetic outflow and circulating catecholamines and in part by activation of the renin-angiotensin system. Endothelin, a potent vasoconstrictor peptide, may also be involved. This sets the stage for the use of drugs that reduce arteriolar tone in heart failure.

3. Contractility: Heart muscle obtained by biopsy from patients with chronic low-output failure demonstrates a reduction in intrinsic contractility. As contractility decreases in the patient, there is a reduction in the velocity of muscle shortening, the rate of intraventricular pressure development (dP/dt), and the stroke output achieved (Figure 13–3). However, the heart is still capable of some increase in all of these measures of contractility in response to inotropic drugs.

4. Heart rate: The heart rate is a major determinant of cardiac output. As the intrinsic function of the heart decreases in failure and stroke volume diminishes, an increase in heart rate—through sympathetic activation of β adrenoceptors—is the first compensatory mechanism that comes into play to maintain cardiac output.

I. BASIC PHARMACOLOGY OF DRUGS USED IN HEART FAILURE

Although digitalis is rarely the first drug used in heart failure, we begin our discussion with this group because other drugs are discussed in more detail in chapters 11, 12, and 15.

DIGITALIS

Digitalis is the genus name for the family of plants that provide most of the medically useful cardiac glycosides, eg, **digoxin.** Such plants have been known for thousands of years but were used erratically and with variable success until 1785, when William Withering, an English physician and botanist, published a monograph describing the clinical effects of an extract of the foxglove plant (*Digitalis purpurea,* a major source of these agents).

Chemistry

All of the cardiac glycosides, or cardenolides—of which digoxin is the prototype—combine a steroid nucleus

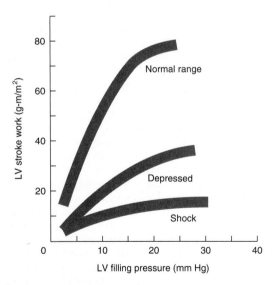

Figure 13–3. Relation of left ventricular (LV) performance to filling pressure in patients with acute myocardial infarction, an important cause of heart failure. The upper line indicates the range for normal, healthy individuals. If acute heart failure occurs, function is shifted down and to the right. Similar depression is observed in patients with chronic heart failure. (Modified and reproduced with permission, from Swan HJC, Parmley WW: Congestive heart failure. In: Sodeman WA Jr, Sodeman TM [editors]. *Pathologic Physiology.* Saunders, 1979.)

linked to a lactone ring at the 17 position and a series of sugars at carbon 3 of the nucleus. Because they lack an easily ionizable group, their solubility is not pH-dependent.

Sources of these drugs include white and purple foxglove (*Digitalis lanata* and *D purpurea*) and numerous other temperate zone and tropical plants. Certain toads have skin glands capable of elaborating **bufadienolides,** which differ only slightly from the cardenolides.

Pharmacokinetics

A. ABSORPTION AND DISTRIBUTION

Cardenolides vary in their absorption, distribution, metabolism, and excretion, as shown by comparison of three representative agents: digoxin, digitoxin, and ouabain (Table 13–2). Of these three, digoxin is the only preparation used in the USA.

Digoxin is fairly well absorbed after oral administration. However, about 10% of individuals harbor enteric bacteria that inactivate digoxin in the gut, greatly reducing bioavailability and requiring higher than average maintenance dosage. Treatment of such patients with antibiotics can result in a sudden increase in bioavailability and digitalis toxicity. Because the safety margin of cardiac glycosides is very narrow, even minor variations in bioavailability can cause serious toxicity or loss of effect.

Once absorbed into the blood, all cardiac glycosides are widely distributed to tissues, including the central nervous system. Their volumes of distribution differ, however, depending on their tendency to bind to plasma proteins versus tissue proteins.

B. METABOLISM AND EXCRETION

Digoxin is not extensively metabolized in humans; almost two thirds is excreted unchanged by the kidneys. Its renal clearance is proportional to creatinine clearance. Equations and nomograms are available for adjusting digoxin dosage in patients with renal impairment.

Table 13–2. Properties of three typical cardiac glycosides.

	Ouabain[1]	Digoxin	Digitoxin[1]
Lipid solubility (oil/water coefficient)	Low	Medium	High
Oral availability (percentage absorbed)	0	75	> 90
Half-life in body (hours)	21	40	168
Plasma protein binding (percentage bound)	0	20–40	> 90
Percentage metabolized	0	< 40	> 80
Volume of distribution (L/kg)	18	6.3	0.6

[1]Ouabain and digitoxin are no longer in use in the USA.

Digitoxin is metabolized in the liver and excreted into the gut via the bile. Cardioactive metabolites (which include digoxin) as well as unchanged digitoxin can then be reabsorbed from the intestine, thus establishing an **enterohepatic circulation** that contributes to the very long half-life of this agent. Renal impairment does not significantly prolong the half-life of digitoxin.

Ouabain must be given parenterally and is excreted, mostly unchanged, in the urine.

Pharmacodynamics

Digitalis has multiple direct and indirect cardiovascular effects, with both therapeutic and toxic consequences. In addition, it has undesirable effects on the central nervous system and gut.

At the molecular level, all therapeutically useful cardiac glycosides **inhibit Na+/K+ ATPase,** the membrane-bound transporter often called the *sodium pump.* This protein consists of α and β subunits. The binding sites for Na+, K+, ATP, and digitalis all appear to reside on the α subunit. Different isoforms of the subunits have been identified, thus providing for different isoforms of the complete enzyme with differing affinities for cardiac glycosides in various tissues. Very low concentrations of these drugs have occasionally been reported to *stimulate* the enzyme. In contrast, inhibition over most of the dose range has been extensively documented in all tissues studied. It is probable that the inhibitory action is largely responsible for the therapeutic effect (positive inotropy) in the heart. Since the sodium pump is necessary for maintenance of normal resting potential in most excitable cells, it is likely that a major portion of the toxicity of digitalis is also caused by this enzyme-inhibiting action. Other molecular-level effects of digitalis have been studied in the heart and are discussed below. The fact that the receptor for cardiac glycosides exists on the sodium pump has prompted some investigators to propose that an endogenous "digitalis-like" agent, possibly ouabain, must exist.

A. CARDIAC EFFECTS

1. Mechanical effects—Cardiac glycosides increase the intensity of the interaction of the actin and myosin filaments of the cardiac sarcomere (Figure 13–1) by increasing the free calcium concentration in the vicinity of the contractile proteins during systole. The increase in calcium concentration is the result of a two-step process: first, an increase of intracellular sodium concentration because of Na^+/K^+ ATPase inhibition (1 in Figure 13–1); and second, a relative reduction of calcium expulsion from the cell by the sodium-calcium exchanger (2 in Figure 13–1) caused by the increase in intracellular sodium. Other mechanisms have been proposed but are not well supported.

The net result of the action of therapeutic concentra-

tions of a cardiac glycoside is a distinctive increase in cardiac contractility (Figure 13–4, bottom trace). In isolated myocardial preparations, the rate of development of tension and of relaxation are both increased, with little or no change in time to peak tension. This effect occurs in both normal and failing myocardium, but in the intact animal or patient the responses are modified by cardiovascular reflexes and the pathophysiology of heart failure.

2. Electrical effects—The effects of digitalis on the electrical properties of the heart are a mixture of direct and autonomic actions. Direct actions on the membranes of cardiac cells follow a well-defined progression: an early, brief prolongation of the action potential, followed by a protracted period of shortening (especially the plateau phase). The decrease in action potential duration is probably the result of increased potassium conductance that is caused by increased intracellular calcium (see Chapter 14). All of these effects can be observed at therapeutic concentrations in the absence of overt toxicity. Shortening of the action potential contributes to the shortening of atrial and ventricular refractoriness (Table 13–3).

At higher concentrations, resting membrane potential is reduced (made less negative) as a result of inhibition of the sodium pump and reduced intracellular potassium. As toxicity progresses, oscillatory depolariz-

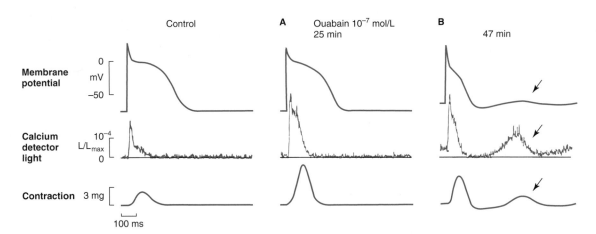

Figure 13–4. Effects of a cardiac glycoside, ouabain, on isolated cardiac tissue. The top tracing shows action potentials evoked during the control period, early in the "therapeutic" phase, and later, when toxicity is present. The middle tracing shows the light (L) emitted by the calcium-detecting protein aequorin (relative to the maximum possible, L_{max}) and is roughly proportionate to the free intracellular calcium concentration. The bottom tracing records the tension elicited by the action potentials. The early phase of ouabain action (**A**) shows a slight shortening of action potential and a marked increase in free intracellular calcium concentration and contractile tension. The toxic phase (**B**) is associated with depolarization of the resting potential, a marked shortening of the action potential, and the appearance of an oscillatory depolarization, calcium increment, and contraction (*arrows*). (Unpublished data kindly provided by P Hess and H Gil Wier.)

Table 13–3. Major actions of digitalis on cardiac electrical functions.

Variable	Tissue		
	Atrial Muscle	**AV Node**	**Purkinje System, Ventricles**
Effective refractory period	↓ (PANS)	↑ (PANS)	↓ (Direct)
Conduction velocity	↑ (PANS)	↓ (PANS)	Negligible
Automaticity	↑ (Direct)	↑ (Direct)	↑(Direct)
Electrocardiogram Before arrhythmias	Negligible	↑ PR interval	↓ QT interval; T wave inversion; ST segment depression
During arrhythmias	Atrial tachycardia, atrial fibrillation	AV nodal tachycardia, AV blockade	Premature ventricular contractions, bigeminy, ventricular tachycardia, ventricular fibrillation

Key:

   (PANS) = parasympathetic actions

   (Direct) = direct membrane actions

ing afterpotentials appear following normally evoked action potentials (Figure 13–4, panel B). The afterpotentials (also known as *delayed afterdepolarizations*) are associated with overloading of the intracellular calcium stores and oscillations in the free intracellular calcium ion concentration. When below threshold, these afterpotentials may interfere with normal conduction because of the further reduction of resting potential. Eventually, an afterpotential may reach threshold, eliciting an action potential (premature depolarization or ectopic "beat") that is coupled to the preceding normal one. If afterpotentials in the Purkinje conducting system regularly reach threshold in this way, bigeminy will be recorded on the electrocardiogram (Figure 13–5). With further intoxication, each afterpotential-evoked action potential will itself elicit a suprathreshold afterpotential, and a self-sustaining tachycardia will be established. If allowed to progress, such a tachycardia may deteriorate into fibrillation; in the case of ventricular fibrillation, the arrhythmia will be rapidly fatal unless corrected.

Autonomic actions of cardiac glycosides on the heart involve both the parasympathetic and the sympathetic systems. In the lower portion of the dose range, cardioselective **parasympathomimetic** effects predominate. In fact, these atropine-blockable effects account for a significant portion of the early electrical effects of digitalis (Table 13–3). This action involves sensitization of the baroreceptors, central vagal stimulation, and facilitation of mus-

carinic transmission at the cardiac muscle cell. Because cholinergic innervation is much richer in the atria, these actions affect atrial and atrioventricular nodal function more than Purkinje or ventricular function. Some of the cholinomimetic effects are useful in the treatment of cer-

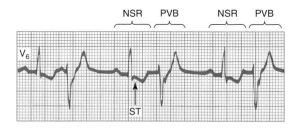

Figure 13–5. Electrocardiographic record showing digitalis-induced bigeminy. The complexes marked NSR are normal sinus rhythm beats; an inverted T wave and depressed ST segment are present. The complexes marked PVB are premature ventricular beats and are the electrocardiographic manifestations of depolarizations evoked by delayed oscillatory afterpotentials as shown in Figure 13–4. (Modified and reproduced, with permission, from Goldman MJ: *Principles of Clinical Electrocardiography,* 12th ed. Lange, 1986.)

tain arrhythmias. At toxic levels, sympathetic outflow is increased by digitalis. This effect is not essential for typical cardenolide toxicity but sensitizes the myocardium and exaggerates all the toxic effects of the drug.

The most common cardiac manifestations of glycoside toxicity include atrioventricular junctional rhythm, premature ventricular depolarizations, bigeminal rhythm, and second-degree atrioventricular blockade. However, it is claimed that digitalis can cause virtually every variety of arrhythmia.

B. EFFECTS ON OTHER ORGANS

Cardiac glycosides affect all excitable tissues, including smooth muscle and the central nervous system. Inhibition of Na^+/K^+ ATPase in these tissues depolarizes and increases spontaneous activity both in neurons and in smooth muscle cells. The gastrointestinal tract is the most common site of digitalis toxicity outside the heart. The effects include anorexia, nausea, vomiting, and diarrhea. This toxicity may be partially caused by direct effects on the gastrointestinal tract but is also the result of central nervous system actions, including chemoreceptor trigger zone stimulation.

Central nervous system effects commonly include vagal and chemoreceptor zone stimulation. Much less often, disorientation and hallucinations—especially in the elderly—and visual disturbances are noted. The latter effect may include aberrations of color perception. Agitation and even convulsions are occasionally reported in patients taking digitalis.

Gynecomastia is a rare effect reported in men taking digitalis; it is not certain whether this effect represents a peripheral estrogenic action of these steroid drugs or a manifestation of hypothalamic stimulation.

C. INTERACTIONS WITH POTASSIUM, CALCIUM, AND MAGNESIUM

Potassium and digitalis interact in two ways. First, they inhibit each other's binding to Na^+/K^+ ATPase; therefore, hyperkalemia reduces the enzyme-inhibiting actions of cardiac glycosides, whereas hypokalemia facilitates these actions. Second, abnormal cardiac automaticity is inhibited by hyperkalemia (see Chapter 14). Moderately increased extracellular K^+ therefore reduces the effects of digitalis, especially the toxic effects.

Calcium ion facilitates the toxic actions of cardiac glycosides by accelerating the overloading of intracellular calcium stores that appears to be responsible for digitalis-induced abnormal automaticity. Hypercalcemia therefore increases the risk of a digitalis-induced arrhythmia. The effects of magnesium ion appear to be opposite to those of calcium. Hypomagnesemia is therefore a risk factor for arrhythmias. These interactions mandate careful evaluation of serum electrolytes in patients with digitalis-induced arrhythmias.

OTHER POSITIVE INOTROPIC DRUGS USED IN HEART FAILURE

Drugs that inhibit **phosphodiesterases,** the family of enzymes that inactivate cAMP and cGMP, have long been used in therapy of heart failure. Although they have positive inotropic effects, most of their benefits appear to derive from vasodilation, as discussed below. Phosphodiesterase inhibitors have been intensively studied for several decades with mixed results. The bipyridines inamrinone and milrinone are the most successful of these agents found to date, but their usefulness is quite limited. Levosimendan, an investigational drug that sensitizes the troponin system to calcium, also appears to inhibit phosphodiesterase and cause some vasodilation in addition to its inotropic effects. Some early clinical trials suggest that this drug may be useful in patients with heart failure (Follath, et al, 2002). A group of β-adrenoceptor stimulants have also been used as digitalis substitutes, but they may increase mortality (see below).

BIPYRIDINES

Inamrinone (previously called amrinone) and **milrinone** are bipyridine compounds that inhibit phosphodiesterase. They are active orally as well as parenterally but are only available in parenteral forms. They have elimination half-lives of 3–6 hours, with 10–40% being excreted in the urine.

Pharmacodynamics

The bipyridines increase myocardial contractility by increasing inward calcium flux in the heart during the action potential; they may also alter the intracellular movements of calcium by influencing the sarcoplasmic reticulum. They also have an important vasodilating effect. These drugs are relatively selective for phosphodiesterase isozyme 3, a form found in cardiac and smooth muscle. Inhibition of this isozyme results in an increase in cAMP and the increase in contractility and vasodilation noted above.

The toxicity of inamrinone includes nausea and vomiting; arrhythmias, thrombocytopenia, and liver enzyme changes have been reported in a significant number of patients. This drug has been withdrawn in some countries. Milrinone appears less likely to cause bone marrow and liver toxicity than inamrinone, but it does cause arrhythmias. Inamrinone and milrinone are now used only intravenously and only for acute heart failure or for an exacerbation of chronic heart failure.

BETA ADRENOCEPTOR STIMULANTS

The general pharmacology of these agents is discussed in Chapter 9. The selective β_1-agonist that has been most widely used in patients with heart failure is **dobutamine**. This drug produces an increase in cardiac output together with a decrease in ventricular filling pressure. Some tachycardia and an increase in myocardial oxygen consumption have been reported. The potential for producing angina or arrhythmias in patients with coronary artery disease must be considered, as well as the tachyphylaxis that accompanies the use of any β stimulant. Intermittent dobutamine infusion may benefit some patients with chronic heart failure.

Dopamine has also been used in acute heart failure and may be particularly helpful if there is a need to raise blood pressure.

DRUGS WITHOUT POSITIVE INOTROPIC EFFECTS USED IN HEART FAILURE

The drugs most commonly used in chronic heart failure are diuretics, ACE inhibitors, angiotensin receptor antagonists, and β-blockers (Table 13–1). In acute failure, diuretics and vasodilators play important roles.

DIURETICS

The diuretics are discussed in detail in Chapter 15. Their major mechanism of action in heart failure is to reduce venous pressure and ventricular preload. These reductions have two useful effects: reduction of edema and its symptoms and reduction of cardiac size, which leads to improved pump efficiency. Spironolactone, the aldosterone antagonist diuretic (see Chapter 15), has the additional benefit of decreasing morbidity and mortality in patients with severe heart failure who are also receiving ACE inhibitors and other standard therapy. One possible mechanism for this benefit lies in accumulating evidence that aldosterone may also cause myocardial and vascular fibrosis and baroreceptor dysfunction in addition to its renal effects.

ANGIOTENSIN-CONVERTING ENZYME INHIBITORS, ANGIOTENSIN RECEPTOR ANTAGONISTS, & RELATED AGENTS

The ACE inhibitors such as **captopril** are introduced in Chapter 11 and discussed again in Chapter 17. These versatile drugs reduce peripheral resistance and thereby reduce afterload; they also reduce salt and water retention (by reducing aldosterone secretion) and in that way reduce preload. The reduction in tissue angiotensin levels also reduces sympathetic activity, probably through diminution of angiotensin's presynaptic effects on norepinephrine release. Finally, these drugs reduce the long-term remodeling of the heart and vessels, an effect that

may be responsible for the observed reduction in mortality and morbidity (see Clinical Pharmacology).

Angiotensin AT_1 receptor-blockers such as **losartan** (see Chapters 11 and 17) appear to have similar but more limited beneficial effects, and clinical trials of these drugs in heart failure continue.

A newer class of drugs that inhibit both ACE and neutral endopeptidase, an enzyme that inactivates bradykinin and natriuretic peptide (see below), has been introduced into clinical trials recently. **Omapatrilat** is the first of these agents and has been shown in early studies to increase exercise tolerance and to reduce morbidity and mortality. Unfortunately, it causes a significant incidence of angioedema.

VASODILATORS

The vasodilators are effective in acute heart failure because they provide a reduction in preload (through venodilation), or reduction in afterload (through arteriolar dilation), or both. Some evidence suggests that long-term use of hydralazine and isosorbide dinitrate can also reduce damaging remodeling of the heart.

A synthetic form of the endogenous peptide **brain natriuretic peptide** (BNP) has recently been approved for use in acute cardiac failure as **nesiritide**. This recombinant product increases cGMP in smooth muscle cells and effectively reduces venous and arteriolar tone in experimental preparations. It also causes diuresis. The peptide has a short half-life of about 18 minutes and is administered as a bolus intravenous dose followed by continuous infusion. Excessive hypotension is the most common adverse effect. Measurement of *endogenous* BNP has been proposed as a diagnostic test because plasma concentrations rise in most patients with heart failure.

Bosentan, an orally active competitive inhibitor of endothelin (see Chapter 17), has been shown to have some benefits in experimental animal models of heart failure, but results in human trials have not been impressive. This drug is approved for use in pulmonary hypertension (see Chapter 11). It has significant teratogenic and hepatotoxic effects.

BETA ADRENOCEPTOR BLOCKERS

Most patients with chronic heart failure respond favorably to certain β-blockers in spite of the fact that these drugs can precipitate acute decompensation of cardiac function (see Chapter 10). Studies with bisoprolol, carvedilol, and metoprolol showed a reduction in mortality in patients with stable severe heart failure but this effect was not observed with another β-blocker, bucindolol. A full understanding of the beneficial action of β-blockade is lacking, but suggested mechanisms include attenuation of the adverse effects of high concentrations of catecholamines (including apoptosis), up-regulation of β-receptors, decreased heart rate, and reduced remodeling through inhibition of the mitogenic activity of catecholamines.

II. CLINICAL PHARMACOLOGY OF DRUGS USED IN HEART FAILURE

In the past, prescription of a diuretic plus digitalis was almost automatic in every case of chronic heart failure, and other drugs were rarely considered. At present, diuretics are still considered as first-line therapy, but digitalis is usually reserved for patients who do not respond adequately to diuretics, ACE inhibitors, and β-blockers (Table 13–1).

MANAGEMENT OF CHRONIC HEART FAILURE

The major steps in the management of patients with chronic heart failure are outlined in Table 13–4. Reduction of cardiac work is helpful in most cases. This can be accomplished by reducing activity and weight, and—especially important—control of hypertension.

SODIUM REMOVAL

Sodium removal is the next important step—by dietary salt restriction or a diuretic—especially if edema is present. In mild failure, it is reasonable to start with a thiazide diuretic, switching to more powerful agents as required. Sodium loss causes secondary loss of potas-

Table 13–4. Steps in the treatment of chronic heart failure.

1. Reduce workload of the heart
   a. Limit activity level
   b. Reduce weight
   c. Control hypertension
2. Restrict sodium
3. Restrict water (rarely required)
4. Give diuretics
5. Give ACE inhibitor or angiotensin receptor blocker
6. Give digitalis if systolic dysfunction with 3rd heart sound or atrial fibrillation is present
7. Give β-blockers to patients with stable class II–IV heart failure
8. Give vasodilators

sium, which is particularly hazardous if the patient is to be given digitalis. Hypokalemia can be treated with potassium supplementation or through the addition of a potassium-sparing diuretic such as spironolactone. As noted above, spironolactone should probably be considered in all patients with moderate or severe heart failure since it appears to reduce both morbidity and mortality.

ACE INHIBITORS & ANGIOTENSIN RECEPTOR BLOCKERS

In patients with left ventricular dysfunction but no edema, an ACE inhibitor should be used first. Several large studies have compared ACE inhibitors with digoxin or with other traditional therapies for chronic heart failure. The results show clearly that ACE inhibitors are superior to both placebo and to vasodilators and must be considered, along with diuretics, as first-line therapy for chronic failure. However, ACE inhibitors cannot replace digoxin in patients already receiving that drug because patients withdrawn from the cardiac glycoside while on ACE inhibitor therapy deteriorate.

Additional studies suggest that ACE inhibitors are also valuable in asymptomatic patients with ventricular dysfunction. By reducing preload and afterload, these drugs appear to slow the rate of ventricular dilation and thus delay the onset of clinical heart failure. Thus, ACE inhibitors are beneficial in all subsets of patients, from those who are asymptomatic to those in severe chronic failure.

It appears that all ACE inhibitors tested to date have beneficial effects in patients with chronic heart failure. Recent studies have documented these beneficial effects with enalapril, captopril, lisinopril, quinapril, and ramipril. Thus, this benefit appears to be a class effect.

The angiotensin II receptor antagonists (eg, losartan, valsartan, etc) produce beneficial hemodynamic effects similar to those of the ACE inhibitors. However, large clinical trials suggest that the angiotensin receptor blockers should only be used in patients who are intolerant of ACE inhibitors (usually because of cough).

VASODILATORS

Vasodilator drugs can be divided into selective arteriolar dilators, venous dilators, and drugs with nonselective vasodilatory effects. For this purpose, the ACE inhibitors may be considered nonselective arteriolar and venous dilators. The choice of agent should be based on the patient's signs and symptoms and hemodynamic measurements. Thus, in patients with high filling pressures in whom the principal symptom is dyspnea, venous dilators such as long-acting nitrates will be most helpful in reducing filling pressures and the symptoms of pulmonary congestion. In patients in whom fatigue due to low left ventricular output is a primary symptom, an arteriolar dilator such as hydralazine may be helpful in increasing forward cardiac output. In most patients with severe chronic failure that responds poorly to other therapy, the problem usually involves both elevated filling pressures and reduced cardiac output. In these circumstances, dilation of both arterioles and veins is required. In one trial, combined therapy with hydralazine (arteriolar dilation) and isosorbide dinitrate (venous dilation) prolonged life more than placebo in patients already receiving digitalis and diuretics.

BETA BLOCKERS & CALCIUM CHANNEL BLOCKERS

Many trials have evaluated the potential for β-blocker therapy in patients with heart failure. The rationale is based on the hypothesis that excessive tachycardia and adverse effects of high catecholamine levels on the heart contribute to the downward course of heart failure patients. However, such therapy must be initiated very cautiously at low doses, since acutely blocking the supportive effects of catecholamines can worsen heart failure. Several months of therapy may be required before improvement is noted; this usually consists of a slight rise in ejection fraction, slower heart rate, and reduction in symptoms. As noted above, bisoprolol, carvedilol, and metoprolol have been shown to reduce mortality.

The calcium-blocking drugs appear to have no role in the treatment of patients with heart failure. Their depressant effects on the heart may worsen heart failure.

DIGITALIS

Digoxin is indicated in patients with heart failure and atrial fibrillation. It is also most helpful in patients with a dilated heart and third heart sound. It is usually given after ACE inhibitors. Only about 50% of patients with normal sinus rhythm (usually those with documented *systolic* dysfunction) will have documentable relief of heart failure from digitalis. Better results are obtained in patients with atrial fibrillation. If the decision is made to use a cardiac glycoside, digoxin is the one chosen in the great majority of cases (and the only one available in the USA). When symptoms are mild, slow loading (digitalization) (Table 13–3) is safer and just as effective as the rapid method.

Determining the optimal level of digitalis effect may be difficult. In patients with atrial fibrillation, reduction of ventricular rate is the best measure of glycoside effect. In patients in normal sinus rhythm, symptomatic improvement and reductions in heart size, heart rate during exercise, venous pressure, or edema may signify optimum drug levels in the myocardium. Unfortu-

nately, toxic effects may occur before the therapeutic end point is detected. If digitalis is being loaded slowly, simple omission of one dose and halving the maintenance dose will often bring the patient to the narrow range between suboptimal and toxic concentrations. Measurement of plasma digoxin levels is useful in patients who appear unusually resistant or sensitive; a level of 1.1 ng/mL or less is appropriate.

Because it has a moderate but persistent positive inotropic effect, digitalis can, in theory, reverse the signs and symptoms of heart failure. In an appropriate patient, digitalis increases stroke work and cardiac output. The increased output (and possibly a direct action resetting the sensitivity of the baroreceptors) eliminates the stimuli evoking increased sympathetic outflow, and both heart rate and vascular tone diminish. With decreased end-diastolic fiber tension (the result of increased systolic ejection and decreased filling pressure), heart size and oxygen demand decrease. Finally, increased renal blood flow improves glomerular filtration and reduces aldosterone-driven sodium reabsorption. Thus, edema fluid can be excreted, further reducing ventricular preload and the danger of pulmonary edema. Although digitalis had a neutral effect on mortality (Digitalis Investigation Group, 1997), it reduced hospitalization and deaths from progressive heart failure at the expense of an increase in sudden death. It is important to note that the mortality rate was reduced in patients with serum digoxin concentrations of 1 ng/mL or less but increased in those with digoxin levels greater than 1.5 ng/mL.

Administration & Dosage

Long-term treatment with digoxin requires careful attention to pharmacokinetics because of its long half-life. According to the rules set forth in Chapter 3, it will take three to four half-lives to approach steady-state total body load when given at a constant dosing rate, ie, approximately 1 week for digoxin. Typical doses used in adults are given in Table 13–5. A parenteral preparation of digoxin is available but is not used to achieve a faster onset of effect because the time to peak effect is determined mainly by time-dependent ion changes in the tissue. Thus, the parenteral preparation is only suitable for patients who cannot take drugs by mouth.

Interactions

Patients are at risk for developing serious digitalis-induced cardiac arrhythmias if hypokalemia develops, as in diuretic therapy or diarrhea. Furthermore, patients taking digoxin are at risk if given quinidine, which displaces digoxin from tissue binding sites (a minor effect) and depresses renal digoxin clearance (a major effect).

Table 13–5. Clinical use of digoxin.[1]

	Digoxin
Therapeutic plasma concentration	0.5–1.5 ng/mL
Toxic plasma concentration	> 2 ng/mL
Daily dose (slow loading or maintenance)	0.25 (0.125–0.5) mg
Rapid digitalizing dose (rarely used)	0.5–0.75 mg every 8 hours for three doses

[1]These values are appropriate for adults with normal renal and hepatic function.

The plasma level of the glycoside may double within a few days after beginning quinidine therapy, and toxic effects may become manifest. As noted above, antibiotics that alter gastrointestinal flora may increase digoxin bioavailability in about 10% of patients. Finally, agents that release catecholamines may sensitize the myocardium to digitalis-induced arrhythmias.

Other Clinical Uses of Digitalis

Digitalis is useful in the management of atrial arrhythmias because of its cardioselective parasympathomimetic effects. In atrial flutter, the depressant effect of the drug on atrioventricular conduction will help control an excessively high ventricular rate. The effects of the drug on the atrial musculature may convert flutter to fibrillation, with a further decrease in ventricular rate. In atrial fibrillation, the same vagomimetic action helps control ventricular rate, thereby improving ventricular filling and increasing cardiac output. Digitalis has also been used in the control of paroxysmal atrial and atrioventricular nodal tachycardia. At present, calcium channel blockers and adenosine are preferred for this application.

Digitalis should be avoided in the therapy of arrhythmias associated with Wolff-Parkinson-White syndrome because it increases the probability of conduction of arrhythmic atrial impulses through the alternative rapidly conducting atrioventricular pathway. It is explicitly contraindicated in patients with Wolff-Parkinson-White syndrome and atrial fibrillation (see Chapter 14).

Toxicity

In spite of its recognized hazards, digitalis is heavily used and toxicity is common. Therapy of toxicity manifested as visual changes or gastrointestinal disturbances generally requires no more than reducing the dose of the drug. If cardiac arrhythmia is present and can definitely be ascribed to digitalis, more vigorous therapy may be necessary. Serum digitalis and potassium levels and the ECG should be monitored during therapy of significant digitalis toxicity. Electrolyte status should be corrected if abnormal (see above). For patients who do not respond promptly (within one to two half-lives), calcium and magnesium as well as potassium levels should be checked. For occasional premature ventricular depolarizations or brief runs of bigeminy, oral potassium supplementation and withdrawal of the glycoside may be sufficient. If the arrhythmia is more serious, parenteral potassium and antiarrhythmic drugs may be required. Of the available antiarrhythmic agents, lidocaine is favored.

In severe digitalis intoxication (which usually involves young children or suicidal overdose), serum potassium will already be elevated at the time of diagnosis (because of potassium loss from the intracellular compartment of skeletal muscle and other tissues). Furthermore, automaticity is usually depressed, and antiarrhythmic agents administered in this setting may lead to cardiac arrest. Such patients are best treated with insertion of a temporary cardiac pacemaker catheter and administration of digitalis antibodies (**digoxin immune fab**). These antibodies are produced in sheep, and although they are raised to digoxin they also recognize digitoxin and cardiac glycosides from many other plants. They are extremely useful in reversing severe intoxication with most glycosides.

Digitalis-induced arrhythmias are frequently made worse by cardioversion; this therapy should be reserved for ventricular fibrillation if the arrhythmia is glycoside-induced.

MANAGEMENT OF ACUTE HEART FAILURE

Acute heart failure occurs frequently in patients with chronic failure. Such episodes are usually associated with increased exertion, emotion, salt in the diet, noncompliance with medical therapy, or increased metabolic demand occasioned by fever, anemia, etc. A particularly common and important cause of acute failure—with or without chronic failure—is acute myocardial infarction.

Patients with acute myocardial infarction are best treated with emergency revascularization with either coronary angioplasty and a stent or a thrombolytic agent. Even with revascularization, acute failure may develop in such patients. Many of the signs and symptoms of acute and chronic failure are identical, but their therapies diverge because of the need for more rapid response and the relatively greater frequency and sever-

Table 13–6. Therapeutic classification of subsets in acute myocardial infarction.[1]

Subset	Systolic Arterial Pressure (mm Hg)	Left Ventricular Filling Pressure (mm Hg)	Cardiac Index (L/min/m²)	Therapy
1. Hypovolemia	< 100	< 10	< 2.5	Volume replacement
2. Pulmonary congestion	100–150	> 20	> 2.5	Diuretics
3. Peripheral vasodilation	< 100	10–20	> 2.5	None, or vasoactive drugs
4. Power failure	< 100	> 20	< 2.5	Vasodilators, inotropic drugs
5. Severe shock	< 90	> 20	< 2.0	Vasoactive drugs, inotropic drugs, vasodilators, circulatory assist
6. Right ventricular infarct	< 100	RVFP > 10 LVFP < 15	< 2.5	Provide volume replacement for LVFP, inotropic drugs. Avoid diuretics.
7. Mitral regurgitation, ventricular septal defect	< 100	> 20	< 2.5	Vasodilators, inotropic drugs, circulatory assist, surgery

[1]The numerical values are intended to serve as general guidelines and not as absolute cutoff points. Arterial pressures apply to patients who were previously normotensive and should be adjusted upward for patients who were previously hypertensive. (RVFP and LVFP = right and left ventricular filling pressure.)

ity of pulmonary vascular congestion in the acute form.

Measurements of arterial pressure, cardiac output, stroke work index, and pulmonary capillary wedge pressure are particularly useful in patients with acute myocardial infarction and acute heart failure. Such patients can be usefully characterized on the basis of three hemodynamic measurements: arterial pressure, left ventricular filling pressure, and cardiac index. One such classification and therapies that have proved most effective are set forth in Table 13–6. When filling pressure is greater than 15 mm Hg and stroke work index is less than 20 g-m/m², the mortality rate is high (Figure 13–3). Intermediate levels of these two variables imply a much better prognosis.

REFERENCES

BASIC PHARMACOLOGY

Katz AM: Effects of digitalis on cell biochemistry: Sodium pump inhibition. J Am Coll Cardiol 1985;5(Suppl A):16A.

Kelly RA, Smith TW: Recognition and management of digitalis toxicity. Am J Cardiol 1992;69:108G.

Lindenbaum J et al: Inactivation of digoxin by the gut flora: Reversal by antibiotic therapy. N Engl J Med 1981;305:789.

Post SR, Hammond HK, Insel PA: β-Adrenergic receptors and receptor signaling in heart failure. Annu Rev Pharmacol Toxicol 1999;39:343.

Wenger TL et al: Treatment of 63 severely digitalis-toxic patients with digoxin-specific antibody fragments. J Am Coll Cardiol 1985;5(Suppl A):118A.

Zimmermann N et al: Positive inotropic effects of the calcium sensitizer CGP 48506 in guinea pig myocardium. J Pharmacol Exp Ther 1996;277:1572.

PATHOPHYSIOLOGY OF HEART FAILURE

Ferguson DW: Digitalis and neurohormonal abnormalities in heart failure and implications for therapy. Am J Cardiol 1992;69:24G.

Schrier RW, Abraham WT: Hormones and hemodynamics in heart failure. N Engl J Med 1999;341:577.

Torre-Amione G: Tumor necrosis factor-α and tumor necrosis factor receptors in the failing human heart. Circulation 1996;93:704.

ACUTE MYOCARDIAL INFARCTION

Hennekens CH et al: Adjunctive drug therapy of acute myocardial infarction: Evidence from clinical trials. N Engl J Med 1996;335:1660.

Ryan TJ et al: 1999 Update ACC/AHA Guidelines for the management of acute myocardial infarction. Circulation 1999;100:1016.

PREPARATIONS AVAILABLE

(DIURETICS: SEE CHAPTER 15.)

DIGITALIS
Digoxin (generic, Lanoxicaps, Lanoxin)
Oral: 0.125, 0.25 mg tablets; 0.05, 0.1, 0.2 mg capsules*; 0.05 mg/mL elixir
Parenteral: 0.1, 0.25 mg/mL for injection

DIGITALIS ANTIBODY
Digoxin immune fab (ovine) (digibind, digifab)
Parenteral: 38 or 40 mg per vial with 75 mg sorbitol lyophilized powder to reconstitute for IV injection. Each vial will bind approximately 0.5 mg digoxin or digitoxin.

SYMPATHOMIMETICS MOST COMMONLY USED IN CONGESTIVE HEART FAILURE
Dobutamine (generic, Dobutrex)
Parenteral: 12.5 mg/mL for IV infusion
Dopamine (generic, Intropin)
Parenteral: 40, 80, 160 mg/mL for IV injection; 80, 160, 320 mg/dL in 5% dextrose for IV infusion

ANGIOTENSIN-CONVERTING ENZYME INHIBITORS LABELED FOR USE IN CONGESTIVE HEART FAILURE
Captopril (generic, Capoten)
Oral: 12.5, 25, 50, 100 mg tablets
Enalapril (Vasotec, Vasotec I.V.)
Oral: 2.5, 5, 10, 20 mg tablets
Parenteral: 1.25 mg enalaprilat/mL
Fosinopril (Monopril)
Oral: 10, 20, 40 mg tablets
Lisinopril (Prinivil, Zestril)
Oral: 2.5, 5, 10, 20, 40 mg tablets
Quinapril (Accupril)
Oral: 5, 10, 20, 40 mg tablets
Ramipril (Altace)
Oral: 1.25, 2.5, 5, 10 mg capsules

Trandolapril (Mavik)
Oral: 1, 2, 5 mg tablets

ANGIOTENSIN RECEPTOR BLOCKERS
Candesartan (Atacand)
Oral: 4, 8, 16, 32 mg tablets
Eprosartan (Teveten)
Oral: 400, 800 mg tablets
Irbesartan (Avapro)
Oral: 75, 150, 300 mg tablets
Losartan (Cozaar)
Oral: 25, 50, 100 mg tablets
Olmesartan (Benicar)
Oral: 5, 20, 40 mg tablets
Telmisartan (Micardis)
Oral: 20, 40, 80 mg tablets
Valsartan (Diovan)
Oral: 40, 80, 160, 320 mg tablets

BETA-BLOCKERS THAT HAVE REDUCED MORTALITY IN HEART FAILURE
Bisoprolol (Zebeta, unlabeled use)
Oral: 5, 10 mg tablets
Carvedilol (Coreg)
Oral: 3.125, 6.25, 12.5, 25 mg tablets
Metoprolol (Lopressor, Toprol XL)
Oral: 50, 100 mg tablets; 25, 50, 100, 200 mg extended-release tablets
Parenteral: 1 mg/mL for IV injection

OTHER DRUGS
Inamrinone
Parenteral: 5 mg/mL for IV injection
Milrinone (generic, Primacor)
Parenteral: 1 mg/mL for IV injection; 200 μg/mL premixed for IV infusion
Nesiritide (Natrecor)
Parenteral: 1.58 mg powder for IV injection
Bosentan (Tracleer)
Oral: 62.5, 125 mg tablets

---

* Digoxin capsules (Lanoxicaps) have greater bioavailability than digoxin tablets.

CHRONIC HEART FAILURE

Cohn J et al: A randomized trial of the angiotensin receptor blocker valsartan in heart failure. N Engl J Med 2002;345:1667.

CONSENSUS Trial Study Group: Effects of enalapril on mortality in severe congestive heart failure. N Engl J Med 1987;316:1429.

Digitalis Investigation Group: The effect of digoxin on mortality and morbidity in patients with heart failure. N Engl J Med 1997;336:525.

Follath F et al: Efficacy and safety of intravenous levosimendan compared with dobutamine in severe low-output heart failure (the LIDO study): a randomized double-blind trial. Lancet 2002;360:196.

Fonarow GC et al: Effect of direct vasodilation with hydralazine versus angiotensin-converting enzyme inhibition with captopril on mortality in advanced heart failure: The Hy-C Trial. J Am Coll Cardiol 1992;19:842.

Foody JM, Farrell MH, Krumholtz H: Beta blocker therapy in heart failure. JAMA 2002;287:883.

Francis GS, McDonald KM, Cohn JN: Neurohumoral activation in preclinical heart failure: Remodeling and the potential for intervention. Circulation 1993; 87(Suppl 1V):1V–90.

Garg R, Yusuf S: Overview of randomized trials of angiotensin-converting enzyme inhibitors on mortality and morbidity in patients with heart failure. JAMA 1995;273:1450.

Goodley E: Newer drug therapy for congestive heart failure. Arch Intern Med 1999;159:1177.

Klein L et al: Pharmacologic therapy for patients with chronic heart failure and reduced systolic function: review of trials and practical considerations. Am J Cardiol 2003;91(Supple 9A):18F.

Mann DL et al: New therapeutics for chronic heart failure. Annu Rev Med 2002;53:59.

Newton GE, Parker JD: Acute effects of β_1-selective and nonselective β-adrenergic receptor blockade on cardiac sympathetic activity in congestive heart failure. Circulation 1996;94:353.

Packer M et al: The effect of carvedilol on morbidity and mortality in patients with chronic heart failure. N Engl J Med 1996; 334:334.

Pitt B et al: The effect of spironolactone on morbidity and mortality in patients with severe heart failure. N Engl J Med 1999;341:709.

Pitt B et al: Effect of losartan compared to captopril on mortality in patients with symptomatic heart failure: randomized trial—The Losartan Heart Failure Survival Study, Elite II. Lancet 2000;355:1582.

Pitt B et al: Randomized trial of losartan versus captopril in patients over 65 with heart failure. (Evaluation of Losartan in the Elderly Study, ELITE.) Lancet 1997;349:747.

Stevenson WG et al: Improving survival for patients with advanced heart failure: A study of 737 consecutive patients. J Am Coll Cardiol 1995;26:1417.

Agents Used in Cardiac Arrhythmias

Joseph R. Hume, PhD, & Augustus O. Grant, MD, PhD*

Cardiac arrhythmias are a frequent problem in clinical practice, occurring in up to 25% of patients treated with digitalis, 50% of anesthetized patients, and over 80% of patients with acute myocardial infarction. Arrhythmias may require treatment because rhythms that are too rapid, too slow, or asynchronous can reduce cardiac output. Some arrhythmias can precipitate more serious or even lethal rhythm disturbances—eg, early premature ventricular depolarizations can precipitate ventricular fibrillation. In such patients, antiarrhythmic drugs may be lifesaving. On the other hand, the hazards of antiarrhythmic drugs—and in particular the fact that they can *precipitate* lethal arrhythmias in some patients—has led to a reevaluation of their relative risks and benefits. In general, treatment of asymptomatic or minimally symptomatic arrhythmias should be avoided for this reason.

Arrhythmias can be treated with the drugs discussed in this chapter and with nonpharmacologic therapies such as pacemakers, cardioversion, catheter ablation, and surgery. This chapter describes the pharmacology of drugs that suppress arrhythmias by a direct action on the cardiac cell membrane. Other modes of therapy are discussed briefly.

ELECTROPHYSIOLOGY OF NORMAL CARDIAC RHYTHM

The electrical impulse that triggers a normal cardiac contraction originates at regular intervals in the sinoatrial node (Figure 14–1), usually at a frequency of 60–100 beats per minute. This impulse spreads rapidly through the atria and enters the atrioventricular node, which is normally the only conduction pathway between the atria and ventricles. Conduction through the atrioventricular node is slow, requiring about 0.15 s. (This delay provides time for atrial contraction to propel blood into the ventricles.) The impulse then propagates over the His-Purkinje system and invades all parts of the ventricles. Ventricular activation is complete in less than 0.1 s; therefore, contraction of all of the ventricular muscle is synchronous and hemodynamically effective.

Arrhythmias consist of cardiac depolarizations that deviate from the above description in one or more aspects—ie, there is an abnormality in the site of origin of the impulse, its rate or regularity, or its conduction.

Ionic Basis of Membrane Electrical Activity

The transmembrane potential of cardiac cells is determined by the concentrations of several ions—chiefly sodium (Na^+), potassium (K^+), calcium (Ca^{2+}), and chloride (Cl^-)—on either side of the membrane and the permeability of the membrane to each ion. These water-soluble ions are unable to freely diffuse across the lipid cell membrane in response to their electrical and concentration gradients; they require aqueous channels (specific pore-forming proteins) for such diffusion. Thus, ions move across cell membranes in response to their gradients only at specific times during the cardiac cycle when these ion channels are open. The movements of these ions produce currents that form the basis of the cardiac action potential. Individual channels are relatively ion-specific, and the flux of ions through them is thought to be controlled by "gates" (probably flexible peptide chains or energy barriers). Each type of channel has its own type of gate (sodium, calcium, and some potassium channels are each thought to have two types of gates), and each type of gate is opened and closed by specific transmembrane voltage, ionic, or metabolic conditions.

At rest, most cells are not significantly permeable to sodium, but at the start of each action potential, they become quite permeable (see below). Similarly, calcium enters and potassium leaves the cell with each action potential. Therefore, the cell must have a mechanism to maintain stable transmembrane ionic conditions by establishing and maintaining ion gradients. The most

---

* The authors acknowledge the contributions of the previous authors of this chapter, Drs L Hondeghem and D Roden.

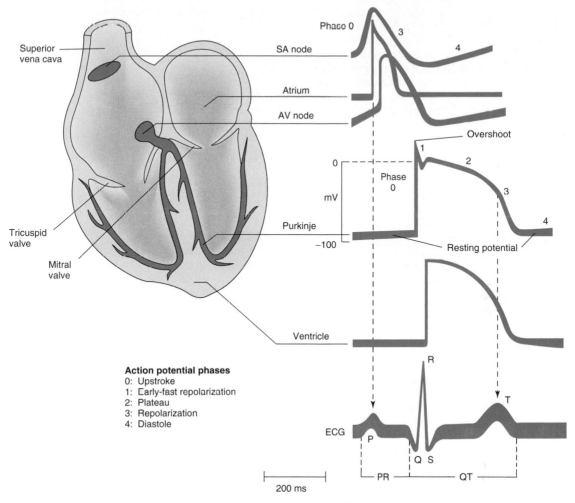

Action potential phases
0: Upstroke
1: Early-fast repolarization
2: Plateau
3: Repolarization
4: Diastole

Figure 14–1. Schematic representation of the heart and normal cardiac electrical activity (intracellular recordings from areas indicated and ECG). Sinoatrial node, atrioventricular node, and Purkinje cells display pacemaker activity (phase 4 depolarization). The ECG is the body surface manifestation of the depolarization and repolarization waves of the heart. The P wave is generated by atrial depolarization, the QRS by ventricular muscle depolarization, and the T wave by ventricular repolarization. Thus, the PR interval is a measure of conduction time from atrium to ventricle, and the QRS duration indicates the time required for all of the ventricular cells to be activated (ie, the intraventricular conduction time). The QT interval reflects the duration of the ventricular action potential.

important of these active mechanisms is the sodium pump, Na$^+$/K$^+$ ATPase, described in Chapter 13. This pump and other active ion carriers contribute indirectly to the transmembrane potential by maintaining the gradients necessary for diffusion through channels. In addition, some pumps and exchangers produce net current flow (eg, by exchanging three Na$^+$ for two K$^+$ ions) and hence are termed "electrogenic."

When the cardiac cell membrane becomes permeable to a specific ion (ie, when the channels selective for that

ion are open), movement of that ion across the cell membrane is determined by Ohm's law: current = voltage ÷ resistance, or current = voltage × conductance. Conductance is determined by the properties of the individual ion channel protein. The voltage term is the difference between the actual membrane potential and the reversal potential for that ion (the membrane potential at which no current would flow even if channels were open). For example, in the case of sodium in a cardiac cell at rest, there is a substantial concentration gradient (140 mmol/L Na$^+$ outside; 10–15 mmol/L Na$^+$ inside) and electrical gradient (0 mV outside; −90 mV inside) that would drive Na$^+$ into cells. Sodium does not enter the cell at rest because sodium channels are closed; when sodium channels open, the very large influx of Na$^+$ ions accounts for phase 0 depolarization. The situation for K$^+$ ions in the resting cardiac cell is quite different. Here, the concentration gradient (140 mmol/L inside; 4 mmol/L outside) would drive the ion out of the cell, but the electrical gradient would drive it in, ie, the inward gradient is in equilibrium with the outward gradient. In fact, certain potassium channels ("inward rectifier" channels) are open in the resting cell, but little current flows through them because of this balance. The equilibrium, or **reversal potential**, for ions is determined by the **Nernst equation:**

$$E_{ion} = 61 \times log \left(\frac{C_e}{C_i} \right)$$

where C_e and C_i are the extracellular and intracellular concentrations, respectively, multiplied by their activity coefficients. Note that raising extracellular potassium makes E_K less negative. When this occurs, the membrane depolarizes until E_K is reached. Thus, extracellular potassium concentration and inward rectifier channel function are the major factors determining the membrane potential of the resting cardiac cell. The conditions required for application of the Nernst equation are approximated at the peak of the overshoot and during rest in most nonpacemaker cardiac cells. If the permeability is significant for both potassium and sodium, the Nernst equation is

not a good predictor of membrane potential, but the **Goldman-Hodgkin-Katz equation** may be used.

$$E_{mem} = 61 \times log \left(\frac{P_K \times K_e + P_{Na} \times Na_e}{P_K \times K_i + P_{Na} \times Na_i} \right)$$

In pacemaker cells (whether normal or ectopic), spontaneous depolarization (the pacemaker potential) occurs during diastole (phase 4, Figure 14–1). This depolarization results from a gradual increase of depolarizing current through special hyperpolarization-activated ion channels in pacemaker cells. The effect of changing extracellular potassium is more complex in a pacemaker cell than it is in a nonpacemaker cell because the effect on permeability to potassium is much more important in a pacemaker (see Box, Effects of Potassium). In a pacemaker—especially an ectopic one—the end result of an increase in extracellular potassium will usually be to slow or stop the pacemaker. Conversely, hypokalemia will often facilitate ectopic pacemakers.

The Active Cell Membrane

In normal atrial, Purkinje, and ventricular cells, the action potential upstroke (phase 0) is dependent on sodium current. From a functional point of view, it is convenient to describe the behavior of the sodium current in terms of three channel states (Figure 14–2). The cardiac sodium channel protein has been cloned, and it is now recognized that these channel states actually represent different protein conformations. In addition, regions of the protein that confer specific behaviors,

---

EFFECTS OF POTASSIUM

The effects of changes in serum potassium on cardiac action potential duration, pacemaker rate, and arrhythmias can appear somewhat paradoxical if changes are predicted based solely on a consideration of changes in the potassium *electrochemical gradient*. In the heart, however, changes in serum potassium concentration have an additional effect to alter potassium *conductance* (increased extracellular potassium increases potassium conductance) independent of simple changes in electrochemical driving force, and this effect often predominates. As a result, the actual observed effects of *hyperkalemia* include reduced action potential duration, slowed conduction, decreased pacemaker rate, and

decreased pacemaker arrhythmogenesis. Conversely, the actual observed effects of *hypokalemia* include prolonged action potential duration, increased pacemaker rate, and increased pacemaker arrhythmogenesis. Furthermore, pacemaker rate and arrhythmias involving ectopic pacemaker cells appear to be more sensitive to changes in serum potassium concentration, compared with cells of the sinoatrial node. These effects of serum potassium on the heart probably contribute to the observed increased sensitivity to potassium channel-blocking antiarrhythmic agents (quinidine or sotalol) during hypokalemia, eg, accentuated action potential prolongation and tendency to cause torsade de pointes.

such as voltage sensing, pore formation, and inactivation, are now being identified. The gates described below and in Figure 14–2 represent such regions.

Depolarization to the threshold voltage results in opening of the activation *(m)* gates of sodium channels (Figure 14–2, middle). If the inactivation *(h)* gates of these channels have not already closed, the channels are now open or activated, and sodium permeability is markedly increased, greatly exceeding the permeability for any other ion. Extracellular sodium therefore diffuses down its electrochemical gradient into the cell, and the membrane potential very rapidly approaches the sodium equilibrium potential, E_{Na} (about +70 mV when Na_e = 140 mmol/L and Na_i = 10 mmol/L). This intense sodium current is very brief because opening of the *m* gates upon depolarization is promptly followed by closure of the *h* gates and inactivation of the sodium channels (Figure 14–2, right).

Most calcium channels become activated and inactivated in what appears to be the same way as sodium channels, but in the case of the most common type of cardiac calcium channel (the "L" type), the transitions occur more slowly and at more positive potentials. The action potential plateau (phases 1 and 2) reflects the turning off of most of the sodium current, the waxing and waning of calcium current, and the slow development of a repolarizing potassium current.

Final repolarization (phase 3) of the action potential results from completion of sodium and calcium channel inactivation and the growth of potassium permeability, so that the membrane potential once again approaches the potassium equilibrium potential. The major potassium currents involved in phase 3 repolarization include a rapidly activating potassium current (I_{Kr}) and a slowly activating potassium current (I_{Ks}). These processes are diagrammed in Figure 14–3.

The Effect of Resting Potential on Action Potentials

A key factor in the pathophysiology of arrhythmias and the actions of antiarrhythmic drugs is the relationship between the resting potential of a cell and the action potentials that can be evoked in it (Figure 14–4, left panel). Because the inactivation gates of sodium channels in the resting membrane close over the potential range −75 to −55 mV, fewer sodium channels are "available" for diffusion of sodium ions when an action potential is evoked from a resting potential of −60 mV than when it is evoked from a resting potential of −80 mV. Important consequences of the reduction in peak sodium permeability include reduced upstroke velocity (called V_{max}, for maximum rate of change of membrane voltage), reduced action potential amplitude, reduced excitability, and reduced conduction velocity.

During the plateau of the action potential, most sodium channels are inactivated. Upon repolarization, recovery from inactivation takes place (in the terminology of Figure 14–2, the *h* gates reopen), making the

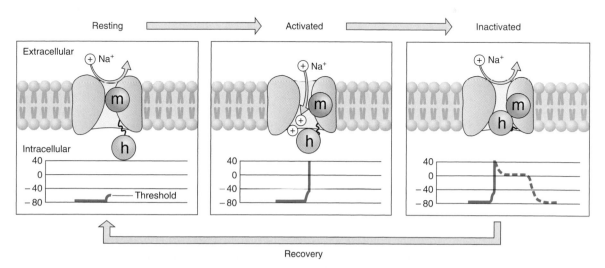

Figure 14–2. A schematic representation of Na⁺ channels cycling through different conformational states during the cardiac action potential. Transitions between resting, activated, and inactivated states are dependent on membrane potential and time. The activation gate is shown as *m* and the inactivation gate as *h*. Potentials typical for each state are shown under each channel schematic as a function of time. The dashed line indicates that part of the action potential during which most Na⁺ channels are completely or partially inactivated and unavailable for reactivation.

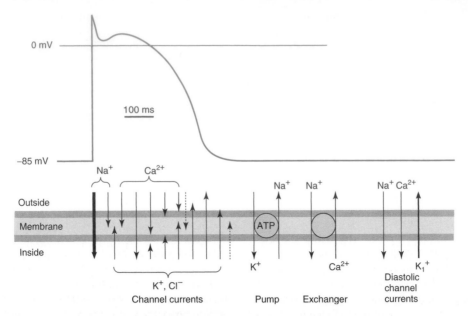

Figure 14–3. Schematic diagram of the ion permeability changes and transport processes that occur during an action potential and the diastolic period following it. The size and weight of the arrows indicate approximate magnitudes of the ion channel currents; arrows pointing down indicate inward (depolarizing) membrane currents, arrows pointing up indicate outward (repolarizing) membrane currents. Multiple subtypes of potassium and calcium currents, with different sensitivities to blocking drugs, have been identified. Chloride currents (dotted arrows) produce both inward and outward membrane currents during the cardiac action potential.

channels again available for excitation. The time between phase 0 and sufficient recovery of sodium channels in phase 3 to permit a new propagated response to external stimulus is the **refractory period.** Changes in refractoriness (determined by either altered recovery from inactivation or altered action potential duration) can be important in the genesis or suppression of certain arrhythmias. Another important effect of less negative resting potential is prolongation of this recovery time, as shown in Figure 14–4 (right panel). The prolongation of recovery time is reflected in an increase in the effective refractory period.

A brief depolarizing stimulus, whether caused by a propagating action potential or by an external electrode arrangement, causes the opening of large numbers of activation gates before a significant number of inactivation gates can close. In contrast, slow reduction (depolarization) of the resting potential, whether brought about by hyperkalemia, sodium pump blockade, or ischemic cell damage, results in depressed sodium currents during the upstrokes of action potentials. Depolarization of the resting potential to levels positive to −55 mV abolishes sodium currents, since all sodium channels are inactivated. However, such severely depolarized cells have been found to support special action potentials under circum-

stances that increase calcium permeability or decrease potassium permeability. These "slow responses"—slow upstroke velocity and slow conduction—depend on a calcium inward current and constitute the normal electrical activity in the sinoatrial and atrioventricular nodes, since these tissues have a normal resting potential in the range of −50 to −70 mV. Slow responses may also be important for certain arrhythmias. Modern techniques of molecular biology and electrophysiology can identify multiple subtypes of calcium and potassium channels. One way in which such subtypes may differ is in sensitivity to drug effects, so drugs targeting specific channel subtypes may be developed in the future.

MECHANISMS OF ARRHYTHMIAS

Many factors can precipitate or exacerbate arrhythmias: ischemia, hypoxia, acidosis or alkalosis, electrolyte abnormalities, excessive catecholamine exposure, autonomic influences, drug toxicity (eg, digitalis or antiarrhythmic drugs), overstretching of cardiac fibers, and the presence of scarred or otherwise diseased tissue. However, all arrhythmias result from (1) disturbances in impulse formation, (2) disturbances in impulse conduction, or (3) both.

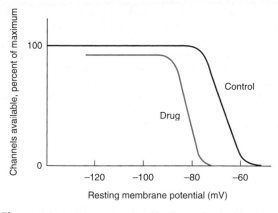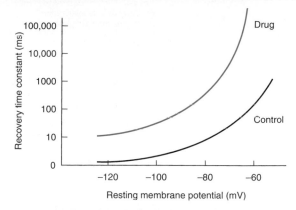

Figure 14–4. Dependence of sodium channel function on the membrane potential preceding the stimulus. **Left:** The fraction of sodium channels available for opening in response to a stimulus is determined by the membrane potential immediately preceding the stimulus. The decrease in the fraction available when the resting potential is depolarized in the absence of a drug (control curve) results from the voltage-dependent closure of *h* gates in the channels. The curve labeled **Drug** illustrates the effect of a typical local anesthetic antiarrhythmic drug. Most sodium channels are inactivated during the plateau of the action potential. **Right:** The time constant for recovery from inactivation after repolarization also depends on the resting potential. In the absence of drug, recovery occurs in less than 10 ms at normal resting potentials (–85 to –95 mV). Depolarized cells recover more slowly (note logarithmic scale). In the presence of a sodium channel-blocking drug, the time constant of recovery is increased, but the increase is far greater at depolarized potentials than at more negative ones.

Disturbances of Impulse Formation

The interval between depolarizations of a pacemaker cell is the sum of the duration of the action potential and the duration of the diastolic interval. Shortening of either duration results in an increase in pacemaker rate. The more important of the two, diastolic interval, is determined primarily by the slope of phase 4 depolarization (pacemaker potential). Vagal discharge and β-receptor-blocking drugs slow normal pacemaker rate by reducing the phase 4 slope (acetylcholine also makes the maximum diastolic potential more negative). Acceleration of pacemaker discharge is often brought about by increased phase 4 depolarization slope, which can be caused by hypokalemia, β-adrenoceptor stimulation, positive chronotropic drugs, fiber stretch, acidosis, and partial depolarization by currents of injury.

Latent pacemakers (cells that show slow phase 4 depolarization even under normal conditions, eg, some Purkinje fibers) are particularly prone to acceleration by the above mechanisms. However, all cardiac cells, including normally quiescent atrial and ventricular cells, may show repetitive pacemaker activity when depolarized under appropriate conditions, especially if hypokalemia is also present.

Afterdepolarizations (Figure 14–5) are depolarizations that interrupt phase 3 (early afterdepolarizations, EADs) or phase 4 (delayed afterdepolarizations, DADs). DADs, discussed in Chapter 13, often occur when intracellular calcium is increased. They are exacerbated by fast heart rates and are thought to be responsible for some arrhythmias related to digitalis excess, to catecholamines, and to myocardial ischemia. EADs, on the other hand, are usually exacerbated at slow heart rates and are thought to contribute to the development of long QT-related arrhythmias (see Box, Molecular & Genetic Bases of Cardiac Arrhythmias).

Disturbances of Impulse Conduction

Severely depressed conduction may result in simple **block,** eg, atrioventricular nodal block or bundle branch block. Because parasympathetic control of atrioventricular conduction is significant, partial atrioventricular block is sometimes relieved by atropine. Another common abnormality of conduction is **reentry** (also known as "circus movement"), in which one impulse reenters and excites areas of the heart more than once (Figure 14–6). The path of the reentering impulse may be confined to very small areas, eg, within or near the atrioventricular node, or it may involve large portions of the atrial or ventricular walls. Some forms of reentry are strictly anatomically determined; for example, in the Wolff-Parkinson-White syndrome, the reentry circuit

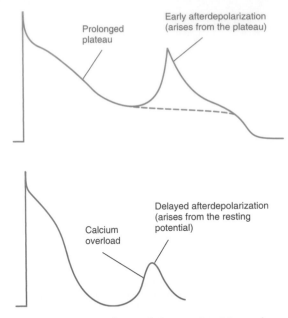

Figure 14–5. Two forms of abnormal activity, early (*top*) and delayed afterdepolarizations (*bottom*). In both cases, abnormal depolarizations arise during or after a normally evoked action potential. They are therefore often referred to as "triggered" automaticity, ie, they require a normal action potential for their initiation.

consists of atrial tissue, the AV node, ventricular tissue, and an accessory atrioventricular connection (a "bypass tract"). In other cases (eg, atrial or ventricular fibrillation), multiple reentry circuits, determined by the properties of the cardiac tissue, may meander through the heart in apparently random paths. Furthermore, the circulating impulse often gives off "daughter impulses" that can spread to the rest of the heart. Depending on how many round trips through the pathway the impulse makes before dying out, the arrhythmia may be manifest as one or a few extra beats or as a sustained tachycardia.

In order for reentry to occur, three conditions must coexist, as indicated in Figure 14–6: (1) There must be an obstacle (anatomic or physiologic) to homogeneous conduction, thus establishing a circuit around which the reentrant wavefront can propagate; (2) there must be unidirectional block at some point in the circuit, ie, conduction must die out in one direction but continue in the opposite direction (as shown in Figure 14–6, the impulse can gradually decrease as it invades progressively more depolarized tissue until it finally blocks—a process known as decremental conduction); and (3) conduction time around the circuit must be long

enough so that the retrograde impulse does not enter refractory tissue as it travels around the obstacle, ie, the conduction time must exceed the effective refractory period. Importantly, reentry depends on conduction that has been depressed by some critical amount, usually as a result of injury or ischemia. If conduction velocity is too slow, bidirectional block rather than unidirectional block occurs; if the reentering impulse is too weak, conduction may fail, or the impulse may arrive so late that it collides with the next regular impulse. On the other hand, if conduction is too rapid, ie, almost normal, bidirectional conduction rather than unidirectional block will occur. Even in the presence of unidirectional block, if the impulse travels around the obstacle too rapidly, it will reach tissue that is still refractory.

Slowing of conduction may be due to depression of sodium current, depression of calcium current (the latter especially in the atrioventricular node), or both. Drugs that abolish reentry usually work by further slowing depressed conduction (by blocking the sodium or calcium current) and causing bidirectional block. In theory, accelerating conduction (by increasing sodium or calcium current) would also be effective, but only under very unusual circumstances does this mechanism explain the action of any available drug.

Lengthening (or shortening) of the refractory period may also make reentry less likely. The longer the refractory period in tissue near the site of block, the greater the chance that the tissue will still be refractory when reentry is attempted. (Alternatively, the shorter the refractory period in the depressed region, the less likely it is that unidirectional block will occur.) Thus, increased dispersion of refractoriness is one contributor to reentry, and drugs may suppress arrhythmias by reducing such dispersion.

I. BASIC PHARMACOLOGY OF THE ANTIARRHYTHMIC AGENTS

Mechanisms of Action

Arrhythmias are caused by abnormal pacemaker activity or abnormal impulse propagation. Thus, the aim of therapy of the arrhythmias is to reduce ectopic pacemaker activity and modify conduction or refractoriness in reentry circuits to disable circus movement. The major mechanisms currently available for accomplishing these goals are (1) sodium channel blockade, (2) blockade of sympathetic autonomic effects in the heart, (3) prolongation of the effective refractory period, and (4) calcium channel blockade.

A. Normal

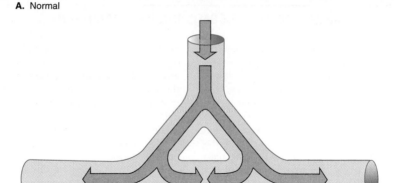

B. Unidirectional block

Block

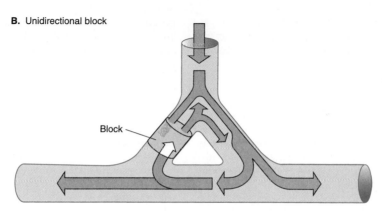

Figure 14–6. Schematic diagram of a reentry circuit that might occur in small bifurcating branches of the Purkinje system where they enter the ventricular wall. **A:** Normally, electrical excitation branches around the circuit, is transmitted to the ventricular branches, and becomes extinguished at the other end of the circuit due to collision of impulses. **B:** An area of unidirectional block develops in one of the branches, preventing anterograde impulse transmission at the site of block, but the retrograde impulse may be propagated through the site of block if the impulse finds excitable tissue, ie, the refractory period is shorter than the conduction time. This impulse will then reexcite tissue it had previously passed through, and a reentry arrhythmia will be established.

Antiarrhythmic drugs decrease the automaticity of ectopic pacemakers more than that of the sinoatrial node. They also reduce conduction and excitability and increase the refractory period to a greater extent in depolarized tissue than in normally polarized tissue. This is accomplished chiefly by selectively blocking the sodium or calcium channels of depolarized cells (Figure 14–8). Therapeutically useful channel-blocking drugs have a high affinity for activated channels (ie, during phase 0) or inactivated channels (ie, during phase 2) but very low affinity for rested channels. Therefore, these drugs block electrical activity when there is a fast tachycardia (many channel activations and inactivations per unit time) or when there is significant loss of resting potential (many inactivated channels during rest). This type of drug action is often described as **use-dependent** or **state-dependent,** ie, channels that are being used frequently, or in an inactivated state, are more susceptible to block. Channels in normal cells that become blocked by a drug during normal activation-inactivation cycles will rapidly lose the drug from the receptors during the resting portion of the cycle (Figure 14–8). Channels in myocardium that is chronically depolarized (ie, has a resting potential more positive than −75 mV) will recover from block very slowly if at all (see also right panel, Figure 14–4).

In cells with abnormal automaticity, most of these drugs reduce the phase 4 slope by blocking either

MOLECULAR & GENETIC BASIS OF CARDIAC ARRHYTHMIAS

During the past decade, molecular biologic, genetic, and biophysical approaches have provided remarkable new insights into the molecular basis of several congenital and acquired cardiac arrhythmias. The best example is the polymorphic ventricular tachycardia known as torsade de pointes (shown in Figure 14–7), which is associated with syncope and sudden death. The electrocardiographic hallmark of both the acquired and congenital syndromes is prolongation of the QT interval, especially at the onset of the tachycardia. As can be inferred from Figure 14–1, this must represent prolongation of the action potential of at least some ventricular cells. This effect can, in theory, be attributed either to increased inward current (gain of function) or decreased outward current (loss of function) during the plateau of the action potential. In fact, recent molecular genetic studies have identified up to 300 different mutations in at least five ion channel genes that produce the congenital long QT (LQT) syndrome (Table 14–1), and each mutation may have different clinical implications. Loss of function mutations in potassium channel genes produce decreases in outward repolarizing current and are responsible for LQT subtypes 1, 2, 5, and 6. *HERG* and *KCNE2* (*MiRP1*) genes encode subunits of the the rapid delayed rectifer potassium curent (I_{Kr}), whereas *KCNQ1* and *KCNE1* (*minK*) encode subunits of the slow delayed rectifier potassium current (I_{Ks}). In contrast, gain of function mutations in the sodium channel gene (*SCN5A*) cause increases in inward plateau current and are responsible for LQT subtype 3.

Molecular genetic studies have identified the reason why congenital and acquired cases of torsades de pointes can be so strikingly similar. The potassium channel gene (*HERG*) that encodes I_{Kr} is blocked or modified by many drugs (eg, quinidine, sotalol) or electrolyte abnormalities (hypokalemia, hypomagnesemia, hypocalcemia) that also produce torsades de pointes. Thus, the identification of the precise molecular mechanisms underlying various forms of the long QT syndromes now raises the possibility that specific therapies may be developed for individuals with defined molecular abnormalities. Indeed, preliminary reports suggest that the sodium channel blocker mexiletine can correct the clinical manifestations of congenital long QT subtype 3 syndrome. In vitro and clinical data demonstrate that most available action potential-prolonging drugs exert greater effects at slow rates (where torsade de pointes is a risk) than at fast rates (where arrhythmia suppression would occur). This "reverse use-dependent" action potential prolongation seems to be absent with amiodarone, which may help explain that drug's apparently greater clinical efficacy with its low rate of torsade de pointes. It is likely that torsade de pointes originates from triggered upstrokes arising from early afterdepolarizations (Figure 14–5). Thus, therapy is directed at correcting hypokalemia, eliminating triggered upstrokes (eg, by using β-blockers or magnesium), or shortening the action potential (eg, by increasing heart rate with isoproterenol or pacing)—or all of these.

The molecular basis of several other congenital cardiac arrhythmias associated with sudden death has also recently been identified. The Brugada syndrome, which is characterized by ventricular fibrillation associated with persistent ST-segment elevation and progressive cardiac conduction disorder (PCCD), characterized by impaired conduction in the His-Purkinje system and right or left bundle block leading to complete atrioventricular block, have both been linked to several loss-of-function mutations in the sodium channel gene, SCN5A. At least one form of familial atrial fibrillation is caused by a gain-of-function mutation in the potassium channel gene, KCNQ1.

---

sodium or calcium channels and thereby reducing the ratio of sodium (or calcium) permeability to potassium permeability. As a result, the membrane potential during phase 4 stabilizes closer to the potassium equilibrium potential. In addition, some agents may increase the threshold (make it more positive). Beta-adrenoceptor-blocking drugs indirectly reduce the phase 4 slope by blocking the positive chronotropic action of norepinephrine in the heart.

In reentry arrhythmias, which depend on critically depressed conduction, most antiarrhythmic agents slow conduction further by one or both of two mechanisms:

(1) steady-state reduction in the number of available unblocked channels, which reduces the excitatory currents to a level below that required for propagation (Figure 14–4, left); and (2) prolongation of recovery time of the channels still able to reach the rested and available state, which increases the effective refractory period (Figure 14–4, right). As a result, early extrasystoles are unable to propagate at all; later impulses propagate more slowly and are subject to bidirectional conduction block.

By these mechanisms, antiarrhythmic drugs can suppress ectopic automaticity and abnormal conduction

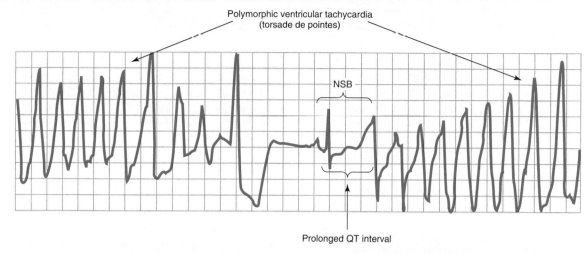

Figure 14–7. Electrocardiogram from a patient with the long QT syndrome during two episodes of torsade de pointes. The polymorphic ventricular tachycardia is seen at the start of this tracing and spontaneously halts at the middle of the panel. A single normal sinus beat (NSB) with an extremely prolonged QT interval follows, succeeded immediately by another episode of ventricular tachycardia of the torsade type. The usual symptoms would be dizziness or transient loss of consciousness.

occurring in depolarized cells—rendering them electrically silent—while minimally affecting the electrical activity in normally polarized parts of the heart. However, as dosage is increased, these agents also depress conduction in normal tissue, eventually resulting in *drug-induced* arrhythmias. Furthermore, a drug concentration that is therapeutic (antiarrhythmic) under the initial circumstances of treatment may become "proar-

Table 14–1. Molecular and genetic basis of some cardiac arrhythmias.

Type	Chromosome Involved	Defective Gene	Ion Channel or Proteins Affected	Result[1]
LQT-1[2]	11	KCNQ1	I_{Ks}	LF
LQT-2	7	HERG	I_{Kr}	LF
LQT-3	3	SCN5A	I_{Na}	GF
LQT-4	4	Ankyrin-B	[3]	LF
LQT-5	21	KCNE1 (minK)	I_{Ks}	LF
LQT-6	21	KCNE2 (MiRP1)	I_{Kr}	LF
Brugada syndrome	3	SCN5A	I_{Na}	LF
PCCD[4]	3	SCN5A	I_{Na}	LF
Familial atrial fibrillation	11	KCNQ1	I_{Ks}	GF

[1]LF, loss of function; GF, gain of function.

[2]LQT, long QT syndrome.

[3]Ankyrins are intracellular proteins that associate with a variety of transport proteins including Na+ channels, Na+/K+ ATPase, Na+/Ca2+ exchange, Ca2+ release channels.

[4]PCCD, progressive cardiac conduction disorder.

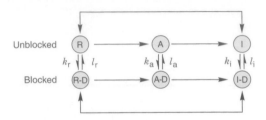

Figure 14–8. Diagram of a mechanism for the selective depressant action of antiarrhythmic drugs on sodium channels. The upper portion of the figure shows the population of channels moving through a cycle of activity during an action potential in the absence of drugs: R (rested) → A (activated) → I (inactivated). Recovery takes place via the I → R pathway. Antiarrhythmic drugs (D) that act by blocking sodium channels can bind to their receptors in the channels, as shown by the vertical arrows, to form drug-channel complexes, indicated as R-D, A-D, and I-D. Affinity of the drugs for the receptor varies with the state of the channel, as indicated by the separate rate constants (*k* and *l*) for the R → R-D, A → A-D, and I → I-D steps. The data available for a variety of sodium channel blockers indicate that the affinity of the drugs for the active and inactivated channel receptor is much higher than the affinity for the rested channel. Furthermore, recovery from the I-D state to the R-D state is much slower than from I to R. As a result, rapid activity (more activations and inactivations) and depolarization of the resting potential (more channels in the I state) will favor blockade of the channels and selectively suppress arrhythmic cells.

rhythmic" (arrhythmogenic) during fast heart rates (more development of block), acidosis (slower recovery from block for most drugs), hyperkalemia, or ischemia.

II. SPECIFIC ANTIARRHYTHMIC AGENTS

The most widely used scheme for the classification of antiarrhythmic drug actions recognizes four classes:

1. Class 1 action is sodium channel blockade. Subclasses of this action reflect effects on the action potential duration (APD) and the kinetics of sodium channel blockade. Drugs with class 1A action prolong the APD and dissociate from the channel with intermediate kinetics; drugs with class 1B action have no significant effects on the APD and dissociate from the channel with rapid kinetics; and drugs with class 1C action have minimal effects on the APD and dissociate from the channel with slow kinetics.

2. Class 2 action is sympatholytic. Drugs with this action reduce β-adrenergic activity in the heart.

3. Class 3 action is manifest by prolongation of the APD. Most drugs with this action block the rapid component of the delayed rectifier potassium current, I_{Kr}.

4. Class 4 action is blockade of the cardiac calcium current. This action slows conduction in regions where the action potential upstroke is calcium dependent, eg, the sinoatrial and atrioventricular nodes.

A given drug may have multiple classes of action. For example, amiodarone shares all four classes of action. Drugs are usually discussed according to the predominant class of action. Certain antiarrhythmic agents, eg, adenosine and magnesium, do not fit readily into this scheme and are described separately.

SODIUM CHANNEL-BLOCKING DRUGS (CLASS 1)

QUINIDINE (SUBGROUP 1A)

Cardiac Effects

Quinidine slows the upstroke of the action potential and conduction, and prolongs the QRS duration of the ECG, by blockade of activated sodium channels. Recovery from block occurs with intermediate kinetics and is slowed further in partially depolarized cells. Sodium channel-blocking concentrations of quinidine also prolong the action potential duration as a result of potassium channel blockade. This action is relatively nonspecific as most types of potassium channels are blocked by therapeutic concentrations of quinidine although the resting potential is not altered. The action potential prolonging action is greatest at slow rates. Its major cardiac effects are excessive QT interval prolongation and induction of torsade de pointes arrhythmia, and syncope. Toxic concentrations of quinidine also produce excessive sodium channel blockade with slowed conduction throughout the heart, increased PR interval, and further QRS duration prolongation.

Quinidine

Table 14–2. Membrane actions of antiarrhythmic drugs.

Drug	Block of Sodium Channels		Refractory Period		Calcium Channel Blockade	Effect on Pacemaker Activity	Sympatholytic Action
	Normal Cells	Depolarized Cells	Normal Cells	Depolarized Cells			
Adenosine	0	0	0	0	0	0	+
Amiodarone	+	+++	↑↑	↑↑	+	↓↓	+
Bretylium	0	0	↑↑↑	↑↑↑	0	↑↓[1]	++
Diltiazem	0	0	0	0	+++	↓↓	0
Disopyramide	+	+++		↑↑	+		0
Dofetilide	0	0	↑	?	0	0	0
Esmolol	0	+	0	NA[2]	0	↓↓	+++
Flecainide	+	+++	0	↑	0	↓↓	0
Ibutilide	0	0	↑	?	0	0	0
Lidocaine	0	+++	↓	↑↑	0	↓↓	0
Mexiletine	0	+++	0	↑↑	0	↓↓	0
Moricizine	+	++	↓	↓	0	↓↓	0
Procainamide	+	+++	↑	↑↑↑	0	↓	+
Propafenone	+	++	↑	↑↑	+	↓↓	+
Propranolol	0	+	↓	↑↑	0	↓↓	+++
Quinidine	+	++	↑	↑↑	0	↓↓	+
Sotalol	0	0	↑↑	↑↑↑	0	↓↓	++
Tocainide	0	+++	0	↑↑	0	↓↓	0
Verapamil	0	+	0	↑	+++	↓↓	+

[1]Bretylium may transiently increase pacemaker rate by causing catecholamine release.

[2]Data not available.

Extracardiac Effects

Gastrointestinal side effects of diarrhea, nausea, and vomiting are observed in one third to half of patients. A syndrome of headache, dizziness, and tinnitus (cinchonism) is observed at toxic drug concentrations. Idiosyncratic reactions including thrombocytopenia, hepatitis, angioneurotic edema, and fever are observed rarely.

Pharmacokinetics

Quinidine is 70–80% bioavailable following oral administration. It is 80% bound to albumin and α_1-acid glycoprotein. It is eliminated primarily by hepatic metabolism. The principal metabolite, 3-hydroxy quinidine is biologically active with half the activity of the parent compound.

Twenty percent of the quinidine dose appears in the unchanged form in the urine. The elimination half-life is 6–8 hours. Quinidine is usually administered in a slow release formulation, eg, that of the gluconate salt.

Therapeutic Use

Quinidine is used for the maintenance of normal sinus rhythm in patients with atrial flutter or fibrillation. It is also used occasionally to treat patients with ventricular tachycardia. Because of its cardiac and extracardiac side effects, its use has decreased considerably in recent years and is now largely restricted to patients with normal (but arrhythmic) hearts. In randomized, controlled clinical trials, quinidine-treated patients are twice as likely

Table 14–3. Clinical pharmacologic properties of antiarrhythmic drugs.

Drug	Effect on SA Nodal Rate	Effect on AV Nodal Refractory Period	PR Interval	QRS Duration	QT Interval	Usefulness in Arrhythmias		Half-Life
						Supra-ventricular	Ventricular	
Adenosine	Little	↑↑↑	↑↑↑	0	0	++++	?	< 10 s
Amiodarone	↓↓[1]	↑↑	↑↑	↑	↑↑↑↑	+++	+++	(weeks)
Bretylium	↑↓[2]	↑↓[2]	0	0	0	0	+	4 h
Diltiazem	↑↓	↑↑	↑	0	0	+++	–	4–8 h
Disopyramide	↑↓[1,3]	↑↓[3]	↑↓[3]	↑↑	↑↑	+	+++	6–8 h
Dofetilide	↓(?)	0	0	0	↑↑	++	None	7 h
Esmolol	↓↓	↑↑	↑↑	0	0	+	+	10 min
Flecainide	None	↑	↑	↑↑↑	0	+[4]	++++	20 h
Ibutilide	↓(?)	0	0	0	↑↑	++	?	6 h
Lidocaine	None[1]	None	0	0	0	None[5]	+++	1–2 h
Mexiletine	None[1]	None	0	0	0	None[6]	+++	12 h
Moricizine	None	None	↑	↑↑	0	None	+++	2–6 h[6]
Procainamide	↓[1]	↑↓[3]	↑↓[3]	↑↑	↑↑	+	+++	3–4 h
Propafenone	0	↑	↑	↑↑↑	0	+	+++	5–7 h
Propranolol	↓↓	↑↑	↑↑	0	0	+	+	8 h
Quinidine	↑↓[1,3]	↑↓[3]	↑↓[3]	↑↑	↑↑	+	+++	6 h
Sotalol	↓↓	↑↑	↑↑	0	↑↑↑	+++	+++	7 h
Tocainide	None[1]	None	0	0	0	None[5]	+++	12 h
Verapamil	↓↓	↑↑	↑↑	0	0	+++	–	7 h

[1]May suppress diseased sinus nodes.
[2]Initial stimulation by release of endogenous norepinephrine followed by depression.
[3]Anticholinergic effect and direct depressant action.
[4]Especially in Wolff-Parkinson-White syndrome.
[5]May be effective in atrial arrhythmias caused by digitalis.
[6]Half-life of active metabolites much longer.

to remain in normal sinus rhythm compared with controls. However, drug treatment was associated with a twofold to threefold increase in mortality.

PROCAINAMIDE (SUBGROUP 1A)

Cardiac Effects

The electrophysiologic effects of procainamide are similar to those of quinidine. The drug may be somewhat less effective in suppressing abnormal ectopic pacemaker activity but more effective in blocking sodium channels in depolarized cells.

Procainamide

Perhaps the most important difference between quinidine and procainamide is the less prominent antimuscarinic action of procainamide. Therefore, the directly depressant actions of procainamide on sinoatrial and atrioventricular nodes are not as effectively counterbalanced by drug-induced vagal block as in the case of quinidine.

Extracardiac Effects

Procainamide has ganglion-blocking properties. This action reduces peripheral vascular resistance and can cause hypotension, particularly with intravenous use. However, in therapeutic concentrations, its peripheral vascular effects are less prominent than those of quinidine. Hypotension is usually associated with excessively rapid procainamide infusion or the presence of severe underlying left ventricular dysfunction.

Toxicity

A. CARDIAC

Procainamide's cardiotoxic effects are similar to those of quinidine. Antimuscarinic and direct depressant effects may occur. New arrhythmias may be precipitated.

B. EXTRACARDIAC

The most troublesome adverse effect of long-term procainamide therapy is a syndrome resembling lupus erythematosus and usually consisting of arthralgia and arthritis. In some patients, pleuritis, pericarditis, or parenchymal pulmonary disease also occurs. Renal lupus is rarely induced by procainamide. During long-term therapy, serologic abnormalities (eg, increased antinuclear antibody titer) occur in nearly all patients, and in the absence of symptoms these are not an indication to stop drug therapy. Approximately one third of patients receiving long-term procainamide therapy develop these reversible lupus-related symptoms.

Other adverse effects include nausea and diarrhea (about 10% of cases), rash, fever, hepatitis (< 5%), and agranulocytosis (approximately 0.2%).

Pharmacokinetics & Dosage

Procainamide can be administered safely by the intravenous and intramuscular routes and is well absorbed orally, with 75% systemic bioavailability. The major metabolite is N-acetylprocainamide (NAPA), which has class III activity. Excessive accumulation of NAPA has been implicated in torsade de pointes during procainamide therapy, especially in patients with renal failure. Some individuals rapidly acetylate procainamide and develop high levels of NAPA. The lupus syndrome appears to be less common in these patients.

Procainamide is eliminated by hepatic metabolism to NAPA and by renal elimination. Its half-life is only 3–4 hours, which necessitates frequent dosing or use of a slow-release formulation (the usual practice). NAPA is eliminated by the kidneys. Thus, procainamide dosage must be reduced in patients with renal failure. The reduced volume of distribution and renal clearance associated with heart failure also require reduction in dosage. The half-life of NAPA is considerably longer than that of procainamide, and it therefore accumulates more slowly. Thus, it is important to measure plasma levels of both procainamide and NAPA, especially in patients with circulatory or renal impairment.

If a rapid procainamide effect is needed, an intravenous loading dose of up to 12 mg/kg can be given at a rate of 0.3 mg/kg/min or less rapidly. This dose is followed by a maintenance dosage of 2–5 mg/min, with careful monitoring of plasma levels. The risk of gastrointestinal or cardiac toxicity rises at plasma concentrations greater than 8 μg/mL or NAPA concentrations greater than 20 μg/mL.

In order to control ventricular arrhythmias, a total procainamide dosage of 2–5 g/d is usually required. In an occasional patient who accumulates high levels of NAPA, less frequent dosing may be possible. This is also possible in renal disease, where procainamide elimination is slowed.

Therapeutic Use

Like quinidine, procainamide is effective against most atrial and ventricular arrhythmias. However, many clinicians attempt to avoid long-term therapy because of the requirement for frequent dosing and the common occurrence of lupus-related effects. Procainamide is the drug of second choice (after lidocaine) in most coronary care units for the treatment of sustained ventricular arrhythmias associated with acute myocardial infarction.

DISOPYRAMIDE (SUBGROUP 1A)

Cardiac Effects

The effects of disopyramide are very similar to those of quinidine. Its cardiac antimuscarinic effects are even more marked than those of quinidine. Therefore, a drug that slows atrioventricular conduction should be administered with disopyramide when treating atrial flutter or fibrillation.

Disopyramide

Toxicity

A. CARDIAC

Toxic concentrations of disopyramide can precipitate all of the electrophysiologic disturbances described under quinidine. As a result of its negative inotropic effect, disopyramide may precipitate heart failure de novo or in patients with preexisting depression of left ventricular function. Because of this effect, disopyramide is not used as a first-line antiarrhythmic agent in the USA. It should not be used in patients with heart failure.

B. EXTRACARDIAC

Disopyramide's atropine-like activity accounts for most of its symptomatic adverse effects: urinary retention (most often, but not exclusively, in male patients with prostatic hyperplasia), dry mouth, blurred vision, constipation, and worsening of preexisting glaucoma. These effects may require discontinuation of the drug.

Pharmacokinetics & Dosage

In the USA, disopyramide is only available for oral use. The usual oral dosage of disopyramide is 150 mg three times a day, but as much as 1 g/d has been used. In patients with renal impairment, dosage must be reduced. Because of the danger of precipitating heart failure, the use of loading doses is not recommended.

Therapeutic Use

Although disopyramide has been shown to be effective in a variety of supraventricular arrhythmias, in the USA it is approved only for the treatment of ventricular arrhythmias.

LIDOCAINE (SUBGROUP 1B)

Lidocaine has a low incidence of toxicity and a high degree of effectiveness in arrhythmias associated with acute myocardial infarction. It is used only by the intravenous route.

Lidocaine

Cardiac Effects

Lidocaine blocks activated and inactivated sodium channels with rapid kinetics (Figure 14–9); the inacti-

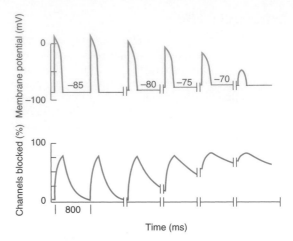

Figure 14–9. Effect of resting membrane potential on the blocking and unblocking of sodium channels by lidocaine. **Upper tracing:** Action potentials in a ventricular muscle cell. **Lower tracing:** Percentage of channels blocked by the drug. As the membrane depolarizes through –80, –75, –70 and –65 mV, an 800 ms time segment is shown. Extra passage of time is indicated by breaks in the traces. **Left side:** At the normal resting potential of –85 mV, the drug combines with open (activated) and inactivated channels during each action potential, but block is rapidly reversed during diastole because the affinity of the drug for its receptor is so low when the channel recovers to the resting state at –85 mV. **Middle:** Metabolic injury has occurred, eg, ischemia due to coronary occlusion, that causes gradual depolarization over time. With subsequent action potentials arising from more depolarized potentials, the fraction of channels blocked increases because more channels remain in the inactivated state at less negative potentials (Figure 14–4, left), and the time constant for unblocking during diastole rapidly increases at less negative resting potentials (Figure 14–4, right). **Right:** Because of marked drug binding, conduction block and loss of excitability in this tissue result, ie, the "sick" (depolarized) tissue is selectively suppressed.

vated state block ensures greater effects on cells with long action potentials such as Purkinje and ventricular cells, compared with atrial cells. The rapid kinetics at normal resting potentials result in recovery from block between action potentials and no effect on conduction. The increased inactivation and slower unbinding kinetics result in the selective depression of conduction in depolarized cells.

Toxicity

A. CARDIAC

Lidocaine is one of the least cardiotoxic of the currently used sodium channel blockers. Proarrhythmic effects, including sinoatrial node arrest, worsening of impaired conduction, and ventricular arrhythmias are uncommon with lidocaine use. In large doses, especially in patients with preexisting heart failure, lidocaine may cause hypotension—partly by depressing myocardial contractility.

B. EXTRACARDIAC

Lidocaine's most common adverse effects—like those of other local anesthetics—are neurologic: paresthesias, tremor, nausea of central origin, lightheadedness, hearing disturbances, slurred speech, and convulsions. These occur most commonly in elderly or otherwise vulnerable patients or when a bolus of the drug is given too rapidly. The effects are dose-related and usually short-lived; seizures respond to intravenous diazepam. In general, if plasma levels above 9 μg/mL are avoided, lidocaine is well tolerated.

Pharmacokinetics & Dosage

Because of its very extensive first-pass hepatic metabolism, only 3% of orally administered lidocaine appears in the plasma. Thus, lidocaine must be given parenterally. Lidocaine has a half-life of 1–2 hours. In adults, a loading dose of 150–200 mg administered over about 15 minutes (as a single infusion or as a series of slow boluses) should be followed by a maintenance infusion of 2–4 mg/min to achieve a therapeutic plasma level of 2–6 μg/mL. Determination of lidocaine plasma levels is of great value in adjusting the infusion rate. Occasional patients with myocardial infarction or other acute illness require (and tolerate) higher concentrations. This may be due to increased plasma α_1-acid glycoprotein, an acute phase reactant protein that binds lidocaine, making less free drug available to exert its pharmacologic effects.

In patients with heart failure, lidocaine's volume of distribution and total body clearance may both be decreased. Thus, both loading and maintenance doses should be decreased. Since these effects counterbalance each other, the half-life may not be increased as much as predicted from clearance changes alone. In patients with liver disease, plasma clearance is markedly reduced and the volume of distribution is often increased; the elimination half-life in such cases may be increased threefold

or more. In liver disease, the maintenance dose should be decreased, but usual loading doses can be given. Elimination half-life determines the time to steady state. Thus, while steady-state concentrations may be achieved in 8–10 hours in normal patients and patients with heart failure, 24–36 hours may be required in those with liver disease. Drugs that decrease liver blood flow (eg, propranolol, cimetidine) reduce lidocaine clearance and so increase the risk of toxicity unless infusion rates are decreased. With infusions lasting more than 24 hours, clearance falls and plasma concentrations rise. Renal disease has no major effect on lidocaine disposition.

Therapeutic Use

Lidocaine is the agent of choice for termination of ventricular tachycardia and prevention of ventricular fibrillation after cardioversion in the setting of acute ischemia. However, routine *prophylactic* use of lidocaine in this setting may actually increase total mortality, possibly by increasing the incidence of asystole and is not the standard of care. Most physicians administer lidocaine only to patients with arrhythmias.

MEXILETINE (SUBGROUP 1B)

Mexiletine is a congener of lidocaine that is resistant to first-pass hepatic metabolism and is effective by the oral route. Its electrophysiologic and antiarrhythmic actions are similar to those of lidocaine. (The anticonvulsant phenytoin [see Chapter 24] also exerts similar electrophysiologic effects and has been used as an antiarrhythmic.) Mexiletine is used in the treatment of ventricular arrhythmias. The elimination half-life is 8–20 hours and permits administration two or three times a day. The usual daily dosage of mexiletine is 600–1200 mg/d. Dose-related adverse effects are seen frequently at therapeutic dosage. These are predominantly neurologic, including tremor, blurred vision, and lethargy. Nausea is also a common effect.

Mexiletine

Mexiletine has also shown significant efficacy in relieving chronic pain, especially pain due to diabetic neuropathy and nerve injury. The usual dosage is 450–750 mg/d orally. This application is unlabeled.

FLECAINIDE (SUBGROUP 1C)

Flecainide is a potent blocker of sodium and potassium channels with slow unblocking kinetics. (Note that although it does block certain potassium channels, it does not prolong the action potential or the QT interval.) It is currently used for patients with otherwise normal hearts who have supraventricular arrhythmias. It has no antimuscarinic effects.

Flecainide

Flecainide is very effective in suppressing premature ventricular contractions. However, it may cause severe exacerbation of arrhythmia even when normal doses are administered to patients with preexisting ventricular tachyarrhythmias and those with a previous myocardial infarction and ventricular ectopy (see Box: The Cardiac Arrhythmia Suppression Trial). The drug is well absorbed and has a half-life of approximately 20 hours. Elimination is both by hepatic metabolism and by the kidney. The usual dosage of flecainide is 100–200 mg twice a day.

PROPAFENONE (SUBGROUP 1C)

Propafenone has some structural similarities to propranolol and possesses weak β-blocking activity. Its spectrum of action is very similar to that of quinidine. Its sodium channel blocking kinetics are similar to that of flecainide. Propafenone is metabolized in the liver, with an average elimination of 5–7 hours except in poor metabolizers (7% of whites), in whom it is as much as 17 hours. The usual daily dosage of propafenone is 450–900 mg in three doses. The drug is used primarily for supraventricular arrhythmias. The most common adverse effects are a metallic taste and constipation; arrhythmia exacerbation can occur.

MORICIZINE (SUBGROUP 1C)

Moricizine is an antiarrhythmic phenothiazine derivative that is used for treatment of ventricular arrhythmias. It is a relatively potent sodium channel blocker that does not prolong action potential duration.

Moricizine has multiple metabolites, some of which are probably active and have long half-lives. Its most common adverse effects are dizziness and nausea. Like other potent sodium channel blockers, it can exacerbate arrhythmias. The usual dosage of moricizine is 200–300 mg by mouth three times a day.

BETA-ADRENOCEPTOR-BLOCKING DRUGS (CLASS 2)

Cardiac Effects

Propranolol and similar drugs have antiarrhythmic properties by virtue of their β-receptor–blocking action and direct membrane effects. As described in Chapter 10, some of these drugs have selectivity for cardiac β_1-receptors; some have intrinsic sympathomimetic activity; some have marked direct membrane effects; and some prolong the cardiac action potential. The relative contributions of the β-blocking and direct membrane effects to the antiarrhythmic effects of these drugs are not fully known. Although β-blockers are fairly well tolerated, their efficacy for suppression of ventricular ectopic depolarizations is lower than that of sodium channel blockers. However, there is good evidence that these agents can prevent recurrent infarction and sudden death in patients recovering from acute myocardial infarction (see Chapter 10).

Esmolol is a short-acting β blocker used primarily as an antiarrhythmic drug for intraoperative and other acute arrhythmias. See Chapter 10 for more information. Sotalol is a nonselective β-blocking drug that prolongs the action potential (class 3 action).

DRUGS THAT PROLONG EFFECTIVE REFRACTORY PERIOD BY PROLONGING ACTION POTENTIAL (CLASS 3)

These drugs prolong action potentials, usually by blocking potassium channels in cardiac muscle or by enhancing inward current, eg, through sodium channels. Action potential prolongation by most of these drugs often exhibits the undesirable property of "reverse use-dependence": action potential prolongation is least marked at fast rates (where it is desirable) and most marked at slow rates, where it can contribute to the risk of torsade de pointes.

AMIODARONE

In the USA, amiodarone is approved for oral and intravenous use to treat serious ventricular arrhythmias. However, the drug is also highly effective for the treat-

---

THE CARDIAC ARRHYTHMIA SUPPRESSION TRIAL

Premature ventricular contractions (PVCs) are commonly recorded in patients convalescing from myocardial infarction. Since such arrhythmias have been associated with an increased risk of sudden cardiac death, it had been the empiric practice of many physicians to treat PVCs, even if asymptomatic, in such patients. In CAST (Cardiac Arrhythmia Suppression Trial [CAST], Echt et al, 1991), an attempt was made to document the efficacy of such therapy in a controlled clinical trial. The effects of several antiarrhythmic drugs on arrhythmia frequency were first evaluated in an open-label fashion. Then, patients in whom antiarrhythmic therapy suppressed PVCs were randomly assigned, in a double-blind fashion, to continue that therapy or its corresponding placebo.

The results showed that mortality among patients treated with the drugs flecainide and encainide (the latter is no longer available) was *increased* more than twofold compared with those treated with placebo. The mechanism underlying this effect is not known, although an interaction between conduction depression by sodium channel block and chronic or acute myocardial ischemia seems likely. Indirect evidence suggests that other sodium channel blockers may produce a similar effect. Whatever the mechanism, the important lesson reinforced by CAST was that the decision to initiate any form of drug therapy (antiarrhythmic or otherwise) should be predicated on the knowledge (or at least a reasonable assumption) that any risk is outweighed by real or potential benefit. Large trials suggest that amiodarone (unlike flecainide) has a slightly beneficial effect on survival of patients with advanced heart disease, while many studies indicate a prominent beneficial effect of β-blockade.

---

ment of supraventricular arrhythmias such as atrial fibrillation. Amiodarone has a broad spectrum of cardiac actions, unusual pharmacokinetics, and important extracardiac side effects.

Amiodarone

Cardiac Effects

Amiodarone markedly prolongs the action potential duration (and the QT interval on the ECG) by blockade of I_{Kr}. During chronic administration, I_{Ks} is also blocked. The action potential duration is prolonged uniformly over a wide range of heart rates, ie, the drug does not have reverse use-dependent action. In spite of its present classification as a class 3 agent, amiodarone also significantly blocks inactivated sodium channels. Its action potential prolonging action reinforces this effect. Amiodarone also has weak adrenergic and calcium channel blocking actions. Consequences of these actions include slowing of the heart rate and atrioventricular node conduction. The broad spectrum of actions may account for its relatively high efficacy and low incidence of torsade de pointes despite significant QT interval prolongation.

Extracardiac Effects

Amiodarone causes peripheral vasodilation. This action is prominent following intravenous administration and may be related to the action of the solvent.

Toxicity

A. CARDIAC

Amiodarone may produce symptomatic bradycardia and heart block in patients with preexisting sinus or atrioventricular node disease.

B. EXTRACARDIAC

Amiodarone accumulates in many tissues, including the heart (10–50 times greater than plasma), lung, liver, and skin, and is concentrated in tears. Dose-related pulmonary toxicity is the most important adverse effect. Even on a low dose of $\leq$ 200 mg/d, fatal pulmonary fibrosis may be observed in 1% of patients. Abnormal liver function tests and hepatitis may develop during amiodarone treatment. The skin deposits result in a photodermatitis and a gray-blue skin discoloration in sun-exposed areas, eg, the malar regions. After a few weeks of treatment, asymptomatic corneal microdeposits are present in virtually all patients treated with amiodarone. Halos develop in the peripheral visual fields of some patients. Drug discontinuation is usually not required. Rarely, an optic neuritis may progress to blindness.

Amiodarone blocks the peripheral conversion of thyroxine (T_4) to triiodothyronine (T_3). It is also a potential source of large amounts of inorganic iodine. Amiodarone may result in hypothyroidism or hyperthyroidism. Thyroid function should be evaluated prior to initiation of treatment and monitored periodically. Because effects have been described in virtually every organ system, amiodarone treatment should be reevaluated whenever new symptoms develop in a patient, including arrhythmia aggravation.

Pharmacokinetics

Amiodarone is variably absorbed with a bioavailability of 35–65%. It undergoes hepatic metabolism, and the major metabolite, desethylamiodarone, is bioactive. The elimination half-life is complex, with a rapid component of 3–10 days (50% of the drug) and a slower component of several weeks. Following discontinuation of the drug, effects are maintained for 1–3 months. Measurable tissue levels may be observed up to 1 year after dosing. A total loading dose of 10 g is usually achieved with 0.8–1.2 g daily doses. The maintenance dose is 200–400 mg daily. Pharmacologic effects may be achieved rapidly by IV loading. QT-prolonging effect is modest with this route of administration, whereas bradycardia and atrioventricular block may be significant.

Amiodarone has many important drug interactions and all medications should be reviewed during drug initiation or dose adjustments. Amiodarone is a substrate for the liver cytochrome metabolizing enzyme CYP3A4 and its levels are increased by drugs that inhibit this enzyme, eg, the histamine H_2 blocker cimetidine. Drugs that induce CYP3A4, eg, rifampin, decrease amiodarone concentration when coadministered. Amiodarone inhibits the other liver cytochrome metabolizing enzymes and may result in high levels of drugs that are substrates for these enzymes eg, digoxin and warfarin.

Therapeutic Use

Low doses (100–200 mg/d) of amiodarone are effective in maintaining normal sinus rhythm in patients with atrial fibrillation. The drug is effective in the prevention of recurrent ventricular tachycardia. Its use is not associated with an increase in mortality in patients with coronary artery disease or heart failure. The implanted cardioverter-defibrillator (ICD) has succeeded drug therapy as the primary treatment modality for ventricular tachycardia, but amiodarone may be used for ventricular tachycardia as adjuvant therapy to decrease the frequency of uncomfortable ICD discharges. The drug increases the pacing and defibrillation threshold and these devices require retesting after a maintenance dose has been achieved.

BRETYLIUM

Bretylium was first introduced as an antihypertensive agent. It interferes with the neuronal release of cate-

cholamines but also has direct antiarrhythmic properties.

Cardiac Effects

Bretylium lengthens the ventricular (but not the atrial) action potential duration and effective refractory period. This effect is most pronounced in ischemic cells, which have shortened action potential durations. Thus, bretylium may reverse the shortening of action potential duration caused by ischemia.

Since bretylium causes an initial release of catecholamines, it has some positive inotropic actions when first administered. This action may also *precipitate* ventricular arrhythmias and must be watched for at the onset of therapy with the drug.

Extracardiac Effects

These result from the drug's sympathoplegic actions. The major adverse effect is postural hypotension. This effect can be almost totally prevented by concomitant administration of a tricyclic antidepressant agent such as protriptyline. Nausea and vomiting may occur after the intravenous administration of a bolus of bretylium.

Pharmacokinetics & Dosage

Bretylium is available only for intravenous use in the USA. In adults, an intravenous bolus of bretylium tosylate, 5 mg/kg, is administered over a 10-minute period. This dosage may be repeated after 30 minutes. Maintenance therapy is achieved by a similar bolus every 4–6 hours or by a constant infusion of 0.5–2 mg/min.

Therapeutic Use

Bretylium is usually used in an emergency setting, often during attempted resuscitation from ventricular fibrillation when lidocaine and cardioversion have failed.

SOTALOL

Sotalol has both β-adrenergic receptor-blocking (class 2) and action potential prolonging (class 3) actions. The drug is formulated as a racemic mixture of d- and l-sotalol. All the beta-adrenergic blocking activity resides in the l-isomer; the d- and l-isomers share action potential prolonging actions. Beta-adrenergic action is noncardioselective and is maximal at doses below those required for action potential prolongation.

$$CH_3SO_2NH - \!\!\!\!\bigcirc\!\!\!\!- \overset{\overset{\displaystyle OH}{|}}{CHCH_2NHCH(CH_3)_2}$$

Sotalol

Sotalol is well absorbed orally with bioavailability of approximately 100%. It is not metabolized in the liver and it is not bound to plasma proteins. Excretion is predominantly by the kidneys in the unchanged form with a half-life of approximately 12 hours. Because of its relatively simple pharmacokinetics, it exhibits few direct drug interactions. Its most significant cardiac adverse effect is an extension of its pharmacologic action: a dose-related incidence of torsade de pointes that approaches 6% at the highest recommended daily dose. Patients with overt heart failure may experience further depression of left ventricular function during treatment with sotalol.

Sotalol is approved for the treatment of life-threatening ventricular arrhythmias and the maintenance of sinus rhythm in patients with atrial fibrillation. It is also approved for treatment of supraventricular and ventricular arrhythmias in the pediatric age group. Sotalol decreases the threshold for cardiac defibrillation.

DOFETILIDE

Dofetilide has class 3 action potential prolonging action. This action is effected by a dose-dependent blockade of the rapid component of the delayed rectifier potassium current, I_{Kr}. Dofetilide block of I_{Kr} increases in hypokalemia. Dofetilide produces no relevant blockade of the other potassium channels or the sodium channel. Because of the slow rate of recovery from blockade, the extent of blockade shows little dependence on stimulation frequency. However, dofetilide does show less action potential prolongation at rapid rates because of the increased importance of other potassium channels such as I_{Ks} at rapid rates.

Dofetilide is 100% bioavailable. Verapamil increases peak plasma dofetilide concentration by increasing intestinal blood flow. Eighty percent of an oral dose is eliminated by the kidneys unchanged; the remainder is eliminated by the kidneys as inactive metabolites. Inhibitors of the renal cation secretion mechanism, eg, cimetidine, prolong the half-life of dofetilide. Since the QT-prolonging effects and risks of ventricular proarrhythmia are directly related to plasma concentration, dofetilide dose must be based on the estimated creatinine clearance. Treatment with dofetilide should be initiated in hospital after baseline measurement of the QT_C and serum electrolytes. A baseline QT_C of > 450 ms (500 ms in the presence of an intraventricular conduction delay), bradycardia of < 50 beats/min, and hypokalemia are relative contraindications to its use.

Dofetilide is approved for the maintenance of normal sinus rhythm in patients with atrial fibrillation. It is also effective in restoring normal sinus rhythm in patients with atrial fibrillation.

IBUTILIDE

Ibutilide slows cardiac repolarization by blockade of the rapid component of the delayed rectifier potassium current. Activation of slow inward sodium current has also been suggested as an additional mechanism of action. After intravenous administration, ibutilide is rapidly cleared from the plasma by hepatic metabolism. The metabolites are excreted by the kidney. The elimination half-life averages 6 hours.

Intravenous ibutilide is used for the acute conversion of atrial flutter and atrial fibrillation to normal sinus rhythm. The drug is more effective in atrial flutter than fibrillation, with a mean time to termination of 20 minutes. The most important adverse effect is excessive QT interval prolongation and torsade de pointes. Patients require continuous ECG monitoring for 4 hours following ibutilide infusion or until QT_C returns to baseline.

CALCIUM CHANNEL-BLOCKING DRUGS (CLASS 4)

These drugs, of which verapamil is the prototype, were first introduced as antianginal agents and are discussed in greater detail in Chapter 12. Verapamil, diltiazem, and bepridil also have antiarrhythmic effects.

VERAPAMIL

Cardiac Effects

Verapamil blocks both activated and inactivated L-type calcium channels. Thus, its effect is more marked in tissues that fire frequently, those that are less completely polarized at rest, and those in which activation depends exclusively on the calcium current, such as the sinoatrial and atrioventricular nodes. Atrioventricular nodal conduction and effective refractory period are invariably prolonged by therapeutic concentrations. Verapamil usually slows the sinoatrial node by its direct action, but its hypotensive action may occasionally result in a small reflex increase of sinoatrial nodal rate.

Verapamil can suppress both early and delayed after-depolarizations and may antagonize slow responses arising in severely depolarized tissue.

Extracardiac Effects

Verapamil causes peripheral vasodilation, which may be beneficial in hypertension and peripheral vasospastic disorders. Its effects upon smooth muscle produce a number of extracardiac effects (see Chapter 12).

Toxicity

A. CARDIAC

Verapamil's cardiotoxic effects are dose-related and usually avoidable. A common error has been to administer intravenous verapamil to a patient with ventricular tachycardia misdiagnosed as supraventricular tachycardia. In this setting, hypotension and ventricular fibrillation can occur. Verapamil's negative inotropic effects may limit its clinical usefulness in diseased hearts (see Chapter 12). Verapamil can lead to atrioventricular block when used in large doses or in patients with atrioventricular nodal disease. This block can be treated with atropine and β-receptor stimulants. In patients with sinus node disease, verapamil can precipitate sinus arrest.

B. EXTRACARDIAC

Adverse effects include constipation, lassitude, nervousness, and peripheral edema.

Pharmacokinetics & Dosage

The half-life of verapamil is approximately 7 hours. It is extensively metabolized by the liver; after oral administration, its bioavailability is only about 20%. Therefore, verapamil must be administered with caution in patients with hepatic dysfunction.

In adult patients without heart failure or sinoatrial or atrioventricular nodal disease, parenteral verapamil can be used to terminate supraventricular tachycardia, although adenosine has become the agent of first choice. Verapamil dosage is an initial bolus of 5 mg administered over 2–5 minutes, followed a few minutes later by a second 5 mg bolus if needed. Thereafter, doses of 5–10 mg can be administered every 4–6 hours, or a constant infusion of 0.4 μg/kg/min may be used.

Effective oral dosages are higher than with intravenous drug because of first-pass metabolism and range from 120 to 640 mg daily, divided into three or four doses.

Therapeutic Use

Supraventricular tachycardia is the major arrhythmia indication for verapamil. Adenosine or verapamil are preferred over older treatments (propranolol, digoxin, edrophonium, vasoconstrictor agents, and cardioversion) for termination. Verapamil can also reduce the ventricular rate in atrial fibrillation and flutter. It only rarely converts atrial flutter and fibrillation to sinus rhythm. Verapamil is occasionally useful in ventricular arrhythmias. However, the use of intravenous verapamil in a patient with sustained ventricular tachycardia can cause hemodynamic collapse.

DILTIAZEM & BEPRIDIL

These agents appear to be similar in efficacy to verapamil in the management of supraventricular arrhythmias, including rate control in atrial fibrillation. An intravenous form of diltiazem is available for the latter indication and causes hypotension or bradyarrhythmias relatively infrequently. Bepridil also has action potential- and QT-prolonging actions that theoretically may make it more useful in some ventricular arrhythmias but also create the risk of torsade de pointes. Bepridil is only rarely used, primarily to control refractory angina.

MISCELLANEOUS ANTIARRHYTHMIC AGENTS

Certain agents used for the treatment of arrhythmias do not fit the conventional class 1–4 organization. These include digitalis (already discussed in Chapter 13), adenosine, magnesium, and potassium.

ADENOSINE

Mechanism & Clinical Use

Adenosine is a nucleoside that occurs naturally throughout the body. Its half-life in the blood is less than 10 seconds. Its mechanism of action involves activation of an inward rectifier K^+ current and inhibition of calcium current. The results of these actions are marked hyperpolarization and suppression of calcium-dependent action potentials. When given as a bolus dose, adenosine directly inhibits atrioventricular nodal conduction and increases the atrioventricular nodal refractory period but has lesser effects on sinoatrial node. Adenosine is currently the drug of choice for prompt conversion of paroxysmal supraventricular tachycardia to sinus rhythm because of its high efficacy (90–95%) and very short duration of action. It is usually given in a bolus dose of 6 mg followed, if necessary, by a dose of 12 mg. An uncommon variant of ventricular tachycardia is adenosine sensitive. It is less effective in the presence of adenosine receptor blockers such as theophylline or caffeine, and its effects are potentiated by adenosine uptake inhibitors such as dipyridamole.

Toxicity

Adenosine causes flushing in about 20% of patients and shortness of breath or chest burning (perhaps related to bronchospasm) in over 10%. Induction of high-grade atrioventricular block may occur but is very short-lived. Atrial fibrillation may occur. Less common toxicities include headache, hypotension, nausea, and paresthesias.

MAGNESIUM

Originally used for patients with digitalis-induced arrhythmias who were hypomagnesemic, magnesium infusion has been found to have antiarrhythmic effects in some patients with normal serum magnesium levels. The mechanisms of these effects are not known, but magnesium is recognized to influence Na^+/K^+ ATPase, sodium channels, certain potassium channels, and calcium channels. Magnesium therapy appears to be indicated in patients with digitalis-induced arrhythmias if hypomagnesemia is present; it is also indicated in some patients with torsade de pointes even if serum magnesium is normal. The usual dosage is 1 g (as sulfate) given intravenously over 20 minutes and repeated once if necessary. A full understanding of the action and indications of magnesium as an antiarrhythmic drug awaits further investigation.

POTASSIUM

The significance of the potassium ion concentrations inside and outside the cardiac cell membrane has been discussed earlier in this chapter. The effects of increasing serum K^+ can be summarized as (1) a resting potential depolarizing action and (2) a membrane potential stabilizing action, caused by increased potassium permeability. Hypokalemia results in an increased risk of early and delayed afterdepolarizations, and ectopic pacemaker activity, especially in the presence of digitalis; hyperkalemia depresses ectopic pacemakers (severe hyperkalemia is required to suppress the sinoatrial node) and slows conduction. Because both insufficient and excess potassium are potentially arrhythmogenic, potassium therapy is directed toward normalizing potassium gradients and pools in the body.

III. PRINCIPLES IN THE CLINICAL USE OF ANTIARRHYTHMIC AGENTS

The margin between efficacy and toxicity is particularly narrow for antiarrhythmic drugs. Therefore, individuals prescribing antiarrhythmic drugs must be thoroughly familiar with the indications, contraindications, risks, and clinical pharmacologic characteristics of each compound they use.

Pretreatment Evaluation

Several important determinations must be made prior to initiation of any antiarrhythmic therapy:

(1) Precipitating factors must be recognized and eliminated if possible. These include not only abnormalities of internal homeostasis, such as hypoxia or electrolyte abnormalities (especially hypokalemia or hypomagnesemia), but also drug therapy and underlying disease states such as hyperthyroidism or underlying cardiac disease. It is important to separate this abnormal substrate from triggering factors, such as

---

THE NONPHARMACOLOGIC THERAPY OF CARDIAC ARRHYTHMIAS

It was recognized at the start of the 20th century that reentry in simple in vitro models (eg, rings of conducting tissues) was permanently interrupted by transecting the reentry circuit. This concept has now been applied to treat clinical arrhythmias that occur as a result of reentry in anatomically delineated pathways. For example, interruption of accessory atrioventricular connections can permanently cure arrhythmias in patients with the Wolff-Parkinson-White syndrome. Such interruption was originally performed at open heart surgery but is now readily accomplished by delivery of radiofrequency energy through an appropriately positioned intracardiac catheter. Since the procedure carries only minimal morbidity, it is being increasingly applied to other reentry arrhythmias with defined pathways, such as atrioventricular nodal reentry, atrial flutter, and some forms of ventricular tachycardia.

Another form of nonpharmacologic therapy is the implantable cardioverter-defibrillator (ICD), a device that can automatically detect and treat potentially fatal arrhythmias such as ventricular fibrillation. ICDs are now widely used in patients who have been resuscitated from such arrhythmias, and several trials have suggested that they should be used in patients with advanced heart disease who have not yet had such arrhythmias but are judged to be at high risk. The increasing use of nonpharmacologic antiarrhythmic therapies reflects both advances in the relevant technologies and an increasing appreciation of the dangers of long-term therapy with currently available drugs.

myocardial ischemia or acute cardiac dilation, which may be treatable and reversible.

(2) A firm arrhythmia diagnosis should be established. For example, the misuse of verapamil in patients with ventricular tachycardia mistakenly diagnosed as supraventricular tachycardia can lead to catastrophic hypotension and cardiac arrest. As increasingly sophisticated methods to characterize underlying arrhythmia mechanisms become available and are validated, it may be possible to direct certain drugs (or other therapies—see Box, The Nonpharmacologic Therapy of Cardiac Arrhythmias) toward specific arrhythmia mechanisms.

(3) It is important to establish a reliable baseline upon which to judge the efficacy of any subsequent antiarrhythmic intervention. A number of methods are now available for such baseline quantitation. These include prolonged ambulatory monitoring, electrophysiologic studies that reproduce a target arrhythmia, reproduction of a target arrhythmia by treadmill exercise, or the use of transtelephonic monitoring for recording of sporadic but symptomatic arrhythmias.

(4) The mere identification of an abnormality of cardiac rhythm does not necessarily require that the arrhythmia be treated. An excellent justification for conservative treatment was provided by the Cardiac Arrhythmia Suppression Trial (CAST) referred to earlier.

Benefits & Risks

The benefits of antiarrhythmic therapy are actually relatively difficult to establish. Two types of benefits can be envisioned: reduction of arrhythmia-related symptoms, such as palpitations, syncope, or cardiac arrest; or reduction in long-term mortality in asymptomatic patients. Among drugs discussed here, only β-blockers have been definitely associated with reduction of mortality in relatively asymptomatic patients, and the mechanism underlying this effect is not established (see Chapter 10).

Antiarrhythmic therapy carries with it a number of risks. In some cases, the risk of an adverse reaction is clearly related to high dosages or plasma concentrations. Examples include lidocaine-induced tremor or quinidine-induced cinchonism. In other cases, adverse reactions are unrelated to high plasma concentrations (eg, procainamide-induced agranulocytosis). For many serious adverse reactions to antiarrhythmic drugs, the *combination* of drug therapy and the underlying heart disease appears important.

Several specific syndromes of arrhythmia provocation by antiarrhythmic drugs have also been identified, each with its underlying pathophysiologic mechanism and risk factors. Drugs such as quinidine, sotalol, ibutilide, and dofetilide, which act—at least in part—by slowing repolarization and prolonging cardiac action potentials, can result in marked QT prolongation and torsade de pointes. Treatment of torsade de pointes requires recognition of the arrhythmia, withdrawal of any offending agent, correction of hypokalemia, and treatment with maneuvers to increase heart rate (pacing or isoproterenol); intravenous magnesium also appears effective, even in patients with normal magnesium levels.

Drugs that markedly slow conduction, such as flecainide, or high concentrations of quinidine, can result in an increased frequency of reentry arrhythmias, notably ventricular tachycardia in patients with prior myocardial infarction in whom a potential reentry circuit may be present. Treatment here consists of recognition, withdrawal of the offending agent, and intravenous sodium. Some patients with this form of arrhythmia aggravation cannot be resuscitated, and deaths have been reported.

Conduct of Antiarrhythmic Therapy

The urgency of the clinical situation determines the route and rate of drug initiation. When immediate drug action is required, the intravenous route is preferred. Therapeutic drug levels can be achieved by administration of multiple intravenous boluses. Drug therapy can be considered effective when the target arrhythmia is suppressed (according to the measure used to quantify at baseline) and toxicities are absent. Conversely, drug therapy should not be considered ineffective unless toxicities occur at a time when arrhythmias are not suppressed. Occasionally, arrhythmias may recur at a time when plasma drug concentrations are relatively high but toxicities have not recurred. Under these conditions, the prescriber must decide whether a judicious increase in dose might suppress the arrhythmia and still leave the patient free of toxicity.

Monitoring plasma drug concentrations can be a useful adjunct to managing antiarrhythmic therapy. Plasma drug concentrations are also important in establishing compliance during long-term therapy as well as in detecting drug interactions that may result in very high concentrations at low drug dosages or very low concentrations at high dosages.

REFERENCES

Antzelevitch C, Shimizu W: Cellular mechanisms underlying the long QT syndrome. Curr Opin Cardiol 2002;17:43.

Bezzina CR, Rook MB, Wilde AA: Cardiac sodium channel and inherited arrhythmia syndromes. Cardiovasc Res 2001;49: 257.

Chen YH et al: KCNQ1 gain-of-function mutation in familial atrial fibrillation. Science 2003;299:251.

PREPARATIONS AVAILABLE

SODIUM CHANNEL BLOCKERS

Disopyramide (generic, Norpace)
Oral: 100, 150 mg capsules
Oral controlled-release (generic, Norpace CR): 100, 150 capsules

Flecainide (Tambocor)
Oral: 50, 100, 150 mg tablets

Lidocaine (generic, Xylocaine)
Parenteral: 100 mg/mL for IM injection; 10, 20 mg/mL for IV injection; 40, 100, 200 mg/mL for IV admixtures; 2, 4, 8 mg/mL premixed IV (5% D/W) solution

Mexiletine (Mexitil)
Oral: 150, 200, 250 mg capsules

Moricizine (Ethmozine)
Oral: 200, 250, 300 mg tablets

Procainamide (generic, Pronestyl, others)
Oral: 250, 375, 500 mg tablets and capsules
Oral sustained-release (generic, Procan-SR): 250, 500, 750, 1000 mg tablets
Parenteral: 100, 500 mg/mL for injection

Propafenone (Rythmol)
Oral: 150, 225, 300 mg tablets

Quinidine sulfate [83% quinidine base] (generic)
Oral: 200, 300 mg tablets
Oral sustained-release (Quinidex Extentabs): 300 mg tablets

Quinidine gluconate [62% quinidine base] (generic)
Oral sustained-release: 324 mg tablets
Parenteral: 80 mg/mL for injection

Quinidine polygalacturonate [60% quinidine base] (Cardioquin)
Oral: 275 mg tablets

β-BLOCKERS LABELED FOR USE AS ANTIARRHYTHMICS

Acebutolol (generic, Sectral)
Oral: 200, 400 mg capsules

Esmolol (Brevibloc)
Parenteral: 10 mg/mL, 250 mg/mL for IV injection

Propranolol (generic, Inderal)
Oral: 10, 20, 40, 60, 80, 90 mg tablets
Oral sustained-release: 60, 80, 120, 160 mg capsules
Oral solution: 4, 8 mg/mL
Parenteral: 1 mg/mL for injection

ACTION POTENTIAL-PROLONGING AGENTS

Amiodarone (Cordarone)
Oral: 200, 400 mg tablets
Parenteral: 150 mg/3 mL for intravenous infusion

Bretylium (generic)
Parenteral: 2, 4, 50 mg/mL for injection

Dofetilide (Tikosyn)
Oral: 125, 250, 500 μg capsules

Ibutilide (Corvert)
Parenteral: 0.1 g/mL solution for IV infusion

Sotalol (generic, Betapace)
Oral: 80, 120, 160, 240 mg capsules

CALCIUM CHANNEL BLOCKERS

Bepridil (Vascor; *not labeled for use in arrhythmias*)
Oral: 200, 300 mg tablets

Diltiazem (generic, Cardizem, Dilacor)
Oral: 30, 60, 90, 120 mg tablets; 60, 90, 120, 180, 240, 300, 340, 420 mg extended- or sustained-release capsules (*not labeled for use in arrhythmias*)
Parenteral: 5 mg/mL for intravenous injection

Verapamil (generic, Calan, Isoptin)
Oral: 40, 80, 120 mg tablets;
Oral sustained-release (Calan SR, Isoptin SR): 100, 120, 180, 240 mg capsules
Parenteral: 5 mg/2 mL for injection

MISCELLANEOUS

Adenosine (Adenocard)
Parenteral: 3 mg/mL for injection

Magnesium sulfate
Parenteral: 125, 500 mg/mL for intravenous infusion

Dumaine R, Antzelevitch C: Molecular mechanisms underlying the long QT syndrome. Curr Opin Cardiol 2002;17:36.

Echt DS et al for the CAST Investigators: Mortality and morbidity in patients receiving encainide, flecainide, or placebo. The Cardiac Arrhythmia Suppression Trial. N Engl J Med 1991; 324:781.

Gollob MH, Seger JJ: Current status of the implantable cardioverter-defibrillator. Chest 2001;119:1210.

Grant AO: Molecular biology of sodium channels and their role in cardiac arrhythmias. Am J Med 2001;110:296.

Hohnloser SH, Woosley RL: Sotalol. N Engl J Med 1994;331:31.

Hondeghem LM: Classification of antiarrhythmic agents and the two laws of pharmacology. Cardiovasc Res 2000;45:57.

Hondeghem LM, Katzung BG: Antiarrhythmic agents: the modulated receptor mechanism of action of sodium and calcium channel-blocking drugs. Annu Rev Pharmacol Toxicol 1984; 24:387.

Hume JR et al: Anion transport in heart. Physiol Rev 2000;80:31.

Keating MT, Sanguinetti MC: Molecular and cellular mechanisms of cardiac arrhythmias. Cell 2001;104:569.

Khan IA: Clinical and therapeutic aspects of congenital and acquired long QT syndrome. Am J Med 2002;112:58.

Members of the Sicilian Gambit: New approaches to antiarrhythmic therapy: emerging therapeutic applications of the cell biology of cardiac arrhythmias. Cardiovasc Res 2001;52:345.

Mohler PJ, Gramolini AO, Bennett V: Ankyrins. J Cell Biol 2002; 115:1565.

Morady F: Radio-frequency ablation as treatment for cardiac arrhythmias. N Engl J Med 1999;340:534.

Murray KT: Ibutilide. Circulation 1998;97:493.

Napolitano C, Priori SG: Genetics of ventricular tachycardia. Curr Opin Cardiol 2002;17:222.

Nattel S: New ideas about atrial fibrillation 50 years on. Nature 2002;415:219.

Roberts R, Brugada R: Genetic aspects of arrhythmias. Am J Med Genet 2000;97:310.

Roden DM: Pharmacogenetics and drug-induced arrhythmias. Cardiovasc Res 2001;50:224.

Splawski I et al: Spectrum of mutations in long-QT syndrome genes. KVLQT1, HERG, SCN5A, KCNE1, and KCNE2. Circulation 2000;102:1178.

Splawski I et al: Variant of SCN5A sodium channel implicated in risk of cardiac arrhythmia. Science 2002;297:1333.

Srivatsa U, Wadhani N, Singh AB: Mechanisms of antiarrhythmic drug actions and their clinical relevance for controlling disorders of cardiac rhythm. Curr Cardiol Rep 2002;4:401.

Towbin JA: Molecular genetic basis of sudden cardiac death. Cardiovasc Pathol 2001;10:283.

Tristani-Firouzi M et al: Molecular biology of K(+) channels and their role in cardiac arrhythmias. Am J Med 2001;110:50.

Woosley RL: Cardiac actions of antihistamines. Annu Rev Pharmacol Toxicol 1996;36:233.

Diuretic Agents

15

Harlan E. Ives, MD, PhD

Abnormalities in fluid volume and electrolyte composition are common and important clinical problems. Drugs that block the transport functions of the renal tubules are valuable clinical tools in the treatment of these disorders. Although various agents that increase urine flow have been described since antiquity, it was not until 1957 that a practical and powerful diuretic agent (chlorothiazide) became available for widespread use. Technically, the term "diuresis" signifies an increase in urine volume, while "natriuresis" denotes an increase in renal sodium excretion. Because natriuretic drugs almost always also increase water excretion, they are usually called diuretics.

Many diuretic agents (loop diuretics, thiazides, amiloride, and triamterene) exert their effects on specific membrane transport proteins in renal tubular epithelial cells. Other diuretics exert osmotic effects that prevent water reabsorption (mannitol), inhibit enzymes (acetazolamide), or interfere with hormone receptors in renal epithelial cells (spironolactone).

Most diuretics act upon a single anatomic segment of the nephron (Figure 15–1). Because these segments have distinctive transport functions, the first section of this chapter is devoted to a review of those features of renal tubule physiology that are relevant to diuretic action. The second section is devoted to the basic pharmacology of diuretics, and the third section discusses the clinical applications of these drugs.

I. RENAL TUBULE TRANSPORT MECHANISMS

PROXIMAL TUBULE

Sodium bicarbonate, sodium chloride, glucose, amino acids, and other organic solutes are reabsorbed via specific transport systems in the early proximal tubule. Water is reabsorbed passively so as to maintain nearly constant osmolality of proximal tubular fluid. As tubule fluid is processed along the length of the proximal tubule, the luminal concentrations of the solutes decrease relative to the concentration of inulin, an experimental marker that is neither secreted nor absorbed by renal tubules (Figure 15–2). Approximately 85% of the filtered sodium bicarbonate, 40% of the sodium chloride, 60% of the water, and virtually all of the filtered organic solutes are reabsorbed in the proximal tubule.

Of the various solutes reabsorbed in the proximal tubule, the most relevant to diuretic action are sodium bicarbonate and sodium chloride. Of the currently available diuretics, only one group (carbonic anhydrase inhibitors, which block $NaHCO_3$ reabsorption) acts predominantly in the proximal tubule. In view of the large quantity of sodium chloride absorbed in the proximal tubule, a drug that specifically blocked reabsorption of this salt at this site might be a particularly powerful diuretic agent. No such drug is currently available.

Sodium bicarbonate reabsorption by the proximal tubule is initiated by the action of a Na^+/H^+ exchanger located in the luminal membrane of the proximal tubule epithelial cell (Figure 15–3). This transport system allows sodium to enter the cell from the tubular lumen in exchange for a proton from inside the cell. As in all portions of the nephron, Na^+/K^+ ATPase in the basolateral membrane pumps the reabsorbed Na^+ into the interstitium so as to maintain the normal intracellular concentration of this ion. Protons secreted into the lumen combine with bicarbonate to form carbonic acid, H_2CO_3. Carbonic acid is rapidly dehydrated to CO_2 and H_2O by carbonic anhydrase. CO_2 produced by dehydration of H_2CO_3 enters the proximal tubule cell by simple diffusion where it is then rehydrated back to H_2CO_3. After dissociation of H_2CO_3, the H^+ is available for transport by the Na^+/H^+ exchanger, and the bicarbonate is transported out of the cell by a basolateral membrane transporter (Figure 15–3). Bicarbonate reabsorption by the proximal tubule is thus dependent on carbonic anhydrase. This enzyme can be inhibited by acetazolamide and related agents.

In the late proximal tubule, as bicarbonate and organic solutes have been largely removed from the tubular fluid, the residual luminal fluid contains predominantly NaCl. Under these conditions, Na^+ reabsorption continues, but the protons secreted by the

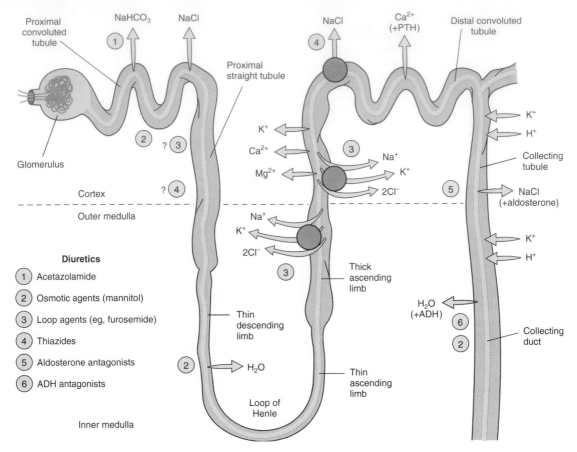

Figure 15–1. Tubule transport systems and sites of action of diuretics.

Na^+/H^+ exchanger can no longer bind to bicarbonate. Free H^+ causes luminal pH to fall, activating a still poorly defined Cl^-/base exchanger (Figure 15–3). The net effect of parallel Na^+/H^+ exchange and Cl^-/base exchange is NaCl reabsorption. As yet, there are no diuretic agents that are known to act on this conjoint process.

Because of the high water permeability of the proximal tubule, water is reabsorbed in direct proportion to salt reabsorption in this segment. Thus, luminal fluid osmolality and sodium concentration remain nearly constant along the length of the proximal tubule (Figure 15–2). An experimental impermeant solute like inulin will rise in concentration as water is reabsorbed (Figure 15–2). If large amounts of an impermeant solute such as mannitol are present in the tubular fluid, water reabsorption will cause the concentration of the solute to rise to a point at which further water reabsorption is prevented. This is the mechanism by which osmotic diuretics act (see below).

Organic acid secretory systems are located in the middle third of the proximal tubule (S_2 segment). These systems secrete a variety of organic acids (uric acid, non-steroidal anti-inflammatory drugs NSAIDs, diuretics, antibiotics, etc) into the luminal fluid from the blood. These systems thus help deliver diuretics to the luminal side of the tubule, where most of them act. Organic base secretory systems (creatinine, choline, etc) are also present, in the early (S_1) and middle (S_2) segments of the proximal tubule.

LOOP OF HENLE

At the boundary between the inner and outer stripes of the outer medulla, the thin limb of Henle's loop begins. Water is extracted from the thin descending limb of the loop of Henle by osmotic forces created in the hypertonic medullary interstitium. As in the proximal tubule, impermeant luminal solutes such as mannitol oppose water extraction.

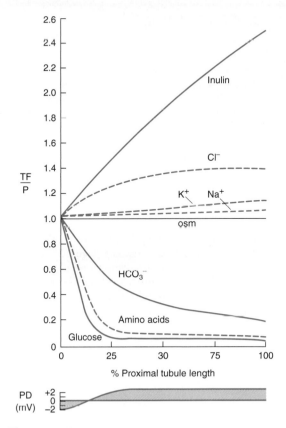

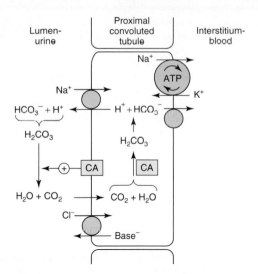

Figure 15–3. Apical membrane Na+/H+ exchange and bicarbonate reabsorption in the proximal convoluted tubule cell. Na+/K+ ATPase is present in the basolateral membrane to maintain intracellular sodium and potassium levels within the normal range. Because of rapid equilibration, concentrations of the solutes shown are approximately equal in the interstitial fluid and the blood. Carbonic anhydrase (CA) is found in other locations in addition to the brush border of the luminal membrane.

Figure 15–2. Reabsorption of various solutes in the proximal tubule in relation to tubule length. (TF/P, tubular fluid to plasma concentration ratio; PD, potential difference across the tubule.) (Reproduced, with permission, from Ganong WF: *Review of Medical Physiology*, 17th ed. Lange, 1993.)

The thick ascending limb of the loop of Henle actively reabsorbs NaCl from the lumen (about 35% of the filtered sodium), but unlike the proximal tubule and the thin limb, it is nearly impermeable to water. Salt reabsorption in the thick ascending limb therefore dilutes the tubular fluid, leading to its designation as a "diluting segment." Medullary portions of the thick ascending limb contribute to medullary hypertonicity and thereby also play an important role in concentration of urine.

The NaCl transport system in the luminal membrane of the thick ascending limb is a Na+/K+/2Cl− cotransporter (Figure 15–4). This transporter is selectively blocked by diuretic agents known as "loop" diuretics (see below). Although the Na+/K+/2Cl− transporter is itself electrically neutral (two cations and two

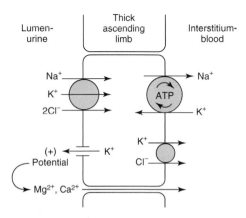

Figure 15–4. Ion transport pathways across the luminal and basolateral membranes of the thick ascending limb cell. The lumen positive electrical potential created by K+ back diffusion drives divalent cation reabsorption via the paracellular pathway.

anions are cotransported), the action of the transporter contributes to excess K^+ accumulation within the cell. This results in back diffusion of K^+ into the tubular lumen and development of a lumen-positive electrical potential. This electrical potential provides the driving force for reabsorption of cations—including Mg^{2+} and Ca^{2+}—via the paracellular pathway (between the cells). Thus, inhibition of salt transport in the thick ascending limb by loop diuretics causes an increase in urinary excretion of divalent cations in addition to NaCl.

DISTAL CONVOLUTED TUBULE

Only about 10% of the filtered NaCl is reabsorbed in the distal convoluted tubule. Like the thick ascending limb, this segment is relatively impermeable to water, and the NaCl reabsorption therefore further dilutes the tubular fluid. The mechanism of NaCl transport in the distal convoluted tubule is electrically neutral Na^+ and Cl^- cotransport (Figure 15–5). This NaCl transporter is blocked by diuretics of the thiazide class.

Because K^+ does not recycle across the apical membrane of the distal convoluted tubule as it does in the loop of Henle, there is no lumen-positive potential in this segment, and Ca^{2+} and Mg^{2+} are not driven out of the tubular lumen by electrical forces. However, Ca^{2+} is actively reabsorbed by the distal convoluted tubule epithelial cell via an apical Ca^{2+} channel and basolateral Na^+/Ca^{2+} exchanger (Figure 15–5). This process is regulated by parathyroid hormone. As will be seen below, the differences in the mechanism of Ca^{2+} transport in the distal convoluted tubule and in the loop of Henle have important implications for the effects of various diuretics on Ca^{2+} transport.

COLLECTING TUBULE

The collecting tubule is responsible for only 2–5% of NaCl reabsorption by the kidney. Despite this small contribution, the collecting tubule plays an important role in renal physiology and in diuretic action. As the final site of NaCl reabsorption, the collecting tubule is responsible for volume regulation and for determining the final Na^+ concentration of the urine. Furthermore, the collecting tubule is a site at which mineralocorticoids exert a significant influence. Lastly, the collecting tubule is the major site of potassium secretion by the kidney and the site at which virtually all diuretic-induced changes in potassium balance occur.

The mechanism of NaCl reabsorption in the collecting tubule is distinct from the mechanisms found in other tubule segments. The **principal cells** are the major sites of Na^+, K^+, and H_2O transport (Figure 15–6), and the **intercalated cells** are the primary sites of proton secretion. Unlike cells in other nephron segments, the principal cells do not contain cotransport systems for Na^+ and other ions in their apical membranes. Rather, principal cell membranes exhibit separate ion channels for Na^+ and K^+. Since these channels exclude anions,

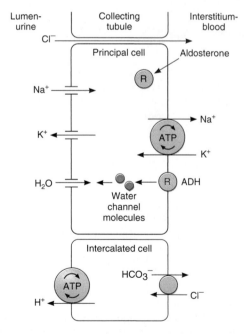

Figure 15–6. Ion and H_2O transport pathways across the luminal and basolateral membranes of collecting tubule and collecting duct cells. Inward diffusion of Na^+ leaves a lumen-negative potential, which drives reabsorption of Cl^- and efflux of K^+. (R, aldosterone or ADH receptor.)

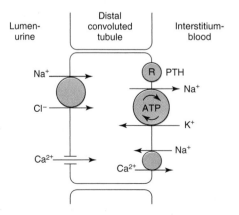

Figure 15–5. Ion transport pathways across the luminal and basolateral membranes of the distal convoluted tubule cell. As in all tubular cells, Na^+/K^+ ATPase is present in the basolateral membrane. (R, PTH receptor.)

transport of Na^+ or K^+ leads to a net movement of charge across the membrane. Because the driving force for Na^+ entry into the principal cell greatly exceeds that for K^+ exit, Na^+ reabsorption predominates, and a 10–50 mV lumen-negative electrical potential develops. Na^+ that enters the principal cell from the urine is then transported back to the blood via the basolateral Na^+/K^+ ATPase (Figure 15–6). The lumen-negative electrical potential drives the transport of Cl^- back to the blood via the paracellular pathway and also pulls K^+ out of the cell through the apical membrane K^+ channel. Thus, there is an important relationship between Na^+ delivery to the collecting tubule and the resulting secretion of K^+. Diuretics that act upstream of the collecting tubule will increase Na^+ delivery to this site and will enhance K^+ secretion. If the Na^+ is delivered with an anion which cannot be reabsorbed as readily as Cl^- (eg, bicarbonate), the lumen-negative potential is increased, and K^+ secretion will be enhanced. This mechanism, combined with enhanced aldosterone secretion due to volume depletion, is the basis for most diuretic-induced K^+ wasting.

Reabsorption of Na^+ via the epithelial Na channel (ENaC) and its coupled secretion of K^+ is regulated by aldosterone. This steroid hormone, through its actions on gene transcription, increases the activity of both apical membrane channels and the basolateral N^+/K^+ ATPase. This leads to an increase in the transepithelial electrical potential and a dramatic increase in both Na^+ reabsorption and K^+ secretion.

A key determinant of the final urine concentration is antidiuretic hormone (ADH; also called vasopressin). In the absence of ADH, the collecting tubule (and duct) is impermeable to water, and dilute urine is produced. However, membrane water permeability of principal cells can be increased by ADH-induced fusion of vesicles containing preformed water channels with the apical membranes (Figure 15–6). ADH secretion is regulated by serum osmolality and by volume status.

II. BASIC PHARMACOLOGY OF DIURETIC AGENTS

CARBONIC ANHYDRASE INHIBITORS

Carbonic anhydrase is present in many nephron sites, but the predominant location of this enzyme is the luminal membrane of the proximal tubule cells (Figure 15–3), where it catalyzes the dehydration of H_2CO_3, a critical step in the reabsorption of bicarbonate. By blocking carbonic anhydrase, inhibitors block sodium bicarbonate reabsorption and cause diuresis.

The carbonic anhydrase inhibitors were the forerunners of modern diuretics. They are unsubstituted sulfonamide derivatives and were discovered when it was found that bacteriostatic sulfonamides caused an alkaline diuresis and hyperchloremic metabolic acidosis. With the development of newer agents, carbonic anhydrase inhibitors are now rarely used as diuretics, but they still have several specific applications that are discussed below. The prototypical carbonic anhydrase inhibitor is **acetazolamide**.

Pharmacokinetics

The carbonic anhydrase inhibitors are well absorbed after oral administration. An increase in urine pH from the bicarbonate diuresis is apparent within 30 minutes, maximal at 2 hours, and persists for 12 hours after a single dose. Excretion of the drug is by secretion in the proximal tubule S_2 segment. Therefore, dosing must be reduced in renal insufficiency.

Pharmacodynamics

Inhibition of carbonic anhydrase activity profoundly depresses bicarbonate reabsorption in the proximal tubule. At its maximal safely administered dosage, 85% of the bicarbonate reabsorptive capacity of the superficial proximal tubule is inhibited. Some bicarbonate can still be absorbed at other nephron sites by carbonic anhydrase–independent mechanisms, and the overall effect of maximal acetazolamide dosage is about 45% inhibition of whole kidney bicarbonate reabsorption. Nevertheless, carbonic anhydrase inhibition causes significant bicarbonate losses and hyperchloremic metabolic acidosis. Because of this and the fact that HCO_3^- depletion leads to enhanced NaCl reabsorption by the remainder of the nephron, the diuretic efficacy of acetazolamide decreases significantly with use over several days.

The major clinical applications of acetazolamide involve carbonic anhydrase–dependent bicarbonate transport at sites other than the kidney. The ciliary body of the eye secretes bicarbonate from the blood into the aqueous humor. Likewise, formation of cerebrospinal fluid by the choroid plexus involves bicarbonate secretion into the cerebrospinal fluid. Although these processes remove bicarbonate from the blood (the direction opposite to that in the proximal tubule), they are significantly inhibited by carbonic anhydrase inhibitors, which in both cases dramatically alter the pH and quantity of fluid produced.

Clinical Indications & Dosage (Table 15–1)

A. GLAUCOMA

The reduction of aqueous humor formation by carbonic anhydrase inhibitors decreases the intraocular pressure. This effect is valuable in the management of severe

Table 15–1. Carbonic anhydrase inhibitors used orally in treatment of glaucoma.

Drug	Usual Oral Dose (1–4 Times Daily)
Acetazolamide	250 mg
Dichlorphenamide	50 mg
Methazolamide	50 mg

forms of glaucoma, making it the most common indication for use of carbonic anhydrase inhibitors. Topically active carbonic anhydrase inhibitors (dorzolamide, brinzolamide) are also available. These topical compounds reduce intraocular pressure, but plasma levels are undetectable. Thus, diuretic and systemic metabolic effects are eliminated.

B. URINARY ALKALINIZATION

Uric acid, cystine, and some other weak acids are relatively insoluble in, and easily reabsorbed from, acidic urine. Renal excretion of these compounds can be enhanced by increasing urinary pH with carbonic anhydrase inhibitors. In the absence of continuous bicarbonate administration, these effects of acetazolamide are of relatively short duration (2–3 days). Prolonged therapy requires bicarbonate administration.

C. METABOLIC ALKALOSIS

Metabolic alkalosis is generally treated by correction of abnormalities in total body K^+, intravascular volume, or mineralocorticoid levels.

However, when the alkalosis is due to excessive use of diuretics in patients with severe heart failure, saline administration may be contraindicated. In these cases, acetazolamide can be useful in correcting the alkalosis as well as producing a small additional diuresis for the correction of heart failure. Acetazolamide has also been used to rapidly correct the metabolic alkalosis that may develop in the setting of respiratory acidosis.

D. ACUTE MOUNTAIN SICKNESS

Weakness, dizziness, insomnia, headache, and nausea can occur in mountain travelers who rapidly ascend above 3000 m. The symptoms are usually mild and last for a few days. In more serious cases, rapidly progressing pulmonary or cerebral edema can be life-threatening. By decreasing cerebrospinal fluid formation and by decreasing the pH of the cerebrospinal fluid and brain, acetazolamide can enhance performance status and diminish symptoms of mountain sickness.

E. OTHER USES

Carbonic anhydrase inhibitors have been used as adjuvants for the treatment of epilepsy, in some forms of hypokalemic periodic paralysis, and to increase urinary phosphate excretion during severe hyperphosphatemia.

Toxicity

A. HYPERCHLOREMIC METABOLIC ACIDOSIS

Acidosis predictably results from chronic reduction of body bicarbonate stores by carbonic anhydrase inhibitors and limits the diuretic efficacy of these drugs to 2 or 3 days.

B. RENAL STONES

Phosphaturia and hypercalciuria occur during the bicarbonaturic response to inhibitors of carbonic anhydrase. Renal excretion of solubilizing factors (eg, citrate) may also decline with chronic use. Calcium salts are relatively insoluble at alkaline pH, which means that the potential for renal stone formation from these salts is enhanced.

C. RENAL POTASSIUM WASTING

Potassium wasting can occur because $NaHCO_3$ presented to the collecting tubule increases the lumen-negative electrical potential in that segment and enhances K^+ secretion. This effect can be counteracted by simultaneous administration of KCl.

D. OTHER TOXICITIES

Drowsiness and paresthesias are common following large doses. Carbonic anhydrase inhibitors may accumulate in patients with renal failure, leading to nervous system toxicity. Hypersensitivity reactions (fever, rashes, bone marrow suppression, and interstitial nephritis) may also occur.

Contraindications

Carbonic anhydrase inhibitor-induced alkalinization of the urine will decrease urinary excretion of NH_4^+ and may contribute to the development of hyperammonemia and hepatic encephalopathy in patients with cirrhosis.

LOOP DIURETICS

Loop diuretics selectively inhibit NaCl reabsorption in the thick ascending limb of the loop of Henle. Due to the large NaCl absorptive capacity of this segment and the fact that diuresis is not limited by development of acidosis, as it is with the carbonic anhydrase inhibitors, these drugs are the most efficacious diuretic agents available.

Chemistry

The two prototypical drugs of this group are **furosemide** and **ethacrynic acid.** The structures of several loop diuretics are shown in Figure 15–7. Like the carbonic anhydrase inhibitors, furosemide, bumetanide, and torsemide are sulfonamide derivatives.

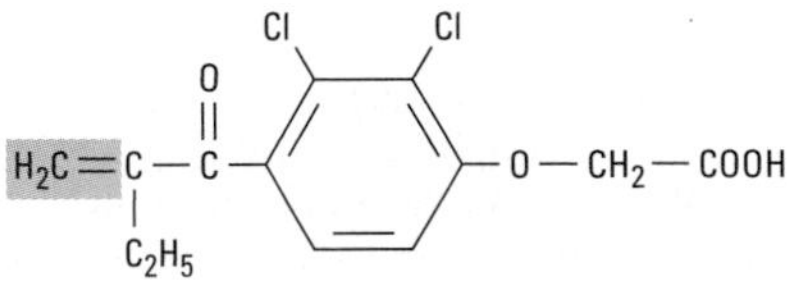

Ethacrynic acid—not a sulfonamide derivative—is a phenoxyacetic acid derivative containing an adjacent ketone and methylene group (Figure 15–7). The methylene group (shaded) forms an adduct with the free sulfhydryl group of cysteine. The cysteine adduct appears to be an active form of the drug.

Organic **mercurial diuretics** also inhibit salt transport in the thick ascending limb but are no longer used because of their high toxicity.

Pharmacokinetics

The loop diuretics are rapidly absorbed. They are eliminated by tubular secretion as well as by glomerular filtration. Absorption of oral torsemide is more rapid (1 hour) than that of furosemide (2–3 hours) and is nearly as complete as with intravenous administration. Diuretic response is extremely rapid following intravenous injection. The duration of effect for furosemide is usually 2–3

Figure 15–7. Some loop diuretics. The shaded methylene group on ethacrynic acid is reactive and may combine with free sulfhydryl groups.

hours and that of torsemide is 4–6 hours. Half-life depends on renal function. Since loop agents act on the luminal side of the tubule, their diuretic activity correlates with their secretion by the proximal tubule. Reduction in the secretion of loop diuretics may result from simultaneous administration of agents such as NSAIDs or probenecid, which compete for weak acid secretion in the proximal tubule. Metabolites of ethacrynic acid and furosemide have been identified, but it is not known if they have any diuretic activity. Torsemide has at least one active metabolite with a half-life considerably longer than that of the parent compound.

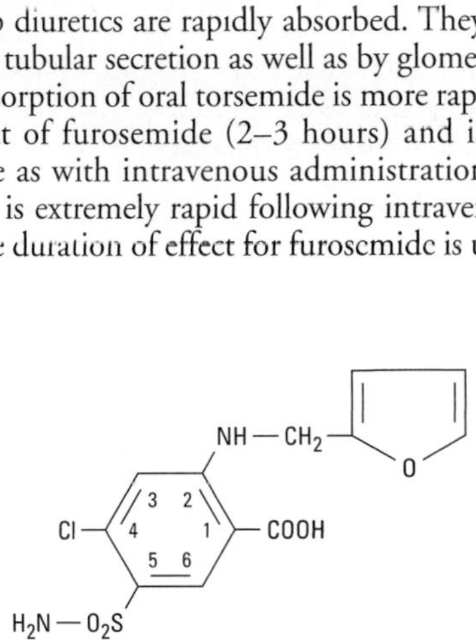

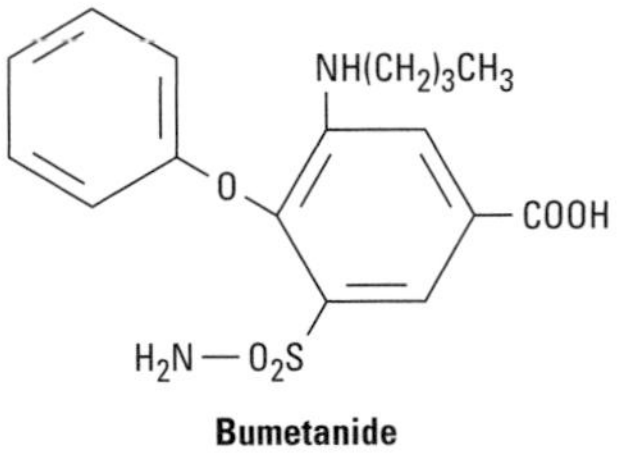

Pharmacodynamics

These drugs inhibit the luminal $Na^+/K^+/2Cl^-$ transporter in the thick ascending limb of Henle's loop. By inhibiting this transporter, the loop diuretics reduce the reabsorption of NaCl and also diminish the lumen-positive potential that derives from K^+ recycling (Figure 15–4). This electrical potential normally drives divalent cation reabsorption in the loop, and by reducing this potential, loop diuretics cause an increase in Mg^{2+} and Ca^{2+} excretion. Prolonged use can cause significant hypomagnesemia in some patients. Since Ca^{2+} is actively reabsorbed in the distal convoluted tubule, loop diuretics do not generally cause hypocalcemia. However, in disorders that cause hypercalcemia, Ca^{2+} excretion can be greatly enhanced by combining loop agents with saline infusions.

Loop diuretics induce renal prostaglandin synthesis, and these prostaglandins participate in the renal actions of these drugs. NSAIDs (eg, indomethacin) can interfere with the actions of the loop diuretics by reducing prostaglandin synthesis in the kidney. This interference is minimal in otherwise normal subjects but may be significant in patients with nephrotic syndrome or hepatic cirrhosis.

In addition to their diuretic activity, loop agents appear to have direct effects on blood flow through several vascular beds. Furosemide increases renal blood flow. Furosemide and ethacrynic acid have also been shown to reduce pulmonary congestion and left ventricular filling pressures in heart failure before a measurable increase in urinary output occurs, and in anephric patients.

Clinical Indications & Dosage (Table 15–2)

The most important indications for the use of the loop diuretics include acute pulmonary edema, other edematous conditions, and acute hypercalcemia. The use of loop diuretics in these conditions is discussed in Section III, Clinical Pharmacology. Other indications for loop diuretics include hyperkalemia, acute renal failure, and anion disease.

Table 15–2. Loop diuretics: Dosages.

Drug	Daily Oral Dose[1]
Bumetanide	0.5–2 mg
Ethacrynic acid	50–200 mg
Furosemide	20–80 mg
Torsemide	2.5–20 mg

[1]As single dose or in two divided doses.

A. HYPERKALEMIA

In mild hyperkalemia—or after acute management of severe hyperkalemia by other measures—loop diuretics can significantly enhance urinary excretion of K^+. This response is enhanced by simultaneous NaCl and water administration.

B. ACUTE RENAL FAILURE

Loop agents can increase the rate of urine flow and enhance K^+ excretion in acute renal failure. However, they do not seem to shorten the duration of renal failure. If a large pigment load has precipitated acute renal failure or threatens to do so, loop agents may help flush out intratubular casts and ameliorate intratubular obstruction. On the other hand, loop agents can theoretically worsen cast formation in myeloma and light chain nephropathy.

C. ANION OVERDOSE

Loop diuretics are useful in treating toxic ingestions of bromide, fluoride, and iodide, which are reabsorbed in the thick ascending limb. Saline solution must be administered to replace urinary losses of Na^+ and to provide Cl^-, so as to avoid extracellular fluid volume depletion.

Toxicity

A. HYPOKALEMIC METABOLIC ALKALOSIS

Loop diuretics increase delivery of salt and water to the collecting duct and thus enhance the renal secretion of K^+ and H^+, causing hypokalemic metabolic alkalosis. This toxicity is a function of the magnitude of the diuretic effect and can be reversed by K^+ replacement and correction of hypovolemia.

B. OTOTOXICITY

Loop diuretics can cause dose-related hearing loss that is usually reversible. It is most common in patients who have diminished renal function or who are also receiving other ototoxic agents such as aminoglycoside antibiotics.

C. HYPERURICEMIA

Loop diuretics can cause hyperuricemia and precipitate attacks of gout. This is caused by hypovolemia-associated enhancement of uric acid reabsorption in the proximal tubule. It may be avoided by using lower doses.

D. HYPOMAGNESEMIA

Magnesium depletion is a predictable consequence of the chronic use of loop agents and occurs most often in patients with dietary magnesium deficiency. It can be reversed by administration of oral magnesium preparations.

E. ALLERGIC REACTIONS

Skin rash, eosinophilia and, less often, interstitial nephritis are occasional side effects of furosemide, bumetanide, and torsemide therapy. These usually resolve rapidly after drug withdrawal. Allergic reactions are much less common with ethacrynic acid.

F. OTHER TOXICITIES

Even more than other diuretics, loop agents can cause severe dehydration. Hyponatremia is less common than with the thiazides (see below), but patients who increase water intake in response to hypovolemia-induced thirst can become severely hyponatremic with loop agents. Loop agents are known for their calciuric effect, but hypercalcemia can occur in patients who have another—previously occult—cause for hypercalcemia, such as an oat cell carcinoma of the lung if they become severely volume-depleted.

Contraindications

Furosemide, bumetanide, and torsemide may demonstrate cross-reactivity in patients who are sensitive to other sulfonamides. Overzealous use of any diuretic is dangerous in hepatic cirrhosis, borderline renal failure, or heart failure (see below).

THIAZIDES

The thiazide diuretics emerged from efforts to synthesize more potent carbonic anhydrase inhibitors. It subsequently became clear that the thiazides inhibit NaCl transport predominantly in the distal convoluted tubule. However, some members of this group retain significant carbonic anhydrase inhibitory activity. The prototypical thiazide is **hydrochlorothiazide.**

Chemistry & Pharmacokinetics

Similar to the carbonic anhydrase inhibitors, all of the thiazides have an unsubstituted sulfonamide group (Figure 15–8).

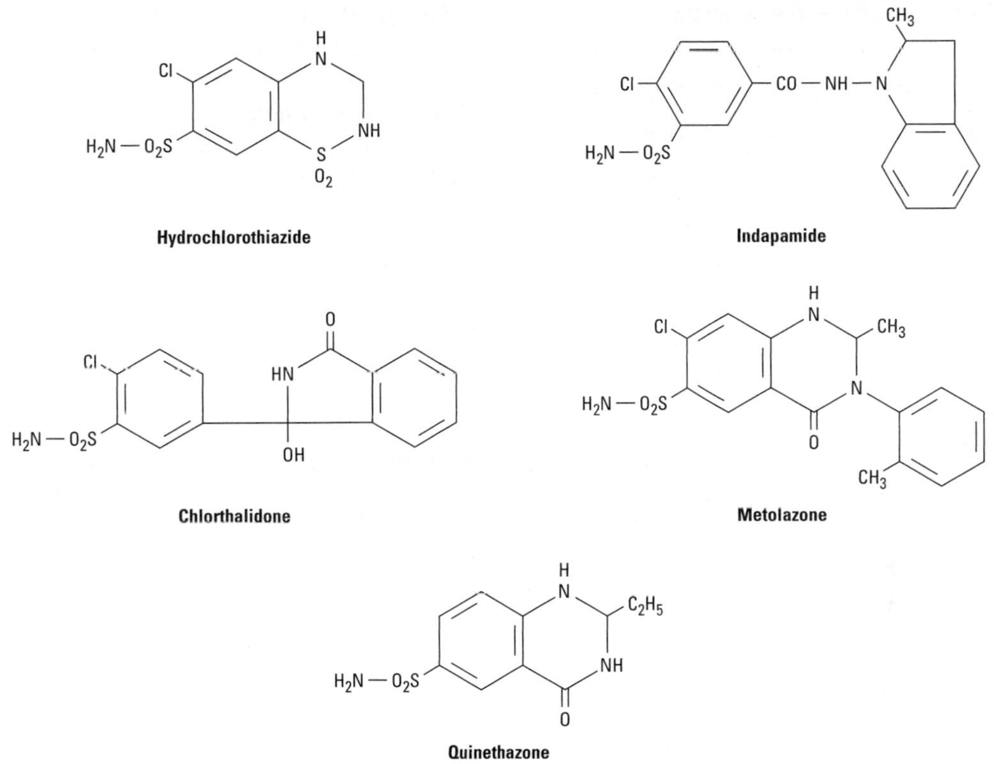

Figure 15–8. Hydrochlorothiazide and related agents.

All of the thiazides can be administered orally, but there are differences in their metabolism. Chlorothiazide, the parent of the group, is not very lipid-soluble and must be given in relatively large doses. It is the only thiazide available for parenteral administration. Chlorthalidone is slowly absorbed and has a longer duration of action. Although indapamide is excreted primarily by the biliary system, enough of the active form is cleared by the kidney to exert its diuretic effect in the distal convoluted tubule.

All of the thiazides are secreted by the organic acid secretory system in the proximal tubule and compete with the secretion of uric acid by that system. As a result, uric acid secretion may be reduced, with an elevation in serum uric acid level.

Pharmacodynamics

Thiazides inhibit NaCl reabsorption from the luminal side of epithelial cells in the distal convoluted tubule by blocking the Na^+/Cl^- transporter. In contrast to the situation in the loop of Henle, where loop diuretics inhibit Ca^{2+} reabsorption, thiazides actually enhance Ca^{2+} reabsorption in the distal convoluted tubule. This enhancement has been postulated to result from a lowering of intracellular Na^+ upon blockade of Na^+ entry by thiazides. The lower cell Na^+ would enhance Na^+/Ca^{2+} exchange in the basolateral membrane (Figure 15–5), increasing overall reabsorption of Ca^{2+}. While thiazides rarely cause hypercalcemia as the result of this enhanced reabsorption, they can unmask hypercalcemia due to other causes (eg, hyperparathyroidism, carcinoma, sarcoidosis). Thiazides are useful in the treatment of kidney stones caused by hypercalciuria.

The action of thiazides depends in part on renal prostaglandin production. As described above for the loop diuretics, the actions of thiazides can also be inhibited by NSAIDs under certain conditions.

Clinical Indications & Dosage (Table 15–3)

The major indications for thiazide diuretics are (1) hypertension, (2) heart failure, (3) nephrolithiasis due to idiopathic hypercalciuria, and (4) nephrogenic diabetes insipidus. Use of the thiazides in each of these conditions is described below in the section on clinical pharmacology.

Table 15–3. Thiazides and related diuretics: Dosages.

Drug	Daily Oral Dose	Frequency of Dosage
Bendroflumethiazide	2.5–10 mg	As single dose
Benzthiazide	25–100 mg	In two divided doses
Chlorothiazide	0.5–1 g	In two divided doses
Chlorthalidone[1]	50–100 mg	As single dose
Hydrochlorothiazide	25–100 mg	As single dose
Hydroflumethiazide	25–100 mg	In two divided doses
Indapamide[1]	2.5–10 mg	As single dose
Methyclothiazide	2.5–10 mg	As single dose
Metolazone[1]	2.5–10 mg	As single dose
Polythiazide	1–4 mg	As single dose
Quinethazone[1]	50–100 mg	As single dose
Trichlormethiazide	2–8 mg	As single dose

[1]Not a thiazide but a sulfonamide qualitatively similar to the thiazides.

Toxicity

A. HYPOKALEMIC METABOLIC ALKALOSIS AND HYPERURICEMIA

These toxicities are similar to those observed with loop diuretics (see above).

B. IMPAIRED CARBOHYDRATE TOLERANCE

Hyperglycemia may occur in patients who are overtly diabetic or who have even mildly abnormal glucose tolerance tests. The effect is due both to impaired pancreatic release of insulin and to diminished tissue utilization of glucose. Hyperglycemia may be partially reversible with correction of hypokalemia.

C. HYPERLIPIDEMIA

Thiazides cause a 5–15% increase in serum cholesterol and increased low-density lipoproteins (LDL). These levels may return toward baseline after prolonged use.

D. HYPONATREMIA

Hyponatremia is an important adverse effect of thiazide diuretics. It is due to a combination of hypovolemia-induced elevation of ADH, reduction in the diluting capacity of the kidney, and increased thirst. It can be prevented by reducing the dose of the drug or limiting water intake.

E. ALLERGIC REACTIONS

The thiazides are sulfonamides and share cross-reactivity with other members of this chemical group. Photosensitivity or generalized dermatitis occurs rarely. Serious allergic reactions are extremely rare but do include hemolytic anemia, thrombocytopenia, and acute necrotizing pancreatitis.

F. OTHER TOXICITIES

Weakness, fatigability, and paresthesias similar to those of carbonic anhydrase inhibitors may occur. Impotence has been reported but is probably related to volume depletion.

Contraindications

Excessive use of any diuretic is dangerous in hepatic cirrhosis, borderline renal failure, or heart failure (see below).

POTASSIUM-SPARING DIURETICS

These diuretics antagonize the effects of aldosterone at the late distal tubule and cortical collecting tubule. Inhibition may occur by direct pharmacologic antagonism of mineralocorticoid receptors (**spironolactone, eplerenone**) or by inhibition of Na^+ influx through ion channels in the luminal membrane (**amiloride, triamterene**).

Chemistry & Pharmacokinetics

Spironolactone is a synthetic steroid that acts as a competitive antagonist to aldosterone. Its onset and duration of action are determined by the kinetics of the aldosterone response in the target tissue. Substantial inactivation of spironolactone occurs in the liver. Overall, spironolactone has a rather slow onset of action, requiring several days before full therapeutic effect is achieved. Eplerenone, a new spironolactone analog with greater selectivity for the aldosterone receptor, has recently been approved for the treatment of hypertension.

Amiloride is excreted unchanged in the urine. Triamterene is metabolized in the liver, but renal excretion is a major route of elimination for the active form and the metabolites. Because triamterene is extensively metabolized, it has a shorter half-life and must be given more frequently than amiloride. The structures of spironolactone, triamterene, and amiloride are shown in Figure 15–9.

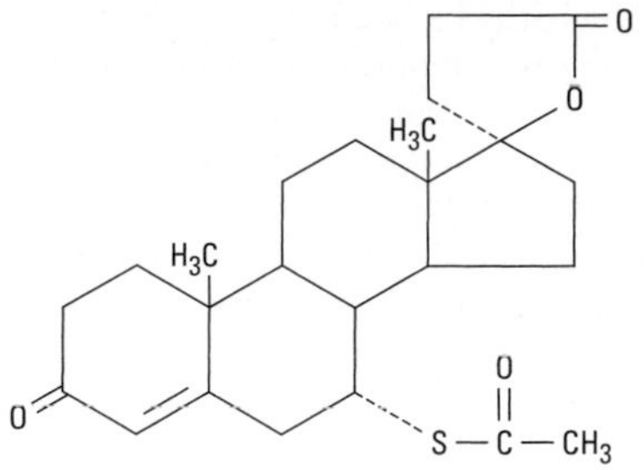

Figure 15–9. Aldosterone antagonists.

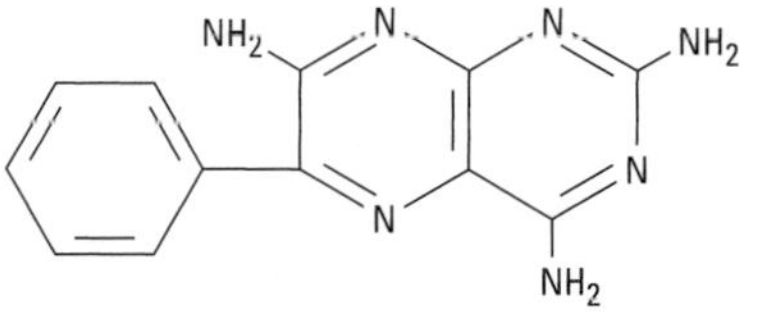

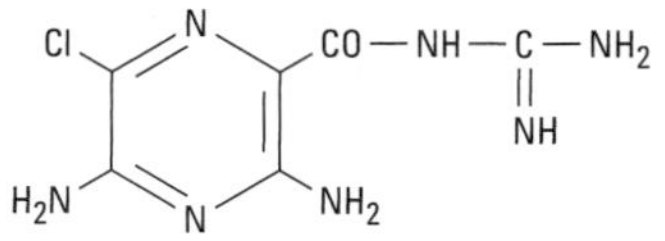

Pharmacodynamics

Potassium-sparing diuretics reduce Na⁺ absorption in the collecting tubules and ducts. Na⁺ absorption (and K⁺ secretion) at this site is regulated by aldosterone, as described above. Aldosterone antagonists interfere with this process. Similar effects are observed with respect to H⁺ handling by the intercalated cells of the collecting tubule, in part explaining the metabolic acidosis seen with aldosterone antagonists.

Spironolactone and eplerenone bind to aldosterone receptors and may also reduce the intracellular formation of active metabolites of aldosterone. Triamterene and amiloride do not block the aldosterone receptor but instead directly interfere with Na⁺ entry through the sodium-selective (ENaC) ion channels in the apical membrane of the collecting tubule. Since K⁺ secretion is coupled with Na⁺ entry in this segment, these agents are also effective potassium-sparing diuretics.

The actions of triamterene and spironolactone depend on renal prostaglandin production. As described above for loop diuretics and thiazides, the actions of triamterene and spironolactone can also be inhibited by NSAIDs under certain conditions.

Clinical Indications & Dosage (Table 15–4)

These agents are most useful in states of mineralocorticoid excess, due either to primary hypersecretion (Conn's syndrome, ectopic ACTH production) or to secondary aldosteronism (from heart failure, hepatic cirrhosis, nephrotic syndrome, and other conditions associated with diminished effective intravascular volume). Use of other diuretics, like thiazides or loop agents, can

Table 15–4. Potassium-sparing diuretics and combination preparations.

Trade Name	Potassium-Sparing Agent	Hydrochlorothiazide	Frequency of Dosage
Aldactazide	Spironolactone 25 mg	25 mg	1–4 times daily
Aldactone	Spironolactone 25 mg	...	1–4 times daily
Dyazide	Triamterene 50 mg	25 mg	1–4 times daily
Dyrenium	Triamterene 50 mg	...	1–3 times daily
Inspra[1]	Eplerenone 25, 50 mg	...	Once or twice daily
Maxzide	Triamterene 75 mg	50 mg	Once daily
Maxzide-25 mg	Triamterene 27.5 mg	25 mg	Once daily
Midamor	Amiloride 5 mg	...	Once daily
Moduretic	Amiloride 5 mg	50 mg	Once or twice daily

[1]Eplerenone is currently approved for use only in hypertension.

cause or exacerbate volume contraction and thus intensify secondary aldosteronism. In the setting of enhanced mineralocorticoid secretion and continuing delivery of Na^+ to distal nephron sites, renal K^+ wasting occurs. Potassium-sparing diuretics of either type may be used in this setting to blunt the K^+ secretory response.

Toxicity

A. HYPERKALEMIA

Unlike other diuretics, these agents can cause mild, moderate, or even life-threatening hyperkalemia. The risk of this complication is greatly increased in the presence of renal disease or of other drugs that reduce renin (β-blockers, NSAIDs) or angiotensin II activity (angiotensin-converting enzyme [ACE] inhibitors, angiotensin receptor inhibitors). Since most other diuretic agents lead to K^+ losses, hyperkalemia is more common when aldosterone antagonists are used as the sole diuretic agent, especially in patients with renal insufficiency. With fixed-dosage combinations of potassium-sparing and thiazide diuretics, the thiazide-induced hypokalemia and metabolic alkalosis are ameliorated by the aldosterone antagonist. However, owing to variations in the bioavailability of the components of fixed-dosage forms, the thiazide-associated adverse effects may predominate. Therefore, it is generally preferable to adjust the doses of the two drugs separately.

B. HYPERCHLOREMIC METABOLIC ACIDOSIS

By inhibiting H^+ secretion in parallel with K^+ secretion, the potassium-sparing diuretics can cause acidosis similar to that seen with type IV renal tubular acidosis.

C. GYNECOMASTIA

Synthetic steroids may cause endocrine abnormalities by effects on other steroid receptors. Gynecomastia, impotence, and benign prostatic hyperplasia have all been reported with spironolactone. Such effects have not been reported with eplerenone.

D. ACUTE RENAL FAILURE

The combination of triamterene with indomethacin has been reported to cause acute renal failure. This has not been reported with other potassium-sparing agents.

E. KIDNEY STONES

Triamterene is poorly soluble and may precipitate in the urine, causing kidney stones.

Contraindications

These agents can cause severe, even fatal hyperkalemia in susceptible patients. Oral K^+ administration should be discontinued if aldosterone antagonists are adminis-

tered. Patients with chronic renal insufficiency are especially vulnerable and should rarely be treated with aldosterone antagonists. Concomitant use of other agents that blunt the renin-angiotensin system (β-blockers or ACE inhibitors) increases the likelihood of hyperkalemia. Patients with liver disease may have impaired metabolism of triamterene and spironolactone, and dosing must be carefully adjusted. Strong CYP3A4 inhibitors (eg, ketoconazole, itraconazole) can markedly increase blood levels of eplerenone.

AGENTS THAT ALTER WATER EXCRETION

1. OSMOTIC DIURETICS

The proximal tubule and descending limb of Henle's loop are freely permeable to water. An osmotic agent that is not reabsorbed causes water to be retained in these segments and promotes a water diuresis. Such agents can be used to reduce increased intracranial pressure and to promote prompt removal of renal toxins. The prototypic osmotic diuretic is **mannitol.**

Pharmacokinetics

Osmotic diuretics are poorly absorbed, which means that they must be given parenterally. If administered orally, mannitol causes osmotic diarrhea. Mannitol is not metabolized and is excreted primarily by glomerular filtration within 30–60 minutes, without any important tubular reabsorption or secretion.

Pharmacodynamics

Osmotic diuretics have their major effect in those segments of the nephron that are freely permeable to water: the proximal tubule and the descending limb of the loop of Henle. They also oppose the action of ADH in the collecting tubule. The presence of a nonreabsorbable solute such as mannitol prevents the normal absorption of water by interposing a countervailing osmotic force. As a result, urine volume increases. The increase in urine flow rate decreases the contact time between fluid and the tubular epithelium, thus reducing Na^+ reabsorption. However, the resulting natriuresis is of lesser magnitude than the water diuresis, leading eventually to hypernatremia.

Clinical Indications & Dosage

A. TO INCREASE URINE VOLUME

Osmotic diuretics are used to increase water excretion in preference to sodium excretion. This effect can be useful when avid Na^+ retention limits the response to conventional agents. It can be used to maintain urine volume and to prevent anuria that might otherwise result from presentation of large pigment loads to the kidney (eg, from hemolysis or rhabdomyolysis). Some oliguric patients do not respond to an osmotic diuretic. Therefore, a test dose of mannitol (12.5 g intravenously) should be given prior to starting a continuous infusion. Mannitol should not be continued unless there is an increase in urine flow rate to more than 50 mL/h during the 3 hours following the test dose. Mannitol (12.5–25 g) can be repeated every 1–2 hours to maintain urine flow rate greater than 100 mL/h. Prolonged use of mannitol is not advised.

B. REDUCTION OF INTRACRANIAL AND INTRAOCULAR PRESSURE

Osmotic diuretics alter Starling forces so that water leaves cells and reduces intracellular volume. This effect is used to reduce intracranial pressure in neurologic conditions and to reduce intraocular pressure before ophthalmologic procedures. A dose of 1–2 g/kg mannitol is administered intravenously. Intracranial pressure, which must be monitored, should fall in 60–90 minutes.

Toxicity

A. EXTRACELLULAR VOLUME EXPANSION

Mannitol is rapidly distributed in the extracellular compartment and extracts water from cells. Prior to the diuresis, this leads to expansion of the extracellular volume and hyponatremia. This effect can complicate heart failure and may produce florid pulmonary edema. Headache, nausea, and vomiting are commonly observed in patients treated with osmotic diuretics.

B. DEHYDRATION AND HYPERNATREMIA

Excessive use of mannitol without adequate water replacement can ultimately lead to severe dehydration, free water losses, and hypernatremia. These complications can be avoided by careful attention to serum ion composition and fluid balance.

2. ANTIDIURETIC HORMONE (ADH) AGONISTS

Vasopressin and desmopressin are used in the treatment of pituitary diabetes insipidus. They are discussed in Chapter 37.

3. ANTIDIURETIC HORMONE (ADH) ANTAGONISTS

A variety of medical conditions cause water retention as the result of ADH excess. Unfortunately, specific ADH antagonists are available only for investigational purposes. Two nonselective agents, lithium and demeclocy-cline (a tetracycline derivative), are of limited use in some situations.

Pharmacokinetics

Both lithium and demeclocycline are orally active. Lithium is excreted by the kidney, and demeclocycline is metabolized in the liver.

Pharmacodynamics

ADH antagonists inhibit the effects of ADH in the collecting tubule. Both lithium and demeclocycline appear to reduce the formation of cyclic adenosine monophospate (cAMP) in response to ADH and also to interfere with the actions of cAMP in the collecting tubule cells.

Clinical Indications & Dosage

A. SYNDROME OF INAPPROPRIATE ADH SECRETION (SIADH)

ADH antagonists are used to manage SIADH when water restriction has failed to correct the abnormality. This generally occurs in the outpatient setting, where water restriction cannot be enforced, or in the hospital when large quantities of intravenous fluid are administered with drugs. Lithium carbonate has been used to treat this syndrome, but the response is unpredictable. Serum levels of lithium must be monitored closely, as serum concentrations greater than 1 mmol/L are toxic. Demeclocycline, in dosages of 600–1200 mg/d, yields a more predictable result and is less toxic. Appropriate plasma levels (2 μg/mL) should be maintained by monitoring.

B. OTHER CAUSES OF ELEVATED ANTIDIURETIC HORMONE (ADH)

ADH is also elevated in response to diminished effective circulating blood volume. When treatment by volume replacement is not possible, as in heart failure or liver disease, hyponatremia may result. As for SIADH, water restriction is the treatment of choice, but if it is not successful, demeclocycline may be used.

Toxicity

A. NEPHROGENIC DIABETES INSIPIDUS

If serum Na+ is not monitored closely, ADH antagonists can cause severe hypernatremia and nephrogenic diabetes insipidus. If lithium is being used for an affective disorder, nephrogenic diabetes insipidus can be treated with a thiazide diuretic or amiloride (see below).

B. RENAL FAILURE

Both lithium and demeclocycline have been reported to cause acute renal failure. Long-term lithium therapy may also cause chronic interstitial nephritis.

C. OTHER

Adverse effects associated with lithium therapy include tremulousness, mental obtundation, cardiotoxicity, thyroid dysfunction, and leukocytosis (see Chapter 29). Demeclocycline should be avoided in patients with liver disease (see Chapter 44) and in children younger than 12 years.

DIURETIC COMBINATIONS

LOOP AGENTS & THIAZIDES

Some patients are refractory to the usual dose of loop diuretics or become refractory after an initial response. Since these agents have a short half-life, refractoriness may be due to an excessively long interval between doses. Renal Na$^+$ retention is enhanced during the time period when the drug is no longer active. After the dosing interval for loop agents is minimized or the dose is maximized, the use of two drugs acting at different nephron sites may exhibit synergy. Loop agents and thiazides in combination will often produce diuresis when neither agent acting alone is even minimally effective. There are several reasons for this phenomenon. First, salt and water reabsorption in either the thick ascending limb or the distal convoluted tubule can increase when the other is blocked. Inhibition of both can therefore produce more than an additive diuretic response. Second, thiazide diuretics may produce a mild natriuresis in the proximal tubule that is usually masked by increased reabsorption in the thick ascending limb. The combination of loop diuretics and thiazides will therefore blunt Na$^+$ reabsorption, to some extent, from all three segments.

Metolazone is the usual choice of thiazide-like drug in patients refractory to loop agents alone, but it is likely that other thiazides would be as effective as metolazone. Moreover, metolazone is available only in an oral preparation, while chlorothiazide can be given parenterally.

The combination of loop diuretics and thiazides can mobilize large amounts of fluid, even in patients who have not responded to single agents. Therefore, close hemodynamic monitoring is essential. Routine outpatient use is not recommended. Furthermore, K$^+$-wasting is extremely common and may require parenteral K$^+$ administration with careful monitoring of fluid and electrolyte status.

POTASSIUM-SPARING DIURETICS & LOOP AGENTS OR THIAZIDES

Hypokalemia eventually develops in many patients who are placed on loop diuretics or thiazides. This can often be managed with dietary NaCl restriction. When hypokalemia cannot be managed in this way, or with dietary KCl supplements, the addition of a potassium-sparing diuretic can significantly lower potassium excretion. While this approach is generally safe, it should be avoided in patients with renal insufficiency in whom life-threatening hyperkalemia can develop in response to potassium-sparing diuretics.

III. CLINICAL PHARMACOLOGY OF DIURETIC AGENTS

This section discusses the clinical use of diuretic agents in edematous and nonedematous states. The effects of these agents on urinary electrolyte excretion are shown in Table 15–5.

EDEMATOUS STATES

The most common reason for diuretic use is for reduction of peripheral or pulmonary edema that has accumulated as a result of cardiac, renal, or vascular diseases, or abnormalities in the blood oncotic pressure. Salt and water retention with edema formation often occurs when diminished blood delivery to the kidney is sensed as insufficient "effective" arterial blood volume. Judicious use of diuretics can mobilize interstitial edema fluid without significant reductions in plasma volume. However, excessive diuretic therapy in this setting may lead to further compromise of the effective arterial blood volume with reduction in perfusion of vital organs. Therefore, the use of diuretics to mobilize edema requires careful monitoring of the patient's hemodynamic status and an understanding of the pathophysiology of the underlying condition.

Table 15–5. Changes in urinary electrolyte patterns in response to diuretic drugs.

Agent	Urinary Electrolyte Patterns		
	NaCl	NaHCO$_3$	K$^+$
Carbonic anhydrase inhibitors	+	+++	+
Loop agents	++++	–	+
Thiazides	++	±	+
Loop agents plus thiazides	+++++	+	++
K$^+$-sparing agents	+	–	–

+, increase; –, decrease.

HEART FAILURE

When cardiac output is reduced by disease, the resultant changes in blood pressure and blood flow to the kidney are sensed as hypovolemia and thus induce renal retention of salt and water. This physiologic response initially expands the intravascular volume and venous return to the heart and may partially restore the cardiac output toward normal (see Chapter 13).

If the underlying disease causes cardiac function to deteriorate despite expansion of plasma volume, the kidney continues to retain salt and water, which then leaks from the vasculature and becomes interstitial or pulmonary edema. At this point, diuretic use becomes necessary to reduce the accumulation of edema, particularly that which is in the lungs. Reduction of pulmonary vascular congestion with diuretics may actually improve oxygenation and thereby improve myocardial function. Edema associated with heart failure is generally managed with loop diuretics. In some instances, salt and water retention may become so severe that a combination of thiazides and loop diuretics is necessary.

In treating the heart failure patient with diuretics, it must always be remembered that cardiac output in these patients is being maintained in part by high filling pressures and that excessive use of diuretics may diminish venous return and thereby impair cardiac output. This issue is especially critical in right ventricular failure. Systemic rather than pulmonary vascular congestion is the hallmark of this disorder. Diuretic-induced volume contraction will predictably reduce venous return and can severely compromise cardiac output if left ventricular filling pressure is reduced below 15 mm Hg.

Diuretic-induced metabolic alkalosis is another adverse effect that may further compromise cardiac function. While this effect is generally treated with replacement of potassium and restoration of intravascular volume with saline, severe heart failure may preclude the use of saline even in patients who have received too much diuretic. In these cases, adjunctive use of acetazolamide can help correct the alkalosis.

Another serious toxicity of diuretic use, particularly in the cardiac patient, is hypokalemia. Hypokalemia can exacerbate underlying cardiac arrhythmias and contribute to digitalis toxicity. This can often be avoided by having the patient reduce sodium intake, thus decreasing sodium delivery to the K^+-secreting collecting tubule. Patients who are noncompliant with a low sodium diet must take oral KCl supplements or a potassium-sparing diuretic or must stop using the thiazide diuretic.

Finally, it should be kept in mind that diuretics can never correct the underlying cardiac disease. Drugs that improve myocardial contractility or reduce peripheral vascular resistance are more direct approaches to the basic problem.

KIDNEY DISEASE

A variety of renal diseases may interfere with the kidney's critical role in volume homeostasis. Although renal disorders will occasionally cause salt wasting, most kidney diseases cause retention of salt and water. When loss of renal function is severe, diuretic agents are of little benefit, because there is insufficient glomerular filtration to sustain a natriuretic response. However, a large number of patients with milder degrees of renal insufficiency can be treated with diuretics when they retain sodium.

Many primary and secondary glomerular diseases, such as those associated with diabetes mellitus or systemic lupus erythematosus, exhibit renal retention of salt and water. The cause of this sodium retention is not precisely known, but it probably involves disordered regulation of the renal microcirculation and tubular function through release of vasoconstrictors, prostaglandins, cytokines, and other mediators. When edema or hypertension develops in these patients, diuretic therapy can be very effective. If heart failure is also present, see the warnings mentioned above.

Certain forms of renal disease, particularly diabetic nephropathy, are frequently associated with development of hyperkalemia at a relatively early stage of renal failure. In these cases, a thiazide or loop diuretic will enhance K^+ excretion by increasing delivery of salt to the K^+-secreting collecting tubule.

Patients with renal diseases leading to the nephrotic syndrome often present complex problems in volume management. These patients may have reduced plasma volume in conjunction with reduced plasma oncotic pressures, especially those with "minimal change" nephropathy. In these patients, diuretic use may cause further reductions in plasma volume that can impair glomerular filtration rate and may lead to orthostatic hypotension. However, most other causes of nephrotic syndrome are associated with a primary retention of salt and water by the kidney, leading to expanded plasma volume and hypertension despite the low plasma oncotic pressure. In these cases, diuretic therapy may be beneficial in controlling the volume-dependent component of hypertension. In choosing a diuretic for the patient with kidney disease, there are a number of important limitations. Acetazolamide and potassium-sparing diuretics must usually be avoided because of their tendency to exacerbate acidosis and hyperkalemia, respectively. Thiazide diuretics are generally ineffective when glomerular filtration rate falls below 30 mL/min. Thus, loop diuretics are often the best choice in treating edema associated with kidney failure. Lastly, excessive use of diuretics will cause renal function to decline in all patients, but the consequences are more serious in those with underlying renal disease.

HEPATIC CIRRHOSIS

Liver disease is often associated with edema and ascites in conjunction with elevated portal hydrostatic pressures and reduced plasma oncotic pressures. The mechanisms for retention of sodium by the kidney are complex. They probably involve a combination of factors, including diminished renal perfusion resulting from systemic vascular alterations, diminished plasma volume as the result of ascites formation, and diminished oncotic pressure from hypoalbuminemia. In addition, there may be primary sodium retention by the kidney. Plasma aldosterone levels are usually high in response to the reduction in effective circulating volume.

When ascites and edema become severe, diuretic therapy can be useful in initiating and maintaining diuresis. Cirrhotic patients are often resistant to loop diuretics, in part because of a decrease in secretion of the drug into the tubular fluid and in part because of high aldosterone levels leading to enhanced collecting duct salt reabsorption. In contrast, cirrhotic edema is unusually responsive to spironolactone. The combination of loop diuretics and spironolactone may be useful in some patients. However, even more than in heart failure, overly aggressive use of diuretics in this setting can be disastrous. Vigorous diuretic therapy can cause marked depletion of intravascular volume, hypokalemia, and metabolic alkalosis. Hepatorenal syndrome and hepatic encephalopathy are the unfortunate consequences of excessive diuretic use in the cirrhotic patient.

IDIOPATHIC EDEMA

Despite intensive study, the pathophysiology of this disorder (fluctuating salt retention and edema) remains obscure. Some studies suggest that intermittent diuretic use may actually contribute to the syndrome. Therefore, idiopathic edema should be managed with mild salt restriction alone if possible.

NONEDEMATOUS STATES

HYPERTENSION

The diuretic and mild vasodilator actions of the thiazides are useful in treating virtually all patients with essential hypertension, and may be completely sufficient in two thirds. Moderate restriction of dietary Na+ intake (60–100 meq/d) has been shown to potentiate the effects of diuretics in essential hypertension and to lessen renal K+ wasting.

A recent very large study (over 30,000 participants) has shown that inexpensive diuretics are similar or superior in outcomes to ACE inhibitor or calcium channel blocker therapy (ALLHAT, 2002). This important result reinforces the importance of thiazide therapy in hypertension.

Diuretics also play an important role in patients who require multiple drugs to control blood pressure. Diuretics enhance the efficacy of many agents, particularly the ACE inhibitors. Patients being treated with powerful vasodilators such as hydralazine or minoxidil usually require diuretics simultaneously because the vasodilators cause significant salt and water retention.

NEPHROLITHIASIS

Approximately two thirds of all renal stones contain calcium phosphate or calcium oxalate. Many patients with such stones exhibit a renal defect in calcium reabsorption that causes hypercalciuria. This can be treated with thiazide diuretics, which enhance calcium reabsorption in the distal convoluted tubule and thus reduce the urinary calcium concentration. Salt intake must be reduced in this setting, as excess dietary NaCl will overwhelm the hypocalciuric effect of thiazides. Calcium stones may also be caused by increased intestinal absorption of calcium, or they may be idiopathic. In these situations, thiazides are also effective, but should be used as adjunctive therapy with decreased calcium intake and other measures.

HYPERCALCEMIA

Hypercalcemia can be a medical emergency. Since the loop of Henle is an important site of calcium reabsorption, loop diuretics can be quite effective in promoting calcium diuresis. However, loop diuretics alone can cause marked volume contraction. If this occurs, loop diuretics are ineffective (and potentially counterproductive) because calcium reabsorption in the proximal tubule is enhanced. Thus, saline must be administered simultaneously with loop diuretics if an effective calcium diuresis is to be achieved. The usual approach is to infuse normal saline and furosemide (80–120 mg) intravenously. Once the diuresis begins, the rate of saline infusion can be matched with the urine flow rate to avoid volume depletion. Potassium may be added to the saline infusion as needed.

DIABETES INSIPIDUS

Thiazide diuretics can reduce polyuria and polydipsia in patients who are not responsive to ADH. This seemingly paradoxic beneficial effect is mediated through plasma volume reduction, with an associated fall in glomerular filtration rate, enhanced proximal reabsorption of NaCl and water, and decreased delivery of fluid to the diluting segments. Thus, the maximum volume of dilute urine that can be produced is lowered and thiazides can significantly reduce urine flow in the polyuric patient. Dietary sodium restriction can potentiate the beneficial effects of thiazides on urine volume in this setting. Lithium, used in the treatment of manic-depressive disorder, is a common cause of drug-induced diabetes insipidus, and thiazide diuretics have been found to be helpful in treating it. Serum lithium levels must be carefully monitored in this situation, since diuretics may *reduce* renal clearance of lithium and raise plasma lithium levels into the toxic range (see Chapter 29). Lithium polyuria can also be partially reversed by amiloride, which appears to block lithium entry into collecting duct cells, much as it blocks Na⁺ entry.

PREPARATIONS AVAILABLE

Acetazolamide (generic, Diamox)
Oral: 125, 250 mg tablets
Oral sustained-release: 500 mg capsules
Parenteral: 500 mg powder for injection
Amiloride (generic, Midamor, combination drugs)
Oral: 5 mg tablets
Bendroflumethiazide (Naturetin)
Oral: 5, 10 mg tablets
Benzthiazide (Exna, combination drugs)
Oral: 50 mg tablets
Brinzolamide (Azopt)
Ophthalmic: 1% suspension
Bumetanide (generic, Bumex)
Oral: 0.5, 1, 2 mg tablets
Parenteral: 0.5 mg/2 mL ampule for IV or IM injection
Chlorothiazide (generic, Diuril, others)
Oral: 250, 500 mg tablets; 250 mg/5 mL oral suspension
Parenteral: 500 mg for injection
Chlorthalidone (generic, Thalitone, combination drugs)
Oral: 15, 25, 50, 100 mg tablets
Demeclocycline (Declomycin)
Oral: 150 mg tablets and capsules; 300 mg tablets
Dichlorphenamide (Daranide)
Oral: 50 mg tablets
Dorzolamide (Trusopt)
Ophthalmic: 2% solution
Eplerenone (Inspra)
Oral: 25, 50, 100 mg tablets
Ethacrynic acid (Edecrin)
Oral: 25, 50 mg tablets
Parenteral: 50 mg IV injection

Furosemide (generic, Lasix, others)
Oral: 20, 40, 80 mg tablets; 8 mg/mL solutions
Parenteral: 10 mg/mL for IM or IV injection
Hydrochlorothiazide (generic, Microzide, Hydro-DIURIL, combination drugs)
Oral: 12.5 mg capsules; 25, 50, 100 mg tablets; 10 mg/mL solution
Hydroflumethiazide (generic, Diucardin)
Oral: 50 mg tablets
Indapamide (generic, Lozol)
Oral: 1.25, 2.5 mg tablets
Mannitol (generic, Osmitrol)
Parenteral: 5, 10, 15, 20, 25% for injection
Methazolamide (generic, Neptazane)
Oral: 25, 50 mg tablets
Methyclothiazide (generic, Aquatensen)
Oral: 2.5, 5 mg tablets
Metolazone (Mykrox, Zaroxolyn) (Note: Bio-Availability of Mykrox is greater than that of Zaroxolyn.)
Oral: 0.5 (Mykrox); 2.5, 5, 10 mg (Zaroxolyn) tablets
Polythiazide (Renese)
Oral: 1, 2, 4 mg tablets
Quinethazone (Hydromox)
Oral: 50 mg tablets
Spironolactone (generic, Aldactone)
Oral: 25, 50, 100 mg tablets
Torsemide (Demadex)
Oral: 5, 10, 20, 100 mg tablets
Parenteral: 10 mg/mL for injection
Triamterene (Dyrenium)
Oral: 50, 100 mg capsules
Trichlormethiazide (generic, Diurese, others)
Oral: 2, 4 mg tablets

REFERENCES

Aiza I, Perez GO, Schiff ER: Management of ascites in patients with chronic liver disease. Am J Gastroenterol 1994;89:1949.

ALLHAT Officers and Coordinators for the ALLHAT Collaborative Research Group: Major outcomes in high-risk hypertensive patients randomized to angiotensin-converting enzyme inhibitor or calcium channel blocker vs diuretic: The Antihypertensive and Lipid-Lowering Treatment to Prevent Heart Attack Trial (ALLHAT). JAMA 2002;288:2981.

Ashraf N, Locksley R, Arieff AI: Thiazide-induced hyponatremia associated with death or neurologic damage in outpatients. Am J Med 1981;70:1163.

Baglin A et al: Metabolic adverse reactions to diuretics: Clinical relevance to elderly patients. Drug Saf 1995;12:161.

Battle DC et al: Amelioration of polyuria by amiloride in patients receiving long-term lithium therapy. N Engl J Med 1985;312:408.

Berkowitz HL: Thiazide diuretics and lithium levels. J Clin Psychiatry 2001;62:57.

Bernardo A et al: Basolateral Na^+/HCO_3^- cotransport activity is regulated by the dissociable Na^+/H^+ exchanger regulatory factor. J Clin Invest 1999;104:195.

Biollaz J et al: Whole-blood pharmacokinetics and metabolic effects of the topical carbonic anhydrase inhibitor dorzolamide. Eur J Clin Pharmacol 1995;47:453.

Blose JS, Adams KF Jr, Patterson JH: Torsemide: a pyridine-sulfonylurea loop diuretic. Ann Pharmacother 1995;29:396.

Brater DC: Diuretic resistance: mechanisms and therapeutic strategies. Cardiology 1994;84(Suppl 2):57.

Brater DC: Pharmacology of diuretics. Am J Med Sci 2000;319:38.

Brenner BM (editor): *The Kidney,* 65th ed. Saunders, 2001.

Brown CB, Ogg CS, Cameron JS: High dose frusemide in acute renal failure: a controlled trial. Clin Nephrol 1981;15:90.

Cotter G et al: Randomized trial of high-dose isosorbide dinitrate plus low-dose furosemide versus high-dose furosemide plus low-dose isosorbide dinitrate in severe pulmonary oedema. Lancet 1998;351:389.

De Marchi S, Ceddhin E: Severe metabolic acidosis and disturbances of calcium metabolism induced by acetazolamide in patients on haemodialysis. Clin Sci 1990;78:295.

DeTroyer A: Demeclocycline: treatment for syndrome of inappropriate antidiuretic hormone secretion. JAMA 1977;237:2723.

Ellison DH: Diuretic drugs and the treatment of edema: from clinic to bench and back again. Am J Kidney Dis 1994;23:623.

Fall PJ: Hyponatremia and hypernatremia. A systematic approach to causes and their correction. Postgrad Med 2000;107:75.

Forns X et al: Management of ascites and renal failure in cirrhosis. Semin Liver Dis 1994;14:82.

Gamba G et al: Molecular cloning, primary structure, and characterization of two members of the mammalian electroneutral sodium-(potassium)-chloride cotransporter family expressed in kidney. J Biol Chem 1994;269:17713.

Giebisch G et al: Renal and extrarenal sites of action of diuretics. Cardiovasc Drugs Ther 1993;7:11.

Greenberg A: Diuretic complications. Am J Med Sci 2000;319:10.

Greene MK et al: Acetazolamide in prevention of acute mountain sickness: a double-blind controlled cross-over study. Br Med J 1981;283:811.

Greger R: Physiology of renal sodium transport. Am J Med Sci 2000;319:51.

Hackett PH, Roach RC: High-altitude illness. N Engl J Med 2001;345:107.

Hollifield JW, Slaton PE: Thiazide diuretics, hypokalemia, and cardiac arrhythmias. Acta Med Scand 1981;647(Suppl):67.

Horisberger J-D, Giebisch G: Potassium-sparing diuretics. Renal Physiol 1987;10:198.

Kalra PR et al: The regulation and measurement of plasma volume in heart failure. J Am Coll Cardiol 2002;39:1901.

Kirchner KA et al: Mechanism of attenuated hydrochlorothiazide response during indomethacin administration. Kidney Int 1987;31:1097.

Loon NR et al: Mechanism of impaired natriuretic response to furosemide during prolonged therapy. Kidney Int 1989;36:682.

Margo KL, Luttermoser G, Shaughnessy AF: Spironolactone in left-sided heart failure: how does it fit in? Am Fam Physician 2001;64:1393.

Mount DB et al: The electroneutral cation-chloride cotransporters. J Exp Biol 1998;201:2091.

Nakahama H et al: Pharmacokinetic and pharmacodynamic interactions between furosemide and hydrochlorothiazide in nephrotic patients. Nephron 1988;49:223.

Pollare T et al: A comparison of the effects of hydrochlorothiazide and captopril on glucose and lipid metabolism in patients with hypertension. N Engl J Med 1989;321:868.

Puschett JB: Pharmacological classification and renal actions of diuretics. Cardiology 1994;84(Suppl 2):4.

Rose BD: Diuretics. Kidney Int 1991;39:336.

Schrot RJ, Muizelaar JP: Mannitol in acute traumatic brain injury. Lancet 2002;359:1633.

Shilliday IR et al: Loop diuretics in the management of acute renal failure: a prospective, double-blind, placebo-controlled, randomized study. Nephrol Dial Transplant 1997;12:2592.

Shimuzu T et al: Effects of PTH, calcitonin, and cAMP on calcium transport in rabbit distal nephron. Am J Physiol 1990;259:F408.

Sorrentino MJ: Drug therapy for congestive heart failure. Postgrad Med 1997;101:83.

Stanton BA: Cellular actions of thiazide diuretics in the distal tubule. J Am Soc Nephrol 1990;1:832.

Strahlman E, Tiping R, Vogel R: A double-masked randomized 1-year study comparing dorzolamide (Trusopt), timolol, and betaxolol. Arch Ophthalmol 1995;113:1009.

Tse CM et al: Cloning and sequencing of a rabbit cDNA encoding an intestinal and kidney-specific Na^+/H^+ exchanger isoform (NHE-3). J Biol Chem 1992;267:9340.

Van Brummelen P, Woerlee M, Schalekamp MA: Long-term versus short-term effects of hydrochlorothiazide on renal haemodynamics in essential hypertension. Clin Sci 1979;56:463.

Vargo DL et al: Bioavailability, pharmacokinetics, and pharmacodynamics of torsemide and furosemide in patients with congestive heart failure. Clin Pharmacol Ther 1995;57:601.

Warren SE, Blantz RC: Mannitol. Arch Intern Med 1981;141:493.

Wollam GL et al: Diuretic potency of combined hydrochlorothiazide and furosemide therapy in patients with azotemia. Am J Med 1982;72:929.

Xu J et al: Molecular cloning and functional expression of the bumetanide-sensitive Na-K-Cl cotransporter. Proc Natl Acad Sci U S A 1994;91:2201.

SECTION IV
Drugs With Important Actions on Smooth Muscle

Histamine, Serotonin, & the Ergot Alkaloids

16

Bertram G. Katzung, MD, PhD

Histamine and serotonin (5-hydroxytryptamine) are biologically active amines that are found in many tissues, have complex physiologic and pathologic effects through multiple receptor subtypes, and are often released locally. Together with endogenous peptides (see Chapter 17), prostaglandins and leukotrienes (see Chapter 18), and cytokines (see Chapter 56), they are sometimes called autacoids (Gk "self-remedy") or local hormones in recognition of these properties.

Because of their broad and largely undesirable effects, neither histamine nor serotonin has any clinical application in the treatment of disease. However, compounds that *selectively* activate certain receptor subtypes or selectively antagonize the actions of these amines are of considerable clinical usefulness. This chapter therefore emphasizes the basic pharmacology of the agonist amines and the clinical pharmacology of the more selective agonist and antagonist drugs. The ergot alkaloids, compounds with partial agonist activity at serotonin and several other receptors, are discussed at the end of the chapter.

I. HISTAMINE

Histamine was synthesized in 1907 and later isolated from mammalian tissues. Early hypotheses concerning the possible physiologic roles of tissue histamine were based on similarities between histamine's actions and the symptoms of anaphylactic shock and tissue injury. Marked species variation is observed, but in humans histamine is an important mediator of immediate allergic and inflammatory reactions; has an important role in gastric acid secretion; and functions as a neurotransmitter and neuromodulator. New evidence indicates that histamine also plays a role in chemotaxis of white blood cells.

BASIC PHARMACOLOGY OF HISTAMINE

Chemistry & Pharmacokinetics

Histamine occurs in plants as well as in animal tissues and is a component of some venoms and stinging secretions.

Histamine is formed by decarboxylation of the amino acid L-histidine, a reaction catalyzed in mammalian tissues by the enzyme histidine decarboxylase. Once formed, histamine is either stored or rapidly inactivated. Very little histamine is excreted unchanged. The major inactivation pathways involve conversion to methylhistamine, methylimidazoleacetic acid, and imidazoleacetic acid. Certain neoplasms (systemic mastocytosis, urticaria pigmentosa, gastric carcinoid, and occasionally myelogenous leukemia) are associated with increased numbers of mast cells or basophils and with increased excretion of histamine and its metabolites.

Histamine

Most tissue histamine is sequestered and bound in granules (vesicles) in mast cells or basophils; the histamine content of many tissues is directly related to their mast cell content. The bound form of histamine is biologically inactive, but many stimuli, as noted below, can trigger the release of mast cell histamine, allowing the free amine to exert its actions on surrounding tissues. Mast cells are especially rich at sites of potential tissue injury—nose, mouth, and feet; internal body surfaces; and blood vessels, particularly at pressure points and bifurcations.

Non-mast cell histamine is found in several tissues, including the brain, where it functions as a neurotransmitter (see Chapter 21). Endogenous neurotransmitter histamine may play a role in many brain functions such as neuroendocrine control, cardiovascular regulation, thermal and body weight regulation, and arousal.

A second important nonneuronal site of histamine storage and release is the enterochromaffin-like (ECL) cell of the fundus of the stomach. These cells release histamine, one of the primary acid secretagogues, to activate the acid-producing parietal cells of the mucosa (see Chapter 63).

Storage & Release of Histamine

The stores of histamine in mast cells can be released through several mechanisms.

A. IMMUNOLOGIC RELEASE

The important pathophysiologic mechanism of mast cell and basophil histamine release is immunologic. These cells, if sensitized by IgE antibodies attached to their surface membranes, degranulate when exposed to the appropriate antigen (see Figure 56–5, effector phase). This type of release also requires energy and calcium. Degranulation leads to the simultaneous release of histamine, ATP, and other mediators that are stored together in the granules. Histamine released by this mechanism is a mediator in immediate (type I) allergic reactions. Substances released during IgG- or IgM-mediated immune reactions that activate the complement cascade also release histamine from mast cells and basophils.

By a negative feedback control mechanism mediated

by H_2 receptors, histamine appears to modulate its own release and that of other mediators from sensitized mast cells in some tissues. In humans, mast cells in skin and basophils show this negative feedback mechanism; lung mast cells do not. Thus, histamine may act to limit the intensity of the allergic reaction in the skin and blood.

Endogenous histamine has a modulating role in a variety of inflammatory and immune responses. Upon injury to a tissue, released histamine causes local vasodilation and leakage of plasma containing mediators of acute inflammation (complement, C-reactive protein), and antibodies. Histamine has an active chemotactic attraction for inflammatory cells (neutrophils, eosinophils, basophils, monocytes, and lymphocytes). Histamine inhibits the release of lysosome contents and several T and B lymphocyte functions. Most of these actions are mediated by H_2 or H_4 receptors acting through increased intracellular cAMP. Release of peptides from nerves in response to inflammation is also probably modulated by histamine, in this case acting through presynaptic H_3 receptors.

B. CHEMICAL AND MECHANICAL RELEASE

Certain amines, including drugs such as morphine and tubocurarine, can displace histamine from the heparin-protein complex within cells. This type of release does not require energy and is not associated with mast cell injury or degranulation. Loss of granules from the mast cell will also release histamine, since sodium ions in the extracellular fluid rapidly displace the amine from the complex. Chemical and mechanical mast cell injury causes degranulation and histamine release. **Compound 48/80**, an experimental diamine polymer, specifically releases histamine from tissue mast cells by an exocytotic degranulation process requiring energy and calcium.

Pharmacodynamics

A. MECHANISM OF ACTION

Histamine exerts its biologic actions by combining with specific cellular receptors located on the surface membrane. The four different histamine receptors thus far characterized are designated H_1–H_4 and are described in Table 16–1. Unlike the other amine transmitter receptors discussed previously, no subfamilies have been found within these major types.

All four receptor types have been cloned and belong to the large superfamily of receptors having seven membrane-spanning regions and intracellular association with G proteins. The structures of the H_1 and H_2 receptors differ significantly and appear to be more closely related to muscarinic and 5-HT$_1$ receptors, respectively, than to each other. The H_4 receptor has about 40% homology with the H_3 receptor but does not seem to be closely related to any other histamine receptor.

Table 16–1. Histamine receptor subtypes.

Receptor Subtype	Distribution	Postreceptor Mechanism	Partially Selective Agonists	Partially Selective Antagonists
H_1	Smooth muscle, endothelium, brain	$\uparrow IP_3$, DAG (G_q)	2-(*m*-Fluorophenyl)-histamine[1]	Mepyramine, triprolidine
H_2	Gastric mucosa, cardiac muscle, mast cells, brain	$\uparrow$ cAMP (G_s)	Dimaprit, impromidine, amthamine	Ranitidine, tiotidine
H_3	Presynaptic: brain, myenteric plexus, other neurons	$\downarrow$ cAMP, Ca_i^{2+} (G_i)	*R*-α-Methylhistamine, imetit, immepip	Thioperamide, iodophenpropit, clobenpropit
H_4	Eosinophils, neutrophils, CD4 T cells	$\downarrow$ cAMP, Ca_i^{2+} (G_i)	Clobenpropit, imetit, clozapine	Thioperamide

[1]Partial agonist.

In the brain, H_1 and H_2 receptors are located on postsynaptic membranes, while H_3 receptors are predominantly presynaptic. Activation of H_1 receptors, which are present in endothelium, smooth muscle cells, and nerve endings, usually elicits an increase in phosphoinositol hydrolysis and an increase in intracellular calcium. Activation of H_2 receptors, present in gastric mucosa, cardiac muscle cells, and some immune cells, increases intracellular cAMP. Like the β_2 adrenoceptor, under certain circumstances the H_2 receptor may couple to G_q, activating the IP_3-DAG cascade. Activation of H_3 receptors decreases transmitter release from histaminergic and other neurons, probably mediated by a decrease in calcium influx through N-type calcium channels in nerve endings. H_4 receptors are mainly found on blood cells in the bone marrow and circulating blood. They may modulate production of these cell types and they may mediate, in part, the previously recognized effects of histamine on cytokine production.

B. TISSUE AND ORGAN SYSTEM EFFECTS OF HISTAMINE

Histamine exerts powerful effects on smooth and cardiac muscle, on certain endothelial and nerve cells, and on the secretory cells of the stomach. However, sensitivity to histamine varies greatly among species. Humans, guinea pigs, dogs, and cats are quite sensitive, while mice and rats are much less so.

1. Nervous system—Histamine is a powerful stimulant of sensory nerve endings, especially those mediating pain and itching. This H_1-mediated effect is an important component of the urticarial response and reactions to insect and nettle stings. Some evidence suggests that local high concentrations can also depolarize efferent (axonal) nerve endings (see ¶ 8, below). In the mouse, and probably in humans, respiratory neurons signaling inspiration and expiration are modulated by H_1 receptors. Presynaptic H_3 receptors play important roles in modulating transmitter release in the nervous system. H_3 agonists reduce the release of acetylcholine, amine, and peptide transmitters in various areas of the brain and in peripheral nerves.

2. Cardiovascular system—In humans, injection or infusion of histamine causes a decrease in systolic and diastolic blood pressure and an increase in heart rate (Figure 16–1). The blood pressure changes are caused by the direct vasodilator action of histamine on arterioles and precapillary sphincters; the increase in heart rate involves both stimulatory actions of histamine on the heart and a reflex tachycardia. Flushing, a sense of warmth, and headache may also occur during histamine administration, consistent with the vasodilation. Histamine-induced vasodilation is mediated primarily by release of nitric oxide (see Chapter 19). Studies with histamine receptor antagonists show that both H_1 and H_2 receptors are involved in these cardiovascular responses to high doses. However, in humans, the cardiovascular effects of small doses of histamine can usually be antagonized by H_1 receptor antagonists alone.

Histamine-induced edema results from the action of the amine on H_1 receptors in the vessels of the microcirculation, especially the postcapillary vessels. The effect is associated with the separation of the endothelial cells, which permits the transudation of fluid and molecules as large as small proteins into the perivascular tissue.

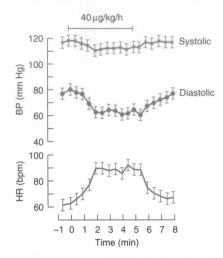

Figure 16–1. Effects of histamine on blood pressure and heart rate in humans. Histamine was infused at 40 μg/kg/h for 5 minutes as shown at the top of the panel. (Modified and reproduced, with permission, from Torsoli A, Lucchelli PE, Brimblecombe RW [editors]: *H-Antagonists: H₂ Receptor Antagonists in Peptic Ulcer Disease and Progress in Histamine Research*. Excerpta Medica, 1980.)

This effect is responsible for the urticaria (hives) that signals the release of histamine in the skin. Studies of endothelial cells suggest that actin and myosin within these cells contract, resulting in separation of the endothelial cells and increased permeability.

Direct cardiac effects of histamine include both increased contractility and increased pacemaker rate. These effects are mediated chiefly by H_2 receptors. In human atrial muscle, histamine can also decrease contractility; this effect is mediated by H_1 receptors. The physiologic significance of these cardiac actions is not clear. Some of the cardiovascular signs and symptoms of anaphylaxis are due to released histamine, though several other mediators are involved and appear to be more important than histamine in humans.

3. Bronchiolar smooth muscle—In both humans and guinea pigs, histamine causes bronchoconstriction mediated by H_1 receptors. In the guinea pig, this effect is the cause of death from histamine toxicity, but in normal humans, bronchoconstriction following small doses of histamine is not marked. However, patients with asthma are very sensitive to histamine. The bronchoconstriction induced in these patients probably represents a hyperactive neural response, since such patients also respond excessively to many other stimuli, and the response to histamine can be blocked by autonomic

blocking drugs such as ganglionic blocking agents as well as by H_1 receptor antagonists (see Chapter 20). Provocative tests using increasing doses of inhaled histamine are of diagnostic value for bronchial hyperreactivity in patients with suspected asthma or cystic fibrosis. Such individuals may be 100- to 1000-fold more sensitive to histamine than are normal subjects. Curiously, a few species (eg, rabbit) respond to histamine with bronchodilation, reflecting the dominance of the H_2 receptor in their airways.

4. Gastrointestinal tract smooth muscle—Histamine causes contraction of intestinal smooth muscle, and histamine-induced contraction of guinea pig ileum is a standard bioassay for this amine. The human gut is not as sensitive as that of the guinea pig, but large doses of histamine may cause diarrhea, partly as a result of this effect. This action of histamine is mediated by H_1 receptors.

5. Other smooth muscle organs—In humans, histamine generally has insignificant effects on the smooth muscle of the eye and genitourinary tract. However, pregnant women suffering anaphylactic reactions may abort as a result of histamine-induced contractions, and in some species the sensitivity of the uterus is sufficient to form the basis for a bioassay.

6. Secretory tissue—Histamine has long been recognized as a powerful stimulant of gastric acid secretion and, to a lesser extent, of gastric pepsin and intrinsic factor production. The effect is caused by activation of H_2 receptors on gastric parietal cells and is associated with increased adenylyl cyclase activity, cAMP concentration, and intracellular Ca^{2+} concentration. Other stimulants of gastric acid secretion such as acetylcholine and gastrin do not increase cAMP even though their maximal effects on acid output can be reduced—but not abolished—by H_2-receptor antagonists. These actions are discussed in detail in Chapter 63. Histamine also stimulates secretion in the small and large intestine. In contrast, H_3-selective histamine agonists *inhibit* acid secretion stimulated by food or pentagastrin in several species.

Histamine has much smaller effects on the activity of other glandular tissue at ordinary concentrations. Very high concentrations can cause adrenal medullary discharge.

7. Metabolic effects—Recent studies of H_3 receptor knockout mice demonstrate that absence of this receptor results in animals with increased food intake, decreased energy expenditure, and obesity. They also show insulin resistance and increased blood levels of leptin and insulin. It is not yet known whether the H_3 receptor has a similar role in humans.

8. The "triple response"—Intradermal injection of histamine causes a characteristic wheal-and-flare response that was first described over 60 years ago. The effect involves three separate cell types: smooth muscle in the microcirculation, capillary or venular endothelium, and sensory nerve endings. At the site of injection, a reddening appears owing to dilation of small vessels, followed soon by an edematous wheal at the injection site and a red irregular flare surrounding the wheal. The flare is said to be caused by an axon reflex. The sensation of itch may also accompany the appearance of these effects. The wheal is due to local edema.

Similar local effects may be produced by injecting histamine liberators (compound 48/80, morphine, etc) intradermally or by applying the appropriate antigens to the skin of a sensitized person. Although most of these local effects can be blocked by prior administration of an H_1 receptor-blocking agent, H_2 and H_3 receptors may also be involved.

9. Other effects possibly mediated by histamine receptors—In addition to the local stimulation of peripheral pain nerve endings via H_3 and H_1 receptors, histamine may play a role in nociception in the central nervous system. **Burimamide,** an early candidate for H_2 blocking action, and **improgan,** a newer analog with no effect on H_1, H_2, or H_3 receptors, have been shown to have significant analgesic action in rodents when administered into the central nervous system. The analgesia is said to be comparable to that produced by opioids, but tolerance, respiratory depression, and constipation have not been reported. Although the mechanism of this action is not known, these compounds may represent an important new class of analgesics.

Other Histamine Agonists

Small substitutions on the imidazole ring of histamine significantly modify the selectivity of the compounds for the histamine receptor subtypes. Some of these are listed in Table 16–1.

CLINICAL PHARMACOLOGY OF HISTAMINE

Clinical Uses

In pulmonary function laboratories, histamine aerosol (in addition to other agents) is sometimes used as a provocative test of **bronchial hyperreactivity.** Histamine has no other current clinical applications.

Toxicity & Contraindications

Adverse effects of histamine release, like those following administration of histamine, are dose-related. Flushing, hypotension, tachycardia, headache, wheals, bron-choconstriction, and gastrointestinal upset are noted. These effects are also observed after the ingestion of spoiled fish (scombroid fish poisoning), and there is evidence that histamine produced by bacterial action in the flesh of the fish is the major causative agent.

Histamine should not be given to asthmatics (except as part of a carefully monitored test of pulmonary function) or to patients with active ulcer disease or gastrointestinal bleeding.

HISTAMINE ANTAGONISTS

The effects of histamine released in the body can be reduced in several ways. **Physiologic antagonists,** especially epinephrine, have smooth muscle actions opposite to those of histamine, but they act at different receptors. This is important clinically because injection of epinephrine can be lifesaving in systemic **anaphylaxis** and in other conditions in which massive release of histamine—and other mediators—occurs.

Release inhibitors reduce the degranulation of mast cells that results from immunologic triggering by antigen-IgE interaction. Cromolyn and nedocromil appear to have this effect (see Chapter 20) and are used in the treatment of asthma, though the molecular mechanism underlying their action is presently unknown. Beta$_2$ adrenoceptor agonists also appear capable of reducing histamine release.

Histamine **receptor antagonists** represent a third approach to the reduction of histamine-mediated responses. For over 60 years, compounds have been available that competitively antagonize many of the actions of histamine on smooth muscle. However, not until the H_2 receptor antagonist burimamide was described in 1972 was it possible to antagonize the gastric acid-stimulating activity of histamine. The development of selective H_2 receptor antagonists has led not only to more precise definition of histamine's actions in terms of receptors involved but also to more effective therapy for peptic ulcer. Selective H_3 antagonists are not yet available for clinical use. However, potent and selective experimental H_3 receptor antagonists, thioperamide and clobenpropit, have been developed.

II. H$_1$ RECEPTOR ANTAGONISTS

Compounds that competitively block histamine at H_1 receptors have been used clinically for many years, and many H_1 antagonists are currently marketed in the USA. Many are available without prescription, both alone and in combination formulations such as "cold pills" and sleep aids (see Chapter 64).

BASIC PHARMACOLOGY OF H₁ RECEPTOR ANTAGONISTS

Chemistry & Pharmacokinetics

The H₁ antagonists are conveniently divided into first-generation and second-generation agents. These groups are distinguished by the relatively strong sedative effects of most of the first-generation drugs. The first-generation agents are also more likely to block autonomic receptors. The relatively less sedating characteristic of the second-generation H₁ blockers is due in part to their less complete distribution into the central nervous system. All of the H₁ antagonists are stable amines with the general structure illustrated in Figure 16–2. There are several chemical subgroups, and the structures of com-

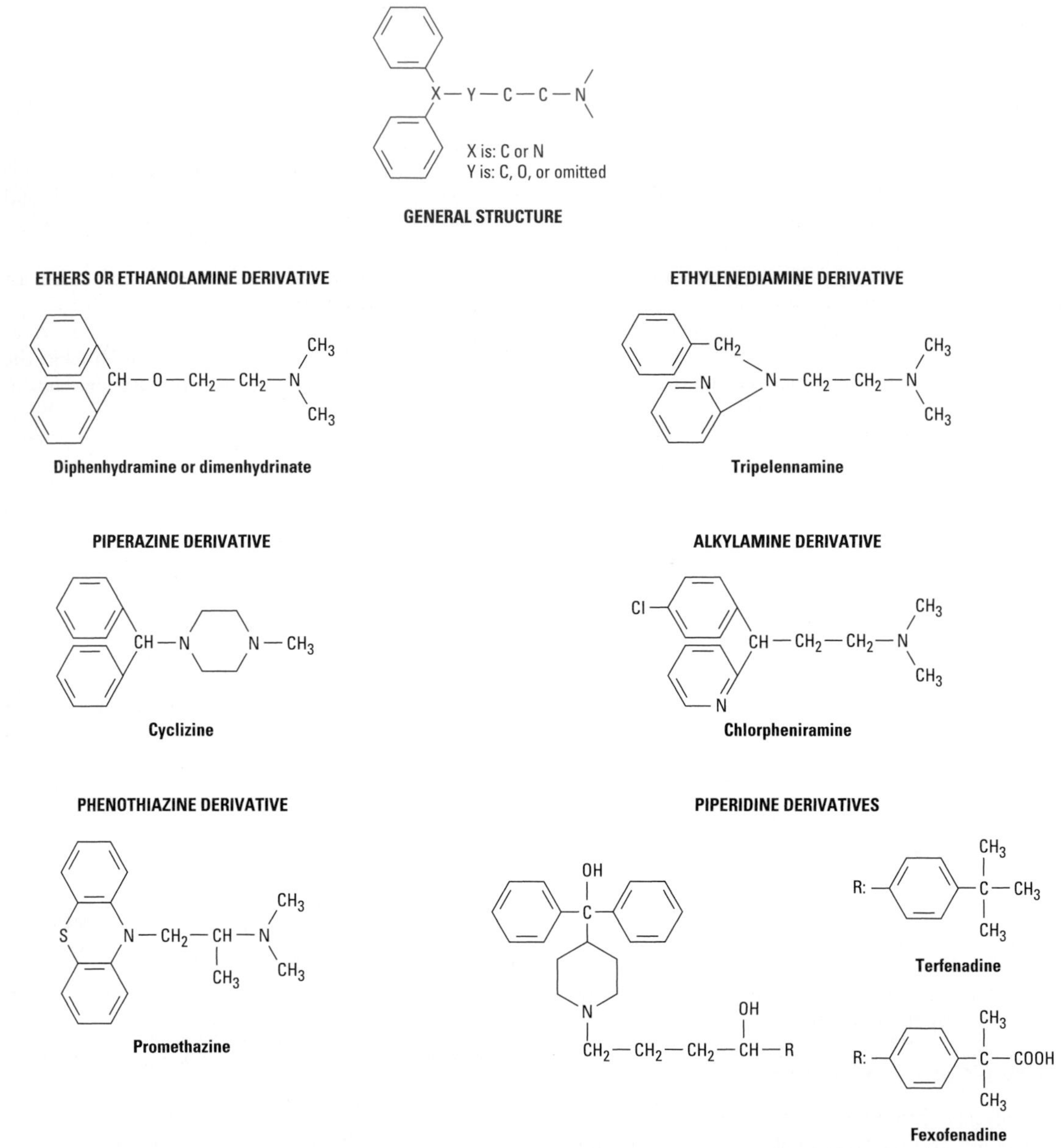

GENERAL STRUCTURE

X is: C or N
Y is: C, O, or omitted

ETHERS OR ETHANOLAMINE DERIVATIVE

Diphenhydramine or dimenhydrinate

ETHYLENEDIAMINE DERIVATIVE

Tripelennamine

PIPERAZINE DERIVATIVE

Cyclizine

ALKYLAMINE DERIVATIVE

Chlorpheniramine

PHENOTHIAZINE DERIVATIVE

Promethazine

PIPERIDINE DERIVATIVES

Terfenadine

Fexofenadine

Figure 16–2. General structure of H₁ antagonist drugs and examples of the major subgroups.

pounds representing different subgroups are shown in the figure. Doses of some of these drugs are given in Table 16–2.

These agents are rapidly absorbed following oral administration, with peak blood concentrations occur-

ring in 1–2 hours. They are widely distributed throughout the body, and the first-generation drugs enter the central nervous system readily. Some of them are extensively metabolized, primarily by microsomal systems in the liver. Several of the second-generation agents are

Table 16–2. Some H_1 antihistaminic drugs in past or current clinical use.

Drugs	Usual Adult Dose	Anti-cholinergic Activity	Comments
FIRST-GENERATION ANTIHISTAMINES			
Ethanolamines			
Carbinoxamine (Clistin)	4–8 mg	+++	Slight to moderate sedation
Dimenhydrinate (salt of diphenhydramine) (Dramamine)	50 mg	+++	Marked sedation; anti-motion sickness activity
Diphenhydramine (Benadryl, etc)	25–50 mg	+++	Marked sedation; anti-motion sickness activity
Doxylamine	1.25–25 mg	nd	Marked sedation; now available only in OTC "sleep aids"
Ethylaminediamines			
Pyrilamine (Neo-Antergan)	25–50 mg	+	Moderate sedation; component of OTC "sleep aids"
Tripelennamine (PBZ, etc)	25–50 mg	+	Moderate sedation
Piperazine derivatives			
Hydroxyzine (Atarax, etc)	15–100 mg	nd	Marked sedation
Cyclizine (Marezine)	25–50 mg	–	Slight sedation; anti-motion sickness activity
Meclizine (Bonine, etc)	25–50 mg	–	Slight sedation; anti-motion sickness activity
Alkylamines			
Brompheniramine (Dimetane, etc)	4–8 mg	+	Slight sedation
Chlorpheniramine (Chlor-Trimeton, etc)	4–8 mg	+	Slight sedation; common component of OTC "cold" medication
Phenothiazine derivatives			
Promethazine (Phenergan, etc)	10–25 mg	+++	Marked sedation; antiemetic
Miscellaneous			
Cyproheptadine (Periactin, etc)	4 mg	+	Moderate sedation; also has antiserotonin activity
SECOND-GENERATION ANTIHISTAMINES			
Piperidines			
Fexofenadine (Allegra)	60 mg	–	Lower risk of arrhythmia
Miscellaneous			
Loratadine (Claritin)	10 mg	–	Longer action
Cetirizine (Zyrtec)	5–10 mg	–	

Nd, no data found.

metabolized by the CYP3A4 system and thus are subject to important interactions when other drugs (such as ketoconazole) inhibit this subtype of P450 enzymes. Most of the drugs have an effective duration of action of 4–6 hours following a single dose, but meclizine and several second-generation agents are longer-acting, with a duration of action of 12–24 hours. The newer agents also are considerably less lipid-soluble and enter the central nervous system with difficulty or not at all. Many H_1 antagonists have active metabolites. The active metabolites of hydroxyzine, terfenadine, and loratadine are available as drugs (cetirizine, fexofenadine, and desloratadine, respectively).

Pharmacodynamics

A. HISTAMINE RECEPTOR BLOCKADE

H_1 receptor antagonists block the actions of histamine by reversible competitive antagonism at the H_1 receptor. They have negligible potency at the H_2 receptor and little at the H_3 receptor. For example, histamine-induced contraction of bronchiolar or gastrointestinal smooth muscle can be completely blocked by these agents, but the effects on gastric acid secretion and the heart are unmodified.

B. ACTIONS NOT CAUSED BY HISTAMINE RECEPTOR BLOCKADE

The first-generation H_1 receptor antagonists have many actions not ascribable to blockade of the actions of histamine. The large number of these actions probably results from the similarity of the general structure (Figure 16–2) to the structure of drugs that have effects at muscarinic cholinoceptor, α-adrenoceptor, serotonin, and local anesthetic receptor sites. Some of these actions are of therapeutic value and some are undesirable.

1. Sedation—A common effect of first-generation H_1 antagonists is sedation, but the intensity of this effect varies among chemical subgroups (Table 16–2) and among patients as well. The effect is sufficiently prominent with some agents to make them useful as "sleep aids" (see Chapter 64) and unsuitable for daytime use. The effect resembles that of some antimuscarinic drugs and is considered very unlike the disinhibited sedation produced by sedative-hypnotic drugs. Compulsive use has not been reported. At ordinary dosages, children occasionally (and adults rarely) manifest excitation rather than sedation. At very high toxic dose levels, marked stimulation, agitation, and even convulsions may precede coma. Second-generation H_1 antagonists have little or no sedative or stimulant actions. These drugs (or their active metabolites) also have far fewer autonomic effects than the first-generation antihistamines.

2. Antinausea and antiemetic actions—Several first-generation H_1 antagonists have significant activity in preventing motion sickness (Table 16–2). They are less effective against an episode of motion sickness already present. Certain H_1 antagonists, notably doxylamine (in Bendectin), were used widely in the past in the treatment of nausea and vomiting of pregnancy (see below).

3. Antiparkinsonism effects—Perhaps because of their anticholinergic effects (cf benztropine, Chapter 28), some of the H_1 antagonists have significant acute suppressant effects on the parkinsonism symptoms associated with certain antipsychotic drugs.

4. Anticholinoceptor actions—Many of the first-generation agents, especially those of the ethanolamine and ethylenediamine subgroups, have significant atropine-like effects on peripheral muscarinic receptors. This action may be responsible for some of the (uncertain) benefits reported for nonallergic rhinorrhea but may also cause urinary retention and blurred vision.

5. Adrenoceptor-blocking actions—Alpha receptor-blocking effects can be demonstrated for many H_1 antagonists, especially those in the phenothiazine subgroup, eg, promethazine. This action may cause orthostatic hypotension in susceptible individuals. Beta receptor blockade is not observed.

6. Serotonin-blocking action—Strong blocking effects at serotonin receptors have been demonstrated for some first-generation H_1 antagonists, notably cyproheptadine. This drug is promoted as an antiserotonin agent and is discussed with that drug group. Nevertheless, its structure resembles that of the phenothiazine antihistamines, and it is a potent H_1 blocking agent.

7. Local anesthesia—Many first-generation H_1 antagonists are potent local anesthetics. They block sodium channels in excitable membranes in the same fashion as procaine and lidocaine. Diphenhydramine and promethazine are actually more potent than procaine as local anesthetics. They are occasionally used to produce local anesthesia in patients allergic to the conventional local anesthetic drugs. A small number of these agents also block potassium channels; this action is discussed below (see Toxicity).

8. Other actions—Certain H_1 antagonists, eg, cetirizine, inhibit mast cell release of histamine and some other mediators of inflammation. This action is not due to H_1 receptor blockade. The mechanism is not understood but could play a role in the beneficial effects of these drugs in the treatment of allergies such as rhinitis. A few H_1 antagonists (eg, terfenadine, acrivastine) have been shown to inhibit the P-glycoprotein transporter found in cancer cells, the epithelium of the gut, and the capillaries of the brain. The significance of this effect is not known.

CLINICAL PHARMACOLOGY OF H₁ RECEPTOR ANTAGONISTS

Clinical Uses

A. ALLERGIC REACTIONS

The H₁ antihistaminic agents are often the first drugs used to prevent or treat the symptoms of allergic reactions. In allergic rhinitis and urticaria, in which histamine is the primary mediator, the H₁ antagonists are the drugs of choice and are often quite effective. However, in bronchial asthma, which involves several mediators, the H₁ antagonists are largely ineffective.

Angioedema may be precipitated by histamine release but appears to be maintained by peptide kinins that are not affected by antihistaminic agents. For atopic dermatitis, antihistaminic drugs such as diphenhydramine are used mostly for their sedative side effects and for some control of the itching.

The H₁ antihistamines used for treating allergic conditions such as hay fever are usually selected with the goal of minimizing sedative effects; in the USA, the drugs in widest use are the alkylamines and the second-generation nonsedating agents. However, the sedative effect and the therapeutic efficacy of different agents vary widely among individuals. In addition, the clinical effectiveness of one group may diminish with continued use, and switching to another group may restore drug effectiveness for as yet unexplained reasons.

The second-generation H₁ antagonists are used mainly for the treatment of allergic rhinitis and chronic urticaria. Several double-blind comparisons with older agents (such as chlorpheniramine) indicated about equal therapeutic efficacy. However, sedation and interference with safe operation of machinery, which occur in about 50% of subjects taking first-generation antihistamines, occurred in only about 7% of subjects taking second generation agents. The newer drugs are much more expensive.

B. MOTION SICKNESS AND VESTIBULAR DISTURBANCES

Scopolamine and certain first-generation H₁ antagonists are the most effective agents available for the prevention of motion sickness. The antihistaminic drugs with the greatest effectiveness in this application are diphenhydramine and promethazine. Dimenhydrinate, which is promoted for the treatment of motion sickness, is a salt of diphenhydramine. The piperazines (cyclizine and meclizine) also have significant activity in preventing motion sickness and are less sedative in most patients. Dosage is the same as that recommended for allergic disorders (Table 16–2). Both scopolamine and the H₁ antagonists are more effective in preventing motion sickness when combined with ephedrine or amphetamine.

It has been claimed that the antihistaminic agents effective in prophylaxis of motion sickness are also useful in Meniere's syndrome, but efficacy in the latter application is not well established.

C. NAUSEA AND VOMITING OF PREGNANCY

Several H₁ antagonist drugs have been studied for possible use in treating "morning sickness." The piperazine derivatives were withdrawn from such use when it was demonstrated that they have teratogenic effects in rodents. Doxylamine, an ethanolamine H₁ antagonist, was promoted for this application as a component of Bendectin, a prescription medication that also contained pyridoxine. Possible teratogenic effects of doxylamine were widely publicized in the lay press after 1978 as a result of a few case reports of fetal malformation associated with maternal ingestion of Bendectin. However, several large prospective studies involving over 60,000 pregnancies, of which more than 3000 involved maternal Bendectin ingestion, disclosed no increase in the incidence of birth defects. However, because of the continuing controversy, adverse publicity, and lawsuits, the manufacturer of Bendectin withdrew the product from the market. Doxylamine is still available over-the-counter as a sleep aid.

Toxicity

The wide spectrum of adverse effects of the H₁ antihistamines is described above. Several of these effects (sedation, antimuscarinic action) have been used for therapeutic purposes, especially in OTC remedies (see Chapter 64). Nevertheless, these two effects constitute the most common undesirable actions when these drugs are used to block histamine receptors.

Less common toxic effects of systemic use include excitation and convulsions in children, postural hypotension, and allergic responses. Drug allergy is relatively common after topical use of H₁ antagonists. The effects of severe systemic overdosage of the older agents resemble those of atropine overdosage and are treated in the same way (see Chapters 8 and 59). Overdosage of astemizole or terfenadine may induce cardiac arrhythmias, but these drugs are no longer marketed in the USA; the same effect may be caused by interaction with enzyme inhibitors (see Drug Interactions, below).

Drug Interactions

Lethal ventricular arrhythmias occurred in several patients taking either of the early second-generation agents, terfenadine or astemizole, in combination with ketoconazole, itraconazole, or macrolide antibiotics such as erythromycin. These antimicrobial drugs inhibit the metabolism of many drugs by CYP3A4 and cause significant increases in blood concentrations of the antihistamines. The mechanism of this toxicity involves blockade of the potassium channels in the heart that are responsible for repolarization of the action potential, the I_K channels (see Chapter 14). The result is prolongation of the action potential, and excessive prolongation leads to arrhythmias. Both terfenadine and astemizole were withdrawn from the United States market in recognition of these problems. Where still available, terfenadine and astemizole should be considered to be contraindicated in patients taking ketoconazole, itraconazole, or macrolides and in patients with liver disease. Grapefruit juice also inhibits CYP3A4 and has been shown to increase terfenadine's blood levels significantly.

For those H_1 antagonists that cause significant sedation, concurrent use of other drugs that cause central nervous system depression produces additive effects and is contraindicated while driving or operating machinery. Similarly, the autonomic blocking effects of older antihistamines are additive with those of muscarinic and α-blocking drugs.

III. H₂ RECEPTOR ANTAGONISTS

The development of H_2 receptor antagonists was based on the observation that H_1 antagonists had no effect on histamine-induced acid secretion in the stomach. Molecular manipulation of the histamine molecule resulted in a compound that blocked rather than stimulated acid production and then a series of drugs with progressive increases in the acid secretion-blocking action and reduction in irrelevant effects. This development led to renewed interest in possible physiologic roles for histamine and to a classification of effects of both agonists and antagonists based upon histamine receptor subtypes. The high incidence of peptic ulcer disease and related gastrointestinal complaints created great interest in the therapeutic potential of H_2 receptor antagonists. Because of the ability of this class of drugs to reduce gastric acid secretion and their low toxicity, they are now among the most frequently used drugs in the USA and have become OTC items. These drugs are discussed in Chapter 63.

IV. SEROTONIN (5-HYDROXY-TRYPTAMINE)

Before the identification of 5-hydroxytryptamine (5-HT), it was known that when blood is allowed to clot, a vasoconstrictor (tonic) substance is released from the clot into the serum; this substance was called serotonin. Independent studies established the existence of a smooth muscle stimulant in intestinal mucosa; this was called enteramine. The synthesis of 5-hydroxytryptamine in 1951 permitted the identification of serotonin and enteramine as the same metabolite of 5-hydroxytryptophan.

Serotonin is thought to play a role in migraine headache. Serotonin is also one of the mediators of the signs and symptoms of carcinoid syndrome, an unusual manifestation of carcinoid tumor, a neoplasm of enterochromaffin cells. In patients whose tumor is not operable, serotonin antagonists may constitute the best treatment.

BASIC PHARMACOLOGY OF SEROTONIN

Chemistry & Pharmacokinetics

Like histamine, serotonin is widely distributed in nature, being found in plant and animal tissues, venoms, and stings. It is an indoleethylamine formed in biologic systems from the amino acid L-tryptophan by hydroxylation of the indole ring followed by decarboxylation of the amino acid (Figure 16–3). Hydroxylation at C5 is the rate-limiting step and can be blocked by p-chlorophenylalanine (PCPA; fenclonine) and by p-chloroamphetamine. These agents have been used experimentally to reduce serotonin synthesis in carcinoid syndrome.

After synthesis, the free amine is stored or is rapidly inactivated, usually by oxidation catalyzed by the enzyme monoamine oxidase. In the pineal gland, serotonin serves as a precursor of melatonin, a melanocyte-stimulating hormone. In mammals (including humans), over 90% of the serotonin in the body is found in enterochromaffin cells in the gastrointestinal tract. In the blood, serotonin is found in platelets, which are able to concentrate the amine by means of an active carrier mechanism similar to that in the vesicles of noradrenergic and serotonergic nerve endings. Serotonin is also found in the raphe nuclei of the brain stem, which contain cell bodies of serotonergic neurons that synthesize, store, and release serotonin as a transmitter. Brain serotonergic neurons are involved in various functions such as mood, sleep, appetite, temperature regulation, the perception of pain, the regulation of blood pressure, and vomiting (see Chapter 21). Serotonin also appears to be involved in conditions such as depression, anxiety, and migraine. Serotonergic neurons are also found in the enteric nervous system of the gastrointestinal tract and around blood vessels. In rodents (but not in humans), serotonin is found in mast cells.

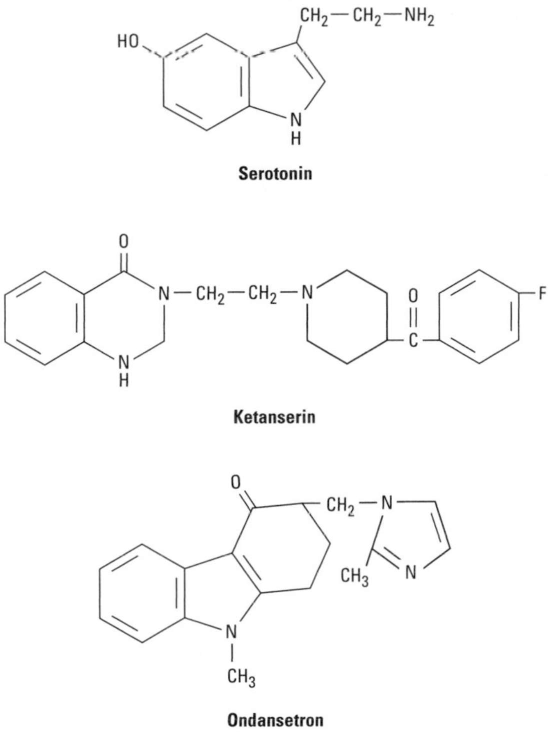

Figure 16–3. Structures of serotonin and two 5-HT-receptor blockers.

The function of serotonin in enterochromaffin cells is not clear. These cells synthesize serotonin, store the amine in a complex with ATP and with other substances in granules, and can release serotonin in response to mechanical and neuronal stimuli. Some of the released serotonin diffuses into blood vessels and is taken up and stored in platelets.

Stored serotonin can be depleted by **reserpine** in much the same manner as this drug depletes catecholamines from vesicles in adrenergic nerves (see Chapter 6).

Serotonin is metabolized by monoamine oxidase, and the intermediate product, 5-hydroxyindoleacetaldehyde, is further oxidized by aldehyde dehydrogenase to 5-hydroxyindoleacetic acid (5-HIAA). In humans consuming a normal diet, the excretion of 5-HIAA is a measure of serotonin synthesis. Therefore, the 24-hour excretion of 5-HIAA can be used as a diagnostic test for tumors that synthesize excessive quantities of serotonin, especially carcinoid tumor. A few foods (eg, bananas) contain large amounts of serotonin or its precursors and must be prohibited during such diagnostic tests.

Pharmacodynamics

A. MECHANISMS OF ACTION

Serotonin exerts many actions and, like histamine, has many species differences, making generalizations difficult. The actions of serotonin are mediated through a remarkably large number of cell membrane receptors. The serotonin receptors that have been characterized thus far are described in Table 16–3. Seven families of 5-HT-receptor subtypes (those given numeric subscripts 1 through 7) have been identified, six involving G protein-coupled receptors and one a ligand-gated ion channel. Among these receptor subtypes, several lack any recognized physiologic function. Discovery of these functions awaits the development of subtype-selective drugs or the mutation or deletion of genes encoding these receptors from the mouse genome.

B. TISSUE AND ORGAN SYSTEM EFFECTS

1. Nervous system—Serotonin is present in a variety of sites in the brain. Its role as a neurotransmitter and its relation to the actions of drugs acting in the central nervous system are discussed in Chapters 21 and 30. Serotonin is also a precursor of melatonin (see Chapter 65).

$5-HT_3$ receptors in the gastrointestinal tract and in the vomiting center of the medulla participate in the vomiting reflex (see Chapter 63). They are particularly important in vomiting caused by chemical triggers such as cancer chemotherapy drugs. $5-HT_{1P}$ and $5-HT_4$ receptors also play a role in enteric nervous system function.

Like histamine, serotonin is a potent stimulant of pain and itch sensory nerve endings and is responsible for some of the symptoms caused by insect and plant stings. In addition, serotonin is a powerful activator of chemosensitive endings located in the coronary vascular bed. Activation of $5-HT_3$ receptors on these afferent vagal nerve endings is associated with the **chemoreceptor reflex** (also known as the Bezold-Jarisch reflex). The reflex response consists of marked bradycardia and hypotension. The bradycardia is mediated by vagal outflow to the heart and can be blocked by atropine. The hypotension is a consequence of the decrease in cardiac output that results from bradycardia. A variety of other agents can activate the chemoreceptor reflex. These include nicotinic cholinoceptor agonists and some cardiac glycosides, eg, ouabain.

2. Airways—Serotonin has a small direct stimulant effect on bronchiolar smooth muscle in normal humans. It also appears to facilitate acetylcholine release from bronchial vagal nerve endings. In patients with carcinoid syndrome, episodes of bronchoconstriction occur in response to elevated levels of the amine or peptides released from the tumor. Serotonin may also cause

Table 16–3. Serotonin receptor subtypes.

Receptor Subtype	Distribution	Postreceptor Mechanism	Partially Selective Agonists	Partially Selective Antagonists
5-HT$_{1A}$	Raphe nuclei, hippocampus	Multiple, G$_i$ coupling dominates	8-OH-DPAT	WAY100635
5-HT$_{1B}$	Substantia nigra, globus pallidus, basal ganglia	G$_i$, ↓ cAMP	CP93129	
5-HT$_{1Da,b}$	Brain	G$_i$, ↓ cAMP	Sumatriptan	
5-HT$_{1E}$	Cortex, putamen	G$_i$, ↓ cAMP		
5-HT$_{1F}$	Cortex, hippocampus	G$_i$, ↓ cAMP		
5-HT$_{1P}$	Enteric nervous system	G$_o$; slow EPSP	5-Hydroxyindalpine	Renzapride
5-HT$_{2A}$	Platelets, smooth muscle, cerebral cortex, skeletal muscle	G$_q$, ↑ IP$_3$	α-Methyl-5-HT	Ketanserin
5-HT$_{2B}$	Stomach fundus	G$_q$, ↑ IP$_3$	α-Methyl-5-HT	SB204741
5-HT$_{2C}$	Choroid, hippocampus, substantia nigra	G$_q$, ↑ IP$_3$	α-Methyl-5-HT	Mesulergine
5-HT$_3$	Area postrema, sensory and enteric nerves	Receptor is a Na$^+$-K$^+$ ion channel	2-Methyl-5-HT, *m*-chlorophenylbiguanide	Tropisetron, ondansetron, granisetron
5-HT$_4$	CNS and myenteric neurons, smooth muscle	G$_s$, ↑ cAMP	5-Methoxytryptamine, renzapride, metoclopramide	
5-HT$_{5A,B}$	Brain	↓ cAMP		
5-HT$_{6,7}$	Brain	G$_s$, ↑ cAMP		Clozapine (5-HT$_7$)

8-OH-DPAT = 8-Hydroxy-2-(di-*n*-propylamine)tetralin; CP93129 = 5-Hydroxy-3(4-1,2,5,6-tetrahydropyridyl)-4-azaindole; SB204741 = *N*-(1-methyl-5-indolyl)-*N'*-(3-methyl-5-isothiazolyl)urea; WAY100635 = *N-tert*-Butyl 3-4-(2-methoxyphenyl) piperazin-1-yl-2-phenylpropanamide

hyperventilation as a result of the chemoreceptor reflex or stimulation of bronchial sensory nerve endings.

3. Cardiovascular system—Serotonin directly causes the contraction of vascular smooth muscle, mainly through 5-HT$_2$ receptors. In humans, serotonin is a powerful vasoconstrictor except in skeletal muscle and heart, where it dilates blood vessels. At least part of this 5-HT-induced vasodilation requires the presence of vascular endothelial cells. When the endothelium is damaged, coronary vessels constrict. As noted previously, serotonin can also elicit reflex bradycardia by activation of 5-HT$_3$ receptors on chemoreceptor nerve endings. A

triphasic blood pressure response is often seen following injection of serotonin. Initially, there is a decrease in heart rate, cardiac output, and blood pressure caused by the chemoreceptor response. Following this decrease, blood pressure increases as a result of vasoconstriction. The third phase is again a decrease in blood pressure attributed to vasodilation in vessels supplying skeletal muscle. Pulmonary and renal vessels seem especially sensitive to the vasoconstrictor action of serotonin.

Serotonin also constricts veins, and venoconstriction with a resulting increased capillary filling appears responsible for the flush that is observed following serotonin administration. Serotonin has small direct positive chronotropic and inotropic effects on the heart that are probably of no clinical significance. However, prolonged elevation of the blood level of serotonin (which occurs in carcinoid syndrome) is associated with pathologic alterations in the endocardium (subendocardial fibroplasia) that may result in valvular or electrical malfunction.

Serotonin causes blood platelets to aggregate by activating surface 5-HT$_2$ receptors. This response, in contrast to aggregation induced during clot formation, is not accompanied by the release of serotonin stored in the platelets. The physiologic role of this effect is unclear.

4. Gastrointestinal tract—Serotonin is a powerful stimulant of gastrointestinal smooth muscle, increasing tone and facilitating peristalsis. This action is caused by the direct action of serotonin on 5-HT$_2$ smooth muscle receptors plus a stimulating action on ganglion cells located in the enteric nervous system (see Chapter 6). Activation of 5-HT$_4$ receptors in the ENS causes increased acetylcholine release and thereby mediates a motility-enhancing or "prokinetic" effect of selective serotonin agonists such as cisapride. These agents are useful in several gastrointestinal disorders (see Chapter 63). Overproduction of serotonin (and other substances) in carcinoid tumor is associated with severe diarrhea. Serotonin has little effect on secretions, and what effects it has are generally inhibitory.

5. Skeletal muscle—5-HT$_2$ receptors are present on skeletal muscle membranes, but their physiologic role is not understood. **Malignant hyperthermia** is a condition precipitated by certain anesthetic and neuromuscular agents that results in severe hyperthermia due to skeletal muscle overactivity and metabolic and autonomic instability. In a genetic porcine model of this condition, administration of serotonin or serotonin agonists can precipitate a typical attack. 5-HT$_2$ blockers such as ketanserin can reduce or prevent many manifestations of the condition when evoked in this way. However, malignant hyperthermia provoked by anesthetic agents in these animals is not effectively prevented by 5-HT$_2$ antagonists. **Serotonin syndrome** is a similar but not identical condition precipitated when MAO inhibitors are given with serotonin agonists, especially antidepressants of the selective serotonin reuptake inhibitor class (SSRIs).

CLINICAL PHARMACOLOGY OF SEROTONIN

SEROTONIN AGONISTS

Serotonin has no clinical applications as a drug. However, several receptor subtype-selective agonists have

---

APPETITE CONTROL THROUGH SEROTONIN?

As noted in the text, serotonin appears to be related to several general behaviors such as sleep, emotion, sex, and appetite, and early studies with the amine suggested that it could reduce food intake in animals, an anorexigenic effect.

Fenfluramine, a racemic chemical more closely related to amphetamine than to serotonin, affects brain levels of serotonin and its metabolites at relatively low doses. It was introduced as an anorexigenic drug almost 20 years ago. Its *d*- isomer, *d*-fenfluramine (**dexfenfluramine, Redux**) was about twice as potent as fenfluramine. After several controlled clinical trials demonstrated that dexfenfluramine could help patients maintain weight loss for at least a year, it was quickly introduced into the market in the USA and became a best-selling drug overnight.

Dexfenfluramine caused serotonin release and inhibited reuptake at moderately low concentrations. It also stimulated 5-HT receptors at relatively low concentrations. Metergoline, an ergot derivative with high affinity for 5-HT receptors, completely blocked the anorexian effect of dexfenfluramine, further suggesting a serotonergic action.

Unfortunately, after the introduction of the drug, several cases of fatal and nonfatal pulmonary hypertension were reported in individuals with no known risk factor for this devastating condition other than consumption of dexfenfluramine. These reports were followed by reports of valvular lesions appearing in young women with a similar lack of risk factors other than the consumption of weight-loss products. Assignment of causality was somewhat slowed by the fact that dexfenfluramine was usually used in combination with a much older amphetamine-like anorexiant, phentermine. (This combination was known as "Fen-Phen.") It soon became clear that the valvular lesions fell into the same class of drug-induced pathology as that caused by chronic ergot treatment for migraine (endocardial fibroplasia, retroperitoneal fibroplasia). These effects appear to be associated with 5-HT agonist action. Dexfenfluramine was withdrawn but not before multiple lawsuits had been filed against the manufacturer. Unfortunately, some weight loss clinics now recommend the combination of the antidepressant fluoxetine (Prozac) with phentermine, a combination known as "Phen-Pro."

proved to be of value. **Buspirone**, a 5-HT$_{1A}$ agonist, has received wide attention for its utility as an effective non-benzodiazepine anxiolytic (see Chapter 22). **Dexfenfluramine**, another selective 5-HT agonist, was widely used as an appetite suppressant (see Box, Appetite Control Through Serotonin?) but was withdrawn because of toxicity. Sumatriptan and its congeners are agonists effective in the treatment of acute migraine and cluster headache attacks (see below).

5-HT$_{1D}$ Agonists

Sumatriptan and several other "triptans" are selective agonists for 5-HT$_{1D}$ and 5-HT$_{1B}$ receptors. These receptor types are found in cerebral and meningeal vessels and mediate vasoconstriction. They are also found on neurons and probably function as presynaptic inhibitory receptors. These drugs have proved to be very effective in the treatment of acute migraine headache. The mechanism of action is discussed in more detail below under Clinical Pharmacology of Ergot Alkaloids.

The bioavailability of sumatriptan is only about 15%, but the other agents in the group have availabilities of 40–80%. Sumatriptan, almotriptan, eletriptan, rizatriptan, and zolmitriptan have half-lives of 2–3 hours, while the half-life of naratriptan is 6 hours and that of frovatriptan more than 25 hours. Sumatriptan can be administered subcutaneously by self-injection, as a nasal spray, or orally. The other members of the group are available only for oral administration.

The efficacy of 5-HT$_1$ agonists in migraine is equal to or greater than that of other drug treatments, eg, parenteral or oral ergot alkaloids. Most adverse effects are mild and include altered sensations (tingling, warmth, etc), dizziness, muscle weakness, neck pain, and injection site reactions. Chest discomfort occurs in 1–5% of patients, and chest pain has been reported, probably because of the ability of these drugs to cause coronary vasospasm. They are therefore contraindicated in patients with coronary artery disease and in patients with angina. Another disadvantage is the fact that their duration of effect (especially that of almotriptan, sumatriptan, rizatriptan, and zolmitriptan) is often shorter than the duration of the headache. As a result, several doses may be required during a prolonged migraine attack. In addition, these drugs are extremely expensive at present. Naratriptan and eletriptan are contraindicated in patients with severe hepatic or renal impairment or peripheral vascular syndromes; frovatriptan in patients with peripheral vascular disease; and zolmitriptan in patients with Wolff-Parkinson-White syndrome.

Other Serotonin Agonists in Clinical Use

Cisapride, a 5-HT$_4$ agonist, was used in the treatment of gastroesophageal reflux and motility disorders. Because of toxicity, it is now available only for compassionate use in the USA. **Tegaserod**, a newer 5-HT$_4$ partial agonist, is used for irritable bowel syndrome with constipation. These drugs are discussed in Chapter 63.

Compounds such as fluoxetine and other serotonin-selective reuptake inhibitors, which modulate serotonergic transmission by blocking reuptake of the transmitter, are among the most widely prescribed drugs for the management of depression and other behavioral disorders. These drugs are discussed in Chapter 30.

SEROTONIN ANTAGONISTS

The actions of serotonin, like those of histamine, can be antagonized in several different ways. Such antagonism is clearly desirable in those rare patients who have carcinoid tumor and may also be valuable in certain other conditions.

As noted above, serotonin synthesis can be inhibited by p-chlorophenylalanine and p-chloroamphetamine. However, these agents are too toxic for general use. Storage of serotonin can be inhibited by the use of reserpine, but the sympatholytic effects of this drug (see Chapter 11) and the high levels of circulating serotonin that result from release prevent its use in carcinoid. Therefore, receptor blockade is the major approach to therapeutic limitation of serotonin effects.

SEROTONIN RECEPTOR ANTAGONISTS

A wide variety of drugs with actions at other receptors (α adrenoceptors, H$_1$ histamine receptors, etc) are also serotonin receptor-blocking agents. **Phenoxybenzamine** (see Chapter 10) has a long-lasting blocking action at 5-HT$_2$ receptors. In addition, the ergot alkaloids discussed in the last portion of the chapter are partial agonists at serotonin receptors.

Cyproheptadine resembles the phenothiazine antihistaminic agents in chemical structure and has potent H$_1$ receptor-blocking as well as 5-HT$_2$-blocking actions. The actions of cyproheptadine are predictable from its H$_1$ histamine and serotonin receptor affinities. It prevents the smooth muscle effects of both amines but has no effect on the gastric secretion stimulated by histamine. It has significant antimuscarinic effects and causes sedation.

The major clinical applications of cyproheptadine are in the treatment of the smooth muscle manifestations of carcinoid tumor and in the postgastrectomy dumping syndrome. It is also the preferred drug in cold-induced urticaria. The usual dosage in adults is 12–16 mg/d in three or four divided doses.

Ketanserin (Figure 16–3) blocks 5-HT$_{1c}$ and 5-HT$_2$ receptors and has little or no reported antagonist activity at other 5-HT or H$_1$ receptors. However, this drug potently blocks vascular α$_1$ adrenoceptors. The drug blocks 5-HT$_2$ receptors on platelets and antagonizes platelet aggregation promoted by serotonin. The mechanism involved in ketanserin's hypotensive action is not clear but probably involves α_1 adrenoceptors more than 5-HT$_2$ receptors. Ketanserin is available in Europe for the treatment of hypertension and vasospastic conditions but has not been approved in the USA.

Ritanserin, another 5-HT$_2$ antagonist, has little or no α-blocking action. It has been reported to alter bleeding time and to reduce thromboxane formation, presumably by altering platelet function.

Ondansetron (Figure 16–3) is the prototypical 5-HT$_3$ antagonist. This drug and its analogs are very important in the prevention of nausea and vomiting associated with surgery and cancer chemotherapy. They are discussed in Chapter 63.

Considering the diverse effects attributed to serotonin and the heterogeneous nature of 5-HT receptors, other selective 5-HT antagonists may prove to be clinically useful.

V. THE ERGOT ALKALOIDS

Ergot alkaloids are produced by *Claviceps purpurea,* a fungus that infects grain—especially rye—under damp growing or storage conditions. This fungus synthesizes histamine, acetylcholine, tyramine, and other biologically active products in addition to a score or more of unique ergot alkaloids. These alkaloids affect α adrenoceptors, dopamine receptors, 5-HT receptors, and perhaps other receptor types. Similar alkaloids are produced by fungi parasitic to a number of other grass-like plants.

The accidental ingestion of ergot alkaloids in contaminated grain can be traced back more than 2000 years from descriptions of epidemics of ergot poisoning (**ergotism**). The most dramatic effects of poisoning are dementia with florid hallucinations; prolonged vasospasm, which may result in gangrene; and stimulation of uterine smooth muscle, which in pregnancy may result in abortion. In medieval times, ergot poisoning was called **St. Anthony's fire** after the saint whose help was sought in relieving the burning pain of vasospastic ischemia. Identifiable epidemics have occurred sporadically up to modern times (see Box, Ergot Poisoning: Not Just an Ancient Disease) and mandate continuous surveillance of all grains used for food. Poisoning of grazing animals is common in many areas because the same and related fungi may grow on pasture grasses.

In addition to the effects noted above, the ergot alkaloids produce a variety of other central nervous system and peripheral effects. Detailed structure-activity analysis and appropriate semisynthetic modifications have yielded a large number of agents with documented or potential clinical value.

BASIC PHARMACOLOGY OF ERGOT ALKALOIDS

Chemistry & Pharmacokinetics

Two major families of compounds that incorporate the tetracyclic **ergoline** nucleus may be identified; the amine alkaloids and the peptide alkaloids (Table 16–4). Drugs of therapeutic and toxicologic importance are found in both groups.

The ergot alkaloids are variably absorbed from the gastrointestinal tract. The oral dose of ergotamine is about ten times larger than the intramuscular dose, but the speed of absorption and peak blood levels after oral administration can be improved by administration with caffeine (see below). The amine alkaloids are also absorbed from the rectum and the buccal cavity and after administration by aerosol inhaler. Absorption after intramuscular injection is slow but usually reliable. Bromocriptine and the amine derivative cabergoline are well absorbed from the gastrointestinal tract.

The ergot alkaloids are extensively metabolized in the body. The primary metabolites are hydroxylated in the A ring, and peptide alkaloids are also modified in the peptide moiety.

Pharmacodynamics

A. MECHANISM OF ACTION

As suggested above, the ergot alkaloids act on several types of receptors. Their effects include agonist, partial agonist, and antagonist actions at α adrenoceptors and serotonin receptors (especially 5-HT$_{1A}$ and 5-HT$_{1D}$; less for 5-HT$_{1C}$, 5-HT$_2$, and 5-HT$_3$); and agonist or partial agonist actions at central nervous system dopamine receptors (Table 16–5). Furthermore, some members of the ergot family have a high affinity for presynaptic receptors, while others are more selective for postjunctional receptors. There is a powerful stimulant effect on the uterus that seems to be most closely associated with agonist or partial agonist effects at 5-HT$_2$ receptors. Structural variations increase the selectivity of certain members of the family for specific receptor types.

B. ORGAN SYSTEM EFFECTS

1. Central nervous system—As indicated by traditional descriptions of ergotism, certain of the naturally occurring alkaloids are powerful hallucinogens. Lysergic acid diethylamide (LSD; "acid") is a synthetic ergot compound that clearly demonstrates this action. The drug has been used in the laboratory as a potent periph-

ERGOT POISONING: NOT JUST AN ANCIENT DISEASE

As noted in the text, epidemics of ergotism, or poisoning by ergot-contaminated grain, are known to have occurred sporadically in ancient times and through the Middle Ages. It is easy to imagine the social chaos that might result if fiery pain, gangrene, hallucinations, convulsions, and abortions occurred simultaneously throughout a community in which all or most of the people believed in witchcraft, demonic possession, and the visitation of supernatural punishments upon humans for their misdeeds. Such beliefs are uncommon in most cultures today. However, ergotism has not disappeared. A most convincing demonstration of ergotism occurred in the small French village of Pont-Saint-Esprit in 1951. It was described in the British Medical Journal in 1951 (Gabbai et al, 1951) and in a later book-length narrative account (Fuller, 1968). Several hundred individuals suffered symptoms of hallucinations, convulsions, and ischemia—and several died—after eating bread made from contaminated flour. Similar events have occurred even more recently when poverty, famine, or incompetence resulted in the consumption of contaminated grain.

Iatrogenic ergot toxicity caused by excessive use of medical ergot preparations is still frequently reported.

Table 16–4. Major ergoline derivatives (ergot alkaloids).

Amine alkaloids							
	R_1	R_8			R_2	R_2'	R_5'
6-Methylergoline	—H	—H					
Lysergic acid	—H	—COOH		Ergotamine[1]	—H	—CH_3	—CH_2—
Lysergic acid diethylamide (LSD)	—H	—C(=O)—$N(CH_2$—$CH_3)_2$		α-Ergocryptine	—H	—$CH(CH_3)_2$	—CH_2—$CH(CH_3)_2$
Ergonovine (ergometrine)	—H	—C(=O)—$NHCHCH_3$ (CH_2OH)		Bromocriptine	—Br	—$CH(CH_3)_2$	—CH_2—$CH(CH_3)_2$
Methysergide	—CH_3	—C(=O)—NH—CH(CH_2OH)—CH_2—CH_3					

[1]Dihydroergotamine lacks the double bond between carbons 9 and 10.

Table 16–5. Effects of ergot alkaloids at several receptors.[1]

Ergot Alkaloid	α Adrenoceptor	Dopamine Receptor	Serotonin Receptor (5-HT$_2$)	Uterine Smooth Muscle Stimulation
Bromocriptine	–	+++	–	0
Ergonovine	+	+	– (PA)	+++
Ergotamine	– – (PA)	0	+ (PA)	+++
Lysergic acid diethylamide (LSD)	0	+++	– – ++ in CNS	+
Methysergide	+/0	+/0	– – – (PA)	+/0

[1]Agonist effects are indicated by +, antagonist by –, no effect by 0. Relative affinity for the receptor is indicated by the number of + or – signs. PA means partial agonist (both agonist and antagonist effects can be detected).

eral 5-HT$_2$ antagonist, but good evidence suggests that its behavioral effects are mediated by *agonist* effects at prejunctional or postjunctional 5-HT$_2$ receptors in the central nervous system. In spite of extensive research, no clinical value has been discovered for LSD's dramatic effects. Abuse of this drug has waxed and waned but is still widespread. It is discussed in Chapter 32.

Dopamine receptors in the central nervous system play important roles in extrapyramidal motor control and the regulation of prolactin release. The actions of the peptide ergoline **bromocriptine** on the extrapyramidal system are discussed in Chapter 28. Of all the currently available ergot derivatives, bromocriptine, **cabergoline,**

and **pergolide** have the highest selectivity for the pituitary dopamine receptors. These drugs directly suppress prolactin secretion from pituitary cells by activating regulatory dopamine receptors (Chapter 37). They compete for binding to these sites with dopamine itself and with other dopamine agonists such as apomorphine.

2. Vascular smooth muscle—The action of ergot alkaloids on vascular smooth muscle is drug-, species-, and vessel-dependent, so few generalizations are possible. Ergotamine and related compounds constrict most human blood vessels in a predictable, prolonged, and potent manner (Figure 16–4). This response is partially

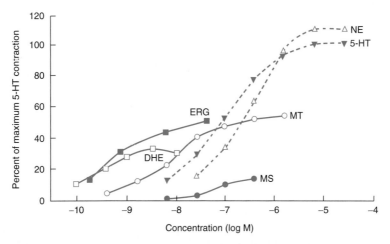

Figure 16–4. Effects of ergot derivatives on contraction of isolated segments of human basilar artery strips removed at surgery. All of the ergot derivatives are partial agonists, and all are more potent than the full agonists, norepinephrine and serotonin. (NE, norepinephrine; 5-HT, serotonin; ERG, ergotamine; MT, methylergometrine; DHE, dihydroergotamine; MS, methysergide.) (Modified and reproduced, with permission, from Müller-Schweinitzer E in: 5-Hydroxytryptamine Mechanisms in Primary Headaches. Oleson J, Saxena PR [editors]. Raven Press, 1992.)

blocked by conventional α-blocking agents. However, ergotamine's effect is also associated with "epinephrine reversal" (see Chapter 10) and with *blockade* of the response to other α agonists. This dual effect represents partial agonist action (Table 16–5). Because ergotamine dissociates very slowly from the α receptor, it produces very long-lasting agonist and antagonist effects at this receptor. There is little or no effect at β adrenoceptors.

While much of the vasoconstriction elicited by ergot alkaloids can be ascribed to partial agonist effects at α adrenoceptors, some may be the result of effects at 5-HT receptors. Ergotamine, ergonovine, and methysergide all have partial agonist effects at 5-HT$_2$ vascular receptors. The remarkably specific antimigraine action of the ergot derivatives was originally thought to be related to their actions on vascular serotonin receptors. Current hypotheses, however, emphasize their action on prejunctional neuronal 5-HT receptors.

After overdosage with ergotamine and similar agents, vasospasm is severe and prolonged (see Toxicity, below). This vasospasm is not easily reversed by α antagonists, serotonin antagonists, or combinations of both.

Ergotamine is typical of the ergot alkaloids that have a strong vasoconstrictor spectrum of action. The hydrogenation of ergot alkaloids at the 9 and 10 positions (Table 16–4) yields dihydro derivatives that have reduced serotonin partial agonist effects and increased selective α receptor-blocking actions.

3. Uterine smooth muscle—The stimulant action of ergot alkaloids on the uterus, as on vascular smooth muscle, appears to combine α agonist, serotonin, and other effects. Furthermore, the sensitivity of the uterus to the stimulant effects of ergot changes dramatically during pregnancy, perhaps because of increasing dominance of α$_1$ receptors as pregnancy progresses. As a result, the uterus at term is more sensitive than earlier in pregnancy and far more sensitive than the nonpregnant organ.

In very small doses, ergot preparations can evoke rhythmic contraction and relaxation of the uterus. At higher concentrations, these drugs induce powerful and prolonged contracture. Ergonovine is more selective than other ergot alkaloids in affecting the uterus and is the agent of choice in obstetric applications of these drugs.

4. Other smooth muscle organs—In most patients, the ergot alkaloids have no significant effect on bronchiolar smooth muscle. The gastrointestinal tract, on the other hand, is quite sensitive in most patients. Nausea, vomiting, and diarrhea may be induced even by low doses in some patients. The effect is consistent with action on the central nervous system emetic center and on gastrointestinal serotonin receptors.

CLINICAL PHARMACOLOGY OF ERGOT ALKALOIDS

Clinical Uses

A. MIGRAINE

Migraine headache in its "classic" form is characterized by a brief aura that may involve visual scotomas or even hemianopia and speech abnormalities, followed by a severe throbbing unilateral headache that lasts for a few hours to 1–2 days. "Common" migraine lacks the aura phase, but the headache is similar. Although the symptom pattern varies among patients, the severity of migraine headache justifies vigorous therapy in the great majority of cases.

Migraine involves the trigeminal nerve distribution to intracranial (and possibly extracranial) arteries. These nerves appear to release peptide neurotransmitters, especially **calcitonin gene-related peptide** (CGRP; see Chapter 17), an extremely powerful vasodilator. Substance P and neurokinin A may also be involved. Extravasation of plasma and plasma proteins into the perivascular space appears to be a common feature of animal migraine models and biopsy specimens from migraine patients and probably represents the effect of the neuropeptides on the vessels. The mechanical stretching caused by this perivascular edema may be the immediate cause of activation of pain nerve endings in the dura. The onset of headache is sometimes associated with a marked increase in amplitude of temporal artery pulsations, and relief of pain by administration of ergotamine is sometimes accompanied by diminution of the arterial pulsations.

The mechanisms of action of drugs used in migraine are poorly understood because they include such a wide variety of drug groups and actions. These include ergot alkaloids and synthetic 5-HT agonists (triptans), nonsteroidal anti-inflammatory analgesic agents, β-adrenoceptor blockers, tricyclic and serotonin-selective reuptake-inhibiting antidepressants, and several antiseizure agents. Furthermore, some of these drug groups are effective only for prophylaxis and not for the acute attack.

Two primary hypotheses have been proposed to explain the actions of these drugs. First, 5-HT agonists, such as ergot alkaloids, the triptans, and antidepressants may activate 5-HT$_1$ receptors on presynaptic trigeminal nerve endings to inhibit the release of vasodilating peptides, and antiseizure agents may suppress excessive firing of these nerve endings. Second, the vasoconstrictor actions of direct 5-HT agonists (ergot and the triptans) may prevent vasodilation and stretching of the pain endings. It is possible that both mechanisms contribute in the case of some drugs. **Sumatriptan** and its congeners, discussed above, are currently first-line therapy for acute severe migraine attacks in most patients. However, they should not be used in patients at risk for coronary artery disease. Anti-inflammatory analgesics such as aspirin and ibuprofen are often helpful in controlling the pain of migraine. Rarely, parenteral opioids may be needed in refractory cases. For patients with very severe nausea and vomiting, parenteral metoclopramide may be helpful.

Ergot derivatives are highly specific for migraine pain; they are not analgesic for any other condition. Although the triptan drugs discussed above are preferred by most clinicians and patients, traditional therapy with **ergotamine** can also be quite effective when given during the prodrome of an attack; it becomes progressively less effective if delayed. Ergotamine tartrate is available for oral, sublingual, rectal suppository, and inhaler use. It is often combined with caffeine (100 mg caffeine for each 1 mg ergotamine tartrate) to facilitate absorption of the ergot alkaloid.

The vasoconstriction induced by ergotamine is long-lasting and cumulative when the drug is taken repeatedly, as in a severe migraine attack. Therefore, patients must be carefully informed that no more than 6 mg of the oral preparation may be taken for each attack and no more than 10 mg per week. For very severe attacks, ergotamine tartrate, 0.25–0.5 mg, may be given intravenously or intramuscularly. **Dihydroergotamine,** 0.5–1 mg intravenously, is favored by some clinicians for treatment of intractable migraine. Intranasal dihydroergotamine may also be effective.

Because of the cumulative toxicity of ergotamine, safer agents useful for the prophylaxis of migraine have been sought. **Methysergide,** a derivative of the amine subgroup (Table 16–5), was shown to be effective in this application in about 60% of patients. Unfortunately, significant toxicity (discussed below) occurred in almost 40% of patients. Furthermore, methysergide was relatively *ineffective* in treatment of impending or active episodes of migraine. Although relatively free of the rapidly cumulative vasospastic toxicity of ergotamine, chronic use of methysergide was sometimes associated with retroperitoneal fibroplasia and subendocardial fibrosis, possibly through its vascular effects.

Propranolol and **amitriptyline** have also been found to be effective for the prophylaxis of migraine in some patients. Like methysergide, they are of no value in the treatment of acute migraine. The anticonvulsant valproic acid in the form of divalproex (see Chapter 24) has recently been found to have good prophylactic efficacy in many migraine patients. **Flunarizine,** a calcium channel blocker used in Europe, has been reported in clinical trials to effectively reduce the severity of the acute attack and to prevent recurrences. **Verapamil** appears to have modest efficacy as prophylaxis against migraine.

B. HYPERPROLACTINEMIA

Increased serum levels of the anterior pituitary hormone prolactin are associated with secreting tumors of the gland and also with the use of centrally acting dopamine antagonists, especially the antipsychotic drugs. Because of negative feedback effects, hyperprolactinemia is associated with amenorrhea and infertility in women as well as galactorrhea in both sexes.

Bromocriptine is extremely effective in reducing the high levels of prolactin that result from pituitary tumors and has even been associated with regression of the tumor in some cases. The usual dosage of bromocriptine is 2.5 mg two or three times daily. **Cabergoline** is similar but more potent. Bromocriptine has also been used in the same dosage to suppress physiologic lactation. However, serious postpartum cardiovascular toxicity has been reported in association with the latter use of bromocriptine or pergolide, and this application is discouraged (Chapter 37).

C. POSTPARTUM HEMORRHAGE

The uterus at term is extremely sensitive to the stimulant action of ergot, and even moderate doses produce a prolonged and powerful spasm of the muscle quite unlike natural labor. This was not appreciated when the drugs were introduced into obstetrics in the 18th century. Their use at that time to accelerate labor caused a dramatic *increase* in fetal and maternal mortality rates. Therefore, ergot derivatives are useful only for control of late uterine bleeding and should never be given before delivery. Oxytocin is the preferred agent for control of postpartum hemorrhage, but if this peptide agent is ineffective, ergonovine maleate, 0.2 mg usually given intramuscularly, can be tried. It is usually effective within 1–5 minutes and is less toxic than other ergot derivatives for this application. It is given at the time of delivery of the placenta or immediately afterward if bleeding is significant.

D. DIAGNOSIS OF VARIANT ANGINA

Ergonovine produces prompt vasoconstriction during coronary angiography to diagnose variant angina.

E. SENILE CEREBRAL INSUFFICIENCY

Dihydroergotoxine, a mixture of dihydro-α-ergocryptine and three similar dihydrogenated peptide ergot alkaloids (ergoloid mesylates), has been promoted for many years for the relief of senility and more recently for the treatment of Alzheimer's dementia. There is no evidence of significant benefit.

Toxicity & Contraindications

The most common toxic effects of the ergot derivatives are gastrointestinal disturbances, including diarrhea, nausea, and vomiting. Activation of the medullary vomiting center and of the gastrointestinal serotonin receptors is involved. Since migraine attacks are often associated with these symptoms before therapy is begun, these adverse effects are rarely contraindications to the use of ergot.

A more dangerous toxic effect of overdosage with agents like ergotamine and ergonovine is prolonged vasospasm. As described above, this sign of vascular smooth muscle stimulation may result in gangrene and require amputation. Most cases involve the circulation to the arms and legs. However, bowel infarction resulting from mesenteric artery vasospasm has also been reported. Peripheral vascular vasospasm caused by ergot is refractory to most vasodilators, but infusions of large doses of nitroprusside or nitroglycerin have been successful in some cases.

Chronic therapy with methysergide was associated with connective tissue proliferation in the retroperitoneal space, the pleural cavity, and the endocardial tissue of the heart. These changes occurred insidiously over months and presented as hydronephrosis (from

obstruction of the ureters) or a cardiac murmur (from distortion of the valves of the heart). In some cases, valve damage required surgical replacement. As a result, this drug was withdrawn.

Other toxic effects of the ergot alkaloids include drowsiness and, in the case of methysergide, occasional instances of central stimulation and hallucinations. In fact, methysergide was sometimes used as a substitute for LSD by members of the "drug culture."

Contraindications to the use of ergot derivatives consist of the obstructive vascular diseases and collagen diseases.

There is no evidence that ordinary use of ergotamine for migraine is hazardous in pregnancy. However, most clinicians counsel restraint in the use of the ergot derivatives by pregnant patients.

PREPARATIONS AVAILABLE

ANTIHISTAMINES (H₁ BLOCKERS)*

Azelastine (Astelin)
Nasal: 137 µg/puff nasal spray
Ophthalmic: 0.5 mg/mL solution

Brompheniramine (Brovex)
Oral: 12 mg tablets; 12 mg/5 mL suspension

Buclizine (Bucladin-S Softabs)
Oral: 50 mg tablets

Carbinoxamine (Histex, Pediatex)
Oral: 8 mg timed-release tablets; 1.75, 4 mg/5 mL liquid

Cetirizine (Zyrtec)
Oral: 5, 10 mg tablets; 5 mg/5 mL syrup

Chlorpheniramine (generic, Chlor-Trimeton, Teldrin, others)
Oral: 2 mg chewable tablets; 4 mg tablets; 2 mg/5 mL syrup
Oral sustained-release: 8, 12, 16 mg tablets; 8, 12 mg capsules

Clemastine (generic, Tavist)
Oral: 1.34, 2.68 mg tablets; 0.67 mg/5 mL syrup

Cyclizine (Marezine)
Oral: 50 mg tablets

Cyproheptadine (generic)
Oral: 4 mg tablets; 2 mg/5 mL syrup

Desloratadine (Clarinex)
Oral: 5 mg regular or rapidly disintegrating tablets

Dimenhydrinate† (Dramamine, others)

Oral: 50 mg tablets; 50 mg chewable tablets; 12.5/5 mL, 12.5 mg/4 mL, 15.62 mg/5 mL liquid

Diphenhydramine (generic, Benadryl)
Oral: 12.5 mg chewable tablets; 25, 50 mg capsules; 25, 50 mg tablets; 12.5 mg/5 mL elixir and syrup
Parenteral: 50 mg/mL for injection

Emedastine (Emadine)
Ophthalmic: 0.05% solution

Fexofenadine (Allegra)
Oral: 30, 60, 180 mg tablets; 60 mg capsules

Hydroxyzine (generic, Atarax, Vistaril)
Oral: 10, 25, 50, 100 mg tablets; 25, 50, 100 mg capsules; 10 mg/5 mL syrup; 25 mg/5 mL suspension
Parenteral: 25, 50 mg/mL for injection

Ketotifen (Zaditor)
Ophthalmic: 0.025% solution

Levocabastine (Livostin)
Ophthalmic: 0.05% solution

Loratadine (Claritin)
Oral: 10 mg tablets; 10 mg rapidly disintegrating tablets; 1 mg/mL syrup

Meclizine (generic, Antivert, others)
Oral: 12.5, 25, 50 mg tablets; 25, 30 mg capsules; 25 mg chewable tablets

Olopatadine (Patanol)
Ophthalmic: 0.1% solution

Phenindamine (Nolahist)
Oral: 25 mg tablets

Promethazine (generic, Phenergan, others)
Oral: 12.5, 25, 50 mg tablets; 6.25 mg/5 mL syrups

---

* Several other antihistamines are available only in combination products with, for example, pseudoephedrine.
† Dimenhydrinate is the chlorotheophylline salt of diphenhydramine.

Parenteral: 25 mg/mL for injection; 50 mg/mL for IM injection
Rectal: 12.5, 25, 50 mg suppositories

H₂ BLOCKERS
See Chapter 63.

5-HT AGONISTS
Almotriptan (Axert)
Oral: 6.25, 12.5 mg tablets
Eletriptan (Relpax)
Oral: 24.2, 48.5 mg tablets
Frovatriptan (Frova)
Oral: 2.5 mg tablets
Naratriptan (Amerge)
Oral: 1, 2.5 mg tablets
Rizatriptan
Oral: 5, 10 mg tablets (Maxalt); 5, 10 mg orally disintegrating tablets (Maxalt-MLT)
Sumatriptan (Imitrex)
Oral: 25, 50, 100 mg tablets
Nasal: 5, 20 mg unit dose spray devices
Parenteral: 6 mg/0.5 mL in *SELFdose* autoinjection units for subcutaneous injection

Zolmitriptan (Zomig)
Oral: 2.5, 5 mg tablets; 2.5 mg orally disintegrating tablets

5-HT ANTAGONISTS
See Chapter 63.

ERGOT ALKALOIDS
Dihydroergotamine
Nasal (Migranal): 4 mg/mL nasal spray
Parenteral (D.H.E. 45): 1 mg/mL for injection
Ergonovine (Ergotrate maleate)
Parenteral: 0.2 mg/mL for injection
Ergotamine [mixtures] (generic, Cafergot, others)
Oral: 1 mg ergotamine/100 mg caffeine tablets
Rectal: 2 mg ergotamine/100 mg caffeine suppositories
Ergotamine tartrate (Ergomar)
Sublingual: 2 mg sublingual tablets
Methylergonovine (Methergine)
Oral: 0.2 mg tablets
Parenteral: 0.2 mg/mL for injection

REFERENCES

HISTAMINE

Barnes PJ: Histamine and serotonin. Pulm Pharmacol Ther 2001;14:329.

Bochner BS, Lichtenstein LM: Anaphylaxis. N Engl J Med 1991;324:1785.

Blandizzi C et al: Histamine H₃ receptors mediate inhibition of noradrenaline release from intestinal sympathetic nerves. Br J Pharmacol 2000;129:1387.

Cuss FM: Beyond the histamine receptor: Effect of antihistamines on mast cells. Clin Exper Allergy 1999;29(Suppl 3):54.

Del Valle J, Gantz I: Novel insights into histamine H₂ receptor biology. Am J Physiol 1997;273:G987.

Desager J-P, Horsmans Y: Pharmacokinetic-pharmacodynamic relationships of H₁-antihistamines. Clin Pharmacokinet 1995;28:418.

Dutschmann M et al: Histaminergic modulation of the intact respiratory network of adult mice. Pflugers Arch 2003;445:570.

Esbenshade TA et al: Differential activation of dual signaling responses by human H₁ and H₂ histamine receptors. J Recept Sig Transduct 2003;23:17.

Gantner F et al: Histamine H₄ and H₂ receptors control histamine-induced interleukin-16 release from human CD8+ T cells. J Pharmacol Exp Ther 2002;303:300.

Haaksma EEJ, Leurs R, Timmerman H: Histamine receptors: Subclasses and specific ligands. Pharmacol Ther 1990;47:73.

Harper EA, Shankley NP, Black JW: Evidence that histamine homologues discriminate between H₃ receptors in guinea-pig cerebral cortex and ileum longitudinal muscle myenteric plexus. Br J Pharmacol 1999;128:751.

Holgate ST (editor): Antihistamines: Back to the future. Clin Exper Allergy 1999;29(Suppl 3). [Entire issue.]

Horak F, Stübner UP: Comparative tolerability of second generation antihistamines. Drug Saf 1999;20:385.

Hough LB et al: Antinociceptive activity of derivatives of improgran and burimamide. Pharmacol Biochem Behav 2000;65:61.

Izzo AA et al: The role of histamine H₁, H₂, and H₃ receptors on enteric ascending synaptic transmission in the guinea pig ileum. J Pharmacol Exp Ther 1998;287:952.

Leurs R et al: Therapeutic potential of histamine H₃-receptor agonists and antagonists. Trends Pharmacol Sci 1998;19:177.

Nemmar A et al: Modulatory effect of imetit, a histamine H₃ receptor antagonist, on C-fibers, cholinergic fibers, and mast cells in rabbit lungs in vitro. Eur J Pharmacol 1999;371:23.

Pauls JD et al: Mastocytosis. Diverse presentations and outcomes. Arch Intern Med 1999;159:401.

Rascol O et al: Antivertigo medications and drug-induced vertigo: A pharmacological review. Drugs 1995; 50:777.

Sachs G, Prinz C: Gastric enterochromaffin-like cells and the regulation of acid secretion. News Physiol Sci 1996;11:57.

Schneider E et al: Trends in histamine research: new functions during immune responses and hematopoiesis. Trends Immunol 2002;23:255.

Shin N et al: Molecular modeling and site-specific mutagenesis of the histamine-binding site of the histamine H₄ receptor. Mol Pharmacol 2002;62:38.

Simons FE, Simons KJ: Clinical pharmacology of new histamine H₁ receptor antagonists. Clin Pharmacokinet 1999;36:329.

Smit MJ et al: Molecular properties and signalling pathways of the histamine H_1 receptor. Clin Exper Allergy 1999;29(Suppl 3): 19.

Takahashi K et al: Targeted disruption of H3 receptors results in changes in brain histamine tone leading to an obese phenotype. J Clin Invest 2002;110:1791.

Timm J et al: H_2 receptor-mediated facilitation and H_3 receptor-mediated inhibition of noradrenaline release in the guinea-pig brain. Naunyn-Schmiedebergs Arch Pharmacol 1998;357: 232.

Timmerman H: Why are non-sedating antihistamines non-sedating? Clin Exper Allergy 1999;29(Suppl 3):13.

Woosley RL: Cardiac actions of antihistamines. Annu Rev Pharmacol Toxicol 1996;36:233.

SEROTONIN

Abenheim L et al: Appetite-suppressant drugs and the risk of primary pulmonary hypertension. N Engl J Med 1996;335:609.

Cacoub P et al: Pulmonary hypertension and dexfenfluramine. Eur J Clin Pharmacol 1995;48:81.

Durham PL, Russo AF: New insights into the molecular actions of serotonergic antimigraine drugs. Pharmacol Ther 2002;94:77.

Egermayer P: Epidemics of vascular toxicity and pulmonary hypertension: what can be learned? J Intern Med 2000;247:11.

Gershon MD: Review article: Roles played by 5-hydroxytryptamine in the physiology of the bowel. Aliment Pharmacol Ther 1999;13(Suppl 2):15.

MacLean MR: Pulmonary hypertension, anorexigens and 5-HT: Pharmacological synergism in action? Trends Pharmacol Sci 1999;20:490.

Michel K et al: Subpopulations of gastric myenteric neurons are differentially activated via distinct serotonin receptors: projection, neurochemical coding, and functional implications. J Neurosci 1997;17:8009.

Peroutka SJ: Serotonin receptor subtypes. Their evolution and clinical relevance. CNS Drugs 1995;4:19.

Raymond JR et al: Multiplicity of mechanisms of serotonin receptor signal transduction. Pharmacol Therap 2001;92:179.

Wappler F, Fiege M, Schulte an Esch J: Pathophysiological role of the serotonin system in malignant hyperthermia. Br J Anaesthesia 2001;87:794.

ERGOT ALKALOIDS: HISTORICAL

Fuller JG: *The Day of St. Anthony's Fire.* Macmillan, 1968; Signet, 1969.

Gabbai Dr, Lisbonne Dr, Pourquier Dr: Ergot poisoning at Pont St. Esprit. Br Med J (Sept 15) 1951;650.

ERGOT ALKALOIDS: PHARMACOLOGY

Andersen PK et al: Sodium nitroprusside and epidural blockade in the treatment of ergotism. N Engl J Med 1977;296:1271.

Berde B: Ergot compounds: A synopsis. Adv Biochem Psychopharmacol 1980;23:3.

Buzzi MG, Moskowitz MA: The antimigraine drug, sumatriptan (GR43175) selectively blocks neurogenic plasma extravasation from blood vessels in dura mater. Br J Pharmacol 1990;99:202.

DeGroot ANJA et al: Ergot alkaloids. Current status and review of clinical pharmacology and therapeutic use compared with other oxytocics in obstetrics and gynaecology. Drugs 1998;56:523.

Dierckx RA et al: Intraarterial sodium nitroprusside infusion in the treatment of severe ergotism. Clin Neuropharmacol 1986;9:542.

Dildy GA: Postpartum hemorrhage: new management options. Clin Obstet Gynecol 2002;45:330.

Lake AE, Saper JR: Chronic headache. New advances in treatment strategies. Neurology 2002;59:S8

Mantegani S, Brambilla E, Varasi M: Ergoline derivatives: receptor affinity and selectivity. Farmaco 1999;54:288.

Porter JK, Thompson FN Jr: Effects of fescue toxicosis on reproduction in livestock. J Animal Sci 1992;70:1594.

Redfield MM et al: Valve disease associated with ergot alkaloid use: Echocardiographic and pathologic correlations. Ann Intern Med 1992;117:50.

Sadzot B et al: Hallucinogenic drug interactions at human brain 5-HT_2 receptors: Implications for treating LSD-induced hallucinogenesis. Psychopharmacology 1989;98:495.

Silberstein SD: Methysergide. Cephalalgia 1998;18:421.

Snow V et al: Pharmacologic management of acute attacks of migraine and prevention of migraine headache. Ann Intern Med 2002;137:840.

Williamson DJ, Hargreaves RJ: Neurogenic inflammation in the context of migraine. Microsc Res Tech 2001;53:167.

Young WB, Silberstein SD, Dayno JM: Migraine treatment. Semin Neurol 1997;17:325.

Vasoactive Peptides

Ian A. Reid, PhD

Peptides are used by most tissues for cell-to-cell communication. As noted in Chapters 6 and 21, they play important roles in the autonomic and central nervous systems. Several peptides exert important direct effects on vascular and other smooth muscles. These peptides include vasoconstrictors (**angiotensin II, vasopressin, endothelins, neuropeptide Y,** and **urotensin**) and vasodilators (**bradykinin** and related **kinins, natriuretic peptides, vasoactive intestinal peptide, substance P, neurotensin, calcitonin gene-related peptide,** and **adrenomedullin**). This chapter focuses on the smooth muscle actions of the peptides.

ANGIOTENSIN

BIOSYNTHESIS OF ANGIOTENSIN

The pathway for the formation and metabolism of angiotensin II is summarized in Figure 17–1. The principal steps include enzymatic cleavage of angiotensin I from angiotensinogen by renin, conversion of angiotensin I to angiotensin II by converting enzyme, and degradation of angiotensin II by several peptidases.

Renin & Factors Controlling Renin Secretion

Renin is an aspartyl protease that specifically catalyzes the hydrolytic release of the decapeptide angiotensin I from angiotensinogen. It is synthesized as a preprohormone that is processed to prorenin, which is inactive, and then to active renin, a glycoprotein consisting of 340 amino acids.

Renin in the circulation originates in the kidneys. Enzymes with renin-like activity are present in several extrarenal tissues, including blood vessels, uterus, salivary glands, and adrenal cortex, but no physiologic role for these enzymes has been established. Within the kidney, renin is synthesized and stored in the juxtaglomerular apparatus of the nephron. Specialized granular cells called juxtaglomerular cells are the site of synthesis, stor-

age, and release of renin. The macula densa is a specialized tubular segment closely associated with the vascular components of the juxtaglomerular apparatus. The vascular and tubular components of the juxtaglomerular apparatus, including the juxtaglomerular cells, are innervated by noradrenergic neurons.

The rate at which renin is secreted by the kidney is the primary determinant of activity of the renin-angiotensin system. Renin secretion is controlled by a variety of factors, including a renal vascular receptor, the macula densa, the sympathetic nervous system, and angiotensin II.

A. RENAL VASCULAR RECEPTOR

The renal vascular receptor functions as a stretch receptor, decreased stretch leading to increased renin release and vice versa. The receptor is apparently located in the afferent arteriole, possibly in the juxtaglomerular cells. Stretch-induced changes in renin release are mediated by changes in Ca^{2+} concentration in the juxtaglomerular cells.

B. MACULA DENSA

The macula densa contains a different type of receptor, sensitive to changes in the rate of delivery of sodium or chloride to the distal tubule. Decreases in distal delivery result in stimulation of renin secretion and vice versa. Potential candidates for signal transmission between the macula densa and the juxtaglomerular cells include adenosine, prostaglandins, and nitric oxide.

C. SYMPATHETIC NERVOUS SYSTEM

Maneuvers that increase renal nerve activity cause stimulation of renin secretion, while renal denervation results in suppression of renin secretion. Norepinephrine stimulates renin secretion by a direct action on the juxtaglomerular cells. In humans, this effect is mediated by β_1 adrenoceptors.

Circulating epinephrine and norepinephrine may act via the same mechanisms as the norepinephrine released locally from the renal sympathetic nerves, but there is evidence that a major component of the renin secretory response to circulating catecholamines is mediated by extrarenal β receptors.

D. Angiotensin

Angiotensin II inhibits renin secretion. The inhibition, which results from a direct action of the peptide on the juxtaglomerular cells, forms the basis of a short-loop negative feedback mechanism controlling renin secretion. Interruption of this feedback with inhibitors of the renin-angiotensin system (see below) results in stimulation of renin secretion.

E. Pharmacologic Alteration of Renin Release

The release of renin is altered by a wide variety of pharmacologic agents. Renin release is stimulated by vasodilators (hydralazine, minoxidil, nitroprusside), β-adrenoceptor agonists (isoproterenol), α-adrenoceptor antagonists, phosphodiesterase inhibitors (theophylline, milrinone, rolipram), and most diuretics and anesthetics. This stimulation can be accounted for by the control mechanisms just described. Drugs that inhibit renin release are discussed below in the section on inhibition of the renin-angiotensin system.

Angiotensinogen

Angiotensinogen is the circulating protein substrate from which renin cleaves angiotensin I. It is synthesized in the liver. Human angiotensinogen is a glycoprotein with a molecular weight of approximately 57,000. The 14 amino acids at the amino terminal of the molecule are shown in Figure 17–1. In humans, the concentration of angiotensinogen in the circulation is less than the K_m of the renin-angiotensinogen reaction and is therefore an important determinant of the rate of formation of angiotensin.

The production of angiotensinogen is increased by corticosteroids, estrogens, thyroid hormones, and angiotensin II. It is also elevated during pregnancy and in women taking estrogen-containing oral contraceptives. The increased plasma angiotensinogen concentration is thought to contribute to the hypertension that may occur in these situations. There is also evidence for a genetic linkage between the angiotensinogen gene and essential hypertension (Lalouel et al, 2001).

Angiotensin I

Although angiotensin I contains the peptide sequences necessary for all of the actions of the renin-angiotensin system, it has little or no biologic activity. Instead, it must be converted to angiotensin II by converting enzyme (Figure 17–1). Angiotensin I may also be acted on by plasma or tissue aminopeptidases to form [des-Asp[1]]angiotensin I; this in turn is converted to [des-Asp[1]]angiotensin II (commonly known as angiotensin III) by converting enzyme.

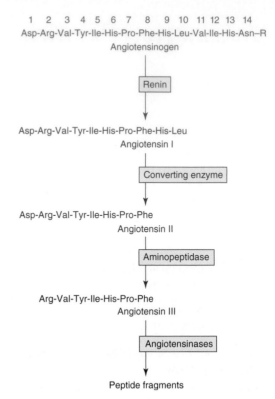

Figure 17–1. Chemistry of the renin-angiotensin system. The amino acid sequence of the amino terminal of human angiotensinogen is shown. R denotes the remainder of the protein molecule.

Converting Enzyme (Peptidyl Dipeptidase [PDP], Kininase II)

Converting enzyme is a dipeptidyl carboxypeptidase that catalyzes the cleavage of dipeptides from the carboxyl terminal of certain peptides. Its most important substrates are angiotensin I, which it converts to angiotensin II, and bradykinin, which it inactivates (see below). It also cleaves enkephalins and substance P, but the physiologic significance of these effects has not been established. The action of converting enzyme is prevented by a penultimate prolyl residue, and angiotensin II is therefore not hydrolyzed by converting enzyme. Converting enzyme is distributed widely in the body. In most tissues, converting enzyme is located on the luminal surface of vascular endothelial cells and is thus in close contact with the circulation.

Angiotensinase

Angiotensin II, which has a plasma half-life of 15–60 seconds, is removed rapidly from the circulation by a variety of peptidases collectively referred to as angiotensinase. It is metabolized during passage through most vascular beds (a notable exception being the lung). Most metabolites of angiotensin II are biologically inactive, but the initial product of aminopeptidase action—[des-Asp^1]angiotensin II—retains considerable biologic activity.

ACTIONS OF ANGIOTENSIN II

Angiotensin II exerts important actions at several sites in the body, including vascular smooth muscle, adrenal cortex, kidney, and brain. Through these actions, the renin-angiotensin system plays a key role in the regulation of fluid and electrolyte balance and arterial blood pressure. Excessive activity of the renin-angiotensin system can result in hypertension and disorders of fluid and electrolyte homeostasis.

Blood Pressure

Angiotensin II is a very potent pressor agent—on a molar basis, approximately 40 times more potent than norepinephrine. The pressor response to intravenous angiotensin II is rapid in onset (10–15 seconds) and sustained during long-term infusions of the peptide. A large component of the pressor response to intravenous angiotensin II is due to direct contraction of vascular—especially arteriolar—smooth muscle. In addition, however, angiotensin II can also increase blood pressure through actions on the brain and autonomic nervous system. The pressor response to angiotensin is usually accompanied by little or no reflex bradycardia because the peptide acts on the brain to reset the baroreceptor reflex control of heart rate to a higher pressure.

Angiotensin II also interacts with the autonomic nervous system. It stimulates autonomic ganglia, increases the release of epinephrine and norepinephrine from the adrenal medulla, and—what is most important—facilitates sympathetic transmission by an action at adrenergic nerve terminals. The latter effect involves both increased release and reduced reuptake of norepinephrine. Angiotensin II also has a less important direct positive inotropic action on the heart.

Adrenal Cortex

Angiotensin II acts directly on the zona glomerulosa of the adrenal cortex to stimulate aldosterone biosynthesis. At higher concentrations, angiotensin II also stimulates glucocorticoid biosynthesis.

Kidney

Angiotensin II acts on the kidney to cause renal vasoconstriction, increase proximal tubular sodium reabsorption, and inhibit the secretion of renin.

Central Nervous System

In addition to its central effects on blood pressure, angiotensin II acts on the central nervous system to stimulate drinking (dipsogenic effect) and increase the secretion of vasopressin and adrenocorticotropic hormone (ACTH). The physiologic significance of the effects of angiotensin II on drinking and pituitary hormone secretion is not known.

Cell Growth

Angiotensin II is mitogenic for vascular and cardiac muscle cells and may contribute to the development of cardiovascular hypertrophy. Considerable evidence now indicates that angiotensin-converting enzyme (ACE) inhibitors and angiotensin II receptor antagonists (see below) slow or prevent morphologic changes (remodeling) following myocardial infarction that would otherwise lead to heart failure.

ANGIOTENSIN RECEPTORS & MECHANISM OF ACTION

Angiotensin II receptors are widely distributed in the body. Like the receptors for other peptide hormones, angiotensin II receptors are located on the plasma membrane of target cells, and this permits rapid onset of the various actions of angiotensin II.

Two distinct subtypes of angiotensin II receptors, termed **AT$_1$** and **AT$_2$**, have been identified on the basis of their differential affinity for antagonists, and their sensitivity to sulfhydryl-reducing agents. AT$_1$ receptors have a high affinity for losartan and a low affinity for PD 123177 (an experimental nonpeptide antagonist), while AT$_2$ receptors have a high affinity for PD 123177 and a low affinity for losartan. Angiotensin II and saralasin (see below) bind equally to both subtypes. The relative proportion of the two subtypes varies from tissue to tissue: AT$_1$ receptors predominate in vascular smooth muscle.

Most of the known actions of angiotensin II are mediated by the AT$_1$ receptor, a G protein-coupled receptor. Binding of angiotensin II to AT$_1$ receptors in vascular smooth muscle results in activation of phospholipase C and generation of inositol trisphosphate and diacylglycerol (see Chapter 2). These events, which occur within seconds, result in smooth muscle contraction.

The stimulation of vascular and cardiac growth by angiotensin II is mediated by other pathways, probably receptor and nonreceptor tyrosine kinases such as the Janus tyrosine kinase Jak2 and increased transcription of specific genes (see Chapter 2).

The AT$_2$ receptor has a structure and affinity for angiotensin II similar to those of the AT$_1$ receptor.

However, signal transduction by the AT_2 receptor differs from transduction by the AT_1 receptor, and current evidence suggests that serine and tyrosine phosphatases, phospholipase A_2, nitric oxide, and cyclic guanosine monophosphate (cGMP) are involved. AT_2 receptors are present at high density in all tissues during fetal development, but they are much less abundant in the adult where they are expressed at high concentration only in the adrenal medulla, reproductive tissues, vascular endothelium and parts of the brain. AT_2 receptors are upregulated in pathologic conditions including heart failure and myocardial infarction. The functions of the AT_2 receptor appear to include fetal tissue development, inhibition of growth and proliferation, cell differentiation, apoptosis, and possibly, vasodilation.

INHIBITION OF THE RENIN-ANGIOTENSIN SYSTEM

A wide variety of agents are now available that block the formation or actions of angiotensin II. These drugs may block renin secretion, the enzymatic action of renin, the conversion of angiotensin I to angiotensin II, or angiotensin II receptors.

Drugs That Block Renin Secretion

Several drugs that interfere with the sympathetic nervous system inhibit the secretion of renin. Examples are clonidine and propranolol. Clonidine inhibits renin secretion by causing a centrally mediated reduction in renal sympathetic nerve activity, and it may also exert a direct intrarenal action. Propranolol and other β-adrenoceptor-blocking drugs act by blocking the intrarenal and extrarenal β receptors involved in the neural control of renin secretion.

Renin Inhibitors

Several orally active renin inhibitors have been developed. Two inhibitors that have been tested in humans are **remikiren** and **enalkiren.** They have a high specificity for renin, cause marked suppression of plasma renin activity and plasma angiotensin II concentration, and lower blood pressure in hypertensive patients. However, the bioavailability of these inhibitors is generally poor, mainly because of poor absorption and a considerable first pass effect. They also increase plasma renin concentrations because of interruption of the negative feedback effect of angiotensin II on renin secretion, and this further limits the reduction in plasma renin activity that can be achieved. Renin inhibitors have the potential to be as effective as converting enzyme inhibitors in inhibiting the renin-angiotensin system, but further improvement of their bioavailability and efficacy is needed.

Converting Enzyme Inhibitors

An important class of orally active **ACE** inhibitors, directed against the active site of ACE, is now extensively used. **Captopril** and **enalapril** (Figure 17–2) are examples of the many potent ACE inhibitors that are available. These drugs differ in their structure and pharmacokinetics, but in clinical use, they are interchangeable. ACE inhibitors decrease systemic vascular resistance without increasing heart rate, and they promote natriuresis. As described in Chapters 11 and 13, they are effective in the treatment of hypertension, decrease morbidity and mortality in heart failure and left ventricular dysfunction after myocardial infarction, and delay the progression of diabetic nephropathy.

ACE inhibitors not only block the conversion of angiotensin I to angiotensin II but also inhibit the degradation of other substances, including bradykinin, substance P, and enkephalins. The action of ACE inhibitors to inhibit bradykinin metabolism contributes significantly to their hypotensive action (Figure 11–6) and is apparently responsible for some adverse side effects, including cough and angioedema.

Angiotensin Antagonists

Substitution of certain amino acids, especially sarcosine, for the phenylalanine in position 8 of angiotensin II results in the formation of potent peptide antagonists of the action of angiotensin II. The best-known of these antagonists is **saralasin.**

Saralasin exhibits some agonist activity and may elicit pressor responses, particularly when circulating angiotensin II levels are low. Saralasin must be administered intravenously, and this severely restricts its use as an antihypertensive agent. However, it has been used for

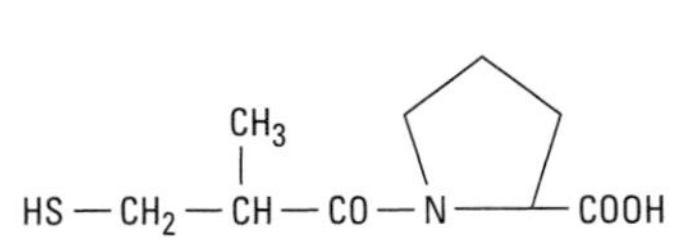

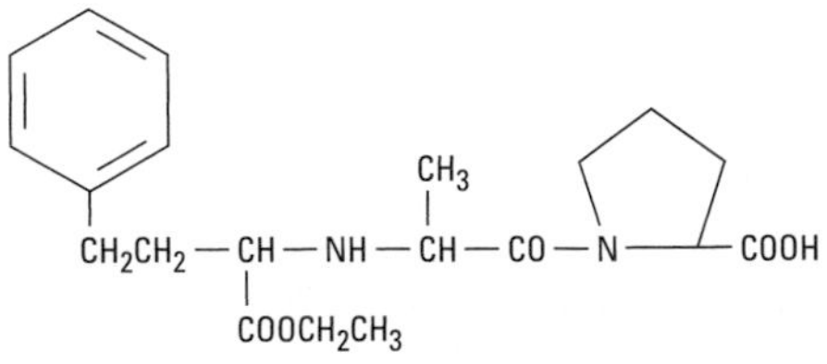

Figure 17–2. Two orally active converting enzyme inhibitors. Enalapril is a prodrug ethyl ester that is hydrolyzed in the body.

the detection of renin-dependent hypertension and other hyperreninemic states.

The *non*peptide angiotensin II antagonists are of much greater interest. **Losartan**, **valsartan** (Figure 17–3), **eprosartan**, **irbesartan**, **candesartan**, and **telmesartan** are orally active, potent, and specific competitive antagonists of angiotensin AT_1 receptors. The blood pressure-lowering efficacy of these drugs is similar to that of enalapril, a typical ACE inhibitor, but associated with a lower incidence of cough. Like the ACE inhibitors, they are well tolerated but should not be used by patients with nondiabetic renal disease or in pregnancy.

The current angiotensin II receptor antagonists are selective for the AT_1 receptor. Since prolonged treatment with the drugs disinhibits renin secretion and increases circulating angiotensin II levels, there may be increased stimulation of AT_2 receptors. This may be significant in view of the evidence that activation of the AT_2 receptor causes vasodilation and other beneficial effects. AT_2 receptor antagonists such as PD 123177 are available for research but have no clinical applications at this time.

The clinical benefits of AT_1 receptor antagonists are similar to those of ACE inhibitors, and it is currently not clear if one group of drugs has significant advantages over the other.

KININS

BIOSYNTHESIS OF KININS

Kinins are a group of potent vasodilator peptides. They are formed enzymatically by the action of enzymes known as kallikreins or kininogenases acting on protein substrates called kininogens. From the biochemical point of view, the kallikrein-kinin system has several features in common with the renin-angiotensin system.

Kallikreins

Kallikreins are glycoprotein enzymes produced in the liver as prekallikreins and present in plasma and in several tissues, including the kidneys, pancreas, intestine, sweat glands, and salivary glands. They are serine proteases with active sites and catalytic properties similar to those of enzymes such as trypsin, chymotrypsin, elastase, thrombin, plasmin, and other serine proteases. Plasma prekallikrein can be activated to kallikrein by trypsin, Hageman factor, and possibly kallikrein itself. In general, the biochemical properties of glandular kallikreins are quite different from those of plasma kallikreins. Kallikreins can convert prorenin to active renin, but the physiologic significance of this action has not been established.

Kininogens

Kininogens—the precursors of kinins and substrates of kallikreins—are present in plasma, lymph, and interstitial fluid. Two kininogens are known to be present in plasma: a low-molecular-weight form (LMW kininogen) and a high-molecular-weight form (HMW kininogen). About 15–20% of the total plasma kininogen is in the HMW form. It is thought that LMW kininogen crosses capillary walls and serves as the substrate for tissue kallikreins, while HMW kininogen is confined to the bloodstream and serves as the substrate for plasma kallikrein.

FORMATION OF KININS IN PLASMA & TISSUES

The pathway for the formation and metabolism of kinins is shown in Figure 17–4. Three kinins have been identified in mammals: bradykinin, lysylbradykinin

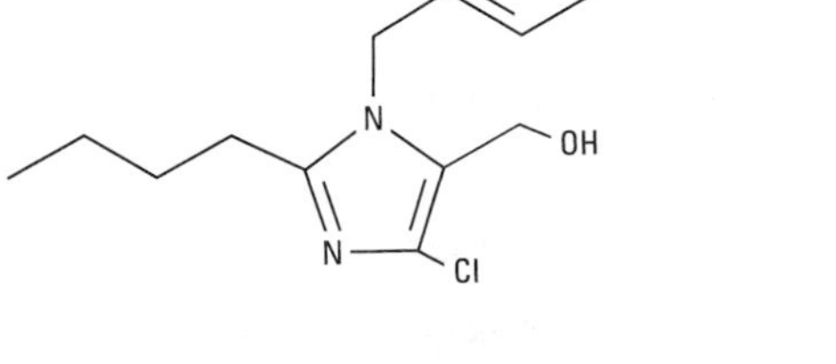

Losartan

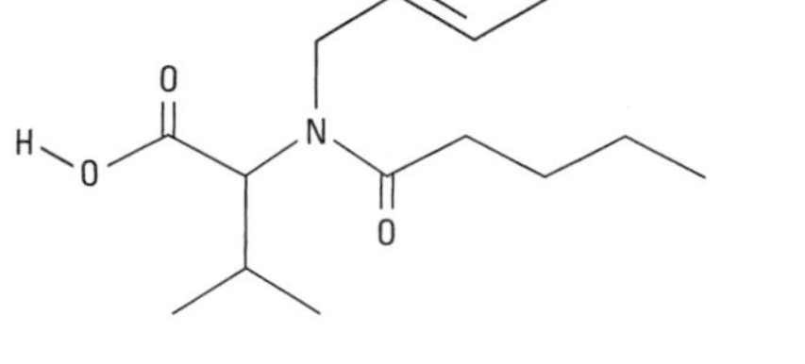

Valsartan

Figure 17–3. Structures of two angiotensin AT_1 receptor antagonists.

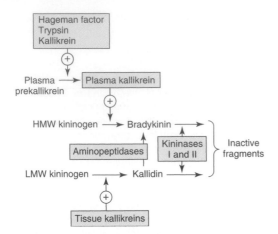

Figure 17–4. The kallikrein-kinin system. Kininase II is identical to converting enzyme peptidyl dipeptidase.

(also known as kallidin), and methionyllysylbradykinin. Their structures are shown below:

Arg-Pro-Pro-Gly-Phe-Ser-Pro-Phe-Arg
 1   2   3   4   5   6   7   8   9
Bradykinin

Lys-Arg-Pro-Pro-Gly-Phe-Ser-Pro-Phe-Arg
Lysylbradykinin (kallidin; Lys-bradykinin)

Met-Lys-Arg-Pro-Pro-Gly-Phe-Ser-Pro-Phe-Arg
Methionyllysylbradykinin (Met-Lys-bradykinin)

Note that each kinin contains bradykinin in its structure. Each kinin is formed from a kininogen by the action of a different enzyme. Bradykinin is released by plasma kallikrein, lysylbradykinin by glandular kallikrein, and methionyllysylbradykinin by pepsin and pepsin-like enzymes. The three kinins have been found in plasma and urine. Bradykinin is the predominant kinin in plasma, while lysylbradykinin is the major urinary form.

ACTIONS OF KININS

Effects on the Cardiovascular System

Kinins produce marked vasodilation in several vascular beds, including the heart, kidney, intestine, skeletal muscle, and liver. In this respect, kinins are approximately 10 times more potent on a molar basis than histamine. The vasodilation may result from a direct inhibitory effect of kinins on arteriolar smooth muscle or may be mediated by the release of endothelium-derived relaxing factor (EDRF, nitric oxide) or vasodilator prostaglandins such as PGE_2 and PGI_2. In contrast,

the predominant effect of kinins on veins is contraction; again, this may result from direct stimulation of venous smooth muscle or from the release of venoconstrictor prostaglandins such as $PGF_{2\alpha}$. Kinins also produce contraction of most visceral smooth muscle.

When injected intravenously, kinins produce a rapid fall in blood pressure that is due to their arteriolar vasodilator action. The hypotensive response to bradykinin is of very brief duration. Intravenous infusions of the peptide fail to produce a sustained decrease in blood pressure; prolonged hypotension can only be produced by progressively increasing the rate of infusion. The rapid reversibility of the hypotensive response to kinins is due primarily to reflex increases in heart rate, myocardial contractility, and cardiac output. In some species, bradykinin produces a biphasic change in blood pressure—an initial hypotensive response followed by an increase above the preinjection level. The increase in blood pressure may be due to a reflex activation of the sympathetic nervous system, but under some conditions, bradykinin can directly release catecholamines from the adrenal medulla and stimulate sympathetic ganglia. Bradykinin also increases blood pressure when injected into the central nervous system, but the physiologic significance of this effect is not clear, since it is unlikely that kinins cross the blood-brain barrier. Kinins have no consistent effect on sympathetic or parasympathetic nerve endings.

The arteriolar dilation produced by kinins causes an increase in pressure and flow in the capillary bed, thus favoring efflux of fluid from blood to tissues. This effect may be facilitated by increased capillary permeability resulting from contraction of endothelial cells and widening of intercellular junctions, and by increased venous pressure secondary to constriction of veins. As a result of these changes, water and solutes pass from the blood to the extracellular fluid, lymph flow increases, and edema may result.

Effects on Endocrine & Exocrine Glands

As noted earlier, prekallikreins and kallikreins are present in several glands, including the pancreas, kidney, intestine, salivary glands, and sweat glands, and can be released into the secretory fluids of these glands. The function of the enzymes in these tissues is not known. The enzymes (or active kinins) may diffuse from the organs to the blood and act as local modulators of blood flow. Since kinins have such marked effects on smooth muscle, they may also modulate the tone of salivary and pancreatic ducts and help regulate gastrointestinal motility. Kinins also influence the transepithelial transport of water, electrolytes, glucose, and amino acids, and may regulate the transport of these substances in the gastrointestinal tract and kidney. Finally, kallikreins may play a role in the physiologic activation of various prohormones, including proinsulin and prorenin.

Role in Inflammation

Kinins play an important role in the inflammatory process. Kallikreins and kinins can produce redness, local heat, swelling, and pain, and the production of kinins is increased in inflammatory lesions produced by a variety of methods.

Effects on Sensory Nerves

Kinins are potent pain-producing substances when applied to a blister base or injected intradermally. They elicit pain by stimulating nociceptive afferents in the skin and viscera.

KININ RECEPTORS & MECHANISMS OF ACTION

The biologic actions of kinins are mediated by specific receptors located on the membranes of the target tissues. Two types of kinin receptors, termed B_1 and B_2, have been defined based on the rank orders of agonist potencies: for B_1 receptors, [des-Arg^9]bradykinin > [Tyr(Me)^8] bradykinin > bradykinin. For B_2 receptors, [Tyr(Me)^8] bradykinin > bradykinin > [des-Arg^9]bradykinin. (Note that *B* here stands for bradykinin, not for β-adrenoceptor.) Bradykinin displays the highest affinity in most B_2 receptor systems, followed by Lys-bradykinin and then by Met-Lys-bradykinin. One exception is the B_2 receptor that mediates contraction of venous smooth muscle; this appears to be most sensitive to Lys-bradykinin. Recent evidence suggests the existence of two B_2 receptor subtypes, which have been termed B_{2A} and B_{2B}.

B_1 receptors appear to have a very limited distribution in mammalian tissues. Known functional roles for B_1 receptors are limited. Studies with knockout mice that lack functional B_1 receptors have provided evidence that these receptors participate in the inflammatory response (Pesquero, 2000). B_1 receptors may also be important in long-lasting kinin effects such as collagen synthesis and cell multiplication. By contrast, B_2 receptors have a widespread distribution that is consistent with the multitude of biologic effects that are mediated by this receptor type. B_2 receptors belong to the G protein–coupled family of receptors. Receptor binding sets in motion multiple signal transduction events, including calcium mobilization, chloride transport, formation of nitric oxide, and activation of phospholipase C, phospholipase A_2, and adenylyl cyclase.

METABOLISM OF KININS

Kinins are metabolized rapidly (half-life < 15 seconds) by nonspecific exopeptidases or endopeptidases, commonly referred to as kininases. Two plasma kininases have been well characterized. Kininase I, apparently synthesized in the liver, is a carboxypeptidase that releases the carboxyl terminal arginine residue. Kininase II is present in plasma and vascular endothelial cells throughout the body. It is identical to angiotensin-converting enzyme (ACE, peptidyl dipeptidase), discussed above. Kininase II inactivates kinins by cleaving the carboxyl terminal dipeptide phenylalanyl-arginine. Like angiotensin I, bradykinin is almost completely hydrolyzed during a single passage through the pulmonary vascular bed.

DRUGS AFFECTING THE KALLIKREIN-KININ SYSTEM

Drugs that modify the activity of the kallikrein-kinin system are available, though none are in wide clinical use. Considerable effort has been directed toward developing kinin receptor antagonists, since such drugs have considerable therapeutic potential as anti-inflammatory and antinociceptive agents. Competitive antagonists of both B_1 and B_2 receptors are available for research use. Examples of B_1 receptor antagonists are the peptides [Leu^8-des-Arg^9]bradykinin and Lys[Leu^8-des Arg^9]bradykinin. Nonpeptide B_1 receptor antagonists are not yet available. The first B_2 receptor antagonists to be discovered were also peptide derivatives of bradykinin. These first-generation antagonists were used extensively in animal studies of kinin receptor pharmacology. However, their half-life is short, and they are almost inactive on the human B_2 receptor.

Icatibant is a second generation B_2 receptor antagonist. It is orally active, potent, and selective, has a long duration of action (> 60 minutes), and displays high B_2 receptor affinity in humans and all other species in which it has been tested. Icatibant has been used extensively in animal studies to block exogenous and endogenous bradykinin and in human studies to evaluate the role of kinins in pain, hyperalgesia, and inflammation.

Recently, a third generation of B_2 receptor antagonists was developed; examples are FR 173657, FR 172357, and NPC 18884. These antagonists block both human and animal B_2 receptors and are orally active. They have been reported to inhibit bradykinin-induced bronchoconstriction in guinea pigs, carrageenin-induced inflammatory responses in rats, and capsaicin-induced nociception in mice.

The synthesis of kinins can be inhibited with the kallikrein inhibitor aprotinin. Actions of kinins mediated by prostaglandin generation can be blocked nonspecifically with inhibitors of prostaglandin synthesis such as aspirin. Conversely, the actions of kinins can be enhanced with ACE inhibitors, which block the degradation of the peptides. Indeed, as noted above, inhibition of bradykinin metabolism by ACE inhibitors contributes significantly to their antihypertensive action.

There is evidence that by acting on B_2 receptors, bradykinin may play a beneficial, protective role in cardiovascular disease. Selective B_2 agonists are available and have been shown to be effective in some animal models of human cardiovascular disease. These drugs may have potential for the treatment of hypertension and myocardial hypertrophy.

VASOPRESSIN

Vasopressin (antidiuretic hormone, ADH) plays an important role in the long-term control of blood pressure through its action on the kidney to increase water reabsorption. This and other aspects of the physiology of vasopressin are discussed in Chapters 15 and 37 and will not be reviewed here.

Vasopressin also plays an important role in the short-term regulation of arterial pressure by its vasoconstrictor action. It increases total peripheral resistance when infused in doses less than those required to produce maximum urine concentration. Such doses do not normally increase arterial pressure because the vasopressor activity of the peptide is buffered by a reflex decrease in cardiac output. When the influence of this reflex is removed, eg, in shock, pressor sensitivity to vasopressin is greatly increased. Pressor sensitivity to vasopressin is also enhanced in patients with idiopathic orthostatic hypotension. Higher doses of vasopressin increase blood pressure even when baroreceptor reflexes are intact.

VASOPRESSIN RECEPTORS & ANTAGONISTS

Three subtypes of vasopressin receptors have been identified. V_{1a} **receptors** mediate the vasoconstrictor action of vasopressin; V_{1b} **receptors** potentiate the release of ACTH by pituitary corticotropes; and V_2 **receptors** mediate the antidiuretic action. V_{1a} effects are mediated by activation of phospholipase C, formation of inositol trisphosphate, and increased intracellular calcium concentration. V_2 effects are mediated by activation of adenylyl cyclase.

Vasopressin-like peptides selective for either vasoconstrictor or antidiuretic activity have been synthesized. The most specific V_1 vasoconstrictor agonist synthesized to date is [Phe[2], Ile[3], Orn[8]]vasotocin. Selective V_2 antidiuretic analogs include 1-deamino[D-Arg[8]]arginine vasopressin (dDAVP) and 1-deamino[Val[4],D-Arg[8]]arginine vasopressin (dVDAVP).

Specific antagonists of the vasoconstrictor action of vasopressin are also available. The peptide antagonist [1-(β-mercapto-β,β-cyclopentamethylenepropionic acid)-2-(O-methyl)tyrosine] arginine vasopressin also has antioxytocic activity but does not antagonize the antidiuretic action of vasopressin. Recently, nonpeptide, orally active V_{1a} receptor antagonists have been discovered,

examples being OPC-21268 and SR-49059 (Thibonnier et al, 2001).

The vasopressor antagonists have been particularly useful in revealing the important role that vasopressin plays in blood pressure regulation in situations such as dehydration and hemorrhage. They have potential for the treatment of hypertension and heart failure.

NATRIURETIC PEPTIDES

Synthesis & Structure

The atria and other tissues of mammals contain a family of peptides with natriuretic, diuretic, vasorelaxant and other properties. The family consists of atrial natriuretic peptide (ANP), brain natriuretic peptide (BNP) and C-type natriuretic peptide (CNP). The structures of the three peptides are similar (Figure 17–5), but there are differences in their biologic effects. ANP is derived from the carboxyl terminal end of a common precursor termed preproANP which, in humans, is a 151-amino-acid peptide. ANP is synthesized primarily in cardiac atrial cells, but small amounts are syn-

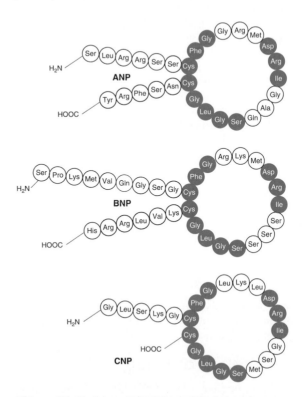

Figure 17–5. Structures of the atrial natriuretic peptide (ANP), brain natriuretic peptide (BNP), and C-type natriuretic peptide (CNP). Sequences common to the peptides are indicated in blue.

thesized in ventricular cells. It is also synthesized by neurons in the central and peripheral nervous systems and in the lungs. ANP circulates as a 28-amino-acid peptide with a single disulfide bridge that forms a 17-residue ring.

Several factors increase the release of ANP from the heart, but the most important one appears to be atrial stretch via mechanosensitive ion channels (Thibault et al, 1999). ANP release is also increased by volume expansion, head-out water immersion, changing from the standing to the supine position, and exercise. In each case, the increase in ANP release is probably due to increased atrial stretch. ANP release can also be increased by sympathetic stimulation via α_{1A}-adrenoceptors, endothelins (see below) via the ET_A receptor subtype, glucocorticoids, and vasopressin. Finally, plasma ANP concentration increases in various pathologic states, including heart failure, primary aldosteronism, chronic renal failure, and inappropriate ADH secretion syndrome.

Administration of ANP produces prompt and marked increases in sodium excretion and urine flow. Glomerular filtration rate increases, with little or no change in renal blood flow, so that the filtration fraction increases. The ANP-induced natriuresis is apparently due to both the increase in glomerular filtration rate and a decrease in proximal tubular sodium reabsorption. ANP also inhibits the secretion of renin, aldosterone, and vasopressin; these changes may also increase sodium and water excretion. Finally, ANP decreases arterial blood pressure. This hypotensive action is due to vasodilation, which results from stimulated particulate guanylyl cyclase activity, increased cGMP levels, and decreased cytosolic free calcium concentration. ANP also reduces sympathetic tone to the peripheral vasculature and antagonizes the vasoconstrictor action of angiotensin II and other vasoconstrictors. These actions may contribute to the hypotensive action of the peptide.

There is considerable evidence that ANP participates in the physiologic regulation of sodium excretion and blood pressure. For example, suppression of ANP production or blockade of its action impairs the natriuretic response to volume expansion, and increases blood pressure.

BNP was originally isolated from porcine brain but, like ANP, it is synthesized primarily in the heart. It exists in two forms, having either 26 or 32 amino acids (Figure 17–5). Like ANP, the release of BNP appears to be volume-related; indeed, the two peptides may be cosecreted. BNP exhibits natriuretic, diuretic, and hypotensive activities similar to those of ANP but circulates at a lower concentration.

CNP consists of 22 amino acids (Figure 17–5). It is located predominantly in the central nervous system but is also present in several tissues including the vascular endothelium, kidneys, and intestine. It has not been found in significant concentrations in the circulation. CNP has less natriuretic and diuretic activity than ANP and BNP but is a potent vasodilator. Its physiologic role is unclear.

Pharmacodynamics & Pharmacokinetics

The biologic actions of the natriuretic peptides are mediated through association with specific high-affinity receptors located on the surface of the target cells. Three receptor subtypes termed ANP_A, ANP_B, and ANP_C have been identified. The ANP_A receptor consists of a 120 kDa protein; its primary ligands are ANP and BNP. The ANP_B receptor is similar in structure to the ANP_A receptor, but its primary ligand appears to be CNP. The ANP_A and ANP_B receptors, but not the ANP_C receptor, are coupled to guanylyl cyclase.

The natriuretic peptides have a short half-life in the circulation. They are metabolized in the kidneys, liver, and lungs by the neutral endopeptidase NEP 24.11. Inhibition of this endopeptidase results in increases in circulating levels of the natriuretic peptides, natriuresis, and diuresis. The peptides are also removed from the circulation by binding to ANP_C receptors in the vascular endothelium. This receptor binds the three natriuretic peptides with equal affinity. The receptor and bound peptide are internalized, the peptide is degraded enzymatically, and the receptor is returned to the cell surface.

Administration of BNP as **nesiritide** (see Chapter 13) in patients with severe heart failure increases sodium excretion and improves hemodynamics. However, the peptide has to be given by constant intravenous infusion. A more promising approach may be the use of drugs that inhibit the neutral endopeptidase responsible for the breakdown of ANP. This is discussed below under Vasopeptidase Inhibitors.

Pathophysiology

Patients with heart failure have high plasma levels of ANP and BNP, which have emerged as important diagnostic and prognostic markers in this condition. Thus, plasma ANP concentration has been shown to be closely correlated with the New York Heart Association functional class of symptomatic heart failure (Boomsma, 2001). Through the actions described above, the peptides reduce salt and water retention. However, renal responsiveness to the peptides decreases as heart failure worsens. The natriuretic peptides may also play a role in preventing the development of hypertension. For example, studies in experimental animals have identified an important role of the peptides in helping prevent mineralocorticoid-induced and salt-induced hypertension.

VASOPEPTIDASE INHIBITORS

Vasopeptidase inhibitors are a new class of cardiovascular drugs that inhibit two metalloprotease enzymes,

NEP 24.11 and ACE. They thus simultaneously increase the levels of natriuretic peptides and decrease the formation of angiotensin II. As a result, they enhance vasodilation, reduce vasoconstriction, and increase sodium excretion, in turn reducing peripheral vascular resistance and blood pressure.

Recently developed vasopeptidase inhibitors include **omapatrilat**, **sampatrilat**, and **fasidotrilat**. Of these, omapatrilat is at the most advanced stage of clinical development. It lowers blood pressure in animal models of hypertension as well as in hypertensive patients and improves cardiac function in patients with heart failure. Unfortunately, omapatrilat causes a significant incidence of angioedema in addition to cough and dizziness. Nevertheless, combined inhibition of neutral endopeptidase NEP 24.11 and ACE with this new class of drugs may be a promising approach to treat cardiovascular disease and further clinical trials are underway.

ENDOTHELINS

The endothelium is the source of a variety of substances with vasodilator (PGI$_2$ and nitric oxide) and vasoconstrictor activities. The latter include the endothelin family, potent vasoconstrictor peptides that were first isolated from aortic endothelial cells.

Biosynthesis, Structure, & Clearance

Three isoforms of endothelin have been identified: the originally described endothelin (**ET-1**) and two similar peptides, **ET-2** and **ET-3**. Each isoform is a product of a different gene and is synthesized as a prepro form that is processed to a propeptide and then to the mature peptide. Processing to the mature peptides occurs through the action of endothelin-converting enzyme. Each endothelin is a 21-amino-acid peptide containing two disulfide bridges (Figure 17–6).

Endothelins are widely distributed in the body. ET-1 is the predominant endothelin secreted by the vascular endothelium. It is also produced by neurons and astrocytes in the central nervous system and in endometrial, renal mesangial, Sertoli, breast epithelial, and other cells. ET-2 is produced predominantly in the kidneys and intestine, while ET-3 is found in highest concentration in the brain but is also present in the gastrointestinal tract, lungs, and kidneys. Endothelins are present in the blood but in low concentration; they apparently act locally in a paracrine or autocrine fashion rather than as circulating hormones.

The expression of the ET-1 gene is increased by

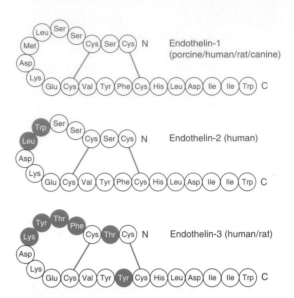

Figure 17–6. Structures of the endothelin peptides endothelin-1, endothelin-2, and endothelin-3. Sequences different in the three peptides are shown in blue.

growth factors and cytokines, including transforming growth factor-β (TGF-β) and interleukin 1 (IL-1), vasoactive substances including angiotensin II and vasopressin, and mechanical stress. Expression is inhibited by nitric oxide, prostacyclin, and atrial natriuretic peptide.

Clearance of endothelins from the circulation is rapid, and involves both enzymatic degradation by NEP 24.11 and clearance by the ET$_B$ receptor.

Actions

Endothelins exert widespread actions in the body. In particular, they cause dose-dependent vasoconstriction in most vascular beds. Intravenous administration of ET-1 causes a rapid and transient decrease in arterial blood pressure followed by a prolonged increase. The depressor response results from release of prostacyclin and nitric oxide from the vascular endothelium, while the pressor response is due to direct constriction of vascular smooth muscle. Endothelins also exert direct positive inotropic and chronotropic actions on the heart and are potent coronary vasoconstrictors. They act on the kidneys to cause vasoconstriction and decrease glomerular filtration rate and sodium and water excretion. In the respiratory system, they cause potent constriction of tracheal and bronchial smooth muscle. Endothelins interact with several endocrine systems, increasing the secretion of renin, aldosterone, vasopressin, and atrial natriuretic peptide. They exert a variety of actions on the central and peripheral nervous systems, the gastrointestinal system, the liver, the urinary tract, the male and female reproductive systems, the eye, the skeletal system, and the skin. Finally, ET-1 is a potent mitogen for vascular smooth muscle cells, cardiac myocytes, and glomerular mesangial cells.

Endothelin receptors are present in many tissues and organs, including the blood vessel wall, cardiac muscle, central nervous system, lung, kidney, adrenal, spleen, and intestine. Two receptor subtypes, termed **ET**$_A$ and **ET**$_B$, have been cloned and sequenced. ET$_A$ receptors have a high affinity for ET-1 and a low affinity for ET-3 and are located on smooth muscle cells, where they mediate vasoconstriction. ET$_B$ receptors have approximately equal affinities for ET-1 and ET-3 and are located on vascular endothelial cells, where they mediate release of PGI$_2$ and nitric oxide. Both receptor subtypes belong to the G protein-coupled seven-transmembrane domain family of receptors.

The signal transduction mechanisms triggered by binding of ET-1 to its receptors are summarized in Figure 17–7. Major effects include stimulation of phospholipase C, formation of inositol trisphosphate, and release of calcium from the endoplasmic reticulum, which results in vasoconstriction. Stimulation of PGI$_2$ and nitric oxide synthesis results in decreased intracellular calcium concentration and vasodilation.

INHIBITORS OF ENDOTHELIN SYNTHESIS & ACTION

The endothelin system can be blocked with receptor antagonists and drugs that block endothelin-converting enzyme. Endothelin ET$_A$ or ET$_B$ receptors can be blocked selectively, or both can be blocked with nonselective ET$_A$-ET$_B$ antagonists.

An example of a nonselective antagonist is **bosentan.** This drug is active both intravenously and orally, and blocks both the initial transient depressor (ET$_B$) and the prolonged pressor (ET$_A$) responses to intravenous endothelin. Many orally active endothelin receptor antagonists with increased selectivity have been developed and are available for research use.

The formation of endothelins can be blocked by inhibiting endothelin-converting enzyme with phosphoramidon. This compound is not specific for endothelin-converting enzyme, but several potent and more selective inhibitors are now available. The therapeutic potential of these drugs may be similar to that of the endothelin receptor antagonists (see below).

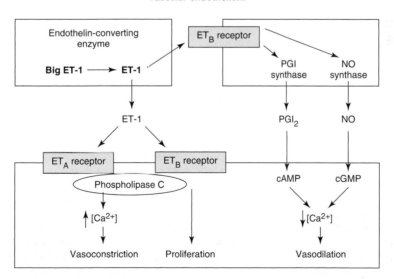

Vascular endothelium

Smooth muscle

Figure 17–7. Signal transduction mechanisms mediating the effects of ET-1 on vascular smooth muscle.

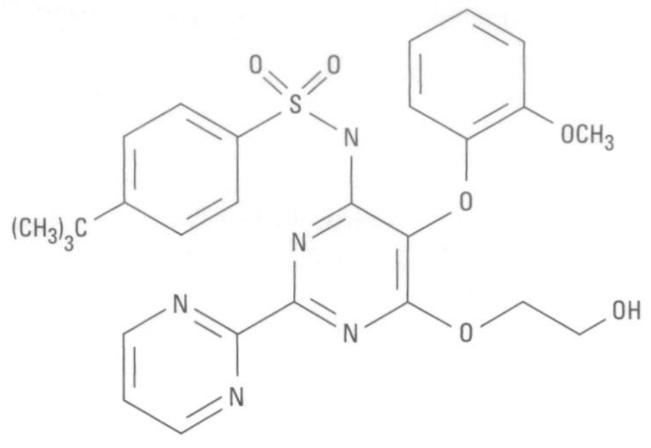

Bosentan

PHYSIOLOGIC & PATHOLOGIC ROLES OF ENDOTHELIN: EFFECTS OF ENDOTHELIN ANTAGONISTS

Systemic administration of endothelin receptor antagonists or endothelin-converting enzyme inhibitors causes vasodilation and decreases arterial pressure in humans and experimental animals. Intra-arterial administration of the drugs also causes slow-onset forearm vasodilation in humans. These observations provide evidence that the endothelin system participates in the regulation of vascular tone, even under resting conditions.

There is increasing evidence that endothelins participate in a variety of cardiovascular diseases, including hypertension, cardiac hypertrophy, heart failure, atherosclerosis, coronary artery disease, and myocardial infarction. Endothelins have also been implicated in pulmonary diseases, including asthma and pulmonary hypertension, as well as in several renal diseases. This evidence includes findings of increased endothelin levels in the blood, increased expression of endothelin mRNA in endothelial or vascular smooth muscle cells, and the responses to administration of endothelin antagonists.

Endothelin antagonists have considerable potential in the treatment of these diseases. In clinical trials, bosentan and other nonselective antagonists as well as ET_A-selective antagonists have produced beneficial effects on hemodynamics and other symptoms in heart failure, pulmonary hypertension, and essential hypertension. Bosentan is currently approved for use in pulmonary hypertension (see Chapter 11).

Endothelin antagonists occasionally cause systemic hypotension, increased heart rate, facial flushing or edema, and headaches. Potential gastrointestinal effects include nausea, vomiting, and constipation. Because of their teratogenic effects, ET antagonists are contraindicated in pregnancy. Thus, despite their considerable potential, additional research is needed before these drugs can be considered safe for more extensive clinical use.

VASOACTIVE INTESTINAL PEPTIDE

Vasoactive intestinal peptide (VIP) is a 28-amino-acid peptide related structurally to secretin and glucagon. Its structure is shown below.

His-Ser-Asp-Ala-Val-Thr-Asp-Asn-Tyr-Thr-Arg-Leu-Arg-
Lys-Gln-Met-Ala-Val-Lys-Lys-Tyr-Leu-Asn-Ser-Ile-Leu-Asn-NH$_2$

Vasoactive intestinal peptide (VIP)

VIP is widely distributed in the central and peripheral nervous systems where it functions as a neurotransmitter or neuromodulator. It is also present in several organs including the gastrointestinal tract, heart, lungs, kidneys, and thyroid gland. Many blood vessels are innervated by VIP neurons. VIP is present in the circulation but does not appear to function as a hormone.

VIP exerts marked effects on the cardiovascular system. It produces marked vasodilation in most vascular beds and in this regard is more potent on a molar basis than acetylcholine. In the heart, VIP causes coronary vasodilation and exerts positive inotropic and chronotropic effects. It may thus participate in the regulation of coronary blood flow, cardiac contraction, and heart rate.

The effects of VIP are mediated by G protein-coupled receptors, of which two subtypes termed **VPAC1** and **VPAC2** have been cloned from human tissues. Both subtypes are widely distributed in the central nervous system and in the heart, blood vessels, and other tissues. Binding of VIP to its receptors results in activation of adenylyl cyclase and formation of cAMP, which is responsible for the vasodilation and many other effects of the peptide. Other actions may be mediated by nitric oxide and cGMP.

Specific VIP receptor agonists and antagonists are currently available for research use.

SUBSTANCE P

Substance P belongs to the **tachykinin** family of peptides, which share the common carboxyl terminal sequence Phe-X-Gly-Leu-Met. Other members of this family are **neurokinin A** and **neurokinin B**. Substance P is an undecapeptide, while neurokinins A and B are decapeptides. They have the following structures:

Arg-Pro-Lys-Pro-Gln-Gln-Phe-Phe-Gly-Leu-Met

Substance P

His-Lys-Thr-Asp-Ser-Phe-Val-Gly-Leu-Met

Neurokinin A

Asp-Met-His-Asp-Phe-Phe-Val-Gly-Leu-Met

Neurokinin B

The amino terminal of substance P is not essential for biologic activity, but the carboxyl terminal is. The minimum fragment of substance P with significant activity is the carboxyl terminal hexapeptide.

Substance P is present in the central nervous system, where it is a neurotransmitter (see Chapter 21), and in the gastrointestinal tract, where it may play a role as a transmitter in the enteric nervous system and as a local hormone (see Chapter 6).

Substance P exerts a variety of incompletely understood central actions that implicate the peptide in behavior, anxiety, depression, nausea, and emesis. It is a potent vasodilator, producing marked hypotension in humans and several animal species. The vasodilation is mediated by release of nitric oxide from the endothelium. Conversely, substance P causes contraction of venous, intestinal, and bronchial smooth muscle. It also stimulates secretion by the salivary glands and causes diuresis and natriuresis by the kidneys.

The actions of substance P and neurokinins A and B are mediated by three G protein-coupled receptors designated NK_1, NK_2, and NK_3. Substance P is the preferred ligand for the NK_1 receptor, the predominant tachykinin receptor in the human brain. However, neurokinins A and B also possess considerable affinity for this receptor. In humans, the majority of the central and peripheral effects of substance P are mediated by NK_1 receptors.

Several nonpeptide NK_1 receptor antagonists have been developed. These compounds are highly selective, orally active, and enter the brain. Recent clinical trials have shown that these antagonists may be useful in treating depression and other disorders, and in preventing chemotherapy-induced emesis. The first of these to be approved for the prevention of chemotherapy-induced nausea and vomiting is **aprepitant.**

NEUROTENSIN

Neurotensin is a tridecapeptide that was first isolated from the central nervous system but subsequently was found to be present in the gastrointestinal tract and in the circulation. It is synthesized as part of a larger precursor that also contains **neuromedin N**, a six-amino-acid neurotensin-like peptide. Neurotensin and neuromedin N have the following structures:

Glu-Leu-Tyr-Glu-Asn-Lys-Pro-Arg-Arg-Pro-Tyr-Ile-Leu

Neurotensin

Lys-Ile-Pro-Tyr-Ile-Leu

Neuromedin N

In the brain, processing of the precursor leads primarily to the formation of neurotensin and neuromedin N; these are released together from nerve endings. In the gut, processing leads mainly to the formation of neurotensin and a larger peptide that contains the neuromedin N sequence at the carboxyl terminal. Both peptides are secreted into the circulation after ingestion of food.

Like many other neuropeptides, neurotensin serves a dual function as a neurotransmitter or neuromodulator in the central nervous system and as a local hormone in the periphery. When administered centrally, neurotensin exerts potent effects including hypothermia, antinociception and modulation of dopamine neurotransmission. When administered into the peripheral circulation, it causes vasodilation, hypotension, increased vascular permeability, increased secretion of several anterior pituitary hormones, hyperglycemia, inhibition of gastric acid and pepsin secretion, and inhibition of gastric motility.

Three subtypes of neurotensin receptors designated NT_1, NT_2, and NT_3 have been cloned. NT_1 and NT_2 receptors belong to the G protein-coupled superfamily; NT_3 receptors are structurally different.

Neurotensin agonists that cross the blood-brain barrier have been developed and have potential as potential therapeutic agents for diseases such as schizophrenia and Parkinson's disease (McMahon, 2002).

Neurotensin receptors can be blocked with the nonpeptide antagonists SR142948A and SR48692. SR142948A is a potent antagonist of the hypothermia and analgesia produced by centrally administered neurotensin. It also blocks the cardiovascular effects of systemic neurotensin.

CALCITONIN GENE-RELATED PEPTIDE

Calcitonin gene-related peptide (**CGRP**) is a member of the calcitonin family of peptides, which also includes calcitonin, adrenomedullin (see below) and amylin. CGRP consists of 37 amino acids and displays approximately 30% structural homology with salmon calcitonin.

Like calcitonin, CGRP is present in large quantities in the C cells of the thyroid gland. It is also distributed widely in the central and peripheral nervous systems, in the cardiovascular system, the gastrointestinal tract, and the urogenital system. CGRP is found with substance P (see above) in some of these regions and with acetylcholine in others.

When CGRP is injected into the central nervous system, it produces a variety of effects, including hypertension and suppression of feeding. When injected into the systemic circulation, the peptide causes hypotension and tachycardia. The hypotensive action of CGRP results from the potent vasodilator action of the peptide; indeed, CGRP is the most potent vasodilator yet discovered.

ADRENOMEDULLIN

Adrenomedullin is a 52-amino-acid peptide that was discovered in human adrenal medullary pheochromocytoma tissue. Like CGRP, it is a member of the calcitonin family of peptides. Adrenomedullin is present in several organs including the adrenals, lungs, heart, vascular tissue, and kidneys. It also circulates in the blood.

In animals, adrenomedullin dilates resistance vessels in the kidney, brain, lung, hind limbs, and mesentery, resulting in a marked, long-lasting hypotension. The hypotension in turn causes reflex increases in heart rate and cardiac output. Adrenomedullin also acts on the kidneys to increase sodium excretion, and exerts several endocrine effects including inhibition of aldosterone and insulin secretion. Finally it acts on the central nervous system to increase sympathetic outflow. These diverse actions of adrenomedullin are mediated both by CGRP receptors and unique adrenomedullin receptors, the properties of which are incompletely defined. The major second messenger for both receptors is cAMP.

Circulating adrenomedullin levels increase during intense exercise. Levels are also elevated in patients with hypertension, as well as in patients with renal failure, heart failure, and septic shock.

NEUROPEPTIDE Y

Neuropeptide Y is a member of the family that also includes peptide YY and pancreatic polypeptide. Each peptide consists of 36 amino acids. The amino acid sequence of neuropeptide Y is shown below.

Tyr-Pro-Ser-Lys-Pro-Asp-Asn-Pro-Gly-Glu-Asp-Ala-
Pro-Ala-Glu-Asp-Met-Ala-Arg-Tyr-Tyr-Ser-Ala-Leu-
Arg-His-Tyr-Ile-Asn-Leu-Ile-Thr-Arg-Gln-Arg-Tyr-NH$_2$

Neuropeptide Y

Neuropeptide Y is one of the most abundant neuropeptides in both the central and peripheral nervous systems. In the sympathetic nervous system, neuropeptide Y is frequently localized in noradrenergic neurons and apparently functions both as a vasoconstrictor and as a cotransmitter with norepinephrine. Peptide YY and pancreatic polypeptide are both gut endocrine peptides.

Neuropeptide Y produces a variety of central nervous system effects, including increased feeding (it is one of the most potent orexigenic molecules in the brain), hypotension, hypothermia, and respiratory depression. Other effects include vasoconstriction of cerebral blood vessels, positive chronotropic and inotropic actions on the heart, and hypertension. The peptide is a potent renal vasoconstrictor and suppresses renin secretion, but can cause diuresis and natriuresis. Prejunctional actions include inhibition of transmitter release from sympathetic and parasympathetic nerves; vascular actions include direct vasoconstriction, potentiation of the action of vasoconstrictors, and inhibition of the action of vasodilators.

These diverse effects are mediated by multiple receptors designated Y_1 through Y_6. All receptors except Y_3 have been cloned and shown to be G protein-coupled receptors coupled to mobilization of Ca^{2+} and inhibition of adenylyl cyclase. Y_1 and Y_2 receptors are of major importance in the cardiovascular and other peripheral effects of the peptide. Y_4 receptors have a high affinity for pancreatic polypeptide and may be a receptor for this peptide rather than for neuropeptide Y. Y_5 receptors are found mainly in the central nervous system and may be involved in the control of food intake. Y_6 receptors do not appear to contribute significantly to the physiologic effects of neuropeptide Y in humans.

Selective nonpeptide neuropeptide Y receptor antagonists are now available. The first nonpeptide Y_1 receptor antagonist, BIBP3226, is also the most thoroughly studied. In animal models, it blocks the vasoconstrictor and pressor responses to neuropeptide Y. It has a short half-life in vivo. Structurally related Y_1 antagonists include BIB03304 and H 409/22, which has been tested in humans. SR120107A and SR120819A are orally active Y_1 antagonists and have a long duration of action. BIIE0246 is the first nonpeptide antagonist selective for the Y_2 receptor.

These antagonists have been useful in analyzing the role of neuropeptide Y in cardiovascular regulation. It now appears that the peptide is not important in the regulation of hemodynamics under resting conditions, but may be of increased importance in cardiovascular disorders including hypertension and heart failure. Other studies have implicated neuropeptide Y in feeding disorders, seizures, anxiety, and diabetes, and Y_1 and Y_5 receptor antagonists have potential as anti-obesity agents (Parker, 2002).

UROTENSIN

Urotensin II was originally identified in fish, but isoforms are now known to be present in mammalian species including the mouse, rat, pig, and human. The structure of human urotensin II is shown below.

Glu-Thr-Pro-Asp-Cys-Phe-Trp-Lys-Tyr-Cys-Val

Urotensin II

There are species differences in the structure of urotensin II but the cyclic hexapeptide is conserved in all known isoforms. Major sites of urotensin II expression in humans are the brain, spinal cord, and kidneys. The kidneys may be the major source of circulating urotensin II.

In vitro, urotensin II is a potent constrictor of vascular smooth muscle; its activity depends on the type of blood vessel and the species from which it was obtained. Vasoconstriction occurs primarily in arterial vessels, where urotensin II can be more potent than endothelin 1, making it the most potent known vasoconstrictor. In vivo, urotensin II has complex hemodynamic effects, the most prominent being regional vasoconstriction and cardiac depression. The extent to which the peptide is involved in the regulation of vascular tone and blood pressure in humans is not clear; recent studies have produced conflicting results. The actions of urotensin II are mediated by G protein-coupled receptors that are widely distributed in the brain, spinal cord, heart, vascular smooth muscle, skeletal muscle, and pancreas. Some effects of the peptide including vasoconstriction are mediated by the phospholipase $C/IP_3/DAG$ signal transduction pathway.

It has been reported that the expression of urotensin II is upregulated in the heart of humans with end-stage heart failure, but it is not clear if the increase was a cause or consequence of the disease.

 PREPARATIONS AVAILABLE[1]

Aprepitant (Emend)
Oral: 80, 125 mg capsules
Bosentan (Tracleer)
Oral: 62.5, 125 mg tablets

[1]Preparations of angiotensin-converting enzyme inhibitors and angiotensin receptor antagonists are found in Chapter 11; preparations of vasopressin are found in Chapter 37.

REFERENCES

ANGIOTENSIN

Akishita M et al: Increased vasoconstrictor response of the mouse lacking angiotensin II type 2 receptor. Biochem Biophys Res Commun 1999;261:345.

Burnier M: Angiotensin II type 1 receptor blockers. Circulation 2001;103:904.

de Gasparo M et al: International union of pharmacology. XXIII. The angiotensin II receptors. Pharmacol Rev 2000;52:415.

Dina R, Jafari M: Angiotensin II-receptor antagonists: an overview. Am J Health Syst Pharm 2000;57:1231.

Dinh DT et al: Angiotensin receptors: distribution, signalling and function. Clin Sci 2001;100:481.

Kang AK et al: Effect of oral contraceptives on the renin-angiotensin system and renal function. Am J Physiol 2001;280:R807.

Klett CP, Granger JP: Physiological elevation in plasma angiotensinogen increases blood pressure. Am J Physiol 2001;281:R1437.

Lalouel J-M et al: Angiotensinogen in essential hypertension: from genetics to nephrology. J Am Soc Nephrol 2001;12:606.

Markham A, Spencer CM, Jarvis B: Irbesartan: an updated review of its use in cardiovascular disorders. Drugs 2000;59:1187.

Matsusaka T, Miyazaki Y, Ichikawa I: The renin-angiotensin system and kidney development. Annu Rev Physiol 2002;64:551.

McConnaughey MM, McConnaughey JS, Ingenito AJ: Practical considerations of the pharmacology of angiotensin receptor blockers. J Clin Pharmacol 1999;39:547.

Menard J, Patchett AA: Angiotensin-converting enzyme inhibitors. Advances in Protein Chemistry 2001;56:13.

Nouet S, Nahmias C: Signal transduction from the angiotensin II AT2 receptor. Trends Endocrinol Metab 2000;11:1.

Plosker GL, Foster RH: Eprosartan: a review of its use in the management of hypertension. Drugs 2000;60:177.

Reid IA: Role of phosphodiesterase isoenzymes in the control of renin secretion: effects of selective enzyme inhibitors. Curr Pharm Design 1999;5:725.

Touyz RM, Schiffrin EL: Signal transduction mechanisms mediating the physiological and pathophysiological actions of angiotensin II in vascular smooth muscle cells. Pharmacol Rev 2000;52:639.

Unger T: The role of the renin-angiotensin system in the development of cardiovascular disease. Am J Cardiol 2002;89:3A.

KININS

Blais C Jr et al: The kallikrein-kininogen-kinin system: lessons from the quantification of endogenous kinins. Peptides 2000;21:1903.

Bock MG, Longmore J: Bradykinin antagonists: new opportunities. Curr Opin Chem Biol 2000;4:401.

Calixto JB et al: Kinins in pain and inflammation. Pain 2000;87:1.

Couture R et al: Kinin receptors in pain and inflammation. Eur J Pharmacol 2001;429:161.

Griesbacher T, Legat FJ: Effects of the non-peptide B_2 receptor antagonist FR173657 in models of visceral and cutaneous inflammation. Inflamm Research 2000;49:535.

McLean PG, Perretti M, Ahluwalia A: Kinin B$_1$ receptors and the cardiovascular system: regulation of expression and function. Cardiovasc Res 2000;48:194.

Ozturk Y: Kinin receptors and their antagonists as novel therapeutic agents. Curr Pharm Design 2001;7:135.

Pesquero JB et al: Hypoalgesia and altered inflammatory responses in mice lacking kinin B$_1$ receptors. Proc Nat Acad Sci USA 2000;97:8140.

Stewart JM et al: Bradykinin antagonists: present progress and future prospects. Immunopharmacology 1999;43:155.

VASOPRESSIN

Birnbaumer M: Vasopressin receptors. Trends Endocrinol Metab 2000;V11:406.

Holmes CL et al: Physiology of vasopressin relevant to management of septic shock. Chest 2001;120:989.

Mayinger B, Hensen J: Nonpeptide vasopressin antagonists: a new group of hormone blockers entering the scene. Exp Clin Endocrinol Diabetes 1999;107:157.

Thibonnier M et al: The basic and clinical pharmacology of nonpeptide vasopressin receptor antagonists. Annu Rev Pharmacol Toxicol 2001;41:175.

NATRIURETIC PEPTIDES

Boomsma F, van den Meiracker AH: Plasma A- and B-type natriuretic peptides: physiology, methodology and clinical use. Cardiovasc Res 2001;51:442.

Chen HH, Burnett JC: The natriuretic peptides in heart failure: diagnostic and therapeutic potentials. Proc Assoc Am Physicians 1999;111:406.

de Bold AJ et al: The physiological and pathophysiological modulation of the endocrine function of the heart. Can J Physiol Pharmacol 2001;79:705.

Melo LG, Pang SC, Ackermann U: Atrial natriuretic peptide: regulator of chronic arterial blood pressure. News Physiol Sci 2000;15:143.

Thibault G, Amiri F, Garcia R: Regulation of natriuretic peptide secretion by the heart. Annu Rev Physiol 1999;61:193.

Vesely DL: Atrial natriuretic peptides in pathophysiological diseases. Cardiovasc Res 2001;51:647.

VASOPEPTIDASE INHIBITORS

Cataliotti A et al: Differential actions of vasopeptidase inhibition versus angiotensin-converting enzyme inhibition on diuretic therapy in experimental congestive heart failure. Circulation 2002;105:639.

Corti R et al: Vasopeptidase inhibitors: a new therapeutic concept in cardiovascular disease? Circulation 2001;104:1856.

Weber MA: Vasopeptidase inhibitors. Lancet 2001;358:1525.

ENDOTHELINS

Channick RN et al: Effects of the dual endothelin-receptor antagonist bosentan in patients with pulmonary hypertension: a randomised placebo-controlled study. Lancet 2001;358:1119.

Giannessi D, Del Ry S, Vitale RL: The role of endothelins and their receptors in heart failure. Pharmacol Res 2001;43:111.

Kedzierski RM, Yanagisawa M: Endothelin system: the double-edged sword in health and disease. Annu Rev Pharmacol Toxicol 2001;41:851.

Luscher TF, Barton M: Endothelins and endothelin receptor antagonists: therapeutic considerations for a novel class of cardiovascular drugs. Circulation 2000;102:2434.

Miyauchi T, Masaki T: Pathophysiology of endothelin in the cardiovascular system. Annu Rev Physiol 1999;61:391.

Naicker S, Bhoola KD: Endothelins: vasoactive modulators of renal function in health and disease. Pharmacol Ther 2001;90:61.

Roux S et al: Endothelin antagonism with bosentan: a review of potential applications. J Mol Med 1999;77:364.

Schalcher C et al: The dual endothelin receptor antagonist tezosentan acutely improves hemodynamic parameters in patients with advanced heart failure. Am Heart J 2001;142:340.

Spieker LE et al: Endothelin receptor antagonists in congestive heart failure: a new therapeutic principle for the future? J Am Coll Cardiol 2001;37:1493.

Wada A et al: Effects of a specific endothelin-converting enzyme inhibitor on cardiac, renal, and neurohumoral functions in congestive heart failure: comparison of effects with those of endothelin A receptor antagonism. Circulation 1999;99:570.

VASOACTIVE INTESTINAL PEPTIDE

Henning RJ, Sawmiller DR: Vasoactive intestinal peptide: cardiovascular effects. Cardiovasc Res 2001;49:27.

SUBSTANCE P

Aprepitant (emend) for prevention of nausea and vomiting due to cancer chemotherapy. Med Lett Drug Ther 2003;45:620.

Harrison S, Geppetti P: Substance P. Int J Biochem Cell Biol 2001;33:555.

Hokfelt T, Pernow B, Wahren J: Substance P: a pioneer amongst neuropeptides. J Intern Med 2001;249:27.

Newby D et al: Substance P-induced vasodilatation is mediated by the neurokinin type I receptor but does not contribute to basal vascular tone in man. Br J Clin Pharmacol 1999;48:336.

Saria A: The tachykinin NK1 receptor in the brain: pharmacology and putative functions. Eur J Pharmacol 1999;375:51.

Seward E, Swain C: Neurokinin receptor antagonists. Expert Opin Ther Patents 1999;9:571.

NEUROTENSIN

Binder EB et al: Neurotensin and dopamine interactions. Pharmacol Rev 2001;53:453.

McMahon BM et al: Neurotensin analogs indications for use as potential antipsychotic compounds. Life Sci 2002;70:1101.

Vincent JP, Mazella J, Kitabgi P: Neurotensin and neurotensin receptors. Trends Pharmacol Sci 1999;20:302.

CALCITONIN GENE-RELATED PEPTIDE

Goodman EC, Iversen LL: Calcitonin gene-related peptide: novel neuropeptide. Life Sci 1986;38:2169.

Zaidi M, Breimer LH, MacIntyre I: Biology of peptides from the calcitonin genes. Quart J Exp Physiol 1987;72:371.

ADRENOMEDULLIN

Kitamura K, Kangawa K, Eto T: Adrenomedullin and PAMP: discovery, structures, and cardiovascular functions. Microsc Res Tech 2002;57:3.

Minamino N, Kikumoto K, Isumi Y: Regulation of adrenomedullin expression and release. Microsc Res Tech 2002;57:28.

Poyner DR et al: International Union of Pharmacology. XXXII. The mammalian calcitonin gene-related peptides, adrenomedullin, amylin, and calcitonin receptors. Pharmacol Rev 2002;54:233.

Smith DM et al: Adrenomedullin: receptor and signal transduction. Biochem Soc Trans 2002;30:432.

NEUROPEPTIDE Y

Balasubramaniam A: Clinical potentials of neuropeptide Y family of hormones. Am J Surg 2002;183:430.

DiBona GF: Neuropeptide Y. Am J Physiol 2002;282:R635.

Malmstrom RE: Pharmacology of neuropeptide Y receptor antagonists: focus on cardiovascular functions. Eur J Pharmacol 2002;447:11.

Parker E, Van Heek M, Stamford A: Neuropeptide Y receptors as targets for anti-obesity drug development: perspective and current status. Eur J Pharmacol 2002;440:173.

UROTENSIN

Bohm F, Pernow J: Urotensin II evokes potent vasoconstriction in humans in vivo. Br J Pharmacol 2002;135:25.

Douglas SA et al: Congestive heart failure and expression of myocardial urotensin II. Lancet 2002;359:1990.

Wilkinson IB et al: High plasma concentrations of human urotensin II do not alter local or systemic hemodynamics in man. Cardiovasc Res 2002;53:341.

The Eicosanoids: Prostaglandins, Thromboxanes, Leukotrienes, & Related Compounds

Marie L. Foegh, MD, DSc, & Peter W. Ramwell, PhD

18

The eicosanoids are oxygenation products of polyunsaturated long chain fatty acids. They are ubiquitous in the animal kingdom and are also found—together with their precursor oils—in a variety of plants. They constitute a very large family of compounds that are not only highly potent but also display an extraordinarily wide spectrum of biologic activity. Because of their biologic activity, the eicosanoids, their specific receptor and enzyme inhibitors, and their plant and fish oil precursors have great therapeutic potential. Their short half-lives—seconds to minutes—make special delivery systems or synthesis of stable analogs mandatory for their clinical use.

ARACHIDONIC ACID & OTHER POLYUNSATURATED PRECURSORS

Arachidonic acid is the most abundant and the most important of the precursors of the eicosanoids. Arachidonic acid is a 20-carbon (C20) fatty acid that contains four double bonds beginning at the omega-6 position to yield a 5,8,11,14-eicosatetraenoic acid (designated C20:4–6). For eicosanoid synthesis to occur, arachidonate must first be released or mobilized from membrane phospholipids by one or more lipases of the phospholipase A_2 (PLA_2) type (Figure 18–1). At least three phospholipases mediate arachidonate release from membrane lipids: cardiac PLA_2 ($cPLA_2$), cytosolic PLA_2, and secretory PLA_2. In addition, arachidonate is also released by a combination of phospholipase C and diglyceride lipase. These lipase pathways are interdicted by corticosteroids. The precise mechanisms are still conjectural.

Following mobilization, arachidonic acid is oxygenated by four separate routes: the cyclooxygenase (COX), lipoxygenase, P450 epoxygenase, and isoprostane pathways (Figure 18–1). A number of factors determine the type of eicosanoid synthesized: (1) the species, (2) the type of cell, and (3) the cell's particular phenotype. The pattern of eicosanoids synthesized also frequently reflects (4) the manner in which the cell is stimulated. Finally, an important factor governing the pattern of eicosanoid release is (5) the nature of the precursor polyunsaturated fatty acid that has been esterified in specific membrane phospholipids. For example, homo-γ-linoleic acid (C20:3–6), which is trienoic, yields products that differ from those derived from arachidonate (C20:4–6), which has four double bonds. Similarly, the products derived from eicosapentaenoic acid (C20:5–3), which has five double bonds, are also quantitatively different. This is the basis for using as nutritional supplements in humans the structurally different fatty acids obtained from cold water fish or from plants. An example of the significance of the polyunsaturated fatty acid precursors is evident when one considers thromboxane A (TXA) derived from the COX pathway. TXA_2 is synthesized from arachidonate, a tetraenoic acid and is a powerful vasoconstrictor and aggregator of platelets. However 5,8,11,14,17-eicosapentaenoic acid yields TXA_3, which is relatively inactive. In theory, dietary eicosapentaenoate substitution for arachidonate should minimize thrombotic events due to the displacement of tetraenoic arachidonate in the membrane by a pentaenoic acid.

SYNTHESIS OF EICOSANOIDS

Products of Prostaglandin Endoperoxide Synthases (Cyclooxygenases)

Two unique COX isozymes convert arachidonic acid into prostaglandin endoperoxide. PGH synthase-1 (COX-1) is constitutively expressed, ie, it is always present. In contrast, PGH synthase-2 (COX-2) is inducible, ie, its expression varies markedly depending on the stimulus. The two isozymes also differ in function in that COX-1 is widely distributed and has "housekeeping" functions, eg, gastric cytoprotection.

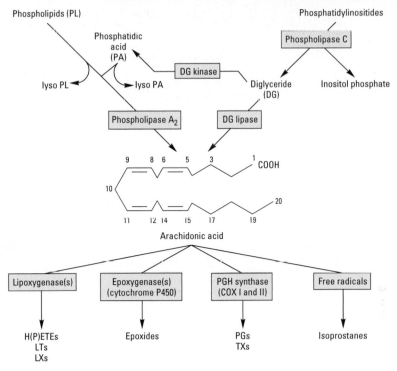

Figure 18–1. Pathways of arachidonic acid release and metabolism.

Two-fold to four-fold increases occur following humoral stimulation. In contrast, COX-2 is an immediate early response gene product in inflammatory and immune cells and expression is stimulated ten-fold to eighteen-fold by growth factors, tumor promoters, and cytokines. Lipopolysaccharide (endotoxin) is particularly potent in this respect. However, COX-2 is also involved in normal renal development and vascular prostacyclin production. Several additional COX isoforms have been described recently (Chandrasekharan, 2002).

The synthases are important because it is at this step that the nonsteroidal anti-inflammatory drugs (NSAIDs) exert their therapeutic effects (see Chapter 36). Indomethacin and sulindac are slightly selective for COX-1. Meclofenamate and ibuprofen are approximately equipotent on COX-1 and COX-2, while celecoxib and rofecoxib preferentially inhibit COX-2. The steroidal anti-inflammatory drugs such as dexamethasone can inhibit COX-2 gene expression. Aspirin acetylates and inhibits both enzymes to different extents.

Both COXs promote the uptake of two molecules of oxygen by cyclization of arachidonic acid to yield a C_9–C_{11} endoperoxide C_{15} hydroperoxide (Figure 18–2). This product is PGG_2, which is then rapidly modified by the peroxidase moiety of the COX enzyme to add a 15-hydroxyl group that is essential for biologic activity. This product is PGH_2. Both endoperoxides are highly unstable. Analogous families—PGH_1 and PGH_3 and all their subsequent products—are derived from homo-γ-linolenic acid and eicosapentaenoic acid, respectively.

PGH_2 then yields the prostaglandins, thromboxane, and prostacyclin by separate pathways. The prostaglandins differ from each other in two ways: (1) in the substituents of the pentane ring (indicated by the last letter, eg, E and F in PGE and PGF) and (2) in the number of double bonds in the side chains (indicated by the subscript, eg, PGE_1, PGE_2). Several products of the arachidonate series are of current clinical importance. **Alprostadil** (PGE_1) is used for its smooth muscle relaxing effects. **Misoprostol,** a PGE_1 derivative, is a cytoprotective prostaglandin used in preventing peptic ulcer and in combination with mifepristone for terminating early pregnancies. **PGE_2** and **$PGF_{2\alpha}$** are used in obstetrics. **Latanoprost** and several similar compounds are topically active $PGF_{2\alpha}$ derivatives used in ophthalmology. **Prostacyclin** (PGI_2, epoprostenol) is synthesized mainly by the vascular endothelium and is a powerful vasodilator and inhibitor of platelet aggregation. In con-

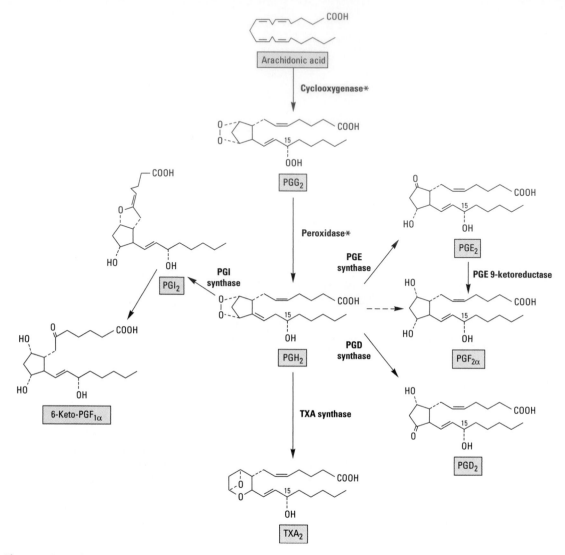

Figure 18–2. Prostaglandin and thromboxane biosynthesis. Compound names are enclosed in boxes. The asterisks indicate that both cyclooxygenase and peroxidase steps are catalyzed by the single enzyme prostaglandin endoperoxide (PGH) synthase.

trast, **thromboxane (TXA$_2$)** has undesirable properties (aggregation of platelets, vasoconstriction). Therefore TXA$_2$ receptor antagonists and synthesis inhibitors are developed for cardiovascular indications.

All the naturally occurring COX products rapidly undergo metabolism by β-oxidation, ω-oxidation, and oxidation of the key 15-hydroxyl group to the corresponding ketone. These inactive metabolites can be determined in blood and urine by immunoassay or mass spectrometry as a measure of the in vivo synthesis of their parent compounds.

Products of Lipoxygenase

The metabolism of arachidonic acid by the 5-, 12-, and 15-lipoxygenases results in the production of hydroperoxyeicosatetraenoic acids (HPETEs), which rapidly convert to hydroxy derivatives (HETEs) and leukotrienes (Figure 18–3). The most actively investigated leukotrienes are those produced by the 5-lipoxygenase present in inflammatory cells (PMNs, basophils, mast cells, eosinophils, macrophages). This pathway is of great interest since it is associated with asthma and

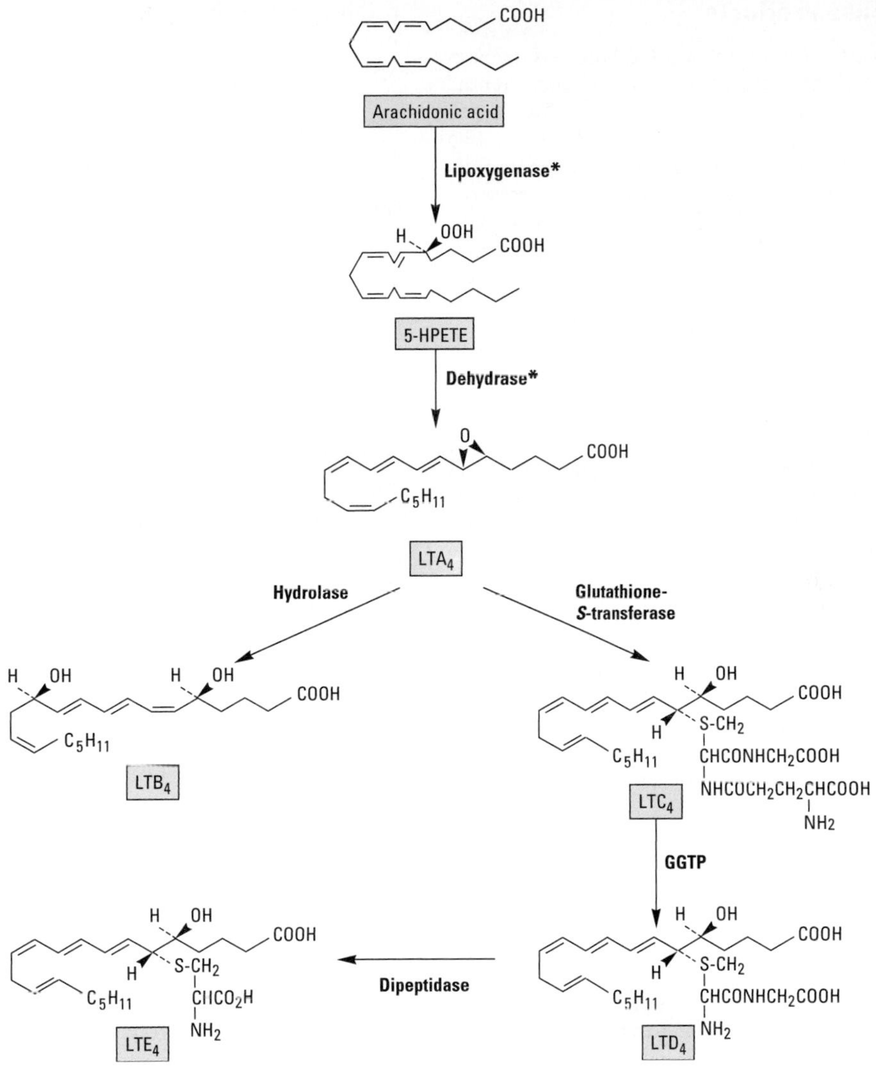

Figure 18–3. Leukotriene biosynthesis. The asterisks indicate that both the lipoxygenase and dehydrase reactions are driven by the single enzyme 5-lipoxygenase. (GGTP, γ-glutamyltranspeptidase.)

anaphylactic shock. Stimulation of these cells elevates intracellular Ca^{2+}, and releases arachidonate; incorporation of molecular oxygen by 5-lipoxygenase then yields the unstable epoxide leukotriene A_4 (LTA_4). This intermediate either converts to the dihydroxy leukotriene B_4 (LTB_4) or conjugates with glutathione to yield leukotriene C_4 (LTC_4), which undergoes sequential degradation of the glutathione moiety by peptidases to yield LTD_4 and LTE_4. These three products are called cysteinyl leukotrienes or peptidoleukotrienes.

LTC_4 and **LTD_4** are potent bronchoconstrictors and are recognized as the primary components of the **slow-**reacting substance of anaphylaxis (SRS-A) that is secreted in asthma and anaphylaxis. There are four current approaches to anti-leukotriene drug development: 5-lipoxygenase enzyme inhibitors, leukotriene receptor antagonists, inhibitors of an important membrane-bound 5-lipoxygenase activating protein (FLAP), and phospholipase A_2 inhibitors. Two selective leukotriene receptor antagonists are currently used for treatment of asthma.

Another group of 5-lipoxygenase products are the **lipoxins** LXA and LXB. Their biologic roles are still to be defined.

Epoxygenase Products

Specific isozymes of microsomal P450 monooxygenases convert arachidonic acid to four epoxyeicosatrienoic acids (EETs) (Figure 18–1). These are the 5,6-, 6,9-, 11,12-, and 14,15-oxido products. Each EET has two stereoisomers. These epoxides are unstable and rapidly form the corresponding dihydroxyeicosatrienoic (DHET) acid, eg, 5,6-DHET. Unlike the prostaglandins, both the EETs and the DHETs can be incorporated into phospholipids that then act as storage sites. The epoxygenase products are active on smooth muscle cells and in cell signaling pathways and are thought to have important roles in renal function.

Isoprostanes

The generation of isoprostanes from arachidonic acid is another potentially important pathway. The isoprostanes are prostaglandin stereoisomers. Because prostaglandins have many asymmetric centers, they have a large number of potential stereoisomers. Prostaglandin synthase (COX) is not needed for the formation of the isoprostanes, and aspirin and other nonsteroidal inhibitors of COX should not affect the isoprostane pathway. The primary epimerization mechanism is peroxidation of arachidonate by free radicals. Peroxidation occurs while arachidonic acid is still esterified to the membrane phospholipids. Thus, unlike prostaglandins, these stereoisomers are "stored" as part of the membrane. The importance of the isoprostane

pathway lies in the relatively large amounts of these products (ten-fold greater in blood and urine than the COX-derived prostaglandins) and their potent vasoconstrictor effects in the renal and other vascular beds. It has been proposed that isoprostanes play an important role in the hepatorenal syndrome.

I. BASIC PHARMACOLOGY OF EICOSANOIDS

MECHANISMS & EFFECTS OF EICOSANOIDS

Receptor Mechanisms

The eicosanoids act in an autocrine and paracrine fashion. These ligands bind to receptors on the cell surface, and pharmacologic specificity is determined by receptor density and type on different cells. A number of the membrane receptors and their subtypes have been cloned. All of these receptors appear to be G protein-linked; properties of the best-studied receptors are listed in Table 18–1.

Binding of PGI_2, PGE_1, and PGD_2 to their platelet receptors inhibits platelet aggregation by activating adenylyl cyclase. This leads to increased intracellular cAMP levels, which in turn activates specific protein kinases. These kinases phosphorylate internal calcium

Table 18–1. Some properties of prostanoid membrane receptors.

Receptor Type	Endogenous Agonist	G protein, Second Messenger	Smooth Muscle Tone	Result of Receptor Knockout
DP	PGD_2	G_s, inc cAMP	+/–	Dec allergic bronchial responses
EP_1	PGE_2	G_q, inc IP_3, DAG	+	Dec response to colon carcinogens
EP_2	PGE_2	G_s, inc cAMP	–	Impaired ovulation and fertilization; salt-sensitive HTN, dec bronchodilation to EP_2
EP_3	PGE_2	G_i, G_s, G_q, inc or dec cAMP, IP_3, DAG	+/–	Dec febrile response; inc hypotensive response to PGE_2
EP_4	PGE_2	G_s, inc cAMP	–	Patent ductus; dec bone inflammatory resorption response
FP	$PGF_{2\alpha}$	G_q, inc IP_3, DAG	+	Loss of labor, delivery
IP	PGI_2	G_s, inc cAMP	–	Inc thrombosis, dec pain responses to chemical stimuli
TP	TXA_2	G_q, inc IP_3, DAG	+	Inc bleeding; dec thrombosis

inc, increased; dec, decreased; HTN, hypertension.

pump proteins, an action that decreases free intracellular calcium concentration. In contrast, the binding of TXA_2 to its specific receptors activates phosphatidylinositol metabolism, leading to the formation of IP_3. IP_3 causes mobilization of Ca^{2+} stores and an increase of free intracellular calcium. LTB_4 also generates IP_3 release and causes activation, degranulation, and superoxide anion generation in polymorphonuclear leukocytes.

Subtypes are described for PGE_2 receptors (EP_1, EP_2, EP_3, and EP_4), each of which activates distinct signaling pathways. EP_1 is coupled to activation of phospholipase C, EP_2 and EP_4 to stimulation of adenylyl cyclase. EP_3 appears to have multiple effects depending on concentration. The recent description of isoforms of receptor subtypes with coupling to different G proteins makes the issue of second messenger activation more complex. However this multiplicity of pathways may help clarify seemingly paradoxical experimental results.

The contractile effects of eicosanoids on smooth muscle are mediated by the release of calcium, while their relaxing effects are mediated by the generation of cAMP. The effects of eicosanoids on many target systems, including the immune system, can be similarly explained (see below). Many of the eicosanoids' contractile effects on smooth muscle can be inhibited by lowering extracellular calcium or by using calcium channel blocking drugs.

Action on nuclear PPAR receptors has also been proposed but the physiologic role of this interaction has not been determined.

Effects of Prostaglandins & Thromboxanes

The prostaglandins and thromboxanes have major effects on four types of smooth muscle: airway, gastrointestinal, reproductive, and vascular. Other important targets include platelets and monocytes, kidneys, the central nervous system, autonomic presynaptic nerve terminals, sensory nerve endings, endocrine organs, adipose tissue, and the eye (the effects on the eye may involve smooth muscle).

A. SMOOTH MUSCLE

1. Vascular—TXA_2 is a smooth muscle cell mitogen and is the only eicosanoid that has convincingly been shown to have this effect. The mitogenic effect is potentiated by exposure of smooth muscle cells to testosterone, which up-regulates smooth muscle cell TXA_2 receptors. In addition to its mitogenic effect, TXA_2 is a potent vasoconstrictor. $PGF_{2\alpha}$ is also a vasoconstrictor (via FP receptors) but is not a mitogen for smooth muscle cells. Another potent vasoconstrictor is 8-*epi*-$PGF_{2\alpha}$. In patients with cirrhosis, it is produced in large amounts in the liver and is thought to play a pathophysiologic role as an important vasoconstrictor substance in the hepatorenal syndrome.

Vasodilator prostaglandins, especially PGI_2 and PGE_2, promote vasodilation by increasing cAMP and decreasing smooth muscle intracellular calcium, primarily via IP and EP_4 receptors. Vascular prostacyclin is synthesized by both smooth muscle and endothelial cells, with the latter as the major contributor. PGI_2 undergoes rapid metabolism in a few seconds to more stable but inactive products. In the microcirculation, PGE_2 is an endothelial vasodilator product.

2. Gastrointestinal tract—Most of the prostaglandins and thromboxanes activate gastrointestinal smooth muscle. Longitudinal muscle is contracted by PGE_2 (via EP_3) and $PGF_{2\alpha}$ (via FP), while circular muscle is contracted strongly by $PGF_{2\alpha}$ and weakly by PGI_2, and relaxed by PGE_2 (via EP_4). Administration of either PGE_2 or $PGF_{2\alpha}$ results in colicky cramps (see Clinical Pharmacology of Eicosanoids, below).

3. Airways—Respiratory smooth muscle is relaxed by PGD_2, PGE_1, PGE_2, and PGI_2 and contracted by TXA_2 and $PGF_{2\alpha}$. Although PGD_2 is less well-studied than the other prostaglandins, studies of PGD_2 receptor knockout mice suggest an important role of this receptor in asthma.

B. PLATELETS AND BLOOD CELLS

Platelet aggregation is markedly affected by eicosanoids. PGE_1 and especially PGI_2 effectively inhibit aggregation, while TXA_2 is a potent platelet aggregator. Platelets release TXA_2 during activation and aggregation, suggesting that thrombotic events such as myocardial infarction may result in the release of TXA_2. In fact, urinary metabolites of TXA_2 increase in patients experiencing a myocardial infarction even if they are receiving low-dosage aspirin. At this aspirin dosage, thromboxane synthesis is significantly inhibited only in platelets. This suggests that other cells may contribute to the increase in TXA_2; these other cells may be monocytes, since monocytes have a high capacity for sustained release of TXA_2. Neutrophils and lymphocytes synthesize little if any prostaglandins, while monocytes have a substantial capacity for prostaglandin and thromboxane synthesis through both constitutive and inducible COXs. Human eosinophils also seem to have a high capacity for prostaglandin and thromboxane synthesis.

C. KIDNEY

Both the renal medulla and the renal cortex synthesize prostaglandins, the medulla substantially more than the cortex. The kidney also synthesizes several hydroxyeicosatetraenoic acids, leukotrienes, cytochrome P450 products, and epoxides. These compounds play important autoregulatory roles in renal function by modifying renal hemodynamics and glomerular and tubular function. This regulatory role is especially important in marginally functioning kidneys, as shown by the decline in kidney function caused by COX inhibitors in elderly patients and those with renal disease.

The major eicosanoid products of the renal cortex are PGE_2 and PGI_2. Both compounds increase renin release; normally, however, renin release is more directly under β_1 adrenoceptor control. The glomeruli synthesize small amounts of TXA_2 but this potent vasoconstrictor does not appear to be responsible for regulating glomerular function in healthy humans.

PGE_1, PGE_2, and PGI_2 increase glomerular filtration through their vasodilating effects. These prostaglandins also increase water and sodium excretion. The increase in water clearance probably results from an attenuation of the action of antidiuretic hormone on adenylyl cyclase. It is uncertain whether the natriuretic effect is caused by the direct inhibition of sodium resorption in the distal tubule or by increased medullary blood flow. Loop diuretics, eg, furosemide, produce some of their effect by stimulating COX activity. In the normal kidney, this increases the synthesis of the vasodilator prostaglandins. Therefore, patient response to a loop diuretic will be diminished if a COX inhibitor is administered concurrently (see Chapter 15).

TXA_2 causes intrarenal vasoconstriction (and perhaps an ADH-like effect), resulting in a decline in renal function. The normal kidney synthesizes only small amounts of TXA_2. However, in renal conditions involving inflammatory cell infiltration (such as glomerulonephritis and renal transplant rejection), the inflammatory cells (monocyte-macrophages) release substantial amounts of TXA_2. Theoretically, TXA_2 synthase inhibitors or receptor antagonists should improve renal function in these patients, but no such drug is clinically available.

Hypertension is associated with increased TXA_2 and decreased PGE_2 and PGI_2 synthesis in some animal models, eg, the Goldblatt kidney model. It is not known whether these changes are primary contributing factors or secondary responses. Similarly, increased TXA_2 formation has been reported in cyclosporine-induced nephrotoxicity, but no causal relationship has been established.

PGE_2 may also be involved in renal phosphate excretion, because exogenous PGE_2 antagonizes the inhibition of phosphate resorption by parathyroid hormone in the proximal tubule. However, the physiologic role of this eicosanoid may be limited because the proximal tubule, the major site for phosphate transport, produces few prostaglandins.

D. Reproductive Organs

1. Female reproductive organs—The effects of prostaglandins on uterine function are of great clinical importance. They are discussed below. (See Clinical Pharmacology of Eicosanoids.)

2. Male reproductive organs—The role of prostaglandins in semen is still conjectural. The major source of these prostaglandins is the seminal vesicle; the prostate and the testes synthesize only small amounts. Thus, the term prostaglandin (referring to the prostate gland) is now known to be a misnomer. Semen from fertile men contains about 400 μg/mL of PGE and PGF and their 19-hydroxy metabolites. There is about 20 times more PGE than PGF in fertile semen, although this ratio varies greatly among individuals. However, within individuals, this ratio remains fairly constant as long as the sperm characteristics are unchanged. The factors that regulate the concentration of prostaglandins in human seminal plasma are not known in detail, but testosterone does promote prostaglandin production. Thromboxane and leukotrienes have not been found in seminal plasma. Men with a low seminal fluid concentration of prostaglandins are relatively infertile. Large doses of aspirin reduce the prostaglandin content of seminal plasma.

Smooth muscle–relaxing prostaglandins such as PGE_1 enhance penile erection by relaxing the smooth muscle of the corpora cavernosa. (See Clinical Pharmacology of the Eicosanoids.)

E. Central and Peripheral Nervous Systems

1. Fever—PGE_1 and PGE_2 increase body temperature, probably via EP_3 receptors, especially when administered into the cerebral ventricles. Pyrogens release interleukin-1, which in turn promotes the synthesis and release of PGE_2. This synthesis is blocked by aspirin and other antipyretic compounds.

2. Sleep—When infused into the cerebral ventricles, PGD_2 induces natural sleep (as determined by electroencephalographic analysis) in a number of species, including primates.

3. Neurotransmission—PGE compounds inhibit the release of norepinephrine from postganglionic sympathetic nerve endings. Moreover, NSAIDs increase norepinephrine release in vivo, suggesting that the prostaglandins play a physiologic role in this process. Thus, vasoconstriction observed during treatment with COX inhibitors may be due to increased release of norepinephrine as well as to inhibition of the endothelial synthesis of the vasodilators PGE_2 and PGI_2.

F. Neuroendocrine Organs

Both in vitro and in vivo tests have shown that some of the eicosanoids affect the secretion of anterior pituitary hormones. PGE compounds promote the release of growth hormone, prolactin, TSH, ACTH, FSH, and LH. However, endocrine changes reflecting significant release of these hormones have not been reported in patients receiving PGE compounds. LTC_4 and LTD_4 stimulate LHRH and LH secretion (see below).

G. BONE METABOLISM

Prostaglandins are abundant in skeletal tissue and are produced by the osteoblasts and the adjacent hematopoietic cells. The major effect of prostaglandins (especially PGE_2, acting on EP_4 receptors) in vivo is to increase bone turnover, ie, stimulation of bone resorption and formation. Prostaglandins may mediate the effects of mechanical forces on bones and some of the changes that occur in bones with inflammation. Finally, prostaglandins may play a role in the bone loss that occurs at menopause.

H. EYE

PGE and PGF derivatives lower the intraocular pressure. The mechanism of this action is unclear but probably involves increased outflow of aqueous humor from the anterior chamber via the uveoscleral pathway (see Clinical Applications).

Effects of Lipoxygenase & Cytochrome P450-Derived Metabolites

The actions of lipoxygenases generate compounds that can regulate specific cellular responses important in inflammation and immunity. Cytochrome P450-derived metabolites affect nephron transport functions either directly or via metabolism to active compounds (see below). The biologic functions of the various forms of hydroxy- and hydroperoxyeicosaenoic acids are largely unknown, but their pharmacologic potency is impressive.

A. BLOOD CELLS AND INFLAMMATION

LTB_4 is a potent chemoattractant for neutrophils; LTC_4 and LTD_4 are potent chemoattractants for eosinophils. These leukotrienes also promote eosinophil adherence, degranulation, and oxygen radical formation. The leukotrienes have been strongly implicated in the pathogenesis of inflammation, especially in chronic diseases such as asthma and inflammatory bowel disease. Lipoxin A seems to exert effects similar to those of LTB_4 on neutrophils. Lymphocyte proliferation and differentiation are modified by LTB_4. Both lipoxin A and lipoxin B inhibit natural killer cell cytotoxicity.

B. HEART AND SMOOTH MUSCLE

1. Cardiovascular—12(S)-HETE is a potent chemoattractant for smooth muscle cells, causing migration at concentrations as low as 1 fmol/L; it may play a role in myointimal proliferation that occurs after vascular injury such as that caused by angioplasty. Its stereoiso-

mer, 12(R)-HETE, is not a chemoattractant but is a potent inhibitor of the Na^+/K^+ ATPase in the cornea. LTC_4 and LTD_4 reduce myocardial contractility and coronary blood flow, leading to cardiac depression. Lipoxin A and lipoxin B seem to exert coronary vasoconstrictor effects.

2. Gastrointestinal—Human colonic epithelial cells synthesize LTB_4, a chemoattractant for neutrophils. The colonic mucosa of patients with inflammatory bowel disease contains substantially increased amounts of LTB_4.

3. Airways—The peptidoleukotrienes, particularly LTC_4 and LTD_4, are potent bronchoconstrictors and cause increased microvascular permeability, plasma exudation, and mucus secretion in the airways. Controversies exist over whether the pattern and specificity of the leukotriene receptors differ in animal models and humans. LTC_4-specific receptors have not been found in human lung tissue, whereas both high- and low-affinity LTD_4 receptors are present.

C. RENAL SYSTEM

The roles of leukotrienes and cytochrome P450 products in the human kidney are currently speculative. Recently, the 5,6-epoxide has been shown to be a powerful vasodilator in animal experiments. Another recent discovery is that free radicals attack arachidonic acid-containing phospholipids to yield an 8-epi-$PGF_{2\alpha}$ that has powerful thromboxane-like properties. Synthesis is not blocked by COX inhibitors but can be blocked by antioxidants. This vasoconstrictor, which is present in humans, is thought to be another important mediator causing renal failure in the hepatorenal syndrome.

D. MISCELLANEOUS

The effects of these products on the reproductive organs remain to be elucidated. Similarly, actions on the nervous system have been suggested (recent data indicate that 12-HPETE acts as a neurotransmitter in *Aplysia* neurons), but this has not been confirmed in higher organisms. Very low concentrations of LTC_4 increase and higher concentrations of arachidonate-derived epoxides augment LH and LHRH release from isolated rat anterior pituitary cells.

INHIBITION OF EICOSANOID SYNTHESIS

Corticosteroids block all the known pathways of eicosanoid synthesis, perhaps by stimulating the synthesis of several inhibitory proteins collectively called **annexins** or **lipocortins**. They inhibit phospholipase A_2 activity, probably by interfering with phospholipid binding and thus preventing the release of arachidonic acid.

The NSAIDs (eg, aspirin, indomethacin, ibuprofen) block both prostaglandin and thromboxane formation by inhibiting COX activity. For example, aspirin is a long-lasting inhibitor of platelet COX and of TXA$_2$ biosynthesis because it irreversibly acetylates the enzyme. Once acetylated, platelet COX cannot be restored via protein biosynthesis because platelets lack a nucleus.

The development of selective thromboxane synthase inhibitors and TXA$_2$ receptor antagonists has required considerable effort. The resulting compounds, eg, **sulotroban,** have been useful for characterizing TXA$_2$-related effects in vitro and in vivo. They are being tested in the treatment of thromboembolism, pulmonary hypertension, and preeclampsia-eclampsia.

Selective inhibitors of the lipoxygenase pathway are also mainly investigational. With a few exceptions, NSAIDs do not inhibit lipoxygenase activity at concentrations that markedly inhibit COX activity. In fact, by preventing arachidonic acid conversion via the COX pathway, NSAIDs may cause more substrate to be metabolized through the lipoxygenase pathways, leading to an increased formation of the inflammatory leukotrienes. Even among the COX-dependent pathways, inhibiting the synthesis of one derivative may increase the synthesis of an enzymatically related product. Therefore, researchers are attempting to develop drugs that inhibit both COX and lipoxygenase.

II. CLINICAL PHARMACOLOGY OF EICOSANOIDS

Several approaches have been used in the clinical application of eicosanoids. First, stable oral or parenteral long-acting analogs of the naturally occurring prostaglandins have been developed. Several such compounds have been approved for clinical use overseas and are being introduced in the USA (Figure 18–4). Second, enzyme inhibitors and receptor antagonists have been developed to interfere with the synthesis or effects of the "pathologic" eicosanoids (ie, thromboxanes and leukotrienes). For example, knowledge of eicosanoid synthesis and metabolism has led to the development of

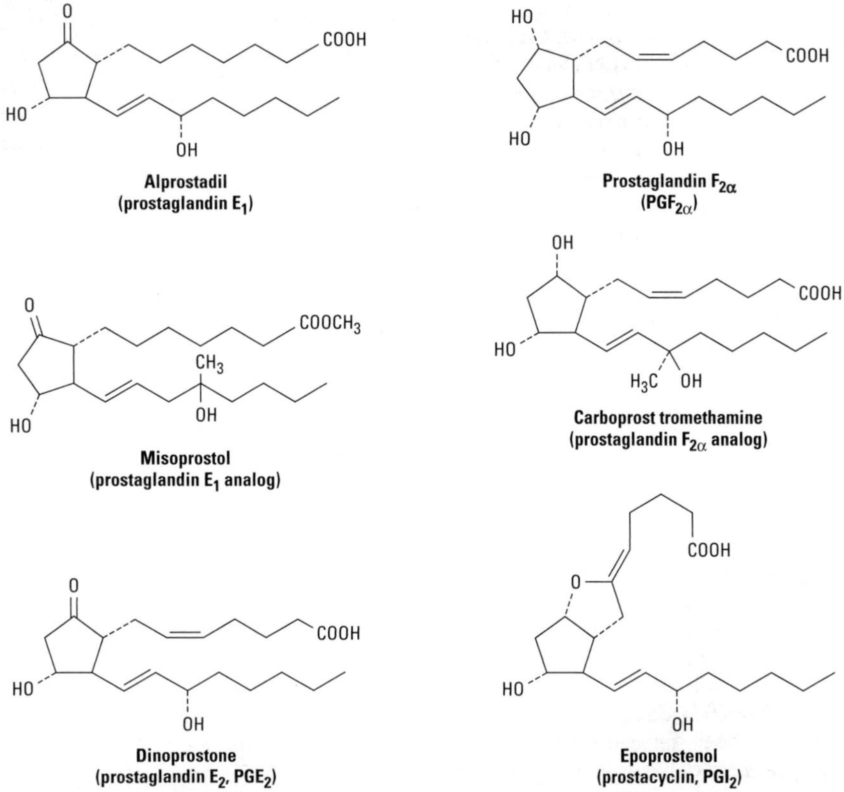

Alprostadil
(prostaglandin E$_1$)

Prostaglandin F$_{2\alpha}$
(PGF$_{2\alpha}$)

Misoprostol
(prostaglandin E$_1$ analog)

Carboprost tromethamine
(prostaglandin F$_{2\alpha}$ analog)

Dinoprostone
(prostaglandin E$_2$, PGE$_2$)

Epoprostenol
(prostacyclin, PGI$_2$)

Figure 18–4. Chemical structures of some prostaglandins and prostaglandin analogs currently in clinical use.

new NSAIDs that inhibit COX (especially COX-2), with improved pharmacokinetic and pharmacodynamic characteristics. One objective, described earlier, is to develop dual inhibitors that block both the COX (especially COX-2) and lipoxygenase pathways. Another goal is to decrease gastrointestinal and renal toxicity. Third, dietary manipulation—to change the polyunsaturated fatty acid precursors in the cell membrane phospholipids and so change eicosanoid synthesis—is used extensively in over-the-counter products and in diets emphasizing increased consumption of cold water fish.

Female Reproductive System

The physiologic role of prostaglandins in reproduction has been intensively studied since the discovery of prostaglandins in the seminal plasma of primates and sheep. It has been suggested that the prostaglandins in seminal plasma facilitate blastocyst implantation or egg transport and that uterine secretion of prostaglandins causes luteolysis. The latter is not true in humans but appears to be true in cattle and pigs. This finding has led to the marketing of veterinary preparations of $PGF_{2\alpha}$ and its analogs for synchronizing ovulation in animals.

A. ABORTION

PGE_2 and $PGF_{2\alpha}$ have potent oxytocic actions. The ability of the E and F prostaglandins and their analogs to terminate pregnancy at any stage by promoting uterine contractions has been adapted to routine clinical use. Many studies worldwide have established that prostaglandin administration efficiently terminates pregnancy. The drugs are used for first- and second-trimester abortion and for priming or ripening the cervix before abortion. These prostaglandins appear to soften the cervix by increasing proteoglycan content and changing the biophysical properties of collagen.

Early studies found that intravenous PGE_2 and $PGF_{2\alpha}$ produced abortion in about 80% of cases. The success rate is dependent on the dose, the duration of the infusion, and parity of the woman. Dose-limiting adverse effects include vomiting, diarrhea, fever, and bronchoconstriction. Hypotension, hypertension, syncope, dizziness, and flushing can occur and may be related to the vasomotor and vasovagal effects of PGE_2.

In current practice, **dinoprostone,** a synthetic preparation of PGE_2, is administered vaginally for oxytocic use. In the USA, it is approved for inducing abortion in the second trimester of pregnancy, for missed abortion, for benign hydatidiform mole, and for ripening of the cervix for induction of labor in patients at or near term.

Dinoprostone stimulates the contraction of the uterus throughout pregnancy. As the pregnancy progresses, the uterus increases its contractile response, and the contractile effect of oxytocin is potentiated as well.

Dinoprostone also directly affects the collagenase of the cervix, resulting in softening. The vaginal dose enters the maternal circulation, and a small amount is absorbed directly by the uterus via the cervix and the lymphatic system. Dinoprostone is metabolized in local tissues and on the first pass through the lungs (about 95%). The metabolites are mainly excreted in the urine. The plasma half-life is 2.5–5 minutes.

For the induction of labor, dinoprostone is available either as a gel (0.5 mg PGE_2) or as a controlled-release formulation (10 mg PGE_2) that releases PGE_2 in vivo at a rate of about 0.3 mg/h over 12 hours. An advantage of the controlled-release formulation is a lower incidence of gastrointestinal side effects (< 1%). A further advantage of this delivery system is that the medication is contained within a vaginal insert that can be retrieved at any time.

For abortifacient purposes, the recommended dosage is a 20 mg dinoprostone vaginal suppository repeated at 3- to 5-hour intervals depending on the response of the uterus. The mean time to abortion is 17 hours, but in more than 25% of cases the abortion is incomplete and requires additional intervention.

For softening of the cervix at term, the preparations used are either a single vaginal insert containing 10 mg PGE_2 or a vaginal gel containing 0.5 mg PGE_2 administered every 6 hours. The softening of the cervix for induction of labor substantially shortens the time to onset of labor and the delivery time.

The use of PGE analogs for "menstrual regulation" or very early abortions—within 1–2 weeks after the last menstrual period—has been explored extensively. There are two problems: prolonged vaginal bleeding and severe menstrual cramps.

Antiprogestins (eg, **mifepristone**) have been combined with an oral oxytocic prostaglandin (eg, **misoprostol**) to produce early abortion. This regimen is now available in the USA (see Chapter 39). The ease of use and the effectiveness of the combination have aroused considerable opposition in some quarters. The major toxicities are cramping pain and diarrhea.

$PGF_{2\alpha}$ is available for clinical gynecologic use. This drug, **carboprost tromethamine** (15-methyl-$PGF_{2\alpha}$; the 15-methyl group prolongs the duration of action) was withdrawn from the United States market. Carboprost is used to induce second-trimester abortions and is usually administered as a single 2.5 mg intra-amniotic injection. The abortion is normally completed in less than 20 hours. The most serious adverse effects of this route of administration involve cardiovascular collapse. Most of the reported cases have been diagnosed as anaphylactic shock, but others may have been due to the drug escaping into the circulation and causing severe pulmonary hypertension. In pregnant anesthetized women, $PGF_{2\alpha}$, 300 µg/min intravenously, doubles pulmonary resistance and increases the work of the right side of the heart three-fold. Thus, only minimal amounts of the 40 mg intra-amniotic dose need to reach the circulation to cause cardiovascular effects. This problem may be avoided by instilling the drug under ultrasonic guidance.

Intramuscular injection of carboprost tromethamine can also be used to induce abortion. Unlike the one-time intrauterine instillation of dinoprost, carboprost is given repeatedly up to the total dose of 2.6 mg normally required to cause abortion. Intra-amniotic administration has close to a 100% success rate, with fewer and less severe adverse effects than intravenous administration.

B. Facilitation of Labor

Numerous studies have shown that PGE_2, $PGF_{2\alpha}$, and their analogs effectively initiate and stimulate labor. However, this is an unlabeled use. There appears to be no difference in the efficacy of the two drugs when they are administered intravenously, but $PGF_{2\alpha}$ is one tenth as potent as PGE_2. These agents and oxytocin have similar success rates and comparable induction-to-delivery intervals. The adverse effects of the prostaglandins are moderate, with a slightly higher incidence of nausea, vomiting, and diarrhea than that produced by oxytocin. $PGF_{2\alpha}$ has more gastrointestinal toxicity than PGE_2. Neither drug has significant maternal cardiovascular toxicity in the recommended doses. In fact, PGE_2 must be infused at a rate about 20 times faster than that used for induction of labor to decrease blood pressure and increase heart rate. $PGF_{2\alpha}$ is a bronchoconstrictor and should be used with caution in persons with asthma; however, neither asthma attacks nor bronchoconstriction have been observed during the induction of labor. Although both PGE_2 and $PGF_{2\alpha}$ pass the fetoplacental barrier, fetal toxicity is uncommon.

The effects of oral PGE_2 administration (0.5–1.5 mg/h) have been compared with those of intravenous oxytocin and oral demoxytocin, an oxytocin derivative, in the induction of labor. Oral PGE_2 is superior to the oral oxytocin derivative and in most studies is as efficient as intravenous oxytocin. However, the only available form of PGE_2 in the USA at present is dinoprostone for vaginal administration, and by this route of administration the drug is slightly less effective than oxytocin. Vaginal PGE_2 is also used to soften the cervix before inducing labor. Oral $PGF_{2\alpha}$ causes too much gastrointestinal toxicity to be useful by this route.

Theoretically, PGE_2 and $PGF_{2\alpha}$ should be superior to oxytocin for inducing labor in women with preeclampsia-eclampsia or cardiac and renal diseases because, unlike oxytocin, they have no antidiuretic effect. In addition, PGE_2 has natriuretic effects. However, the clinical benefits of these effects have not been documented. In cases of intrauterine fetal death, the

prostaglandins alone or with oxytocin seem to cause delivery effectively. In some cases of postpartum bleeding, 15-methyl-$PGF_{2\alpha}$ will successfully control hemorrhage when oxytocin and methylergonovine fail to do so.

C. Dysmenorrhea

Primary dysmenorrhea is attributable to increased endometrial synthesis of PGE_2 and $PGF_{2\alpha}$ during menstruation, with contractions of the uterus that lead to ischemic pain. NSAIDs successfully inhibit the formation of these prostaglandins (see Chapter 36) and so relieve dysmenorrhea in 75–85% of cases. Some of these drugs are available over the counter. Aspirin is also effective in dysmenorrhea, but because it has low potency and is quickly hydrolyzed, large doses and frequent administration are necessary. In addition, the acetylation of platelet COX, causing irreversible inhibition of platelet TXA_2 synthesis, may have an adverse effect on the amount of menstrual bleeding.

Male Reproductive System

Intracavernosal injection or urethral suppository therapy with **alprostadil** (PGE_1) is useful in the treatment of erectile dysfunction, especially in spinal cord injury. Doses of 2.5–25 µg are used. Penile pain is a frequent side effect that may be related to the algesic effects of PGE derivatives; however, only a few patients discontinue the use due to pain. Prolonged erection and priapism are less frequent side effects that occur in fewer than 4% of patients and are minimized by careful titration to the minimal effective dose. When given by injection, alprostadil may be used as monotherapy or in combination with either papaverine or phentolamine.

Cardiovascular System

The vasodilator effects of PGE compounds have been studied extensively in hypertensive patients. These compounds also promote sodium diuresis. Practical application will require derivatives with oral activity, longer half-lives, and fewer adverse effects.

A. Pulmonary Hypertension

Prostacyclin lowers peripheral, pulmonary, and coronary resistance. It has been used to treat both primary pulmonary hypertension and secondary pulmonary hypertension, which sometimes occurs after mitral valve surgery. A commercial preparation of prostacyclin (epoprostenol) is approved for treatment of primary pulmonary hypertension, in which it appears to improve symptoms and prolong survival. However, because of its extremely short plasma half-life, the drug must be administered as a continuous intravenous infusion through a central line. Several prostacyclin analogs with longer half-lives have been developed and **treprostinil** was recently approved for use in pulmonary hypertension (Horn, 2002). This drug is administered by continuous subcutaneous infusion.

B. PERIPHERAL VASCULAR DISEASE

A number of studies have investigated the use of PGE and PGI_2 compounds in Raynaud's phenomenon and peripheral atherosclerosis. In the latter case, prolonged infusions have been used to permit remodeling of the vessel wall and to enhance regression of ischemic ulcers.

C. PATENT DUCTUS ARTERIOSUS

Patency of the fetal ductus arteriosus is now generally believed to depend on local PGE_2 and PGI_2 synthesis. In certain types of congenital heart disease (eg, transposition of the great arteries, pulmonary atresia, pulmonary artery stenosis), it is important to maintain the patency of the neonate's ductus arteriosus before surgery. This is done with alprostadil, PGE_1. Like PGE_2, PGE_1 is a vasodilator and an inhibitor of platelet aggregation, and it contracts uterine and intestinal smooth muscle. Adverse effects include apnea, bradycardia, hypotension, and hyperpyrexia. Because of rapid pulmonary clearance, the drug must be continuously infused at an initial rate of 0.05–0.1 µg/kg/min, which may be increased to 0.4 µg/kg/min. Prolonged treatment has been associated with ductal fragility and rupture.

In delayed closure of the ductus arteriosus, COX inhibitors are often used to inhibit synthesis of PGE_2 and PGI_2 and so close the ductus. Premature infants in whom respiratory distress develops due to failure of ductus closure can be treated with a high degree of success with indomethacin. This treatment often precludes the need for surgical closure of the ductus.

Blood

As noted above, eicosanoids are involved in thrombosis because TXA_2 promotes platelet aggregation and PGI_2 inhibits it. Aspirin inhibits platelet COX to produce a mild clotting defect. The mildness of this defect is supported by the fact that very modest hemostatic defects are noted in patients with diseases involving deficiencies of platelet COX and thromboxane synthase—eg, these patients have no history of increased or decreased bleeding. Blockade of either of these two enzymes inhibits secondary aggregation of platelets induced by ADP, by low concentrations of thrombin and collagen, or by epinephrine. Thus, these platelet enzymes are not necessary for platelet function but may amplify an aggregating stimulus.

Epidemiologic studies in the USA and United Kingdom indicate that low doses of aspirin reduce the risk of death due to infarction but may *increase* overall mortality rates due to hemorrhagic stroke (see Chapter 34). It is now difficult to find patients at risk for thromboembolism—as in orthopedic surgery or angioplasty for coronary artery stenosis—who do not take aspirin. The beneficial effects of aspirin are discussed in greater detail in Chapter 34.

Respiratory System

PGE_2 is a powerful bronchodilator when given in aerosol form. Unfortunately, it also promotes coughing, and an analog that possesses only the bronchodilator properties has been difficult to obtain.

$PGF_{2\alpha}$ and TXA_2 are both strong bronchoconstrictors and were once thought to be primary mediators in asthma. However, the identification of the peptidoleukotrienes—LTC_4, LTD_4, and LTE_4—expanded the role of eicosanoids as important mediators in asthma and other immune responses. As described in Chapter 20, leukotriene receptor inhibitors (eg, **zafirlukast**, **montelukast**) are effective in asthma. A lipoxygenase inhibitor (**zileuton**) has also been used in asthma but is not as popular as the receptor inhibitors. It remains unclear whether leukotrienes are partially responsible for the acute respiratory distress syndrome.

Corticosteroids and cromolyn are also useful in asthma. Corticosteroids inhibit eicosanoid synthesis and thus limit the amounts of eicosanoid mediator available for release. Cromolyn appears to inhibit the release of eicosanoids and other mediators such as histamine and platelet-activating factor from mast cells.

Gastrointestinal System

The word "cytoprotection" was coined to signify the remarkable protective effect of the E prostaglandins against peptic ulcers in animals at doses that do not reduce acid secretion. These prostaglandins were independently discovered also to inhibit gastric acid secretion (at higher doses). Since then, numerous experimental and clinical investigations have shown that the PGE compounds and their analogs protect against peptic ulcers produced by either steroids or NSAIDs. **Misoprostol** is an orally active synthetic analog of PGE_1 available in Europe and the USA for ulcer treatment. The FDA-approved indication is for prevention of NSAID-induced peptic ulcers. The drug is administered at a dosage of 200 µg four times daily. This and other PGE analogs (eg, enprostil) are cytoprotective at low doses and inhibit gastric acid secretion at higher doses. The adverse effects are abdominal discomfort and occasional diarrhea; both effects are dose-related. More recently, dose-dependent bone pain and hyperostosis have been described in patients with liver disease who were given long-term PGE treatment. This adverse effect can be explained by a PGE-induced, EP_4-mediated acceleration of osteoclast and osteoblast activity. Recurrent calcium oxalate kidney stones were described in the same group of patients. This may be related to PGE-induced hypercalciuria.

Gastrointestinal side effects seen in many patients using NSAIDs may be reduced by the recent introduction of selective inhibitors of COX-2 that spare gastric COX-1 so that the natural cytoprotection by locally synthesized PGE_2 is undisturbed (see Chapter 36).

Immune System

Monocyte-macrophages are the only principal cells of the immune system that can synthesize all the eicosanoids. T and B lymphocytes are interesting exceptions to the general rule that all nucleated cells produce eicosanoids. However, in a B lymphoma cell line, there is non-receptor-mediated uptake of LTB_4 and 5-HETE. Interaction between lymphocytes and monocyte-macrophages may cause the lymphocytes to release arachidonic acid from their cell membranes. The arachidonic acid is then used by the monocyte-macrophages for eicosanoid synthesis. In addition to these cells, there is evidence for eicosanoid-mediated cell-cell interaction by platelets, erythrocytes, PMNs, and endothelial cells.

The eicosanoids modulate the effects of the immune system, as illustrated by the cell-mediated immune response. As shown in Figure 18–5, PGE_2 and PGI_2 affect T cell proliferation in vitro as corticosteroids do. T cell clonal expansion is attenuated through inhibition of interleukin-1 and interleukin-2 and class II antigen expression by macrophages or other antigen-presenting cells. The leukotrienes, TXA_2, and platelet-activating factor stimulate T cell clonal expansion. These compounds stimulate the formation of interleukin-1 and interleukin-2 as well as the expression of interleukin-2 receptors. The leukotrienes also promote interferon-γ release and can replace interleukin-2 as a stimulator of interferon-γ. These in vitro effects of the eicosanoids agree with in vivo findings in animals with acute organ transplant rejection, as described below.

A. CELL-MEDIATED ORGAN TRANSPLANT REJECTION

Acute organ transplant rejection is a cell-mediated immune response. Administration of PGI_2 to renal transplant patients has reversed the rejection process in some cases. Experimental in vitro and in vivo data show that PGE_2 and PGI_2 can attenuate T cell proliferation and rejection, which can also be seen with drugs that inhibit TXA_2 and leukotriene formation. In organ transplant patients, urinary excretion of TXB_2, a metabolite of TXA_2, increases during acute rejection. Corticosteroids, the primary drugs used for treatment of acute

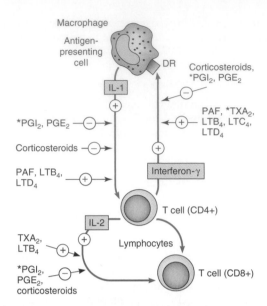

Figure 18–5. Modulation of macrophage and lymphocyte interactions by eicosanoids, platelet-activating factor, and corticosteroids. Corticosteroids, PGE_2, and possibly PGI_2 inhibit the expression of interleukin-1 (IL-1) and its effect on T lymphocytes. Platelet-activating factor (PAF), LTB_4, and LTD_4 increase IL-1 expression. Similar inhibitory and stimulant effects are exerted on the action of interferon-γ on the macrophage and on the action of interleukin-2 (IL-2). Agents marked with an asterisk are suspected, but not yet proved, to have the effects indicated. (DR, class II MHC [major histocompatibility complex] receptor; T, T lymphocytes.) (Modified and reproduced, with permission, from Foegh ML, Ramwell PW: PAF and transplant immunology. In: Braquet P [editor]: *The Role of Platelet Activating Factor in Immune Disorders.* Karger, 1988.)

rejection due to their effects on lymphocytes, inhibit both phospholipase and COX-2 activity.

B. INFLAMMATION

Aspirin has been used to treat arthritis for nearly a century, but its mechanism of action—inhibition of COX activity—was not discovered until 1971. Aspirin and other anti-inflammatory agents that inhibit COX are discussed in Chapter 36. COX-2 appears to be the form of the enzyme associated with cells involved in the inflammatory process. The prostaglandins are not chemoattractants, but the leukotrienes and some of the HETEs (eg, 12-HETE) are strong chemoattractants. PGE_2 inhibits both antigen-driven and mitogen-induced B lymphocyte proliferation and differentiation to plasma cells, resulting in inhibition of IgM synthesis. The concomitant elevation of serum IgE and monocyte PGE_2 synthesis, seen in patients with severe trauma and patients with Hodgkin's disease, is explained by PGE_2 ability to enhance immunoglobulin class switching to IgE.

C. Rheumatoid Arthritis

In rheumatoid arthritis, immune complexes are deposited in the affected joints, causing an inflammatory response that is amplified by eicosanoids. Lymphocytes and macrophages accumulate in the synovium, while PMNs localize mainly in the synovial fluid. The major eicosanoids produced by PMNs are leukotrienes, which facilitate T cell proliferation and act as chemoattractants. Human macrophages synthesize the COX products PGE_2 and TXA_2 and large amounts of leukotrienes.

D. Infection

The relationship of eicosanoids to infection is not well defined. The association between the use of the anti-inflammatory steroids and increased risk of infection is well established. However, the NSAIDs do not seem to alter patient responses to infection.

Glaucoma

Latanoprost, a stable long-acting $PGF_{2\alpha}$ derivative, was the first prostanoid used for glaucoma. The success of latanoprost has stimulated development of similar prostanoids with ocular hypotensive effects, and **bimatoprost, travaprost,** and **unoprostone** are now available. These drugs act at the FP receptor and are administered as drops into the conjunctival sac once or twice daily. Adverse effects include irreversible brown pigmentation of the iris and eyelashes, drying of the eyes, and conjunctivitis.

DIETARY MANIPULATION OF ARACHIDONIC ACID METABOLISM

Because arachidonic acid is derived from dietary linoleic and α-linolenic acids, which are essential fatty acids, the effects of dietary manipulation on arachidonic acid metabolism have been extensively studied. Two approaches have been used. The first adds corn, safflower, and sunflower oils, which contain linoleic acid (C18:2), to the diet. The second approach adds oils containing eicosapentaenoic (C20:5) and docosahexaenoic acids (C22:6), so-called omega-3 fatty acids, from cold water fish. Both types of diet change the phospholipid composition of cell membranes by replacing arachidonic acid with the dietary fatty acids. It has been claimed that the synthesis of both TXA_2 and PGI_2 is reduced and that changes in platelet aggregation, vasomotor spasm, and cholesterol metabolism follow.

As indicated above, there are many possible oxidation products of the different polyenoic acids. It is prob-

---

PREPARATIONS AVAILABLE

Nonsteroidal anti-inflammatory drugs are listed in Chapter 36.
  Alprostadil
    Penile injection (Caverject, Edex): 5, 10, 20, 40 µg sterile powder for reconstitution
    Penile pellet (Muse): 125, 250, 500, 1000 µg
    Parenteral (Prostin VR Pediatric): 500 µg/mL ampules
  Bimatoprost (Lumigan)
    Ophthalmic drops: 0.03% solution
  Carboprost tromethamine (Hemabate)
    Parenteral: 250 µg carboprost and 83 µg tromethamine per mL ampules
  Dinoprostone [prostaglandin E2] (Prostin E2, Prepidil, Cervidil)
    Vaginal: 20 mg suppositories, 0.5 mg gel, 10 mg controlled release system
  Epoprostenol [prostacyclin] (Flolan)
    Intravenous: powder to make 3, 5, 10, 15 µg/mL

Latanoprost (Xalatan)
  Topical: 50 µg/mL ophthalmic solution
Misoprostol (Cytotec)
  Oral: 100 and 200 µg tablets
Monteleukast (Singulair)
  Oral: 5 mg chewable, 10 mg tablets
Travaprost (Travatan)
  Ophthalmic solution: 0.0004%
Treprostinil (Remodulin)
  Parenteral: 1, 2.5, 5, 10 mg/mL for continuous subcutaneous infusion
Unoprostone (Rescula)
  Ophthalmic solution 0.15%
Zafirleukast (Accolate)
  Oral: 10, 20 mg tablets
Zileuton (Zyflo))
  Oral: 600 mg tablets

ably naive to ascribe the effects of dietary intervention reported thus far to such metabolites. Carefully controlled clinical studies will be needed before these questions can be satisfactorily answered. However, subjects on diets containing highly saturated fatty acids clearly show increased platelet aggregation when compared with other study groups. Such diets (eg, in Finland and the USA) are associated with higher rates of myocardial infarction than are more polyunsaturated diets (eg, in Italy).

REFERENCES

Berger J, Moller DE: The mechanisms of action of PPARs. Annu Rev Med 2002;53:409.

Breyer RM, Bagdassarian CK, Myers SA, Breyer MD: Prostanoid receptors: subtypes and signaling. Annu Rev Pharmacol Toxicol 2001;41:661.

Chandrasekharan NV et al: COX-3, a cyclooxygenase-1 variant inhibited by acetaminophen and other analgesic/antipyretic drugs: cloning, structure and expression. Proc Natl Acad Sci U S A 2002;99:13926.

Claesson HE, Dahlen SE: Asthma and leukotrienes: antileukotrienes as novel antiasthmatic drugs. J Intern Med 1999; 245:205.

DuBois A: Special Issue. The role of prostaglandins and leukotrienes in the physiology and pathology of the digestive tract. Prostaglandins & Other Lipid Mediators 2000;61:89.

FitzGerald GA, Patrono C: The COXIBs, selective inhibitors of cyclooxygenase-2. N Engl J Med 2001;345:433.

Horn EM, Barst RJ: Treprostinil therapy for pulmonary artery hypertension. Expert Opin Investig Drugs 2002;11:1615.

Leonhardt A et al: Expression of prostanoid receptors in human ductus arteriosus. Br J Pharmacol 2003;138:655.

Maxey KM: Eicosanoids acting via nuclear receptors: the 15-deoxy PGJ compounds and congeners. Prostaglandins & other Lipid Mediators 2000;62:1.

Narumiya S, FitzGerald GA: Genetic and pharmacological analysis of prostanoid receptor function. J Clin Invest 2001;108:25.

Olschewski H et al: Inhaled Iloprost for severe pulmonary hypertension. N Engl J Med 2002;347:322.

Roviezzo F et al: The annexin-1 knockout mouse: what it tells us about the inflammatory response. J Physiol Pharmacol 2002;53:541.

Smith WL, Dewitt DL, Garavito MR: Cyclooxygenases: Structural, cellular, and molecular biology. Annu Rev Biochem 2000;69:145.

Turini ME, DuBois RN: Cyclooxygenase-2: a therapeutic target. Annu Rev Med 2002;53:35.

Wright DH et al: Prostanoid receptors: ontogeny and implications in vascular physiology. Am J Physiol 2001;281:R1343.

Yamamoto S, Smith WL: Molecular biology of the arachidonate cascade. Prostaglandins & Other Lipid Mediators 2002;68-69:1.

Nitric Oxide, Donors, & Inhibitors

19

George Thomas, PhD, & Peter W. Ramwell, PhD

Nitric oxide (NO) is a gaseous signaling molecule that readily diffuses across cell membranes and regulates a wide range of physiologic and pathophysiologic processes including cardiovascular, inflammation, immune and neuronal functions.

DISCOVERY OF ENDOGENOUS NITRIC OXIDE

Early observations of the biologic role of endogenously generated NO were made in rodent macrophages and neutrophils: In vitro exposure of these cells to endotoxin lipopolysaccharide released significant amounts of nitrite and nitrate into the cell culture medium. Furthermore, injection of endotoxin in vivo elevated urinary nitrite and nitrate, the two oxidation products of nitric oxide. This nitric oxide was found to originate from oxidation of the guanidino group of L-arginine.

The second observation was made by Furchgott and Zawadzki in 1980 using isolated vascular smooth muscle preparations. They discovered that following stimulation with acetylcholine or carbachol, the endothelium released a short-lived vasodilator, which—unlike endothelium-derived prostacyclin—was not blocked by cyclooxygenase inhibitors. They named this vasodilator **endothelium-derived relaxing factor** (**EDRF**) since it promoted relaxation of precontracted smooth muscle preparations. Other workers confirmed and extended these findings. In 1987, by comparing the pharmacologic and biochemical properties of the suspect molecule, three independent groups reported that EDRF and nitric oxide are the same molecule. It was later reported that other vasodilator molecules may be a part of EDRF, but it appears clear that nitric oxide provides the major part of its activity. Subsequent studies revealed that nitric oxide was generated by many cells and was, like the eicosanoids (see Chapter 18), found in almost all tissues. The major exogenous donors of nitric oxide (nitrates, nitrites, nitroprusside) have been discussed (see Chapters 11 and 12).

BIOLOGIC SYNTHESIS & INACTIVATION OF NITRIC OXIDE

Synthesis

Nitric oxide, written as NO˙ or simply NO, is a highly diffusible stable gas composed of one atom each of nitrogen and oxygen. It is synthesized by a family of enzymes that are collectively called **nitric oxide synthase, NOS** (EC 1.14.13.49). Three isoforms of NOS have been identified (Table 19–1). These isoforms are heme-containing flavoproteins employing L-arginine as a substrate and requiring NADPH, flavin adenine dinucleotide, and tetrahydrobiopterin as cofactors. Phosphorylation also has differential regulatory effects on the activity of NOS. For example, phosphorylation significantly reduces the activity of NOS-1, whereas phosphorylation of NOS-3 by a serine-threonine protein kinase activates the enzyme. Furthermore, NOS-2 expression is tightly controlled by several transcription factors.

Formation of nitric oxide from L-arginine and several nitric oxide donors is shown in Figure 19–1. Activation of NOS by the influx of extracellular calcium and binding of calmodulin, as in the case of the constitutive enzyme, or following the activation of the inducible NOS (NOS-2) by cytokines, results in the metabolism of L-arginine to L-citrulline and nitric oxide. The conversion of L-arginine to nitric oxide and L-citrulline is inhibited by several arginine competitors such as N^G-monomethyl-L-arginine (below). Some nitric oxide donors, eg, oxygenated nitroprusside, spontaneously generate nitric oxide in aqueous solutions whereas others, such as furoxans and organic nitrates and nitrites such as nitroglycerin, require the presence of a thiol compound such as cysteine. Once generated, nitric oxide interacts with the heme moiety of soluble guanylyl

Table 19–1. Properties of the three isoforms of nitric oxide synthase (NOS).

Property	Isoform Names		
	NOS-1	**NOS-2**	**NOS-3**
Other names	nNOS (neuronal NOS)	iNOS (inducible NOS)	eNOS (endothelial NOS)
Tissue	Neuronal, epithelial cells	Macrophages, smooth muscle cells	Endothelial cells
Expression	Constitutive	Transcriptional induction	Constitutive
Calcium requirement	Yes	No	Yes
Chromosome	12	17	7
Approximate mass	150–160 kDa	125–135 kDa	133 kDa

cyclase in the cytoplasm of cells (Figure 19–1, right). This results in allosteric transformation and activation of the enzyme and leads to the formation of 3′,5′-cyclic-guanosine monophosphate (cGMP) from GTP. Activation of the soluble guanylyl cyclase by nitric oxide can be inhibited by methylene blue. The affinity of nitric oxide for iron is also responsible for its inhibitory effect on several enzymes by interacting with the iron-sulfur centers of these enzymes. Inhibition of enzymes such as cytochrome P450 by nitric oxide is a major problem in inflammatory liver disease and can be reversed by NO synthase inhibitors. Carbon monoxide, another gaseous compound produced endogenously from the catabolism of heme, shares many of the properties of nitric oxide

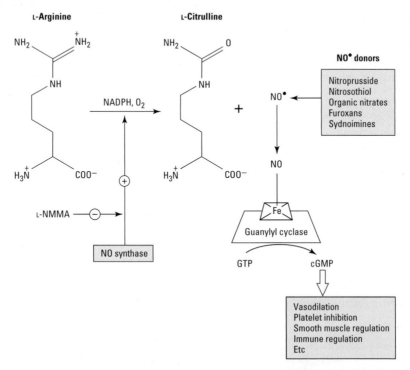

Figure 19–1. Nitric oxide generation from L-arginine and nitric oxide donors and the formation of cGMP. L-NMMA inhibits nitric oxide synthase. Some of the nitric oxide donors such as furoxans and organic nitrates and nitrites require a thiol cofactor such as cysteine or glutathione to form nitric oxide.

such as activation of soluble guanylyl cyclase. However, unlike nitric oxide, which has an extra electron, carbon monoxide is a stable molecule in the presence of oxygen. The affinity of nitric oxide for hemoglobin is several orders of magnitude greater than that of carbon monoxide. Nitric oxide undergoes both oxidative and reductive reactions, resulting in the formation of a variety of oxides of nitrogen (Table 19–2).

Inactivation

Nitric oxide is inactivated by heme and by the free radical, superoxide. Thus, scavengers of superoxide anion such as superoxide dismutase may protect nitric oxide, enhancing its potency and prolonging its duration of action. Conversely, interaction of nitric oxide with superoxide may generate the potent tissue-damaging moiety, peroxynitrite ($ONOO^-$), which has a high affinity for sulfhydryl groups and thus inactivates several key sulfhydryl-bearing enzymes. This effect of peroxynitrite is regulated by the cellular content of glutathione. Since glutathione is the major intracellular soluble sulfhydryl-containing compound, factors that regulate the biosynthesis and decomposition of glutathione may have important consequences.

Glutathione also interacts with nitric oxide under physiologic conditions to generate *S*-nitrosoglutathione, a more stable form of nitric oxide. Nitrosoglutathione may serve as an endogenous long-lived adduct or carrier of nitric oxide. Vascular glutathione is decreased in diabetes mellitus and atherosclerosis, and this may account for the increased incidence of cardiovascular complications in these conditions. Ischemia followed by reperfusion is another situation in which endothelial function is compromised owing to increased production of free radicals, resulting in reduced nitric oxide formation.

INHIBITORS OF NITRIC OXIDE

In theory, several methods are available for reducing nitric oxide levels in tissues and thus inhibiting its actions. Drugs may inhibit the uptake of L-arginine into cells, thus depriving the NOS isoforms of substrate. Other methods include deprivation of the cofactors and calmodulin antagonists; inhibitors of NOS synthesis; inhibitors of binding of arginine to NOS, and scavengers of nitric oxide. The most important thus far have been inhibitors of NOS. Unfortunately, the selectivity of these inhibitors for the individual isoforms is incomplete. Most of these inhibitors are substrate analogs (Table 19–3).

EFFECTS OF NITRIC OXIDE

Nitric oxide has major effects that are mediated by activation of cytoplasmic **soluble guanylyl cyclase** and stimulated production of **cGMP**, an important second messenger. In addition, nitric oxide can produce several reactive nitrogen derivatives by interaction with molecular oxygen and superoxide radicals (Table 19–2). These highly unstable molecules react with a variety of proteins, lipids, nucleic acids, and metals (especially iron) in cells (Davis, 2001). The remainder of this chapter discusses some of the second messenger-mediated effects of nitric oxide and the effects of inhibition of its production.

VASCULAR EFFECTS

Nitric oxide has a significant effect on vascular smooth muscle tone and blood pressure. As stated previously, it

Table 19–2. Oxides of nitrogen.

Name	Symbol	Known Function
Nitric oxide	$NO^{\cdot}$	Vasodilator, platelet inhibitor, immune regulator, neurotransmitter
Nitroxyl anion	NO^-	Smooth muscle relaxant
Nitrogen dioxide	$NO_2^{\cdot}$	Free radical, nitrosating agent, lung irritant
Nitrous oxide	N_2O	Anesthetic
Dinitrogen trioxide	N_2O_3	Nitrosating agent
Dinitrogen tetraoxide	N_2O_4	Nitrosating agent
Nitrite	NO_2^-	Produce $NO^{\cdot}$ at acidic pH
Nitrate	NO_3^-	Stable oxidation product of $NO^{\cdot}$

Table 19–3. Some inhibitors of nitric oxide synthesis or action.

Inhibitor	Mechanism	Comment
N^G–Monomethyl–L–arginine (L–NMMA)	NOS inhibition	May act as substrate in some tissues
N^G–Nitro–L–arginine methyl ester (L–NAME)	NOS inhibition	Less selective NOS inhibitor
7–Nitroindazole	NOS inhibition	Markedly selective for NOS–1 in vivo
S–Methylthiocitrulline	NOS inhibition	Partially selective for NOS–1
Heme	Nitric oxide scavenger	
Protein inhibitor of NOS	Unknown mechanism	Endogenous inhibitor found in brain

NOS, nitric oxide synthase.

is released by acetylcholine and other endothelium-dependent vasodilators. It may play a role in the normal regulation of vascular tone as suggested by the fact that a reduction of nitric oxide synthesis (caused by knockout mutations, infusion of NOS inhibitors such as L-NMMA, or by injury to the vascular endothelium) increases vascular tone and elevates mean arterial pressure. The effects of vasopressor drugs are increased by inhibition of NOS. As described in Chapter 12 and shown in Figure 12–2, increased cGMP synthesis by guanylyl cyclase results in smooth muscle relaxation.

Apart from being a vasodilator, nitric oxide is also a potent inhibitor of neutrophil adhesion to the vascular endothelium. This is due to the inhibitory effect of nitric oxide on the expression of adhesion molecules on the endothelial surface. The role of nitric oxide in protecting the endothelium has been demonstrated by studies that showed that treatment with nitric oxide donors protects against ischemia- and reperfusion-mediated endothelial dysfunction.

RESPIRATORY DISORDERS

Nitric oxide has been shown to improve cardiopulmonary function in adult patients with pulmonary artery hypertension and is approved for this indication (see Preparations Available). It is administered by inhalation. It has also been administered by inhalation to newborns with pulmonary hypertension and acute respiratory distress syndrome. The current treatment for severely defective gas exchange in the newborn is with extracorporeal membrane oxygenation (ECMO), which does not directly affect pulmonary vascular pressures. Nitric oxide inhalation decreases pulmonary arterial pressure and improves blood oxygenation. Thus, when pulmonary resistance is elevated, it is possible to exploit the vasodilator properties of nitric oxide by administering it via inhalation of a few parts per million. Adults

with respiratory distress syndrome also appear—in open trials—to benefit from nitric oxide inhalation. Nitric oxide may have an additional role in relaxing airway smooth muscle and thus acting as a bronchodilator. For these reasons, nitric oxide inhalation therapy is being widely tested in both infants and adults with acute respiratory distress syndrome. The adverse effects of this use of nitric oxide are being assessed.

SEPTIC SHOCK

As mentioned previously, increased urinary excretion of nitrate, the oxidative product of nitric oxide, is reported in gram-negative bacterial infection. Lipopolysaccharide components from the bacterial wall activate the inducible NOS (NOS-2), resulting in exaggerated hypotension, shock, and possible death. This hypotension is reversed by NOS inhibitors such as L-NMMA (Table 19–3) in humans as well as animal models and by compounds such as methylene blue, which prevent the action of nitric oxide, as well as by scavengers of nitric oxide such as hemoglobin. Furthermore, knockout mice lacking a functional NOS-2 gene are more resistant to endotoxin than wild-type mice. However, there has been no correlation between the hemodynamic effects of the nitric oxide inhibitors and survival rate in gram-negative sepsis thus far.

ATHEROSCLEROSIS

Vascular plaque formation in hypercholesterolemia leads to reduced nitric oxide formation and endothelium-dependent vasodilator responses. In vitro, nitric oxide carriers and donors and cGMP analogs inhibit smooth muscle cell proliferation. In animal models, myointimal proliferation following angioplasty can be blocked by feeding arginine, by using nitric oxide donors, by NOS gene transfer, and by nitric oxide inhalation. In addition, nitric oxide may act as an antioxidant, blocking the oxidation of low-density lipoproteins (LDL) and thus preventing the formation of foam cells in the vascular wall.

PLATELETS

Abnormal activation of platelets is associated with increased platelet adhesion and aggregation and therefore a higher incidence of thrombotic events. Platelet activation also leads to release of smooth muscle mitogens such as growth factors and thromboxane. Nitric oxide is a potent inhibitor of platelet adhesion and aggregation. Thus, endothelial dysfunction and the associated decrease in nitric oxide generation may result in abnormal platelet function. Platelets also contain both constitutive and inducible NOS, although to a much lesser extent than endothelial cells. As in vascular smooth muscle, cGMP mediates the protective effect of nitric oxide in platelets. Nitric oxide may have an additional beneficial effect on blood coagulation by enhancing fibrinolysis via an effect on plasminogen.

ORGAN TRANSPLANTATION

Accelerated graft atherosclerosis following organ transplantation is a chronic condition and is a major cause of transplant failure, leading to retransplantation or death. Continuous vascular smooth muscle proliferation occurs within the vasculature of most grafts and is a central event in luminal narrowing. Ischemic and reperfusion injuries at the time of organ harvesting, preservation, and revascularization initiate myointimal proliferation, which is also promoted by the continuous immune response to the allogeneic organ graft. By reducing free radical toxicity under these conditions, nitric oxide may act as a cytoprotective agent, inhibiting platelet and neutrophil aggregation and adhesion to the vascular wall. Dietary L-arginine supplementation increases plasma nitrite and nitrate formation and has been shown to attenuate accelerated graft atherosclerosis. However, excessively high concentrations of nitric oxide may be detrimental during *acute* organ rejection due to up-regulation of inducible NOS by cytokines; under these circumstances, *inhibition* of nitric oxide synthesis has been shown to prolong graft survival in experimental animals.

THE CENTRAL NERVOUS SYSTEM

Nitric oxide has been proposed to have a major role in the central nervous system—as a neurotransmitter, as a modulator of ligand-gated receptors, or both. In addition, nitric oxide probably plays a role in neuronal degeneration in some conditions. The likely cellular targets of nitric oxide in the central nervous system include presynaptic and postsynaptic nerve terminals. Nitric oxide modifies neurotransmitter release in different areas of the brain. Postsynaptic release of nitric oxide following activation of the NMDA receptor may initiate presynaptic transmitter release of glutamate, ie, nitric oxide may function as a *retrograde* messenger that is synthesized in postsynaptic sites following opening of the Ca^{2+} channels and activation of NOS. It is proposed that the nitric oxide thus produced rapidly diffuses to the presynaptic nerve terminal where guanylyl cyclase is activated to yield cGMP and thus facilitate transmitter release. In the cerebellum and in neuroblastoma cells, this effect is blocked by NOS inhibitors such as L-NMMA and is enhanced by L-arginine. It has been suggested that nitric oxide (like many other substances) may have a role in short- and long-term potentiating effects on excitatory amino acids in brain development and learning.

7-Nitroindazole, an inhibitor of NOS-1, and L-NAME, a less selective inhibitor of neuronal NOS, have significant antinociceptive effects in humans and animals and 7-nitroindazol reduces the signs of opioid withdrawal and cocaine action in animal models. This inhibitor also reduces cerebral blood flow. Nevertheless, 7-nitroindazole can reduce the size of cerebral infarcts in animal models. In contrast, NOS-3-deficient mice are more susceptible to ischemic cerebral damage. NOS-1 inhibition by 7-nitroindazole also reduces the neurotoxicity of MPTP and MPP^+ (see Chapter 28) in several animal models.

It is well known that prolonged NMDA glutamate receptor activation results in degeneration of neurons (excitotoxicity). This has been attributed to a large increase in calcium influx, which activates the calmodulin-dependent NOS-1 and leads to sustained elevation of nitric oxide concentrations. The increase in neurodegeneration caused by excitatory amino acids may be due to enhanced oxygen radical formation since superoxide dismutase has a beneficial effect in experimental models. The damage may also be mediated by the generation of secondary radicals such as peroxynitrite, which has a high affinity for sulfhydryl-containing enzymes such as calcium ATPase. Inhibition of calcium ATPases by peroxynitrite may in turn lead to enhanced Ca^{2+} accumulation and associated neurodegeneration. NOS-2 has been implicated in several other degenerative neurologic conditions, eg, Alzheimer's disease, multiple sclerosis, and Huntington's disease.

High levels of nitric oxide have also been shown to cause destruction of photoreceptor cells in the retina. This is believed to be due to a prolonged increase in cGMP formation. Finally, nitric oxide and cGMP have been reported to have a role in epileptic seizures.

THE PERIPHERAL NERVOUS SYSTEM

Nonadrenergic, noncholinergic (NANC) neurons are widely distributed in peripheral tissues, especially the gastrointestinal and reproductive tracts (see Chapter 6). Considerable evidence implicates nitric oxide as a mediator of certain NANC actions, and some NANC neurons appear to release nitric oxide. Penile erection is thought to be caused by the release of nitric oxide from NANC neurons; it is well documented that nitric oxide promotes relaxation of the smooth muscle in the corpora cavernosa—the initiating factor in penile erection—and inhibitors of NOS have been shown to prevent erection caused by pelvic nerve stimulation in the rat. Thus, impotence is a possible clinical indication for the use of a nitric oxide donor, and trials have been carried out with nitroglycerin ointment and the nitroglycerin patch. Another approach is to inhibit the breakdown of cGMP by the phosphodiesterase (PDE isoform 5) present in the smooth muscle of the corpora cavernosa with drugs such as sildenafil (see Chapter 12).

INFLAMMATION

Nitric oxide has a role in both acute and chronic inflammation. NOS-3 is involved in the vasodilation associated with acute inflammation. In experimental models of acute inflammation, inhibitors of NOS-3 have a dose-dependent protective effect, suggesting that nitric oxide promotes edema and vascular permeability. Nitric oxide has a detrimental effect in chronic models of arthritis; dietary L-arginine supplementation exacerbates arthritis whereas protection is seen with NOS-2 inhibitors. Psoriasis lesions, airway epithelium in asthma, and inflammatory bowel lesions in humans all demonstrate elevated levels of nitric oxide and NOS-2. Synovial fluid from patients with arthritis contains increased oxidation products of nitric oxide, particularly peroxynitrite. Recent studies have shown that nitric oxide stimulates the synthesis of inflammatory prostaglandins by activating cyclooxygenase isoenzyme II (COX-2). Thus, inhibition of the nitric oxide pathway may have a beneficial effect on inflammatory diseases, including joint diseases. Studies using inhibitors of NOS-2 have shown that nitric oxide is required for maintaining COX-2 gene expression.

Nitric oxide also appears to play an important protective role in the body via immune cell function. When challenged with foreign antigens, TH1 cells (see Chapter 56) respond by synthesizing nitric oxide. Inhibition of NOS and knockout of the NOS-2 gene can markedly impair the protective response to injected parasites in animal models.

PREPARATIONS AVAILABLE

Nitric Oxide (INOmax)
Inhalation: 100, 800 ppm gas

REFERENCES

Blum A et al: Oral L-arginine in patients with coronary artery disease on medical management. Circulation 2000;101:2160.

Davis KL et al: Novel effects of nitric oxide. Annu Rev Pharmacol Toxicol 2001;41:203.

Derry F et al: Efficacy and safety of sildenafil citrate (Viagra) in men with erectile dysfunction and spinal cord injury: a review. Urology 2002;20(2 Suppl 2):49.

Furchgott RF: Endothelium-derived relaxing factor: discovery, early studies, and identification as nitric oxide. Biosci Rep 1999;19:235.

Hamilton LC, Warner TD: Interactions between inducible isoforms of nitric oxide synthase and cyclooxygenase in vivo; investigations using the selective inhibitors 1400W and celecoxib. Br J Pharmacol 1998;125:335.

Hobbs AJ, Higgs A, Moncada S: Inhibition of nitric oxide synthesis as a potential therapeutic target. Annu Rev Pharmacol Toxicol 1999;39:191.

Hofseth LJ et al: Nitric oxide-induced cellular stress and p53 activation in chronic inflammation. Proc Natl Acad Sci U S A 2003;100:143.

Ignarro LJ et al: Nitric oxide as a signaling molecule in the vascular system: an overview. J Cardiovasc Pharmacol 1999;34:879.

Moncada S, Palmer RM, Higgs EA: Nitric oxide: physiology, pathophysiology, and pharmacology. Pharmacol Rev 1991;43:109.

Muscara MN, Wallace JL: Nitric oxide V. Therapeutic potential of nitric oxide donors and inhibitors. Am J Physiol 1999; 276:1313.

Napoli C, Ignarro LJ: Nitric oxide-releasing drugs. Annu Rev Pharmacol Toxicol 2003;43:97.

Perkins DJ, Kniss DA: Blockade of nitric oxide formation downregulates cyclooxygenase-2 and decreases PGE2 biosynthesis in macrophages. J Leukoc Biol 1999;65:792.

Steudel W, Hurford WE, Zaploi WM: Inhaled nitric oxide. Basic biology and clinical applications. Anesthesiology 1999;91:1090.

Toda N, Okamura T: The pharmacology of nitric oxide in the peripheral nervous system of blood vessels. Pharmacol Rev 2003;55:271.

Drugs Used in Asthma

Homer A. Boushey, MD, & Bertram G. Katzung, MD, PhD

The clinical hallmarks of asthma are recurrent, episodic bouts of coughing, shortness of breath, chest tightness, and wheezing. In mild asthma, symptoms occur only occasionally, eg, on exposure to allergens or certain pollutants, on exercise, or after a viral upper respiratory infection. More severe forms of asthma are associated with frequent attacks of wheezing dyspnea, especially at night, and even chronic limitation of activity. Asthma is the most common chronic disabling disease of childhood, but it affects all age groups.

Asthma is physiologically characterized by increased responsiveness of the trachea and bronchi to various stimuli and by widespread narrowing of the airways that changes in severity either spontaneously or as a result of therapy. Its pathologic features are contraction of airway smooth muscle, mucosal thickening from edema and cellular infiltration, and inspissation in the airway lumen of abnormally thick, viscid plugs of mucus. Of these causes of airway obstruction, contraction of smooth muscle is most easily reversed by current therapy; reversal of the edema and cellular infiltration requires sustained treatment with anti-inflammatory agents. Asthma therapies are thus sometimes divided into two categories: "short-term relievers" and "long-term controllers."

Short-term relief is most effectively achieved with bronchodilators, agents that increase airway caliber by relaxing airway smooth muscle, and of these the β-adrenoceptor stimulants (see Chapter 9) are the most widely used. Theophylline, a methylxanthine drug, and antimuscarinic agents (see Chapter 8) are also used for reversal of airway constriction. Long-term control is most often achieved with an anti-inflammatory agent such as an inhaled corticosteroid, with a leukotriene antagonist, or with an inhibitor of mast cell degranulation, eg, cromolyn or nedocromil. The distinction between "short-term relievers" and "long-term controllers" has become blurred by the finding that theophylline inhibits some lymphocyte functions and modestly reduces airway mucosal inflammation and that budesonide, an inhaled corticosteroid, produces modest immediate bronchodilation. Similarly, two recently released long-acting β-adrenoceptor stimulants, salmeterol and formoterol, appear to be effective in improving

asthma control when taken regularly. Finally, clinical trials are demonstrating the efficacy of specifically targeting a mechanism thought to be fundamental to asthma's pathogenesis by repeated treatment with a humanized monoclonal anti-IgE antibody.

This chapter presents the basic pharmacology of the methylxanthines, cromolyn, leukotriene pathway inhibitors, and monoclonal anti-IgE antibody—agents whose medical use is almost exclusively for pulmonary disease. The other classes of drugs listed above are discussed in relation to the therapy of asthma.

PATHOGENESIS OF ASTHMA

A rational approach to the pharmacotherapy of asthma depends on an understanding of the disease's pathogenesis. In the classic immunologic model, asthma is a disease mediated by reaginic (IgE) antibodies bound to mast cells in the airway mucosa (Figure 20–1). On reexposure to an antigen, antigen-antibody interaction on the surface of the mast cells triggers both the release of mediators stored in the cells' granules and the synthesis and release of other mediators. The agents responsible for the early reaction—immediate bronchoconstriction—include histamine, tryptase and other neutral proteases, leukotrienes C_4 and D_4, and prostaglandins. These agents diffuse throughout the airway wall and cause muscle contraction and vascular leakage. Other mediators are responsible for the more sustained bronchoconstriction, cellular infiltration of the airway mucosa, and mucus hypersecretion of the late asthmatic reaction that occurs 2–8 hours later. These mediators are thought to be cytokines characteristically produced by TH2 lymphocytes, especially GM-CSF and interleukins 4, 5, 9, and 13, which attract and activate eosinophils and stimulate IgE production by B lymphocytes. It is not clear whether lymphocytes or mast cells in the airway mucosa are the primary source of the cytokines and other mediators responsible for the late inflammatory response, but it is now thought that the benefits of corticosteroid therapy may result from their inhibition of cytokine production in the airways.

Not all of the features of asthma can be accounted for by the antigen challenge model. Some adults with

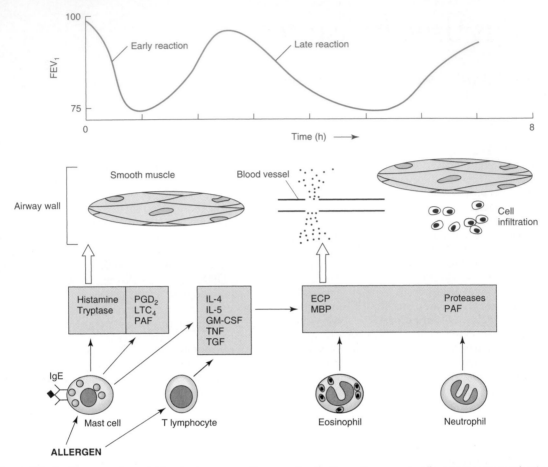

Figure 20–1. Conceptual model for the immunopathogenesis of asthma. Exposure to allergen causes synthesis of IgE, which binds to mast cells in the airway mucosa. On reexposure to allergen, antigen-antibody interaction on mast cell surfaces triggers release of mediators of anaphylaxis: histamine, tryptase, prostaglandin D_2 (PGD_2), leukotriene C_4, and platelet-activating factor (PAF). These agents provoke contraction of airway smooth muscle, causing the immediate fall in FEV_1. Reexposure to allergen also causes the synthesis and release of a variety of cytokines: interleukins 4 and 5, granulocyte-macrophage colony stimulating factor (GM-CSF), tumor necrosis factor (TNF), and tissue growth factor (TGF) from T cells and mast cells. These cytokines in turn attract and activate eosinophils and neutrophils, whose products include eosinophil cationic protein (ECP), major basic protein (MBP), proteases, and platelet-activating factor. These mediators cause the edema, mucus hypersecretion, smooth muscle contraction, and increase in bronchial reactivity associated with the late asthmatic response, indicated by a fall in FEV_1 2–8 hours after the exposure.

asthma have no evidence of immediate hypersensitivity to antigens, most severe exacerbations of asthma appear to be provoked by viral respiratory infection, the severity of symptoms correlates poorly with the quantity of antigen in the atmosphere, and in many patients bronchospasm can be provoked by nonantigenic stimuli such as distilled water, exercise, cold air, sulfur dioxide, and rapid respiratory maneuvers.

This tendency to develop bronchospasm upon encountering stimuli that do not affect healthy nonasthmatic airways is characteristic of asthma and is sometimes called "nonspecific bronchial hyperreactivity" to distinguish it from bronchial responsiveness to specific antigens. Bronchial hyperreactivity is quantitated by measuring the fall in forced expiratory volume in 1 second (FEV_1) provoked by inhaling serially increasing concentrations of aerosolized histamine or methacholine. This exaggerated sensitivity of the airways appears to be fundamental to asthma's pathogenesis, for it is nearly ubiquitous in patients with asthma and its degree correlates with the symptomatic severity of the disease.

The mechanisms underlying bronchial hyperreactivity are somehow related to inflammation of the airway mucosa. The agents that increase bronchial reactivity, such as ozone exposure, allergen inhalation, and infection with respiratory viruses, also cause airway inflammation. In both dogs and humans, the increase in bronchial reactivity induced by ozone is associated with an increase in the number of polymorphonuclear leukocytes found in fluid obtained by bronchial lavage or from bronchial mucosal biopsies. The increase in reactivity due to allergen inhalation is associated with an increase in both eosinophils and polymorphonuclear leukocytes in bronchial lavage fluid. The increase in reactivity that is associated with the late asthmatic response to allergen inhalation (Figure 20–1) is sustained and, because it is prevented by treatment with inhaled corticosteroids immediately before antigen challenge, is thought to be caused by airway inflammation.

How the increase in airway reactivity is linked to inflammation is uncertain. Much evidence points to the eosinophil. The most consistent difference in bronchial mucosal biopsies obtained from asthmatic and healthy subjects is an increase in the number of eosinophils found beneath the airway epithelium. Immunohistochemical staining shows increased levels of eosinophil cationic protein, indicating activation of the cells. The number of eosinophils in expectorated sputum or in fluid lavaged from the lungs correlates roughly with the degree of bronchial hyperreactivity. Eosinophil products have in turn been shown to cause epithelial sloughing and an increase in contractile responsiveness of airway smooth muscle. The importance of the eosinophil has been challenged, however, by a study showing that treatment with an anti-IL-5 monoclonal antibody effectively blocks airway eosinophilia caused by allergen challenge but does not prevent bronchoconstriction or any further increase in bronchial hyperactivity (Leckie, 2000).

The products of other cells in the airways, such as lymphocytes, macrophages, mast cells, sensory nerves, and epithelial cells, have also been shown to alter airway smooth muscle function, so a specific antagonist to a single mediator or class of mediators might not prove wholly effective as asthma therapy. Other evidence suggests a role for sensitization of sensory nerves in the airways as a mechanism for hyperreactivity (see Box, Pharmacologic Significance of Lung Innervation).

Whatever the mechanisms responsible for bronchial hyperreactivity, bronchoconstriction itself seems to result not simply from the direct effect of the released mediators but also from their activation of neural or humoral pathways. Evidence for the importance of neural pathways stems largely from studies of laboratory animals. Thus, the bronchospasm provoked in dogs by histamine can be greatly reduced by pretreatment with an inhaled topical anesthetic agent, by transection of the vagus nerves, and by pretreatment with atropine. Studies of asthmatic humans, however, have shown that treatment with atropine causes only a reduction in—not abolition of—the bronchospastic responses to antigens and to nonantigenic stimuli. While it is possible that activity in some other neural pathway (eg, the nonadrenergic, noncholinergic system; see Box, Pharmacologic Significance of Lung Innervation) contributes to

---

PHARMACOLOGIC SIGNIFICANCE OF LUNG INNERVATION

As noted previously, the airways are richly supplied with afferent and efferent vagal nerves. The cholinergic motor fibers are clearly responsible in some patients for a portion of the bronchoconstriction characteristic of acute asthma. Such fibers innervate M_3 receptors on the smooth muscle and contain modulatory M_2 receptors on the nerve terminals. Selective inhibition of M_2 receptors can increase bronchoconstrictor responses to a variety of stimuli, while M_3 inhibitors can produce dilation of constricted airways.

In contrast, noradrenergic sympathetic innervation of the airways is sparse, and these fibers do not appear to play a major role in controlling airway diameter. Bronchodilation may be brought about by nonadrenergic, noncholinergic nerves releasing nitric oxide since nitric oxide synthase inhibitors have been shown to reduce bronchodilation produced by electrical field stimulation in vitro.

The role of peptidergic neurons is not so clear. Capsaicin, the hot chile pepper chemical that evokes release of peptide transmitters from several types of sensory nerves, has been shown to reproduce some of the signs of bronchial hyperreactivity in animal and human experiments. These findings led to the proposal that sensitization of afferent nerve endings played a major role in chronic airway hyperreactivity. However, peptide transmitter antagonists have not been able to prevent bronchoconstriction in several models. Clearly, much remains to be learned about airway pharmacology.

bronchomotor responses to nonspecific nonantigenic stimuli, their inhibition by cromolyn, a drug that appears to inhibit mast cell degranulation, suggests that both antigenic and nonantigenic stimuli may provoke the release from mast cells of mediators that stimulate smooth muscle contraction by direct and indirect mechanisms (Figure 20–2).

The hypothesis suggested by these studies—that asthmatic bronchospasm results from a combination of release of mediators and an exaggeration of responsiveness to their effects—predicts that asthma may be effectively treated by drugs with different modes of action. Asthmatic bronchospasm might be reversed or prevented, for example, by drugs that reduce the amount of IgE bound to mast cells (anti-IgE antibody), prevent mast cell degranulation (cromolyn or nedocromil, sympathomimetic agents, calcium channel blockers), block the action of the products released (antihistamines and leukotriene receptor antagonists), inhibit the effect of acetylcholine released from vagal motor nerves (muscarinic antagonists), or directly relax airway smooth muscle (sympathomimetic agents, theophylline).

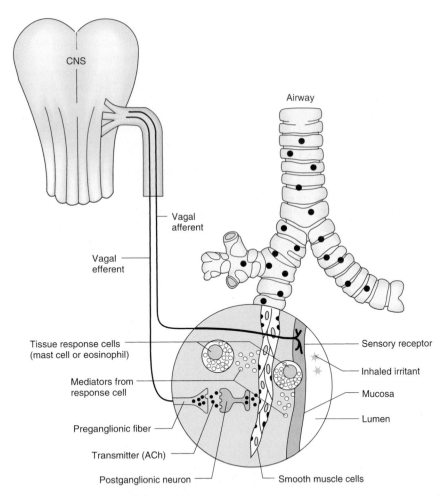

Figure 20–2. Mechanisms of response to inhaled irritants. The airway is represented microscopically by a cross-section of the wall with branching vagal sensory endings lying adjacent to the lumen. Afferent pathways in the vagus nerves travel to the central nervous system; efferent pathways from the central nervous system travel to efferent ganglia. Postganglionic fibers release acetylcholine (ACh), which binds to muscarinic receptors on airway smooth muscle. Inhaled materials may provoke bronchoconstriction by several possible mechanisms. First, they may trigger the release of chemical mediators from mast cells. Second, they may stimulate afferent receptors to initiate reflex bronchoconstriction or to release tachykinins (eg, substance P) that directly stimulate smooth muscle contraction.

The second approach to the treatment of asthma is aimed not just at preventing or reversing acute bronchospasm but at reducing the level of bronchial responsiveness. Because increased responsiveness appears to be linked to airway inflammation and because airway inflammation is a feature of late asthmatic responses, this strategy is implemented both by reducing exposure to the allergens that provoke inflammation and by prolonged therapy with anti-inflammatory agents, especially inhaled corticosteroids.

I. BASIC PHARMACOLOGY OF AGENTS USED IN THE TREATMENT OF ASTHMA

The drugs most used for management of asthma are adrenoceptor agonists (used as "relievers" or bronchodilators) and inhaled corticosteroids (used as "controllers" or anti-inflammatory agents). Their basic pharmacology is presented elsewhere (see Chapters 9 and 39). In this chapter, we review their pharmacology relevant to asthma.

SYMPATHOMIMETIC AGENTS

The adrenoceptor agonists have several pharmacologic actions important in the treatment of asthma. They relax airway smooth muscle and inhibit release of some bronchoconstricting substances from mast cells. They may also inhibit microvascular leakage and increase mucociliary transport by increasing ciliary activity or by affecting the composition of mucous secretions. As in other tissues, the β agonists stimulate adenylyl cyclase and increase the formation of cAMP in the airway tissues (Figure 20–3).

The best-characterized action of the adrenoceptor agonists on airways is relaxation of airway smooth muscle that results in bronchodilation. Although there is no evidence for significant sympathetic innervation of human airway smooth muscle, there is ample evidence for the presence of adrenoceptors on airway smooth muscle. In general, stimulation of β_2 receptors relaxes airway smooth muscle, inhibits mediator release, and causes tachycardia and skeletal muscle tremor as toxic effects.

The sympathomimetic agents that have been widely used in the treatment of asthma include epinephrine, ephedrine, isoproterenol, and a number of β_2-selective agents (Figure 20–4). Because epinephrine and isoproterenol cause more cardiac stimulation (mediated mainly by β_1 receptors), they should probably be reserved for special situations (see below).

Epinephrine is an effective, rapidly acting bronchodilator when injected subcutaneously (0.4 mL of 1:1000 solution) or inhaled as a microaerosol from a pressurized canister (320 µg per puff). Maximal bronchodilation is achieved 15 minutes after inhalation and lasts 60–90 minutes. Because epinephrine stimulates β_1 as well as β_2 receptors, tachycardia, arrhythmias, and worsening of angina pectoris are troublesome adverse effects. Epinephrine is the active agent in many nonprescription inhalants (eg, Primatene Mist) but is now rarely prescribed.

Ephedrine was used in China for more than 2000 years before its introduction into Western medicine in

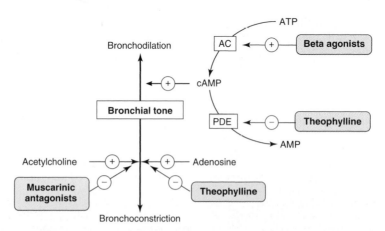

Figure 20–3. Bronchodilation is promoted by cAMP. Intracellular levels of cAMP can be increased by β-adrenoceptor agonists, which increase the rate of its synthesis by adenylyl cyclase (AC); or by phosphodiesterase (PDE) inhibitors such as theophylline, which slow the rate of its degradation. Bronchoconstriction can be inhibited by muscarinic antagonists and possibly by adenosine antagonists.

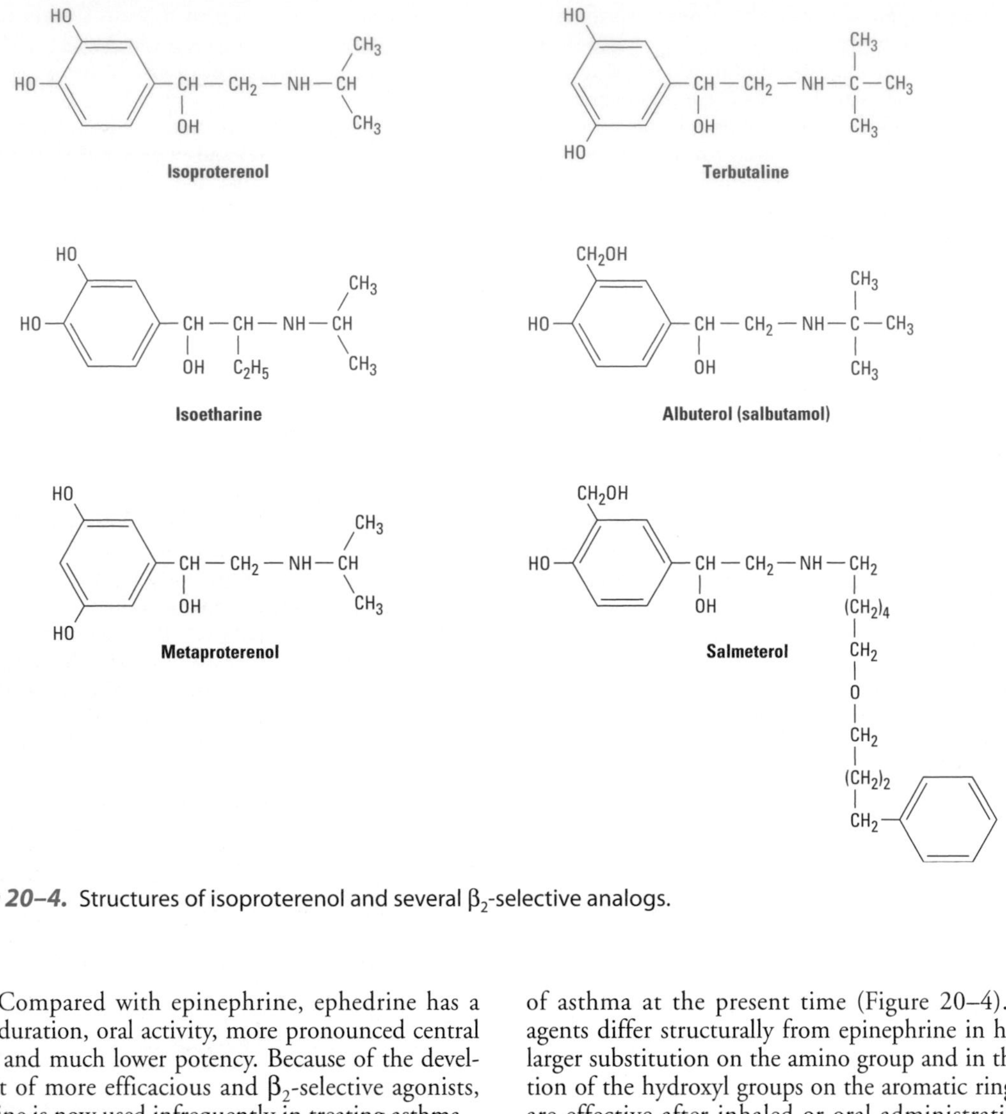

Figure 20–4. Structures of isoproterenol and several β_2-selective analogs.

1924. Compared with epinephrine, ephedrine has a longer duration, oral activity, more pronounced central effects, and much lower potency. Because of the development of more efficacious and β_2-selective agonists, ephedrine is now used infrequently in treating asthma.

Isoproterenol is a potent bronchodilator; when inhaled as a microaerosol from a pressurized canister, 80–120 μg causes maximal bronchodilation within 5 minutes. Isoproterenol has a 60- to 90-minute duration of action. An increase in the asthma mortality rate that occurred in the United Kingdom in the mid 1960s was attributed to cardiac arrhythmias resulting from the use of high doses of inhaled isoproterenol, though this attribution remains a subject of controversy.

Beta$_2$ Selective Drugs

The β_2-selective adrenoceptor agonist drugs are the most widely used sympathomimetics for the treatment of asthma at the present time (Figure 20–4). These agents differ structurally from epinephrine in having a larger substitution on the amino group and in the position of the hydroxyl groups on the aromatic ring. They are effective after inhaled or oral administration and have a long duration of action and significant β_2 selectivity.

Albuterol, terbutaline, metaproterenol, and **pirbuterol** are available as metered-dose inhalers. Given by inhalation, these agents cause bronchodilation equivalent to that produced by isoproterenol. Bronchodilation is maximal by 30 minutes and persists for 3–4 hours. Albuterol, levalbuterol, bitolterol, and metaproterenol can be diluted in saline for administration from a hand-held nebulizer. Because the particles generated by a nebulizer are much larger than those from a metered-dose inhaler, much higher doses must be given (15 mg vs 2.5–5 mg) but are no more effective. Nebulized therapy should thus be reserved for patients unable to coordinate inhalation from a metered-dose inhaler.

Albuterol and terbutaline are also prepared in tablet form. One tablet two or three times daily is the usual regimen; the principal adverse effects of skeletal muscle tremor, nervousness, and occasional weakness may be reduced by starting the patient on half-strength tablets for the first 2 weeks of therapy.

Of these agents, only terbutaline is available for subcutaneous injection (0.25 mg). The indications for this route are similar to those for subcutaneous epinephrine—severe asthma requiring emergency treatment when aerosolized therapy is not available or has been ineffective—but it should be remembered that terbutaline's longer duration of action means that cumulative effects may be seen after repeated injections.

A new generation of long-acting β_2-selective agonists includes **salmeterol** and **formoterol**. Both drugs are potent selective β_2 agonists that appear to achieve their long duration of action (12 hours or more) as a result of high lipid solubility, which permits them to dissolve in the smooth muscle cell membrane in high concentration or, possibly, attach to "mooring" molecules in the vicinity of the adrenoceptor. It is postulated that this local drug functions as a slow-release depot that provides drug to adjacent β receptors over a long period. These drugs appear to interact with inhaled corticosteroids to improve asthma control. They are not recommended as the sole therapy for asthma.

Although adrenoceptor agonists may be administered by inhalation or by the oral or parenteral routes, delivery by inhalation results in the greatest local effect on airway smooth muscle with the least systemic toxicity. Aerosol deposition depends on the particle size, the pattern of breathing (tidal volume and rate of airflow), and the geometry of the airways. Even with particles in the optimal size range of 2–5 μm, 80–90% of the total dose of aerosol is deposited in the mouth or pharynx. Particles under 1–2 μm in size remain suspended and may be exhaled. Deposition can be increased by holding the breath in inspiration.

Toxicities

The use of sympathomimetic agents by inhalation at first raised fears about possible tachyphylaxis or tolerance to β agonists, cardiac arrhythmias, and hypoxemia. The concept that β-agonist drugs cause worsening of clinical asthma by inducing tachyphylaxis to their own action remains unestablished. Most studies have shown only a small change in the bronchodilator response to β stimulation after prolonged treatment with β-agonist drugs, but other studies have shown a loss in the ability of β-agonist treatment to inhibit the response to subsequent challenge with exercise, methacholine, or antigen challenge (referred to as a loss of bronchoprotective action).

Other experiments have demonstrated that arterial oxygen tension (PaO₂) may decrease after administration of β agonists if ventilation/perfusion ratios in the lung worsen. This effect is usually small, however, and may occur with any bronchodilator drug; the significance of such an effect will depend on the initial PaO₂ of the patient. Supplemental oxygen may be necessary if the initial PaO₂ is decreased markedly or if there is a large decrease in PaO₂ during treatment with bronchodilators. Finally, there is concern over myocardial toxicity from Freon propellants contained in all of the commercially available metered-dose canisters. While fluorocarbons may sensitize the heart to toxic effects of catecholamines, such an effect occurs only at very high myocardial concentrations, which are not achieved if inhalers are used as recommended. Under the terms of an international agreement, fluorocarbon-free inhalers will soon replace existing preparations.

Fears that heavy use of β-agonist inhalers could actually increase morbidity and mortality have not been borne out by careful epidemiologic investigations. Heavy use most often indicates that the patient should be receiving more effective prophylactic therapy with corticosteroids. In general, β_2-adrenoceptor agonists are safe and effective bronchodilators when given in doses that avoid systemic adverse effects.

METHYLXANTHINE DRUGS

The three important methylxanthines are **theophylline**, **theobromine**, and **caffeine**. Their major source is beverages (tea, cocoa, and coffee, respectively). The importance of theophylline as a therapeutic agent in the treatment of asthma has waned as the greater effectiveness of inhaled adrenoceptor agents for acute asthma and of inhaled anti-inflammatory agents for chronic asthma has been established, but theophylline's very low cost is an important advantage for economically disadvantaged patients in societies where health care resources are limited.

Chemistry

As shown below, theophylline is 1,3-dimethylxanthine; theobromine is 3,7-dimethylxanthine; and caffeine is 1,3,7-trimethylxanthine. A theophylline preparation commonly used for therapeutic purposes is **aminophylline**, a theophylline-ethylenediamine complex. A synthetic analog of theophylline (dyphylline) is both less potent and shorter-acting than theophylline. The pharmacokinetics of theophylline are discussed below (see Clinical Use of Methylxanthines). The metabolic products, partially demethylated xanthines (not uric acid), are excreted in the urine.

Xanthine

Theobromine

Caffeine

Theophylline

Mechanism of Action

Theophylline produces direct bronchodilation and has some anti-inflammatory actions in the airway as well. Several mechanisms have been proposed for these actions, but none have been firmly established. At high concentrations, the methylxanthines can be shown in vitro to inhibit several members of the phosphodiesterase (PDE) enzyme family (Figure 20–3). Since the phosphodiesterases hydrolyze cyclic nucleotides, this inhibition results in higher concentrations of intracellular cAMP and, in some tissues, cGMP. This effect could explain the cardiac stimulation and smooth muscle relaxation produced by these drugs as well as decreased release of inflammatory mediators from mast cells. PDE4 appears to be the isoform most directly involved in the airway actions of methylxanthines. More selective inhibitors of PDE4 have been developed in an effort to reduce toxicity while maintaining therapeutic efficacy. Thus far, such selective PDE4 inhibitors have proved more effective in chronic obstructive pulmonary disease (COPD) than in asthma. A major adverse effect of the PDE4-selective drugs is nausea and vomiting.

Another proposed mechanism is the inhibition of cell surface receptors for adenosine. These receptors modulate adenylyl cyclase activity, and adenosine has been shown to cause contraction of isolated airway smooth muscle and to provoke histamine release from airway mast cells. These effects are antagonized by theophylline, which blocks cell surface adenosine receptors. It has also been shown, however, that xanthine derivatives devoid of adenosine-antagonistic properties (eg, enprofylline) may be more potent than theophylline in inhibiting bronchoconstriction in asthmatic subjects.

Pharmacodynamics of Methylxanthines

The methylxanthines have effects on the central nervous system, kidney, and cardiac and skeletal muscle as well as smooth muscle. Of the three agents, theophylline is most selective in its smooth muscle effects, while caffeine has the most marked central nervous system effects.

A. CENTRAL NERVOUS SYSTEM EFFECTS

In low and moderate doses, the methylxanthines—especially caffeine—cause mild cortical arousal with increased alertness and deferral of fatigue. The caffeine contained in beverages—eg, 100 mg in a cup of coffee—is sufficient to cause nervousness and insomnia in unusually sensitive individuals and slight bronchodilation in patients with asthma. At very high doses, medullary stimulation and convulsions may occur and can lead to death; theophylline has been used successfully in suicide attempts. Nervousness and tremor are primary side effects in patients taking large doses of aminophylline for asthma.

B. CARDIOVASCULAR EFFECTS

The methylxanthines have direct positive chronotropic and inotropic effects on the heart. At low concentrations, these effects appear to result from increased catecholamine release that is caused by inhibition of presynaptic adenosine receptors. At higher concentrations (> 10 μmol/L), calcium influx may be increased directly through the increase in cAMP that results from inhibition of phosphodiesterase. At very high concentrations (> 100 μmol/L), sequestration of calcium by the sarcoplasmic reticulum is impaired. In unusually sensitive individuals, consumption of a few cups of coffee may result in arrhythmias, but in most people even parenteral administration of higher doses of the methylxanthines produces only sinus tachycardia and increased cardiac output. In large doses, these agents also relax vascular smooth muscle except in cerebral blood vessels, where they cause contraction. Ordinary consumption of coffee and other methylxanthine-containing beverages, however, usually raises the peripheral vascular resistance and blood pressure slightly, probably through the release of catecholamines.

Methylxanthines decrease blood viscosity and may improve blood flow under certain conditions. The mechanism of this action is not well defined, but the effect is exploited in the treatment of intermittent claudication with **pentoxifylline,** a dimethylxanthine agent. However, no evidence suggests that this therapy is superior to other approaches.

C. EFFECTS ON GASTROINTESTINAL TRACT

The methylxanthines stimulate secretion of both gastric acid and digestive enzymes. However, even decaffeinated coffee has a potent stimulant effect on secretion, which means that the primary secretagogue in coffee is not caffeine.

D. Effects on Kidney

The methylxanthines—especially theophylline—are weak diuretics. This effect may involve both increased glomerular filtration and reduced tubular sodium reabsorption. The diuresis is not of sufficient magnitude to be therapeutically useful.

E. Effects on Smooth Muscle

The bronchodilation produced by the methylxanthines is the major therapeutic action in asthma. Tolerance does not develop, but adverse effects, especially in the central nervous system, may limit the dose (see below). In addition to this direct effect on the airway smooth muscle, these agents—in sufficient concentration—inhibit antigen-induced release of histamine from lung tissue; their effect on mucociliary transport is unknown.

F. Effects on Skeletal Muscle

The therapeutic actions of the methylxanthines may not be confined to the airways, for they also strengthen the contractions of isolated skeletal muscle in vitro and have potent effects in improving contractility and in reversing fatigue of the diaphragm in patients with chronic obstructive lung diseases. This effect on diaphragmatic performance—rather than an effect on the respiratory center—may account for theophylline's ability to improve the ventilatory response to hypoxia and to diminish dyspnea even in patients with irreversible airflow obstruction.

Clinical Use of Methylxanthines

Of the xanthines, theophylline is the most effective bronchodilator, and it has been shown repeatedly both to relieve airflow obstruction in acute asthma and to reduce the severity of symptoms and time lost from work or school in patients with chronic asthma. Theophylline base is only slightly soluble in water, so it has been administered as several salts containing varying amounts of theophylline base. Most preparations are well absorbed from the gastrointestinal tract, but absorption of rectal suppositories is unreliable.

Improvements in theophylline preparations have come from alterations in the physical state of the drugs rather than from new chemical formulations. For example, several companies now provide anhydrous theophylline in a microcrystalline form in which the increased surface area facilitates solubilization for complete and rapid absorption after oral administration. In addition, several sustained-release preparations (eg, Slo-Phyllin, Theo-Dur) are available and can produce therapeutic blood levels of theophylline for 12 hours or more. These preparations offer the advantages of less frequent drug administration, less fluctuation of theophylline blood levels, and, in many cases, more effective treatment of nocturnal bronchospasm.

Theophylline should only be used where methods to measure theophylline blood levels are available because it has a narrow therapeutic window and its therapeutic and toxic effects are related to its plasma concentrations. Improvement in pulmonary function is correlated with plasma concentration in the range of 5–20 mg/L. Anorexia, nausea, vomiting, abdominal discomfort, headache, and anxiety occur at concentrations of 15 mg/L in some patients and become common at concentrations greater than 20 mg/L. Higher levels (> 40 mg/L) may cause seizures or arrhythmias; these may not be preceded by gastrointestinal or neurologic warning symptoms.

The plasma clearance of theophylline varies widely. Theophylline is metabolized by the liver, so usual doses may lead to toxic concentrations of the drug in patients with liver disease. Conversely, clearance may be increased through the induction of hepatic enzymes by cigarette smoking or by changes in diet. In normal adults, the mean plasma clearance is 0.69 mL/kg/min. Children clear theophylline faster than adults (1–1.5 mL/kg/min). Neonates and young infants have the slowest clearance (see Chapter 60). Even when maintenance doses are altered to correct for the above factors, plasma concentrations vary widely.

Theophylline improves long-term control of asthma when taken as the sole maintenance treatment or when added to inhaled corticosteroids. It is inexpensive, and it can be taken orally. Its use, however, also requires occasional measurement of plasma levels; it often causes unpleasant minor side effects (especially insomnia); and accidental or intentional overdose can result in severe toxicity or death. For oral therapy with the prompt-release formulation, the usual dose is 3–4 mg/kg of theophylline every 6 hours. Changes in dosage will result in a new steady state concentration of theophylline in 1–2 days, so the dose may be increased at intervals of 2–3 days until therapeutic plasma concentrations are achieved (10–20 mg/L) or until adverse effects develop.

ANTIMUSCARINIC AGENTS

Leaves from *Datura stramonium* have been used in treating asthma for hundreds of years. Interest in the potential value of antimuscarinic agents increased with demonstration of the importance of the vagus in bronchospastic responses of laboratory animals and by the development of a potent antimuscarinic agent that is poorly absorbed after aerosol administration to the airways and is therefore not associated with systemic atropine effects.

Mechanism of Action

Muscarinic antagonists competitively inhibit the effect of acetylcholine at muscarinic receptors (see Chapter 8). In the airways, acetylcholine is released from efferent endings of the vagus nerves, and muscarinic antagonists can effectively block the contraction of airway smooth muscle and the increase in secretion of mucus that occurs in response to vagal activity (Figure 20–2). Very high concentrations—well above those achieved even with maximal therapy—are required to inhibit the response of airway smooth muscle to nonmuscarinic stimulation. This selectivity of muscarinic antagonists accounts for their usefulness as investigative tools in examining the role of parasympathetic pathways in bronchomotor responses but limits their usefulness in preventing bronchospasm. In the doses given, antimuscarinic agents inhibit only that portion of the response mediated by muscarinic receptors, and the involvement of parasympathetic pathways in bronchospastic responses appears to vary among individuals.

Clinical Use of Muscarinic Antagonists

Antimuscarinic agents are effective bronchodilators. When given intravenously, atropine, the prototypical muscarinic antagonist, causes bronchodilation at a lower dose than that needed to cause an increase in heart rate. The selectivity of atropine's effect can be increased further by administering the drug by inhalation or by use of a more selective quaternary ammonium derivative of atropine, **ipratropium bromide.** Ipratropium can be delivered in high doses to muscarinic receptors in the airways because this compound is poorly absorbed and does not readily enter the central nervous system. Studies with this agent have shown that the degree of involvement of parasympathetic pathways in bronchomotor responses varies among subjects. In some, bronchoconstriction is inhibited effectively; in others, only modestly. The failure of higher doses of the muscarinic antagonist to further inhibit the response in these individuals indicates that mechanisms other than parasympathetic reflex pathways must be involved.

Even in the subjects least protected by this antimuscarinic agent, however, the bronchodilation and partial inhibition of provoked bronchoconstriction are of potential clinical value, and antimuscarinic agents are valuable for patients intolerant of inhaled β-agonist agents. While antimuscarinic drugs appear to be slightly less effective than β-agonist agents in reversing asthmatic bronchospasm, the addition of ipratropium enhances the bronchodilation produced by nebulized albuterol in acute severe asthma.

Ipratropium appears to be at least as effective in patients with chronic obstructive pulmonary disease that includes a partially reversible component. A longer-acting, selective antimuscarinic agent, **tiotropium,** is in clinical trials as treatment for COPD. This drug's 24-hour duration of action is a potentially important advantage.

CORTICOSTEROIDS

Mechanism of Action

Corticosteroids have been used to treat asthma since 1950 and are presumed to act by their broad anti-inflammatory efficacy, mediated in part by inhibition of production of inflammatory cytokines (see Chapter 39). They do not relax airway smooth muscle directly but reduce bronchial reactivity and reduce the frequency of asthma exacerbations if taken regularly. Their effect on airway obstruction may be due in part to their potentiation of the effects of β-receptor agonists, but their most important action is their inhibition of the lymphocytic, eosinophilic airway mucosal inflammation of asthmatic airways.

Clinical Use of Corticosteroids

Clinical studies of corticosteroids consistently show them to be effective in improving all indices of asthma control—severity of symptoms, tests of airway caliber and bronchial reactivity, frequency of exacerbations, and quality of life. Because of severe adverse effects when given chronically, oral and parenteral corticosteroids are reserved for patients who require urgent treatment, ie, those who have not improved adequately with bronchodilators or who experience worsening symptoms despite maintenance therapy. Regular or "controller" therapy is maintained with aerosol corticosteroids.

Urgent treatment is often begun with an oral dose of 30–60 mg of prednisone per day or an intravenous dose of 1 mg/kg of methylprednisolone every 6 hours; the daily dose is decreased gradually after airway obstruction has improved. In most patients, systemic corticosteroid therapy can be discontinued in a week or 10 days, but in other patients symptoms may worsen as the dose is decreased to lower levels. Because adrenal suppression by corticosteroids is related to dose and because secretion of corticosteroids has a diurnal variation, it has become customary to administer corticosteroids early in the morning, after endogenous ACTH secretion has peaked. For prevention of nocturnal asthma, however, oral or inhaled corticosteroids are most effective when given in the late afternoon.

Aerosol treatment is the most effective way to decrease the systemic adverse effects of corticosteroid therapy. The introduction of lipid-soluble corticosteroids such as **beclomethasone, budesonide, flunisolide, fluticasone,** and **triamcinolone** makes it possible to deliver corticosteroids to the airways with minimal systemic absorption. An average daily dose of four puffs twice daily of beclomethasone (400 μg/d) is equivalent to about 10–15 mg/d of oral prednisone for the control of asthma, with far fewer systemic effects. Indeed, one of the cautions in switching patients from oral to inhaled corticosteroid therapy is to taper oral therapy slowly to avoid precipitation of adrenal insufficiency. In patients requiring continued prednisone treatment despite inhalation of standard doses of an aerosol corticosteroid, higher doses appear to be more effective; inhaled dosages up to 2000 μg/d of fluticasone are effective in weaning patients from chronic prednisone therapy. While these high doses of inhaled steroids may cause adrenal suppression, the risks of systemic toxicity from chronic use appear negligible compared with those of the oral corticosteroid therapy they replace. A special problem caused by inhaled topical corticosteroids is the occurrence of oropharyngeal candidiasis. The risk of this complication can be reduced by having patients gargle water and spit after each inhaled treatment. Hoarseness can also result from a direct local effect of inhaled corticosteroids on the vocal cords. These agents are remarkably free of other short-term complications in adults but may increase the risks of osteoporosis and cataracts over the long term. In children, inhaled corticosterone therapy has been shown to slow the rate of growth, but asthma itself delays puberty, and there is no evidence that inhaled corticosteroid therapy influences adult height.

Chronic use of inhaled corticosteroids effectively reduces symptoms and improves pulmonary function in patients with mild asthma. Such use also reduces or eliminates the need for oral corticosteroids in patients with more severe disease. In contrast to β-stimulant agents and theophylline, chronic use of inhaled corticosteroids reduces bronchial reactivity. Because of the efficacy and safety of inhaled corticosteroids, they are now routinely prescribed for patients who require more than occasional inhalations of a β agonist for relief of symptoms. This therapy is continued for 10–12 weeks and then withdrawn to determine if more prolonged therapy is needed.

Inhaled corticosteroids are not curative. In most patients, the manifestations of asthma return within a few weeks after stopping therapy even if they have been taken in high doses for 2 years or longer.

CROMOLYN & NEDOCROMIL

Cromolyn sodium (disodium cromoglycate) and nedocromil sodium are stable but extremely insoluble salts (see structures below). When used as aerosols (metered-dose inhalers), they effectively inhibit both antigen- and exercise-induced asthma, and chronic use (four times daily) slightly reduces the overall level of bronchial reactivity. However, these drugs have no effect on airway smooth muscle tone and are ineffective in reversing asthmatic bronchospasm; they are only of value when taken prophylactically.

Cromolyn sodium

Nedocromil sodium

Cromolyn is poorly absorbed from the gastrointestinal tract and must be inhaled as a microfine powder or aerosolized solution. Nedocromil also has a very low bioavailability and is available only in metered-dose aerosol form.

Mechanism of Action

Cromolyn and nedocromil differ structurally but are thought to share a common mechanism of action, an alteration in the function of delayed chloride channels in the cell membrane, inhibiting cellular activation. This action on airway nerves is thought to be responsible for nedocromil's inhibition of cough; on mast cells, for inhibition of the early response to antigen challenge; and on eosinophils, for inhibition of the inflammatory response to inhalation of allergens. The inhibitory effect on mast cells appears to be specific for cell type, since cromolyn has little inhibitory effect on mediator release from human basophils. It may also be specific for different organs, since cromolyn inhibits mast cell degranulation in human and primate lung but not in skin. This in turn may reflect known differences in mast cells found in different sites, as in their neutral protease content.

Until recently, the idea that cromolyn inhibits mast cell degranulation was so well accepted that the inhibition of a response by cromolyn was thought to indicate the involvement of mast cells in the response. This simplistic idea has been overturned in part by the finding that cromolyn and nedocromil inhibit the function of cells other than mast cells and in part by the finding that nedocromil inhibits appearance of the late response even when given after the early response to antigen challenge, ie, after mast cell degranulation has occurred.

Clinical Use of Cromolyn & Nedocromil

In short-term clinical trials, pretreatment with cromolyn or nedocromil blocks the bronchoconstriction caused by antigen inhalation, by exercise, by aspirin, and by a variety of causes of occupational asthma. This acute protective effect of a single treatment makes cromolyn useful for administration shortly before exercise or before unavoidable exposure to an allergen.

When taken regularly (two to four puffs two to four times daily) by patients with perennial asthma, both agents reduce symptomatic severity and the need for bronchodilator medications. These drugs are neither as potent nor as predictably effective as inhaled corticosteroids. In general, young patients with extrinsic asthma are most likely to respond favorably. At present, the only way of determining whether a patient will respond is by a therapeutic trial for 4 weeks. The addition of nedocromil to a standard dose of an inhaled corticosteroid appears to improve asthma control.

Cromolyn solution is also useful in reducing symptoms of **allergic rhinoconjunctivitis.** Applying the solution by nasal spray or eye drops several times a day is effective in about 75% of patients, even during the peak pollen season.

Because the drugs are so poorly absorbed, adverse effects of cromolyn and nedocromil are minor and are localized to the sites of deposition. These include such symptoms as throat irritation, cough, mouth dryness, chest tightness, and wheezing. Some of these symptoms can be prevented by inhaling a β_2-adrenoceptor agonist before cromolyn or nedocromil treatment. Serious adverse effects are rare. Reversible dermatitis, myositis, or gastroenteritis occurs in fewer than 2% of patients, and a very few cases of pulmonary infiltration with eosinophilia and anaphylaxis have been reported. This lack of toxicity accounts for cromolyn's widespread use in children, especially those at ages of rapid growth. For children who have difficulty coordinating the use of the inhaler device, cromolyn may be given by aerosol of a 1% solution.

LEUKOTRIENE PATHWAY INHIBITORS

Because of the evidence of leukotriene involvement in many inflammatory diseases (see Chapter 18) and in anaphylaxis, considerable effort has been expended on the development of drugs that block the synthesis of these arachidonic acid derivatives or their receptors. Leukotrienes result from the action of 5-lipoxygenase on arachidonic acid and are synthesized by a variety of inflammatory cells in the airways, including eosinophils,

mast cells, macrophages, and basophils. Leukotriene B_4 is a potent neutrophil chemoattractant, and LTC_4 and LTD_4 exert many effects known to occur in asthma, including bronchoconstriction, increased bronchial reactivity, mucosal edema, and mucus hypersecretion. Early studies established that antigen challenge of sensitized human lung tissue results in the generation of leukotrienes, while other studies of human subjects have shown that inhalation of leukotrienes causes not only bronchoconstriction but also an increase in bronchial reactivity to histamine that persists for several days.

Two approaches to interrupting the leukotriene pathway have been pursued: inhibition of 5-lipoxygenase, thereby preventing leukotriene synthesis; and inhibition of the binding of leukotriene D_4 to its receptor on target tissues, thereby preventing its action. Efficacy in blocking airway responses to exercise and to antigen challenge has been shown for drugs in both categories: **zileuton,** a 5-lipoxygenase inhibitor, and **zafirlukast** and **montelukast,** LTD_4-receptor antagonists. All have been shown to be effective when taken regularly in outpatient clinical trials. Their effects on symptoms, airway caliber, bronchial reactivity, and airway inflammation are less marked than the effects of inhaled corticosteroids, but they are almost equally effective in reducing the frequency of exacerbations. Their principal advantage is that they are taken orally; some patients—especially children—comply poorly with inhaled therapies. Montelukast is approved for children as young as 6 years of age.

Zafirlukast

Montelukast

Zileuton

Some patients appear to have particularly favorable responses, but no clinical features allow identification of "responders" before a trial of therapy. In the USA, zileuton is approved for use in an oral dosage of 600 mg given four times daily; zafirlukast, 20 mg twice daily; and montelukast, 10 mg once daily.

Trials with leukotriene inhibitors have demonstrated an important role for leukotrienes in aspirin-induced asthma. It has long been known that 5–10% of asthmatics are exquisitely sensitive to aspirin, so that ingestion of even a very small dose causes profound bronchoconstriction and symptoms of systemic release of histamine, such as flushing and abdominal cramping. Because this reaction to aspirin is not associated with any evidence of allergic sensitization to aspirin or its metabolites, and because it is produced by any of the nonsteroidal anti-inflammatory agents, it is thought to result from inhibition of prostaglandin synthetase, shifting arachidonic acid metabolism from the prostaglandin to the leukotriene pathway. Support for this idea was provided by the demonstration that leukotriene pathway inhibitors impressively reduce the response to aspirin challenge and improve overall control of asthma on a day-to-day basis.

Of these agents, zileuton is the least prescribed because of the requirement of four times daily dosing and because of occasional liver toxicity. The receptor antagonists appear to be safe to use. Reports of Churg-Strauss syndrome (a systemic vasculitis characterized by worsening asthma, pulmonary infiltrates, and eosinophilia) appear to have been coincidental, with the syndrome unmasked by the reduction in prednisone dosage made possible by the addition of zafirlukast or montelukast.

OTHER DRUGS IN THE TREATMENT OF ASTHMA

Anti-IgE Monoclonal Antibodies

An entirely new approach to the treatment of asthma exploits advances in molecular biology to target IgE antibody. From a collection of monoclonal antibodies raised in mice against IgE antibody itself, a monoclonal antibody was selected that appeared to be targeted against the portion of IgE that binds to its receptors (FCe-R1 and -R2 receptors) on mast cells and other inflammatory cells. **Omalizumab** (anti-IgE Mab) inhibits the binding of IgE to mast cells but does not activate IgE already bound to these cells and thus does not provoke mast cell degranulation. In mice, it also appears to inhibit IgE synthesis by B lymphocytes. The murine antibody has been genetically "humanized" by replacing all but a small fraction of its amino acids with those found in human proteins, and it does not appear to cause sensitization when given to human subjects.

Studies of omalizumab in asthmatic volunteers showed that its administration over 10 weeks lowered plasma IgE to undetectable levels and significantly reduced the magnitude of both the early and the late bronchospastic responses to antigen challenge. Clinical trials have shown repeated intravenous or subcutaneous injection of anti-IgE MAb to lessen asthma severity and reduce the corticosteroid requirement in patients with moderate to severe disease, especially those with a clear environmental antigen precipitating factor, and to improve nasal and conjunctival symptoms in patients with perennial or seasonal allergic rhinitis.

Calcium Channel Blockers

Each of the cell functions that may become abnormal in patients with asthma depends to some degree on the movement of calcium into cells. The calcium channel blockers have no effect on baseline airway diameter but do significantly inhibit the airway narrowing that is induced by various stimuli. In patients, both **nifedipine** and **verapamil** given by inhalation significantly inhibited the bronchoconstriction induced by a variety of stimuli. However, both drugs were much less effective than inhaled albuterol.

Nitric Oxide Donors

Preliminary studies in animals suggest that airway smooth muscle, like that in the vasculature, is effectively relaxed by nitric oxide. This very lipophilic drug can be inhaled as a gas in acute asthma and dilates the pulmonary blood vessels as well as the airway smooth muscle. Although nitric oxide itself—or nitric oxide donors—may prove of value in acute severe asthma, it appears likely that they will be more useful in pulmonary hypertension (for which nitric oxide is already approved).

Possible Future Therapies

The rapid advance in the scientific description of the immunopathogenesis of asthma has spurred the development of many new therapies targeting different sites in the immune cascade. These include monoclonal antibodies directed against cytokines (IL-4, IL-5, IL-8), antagonists of cell adhesion molecules, protease inhibitors, and immunomodulators aimed at shifting CD4 lymphocytes from the TH2 to the TH1 phenotype. There is evidence that asthma may be aggravated—or even caused—by chronic airway infection with *Chlamydia pneumoniae* or *Mycoplasma pneumoniae*. This may explain the reports of benefit from treatment with macrolide antibiotics and, if confirmed, would stimulate the development of new diagnostic methods and antimicrobial therapies.

II. CLINICAL PHARMACOLOGY OF DRUGS USED IN THE TREATMENT OF ASTHMA

BRONCHODILATORS

Patients with mild asthma and only occasional symptoms require no more than an inhaled β-receptor agonist (eg, albuterol) on an "as-needed" basis. If symptoms require frequent inhalations (more often than twice a week), or if nocturnal symptoms occur, additional treatment is needed, preferably with an inhaled anti-inflammatory agent such as a corticosteroid or cromolyn, or with oral therapy with a leukotriene receptor antagonist. Theophylline is now largely reserved for patients in whom symptoms remain poorly controlled despite the combination of regular treatment with an inhaled anti-inflammatory agent and as-needed use of a β_2 agonist. If the addition of theophylline fails to improve symptoms or if adverse effects become bothersome, it is important to check the plasma level of theophylline to be sure it is in the therapeutic range (10–20 mg/L).

CORTICOSTEROIDS

If asthmatic symptoms occur frequently or if significant airflow obstruction persists despite bronchodilator therapy, inhaled corticosteroids should be started. For patients with severe symptoms or severe airflow obstruction (eg, FEV_1 < 1.5 L), initial treatment with oral corticosteroid (eg, 30 mg/d of prednisone for 3 weeks) is appropriate. Once clinical improvement is noted, inhaled corticosteroid treatment should be started and the oral dose reduced to the minimum necessary to control symptoms. For patients with milder symptoms but still inadequately controlled by as-needed use of an inhaled bronchodilator, corticosteroids may be initiated by the inhaled route.

In patients whose symptoms are inadequately controlled by a standard dose of an inhaled corticosteroid, the addition of a long-acting inhaled β-receptor agonist (salmeterol, formoterol) is more effective than is doubling the dose of the inhaled corticosteroid. The improvement in clinical symptoms and peak flow is usually prompt and sustained. In patients on such a combined treatment regimen, it is important to provide explicit instructions that a standard, short-acting inhaled β agonist, like albuterol, be used for relief of acute symptoms. It is also important that the patient not stop the inhaled corticosteroid, continuing only the long-acting β agonist, because exacerbations are not prevented by this monotherapy. For this reason—and

because long-acting β agonists appear to enhance the local but not the systemic actions of inhaled corticosteroids—inhalers containing both agents have been developed (see Preparations Available).

CROMOLYN & NEDOCROMIL

Cromolyn or nedocromil may be considered as an alternative to inhaled corticosteroids in patients with symptoms occurring more than twice a week or who are wakened from sleep by asthma. They may also be useful in patients whose symptoms occur seasonally or after clear-cut inciting stimuli such as exercise or exposure to animal danders or irritants. In patients whose symptoms are continuous or occur without an obvious inciting stimulus, the value of these drugs can only be established with a therapeutic trial of inhaled drug four times a day for 4 weeks. If the patient responds to this therapy, the dose can be reduced. Maintenance therapy with cromolyn appears to be as effective as maintenance therapy with theophylline and, because of concerns over the possible long-term toxicity of systemic absorption of inhaled corticosteroids, has become widely used for treating children in the USA.

MUSCARINIC ANTAGONISTS

Inhaled muscarinic antagonists have so far earned a limited place in the treatment of asthma. When adequate doses are given, their effect on baseline airway resistance is nearly as great as that of the sympathomimetic drugs. The airway effects of antimuscarinic and sympathomimetic drugs given in full doses have been shown to have significant additive effects only in patients with severe airflow obstruction who present for emergency care. Antimuscarinic agents appear to be of significant value in chronic obstructive pulmonary disease—perhaps more so than in asthma. They are useful as alternative therapies for patients intolerant of β-adrenoceptor agonists.

When muscarinic antagonists are used for long-term treatment, they appear to be effective bronchodilators. Although it was predicted that muscarinic antagonists might dry airway secretions, direct measurements of fluid volume secretion from single airway submucosal glands in animals show that atropine decreases secretory rates only slightly; however, the drug does prevent excessive secretion caused by vagal reflex stimulation. No cases of inspissation of mucus have been reported following administration of these drugs.

OTHER ANTI-INFLAMMATORY THERAPIES

Some recent reports suggest that agents commonly used to treat rheumatoid arthritis might also be used to treat patients with chronic steroid-dependent asthma. The development of an alternative treatment is important, since chronic treatment with oral corticosteroids may cause osteoporosis, cataracts, glucose intolerance, worsening of hypertension, and cushingoid changes in appearance. Initial studies suggested that oral methotrexate or gold salt injections were beneficial in prednisone-dependent asthmatics, but subsequent studies did not confirm this promise. The benefit from treatment with cyclosporine seems real. However, this drug's great toxicity makes this finding only a source of hope that other immunomodulatory therapies will ultimately be developed for the small proportion of patients whose asthma can be managed only with high oral doses of prednisone.

MANAGEMENT OF ACUTE ASTHMA

The treatment of acute attacks of asthma in patients reporting to the hospital requires more continuous assessment and repeated objective measurement of lung function. For patients with mild attacks, inhalation of a β-receptor agonist is as effective as subcutaneous injection of epinephrine. Both of these treatments are more effective than intravenous administration of aminophylline. Severe attacks require treatment with oxygen, frequent or continuous administration of aerosolized albuterol, and systemic treatment with prednisone or methylprednisolone (0.5 mg/kg every 6 hours). Even this aggressive treatment is not invariably effective, and patients must be watched closely for signs of deterioration. Intubation and mechanical ventilation of asthmatic patients cannot be undertaken lightly but may be lifesaving if respiratory failure supervenes.

PREPARATIONS AVAILABLE

Sympathomimetics Used in Asthma
Albuterol (generic, Proventil, Ventolin, others)
Inhalant: 90 µg/puff aerosol; 0.083, 0.5% solution for nebulization
Oral: 2, 4 mg tablets; 2 mg/5 mL syrup
Oral sustained-release: 4, 8 mg tablets
Albuterol/Ipratropium (Combivent, DuoNeb)
Inhalant: 103 µg albuterol + 18 µg ipratropium/puff; 3 mg albuterol + 0.5 mg ipratropium/3 mL solution for nebulization
Bitolterol (Tornalate)
Inhalant: 0.2% solution for nebulization
Ephedrine (generic)
Oral: 25 mg capsules
Parenteral: 50 mg/mL for injection
Epinephrine (generic, Adrenalin, others)
Inhalant: 1, 10 mg/mL for nebulization; 0.22 mg epinephrine base aerosol
Parenteral: 1:10,000 (0.1 mg/mL), 1:1000 (1 mg/mL)
Formoterol (Foradil)
Inhalant: 12 µg/puff aerosol; 12 µg/unit inhalant powder
Isoetharine (generic)
Inhalant: 1% solution for nebulization
Isoproterenol (generic, Isuprel, others)
Inhalant: 0.5, 1% for nebulization; 80, 131 µg/puff aerosols
Parenteral: 0.02, 0.2 mg/mL for injection
Levalbuterol (Xenopex)
Inhalant: 0.31, 0.63, 1.25 mg/3 mL solution
Metaproterenol (Alupent, generic)

Inhalant: 0.65 mg/puff aerosol in 7, 14 g containers; 0.4, 0.6, 5% for nebulization
Pirbuterol (Maxair)
Inhalant: 0.2 mg/puff aerosol in 80 and 300 dose containers
Salmeterol (Serevent)
Inhalant aerosol: 25 µg salmeterol base/puff in 60 and 120 dose containers
Inhalant powder: 50 µg/unit
Salmeterol/Fluticasone (Advair Diskus)
Inhalant: 100, 250, 500 µg fluticasone + 50 µg salmeterol/unit
Terbutaline (Brethine, Bricanyl)
Inhalant: 0.2 mg/puff aerosol
Oral: 2.5, 5 mg tablets
Parenteral: 1 mg/mL for injection

Aerosol Corticosteroids (see also Chapter 39.)
Beclomethasone (QVAR, Vanceril)
Aerosol: 40, 80 µg/puff in 200 dose containers
Budesonide (Pulmicort)
Aerosol powder: 160 µg/activation
Flunisolide (AeroBid)
Aerosol: 250 µg/puff in 100 dose container
Fluticasone (Flovent)
Aerosol: 44, 110, and 220 µg/puff in 120 dose container; powder, 50, 100, 250 µg/activation
Fluticasone/Salmeterol (Advair Diskus)
Inhalant: 100, 250, 500 µg fluticasone + 50 µg salmeterol/unit
Triamcinolone (Azmacort)
Aerosol: 100 µg/puff in 240 dose container

LEUKOTRIENE INHIBITORS
Montelukast (Singulair)
Oral: 10 mg tablets; 4, 5 mg chewable tablets; 4 mg/packet granules
Zafirlukast (Accolate)
Oral: 10, 20 mg tablets
Zileuton (Zyflo)
Oral: 600 mg tablets

CROMOLYN SODIUM & NEDOCROMIL SODIUM
Cromolyn sodium
Pulmonary aerosol (generic, Intal): 800 µg/puff in 200 dose container; 20 mg/2 mL for nebulization (for asthma)
Nasal aerosol (Nasalcrom):* 5.2 mg/puff (for hay fever)
Oral (Gastrocrom): 100 mg/5 mL concentrate (for gastrointestinal allergy)
Nedocromil sodium (Tilade)
Pulmonary aerosol: 1.75 mg/puff in 112 metered-dose container

METHYLXANTHINES: THEOPHYLLINE & DERIVATIVES
Aminophylline (theophylline ethylenediamine, 79% theophylline) (generic, others)
Oral: 105 mg/5 mL liquid; 100, 200 mg tablets
Oral sustained-release: 225 mg tablets
Rectal: 250, 500 mg suppositories
Parenteral: 250 mg/10 mL for injection
Theophylline (generic, Elixophyllin, Slo-Phyllin, Uniphyl, Theo-Dur, Theo-24, others)
Oral: 100, 125, 200, 250, 300 mg tablets; 100, 200 mg capsules; 26.7, 50 mg/5 mL elixirs, syrups, and solutions

Oral sustained-release, 8–12 hours: 50, 60, 75, 100, 125, 130, 200, 250, 260, 300 mg capsules
Oral sustained-release, 8–24 hours: 100, 200, 300, 450 mg tablets
Oral sustained-release, 12 hours: 100, 125, 130, 200, 250, 260, 300 mg capsules
Oral sustained-release, 12–24 hours: 100, 200, 300 tablets
Oral sustained-release, 24 hours: 100, 200, 300 mg tablets and capsules; 400, 600 mg tablets
Parenteral: 200, 400, 800 mg/container, theophylline and 5% dextrose for injection

OTHER METHYLXANTHINES
Dyphylline (generic, other)
Oral: 200, 400 mg tablets; 33.3, 53.3 mg/5 mL elixir
Parenteral: 250 mg/mL for injection
Oxtriphylline (generic, Choledyl)
Oral: equivalent to 64, 127, 254, 382 mg theophylline tablets; 32, 64 mg/5 mL syrup
Pentoxifylline (generic, Trental)
Oral: 400 mg tablets and controlled-release tablets
Note: Pentoxifylline is labeled for use in intermittent claudication only.

ANTIMUSCARINIC DRUGS USED IN ASTHMA
Ipratropium (generic, Atrovent)
Aerosol: 18 µg/puff in 200 metered-dose inhaler; 0.02% (500 µg/vial) for nebulization
Nasal spray: 21, 42 µg/spray

ANTIBODY
Omalizumab (Xolair)
Powder for SC injection, 202.5 mg

---

* OTC preparation.

REFERENCES

PATHOPHYSIOLOGY OF AIRWAY DISEASE

Belvisi MG: Overview of the innervation of the lung. Curr Opin Pharmacol 2002;2:211.

Bousquet J et al: Eosinophilic inflammation in asthma. N Engl J Med 1990;323:1033.

Mazzone SB, Canning BJ: Central nervous system control of the airways: pharmacological implications. Curr Opin Pharmacol 2002;2:220.

Spina D, Page CP: Pharmacology of airway irritability. Curr Opin Pharmacol 2002;2:264.

METHYLXANTHINES

Kidney J et al: Immunomodulation by theophylline in asthma: Demonstration by withdrawal of therapy. Am J Respir Crit Care Med 1995;151:1907.

Murciano D et al: Effects of theophylline on diaphragmatic strength and fatigue in patients with chronic obstructive pulmonary disease. N Engl J Med 1984;311:349.

Page CP: Recent advances in our understanding of the use of theophylline in the treatment of asthma. J Clin Pharmacol 1999; 39:237.

Ward AJ et al: Theophylline—an immunomodulating role in asthma? Am Rev Resp Dis 1993;147:518.

CROMOLYN & NEDOCROMIL

Aalbers R et al: The effect of nedocromil sodium on the early and late reaction and allergen-induced bronchial hyperresponsiveness. J Allergy Clin Immunol 1991; 87:993.

Barnes PJ et al: Asthma mechanisms, determinants of severity and treatment: The role of nedocromil sodium. Clin Exper Allergy 1995;25:771.

Pelikan Z, Knotterus I: Inhibition of the late response asthmatic response by nedocromil sodium administered more than two hours after antigen challenge. J Allergy Clin Immunol 1993;92:19.

CORTICOSTEROIDS

Juniper EF et al: Effect of long-term treatment with an inhaled corticosteroid (budesonide) on airway hyperresponsiveness and clinical asthma in nonsteroid-dependent asthmatics. Am Rev Respir Dis 1990;142:832.

Noonan M et al: Fluticasone propionate reduces oral prednisone use while it improves asthma control and quality of life. Am J Respir Crit Care Med 1995;152:1467.

Robinson DS, Geddes DM: Inhaled corticosteroids: Benefits and risks. J Asthma 1996;33:5.

Stein LM, Cole RP: Early administration of corticosteroids in emergency room treatment of acute asthma. Ann Intern Med 1990;112:822.

Suissa S et al: Low-dose inhaled corticosteroids and the prevention of death from asthma. N Engl J Med 2000;343:332.

BETA AGONISTS

Anderson GP: Formoterol: Pharmacology, molecular basis of agonism, and mechanism of long duration of a highly potent and selective β_2-adrenoceptor agonist bronchodilator. Life Sci 1993;52:2145.

Greening AP et al: Added salmeterol versus higher-dose corticosteroid in asthma patients with symptoms on existing inhaled corticosteroid. Lancet 1994;344:219.

Mullen M, Mullen B, Carey M: The association between β-agonist use and death from asthma. A meta-analytic integration of case-control studies. JAMA 1993;270:1842.

Spitzer WO et al: The use of β-agonists and the risk of death and near death from asthma. N Engl J Med 1992;326:501.

Svedmyr N: The current place of β_2-agonists in the management of asthma. Lung 1990;168(Suppl):105.

Ullman A, Svedmyr N: Salmeterol, a new long acting inhaled β_2-adrenoceptor agonist: Comparison with salbutamol in adult asthmatic patients. Thorax 1988;43:674.

ANTIMUSCARINIC DRUGS

Barnes PJ et al: Tiotropium bromide (ba 679 br), a novel long-acting muscarinic antagonist for the treatment of obstructive airways disease. Life Sci 1995;56:853.

Lee AM, Jacoby DB, Fryer AD: Selective muscarinic receptor antagonists for airway diseases. Curr Opin Pharmacol 2001;1:223.

LEUKOTRIENE PATHWAY INHIBITORS

Calhoun WJ: Anti-leukotrienes for asthma. Curr Opin Pharmacol 2001;1:230.

Drazen JM et al: Treatment of asthma with drugs modifying the leukotriene pathway. N Engl J Med 1999;340:197.

Holgate ST, Bradding P, Sampson AP: Leukotriene antagonists and synthesis inhibitors: New directions in asthma therapy. J Allergy Clin Immunol 1996;98:1.

Krawiec ME, Wenzel SE: Leukotriene inhibitors and non-steroidal therapies in the treatment of asthma. Exp Opin Invest Drugs 2001;2:47.

Malmstrom K et al: Oral montelukast, inhaled beclomethasone, and placebo for chronic asthma. A randomized, controlled trial. Montelukast/Beclomethasone Study Group. Ann Intern Med 1999;130:487.

OTHER DRUGS FOR ASTHMA

Bryan SA et al: Novel therapy for asthma. Exp Opin Invest Drugs 2000;9:25.

Fahy JV et al: The effect of anti-IgE recombinant humanized monoclonal antibody-E25 on the early and late phase response to airway challenge with allergen in asthmatic subjects. Am J Respir Crit Care Med 1997;155:1828.

Leckie MJ et al: A humanized anti-IL5 monoclonal antibody. Initial single dose safety and activity in patients with asthma. Am J Respir Crit Care Med 1999;159(3 Part 2):A624.

Leckie MJ et al: Effects of an interleukin-5 blocking monoclonal antibody on eosinophils, airway hyper-responsiveness, and the late asthmatic response. Lancet 2000;456:2144.

Lock SH et al: Double-blind, placebo-controlled study of cyclosporin A as a corticosteroid-sparing agent in corticosteroid-dependent asthma. Am J Respir Crit Care Med 1996;153:509.

Milgrom H et al: Treatment of allergic asthma with monoclonal anti-IgE antibody. rhuMAb-E25 Study Group. N Engl J Med 1999;341:1966.

Patacchini R, Maggi CA: Peripheral tachykinin receptors as targets for new drugs. Eur J Pharmacol 2001;429:13.

CLINICAL MANAGEMENT OF AIRWAY DISEASE

Barnes PJ: Current therapies for asthma. Promise and limitations. Chest 1997;111(2 suppl):17s.

Corbridge TC, Hall JB: The assessment and management of adults with status asthmaticus. Am J Respir Crit Care Med 1995;151:1296.

Guidelines for the diagnosis and management of asthma: National Heart, Lung, and Blood Institute National Asthma Education Program Expert Panel Report. J Allergy Clin Immunol 1991;88:425.

Tattersfield AE et al: Asthma. Lancet 2002;360:1313.

SECTION V
Drugs That Act in the Central Nervous System

Introduction to the Pharmacology of CNS Drugs

21

Roger A. Nicoll, MD

Drugs acting in the central nervous system (CNS) were among the first to be discovered by primitive humans and are still the most widely used group of pharmacologic agents. In addition to their use in therapy, many drugs acting on the CNS are used without prescription to increase one's sense of well-being.

The mechanisms by which various drugs act in the CNS have not always been clearly understood. Since the causes of many of the conditions for which these drugs are used (schizophrenia, anxiety, etc) are themselves poorly understood, it is not surprising that in the past much of CNS pharmacology has been purely descriptive. In the last 3 decades, however, dramatic advances have been made in the methodology of CNS pharmacology. It is now possible to study the action of a drug on individual cells and even single ion channels within synapses. The information obtained from such studies is the basis for several major developments in studies of the CNS.

First, it is clear that nearly all drugs with CNS effects act on specific receptors that modulate synaptic transmission. A very few agents such as general anesthetics and alcohol may have nonspecific actions on membranes (although these exceptions are not fully accepted), but even these non-receptor-mediated actions result in demonstrable alterations in synaptic transmission.

Second, drugs are among the most important tools for studying all aspects of CNS physiology, from the mechanism of convulsions to the laying down of long-term memory. As will be described below, agonists that mimic natural transmitters (and in many cases are more selective than the endogenous substances) and antagonists are extremely useful in such studies. The Box, Natural Toxins: Tools for Characterizing Ion Channels, page 337, describes the uses of some of these substances.

Third, unraveling the actions of drugs with known clinical efficacy has led to some of the most fruitful hypotheses regarding the mechanisms of disease. For example, information on the action of antipsychotic drugs on dopamine receptors has provided the basis for important hypotheses regarding the pathophysiology of schizophrenia. Studies of the effects of a variety of agonists and antagonists on γ-aminobutyric acid (GABA) receptors are resulting in new concepts pertaining to the pathophysiology of several diseases, including anxiety and epilepsy.

This chapter provides an introduction to the functional organization of the CNS and its synaptic transmitters as a basis for understanding the actions of the drugs described in the following chapters.

NATURAL TOXINS: TOOLS FOR CHARACTERIZING ION CHANNELS

Evolution is a tireless chemist when it comes to inventing toxins. A vast number of variations are possible with even a small number of amino acids in peptides, and peptides are only one of a broad array of toxic compounds. For example, the predatory marine snail genus *Conus* is estimated to include at least 500 different species. Each species kills or paralyzes its prey with a venom that contains 50–200 different peptides or proteins. Furthermore, there is little duplication of peptides among *Conus* species. Other animals with useful toxins include snakes, frogs, spiders, bees, wasps, and scorpions. Plant species with toxic (or therapeutic) substances are too numerous to mention here; they are referred to in many chapters of this book.

Since many toxins act on ion channels, they provide a wealth of chemical tools for studying the function of these channels. In fact, much of our current understanding of the properties of ion channels comes from studies utilizing only a small fraction of the highly potent and selective toxins that are now available. The toxins typically target voltage-sensitive ion channels, but a number of very useful toxins block ionotropic neurotransmitter receptors. Table 21–1 lists some of the toxins most commonly used in research, their mode of action, and their source.

Methods for the Study of CNS Pharmacology

Although scientists (and the public) have always been interested in the action of drugs in the CNS, a detailed description of synaptic transmission was not possible until glass microelectrodes, which permit intracellular recording, were developed. Detailed electrophysiologic studies of the action of drugs on both voltage- and transmitter-operated channels were further facilitated by the introduction of the patch clamp technique, which permits the recording of current through single channels. Histochemical, immunologic, and radioisotopic methods are widely used to map the distribution of specific transmitters, their associated enzyme systems, and their receptors. Molecular cloning has had a major impact on our understanding of CNS receptors. These techniques make it possible to determine the precise molecular structure of the receptors and their associated channels. Finally, mice with mutated genes for specific receptors or enzymes (knockout mice) can provide important information regarding the physiologic and pharmacologic roles of these components.

ION CHANNELS & NEUROTRANSMITTER RECEPTORS

The membranes of nerve cells contain two types of channels defined on the basis of the mechanisms controlling their gating (opening and closing): **voltage-gated** and **ligand-gated** channels (Figures 21–1A and 21–1B). Voltage-gated channels respond to changes in the membrane potential of the cell. The voltage-gated sodium channel described in Chapter 14 for the heart is an example of the first type and is very important in the CNS. In nerve cells, these channels are concentrated on the initial segment and the axon and are responsible for the fast action potential, which transmits the signal from cell body to nerve terminal. There are many types of voltage-sensitive calcium and potassium channels on the cell body, dendrites, and initial segment, which act on a much slower time scale and modulate the rate at which the neuron discharges. For example, some types of potassium channels opened by depolarization of the cell result in slowing of further depolarization and act as a brake to limit further action potential discharge.

Ligand-gated channels, also called **ionotropic receptors,** are opened by the binding of neurotransmitters to the channel. The receptor is formed of subunits, and the channel is an integral part of the receptor complex. These channels are insensitive or only weakly sensitive to membrane potential. Activation of these channels typically results in a brief (a few milliseconds to tens of milliseconds) opening of the channel. Ligand-gated channels are responsible for fast synaptic transmission typical of hierarchical pathways in the CNS (see below).

It is now well established that the traditional view of completely separate voltage-gated and ligand-gated channels requires substantial modifications. As discussed in Chapter 2, most neurotransmitters, in addition to binding to ionotropic receptors, also bind to G protein-coupled receptors, often referred to as **metabotropic** receptors. Metabotropic receptors, via G proteins, modulate voltage-gated channels. This interaction can occur entirely within the membrane and is referred to as a **membrane delimited** pathway (Figure 21–1C). In this case the G protein interacts directly with the voltage-gated ion channel. In general, two types of voltage-gated ion channel are involved in this type of signaling: calcium channels and potassium channels. When G proteins interact with calcium channels, they inhibit channel function. This mechanism accounts for the

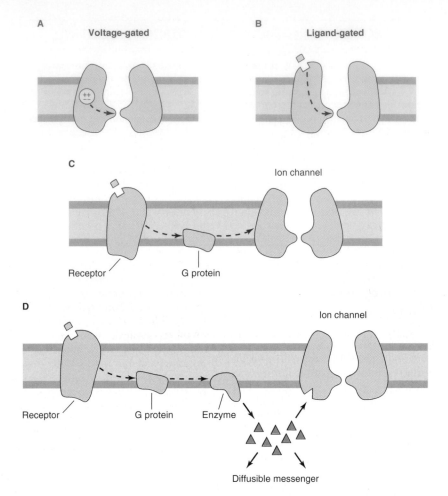

Figure 21–1. Types of ion channels and neurotransmitter receptors in the CNS. **A** shows a voltage-gated channel in which a voltage sensor controls the gating (broken arrow) of the channel. **B** shows a ligand-gated channel in which the binding of the neurotransmitter to the channel controls the gating (broken arrow) of the channel. **C** shows a G protein coupled receptor, which when bound, activates a G protein which then interacts directly with an ion channel. **D** shows a G protein coupled receptor, which when bound, activates a G protein which then activates an enzyme. The activated enzyme generates a diffusible second messenger that interacts with an ion channel.

presynaptic inhibition that occurs when presynaptic metabotropic receptors are activated. In contrast, when these receptors are postsynaptic, they activate (cause the opening of) potassium channels, resulting in a slow post-synaptic inhibition. Metabotropic receptors can also modulate voltage-gated channels less directly by the generation of **diffusible second messengers** (Figure 21–1D). A classic example of this type of action is provided by the β adrenoceptor, which generates cAMP via the activation of adenylyl cyclase (see Chapter 2). Whereas membrane-delimited actions occur within microdomains in the membrane, second messenger-mediated effects can occur over considerable distances. Finally, an important conse-

quence of the involvement of G proteins in receptor signaling is that, in contrast to the brief effect of ionotropic receptors, the effects of metabotropic receptor activation can last tens of seconds to minutes. Metabotropic receptors predominate in the diffuse neuronal systems in the CNS (see below).

THE SYNAPSE & SYNAPTIC POTENTIALS

The communication between neurons in the CNS occurs through chemical synapses in the vast majority of cases. (A few instances of electrical coupling between neurons have been documented, and such coupling may play a role in synchronizing neuronal discharge. However, it is unlikely that these electrical synapses are an important site of drug action.) The events involved in the release of transmitter from the presynaptic terminal have been studied most extensively at the vertebrate neuromuscular junction and at the giant synapse of the squid. More recently, the calix of Held synapse, a specialized synapse in the brain stem with a large presynaptic terminal, has served as a model for the study of transmitter release from CNS synapses.

An action potential in the presynaptic fiber propagates into the synaptic terminal and activates voltage-sensitive calcium channels in the membrane of the terminal (Figure 6–3). The calcium channels responsible for the release of transmitter are generally resistant to the calcium channel-blocking agents discussed in Chapter 12 (verapamil, etc) but are sensitive to blockade by certain marine toxins and metal ions (Tables 12–4 and

21–1). Calcium flows into the terminal, and the increase in intraterminal calcium concentration promotes the fusion of synaptic vesicles with the presynaptic membrane. The transmitter contained in the vesicles is released into the synaptic cleft and diffuses to the receptors on the postsynaptic membrane. Binding of the transmitter to its receptor causes a brief change in membrane conductance (permeability to ions) of the postsynaptic cell. The time delay from the arrival of the presynaptic action potential to the onset of the postsynaptic response is approximately 0.5 ms. Most of this delay is consumed by the release process, particularly the time required for calcium channels to open.

The first systematic analysis of synaptic potentials in the CNS was in the early 1950s by Eccles and associates, who recorded intracellularly from spinal motoneurons. When a microelectrode enters a cell, there is a sudden change in the potential recorded by the electrode, which is typically about −70 mV (Figure 21–2). This is the

Table 21–1. Some toxins used to characterize ion channels.

Channel Types	Mode of Toxin Action	Source
Voltage-gated		
Sodium channels		
Tetrodotoxin (TTX)	Blocks from outside	Puffer fish
α-Scorpion toxin	Slows inactivation	Scorpion
Batrachotoxin (BTX)	Slows inactivation, shifts activation	Colombian frog
Potassium channels		
Apamin	Blocks "small Ca^{2+}-activated" K^+ channel	Honeybee
Charybdotoxin	Blocks "big Ca^{2+}-activated" K^+ channel	Scorpion
Dendrotoxin	Blocks delayed rectifier	Snake
Calcium channels		
Omega conotoxin (ω-CTX-GVIA)	Blocks N-type channel	Pacific cone snail
Agatoxin (ω-AGA-IVA)	Blocks P-type channel	Funnel web spider
Ligand-gated		
Nicotinic ACh receptor		
α-Bungarotoxin	Irreversible antagonist	Marine snake
d-Tubocurarine	Competitive antagonist	Amazon plant
GABA$_A$ receptor		
Picrotoxin	Blocks channel	South Pacific plant
Bicuculline	Competitive antagonist	Plant
Glycine receptor		
Strychnine	Competitive antagonist	Indian plant
AMPA receptor		
Philanthotoxin	Blocks channel	Wasp

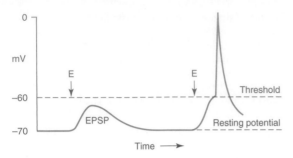

Figure 21–2. Excitatory synaptic potentials and spike generation. The figure shows a resting membrane potential of –70 mV in a postsynaptic cell. Stimulation of an excitatory pathway (*E*) generates transient depolarization. Increasing the stimulus strength (second *E*) increases the size of the depolarization, so that the threshold for spike generation is reached.

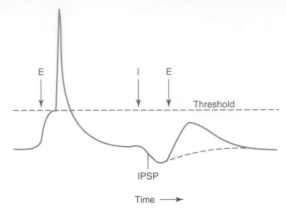

Figure 21–3. Interaction of excitatory and inhibitory synapses. On the left, a suprathreshold stimulus is given to an excitatory pathway (*E*). On the right, this same stimulus is given shortly after stimulating an inhibitory pathway (*I*), which prevents the excitatory potential from reaching threshold.

resting membrane potential of the neuron. Two types of pathways, excitatory and inhibitory, impinge on the motoneuron. When an excitatory pathway is stimulated, a small depolarization or excitatory postsynaptic potential (EPSP) is recorded. This potential is due to the excitatory transmitter acting on an ionotropic receptor, causing an increase in sodium and potassium permeability. The duration of these potentials is quite brief, usually less than 20 ms. Changing the stimulus intensity to the pathway and therefore the number of presynaptic fibers activated results in a graded change in the size of the depolarization. This indicates that the contribution a single fiber makes to the EPSP is quite small. When a sufficient number of excitatory fibers are activated, the EPSP depolarizes the postsynaptic cell to threshold, and an all-or-none action potential is generated.

When an inhibitory pathway is stimulated, the postsynaptic membrane is hyperpolarized, producing an inhibitory postsynaptic potential (IPSP) (Figure 21–3). A number of inhibitory synapses must be activated simultaneously to appreciably alter the membrane potential. This hyperpolarization is due to a selective increase in membrane permeability to chloride ions that flow into the cell during the IPSP. If an EPSP that under resting conditions would evoke an action potential in the postsynaptic cell (Figure 21–3) is elicited during an IPSP, it no longer evokes an action potential, because the IPSP has moved the membrane potential farther away from the threshold for action potential generation. A second type of inhibition is termed presynaptic inhibition. It was first described for sensory fibers entering the spinal cord, where excitatory synaptic terminals receive synapses called axoaxonic synapses (Figure 21–5B). When activated, axoaxonic synapses reduce the amount of transmitter released from the synapses of sensory fibers. Interestingly, presynaptic inhibitory receptors are present on virtually all presynaptic terminals in the brain even though axoaxonic synapses appear to be restricted to the spinal cord. In this case, transmitter spills over to neighboring synapses to activate those presynaptic receptors.

SITES OF DRUG ACTION

Virtually all of the drugs that act in the CNS produce their effects by modifying some step in chemical synaptic transmission. Figure 21–4 illustrates some of the steps that can be altered. These transmitter-dependent actions can be divided into presynaptic and postsynaptic categories.

Drugs acting on the synthesis, storage, metabolism, and release of neurotransmitters fall into the presynaptic category. Synaptic transmission can be depressed by blockade of transmitter synthesis or storage. For example, *p*-chlorophenylalanine blocks the synthesis of serotonin, and reserpine depletes the synapses of monoamines by interfering with intracellular storage. Blockade of transmitter catabolism can increase transmitter concentrations and has been reported to increase the amount of transmitter released per impulse. Drugs can also alter the release of transmitter. The stimulant amphetamine induces the release of catecholamines from adrenergic synapses. Capsaicin causes the release of the peptide substance P from sensory neurons, and tetanus toxin blocks the release of transmitters. After a

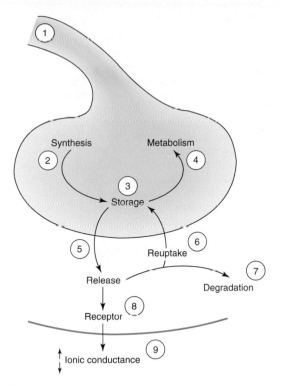

Figure 21–4. Sites of drug action. Schematic drawing of steps at which drugs can alter synaptic transmission. (*1*) Action potential in presynaptic fiber; (*2*) synthesis of transmitter; (*3*) storage; (*4*) metabolism; (*5*) release; (*6*) reuptake; (*7*) degradation; (*8*) receptor for the transmitter; (*9*) receptor-induced increase or decrease in ionic conductance.

transmitter has been released into the synaptic cleft, its action is terminated either by uptake or degradation. For most neurotransmitters, there are uptake mechanisms into the synaptic terminal and also into surrounding neuroglia. Cocaine, for example, blocks the uptake of catecholamines at adrenergic synapses and thus potentiates the action of these amines. However, acetylcholine is inactivated by enzymatic degradation. Anticholinesterases block the degradation of acetylcholine and thereby prolong its action. In contrast, no uptake mechanism has been found for any of the numerous CNS peptides, and it has yet to be demonstrated whether specific enzymatic degradation terminates the action of peptide transmitters.

In the postsynaptic region, the transmitter receptor provides the primary site of drug action. Drugs can act either as neurotransmitter agonists, such as the opioids, which mimic the action of enkephalin, or they can

block receptor function. Receptor antagonism is a common mechanism of action for CNS drugs. An example is strychnine's blockade of the receptor for the inhibitory transmitter glycine. This block, which underlies strychnine's convulsant action, illustrates how the blockade of inhibitory processes results in excitation. Drugs can also act directly on the ion channel of ionotropic receptors. For example, barbiturates can enter and block the channel of many excitatory ionotropic receptors. In the case of metabotropic receptors, drugs can act at any of the steps downstream of the receptor. Perhaps the best example is provided by the methylxanthines, which can modify neurotransmitter responses mediated through the second-messenger cAMP. At high concentrations, the methylxanthines elevate the level of cAMP by blocking its metabolism and thereby prolong its action in the postsynaptic cell.

The selectivity of CNS drug action is based almost entirely on the fact that different transmitters are used by different groups of neurons. Furthermore, these transmitters are often segregated into neuronal systems that subserve broadly different CNS functions. Without such segregation, it would be impossible to selectively modify CNS function even if one had a drug that operated on a single neurotransmitter system. It is not entirely clear why the CNS has relied on so many neurotransmitters and segregated them into different neuronal systems, since the primary function of a transmitter is either excitation or inhibition; this could be accomplished with two transmitter substances or perhaps even one. That such segregation does occur has provided neuroscientists with a powerful pharmacologic approach for analyzing CNS function and treating pathologic conditions.

IDENTIFICATION OF CENTRAL NEUROTRANSMITTERS

Since drug selectivity is based on the fact that different pathways utilize different transmitters, it is a primary goal of neuropharmacologists to identify the transmitters in CNS pathways. Establishing that a chemical substance is a transmitter has been far more difficult for central synapses than for peripheral synapses. In theory, to identify a transmitter it is sufficient to show that stimulation of a pathway releases enough of the substance to produce the postsynaptic response. In practice, this experiment cannot be done satisfactorily for at least two reasons. First, the anatomic complexity of the CNS prevents the selective activation of a single set of synaptic terminals. Second, available techniques for measuring the released transmitter and applying the transmitter are not sufficiently precise to satisfy the quantitative requirements. Therefore, the following criteria have been established for transmitter identification.

Localization

A number of approaches have been used to prove that a suspected transmitter resides in the presynaptic terminal of the pathway under study. These include biochemical analysis of regional concentrations of suspected transmitters, often combined with interruption of specific pathways, and microcytochemical techniques. Immunocytochemical techniques have proved very useful in localizing peptides and enzymes that synthesize or degrade nonpeptide transmitters.

Release

To determine whether the substance can be released from a particular region, local collection (in vivo) of the extracellular fluid can sometimes be accomplished. In addition, slices of brain tissue can be electrically or chemically stimulated in vitro and the released substances measured. To determine if the release is relevant to synaptic transmission, it is important to establish that the release is calcium-dependent. As mentioned above, anatomic complexity often prevents identification of the synaptic terminals responsible for the release, and the amount collected in the perfusate is a small fraction of the amount actually released.

Synaptic Mimicry

Finally, application of the suspected substance should produce a response that mimics the action of the transmitter released by nerve stimulation. Microiontophoresis, which permits highly localized drug administration, has been a valuable technique in assessing the action of suspected transmitters. In practice, this criterion has two parts: physiologic and pharmacologic identity. To establish physiologic identity of action, the substance must be shown to initiate the same change in ionic conductance in the postsynaptic cell as synaptically released transmitter. This requires intracellular recording and determination of the reversal potential and ionic dependencies of the responses. However, since different transmitters can elicit identical ionic conductance changes, this finding is not sufficient. Thus, selective pharmacologic antagonism is used to further establish that the suspected transmitter is acting in a manner identical to synaptically released transmitter. Because of the complexity of the CNS, specific pharmacologic antagonism of a synaptic response provides a particularly powerful technique for transmitter identification.

CELLULAR ORGANIZATION OF THE BRAIN

Most of the neuronal systems in the CNS can be divided into two broad categories: hierarchical systems and nonspecific or diffuse neuronal systems.

Hierarchical Systems

These systems include all of the pathways directly involved in sensory perception and motor control. The pathways are generally clearly delineated, being composed of large myelinated fibers that can often conduct action potentials at a rate in excess of 50 m/s. The information is typically phasic, and in sensory systems the information is processed sequentially by successive integrations at each relay nucleus on its way to the cortex. A lesion at any link will incapacitate the system. Within each nucleus and in the cortex, there are two types of cells: relay or projection neurons and local circuit neurons (Figure 21–5A). The projection neurons that form the interconnecting pathways transmit signals over long distances. The cell bodies are relatively large, and their axons emit collaterals that arborize extensively in the vicinity of the neuron. These neurons are excitatory, and their synaptic influences, which involve ionotropic receptors, are very short-lived. The excitatory transmitter released from these cells is, in most instances, glutamate. Local circuit neurons are typically smaller than projection neurons, and their axons arborize in the immediate vicinity of the cell body. The vast majority of these neurons are inhibitory, and they release either GABA or glycine. They synapse primarily on the cell body of the projection neurons but can also synapse on the dendrites of projection neurons as well as with each other. A special class of local circuit neurons in the spinal cord forms axoaxonic synapses on the terminals of sensory axons (Figure 21–5B). Two common types of pathways for these neurons (Figure 21–5A) include recurrent feedback pathways and feed-forward pathways. In some sensory pathways such as the retina and olfactory bulb, local circuit neurons may actually lack an axon and release neurotransmitter from dendritic synapses in a graded fashion in the absence of action potentials. Some pathways involving presynaptic dendrites of local circuit neurons are shown in Figure 21–5C.

Although there is a great variety of synaptic connections in these hierarchical systems, the fact that a limited number of transmitters are utilized by these neurons indicates that any major pharmacologic manipulation of this system will have a profound effect on the overall excitability of the CNS. For instance, selectively blocking GABA receptors with a drug such as picrotoxin results in generalized convulsions. Thus, while the mechanism of action of picrotoxin is quite specific in blocking the effects of GABA, the overall functional effect appears to be quite nonspecific, since GABA-mediated synaptic inhibition is so widely utilized in the brain.

Nonspecific or Diffuse Neuronal Systems

Neuronal systems that contain one of the monoamines—norepinephrine, dopamine, or 5-hydroxy-

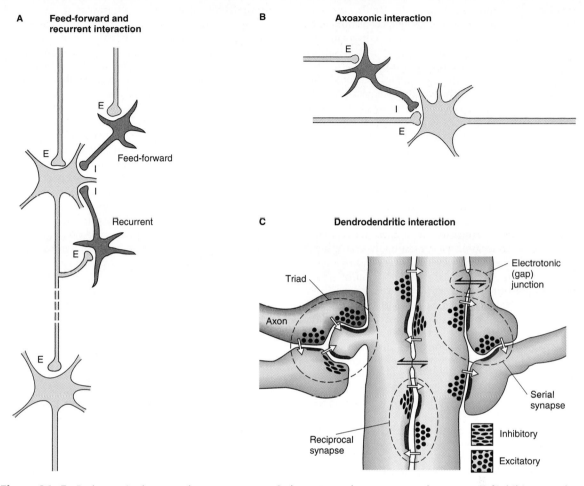

Figure 21–5. Pathways in the central nervous system. **A** shows two relay neurons and two types of inhibitory pathways, recurrent and feed-forward. The inhibitory neurons are shown in black. **B** shows the pathway responsible for presynaptic inhibition in which the axon of an inhibitory neuron synapses on the axon terminal of an excitatory fiber. **C:** Diagram illustrating that dendrites may be both pre- and postsynaptic to each other, forming reciprocal synapses, two of which are shown between the same dendrite pair. In triads, an axon synapses on two dendrites, and one of these dendrites synapses on the second. In serial synapses, a dendrite may be postsynaptic to one dendrite and presynaptic to another, thus connecting a series of dendrites. Dendrites also interact through low-resistance electrotonic ("gap") junctions (two of which are shown). Except for one axon, all structures shown in *C* are dendrites. (Reproduced, with permission, from Schmitt FO, Dev P, Smith BH: Electrotonic processing of information by brain cells. Science 1976;193:114. Copyright © 1976 by the American Association for the Advancement of Science.)

tryptamine (serotonin)—provide examples in this category. Certain other pathways emanating from the reticular formation and possibly some peptide-containing pathways also fall into this category. These systems differ in fundamental ways from the hierarchical systems, and the noradrenergic systems will serve to illustrate the differences.

Noradrenergic cell bodies are found primarily in a compact cell group called the locus ceruleus located in the caudal pontine central gray matter. The number of neurons in this cell group is quite small, approximately 1500 on each side of the brain in the rat. The axons of these neurons are very fine and unmyelinated. Indeed, they were entirely missed with classic anatomic techniques. It was not until the mid 1960s, when the formaldehyde fluorescence histochemical technique was applied to the study of CNS tissues, that the anatomy of the monoamine-containing systems was described. Because these axons are fine and unmyelinated, they conduct very slowly, at about 0.5 m/s. The axons branch repeatedly and are extraordinarily divergent. Branches from the same neuron can innervate several functionally different parts of the CNS. In the neocortex, these fibers have a tangential organization and therefore can monosynaptically influence large areas of cortex. The pattern of innervation in the cortex and nuclei of the hierarchical systems is diffuse, and the noradrenergic fibers form a very small percentage of the total number in the area. In addition, the axons are studded with periodic enlargements called varicosities that contain large numbers of vesicles. In some instances, these varicosities do not form synaptic contacts, suggesting that norepinephrine may be released in a rather diffuse manner, as occurs with the noradrenergic innervation of smooth muscle. This indicates that the cellular targets of these systems will be determined largely by the location of the receptors rather than the location of the release sites. Finally, most neurotransmitters utilized by diffuse neuronal systems, including norepinephrine, act—perhaps exclusively—on metabotropic receptors and therefore initiate long-lasting synaptic effects. Based on all of these observations, it is clear that the monoamine systems cannot be conveying specific topographic types of information—rather, vast areas of the CNS must be affected simultaneously and in a rather uniform way. It is not surprising, then, that these systems have been implicated in such global functions as sleeping and waking, attention, appetite, and emotional states.

CENTRAL NEUROTRANSMITTERS

A vast number of small molecules have been isolated from brain, and studies using a variety of approaches suggest that the agents listed in Table 21–2 are neurotransmitters. A brief summary of the evidence for some of these compounds follows.

Amino Acids

The amino acids of primary interest to the pharmacologist fall into two categories: the neutral amino acids **glycine** and **GABA** and the acidic amino acid **glutamate.** All of these compounds are present in high concentrations in the CNS and are extremely potent modifiers of neuronal excitability.

A. NEUTRAL AMINO ACIDS

The neutral amino acids are inhibitory and increase membrane permeability to chloride ions, thus mimick-

ing the IPSP. Glycine concentrations are particularly high in the gray matter of the spinal cord, and strychnine, which is a potent spinal cord convulsant and has been used in some rat poisons, selectively antagonizes both the action of glycine and the IPSPs recorded in spinal cord neurons. Thus, it is generally agreed that glycine is released from spinal cord inhibitory local circuit neurons involved in postsynaptic inhibition.

GABA receptors are divided into two types: $GABA_A$ and $GABA_B$. $GABA_A$ receptors open chloride channels and are antagonized by picrotoxin and bicuculline, which both cause generalized convulsions. $GABA_B$ receptors, which can be selectively activated by the antispastic drug baclofen, are coupled to G proteins that either inhibit calcium channels or activate potassium channels. In most regions of the brain, IPSPs have a fast and slow component mediated by $GABA_A$ and $GABA_B$ receptors, respectively. Immunohistochemical studies indicate that a large majority of the local circuit neurons synthesize GABA. A special class of local circuit neuron localized in the dorsal horn of the spinal cord also synthesizes GABA. These neurons form axoaxonic synapses with primary sensory nerve terminals and are responsible for presynaptic inhibition (Figure 21–5B).

B. ACIDIC AMINO ACIDS

Glutamate is present in very high concentrations in the CNS. Virtually all neurons that have been tested are strongly excited by this amino acid. This excitation is caused by the activation of both ionotropic and metabotropic receptors, which have been extensively characterized by molecular cloning. The ionotropic receptors can be further divided into three subtypes based on the action of the selective agonists: kainate (KA), α-amino-3-hydroxy-5-methylisoxazole-4-propionate (AMPA), and *N*-methyl-D-aspartate (NMDA). The AMPA- and KA-activated channels are permeable to sodium and potassium ions and, for certain subtypes, calcium as well. They are often grouped together and referred to as non-NMDA channels. The NMDA-activated channel is highly permeable to sodium, potassium, and calcium ions.

The metabotropic glutamate receptors act indirectly on ion channels via G proteins. They are selectively activated by *trans*-1-amino-cyclopentyl-1,3-dicarboxylate (ACPD). These G protein-coupled receptors are either positively coupled to (ie, stimulate) phospholipase C or negatively coupled to adenylyl cyclase. Depending on the type of synapse, metabotropic glutamate receptors can initiate a slow postsynaptic excitation or a presynaptic inhibition. Although the presence of metabotropic receptors at excitatory synapses varies, most excitatory synapses contain both NMDA receptors and non-NMDA receptors in the postsynaptic membrane.

The role of NMDA receptors has received consider-

Table 21–2. Summary of neurotransmitter pharmacology in the central nervous system.

Transmitter	Anatomy	Receptor Subtypes and Preferred Agonists	Receptor Antagonists	Mechanisms
Acetylcholine	Cell bodies at all levels; long and short connections	Muscarinic (M_1): muscarine, McN-A-343	Pirenzepine, atropine	Excitatory: $\downarrow$ in K^+ conductance; $\uparrow IP_3$, DAG
		Muscarinic (M_2): muscarine, bethanechol	Atropine, methoctramine	Inhibitory: $\uparrow K^+$ conductance; $\downarrow$ cAMP
	Motoneuron-Renshaw cell synapse	Nicotinic: nicotine	Dihydro-β-erythroidine, α-bungarotoxin	Excitatory: $\uparrow$ cation conductance
Dopamine	Cell bodies at all levels; short, medium, and long connections	D_1: SKF 38393	Phenothiazines, SCH 23390	Inhibitory (?): $\uparrow$ cAMP
		D_2: quinpirole, bromocriptine	Phenothiazines, butyrophenones	Inhibitory (presynaptic): $\downarrow Ca^{2+}$ Inhibitory (postsynaptic): $\uparrow$ in K^+ conductance, $\downarrow$ cAMP
GABA	Supraspinal interneurons involved in pre- and postsynaptic inhibition	$GABA_A$: muscimol	Bicuculline, picrotoxin	Inhibitory: $\uparrow Cl^-$ conductance
		$GABA_B$: baclofen	2-OH saclofen, CGP 35348, CGP55845	Inhibitory (presynaptic): $\downarrow Ca^{2+}$ conductance Inhibitory (postsynaptic): $\uparrow K^+$ conductance
Glutamate	Relay neurons at all levels and some interneurons	*N*-Methyl-D-aspartate (NMDA): NMDA	2-Amino-5-phosphonovalerate, CPP, MK-801	Excitatory: $\uparrow$ cation conductance, particularly Ca^{2+}
		AMPA: AMPA	CNQX, GYKI52466	Excitatory: $\uparrow$ cation conductance
		Kainate: kainate, domoic acid	CNQX	
		Metabotropic: ACPD, quisqualate	MCPG	Inhibitory (presynaptic): $\downarrow Ca^{2+}$ conductance; $\downarrow$ cAMP Excitatory: $\downarrow K^+$ conductance, $\uparrow IP_3$, DAG
Glycine	Spinal interneurons and some brain stem interneurons	Taurine, β-alanine	Strychnine	Inhibitory: $\uparrow Cl^-$ conductance

(continued)

Table 21–2. Summary of neurotransmitter pharmacology in the central nervous system (continued).

Transmitter	Anatomy	Receptor Subtypes and Preferred Agonists	Receptor Antagonists	Mechanisms
5-Hydroxytryptamine (serotonin)	Cell bodies in midbrain and pons project to all levels	5-HT$_{1A}$: LSD, 8-OH-DPAT	Metergoline, spiperone	Inhibitory: $\uparrow$ K$^+$ conductance, $\downarrow$ cAMP
		5-HT$_{2A}$: LSD, DOB	Ketanserin	Excitatory: $\downarrow$ K$^+$ conductance, $\uparrow$IP$_3$, DAG
		5-HT$_3$: 2-methyl-5-HT, phenylbiguanide	ICS 205930, ondansetron	Excitatory: $\uparrow$ cation conductance
		5-HT$_4$: BIMU8	GR 1138089	Excitatory: $\downarrow$ K$^+$ conductance
Norepinephrine	Cell bodies in pons and brain stem project to all levels	α_1: phenylephrine	Prazosin	Excitatory: $\downarrow$ K$^+$ conductance, $\uparrow$ IP$_3$, DAG
		α_2: clonidine	Yohimbine	Inhibitory (presynaptic): $\downarrow$ Ca^{2+} conductance Inhibitory: $\uparrow$ K$^+$ conductance, $\downarrow$ cAMP
		β_1: isoproterenol, dobutamine	Atenolol, practolol	Excitatory: $\downarrow$ K$^+$ conductance, $\uparrow$ cAMP
		β_2: salbutamol	Butoxamine	Inhibitory: may involve $\uparrow$ in electrogenic sodium pump; $\uparrow$ cAMP
Histamine	Cells in ventral posterior hypothalamus	H$_1$: 2(m-fluorophenyl)-histamine phenyl-histamine	Mepyramine	Excitatory: $\downarrow$ K$^+$ conductance, $\uparrow$ IP$_3$, DAG
		H$_2$: dimaprit	Ranitidine	Excitatory: $\downarrow$ K$^+$ conductance, $\uparrow$ cAMP
Opioid peptides	Cell bodies at all levels; long and short connections	Mu: bendorphin, DAMGO	Naloxone, CTOP	Inhibitory (presynaptic): $\downarrow$ Ca^{2+} conductance, $\downarrow$ cAMP
		Delta: enkephalin, DPDPE	Naloxone	Inhibitory (postsynaptic): $\uparrow$ K$^+$ conductance, $\downarrow$ cAMP
		Kappa: dynorphin, U-69593	Naloxone, nor-BNI	
Tachykinins	Primary sensory neurons, cell bodies at all levels; long and short connections	NK1: Substance P methylester	CP99994	Excitatory: $\downarrow$ K$^+$ conductance, $\uparrow$ IP$_3$, DAG
		NK2: β-[Ala^8] NKA$_{4-10}$	SR48968	
		NK3: GR138676	[Pro^7]NKB	

(continued)

Table 21–2. Summary of neurotransmitter pharmacology in the central nervous system *(continued)*.

Transmitter	Anatomy	Receptor Subtypes and Preferred Agonists	Receptor Antagonists	Mechanisms
Endocannabinoids (anandamide, 2-arachidonylglycerol	Widely distributed	CB1: WIN55212-2 methylester	SR141716	Inhibitory (presynaptic): ↓ Ca^{2+} conductance, ↓ cAMP

8-OH DPAT, 8-hydroxy-2(di-*n*-propylamino)tetralin; ACPD, *trans*-1-amino-cyclopentyl-1,3-dicarboxylate; AMPA, DL-α-amino-3-hydroxy-5-methylisoxazole-4-propionate; BIMU8, [endo-*N*-8-methyl-8-azabicyclo(3.2.1)oct-3-yl]-2,3-dihydro-3-isopropyl-2-oxo-1*H*-benzimidazol-1-carboxamide hydrochloride; CGP 35348, 3-aminopropyl(diethoxymethyl)phosphinic acid; CNQX, 6-cyano-7-nitroquinoxaline-2,3-dione; CP 99994, (+)-(2*S*, 3*S*)-3-(2-methoxybenzylamino)-2-phenylpiperidine; CPP, 3-(2-carboxypiperazin-4-yl)propyl-1-phosphonic acid; CTOP, D-Phe-Cys-Tyr-D-Trp-Orn-Thr-Pen-Thr-NH_2; DAG, diacylglycerol; DAMGO, D-ala-2,Me-Phe[1],Gly[1]-enkephalin; DOB, 5-bromo-2,5-dimethoxyamphetamine; DPDPE, D-pen[2]D-pen[5](-enkephalin); GR 113808, (1-{2-[(methylsulfonyl)amino]ethyl}-4-piperidinyl)methyl-1-methyl-1*H*-indole-3-carboxylate; GYKI 52466, 1-(4-aminophenyl)-4-methyl-7,8-methylenedioxy-5*H*-2,3-benzodiazepine; IP_3, inositol trisphosphate; MCPG, α-methyl-4-carboxyphenylglycine; MK-801, (dizocilpine), 10,11-dihydro-5-methyl-5*H*-dibenzo(a,d)cyclohepten-5,10-imine; NK1,2,3, neurokinin and derivatives; nor-BNI, nor-binaltorphimine; SR 141716, *N*-(piperidine-1yl)-5-(4-chlorophenyl)-1-(2,4-dichlorophenyl)-4-methyl-1*H*-pyrazole-3-carboxamide; SR 48968, (*S*)-*N*-methyl-*N*-(4-acetylamino-4-phenylpiperidino)-2-(3,4-dichlorophenyl)butylbenzamide; U-69593, (+)-(5α,7α,8β)-*N*-methyl-*N*-[7-(1-pyrrolidinyl)]-1-oxaspiro(4,5)dec-8-yl-benzenacetamide; WIN 55212-2, (*R*)-(+)-[2,3-dihydro-5-methyl-3-[(morpholino)methyl]pyrrolo-[1,2,3-*de*]-1,4-benzoxazin-6-yl] (1-naphthyl)methanone

able attention. These receptors play a critical role in synaptic plasticity, which is thought to underlie certain forms of learning and memory. They are selectively blocked by the dissociative anesthetic ketamine and the hallucinogenic drug phencyclidine. These drugs exert their effects by entering and blocking the open channel. Some drugs that block this receptor channel have potent antiepileptic activity in animal models, though these drugs have yet to be tested clinically. Considerable evidence exists that the release of glutamate during neuronal injury can, by activating the NMDA receptor, cause further cell injury and death. Thus, a particularly exciting finding is that blocking the NMDA receptor can attenuate the neuronal damage caused by anoxia in experimental animals. The potential therapeutic benefits of this action are considerable, although clinical trials to date have been disappointing.

C. ACETYLCHOLINE

Acetylcholine was the first compound to be identified pharmacologically as a transmitter in the CNS. Eccles showed in the early 1950s that excitation of Renshaw cells by motor axon collaterals was blocked by nicotinic antagonists. Furthermore, Renshaw cells were extremely sensitive to nicotinic agonists. These experiments were remarkable for two reasons. First, this early success at identifying a transmitter for a central synapse was followed by disappointment, because it remained the sole central synapse for which the transmitter was known until the late 1960s, when comparable data became available for the neutral amino acids. Second, the motor axon collateral synapse remains one of the best-documented examples of a cholinergic nicotinic synapse in the mammalian CNS, despite the rather widespread distribution of nicotinic receptors as defined by in situ hybridization studies. Most CNS responses to acetylcholine are mediated by a large family of G protein-coupled muscarinic receptors. At a few sites, acetylcholine causes slow inhibition of the neuron by activating the M_2 subtype of receptor, which opens potassium channels. A far more widespread muscarinic action in response to acetylcholine is a slow excitation that in some cases is mediated by M_1 receptors. These muscarinic effects are much slower than either nicotinic effects on Renshaw cells or the effect of amino acids. Furthermore, this muscarinic excitation is unusual in that acetylcholine produces it by *decreasing* the membrane permeability to potassium, ie, the opposite of conventional transmitter action.

A number of pathways contain acetylcholine, including neurons in the neostriatum, the medial septal nucleus, and the reticular formation. Cholinergic pathways appear to play an important role in cognitive functions, especially memory. Presenile dementia of the Alzheimer type is reportedly associated with a profound loss of cholinergic neurons. However, the specificity of this loss has been questioned since the levels of other putative transmitters, eg, somatostatin, are also decreased.

Monoamines

Monoamines include the catecholamines (dopamine and norepinephrine) and 5-hydroxytryptamine. Although these compounds are present in very small amounts in the CNS, they can be localized using extremely sensitive histochemical methods. These pathways are the site of action of many drugs; for example, the CNS stimulants cocaine and amphetamine are believed to act primarily at catecholamine synapses. Cocaine blocks the reuptake of dopamine and norepinephrine, while amphetamines cause presynaptic terminals to release these transmitters.

A. Dopamine

The major pathways containing dopamine are the projection linking the substantia nigra to the neostriatum and the projection linking the ventral tegmental region to limbic structures, particularly the limbic cortex. The therapeutic action of the antiparkinsonism drug levodopa is associated with the former area, whereas the therapeutic action of the antipsychotic drugs is thought to be associated with the latter area. Dopamine-containing neurons in the tuberobasal ventral hypothalamus play an important role in regulating hypothalamohypophysial function. A number of dopamine receptors have been identified, and they fall into two categories: D_1-like and D_2-like. All dopamine receptors are metabotropic. Dopamine generally exerts a slow inhibitory action on CNS neurons. This action has been best characterized on dopamine-containing substantia nigra neurons, where D_2 receptor activation opens potassium channels.

B. Norepinephrine

This system has already been discussed. Most noradrenergic neurons are located in the locus ceruleus or the lateral tegmental area of the reticular formation. Although the density of fibers innervating various sites differs considerably, most regions of the central nervous system receive diffuse noradrenergic input. All noradrenergic receptor subtypes are metabotropic. When applied to neurons, norepinephrine can hyperpolarize them by increasing potassium conductance. This effect is mediated by α_2 receptors and has been characterized most thoroughly on locus ceruleus neurons. In many regions of the CNS, norepinephrine actually enhances excitatory inputs by both indirect and direct mechanisms. The indirect mechanism involves disinhibition, ie, inhibitory local circuit neurons are inhibited. The direct mechanism is blockade of potassium conductances that slow neuronal discharge. Depending on the type of neuron, this effect is mediated by either α_1 or β receptors. Facilitation of excitatory synaptic transmission is in accordance with many of the behavioral processes thought to involve noradrenergic pathways, eg, attention and arousal.

C. 5-Hydroxytryptamine

Most 5-hydroxytryptamine (5-HT, serotonin) pathways originate from neurons in the raphe or midline regions of the pons and upper brain stem. 5-HT is contained in unmyelinated fibers that diffusely innervate most regions of the CNS, but the density of the innervation varies. 5-HT acts on more than a dozen receptor subtypes. Except for the $5-HT_3$ receptor, all of these receptors are metabotropic. The ionotropic $5-HT_3$ receptor exerts a rapid excitatory action at a very limited number of sites in the CNS. In most areas of the central nervous system, 5-HT has a strong inhibitory action. This action is mediated by $5-HT_{1A}$ receptors and is associated with membrane hyperpolarization caused by an increase in potassium conductance. It has been found that $5-HT_{1A}$ receptors and $GABA_B$ receptors share the same potassium channels. Some cell types are slowly excited by 5-HT owing to its blockade of potassium channels via $5-HT_2$ or $5-HT_4$ receptors. Both excitatory and inhibitory actions can occur on the same neurons. It has often been speculated that 5-HT pathways may be involved in the hallucinations induced by LSD, since this compound can antagonize the peripheral actions of 5-HT. However, LSD does not appear to be a 5-HT antagonist in the central nervous system, and typical LSD-induced behavior is still seen in animals after raphe nuclei are destroyed. Other proposed regulatory functions of 5-HT-containing neurons include sleep, temperature, appetite, and neuroendocrine control.

Peptides

A great many CNS peptides have been discovered that produce dramatic effects both on animal behavior and on the activity of individual neurons. Many of the peptides have been mapped with immunohistochemical techniques and include opioid peptides (enkephalins, endorphins, etc), neurotensin, substance P, somatostatin, cholecystokinin, vasoactive intestinal polypeptide, neuropeptide Y, and thyrotropin-releasing hormone. As in the peripheral autonomic nervous system, peptides often coexist with a conventional nonpeptide transmitter in the same neuron. A good example of the approaches used to define the role of these peptides in the central nervous system comes from studies on substance P and its association with sensory fibers. Substance P is contained in and released from small unmyelinated primary sensory neurons of the spinal cord and brain stem and causes a slow EPSP in target neurons. These sensory fibers are known to transmit noxious stimuli, and it is therefore surprising that—while substance P receptor antagonists can modify responses to certain types of pain—they do not block the response. Glutamate, which is released with substance P from these synapses, presumably plays an important role in transmitting pain stimuli. Substance P is certainly involved in many other functions, since it is found in many areas of the central nervous system that are unrelated to pain pathways.

Many of these peptides are also found in peripheral structures, including peripheral synapses. They are described in Chapters 6 and 17.

Nitric Oxide

The CNS contains a substantial amount of nitric oxide synthase (NOS), which is found within certain classes of neurons. This neuronal NOS is an enzyme activated by calcium-calmodulin, and activation of NMDA receptors, which increases intracellular calcium, results in the generation of nitric oxide. While a physiologic role for nitric oxide has been clearly established for vascular smooth muscle, its role in synaptic transmission and synaptic plasticity remains controversial.

Endocannabinoids

The primary psychoactive ingredient in cannabis, Δ^9-tetrahydrocannabinol (Δ^9-THC), affects the brain mainly by activating a specific cannabinoid receptor, CB1. CB1 is expressed at high levels in many brain regions, and several endogenous brain lipids, including anandamide and 2-arachidonylglycerol, have been identified as CB1 ligands. These ligands are not stored, as are classic neurotransmitters, but instead are rapidly synthesized by neurons in response to depolarization and consequent calcium influx. In further contradistinction to classic neurotransmitters, endogenous cannabinoids can function as retrograde synaptic messengers: they are released from postsynaptic neurons and travel backward across synapses, activating CB1 receptors on presynaptic neurons and suppressing transmitter release. Cannabinoids may affect memory, cognition, and pain perception by this mechanism.

REFERENCES

Bettler B, Kaupmann K, Bowery N: GABA$_B$ receptors: Drugs meet clones. Curr Opin Neurobiol 1998;8:345.

Bettler B, Mulle C: Review: Neurotransmitter receptors 11. AMPA and kainate receptors. Neuropharmacology 1995;34:123.

Betz H: Structure and function of inhibitory glycine receptors. Q Rev Biophys 1992;25:381.

Bliss TVP, Collingridge GL: A synaptic model of memory: Long-term potentiation in the hippocampus. Nature 1993;361:31.

Bourne HR, Nicoll R: Molecular machines integrate coincident synaptic signals. Cell 1993;72(Suppl):65.

Catterall WA: From ionic currents to molecular mechanisms: the structure and function of voltage-gated sodium channels. Neuron 2000;26:13.

Catterall WA: Structure and function of voltage-gated ion channels. Trends Neurosci 1993;16:500.

Catterall WA: Structure and regulation of voltage-gated Ca^{2+} channels. Annu Rev Cell Dev Biol 2000;16:521.

Conn PJ, Pin JP: Pharmacology and functions of metabotropic glutamate receptors. Annu Rev Pharmacol Toxicol 1997;37:205.

Costa E: From GABA$_A$ receptor diversity emerges a unified vision of GABAergic inhibition. Annu Rev Pharmacol Toxicol 1998;38:321.

Dingledine R et al: The glutamate receptor ion channels. Pharmacol Rev 1999;51:7.

Eccles JC: In: *The Physiology of Synapses.* Springer, 1964.

Hall ZW: In: *An Introduction to Molecular Neurobiology.* Sinauer, 1992.

Hille B: *Ionic Channels of Excitable Membranes.* 3rd ed. Sinauer, 2001.

Hokfelt T et al: Neuropeptides—an overview. Neuropharmacology 2000;39:1337.

Jahn R, Südhof TC: Membrane fusion and exocytosis. Annu Rev Biochem 1999;68:863.

Laube B et al: Modulation of glycine receptor function: a novel approach for therapeutic intervention at inhibitory synapses? Trends Pharmacol Sci 2002;23:519.

Linden DJ: Long-term synaptic depression in the mammalian brain. Neuron 1994;12:457.

Liu Y et al: Membrane trafficking of neurotransmitter transporters in the regulation of synaptic transmission. Trends Cell Biol 1999;9:356.

Llinas RR: The intrinsic electrophysiological properties of mammalian neurons: Insights into central nervous system function. Science 1988;242:1654.

Macdonald RL, Olsen, RW: GABA$_A$ receptor channels. Annu Rev Neurosci 1994;17:569.

Malenka RC, Nicoll RA: Long-term potentiation—A decade of progress? Science 1999;285:1870.

Martin GR et al: The structure and signaling properties of 5-HT receptors: An endless diversity? Trends Pharmacol Sci 1998;19:2.

McIntosh JM, Olivera BM, Cruz LJ: *Conus* peptides as probes for ion channels. Methods Enzymol 1999; 294:605.

Miller RJ: Presynaptic receptors. Annu Rev Pharmacol Toxicol 1998;38:201.

Missale C et al: Dopamine receptors: From structure to function. Physiol Rev 1998;78:189.

Nakanishi S: Metabotropic glutamate receptors: Synaptic transmission, modulation, and plasticity. Neuron 1994;13:1031.

Nakanishi S: Molecular diversity of glutamate receptors and implications for brain function. Science 1992;258:597.

Nestler EJ, Hyman SE, Malenka RC: *Molecular Neuropharmacology.* McGraw-Hill, 2001.

Nicoll RA: The coupling of neurotransmitter receptors to ion channels in the brain. Science 1988;241:545.

North RA: Molecular physiology of P2X receptors. Physiol Rev 2002;82:1013.

Seal RP, Amara SG: Excitatory amino acid transporters: A family in flux. Annu Rev Pharmacol Toxicol 1999;39: 431.

Seeburg PH: The TiNS/TiPS Lecture. The molecular biology of mammalian glutamate receptor channels. Trends Neurosci 1993;16:359.

Südhof TC: The synaptic vesicle cycle: A cascade of protein-protein interactions. Nature 1995;375:645.

Walmsley B, Alvarez FJ, Fyffe RE: Diversity of structure and function at mammalian central synapses. Trends Neurosci 1998;21:81.

Wilson RI, Nicoll RA: Endocannabinoid signaling in the brain. Science 2002;296:678.

Sedative-Hypnotic Drugs

22

Anthony J. Trevor, PhD, & Walter L. Way, MD

Assignment of a drug to the sedative-hypnotic class indicates that its major therapeutic use is to cause sedation (with concomitant relief of anxiety) or to encourage sleep. Because there is considerable chemical variation within this group, this drug classification is based on clinical uses rather than on similarities in chemical structure. Anxiety states and sleep disorders are common problems, and sedative-hypnotics are among the most widely prescribed drugs worldwide.

I. BASIC PHARMACOLOGY OF SEDATIVE-HYPNOTICS

An effective **sedative** (anxiolytic) agent should reduce anxiety and exert a calming effect. The degree of central nervous system depression caused by a sedative should be the minimum consistent with therapeutic efficacy. A **hypnotic** drug should produce drowsiness and encourage the onset and maintenance of a state of sleep. Hypnotic effects involve more pronounced depression of the central nervous system than sedation, and this can be achieved with most drugs in this class simply by increasing the dose. Graded dose-dependent depression of central nervous system function is a characteristic of sedative-hypnotics. However, individual drugs differ in the relationship between the dose and the degree of central nervous system depression. Two examples of such dose-response relationships are shown in Figure 22–1. The linear slope for drug A is typical of many of the older sedative-hypnotics, including the barbiturates and alcohols. With such drugs, an increase in dose above that needed for hypnosis may lead to a state of general anesthesia. At still higher doses, sedative-hypnotics may depress respiratory and vasomotor centers in the medulla, leading to coma and death. Deviations from a linear dose-response relationship, as shown for drug B,

will require proportionately greater dosage increments in order to achieve central nervous system depression more profound than hypnosis. This appears to be the case for benzodiazepines and certain newer hypnotics; the greater margin of safety this offers is an important reason for their widespread use to treat anxiety states and sleep disorders.

CHEMICAL CLASSIFICATION

The benzodiazepines (Figure 22–2) are the most widely used sedative-hypnotics. All of the structures shown are 1,4-benzodiazepines, and most contain a carboxamide group in the 7-membered heterocyclic ring structure. A substituent in the 7 position, such as a halogen or a nitro group, is required for sedative-hypnotic activity. The structures of triazolam and alprazolam include the addition of a triazole ring at the 1,2-position, and such drugs are sometimes referred to as triazolobenzodiazepines.

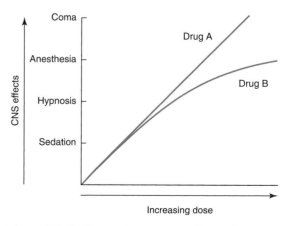

Figure 22–1. Dose-response curves for two hypothetical sedative-hypnotics.

351

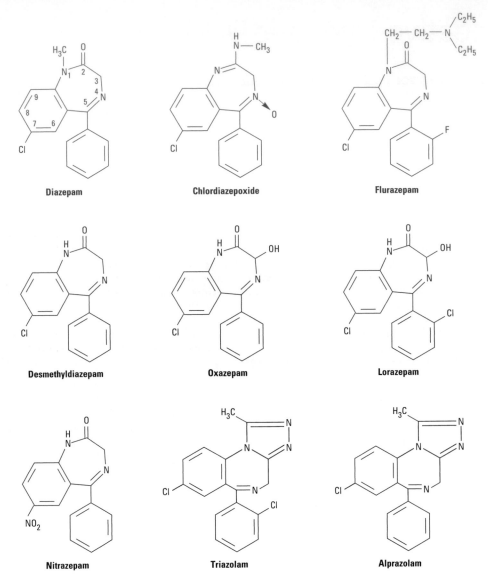

Figure 22–2. Chemical structures of benzodiazepines.

The chemical structures of some older and less commonly used sedative-hypnotics, including several barbiturates, are shown in Figure 22–3. Glutethimide (a piperidinedione) and meprobamate (a carbamate) are of distinctive chemical structure but are practically equivalent to barbiturates in their pharmacologic effects, and their clinical use is rapidly declining. The sedative-hypnotic class also includes compounds of simple chemical structure, including ethanol (see Chapter 23), chloral hydrate, trichloroethanol, and paraldehyde (not shown).

Several drugs with novel chemical structures have been introduced recently. Buspirone is an anxiolytic agent that has actions different from those of conventional sedative-hypnotic drugs. Zolpidem and zaleplon, while structurally unrelated to benzodiazepines, share a similar mechanism of action.

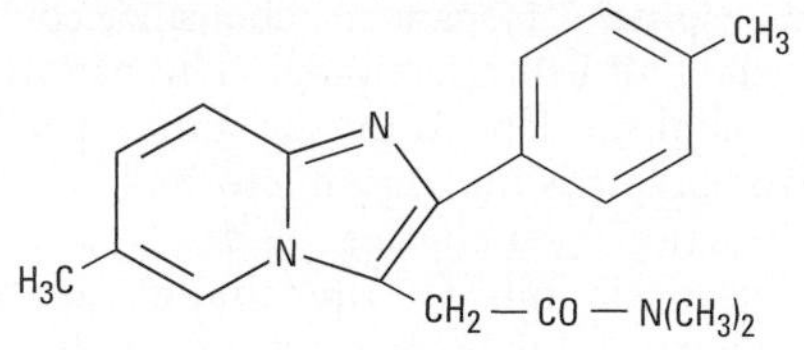

Zolpidem

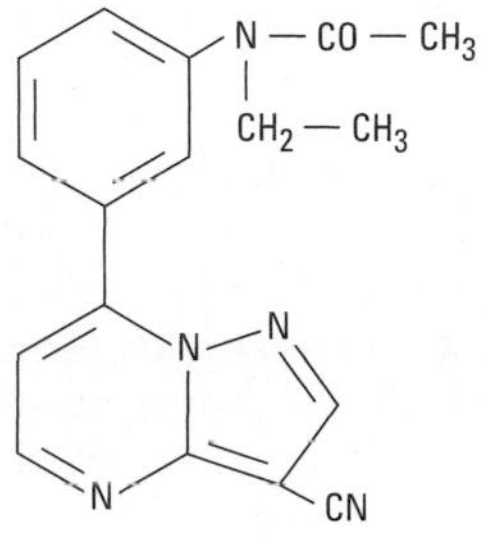

Zaleplon

Other classes of drugs not included in Figure 22–3 that may exert sedative effects include most antipsychotic and many antidepressant drugs and certain antihistaminic agents (eg, hydroxyzine, promethazine). As discussed in other chapters, these agents differ from conventional sedative-hypnotics in both their effects and their major therapeutic uses. Since they commonly exert marked effects on the peripheral autonomic nervous system, they are sometimes referred to as "**sedative-autonomic**" drugs. Certain antihistaminics with sedative effects are available in over-the-counter sleep aids. Their autonomic properties and their long durations of action can result in adverse effects.

THE BENZODIAZEPINES & BARBITURATES

Pharmacokinetics

A. ABSORPTION AND DISTRIBUTION

The rates of oral absorption of benzodiazepines differ depending on a number of factors, including lipophilicity. Oral absorption of triazolam is extremely rapid, and that of diazepam and the active metabolite of clorazepate is more rapid than other commonly used benzodiazepines. Clorazepate is converted to its active form, desmethyldiazepam (nordiazepam), by acid hydrolysis in the stomach. Oxazepam, lorazepam, and temazepam are absorbed from the gut at slower rates than other benzodiazepines. The bioavailability of several benzodiazepines, including chlordiazepoxide and diazepam, may be unreliable after intramuscular injection. Most of the barbiturates and other older sedative-hypnotics are absorbed rapidly into the blood following their oral administration.

Lipid solubility plays a major role in determining the rate at which a particular sedative-hypnotic enters the central nervous system. For example, diazepam and triazolam are more lipid-soluble than chlordiazepoxide

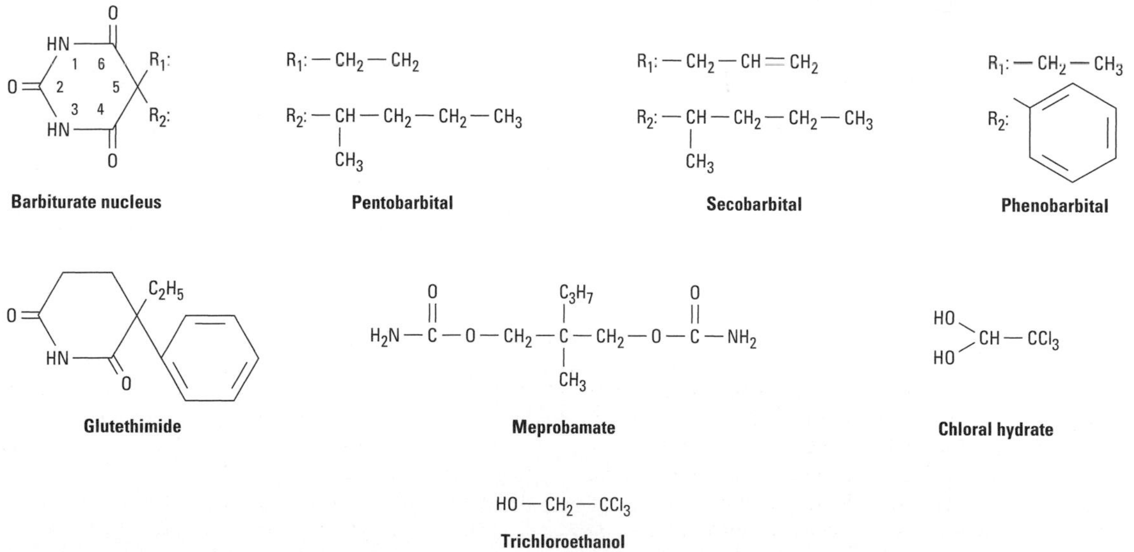

Barbiturate nucleus

Pentobarbital

Secobarbital

Phenobarbital

Glutethimide

Meprobamate

Chloral hydrate

Trichloroethanol

Figure 22–3. Chemical structures of barbiturates and other sedative-hypnotics.

and lorazepam; thus, the central nervous system actions of the former drugs are more rapid in onset. The thiobarbiturates (eg, thiopental), in which the oxygen on C_2 is replaced by sulfur, are very lipid-soluble, and a high rate of entry into the central nervous system contributes to the rapid onset of their central effects (see Chapter 25). In contrast, phenobarbital and meprobamate have quite low lipid solubility and penetrate the brain slowly.

All sedative-hypnotics cross the placental barrier during pregnancy. If sedative-hypnotics are given in the predelivery period, they may contribute to the depression of neonatal vital functions. Sedative-hypnotics are detectable in breast milk and may exert depressant effects in the nursing infant.

Although sedative-hypnotic drugs, including benzodiazepines, bind to plasma proteins, few clinically significant interactions involving these drugs appear to be based on such protein binding. One exception is chloral hydrate, which transiently increases the anticoagulant effects of warfarin by displacement of the anticoagulant drug from such binding sites.

B. Biotransformation

Metabolic transformation to more water-soluble metabolites is necessary for clearance of sedative-hypnotics from the body. The microsomal drug-metabolizing enzyme systems of the liver are most important in this regard. Few sedative-hypnotics are excreted from the body in unchanged form, so elimination half-life depends mainly on the rate of metabolic transformation.

1. Benzodiazepines—Hepatic metabolism accounts for the clearance of all benzodiazepines. The patterns and rates of metabolism depend on the individual drugs. Most benzodiazepines undergo microsomal oxidation (phase I reactions), including *N*-dealkylation and aliphatic hydroxylation. The metabolites are subsequently conjugated (phase II reactions) to form glucuronides that are excreted in the urine. However, many phase I metabolites of benzodiazepines are pharmacologically active, with long half-lives.

As shown in Figure 22–4, desmethyldiazepam, which has an elimination half-life of more than 40 hours, is an active metabolite of chlordiazepoxide, diazepam, prazepam, and clorazepate. Desmethyldiazepam in turn is biotransformed to the active compound, oxazepam. Other active metabolites of chlordiazepoxide include desmethylchlordiazepoxide and demoxepam. While diazepam is metabolized mainly to desmethyldiazepam, it is also converted to temazepam (not shown in Figure 22–4), which is further metabolized in part to oxazepam. Flurazepam, which is used mainly for hypnosis, is oxidized by hepatic enzymes to three active metabolites, desalkylflurazepam, hydroxyethylflurazepam, and flurazepam aldehyde (not shown), which have elimination half-lives ranging from 30 to 100 hours. Alprazolam and triazolam undergo α-hydroxylation, and the resulting metabolites appear to exert short-lived pharmacologic effects since they are rapidly conjugated to form inactive glucuronides.

The formation of active metabolites has complicated

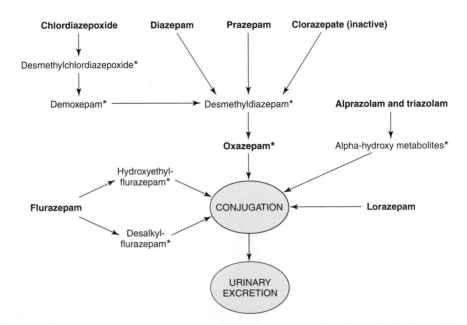

Figure 22–4. Biotransformation of benzodiazepines. (Boldface, drugs available for clinical use; *, active metabolite.)

studies on the pharmacokinetics of the benzodiazepines in humans because the elimination half-life of the parent drug may have little relationship to the time course of pharmacologic effects. Those benzodiazepines for which the parent drug or active metabolites have long half-lives are more likely to cause cumulative effects with multiple doses. Cumulative and residual effects such as excessive drowsiness appear to be less of a problem with such drugs as estazolam, oxazepam, and lorazepam, which have shorter half-lives and are metabolized directly to inactive glucuronides. Some pharmacokinetic properties of selected benzodiazepines are listed in Table 22–1.

2. Barbiturates—With the exception of phenobarbital, only insignificant quantities of the barbiturates are excreted unchanged. The major metabolic pathways involve oxidation by hepatic enzymes of chemical groups attached to C_5, which are different for the individual barbiturates. The alcohols, acids, and ketones formed appear in the urine as glucuronide conjugates. With very few exceptions, the metabolites of the barbiturates lack pharmacologic activity. The overall rate of hepatic metabolism in humans depends on the individual drug but (with the exception of the thiobarbiturates) is usually slow. The elimination half-lives of secobarbital

and pentobarbital range from 18 to 48 hours in different individuals. The elimination half-life of phenobarbital in humans is 4–5 days. Multiple dosing with these agents can lead to cumulative effects.

C. EXCRETION

The water-soluble metabolites of benzodiazepines and other sedative-hypnotics are excreted mainly via the kidney. In most cases, changes in renal function do not have a marked effect on the elimination of parent drugs. Phenobarbital is excreted unchanged in the urine to a certain extent (20–30% in humans), and its elimination rate can be increased significantly by alkalinization of the urine. This is partly due to increased ionization at alkaline pH, since phenobarbital is a weak acid with a pK_a of 7.4. Only trace amounts of the benzodiazepines appear in the urine unchanged.

D. FACTORS AFFECTING BIODISPOSITION

The biodisposition of sedative-hypnotics can be influenced by several factors, particularly alterations in hepatic function resulting from disease or drug-induced increases or decreases in microsomal enzyme activities (see Chapter 4).

Table 22–1. Pharmacokinetic properties of benzodiazepines in humans.

Drug	Peak Blood Level (hours)	Elimination Half-Life[1] (hours)	Comments
Alprazolam	1–2	12–15	Rapid oral absorption
Chlordiazepoxide	2–4	15–40	Active metabolites; erratic bioavailability from IM injection
Clorazepate	1–2 (nordiazepam)	50–100	Prodrug; hydrolyzed to active form in stomach
Diazepam	1–2	20–80	Active metabolites; erratic bioavailability from IM injection
Estazolam	2	10–24	No active metabolites
Flurazepam	1–2	40–100	Active metabolites with long half-lives
Lorazepam	1–6	10–20	No active metabolites
Oxazepam	2–4	10–20	No active metabolites
Prazepam	1–2	50–100	Active metabolites with long half-lives
Quazepam	2	30–100	Active metabolites with long half-lives
Temazepam	2–3	10–40	Slow oral absorption
Triazolam	1	2–3	Rapid onset; short duration of action

[1]Includes half-lives of major metabolites.

In very old patients and in patients with severe liver disease, the elimination half-lives of these drugs are often increased significantly. In such cases, multiple normal doses of these sedative-hypnotics often result in excessive central nervous system effects.

The activity of hepatic microsomal drug-metabolizing enzymes may be increased in patients exposed to certain older sedative-hypnotics on a chronic basis (enzyme induction; see Chapter 4). Barbiturates (especially phenobarbital) and meprobamate are most likely to cause this effect, which may result in an increase in their hepatic metabolism as well as that of other drugs. Increased biotransformation of other pharmacologic agents as a result of enzyme induction by barbiturates is a potential mechanism underlying drug interactions (Appendix II). In contrast, the benzodiazepines do not change hepatic drug-metabolizing enzyme activity with continuous use.

Pharmacodynamics of Benzodiazepines & Barbiturates

A. MOLECULAR PHARMACOLOGY OF THE GABA$_A$ RECEPTOR

The benzodiazepines, the barbiturates, zolpidem, and many other drugs bind to molecular components of the GABA$_A$ receptor present in neuronal membranes in the central nervous system. This receptor, which functions as a chloride ion channel, is activated by the inhibitory neurotransmitter GABA (see Chapter 21).

The GABA$_A$ receptor has a pentameric structure assembled from five subunits (each with four transmembrane-spanning domains) selected from multiple polypeptide classes (α, β, γ, δ, ε, π, ρ, etc). Different subunits of several of these classes have been characterized, eg, six different α, four β, and three γ. A major isoform of the GABA$_A$ receptor found in many regions of the brain consists of two α_1 and two β_2 subunits and one γ_2 subunit. In this receptor isoform, the binding site for GABA is located between an α_1 and a β_2 subunit and the binding pocket for benzodiazepines (a benzodiazepine receptor subtype, BZ$_1$ or ω_1) is between an α_1 and the γ_2 subunit. However, GABA$_A$ receptors in different areas of the central nervous system consist of various combinations of the essential subunits, and the benzodiazepines bind to many of these, including receptor isoforms containing α_2, α_3, and α_5 subunits. Barbiturates also bind to multiple isoforms of the GABA$_A$ receptor but at different sites from those with which benzodiazepines interact. In contrast to benzodiazepines, zolpidem and zaleplon bind more selectively since these drugs only interact with GABA$_A$ receptor isoforms that contain α_1 subunits (BZ$_1$ subtype). The heterogeneity of GABA$_A$ receptors may constitute the molecular basis for the varied pharmacologic actions of benzodiazepines and related drugs (see Box, GABA Receptor Heterogeneity & Pharmacologic Selectivity).

A model of the hypothetical GABA-BZ receptor-chloride ion channel macromolecular complex is shown in Figure 22–5.

B. NEUROPHARMACOLOGY

Gamma-aminobutyric acid (GABA) is the major inhibitory neurotransmitter in the central nervous system. Electrophysiologic studies have shown that benzodiazepines potentiate GABAergic inhibition at all levels

---

GABA RECEPTOR HETEROGENEITY & PHARMACOLOGIC SELECTIVITY

Studies involving genetically engineered mice have demonstrated that the specific pharmacologic actions elicited by benzodiazepines and other drugs that modulate GABA actions are influenced by the composition of the subunits assembled to form the GABA$_A$ receptor. Benzodiazepines only interact with brain GABA$_A$ receptors in which the α subunits (1,2,3, and 5) have a conserved histidine residue in the N-terminal domain. Strains of mice in which a point mutation has been inserted ("knock-in" strategy), converting histidine to arginine in the α_1 subunit, show resistance to both the sedative and amnestic effects of benzodiazepines, but anxiolytic and muscle relaxing effects are largely unchanged. These animals are also unresponsive to the hypnotic actions of zolpidem and zaleplon, drugs that bind selectively to GABA$_A$ receptors containing α_1 subunits. In contrast, mice with selective histidine-arginine mutations in the α_2 subunit of GABA$_A$ receptors show selective resistance to the antianxiety effects of benzodiazepines. Based on studies of this type it has been suggested that α_1 subunits in GABA$_A$ receptors mediate sedation, amnesia and possibly antiseizure effects of benzodiazepines, while α_2 subunits are involved in their anxiolytic and muscle-relaxing actions. Other transgenic studies have led to suggestions that an α_5 subtype is involved in at least some of the memory impairment caused by benzodiazepines. It should be noted that these studies involving genetic manipulations of the GABA$_A$ receptor utilize rodent models of the anxiolytic and amnestic actions of drugs.

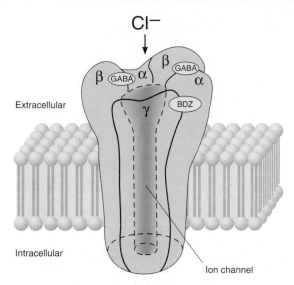

Cl^-

Extracellular

β   β
 GABA α   GABA
              α
        γ   BDZ

Intracellular

Ion channel

Figure 22–5. A model of the $GABA_A$ receptor-chloride ion channel macromolecular complex (many others could be proposed). A heteroligomeric glycoprotein, the complex consists of five or more membrane-spanning subunits. Multiple forms of α, β, and γ subunits are arranged in different pentameric combinations so that $GABA_A$ receptors exhibit molecular heterogeneity. GABA appears to interact with α or β subunits triggering chloride channel opening with resultant membrane hyperpolarization. Binding of benzodiazepines to γ subunits or to an area of the α unit influenced by the γ unit facilitates the process of channel opening but does not directly initiate chloride current. (Modified and reproduced, with permission, from Zorumsky CF, Isenberg KE: Insights into the structure and function of GABA-benzodiazepine receptors: Ion channels and psychiatry. Am J Psychiatry 1991;148:162.)

of the neuraxis, including the spinal cord, hypothalamus, hippocampus, substantia nigra, cerebellar cortex, and cerebral cortex. Benzodiazepines appear to increase the efficiency of GABAergic synaptic inhibition. The benzodiazepines do not substitute for GABA but appear to enhance GABA's effects without directly activating GABA receptors or opening the associated chloride channels. The enhancement in chloride ion conductance induced by the interaction of benzodiazepines with GABA takes the form of an increase in the *frequency* of channel-opening events

Barbiturates also facilitate the actions of GABA at multiple sites in the central nervous system, but—in contrast to benzodiazepines—they appear to increase the *duration* of the GABA-gated chloride channel openings.

At high concentrations, the barbiturates may also be GABA-mimetic, directly activating chloride channels. These effects involve a binding site or sites distinct from the benzodiazepine binding sites. Barbiturates are less selective in their actions than benzodiazepines, since they also depress the actions of excitatory neurotransmitters (eg, glutamic acid) and exert nonsynaptic membrane effects in parallel with their effects on GABA neurotransmission. This multiplicity of sites of action of barbiturates may be the basis for their ability to induce full surgical anesthesia (see Chapter 25) and for their more pronounced central depressant effects (which result in their low margin of safety) compared to benzodiazepines.

C. BENZODIAZEPINE RECEPTOR LIGANDS

The components of the $GABA_A$ receptor-chloride ion channel macromolecule that function as benzodiazepine receptors exhibit heterogeneity and include BZ_1 (ω_1) and BZ_2 (ω_2) subtypes (see Box, The Versatility of the Chloride Channel GABA Receptor Complex). Three types of ligand-benzodiazepine receptor interactions have been reported: (1) **Agonists** facilitate GABA actions, and this occurs at multiple BZ receptor sites in the case of the benzodiazepines. The nonbenzodiazepines zolpidem and zaleplon are selective agonists at the BZ_1 (ω_1) receptor subtype. Endogenous agonist ligands for the BZ receptors have been proposed, since benzodiazepine-like chemicals have been isolated from brain tissue of animals never exposed to these drugs. Nonbenzodiazepine molecules that have affinity for benzodiazepine receptors have also been detected in human brain. Such "endozepines" facilitate GABA-mediated chloride channel gating in cultured neurons. (2) **Antagonists** are typified by the synthetic benzodiazepine derivative flumazenil, which blocks the actions of benzodiazepines and zolpidem but does not antagonize the actions of barbiturates, meprobamate, or ethanol. Certain endogenous compounds, eg, diazepam-binding inhibitor (DBI), are also capable of blocking the interaction of benzodiazepines with benzodiazepine receptors. (3) **Inverse agonists** act as negative allosteric modulators of GABA receptor function. Their interaction with benzodiazepine receptors can produce anxiety and seizures, an action that has been demonstrated for several compounds, especially the β-carbolines, eg, *n*-butyl-β-carboline-3-carboxylate (β-CCB). In addition to their direct actions, these molecules can block the effects of benzodiazepines.

The physiologic significance of endogenous modulators of the functions of GABA in the central nervous system remains unclear. To date it has not been established that the putative endogenous ligands of BZ receptors play a role in the control of states of anxiety, sleep patterns, or any other characteristic behavioral expression of central nervous system function.

THE VERSATILITY OF THE CHLORIDE CHANNEL GABA RECEPTOR COMPLEX

The GABA$_A$-chloride channel macromolecular complex is one of the most versatile drug-responsive machines in the body. In addition to the benzodiazepines, barbiturates and zolpidem, many other drugs with central nervous system effects can modify the function of this important ionotropic receptor. These include alcohol, alphaxolone (a steroid anesthetic), etomidate and propofol (intravenous anesthetics), volatile anesthetics (eg, halothane), several anticonvulsants (eg, gabapentin, vigabatrin), and

ivermectin (an anthelmintic agent). Most of these agents facilitate or mimic the action of GABA. (It must be noted that it has not been shown that these drugs act exclusively or even primarily by this mechanism.) Central nervous system excitatory agents that act on the chloride channel include picrotoxin and bicuculline. These convulsant drugs block the channel directly (picrotoxin) or interfere with GABA binding (bicuculline).

D. ORGAN LEVEL EFFECTS

1. Sedation—Benzodiazepines, barbiturates, and most older sedative-hypnotic drugs exert calming effects with concomitant reduction of anxiety at relatively low doses. In most cases, however, the anxiolytic actions of sedative-hypnotics are accompanied by some decremental effects on psychomotor and cognitive functions. In experimental animal models, sedative-hypnotic drugs are able to disinhibit punishment-suppressed behavior. This disinhibition has been equated with antianxiety effects of sedative-hypnotics, and it is not a characteristic of all drugs that have sedative effects, eg, the tricyclic antidepressants and antihistamines. However, the disinhibition of previously suppressed behavior may be more related to behavioral disinhibitory effects of sedative-hypnotics, including euphoria, impaired judgment, and loss of self-control, which can occur at dosages in the range of those used for management of anxiety. The benzodiazepines also exert dose-dependent anterograde amnesic effects (inability to remember events occurring during the drug's duration of action).

2. Hypnosis—By definition, all of the sedative-hypnotics will induce sleep if high enough doses are given. The effects of sedative-hypnotics on the stages of sleep depend on several factors, including the specific drug, the dose, and the frequency of its administration. The effects of benzodiazepines and older sedative-hypnotics on patterns of normal sleep are as follows: (1) the latency of sleep onset is decreased (time to fall asleep); (2) the duration of stage 2 NREM sleep is increased; (3) the duration of REM sleep is decreased; and (4) the duration of stage 4 NREM slow-wave sleep is decreased. Zolpidem also decreases REM sleep but has minimal effect on slow-wave sleep. Zaleplon decreases the latency of sleep onset with little effect on total sleep time, NREM, or REM sleep.

More rapid onset of sleep and prolongation of stage 2 are presumably clinically useful effects. However, the

significance of sedative-hypnotic drug effects on REM and slow-wave sleep is not clear. Deliberate interruption of REM sleep causes anxiety and irritability followed by a rebound increase in REM sleep at the end of the experiment. A similar pattern of "REM rebound" can be detected following abrupt cessation of drug treatment with sedative-hypnotics, especially when drugs with short durations of action are used at high doses. Despite possible reductions in slow-wave sleep, there are no reports of disturbances in the secretion of pituitary or adrenal hormones when either barbiturates or benzodiazepines are used as hypnotics. The use of sedative-hypnotics for more than 1–2 weeks leads to some tolerance to their effects on sleep patterns.

3. Anesthesia—As shown in Figure 22–1, certain sedative-hypnotics in high doses will depress the central nervous system to the point known as stage III of general anesthesia (see Chapter 25). However, the suitability of a particular agent as an adjunct in anesthesia depends mainly on the physicochemical properties that determine its rapidity of onset and duration of effect. Among the barbiturates, thiopental and methohexital are very lipid-soluble, penetrating brain tissue rapidly following intravenous administration, a characteristic favoring their use for induction of the anesthetic state. Rapid tissue redistribution accounts for the short duration of action of these drugs, a feature useful in recovery from anesthesia.

Benzodiazepines—including diazepam, lorazepam, and midazolam—are used intravenously in anesthesia (see Chapter 25), often in combination with other agents. Not surprisingly, benzodiazepines given in large doses as adjuncts to general anesthetics may contribute to a persistent postanesthetic respiratory depression. This is probably related to their relatively long half-lives and the formation of active metabolites.

4. Anticonvulsant effects—Most of the sedative-hypnotics are capable of inhibiting the development and spread of epileptiform activity in the central nervous system. Some selectivity exists in that some members of the group can exert anticonvulsant effects without marked central nervous system depression (although psychomotor function may be impaired). Several benzodiazepines—including clonazepam, nitrazepam, lorazepam, and diazepam—are sufficiently selective to be clinically useful in the management of seizure states (see Chapter 24). Of the barbiturates, phenobarbital and metharbital (converted to phenobarbital in the body) are effective in the treatment of generalized tonic-clonic seizures.

5. Muscle relaxation—Some sedative-hypnotics, particularly members of the carbamate and benzodiazepine groups, exert inhibitory effects on polysynaptic reflexes and internuncial transmission and at high doses may also depress transmission at the skeletal neuromuscular junction. Somewhat selective actions of this type that lead to muscle relaxation can be readily demonstrated in animals and have led to claims of usefulness for relaxing contracted voluntary muscle in joint disease or muscle spasm (see Clinical Pharmacology).

6. Effects on respiration and cardiovascular function—At hypnotic doses in healthy patients, the effects of sedative-hypnotics on respiration are comparable to changes during natural sleep. However, even at therapeutic doses, sedative-hypnotics can produce significant respiratory depression in patients with pulmonary disease. Effects on respiration are dose-related, and depression of the medullary respiratory center is the usual cause of death due to overdose of sedative-hypnotics.

At doses up to those causing hypnosis, no significant effects on the cardiovascular system are observed in healthy patients. However, in hypovolemic states, heart failure, and other diseases that impair cardiovascular function, normal doses of sedative-hypnotics may cause cardiovascular depression, probably as a result of actions on the medullary vasomotor centers. At toxic doses, myocardial contractility and vascular tone may both be depressed by central and peripheral effects, leading to circulatory collapse. Respiratory and cardiovascular effects are more marked when sedative-hypnotics are given intravenously.

Tolerance; Psychologic & Physiologic Dependence

Tolerance—decreased responsiveness to a drug following repeated exposure—is a common feature of sedative-hypnotic use. It may result in an increase in the dose needed to maintain symptomatic improvement or to promote sleep. It is important to recognize that partial cross-tolerance occurs between the sedative-hypnotics described here and also with ethanol (Chapter 23)—a feature of some clinical importance, as explained below. The mechanisms responsible for tolerance to sedative-hypnotics are not well understood. An increase in the rate of drug metabolism (metabolic tolerance) may be partly responsible in the case of chronic administration of barbiturates, but changes in responsiveness of the central nervous system (pharmacodynamic tolerance) are of greater importance for most sedative-hypnotics. In the case of benzodiazepines, the development of tolerance in animals is associated with down-regulation of brain benzodiazepine receptors.

The perceived desirable properties of relief of anxiety, euphoria, disinhibition, and promotion of sleep have led to the compulsive misuse of virtually all sedative-hypnotics. For this reason, most sedative-hypnotic drugs are classified as Schedule III or Schedule IV drugs for prescribing purposes. (See Chapter 32 for a detailed discussion.) The consequences of abuse of these agents can be defined in both psychologic and physiologic terms. The psychologic component may initially parallel simple neurotic behavior patterns difficult to differentiate from those of the inveterate coffee drinker or cigarette smoker. When the pattern of sedative-hypnotic use becomes compulsive, more serious complications develop, including physiologic dependence and tolerance.

Physiologic dependence can be described as an altered physiologic state that requires continuous drug administration to prevent the appearance of an abstinence or withdrawal syndrome. In the case of sedative-hypnotics, this syndrome is characterized by states of increased anxiety, insomnia, and central nervous system excitability that may progress to convulsions. Most sedative-hypnotics—including benzodiazepines—are capable of causing physiologic dependence when used on a chronic basis. However, the severity of withdrawal symptoms differs between individual drugs and depends also on the magnitude of the dose used immediately prior to cessation of use. When higher doses of sedative-hypnotics are used, abrupt withdrawal leads to more serious withdrawal signs. Differences in the severity of withdrawal symptoms between individual sedative-hypnotics relate in part to half-life, since drugs with long half-lives are eliminated slowly enough to accomplish gradual withdrawal with few physical symptoms. The use of drugs with very short half-lives for hypnotic effects may lead to signs of withdrawal even between doses. For example, triazolam, a benzodiazepine with a half-life of about 4 hours, has been reported to cause daytime anxiety when used to treat sleep disorders.

BENZODIAZEPINE ANTAGONISTS: FLUMAZENIL

Flumazenil is one of several 1,4-benzodiazepine derivatives with high affinity for the benzodiazepine receptor that act as competitive antagonists. It is the only benzodiazepine receptor antagonist available for clinical use at present. It blocks many of the actions of benzodiazepines (and imidazopyridines) but does not antagonize the central nervous system effects of other sedative-hypnotics, ethanol, opioids, or general anesthetics. Flumazenil is approved for use in reversing the central nervous system depressant effects of benzodiazepine overdose and to hasten recovery following use of these drugs in anesthetic and diagnostic procedures. While the drug reverses the sedative effects of benzodiazepines, antagonism of benzodiazepine-induced respiratory depression is less predictable. When given intravenously, flumazenil acts rapidly but has a short half-life (0.7–1.3 hours) due to rapid hepatic clearance. Since all benzodiazepines have a longer duration of action than flumazenil, sedation commonly recurs, requiring repeated administration of the antagonist.

Adverse effects of flumazenil include agitation, confusion, dizziness, and nausea. Flumazenil may cause a severe precipitated abstinence syndrome in patients who have developed physiologic benzodiazepine dependence. In patients who have ingested benzodiazepines with tricyclic antidepressants, seizures and cardiac arrhythmias may occur following flumazenil administration. Transient improvement in mental status has been reported with flumazenil when used in patients with hepatic encephalopathy.

NEWER DRUGS FOR ANXIETY & SLEEP DISORDERS

Although the benzodiazepines continue to be widely used in the treatment of anxiety states and for insomnia, their adverse effects include daytime sedation and drowsiness, synergistic depression of the central nervous system with other drugs (especially alcohol), and the possibility of psychologic and physiologic dependence with repeated use. Anxiolytic drugs that act through non-GABAergic systems might have a reduced propensity for such actions. Several nonbenzodiazepines, including buspirone, have such characteristics. In addition, the newer hypnotics zolpidem and zaleplon are more selective in their central actions even though they appear to act through benzodiazepine receptors.

Buspirone

Buspirone has selective anxiolytic effects, and its pharmacologic characteristics are quite different from those of other drugs described in this chapter. Buspirone relieves anxiety without causing marked sedative or euphoric effects. Unlike benzodiazepines, the drug has no hypnotic, anticonvulsant, or muscle relaxant properties. Buspirone does not interact directly with GABA-ergic systems. It may exert its anxiolytic effects by acting as a partial agonist at brain $5-HT_{1A}$ receptors, but it also has affinity for brain dopamine D_2 receptors. Buspirone-treated patients show no rebound anxiety or withdrawal signs on abrupt discontinuance. The drug is not effective in blocking the acute withdrawal syndrome resulting from abrupt cessation of use of benzodiazepines or other sedative-hypnotics. Buspirone has minimal abuse liability. In marked contrast to the benzodiazepines, the anxiolytic effects of buspirone may take more than a week to become established, making the drug unsuitable for management of acute anxiety states. The drug is used in generalized anxiety states but is not very effective in panic disorders.

Buspirone is rapidly absorbed orally but undergoes extensive first-pass metabolism via hydroxylation and dealkylation reactions to form several active metabolites. The major metabolite is 1-(2-pyrimidyl)-piperazine (1-PP), which has α_2-adrenoceptor-blocking actions and which enters the central nervous system to reach higher levels than the parent drug. It is not known what role (if any) 1-PP plays in the central actions of buspirone. The elimination half-life of buspirone is 2–4 hours, and liver dysfunction may decrease its clearance. Rifampin, an inducer of cytochrome P450, decreases the half-life of buspirone; inhibitors of CYP3A4 (eg, erythromycin, ketoconazole) increase plasma levels of buspirone.

Buspirone causes less psychomotor impairment than diazepam and does not affect driving skills. The drug does not potentiate the central nervous system depressant effects of conventional sedative-hypnotic drugs, ethanol, or tricyclic antidepressants, and elderly patients do not appear to be more sensitive to its actions. Tachycardia, palpitations, nervousness, gastrointestinal distress, and paresthesias may occur more frequently than with benzodiazepines. Buspirone also causes a dose-dependent pupillary constriction. Blood pressure may be elevated in patients receiving MAO inhibitors. A number of buspirone analogs have been developed (eg, **ipsapirone, gepirone, tandospirone**) and are under study.

Zolpidem

Zolpidem, an imidazopyridine derivative structurally unrelated to benzodiazepines, has hypnotic actions. The drug binds selectively to the BZ_1 (ω_1) subtype of benzodiazepine receptors that contain α_1 subunits and facilitates GABA-mediated neuronal inhibition. Like the benzodiazepines, the actions of zolpidem are antagonized by flumazenil. Unlike benzodiazepines, zolpidem has minimal muscle relaxing and anticonvulsant effects. However, amnestic effects have been reported with use of doses greater than recommended. The drug has a rapid onset of action, and its duration of hypnotic action is close to that of triazolam. Zolpidem causes minor effects on sleep patterns at the recommended hypnotic dose but can suppress REM sleep at higher doses. Rebound insomnia may occur on abrupt discontinuance of higher doses. Respiratory depression occurs if large doses of zolpidem are ingested with other CNS depressants, including ethanol.

The risk of development of tolerance and dependence with extended use of zolpidem appears to be less than with the use of hypnotic benzodiazepines. Zolpidem is rapidly metabolized to inactive metabolites by the liver via oxidation and hydroxylation. The elimination half-life of the drug is 1.5–3.5 hours, with clearance decreased in elderly patients. Dosage reductions are recommended in patients with hepatic dysfunction, in elderly patients, and in patients taking cimetidine. Rifampin, an inducer of hepatic cytochrome P450, decreases the half-life of zolpidem.

Zaleplon

Zaleplon binds selectively to the BZ_1 receptor subtype, facilitating the inhibitory actions of GABA. Zaleplon is rapidly absorbed from the gastrointestinal tract and has an elimination half-life of about 1 hour. The drug is metabolized to inactive metabolites mainly by hepatic aldehyde oxidase and partly by the cytochrome P450 isoform CYP3A4. Dosage should be reduced in patients with hepatic impairment and in the elderly. Metabolism of zaleplon is inhibited by cimetidine; drugs that induce hepatic CYP3A4 increase the clearance of zaleplon.

Zaleplon decreases sleep latency but has little effect on total sleep time or on sleep architecture. Rapid onset and short duration of action are favorable properties for those patients who have difficulty falling asleep. Amnestic effects and next-day impairment of psychomotor performance may occur, but less commonly than in the case of hypnotic benzodiazepines or zolpidem. The risk of development of tolerance and of withdrawal symptoms indicative of physiologic dependence appears to be low, but the use of high doses (twice the recommended dose) has caused rebound insomnia. Zaleplon potentiates the CNS depressant effects of ethanol and other sedative-hypnotics.

OLDER SEDATIVE-HYPNOTICS

These drugs include alcohols (**ethchlorvynol, chloral hydrate**), piperidinediones (**glutethimide, methyprylon**), and carbamates (**meprobamate**). They are rarely used in therapy, though the low cost of chloral hydrate makes it attractive for institutional use. Little is known about their molecular mechanisms of action. Most of these drugs are biotransformed to more water-soluble compounds by hepatic enzymes. Trichloroethanol is the pharmacologically active metabolite of chloral hydrate and has a half-life of 6–10 hours. However, its toxic metabolite, trichloroacetic acid, is cleared very slowly and can accumulate with the nightly administration of chloral hydrate.

II. CLINICAL PHARMACOLOGY OF SEDATIVE-HYPNOTICS

TREATMENT OF ANXIETY STATES

The psychologic, behavioral, and physiologic responses that characterize anxiety can take many forms. Typically, the psychic awareness of anxiety is accompanied by enhanced vigilance, motor tension, and autonomic hyperactivity. Before prescribing sedative-hypnotics, one should analyze the patient's symptoms carefully. Anxiety is in many cases secondary to organic disease states—acute myocardial infarction, angina pectoris, gastrointestinal ulcers, etc—which themselves require specific therapy. Another class of secondary anxiety states (situational anxiety) results from circumstances that may have to be dealt with only once or a few times, including anticipation of frightening medical or dental procedures and family illness or other tragedy. Even though situational anxiety tends to be self-limiting, the short-term use of sedative-hypnotics may be appropriate for the treatment of this and certain disease-associated anxiety states. Similarly, the use of a sedative-hypnotic as premedication prior to surgery or some unpleasant medical procedure is rational and proper (Table 22–2). If the patient presents with chronic anxiety as the primary complaint, it may be appropriate to review the diagnostic criteria set forth in the *Diagnostic & Statistical Manual of Mental Disorders (DSM IV)* to determine whether the diagnosis is correct and if treatment should

Table 22–2. Clinical uses of sedative-hypnotics.

For relief of anxiety
For insomnia
For sedation and amnesia before medical and surgical procedures
For treatment of epilepsy and seizure states
As a component of balanced anesthesia (intravenous administration)
For control of ethanol or other sedative-hypnotic withdrawal states
For muscle relaxation in specific neuromuscular disorders
As diagnostic aids or for treatment in psychiatry

include drug therapy. For example, excessive or unreasonable anxiety about life circumstances (generalized anxiety disorder), panic disorders, and agoraphobia are amenable to drug therapy, usually in conjunction with psychotherapy. In many cases, anxiety is a symptom of psychiatric problems that may warrant the use of antidepressant or antipsychotic drugs.

The benzodiazepines continue to be widely used for the management of anxiety states. Since anxiety symptoms may be relieved by many benzodiazepines, it is not always easy to demonstrate the superiority of one drug over another. However, alprazolam is particularly effective in the treatment of panic disorders and agoraphobia and is more selective in this regard than other benzodiazepines. The choice of benzodiazepines for anxiety is based on several sound pharmacologic principles: (1) a relatively high therapeutic index (see drug B in Figure 22–1), plus availability of flumazenil for treatment of overdose; (2) a low risk of drug interactions based on liver enzyme induction; (3) slow elimination rates, which may favor persistence of useful CNS effects.

Disadvantages of the benzodiazepines include the risk of psychologic dependence, the formation of active metabolites, amnestic effects, and their cost. In addition, the benzodiazepines exert additive central nervous system depression when administered with other drugs, including ethanol. The patient should be warned of this possibility to avoid impairment of performance of any task requiring mental alertness and motor coordination. Many of the disadvantages of benzodiazepines are not shared by buspirone, which appears to be a more selective drug. However, limitations of buspirone include the slow onset of its anxiolytic actions—confining its use to generalized anxiety—and its limited efficacy in anxiety states that feature panic attacks and phobic characteristics. In the treatment of generalized anxiety disorders and certain phobias, newer antidepressants such as paroxetine and venlafaxine are now considered by many authorities to be drugs of first choice (see Chapter 30). However, these agents have minimal effectiveness in acute anxiety states.

Sedative-hypnotics should be used with appropriate caution so as to minimize adverse effects. A dose should be prescribed that does not impair mentation or motor functions during waking hours. Some patients may tolerate the drug better if most of the daily dose is given at bedtime, with smaller doses during the day. Prescriptions should be written for short periods, since there is little justification for long-term therapy. The physician should make an effort to assess the efficacy of therapy from the patient's subjective responses. Combinations of antianxiety agents should be avoided, and people taking sedatives should be cautioned about the consumption of alcohol and the concurrent use of over-the-counter medications containing antihistaminic or anticholinergic drugs (see Chapter 64).

Phenobarbital, meprobamate, and sedative-autonomic drugs are used occasionally as antianxiety agents. The antihistaminics (diphenhydramine, hydroxyzine, promethazine) continue to be used presurgically for their sedative and muscarinic receptor blocking actions.

Beta-blocking drugs (eg, propranolol) may be used as antianxiety agents in situations such as performance anxiety. The sympathetic nervous system overactivity associated with anxiety appears to be satisfactorily relieved by the β blockers, and a slight improvement in the nonsomatic components of anxiety may also occur. Adverse central nervous system effects of propranolol include lethargy, vivid dreams, and hallucinations.

TREATMENT OF SLEEP PROBLEMS

Nonpharmacologic therapies that are sometimes useful for sleep problems include proper diet and exercise, avoiding stimulants before retiring, ensuring a comfortable sleeping environment, and retiring at a regular time each night. In some cases, however, the patient will need and should be given a sedative-hypnotic for a limited period. It should be noted that the abrupt discontinuance of most drugs in this class can lead to rebound insomnia.

Benzodiazepines can cause a dose-dependent decrease in both REM and slow wave sleep, though to a lesser extent than the barbiturates. Zolpidem and zaleplon are less likely than the benzodiazepines to change sleep patterns. However, so little is known about the clinical impact of these effects that statements about the desirability of a particular drug based on its effects on sleep architecture have more theoretical than practical significance. Clinical criteria of efficacy in alleviating a particular sleeping problem are more useful. The drug selected should be one that provides sleep of fairly rapid onset (decreased sleep latency) and sufficient duration, with minimal "hangover" effects such as drowsiness, dysphoria, and mental or motor depression the following day. Older drugs such as chloral hydrate, secobarbital, and pentobarbital continue to be used, but benzodiazepines, zolpidem, or zaleplon are generally preferred. Daytime sedation is more common with benzodiazepines that have slow elimination rates (eg, lorazepam) and those that are biotransformed to active metabolites (eg, flurazepam, quazepam). If hypnotics are used nightly, tolerance can occur, which may lead to dose increases by the patient to produce the desired effect.

Anterograde amnesia occurs to some degree with all hypnotic benzodiazepines. Zaleplon and zolpidem have efficacies similar to those of the hypnotic benzodiazepines in the management of sleep disorders. Favorable clinical features of zolpidem include modest day-after psychomotor depression with few amnestic effects.

Zolpidem is currently the most frequently prescribed hypnotic drug in the United States. Zaleplon acts rapidly, and because of its short half-life the drug appears to have value in the management of patients who awaken early in the sleep cycle. At recommended doses, zaleplon appears to cause less amnesia or day-after somnolence than zolpidem or benzodiazepines. The drugs commonly used for sedation and hypnosis are listed in Table 22–3 together with recommended doses. *Note:* Long-term use of hypnotics is irrational and dangerous medical practice.

OTHER THERAPEUTIC USES

Table 22–2 summarizes several other important clinical uses of drugs in the sedative-hypnotic class. Drugs used in the management of seizure disorders and as intravenous agents in anesthesia are discussed in Chapters 24 and 25.

For sedative and possible amnestic effects during medical or surgical procedures such as endoscopy and bronchoscopy—as well as for premedication prior to anesthesia—oral formulations of shorter-acting drugs are preferred.

Long-acting drugs such as chlordiazepoxide and diazepam and, to a lesser extent, phenobarbital are administered in progressively decreasing doses to patients during withdrawal from physiologic dependence on ethanol or other sedative-hypnotics.

Meprobamate and, more recently, the benzodiazepines have frequently been used as central muscle relaxants, though evidence for general efficacy without accompanying sedation is lacking. A possible exception is diazepam, which has useful relaxant effects in skeletal muscle spasticity of central origin (see Chapter 27).

Psychiatric uses of benzodiazepines other than treatment of anxiety states include the initial management of mania, the control of drug-induced hyperexcitability states (eg, phencyclidine intoxication), and possibly the treatment of major depressive disorders with alprazolam. Sedative-hypnotics are also used occasionally as diagnostic aids in neurology and psychiatry.

CLINICAL TOXICOLOGY OF SEDATIVE-HYPNOTICS

Direct Toxic Actions

Many of the common adverse effects of drugs in this class are those resulting from dose-related depression of central nervous system functions. Relatively low doses may lead to drowsiness, impaired judgment, and diminished motor skills, sometimes with a significant impact on driving ability, job performance, and personal relationships. Benzodiazepines may cause a significant dose-related anterograde amnesia; they can significantly impair ability to learn new information, particularly that involving effortful cognitive processes, while leaving the retrieval of previously learned information intact. This effect is utilized to clinical advantage in uncomfortable procedures, eg, endoscopy, since the appropriate dose leaves the patient able to cooperate during the procedure but amnesic regarding it afterward. The criminal use of benzodiazepines in cases of

Table 22–3. Dosages of drugs used commonly for sedation and hypnosis.

Sedation		Hypnosis	
Drug	**Dosage**	**Drug**	**Dosage (at Bedtime)**
Alprazolam (Xanax)	0.25–0.5 mg 2–3 times daily	Chloral hydrate	500–1000 mg
Buspirone (BuSpar)	5–10 mg 2–3 times daily	Estazolam (ProSom)	0.5–2 mg
Chlordiazepoxide (Librium)	10–20 mg 2–3 times daily	Flurazepam (Dalmane)	15–30 mg
Clorazepate (Tranxene)	5–7.5 mg twice daily	Lorazepam (Ativan)	2–4 mg
Diazepam (Valium)	5 mg twice daily	Quazepam (Doral)	7.5–15 mg
Halazepam (Paxipam)	20–40 mg 3–4 times daily	Secobarbital	100–200 mg
Lorazepam (Ativan)	1–2 mg once or twice daily	Temazepam (Restoril)	7.5–30 mg
Oxazepam (Serax)	15–30 mg 3–4 times daily	Triazolam (Halcion)	0.125–0.5 mg
Phenobarbital	15–30 mg 2–3 times daily	Zaleplon (Sonata)	5–20 mg
Prazepam (Centrax)	10–20 mg 2–3 times daily	Zolpidem (Ambien)	5–10 mg

"date rape" is based on their dose-dependent amnestic effects. Hangover effects are not uncommon following use of hypnotic drugs with long elimination half-lives. Because elderly patients are more sensitive to the effects of sedative-hypnotics, doses approximately half of those used in younger adults are safer and usually as effective. The most common reversible cause of confusional states in the elderly is overuse of sedative-hypnotics. At higher doses, toxicity may present as lethargy or a state of exhaustion or, alternatively, in the form of gross symptoms equivalent to those of ethanol intoxication. The titration of useful therapeutic effects against such unwanted effects is usually more difficult with sedative-hypnotics that exhibit steep dose-response relationships of the type shown in Figure 22–1 (drug A), including the barbiturates, chloral hydrate, and piperidinediones. The physician should be aware of variability among patients in terms of doses causing adverse effects. An increased sensitivity to sedative-hypnotics is more common in patients with cardiovascular disease, respiratory disease, or hepatic impairment and in older patients. Sedative-hypnotics can exacerbate breathing problems in patients with chronic pulmonary disease and in those with symptomatic sleep apnea.

Sedative-hypnotics are the drugs most frequently involved in deliberate overdoses, in part because of their general availability as very commonly prescribed pharmacologic agents. The benzodiazepines are considered to be "safer" drugs in this respect, since they have flatter dose-response curves. Epidemiologic studies on the incidence of drug-related deaths support this general assumption—eg, 0.3 deaths per million tablets of diazepam prescribed versus 11.6 deaths per million capsules of secobarbital in one study. Of course, many factors other than the specific sedative-hypnotic could influence such data—particularly the presence of other central nervous system depressants, including ethanol. In fact, most serious cases of drug overdosage, intentional or accidental, do involve polypharmacy; and when combinations of agents are taken, the practical safety of benzodiazepines may be less than the foregoing would imply.

The lethal dose of any sedative-hypnotic varies with the patient and the circumstances (see Chapter 59). If discovery of the ingestion is made early and a conservative treatment regimen is started, the outcome is rarely fatal, even following very high doses. On the other hand, for most sedative-hypnotics—with the exception of benzodiazepines—a dose as low as ten times the hypnotic dose may be fatal if the patient is not discovered or does not seek help in time. With severe toxicity, the respiratory depression from central actions of the drug may be complicated by aspiration of gastric contents in the unattended patient—an even more likely occurrence if ethanol is present. Loss of brain stem vasomotor con-

trol, together with direct myocardial depression, further complicates successful resuscitation. In such patients, treatment consists of ensuring a patent airway, with mechanical ventilation if needed, and maintenance of plasma volume, renal output, and cardiac function. Use of a positive inotropic drug such as dopamine, which preserves renal blood flow, is sometimes indicated. Hemodialysis or hemoperfusion may be used to hasten elimination of some of these drugs.

Flumazenil reverses the sedative actions of benzodiazepines. However, its duration of action is short and its antagonism of respiratory depression unpredictable. Therefore, the use of flumazenil in benzodiazepine overdose *must* be accompanied by adequate monitoring and support of respiratory function.

The extensive clinical use of triazolam has led to reports of serious central nervous system effects including behavioral disinhibition, delirium, aggression, and violence. While behavioral disinhibition may occur with sedative-hypnotic drugs, it does not appear to be more prevalent with triazolam than with other benzodiazepines. Disinhibitory reactions during benzodiazepine treatment are more clearly associated with the use of very high doses and the pretreatment level of patient hostility.

Adverse effects of the sedative-hypnotics that are not referable to their CNS actions occur infrequently. Hypersensitivity reactions, including skin rashes, occur only occasionally with most drugs of this class. Reports of teratogenicity leading to fetal deformation following use of piperidinediones and certain benzodiazepines justify caution in the use of these drugs during pregnancy. Because barbiturates enhance porphyrin synthesis, they are *absolutely contraindicated* in patients with a history of acute intermittent porphyria, variegate porphyria, hereditary coproporphyria, or symptomatic porphyria.

Alterations in Drug Response

Depending on the dosage and the duration of use, tolerance occurs in varying degrees to many of the pharmacologic effects of sedative-hypnotics. However, it should not be assumed that the degree of tolerance achieved is identical for all pharmacologic effects. There is evidence that the lethal dose range is not altered significantly by the chronic use of sedative-hypnotics. Cross-tolerance between the different sedative-hypnotics, including ethanol, can lead to an unsatisfactory therapeutic response when standard doses of a drug are used in a patient with a recent history of excessive use of these agents. However, there have been few reports of tolerance development when zolpidem or zaleplon was used for less than 4 weeks.

With the chronic use of sedative-hypnotics, especially if doses are increased, a state of physiologic dependence can occur. This may develop to a degree unparalleled by any other drug group, *including the opioids.* Withdrawal from a sedative-hypnotic can have severe and life-threatening manifestations. Withdrawal symptoms range from restlessness, anxiety, weakness, and orthostatic hypotension to hyperactive reflexes and generalized seizures. The severity of withdrawal symptoms depends to a large extent on the dosage range used immediately prior to discontinuance but also on the particular drug. Symptoms of withdrawal are usually more severe following discontinuance of sedative-hypnotics with shorter half-lives. (Zolpidem and zaleplon appear to be exceptions to this, because withdrawal symptoms are minimal following abrupt discontinuance of these newer short-acting agents.) Symptoms are less pronounced with longer-acting drugs, which may partly accomplish their own "tapered" withdrawal by virtue of their slow elimination. Cross-dependence, defined as the ability of one drug to suppress abstinence symptoms from discontinuance of another drug, is quite marked among sedative-hypnotics. This provides the rationale for therapeutic regimens in the management of withdrawal states: Longer-acting drugs such as chlor-

diazepoxide, diazepam, and phenobarbital can be used to alleviate withdrawal symptoms of shorter-acting drugs, including ethanol.

Drug Interactions

The most frequent drug interactions involving sedative-hypnotics are interactions with other central nervous system depressant drugs, leading to additive effects. These interactions have some therapeutic utility with respect to the use of these drugs as premedicants or anesthetic adjuvants. However, if not anticipated, they can lead to serious consequences, including enhanced depression with concomitant use of many other drugs. Additive effects can be predicted with concomitant use of alcoholic beverages, opioid analgesics, anticonvulsants, and phenothiazines. Less obvious but just as important is enhanced central nervous system depression with a variety of antihistamines, antihypertensive agents, and antidepressant drugs of the tricyclic class.

Interactions involving changes in the activity of hepatic drug-metabolizing enzyme systems have been discussed (see also Chapter 4 and Appendix II).

PREPARATIONS AVAILABLE

BENZODIAZEPINES
Alprazolam (generic, Xanax)
Oral: 0.25, 0.5, 1, 2 mg tablets; 0.1, 1.0 mg/mL solution
Chlordiazepoxide (generic, Librium)
Oral: 5, 10, 25 mg capsules; 10, 25 mg tablets
Parenteral: 100 mg powder for injection
Clorazepate (generic, Tranxene)
Oral: 3.75, 7.5, 15 mg tablets and capsules
Oral sustained-release: 11.25, 22.5 mg tablets
Clonazepam (Klonopin)
Oral: 0.5, 1, 2 mg tablets
Diazepam (generic, Valium)
Oral: 2, 5, 10 mg tablets; 1, 5 mg/mL solutions
Parenteral: 5 mg/mL for injection
Estazolam (generic, ProSom)
Oral: 1, 2 mg tablets
Flurazepam (generic, Dalmane)
Oral: 15, 30 mg capsules
Halazepam (Paxipam)
Oral: 20, 40 mg tablets
Lorazepam (generic, Ativan, Alzapam)
Oral: 0.5, 1, 2 mg tablets; 2 mg/mL solution
Parenteral: 2, 4 mg/mL for injection
Midazolam (Versed)
Oral: 2 mg/mL syrup
Parenteral: 1, 5 mg/mL in 1, 2, 5, 10 mL vials for injection

Oxazepam (generic, Serax)
Oral: 10, 15, 30 mg capsules, 15 mg tablets
Quazepam (Doral)
Oral: 7.5, 15 mg tablets
Temazepam (generic, Restoril)
Oral: 7.5, 15, 30 mg capsules
Triazolam (generic, Halcion)
Oral: 0.125, 0.25 mg tablets

BENZODIAZEPINE ANTAGONIST
Flumazenil (Romazicon)
Parenteral: 0.1 mg/mL for IV injection

BARBITURATES
Amobarbital (Amytal)
Parenteral: powder in 250, 500 mg vials to reconstitute for injection
Pentobarbital (generic, Nembutal Sodium)
Oral: 50, 100 mg capsules; 4 mg/mL elixir
Rectal: 30, 60, 120, 200 mg suppositories
Parenteral: 50 mg/mL for injection
Phenobarbital (generic, Luminal Sodium)
Oral: 15, 16, 30, 60, 90, 100 mg tablets; 16 mg capsules; 15, 20 mg/5 mL elixirs
Parenteral: 30, 60, 65, 130 mg/mL for injection
Secobarbital (generic, Seconal)
Oral: 100 mg capsules

MISCELLANEOUS DRUGS
  Buspirone (BuSpar)
    Oral: 5, 10, 15 mg tablets
  Chloral hydrate (generic, Aquachloral Supprettes)
    Oral: 500 mg capsules; 250, 500 mg/5 mL syrups
    Rectal: 324, 500, 648 mg suppositories
  Ethchlorvynol (Placidyl)
    Oral: 200, 500, 750 mg capsules
  Hydroxyzine (generic, Atarax, Vistaril)
    Oral: 10, 25, 50, 100 mg tablets; 25, 50, 100 mg capsules; 10 mg/5 mL syrup; 25 mg/5 mL suspension
    Parenteral: 25, 50 mg/mL for injection

Meprobamate (generic, Equanil, Miltown)
  Oral: 200, 400 mg tablets
  Oral sustained-release: 200, 400 mg capsules
Paraldehyde (generic)
  Oral, rectal liquids
Zaleplon (Sonata)
  Oral: 5, 10 mg capsules
Zolpidem (Ambien)
  Oral: 5, 10 mg tablets

REFERENCES

Apter JT, Allen LA: Buspirone: Future directions. J Clin Psychopharmacol 1999;19:86.

Belzung C: The genetic basis of the pharmacological effects of anxiolytics: a review based on rodent models. Behav Pharmacol 2001;12:451.

Blednov YA et al: Deletion of the alpha$_1$ or beta$_2$ subunit of GABA$_A$ receptors reduces actions of alcohol and other drugs. J Pharmacol Exp Ther 2003;304:30.

Chouinard G et al: Metabolism of anxiolytics and hypnotics: Benzodiazepines, buspirone, zopiclone and zolpidem. Cell Mol Neurobiol 1999;19:533.

Crestani F et al: Mechanism of action of the hypnotic zolpidem in vivo. Br J Pharmacol 2000;131:1251.

Crestani F et al: Molecular targets for the myorelaxant action of diazepam. Mol Pharmacol 2001;59:442.

Drover D et al: A pharmacokinetic and psychometric pharmacodynamic comparison of zaleplon and zolpidem. Clin Ther 2000;22:1443.

Fujita M et al: Changes of benzodiazepine receptors during chronic benzodiazepine administration in humans. Eur J Pharmacol 1999;368:161.

Gorman JM: Treating generalized anxiety disorder. J Clin Psychiatry 2003;64(Suppl 2):24.

Gottesmann C: GABA mechanisms and sleep. Neuroscience 2002;111:231.

Holm KJ, Goa KL: Zolpidem: an update of its pharmacology, therapeutic efficacy and tolerability in the treatment of insomnia. Drugs 2000;59:865.

Israel AG, Kramer JA: Safety of zaleplon in the treatment of insomnia. Ann Pharmacother 2002;36:852.

Korpi ER, Grunder G, Luddens H: Drug interactions at GABA(A) receptors. Prog Neurobiol 2002;67:113.

Kralic JE et al: GABA(A) receptor alpha-1 subunit deletion alters receptor subtype assembly, pharmacological and behavioral responses to benzodiazepines and zolpidem. Neuropharmacology 2002;43:685.

Kralic JE et al: Pharmacological characterization of GABA(A) receptor alpha$_1$ subunit knockout mice. J Pharmacol Exp Ther 2002;302:1037.

Mahmood I, Sahalwalla C: Clinical pharmacokinetics and pharmacodynamics of buspirone, an anxiolytic drug. Clin Pharmacokinet 1999;36:277.

McKernan RM et al: Anxiolytic-like action of diazepam: which GABA(A) receptor subtype is involved? Trends Pharmacol Sci 2001;22:402.

Mintzer MZ, Griffiths RR: Triazolam and zolpidem: Effects on human memory and attentional processes. Psychopharmacology (Berl) 1999;144:8.

Mohler H, Fritschy JM, Rudolph U: A new benzodiazepine pharmacology. J Pharmacol Exp Ther 2002;300:2.

Ninan PT: New insights into the diagnosis and pharmacologic management of generalized anxiety disorder. Psychopharmacol Bull 2002;36:105.

Patat A, Paty I, Hindmarch I: Pharmacodynamic profile of Zaleplon, a new non-benzodiazepine hypnotic agent. Hum Psychopharmacol 2001;16:369.

Rickels K, Rynn M: Pharmacotherapy of generalized anxiety disorder. J Clin Psychiatry 2002;63(Suppl 14):9.

Rudolph U, Crestani F, Mohler H: GABA(A) receptor subtypes: dissecting their pharmacological functions. Trends Pharmacol Sci 2001;22:188.

Rush CR et al: Zaleplon and triazolam in humans: Acute behavioral effects and abuse potential. Psychopharmacology (Berl) 1999;145:39.

Smith TA: Type A gamma-aminobutyric acid (GABA$_A$) receptor subunits and benzodiazepine binding: significance to clinical syndromes and their treatment. Br J Biomed Sci 2001;58:111.

Stahl SM: Selective actions on sleep or anxiety by exploiting GABA-A/benzodiazepine receptor subtypes. J Clin Psychiatry 2002;63:179.

Terzano MG et al: New drugs for insomnia: comparative tolerability of zopiclone, zolpidem and zaleplon. Drug Saf 2003;26:261.

van Laar MW, Volkerts ER: Driving and benzodiazepine use: Evidence that they do not mix. CNS Drugs 1998;10:383.

Wagner J, Wagner ML: Non-benzodiazepines for the treatment of insomnia. Sleep Med Rev 2000;4:551.

Wingrove PB et al: Mechanism of alpha-subunit selectivity of benzodiazepine pharmacology at gamma-aminobutyric acid type A receptors. Eur J Pharmacol 2002;437:31.

Yuan R, Flockhart DA, Balian JD: Pharmacokinetic and pharmacodynamic consequences of metabolism-based drug interactions with alprazolam, midazolam, and triazolam. J Clin Pharmacol 1999;39:1109.

The Alcohols

23

Susan B. Masters, PhD

Alcohol, primarily in the form of ethyl alcohol (ethanol), has occupied an important place in the history of humankind for at least 8000 years. In Western society, beer and wine were a main staple of daily life until the 19th century. These relatively dilute alcoholic beverages were preferred over water, which was known to be associated with acute and chronic illness. They provided important calories and nutrients and served as a main source of daily liquid intake. As systems for improved sanitation and water purification were introduced in the 1800s, beer and wine became less important as components of the human diet, and the consumption of alcoholic beverages, including distilled preparations with higher concentrations of alcohol, shifted toward their present-day role (in many societies) as a socially acceptable form of recreation.

Today, alcohol is widely consumed. Like other sedative-hypnotic drugs, alcohol in low to moderate amounts relieves anxiety and fosters a feeling of well-being or even euphoria. However, alcohol is also the most commonly abused drug in the world, a cause of vast medical and societal costs. In the United States, approximately 75% of the adult population drinks alcohol regularly. The majority of this drinking population is able to enjoy the pleasurable effects of alcohol without allowing their alcohol consumption to become a health risk. However, about 10% of the general population in the United States are unable to limit their ethanol consumption, a condition known as alcohol abuse. People who continue to drink alcohol in spite of adverse medical or social consequences related directly to their alcohol consumption suffer from **alcoholism,** a complex disorder that appears to have genetic as well as environmental determinants. The societal and medical costs of alcohol abuse are staggering. It is estimated that about 30% of all people admitted to hospitals have coexisting alcohol problems. Once in the hospital, people with chronic alcoholism generally have poorer outcomes. In addition, each year thousands of children are born in the USA with morphologic and functional defects resulting from prenatal exposure to ethanol. Despite the investment of many resources and much basic research, alcoholism remains a common chronic disease that is difficult to treat.

Ethanol and many other alcohols with potentially toxic effects are used in industry, some in enormous quantities. In addition to ethanol, methanol and ethylene glycol toxicity occur with sufficient frequency to warrant discussion in this chapter.

I. BASIC PHARMACOLOGY OF ETHANOL

Pharmacokinetics

Ethanol is a small water-soluble molecule that is absorbed rapidly from the gastrointestinal tract. After ingestion of alcohol in the fasting state, peak blood alcohol concentrations are reached within 30 minutes. The presence of food in the gut delays absorption by slowing gastric emptying. Distribution is rapid, with tissue levels approximating the concentration in blood. The volume of distribution for ethanol approximates total body water (0.5–0.7 L/kg). For an equivalent oral dose of alcohol, women have a higher peak concentration than men, in part because women have a lower total body water content. In the central nervous system, the concentration of ethanol rises quickly since the brain receives a large proportion of blood flow and ethanol readily crosses biologic membranes.

Over 90% of alcohol consumed is oxidized in the liver; much of the remainder is excreted through the lungs and in the urine. The excretion of a small but consistent proportion of alcohol by the lungs is utilized for breath alcohol tests that serve as a basis for a legal definition of "driving under the influence" in many countries. At levels of ethanol usually achieved in blood, the rate of oxidation follows zero-order kinetics, ie, it is independent of time and concentration of the drug. The typical adult can metabolize 7–10 g (150–220 mmol) of alcohol per hour, the equivalent of approximately 10 oz of beer, 3.5 oz of wine, or 1 oz of distilled 80 proof spirits.

Two major pathways of alcohol metabolism to acetaldehyde have been identified (Figure 23–1).

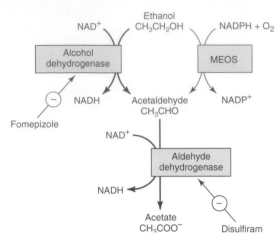

Figure 23–1. Metabolism of ethanol by alcohol dehydrogenase and the microsomal ethanol-oxidizing system (MEOS). Alcohol dehydrogenase and aldehyde dehydrogenase are inhibited by fomepizole and disulfiram, respectively.

Acetaldehyde is then oxidized by a third metabolic process.

A. ALCOHOL DEHYDROGENASE PATHWAY

The primary pathway for alcohol metabolism involves alcohol dehydrogenase (ADH), a cytosolic enzyme that catalyzes the conversion of alcohol to acetaldehyde (Figure 23–1, left). This enzyme is located mainly in the liver, but it is also found in other organs such as brain and stomach.

A significant amount of ethanol metabolism by gastric ADH occurs in the stomach in men, but a smaller amount occurs in women, who appear to have lower levels of the gastric enzyme. This difference in gastric metabolism of alcohol in women probably contributes to the sex-related differences in blood alcohol concentrations noted above.

During conversion of ethanol to acetaldehyde, hydrogen ion is transferred from alcohol to the cofactor nicotinamide adenine dinucleotide (NAD$^+$) to form NADH. As a net result, alcohol oxidation generates an excess of reducing equivalents in the liver, chiefly as NADH. The excess NADH production appears to underlie a number of metabolic disorders that accompany chronic alcoholism.

B. MICROSOMAL ETHANOL OXIDIZING SYSTEM (MEOS)

This enzyme system, also known as the mixed function oxidase system (see Chapter 4), uses NADPH as a cofactor in the metabolism of ethanol (Figure 23–1, right).

At blood concentrations below 100 mg/dL (22 mmol/L), the MEOS system, which has a relatively high K_m for alcohol, contributes little to the metabolism of ethanol. However, when large amounts of ethanol are consumed, the alcohol dehydrogenase system becomes saturated owing to depletion of the required cofactor, NAD$^+$. As the concentration of ethanol increases above 100 mg/dL, there is increased contribution from the MEOS system, which does not rely upon NAD$^+$ as a cofactor.

During chronic alcohol consumption, MEOS activity increases. As a result, chronic alcohol consumption results in significant increases not only in ethanol metabolism but also in the clearance of other drugs eliminated by the MEOS system. Similarly, other inducing drugs such as barbiturates may also enhance the rate of blood alcohol clearance slightly. However, the effect of other enzyme-inducing drugs on ethanol clearance is less important because the MEOS is not the primary pathway for ethanol metabolism.

C. ACETALDEHYDE METABOLISM

Much of the acetaldehyde formed from alcohol appears to be oxidized in the liver in a reaction catalyzed by mitochondrial NAD-dependent aldehyde dehydrogenase. The product of this reaction is acetate (Figure 23–1), which can be further metabolized to CO_2 and water.

Oxidation of acetaldehyde is inhibited by disulfiram, a drug that has been used to deter drinking by alcohol-dependent patients undergoing treatment. When ethanol is consumed in the presence of disulfiram, acetaldehyde accumulates and causes an unpleasant reaction of facial flushing, nausea, vomiting, dizziness, and headache. Several other drugs (eg, metronidazole, cefotetan, trimethoprim) inhibit aldehyde dehydrogenase and can cause a disulfiram-like reaction if combined with ethanol.

Some people, primarily of Asian descent, have a genetic deficiency in the activity of the mitochondrial form of aldehyde dehydrogenase. When these individuals drink alcohol, they develop high blood acetaldehyde concentrations and experience a flushing reaction similar to that seen with the combination of disulfiram and ethanol.

Pharmacodynamics of Acute Ethanol Consumption

A. CENTRAL NERVOUS SYSTEM

The central nervous system is markedly affected by acute alcohol consumption. Alcohol causes sedation and relief of anxiety and, at higher concentrations, slurred speech, ataxia, impaired judgment, and disinhibited behavior, a condition usually called intoxication or drunkenness (Table 23–1). These central nervous system effects are most marked as the blood level is rising, because acute tolerance to the effects of alcohol occurs after a few hours of drinking. For chronic drinkers who are tolerant to the effects of alcohol, much higher concentrations are needed to elicit these central nervous system effects. For example, a chronic alcoholic may appear sober or only slightly intoxicated with a blood alcohol concentration of 300–400 mg/dL, whereas this level is associated with marked intoxication or even coma in a nontolerant individual. The propensity of moderate doses of alcohol to inhibit the attention and information processing skills as well as the motor skills required for operation of motor vehicles has profound effects. Approximately half of all traffic accidents resulting in a fatality in the United States involve at least one person with a blood alcohol near or above the legal level of intoxication, and drunken driving is a leading cause of death in young adults.

Like other sedative-hypnotic drugs, alcohol is a central nervous system depressant. At high blood concentrations, it induces coma, respiratory depression, and death.

No specific receptor for ethanol has been identified. Instead, ethanol has been shown to affect a large number of membrane proteins that participate in signaling pathways, including neurotransmitter receptors for amines, amino acids, and opioids; enzymes such as Na+/K+ ATPase, adenylyl cyclase, phosphoinositide-specific phospholipase C; and ion channels such as those for Ca2+. Much attention has focused on alcohol's effects upon neurotransmission by glutamate and GABA, the main excitatory and inhibitory neurotransmitters in the central nervous system. Acute ethanol exposure enhances the action of GABA at GABAA receptors, which is consistent with the ability of GABA-mimetics to intensify many of the acute effects of alcohol and of GABAA antagonists to attenuate some of the actions of ethanol. Ethanol also inhibits the ability of glutamate to open the cation channel associated with the N-methyl-D-aspartate (NMDA) subtype of glutamate receptors. The NMDA receptor is implicated in many aspects of cognitive function, including learning and memory. "Blackouts"—periods of memory loss that occur with high levels of alcohol—may result from inhibition of NMDA receptor activation.

B. Heart

Significant depression of myocardial contractility has been observed in individuals who acutely consume moderate amounts of alcohol, ie, at a blood concentration above 100 mg/dL. Myocardial biopsies in humans before and after infusion of small amounts of alcohol have shown ultrastructural changes that may be associated with impaired myocardial function. Acetaldehyde is implicated as a cause of cardiac dysfunction by altering myocardial stores of catecholamines.

C. Smooth Muscle

Ethanol is a vasodilator, probably as a result of both central nervous system effects (depression of the vasomotor center) and direct smooth muscle relaxation caused by its metabolite, acetaldehyde. In cases of severe overdose, hypothermia—caused by vasodilation—may be marked in cold environments. Ethanol also relaxes the uterus and—before the introduction of more effective and safer uterine relaxants (eg, calcium blockers, magnesium ion, NSAIDs, and β2-adrenoceptor stimulants)—was used intravenously for the suppression of premature labor.

Consequences of Chronic Alcohol Consumption

Chronic alcohol consumption profoundly affects the function of several vital organs—particularly the liver and skeletal muscle—and the nervous, gastrointestinal, cardiovascular, and immune systems. Since ethanol has low potency, it requires concentrations thousands of times higher than other misused drugs (eg, cocaine, opiates, amphetamines) to produce its intoxicating effects. As a result, ethanol is consumed in quantities that are unusually large for a pharmacologically active drug. The tissue damage caused by chronic alcohol ingestion results directly from toxic effects of ethanol and acetaldehyde and indirectly by making tissues more susceptible to injury. Mechanisms implicated in tissue damage include increased oxidative stress coupled with depletion of glutathione, damage to mitochondria, growth factor dysregulation, and potentiation of cytokine-induced injury.

Table 23–1. Blood alcohol concentration (BAC) and clinical effects in nontolerant individuals.

BAC (mg/dL)[1]	Clinical Effect
50–100	Sedation, subjective "high," increased reaction times
100–200	Impaired motor function, slurred speech, ataxia
200–300	Emesis, stupor
300–400	Coma
>500	Respiratory depression, death

[1]In many parts of the USA, a blood level above 80–100 mg/dL for adults or 10 mg/dL for persons under 21 is sufficient for conviction of driving while "under the influence."

Chronic consumption of large amounts of alcohol is associated with an increased risk of death. Deaths linked to alcohol consumption are caused by liver disease, cancer, accidents, and suicide.

A. LIVER AND GASTROINTESTINAL TRACT

Liver disease is the most common medical complication of alcohol abuse; it is estimated that 15–30% of chronic heavy drinkers eventually develop severe liver disease. Clinically significant alcoholic liver disease may be insidious in onset and progress without evidence of overt nutritional abnormalities. Alcoholic fatty liver, a reversible condition, may progress to alcoholic hepatitis and finally to cirrhosis and liver failure. In the USA, chronic alcohol abuse is the leading cause of liver cirrhosis and of the need for liver transplantation. The risk of developing liver disease is related both to the average amount of daily consumption and to the duration of alcohol abuse. Women appear to be more susceptible to alcohol hepatotoxicity than men. Another factor that increases the risk of severe liver disease is concurrent infection with hepatitis B or C virus.

Other portions of the gastrointestinal tract can also be injured. Chronic alcohol ingestion is by far the most common cause of chronic pancreatitis in the Western world. In addition to its direct toxic effect on pancreatic acinar cells, alcohol alters pancreatic epithelial permeability and promotes the formation of protein plugs and calcium carbonate-containing stones.

Chronic alcoholics are prone to develop gastritis and have increased susceptibility to blood and plasma protein loss during drinking, which may contribute to anemia and protein malnutrition. Alcohol also reversibly injures the small intestine, leading to diarrhea, weight loss, and multiple vitamin deficiencies.

Malnutrition from dietary deficiency and vitamin deficiencies due to malabsorption are common in alcoholic individuals. Malabsorption of water-soluble vitamins is especially severe.

B. NERVOUS SYSTEM

1. Tolerance and physical dependence—The consumption of alcohol in high doses over a long period results in tolerance and in physical and psychologic dependence. Tolerance to the intoxicating effects of alcohol is a complex process involving poorly understood changes in the nervous system as well as the metabolic changes described earlier. As with other sedative-hypnotic drugs, there is a limit to tolerance, so that only a relatively small increase in the lethal dose occurs with increasing alcohol use.

Chronic alcohol drinkers, when forced to reduce or discontinue alcohol, experience a withdrawal syndrome, which indicates the existence of physical dependence. Alcohol withdrawal symptoms classically consist of hyperexcitability in mild cases and seizures, toxic psychosis, and **delirium tremens** in severe ones. The dose, rate, and duration of alcohol consumption determine the intensity of the withdrawal syndrome. When consumption has been very high, merely reducing the rate of consumption may lead to signs of withdrawal.

Psychologic dependence upon alcohol is characterized by a compulsive desire to experience the rewarding effects of alcohol and, for current drinkers, a desire to avoid the negative consequences of withdrawal. People who have recovered from alcoholism and become abstinent still experience periods of intense craving for alcohol that can be set off by environmental cues associated in the past with drinking, such as familiar places, groups of people, or events.

The molecular basis of alcohol tolerance and dependence is not known, nor is it known if the two phenomena reflect opposing effects upon a shared molecular pathway. Tolerance may result from ethanol-induced up-regulation of a pathway in response to the continuous presence of ethanol. Dependence may result from overactivity of that same pathway once the ethanol effect dissipates and before the system has time to return to a normal ethanol-free state. Chronic exposure of animals or cultured cells to alcohol elicits a multitude of adaptive responses involving neurotransmitters and their receptors, ion channels, and enzymes that participate in signal transduction pathways. Up-regulation of the NMDA subtype of glutamate receptors and voltage-sensitive Ca^{2+} channels may underlie the seizures that accompany the alcohol withdrawal syndrome. Based on the ability of sedative-hypnotic drugs that enhance GABAergic neurotransmission to substitute for alcohol during alcohol withdrawal and evidence of down-regulation of $GABA_A$-mediated responses with chronic alcohol exposure, changes in GABA neurotransmission are believed to play a central role in tolerance and withdrawal.

Neurotransmission events involved in the sensation of reward are also important. Alcohol affects local concentrations of serotonin, opioids, and dopamine—neurotransmitters involved in brain reward circuits. Alcohol also has complex effects on the expression of receptors for these neurotransmitters and their signaling pathways. The discovery that naltrexone, a nonselective opioid receptor antagonist, helps patients who are recovering from alcoholism abstain from drinking supports the idea that the neurochemical reward system is shared by drugs associated with physical and psychological dependence.

2. Neurotoxicity—Consumption of large amounts of alcohol over extended periods (usually years) often leads to neurologic deficits. The most frequent neurologic abnormality in chronic alcoholism is generalized symmetric peripheral nerve injury that begins with distal paresthesias of the hands and feet. Chronic alcoholics may also exhibit gait disturbances and ataxia that are due to degenerative changes in the central nervous system. Other neurologic disturbances associated with alcoholism include dementia and, rarely, demyelinating disease.

Wernicke-Korsakoff syndrome is a relatively uncommon but important entity characterized by paralysis of the external eye muscles, ataxia, and a confused state that can progress to coma and death. It is associated with thiamin deficiency but is rarely seen in the absence of alcoholism. Wernicke's encephalopathy represents the acute phase of this disease; it may be difficult to distinguish from the acute confused state created by acute alcohol intoxication, which later blends in with the perceptual and behavioral problems associated with alcohol withdrawal. A distinguishing feature of Wernicke's encephalopathy is the longer duration of confusion and the relative absence of the agitation that would be expected during withdrawal. Because of the importance of thiamin in this pathologic condition, all patients suspected of having Wernicke-Korsakoff syndrome should receive thiamine therapy. Often, the ocular signs, ataxia, and confusion improve upon prompt administration of thiamine. However, most patients are left with a chronic disabling memory disorder known as Korsakoff's psychosis.

Alcohol may also impair visual acuity, with painless blurring that occurs over several weeks of heavy alcohol consumption. Changes are usually bilateral and symmetric and may be followed by optic nerve degeneration. Ingestion of ethanol substitutes such as methanol (see below) causes severe visual disturbances.

C. Cardiovascular System

Alcohol has complex effects upon the cardiovascular system. Heavy alcohol consumption of long duration is associated with a dilated cardiomyopathy with ventricular hypertrophy and fibrosis. In animals and humans, alcohol induces a number of changes in heart cells that may contribute to cardiomyopathy. They include membrane disruption, depressed function of mitochondria and sarcoplasmic reticulum, intracellular accumulation of phospholipids and fatty acids, and up-regulation of voltage-dependent calcium channels. There is evidence that patients with alcohol-induced dilated cardiomyopathy do significantly worse than patients with idiopathic dilated cardiomyopathy, even though cessation of drinking is associated with a reduction in cardiac size and improved function. The poorer prognosis for patients who continue to drink appears to be due in part to interference of ethanol with the beneficial effects of β-blockers and ACE inhibitors.

Heavy drinking—and especially "binge" drinking—are associated with both atrial and ventricular arrhythmias. Patients undergoing alcohol withdrawal syndrome can develop severe arrhythmias that may reflect abnormalities of potassium or magnesium metabolism as well as enhanced release of catecholamines. Seizures, syncope, and sudden death during alcohol withdrawal may be due to these arrhythmias.

A link between heavier alcohol consumption (more than three drinks per day) and hypertension has been firmly established in epidemiologic studies. Alcohol is estimated to be responsible for approximately 5% of cases of hypertension, making it one of the most common causes of reversible hypertension. This association is independent of obesity, salt intake, coffee drinking, or cigarette smoking. The mechanisms responsible for the sustained increase in blood pressure have not been identified. A reduction in alcohol intake appears to be effective in lowering blood pressure in hypertensives who are also heavy drinkers; the hypertension seen in this population is also responsive to standard blood pressure medications.

While the deleterious effects of excessive alcohol use on the cardiovascular system are well established, there is controversy over the effects of moderate drinking (one to three drinks a day) on the incidence of coronary heart disease (CHD). A number of observational studies concluded that moderate alcohol consumption actually prevents CHD and even reduces mortality. This type of relationship between mortality and the dose of a drug is called a "J-shaped" relationship. Results of these clinical studies are supported by ethanol's ability to raise serum levels of high-density lipoprotein (HDL) cholesterol, the form of cholesterol that appears to protect against atherosclerosis (see Chapter 35), its ability to inhibit some of the inflammatory processes that underlie atherosclerosis, and the presence in alcoholic beverages (especially red wine) of antioxidants and other substances that may protect against atherosclerosis. More recently, the relationship between moderate drinking and CHD has been called into question (Corrao et al, 2000) based on further investigation of confounders that affected the outcome of earlier epidemiologic studies. For example, moderate drinkers, especially wine drinkers, come from a higher socioeconomic level and may have healthier dietary habits; consumption tends to decrease with age; abstinence often is associated with ill health; and documenting precise amounts of consumption is difficult. Therefore, definitive conclusions regarding a cardioprotective effect of alcohol must await better clinical evidence.

D. Blood

Alcohol indirectly affects hematopoiesis through metabolic and nutritional effects and may also directly inhibit the proliferation of all cellular elements in bone marrow. The most common hematologic disorder seen in chronic drinkers is mild anemia resulting from alcohol-related folic acid deficiency. Iron deficiency anemia may result from gastrointestinal bleeding. Alcohol has also been implicated as a cause of several hemolytic syndromes, some of which are associated with hyperlipidemia and severe liver disease.

E. Endocrine System and Electrolyte Balance

Chronic alcohol use has important effects on the endocrine system and on fluid and electrolyte balance. Clinical reports of gynecomastia and testicular atrophy in alcoholics with or without cirrhosis suggest a derangement in steroid hormone balance.

Alcoholics with chronic liver disease may have disorders of fluid and electrolyte balance, including ascites, edema, and effusions. These factors may be related to decreased protein synthesis and portal hypertension. Alterations of whole body potassium induced by vomiting and diarrhea, as well as severe secondary aldosteronism, may contribute to muscle weakness and can be worsened by diuretic therapy. Some alcoholic patients develop hypoglycemia, probably as a result of impaired hepatic gluconeogenesis. Some alcoholics also develop ketosis, caused by excessive lipolytic factors, especially increased cortisol and growth hormone.

F. Fetal Alcohol Syndrome

Chronic maternal alcohol abuse during pregnancy is associated with teratogenic effects, and alcohol appears to be a leading cause of mental retardation and congenital malformation. The abnormalities that have been characterized as fetal alcohol syndrome include (1) intrauterine growth retardation, (2) microcephaly, (3) poor coordination, (4) underdevelopment of midfacial region (appearing as a flattened face), and (5) minor joint anomalies. More severe cases may include congenital heart defects and mental retardation. Heavy drinking in the first trimester of pregnancy produces the facial features associated with fetal alcohol syndrome. The consequences of heavy drinking in the second and third trimesters are not well defined, but animal studies suggest that the brain is vulnerable to ethanol throughout development. While the level of alcohol intake required for causing serious neurologic deficits appears quite high, the threshold for causing more subtle neurologic deficits is uncertain.

The mechanisms that underlie ethanol's teratogenic effects are unknown. Ethanol rapidly crosses the placenta and reaches concentrations in the fetus that are similar to those in maternal blood. The fetal liver has little or no alcohol dehydrogenase activity, so the fetus must rely upon maternal and placental enzymes for elimination of alcohol.

The neuropathologic abnormalities seen in humans and in animal models of fetal alcohol syndrome indicate that ethanol triggers apoptotic neurodegeneration and also causes aberrant neuronal and glial migration in the developing nervous system. In tissue culture systems, ethanol causes a striking reduction in neurite outgrowth. Alcohol's toxicity to the developing brain may be due to selective interference with the synthesis or function of molecules that are critical for cell recognition and migration, such as L1, an immunoglobulin cell adhesion molecule and gangliosides, major structural components of neuronal plasma membranes.

G. Immune System

The effects of alcohol on the immune system are complex—immune function in some tissues is inhibited (eg, the lung), while immune function in other tissues is enhanced (eg, liver, pancreas). In addition, acute and chronic exposure to alcohol have widely different effects on immune function. The types of immunologic changes reported include suppression of the function of alveolar macrophages, inhibition of chemotaxis of granulocytes, and reduced number and function of T cells. In the liver, there is enhanced function of Kupffer cells. What is clear is that chronic heavy alcohol use predisposes to the development of infections, especially of the lung, and that it worsens the morbidity and increases the mortality risk of patients with pneumonia.

H. Increased Risk of Cancer

Chronic alcohol use increases the risk for cancer of the mouth, pharynx, larynx, esophagus, and liver. Evidence also points to a small increase in the risk of breast cancer in women. Although the methodologic problems of studies relating cancer to alcohol use have been formidable, the consistency of results showing an increase in the risk of gastrointestinal tract cancer is impressive. Much more information is required before a threshold level for alcohol consumption as it relates to cancer can be established. In fact, alcohol itself does not appear to be a carcinogen in most test systems. However, alcoholic beverages may carry potential carcinogens produced in fermentation or processing and may alter liver function so that the activity of potential carcinogens is increased.

Alcohol-Drug Interactions

Interactions between ethanol and other drugs can have important clinical effects that result from alterations in the pharmacokinetics or pharmacodynamics of the second drug.

The most frequent pharmacokinetic alcohol-drug interactions occur as a result of alcohol-induced increases of drug-metabolizing enzymes in liver cells as described in Chapter 4. Thus, prolonged intake of alcohol without damage to the liver may enhance the metabolic biotransformation of other drugs. Ethanol-mediated induction of hepatic cytochrome P450 enzymes is particularly important with regard to acetaminophen. Chronic consumption at the level of three or more drinks per day increases the risk of hepatotoxicity due to toxic or even high therapeutic levels of acetaminophen. This is probably due to increased P450-mediated conversion of acetaminophen to reactive hepatotoxic metabolites (see Chapter 4). In 1998, the FDA announced that all OTC products containing acetaminophen must carry a warning about the relationship between chronic ethanol consumption and acetaminophen-induced hepatotoxicity.

In contrast, *acute* alcohol use may inhibit metabolism of other drugs. This inhibition may be due to decreased enzyme activity or decreased liver blood flow. This acute alcohol effect may contribute to the commonly recognized danger of mixing alcohol with other drugs when performing activities requiring some skill, especially driving. Phenothiazines, tricyclic antidepressants, and sedative-hypnotic drugs are the most important drugs that may interact with alcohol by this pharmacokinetic mechanism.

Pharmacodynamic alcohol interactions are also of great clinical significance. Additive central nervous system depression with other sedative-hypnotics is most important. Alcohol also potentiates the pharmacologic effects of many nonsedative drugs, including vasodilators and oral hypoglycemic agents. There is some evidence that alcohol also enhances the antiplatelet action of aspirin.

II. CLINICAL PHARMACOLOGY OF ETHANOL

Ethanol is the cause of more preventable morbidity and mortality than all other drugs combined with the exception of tobacco. The search for specific etiologic factors or the identification of significant predisposing variables for alcohol abuse has generally led to disappointing results. Personality type, severe life stresses, psychiatric disorders, and parental role models are not reliable predictors of alcohol abuse. While environmental factors clearly play a role, evidence suggests that there is a large genetic contribution to the development of alcoholism. Using new genetic markers for humans and animals, an intensive search for genes that predispose toward alcohol dependence is under way (Crabbe, 1999). Not surprisingly, polymorphisms in alcohol dehydrogenase and aldehyde dehydrogenase that lead to increased aldehyde accumulation (and therefore more severe hangover symptoms) appear to protect against alcoholism. Much attention in genetic mapping experiments has focused on membrane-signaling proteins known to be affected by ethanol and on protein constituents of reward pathways in the brain. Early reports of an association of an allele of the dopamine D_2 receptor with alcohol dependence have not been confirmed. Other candidate genes for susceptibility to alcoholism identified in genome-wide screens in humans include the dopamine D_4 receptor, the β_1 subunit of the $GABA_A$ receptor, and tyrosine hydroxylase, an enzyme involved in the synthesis of dopamine, norepinephrine, and epinephrine (see Chapter 6).

Genetic mapping studies have also been performed in rodents selectively bred to exhibit high or low voluntary alcohol consumption and to show differences in the severity of alcohol withdrawal seizures. A number of candidate genes have been identified, including neurotransmitter receptors, ion channels, amino acid transporters, and enzymes involved in neurotransmitter synthesis and metabolism. One intriguing candidate is neuropeptide Y (NPY), a small protein expressed in the brain and implicated in the regulation of a variety of behaviors. The role of NPY in behavior related to ethanol has been explored by development of a strain of mice that lack the gene for NPY—NPY knockout mice—and a strain of mice that overexpress NPY. The NPY knockout mice voluntarily consume more ethanol than control mice and are less sensitive to the sedative effects of ethanol. In contrast, mice overexpressing NPY drink less alcohol than the controls even though their total consumption of food and liquid is normal. Much more work is needed to investigate the role of NPY in animal models and in human alcoholism, but these findings illustrate the application of modern genetic techniques for the study of differences in behavioral responses to drugs.

MANAGEMENT OF ACUTE ALCOHOL INTOXICATION

Nontolerant individuals who consume alcohol in large quantities develop typical effects of acute sedative-hypnotic drug overdose along with the cardiovascular effects described above (vasodilation, tachycardia) and gastrointestinal irritation. Since tolerance is not absolute, even chronic alcoholics may become severely intoxicated. The degree of intoxication depends upon three factors: the blood ethanol concentration, the rapidity of the rise of the alcohol level, and the time during which the blood level is maintained. The pattern of drinking, the state of the absorptive surface of the gastrointestinal tract, and the presence in the body of other medications also affect the apparent degree of intoxication.

The most important goals in the treatment of acute alcohol intoxication are to prevent severe respiratory depression and aspiration of vomitus. Even with very high blood ethanol levels, survival is probable as long as the respiratory and cardiovascular systems can be supported. The average blood alcohol concentration in fatal cases is above 400 mg/dL; however, the lethal dose of alcohol varies because of varying degrees of tolerance.

Metabolic alterations may require treatment of hypoglycemia and ketosis by administration of glucose. Thiamine is given to protect against the Wernicke-Korsakoff syndrome. Alcoholic patients who are dehydrated and vomiting should also receive electrolyte solutions. If vomiting is severe, large amounts of potassium may be required as long as renal function is normal. Especially important is recognition of decreased serum concentrations of phosphate, which may be aggravated by glucose administration. Low phosphate stores may contribute to poor wound healing, neurologic deficits, and an increased risk of infection.

MANAGEMENT OF ALCOHOL WITHDRAWAL SYNDROME

Abrupt alcohol withdrawal leads to a characteristic syndrome of motor agitation, anxiety, insomnia, and reduction of seizure threshold. The severity of the syndrome is usually proportionate to the degree and duration of alcohol abuse. However, this can be greatly modified by the use of other sedatives as well as by associated factors (eg, diabetes, injury). In its mildest form, the alcohol withdrawal syndrome of tremor, anxiety, and insomnia occurs 6–8 hours after alcohol is stopped. These effects usually abate in 1–2 days. In some patients, more severe withdrawal reactions occur in which visual hallucinations, total disorientation, and marked abnormalities of vital signs occur. Alcohol withdrawal is one of the most common causes of seizures in adults. The more severe the withdrawal syndrome, the greater the need for meticulous investigation of possible underlying medical complications. The mortality risks of severe alcohol withdrawal have been overstated in the past. The prognosis is probably related chiefly to the underlying medical complications.

The major objective of drug therapy in the alcohol withdrawal period is prevention of seizures, delirium, and arrhythmias. Potassium, magnesium, and phosphate balance should be restored as rapidly as is consistent with renal function. Thiamine therapy is initiated in all cases. Persons in mild alcohol withdrawal do not need any other pharmacologic assistance.

Specific drug treatment for detoxification in severe cases involves two basic principles: substituting a long-acting sedative-hypnotic drug for alcohol and then gradually reducing ("tapering") the dose of the long-acting drug. Because of their wide margin of safety, benzodiazepines are preferred for treatment of alcohol withdrawal syndrome, though barbiturates such as pheno-

barbital were used in the past. Since any benzodiazepine will prevent symptoms of alcohol withdrawal, the choice of a specific agent in this class is generally based upon pharmacokinetic or economic considerations. Long-acting benzodiazepines, including chlordiazepoxide, clorazepate, and diazepam, have the advantage of requiring less frequent dosing. Since their pharmacologically active metabolites are eliminated slowly, the long-acting drugs provide a built-in tapering effect. A disadvantage of the long-acting drugs is that they and their pharmacologically active metabolites may accumulate, especially in patients with compromised liver function. Short-acting drugs such as lorazepam and oxazepam are rapidly converted to inactive water-soluble metabolites that will not accumulate, and for this reason the short-acting drugs are especially useful in alcoholic patients with liver disease. Benzodiazepines can be administered orally in mild or moderate cases, or parenterally for patients with more severe withdrawal reactions.

Phenothiazine medications for alcohol withdrawal have potentially serious adverse effects (eg, increasing seizures) that probably outweigh their benefits. Antihistamines have been used but with little justification.

After the alcohol withdrawal syndrome has been treated acutely, sedative-hypnotic medications must be tapered slowly over several weeks. Complete detoxification is not achieved with just a few days of alcohol abstinence. Several months may be required for restoration of normal nervous system function, especially sleep.

PHARMACOTHERAPY OF ALCOHOLISM

Following detoxification, psychosocial therapy either in intensive inpatient or in outpatient rehabilitation programs serves as the primary treatment for alcohol dependence. Since these programs have been only moderately successful, with about 50% of patients relapsing within the first year, there is much interest in finding drugs that can be useful adjuncts to psychosocial counseling. The first approach to pharmacotherapy was to deter drinking with drugs that cause a noxious reaction to alcohol by blocking its metabolism. Disulfiram, an inhibitor of aldehyde dehydrogenase, is the drug most commonly used for this purpose in the USA. More recently, research has focused on identifying drugs that alter brain responses to alcohol, eg, by decreasing the craving of abstinent alcoholics for alcohol or by blunting the pleasurable "high" that comes with renewed drinking. Naltrexone, an inhibitor of opioid receptors, was the first drug of this type to be approved by the FDA for treatment of alcohol dependence.

Other psychiatric problems, most commonly depressive or anxiety disorders, often coexist with alcoholism and, if untreated, can contribute to the tendency of detoxified alcoholics to relapse. Treatment of these associated disorders with counseling and drugs can help decrease the rate of relapse for alcoholic patients.

Disulfiram

Disulfiram (tetraethylthiuram), a widely used antioxidant in the rubber industry, causes extreme discomfort to patients who drink alcoholic beverages. Disulfiram given by itself to nondrinkers has little effect; however, flushing, throbbing headache, nausea, vomiting, sweating, hypotension, and confusion occur within a few minutes after drinking alcohol. The effect may last 30 minutes in mild cases or several hours in severe ones. Disulfiram acts by inhibiting aldehyde dehydrogenase. Thus, alcohol is metabolized as usual, but acetaldehyde accumulates.

Disulfiram is rapidly and completely absorbed from the gastrointestinal tract; however, a period of 12 hours is required for its full action. Its elimination rate is slow, so that its action may persist for several days after the last dose. The drug inhibits the metabolism of many other therapeutic agents, including phenytoin, oral anticoagulants, and isoniazid.

Compliance with disulfiram therapy is often low, and both compliance and clinical outcome can be improved by supervised administration. When the drug is prescribed, the alcohol content of common nonprescription medications should be communicated to the patient; some of these are listed in Table 64–3. Management with disulfiram should be initiated only when the patient has been free of alcohol for at least 24 hours. The drug may cause mild changes in liver function tests. The safety of disulfiram in pregnancy has not been demonstrated. The duration of disulfiram treatment should be individualized and determined by the patient's responsiveness and clinical improvement. The usual oral dose is 250 mg daily taken at bedtime.

Several other drugs, eg, metronidazole, certain cephalosporins, sulfonylurea hypoglycemic drugs, and chloral hydrate, have disulfiram-like effects on ethanol metabolism. Patients should be warned to avoid drinking ethanol while taking these drugs and for several days after they discontinue them.

Naltrexone

Naltrexone is an orally available opioid receptor antagonist that blocks the effects of exogenous and, presumably, endogenous opioids (see Chapter 31). Studies in experimental animals first suggested a link between alcohol consumption and opioids. Injection of small amounts of opioids was followed by an increase in alcohol drinking, whereas administration of opioid antagonists inhibited self-administration of alcohol. Several double-blind, placebo-controlled clinical trials showed that the combination of naltrexone with psychosocial therapy decreased the rate of relapse and reduced alcohol craving (see Box, Manipulating Brain Neurotransmitter Systems to Treat Alcoholism). The subjects taking naltrexone who "slipped," that is, who sampled alcohol during the trial, were better able to control their drinking and avoid relapsing into heavy drinking. The lower alcohol consumption in naloxone-treated subjects was associated with a diminution of the subjective "high" associated with alcohol (Volpicelli et al, 1995). The durability of naltrexone's effect in alcoholism is not clear, since the initial clinical trials were only for 12 weeks. In a follow-up study, the decrease in relapse after 12 weeks of treatment continued for only one month after discontinuation of the naltrexone (O'Malley et al, 1996).

Naltrexone is taken once a day in a dose of 50 mg for treatment of alcoholism. The drug should be used with caution in alcoholic patients with evidence of mild abnormalities in serum aminotransferase activity. The combination of naltrexone plus disulfiram should be avoided since both drugs are potential hepatotoxins. Administration of naltrexone to patients who are physically dependent upon opioids will precipitate an acute withdrawal syndrome so patients must be opioid-free before initiating naltrexone therapy. Naltrexone also blocks the therapeutic effects of usual doses of opioids.

Other Drugs

Preliminary evidence suggests that topiramate, a drug used for partial and generalized tonic-clonic seizures (Chapter 24), may be effective in reducing craving in chronic alcoholics.

III. PHARMACOLOGY OF OTHER ALCOHOLS

Other alcohols related to ethanol have wide applications as industrial solvents and occasionally cause severe poisoning. Of these, **methanol** and **ethylene glycol** are two of the most common causes of intoxication.

Methanol

Methanol (methyl alcohol, wood alcohol) is widely used in the industrial production of synthetic organic compounds and as a constituent of many commercial solvents. In the home, methanol is most frequently found in the form of "canned heat" or in windshield-washing products. Poisonings occur from accidental ingestion of methanol-containing products or when it is used by alcoholics as an ethanol substitute.

MANIPULATING BRAIN NEUROTRANSMITTER SYSTEMS TO TREAT ALCOHOLISM

Advances in knowledge about the neurochemistry of the brain's reward system have increased the hope that pharmacologic manipulation of brain neurotransmitter systems can help people who become addicted to alcohol and other drugs. The apparent utility of naltrexone, an opioid antagonist, in reducing craving and the incidence of relapse in alcoholic patients provides evidence that the opioid system is an important player in the alcohol response system. The glutamate neurotransmitter system also appears to be important. **Acamprosate,** a competitive inhibitor of the NMDA glutamate receptor, reduces the incidence of relapse and prolongs abstinence. It is widely available in Europe and is being tested in the USA.

Several other neurotransmitter systems are leading targets in studies of pharmacotherapy for alcoholism. Considerable evidence from animal studies indicates that serotonergic and dopaminergic systems participate in the regulation of alcohol consumption. One intriguing clinical trial found that ondansetron reduced drinking in patients with early-onset alcoholism (Johnson et al, 2000). Ondansetron is an antagonist of 5-HT$_3$ serotonin receptors and a commonly used antiemetic (see Chapters 16 and 63)

Other clinical trials are focusing on selective serotonin reuptake inhibitors (SSRI) such as fluoxetine as well as selective serotonin receptor ligands such as buspirone, a 5-HT$_{1A}$ receptor partial agonist; and ritanserin, a 5-HT$_2$ receptor antagonist. Of these other drugs, the SSRI drugs have been most thoroughly studied. Results from clinical trials have been mixed, with some studies showing favorable results and others failing to find that SSRIs attenuate alcohol consumption in nondepressed heavy drinkers. A number of dopamine receptor antagonists are also being studied, including selective antagonists of D$_1$ and D$_2$ dopamine receptors. Because of their importance in alcohol-related effects, drugs that modify neurotransmission through GABA and glutamate systems are also under investigation. Alcoholism is a heterogeneous disorder. As efforts to classify alcoholic patients into specific subtypes become more sophisticated, it may be possible to identify the subtypes that respond best to specific pharmacotherapies.

Methanol can be absorbed through the skin or from the respiratory or gastrointestinal tract and is then distributed in body water. The primary mechanism of elimination of methanol in humans is by oxidation to formaldehyde, formic acid, and CO_2:

$$CH_3OH \xrightarrow{\text{Alcohol dehydrogenase}} H_2CO \longrightarrow HCOO^- \longrightarrow CO_2 + H_2O$$

Methanol **Formaldehyde** **Formate**

Animal species show great variability in mean lethal doses of methanol. The special susceptibility of humans to methanol toxicity is probably due to folate-dependent production of formate and not to methanol itself or to formaldehyde, the intermediate metabolite.

The most characteristic symptom in methanol poisoning is a visual disturbance, frequently described as "like being in a snowstorm." A complaint of blurred vision with a relatively clear sensorium should strongly suggest the diagnosis of methanol poisoning. Since much of the toxicity is due to metabolites of methanol, there is often a delay of up to 30 hours before development of visual disturbances and other signs of severe intoxication.

Physical findings in methanol poisoning are generally nonspecific. In severe cases, the odor of formalde-hyde may be present on the breath or in the urine. Changes in the retina may sometimes be detected on examination, but these are usually late. The development of bradycardia, prolonged coma, seizures, and resistant acidosis all imply a poor prognosis. The cause of death in fatal cases is sudden cessation of respiration.

It is critical that the blood methanol level be determined as soon as possible if the diagnosis is suspected. Methanol concentrations in excess of 50 mg/dL are thought to be an absolute indication for hemodialysis and ethanol treatment, though formate blood levels are a better indication of clinical pathology. Additional laboratory evidence includes metabolic acidosis with an elevated anion gap and osmolar gap (see Chapter 59). A decrease in serum bicarbonate is a uniform feature of severe methanol poisoning.

The first treatment for methanol poisoning, as in all critical poisoning situations, is support of respiration. For hospitalized patients, gastric lavage should be carried out after the airway has been protected by endotracheal intubation. Activated charcoal is not useful.

There are three specific modalities of treatment for severe methanol poisoning: suppression of metabolism by alcohol dehydrogenase to toxic products, dialysis to enhance removal of methanol and its toxic products, and alkalinization to counteract metabolic acidosis.

The enzyme chiefly responsible for methanol oxidation in the liver is alcohol dehydrogenase. Ethanol has a higher affinity than methanol for alcohol dehydrogenase; thus, saturation of the enzyme with ethanol reduces formate production. Ethanol is often used intravenously as treatment for methanol poisoning. The dose-dependent characteristics of ethanol metabolism and the variability of ethanol metabolism require frequent monitoring of blood ethanol levels to ensure appropriate alcohol concentration. **Fomepizole,** an alcohol dehydrogenase inhibitor, is approved for the treatment of ethylene glycol poisoning (see below) and methanol poisoning.

Hemodialysis rapidly eliminates both methanol and formate. However, ethanol will also be eliminated in the dialysate, requiring alterations in the dose of ethanol. Hemodialysis is discussed in Chapter 59.

Two other measures are commonly taken. Because of profound metabolic acidosis in methanol poisoning, treatment with bicarbonate often is necessary. Since folate-dependent systems are responsible for the oxidation of formic acid to CO_2 in humans, it is probably useful to administer folic acid to patients poisoned with methanol, though this has never been fully tested in clinical studies.

Ethylene Glycol

Polyhydric alcohols such as ethylene glycol (CH_2OHCH_2OH) are used as heat exchangers, in antifreeze formulations, and as industrial solvents. Young children and animals are sometimes attracted by the sweet taste of ethylene glycol and, rarely, it is ingested intentionally as an ethanol substitute or in attempted suicide. While ethylene glycol itself is relatively harmless and eliminated by the kidney, it is metabolized to toxic aldehydes and oxalate.

Three stages of ethylene glycol overdose occur. Within the first few hours after ingestion, there is transient excitation followed by central nervous system depression. After a delay of 4–12 hours, severe metabolic acidosis develops from accumulation of acid metabolites and lactate. Finally, delayed renal insufficiency follows deposition of oxalate in renal tubules. The key to the diagnosis of ethylene glycol poisoning is recognition of anion gap acidosis, osmolar gap, and oxalate crystals in the urine in a patient without visual symptoms.

As with methanol poisoning, early ethanol infusion and hemodialysis are standard treatments for ethylene glycol poisoning. Fomepizole, an inhibitor of alcohol dehydrogenase, has FDA approval for treatment of ethylene glycol poisoning in adults based on its ability to decrease concentrations of toxic metabolites in blood and urine and to prevent renal injury. Intravenous treatment with fomepizole is initiated immediately and continued until the patient's serum ethylene glycol concentration drops below a toxic threshold (20 mg/dL). Adverse effects associated with fomepizole are not severe. Headache, nausea, and dizziness are the ones most frequently reported, and a few patients experience minor allergic reactions. Fomepizole is classified as an orphan drug (see Chapter 5) because ethylene glycol poisoning is relatively uncommon. Its cost—estimated to be $4000 per patient—is much higher than the cost of infusible ethanol, but fomepizole offers some advantages over ethanol as an antidote for this potentially fatal poisoning.

PREPARATIONS AVAILABLE

DRUGS FOR THE TREATMENT OF ACUTE ALCOHOL WITHDRAWAL SYNDROME
Diazepam (generic, Valium, others)
  Oral: 2, 3, 10 mg tablets; 5 mg/5 mL solutions (see also Chapter 22)
  Parenteral: 5 mg/mL for injection
Lorazepam (generic, Alzapam, Ativan)
  Oral: 0.5, 1, 2 mg tablets
  Parenteral: 2, 4 mg/mL for injection
Oxazepam (generic, Serax)
  Oral: 10, 15, 30 mg capsules, 15 mg tablets
Thiamine (generic)
  Parenteral: 100 mg/mL for IV injection

DRUGS FOR THE PREVENTION OF ALCOHOL ABUSE
Disulfiram (generic, Antabuse)
  Oral: 250, 500 mg tablets
Naltrexone (ReVia)
  Oral: 50 mg tablets

DRUGS FOR THE TREATMENT OF ACUTE METHANOL OR ETHYLENE GLYCOL POISONING
Ethanol (generic)
  Parenteral: 5% or 10% ethanol and 5% dextrose in water for IV infusion
Fomepizole (Antizol)
  Parenteral: 1 g/mL for IV injection

REFERENCES

Brent J et al: Fomepizole for the treatment of ethylene glycol poisoning. Methylpyrazole for Toxic Alcohols Study Group. N Engl J Med 1999;340,832.

CDC Fetal Alcohol Syndrome Website: http://www.cdc.gov/ncbddd/fas/

Corrao G et al: Alcohol and coronary heart disease: a meta-analysis. Addiction 2000;95:1505.

Crabbe JC et al: Identifying genes for alcohol and drug sensitivity: recent progress and future directions. Trends Neurosci 1999;22:173.

Hoffman PL et al: Transgenic and gene "knockout" models in alcohol research. Alcohol Clin Exp Res 2001;25(Suppl):606.

Jacobsen D: New treatment for ethylene glycol poisoning. N Engl J Med 1999;340:879.

Johnson BA et al: Ondansetron for reduction of drinking among biologically predisposed alcoholic patients: A randomized controlled trial. JAMA 2000;284:963.

Key TJ et al: The effect of diet on risk of cancer. Lancet 2002; 360:861.

Li TK: Pharmacogenetics of responses to alcohol and genes that influence alcohol drinking. J Stud Alcohol 2000; 61:5.

Lieber CS: Medical disorders of alcoholism. N Engl J Med 1995;333:1058.

Littleton J: Receptor regulation as a unitary mechanism for drug tolerance and physical dependence-not quite as simple as it seemed. Addiction 2001;96:87.

National Institute on Drug Abuse (NIDA) Website on Alcohol: http://www.nida.nih.gov/DrugPages/Alcohol.html

Nelson S, Knolls JK: Alcohol, host defence and society. Nat Rev Immunology 2002;2:205.

Olney JW et al: The enigma of fetal alcohol neurotoxicity. Ann Med 2002;34:109.

O'Malley SS et al: Six-month follow-up of naltrexone and psychotherapy for alcohol dependence. Arch Gen Psychiatry 1996;53:217.

Spies CD et al: Effects of alcohol on the heart. Curr Opin Crit Care 2001;7:337.

Swift RM: Drug therapy for alcohol dependence. N Engl J Med 1999;340:1482.

Volpicelli JR et al: Effect of naltrexone on alcohol "high" in alcoholics. Am J Psychiatry 1995;152:613.

Antiseizure Drugs*

Roger J. Porter, MD, & Brian S. Meldrum, MB, PhD

Approximately 1% of the world's population has epilepsy, the second most common neurologic disorder after stroke. Although standard therapy permits control of seizures in 80% of these patients, millions (500,000 people in the USA alone) have uncontrolled epilepsy. Epilepsy is a heterogeneous symptom complex—a chronic disorder characterized by recurrent seizures. Seizures are finite episodes of brain dysfunction resulting from abnormal discharge of cerebral neurons. The causes of seizures are many and include the full range of neurologic diseases, from infection to neoplasm and head injury. In some subgroups, heredity has proved to be a major contributing factor.

The antiseizure drugs described in this chapter are also used in patients with febrile seizures or with seizures occurring as part of an acute illness such as meningitis. The term "epilepsy" is not usually applied to such patients unless chronic seizures develop later. Seizures are occasionally caused by an acute underlying toxic or metabolic disorder, in which case appropriate therapy should be directed toward the specific abnormality, eg, hypocalcemia. In most cases of epilepsy, however, the choice of medication depends on the empiric seizure classification.

Drug Development for Epilepsy

For a long time it was assumed that a single drug could be developed for the treatment of all forms of epilepsy, but the causes of epilepsy are extremely diverse, encompassing genetic and developmental defects and infective, traumatic, neoplastic, and degenerative disease processes, and drug therapy to date shows little evidence of etiologic specificity. There is, however, some specificity according to seizure type. This is most clearly seen with generalized seizures of the absence type (see Table 24–1), typically with 2–3 Hz spike-and-wave discharges on the electroencephalogram, which respond to etho-

suximide and valproate but can be exacerbated by phenytoin and carbamazepine. Drugs acting selectively on absence seizures can be identified by animal screens, using either threshold pentylenetetrazol clonic seizures in mice or rats or mutant mice showing absence-like episodes (so-called lethargic, star-gazer, or tottering mutants). In contrast, the maximal electroshock (MES) test, with suppression of the tonic extensor phase, identifies drugs such as phenytoin, carbamazepine, and lamotrigine that are active against generalized tonic-clonic seizures or complex partial seizures. Use of the maximal electroshock test as the major primary screen for new drugs has probably led to the identification of drugs with a common mechanism of action involving prolonged inactivation of the voltage-sensitive sodium channel. Limbic seizures induced in rats by the process of electrical kindling (involving repeated episodes of focal electrical stimulation) probably provides a better screen for predicting efficacy in complex partial seizures.

Existing antiseizure drugs provide adequate seizure control in about two thirds of patients. A fraction of the epileptic population is resistant to all available drugs and this may be due to increased expression of the multidrug transporter P-glycoprotein 170, a product of the *ABCB1* gene (Siddiqui, 2003). In children, some severe seizure syndromes associated with progressive brain damage are very difficult to treat. In adults, some focal seizures are refractory to medications. Some, particularly in the temporal lobe, are amenable to surgical resection. Some of the drug-resistant population may respond to vagus-nerve stimulation (VNS), a nonpharmacologic treatment for epilepsy, that is now widely approved for treatment of patients with partial seizures. VNS is indicated for refractory cases or for patients in whom antiseizure drugs are poorly tolerated. Stimulating electrodes are implanted in the left vagus nerve and the pacemaker is implanted in the chest wall or axilla. Use of this device may permit seizure control with lower doses of drugs. New antiseizure drugs are being sought not only by the screening tests noted above but also by more rational approaches. Compounds are sought that

---

* The authors wish to thank Philip Mayer, PhD, for his assistance in reviewing the pharmacokinetic data in this chapter.

Table 24–1. Classification of seizure types.

Partial seizures
Simple partial seizures
Complex partial seizures
Partial seizures secondarily generalized
Generalized seizures
Generalized tonic-clonic (grand mal) seizures
Absence (petit mal) seizures
Tonic seizures
Atonic seizures
Clonic and myoclonic seizures
Infantile spasms[1]

[1]An epileptic syndrome rather than a specific seizure type; drugs useful in infantile spasms will be reviewed separately.

act by one of three mechanisms: (1) enhancement of GABAergic (inhibitory) transmission, (2) diminution of excitatory (usually glutamatergic) transmission, or (3) modification of ionic conductances.

I. BASIC PHARMACOLOGY OF ANTISEIZURE DRUGS

Chemistry

Up to 1990, approximately 16 antiseizure drugs were available, and 13 of them can be classified into five very similar chemical groups: barbiturates, hydantoins, oxazolidinediones, succinimides, and acetylureas. These groups have in common a similar heterocyclic ring structure with a variety of substituents (Figure 24–1). For drugs with this basic structure, the substituents on the heterocyclic ring determine the pharmacologic class, either anti-MES or antipentylenetetrazol. Very small changes in structure can dramatically alter the mechanism of action and clinical properties of the compound. The remaining drugs—carbamazepine, valproic acid,

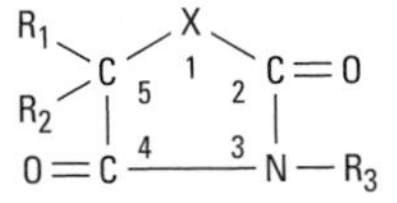

Figure 24–1. Antiseizure heterocyclic ring structure. The "X" varies as follows: hydantoin derivatives, –N–; barbiturates, –C–N–; oxazolidinediones, –O–; succinimides, –C–; acetylureas, –NH$_2$ (N connected to C$_2$). R$_1$, R$_2$, and R$_3$ vary within each subgroup.

and the benzodiazepines—are structurally dissimilar, as are the newer compounds marketed since 1990, ie, felbamate, gabapentin, lamotrigine, oxcarbazepine, tiagabine, topiramate, vigabatrin, and levetiracetam.

Pharmacokinetics

The antiseizure drugs exhibit many similar pharmacokinetic properties—even those whose structural and chemical properties are quite diverse. Although many of these compounds are only slightly soluble, absorption is usually good, with 80–100% of the dose reaching the circulation. Most antiseizure drugs are not highly bound to plasma proteins.

Antiseizure drugs are cleared chiefly by hepatic mechanisms, although they have low extraction ratios (see Chapter 3). Many are converted to active metabolites that are also cleared by the liver. These drugs are predominantly distributed into total body water. Plasma clearance is relatively slow; many anticonvulsants are therefore considered to be medium- to long-acting. For most, half-lives are greater than 12 hours. Phenobarbital and carbamazepine are potent inducers of hepatic microsomal enzyme activity.

DRUGS USED IN PARTIAL SEIZURES & GENERALIZED TONIC-CLONIC SEIZURES

The major drugs for partial and generalized tonic-clonic seizures are phenytoin (and congeners), carbamazepine, valproate, and the barbiturates. However, the availability of newer drugs—lamotrigine, gabapentin, oxcarbazepine, topiramate, vigabatrin, and levetiracetam—is altering clinical practice in countries where these compounds are available.

PHENYTOIN

Phenytoin is the oldest nonsedative antiseizure drug, introduced in 1938 following a systematic evaluation of compounds such as phenobarbital that altered electrically induced seizures in laboratory animals. It was known for decades as **diphenylhydantoin.**

Chemistry

Phenytoin is a diphenyl-substituted hydantoin with the structure shown below. It has much lower sedative properties than compounds with alkyl substituents at the 5 position. A more soluble prodrug of phenytoin, **fosphenytoin,** is available for parenteral use. This phosphate ester compound is rapidly converted to phenytoin in the plasma.

Phenytoin

Mechanism of Action

Phenytoin has major effects on several physiologic systems. It alters Na⁺, K⁺, and Ca²⁺ conductance, membrane potentials, and the concentrations of amino acids and the neurotransmitters norepinephrine, acetylcholine, and γ-aminobutyric acid (GABA). Studies with neurons in cell culture show that phenytoin blocks sustained high-frequency repetitive firing of action potentials (Figure 24–2). This effect is seen at therapeutically relevant concentrations. It is a use-dependent effect (see Chapter 14) on Na⁺ conductance, arising from preferential binding to—and prolongation of—the inactivated state of the Na⁺ channel. This effect is also seen with therapeutically relevant concentrations of carbamazepine and valproate and probably contributes to their antiseizure action in the electroshock model and in partial seizures.

At high concentrations, phenytoin also inhibits the release of serotonin and norepinephrine, promotes the uptake of dopamine, and inhibits monoamine oxidase activity. The drug interacts with membrane lipids; this binding might promote the stabilization of the membrane. In addition, phenytoin paradoxically causes excitation in some cerebral neurons. A reduction of calcium permeability, with inhibition of calcium influx across the cell membrane, may explain the ability of phenytoin to inhibit a variety of calcium-induced secretory processes, including release of hormones and neurotransmitters. The significance of these biochemical actions and their relationship to phenytoin's clinical activity are unclear.

The mechanism of phenytoin's action probably involves a combination of actions at several levels. At therapeutic concentrations, the major action of phenytoin is to block sodium channels and inhibit the generation of repetitive action potentials.

Clinical Use

Phenytoin is one of the most effective drugs against partial seizures and generalized tonic-clonic seizures. In the latter, it appears to be effective against attacks that are either primary or secondary to another seizure type.

Pharmacokinetics

Absorption of phenytoin is highly dependent on the formulation of the dosage form. Particle size and pharmaceutical additives affect both the rate and the extent of absorption. Absorption of phenytoin sodium from the gastrointestinal tract is nearly complete in most patients, although the time to peak may range from 3 hours to 12 hours. Absorption after intramuscular injection is unpredictable, and some drug precipitation in the muscle occurs; this route of administration is not recommended for phenytoin. In contrast, fosphenytoin, a more soluble phosphate prodrug of phenytoin, is well absorbed after intramuscular administration.

Phenytoin is highly bound to plasma proteins. It appears certain that the total plasma level decreases

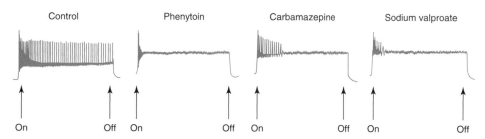

Figure 24–2. Effects of three antiseizure drugs on sustained high-frequency firing of action potentials by cultured neurons. Intracellular recordings were made from neurons while depolarizing current pulses, approximately 0.75 s in duration, were applied (on-off step changes indicated by arrows). In the absence of drug, a series of high-frequency repetitive action potentials filled the entire duration of the current pulse. Phenytoin, carbamazepine, and sodium valproate all markedly reduced the number of action potentials elicited by the current pulses. (Modified and reproduced, with permission, from Macdonald RL, Meldrum BS: Principles of antiepileptic drug action. In: Levy RH, et al [editors]. *Antiepileptic Drugs,* 4th ed. Raven Press, 1995.)

when the percentage that is bound decreases, as in uremia or hypoalbuminemia, but correlation of free levels with clinical states remains uncertain. Drug concentration in cerebrospinal fluid is proportionate to the free plasma level. Phenytoin accumulates in brain, liver, muscle, and fat.

Phenytoin is metabolized to inactive metabolites that are excreted in the urine. Only a very small portion of phenytoin is excreted unchanged.

The elimination of phenytoin is dose-dependent. At very low blood levels, phenytoin metabolism follows first-order kinetics. However, as blood levels rise within the therapeutic range, the maximum capacity of the liver to metabolize phenytoin is approached (Figure 24–3). Further increases in dose, even though relatively small, may produce very large changes in phenytoin concentrations. In such cases, the half-life of the drug increases markedly, steady state is not achieved in routine fashion (since the plasma level continues to rise), and patients quickly develop symptoms of toxicity.

The half-life of phenytoin varies from 12 hours to 36 hours, with an average of 24 hours for most patients in the low to mid therapeutic range. Much longer half-lives are observed at higher concentrations. At low blood levels, it takes 5–7 days to reach steady-state blood levels

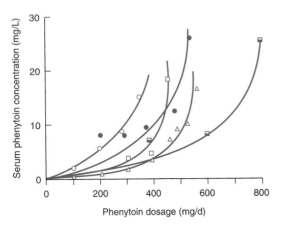

Figure 24–3. Nonlinear relationship of phenytoin dosage and plasma concentrations. Five different patients (identified by different symbols) received increasing dosages of phenytoin by mouth, and the steady-state serum concentration was measured at each dosage. The curves are not linear, since, as the dosage increases, the metabolism is saturable. Note also the marked variation among patients in the serum levels achieved at any dosage. (Modified, with permission, from Jusko WJ: Bioavailability and disposition kinetics of phenytoin in man. In: Kellaway P, Peterson I [editors]. *Quantitative Analytic Studies in Epilepsy.* Raven Press, 1977.)

after every dosage change; at higher levels, it may be 4–6 weeks before blood levels are stable.

Therapeutic Levels & Dosage

The therapeutic plasma level of phenytoin for most patients is between 10 and 20 µg/mL. A loading dose can be given either orally or intravenously; the latter, using fosphenytoin, is the method of choice for convulsive status epilepticus (discussed later). When oral therapy is started, it is common to begin adults at a dosage of 300 mg/d regardless of body weight. While this may be acceptable in some patients, it frequently yields steady-state blood levels below 10 µg/mL, the minimum therapeutic level for most patients. If seizures continue, higher doses are usually necessary to achieve plasma levels in the upper therapeutic range. Because of its dose-dependent kinetics, some toxicity may occur with only small increments in dose; the phenytoin dosage should be increased each time by only 25–30 mg in adults, and ample time should be allowed for the new steady state to be achieved before further increasing the dose. A common clinical error is to increase the dosage directly from 300 mg/d to 400 mg/d; toxicity frequently occurs at a variable time thereafter. In children, a dosage of 5 mg/kg/d should be followed by readjustment after steady-state plasma levels are obtained.

Two types of oral phenytoin sodium are currently available in the USA, differing in their respective rates of dissolution; one is absorbed rapidly and one more slowly. Only the slow-release extended action formulation can be given in a single daily dosage, and care must be used when changing brands (see Preparations Available). Although a few patients being given phenytoin on a chronic basis have been proved to have low blood levels from poor absorption or rapid metabolism, the most common cause of low levels is poor compliance. Fosphenytoin sodium is available for intravenous or intramuscular use and replaces intravenous phenytoin sodium, a much less soluble form of the drug.

Drug Interactions & Interference With Laboratory Tests

Drug interactions involving phenytoin are primarily related to protein binding or to metabolism. Since phenytoin is 90% bound to plasma protein, other highly bound drugs, such as phenylbutazone or sulfonamides, can displace phenytoin from its binding site. In theory, such displacement may cause a transient increase in free drug. A decrease in protein binding—eg, from hypoalbuminemia—results in a decrease in the total plasma concentration of drug but not the free concentration; intoxication may occur if efforts are made to maintain total drug levels in the therapeutic range by increasing the dose. The protein binding of phenytoin is decreased in the presence of renal disease. The drug has an affinity for thyroid-binding globulin, which confuses some tests of thyroid function; the most reliable screening test of thyroid function in patients taking phenytoin appears to be measurement of TSH.

Phenytoin has been shown to induce microsomal enzymes responsible for the metabolism of a number of drugs. Autostimulation of its own metabolism, however, appears to be insignificant. Other drugs, notably phenobarbital and carbamazepine, cause decreases in phenytoin steady-state concentrations through induction of hepatic microsomal enzymes. On the other hand, isoniazid inhibits the metabolism of phenytoin, resulting in increased steady-state concentrations when the two drugs are given together.

Toxicity

Dose-related adverse effects caused by phenytoin are unfortunately similar to other antiseizure drugs in this group, making differentiation difficult in patients receiving multiple drugs. Nystagmus occurs early, as does loss of smooth extraocular pursuit movements, but neither is an indication for decreasing the dose. Diplopia and ataxia are the most common dose-related adverse effects requiring dosage adjustment; sedation usually occurs only at considerably higher levels. Gingival hyperplasia and hirsutism occur to some degree in most patients; the latter can be especially unpleasant in women. Long-term use is associated in some patients with coarsening of facial features and with mild peripheral neuropathy, usually manifested by diminished deep tendon reflexes in the lower extremities. Long-term use may also result in abnormalities of vitamin D metabolism, leading to osteomalacia. Low folate levels and megaloblastic anemia have been reported, but the clinical importance of this observation is unknown.

Idiosyncratic reactions to phenytoin are relatively rare. A skin rash may indicate hypersensitivity of the patient to the drug. Fever may also occur, and in rare cases the skin lesions may be severe and exfoliative. Lymphadenopathy may be difficult to distinguish from malignant lymphoma, and although some studies suggest a causal relationship between phenytoin and Hodgkin's disease, the data are far from conclusive. Hematologic complications are exceedingly rare, although agranulocytosis has been reported in combination with fever and rash.

MEPHENYTOIN, ETHOTOIN, & PHENACEMIDE

Many congeners of phenytoin have been synthesized, but only three have been marketed recently in the USA, and one of these (phenacemide) has been withdrawn from the market. The first two congeners, mephenytoin

and ethotoin, like phenytoin, appear to be most effective against generalized tonic-clonic seizures and partial seizures. No well-controlled clinical trials have documented their effectiveness. The incidence of severe reactions such as dermatitis, agranulocytosis, or hepatitis is higher for mephenytoin than for phenytoin.

Ethotoin may be recommended for patients hypersensitive to phenytoin, but larger doses are required. The adverse effects and toxicity are generally less severe than those associated with phenytoin, but the drug appears to be less effective.

Both ethotoin and mephenytoin share with phenytoin the property of saturable metabolism within the therapeutic dosage range. Careful monitoring of the patient during dosage alterations with either drug is essential. Mephenytoin is metabolized to 5,5-ethylphenylhydantoin via demethylation. This metabolite, **nirvanol**, contributes most of the antiseizure activity of mephenytoin. Both mephenytoin and nirvanol are hydroxylated and undergo subsequent conjugation and excretion. Therapeutic levels for mephenytoin range from 5 μg/mL to 16 μg/mL, and levels above 20 μg/mL are considered toxic.

Therapeutic blood levels of nirvanol are between 25 and 40 μg/mL. A therapeutic range for ethotoin has not been established.

The third congener of phenytoin, phenacemide, is a straight-chain analog of phenytoin. It is a toxic drug of last resort for refractory partial seizures.

CARBAMAZEPINE

Closely related to imipramine and other antidepressants, carbamazepine is a tricyclic compound effective in treatment of bipolar depression. It was initially marketed for the treatment of trigeminal neuralgia but has proved useful for epilepsy as well.

Chemistry

Although not obvious from a two-dimensional representation of its structure, carbamazepine has many similarities to phenytoin. The ureide moiety (−N−CO−NH$_2$) present in the heterocyclic ring of most antiseizure drugs is also present in carbamazepine. Three-dimensional structural studies indicate that its spatial conformation is similar to that of phenytoin.

Carbamazepine

Mechanism of Action

The mechanism of action of carbamazepine appears to be similar to that of phenytoin. Like phenytoin, carbamazepine shows activity against maximal electroshock seizures. Carbamazepine, like phenytoin, blocks sodium channels at therapeutic concentrations and inhibits high-frequency repetitive firing in neurons in culture (Figure 24–2). It also acts presynaptically to decrease synaptic transmission. These effects probably account for the anticonvulsant action of carbamazepine. Binding studies show that carbamazepine interacts with adenosine receptors, but the functional significance of this observation is not known. Carbamazepine also inhibits uptake and release of norepinephrine from brain synaptosomes but does not influence GABA uptake in brain slices. Recent evidence suggests that the postsynaptic action of GABA can be potentiated by carbamazepine.

Clinical Use

Carbamazepine is considered the drug of choice for partial seizures, and many physicians also use it first for generalized tonic-clonic seizures. It can be used with phenytoin in many patients who are difficult to control. Carbamazepine is not sedative in its usual therapeutic range. The drug is also very effective in some patients with trigeminal neuralgia, although older patients may tolerate higher doses poorly, with ataxia and unsteadiness. Carbamazepine is also useful in some patients with mania (bipolar disorder).

Pharmacokinetics

The rate of absorption of carbamazepine varies widely among patients, although almost complete absorption apparently occurs in all. Peak levels are usually achieved 6–8 hours after administration. Slowing absorption by giving the drug after meals helps the patient tolerate larger total daily doses.

Distribution is slow, and the volume of distribution is roughly 1 L/kg. The drug is only 70% bound to plasma proteins; no displacement of other drugs from protein binding sites has been observed.

Carbamazepine has a very low systemic clearance of approximately 1 L/kg/d at the start of therapy. The drug has a notable ability to induce microsomal enzymes. Typically, the half-life of 36 hours observed in subjects following an initial single dose decreases to much less than 20 hours in subjects receiving continuous therapy. Considerable dosage adjustments are thus to be expected during the first weeks of therapy. Carbamazepine also alters the clearance of other drugs (see below).

Carbamazepine is completely metabolized in humans to several derivatives. One of these, carbamazepine-10,11-epoxide, has been shown to have anticonvulsant activity. The contribution of this and other metabolites to the clinical activity of carbamazepine is unknown.

Therapeutic Levels & Dosage

Carbamazepine is considered the drug of choice in partial seizures. It is available only in oral form. The drug is effective in children, in whom a dosage of 15–25 mg/kg/d is appropriate. In adults, daily doses of 1 g or even 2 g are tolerated. Higher dosage is achieved by giving multiple divided doses daily. An extended-release preparation permits twice-daily dosing for most patients. In patients in whom the blood is drawn just before the morning dose (trough level), the therapeutic level is usually 4–8 μg/mL; although many patients complain of diplopia at drug levels above 7 μg/mL, others can tolerate levels above 10 μg/mL, especially with monotherapy.

Drug Interactions

Drug interactions involving carbamazepine are almost exclusively related to the drug's enzyme-inducing properties. As noted previously, the increased metabolic capacity of the hepatic enzymes may cause a reduction in steady-state carbamazepine concentrations and an increased rate of metabolism of other drugs, eg, primidone, phenytoin, ethosuximide, valproic acid, and clonazepam. Other drugs such as propoxyphene, troleandomycin, and valproic acid may inhibit carbamazepine clearance and increase steady-state carbamazepine blood levels. Other anticonvulsants, however, such as phenytoin and phenobarbital, may decrease steady-state concentrations of carbamazepine through enzyme induction. No clinically significant protein-binding interactions have been reported.

Toxicity

The most common dose-related adverse effects of carbamazepine are diplopia and ataxia. The diplopia often occurs first and may last less than an hour during a particular time of day. Rearrangement of the divided daily dose can often remedy this complaint. Other dose-related complaints include mild gastrointestinal upsets, unsteadiness, and, at much higher doses, drowsiness. Hyponatremia and water intoxication have occasionally occurred and may be dose-related.

Considerable concern exists regarding the occurrence of idiosyncratic blood dyscrasias with carbamazepine, including fatal cases of aplastic anemia and agranulocytosis. Most of these have been in elderly patients with trigeminal neuralgia, and most have occurred within the first 4 months of treatment. The mild and persistent leukopenia seen in some patients is not necessarily an indication to stop treatment but requires careful monitoring. The most common idiosyncratic reaction is an erythematous skin rash; other responses such as hepatic dysfunction are unusual.

OXCARBAZEPINE

Oxcarbazepine is closely related to carbamazepine and useful in the same seizure types, but it may have an improved toxicity profile. Oxcarbazepine has a half-life of only 1–2 hours. Its activity, therefore, resides almost exclusively in the 10-hydroxy metabolite, to which it is rapidly converted and which has a half-life similar to that of carbamazepine, ie, 8–12 hours. The drug is mostly excreted as the glucuronide of the 10-hydroxy metabolite. Oxcarbazepine is less potent than carbamazepine, both in animal models of epilepsy and in epileptic patients; clinical doses of oxcarbazepine may need to be 50% higher than those of carbamazepine to obtain equivalent seizure control. Some studies report fewer hypersensitivity reactions to oxcarbazepine, and cross-reactivity with carbamazepine does not always occur. Furthermore, the drug appears to induce hepatic enzymes to a lesser extent than carbamazepine, minimizing drug interactions. Those adverse effects—such as hyponatremia—that do occur with oxcarbazepine are similar in character to reactions reported with carbamazepine.

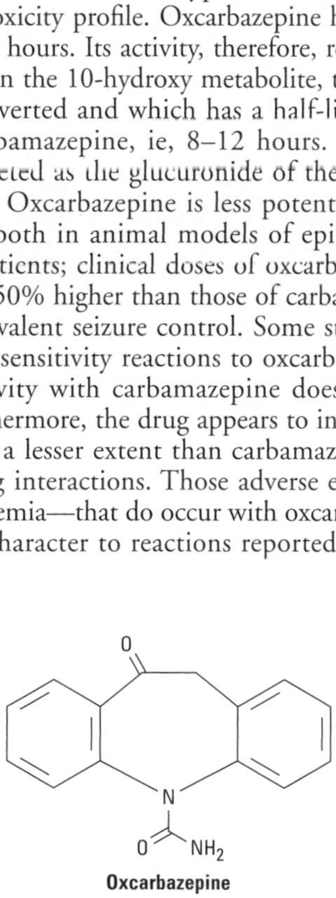

Oxcarbazepine

PHENOBARBITAL

Aside from the bromides, phenobarbital is the oldest of the currently available antiseizure drugs. Although it has long been considered one of the safest of the antiseizure agents, the use of other medications with lesser sedative effects has been urged. Many consider the barbiturates the drugs of choice for seizures only in infants.

Chemistry

The four derivatives of barbituric acid clinically useful as antiseizure drugs are phenobarbital, mephobarbital, metharbital, and primidone (Figure 24–4). The first

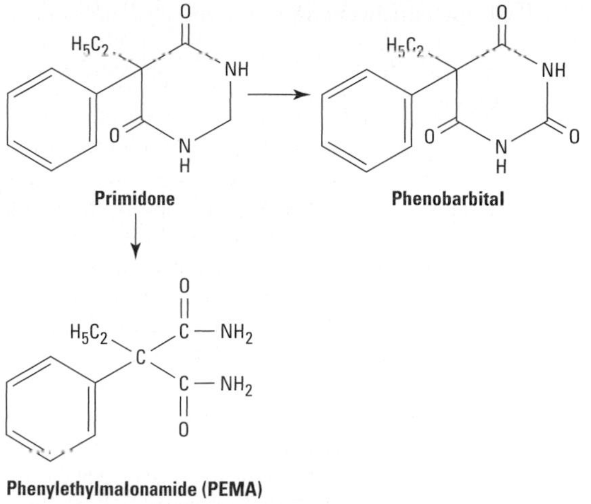

Figure 24–4. Primidone and its active metabolites.

three are so similar that they will be considered together. Metharbital is methylated barbital, and mephobarbital is methylated phenobarbital; both are demethylated in vivo. The pKa's of these three weak acid compounds range from 7.3 to 7.9. Slight changes in the normal acid-base balance, therefore, can cause significant fluctuation in the ratio of the ionized to the un-ionized species. This is particularly important for phenobarbital, the most commonly used barbiturate, whose pKa is similar to the plasma pH of 7.4.

The three-dimensional conformations of phenobarbital and N-methylphenobarbital are similar to that of phenytoin. Both compounds possess a phenyl ring and are active against partial seizures.

Mechanism of Action

The exact mechanism of action of phenobarbital is unknown, but enhancement of inhibitory processes and diminution of excitatory transmission probably contribute importantly. Recent data indicate that phenobarbital may selectively suppress abnormal neurons, inhibiting the spread and suppressing firing from the foci. Like phenytoin, phenobarbital suppresses high-frequency repetitive firing in neurons in culture through an action on Na^+ conductance, but only at high concentrations. Also at high concentrations, barbiturates block some Ca^{2+} currents (L-type and N-type). Phenobarbital binds to an allosteric regulatory site on the GABA-benzodiazepine receptor, and it enhances the GABA receptor-mediated current by prolonging the openings of the Cl^- channels. Phenobarbital also blocks excitatory responses induced by glutamate, principally those mediated by activation of the AMPA receptor (see Chapter

21). Both the enhancement of GABA-mediated inhibition and the reduction of glutamate-mediated excitation are seen with therapeutically relevant concentrations of phenobarbital.

Clinical Use

Phenobarbital is useful in the treatment of partial seizures and generalized tonic-clonic seizures, although the drug is often tried for virtually every seizure type, especially when attacks are difficult to control. There is little evidence for its effectiveness in generalized seizures such as absence, atonic attacks, or infantile spasms; it may worsen certain patients with these seizure types.

Some physicians prefer either metharbital or mephobarbital—especially the latter—to phenobarbital because of supposed decreased adverse effects. Only anecdotal data are available to support such comparisons.

Pharmacokinetics

See Chapter 22.

Therapeutic Levels & Dosage

The therapeutic levels of phenobarbital in most patients range from 10 μg/mL to 40 μg/mL. Documentation of effectiveness is best in febrile seizures, and levels below 15 μg/mL appear ineffective for prevention of febrile seizure recurrence. The upper end of the therapeutic range is more difficult to define, as many patients appear to tolerate chronic levels above 40 μg/mL.

Drug Interactions & Toxicity

See Chapter 22.

PRIMIDONE

Primidone, or 2-desoxyphenobarbital (Figure 24–4), was first marketed in the early 1950s. It was later reported that primidone was metabolized to phenobarbital and phenylethylmalonamide (PEMA). All three compounds are active anticonvulsants.

Mechanism of Action

Although primidone is converted to phenobarbital, the mechanism of action of primidone itself may be more like that of phenytoin.

Clinical Use

Primidone, like its metabolites, is effective against partial seizures and generalized tonic-clonic seizures and may be more effective than phenobarbital. It was previously considered to be the drug of choice for complex partial seizures, but the latest studies of partial seizures in adults strongly suggest that carbamazepine and phenytoin are superior to primidone. Attempts to determine the relative potencies of the parent drug and its two metabolites have been conducted in newborn infants, in whom drug-metabolizing enzyme systems are very immature and in whom primidone is only slowly metabolized. Primidone has been shown to be effective in controlling seizures in this group and in older patients beginning treatment with primidone; the latter show seizure control before phenobarbital concentrations reach the therapeutic range. Finally, studies of maximal electroshock seizures in animals suggest that primidone has an anticonvulsant action independent of its conversion to phenobarbital and PEMA (the latter is relatively weak).

Pharmacokinetics

Primidone is completely absorbed, usually reaching peak concentrations about 3 hours after oral administration, although considerable variation has been reported. Primidone is generally confined to total body water, with a volume of distribution of 0.6 L/kg. It is not highly bound to plasma proteins; approximately 70% circulates as unbound drug.

Primidone is metabolized by oxidation to phenobarbital, which accumulates very slowly, and by scission of the heterocyclic ring to form PEMA (Figure 24–4). Both primidone and phenobarbital also undergo subsequent conjugation and excretion.

Primidone has a larger clearance than most other antiseizure drugs (2 L/kg/d), corresponding to a half-life of 6–8 hours. PEMA clearance is approximately half that of primidone, but phenobarbital has a very low clearance. The appearance of phenobarbital corresponds to the disappearance of primidone. Phenobarbital therefore accumulates very slowly but eventually reaches therapeutic concentrations in most patients when therapeutic doses of primidone are administered. During chronic therapy, phenobarbital levels derived from primidone are usually two to three times higher than primidone levels. PEMA, which probably makes a minimal contribution to the efficacy of primidone, has a half-life of 8–12 hours and therefore reaches steady state more rapidly than phenobarbital.

Therapeutic Levels & Dosage

Primidone is most efficacious when plasma levels are in the range of 8–12 μg/mL. Concomitant levels of its metabolite, phenobarbital, at steady state will usually vary from 15 μg/mL to 30 μg/mL. Dosages of 10–20 mg/kg/d are necessary to obtain these levels. It is very important, however, to start primidone at low doses and gradually increase over days to a few weeks to avoid prominent sedation and gastrointestinal complaints. When adjusting doses of the drug, it is important to remember that the parent drug will rapidly reach steady state (30–40 hours), but the active metabolites phenobarbital (20 days) and PEMA (3–4 days) will reach steady state much more slowly.

Toxicity

The dose-related adverse effects of primidone are similar to those of its metabolite, phenobarbital, except that drowsiness occurs early in treatment and may be prominent if the initial dose is too large; gradual increments are indicated when starting the drug in either children or adults.

VIGABATRIN

Current investigations that seek drugs to enhance the effects of GABA include efforts to find GABA agonists and prodrugs, GABA transaminase inhibitors, and GABA uptake inhibitors. Vigabatrin (γ-vinyl-GABA) is one of these new drugs and has been registered in Europe and South America.

Vigabatrin

Mechanism of Action

Vigabatrin is an irreversible inhibitor of GABA aminotransferase (GABA-T), the enzyme responsible for the degradation of GABA. It apparently acts by increasing the amount of GABA released at synaptic sites, thereby enhancing inhibitory effects. Vigabatrin may also potentiate GABA by inhibiting the GABA transporter. It is effective in a wide range of seizure models. Vigabatrin is marketed as a racemate; the $S(+)$ enantiomer is active and the $R(-)$ enantiomer appears to be inactive.

Clinical Use

Vigabatrin is useful in the treatment of partial seizures and West's syndrome. The half-life is approximately 6–8 hours, but considerable evidence suggests that the pharmacodynamic activity of the drug is more prolonged and not well correlated with the plasma half-life. In adults, vigabatrin should be started at an oral dosage of 500 mg twice daily; a total of 2–3 g (rarely more) daily

may be required for full effectiveness. Typical toxicities include drowsiness, dizziness, and weight gain. Less common but more troublesome adverse reactions are agitation, confusion, and psychosis; preexisting mental illness is a relative contraindication. The drug was delayed in its worldwide introduction by the appearance in rats and dogs of a reversible intramyelinic edema; this phenomenon has not been observed in any patient to date. More recently, unfortunately, long-term therapy with vigabatrin has been associated with development of visual field defects in up to one third of patients. This adverse effect may not be reversible, and vigabatrin may therefore be relegated to use in patients—such as those with infantile spasms—who are refractory to other treatments.

LAMOTRIGINE

Lamotrigine was developed when some investigators thought that the antifolate effects of certain antiseizure drugs (eg, phenytoin) may contribute to their effectiveness. Several phenyltriazines were developed, and although their antifolate properties were weak, some were active in seizure screening tests.

Lamotrigine

Mechanism of Action

Lamotrigine, like phenytoin, suppresses sustained rapid firing of neurons and produces a voltage- and use-dependent inactivation of sodium channels. This action probably explains lamotrigine's efficacy in focal epilepsy. It appears likely that lamotrigine has another mechanism of action to account for its efficacy in primary generalized seizures in childhood, including absence attacks; this mechanism may involve actions on voltage-activated Ca^{2+} channels.

Clinical Use

Although most controlled studies have evaluated lamotrigine as add-on therapy, some also suggest that the drug is effective as monotherapy for partial seizures. Some authorities feel that the drug is also active against absence and myoclonic seizures in children. Adverse effects include dizziness, headache, diplopia, nausea, somnolence, and skin rash. The rash is considered a typical hypersensitivity reaction. Although the risk of rash may be diminished by introducing the drug slowly, pediatric patients are at high risk; some studies suggest that a potentially life-threatening dermatitis will develop in 1–2% of pediatric patients.

Pharmacokinetics & Dosage

Lamotrigine is almost completely absorbed and has a volume of distribution in the range of 1–1.4 L/kg. Protein binding is only about 55%. The drug has linear kinetics and is metabolized primarily by glucuronidation to the 2-*N*-glucuronide, which is excreted in the urine. Lamotrigine has a half-life of approximately 24 hours in normal volunteers; this decreases to 13–15 hours in patients taking enzyme-inducing drugs. Lamotrigine is effective against partial seizures in adults, with dosages typically between 100 mg/d and 300 mg/d and with a therapeutic blood level near 3 μg/mL. Valproate causes a twofold increase in the drug's half-life; in patients receiving valproate, the initial dosage of lamotrigine must be reduced to 25 mg every other day.

FELBAMATE

Felbamate has been approved and marketed in the USA and in some European countries. Although it is effective in some patients with partial seizures, the drug causes aplastic anemia and severe hepatitis at unexpectedly high rates and has been relegated to the status of a third-line drug for refractory cases.

Felbamate

The mechanism of action of felbamate is not established. The strongest evidence suggests NMDA receptor blockade via the glycine binding site. Felbamate has a half-life of 20 hours (somewhat shorter when administered with either phenytoin or carbamazepine) and is metabolized by hydroxylation and conjugation; a significant percentage of the drug is excreted unchanged in the urine. When added to treatment with other antiseizure drugs, felbamate increases plasma phenytoin and valproic acid levels but decreases levels of carbamazepine.

In spite of the seriousness of the adverse effects, more than 10,000 patients worldwide remain on the medica-

tion. Usual dosages are 2000–4000 mg/d in adults, and effective plasma levels range from 30 μg/mL to 100 μg/mL. In addition to its usefulness in partial seizures, felbamate has proved effective against the seizures that occur in Lennox-Gastaut syndrome.

GABAPENTIN

Gabapentin is an amino acid, an analog of GABA, that is effective against partial seizures. Originally planned as a spasmolytic, it was found to be more effective as an antiseizure drug.

GABA   **Gabapentin**

Mechanism of Action

In spite of its close structural relationship to GABA, gabapentin appears not to act on GABA receptors. It may, however, alter GABA metabolism, its nonsynaptic release, or its reuptake by GABA transporters. An increase in brain GABA concentration is observed in man. Gabapentin is transported into the brain by the L-amino acid transporter. Its anticonvulsant effect in the electroshock model is delayed relative to its peak plasma concentration. The drug also binds to the α2δ subunit of voltage-sensitive Ca^{2+} channels.

Clinical Use & Dosage

Gabapentin is effective as an adjunct against partial seizures and generalized tonic-clonic seizures at dosages that range up to 2400 mg/d in controlled clinical trials. Open follow-on studies permitted dosages up to 4800 mg/d, but data are inconclusive on the effectiveness or tolerability of such doses. Monotherapy studies also document some efficacy. Very high dosages have been needed by some clinicians to achieve improvement in seizure control. Effectiveness in other seizure types has not been well demonstrated. Gabapentin has also been found effective in the treatment of neuropathic pain and is now indicated for postherpetic neuralgia in adults at doses of 1800 mg and above. The most common adverse effects are somnolence, dizziness, ataxia, headache, and tremor.

Pharmacokinetics

Gabapentin is not metabolized and does not induce hepatic enzymes. Absorption is nonlinear and dose-dependent at very high doses, but otherwise the elimination kinetics are linear. The drug is not bound to plasma proteins. Drug-drug interactions are negligible. Elimination is via renal mechanisms; the drug is excreted unchanged. The half-life is short, ranging from 5 hours to 8 hours; the drug is typically administered two or three times per day.

TOPIRAMATE

Topiramate is a substituted monosaccharide that is structurally different from all other antiseizure drugs.

Topiramate

Mechanism of Action

Topiramate blocks repetitive firing of cultured spinal cord neurons, as do phenytoin and carbamazepine. Its mechanism of action, therefore, is likely to involve blocking of voltage-dependent sodium channels. Topiramate also appears to potentiate the inhibitory effect of GABA, acting at a site different from the benzodiazepine or barbiturate sites. Topiramate also depresses the excitatory action of kainate on AMPA receptors. It is possible that all three of these actions contribute to topiramate's anticonvulsant effect.

Clinical Use

Clinical trials of topiramate demonstrated a dose-response relationship, and monotherapy trials (using a pseudoplacebo) showed the drug to be effective against partial and generalized tonic-clonic seizures. Some evidence suggests that the drug has a broader spectrum, with effectiveness against Lennox-Gestaut syndrome, West's syndrome, and even absence seizures. Dosages typically ranged from 200 mg/d to 600 mg/d, with a few patients tolerating dosages greater than 1000 mg/d. Most clinicians begin slowly (50 mg/d) and increase slowly to avoid adverse effects. Although no idiosyncratic reactions have been noted, dose-related side effects occur most frequently in the first 4 weeks and include somnolence, fatigue, dizziness, cognitive slowing, paresthesias, nervousness, and confusion. Acute myopia and glaucoma may require prompt drug withdrawal. Urolithiasis has also been reported. However, the discontinuation rate is apparently only about 15%. The drug is teratogenic in animal models, but no human fetal deformities have been noted in the very few pregnancies that have occurred during the course of topiramate administration.

Pharmacokinetics

Topiramate is rapidly absorbed (about 2 hours) and is 80% bioavailable. There is no food effect on absorption, minimal (15%) plasma protein binding, and only moderate (20–50%) metabolism; no active metabolites are formed. The drug is primarily excreted unchanged in the urine. The half-life is about 20–30 hours. Although increased levels are seen with renal failure and hepatic impairment, there is no age or gender effect, no autoinduction, no inhibition of metabolism, and kinetics are linear. Drug interactions do occur and can be complex, but the major effect is on topiramate levels rather than on the levels of other antiseizure drugs. Birth control pills may be less effective in the presence of topiramate, and higher estrogen doses may be required.

TIAGABINE

Tiagabine is a derivative of nipecotic acid and was "rationally designed" as an inhibitor of GABA uptake (as opposed to discovery through random screening).

Tiagabine

Mechanism of Action

Tiagabine is an inhibitor of GABA uptake in both neurons and glia. It preferentially inhibits the transporter isoform 1 (GAT-1) rather than GAT-2 or GAT-3 and increases extracellular GABA levels in the forebrain and hippocampus. It prolongs the inhibitory action of synaptically released GABA. In rodents it is potent against kindled seizures but weak against the maximum electroshock model.

Clinical Use

Tiagabine is indicated for the adjunctive treatment of partial seizures and is effective in doses ranging from 16 mg/d to 56 mg/d. Divided doses as often as four times per day are sometimes required. Some patients appear to do well with tiagabine monotherapy, which is generally well tolerated. Minor adverse events are dose-related and include nervousness, dizziness, tremor, difficulty in concentrating, and depression. Excessive confusion, somnolence, or ataxia may require discontinuation. Psychosis occurs rarely. Rash is an uncommon idiosyncratic adverse effect. Laboratory studies are usually normal.

Pharmacokinetics

Tiagabine is 90–100% bioavailable, has linear kinetics, and is highly protein-bound. The half-life is 5–8 hours and decreases in the presence of enzyme-inducing drugs. Food decreases the peak plasma concentration but not the area under the concentration curve (see Chapter 3). Hepatic impairment causes a slight decrease in clearance (and may necessitate a lower dose), but the drug does not cause inhibition or induction of hepatic enzymes. The drug is oxidized in the liver by CYP3A. Elimination is primarily in the feces (60–65%) and urine (25%).

ZONISAMIDE

Zonisamide is a sulfonamide derivative. Its primary site of action appears to be on the sodium channel; it may also act on voltage-dependent calcium channels. The drug is effective against partial and generalized tonic-clonic seizures and may also be useful against infantile spasms and certain myoclonias. It has good bioavailability, linear kinetics, low protein-binding, renal excretion, and a half-life of 1–3 days. Doses range from 100 mg/d to 600 mg/d in adults and from 4 mg/d to 12 mg/d in children. Adverse effects include drowsiness, cognitive impairment, and potentially serious skin rashes. Zonisamide does not interact with other antiseizure drugs.

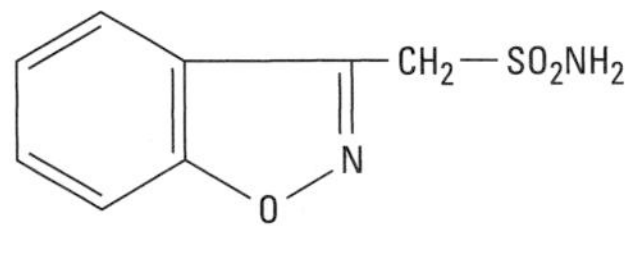

Zonisamide

LEVETIRACETAM

Levetiracetam is a piracetam analog that is ineffective against seizures induced by maximum electroshock or pentylenetetrazol but has prominent activity in the kindling model. Its mechanism of action is unknown. It has a brain-specific binding site and affects allosteric modulations of GABA receptors, high-voltage activated Ca^{2+} channels and some K^+ channels. The drug is marketed for the treatment of partial seizures. Oral absorption is nearly complete; it is rapid and unaffected by food, with peak plasma concentrations in 1.3 hours. Kinetics are linear. Protein binding is less than 10%. The plasma half-life is 6–8 hours, and may be longer in the elderly. Two thirds of the drug is excreted unchanged in the urine. Drug interactions are minimal; levetiracetam is not metabolized by cytochrome P450. Dosing can begin with 500 mg orally twice daily; some patients require up to 3000 mg/d. Adverse effects include somnolence, asthenia, and dizziness. Idiosyncratic reactions are rare.

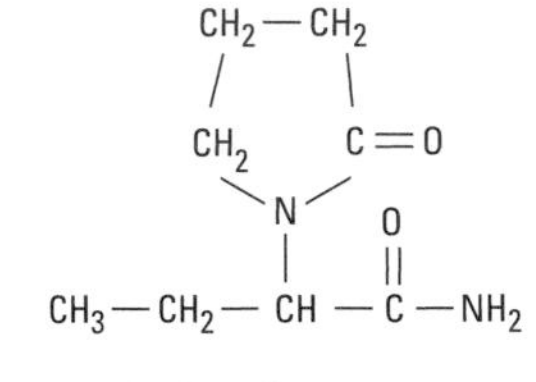

Levetiracetam

DRUGS USED IN GENERALIZED SEIZURES

ETHOSUXIMIDE

Ethosuximide was introduced in 1960 as the third of three marketed succinimides in the USA. Ethosuximide has very little activity against maximal electroshock but considerable efficacy against pentylenetetrazol seizures and was introduced as a "pure petit mal" drug. Its continued popularity is based on its safety and efficacy, and its role as the first choice anti-absence drug remains undiminished—in part because of the idiosyncratic hepatotoxicity of the alternative drug, valproic acid.

Chemistry

Ethosuximide is the last antiseizure drug to be marketed whose origin is in the cyclic ureide structure. The three antiseizure succinimides marketed in the USA are ethosuximide, phensuximide, and methsuximide. All three are substituted at the 2 position. (See structure below, and note the difference in numbering relative to Figure 24–1.) Methsuximide and phensuximide have phenyl substituents, while ethosuximide is 2-ethyl-2-methyl-succinimide.

Ethosuximide

Mechanism of Action

Ethosuximide has an important effect on Ca^{2+} currents, reducing the low-threshold (T-type) current. This effect is seen at therapeutically relevant concentrations in thalamic neurons. The T-type calcium currents are thought to provide a pacemaker current in thalamic neurons responsible for generating the rhythmic cortical discharge of an absence attack. Inhibition of this current could therefore account for the specific therapeutic action of ethosuximide. Ethosuximide also inhibits Na^+/K^+ ATPase, depresses the cerebral metabolic rate, and inhibits GABA aminotransferase. However, none of these actions are seen at therapeutic concentrations.

Clinical Use

As predicted from its activity in laboratory models, ethosuximide is particularly effective against absence seizures. Documentation of its effectiveness required specific advances in quantitation of absence seizures; this was accomplished in the 1970s, when the characteristic generalized 3/s spike-wave electroencephalographic abnormality was correlated with a decrement in consciousness even when the abnormality occurs for only a few seconds. Long-term electroencephalographic recordings, therefore, provided the necessary quantitative method for determining the frequency of absence attacks and allowed rapid and effective evaluation of the efficacy of anti-absence drugs. Although ethosuximide was marketed in advance of the federal requirements for efficacy, these techniques were applied to later drugs such as clonazepam and valproic acid in documentation of their efficacy. This was accomplished by comparison with ethosuximide.

Pharmacokinetics

Absorption is complete following administration of the oral dosage forms. Peak levels are observed 3–7 hours after oral administration of the capsules. Animal studies indicate that chronic administration of the solution may prove irritating to the gastric mucosa. Ethosuximide is uniformly distributed in total body water, ie, 0.7 L/kg and does not penetrate fat. Ethosuximide is not protein-bound, and spinal fluid concentrations are therefore equal to plasma concentrations.

Ethosuximide is completely metabolized, principally by hydroxylation, to inactive metabolites. The drug has a very low total body clearance (0.25 L/kg/d). This corresponds to a half-life of approximately 40 hours, although values from 18 to 72 hours have been reported.

Therapeutic Levels & Dosage

Therapeutic levels of 60–100 µg/mL can be achieved in adults with dosages of 750–1500 mg/d, although lower or higher dosages and blood levels may be necessary and tolerated (up to 125 µg/mL) in some patients. Ethosuximide has a linear relationship between dose and steady-state plasma levels. The drug might be administered as a single daily dose were it not for its adverse gastrointestinal effects; twice-a-day dosage is common.

Drug Interactions

Administration of ethosuximide with valproic acid results in a decrease in ethosuximide clearance and higher steady-state concentrations owing to inhibition of metabolism. No other important drug interactions have been reported for the succinimides.

Toxicity

The most common dose-related adverse effect of ethosuximide is gastric distress, including pain, nausea, and vomiting. This can often be avoided by starting therapy at a low dose, with gradual increases into the therapeutic range. When the adverse effect does occur, temporary dosage reductions may allow adaptation. Ethosuximide is a highly efficacious and safe drug for absence seizures; the appearance of relatively mild, dose-related adverse effects should not immediately call for its abandonment. Other dose-related adverse effects include transient lethargy or fatigue and, much less commonly, headache, dizziness, hiccup, and euphoria. Behavioral changes are usually in the direction of improvement.

Non-dose-related or idiosyncratic adverse effects of ethosuximide are extremely uncommon. Skin rashes have been reported, including at least one case of Stevens-Johnson syndrome. A few patients have had eosinophilia, thrombocytopenia, leukopenia, or pancytopenia; it is not entirely certain that ethosuximide was the causal agent. The development of systemic lupus erythematosus has also been reported, but other drugs may have been involved.

PHENSUXIMIDE & METHSUXIMIDE

Phensuximide and methsuximide are phenylsuccinimides that were developed and marketed before ethosuximide. They are used primarily as anti-absence drugs. Methsuximide is generally considered more toxic, and phensuximide less effective, than ethosuximide. Unlike ethosuximide, these two compounds have some activity against maximal electroshock seizures, and methsuximide has been used for partial seizures by some investigators. The desmethyl metabolite of methsuximide has a half-life of 25 hours or more and exerts the major antiseizure effect. The toxicity and reduced effectiveness of phensuximide when compared with methsuximide has been investigated, and the failure of the desmethyl metabolite to accumulate in the former probably explains its relatively weak effect.

VALPROIC ACID & SODIUM VALPROATE

Sodium valproate, also used as the free acid, valproic acid, was found to have antiseizure properties when it was used as a solvent in the search for other drugs effective against seizures. It was marketed in France in 1969 but was not licensed in the USA until 1978. Valproic acid is fully ionized at body pH, and for that reason the active form of the drug may be assumed to be the valproate ion regardless of whether valproic acid or a salt of the acid is administered.

Chemistry

Valproic acid is one of a series of fatty carboxylic acids that have antiseizure activity; this activity appears to be greatest for carbon chain lengths of five to eight atoms. Branching and unsaturation do not significantly alter the drug's activity but may increase its lipophilicity, thereby increasing its duration of action. The amides and esters of valproic acid are also active antiseizure agents.

$$CH_3-CH_2-CH_2 \atop CH_3-CH_2-CH_2 \Big\rangle CH-COOH$$

Valproic acid

Mechanism of Action

The time course of valproate's anticonvulsant activity appears to be poorly correlated with blood or tissue levels of the parent drug, an observation giving rise to considerable speculation regarding both the active species and the mechanism of action of valproic acid. Valproate is active against both pentylenetetrazol and maximal electroshock seizures. Like phenytoin and carbamazepine, valproate blocks sustained high-frequency repetitive firing of neurons in culture at therapeutically relevant concentrations. Its action against partial seizures may be a consequence of this effect on Na^+ currents. Blockade of NMDA receptor-mediated excitation may also be important. Much attention has been paid to

the effects of valproate on GABA. Several studies have shown increased levels of GABA in the brain after administration of valproate, although the mechanism for this increase remains unclear. An effect of valproate to facilitate glutamic acid decarboxylase (GAD), the enzyme responsible for GABA synthesis, has been described. An inhibitory effect on the GABA transporter GAT-1 may contribute. At very high concentrations, valproate inhibits GABA-T in the brain, thus blocking degradation of GABA. However, at the relatively low doses of valproate needed to abolish pentylenetetrazol seizures, brain GABA levels may remain unchanged. Valproate produces a reduction in the aspartate content of rodent brain, but the relevance of this effect to its anticonvulsant action is not known.

At high concentrations, valproate has been shown to increase membrane potassium conductance. Furthermore, low concentrations of valproate tend to hyperpolarize membrane potentials. These findings have led to speculation that valproate may exert an action through a direct effect on the potassium channels of the membrane.

Valproate probably owes its broad spectrum of action to more than one molecular mechanism. Its action against absence attacks remains to be explained.

Clinical Use

Valproate is very effective against absence seizures. Although ethosuximide is the drug of choice when absence seizures occur alone, valproate is preferred if the patient has concomitant generalized tonic-clonic attacks. The reason for preferring ethosuximide for uncomplicated absence seizures is valproate's idiosyncratic hepatotoxicity, described below. Valproate is unique in its ability to control certain types of myoclonic seizures; in some cases the effect is very dramatic. The drug is effective in generalized tonic-clonic seizures, especially those which are primarily generalized. A few patients with atonic attacks may also respond, and some evidence suggests that the drug is effective in partial seizures.

Other uses of valproate include management of bipolar disorder and migraine prophylaxis.

Pharmacokinetics

Valproate is well absorbed following an oral dose, with bioavailability greater than 80%. Peak blood levels are observed within 2 hours. Food may delay absorption, and decreased toxicity may result if the drug is given after meals.

Valproic acid is 90% bound to plasma proteins, although the fraction bound is somewhat reduced at blood levels greater than 150 μg/mL. Since valproate is both highly ionized and highly protein-bound, its distribution is essentially confined to extracellular water, with a volume of distribution of approximately 0.15 L/kg.

Clearance for valproate is low; its half-life varies from 9 hours to 18 hours. At very high blood levels, the clearance of valproate is dose-dependent. There appear to be offsetting changes in the intrinsic clearance and protein binding at higher doses. Approximately 20% of the drug is excreted as a direct conjugate of valproate.

The sodium salt of valproate is marketed in Europe as a tablet protected by aluminum foil, as it is quite hygroscopic. In Central and South America, the magnesium salt is available, which is considerably less hygroscopic. The free acid of valproate was first marketed in the USA in a capsule containing corn oil; the sodium salt is also available in syrup, primarily for pediatric use. An enteric-coated tablet of divalproex sodium is also marketed in the USA. This improved product, a 1:1 coordination compound of valproic acid and sodium valproate, is as bioavailable as the capsule but is absorbed much more slowly and is preferred by most patients. Peak concentrations following administration of the enteric-coated tablets are seen in 3–4 hours.

Therapeutic Levels & Dosage

Dosages of 25–30 mg/kg/d may be adequate in some patients, but others may require 60 mg/kg/d or even more. Therapeutic levels of valproate range from 50 μg/mL to 100 μg/mL. In testing efficacy, this drug should not be abandoned until morning trough levels of at least 80 μg/mL have been attained; some patients may require and tolerate trough levels in excess of 100 μg/mL.

Drug Interactions

As noted above, the clearance of valproate is dose-dependent, caused by changes in both the intrinsic clearance and protein binding. Valproate inhibits its own metabolism at low doses, thus decreasing intrinsic clearance. At higher doses, there is an increased free fraction of valproate, resulting in lower total drug levels than expected. It may be clinically useful, therefore, to measure both total and free drug levels. Valproate also displaces phenytoin from plasma proteins. In addition to binding interactions, valproate inhibits the metabolism of several drugs, including phenobarbital, phenytoin, and carbamazepine, leading to higher steady-state concentrations of these agents. The side effects and toxicity of phenytoin are enhanced. The inhibition of phenobarbital metabolism may cause levels of the barbiturate to rise precipitously, causing stupor or coma.

Toxicity

The most common dose-related adverse effects of valproate are nausea, vomiting, and other gastrointestinal complaints such as abdominal pain and heartburn. The drug should be started gradually to avoid these symptoms; a temporary reduction in dose can usually alleviate the problems, and the patient will eventually tolerate higher doses. Sedation is uncommon with valproate alone but may be striking when valproate is added to phenobarbital. A fine tremor is frequently seen at higher levels. Other reversible adverse effects, seen in a small number of patients, include weight gain, increased appetite, and hair loss.

The idiosyncratic toxicity of valproate is largely limited to hepatotoxicity, but this may be severe; there seems little doubt that the hepatotoxicity of valproate has been responsible for more than 50 fatalities in the USA alone. The risk is greatest for patients under the age of 2 years and for those taking multiple medications. Initial aspartate aminotransferase values may not be elevated in susceptible patients, although these levels do eventually become abnormal. Most fatalities have occurred within 4 months after initiation of therapy. Careful monitoring of liver function is recommended when starting the drug; the hepatotoxicity is reversible in some cases if the drug is withdrawn. The other observed idiosyncratic response with valproate is thrombocytopenia, although documented cases of abnormal bleeding are lacking. It should be noted that valproate is an effective and popular antiseizure drug and that only a very small number of patients have had severe toxic effects from its use.

Epidemiologic studies of valproate suggest an increased incidence of spina bifida in the offspring of women who took the drug during pregnancy. In addition, an increased incidence of cardiovascular, orofacial, and digital abnormalities has been reported. These observations, although based on a small number of cases, must be strongly considered in the choice of drugs during pregnancy.

OXAZOLIDINEDIONES

Trimethadione, the first oxazolidinedione, was introduced as an antiseizure drug in 1945 and remained the drug of choice for absence seizures until the introduction of succinimides in the 1950s. The use of the oxazolidinediones (trimethadione, paramethadione, and dimethadione) is now very limited.

Chemistry

The oxazolidinediones contain an oxazolidine heterocyclic ring (Figure 24–1) and are similar in structure to other antiseizure drugs introduced before 1960. The structure includes only short-chain alkyl substituents on the heterocyclic ring, with no attached phenyl group.

Trimethadione

Mechanism of Action

These compounds are active against pentylenetetrazol-induced seizures. Trimethadione raises the threshold for seizure discharges following repetitive thalamic stimulation. It—or, more notably, its active metabolite dimethadione—has the same effect on thalamic Ca^{2+} currents as ethosuximide (reducing the T-type calcium current). Thus, suppression of absence seizures is likely to depend on inhibiting the pacemaker action of thalamic neurons.

Pharmacokinetics

Trimethadione is rapidly absorbed, with peak levels reached within an hour after drug administration. It is distributed to all perfused tissues, with a volume of distribution that approximates that of total body water. It is not bound to plasma proteins. Trimethadione is completely metabolized in the liver by demethylation to 5,5-dimethyl-2,4-oxazolidinedione (dimethadione), which may exert the major antiseizure activity. The clearance of dimethadione is 0.08 L/kg/d; this metabolite has an extremely long half-life (240 hours).

Therapeutic Levels & Dosage

The therapeutic plasma level range for trimethadione has never been established, although trimethadione blood levels above 20 μg/mL and dimethadione levels above 700 μg/mL have been suggested. A dosage of 30 mg/kg/d of trimethadione is necessary to achieve these levels in adults.

Drug Interactions

Relatively few drug interactions involving the oxazolidinediones have been reported, although trimethadione may competitively inhibit the demethylation of other drugs such as metharbital.

Toxicity

The most common and bothersome dose-related adverse effect of the oxazolidinediones is sedation. An unusual adverse effect is hemeralopia, a glare effect in which visual adaptation is impaired; it is reversible upon withdrawal of the drug. Accumulation of dimethadione has been reported to cause a very mild metabolic acidosis. Trimethadione has been associated with many other toxic adverse effects, some of which are severe. These drugs should not be used during pregnancy.

OTHER DRUGS USED IN MANAGEMENT OF EPILEPSY

Some drugs not classifiable by application to seizure type are discussed in this section.

BENZODIAZEPINES

Six benzodiazepines play prominent roles in the therapy of epilepsy (see also Chapter 22). Although many benzodiazepines are quite similar chemically, subtle structural alterations result in differences in activity. They have two different mechanisms of antiseizure action, which are shown to different degrees by the six compounds. This is evident from the fact that diazepam is relatively more potent against electroshock and clonazepam against pentylenetetrazol (the latter effect correlating with an action at the GABA-benzodiazepine allosteric receptor site). Possible mechanisms of action are discussed in Chapter 22.

Diazepam given intravenously or rectally is highly effective for stopping continuous seizure activity, especially generalized tonic-clonic status epilepticus (see below). The drug is occasionally given orally on a chronic basis, although it is not considered very effective in this application, probably because of the rapid development of tolerance. A rectal gel is available for refractory patients who need acute control of bouts of seizure activity. **Lorazepam** appears in some studies to be more effective and longer-acting than diazepam in the treatment of status epilepticus.

Clonazepam is a long-acting drug with documented efficacy against absence seizures; it is one of the most potent antiseizure agents known. It is also effective in some cases of myoclonic seizures and has been tried in infantile spasms. Sedation is prominent, especially on initiation of therapy; starting doses should be small. Maximal tolerated doses are usually in the range of 0.1–0.2 mg/kg, but many weeks of gradually increasing daily dosage may be needed to achieve these doses in some patients. Therapeutic blood levels are usually less than 0.1 μg/mL and are not routinely measured in most laboratories. **Nitrazepam** is not marketed in the USA but is used in many other countries, especially for infantile spasms and myoclonic seizures. It is less potent than clonazepam, and its clinical advantages over that drug have not been documented.

Clorazepate dipotassium is approved in the USA as an adjunct to treatment of complex partial seizures in adults. Drowsiness and lethargy are common adverse effects, but as long as the drug is increased gradually, dosages as high as 45 mg/d can be given.

Clobazam is not available in the USA but is marketed in most countries and is widely used in a variety of seizure types. It is a 1,5-benzodiazepine (all other marketed benzodiazepines are 1,4-benzodiazepines) and reportedly has less sedative potential than benzodiazepines marketed in the USA. Whether the drug has significant clinical advantages is not clear. It has a half-life of 18 hours and is effective at dosages of 0.5–1 mg/kg/d. It does interact with some other antiseizure drugs and causes adverse effects typical of the benzodiazepines; efficacy, in some patients, is limited by the development of tolerance.

Pharmacokinetics

The pharmacokinetic properties of the benzodiazepines in part determine their clinical use. In general, the drugs are well absorbed, widely distributed, and extensively metabolized, with many active metabolites. The rate of distribution of benzodiazepines within the body is different from that of other antiseizure drugs. Diazepam and lorazepam in particular are rapidly and extensively distributed to the tissues, with volumes of distribution between 1 L/kg and 3 L/kg. The onset of action is very rapid. Total body clearances of the parent drug and its metabolites are low, corresponding to half-lives of 20–40 hours.

Limitations

Two prominent aspects of benzodiazepines limit their usefulness. The first is their pronounced sedative effect, which is unfortunate both in the treatment of status epilepticus and in chronic therapy. Children may manifest a paradoxical hyperactivity, as with barbiturates. The second problem is tolerance, in which seizures may respond initially but recur within a few months. The remarkable antiseizure potency of these compounds often cannot be realized because of these limiting factors.

ACETAZOLAMIDE

Acetazolamide is a diuretic whose main action is the inhibition of carbonic anhydrase (see Chapter 15). Mild acidosis in the brain may be the mechanism by which the drug exerts its antiseizure activity; alternatively, the depolarizing action of bicarbonate ions moving out of neurons via GABA receptor ion channels will be diminished by carbonic anhydrase inhibition. Acetazolamide has been used for all types of seizures but is severely limited by the rapid development of tolerance, with return of seizures usually within a few weeks. The drug may have a special role in epileptic women who experience seizure exacerbations at the time of menses; seizure control may be improved and tolerance may not develop because the drug is not administered continuously. The usual dosage is approximately 10 mg/kg/d up to a maximum of 1000 mg/d.

Another carbonic anhydrase inhibitor, **sulthiame,** was not found to be effective as an anticonvulsant in clinical trials in the USA. It is marketed in some other countries.

II. CLINICAL PHARMACOLOGY OF ANTISEIZURE DRUGS

SEIZURE CLASSIFICATION

The type of medication utilized for epilepsy depends on the empiric nature of the seizure. For this reason, considerable effort has been expended to classify seizures so that clinicians will be able to make a "seizure diagnosis" and on that basis prescribe appropriate therapy. Errors in seizure diagnosis cause use of the wrong drugs, and an unpleasant cycle ensues in which poor seizure control is followed by increasing drug doses and medication toxicity. As noted above, seizures are divided into two groups: partial and generalized. Drugs used for partial seizures are more or less the same for the entire group, but drugs used for generalized seizures are determined by the individual seizure type. A summary of the international classification of epileptic seizures is presented in Table 24–1.

Partial Seizures

Partial seizures are those in which a localized onset of the attack can be ascertained, either by clinical observation or by electroencephalographic recording; the attack begins in a specific locus in the brain. There are three types of partial seizures, determined to some extent by the degree of brain involvement by the abnormal discharge.

The least complicated partial seizure is the **simple partial seizure,** characterized by minimal spread of the abnormal discharge such that normal consciousness and awareness are preserved. For example, the patient may have a sudden onset of clonic jerking of an extremity lasting 60–90 seconds; residual weakness may last for 15–30 minutes after the attack. The patient is completely aware of the attack and can describe it in detail. The electroencephalogram may show an abnormal discharge highly localized to the involved portion of the brain.

The **complex partial seizure** also has a localized onset, but the discharge becomes more widespread (usually bilateral) and almost always involves the limbic system. Most (not all) complex partial seizures arise from one of the temporal lobes, possibly because of the susceptibility of this area of the brain to insults such as hypoxia or infection. Clinically, the patient may have a brief warning followed by an alteration of consciousness during which some patients may stare and others may stagger or even fall. Most, however, demonstrate fragments of integrated motor behavior called automatisms for which the patient has no memory. Typical automatisms are lip smacking, swallowing, fumbling, scratching, or even walking about. After 30–120 seconds, the patient makes a gradual recovery to normal consciousness but may feel tired or ill for several hours after the attack.

The last type of partial seizure is the **secondarily generalized attack,** in which a partial seizure immediately precedes a generalized tonic-clonic (grand mal) seizure. This seizure type is described below.

Generalized Seizures

Generalized seizures are those in which there is no evidence of localized onset. The group is quite heterogeneous.

Generalized tonic-clonic (grand mal) seizures are the most dramatic of all epileptic seizures and are characterized by tonic rigidity of all extremities, followed in 15–30 seconds by a tremor that is actually an interruption of the tonus by relaxation. As the relaxation phases become longer, the attack enters the clonic phase, with massive jerking of the body. The clonic jerking slows over 60–120 seconds, and the patient is usually left in a stuporous state. The tongue or cheek may be bitten, and urinary incontinence is common. Primary generalized tonic-clonic seizures begin without evidence of localized onset, whereas secondary generalized tonic-clonic seizures are preceded by another seizure type, usually a partial seizure. The medical treatment of both primary and secondary generalized tonic-clonic seizures is the same and uses drugs appropriate for *partial* seizures.

The **absence (petit mal) seizure** is characterized by both sudden onset and abrupt cessation. Its duration is usually less than 10 seconds and rarely more than 45 seconds. Consciousness is altered; the attack may also be associated with mild clonic jerking of the eyelids or extremities, with postural tone changes, autonomic phenomena, and automatisms. The occurrence of automatisms can complicate the clinical differentiation from complex partial seizures in some patients. Absence attacks begin in childhood or adolescence and may occur up to hundreds of times a day. The electroencephalogram during the seizure shows a highly characteristic 2.5–3.5 Hz spike-and-wave pattern. Atypical absence patients have seizures with postural changes that are more abrupt, and such patients are often men-

tally retarded; the electroencephalogram may show a slower spike-and-wave discharge, and the seizures may be more refractory to therapy.

Myoclonic jerking is seen, to a greater or lesser extent, in a wide variety of seizures, including generalized tonic-clonic seizures, partial seizures, absence seizures, and infantile spasms. Treatment of seizures that include myoclonic jerking should be directed at the primary seizure type rather than at the myoclonus. Some patients, however, have myoclonic jerking as the major seizure type, and some have frequent myoclonic jerking and occasional generalized tonic-clonic seizures without overt signs of neurologic deficit. Many kinds of myoclonus exist, and much effort has gone into attempts to classify this entity.

Atonic seizures are those in which the patient has sudden loss of postural tone. If standing, the patient falls suddenly to the floor and may be injured. If seated, the head and torso may suddenly drop forward. Although most often seen in children, this seizure type is not unusual in adults. Many patients with atonic seizures wear helmets to prevent head injury.

Infantile spasms are an epileptic syndrome and not a seizure type. The attacks, although sometimes fragmentary, are most often bilateral and are included for pragmatic purposes with the generalized seizures. These attacks are most often characterized clinically by brief, recurrent myoclonic jerks of the body with sudden flexion or extension of the body and limbs; the forms of infantile spasms are, however, quite heterogeneous. Ninety percent of affected patients have their first attack before the age of 1 year. Most patients are mentally retarded, presumably from the same cause as the spasms. The cause is unknown in many patients, but such widely disparate disorders as infection, kernicterus, tuberous sclerosis, and hypoglycemia have been implicated. In some cases, the electroencephalogram is characteristic. Drugs used to treat infantile spasms are effective only in some patients; there is little evidence that the mental retardation is alleviated by therapy, even when the attacks disappear.

THERAPEUTIC STRATEGY

For most antiseizure drugs, relationships between blood levels and therapeutic effects have been characterized to a high degree. The same is true for the pharmacokinetics of these drugs. These relationships provide significant advantages in the development of therapeutic strategies for the treatment of epilepsy. The therapeutic index for most antiseizure drugs is low, and toxicity is not uncommon. Thus, effective treatment of seizures requires an awareness of the therapeutic levels and pharmacokinetic properties as well as the characteristic toxicities of each agent. Measurements of antiseizure drug plasma levels are extremely useful when combined with clinical observations and pharmacokinetic data (Table 24–2).

MANAGEMENT OF EPILEPSY

PARTIAL SEIZURES & GENERALIZED TONIC-CLONIC SEIZURES

Until recently, the choice of drugs was usually limited to phenytoin, carbamazepine, or barbiturates. There has been a strong tendency in the past few years to limit the use of sedative antiseizure drugs such as barbiturates and benzodiazepines to patients who cannot tolerate other medications. In the 1980s, the trend was to increase the use of carbamazepine. Although the choice now appears to be divided between carbamazepine and phenytoin, all of the newer drugs have shown effectiveness against these seizures. The exact role of these drugs remains to be determined, making decisions for the individual patient more complex.

GENERALIZED SEIZURES

The drugs used for generalized tonic-clonic seizures are the same as for partial seizures; in addition, valproate is clearly useful.

Three drugs are effective against absence seizures. Two are nonsedating and therefore preferred: ethosuximide and valproate. Clonazepam is also highly effective

Table 24–2. Effective plasma levels of six antiseizure drugs.[1]

Drug	Effective Level (μg/mL)	High Effective Level[2] (μg/mL)	Toxic Level (μg/mL)
Carbamazepine	4–12	7	> 8
Primidone	5–15	10	< 12
Phenytoin	10–20	18	> 20
Phenobarbital	10–40	35	> 40
Ethosuximide	50–100	80	> 100
Valproate	50–100	80	> 100

[1]Reprinted, with permission, from Porter RJ: *Epilepsy: 100 Elementary Principles,* 2nd ed. Saunders, 1989.

[2]Level that should be achieved, if possible, in patients with refractory seizures, assuming that the blood samples are drawn before administration of the morning medication. Higher levels are often possible—without toxicity—when the drugs are used alone, ie, as monotherapy.

but has disadvantages of dose-related adverse effects and development of tolerance. The drug of choice is ethosuximide, although valproate is effective in some ethosuximide-resistant patients. Lamotrigine and topiramate may also be useful.

Specific myoclonic syndromes are usually treated with valproate; an intravenous formulation can be used acutely as needed. It is nonsedating and can be dramatically effective. Other patients respond to clonazepam, nitrazepam, or other benzodiazepines, although high doses may be necessary, with accompanying sedation and drowsiness. Zonisamide and levetiracetam may be useful. Another specific myoclonic syndrome, juvenile myoclonic epilepsy, can be aggravated by phenytoin or carbamazepine; valproate is the drug of choice followed by lamotrigine and topiramate.

Atonic seizures are often refractory to all available medications, although some reports suggest that valproate may be beneficial, as may lamotrigine. Benzodiazepines have been reported to improve seizure control in some of these patients but may worsen the attacks in others. Felbamate has been demonstrated to be effective in some patients, although the drug's idiosyncratic toxicity limits its use. If the loss of tone appears to be part of another seizure type (such as absence or complex partial seizures), every effort should be made to treat the other seizure type vigorously, hoping for simultaneous alleviation of the atonic component of the seizure. The ketogenic diet may also be useful.

DRUGS USED IN INFANTILE SPASMS

The treatment of infantile spasms is unfortunately limited to improvement of control of the seizures rather than other features of the disorder, such as retardation. Most patients receive a course of intramuscular corticotropin, although some clinicians note that prednisone may be equally effective and can be given orally. Clinical trials have been unable to settle the matter. In either case, therapy must often be discontinued because of adverse effects. If seizures recur, repeat courses of corticotropin or corticosteroids can be given, or other drugs may be tried. Other drugs widely used are the benzodiazepines such as clonazepam or nitrazepam; their efficacy in this heterogeneous syndrome may be nearly as good as that of corticosteroids. Vigabatrin may also be effective. The mechanism of action of corticosteroids or corticotropin in the treatment of infantile spasms is unknown. Further details may be sought in more specialized texts.

STATUS EPILEPTICUS

There are many forms of status epilepticus. The most common, generalized tonic-clonic status epilepticus, is a life-threatening emergency, requiring immediate cardiovascular, respiratory, and metabolic management as well as pharmacologic therapy. The latter virtually always requires intravenous administration of antiseizure medications. Diazepam is the most effective drug in most patients for stopping the attacks and is given directly by intravenous push to a maximum total dose of 20–30 mg in adults. Intravenous diazepam may depress respiration (less frequently, cardiovascular function), and facilities for resuscitation must be immediately at hand during its administration. The effect of diazepam is not lasting, but the 30- to 40-minute seizure-free interval allows more definitive therapy to be initiated. For patients who are not actually in the throes of a seizure, diazepam therapy can be omitted and the patient treated at once with a long-acting drug such as phenytoin. Some physicians prefer lorazepam, which is equivalent to diazepam in effect and perhaps somewhat longer-acting.

Until the introduction of fosphenytoin, the mainstay of continuing therapy for status epilepticus was intravenous phenytoin, which is effective and nonsedating. It should be given as a loading dose of 13–18 mg/kg in adults; the usual error is to give too little. Administration should be at a maximum rate of 50 mg/min. It is safest to give the drug directly by intravenous push, but it can also be diluted in saline; it precipitates rapidly in the presence of glucose. Careful monitoring of cardiac rhythm and blood pressure is necessary, especially in elderly people. At least part of the cardiotoxicity is from the propylene glycol in which the phenytoin is dissolved. Fosphenytoin, which is freely soluble in intravenous solutions without the need for propylene glycol or other solubilizing agents, is a better parenteral agent. Because of its greater molecular weight, this prodrug is two thirds to three quarters as potent as phenytoin on a milligram basis.

In previously treated epileptic patients, the administration of a large loading dose of phenytoin may cause some dose-related toxicity such as ataxia. This is usually a relatively minor problem during the acute status episode and is easily alleviated by later adjustment of plasma levels.

For patients who do not respond to phenytoin, phenobarbital can be given in large doses: 100–200 mg intravenously to a total of 400–800 mg. Respiratory depression is a common complication, especially if benzodiazepines have already been given, and there should be no hesitation in instituting intubation and ventilation.

Although other drugs such as lidocaine have been recommended for the treatment of generalized tonic-clonic status epilepticus, general anesthesia is usually necessary in highly resistant cases.

For patients in absence status, benzodiazepines are still drugs of first choice. Rarely, intravenous valproate may be required.

SPECIAL ASPECTS OF THE TOXICOLOGY OF ANTISEIZURE DRUGS

TERATOGENICITY

The potential teratogenicity of antiseizure drugs is controversial and important. It is important because teratogenicity resulting from long-term drug treatment of millions of people throughout the world may have a profound effect even if the effect occurs in only a small percentage of cases. It is controversial because both epilepsy and antiseizure drugs are heterogeneous, and few epileptic patients are available for study who are not receiving these drugs. Furthermore, patients with severe epilepsy, in whom genetic factors rather than drug factors may be of greater importance in the occurrence of fetal malformations, are often receiving multiple antiseizure drugs in high doses.

In spite of these limitations, it appears—from whatever cause—that children born to mothers taking antiseizure drugs have an increased risk, perhaps twofold, of congenital malformations. Phenytoin has been implicated in a specific syndrome called **fetal hydantoin syndrome,** although not all investigators are convinced of its existence and a similar syndrome has been attributed both to phenobarbital and to carbamazepine. Valproate, as noted above, has also been implicated in a specific malformation, spina bifida. It is estimated that a pregnant woman taking valproic acid or sodium valproate has a 1–2% risk of having a child with spina bifida. Topiramate has shown some teratogenicity in animal testing.

In dealing with the clinical problem of a pregnant woman with epilepsy, most epileptologists agree that while it is important to minimize exposure to antiseizure drugs, both in numbers and dosages, it is also important not to allow maternal seizures to go unchecked.

WITHDRAWAL

Withdrawal of antiseizure drugs, whether by accident or by design, can cause increased seizure frequency and severity. There are two factors to consider: the effects of the withdrawal itself and the need for continued drug suppression of seizures in the individual patient. In many patients, both factors must be considered. It is important to note, however, that the abrupt discontinuance of antiseizure drugs ordinarily does not cause seizures in nonepileptic patients provided the drug levels are not above the usual therapeutic range when the drug is stopped.

Some drugs are more easily withdrawn than others.

In general, withdrawal of anti-absence drugs is easier than withdrawal of drugs needed for partial or generalized tonic-clonic seizures. Barbiturates and benzodiazepines are the most difficult to discontinue; weeks or months may be required, with very gradual dosage decrements, to accomplish their complete removal, especially if the patient is not hospitalized.

Because of the heterogeneity of epilepsy, complete discontinuance of antiseizure drug administration is an especially difficult problem. If a patient is seizure-free for 3 or 4 years, gradual discontinuance is usually warranted.

OVERDOSE

Antiseizure drugs are central nervous system depressants but are rarely lethal. Very high blood levels are usually necessary before overdoses can be considered life-threatening. The most dangerous effect of antiseizure drugs after large overdoses is respiratory depression, which may be potentiated by other agents, such as alcohol. Treatment of antiseizure drug overdose is supportive; stimulants should not be used. Efforts to hasten removal of antiseizure drugs, such as alkalinization of the urine (phenytoin is a weak acid), are usually ineffective.

PREPARATIONS AVAILABLE

Carbamazepine (generic, Tegretol)
Oral: 200 mg tablets; 100 mg chewable tablets; 100 mg/5 mL suspension
Oral extended-release: 100, 200, 400 mg tablets; 200, 300 mg capsules

Clonazepam (generic, Klonopin)
Oral: 0.5, 1, 2 mg tablets

Clorazepate dipotassium (generic, Tranxene)
Oral: 3.75, 7.5, 15 mg tablets, capsules
Oral sustained-release (Tranxene-SD): 11.25, 22.5 mg tablets

Diazepam (generic, Valium, others)
Oral: 2, 5, 10 mg tablets; 5 mg/5 mL, 5 mg/mL solutions
Parenteral: 5 mg/mL for IV injection
Rectal: 2.5, 5, 10, 15, 20 mg diazepam viscous rectal solution

Ethosuximide (generic, Zarontin)
Oral: 250 mg capsules; 250 mg/5 mL syrup

Ethotoin (Peganone)
Oral: 250, 500 mg tablets

Felbamate (Felbatol)
Oral: 400, 600 mg tablets; 600 mg/5 mL suspension

Fosphenytoin (Cerebyx)
Parenteral: 75 mg/mL for IV or IM injection

Gabapentin (Neurontin)
Oral: 100, 300, 400 mg capsules; 600, 800 mg filmtabs; 50 mg/mL solution

Lamotrigine (Lamictal)
Oral: 25, 100, 150, 200 mg tablets; 2, 5, 25 mg chewable tablets

Levetiracetam (Keppra)
Oral: 250, 500, 750 mg tablets

Lorazepam (generic, Ativan)
Oral: 0.5, 1, 2 mg tablets; 2 mg/mL solution
Parenteral: 2, 4 mg/mL for IV or IM injection

Mephenytoin (Mesantoin)
Oral: 100 mg tablets

Mephobarbital (Mebaral)
Oral: 32, 50, 100 mg tablets

Oxycarbazepine (Trileptal)
Oral: 100, 300, 600 mg tablets; 60 mg/mL suspension

Pentobarbital sodium (generic, Nembutal)
Parenteral: 50 mg/mL for IV or IM injection

Phenobarbital (generic, Luminal Sodium, others)
Oral: 15, 16, 30, 60, 90, 100 mg tablets; 16 mg capsules; 15, 20 mg/5 mL elixirs
Parenteral: 30, 60, 65, 130 mg/mL for IV or IM injection

Phenytoin (generic, Dilantin, others)
Oral (prompt release): 100 mg capsules; 50 mg chewable tablets; 30, 125 mg/5 mL suspension
Oral extended-action: 30, 100 mg capsules
Oral slow release (Phenytek): 200, 300 mg capsules
Parenteral: 50 mg/mL for IV injection

Primidone (generic, Mysoline)
Oral: 50, 250 mg tablets; 250 mg/5 mL suspension

Tiagabine (Gabitril)
Oral: 4, 12, 16, 20 mg tablets

Topiramate (Topamax)
Oral: 25, 100, 200 mg tablets; 15, 25 mg sprinkle capsules

Trimethadione (Tridione)
Oral: 150 mg chewable tablets; 300 mg capsules; 40 mg/mL solution

Valproic acid (generic, Depakene)
Oral: 250 mg capsules; 250 mg/5 mL syrup (sodium valproate)
Oral sustained-release (Depakote): 125, 250, 500 mg tablets (as divalproex sodium)
Parenteral (Depacon): 100 mg/mL in 5 mL vial for IV injection

REFERENCES

Backonja MM: Use of anticonvulsants for treatment of neuropathic pain. Neurology 2002;59(5 Suppl 2):S14.

Ben-Menachem E: Vagus-nerve stimulation for the treatment of epilepsy. The Lancet-Neurology 2002;1:477.

Beydoun A, Kutluay E: Oxcarbazepine. Expert Opin Pharmacother 2002;3:59.

Bialer M et al: Progress report on new antiepileptic drugs: a summary of the Fifth Eiliat Conference. Epilepsy Res 2001;43:11.

Delgado-Escueta AV et al: *Jasper's Basic Mechanisms of the Epilepsies,* Lippincott Williams & Wilkins, 1999.

DeToledo JC, Ramsay RE: Fosphenytoin and phenytoin in patients with status epilepticus: improved tolerability versus increased costs. Drug Saf 2000;22:459.

Duncan JS: The promise of new antiepileptic drugs. Br J Clin Pharmacol 2002;53:123.

Elterman RD et al: Randomized trial of vigabatrin in patients with infantile spasms. Neurology 2001;57:1416.

Faught E et al: Randomized controlled trial of zonisamide for the treatment of refractory partial-onset seizures. Neurology 2001;57:1774.

Fisher RS et al: Rapid initiation of gabapentin: a randomized controlled trial. Neurology 2001;56:743.

Hachad H et al: New antiepileptic drugs: review on drug interactions. Ther Drug Monit 2002;24:91.

Levy RH et al: *Antiepileptic Drugs, 5th Edition,* Lippincott Williams & Wilkins, 2002.

Limdi NA, Faught E: The safety of rapid valproic acid infusion. Epilepsia 2000;41:1342.

Löscher W: Basic pharmacology of valproate: a review after 35 years of clinical use for the treatment of epilepsy. CNS Drugs 2002;16:669.

Marson AG et al: Levetiracetam, oxcarbazepine, remacemide and zonisamide for drug resistant localization-related epilepsy: a systematic review. Epilepsy Res 2001;46:259.

McAuley JW, Anderson GD: Treatment of epilepsy in women of reproductive age: pharmacokinetic considerations. Clin Pharmacokinet 2002;41:559.

Petroff OAC et al: Effects of gabapentin on brain GABA, homocarnosine, and pyrrolidinone in epilepsy patients. Epilepsia 2000;41:675.

Privitera M: Efficacy of levetiracetam: a review of three pivotal trials. Epilepsia 2001;42(Suppl 4):31.

Pryor FM et al: Fosphenytoin: pharmacokinetics and tolerance of intramuscular loading. Epilepsia 2001;42;245.

Siddiqui A et al: Association of multidrug resistance in epilepsy with a polymorphism in the drug-transporter gene *ABCB1*. N Engl J Med 2002;348:15.

Treiman DM et al: A comparison of four treatments for generalized convulsive status epilepticus. N Engl J Med 1998;339:792.

Wallace SJ: Newer antiepileptic drugs: advantages and disadvantages. Brain Dev 2001;23:277.

Willmore LJ: Lamotrigine. Expert Review of Neurotherapeutics 2001;1:33.

General Anesthetics

25

Anthony J. Trevor, PhD, & Paul F. White, PhD, MD

The physiologic state of general anesthesia typically includes analgesia, amnesia, loss of consciousness, inhibition of sensory and autonomic reflexes, and skeletal muscle relaxation. The extent to which any individual anesthetic drug can exert these effects varies with the drug, the dosage, and the clinical situation.

An ideal anesthetic drug would induce anesthesia smoothly and rapidly while allowing for prompt recovery after its administration is discontinued. The drug would also possess a wide margin of safety and be devoid of adverse effects. No single anesthetic agent is capable of achieving all of these desirable effects without some disadvantages when used alone. The modern practice of anesthesiology most commonly involves the use of combinations of intravenous and inhaled drugs, taking advantage of their individual favorable properties while attempting to minimize their potential for causing adverse reactions.

The anesthetic technique will vary depending on the proposed type of diagnostic, therapeutic, or surgical intervention. For minor procedures, so-called monitored anesthesia care or conscious sedation is used, employing oral or parenteral sedatives in conjunction with local anesthetics (see Chapter 26). These techniques provide profound analgesia, but with retention of the patient's ability to maintain a patent airway and to respond to verbal commands. For more extensive surgical procedures, anesthesia frequently includes the use of preoperative benzodiazepines, induction of anesthesia with intravenous thiopental or propofol, and maintenance of anesthesia with a combination of inhaled and intravenous anesthetic drugs. Such protocols also often include the use of neuromuscular blocking drugs (see Chapter 27).

TYPES OF GENERAL ANESTHETICS

General anesthetics are usually given by inhalation or by intravenous injection.

Inhaled Anesthetics

The chemical structures of the currently available inhaled anesthetics are shown in Figure 25–1. Nitrous oxide, a gas at ambient temperature and pressure, contin-ues to be an important component of many anesthesia regimens. Halothane, enflurane, isoflurane, desflurane, sevoflurane, and methoxyflurane are volatile liquids.

Intravenous Anesthetics

Several drugs are used intravenously, alone or in combination with other drugs, to achieve an anesthetic state (as components of balanced anesthesia) or to sedate patients in intensive care units who must be mechanically ventilated. These drugs include the following: (1) barbiturates (thiopental, methohexital); (2) benzodiazepines (midazolam, diazepam); (3) opioid analgesics (morphine, fentanyl, sufentanil, alfentanil, remifentanil); (4) propofol; (5) ketamine; and (6) miscellaneous drugs (droperidol, etomidate, dexmedetomidine). Figure 25–2 shows the structures of commonly used intravenous anesthetics.

SIGNS & STAGES OF ANESTHESIA

The traditional description of the signs and stages of anesthesia (Guedel's signs) were derived from observations of the effects of diethyl ether, which has a slow onset of central action owing to its high solubility in blood. With these signs, anesthetic effects can be divided into four stages of increasing depth of central nervous system depression.

I. Stage of Analgesia: The patient initially experiences analgesia without amnesia. Later in stage I, both analgesia and amnesia are produced.

II. Stage of Excitement: During this stage, the patient often appears to be delirious and excited but definitely is amnesic. Respiration is irregular both in volume and rate, and retching and vomiting may occur. The patient may struggle and is sometimes incontinent. For these reasons, efforts are made to limit the duration and severity of this stage, which ends with the reestablishment of regular breathing.

III. Stage of Surgical Anesthesia: This stage begins with the recurrence of regular respiration and extends to complete cessation of spontaneous respiration. Four planes of stage III have been described in terms of changes in ocular movements, eye reflexes, and pupil

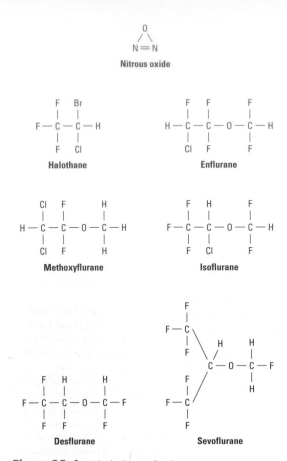

Figure 25–1. Inhaled anesthetics.

piration. The most reliable indication that stage III (surgical anesthesia) has been achieved is loss of the eyelash reflex and establishment of a regular respiratory pattern. The adequacy of depth of anesthesia for the specific surgical requirements is assessed by changes in respiratory and cardiovascular responses with surgical stimulation.

While vital sign monitoring remains a common method of assessing depth of anesthesia during surgery, newer techniques involving computer-assisted monitoring of cerebral function appear to offer some advantages. Automated techniques available include those based on the bispectral index (BIS), the physical state index (PSI) and the middle-latency auditory evoked potential (MLAEP), all of which are processed variables derived from established effects of anesthetics on the electroencephalogram. The application of such real-time cerebral monitoring techniques has been shown to reduce the volatile anesthetic requirement, contributing to a more rapid recovery from general anesthesia.

INHALED ANESTHETICS

PHARMACOKINETICS

Depth of anesthesia is dependent upon the concentration of anesthetic in the central nervous system. The rate at which an effective brain concentration is reached (the rate of induction of anesthesia) depends on multiple pharmacokinetic factors that influence the uptake and distribution of the anesthetic. Certain of these factors also influence the rate of recovery from anesthesia when the anesthetic is discontinued.

Uptake & Distribution

The concentration of an individual gas in a mixture of gases is proportionate to its **partial pressure** or **tension.** These terms are often used interchangeably in discussing the various transfer processes of anesthetic gases in the body. Achievement of a brain concentration of an inhaled anesthetic adequate to cause anesthesia requires transfer of that anesthetic from the alveolar air to blood and then to brain. The rate at which a given concentration of anesthetic in the brain is reached depends on the solubility properties of the anesthetic, its concentration in the inspired air, pulmonary ventilation rate, pulmonary blood flow, and the partial pressure gradient of the anesthetic between arterial and mixed venous blood.

A. SOLUBILITY

One of the most important factors influencing the transfer of an anesthetic from the lungs to the arterial blood is its solubility. The blood:gas partition coefficient

size, which under specified conditions may represent signs of increasing depth of anesthesia.

IV. Stage of Medullary Depression: This stage of anesthesia includes severe depression of the vasomotor center in the medulla as well as the respiratory center. Without full circulatory and respiratory support, death rapidly ensues.

In modern anesthesia practice, the distinctive signs of each of the four stages described above are usually obscured. Reasons for this include the relatively rapid onset of action of many intravenous and inhaled anesthetics compared with ether and the fact that respiratory activity is often controlled mechanically with muscle relaxants. In addition, the practice of administering other pharmacologic agents preoperatively or intraoperatively can also alter the clinical signs of anesthesia. Atropine and glycopyrrolate are used to decrease secretions; however, they also dilate the pupils. Drugs such as tubocurarine and succinylcholine affect muscle tone, and the opioid analgesics exert depressant effects on res-

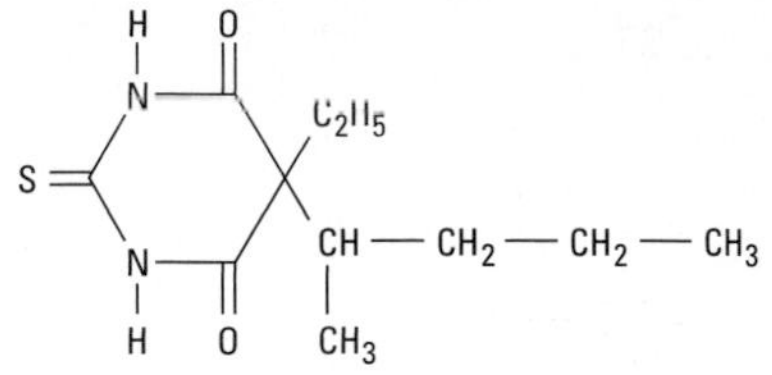

Thiopental

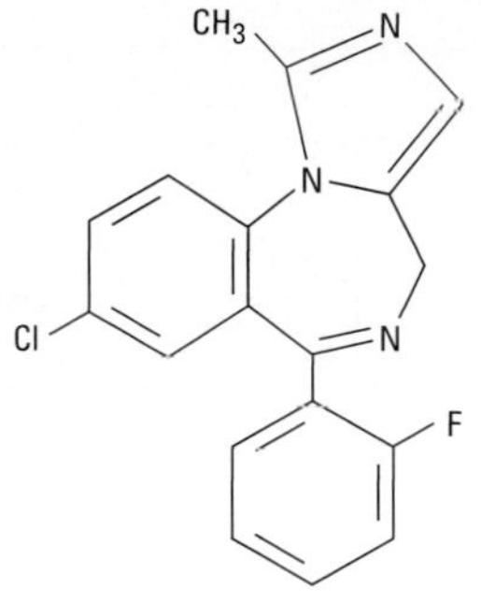

Midazolam

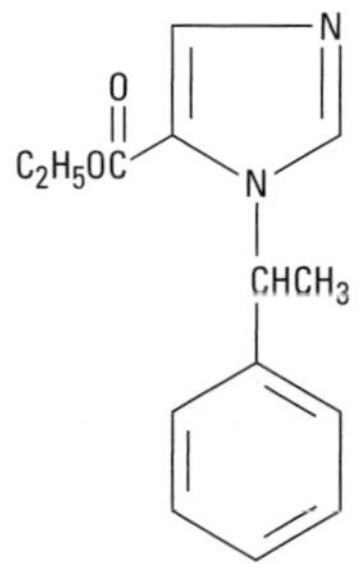

Etomidate

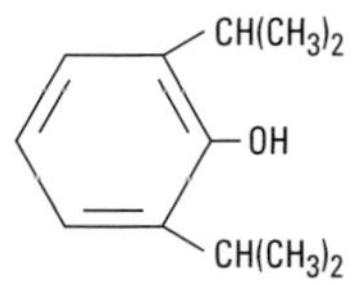

Propofol

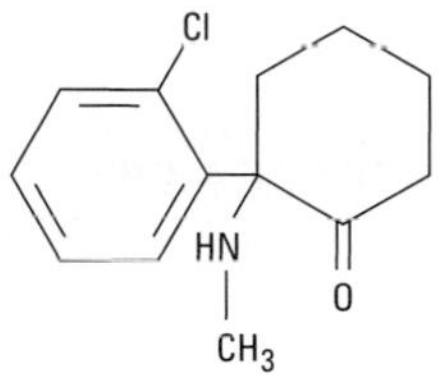

Ketamine

Figure 25–2. Intravenous anesthetics.

is a useful index of solubility and defines the relative affinity of an anesthetic for the blood compared to air. The partition coefficients for desflurane and nitrous oxide, which are not very soluble in the blood, are low (< 0.5). Halothane has a value greater than 2, and methoxyflurane, which is rarely used, has a coefficient of more than 10 (Table 25–1). When an anesthetic with low blood solubility diffuses from the lung into the arterial blood, relatively few molecules are required to raise its partial pressure, and therefore the arterial tension

Table 25–1. Properties of inhaled anesthetics.

Anesthetic	Blood:Gas Partition Coefficient[1]	Brain:Blood Partition Coefficient[1]	Minimal Alveolar Conc (MAC) (%)[2]	Metabolism	Comments
Nitrous oxide	0.47	1.1	> 100	None	Incomplete anesthetic; rapid onset and recovery
Desflurane	0.42	1.3	6–7	< 0.05%	Low volatility; poor induction agent; rapid recovery
Sevoflurane	0.69	1.7	2.0	2–5% (fluoride)	Rapid onset and recovery; unstable in soda-lime
Isoflurane	1.40	2.6	1.4	< 2%	Medium rate of onset and recovery
Enflurane	1.80	1.4	1.7	8%	Medium rate of onset and recovery
Halothane	2.30	2.9	0.75	> 40%	Medium rate of onset and recovery
Methoxyflurane	12	2.0	0.16	> 70% (fluoride)	Slow onset and recovery

[1]Partition coefficients (at 37 °C) are from multiple literature sources.

[2]MAC is the anesthetic concentration that produces immobility in 50% of patients exposed to a noxious stimulus.

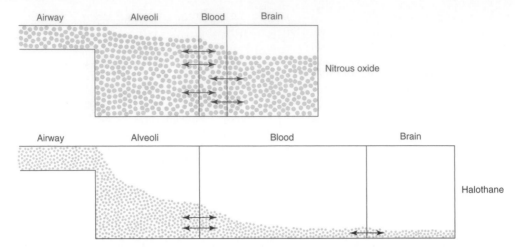

Figure 25–3. Why induction of anesthesia is slower with more soluble anesthetic gases. In this schematic diagram, solubility in blood is represented by the relative size of the blood compartment (the more soluble, the larger the compartment). Relative partial pressures of the agents in the compartments are indicated by the degree of filling of each compartment. For a given concentration or partial pressure of the two anesthetic gases in the inspired air, it will take much longer for the blood partial pressure of the more soluble gas (halothane) to rise to the same partial pressure as in the alveoli. Since the concentration of the anesthetic agent in the brain can rise no faster than the concentration in the blood, the onset of anesthesia will be slower with halothane than with nitrous oxide.

rises quickly (Figure 25–3, top, nitrous oxide). Conversely, for anesthetics with moderate to high solubility, more molecules dissolve before partial pressure changes significantly, and arterial tension of the gas increases less rapidly (Figure 25–3, bottom, halothane). This inverse relationship between the blood solubility of an anesthetic and the rate of rise of its tension in arterial blood is illustrated in Figure 25–4. Nitrous oxide with low solubility in blood, reaches high arterial tensions rapidly, which in turn results in rapid equilibration with the brain and fast onset of action. A rapid onset of anesthetic action is also characteristic of desflurane and sevoflurane, compounds that also have a low blood:gas partition coefficient.

B. ANESTHETIC CONCENTRATION IN THE INSPIRED AIR

The concentration of an inhaled anesthetic in the inspired gas mixture has direct effects on both the maximum tension that can be achieved in the alveoli and the rate of increase in its tension in arterial blood. Increases in the inspired anesthetic concentration will increase the rate of induction of anesthesia by increasing the rate of transfer into the blood according to Fick's law (see Chapter 1). Advantage is taken of this effect in anesthetic practice with inhaled anesthetics of moderate blood solubility such as enflurane, isoflurane, and halothane, which have a relatively slow onset of anesthetic effect. For example, a 3–4% concentration of

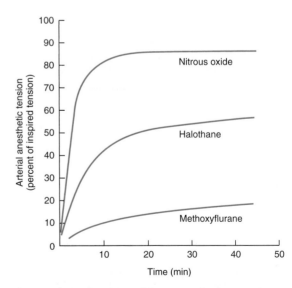

Figure 25–4. Tensions of three anesthetic gases in arterial blood as a function of time after beginning inhalation. Nitrous oxide is relatively insoluble (blood:gas partition coefficient = 0.47); methoxyflurane is much more soluble (coefficient = 12); and halothane is intermediate (2.3).

halothane may be administered initially to increase the rate of induction; this is reduced to 1–2% for maintenance when adequate anesthesia is achieved. In addition, these anesthetics are often administered in combination with a less soluble agent (eg, nitrous oxide) to reduce the time required for loss of consciousness.

C. PULMONARY VENTILATION

The rate of rise of anesthetic gas tension in arterial blood is directly dependent on both the rate and depth of ventilation (ie, minute ventilation). The magnitude of the effect varies according to the blood:gas partition coefficient. An increase in pulmonary ventilation is accompanied by only a slight increase in arterial tension of an anesthetic with low blood solubility or low coefficient but can significantly increase tension of agents with moderate or high blood solubility (Figure 25–5). For example, a fourfold increase in ventilation rate almost doubles the arterial tension of halothane during the first 10 minutes of anesthesia but increases the arterial tension of nitrous oxide by only 15%. Therefore, hyperventilation increases the speed of induction of anesthesia with inhaled anesthetics that would normally have a slow onset. Depression of respiration by opioid analgesics will slow the onset of anesthesia of some inhaled anesthetics if ventilation is not assisted.

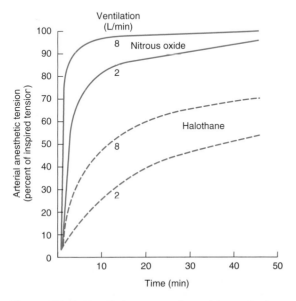

Figure 25–5. Ventilation rate and arterial anesthetic tensions. Increased ventilation (8 versus 2 L/min) has a much greater effect on equilibration of halothane than nitrous oxide.

D. PULMONARY BLOOD FLOW

Changes in blood flow to and from the lungs influence transfer processes of the anesthetic gases. An increase in pulmonary blood flow (increased cardiac output) slows the rate of rise in arterial tension, particularly for those anesthetics with moderate to high blood solubility. This is because increased pulmonary blood flow exposes a larger volume of blood to the anesthetic; thus, blood "capacity" increases and the anesthetic tension rises slowly. A decrease in pulmonary blood flow has the opposite effect and increases the rate of rise of arterial tension of inhaled anesthetics. In a patient with circulatory shock, the combined effects of decreased cardiac output (resulting in decreased pulmonary flow) and increased ventilation will accelerate the induction of anesthesia with halothane and isoflurane. This is not likely to occur with nitrous oxide, desflurane, or sevoflurane because of their low blood solubility.

E. ARTERIOVENOUS CONCENTRATION GRADIENT

The anesthetic concentration gradient between arterial and mixed venous blood is dependent mainly on uptake of the anesthetic by the tissues, including nonneural tissues. Depending on the rate and extent of tissue uptake, venous blood returning to the lungs may contain significantly less anesthetic than arterial blood. The greater this difference in anesthetic tensions, the more has been taken up by viscera, muscle, etc, and the more time it will take to achieve equilibrium with brain tissue. Anesthetic entry into tissues is influenced by factors similar to those that determine transfer from lung to blood, including tissue:blood partition coefficient, rates of blood flow to the tissues, and concentration gradients.

During the induction phase of anesthesia, the tissues that exert greatest influence on the arterial-venous anesthetic concentration gradient are those which are highly perfused. These include the brain, heart, liver, kidneys, and splanchnic bed, which together receive over 75% of the resting cardiac output. In the case of anesthetics with relatively high solubility in these tissues, venous blood concentration will initially be very low, and equilibrium with arterial blood is achieved slowly.

During maintenance of anesthesia with inhaled anesthetics, these drugs may continue to be transferred between various tissues at rates dependent on solubility and blood flow. Muscle and skin, which together constitute 50% of body mass, accumulate anesthetics more slowly than the highly vascularized tissues (eg, brain), since they receive only one-fifth the blood flow of the latter groups. Although most anesthetic gases have high solubility in adipose tissues, low blood perfusion rates to these tissues delay accumulation, and equilibrium is unlikely to occur with most anesthetics during the time usually required for surgery.

Elimination

The time to recovery from inhalation anesthesia depends on the rate of elimination of anesthetics from the brain after the inspired concentration of anesthetic has been decreased. Many of the processes of anesthetic transfer during recovery are similar to those that occur during induction of anesthesia. One of the most important factors governing rate of recovery is the blood:gas partition coefficient of the anesthetic agent (see below). Other factors controlling rate of recovery include the pulmonary blood flow, the magnitude of ventilation, and the solubility of the anesthetic in the tissues. Two features of recovery, however, are quite different from what happens during induction of anesthesia. First, while transfer of an anesthetic from the lungs to blood can be enhanced by increasing its concentration in inspired air, the reverse transfer process cannot be enhanced, since the concentration in the lungs cannot be reduced below zero. Second, at the beginning of recovery, the anesthetic gas tension in different tissues may be quite variable, depending on the specific agent and the duration of anesthesia. With induction of anesthesia, the initial anesthetic tension in all tissues is zero.

Inhaled anesthetics that are relatively insoluble in blood (low blood:gas partition coefficient) and brain are eliminated at faster rates than more soluble anesthetics. The washout of nitrous oxide, desflurane, and sevoflurane occurs at a rapid rate, which leads to a more rapid recovery from their anesthetic effects compared to halothane and isoflurane. Halothane is approximately twice as soluble in brain tissue and five times more soluble in blood than nitrous oxide and desflurane; its elimination therefore takes place more slowly, and recovery from halothane anesthesia is predictably less rapid. The duration of exposure to the anesthetic can also have a marked effect on the time of recovery, especially in the case of more soluble anesthetics. Accumulation of anesthetics in tissues, including muscle, skin, and fat, increases with continuous inhalation (especially in obese patients), and blood tension may decline slowly during recovery as the anesthetic is gradually eliminated from these tissues. Thus, if exposure to the anesthetic is short, recovery may be rapid even with the more soluble agents. However, after prolonged anesthesia, recovery may be delayed even with anesthetics of moderate solubility such as isoflurane.

Clearance of inhaled anesthetics by the lungs into the expired air is the major route of their elimination from the body. However, metabolism by enzymes of the liver and other tissues may also contribute to the elimination of volatile anesthetics. For example, the elimination of halothane during recovery is more rapid than that of enflurane, which would not be predicted from their respective solubilities. However, over 40% of inspired halothane is metabolized during an average anesthetic procedure, while less than 10% of enflurane is metabolized over the same period. Oxidative metabolism of halothane results in the formation of trifluoroacetic acid and release of bromide and chloride ions. Under conditions of low oxygen tension, halothane is metabolized to the chlorotrifluoroethyl free radical, which is capable of reacting with hepatic membrane components. Isoflurane and desflurane are the least metabolized of the fluorinated anesthetics, only traces of trifluoroacetic acid appearing in the urine even after prolonged administration. The metabolism of enflurane and sevoflurane results in the formation of fluoride ion, which does not appear to reach toxic levels under normal circumstances. In addition, sevoflurane is degraded by contact with the carbon dioxide absorbent in anesthesia machines, yielding a vinyl ether called "compound A" that can cause renal damage if high concentrations are absorbed. (See Box, Do We Need Another Inhaled Anesthetic?) Over 70% of absorbed methoxyflurane is metabolized by the liver with the release of fluoride ions at concentrations that can be nephrotoxic. In terms of the extent of metabolism of inhaled anesthetics, the rank order is: methoxyflurane > halothane > enflurane > sevoflurane > isoflurane > desflurane > nitrous oxide (Table 25–1). Nitrous oxide is probably not metabolized by human tissues.

PHARMACODYNAMICS

Mechanism of Action

The inhaled anesthetics—and most of the intravenous agents—depress spontaneous and evoked activity of neurons in many regions of the brain. Older concepts of the mechanism of anesthesia invoked nonspecific interactions of these agents with the lipid matrix of the nerve membrane (the Meyer-Overton principle)—interactions that were thought to lead to secondary changes in ion flux. More recently, evidence has accumulated suggesting that the modification of ion currents by anesthetics results from more specific interactions with nerve membrane components. The ionic mechanisms involved for different anesthetics may vary, but at clinically relevant concentrations they appear to involve interactions with members of the ligand-gated ion channel family.

In the past decade, considerable evidence has accumulated that a primary molecular target of many general anesthetics is the $GABA_A$ receptor-chloride channel, a major mediator of inhibitory synaptic transmission. Inhaled anesthetics, barbiturates, benzodiazepines, etomidate, and propofol facilitate GABA-mediated inhibition at $GABA_A$ receptor sites. These receptors are sensitive to clinically relevant concentrations of the

---

DO WE NEED ANOTHER INHALED ANESTHETIC?

For almost 30 years, from its introduction in 1956, halothane was the standard of comparison for inhaled anesthetics. However, the onset of its anesthetic action is slow compared with many intravenous agents, and the rate of recovery from its anesthetic effects is not rapid. In addition, its hepatic metabolism to a reactive compound may lead to development of halothane-associated hepatitis.

The newer inhaled anesthetics, desflurane and sevoflurane, have physicochemical characteristics (low blood:gas partition coefficients) favorable to a more rapid onset and a shorter duration of anesthetic actions than older agents such as isoflurane and halothane. However, both of these newer agents also have certain limitations. The low volatility of desflurane necessitates the use of a specialized vaporizer, and the pungency of the drug leads to a high incidence of coughing—and sometimes laryngospasm—such that it cannot be used for induction of anesthesia. In addition, desflurane causes a centrally mediated sympathetic activation leading to elevations of blood pressure and heart rate.

In the case of the newest agent, sevoflurane, induction of anesthesia is achieved rapidly and smoothly, and recovery is more rapid than most other inhaled anesthetics including isoflurane. However, sevoflurane is chemically unstable when exposed to carbon dioxide absorbents, degrading to an olefinic compound (fluoromethyl-2,2-difluoro-1-[trifluoromethyl]vinyl ether, compound A) that is potentially nephrotoxic. In addition, sevoflurane is metabolized by the liver to release fluoride ions, raising concerns about possible renal damage similar to that caused by methoxyflurane. Sevoflurane comes close to having the characteristics of an ideal gas anesthetic, but a relatively insoluble compound that has greater chemical stability could be a useful alternative in the future.

---

anesthetic agents and exhibit the appropriate stereospecific effects in the case of enantiomeric drugs. The $GABA_A$ receptor-chloride channel is a pentameric assembly of five proteins derived from several polypeptide subclasses (see Chapter 22). Combinations of three major subunits—α, β, and γ—are necessary for normal physiologic and pharmacologic functions. $GABA_A$ receptors in different areas of the central nervous system contain different subunit combinations conferring different pharmacologic properties on each receptor subtype. Inhaled anesthetics and intravenous agents with general anesthetic properties directly activate $GABA_A$ receptors, but at low concentrations they can also facilitate the action of GABA to increase chloride ion flux. In contrast, sedative benzodiazepines lacking general anesthetic properties (eg, midazolam) facilitate GABA action but have no direct actions on $GABA_A$ receptors even at high concentrations in the absence of GABA.

Reconstitution studies with transfected cells utilizing chimeric and mutated $GABA_A$ receptors reveal that anesthetic molecules do not interact directly with the GABA binding site but with specific sites in the transmembrane domains of both α and β subunits. Two specific amino acid residues in transmembrane segments 2 and 3 of the $GABA_A$ receptor α_2 subunit, Ser270 and Ala291, are critical for the enhancement of $GABA_A$ receptor function by inhaled anesthetics. One consequence of the interaction of isoflurane with this domain is an alteration in the gating of the chloride ion channel. However, differences occur in the precise binding sites of individual anesthetics. For example, a specific aspartate residue within transmembrane segment 2 of the $GABA_A$ receptor α_2 subunit is required for etomidate activity but is not essential for the activity of barbiturates or propofol.

Ketamine does not produce its effects via facilitation of $GABA_A$ receptor functions, but it may function via antagonism of the action of the excitatory neurotransmitter glutamic acid on the NMDA receptor.

In addition to actions on $GABA_A$ chloride channels, inhaled anesthetics have been reported to cause membrane hyperpolarization (an inhibitory action) via their activation of ligand-gated potassium channels. These channels are ubiquitous in the central nervous system and are linked to several neurotransmitters, including acetylcholine, dopamine, norepinephrine, and serotonin. Electrophysiologic analyses of membrane ion flux in cultured cells have shown that inhaled anesthetics decrease the duration of opening of nicotinic receptor-activated cation channels—an action that decreases the excitatory effects of acetylcholine at cholinergic synapses. Most inhaled anesthetics inhibit nicotinic acetylcholine receptor isoforms, particularly those containing the α_4 subunit, though such actions do not appear to be involved in their immobilizing actions. The strychnine-sensitive glycine receptor is another ligand-gated ion channel that may function as a target for inhaled anesthetics which can elicit channel opening directly and independently of their facilitatory effects on neurotransmitter binding.

The neuropharmacologic basis for the effects that characterize the stages of anesthesia appears to be differential sensitivity of specific neurons or neuronal pathways to the anesthetic drugs. Neurons in the substantia gelatinosa of the dorsal horn of the spinal cord are very sensitive to relatively low anesthetic concentrations. Interaction with neurons in this region interrupts sensory transmission in the spinothalamic tract, including transmission of nociceptive (pain) stimuli. These effects contribute to stage I analgesia and conscious sedation. The disinhibitory effects of general anesthetics (stage II), which occur at higher brain concentrations, result from complex neuronal actions including blockade of many small inhibitory neurons such as Golgi type II cells, together with a paradoxical facilitation of excitatory neurotransmitters. A progressive depression of ascending pathways in the reticular activating system occurs during stage III of anesthesia, together with suppression of spinal reflex activity, which contributes to muscle relaxation. Neurons in the respiratory and vasomotor centers of the medulla are relatively insensitive to the effects of the general anesthetics, but at high concentrations their activity is depressed, leading to cardiorespiratory collapse (stage IV). It remains to be determined whether regional variation in anesthetic actions corresponds with the regional variation in the subtypes of $GABA_A$ receptor. The differential sensitivity of specific neurons or neuronal pathways to anesthetics could reflect their interactions with other molecules in the fast ligand-gated ion channel family or could represent the existence of other molecular targets that have yet to be characterized.

Dose-Response Characteristics: The Minimum Alveolar Anesthetic Concentration (MAC)

Inhaled anesthetics are delivered to the lungs in gas mixtures in which concentrations and flow rates are easy to measure and control. However, dose-response characteristics of gaseous anesthetics are difficult to measure. Although achievement of an anesthetic state depends on the concentration of the anesthetic in the brain, that concentration is impossible to measure under clinical conditions. Furthermore, neither the lower nor the upper ends of the graded dose-response curve can be ethically determined, since at very low concentrations severe pain might be experienced while at high concentrations there would be a high risk of fatal cardiovascular and respiratory depression. Nevertheless, a useful estimate of anesthetic potency can be obtained using quantal dose-response principles.

During general anesthesia, the partial pressure of an inhaled anesthetic in the brain equals that in the lung when steady state is reached. Therefore, at a given level of anesthesia, the measurement of the steady-state alveolar concentrations of different anesthetics provides a comparison of their relative potencies. The minimum alveolar anesthetic concentration (MAC) is defined as the median concentration (ie, the percentage of the alveolar gas mixture, or partial pressure of the anesthetic as a percentage of 760 mm Hg) that results in immobility in 50% of patients when exposed to a noxious stimulus (eg, surgical incision). Therefore, MAC represents one point (the ED_{50}) on a conventional quantal dose-response curve (see Figure 2–16). Table 25–1 shows some properties of the common inhaled anesthetics, permitting comparison of their relative anesthetic potencies. The MAC value greater than 100% for nitrous oxide demonstrates that it is the least potent anesthetic, since at normal barometric pressure even 760 mm Hg partial pressure of nitrous oxide (100% of the inspired gas) is still not equal to 1 MAC.

The dose of anesthetic gas that is being administered can be stated in multiples of MAC. While a dose of 1 MAC of any anesthetic prevents movement in response to surgical incision in 50% of patients, individual patients may require 0.5–1.5 MAC. Unfortunately, the MAC gives no information about the slope of the dose-response curve. In general, however, the dose-response relationship for inhaled anesthetics is very steep. Therefore, over 95% of patients may fail to respond to a noxious stimulus at 1.1 MAC. The measurement of MAC values under controlled conditions has permitted quantitation of the effects of a number of variables on anesthetic requirements. For example, MAC values decrease in elderly patients and with hypothermia, but are not affected greatly by sex, height, and weight. Of particular importance is the presence of adjuvant drugs, which can change anesthetic requirement. For example, when drugs such as the opioid analgesics, sympatholytics, or sedative-hypnotics are present, the MAC is decreased in a dose-related fashion. The inspired concentration of anesthetic should be decreased in these situations. MAC values of the inhaled anesthetics are additive. For example, nitrous oxide can be used as a "carrier" gas at 40% of its MAC, decreasing the anesthetic requirement of other inhaled anesthetics; 70% of their MAC would yield a total of 110% of one MAC, which is sufficient for surgical anesthesia in most patients.

Organ System Effects of Inhaled Anesthetics

A. EFFECTS ON CARDIOVASCULAR SYSTEM

Halothane, desflurane, enflurane, sevoflurane, and isoflurane all decrease mean arterial pressure in direct proportion to their alveolar concentration. With halothane and enflurane, the reduced arterial pressure appears to be caused by a reduction in cardiac output because there is little change in systemic vascular resistance despite marked changes in individual vascular beds (eg, increase in cerebral blood flow). In contrast, isoflurane, desflurane, and sevoflurane have a depressant effect on arterial pressure as a result of a decrease in systemic vascular resistance with minimal effect on cardiac output.

Inhaled anesthetics change heart rate either directly by altering the rate of sinus node depolarization or indirectly by shifting the balance of autonomic nervous system activity. Bradycardia is often seen with halothane, probably through vagal stimulation. In contrast, enflurane, and sevoflurane have little effect, and both desflurane and isoflurane increase heart rate. In the case of desflurane, cardiovascular responses include a transient sympathetic activation that can lead to marked increases in heart rate and blood pressure when high inspired gas concentrations are administered.

All inhaled anesthetics tend to increase right atrial pressure in a dose-related fashion, which reflects depression of myocardial function. In general, enflurane and halothane have greater myocardial depressant effects than isoflurane and the newer less soluble halogenated anesthetics. Inhaled anesthetics reduce myocardial oxygen consumption, primarily by decreasing the variables that control oxygen demand, such as arterial blood pressure and contractile force. Although certainly less depressant than the other inhaled anesthetics, nitrous oxide has also been found to depress the myocardium in a dose-dependent manner. However, nitrous oxide in combination with potent inhaled anesthetics produces sympathetic stimulation that minimizes cardiac depressant effects. The combination of nitrous oxide with halothane or enflurane, for example, appears to produce less cardiac depression at a given depth of anesthesia than either of the more potent anesthetics given alone.

Several factors influence the cardiovascular effects of inhaled anesthetics. Surgical stimulation, volume status, ventilatory status, and duration of anesthesia will alter the depressant effects of these drugs. Hypercapnia releases catecholamines, which attenuate the decrease in blood pressure. The blood pressure decrease after 5 hours of anesthesia is less than it is after 1 hour; concomitant use of beta-blockers reduces this adaptive effect. Halothane (and, to a lesser extent, isoflurane) sensitizes the myocardium to catecholamines. Ventricular arrhythmias may occur in patients with cardiac disease who are given sympathomimetic drugs or have high circulating levels of endogenous catecholamines (eg, anxious patients, patients with pheochromocytoma). The newer, less soluble inhaled anesthetics appear to be less arrhythmogenic.

B. Effects on the Respiratory System

With the exception of nitrous oxide, all inhaled anesthetics in current use cause a dose-dependent decrease in tidal volume and an increase in respiratory rate. However, the increase in rate is insufficient to compensate for the decrease in volume, resulting in a decrease in minute ventilation. All inhaled anesthetics are respiratory depressants, as indicated by a reduced response to increased levels of carbon dioxide. The degree of ventilatory depression varies among the volatile agents, with isoflurane and enflurane being the most depressant. All inhaled anesthetics in current use increase the resting level of $PaCO_2$ (the partial pressure of carbon dioxide in arterial blood).

Inhaled anesthetics increase the apneic threshold ($PaCO_2$ level below which apnea occurs through lack of CO_2-driven respiratory stimulation) and decrease the ventilatory response to hypoxia. The latter effect is especially important because subanesthetic concentrations (ie, those that exist during recovery) depress the normal compensating increase in ventilation that occurs during hypoxia. Respiratory depressant effects of anesthetics are overcome by assisting or controlling ventilation mechanically. Furthermore, the ventilatory depressant effects of the inhaled anesthetics are lessened by surgical stimulation.

Inhaled anesthetics also depress mucociliary function in the airway. Thus, prolonged anesthesia may lead to pooling of mucus and then result in atelectasis and postoperative respiratory infections. However, inhaled anesthetics tend to be bronchodilators, an effect of value in the treatment of status asthmaticus. The bronchodilating action of halothane and sevoflurane makes them the induction agents of choice in patients with underlying airway problems. Airway irritation, which may provoke coughing or breath holding, is rarely a problem with most inhaled anesthetics. However, it is relatively common with desflurane, making induction of anesthesia more difficult to accomplish with this anesthetic despite its low blood:gas partition coefficient. Similarly, the pungency of enflurane may elicit breath holding, which can decrease the speed of induction.

C. Effects on Brain

Inhaled anesthetics decrease the metabolic rate of the brain. Nevertheless, most volatile agents increase cerebral blood flow because they decrease cerebral vascular resistance. The increase in cerebral blood flow is often clinically undesirable. For example, in patients who have an increased intracranial pressure because of a brain tumor or head injury, administration of a volatile anesthetic may increase cerebral blood flow, which in turn will increase cerebral blood volume and further increase intracranial pressure.

Of the inhaled anesthetics, nitrous oxide increases cerebral blood flow the least. However, when 60% nitrous oxide is added to halothane anesthesia, cerebral blood flow usually increases more than with halothane alone. At low doses, all of the halogenated agents have similar effects on cerebral blood flow. At larger doses, enflurane and isoflurane increase cerebral blood flow less than halothane. If the patient is hyperventilated before the anesthetic is given (reducing $PaCO_2$), the increase in intracranial pressure from inhaled anesthetics can be minimized.

Halothane, isoflurane, and enflurane have similar effects (eg, burst suppression) on the EEG up to doses of 1–1.5 MAC. At higher doses, the cerebral irritant effects of enflurane may lead to development of a spike-and-wave pattern during which auditory stimuli can precipitate mild generalized muscle twitching that is augmented by hyperventilation. Enflurane-induced EEG seizure activity has never been shown to have any adverse clinical consequences, though it may be prudent to avoid the use of enflurane in patients with a history of seizure disorders. This effect is not seen clinically with the newer volatile anesthetics. Although nitrous oxide has low anesthetic potency, it does exert analgesic and amnesic actions, desirable properties when used in combination with other agents in general anesthesia and dental anesthesia.

D. Effects on the Kidney

To varying degrees, all inhaled anesthetics decrease glomerular filtration rate and effective renal plasma flow and increase filtration fraction. All the anesthetics tend to increase renal vascular resistance. Since renal blood flow decreases during general anesthesia in spite of well-maintained or even increased perfusion pressures, autoregulation of renal flow is probably impaired.

E. Effects on the Liver

All volatile anesthetics cause a decrease in hepatic blood flow, ranging from 15% to 45% of the preanesthetic flow rate. Despite transient intraoperative changes in liver function tests, permanent changes in liver function rarely occur from the use of these agents. The hepatotoxicity of halothane is discussed below.

F. Effects on Uterine Smooth Muscle

Nitrous oxide appears to have little effect on uterine musculature. However, the halogenated hydrocarbon anesthetics are potent uterine muscle relaxants. This pharmacologic effect can be used to advantage when profound uterine relaxation is required for intrauterine fetal manipulation or manual extraction of a retained placenta during delivery.

Toxicity

A. Hepatotoxicity (Halothane)

Postoperative hepatic dysfunction is usually associated with factors such as blood transfusions, hypovolemic shock, and other surgical stresses rather than anesthetic toxicity. However, a very small subset of individuals exposed to halothane may develop a potentially severe and life-threatening hepatitis. The incidence of severe hepatotoxicity following exposure to halothane is probably in the range of one in 20,000–35,000. Obese patients having more than one exposure to halothane during a short time interval may be more susceptible. There is no specific treatment for halothane hepatitis, and liver transplantation may ultimately be required.

The mechanisms underlying hepatotoxicity from halothane remain unclear, but studies in animals have implicated the formation of reactive metabolites that either cause direct hepatocellular damage (eg, free radical intermediates) or initiate immune-mediated responses. With regard to the latter mechanism, serum from patients with halothane hepatitis contains a variety of autoantibodies against hepatic proteins, many of which are in a trifluoroacetylated form. These trifluoroacetylated proteins could be formed in the hepatocyte during the biotransformation of halothane by liver drug-metabolizing enzymes. However, TFA proteins have also been identified in the sera of patients who did not develop hepatitis after halothane anesthesia.

B. Nephrotoxicity

Metabolism of enflurane and sevoflurane leads to the formation of fluoride ions, and this has raised questions concerning the potential nephrotoxicity of these anesthetics. Changes in renal concentrating ability have been observed with prolonged exposure to enflurane but not sevoflurane. Differences between the two agents may be related to the fact that enflurane (but not sevoflurane) is metabolized in part by renal enzymes, generating fluoride ions intrarenally. Sevoflurane degradation by carbon dioxide absorbents in anesthesia machines leads to formation of a haloalkene, compound A, that causes a proximal tubular necrosis when administered to rats. However, there have been no reports of renal injury in humans undergoing sevoflurane anesthesia, and the anesthetic does not appear to change standard markers of renal function. Renal dysfunction following methoxyflurane is caused by inorganic fluoride released during the extensive metabolism of this anesthetic by hepatic and renal enzymes. As a result, methoxyflurane is considered obsolete for most purposes.

C. Malignant Hyperthermia

Malignant hyperthermia is an autosomal dominant genetic disorder of skeletal muscle that occurs in susceptible individuals undergoing general anesthesia with inhaled agents and muscle relaxants (eg, succinylcholine). The malignant hyperthermia syndrome consists of the rapid onset of tachycardia and hypertension, severe muscle rigidity, hyperthermia, hyperkalemia, and acid-base imbalance with acidosis, following exposure to a triggering agent. Malignant hyperthermia is a rare but important cause of anesthetic morbidity and mortality. The specific biochemical abnormality is an increase in free calcium concentration in skeletal muscle cells. Treatment includes administration of dantrolene (which prevents calcium release from the sarcoplasmic reticulum) and appropriate measures to reduce body temperature and restore electrolyte and acid-base balance.

Malignant hyperthermia susceptibility is characterized by genetic heterogeneity, and several predisposing clinical myopathies have been identified. It has been associated with mutations in the gene loci corresponding to the skeletal muscle ryanodine receptor (RYRl), the calcium release channel of the sarcoplasmic reticulum. Mutations in the ryanodine receptor gene are inherited as mendelian dominant characteristics. Other chromosomal loci for malignant hyperthermia susceptibility include mutant alleles of the gene encoding the α_1 subunit of the human skeletal muscle dihydropyridine-sensitive L-type voltage-dependent calcium channel. However, the genetic loci identified to date account for no more than 50% of malignant hyperthermia-susceptible individuals. Given such genetic heterogeneity, it seems premature to utilize genetic testing methods for malignant hyperthermia susceptibility at this time. Currently, the most reliable test to establish such susceptibility is the in vitro caffeine-halothane contracture test utilizing skeletal muscle biopsy tissue.

D. CHRONIC TOXICITY

1. Mutagenicity—Under normal conditions, most modern and many older inhaled anesthetics are neither mutagens nor carcinogens.

2. Carcinogenicity—Some epidemiologic studies have suggested an increase in the cancer rate in operating room personnel who have been exposed to trace concentrations of anesthetic agents. However, no study has demonstrated the existence of a cause-and-effect relationship between anesthetics and cancer. Many other factors might account for the questionably positive results seen after a careful review of epidemiologic data. Most operating room theaters remove trace concentrations of anesthetics released from anesthetic machines via vents to the outdoors.

3. Effects on reproduction—The most consistent finding reported from surveys conducted to determine the reproductive performance of female operating room personnel has been a higher than expected incidence of miscarriages. However, there are several problems in interpreting these studies, and the evidence is not strong.

The association of obstetric problems with surgery and anesthesia in pregnant patients is an important consideration. In the USA, at least 50,000 pregnant women each year undergo anesthesia and surgery for indications unrelated to pregnancy. The risk of abortion is clearly higher following this experience. It is not obvious whether the underlying disease, surgery, anesthesia, or a combination of these factors is the cause of the increased risk. Another concern is that anesthesia during pregnancy may lead to an increased incidence of congenital anomalies. Since anesthetics do not appear to be teratogenic, the risk must be very small.

4. Hematotoxicity—Prolonged exposure to nitrous oxide decreases methionine synthase activity and causes megaloblastic anemia. This is a potential occupational hazard for staff working in poorly ventilated dental operating suites.

Clinical Use of Inhaled Anesthetics

Volatile anesthetics are rarely used as the sole agents for both induction and maintenance of anesthesia. Most commonly, they are combined with intravenous agents in regimens of so-called balanced anesthesia. Of the inhaled anesthetics, nitrous oxide, desflurane, sevoflurane, and isoflurane are the most commonly used in the USA. Use of the more soluble volatile anesthetics has declined during the last decade as more surgical procedures are performed on an outpatient ("short-stay") basis. The low blood:gas coefficients of desflurane and sevoflurane afford more rapid recovery and fewer postoperative adverse effects than halothane or isoflurane. Although halothane is still used in pediatric anesthesia, sevoflurane is rapidly replacing halothane in this setting. As indicated previously, nitrous oxide lacks sufficient potency to produce surgical anesthesia by itself and therefore is used with volatile or intravenous anesthetics to produce a general anesthetic state.

Despite the advantages of the inhaled anesthetics now available, there is reason to believe that better ones might be developed. (See Box, Do We Need Another Inhaled Anesthetic?)

INTRAVENOUS ANESTHETICS

In the last 2 decades there has been increasing use of intravenous drugs in anesthesia, both as adjuncts to inhaled anesthetics and in techniques that do not include inhaled anesthetics (eg, total intravenous anesthesia). Unlike inhaled anesthetics, intravenous agents do not require specialized vaporizer equipment for their delivery or expensive facilities for the recovery and disposal of exhaled gases. Intravenous drugs such as thiopental, etomidate, ketamine, and propofol have an onset of anesthetic action faster than the fastest of the inhaled gaseous agents such as desflurane and sevoflurane. Therefore, intravenous agents are commonly used for induction of anesthesia. Recovery is sufficiently rapid with many intravenous drugs to permit their extensive use for short ambulatory (outpatient) surgical procedures. In the case of propofol, recovery times are similar to those seen with the shortest-acting inhaled anesthetics. The anesthetic potency of intravenous anesthetics, including thiopental, ketamine, and propofol, is adequate to permit their use as the sole anesthetic in short surgical procedures when combined with nitrous oxide and opioid analgesics. Adjunctive use of potent opioids (eg, fentanyl and related compounds) contributes cardiovascular stability, enhanced sedation, and profound analgesia. Other intravenous agents such as the benzodiazepines (eg, midazolam, diazepam) have slower onset and recovery features and are rarely used for induction of anesthesia. However, preanesthetic administration of benzodiazepines can be used to provide a basal level of sedation and amnesia when used in conjunction with other anesthetic agents.

Pharmacokinetic properties of the intravenous anesthetics are summarized in Table 25–2.

SHORT-ACTING BARBITURATES

Thiopental is a short-acting barbiturate commonly used for induction of anesthesia. The general pharmacology of the barbiturates is discussed in Chapter 22.

Following an intravenous bolus injection, thiopental rapidly crosses the blood-brain barrier and, if given in sufficient dosage, produces loss of consciousness (hypnosis) in one circulation time. Similar effects occur with another short-acting barbiturate, methohexital. With these barbiturates, plasma:brain equilibrium occurs rapidly (< 1 minute) because of their high lipid solubility. Thiopental rapidly diffuses out of the brain and other highly vascular tissues and is redistributed to muscle, fat, and eventually all body tissues (Figure 25–6). It is because of this rapid removal from brain tissue that a single dose of thiopental is so short-acting. Thiopental is metabolized at the rate of 12–16% per hour in humans following a single dose. Less than 1% of an administered dose of thiopental is excreted unchanged by the kidney.

With large doses, thiopental causes dose-dependent decreases in arterial blood pressure, stroke volume, and cardiac output. This is due primarily to its myocardial depressant effect and increased venous capacitance; there is little change in total peripheral resistance. Thiopental is also a potent respiratory depressant, lowering the sensitivity of the medullary respiratory center to carbon dioxide.

Cerebral metabolism and oxygen utilization are decreased after thiopental administration in proportion to the degree of cerebral depression. Cerebral blood flow is also decreased, but much less so than oxygen consumption. This makes thiopental a desirable drug for use in patients with cerebral swelling (eg, head trauma, brain tumors), since intracranial pressure and blood volume are not increased (in contrast to the volatile anesthetics).

Thiopental may reduce hepatic blood flow and glomerular filtration rate, but it produces no lasting effects on hepatic and renal function. Barbiturates may exacerbate acute intermittent porphyria by inducing the synthesis of hepatic ALA synthase (see Chapter 22). Thiopental has precipitated porphyric crisis when used as an induction agent in susceptible individuals.

Table 25–2. Characteristics of intravenous anesthetics.

Drug	Induction and Recovery	Comments
Etomidate	Rapid onset and moderately fast recovery	Cardiovascular stability; decreased steroidogenesis; involuntary muscle movements
Ketamine	Moderately rapid onset and recovery	Cardiovascular stimulation; increased cerebral blood flow; emergence reactions impair recovery
Midazolam	Slow onset and recovery; flumazenil reversal available	Used in balanced anesthesia and conscious sedation; cardiovascular stability; marked amnesia
Propofol	Rapid onset and rapid recovery	Used in induction and for maintenance; hypotension; useful antiemetic action
Thiopental	Rapid onset and rapid recovery (bolus dose)— slow recovery following infusion	Standard induction agent; cardiovascular depression; avoid in porphyrias
Fentanyl	Slow onset and recovery; naloxone reversal available	Used in balanced anesthesia and conscious sedation; marked analgesia

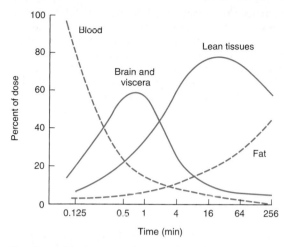

Figure 25–6. Redistribution of thiopental after an intravenous bolus administration. Note that the time axis is not linear.

BENZODIAZEPINES

Diazepam, lorazepam, and midazolam are used in anesthetic procedures. The primary indication is for premedication because of their sedative and amnestic properties. (The basic pharmacology of benzodiazepines is discussed in Chapter 22.) Diazepam and lorazepam are not water-soluble, and their intravenous use necessitates nonaqueous vehicles, which may cause local irritation. Midazolam formulations are water-soluble and thus produce less irritation, but the drug becomes lipid-soluble at physiologic pH and readily crosses the blood-brain barrier.

Compared with intravenous barbiturates, benzodiazepines produce a slower onset of central nervous system effects and induce a plateau of central depression less than that required for a true anesthetic state. Large doses of benzodiazepines can prolong the postanesthetic recovery period (an undesirable effect), but they can produce a high incidence of anterograde amnesia which is clinically useful. Because it causes a high incidence of amnesia (> 50%), midazolam is frequently given intravenously before induction of general anesthesia. Midazolam has a more rapid onset, a shorter elimination half-life (2–4 hours), and a steeper dose-response curve than do the other benzodiazepines used in anesthesia.

The benzodiazepine antagonist flumazenil is sometimes used to accelerate recovery from excessive sedative actions of intravenous benzodiazepines, but reversal of respiratory depression by flumazenil is less predictable. Its short duration of action (< 90 minutes) may necessitate multiple doses to prevent recurrence of central nervous system depressant effects of longer-acting benzodiazepines.

OPIOID ANALGESICS

Large doses of opioid analgesics have been used to achieve general anesthesia, particularly in patients undergoing cardiac surgery or other major surgery when their circulatory reserve is minimal. Intravenous morphine, 1–3 mg/kg, or the high-potency opioid fentanyl, 100–150 µg/kg, have been used in such situations with minimal evidence of cardiovascular deterioration. More recently, several congeners of fentanyl, namely sufentanil, alfentanil, and remifentanil, have also been used. Despite the use of high doses of these potent opioids (see Table 31–2 for conventional analgesic doses), awareness during anesthesia and unpleasant postoperative recall have occurred.

Furthermore, high intravenous doses of opioids can cause chest wall rigidity, thereby acutely impairing ventilation, as well as postoperative respiratory depression requiring prolonged assisted ventilation and the administration of opioid antagonists (eg, naloxone). Low doses of fentanyl have been used as premedication and as an adjunct to both intravenous and inhaled anesthetics. Alfentanil and remifentanil have been used as induction agents since they both have a rapid onset of action. Remifentanil has an extremely short duration of action because it is rapidly metabolized by esterases in the blood (not plasma cholinesterase) and muscle tissues. The metabolism of remifentanil is not subject to genetic variability, and the drug does not interfere with the clearance of compounds metabolized by plasma cholinesterase (eg, esmolol, mivacurium, or succinylcholine. Rapid recovery following remifentanil is important regarding its potential utility in anesthesia regimens for ambulatory surgery. Fentanyl and droperidol (a butyrophenone related to haloperidol) together produce analgesia and amnesia and are sometimes used with nitrous oxide to provide a state of **neuroleptanesthesia**.

Opioid analgesics can also be used at low doses by the epidural and spinal routes of administration to produce excellent postoperative analgesia.

PROPOFOL

Propofol (2,6-diisopropylphenol) is an extremely popular intravenous anesthetic. Its rate of onset of action is similar to that of the intravenous barbiturates; recovery is more rapid; and patients are able to ambulate sooner after propofol. Furthermore, patients subjectively "feel better" in the immediate postoperative period after propofol as compared with other intravenous anesthetics. Postoperative nausea and vomiting is less common because propofol has antiemetic actions. Propofol is used for both induction and maintenance of anesthesia; however, cumulative effects can delay arousal following prolonged infusion. These favorable properties are responsible for the extensive use of propofol as a component of balanced anesthesia and for its great popularity as an anesthetic for use in day surgery outpatient procedures. The drug is also effective in producing prolonged sedation in patients in critical care settings (see Box, Conscious Sedation and Deep Sedation). However, use of propofol for the sedation of children under intensive care has led to severe acidosis in the presence of respiratory infections and possible neurological sequelae on withdrawal.

After intravenous administration of propofol, the distribution half-life is 2–8 minutes; the elimination half-life is approximately 30–60 minutes. The drug is rapidly metabolized in the liver (ten times faster than thiopental) and excreted in the urine as glucuronide and sulfate conjugates. Less than 1% of the drug is excreted unchanged. Total body clearance of the anesthetic is greater than hepatic blood flow, suggesting that its elimination includes extrahepatic mechanisms in addition to metabolism by liver enzymes. This property is useful in patients with impaired ability to metabolize other sedative-anesthetic drugs.

Effects on respiration are similar to those of thiopental at usual anesthetic doses. However, propofol causes a marked decrease in systemic blood pressure during induction of anesthesia, primarily through decreased peripheral resistance. In addition, propofol has greater negative inotropic effects on the heart than etomidate and thiopental. Apnea and pain at the site of injection are common adverse effects of bolus administration. Muscle movements, hypotonus, and (rarely) tremors have also been reported following its use. Clinical infections due to bacterial contamination of the propofol emulsion have led to the addition of antimicrobial adjuvants (eg, ethylenediaminetetraacetic acid and metabisulfite).

ETOMIDATE

Etomidate is a carboxylated imidazole that can be used for induction of anesthesia in patients with limited cardiovascular reserve. Its major advantage over other intravenous agents is that it causes minimal cardiovascular and respiratory depression. Etomidate produces a rapid loss of consciousness, with minimal hypotension. The heart rate is usually unchanged, and the incidence of apnea is low. The drug has no analgesic effects, and coadministration of opioids may be required to decrease cardiac responses during tracheal intubation and to lessen spontaneous muscle movements. Following an induction dose, recovery is rapid (< 5 minutes).

CONSCIOUS SEDATION & DEEP SEDATION

Many diagnostic, therapeutic, and minor surgical procedures require neither general anesthesia nor the availability of specialized equipment and facilities necessary for inhaled anesthesia. In this setting, regional or local anesthesia supplemented with midazolam or propofol and opioid analgesics may be a more appropriate and safer approach than general anesthesia.

Another approach has been the development of protocols to provide a state of **conscious sedation** or drug-induced alleviation of anxiety and pain in combination with an altered level of consciousness, but with retention of the ability of the patient to maintain a patent airway and to respond to verbal commands. A wide variety of intravenous anesthetic agents have proved to be useful drugs in conscious sedation techniques. For example, intravenous benzodiazepines, propofol, and opioid analgesics can provide amnestic, sedative, and analgesic effects without loss of consciousness. Use of benzodiazepines and opioid analgesics in conscious sedation protocols has the advantage of being reversible by the specific receptor antagonist drugs (eg, flumazenil and naloxone, respectively).

A special form of conscious sedation is sometimes needed in the ICU, when patients are under severe stress and often require mechanical ventilation for long periods (days) with an endotracheal tube in place. In this situation, sedative drugs or intravenous anesthetics in low dosage, neuromuscular blockers, and **dexmedetomidine** may be combined. Dexmedetomidine is an α_2 agonist with strong sedative properties. It has a half-life of 2–3 hours and is metabolized in the liver and excreted, mainly as metabolites, in the urine.

Deep sedation is a controlled state of anesthesia involving decreased consciousness from which the patient is not easily aroused. Since deep sedation is often accompanied by a loss of protective reflexes, an inability to maintain a patent airway, and lack of response to surgical stimuli, the state may be indistinguishable from that of general anesthesia. Intravenous agents used in deep sedation protocols include thiopental, ketamine, propofol, and certain intravenous opioid analgesics.

PREPARATIONS AVAILABLE[1]

Desflurane (Suprane)
Liquid: 240 mL for inhalation
Dexmedetomidine (Precedex)
Parenteral: 100 µg/mL for IV infusion
Diazepam (generic, Valium)
Oral: 2, 5, 10 mg tablets; 5 mg/5 mL and 5 mg/mL
solution
Oral sustained-release: 15 mg capsules
Parenteral: 5 mg/mL for injection
Droperidol (generic, Inapsine)
Parenteral: 2.5 mg/mL for IV or IM injection
Enflurane (Enflurane, Ethrane)
Liquid: 125, 250 mL for inhalation
Etomidate (Amidate)
Parenteral: 2 mg/mL for injection
Halothane (generic, Fluothane)
Liquid: 125, 250 mL for inhalation
Isoflurane (Isoflurane, Forane)
Liquid: 100 mL for inhalation

Ketamine (generic, Ketalar)
Parenteral: 10, 50, 100 mg/mL for injection
Lorazepam (generic, Ativan)
Oral: 0.5, 1, 2 mg tablets; 2 mg/mL solution
Parenteral: 2, 4 mg/mL for injection
Methohexital (Brevital Sodium)
Parenteral: 0.5, 2.5, 5 g powder to reconstitute for
injection
Methoxyflurane (Penthrane)
Liquid: 15, 125 mL for inhalation
Midazolam (generic, Versed)
Parenteral: 1, 5 mg/mL for injection in 1, 2, 5, 10 mL
vials
Oral: 2 mg/mL syrup
Nitrous oxide (gas, supplied in blue cylinders)
Propofol (generic, Diprivan)
Parenteral: 10 mg/mL for IV injection
Sevoflurane (Ultane)
Liquid: 250 mL for inhalation
Thiopental (generic, Pentothal)
Parenteral: powder to reconstitute 20, 25 mg/mL
for IV injection

[1]See Chapter 31 for formulations of opioid agents used in anesthesia.

Distribution of etomidate is rapid, with a biphasic plasma concentration curve showing distribution half-lives of 3 and 29 minutes. Redistribution of the drug from brain to highly perfused tissues appears to be responsible for the short duration of its anesthetic effects. Etomidate is extensively metabolized in the liver and plasma to inactive metabolites with only 2% of the drug excreted unchanged in the urine.

Etomidate causes a high incidence of pain on injection, myoclonus, and postoperative nausea and vomiting. The involuntary muscle movements are not associated with electroencephalographic epileptiform activity. Etomidate may also cause adrenocortical suppression via inhibitory effects on steroidogenesis, with decreased plasma levels of hydrocortisone after a single dose. Prolonged infusion of etomidate in critically ill patients may result in hypotension, electrolyte imbalance, and oliguria due to its adrenal suppressive effects.

KETAMINE

Ketamine (Figure 25–2) produces **dissociative anesthesia,** which is characterized by catatonia, amnesia, and analgesia, with or without actual loss of consciousness. The drug is an arylcyclohexylamine chemically related to phencyclidine (PCP), a drug frequently abused because of its psychoactive properties. The mechanism of action of ketamine may involve blockade of the membrane effects of the excitatory neurotransmitter glutamic acid at the NMDA (N-methyl-D-aspartate) receptor subtype (see Chapter 21).

Ketamine is a highly lipophilic drug and is rapidly distributed into highly vascular organs, including the brain, and subsequently redistributed to less well perfused tissues with concurrent hepatic metabolism and both urinary and biliary excretion.

Ketamine is the only intravenous anesthetic that possesses analgesic properties and produces cardiovascular stimulation. Heart rate, arterial blood pressure, and cardiac output are usually significantly increased. The peak increases in these variables occur 2–4 minutes after intravenous injection and then slowly decline to normal over the next 10–20 minutes. Ketamine produces its cardiovascular stimulation by excitation of the central sympathetic nervous system and possibly by inhibition of the reuptake of norepinephrine at sympathetic nerve terminals. Increases in plasma epinephrine and norepinephrine levels occur as early as 2 minutes after intravenous ketamine and return to baseline levels 15 minutes later.

Ketamine markedly increases cerebral blood flow, oxygen consumption, and intracranial pressure. In this regard ketamine resembles the volatile anesthetics as a potentially dangerous drug when intracranial pressure is elevated. In most patients, ketamine decreases the respiratory rate. However, upper airway muscle tone is well maintained, and airway reflexes are usually preserved.

Although it is a desirable anesthetic in many respects, ketamine has been associated with postoperative disorientation, sensory and perceptual illusions, and vivid dreams (so-called emergence phenomena). Diazepam, 0.2–0.3 mg/kg, or midazolam, 0.025–0.05 mg intravenously, given prior to the administration of ketamine reduces the incidence of these adverse effects. Because of the high incidence of postoperative psychic phenomena associated with its use, ketamine is not commonly used in general surgery in the USA. It is considered useful for poor-risk geriatric patients and in unstable patients (eg, cardiogenic or septic shock) because of its cardiostimulatory properties. It is also used in low doses for outpatient anesthesia in combination with propofol and in children undergoing painful procedures (eg, dressing changes for burns).

REFERENCES

Abraham RB et al: Malignant hyperthermia. Postgrad Med J 1998;74:11.

Beaussier M et al: Comparative effects of desflurane and isoflurane on recovery after long lasting anaesthesia. Can J Anaesth 1998;45:429.

Angelini G, Ketzler JT, Coursin DB: Use of propofol and other nonbenzodiazepine sedatives in the intensive care unit. Crit Care Clin 2001;17:863.

Behne M, Wilke HJ, Harder S: Clinical pharmacokinetics of sevoflurane. Clin Pharmacokinet 1999;36:13.

Bissonnette B et al: Neuroleptanesthesia: Current status. Can J Anaesth 1999;46:154.

Bowdle TA: Adverse effects of opioid agonists and agonist-antagonists in anaesthesia. Drug Saf 1998;19:173.

Campagna JA, Miller KW, Forman SA: Mechanisms of actions of inhaled anesthetics. N Engl J Med 2003;348:2110.

Delgado-Herrera L, Ostroff RD, Rogers SA: Sevoflurane: approaching the ideal inhalational anesthetic. a pharmacologic, pharmacoeconomic, and clinical review. CNS Drug Rev 2001;7:48.

Dickinson R: Selective synaptic actions of thiopental and its enantiomers. Anesthesiology 2002;96:884.

Dilger JP: The effects of general anaesthetics on ligand-gated ion channels. Br J Anaesth 2002;89:41.

Ebert TJ et al: Recovery from sevoflurane anesthesia: A comparison to isoflurane and propofol anesthesia. Anesthesiology 1998;89:1524.

Eger EI II, Saidman LJ, Brandstater B: Minimum alveolar anesthetic concentration: A standard of anesthetic potency. Anesthesiology 1965;26:756.

Eger EI II: Uptake and distribution. In: *Anesthesia*, 4th ed. Miller RD (editor). Churchill Livingstone, 1994.

Gentz BA, Malan TP Jr: Renal toxicity with sevoflurane: a storm in a teacup? Drugs 2001;61:2155.

Glass PSA, Gan TJ, Howell S: A review of the pharmacokinetics and pharmacodynamics of remifentanil. Anesth Analg 1999;89(4 Suppl):S7.

Jenkins A et al: Evidence for a common binding cavity for three general anesthetics within the GABA$_A$ receptor. J Neurosci 2001;21:RC136 (1–4).

Jurd R et al: General anesthetic actions in vivo strongly attenuated by a point mutation in the GABA$_A$ receptor beta$_3$ subunit. FASEB J 2003;17:250.

Kang TM: Propofol infusion syndrome in critically ill patients. Ann Pharmacother 2002;36:1453.

Kharasch ED et al: Compound A uptake and metabolism to mercapturic acids and 3,3,3-trifluoro-2-fluoromethoxypropanoic acid during low-flow sevoflurane anesthesia: Biomarkers for exposure, risk assessment, and interspecies comparison. Anesthesiology 1999;91:1267.

Kohrs R, Durieu ME: Ketamine: Teaching an old dog new tricks. Anesth Analg 1998;87:1186.

Krasowski MD, Harrison NL: General anaesthetic actions on ligand-gated ion channels. Cell Mol Life Sci 1999;55:1278.

Nelson LE et al: The sedative component of anesthesia is mediated by GABA$_A$ receptors in an endogenous sleep pathway. Nat Neurosci 2002;5:979.

Nishikawa K et al: Volatile anesthetic actions on the GABA$_A$ receptors: contrasting effects of alpha 1(S270) and beta 2(N265) point mutations. Neuropharmacology 2002;42:337.

O'Keeffe NJ, Healy TE: The role of new anesthetic agents. Pharmacol Ther 1999;84:233.

Park KW: Cardiovascular effects of inhalational anesthetics. Int Anesthesiol Clin 2002;40:1.

Patel S: Cardiovascular effects of intravenous anesthetics. Int Anesthesiol Clin 2002;40:15.

Robinson BJ, Uhrich TD, Ebert TJ: A review of recovery from sevoflurane anaesthesia: Comparisons with isoflurane and propofol including meta-analysis. Acta Anaesthesiol Scand 1999;43:185.

Rosen MA: Management of anesthesia for the pregnant surgical patient. Anesthesiology 1999;91:1159.

Russo H, Bressolle F: Pharmacodynamics and pharmacokinetics of thiopental. Clin Pharmacokinet 1998;35:95.

Siegwart R, Jurd R, Rudolph U: Molecular determinants for the action of general anesthetics at recombinant alpha(2)beta(3) gamma(2)gamma-aminobutyric acid(A) receptors. J Neurochem 2002;80:140.

Tang J et al: Recovery profile, cost and patient satisfaction with propofol and sevoflurane for fast-track office-based anesthesia. Anesthesiology 1999;91:253.

Tassonyi E et al: The role of nicotinic acetylcholine receptors in the mechanisms of anesthesia. Brain Res Bull 2002;57:133.

Topf N et al: Effects of isoflurane on gamma-aminobutyric acid type A receptors activated by full and partial agonists. Anesthesiology 2003;98:306.

Trapani G et al: Propofol in anesthesia. Mechanism of action, structure-activity relationships, and drug delivery. Curr Med Chem 2000;7:249.

Trudell JR, Bertaccini E: Molecular modelling of specific and nonspecific anaesthetic interactions. Br J Anaesth 2002;89:32.

White PF, Way WL, Trevor AJ: Ketamine—its pharmacology and therapeutic uses. Anesthesiology 1982;56:119.

White PF (editor): *Textbook of Intravenous Anesthesia.* Williams & Wilkins, 1997.

Local Anesthetics

26

Paul F. White, PhD, MD, & Bertram G. Katzung, MD, PhD

Local anesthetics reversibly block impulse conduction along nerve axons and other excitable membranes that utilize sodium channels as the primary means of action potential generation. This action can be used clinically to block pain sensation from—or sympathetic vasoconstrictor impulses to—specific areas of the body. Cocaine, the first such agent, was isolated by Niemann in 1860. It was introduced into clinical use by Koller in 1884 as an ophthalmic anesthetic. Cocaine was soon found to be strongly addicting but was widely used, nevertheless, for 30 years, since it was the only local anesthetic drug available. In an attempt to improve the properties of cocaine, Einhorn in 1905 synthesized procaine, which became the dominant local anesthetic for the next 50 years. Since 1905, many local anesthetic agents have been synthesized. The goals of these efforts were reduction of local irritation and tissue damage, minimization of systemic toxicity, faster onset of action, and longer duration of action. Lidocaine, still a popular agent, was synthesized in 1943 by Löfgren and may be considered the prototype local anesthetic agent.

None of the currently available local anesthetics are ideal, and development of newer agents continues. However, while it is relatively easy to synthesize a chemical with local anesthetic effects, it is very difficult to reduce the toxicity significantly below that of the current agents. The major reason for this difficulty is the fact that the much of the serious toxicity of local anesthetics represents extensions of the therapeutic effect on the brain and the circulatory system. However, new research into the mechanisms of cardiac and spinal toxicity and alternative drug targets for spinal analgesia (eg, α_2 receptors) suggest that it may be possible to find better drugs, at least for spinal anesthesia. In an attempt to extend the duration of the local anesthetic action, a variety of novel delivery systems are in development (eg, polymers). Transdermal local anesthetic delivery systems are also being investigated.

I. BASIC PHARMACOLOGY OF LOCAL ANESTHETICS

Chemistry

Most local anesthetic agents consist of a lipophilic group (frequently an aromatic ring) connected by an intermediate chain (commonly including an ester or amide) to an ionizable group (usually a tertiary amine; Table 26–1). In addition to the general physical properties of the molecules, specific stereochemical configurations are associated with differences in the potency of stereoisomers for a few compounds, eg, bupivacaine, ropivacaine. Since ester links (as in procaine) are more prone to hydrolysis than amide links, esters usually have a shorter duration of action.

Local anesthetics are weak bases. For therapeutic application, they are usually made available as salts to increase solubility and stability. In the body, they exist either as the uncharged base or as a cation. The relative proportions of these two forms is governed by their pK_a and the pH of the body fluids according to the Henderson-Hasselbalch equation:

$$\log \frac{\text{Cationic form}}{\text{Uncharged form}} = pK_a - pH$$

Since the pK_a of most local anesthetics is in the range of 8.0–9.0, the larger fraction in the body fluids at physiologic pH will be the charged, cationic form. The cationic form is thought to be the most active form at the receptor site (cationic drug cannot readily leave closed channels), but the uncharged form is very important for rapid penetration of biologic membranes. The local anesthetic receptor is not readily accessible from

Table 26–1. Structure and properties of some ester and amide local anesthetics.[1]

	Lipophilic Group	Intermediate Chain	Amine Substituents	Potency (Procaine = 1)	Duration of Action
Esters					
Cocaine				2	Medium
Procaine (Novocain)				1	Short
Tetracaine (Pontocaine)				16	Long
Benzocaine				Surface use only	
Amides					
Lidocaine (Xylocaine)				4	Medium
Mepivacaine (Carbocaine, Isocaine)				2	Medium
Bupivacaine (Marcaine), levobupivacaine (Chirocaine)				16	Long
Etidocaine (Duranest)				16	Long
Prilocaine (Citanest)				3	Medium
Ropivacaine (Naropin)				16	Long

[1]Other chemical types are available including ethers (pramoxine), ketones (dyclonine), and phenetidin derivatives (phenacaine).

the external side of the cell membrane (see Mechanism of Action, below). This partly explains why dentists and surgeons observe that local anesthetics are much less effective when they are injected into infected tissues. Because infected tissues have a low extracellular pH, a very low fraction of nonionized local anesthetic is available for diffusion into the cell.

Pharmacokinetics

Local anesthetics are usually administered by injection into the area of the nerve fibers to be blocked. Thus, absorption and distribution are not as important in controlling the onset of effect as in determining the rate of offset of local analgesia and the likelihood of central nervous system and cardiac toxicity. Topical application of local anesthetics, however, requires drug diffusion for both onset and offset of anesthetic effect.

A. Absorption

Systemic absorption of injected local anesthetic from the site of administration is modified by several factors, including dosage, site of injection, drug-tissue binding, the presence of vasoconstricting substances (eg, epinephrine), and the physicochemical properties of the drug. Application of a local anesthetic to a highly vascular area such as the tracheal mucosa results in more rapid absorption and thus higher blood levels than if the local anesthetic had been injected into a poorly perfused area, such as tendon or subcutaneous fat. For regional anesthesia involving block of large nerves, maximum blood levels of local anesthetic decrease according to site of administration in the following order: intercostal (highest blood level) > caudal > epidural > brachial plexus > sciatic nerve (lowest).

Vasoconstrictor substances such as epinephrine reduce systemic absorption of local anesthetics from the injection site by decreasing blood flow in these areas. This is especially true for drugs with intermediate or short durations of action such as procaine, lidocaine, and mepivacaine (but not prilocaine). Neuronal uptake of the drug is presumably enhanced by the higher local drug concentration, and the systemic toxic effects of the drug are reduced, since blood levels are lowered by as much as one-third. Furthermore, when used in spinal anesthesia, epinephrine acts directly on the cord to both enhance and prolong local anesthetic-induced spinal anesthesia by acting on α_2 adrenoceptors, which inhibit release of substance P and reduce sensory neuron firing. The recognition of this fact has led to the use of clonidine not only to augment local anesthetic effect in the subarachnoid space but also to produce local analgesia. The combination of reduced systemic absorption, enhanced neuronal local anesthetic uptake, and α_2 activation by epinephrine in the central nervous system is responsible for prolonging the local anesthetic effect by up to 50%. Vasoconstrictors are less effective in prolonging anesthetic properties of the more lipid-soluble, long-acting drugs (eg, bupivacaine), possibly because these molecules are highly tissue-bound. As noted below, cocaine is unique owing to its sympathomimetic properties.

B. Distribution

The amide local anesthetics are widely distributed after intravenous bolus administration. There is evidence that sequestration occurs in storage sites, including fatty tissue. After an initial rapid distribution phase, which consists of uptake into highly perfused organs such as the brain, liver, kidney, and heart, a slower distribution phase occurs with uptake into moderately well perfused tissues, such as muscle and the gastrointestinal tract. Because of the extremely short plasma half-lives of the ester type agents (see below), their tissue distribution has not been extensively studied.

C. Metabolism and Excretion

The local anesthetics are converted in the liver or in plasma to more water-soluble metabolites and then excreted in the urine. Since local anesthetics in the uncharged form diffuse readily through lipid membranes, little or no urinary excretion of the neutral form occurs. Acidification of urine will promote ionization of the tertiary base to the more water-soluble charged form, which is more readily excreted since it is not so easily reabsorbed by renal tubules.

Ester type local anesthetics are hydrolyzed very rapidly in the blood by butyrylcholinesterase (pseudocholinesterase). Therefore, procaine and chloroprocaine have very short plasma half-lives (eg, < 1 minute).

The amide linkage of amide local anesthetics is hydrolyzed by liver microsomal cytochrome P450. There is considerable variation in the rate of liver metabolism of individual amide compounds, the approximate order being prilocaine (fastest) > etidocaine > lidocaine > mepivacaine > ropivacaine > bupivacaine and levobupivacaine (slowest). As a result, toxicity from the amide type of local anesthetic is more likely to occur in patients with liver disease. For example, the average half-life of lidocaine may be increased from 1.8 hours in normal patients to over 6 hours in patients with severe liver disease. Many other drugs used in anesthesia are metabolized by the same P450 isozymes as the local anesthetics. Concomitant use of the other agents may slow the metabolism of the local anesthetics.

Decreased hepatic removal of local anesthetics should also be anticipated in patients with reduced hepatic blood flow. For example, the hepatic elimination of lidocaine in patients anesthetized with halothane is slower than that measured in patients anesthetized with a non-volatile anesthetic. The reduced elimination may be related to decreased hepatic blood flow and to halothane-induced depression of hepatic microsomal enzymes.

Pharmacodynamics

A. Mechanism of Action

The primary mechanism of action of local anesthetics is **blockade of voltage-gated sodium channels.** The excitable membrane of nerve axons, like the membrane of cardiac muscle (see Chapter 14) and neuronal cell bodies (see Chapter 21), maintains a resting transmembrane potential of −90 to −60 mV. During excitation, the sodium channels open, and a fast inward sodium current quickly depolarizes the membrane toward the sodium equilibrium potential (+40 mV). As a result of depolarization, the sodium channels close (inactivate) and the potassium channels open. The outward flow of potassium repolarizes the membrane toward the potassium equilibrium potential (about −95 mV); repolarization returns the sodium channels to the rested state. The transmembrane ionic gradients are maintained by the sodium pump. These characteristics are similar to those of heart muscle, and local anesthetics have similar effects in both tissues.

The function of sodium channels can be disrupted in several ways. Biologic toxins such as **batrachotoxin, aconitine, veratridine,** and some **scorpion venoms** bind to receptors within the channel and prevent inactivation. This results in prolonged influx of sodium through the channel and depolarization of the resting potential rather than block of conduction. The marine toxins **tetrodotoxin** (**TTX**) and **saxitoxin** block these channels by binding to channel receptors near the extracellular surface. Their clinical effects superficially resemble those of local anesthetics (block of conduction without a change in the resting potential) even though their receptor site is quite different. Spinal neurons can be differentiated on the basis of tetrodotoxin effect into TTX-sensitive and TTX-resistant types. Some evidence suggests that the TTX-resistant neurons are responsible for pain transmission and are the primary targets for local anesthetics in spinal anesthesia. Local anesthetics bind to receptors near the intracellular end of the sodium channel and block the channel in a time- and voltage-dependent fashion (see below). The sodium channel has been cloned; its primary structure has been characterized; and mutational analysis has allowed identification of parts of the local anesthetic binding site.

When progressively increasing concentrations of a local anesthetic are applied to a nerve fiber, the threshold for excitation increases, impulse conduction slows, the rate of rise of the action potential declines, action potential amplitude decreases, and, finally, the

ability to generate an action potential is abolished. These progressive effects result from binding of the local anesthetic to more and more sodium channels. If the sodium current is blocked over a critical length of the nerve, propagation across the blocked area is no longer possible. At the minimum dose required to block propagation, the resting potential is not significantly affected.

The blockade of sodium channels by most local anesthetics is both *voltage-* and *time-dependent:* Channels in the rested state (which predominate at more negative membrane potentials) have a much lower affinity for local anesthetics than activated (open state) and inactivated channels (which predominate at more positive membrane potentials; Figure 14–8). Thus, the effect of a given drug concentration is more marked in rapidly firing axons than in resting fibers (Figure 26–1).

Between action potentials, a portion of the sodium channels recover from local anesthetic block (see Figure 14–8). The recovery from drug-induced block is 10–1000 times slower than the recovery of channels from normal inactivation, as shown for the cardiac membrane in Figure 14–4. As a result, the refractory period is lengthened and the nerve can conduct fewer impulses.

Elevated extracellular calcium partially antagonizes the action of local anesthetics. This reversal is caused by

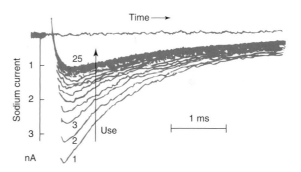

Figure 26–1. Effect of repetitive activity on the block of sodium current produced by a local anesthetic in a myelinated axon. A series of 25 pulses was applied, and the resulting sodium currents (downward deflections) are superimposed. Note that the current produced by the pulses rapidly decreased from the first to the 25th pulse. A long rest period following the train resulted in recovery from block, but the block could be reinstated by a subsequent train. (nA, nanoamperes.) (Modified slightly and reproduced, with permission, from Courtney KR: Mechanism of frequency-dependent inhibition of sodium currents in frog myelinated nerve by the lidocaine derivative GEA. J Pharmacol Exp Ther 1975;195:225.)

the calcium-induced increase of the surface potential on the membrane, which favors the low-affinity rested state. Conversely, increase of extracellular potassium depolarizes the membrane potential and favors the inactivated state. This enhances the effect of local anesthetics.

Local anesthetics can be shown to block a variety of other channels, including nicotinic acetylcholine channels in the spinal cord. However, there is no convincing evidence that such actions play the major role in the clinical effects of any of these drugs. Local anesthetics at high concentrations may interfere with intra-axonal transport and calcium homeostasis in the nerve terminal. These effects may contribute to the spinal toxicity of the local anesthetics.

B. STRUCTURE-ACTIVITY CHARACTERISTICS OF LOCAL ANESTHETICS

The smaller and more lipophilic the local anesthetic, the faster the rate of interaction with the sodium channel receptor. Potency is also positively correlated with lipid solubility as long as the agent retains sufficient water solubility to diffuse to the site of action. Lidocaine, procaine, and mepivacaine are more water-soluble than tetracaine, etidocaine, and bupivacaine. The latter agents are more potent and have longer durations of anesthetic action. They also bind more extensively to proteins and will displace or be displaced from these binding sites by other drugs. In the case of optically active agents, eg, bupivacaine, one isomer can usually be shown to be moderately more potent than the other.

C. OTHER ACTIONS ON NERVES

Since local anesthetics are capable of blocking all nerves, their actions are not usually limited to the desired loss of sensation. Although motor paralysis may at times be desirable, it may also limit the ability of the patient to cooperate, eg, pushing during obstetric delivery. During spinal anesthesia, motor paralysis may impair respiratory activity and autonomic nerve blockade may lead to hypotension. Residual sympathetic nerve blockade may interfere with bladder function (resulting in urinary retention) and early ambulation. However, nerve fibers differ significantly in their susceptibility to local anesthetic blockade on the basis of differences in size and myelination (Table 26–2). Upon direct application of a local anesthetic to a nerve root, the smaller B and C fibers are blocked first, followed by the small type A delta fibers. Thus, pain fibers are blocked first; other sensations disappear next; and motor function is blocked last.

1. Effect of fiber diameter—Local anesthetics preferentially block small fibers because the distance over which such fibers can passively propagate an electrical impulse (related to the space constant) is shorter. During the onset of local anesthesia, when short sections of nerve are blocked, the small-diameter fibers are the first to fail to conduct. For myelinated nerves, at least two and preferably three successive nodes must be blocked by the local anesthetic to halt impulse propagation. The thicker the nerve fiber, the farther apart the nodes tend to be—which explains, in part, the greater resistance to block of large motor fibers. Myelinated nerves tend to become blocked before unmyelinated nerves of the same diameter. For this reason, the preganglionic B fibers may be blocked before the smaller unmyelinated C fibers involved in pain transmission.

2. Effect of firing frequency—Another important reason for preferential blockade of sensory fibers follows directly from the state-dependent mechanism of action of local anesthetics. Block by these drugs is more

Table 26–2. Relative size and susceptibility to block of types of nerve fibers.

Fiber Type	Function	Diameter (μm)	Myelination	Conduction Velocity (m/s)	Sensitivity to Block
Type A					
Alpha	Proprioception, motor	12–20	Heavy	70–120	+
Beta	Touch, pressure	5–12	Heavy	30–70	++
Gamma	Muscle spindles	3–6	Heavy	15–30	++
Delta	Pain, temperature	2–5	Heavy	12–30	+++
Type B	Preganglionic autonomic	< 3	Light	3–15	++++
Type C					
Dorsal root	Pain	0.4–1.2	None	0.5–2.3	++++
Sympathetic	Postganglionic	0.3–1.3	None	0.7–2.3	++++

marked at higher frequencies of depolarization and with longer depolarizations. Sensory fibers, especially pain fibers, have a high firing rate and a relatively long action potential duration (up to 5 ms). Motor fibers fire at a slower rate and have a shorter action potential duration (< 0.5 ms). Type A delta and C fibers are smaller-diameter fibers that participate in high-frequency pain transmission. Therefore these fibers are blocked sooner with lower concentrations of local anesthetics than are the A alpha fibers.

3. Effect of fiber position in the nerve bundle—An anatomic circumstance that sometimes creates exceptions to the above rules for differential nerve block is the location of the fiber in the peripheral nerve bundle. In large nerve trunks, motor nerves are usually located circumferentially, and for that reason they are the first to be exposed to the drug when it is administered by injection into the tissue surrounding the nerve. Therefore, it is not uncommon that motor nerve block occurs before sensory block in large mixed nerves. In the extremities, proximal sensory fibers are located in the outer portion of the nerve trunk, whereas the distal sensory innervation is in the core of the nerve. Thus, during infiltration block of a large nerve, anesthesia first develops proximally and then spreads distally as the drug penetrates into the core of the nerve.

D. EFFECTS ON OTHER EXCITABLE MEMBRANES

Local anesthetics have weak neuromuscular blocking effects that are of minimal clinical importance. However, their effects on cardiac cell membranes are of major clinical significance. Some are useful antiarrhythmic agents (see Chapter 14) at concentrations lower than those required to produce nerve block; others (eg, bupivacaine) can *cause* lethal arrhythmias in high enough concentration.

II. CLINICAL PHARMACOLOGY OF LOCAL ANESTHETICS

Local anesthetics can provide highly effective analgesia in well-defined regions of the body. The usual routes of administration include topical application (eg, nasal mucosa, wound margins), injection in the vicinity of peripheral nerve endings and major nerve trunks (infiltration), and injection into the epidural or subarachnoid spaces surrounding the spinal cord (Figure 26–2). Intravenous regional anesthesia of the arm or leg (Bier block) is used for short surgical procedures (< 45 minutes). This is accomplished by intravenous injection of the anesthetic agent into a distal vein while the circulation of the limb is isolated with a proximally placed tourni-

quet. Finally, an infiltration block of autonomic sympathetic fibers can be used to evaluate the role of sympathetic tone in patients with peripheral vasospasm.

The choice of local anesthetic for a specific procedure is usually based on the duration of action required. Procaine and chloroprocaine are short-acting; lidocaine, mepivacaine, and prilocaine have an intermediate duration of action; and tetracaine, bupivacaine, levobupivacaine, etidocaine, and ropivacaine are long-acting drugs (Table 26–1).

The anesthetic effect of the agents with short and intermediate durations of action can be prolonged by increasing the dose or by adding a vasoconstrictor agent (eg, epinephrine or phenylephrine). The vasoconstrictor retards the removal of drug from the injection site. In addition, it decreases the blood level and hence the probability of central nervous system toxicity.

The onset of local anesthesia can be accelerated by the use of solutions saturated with carbon dioxide ("carbonated"). The high tissue level of CO_2 results in intracellular acidosis (CO_2 crosses membranes readily), which in turn results in intracellular accumulation of the cationic form of the local anesthetic.

Repeated injection of local anesthetics can result in loss of effectiveness (ie, tachyphylaxis) due to extracellular acidosis. Local anesthetics are commonly marketed as hydrochloride salts (pH 4.0–6.0). After injection, the salts are buffered in the tissue to physiologic pH, thereby providing sufficient free base for diffusion through axonal membranes. However, repeated injections deplete the buffering capacity of the local tissues. The ensuing acidosis increases the extracellular cationic form, which diffuses poorly into axons. The clinical result is apparent tachyphylaxis, especially in areas of limited buffer reserve, such as the cerebrospinal fluid.

Pregnancy appears to increase susceptibility to local anesthetic toxicity in that median doses required for nerve block or to induce toxicity are reduced. Cardiac arrest leading to death following the epidural administration of 0.75% bupivacaine to women in labor resulted in the temporary withdrawal from the market of the high concentration of this long-acting local anesthetic and subsequent introduction of potentially less cardiotoxic alternatives (ie, ropivacaine and levobupivacaine) for this high-risk population. It is not clear whether the increased sensitivity during pregnancy is due to elevated estrogen, elevated progesterone, or some other factor.

Topical local anesthesia is often used for eye, ear, nose, and throat procedures and for cosmetic surgery. Satisfactory local anesthesia requires an agent capable of rapid penetration of the skin or mucosa and with limited tendency to diffuse away from the site of application. Cocaine, because of its excellent penetration and vasoconstrictor effects, has been used extensively for nose and throat procedures. It is somewhat irritating, however,

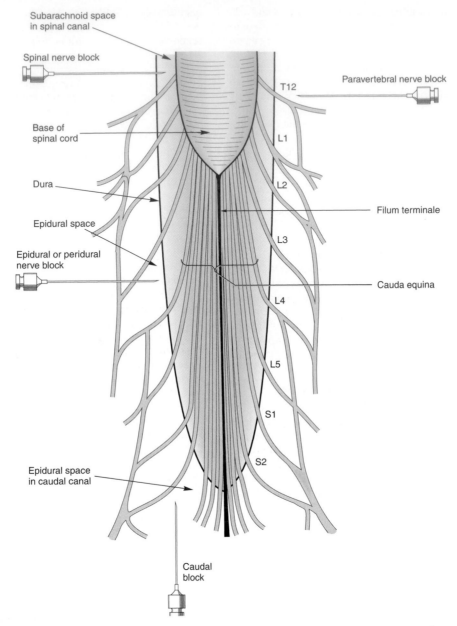

Subarachnoid space
in spinal canal

Spinal nerve block

Paravertebral nerve block

T12

Base of
spinal cord

L1

Dura

L2

Filum terminale

Epidural space

L3

Epidural or peridural
nerve block

Cauda equina

L4

L5

S1

S2

Epidural space
in caudal canal

Caudal
block

Figure 26–2. Schematic diagram of sites of injection of local anesthetics in and near the spinal canal.

and is thus much less popular for ophthalmic procedures. Recent concerns about its potential cardiotoxicity when combined with epinephrine has led most otolaryngologists and plastic surgeons to switch to a combination containing lidocaine and epinephrine. Other drugs used for topical anesthesia include lidocaine, tetracaine, pramoxine, dibucaine, benzocaine, and dyclonine.

Since local anesthetics are membranes-stabilizing drugs, both parenteral (eg, intravenous lidocaine) and oral (eg, mexiletine, tocainide) formulations of these drugs have been used to treat patients with neuropathic pain syndromes. Systemic local anesthetic drugs are commonly used as adjuvants to the combination of a tricyclic antidepressant (eg, amitriptyline) and an anticonvulsant (eg, carbamazepine) in patients who fail to respond to the standard tricyclic plus anticonvulsant combination. One to 3 weeks are required to observe a therapeutic effect after introduction of the local anesthetic in patients with neuropathic pain.

Toxicity

Two major forms of local anesthetic toxicity are recognized: direct neurotoxicity from the local effects of certain agents administered around the cord or other major nerve trunks, and systemic effects, since ultimately, local anesthetic agents are absorbed from the site of administration. If blood levels rise too high, effects on several organ systems may be observed.

A. CENTRAL NERVOUS SYSTEM

1. All local anesthetics—Central nervous system effects at low doses include sleepiness, light-headedness, visual and auditory disturbances, and restlessness. An early symptom of local anesthetic toxicity is circumoral and tongue numbness and a metallic taste. At higher concentrations, nystagmus and muscular twitching occur. Finally, overt tonic-clonic convulsions followed by central nervous system depression and death may occur. Local anesthetics apparently cause depression of cortical inhibitory pathways, thereby allowing unopposed activity of excitatory components. This transitional stage of unbalanced excitation is then followed by generalized central nervous system depression at higher blood levels of local anesthetic.

Convulsions due to excessive blood levels can usually be prevented by administering the smallest dose of local anesthetic required for adequate anesthesia and by avoiding inadvertent intravascular injection or injection into highly perfused tissues. When large doses must be administered, premedication with a benzodiazepine, eg, oral diazepam or midazolam parenterally, appears to provide significant prophylaxis against local anesthetic seizures by raising the seizure threshold. If seizures do occur, it is important to prevent hypoxemia and acidosis. Although administration of oxygen does not prevent seizure activity, hyperoxemia may be beneficial after onset of seizures. Since hypercapnia and acidosis may lower the seizure threshold, hyperventilation is recommended during treatment of seizures. In addition, hyperventilation increases blood pH, which in turn lowers extracellular potassium. This action hyperpolarizes the transmembrane potential of axons, which favors the rested or low-affinity state of the sodium channels, resulting in decreased local anesthetic toxicity.

Seizures induced by local anesthetics can also be treated with small doses (given intravenously) of thiopental 1–2 mg/kg, propofol 0.5–1 mg/kg, midazolam 2–4 mg total dose, or diazepam 0.1 mg/kg. The muscular manifestations of seizures can be suppressed by a short-acting neuromuscular blocking agent (eg, succinylcholine, 0.5–1 mg/kg IV). It should be emphasized that succinylcholine does not obliterate central nervous system manifestations of seizure activity. Rapid tracheal intubation and mechanical ventilation can prevent pulmonary aspiration of gastric contents and facilitate hyperventilation therapy.

2. Cocaine—Since prehistoric times, the natives of Peru have chewed the leaves of the indigenous plant *Erythroxylon coca,* the source of cocaine, to obtain a feeling of well-being and reduce fatigue. Intense central nervous system effects can be achieved by sniffing cocaine powder and smoking cocaine base. Cocaine has become one of the most widely abused drugs (see Chapter 32). High doses of inhaled cocaine as well as injected cocaine have all of the toxicities described for other local anesthetics in general. In addition, cocaine can produce severe cardiovascular toxicity, including hypertension and arrhythmias.

B. NEUROTOXICITY

When applied at excessively high concentrations, all local anesthetics can be toxic to nerve tissue. Chloroprocaine and lidocaine appear to be more neurotoxic than other local anesthetics when used for spinal anesthesia, producing so-called transient radicular irritation. It has been suggested that this toxicity results from pooling of high concentrations of the local anesthetic in the cauda equina. Although the mechanism of this neurotoxic action has not been established, both interference with axonal transport and disruption of calcium homeostasis have been shown to occur and could be responsible. Spinal neurotoxicity does not result from excessive sodium channel blockade.

C. CARDIOVASCULAR SYSTEM

The cardiovascular effects of local anesthetics result partly from direct effects upon the cardiac and smooth muscle membranes and partly from indirect effects upon the autonomic nerves. As described in Chapter 14, local anesthetics block cardiac sodium channels and thus depress abnormal cardiac pacemaker activity, excitability, and conduction. At very high concentrations, they may also block calcium channels. With the notable exception of cocaine, local anesthetics also depress the strength of cardiac contraction and cause arteriolar dilation, both effects leading to severe hypotension. Cardiovascular collapse and death are rare and usually occur only after large doses of 0.75% bupivacaine.

As noted above, cocaine differs from the other local anesthetics in its cardiovascular effects. Cocaine's blockade of norepinephrine reuptake results in vasoconstriction and hypertension. It may also precipitate cardiac

PREPARATIONS AVAILABLE

Articaine (Septocaine)
Parenteral: 4% with 1:100,000 epinephrine
Benzocaine (generic, others)
Topical: 5, 6% creams; 15, 20% gels; 5, 20% ointments; 0.8% lotion; 20% liquid; 20% spray
Bupivacaine (generic, Marcaine, Sensorcaine)
Parenteral: 0.25, 0.5, 0.75% for injection; 0.25, 0.5, 0.75% with 1:200,000 epinephrine
Butamben picrate (Butesin Picrate)
Topical: 1% ointment
Chloroprocaine (generic, Nesacaine)
Parenteral: 1, 2, 3% for injection
Cocaine (generic)
Topical: 40, 100 mg/mL solutions; 5, 25 g powder
Dibucaine (generic, Nupercainal)
Topical: 0.5% cream; 1% ointment
Dyclonine (Dyclone)
Topical: 0.5, 1% solution
Levobupivacaine (Chirocaine)
Parenteral: 2.5, 5, 7.5 mg/mL
Lidocaine (generic, Xylocaine, others)
Parenteral: 0.5, 1, 1.5, 2, 4% for injection; 0.5, 1, 1.5, 2% with 1:200,000 epinephrine; 1, 2% with 1:100,000 epinephrine, 2% with 1:50,000 epinephrine

Topical: 2.5, 5% ointments; 0.5, 4% cream; 0.5, 2.5% gel; 2, 2.5, 4% solutions; 23, 46 mg/2 cm² patch
Lidocaine and etidocaine eutectic mixture (EMLA cream)
Topical: lidocaine 2.5% plus etidocaine 2.5%
Mepivacaine (generic, Carbocaine, others)
Parenteral: 1, 1.5, 2, 3% for injection; 2% with 1:20,000 levonordefrin
Pramoxine (Tronothane, others)
Topical: 1% cream, lotion, spray, and gel
Prilocaine (Citanest)
Parenteral: 4% for injection; 4% with 1:200,000 epinephrine
Procaine (generic, Novocain)
Parenteral: 1, 2, 10% for injection
Proparacaine (generic, Alcain, others)
0.5% solution for ophthalmic use
Ropivacaine (Naropin)
Parenteral: 0.2, 0.5, 0.75, 1.0 % solution for injection
Tetracaine (Pontocaine)
Parenteral: 1% for injection; 0.2, 0.3% with 6% dextrose for spinal anesthesia
Topical: 1% ointment; 0.5% solution (ophthalmic); 1, 2% cream; 2% solution for nose and throat; 2% gel

---

arrhythmias. The vasoconstriction produced by cocaine can lead to ischemia and, in chronic abusers, to ulceration of the mucous membrane and even damage to the nasal septum when "snorted." This vasoconstrictor property of cocaine can be used clinically to decrease bleeding from mucosal damage in the nasopharynx.

Bupivacaine is more cardiotoxic than other local anesthetics. This reflects the fact that bupivacaine block of sodium channels is potentiated by the long action potential duration of cardiac cells (as compared to nerve fibers). Studies have shown that the most common electrocardiographic finding in patients with bupivacaine intoxication is slow idioventricular rhythm with broad QRS complexes and eventually, electromechanical dissociation.

Resuscitation from bupivacaine cardiovascular toxicity is extremely difficult. However, prompt resuscitation has been successful with standard cardiopulmonary support, including the prompt correction of acidosis by hyperventilation and administration of bicarbonate as well as epinephrine, atropine, and bretylium. Local anesthetics, especially bupivacaine, also inhibit basal and epinephrine-stimulated cAMP production. This finding places greater emphasis on aggressive epinephrine therapy during bupivacaine-induced cardiotoxicity.

The (S)-isomer, levobupivacaine, appears to have a lower propensity for cardiovascular toxicity than the racemic mixture or the (R)-isomer and has recently been approved for clinical use. **Ropivacaine,** another newer local anesthetic, has clinical effects similar to those of bupivacaine but may be associated with a lower potential for cardiovascular toxicity. Ropivacaine is available only as the (S)-stereoisomer, which has inherently less affinity for the cardiac sodium channel.

D. HEMATOLOGIC EFFECTS

The administration of large doses (> 10 mg/kg) of prilocaine during regional anesthesia may lead to accumulation of the metabolite *o*-toluidine, an oxidizing agent capable of converting hemoglobin to methemoglobin. When sufficient methemoglobin is present (3–5 mg/dL), the patient may appear cyanotic and the blood chocolate-colored. Although moderate levels of methemoglobinemia are well-tolerated by healthy individuals, they may cause decompensation in patients with cardiac or pulmonary disease. The treatment of methemoglobinemia involves the intravenous administration of reducing agents (eg, methylene blue or ascorbic acid), which rapidly convert methemoglobin to hemoglobin.

E. Allergic Reactions

The ester type local anesthetics are metabolized to *p*-aminobenzoic acid derivatives. These metabolites are responsible for allergic reactions in a small percentage of the population. Amides are not metabolized to *p*-aminobenzoic acid, and allergic reactions to agents of the amide group are extremely rare.

REFERENCES

Albright GA: Cardiac arrest following regional anesthesia with etidocaine or bupivacaine. Anesthesiology 1979;51:285.

Brau ME et al: Effect of drugs used for neuropathic pain management on tetrodotoxin-resistant Na⁺ currents in rat sensory neurons. Anesthesiology 2001;94:137.

Clarkson CW et al: Analysis of the ionic basis for cocaine's biphasic effect on action potential duration in guinea pig ventricular myocytes. J Mol Cell Cardiol 1996;28:667.

Ferreira S et al: Effects of cocaine and its major metabolites on the HERG-encoded potassium channel. J Pharmacol Exp Ther 2001;299:220.

Hille B: Local anesthetics: Hydrophilic and hydrophobic pathways for the drug-receptor reactions. J Gen Physiol 1977;69:497.

Johnson ME et al: Effect of local anesthetic on neuronal cytoplasmic calcium and plasma membrane lysis (necrosis) in a cell culture model. Anesthesiology 2002;97:1466.

Kanai Y, Katsuki H, Takasaki M: Comparisons of the anesthetic potency and intracellular concentrations of S(−) and R(+) bupivacaine and ropivacaine in crayfish giant axon in vitro. Anesth Analg 2000;90:415.

Kanai Y, Katsuki H, Takasaki M: Lidocaine disrupts axonal membrane of rat sciatic nerve in vitro. Anesth Analg 2000;91:944.

Kendig JJ, Courtney KR: New modes of nerve block. Anesthesiology 1991;74:207.

Li YM et al: Local anesthetics inhibit substance P binding and evoked increases in intracellular Ca²⁺. Anesthesiology 1995;82:166.

Miyamoto Y et al: Direct inhibition of microtubule-based kinesin motility by local anesthetics Biophys J 2000;78:940.

Monk TG et al: Effect of topical eutectic mixture of local anesthetics on pain response and analgesic requirement during lithotripsy procedures. Anesth Analg 1994;79:506.

Nau C et al: Point mutations at N434 in D1-S6 of mu1 Na(+) channels modulate binding affinity and stereoselectivity of local anesthetic enantiomers. Mol Pharmacol 1999;56:404.

Oda A et al: Characteristics of ropivacaine block of Na⁺ channels in rat dorsal root ganglion neurons. Anesth Analg 2000;91:1213.

Ragsdale DS et al: Molecular determinants of state-dependent block of Na⁺ channels by local anesthetics. Science 1994;265:1724.

Sakura S et al: Local anesthetic neurotoxicity does not result from blockade of voltage-gated sodium channels. Anesth Analg 1995;81:338.

Scholtz A: Mechanisms of (local) anaesthetics on voltage-gated sodium and other ion channels. Br J Anaesth 2002;89:52.

Sinnott CJ et al: On the mechanism by which epinephrine potentiates lidocaine's peripheral nerve block. Anesthesiology 2003;98:181.

Stoelting RK: Local anesthetics. In: *Pharmacology and Physiology in Anesthetic Practice,* 3rd ed. Lippincott-Raven, 1999.

Tree-Trakarn T, Pirayavaraporn S, Lertakyamanee J: Topical analgesia for relief of post-circumcision pain. Anesthesiology 1987;67:395.

Valenzuela C et al: Stereoselective block of cardiac sodium channels by bupivacaine in guinea pig ventricular myocytes. Circulation 1995;92:3014.

White PF: The role of non-opioid analgesic techniques in the management of pain after ambulatory surgery. Anesth Analg 2002;95:577.

Zapata-Sudo G et al: Is comparative cardiotoxicity of S(-) and R(+) bupivacaine related to enantiomer-selective inhibition of L-type Ca²⁺ channels? Anesth Analg 2001;92:496.

Zhou W et al: Mechanism underlying bupivacaine inhibition of G protein-gated inwardly rectifying K⁺ channels. Proc Natl Acad Sci U S A 2001;98:6482.

Skeletal Muscle Relaxants

Paul F. White, PhD, MD, & Bertram G. Katzung, MD, PhD

Drugs that affect skeletal muscles fall into two major therapeutic groups: those used during surgical procedures and in intensive care units to cause paralysis (ie, **neuromuscular blockers**), and those used to reduce spasticity in a variety of neurologic conditions (ie, **spasmolytics**). Neuromuscular blocking drugs interfere with transmission at the neuromuscular end plate and lack central nervous system activity. These compounds are used primarily as adjuncts to general anesthesia. Drugs in the spasmolytic group have traditionally been called "centrally acting" muscle relaxants. However, at least one of these latter agents (dantrolene) has no significant central effects.

NEUROMUSCULAR BLOCKING DRUGS

History

During the 16th century, European explorers found that natives of the Amazon Basin of South America were using an arrow poison (curare) that produced death by skeletal muscle paralysis. The active compound from curare, *d*-tubocurarine, and its synthetic derivatives have had an enormous influence on the practice of anesthesia and surgery and have been very useful in defining normal neuromuscular physiologic mechanisms.

Normal Neuromuscular Function

The mechanism of neuromuscular transmission at the end plate is similar to that described for preganglionic cholinergic nerves in Chapter 6, with arrival of an impulse at the motor nerve terminal, influx of calcium, and release of acetylcholine. Acetylcholine then diffuses across the synaptic cleft to the nicotinic receptor located on the motor end plate. As noted in Chapter 7, this receptor is composed of five peptides: two alpha peptides, one beta, one gamma, and one delta peptide. Combination of two acetylcholine molecules with receptors on the two α subunits causes opening of the channel. The resulting movements of sodium and potassium are associated with a graded depolarization of the end plate membrane. This change in voltage is termed the motor end plate potential. The magnitude of the end plate potential is directly related to the amount of acetylcholine released. If the potential is small, the permeability and the end plate potential return to normal without an impulse being propagated from the end plate region to the rest of the muscle membrane. However, if the end plate potential is large, the adjacent muscle membrane is depolarized, and an action potential will be propagated along the entire muscle fiber. Muscle contraction is then initiated by excitation-contraction coupling. The released acetylcholine is quickly removed from the end plate region by diffusion and enzymatic destruction by the local acetylcholinesterase enzyme.

At least two additional types of acetylcholine receptors are associated with the neuromuscular apparatus. One is located on the presynaptic motor axon terminal; activation of these receptors mobilizes additional transmitter for subsequent release, perhaps by mobilizing more acetylcholine vesicles within the ending. The second type of receptor is found on perijunctional cells and is not normally involved in neuromuscular transmission. However, under certain conditions (eg, prolonged immobilization, burns), these receptors may proliferate sufficiently to affect subsequent neuromuscular transmission.

Skeletal muscle relaxation and paralysis can occur from interruption of function at several different sites, including the central nervous system, myelinated somatic nerves, unmyelinated motor nerve terminals, nicotinic acetylcholine receptors, the motor end plate, and the muscle membrane or intracellular contractile apparatus itself (Figure 27–1).

In practice, blockade of end plate function is accomplished by two basic mechanisms. Pharmacologic blockade of the physiologic agonist acetylcholine is characteristic of the *antagonist* neuromuscular blocking drugs. These drugs prevent access of the transmitter to its receptor and prevent depolarization. The prototype of this *nondepolarizing* subgroup is *d*-**tubocurarine**. Block of transmission can also be produced by an excess of the depolarizing *agonist*, namely acetylcholine. This paradoxical effect of acetylcholine also occurs at the ganglionic nicotinic acetylcholine receptor. The clinically useful prototypical *depolarizing* blocking drug is **suc-**

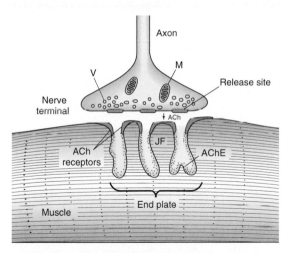

Figure 27–1. Schematic representation of the neuromuscular junction. (V, transmitter vesicle; M, mitochondrion; ACh, acetylcholine; AChE, acetylcholinesterase; JF, junctional folds.) (Reproduced, with permission, from Drachman DB: Myasthenia gravis. N Engl J Med 1978;298:135.)

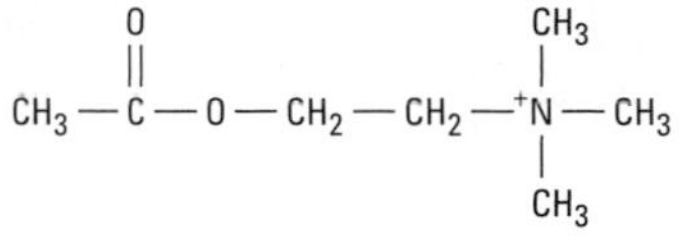

Acetylcholine

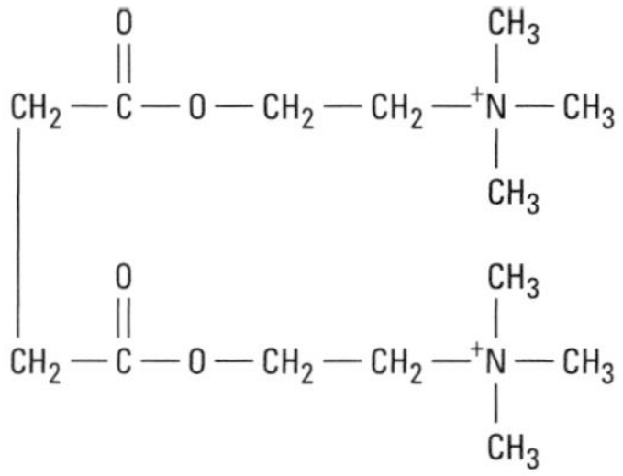

Succinylcholine

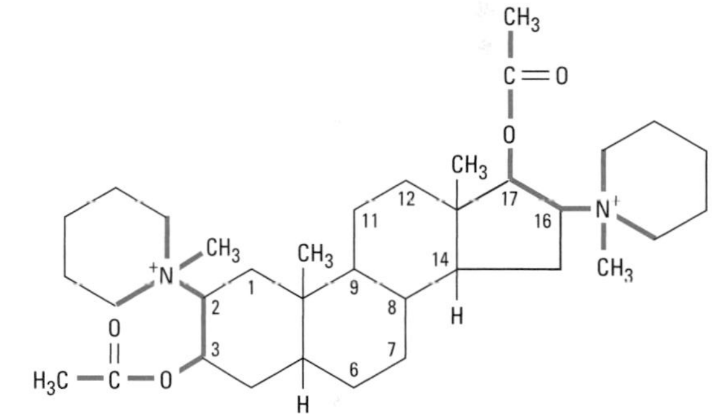

Pancuronium

Figure 27–2. Structural relationship of succinylcholine, a depolarizing agent, and pancuronium, a nondepolarizing agent, to acetylcholine, the neuromuscular transmitter. Succinylcholine, originally called diacetylcholine, is simply two molecules of acetylcholine linked through the acetate methyl groups. Pancuronium may be viewed as two acetylcholine-like fragments (*outlined in color*) oriented on a steroid nucleus.

cinylcholine. A similar depolarizing block can be produced by acetylcholine itself if very high local concentrations are achieved in the synaptic cleft (eg, in cholinesterase inhibitor intoxication), by nicotine, and by other nicotinic agonists. However, because the block produced by these drugs cannot be controlled adequately, they are of no clinical value in this application.

I. BASIC PHARMACOLOGY OF NEUROMUSCULAR BLOCKING DRUGS

Chemistry

All of the available neuromuscular blocking drugs bear a structural resemblance to acetylcholine. In fact, succinylcholine is two acetylcholine molecules linked end-to-end (Figure 27–2). In contrast to the single linear structure of succinylcholine and other depolarizing drugs, the nondepolarizing agents (eg, pancuronium) conceal the "double-acetylcholine" structure in one of two types of bulky, semi-rigid ring systems (Figure 27–2). The two major families of nondepolarizing blocking drugs—the isoquinoline and steroid derivatives—are shown in Figures 27–3 and 27–4. Another feature common to all currently used neuromuscular

blockers is the presence of one or two quaternary nitrogens, which makes them poorly lipid-soluble and limits entry into the central nervous system.

Pharmacokinetics of Neuromuscular Blocking Drugs

All of the neuromuscular blocking drugs are highly polar and inactive when administered by mouth. Therefore, they are always administered intravenously or intramuscularly.

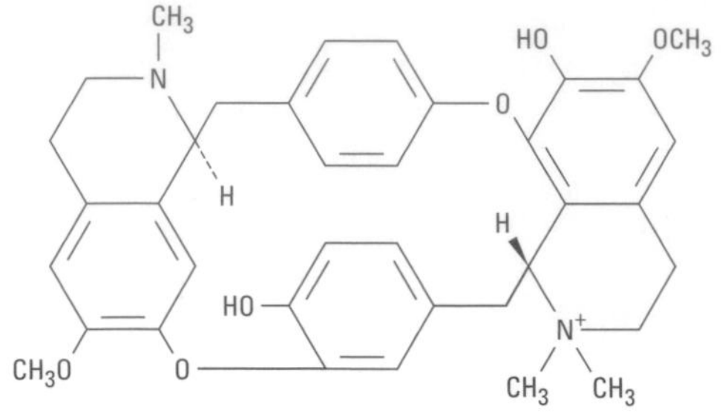

Tubocurarine

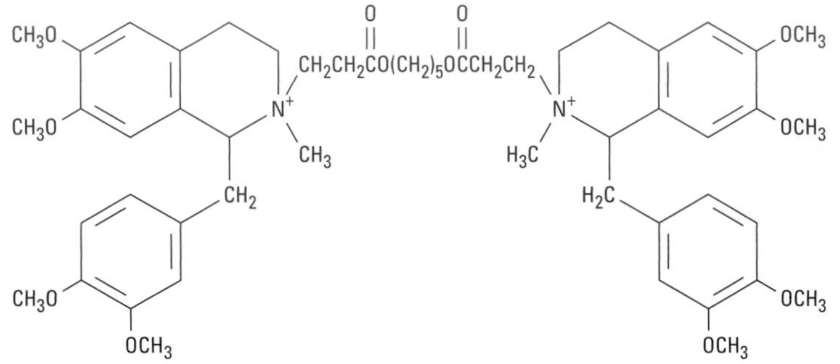

Atracurium

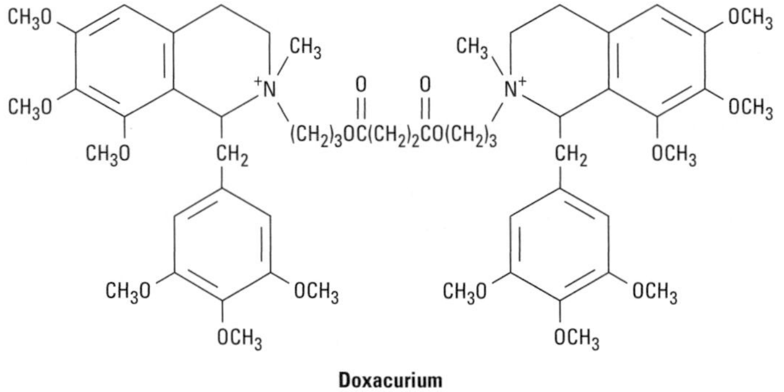

Doxacurium

Figure 27–3. Structures of some isoquinoline neuromuscular blocking drugs. These agents are all nondepolarizing muscle relaxants.

A. Nondepolarizing Drugs

The rate of disappearance of a nondepolarizing neuromuscular blocking drug from blood is characterized by a rapid initial distribution phase followed by a slower elimination phase. Because neuromuscular blocking drugs are highly ionized, they do not readily cross membranes and have a limited volume of distribution of 80–140 mL/kg—only slightly larger than the blood volume.

The route of elimination is strongly correlated with the duration of action of nondepolarizing relaxants. Drugs that are excreted by the kidney typically have longer half-lives, leading to longer durations of action (> 60 minutes). Drugs eliminated by the liver have somewhat shorter half-lives and durations of action (Table 27–1). All steroidal muscle relaxants are metabolized to their 3-hydroxy, 17-hydroxy, or 3,17-dihydroxy products, mainly in the liver. The 3-hydroxy metabo-

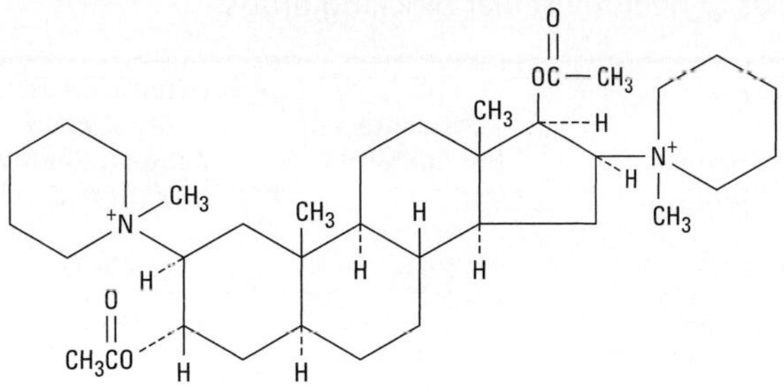

Pancuronium

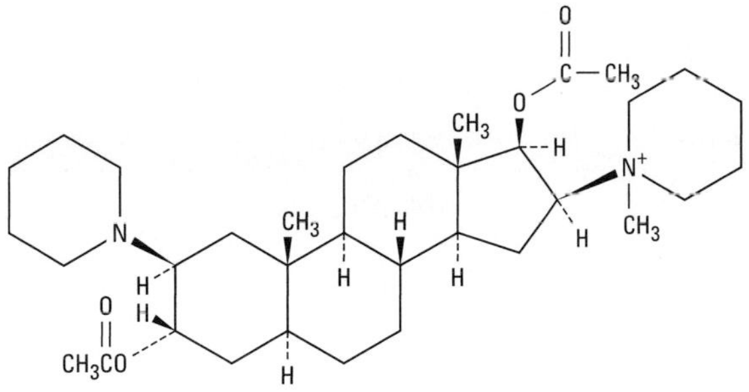

Vecuronium

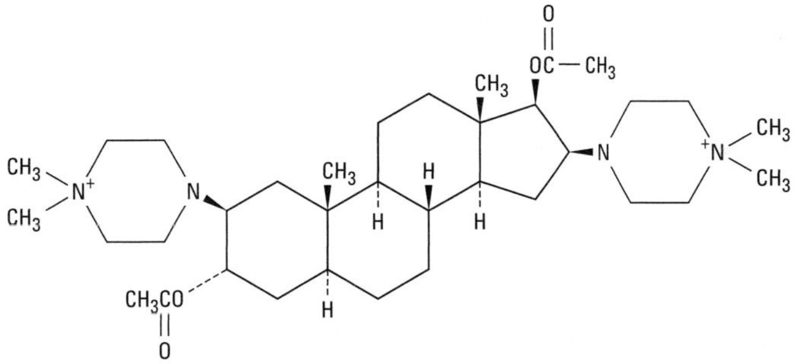

Pipecuronium

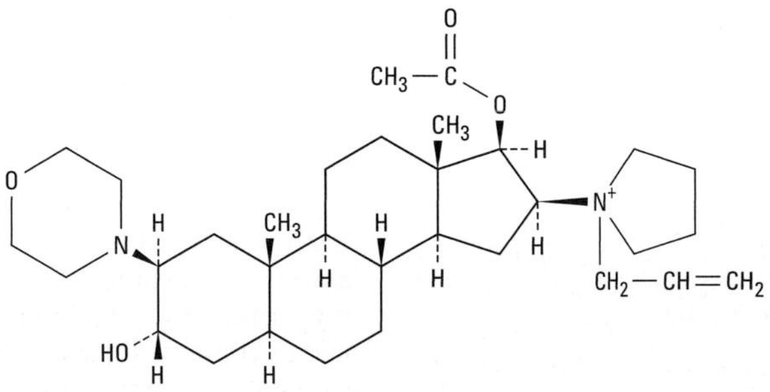

Rocuronium

Figure 27–4. Structures of steroid neuromuscular blocking drugs. These agents are all nondepolarizing muscle relaxants.

Table 27–1. Some properties of neuromuscular blocking drugs.

Drug	Elimination	Clearance (mL/kg/min)	Approximate Duration of Action (minutes)	Approximate Potency Relative to Tubocurarine
Isoquinoline derivatives				
Atracurium	Spontaneous[1]	6.6	20–35	1.5
Cisatracurium	Mostly spontaneous	5–6	25–44	1.5
Doxacurium	Kidney	2.7	> 35	6
Metocurine	Kidney (40%)	1.2	> 35	4
Mivacurium	Plasma ChE[2]	70–95	10–20	4
Tubocurarine	Kidney (40%)	2.3–2.4	> 35	1
Steroid derivatives				
Pancuronium	Kidney (80%)	1.7–1.8	> 35	6
Pipecuronium	Kidney (60%) and liver	2.5–3.0	> 35	6
Rapacuronium[3]	Liver	6–11	10–20	0.4
Rocuronium	Liver (75–90%) and kidney	2.9	20–35	0.8
Vecuronium	Liver (75–90%) and kidney	3–5.3	20–35	6
Depolarizing agent				
Succinylcholine	Plasma ChE[2] (100%)	>100	< 8	0.4

[1]Nonenzymatic and enzymatic hydrolysis of ester bonds.
[2]Butyrylcholinesterase (pseudocholinesterase).
[3]Withdrawn from clinical use.

lites are usually 40–80% as potent as the parent drug. Normally, metabolites are not formed in sufficient quantities to produce significant additional neuromuscular blockade during or after surgical anesthesia. However, if the parent compound is administered for several days, as may occur in the intensive care unit, the 3-hydroxy metabolite may accumulate and cause prolonged paralysis because it is more slowly cleared than the parent compound. Although the remaining metabolites also possess neuromuscular blocking properties, they have a very low potency.

The intermediate-acting steroid muscle relaxants (eg, vecuronium and rocuronium) tend to be more dependent on biliary excretion or hepatic metabolism for their elimination. These drugs are much more commonly used clinically than the long-acting drugs (eg, pancuronium, pipecuronium). Rapacuronium is the newest neuromuscular blocker and has the fastest onset time of any nondepolarizing muscle relaxant and the shortest duration of action. It was expected to be a nondepolariz-ing alternative to succinylcholine for rapid-sequence induction of anesthesia and tracheal intubation. Unfortunately, use of this agent for rapid-sequence intubation was associated with a high incidence of severe bronchospasm, which led to its early withdrawal from clinical practice.

Atracurium (Figure 27–3) is an isoquinoline nondepolarizing muscle relaxant with many of the same pharmacodynamic characteristics as vecuronium. However, atracurium is inactivated primarily by a form of spontaneous breakdown, also known as Hofmann elimination, and to a lesser extent by hepatic mechanisms. The main breakdown products are laudanosine and a related quaternary acid, neither of which has neuromuscular blocking properties. However, laudanosine is very slowly metabolized by the liver and has a long elimination half-life (ie, 150 minutes) compared with its parent compound, atracurium. Laudanosine readily crosses the blood-brain barrier, and high blood concentrations may cause seizures. During surgical procedures in humans, blood levels have ranged from 0.2 to 1 µg/mL. However, with prolonged infusions of atracurium in the intensive care unit, blood levels of laudanosine as high as 5.5 µg/mL have been reported. Even at much lower blood concentrations (0.2–0.8 µg/mL), laudanosine has been reported to produce a 30% increase in the volatile anesthetic requirement.

Atracurium has several stereoisomers, and one of the isomers, **cisatracurium,** has been approved for clinical use. It resembles atracurium but has even less dependence on hepatic inactivation, forms less laudanosine, and releases less histamine. From a clinical perspective, cisatracurium has all the advantages of atracurium with fewer adverse effects. Therefore, cisatracurium has largely replaced atracurium in clinical practice.

Mivacurium has a short duration of action, similar to that of rapacuronium (Table 27–1). However, the onset of action of mivacurium is slower than that of succinylcholine (and rapacuronium). In addition, the use of larger doses to speed the onset can be associated with clinically significant histamine release (eg, hypotension, flushing, and bronchospasm). Clearance by plasma cholinesterase is rapid (Table 27–1) and independent of the liver or kidney. However, because patients with renal failure often have decreased plasma cholinesterase levels, the short duration of action of mivacurium may be prolonged in patients with impaired renal function.

B. Depolarizing Drugs

The extremely brief duration of action of succinylcholine (5–10 minutes) is due chiefly to its rapid hydrolysis by plasma cholinesterase (butyrylcholinesterase, pseudocholinesterase), an enzyme in the liver and plasma. Plasma cholinesterase metabolizes succinylcholine more rapidly than it does mivacurium, and consequently the duration of action of succinylcholine is shorter than both rapacuronium and mivacurium (Table 27–1). The initial metabolite, succinylmonocholine (a weaker neuromuscular blocker), is metabolized to succinic acid and choline. Since plasma cholinesterase has an enormous capacity to rapidly hydrolyze succinylcholine, only a small fraction of the original intravenous dose reaches the neuromuscular junction. There is little or no plasma cholinesterase at the motor end plate, and the neuromuscular blockade of succinylcholine is terminated by its diffusion away from the end plate into extracellular fluid. Circulating levels of plasma cholinesterase, therefore, influence the duration of action of succinylcholine by determining the amount of the drug that actually reaches the motor end plate.

Neuromuscular blockade produced by succinylcholine or mivacurium can be prolonged in patients with a genetically abnormal variant of plasma cholinesterase. The "dibucaine number"—a test of the ability of a patient to metabolize succinylcholine—can be used to identify at-risk patients. Under standardized test conditions, dibucaine inhibits the normal enzyme about 80% and abnormal enzyme only 20%. Many genetic variants of plasma cholinesterase have been identified, though the dibucaine-related variants are the most important. Given the rarity of these genetic variants, plasma cholinesterase testing is not a routine clinical procedure.

Mechanism of Action

The interactions of drugs with the acetylcholine receptor-end plate channel have been described at the molecular level. Several modes of action of drugs on the receptor are possible and are illustrated in Figure 27–5.

A. Nondepolarizing Blocking Drugs

All of the neuromuscular blocking drugs in use in the USA except succinylcholine are classified as nondepolarizing agents. Tubocurarine is considered the prototype neuromuscular blocker. When small doses of nondepolarizing muscle relaxants are administered, they act predominantly at the **nicotinic receptor site** by competing with acetylcholine. The least potent of the nondepolarizing agents (rapacuronium and rocuronium; Table 27–1) have the fastest onset and the shortest duration of action. In larger doses, nondepolarizing drugs also enter the pore of the ion channel to cause a more intense motor blockade. This action further weakens neuromuscular transmission and diminishes the ability of acetylcholinesterase inhibitors (eg, neostigmine, edrophonium, pyridostigmine) to antagonize the effect of nondepolarizing muscle relaxants. Nondepolarizing relaxants can also block prejunctional sodium channels. As a result of this action, these muscle relaxants also interfere with the mobilization of acetylcholine at the nerve ending.

One consequence of the surmountable nature of the postsynaptic blockade produced by nondepolarizing muscle relaxants is the fact that tetanic stimulation, by releasing a large quantity of acetylcholine, is followed by transient posttetanic facilitation of the twitch strength. An important clinical consequence of the same principle is the reversal of residual blockade by cholinesterase inhibitors.

The characteristics of a nondepolarizing neuromuscular blockade are summarized in Table 27–2 and Figure 27–6.

B. Depolarizing Drugs

1. Phase I block (depolarizing)—Succinylcholine is the only depolarizing blocking drug used clinically in the United States. Its neuromuscular effects are like those of acetylcholine except that succinylcholine produces a longer effect at the myoneural junction. Suc-

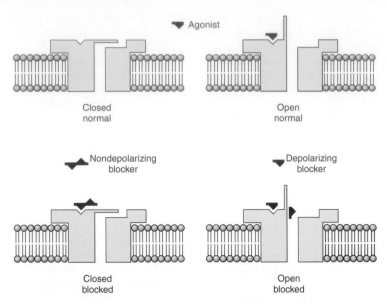

Figure 27–5. Schematic diagram of the interactions of drugs with the acetylcholine receptor on the end plate channel (structures are purely symbolic). **Top:** The action of the normal agonist, acetylcholine, in opening the channel. **Bottom: Left,** A nondepolarizing blocker, eg, rocuronium, is shown as preventing the opening of the channel when it binds to the receptor. **Right,** a depolarizing blocker, eg, succinylcholine, both occupying the receptor and blocking the channel. Normal closure of the channel gate is prevented. Depolarizing blockers may "desensitize" the end plate by occupying the receptor and causing persistent depolarization. An additional effect of drugs on the end plate channel may occur through changes in the lipid environment surrounding the channel (not shown). General anesthetics and alcohols may impair neuromuscular transmission by this mechanism.

cinylcholine reacts with the nicotinic receptor to open the channel and cause depolarization of the motor end plate, and this in turn spreads to the adjacent membranes, causing contractions of muscle motor units. Data from single-channel recordings indicate that depolarizing blockers can enter the channel to produce a prolonged "flickering" of the ion conductance (Figure 27–7). Because succinylcholine is not metabolized effectively at the synapse, the depolarized membranes remain depolarized and unresponsive to subsequent impulses (ie, they are in a state of depolarizing block). Furthermore, because excitation-concentration coupling requires end plate repolarization ("repriming") and repetitive firing to maintain muscle tension, a flaccid paralysis results. As a result, this so-called phase I (depolarizing) block is augmented, not reversed, by cholinesterase inhibitors.

The characteristics of a depolarizing neuromuscular blockade are summarized in Table 27–2 and Figure 27–6.

2. Phase II block (desensitizing)—With continued exposure to succinylcholine, the initial end plate depolarization decreases and the membrane becomes repolar-

ized. Despite this repolarization, the membrane cannot easily be depolarized again (ie, it becomes desensitized). The mechanism for this phase is unclear, but some evidence indicates that channel block may become more important than agonist action at the receptor in phase II of succinylcholine's neuromuscular blocking action. Regardless of the mechanism, the channels behave as if they are in a prolonged closed state (Figure 27–5). Later in phase II, the characteristics of the blockade are nearly identical to those of a nondepolarizing block (ie, a non-sustained response to a tetanic stimulus) (Figure 27–6), with reversal by acetylcholinesterase inhibitors.

II. CLINICAL PHARMACOLOGY OF NEUROMUSCULAR BLOCKING DRUGS

Skeletal Muscle Paralysis

Before the introduction of neuromuscular blocking drugs, profound skeletal muscle relaxation for intracavitary oper-

Table 27–2. Comparison of a typical nondepolarizing muscle relaxant (rocuronium) and a depolarizing muscle relaxant (succinylcholine).

| | | Succinylcholine | |
	Rocuronium	Phase I	Phase II
Administration of tubocurarine	Additive	Antagonistic	Augmented[1]
Administration of succinylcholine	Antagonistic	Additive	Augmented[1]
Effect of neostigmine	Antagonistic	Augmented[1]	Antagonistic
Initial excitatory effect on skeletal muscle	None	Fasciculations	None
Response to a tetanic stimulus	Unsustained (fade)	Sustained[2] (no fade)	Unsustained (fade)
Posttetanic facilitation	Yes	No	Yes
Rate of recovery	30–60 min[3]	4–8 min	> 20 min[3]

[1]It is not known whether this interaction is additive or synergistic (superadditive).
[2]The amplitude is decreased, but the response is sustained.
[3]The rate depends on the dose and on the completeness of neuromuscular blockade.

ations could be achieved only by producing deep levels of anesthesia that was often associated with profound depressant effects on the cardiovascular and respiratory systems. The adjunctive use of neuromuscular blocking drugs makes it possible to achieve adequate muscle relaxation for all types of surgical procedures without the cardiorespiratory depressant effects of deep anesthesia.

Assessment of Neuromuscular Transmission

Monitoring the effect of muscle relaxants during surgery (and recovery following the use of cholinesterase inhibitors) typically involves the use of a device that produces transdermal electrical stimulation of one of the peripheral nerves to the hand and recording of the evoked contractions (twitches; Figure 27–6). The motor responses to different patterns of peripheral nerve stimulation are measured. The three most commonly used patterns of include (1) single-twitch stimulation, (2) train-of-four (TOF) stimulation, and (3) tetanic stimulation. Two newer modalities are also available to monitor neuromuscular transmission: double-burst stimulation and posttetanic count.

With single-twitch stimulation, a single supramaximal electrical stimulus is applied to a peripheral nerve at frequencies from 0.1 Hz to 1.0 Hz. The higher frequency is often used during induction and reversal to more accurately determine the peak (maximal) drug effect. TOF stimulation involves four successive supramaximal stimuli given at intervals of 0.5 second (2 Hz). Each stimulus in the TOF causes the muscle to contract, and the relative magnitude of the response of the fourth twitch compared to the first twitch is the TOF ratio. With a depolarizing block, all four twitches are reduced in a dose-related fashion. With a nondepolarizing block, the TOF ratio decreases ("fades") and is inversely proportionate to the degree of blockade. During recovery from nondepolarizing block, the amount of fade decreases as the TOF ratio approaches 1.0. Fade in the TOF response after administration of succinylcholine signifies the development of a phase II block.

Finally, tetanic stimulation consists of very rapid (30–100 Hz) delivery of electrical stimuli for several seconds. During a nondepolarizing block and a phase II block after succinylcholine, the response will not be sustained and fade is observed. Fade in response to tetanic stimulation is normally considered a presynaptic event. However, the degree of fade depends primarily on the degree of neuromuscular blockade. During a partial nondepolarizing blockade, tetanic nerve stimulation is followed by a posttetanic increase in the twitch response, a manifestation of so-called posttetanic facilitation of neuromuscular transmission. During very intense neuromuscular blockade, there is no response to either tetanic or posttetanic stimulation. As the intensity

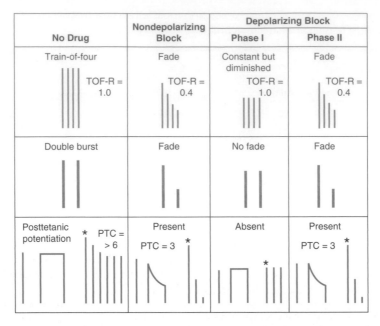

Figure 27–6. Muscle responses to different patterns of nerve stimulation used in monitoring skeletal muscle relaxation. The alterations produced by a nondepolarizing blocker and depolarizing and desensitizing blockade by succinylcholine are shown. In the train of four (TOF) pattern, four stimuli are applied at 2 Hz. The TOF ratio (TOF-R) is calculated from the strength of the fourth contraction divided by that of the first. In the double burst pattern, three stimuli are applied at 50 Hz, followed by a 700 ms rest period and then repeated. In the posttetanic potentiation pattern, several seconds of 50 Hz stimulation are applied followed by several seconds rest and then by single stimuli at a slow rate (eg, 0.5 Hz). The number of detectable posttetanic twitches is the posttetanic count (PTC). (*, first posttetanic contraction.)

of the block diminishes, the response to posttetanic twitch stimulation reappears. The time to reappearance of the first response to TOF stimulation is related to the posttetanic count.

The double-burst stimulation pattern is a newer mode of electrical nerve stimulation developed with the goal of allowing for manual detection of residual neuromuscular blockade when it is not possible to record the responses to single-twitch, TOF, or tetanic stimulation. In this pattern, three nerve stimuli are delivered at 50 Hz followed by a 700 ms rest period and then by two or three additional stimuli at 50 Hz. It is easier to detect fade in the responses to double-burst stimulation than in the responses to TOF stimulation. Note that the absence of fade in the responses to double-burst stimulation implies that clinically significant residual neuromuscular blockade does not exist.

A. NONDEPOLARIZING DRUGS

During anesthesia, the intravenous administration of tubocurarine, 0.1–0.4 mg/kg, will initially cause motor weakness, followed by the skeletal muscles becoming totally flaccid and inexcitable to electrical stimulation

(Figure 27–8). In general, larger muscles (eg, abdominal, trunk, paraspinous, diaphragm) are more resistant to blockade and recover more rapidly than smaller muscles (eg, facial, foot, hand). The diaphragm is usually the last muscle to be paralyzed. Assuming that ventilation is adequately maintained, no adverse effects occur. When administration of muscle relaxants is discontinued, recovery of muscles usually occurs in reverse order, with the diaphragm regaining function first, depending on the relaxant's elimination half-life. The pharmacologic effect of tubocurarine, 0.3 mg/kg IV, usually lasts 45–60 minutes. However, subtle evidence of residual muscle paralysis detected using a neuromuscular monitor may last for another hour. Potency and duration of action of the other nondepolarizing drugs are shown in Table 27–1. In addition to the duration of action, the most important property distinguishing the nondepolarizing relaxants is the time to onset of effect, which determines how rapidly the patient's trachea can be intubated with a tracheal tube. Of the nondepolarizing drugs, rapacuronium has the fastest onset of effect (45–90 seconds) followed by rocuronium (60–120 seconds). As earlier noted, rapacuronium is no longer available.

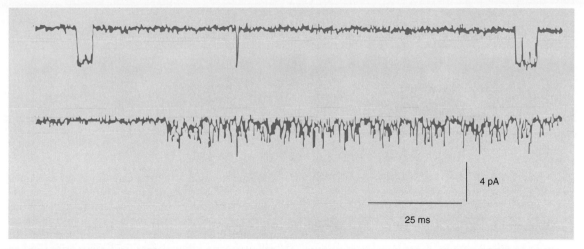

Figure 27–7. Action of succinylcholine on single-channel end plate receptor currents in frog muscle. The upper trace was recorded in the presence of a low concentration of succinylcholine; the downward deflections represent two openings of the channel and passage of inward (depolarizing) current. The lower trace was recorded in the presence of a much higher concentration of succinylcholine and shows prolonged "flickering" of the channel as it repetitively opens and closes or is "plugged" by the drug. (Reproduced, with permission, from Marshall CG, Ogden DC, Colquhoun D: The actions of suxamethonium (succinyldicholine) as an agonist and channel blocker at the nicotinic receptor of frog muscle. J Physiol [Lond] 1990;428:155.)

B. DEPOLARIZING DRUGS

Following the intravenous administration of succinylcholine, 0.75–1.5 mg/kg, transient muscle fasciculations occur, especially over the chest and abdomen, though general anesthesia tends to attenuate them. As complete paralysis develops, the arm, neck, and leg muscles are involved at a time when there is only slight weakness of the facial and pharyngeal muscles. However, respiratory muscle weakness follows rapidly, usually within 60 seconds (Figure 27–9). As a result of succinylcholine's rapid hydrolysis by cholinesterase in the

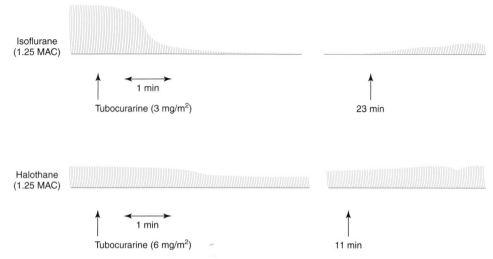

Figure 27–8. Neuromuscular blockade from tubocurarine during isoflurane and halothane anesthesia in patients. Note that at equivalent levels of anesthesia, isoflurane augments the block far more than does halothane.

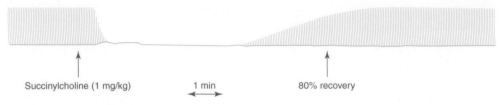

Figure 27–9. Neuromuscular blockade from succinylcholine during anesthesia in patients. Fasciculations were not seen, because the anesthetic obliterated them.

plasma and liver, the duration of neuromuscular block typically lasts 5–10 minutes (Table 27–1).

Cardiovascular Effects

Vecuronium, pipecuronium, doxacurium, cisatracurium, and rocuronium have minimal cardiovascular effects. The other currently used nondepolarizing muscle relaxants (pancuronium, atracurium, mivacurium) produce some cardiovascular effects that are mediated by autonomic or histamine receptors or both (Table 27–3).

Tubocurarine and, to a lesser extent, metocurine, mivacurium, and atracurium, can produce hypotension as a result of systemic histamine release, and with larger doses ganglionic blockade may occur with tubocurarine and metocurine. Premedication with an antihistamine drug will attenuate tubocurarine- and mivacurium-induced hypotension. Pancuronium causes a moderate increase in heart rate and a smaller increase in cardiac output, with little or no change in systemic vascular resistance. Although pancuronium-induced tachycardia is primarily due to a vagolytic action, release of norepinephrine from

Table 27–3. Effects of neuromuscular blocking drugs on other tissues.

Drug	Effect on Autonomic Ganglia	Effect on Cardiac Muscarinic Receptors	Tendency to Cause Histamine Release
Isoquinoline derivatives			
Atracurium	None	None	Slight
Cisatracurium	None	None	None
Doxacurium	None	None	None
Metocurine	Weak block	None	Slight
Mivacurium	None	None	Moderate
Tubocurarine	Weak block	None	Moderate
Steroid derivatives			
Pancuronium	None	Moderate block	None
Pipecuronium	None	None	None
Rapacuronium[1]	None	Very slight block	None
Rocuronium[2]	None	Slight	None
Vecuronium	None	None	None
Other agents			
Gallamine	None	Strong block	None
Succinylcholine	Stimulation	Stimulation	Slight

[1]Withdrawn from clinical use.
[2]Allergic reactions have been reported.

adrenergic nerve endings and blockade of neuronal uptake of norepinephrine have been suggested as secondary mechanisms. Effects of nondepolarizing blockers on the airways are discussed in the Box, Bronchospasm Induced by Neuromuscular Blockers.

Succinylcholine can cause cardiac arrhythmias when administered during halothane anesthesia. The drug stimulates all autonomic cholinoceptors, including the nicotinic receptors in both sympathetic and parasympathetic ganglia and muscarinic receptors in the heart (eg, sinus node). The negative inotropic and chronotropic responses to succinylcholine can be attenuated by administration of an anticholinergic drug (eg, glycopyrrolate, atropine). With large doses of succinylcholine, positive inotropic and chronotropic effects may result. On the other hand, bradycardia has been repeatedly observed when a second dose of succinylcholine is given less than 5 minutes after the first dose. This transient bradycardia can be prevented by thiopental, atropine, ganglionic-blocking drugs, and even nondepolarizing muscle relaxants. Direct myocardial effects, increased muscarinic stimulation, and ganglionic stimulation may all be involved in this bradycardic response.

Other Adverse Effects of Depolarizing Blockade

A. HYPERKALEMIA

Patients with burns, nerve damage or neuromuscular disease, closed head injury, and other trauma can respond to succinylcholine by an exaggerated release of potassium into the blood, occasionally resulting in cardiac arrest. As a result of the cardiac arrests (presumably caused by hyperkalemia), the Food and Drug Administration recommended in 1993 that succinylcholine no longer be used in children. However, this highly controversial contraindication was subsequently modified to a simple

warning because no acceptable alternative to succinylcholine was available for rapid-sequence inductions.

B. INCREASED INTRAOCULAR PRESSURE

Administration of succinylcholine is followed by a transient increase in intraocular pressure that is manifested less than 60 seconds after intravenous injection, peaks at 2–4 minutes, and declines after 5 minutes. The mechanism for this effect has not been clearly defined, but it may involve contraction of tonic myofibrils or transient dilation of choroidal blood vessels. Despite the increase in intraocular pressure, the use of succinylcholine for ophthalmologic operations is not contraindicated unless the anterior chamber is to be opened.

C. INCREASED INTRAGASTRIC PRESSURE

In heavily muscled patients, the fasciculations associated with succinylcholine will cause an increase in intragastric pressure ranging from 5 cm to 40 cm H_2O. This may make emesis more likely, with the potential hazard of aspiration of gastric contents. This complication is more likely to occur in patients with delayed gastric emptying (eg, diabetes, esophageal dysfunction, obesity).

D. MUSCLE PAIN

This is a common postoperative complaint of heavily muscled patients and those who have received large doses of succinylcholine. The true incidence of this symptom is difficult to establish because of subjective factors and differences in study design, but it has been reported in 0.2–20% of patients in different studies. It occurs more frequently in ambulatory than in bedridden patients. The pain is thought to be secondary to the unsynchronized contractions of adjacent muscle fibers just before the onset of paralysis. However, there is controversy over whether the incidence of muscle pain following succinylcholine is really higher than that following nondepolarizing muscle relaxants when other potentially confounding factors are considered.

BRONCHOSPASM INDUCED BY NEUROMUSCULAR BLOCKERS

Skeletal muscle relaxants have no direct effect on bronchial smooth muscle, but tubocurarine and mivacurium have been known to cause bronchoconstriction through the release of histamine. It was therefore unexpected that rapacuronium, which does not release histamine, caused severe bronchospasm in a significant number of patients during rapid-sequence induction for intubation. This dangerous (and in several cases fatal) effect was associated with young age (especially infants and children) and a history of reactive airway disease. Research indicates that rapacuronium blocks presynaptic M_2 muscarinic receptors (which modulate acetylcholine release) more effectively than postsynaptic M_3 receptors (which evoke bronchial smooth muscle contraction). This suggests that in reactive airways, rapacuronium might greatly enhance the release of acetylcholine onto inadequately blocked postsynaptic muscarinic receptors.

Interactions With Other Drugs

A. ANESTHETICS

Inhaled anesthetics augment the neuromuscular blockade produced by nondepolarizing muscle relaxants in a dose-dependent fashion. Of the anesthetics that have been studied, inhaled anesthetics augment the effects of muscle relaxants in the following order: isoflurane (most); then sevoflurane, desflurane, enflurane, and halothane (Figure 27–8); and finally nitrous oxide (least). The most important factors involved in this interaction are the following: (1) nervous system depression at sites proximal to the neuromuscular junction (ie, central nervous system); (2) increased muscle blood flow (ie, due to peripheral vasodilation), which allows a larger fraction of the injected muscle relaxant to reach the neuromuscular junction; and (3) decreased sensitivity of the postjunctional membrane to depolarization.

B. ANTIBIOTICS

Numerous reports have appeared describing enhancement of neuromuscular blockade by antibiotics, especially the aminoglycosides. Many of the antibiotics have been shown to cause a depression of evoked release of acetylcholine similar to that caused by magnesium. The mechanism of this prejunctional effect appears to be blockade of specific P-type calcium channels. These antibiotics also have postjunctional activity.

C. LOCAL ANESTHETICS AND ANTIARRHYTHMIC DRUGS

In large doses, most local anesthetics block neuromuscular transmission. However, in smaller doses, they enhance the neuromuscular block produced by both nondepolarizing and depolarizing muscle relaxants. In small doses, local anesthetics depress posttetanic potentiation, and this is thought to be a prejunctional neural effect. With higher doses, local anesthetics block acetylcholine-induced muscle contractions. This stabilizing effect is the result of blockade of the nicotinic receptor ion channels. Experimentally, similar effects can be demonstrated with sodium channel-blocking antiarrhythmic drugs such as quinidine. However, at the doses used for cardiac arrhythmias, this interaction is of little or no clinical significance. Higher concentrations of bupivacaine (0.75%) have been associated with cardiac arrhythmias independent of the muscle relaxant used.

D. OTHER NEUROMUSCULAR BLOCKING DRUGS

The end plate-depolarizing effect of succinylcholine can be antagonized by administering a small dose of a nondepolarizing blocker. To prevent the fasciculations associated with succinylcholine administration, a small nonparalyzing dose of a nondepolarizer can be given before succinylcholine (eg, *d*-tubocurarine 2 mg intravenously or pancuronium 0.5 mg intravenously). While this dose usually reduces fasciculations and postoperative pain, it can increase the amount of succinylcholine required for relaxation by 50–90% and may produce a feeling of weakness in awake patients. Therefore, preventive curarization prior to succinylcholine is no longer widely practiced.

Effects of Diseases & Aging on the Neuromuscular Response

Several diseases can diminish or augment the neuromuscular blockade produced by nondepolarizing muscle relaxants. Myasthenia gravis strongly enhances the neuromuscular blockade produced by these drugs. Advanced age (> 70 years) is associated with a prolonged duration of action from nondepolarizing relaxants as a result of decreased clearance of the drugs by the liver and kidneys. As a result, the dose of neuromuscular blocking drugs should be reduced in elderly patients.

Conversely, patients with severe burns and those with upper motor neuron disease are resistant to nondepolarizing muscle relaxants. This "desensitization" is probably caused by proliferation of extrajunctional receptors, which results in an increased dose requirement for the nondepolarizing relaxant to block a sufficient number of receptors.

Reversal of Nondepolarizing Neuromuscular Blockade

The cholinesterase inhibitors effectively antagonize the neuromuscular blockade caused by nondepolarizing drugs. Their general pharmacology is discussed in Chapter 7. Neostigmine and pyridostigmine antagonize nondepolarizing neuromuscular blockade by increasing the availability of acetylcholine at the motor end plate, mainly by inhibition of acetylcholinesterase. To a lesser extent, these cholinesterase inhibitors also increase release of transmitter from the motor nerve terminal. In contrast, edrophonium antagonizes neuromuscular blockade purely by inhibiting acetylcholinesterase. Edrophonium may be less effective than neostigmine in reversing the effects of most nondepolarizing blockers in the presence of a more profound degree of neuromuscular blockade. These differences are important in determining recovery from "residual block," the neuromuscular blockade remaining after completion of surgery and movement of the patient to the recovery room. Unsuspected residual block may result in hypoxia and even apnea, especially if patients receive other depressant medications during the recovery period.

Since mivacurium is metabolized by plasma cholinesterase, the interaction with the reversal drugs is unpredictable. On one hand, the neuromuscular blockade is antagonized because of increased acetylcholine concentrations in the synapse. On the other hand, mivacurium concentration may be higher because of decreased plasma cholinesterase breakdown of the muscle relaxant. The former effect usually dominates clinically, and mivacurium block is reversed by neostigmine.

Uses of Neuromuscular Blocking Drugs

A. SURGICAL RELAXATION

By far the most important application of the neuromuscular blockers is in facilitating surgery. This is especially important in intra-abdominal and intrathoracic procedures.

B. CONTROL OF VENTILATION

In critically ill patients who have ventilatory failure from various causes (eg, severe bronchospasm, pneumonia, chronic obstructive airway disease), it may be necessary to control ventilation to provide adequate gas exchange and to prevent atelectasis. Muscle paralysis is produced by administration of neuromuscular blocking drugs to eliminate chest wall resistance and ineffective spontaneous ventilation.

C. TREATMENT OF CONVULSIONS

Neuromuscular blocking drugs are sometimes used to attenuate or eliminate the peripheral manifestations of convulsions associated with epilepsy or local anesthetic toxicity. Although this approach is effective in eliminating the muscular manifestations of the seizures, it has no effect on the central processes involved since neuromuscular blocking drugs do not cross the blood-brain barrier.

SPASMOLYTIC DRUGS

Spasticity is characterized by an increase in tonic stretch reflexes and flexor muscle spasms (ie, increased basal muscle tone), together with muscle weakness. It is often associated with cerebral palsy, multiple sclerosis, and stroke. These conditions often involve abnormal function of the bowel and bladder as well as skeletal muscle. The mechanisms underlying clinical spasticity appear to involve not only the stretch reflex arc itself but also higher centers in the central nervous system (upper motor neuron lesion), with damage to descending pathways in the spinal cord, resulting in hyperexcitability of the alpha motoneurons in the cord. Nevertheless, pharmacologic therapy may ameliorate some of the symptoms of spasticity by modifying the stretch reflex arc or by interfering directly with skeletal muscle (ie, excitation-contraction coupling). The important components involved in these processes are shown in Figure 27–10.

Drugs that modify this reflex arc may modulate excitatory or inhibitory synapses (Chapter 21). Thus, to reduce the hyperactive stretch reflex, it is desirable to reduce the activity of the Ia fibers that excite the primary motoneuron or to enhance the activity of the inhibitory internuncial neurons. These structures are shown in greater detail in Figure 27–11.

A variety of pharmacologic agents described as depressants of the spinal "polysynaptic" reflex arc (eg, barbiturates [phenobarbital] and glycerol ethers [mephenesin]) have been used to treat these conditions of excess skeletal tone. However, as illustrated in Figure 27–11, nonspecific depression of synapses involved in the stretch reflex could reduce the desired inhibitory activity as well as the excitatory transmission. During the past several decades, more specific therapies have become available. Unfortunately, the lack of convenient and quantifiable measures of clinical response and of appropriate experimental models has hampered development of better agents for this heterogeneous group of medical conditions. Furthermore, while currently available drugs do provide significant relief from painful muscle spasms, they are all less effective in improving meaningful function (eg, mobility and return to work).

DIAZEPAM

As described in Chapter 22, benzodiazepines facilitate the action of γ-aminobutyric acid (GABA) in the central nervous system. Diazepam acts at all $GABA_A$ synapses, but its action in reducing spasticity is at least partly mediated in the spinal cord because it is somewhat effective in patients with cord transection. It can be used in patients with muscle spasm of almost any origin, including local muscle trauma. However, it produces sedation in most patients at the doses required to significantly reduce muscle tone. Dosage is usually begun at 4 mg/d and gradually increased to a maximum of 60 mg/d. Other benzodiazepines have been used as spasmolytics, but experience with them is much more limited.

BACLOFEN

Baclofen (p-chlorophenyl-GABA) was designed to be an orally active GABA-mimetic agent. The structure is shown below.

Baclofen

Baclofen exerts its spasmolytic activity at $GABA_B$ receptors. Activation of these receptors in the brain by baclofen results in hyperpolarization, probably by increased K^+ conductance. It has been suggested that hyperpolarization (in the spinal cord as well as in the

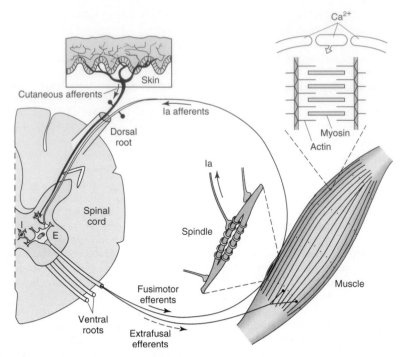

Figure 27–10. Diagram of the structures involved in the stretch reflex arc. *I* is an inhibitory interneuron; *E* indicates an excitatory presynaptic terminal; *Ia* is a primary intrafusal afferent fiber; *Ca²⁺* denotes activator calcium stored in the sarcoplasmic reticulum of skeletal muscle. (Reproduced, with permission, from Young RR, Delwaide PJ: Drug therapy: Spasticity. N Engl J Med 1981;304:28.)

brain) causes presynaptic inhibition by reducing calcium influx (Figure 27–11) and reduces the release of excitatory transmitters in both the brain and the spinal cord. Baclofen may also reduce pain in patients with spasticity, perhaps by inhibiting the release of substance P in the spinal cord.

Baclofen is at least as effective as diazepam in reducing spasticity and produces much less sedation. In addition, baclofen does not reduce overall muscle strength as much as dantrolene. It is rapidly and completely absorbed after oral administration and has a plasma half-life of 3–4 hours. Dosage is started at 15 mg twice daily, increasing as tolerated to 100 mg daily. Adverse effects of this drug include drowsiness, to which the patient may become tolerant with chronic administration. Increased seizure activity has been reported in epileptic patients. Therefore, withdrawal of baclofen must be done very slowly.

Studies have confirmed that intrathecal administration of baclofen can control severe spasticity and muscle pain that is not responsive to medication by other routes of administration. Owing to the poor egress of baclofen from the spinal cord, peripheral symptoms are rare.

Therefore, higher central concentrations of the drug may be tolerated. Partial tolerance to the effect of the drug may occur after several months of therapy but can be overcome by upward dosage adjustments to maintain the beneficial effect. Several cases of excessive somnolence, respiratory depression, and even coma have been reported. Although a major disadvantage of this therapeutic approach is the difficulty of maintaining the drug delivery catheter in the subarachnoid space, long-term intrathecal baclofen therapy can improve the quality of life for patients with severe spastic disorders.

Oral baclofen has been studied in several other medical conditions. Preliminary studies suggest that it may be effective in reducing craving in recovering alcoholics. It has also been found effective in preventing migraine attacks in some patients.

TIZANIDINE

As noted in Chapter 11, α agonists such as clonidine and other imidazoline compounds have a variety of effects on the central nervous system that are not fully understood. Among these effects is the ability to reduce

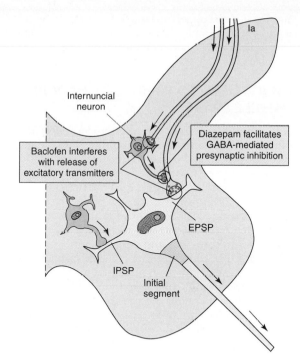

Figure 27–11. Postulated sites of spasmolytic action of diazepam and baclofen in the spinal cord. (Reproduced, with permission, from Young RR, Delwaide PJ: Drug therapy: Spasticity. N Engl J Med 1981;304:28.)

muscle spasm. Tizanidine is a congener of clonidine that has been studied for its spasmolytic actions. Tizanidine has significant α_2-adrenoceptor agonist effects, but it reduces spasticity in experimental models at doses that cause less cardiovascular effect than clonidine. Neurophysiologic studies in animals and humans suggest that tizanidine reinforces both presynaptic and postsynaptic inhibition in the cord. It also inhibits nociceptive transmission in the spinal dorsal horn.

Clinical trials suggest that tizanidine may produce a significant benefit in patients with spasticity. These trials report comparable efficacy in relieving muscle spasm to diazepam, baclofen, and dantrolene. However, tizanidine produces a different spectrum of adverse effects, including drowsiness, hypotension, dry mouth, and asthenia. The dosage requirements vary markedly among patients, suggesting that individual dosage titration is necessary to achieve an optimal effect.

OTHER CENTRALLY ACTIVE SPASMOLYTIC DRUGS

Gabapentin is an antiepileptic drug (see Chapter 24) that has shown considerable promise as a spasmolytic

agent in several studies involving patients with multiple sclerosis. **Progabide** and **glycine** have also been found in preliminary studies to reduce spasticity. Progabide is a $GABA_A$ and $GABA_B$ agonist and has active metabolites, including GABA itself. **Glycine** is another inhibitory amino acid neurotransmitter (see Chapter 21). It appears to possess pharmacologic activity when given orally and readily passes the blood-brain barrier. **Idrocilamide** and **riluzole** are newer drugs for the treatment of amyotrophic lateral sclerosis that appear to have spasm-reducing effects, possibly through inhibition of glutamatergic transmission in the central nervous system.

DANTROLENE

Dantrolene is a hydantoin derivative related to phenytoin that has a unique mechanism of spasmolytic activity. In contrast to the centrally active drugs, dantrolene reduces skeletal muscle strength by interfering with excitation-contraction coupling in the muscle fibers. The normal contractile response involves release of calcium from its stores in the sarcoplasmic reticulum (see Figures 13–1 and 27–10). This activator calcium brings about the tension-generating interaction of actin with myosin. Calcium is released from the sarcoplasmic reticulum via a calcium channel, sometimes called the ryanodine receptor channel because the plant alkaloid **ryanodine** combines with a receptor on the channel protein and, in the case of the skeletal muscle channel, locks it in the open position.

Dantrolene

Dantrolene interferes with the release of activator calcium through this sarcoplasmic reticulum calcium channel by binding to the ryanodine receptor. Motor units that contract rapidly are more sensitive to the drug's effects than are slower-responding units. Cardiac muscle and smooth muscle are depressed only slightly, perhaps because the release of calcium from their sarcoplasmic reticulum involves a somewhat different process.

Treatment with dantrolene is usually initiated with 25 mg daily as a single dose, increasing to a maximum of 100 mg four times daily as tolerated. Only about one third of an oral dose of dantrolene is absorbed, and the elimination half-life of the drug is about 8 hours. Major adverse effects are generalized muscle weakness, sedation, and occasionally hepatitis.

A special application of dantrolene is in the treatment of **malignant hyperthermia**, a rare heritable disorder that can be triggered by a variety of stimuli, including general anesthetics (eg, volatile anesthetics) and neuromuscular blocking drugs (eg, succinylcholine). Patients at risk for this condition have a hereditary impairment in the ability of the sarcoplasmic reticulum to sequester calcium. Following administration of one of the triggering agents, there is a sudden and prolonged release of calcium, with massive muscle contraction, lactic acid production, and increased body temperature. Prompt treatment is essential to control acidosis and body temperature and to reduce calcium release. The latter is accomplished with intravenous dantrolene, starting with a dose of 1 mg/kg intravenously and repeating as necessary to a maximum dose of 10 mg/kg.

BOTULINUM TOXIN

The therapeutic use of botulinum toxin for ophthalmic purposes and for local muscle spasm was mentioned in Chapter 6. Local injection of botulinum toxin has become popular for the treatment of generalized spastic disorders (eg, cerebral palsy). Most clinical studies to date have involved administration in one or two limbs,

and the benefits appear to persist for weeks to several months after a single treatment. Most studies to date have utilized type A botulinum toxin, but type B is also available.

DRUGS USED TO TREAT ACUTE LOCAL MUSCLE SPASM

A large number of drugs (eg, **carisoprodol**, **chlorphenesin**, **chlorzoxazone**, **cyclobenzaprine**, **metaxalone**, **methocarbamol**, and **orphenadrine**) are promoted for the relief of acute muscle spasm caused by local tissue trauma or muscular strains. It has been suggested that these drugs act primarily at the level of the brain stem. Cyclobenzaprine may be regarded as the prototype of the group. Cyclobenzaprine is structurally related to the tricyclic antidepressants and possesses antimuscarinic effects. It is ineffective in treating muscle spasm due to cerebral palsy or spinal cord injury. The drug has strong antimuscarinic actions and may cause significant sedation as well as confusion and transient visual hallucinations. The dosage of cyclobenzaprine for acute injury-related muscle spasm is 20–40 mg/d in divided doses.

PREPARATIONS AVAILABLE

NEUROMUSCULAR BLOCKING DRUGS
Atracurium (Tracrium)
  Parenteral: 10 mg/mL for injection
Cisatracurium (Nimbex)
  Parenteral: 2, 10 mg/mL for IV injection
Doxacurium (Nuromax)
  Parenteral: 1 mg/mL for IV injection
Metocurine (generic, Metubine Iodide)
  Parenteral: 2 mg/mL for injection
Mivacurium (Mivacron)
  Parenteral: 0.5, 2 mg/mL for injection
Pancuronium (generic, Pavulon)
  Parenteral: 1, 2 mg/mL for injection
Pipecuronium (Arduan)
  Parenteral: 1 mg/mL for IV injection
Rocuronium (Zemuron)
  Parenteral: 10 mg/mL for IV injection
Succinylcholine (generic, Anectine)
  Parenteral: 20, 50, 100 mg/mL for injection; 100, 500 mg per vial powders to reconstitute for injection
Tubocurarine (generic)
  Parenteral: 3 mg (20 units)/mL for injection
Vecuronium (generic, Norcuron)
  Parenteral: 10, 20 mg powder to reconstitute for injection

MUSCLE RELAXANTS (SPASMOLYTICS)
Baclofen (generic, Lioresal)
  Oral: 10, 20 mg tablets
  Intrathecal: 0.05, 0.5, 2 mg/mL
Botulinum toxin type A (Botox)
  Parenteral: Powder for solution, 100 units/vial
Botulinum toxin type B (Myobloc)
  Parenteral: 5000 units/mL for injection
Carisoprodol (generic, Soma)
  Oral: 350 mg tablets
Chlorphenesin (Maolate)
  Oral: 400 mg tablets
Chlorzoxazone (generic, Paraflex)
  Oral: 250, 500 mg tablets, caplets
Cyclobenzaprine (generic, Flexeril)
  Oral: 10 mg tablets
Dantrolene (Dantrium)
  Oral: 25, 50, 100 mg capsules
  Parenteral: 20 mg per vial powder to reconstitute for injection
Diazepam (generic, Valium)
  Oral: 2, 5, 10 mg tablets; 5 mg/5 mL, 5 mg/mL solutions
  Parenteral: 5 mg/mL for injection
Gabapentin (Neurontin)
  Oral: 100, 300, 400 mg capsules; 600, 800 mg tablets
  Note: This drug is labeled for use only in epilepsy.

Metaxalone (Skelaxin)
Oral: 400 mg tablets
Methocarbamol (generic, Robaxin)
Oral: 500, 750 mg tablets
Parenteral: 100 mg/mL for IM, IV injection
Orphenadrine (generic, Norflex)
Oral: 100 mg tablets; 100 mg sustained-release tablets
Parenteral: 30 mg/mL for IM, IV injection

Riluzole (Rilutek)
Oral: 50 mg tablets
Note: This drug is labeled only for use in amyotrophic lateral sclerosis.
Tizanidine (Zanaflex)
Oral: 4 mg tablets

REFERENCES

NEUROMUSCULAR BLOCKERS

Adams PR: Acetylcholine receptor kinetics. J Membr Biol 1981;58:161.

Adt M, Baumert J-H, Reimann H-J: The role of histamine in the cardiovascular effects of atracurium. Br J Anaesth 1992;68:155.

Atherton DP, Hunter JM: Clinical pharmacokinetics of the newer neuromuscular blocking drugs. Clin Pharmacokinet 1999;36:169.

Bevan DR et al: Reversal of neuromuscular blockade. Anesthesiology 1992;77:785.

Caldwell JE et al: The pharmacodynamics and pharmacokinetics of the metabolite desacetylvecuronium (ORG 7268) and its parent compound, vecuronium, in human volunteers. J Pharmacol Exp Ther 1994;270:1216.

Duvaldestin P, Slavov V, Rebufat Y: Pharmacokinetics and pharmacodynamics of rapacuronium in patients with cirrhosis. Anesthesiology 1999;91:1305.

Eriksson LI: Residual neuromuscular blockade. Incidence and relevance. Anaesthetist 2000;49(Suppl 1):S18.

Gibb AJ, Marshall IG: Pre- and postjunctional effects of tubocurarine and other nicotinic antagonists during repetitive stimulation in the rat. J Physiol 1984;351:275.

Hansen-Flaschen JH et al: Use of sedating drugs and neuromuscular blocking agents in patients requiring mechanical ventilation for respiratory failure: A national survey. JAMA 1991;266:2870.

Hunter JM: New neuromuscular blocking drugs. N Engl J Med 1995;332:1691.

Jooste E et al: A mechanism for rapacuronium-induced bronchospasm. M2 muscarinic receptor antagonism. Anesthesiology 2003;98:906.

Kaplan RF et al: The potency (ED$_{50}$) and cardiovascular effects of rapacuronium (ORG 9487) during narcotic-nitrous oxide-propofol anesthesia in neonates, infants, and children. Anesth Analg 1999;89:1172.

Kisor DF, Schmith VD: Clinical pharmacokinetics of cisatracurium besilate. Clin Pharmacokinet 1999;36:27.

Lee C: Structure, conformation, and action of neuromuscular blocking drugs. Br J Anaesth 2001;87:755.

Lien CA et al: The pharmacokinetics and pharmacodynamics of the stereoisomers of mivacurium in patients receiving nitrous oxide/opioid/barbiturate anesthesia. Anesthesiology 1994;80:1296.

Marshall CG, Ogden DC, Colquhoun D: The actions of suxamethonium (succinyldicholine) as an agonist and channel blocker at the nicotinic receptor of frog muscle. J Physiol (Lond) 1990;428:155.

Meakin GH: Recent advances in myorelaxant therapy. Paed Anaesthesia 2001;11:523.

Moore EW, Hunter JM: The new neuromuscular blocking agents: do they offer any advantages? Br J Anaesth 2001;87:912.

Savarese JJ et al: Pharmacology of muscle relaxants and their antagonists. In: *Anesthesia,* 5th ed. Miller RD (editor). Churchill Livingstone, 2000.

Morita T et al: Inadequate antagonism of vecuronium-induced neuromuscular blockade by neostigmine during sevoflurane or isoflurane anesthesia. Anesth Analg 1995;80:1175.

Scuka M, Mozrzymas JW: Postsynaptic potentiation and desensitization at the vertebrate end-plate receptors. Prog Neurobiol 1992;38:19.

Smith I et al: Propofol. An update on its clinical uses. Anesthesiology 1994;81:1005.

Szenshradsky J et al: Pharmacokinetics of rocuronium bromide (ORG 9426) in patients with normal renal function or patients undergoing cadaver renal transplantation. Anesthesiology 1992;77:899.

Viby-Mogensen J: Neuromuscular Monitoring. In: *Anesthesia,* 5th ed. Miller RD (editor). Churchill Livingstone, 2000.

Wilson HI, Nicholson GM: Presynaptic snake beta-neurotoxins produce tetanic fade and endplate potential run-down during neuromuscular blockade in mouse diaphragm. Naunyn Schmiedebergs Arch Pharmacol 1997;356:626.

White PF: Rapacuronium: why did it fail as a replacement for succinylcholine? Br J Anaesth 2002;88:163.

SPASMOLYTICS

Albright AL, Cervi A, Singletary J: Intrathecal baclofen for spasticity in cerebral palsy. JAMA 1991;265:1418.

Addolorato G et al: Ability of baclofen in reducing alcohol craving and intake: II. Preliminary clinical evidence. Alcohol Clin Exp Res 2000;24:67.

Bhakta BB et al: Use of botulinum toxin in stroke patients with severe upper limb spasticity. J Neurol Neurosurg Psychiatry 1996;61:30.

Cutter NC et al: Gabapentin effect on spasticity in multiple sclerosis: a placebo-controlled, randomized trial. Arch Phys Med Rehabil 2000;81:164.

Davidoff RA: Antispasticity drugs: Mechanisms of action. Ann Neurol 1985;17:107.

Gracies JM et al: Traditional pharmacological treatments for spasticity. Part II: General and regional treatments. Muscle Nerve Suppl 1997;6:S92.

Groves L, Shellenberger MK, Davis CS: Tizanidine treatment of spasticity: a meta-analysis of controlled, double-blind, comparative studies with baclofen and diazepam. Adv Ther 1998;15:241.

Koman LA et al: Botulinum toxin type A neuromuscular blockade in the treatment of lower extremity spasticity in cerebral palsy: a randomized, double-blind, placebo-controlled trial. BOTOX study group. J Pediatr Orthop 2000;20:108.

Lopez JR et al: Effects of dantrolene on myoplasmic free [Ca^{2+}] measured in vivo in patients susceptible to malignant hyperthermia. Anesthesiology 1992;76:711.

Nance P et al: Intrathecal baclofen therapy for adults with spinal spasticity: Therapeutic efficacy and effect on hospital admissions. Can J Neurol Sci 1995;22:22.

Pierson SH, Katz DI, Tarsy D: Botulinum toxin in the treatment of spasticity: Functional implications and patient selection. Arch Phys Med Rehab 1996;77:717.

Simpson DM et al: Botulinum toxin type A in the treatment of upper extremity spasticity: A randomized, double-blind, placebo-controlled trial. Neurology 1996;46:1306.

Wagstaff AJ, Bryson HM: Tizanidine: A review of its pharmacology, clinical efficacy and tolerability in the management of spasticity associated with cerebral and spinal disorders. Drugs 1997;53:435.

Young RR (editor): Symposium: Role of tizanidine in the treatment of spasticity. Neurology 1994;44(Suppl 9):1. [Entire issue.]

Young RR, Wiegner AW: Spasticity. Clin Orthop 1987;219:50.

Pharmacologic Management of Parkinsonism & Other Movement Disorders

28

Michael J. Aminoff, MD, DSc, FRCP

Several different types of abnormal movement are recognized. **Tremor** consists of a rhythmic oscillatory movement around a joint and is best characterized by its relation to activity. Tremor present at rest is characteristic of parkinsonism, when it is often associated with rigidity and an impairment of voluntary activity. Tremor may occur during maintenance of sustained posture (postural tremor) or during movement (intention tremor). A conspicuous postural tremor is the cardinal feature of benign essential or familial tremor. Intention tremor occurs in patients with a lesion of the brainstem or cerebellum, especially when the superior cerebellar peduncle is involved, and may also occur as a manifestation of toxicity from alcohol or certain other drugs.

Chorea consists of irregular, unpredictable, involuntary muscle jerks that occur in different parts of the body and impair voluntary activity. In some instances, the proximal muscles of the limbs are most severely affected, and because the abnormal movements are then particularly violent, the term ballismus has been used to describe them. Chorea may be hereditary or may occur as a complication of a number of general medical disorders and of therapy with certain drugs.

Abnormal movements may be slow and writhing in character (**athetosis**) and in some instances are so sustained that they are more properly regarded as abnormal postures (**dystonia**). Athetosis or dystonia may occur with perinatal brain damage, with focal or generalized cerebral lesions, as an acute complication of certain drugs, as an accompaniment of diverse neurologic disorders, or as an isolated inherited phenomenon of uncertain cause known as idiopathic torsion dystonia or dystonia musculorum deformans. Its physiologic basis is uncertain, and treatment is unsatisfactory.

Tics are sudden coordinated abnormal movements that tend to occur repetitively, particularly about the face and head, especially in children, and can be suppressed voluntarily for short periods of time. Common tics include, for example, repetitive sniffing or shoulder shrugging. Tics may be single or multiple and transient or chronic. Gilles de la Tourette's syndrome is characterized by chronic multiple tics; its pharmacologic management is discussed at the end of this chapter.

Many of the movement disorders have been attributed to disturbances of the basal ganglia, but the precise function of these anatomic structures is not yet fully understood, and it is not possible to relate individual symptoms to involvement at specific sites.

PARKINSONISM (PARALYSIS AGITANS)

Parkinsonism is characterized by a combination of rigidity, bradykinesia, tremor, and postural instability that can occur for a wide variety of reasons but is usually idiopathic. The pathophysiologic basis of the idiopathic disorder may relate to exposure to some unrecognized neurotoxin or to the occurrence of oxidation reactions with the generation of free radicals. Studies in twins suggest that genetic factors may also be important, especially when the disease occurs in patients under age 50. Parkinson's disease is generally progressive, leading to increasing disability unless effective treatment is provided.

The normally high concentration of dopamine in the basal ganglia of the brain is reduced in parkinsonism, and pharmacologic attempts to restore dopaminergic activity with levodopa and dopamine agonists have been successful in alleviating many of the clinical features of the disorder. An alternative but complementary approach has been to restore the normal balance of cholinergic and dopaminergic influences on the basal ganglia with antimuscarinic drugs. The pathophysiologic basis for these therapies is that in idiopathic parkinsonism, dopaminergic neurons in the substantia nigra that normally inhibit the output of GABAergic cells in the corpus striatum are lost (Figure 28–1). (In

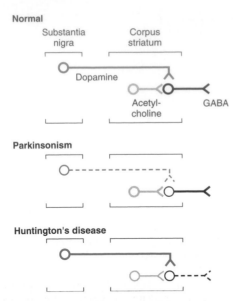

Normal

Substantia nigra   Corpus striatum

Dopamine

Acetyl-choline   GABA

Parkinsonism

Huntington's disease

Figure 28–1. Schematic representation of the sequence of neurons involved in parkinsonism and Huntington's chorea. **Top:** Dopaminergic neurons (color) originating in the substantia nigra normally inhibit the GABAergic output from the striatum, whereas cholinergic neurons (gray) exert an excitatory effect. **Middle:** In parkinsonism, there is a selective loss of dopaminergic neurons (dashed, color). **Bottom:** In Huntington's chorea, some cholinergic neurons may be lost (gray), but even more GABAergic neurons (black, dashed) degenerate.

contrast, Huntington's chorea involves the loss of some cholinergic neurons and an even greater loss of the GABAergic cells that exit the corpus striatum.) Drugs that *induce* parkinsonian syndromes either are dopamine receptor antagonists (eg, antipsychotic agents; see Chapter 29) or lead to the destruction of the dopaminergic nigrostriatal neurons (eg, 1-methyl-4-phenyl-1,2,3,6-tetrahydropyridine [MPTP]; see below).

LEVODOPA

Dopamine does not cross the blood-brain barrier and if given into the peripheral circulation has no therapeutic effect in parkinsonism. However, (–)-3-(3,4-dihydroxyphenyl)-L-alanine (levodopa), the immediate metabolic precursor of dopamine, does penetrate the brain, where it is decarboxylated to dopamine (see Figure 6–5). Several dopamine agonists have also been developed and may lead to clinical benefit, as discussed below.

Dopamine receptors are discussed in detail in Chapters 21 and 29. Dopamine receptors of the D_1 type are located in the zona compacta of the substantia nigra and presynaptically on striatal axons coming from cortical neurons and from dopaminergic cells in the substantia nigra. The D_2 receptors are located postsynaptically on striatal neurons and presynaptically on axons in the substantia nigra belonging to neurons in the basal ganglia. The benefits of dopaminergic antiparkinsonism drugs appear to depend mostly on stimulation of the D_2 receptors, but D_1-receptor stimulation may also be required for maximal benefit. Dopamine agonist or partial agonist ergot derivatives such as lergotrile and bromocriptine that are powerful stimulators of the D_2 receptors have antiparkinsonism properties, whereas certain dopamine blockers that are selective D_2 antagonists can induce parkinsonism.

Chemistry

As discussed in Chapter 6, dopa is the precursor of dopamine and norepinephrine. Its structure is shown in Figure 28–2. Levodopa is the levorotatory stereoisomer of dopa.

Pharmacokinetics

Levodopa is rapidly absorbed from the small intestine, but its absorption depends on the rate of gastric emptying and the pH of the gastric contents. Food will delay

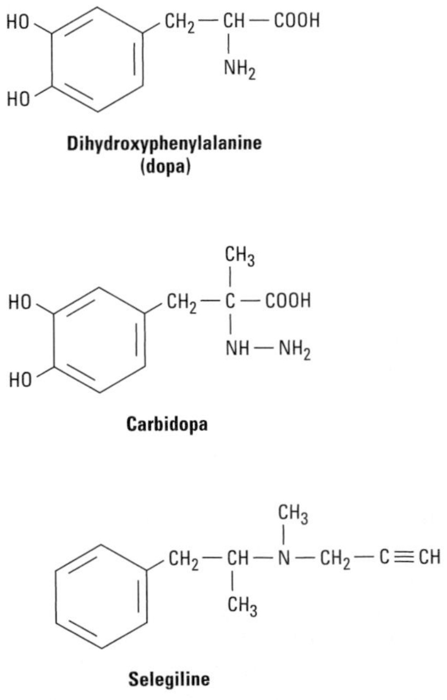

Dihydroxyphenylalanine (dopa)

Carbidopa

Selegiline

Figure 28–2. Some drugs used in the treatment of parkinsonism.

the appearance of levodopa in the plasma. Moreover, certain amino acids from ingested food can compete with the drug for absorption from the gut and for transport from the blood to the brain. Plasma concentrations usually peak between 1 and 2 hours after an oral dose, and the plasma half-life is usually between 1 and 3 hours, although it varies considerably between individuals. About two thirds of the dose appears in the urine as metabolites within 8 hours of an oral dose, the main metabolic products being 3-methoxy-4-hydroxyphenylacetic acid (homovanillic acid, HVA) and dihydroxyphenylacetic acid (DOPAC). Unfortunately, only about 1–3% of administered levodopa actually enters the brain unaltered, the remainder being metabolized extracerebrally, predominantly by decarboxylation to dopamine, which does not penetrate the blood-brain barrier. This means that levodopa must be given in large amounts when it is used alone. However, when it is given in combination with a dopa decarboxylase inhibitor that does not penetrate the blood-brain barrier, the peripheral metabolism of levodopa is reduced, plasma levels of levodopa are higher, plasma half-life is longer, and more dopa is available for entry into the brain (Figure 28–3). Indeed, concomitant administration of a peripheral dopa decarboxylase inhibitor may reduce the daily requirements of levodopa by approximately 75%.

Clinical Use

The best results of levodopa treatment are obtained in the first few years of treatment. This is sometimes because the daily dose of levodopa must be reduced with time in order to avoid side effects at doses that were well tolerated at the outset. The reason that adverse effects develop in this way is unclear, but selective denervation or drug-induced supersensitivity may be responsible. Some patients also become less responsive to levodopa, so that previously effective doses eventually fail to produce any therapeutic benefit. Responsiveness to levodopa may ultimately be lost completely, perhaps because of the disappearance of dopaminergic nigrostriatal nerve terminals or some pathologic process directly involving the striatal dopamine receptors. For such reasons, the benefits of levodopa treatment often begin to diminish after about 3 or 4 years of therapy irrespective of the initial therapeutic response. Although levodopa therapy does not stop the progression of parkinsonism, its early initiation lowers the mortality rate. However, long-term therapy may lead to a number of problems in management such as development of the on-off phenomenon discussed below. The most appropriate time to introduce levodopa therapy must therefore be determined individually.

When levodopa is used, it is generally given in combination with carbidopa (Figure 28–2), a peripheral dopa decarboxylase inhibitor, for the reasons set forth above. **Sinemet** is a dopa preparation containing carbidopa and levodopa in fixed proportion (1:10 or 1:4). Treatment is started with a small dose, eg, Sinemet-25/100 (carbidopa 25 mg, levodopa 100 mg) three times daily, and gradually increased depending on the therapeutic response and development of adverse effects. It should be taken 30–60 minutes before meals. Most patients ultimately require Sinemet-25/250 (carbidopa 25 mg, levodopa 250 mg) three or four times daily. It is generally preferable to keep treatment with this agent at a low level (eg, Sinemet-25/100 three times daily) and to increase dopaminergic therapy by the addition of a dopamine agonist if necessary, in order to reduce the risk of development of response fluctuations, as discussed below. A controlled-release formulation of Sinemet is available and may be helpful in patients with established response fluctuations or as a means of reducing dosing frequency.

Levodopa can ameliorate all of the clinical features of parkinsonism, but it is particularly effective in relieving bradykinesia and any disabilities resulting from it. When it is first introduced, about one third of patients respond very well and one third less well. Most of the remainder either are unable to tolerate the medication or simply do not respond at all.

Adverse Effects

A. GASTROINTESTINAL EFFECTS

When levodopa is given without a peripheral decarboxylase inhibitor, anorexia and nausea and vomiting occur in about 80% of patients. These adverse effects can be minimized by taking the drug in divided doses, with or immediately after meals, and by increasing the total daily dose very slowly; antacids taken 30–60 minutes before levodopa may also be beneficial. The vomiting has been attributed to stimulation of an emetic center located in the brainstem but outside the blood-brain barrier to dopamine and to peripheral decarboxylase inhibitors. Fortunately, tolerance to this emetic effect develops in many patients after several months. Antiemetics such as phenothiazines should be avoided because they reduce the antiparkinsonism effects of levodopa and may exacerbate the disease.

When levodopa is given in combination with carbidopa to reduce its extracerebral metabolism, adverse gastrointestinal effects are much less frequent and troublesome, occurring in fewer than 20% of cases, so that patients can tolerate proportionately higher doses.

B. CARDIOVASCULAR EFFECTS

A variety of cardiac arrhythmias have been described in patients receiving levodopa, including tachycardia, ventricular extrasystoles and, rarely, atrial fibrillation. This

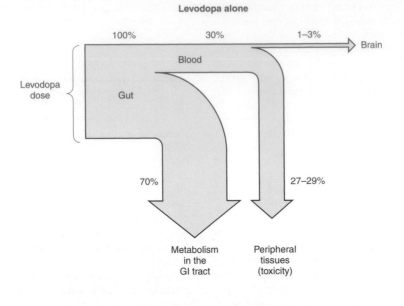

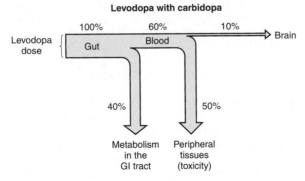

Figure 28–3. Fate of orally administered levodopa and the effect of carbidopa, estimated from animal data. The width of each pathway indicates the absolute amount of the drug present at each site, while the percentages shown denote the relative proportion of the administered dose. The benefits of coadministration of carbidopa include reduction of the amount of levodopa diverted to peripheral tissues and an increase in the fraction of the dose that reaches the brain. (GI, gastrointestinal.) (Data from Nutt JG, Fellman JH: Pharmacokinetics of levodopa. Clin Neuropharmacol 1984;7:35.)

effect has been attributed to increased catecholamine formation peripherally. The incidence of such arrhythmias is low, even in the presence of established cardiac disease, and may be reduced still further if the levodopa is taken in combination with a peripheral decarboxylase inhibitor. In parkinsonism patients who also have heart disease, the anticipated benefits of levodopa, especially when combined with carbidopa, generally outweigh the slight risk of inducing a cardiac arrhythmia.

Postural hypotension is common and often asymptomatic, and tends to diminish with continuing treat-

ment. Hypertension may also occur, especially in the presence of nonselective monoamine oxidase inhibitors or sympathomimetics or when massive doses of levodopa are being taken.

C. DYSKINESIAS

Dyskinesias occur in up to 80% of patients receiving levodopa therapy for long periods. The form and nature of dopa dyskinesias vary widely in different patients but tend to remain constant in character in individual patients. Chorea, ballismus, athetosis, dystonia, myoclonus, tics, and tremor may occur individually or in any combination in the face, trunk, or limbs. Choreoathetosis of the face and distal extremities is the most common presentation. The development of dyskinesias is dose-related, but there is considerable individual variation in the dose required to produce them.

D. BEHAVIORAL EFFECTS

A wide variety of adverse mental effects have been reported including depression, anxiety, agitation, insomnia, somnolence, confusion, delusions, hallucinations, nightmares, euphoria, and other changes in mood or personality. Such adverse effects are more common in patients taking levodopa in combination with a decarboxylase inhibitor rather than levodopa alone, presumably because higher levels are reached in the brain. They may be precipitated by intercurrent illness or operation. It may be necessary to reduce or withdraw the medication. Several atypical antipsychotic agents are now available and may be particularly helpful in countering the behavioral complications of levodopa. Clozapine requires weekly blood counts because it leads to marrow suppression in rare instances. The starting dose is 6.25 mg at bedtime, with subsequent increments depending on response and tolerance; doses of 25–100 mg/d are typical. Olanzapine, quetiapine, and risperidone have also been used; they are less expensive than clozapine and do not cause marrow suppression but sometimes seem less effective.

E. FLUCTUATIONS IN RESPONSE

Certain fluctuations in clinical response to levodopa occur with increasing frequency as treatment continues. In some patients, these fluctuations relate to the timing of levodopa intake, and they are then referred to as wearing-off reactions or end-of-dose akinesia. In other instances, fluctuations in clinical state are unrelated to the timing of doses (on-off phenomenon). In the on-off phenomenon, off-periods of marked akinesia alternate over the course of a few hours with on-periods of improved mobility but often marked dyskinesia. The phenomenon is most likely to occur in patients who responded well to treatment initially. The exact mechanism is unknown.

F. MISCELLANEOUS ADVERSE EFFECTS

Mydriasis may occur and may precipitate an attack of acute glaucoma in some patients. Other reported but rare adverse effects include various blood dyscrasias; a positive Coombs test with evidence of hemolysis; hot flushes; aggravation or precipitation of gout; abnormalities of smell or taste; brownish discoloration of saliva, urine, or vaginal secretions; priapism; and mild—usually transient—elevations of blood urea nitrogen and of serum transaminases, alkaline phosphatase, and bilirubin.

Drug Holidays

A drug holiday (for 3–21 days) may alleviate some of the neurologic and behavioral adverse effects of levodopa but is usually of little help in the management of the on-off phenomenon. Up to two thirds of patients show temporary improved responsiveness to levodopa when the drug is reinstituted, and—because they can be managed on lower doses than before—adverse mental effects and dyskinesias are less troublesome. Fluctuations in response (on-off phenomenon) are reduced in many instances, but any benefit in this regard is usually short-lived. Furthermore, a drug holiday carries the risks of aspiration pneumonia, venous thrombosis, pulmonary embolism, and depression resulting from the immobility accompanying severe parkinsonism. For these reasons and because of the temporary nature of any benefit, drug holidays are no longer recommended.

Drug Interactions

Pharmacologic doses of pyridoxine (vitamin B_6) enhance the extracerebral metabolism of levodopa and may therefore prevent its therapeutic effect unless a peripheral decarboxylase inhibitor is also taken. Levodopa should not be given to patients taking monoamine oxidase A inhibitors or within 2 weeks of their discontinuance, because such a combination can lead to hypertensive crises.

Contraindications

Levodopa should not be given to psychotic patients, as it may exacerbate the mental disturbance. It is also contraindicated in patients with angle-closure glaucoma, but those with chronic open-angle glaucoma may be given levodopa if intraocular pressure is well controlled and can be monitored. It is best given combined with carbidopa to patients with cardiac disease, but even so the risk of cardiac dysrhythmia is slight. Patients with active peptic ulcer must also be managed carefully, since gastrointestinal bleeding has occasionally occurred with levodopa. Because levodopa is a precursor of skin melanin and conceivably may activate malignant melanoma, its use should be avoided in patients with a history of melanoma or with suspicious undiagnosed skin lesions.

DOPAMINE AGONISTS

Drugs acting directly on dopamine receptors may have a beneficial effect additional to that of levodopa. Unlike levodopa, they do not require enzymatic conversion to an active metabolite, have no potentially toxic metabolites, and do not compete with other substances for active transport into the blood and across the blood-brain barrier. Moreover, drugs selectively affecting cer-

Pramipexole

Ropinirole

tain (but not all) dopamine receptors may have more limited adverse effects than levodopa. There are a number of dopamine agonists with antiparkinsonism activity. The older dopamine agonists (bromocriptine and pergolide) are ergot derivatives (see Chapter 16), unlike the newer agents (pramipexole and ropinirole). There is no evidence that one agonist is superior to another; individual patients, however, may respond to one but not another of these agents.

Dopamine agonists have an important role as first-line therapy for Parkinson's disease, and their use is associated with a lower incidence of the response fluctuations and dyskinesias occurring with long-term levodopa therapy. In consequence, dopaminergic therapy may best be initiated with a dopamine agonist. Alternatively, a low dose of carbidopa plus levodopa (eg, Sinemet-25/100 three times daily) is introduced and a dopamine agonist is then added. In either case, the dose of the dopamine agonist is built up gradually depending on response and tolerance. Dopamine agonists may also be given to parkinsonian patients taking levodopa who have end-of-dose akinesia or on-off phenomenon or who are becoming resistant to treatment with levodopa. In such circumstances, it is generally necessary to lower the dose of levodopa to prevent intolerable adverse effects. The response to a dopamine agonist is generally disappointing in patients who have never responded to levodopa.

Bromocriptine

Bromocriptine is a D_2 agonist; its structure is shown in Table 16–4. This drug has been widely used to treat Parkinson's disease and has also been used to treat certain endocrinologic disorders, especially hyperprolactinemia (see Chapter 37), but in lower doses than for parkinsonism. Bromocriptine is absorbed to a variable extent from the gastrointestinal tract; peak plasma levels are reached within 1–2 hours after an oral dose. It is excreted in the bile and feces. The usual daily dose of bromocriptine in the treatment of parkinsonism is between 7.5 and 30 mg, depending on response and tolerance. In order to minimize adverse effects, the dose is built up slowly over 2 or 3 months from a starting level of 1.25 mg twice daily after meals; the daily dose is then

increased by 2.5 mg every 2 weeks depending on the response or the development of adverse reactions.

Pergolide

Pergolide, another ergot derivative, directly stimulates both D_1 and D_2 receptors. It too has been widely used for parkinsonism, and comparative studies suggest that it is more effective than bromocriptine in relieving the symptoms and signs of parkinsonism, increasing "on-time" among response fluctuators, and permitting the levodopa dose to be reduced. The average therapeutic dose is 3 mg daily. Patients are generally started on 0.05 mg daily and the dose is built up over about 4 weeks by increments until benefit occurs or side effects limit further increments.

Pramipexole

Pramipexole, which is not an ergot derivative, has preferential affinity for the D_3 family of receptors. It is effective when used as monotherapy for mild parkinsonism. It is also helpful in patients with advanced disease, permitting the dose of levodopa to be reduced and smoothing out response fluctuations. It may ameliorate affective symptoms. A possible neuroprotective effect has been suggested by its ability to scavenge hydrogen peroxide and enhance neurotrophic activity in mesencephalic dopaminergic cell cultures. Pramipexole is rapidly absorbed, reaching peak plasma concentrations in approximately 2 hours, and is excreted largely unchanged in the urine. It is started at a dose of 0.125 mg three times daily; the dose is doubled after 1 week and again after another week. Further increments in the daily dose are by 0.75 mg at weekly intervals depending on response and tolerance. Most patients require between 0.5 and 1.5 mg three times daily. Renal insufficiency may necessitate dosage adjustment.

Ropinirole

Ropinirole, another nonergoline derivative, is a relatively pure D_2 receptor agonist that is effective as monotherapy in patients with mild disease and as a means of smoothing the response to levodopa in patients with more advanced disease and response fluctuations. It is introduced in a dose of 0.25 mg three times daily, and the total daily dose is then increased by

0.75 mg at weekly intervals until the fourth week and by 1.5 mg thereafter. In most instances, a dose of between 2 and 8 mg three times daily is necessary. Ropinirole is metabolized by CYP1A2; drugs metabolized by the liver may significantly reduce its clearance.

Adverse Effects of Dopamine Agonists

A. GASTROINTESTINAL EFFECTS

Anorexia and nausea and vomiting may occur when a dopamine agonist is introduced and can be minimized by taking the medication with meals. Constipation, dyspepsia, and symptoms of reflux esophagitis may also occur. Bleeding from peptic ulceration has been reported.

B. CARDIOVASCULAR EFFECTS

Postural hypotension may occur, particularly at the initiation of therapy. Painless digital vasospasm is a dose-related complication of long-term treatment with the ergot derivatives (bromocriptine or pergolide). When cardiac arrhythmias occur, they are an indication for discontinuing treatment. Peripheral edema is sometimes problematic.

C. DYSKINESIAS

Abnormal movements similar to those introduced by levodopa may occur and are reversed by reducing the total dose of dopaminergic drugs being taken.

D. MENTAL DISTURBANCES

Confusion, hallucinations, delusions, and other psychiatric reactions are other complications of dopaminergic treatment and are more common and severe with dopamine agonists than levodopa. They clear on withdrawal of the offending medication.

E. MISCELLANEOUS

Headache, nasal congestion, increased arousal, pulmonary infiltrates, pleural and retroperitoneal fibrosis, and erythromelalgia are other reported side effects of the ergot-derived dopamine agonists. Erythromelalgia consists of red, tender, painful, swollen feet and, occasionally, hands, at times associated with arthralgia; symptoms and signs clear within a few days of withdrawal of the causal drug. In rare instances, an uncontrollable tendency to fall asleep at inappropriate times has occurred, particularly in patients receiving pramipexole or ropinirole, requiring the discontinuation of medication.

Contraindications

Dopamine agonists are contraindicated in patients with a history of psychotic illness or recent myocardial infarction, or with active peptic ulceration. The ergot-derived agonists are best avoided in patients with peripheral vascular disease.

MONOAMINE OXIDASE INHIBITORS

Two types of monoamine oxidase have been distinguished. Monoamine oxidase A metabolizes norepinephrine and serotonin; monoamine oxidase B metabolizes dopamine. **Selegiline** (deprenyl) (Figure 28–2), a selective inhibitor of monoamine oxidase B, retards the breakdown of dopamine; in consequence, it enhances and prolongs the antiparkinsonism effect of levodopa (thereby allowing the dose of levodopa to be reduced) and may reduce mild on-off or wearing-off phenomena. It is therefore used as adjunctive therapy for patients with a declining or fluctuating response to levodopa. The standard dose is 5 mg with breakfast and 5 mg with lunch. Selegiline may cause insomnia when taken later during the day. It should not be taken by patients receiving meperidine, tricyclic antidepressants, or serotonin reuptake inhibitors because of the risk of acute toxic interactions. The adverse effects of levodopa may be increased by selegiline. Selegiline has only a minor therapeutic effect on parkinsonism when given alone, but studies in animals suggest that it may reduce disease progression. Such an effect of antioxidative therapy on disease progression may be expected if Parkinson's disease is associated with the oxidative generation of free radicals. However, any neuroprotective effect of selegiline may relate to its metabolite, desmethylselegiline, and involve antiapoptotic mechanisms. Studies to test the effect of selegiline on the progression of parkinsonism in humans have yielded ambiguous results. The findings in a large multicenter study have been taken to suggest a beneficial effect in slowing disease progression but may simply have reflected a symptomatic response.

Rasagiline, another monoamine oxidase B inhibitor, is more potent than selegiline in preventing MPTP-induced parkinsonism and is currently under study as a neuroprotective agent.

The combined administration of levodopa and an inhibitor of both forms of monoamine oxidase must be avoided, since it may lead to hypertensive crises, probably because of the peripheral accumulation of norepinephrine.

CATECHOL-*O*-METHYLTRANSFERASE INHIBITORS

Inhibition of dopa decarboxylase is associated with compensatory activation of other pathways of levodopa metabolism, especially catechol-*O*-methyltransferase (COMT), and this increases plasma levels of 3-*O*-methyldopa (3OMD). Elevated levels of 3OMD have been associated with a poor therapeutic response to levodopa, perhaps in part because 3OMD competes with levodopa for an active carrier mechanism that governs its transport across the intestinal mucosa and the blood-brain barrier. Selective COMT inhibitors such as **tolcapone** and **entacapone** also prolong the action of levodopa by diminishing its peripheral metabolism. Levodopa clearance is decreased, and relative bioavailability of levodopa is thus increased. Neither the time to reach peak concentration nor the maximal concentration of levodopa is increased. These agents may be helpful in patients receiving levodopa who have developed response fluctuations—leading to a smoother response, more prolonged "on-time," and the option of reducing total daily levodopa dose. Tolcapone and entacapone are both widely available, but entacapone is generally preferred because it has not been associated with hepatotoxicity.

The pharmacologic effects of tolcapone and entacapone are similar, and both are rapidly absorbed, bound to plasma proteins, and metabolized prior to excretion. However, tolcapone has both central and peripheral effects, whereas the effect of entacapone is peripheral. The half-life of both drugs is approximately 2 hours, but tolcapone is slightly more potent and has a longer duration of action. Tolcapone is taken in a standard dose of 100 mg three times daily; some patients require a daily dose of twice that amount. By contrast, entacapone (200 mg) needs to be taken with each dose of levodopa, up to five times daily.

Adverse effects of the COMT inhibitors relate in part to increased levodopa exposure and include dyskinesias, nausea, and confusion. It is often necessary to lower the daily dose of levodopa by about 30% in the first 48 hours to avoid or reverse such complications. Other side effects include diarrhea, abdominal pain, orthostatic hypotension, sleep disturbances, and an orange discoloration of the urine. Tolcapone may cause an increase in liver enzyme levels and has been rarely associated with death from acute hepatic failure; accordingly, its use in the USA requires signed patient consent (as provided in the product labeling) plus monitoring of liver function tests every 2 weeks during the first year and less frequently thereafter. No such toxicity has been reported with entacapone.

AMANTADINE

Amantadine, an antiviral agent, was by chance found to have antiparkinsonism properties. Its mode of action in parkinsonism is unclear, but it may potentiate dopaminergic function by influencing the synthesis, release, or reuptake of dopamine. Release of catecholamines from peripheral stores has been documented.

Pharmacokinetics

Peak plasma concentrations of amantadine are reached 1–4 hours after an oral dose. The plasma half-life is between 2 and 4 hours, most of the drug being excreted unchanged in the urine.

Clinical Use

Amantadine is less potent than levodopa and its benefits may be short-lived, often disappearing after only a few weeks of treatment. Nevertheless, during that time it may favorably influence the bradykinesia, rigidity, and tremor of parkinsonism. The standard dose is 100 mg orally twice or three times daily.

Adverse Effects

Amantadine has a number of undesirable central nervous system effects, all of which can be reversed by stopping the drug. These include restlessness, depression, irritability, insomnia, agitation, excitement, hallucinations, and confusion. Overdosage may produce an acute toxic psychosis. With doses several times higher than recommended, convulsions have occurred.

Livedo reticularis sometimes occurs in patients taking amantadine and usually clears within a month after the drug is withdrawn. Other dermatologic reactions have also been described. Peripheral edema, another well-recognized complication, is not accompanied by signs of cardiac, hepatic, or renal disease and responds to diuretics. Other adverse reactions include headache, heart failure, postural hypotension, urinary retention, and gastrointestinal disturbances (eg, anorexia, nausea, constipation, and dry mouth).

Contraindications

Amantadine should be used with caution in patients with a history of seizures or heart failure.

ACETYLCHOLINE-BLOCKING DRUGS

A number of centrally acting antimuscarinic preparations are available that differ in their potency and in their efficacy in different patients.

Clinical Use

Treatment is started with a low dose of one of the drugs in this category, the level of medication gradually being increased until benefit occurs or adverse effects limit further increments. Antimuscarinic drugs may improve the tremor and rigidity of parkinsonism but have little effect on bradykinesia. If patients do not respond to one drug, a trial with another is warranted and may be successful. Some of the more commonly used drugs are listed in Table 28–1.

Adverse Effects

Antimuscarinic drugs have a number of central nervous system effects, including drowsiness, mental slowness,

Table 28–1. Some drugs with antimuscarinic properties used in parkinsonism.

Drug	Usual Daily Dose (mg)
Benztropine mesylate	1–6
Biperiden	2–12
Orphenadrine	150–400
Procyclidine	7.5–30
Trihexyphenidyl	6–20

inattention, restlessness, confusion, agitation, delusions, hallucinations, and mood changes. Other common effects include dryness of the mouth, blurring of vision, mydriasis, urinary retention, nausea and vomiting, constipation, tachycardia, tachypnea, increased intraocular pressure, palpitations, and cardiac arrhythmias. Dyskinesias occur in rare cases. Acute suppurative parotitis sometimes occurs as a complication of dryness of the mouth.

If medication is to be withdrawn, this should be accomplished gradually rather than abruptly in order to prevent acute exacerbation of parkinsonism.

Contraindications

Acetylcholine-blocking drugs should be avoided in patients with prostatic hyperplasia, obstructive gastrointestinal disease (eg, pyloric stenosis or paralytic ileus), or angle-closure glaucoma. In parkinsonism patients receiving antimuscarinic medication, concomitant administration of other drugs with antimuscarinic properties (eg, tricyclic antidepressants or antihistamines) may precipitate some of the complications mentioned above.

SURGICAL PROCEDURES

In patients with advanced disease that is poorly responsive to pharmacotherapy, worthwhile benefit may follow thalamotomy (for conspicuous tremor) or posteroventral pallidotomy. Ablative surgical procedures, however, are being replaced by functional, reversible lesions induced by high-frequency deep-brain stimulation, which has a lower morbidity. Thalamic stimulation by an implanted electrode and stimulator is very effective for the relief of tremor, and stimulation of the subthalamic nucleus or globus pallidus internus has yielded good results for management of the clinical fluctuation occurring in advanced parkinsonism. The anatomic

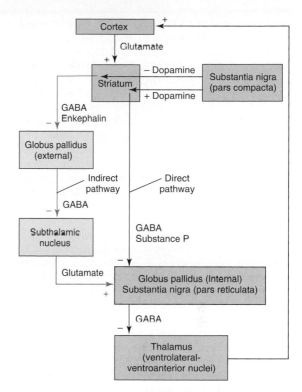

Figure 28–4. Functional circuitry between the cortex, basal ganglia, and thalamus. The involved neurotransmitters are indicated. In Parkinson's disease, there is degeneration of the pars compacta of the substantia nigra, leading to overactivity in the indirect pathway (color) and increased glutamatergic activity by the subthalamic nucleus.

substrate for such therapy is indicated in Figure 28–4. Such procedures are contraindicated in patients with secondary or atypical parkinsonism. Transplantation of dopaminergic tissue (fetal substantia nigra tissue) has been reported to confer benefit in some parkinsonism patients, but the results are conflicting and uncontrollable dyskinesias have occurred in some patients. Such procedures are best regarded as investigational.

NEUROPROTECTIVE THERAPY

A number of different compounds are currently under investigation as potential neuroprotective agents that may slow disease progression. These include antioxidants, antiapoptotic agents, glutamate antagonists, intraparenchymally administered glial-derived neurotrophic factor, coenzyme Q10, and anti-inflammatory drugs. The role of these agents remains to be established, however, and their use for therapeutic purposes is not indicated at this time.

GENERAL COMMENTS ON DRUG MANAGEMENT OF PATIENTS WITH PARKINSONISM

Parkinson's disease generally follows a progressive course. Moreover, the benefits of levodopa therapy often seem to diminish with time and certain adverse effects may complicate long-term levodopa treatment. Nevertheless, evidence is accumulating that dopaminergic therapy at a relatively early stage may be most effective in alleviating symptoms of parkinsonism and may also favorably affect the mortality rate due to the disease. Symptomatic treatment of mild parkinsonism is probably best avoided until there is some degree of disability or until symptoms begin to have a significant impact on the patient's lifestyle. When treatment becomes necessary, a trial of amantadine or an antimuscarinic drug (or both) may be worthwhile. With disease progression, dopaminergic therapy becomes necessary. This can conveniently be initiated with a dopamine agonist, either alone or in combination with low-dose Sinemet therapy. Physical therapy is helpful in improving mobility. In patients with severe parkinsonism and long-term complications of levodopa therapy, such as the on-off phenomena, a trial of treatment with a COMT inhibitor may be worthwhile. Regulation of dietary protein intake may also improve response fluctuations. Pallidotomy or deep-brain stimulation may be helpful in patients who fail to respond adequately to these measures. Treating patients who are young or have mild parkinsonism with selegiline may delay disease progression and merits consideration.

DRUG-INDUCED PARKINSONISM

Reserpine and the related drug tetrabenazine deplete biogenic monoamines from their storage sites, while haloperidol and the phenothiazines block dopamine receptors. These drugs may therefore produce a parkinsonian syndrome, usually within 3 months after introduction, which is related to high dosage and clears over a few weeks or months after withdrawal. If treatment is necessary, antimuscarinic agents are preferred. Levodopa is of no help if neuroleptic drugs are continued and may in fact aggravate the mental disorder for which antipsychotic drugs were prescribed originally.

In 1983, a drug-induced form of parkinsonism was discovered in individuals who attempted to synthesize and use a narcotic drug related to meperidine but actually synthesized and self-administered MPTP, as discussed in the Box, MPTP & Parkinsonism.

OTHER MOVEMENT DISORDERS

Tremor

Tremor consists of rhythmic oscillatory movements. Physiologic postural tremor, which is a normal phenomenon, is enhanced in amplitude by anxiety, fatigue, thy-

---

MPTP & PARKINSONISM

Reports in the early 1980s of a rapidly progressive form of parkinsonism in young persons opened a new area of research in the etiology and treatment of parkinsonism. The initial report described apparently healthy young people who attempted to support their opioid habit with a meperidine analog synthesized by an amateur chemist. They unwittingly self-administered 1-methyl-4-phenyl-1,2,3,6-tetrahydropyridine (MPTP) and subsequently developed a very severe form of parkinsonism.

MPTP is a protoxin that is converted by monoamine oxidase B to N-methyl-4-phenylpyridinium (MPP^+). MPP^+ is selectively taken up by cells in the substantia nigra through an active mechanism normally responsible for dopamine reuptake. MPP^+ inhibits mitochondrial complex I, thereby inhibiting oxidative phosphorylation. The interaction of MPP^+ with complex I probably leads to cell death and thus to striatal dopamine depletion and parkinsonism.

Recognition of the effects of MPTP suggested that spontaneously occurring Parkinson's disease may result from exposure to an environmental toxin that is similarly selective in its target. However, no such toxin has yet been identified. It also suggested a successful means of producing an experimental model of Parkinson's disease in animals, especially nonhuman primates. This model is assisting in the development of new antiparkinsonism drugs. Pretreatment of exposed animals with a monoamine oxidase B inhibitor such as selegiline prevents the conversion of MPTP to MPP^+ and thus protects against the occurrence of parkinsonism. This observation has provided one reason to believe that selegiline may retard the progression of Parkinson's disease in humans.

rotoxicosis, and intravenous epinephrine or isoproterenol. Propranolol reduces its amplitude and, if administered intra-arterially, prevents the response to isoproterenol in the perfused limb, presumably through some peripheral action. Certain drugs—especially the bronchodilators, valproate, tricyclic antidepressants, and lithium—may produce a dose-dependent exaggeration of the normal physiologic tremor that is reversed by discontinuing the drug. Although the tremor produced by sympathomimetics such as terbutaline (a bronchodilator) is blocked by propranolol, which antagonizes both β_1 and β_2 receptors, it is not blocked by metoprolol, a β_1-selective antagonist, suggesting that such tremor is mediated mainly by the β_2 receptors.

Essential tremor is a postural tremor, sometimes familial, that is clinically similar to physiologic tremor. Dysfunction of β_1 receptors has been implicated in some instances, since the tremor may respond dramatically to standard doses of metoprolol as well as to propranolol. The most useful approach is with propranolol, but whether the response depends on a central or peripheral action is unclear. The pharmacokinetics, pharmacologic effects, and adverse reactions of propranolol are discussed in Chapter 10. Daily doses of propranolol on the order of 120 mg (range, 60–240 mg) are usually required, and reported adverse effects have been few. Propranolol should be used with caution in patients with heart failure, heart block, asthma, and hypoglycemia. Patients can be instructed to take their own pulse and call the physician if significant bradycardia develops. Metoprolol is sometimes useful in treating tremor when patients have concomitant pulmonary disease that contraindicates use of propranolol. Primidone (an antiepileptic drug; see Chapter 24), in gradually increasing doses up to 250 mg three times daily, is also effective in providing symptomatic control in some cases. Patients with tremor are very sensitive to primidone and often cannot tolerate the doses used to treat seizures; they should be started on 50 mg once daily and the daily dose increased by 50 mg every 2 weeks depending on response. Topiramate, another antiepileptic drug, may also be helpful in a dose of 400 mg daily, built up gradually. Small quantities of alcohol may suppress essential tremor but only for a short time and by an unknown mechanism. Diazepam, chlordiazepoxide, mephenesin, and antiparkinsonism agents have been advocated in the past but are generally worthless. Alprazolam (in doses up to 3 mg daily) is helpful in some patients. Thalamic stimulation (discussed earlier) is often worthwhile in advanced cases refractory to pharmacotherapy.

Intention tremor is present during movement but not at rest; sometimes it occurs as a toxic manifestation of alcohol or drugs such as phenytoin. Withdrawal or reduction in dosage provides dramatic relief. There is no satisfactory pharmacologic treatment for intention tremor due to other neurologic disorders.

Rest tremor is usually due to parkinsonism.

Huntington's Disease

This dominantly inherited disorder is characterized by progressive chorea and dementia that usually begin in adulthood. The development of chorea seems to be related to an imbalance of dopamine, acetylcholine, GABA, and perhaps other neurotransmitters in the basal ganglia (Figure 28–1). Pharmacologic studies indicate that chorea results from functional overactivity in dopaminergic nigrostriatal pathways, perhaps because of increased responsiveness of postsynaptic dopamine receptors or deficiency of a neurotransmitter that normally antagonizes dopamine. Drugs that impair dopaminergic neurotransmission, either by depleting central monoamines (eg, reserpine, tetrabenazine) or by blocking dopamine receptors (eg, phenothiazines, butyrophenones), often alleviate chorea, whereas dopamine-like drugs such as levodopa tend to exacerbate it.

Both GABA and the enzyme (glutamic acid decarboxylase) concerned with its synthesis are markedly reduced in the basal ganglia of patients with Huntington's disease, and GABA receptors are usually implicated in inhibitory pathways. There is also a significant decline in concentration of choline acetyltransferase, the enzyme responsible for synthesizing acetylcholine, in the basal ganglia of these patients. These findings may be of pathophysiologic significance and have led to attempts to alleviate chorea by enhancing central GABA or acetylcholine activity. Unfortunately, such pharmacologic manipulations have been disappointing, yielding no consistently beneficial response, and as a consequence the most commonly used drugs for controlling dyskinesia in patients with Huntington's disease are still those that interfere with dopamine activity. With all of the latter drugs, however, reduction of abnormal movements may be associated with iatrogenic parkinsonism.

Reserpine depletes cerebral dopamine by preventing intraneuronal storage; it is introduced in low doses (eg, 0.25 mg daily), and the daily dose is then built up gradually (eg, by 0.25 mg every week) until benefit occurs or adverse effects become troublesome. A daily dose of 2–5 mg is often effective in suppressing abnormal movements, but adverse effects may include hypotension, depression, sedation, diarrhea, and nasal congestion. Tetrabenazine resembles reserpine in depleting cerebral dopamine and has less troublesome adverse effects, but it is not available in the USA. Treatment with postsynaptic dopamine receptor blockers such as phenothiazines and butyrophenones may also be helpful. Haloperidol is started in a small dose, eg, 1 mg twice daily, and increased every 4 days depending on the response. If haloperidol is not helpful, treatment with increasing doses of perphenazine up to a total of about 20 mg daily sometimes helps. Several recent reports suggest that olanzapine may also be helpful; the dose varies with the patient, but 10 mg daily is often sufficient although doses as high as 30 mg daily are sometimes required. The pharmacokinetics and clinical properties of these drugs are considered in greater detail elsewhere in this book.

Other Forms of Chorea

Treatment is directed at the underlying cause when chorea occurs as a complication of general medical disorders such as thyrotoxicosis, polycythemia vera rubra, systemic lupus erythematosus, hypocalcemia, and hepatic cirrhosis. Drug-induced chorea is managed by withdrawal of the offending substance, which may be levodopa, an antimuscarinic drug, amphetamine, lithium, phenytoin, or an oral contraceptive. Neuroleptic drugs may also produce an acute or tardive dyskinesia (discussed below). Sydenham's chorea is temporary and usually so mild that pharmacologic management of the dyskinesia is unnecessary, but dopamine-blocking drugs are effective in suppressing it.

Ballismus

The biochemical basis of ballismus is unknown, but the pharmacologic approach to management is the same as for chorea. Treatment with haloperidol, perphenazine, or other dopamine-blocking drugs may be helpful.

Athetosis & Dystonia

The pharmacologic basis of these disorders is unknown, and there is no satisfactory medical treatment for them. Occasional patients with dystonia may respond to diazepam, amantadine, antimuscarinic drugs (in high dosage), levodopa, carbamazepine, baclofen, haloperidol, or phenothiazines. A trial of these pharmacologic approaches is worthwhile even though often not successful. Patients with focal dystonias such as blepharospasm or torticollis may benefit from injection of botulinum toxin into the overactive muscles.

Tics

The pathophysiologic basis of tics is unknown. Chronic multiple tics (Gilles de la Tourette's syndrome) may require treatment if the disorder is severe or is having a significant impact on the patient's life. The most effective pharmacologic approach is with haloperidol, and patients are better able to tolerate this drug if treatment is started with a small dosage (eg, 0.25 or 0.5 mg daily) and then increased very gradually over the following weeks. Most patients ultimately require a total daily dose of 3–8 mg. If haloperidol is not helpful, fluphenazine, clonazepam, clonidine, or carbamazepine should be tried. The pharmacologic properties of these drugs are discussed elsewhere in this book. Pimozide, an oral dopamine blocker, may help patients intolerant or unresponsive to haloperidol. The role of the newer atypical antipsychotic agents, such as risperidone, is unclear.

Drug-Induced Dyskinesias

The pharmacologic basis of the acute dyskinesia or dystonia sometimes precipitated by the first few doses of a phenothiazine is not clear. In most instances, parenteral administration of an antimuscarinic drug such as benztropine (2 mg intravenously), diphenhydramine (50 mg intravenously), or biperiden (2–5 mg intravenously or intramuscularly) is helpful, while in other instances diazepam (10 mg intravenously) alleviates the abnormal movements.

Tardive dyskinesia, a disorder characterized by a variety of abnormal movements, is a common complication of long-term neuroleptic drug treatment (see Chapter 29). Unfortunately, its precise pharmacologic basis is unclear. A reduction in dose of the offending medication, a dopamine receptor blocker, commonly worsens the dyskinesia, while an increase in dose may suppress it. The drugs most likely to provide immediate symptomatic benefit are those interfering with dopaminergic function, either by depletion (eg, reserpine, tetrabenazine) or receptor blockade (eg, phenothiazines, butyrophenones). Paradoxically, the receptor-blocking drugs are the very ones that also cause the dyskinesia, and they are probably best avoided to prevent the development of a spiral phenomenon in which continuing aggravation of the dyskinesia by the drugs used to control it necessitates increasingly higher doses for its temporary suppression.

Because tardive dyskinesia developing in adults is usually irreversible and has no satisfactory treatment, care must be taken to reduce the likelihood of its occurrence. Antipsychotic medication should be prescribed only when necessary and should be withheld periodically to assess the need for continued treatment and to unmask incipient dyskinesia. Thioridazine, a phenothiazine with a piperidine side chain, is an effective antipsychotic that seems less likely than most to cause extrapyramidal reactions, perhaps because it has little effect on dopamine receptors in the striatal system. Finally, antimuscarinic drugs should not be prescribed routinely in patients receiving neuroleptics, since the combination may increase the likelihood of dyskinesia.

Wilson's Disease

Wilson's disease, a recessively inherited disorder of copper metabolism, is characterized biochemically by reduced serum copper and ceruloplasmin concentrations, pathologically by markedly increased concentration of copper in the brain and viscera, and clinically by signs of hepatic and neurologic dysfunction. Treatment involves the removal of excess copper, followed by maintenance of copper balance. A commonly used agent for this purpose is **penicillamine** (dimethylcysteine), a chelating agent that forms a ring complex with copper. It is readily absorbed from the gastrointestinal tract and rapidly excreted in the urine. A common starting dose in adults is 500 mg three or four times daily. After remission occurs, it may be possible to lower the maintenance dose, generally to not less than 1 g daily, which must thereafter be continued indefinitely. Adverse effects include nausea and vomiting, nephrotic syndrome, a lupus-like syndrome, pemphigus, myasthenia, arthropathy, optic neuropathy, and various blood dyscrasias. Treatment should be monitored by frequent urinalysis

and complete blood counts. Dietary copper should also be kept below 2 mg daily. Potassium disulfide, 20 mg three times daily with meals, reduces the intestinal absorption of copper and should also be prescribed.

For those patients who are unable to tolerate penicillamine, **trientine**, another chelating agent, may be used in a daily dose of 1–1.5 g. Trientine appears to have few adverse effects other than mild anemia due to iron deficiency in a few patients. **Zinc acetate** administered orally increases the fecal excretion of copper and is sometimes used for maintenance therapy. The dose is 50 mg three times a day. **Zinc sulfate** (200 mg/d orally) has also been used to decrease copper absorption. Zinc blocks copper absorption from the gastrointestinal tract by induction of intestinal cell metallothionein. Its main advantage is its low toxicity compared with other anticopper agents, although it may cause gastric irritation when first introduced.

PREPARATIONS AVAILABLE

Amantadine (Symmetrel, others)
  Oral: 100 mg capsules; 10 mg/mL syrup
Benztropine (Cogentin, others)
  Oral: 0.5, 1, 2 mg tablets
  Parenteral: 1 mg/mL for injection
Biperiden (Akineton)
  Oral: 2 mg tablets
  Parenteral: 5 mg/mL for injection
Bromocriptine (Parlodel)
  Oral: 2.5 mg tablets; 5 mg capsules
Carbidopa (Lodosyn)
  Oral: 25 mg tablets
Carbidopa/levodopa (Sinemet)
  Oral: 10 mg carbidopa and 100 mg levodopa, 25 mg carbidopa and 100 mg levodopa, 25 mg carbidopa and 250 mg levodopa tablets
  Oral sustained-release (Sinemet CR): 25 mg carbidopa and 100 mg levodopa; 50 mg carbidopa and 200 mg levodopa
Entacapone (Comtan)
  Oral: 200 mg tablets
Levodopa (Dopar, Larodopa)
  Oral: 100, 250, 500 mg tablets, capsules

Orphenadrine (various)
  Oral: 100 mg tablets
  Oral sustained-release: 100 mg tablets
  Parenteral: 30 mg/mL for injection
Penicillamine (Cuprimine, Depen)
  Oral: 125, 250 mg capsules; 250 mg tablets
Pergolide (Permax)
  Oral: 0.05, 0.25, 1 mg tablets
Pramipexole (Mirapex)
  Oral: 0.125, 0.25, 1, 1.5 mg tablets
Procyclidine (Kemadrin)
  Oral: 5 mg tablets
Ropinirole (Requip)
  Oral: 0.25, 0.5, 1, 2, 5 mg tablets
Selegiline (deprenyl) (generic, Eldepryl)
  Oral: 5 mg tablets
Tolcapone (Tasmar)
  Oral: 100, 200 mg tablets
Trientine (Syprine)
  Oral: 250 mg capsules
Trihexyphenidyl (Artane, others)
  Oral: 2, 5 mg tablets; 2 mg/5 mL elixir
  Oral sustained-release (Artane Sequels): 5 mg capsules

REFERENCES

Adler CH et al: Ropinirole for the treatment of early Parkinson's disease. Neurology 1997;49:393.

Biglan KM, Holloway RG: A review of pramipexole and its clinical utility in Parkinson's disease. Expert Opin Pharmacother 2002;3:197.

Bjorklund LM, Isacson O: Regulation of dopamine cell type and transmitter function in fetal and stem cell transplantation for Parkinson's disease. Prog Brain Res 2002;138:411.

Bonelli RM et al: High-dose olanzapine in Huntington's disease. Int Clin Psychopharmacol 2002;17:91.

Bonuccelli U et al: Pergolide in the treatment of patients with early and advanced Parkinson's disease. Clin Neuropharmacol 2002;25:1.

Brewer GJ et al: Diagnosis and treatment of Wilson's disease. Semin Neurol 1999;19:261.

Brewer GJ: Zinc acetate for the treatment of Wilson's disease. Expert Opin Pharmacother 2001;2:1473.

Brewer GJ: Practical recommendations and new therapies for Wilson's disease. Drugs 1995;50:240.

Carter JH et al: Amount and distribution of dietary protein affects clinical response to levodopa in Parkinson's disease. Neurology 1989;39:552.

Clarke CE, Guttman M: Dopamine agonist monotherapy in Parkinson's disease. Lancet 2002;360:1767.

Connor GS: A double-blind placebo-controlled trial of topiramate treatment for essential tremor. Neurology 2002;59:132.

Dawson TM, Dawson VL: Neuroprotective and neurorestorative strategies for Parkinson's disease. Nat Neurosci 2002;5(Suppl):1058.

Deleu D et al: Clinical pharmacokinetic and pharmacodynamic properties of drugs used in the treatment of Parkinson's disease. Clin Pharmacokinet 2002;41:261.

Dunnett SB, Bjorklund A: Prospects for new restorative and neuroprotective treatments in Parkinson's disease. Nature 1999;399:A32.

Etminan M et al: Increased risk of somnolence with the new dopamine agonists in patients with Parkinson's disease: a meta-analysis of randomised controlled trials. Drug Saf 2001;24:863.

Factor SA, Friedman JH: The emerging role of clozapine in the treatment of movement disorders. Mov Disord 1997;12:483.

Foltynie T et al: The genetic basis of Parkinson's disease. J Neurol Neurosurg Psychiatry 2002;73:363.

Hanna PA et al: Switching from pergolide to pramipexole in patients with Parkinson's disease. J Neural Transm 2001;108:63.

Hubble JP et al: Essential tremor. Clin Neuropharmacol 1989;12:453.

Hyde TM, Weinberger DR: Tourette's syndrome: A model neuropsychiatric disorder. JAMA 1995;273:498.

Jankovic J: New and emerging therapies for Parkinson disease. Arch Neurol 1999;56:785.

Koller W et al: High-frequency unilateral thalamic stimulation in the treatment of essential and parkinsonian tremor. Ann Neurol 1997;42:292.

Koller WC, Tolosa E (editors): Current and emerging drug therapies in the management of Parkinson's disease. Neurology 1998;50:Suppl 6. [Entire issue.]

Kurth MC et al: Tolcapone improves motor function and reduces levodopa requirement in patients with Parkinson's disease experiencing motor fluctuations: a multicenter, double-blind, randomized, placebo-controlled trial. Neurology 1997;48:81.

Lambert D, Waters CH: Essential tremor. Curr Treat Options Neurol 1999;1:6.

Lang AE, Lozano AM: Parkinson's disease. (Two parts.) N Engl J Med 1998;339:1044, 1130.

Le WD, Jankovic J: Are dopamine receptor agonists neuroprotective in Parkinson's disease? Drugs Aging 2001;18:389.

Leckman JF: Tourette's syndrome. Lancet 2002;360:1577.

Lieberman A et al: Clinical evaluation of pramipexole in advanced Parkinson's disease: results of a double-blind, placebo-controlled, parallel-group study. Neurology 1997;49:162.

Limousin P et al: Electrical stimulation of the subthalamic nucleus in advanced Parkinson's disease. N Engl J Med 1998;339:1105.

McMurray CT: Huntington's disease: new hope for therapeutics. Trends Neurosci 2001;24(Suppl):S32.

Mehta V et al: Neural transplantation in Parkinson's disease. Can J Neurol Sci 1997;24:292.

Miyasaki JM et al: Practice parameter: initiation of treatment for Parkinson's disease: an evidence-based review. Neurology 2002;58:11.

Mouradian MM et al: Modification of central dopaminergic mechanisms by continuous levodopa therapy for advanced Parkinson's disease. Ann Neurol 1990;27:18.

Muller-Vahl KR: The treatment of Tourette's syndrome: current opinions. Expert Opin Pharmacother 2002;3:899.

Nakanishi T et al: Second interim report of the nation-wide collaborative study on the long-term effects of bromocriptine in the treatment of parkinsonian patients. Eur Neurol 1989;29(Suppl 1):3.

Nygaard TG et al: Dopa-responsive dystonia: Long-term treatment response and prognosis. Neurology 1991;41:174.

Obeso JA et al: Surgery for Parkinson's disease. J Neurol Neurosurg Psychiatry 1997;62:2.

Olanow CW, Koller WC (editors): An algorithm (decision tree) for the management of Parkinson's disease: treatment guidelines. Neurology 1998;50:Suppl 3.

Paleacu D et al: Olanzapine in Huntington's disease. Acta Neurol Scand 2002;105:441.

Parkinson Study Group: A controlled trial of rasagiline in early Parkinson disease: the TEMPO study. Arch Neurol 2002;59:1937.

Parkinson Study Group: Effects of tocopherol and deprenyl on the progression of disability in early Parkinson's disease. N Engl J Med 1993;328:176.

Parkinson Study Group: Entacapone improves motor fluctuations in levodopa-treated Parkinson's disease patients. Ann Neurol 1997;42:747.

Parkinson Study Group: Safety and efficacy of pramipexole in early Parkinson disease. JAMA 1997;278:125.

Quinn N: Drug treatment of Parkinson's disease. Br Med J 1995;310:575.

Reddy S et al: The effect of quetiapine on psychosis and motor function in parkinsonian patients with and without dementia. Mov Disord 2002;17:676.

Riley DE, Lang AK: The spectrum of levodopa-related fluctuations in Parkinson's disease. Neurology 1993;43:1459.

Rinne UK et al: Entacapone enhances the response to levodopa in parkinsonian patients with motor fluctuations. Neurology 1998;51:1309.

Ross RT: Drug-induced parkinsonism and other movement disorders. Can J Neurol Sci 1990;22:155.

Scheinberg IH, Jaffe ME, Sternlieb I: The use of trientine in preventing the effects of interrupting penicillamine therapy in Wilson's disease. N Engl J Med 1987;317:209.

Schilsky ML: Diagnosis and treatment of Wilson's disease. Pediatr Transplant 2002;6:15.

Schneider JS et al: Recovery from experimental parkinsonism in primates with G_{M1} ganglioside treatment. Science 1992;256: 843.

Schulzer M et al: The antiparkinson efficacy of deprenyl derives from transient improvement that is likely to be symptomatic. Ann Neurol 1992;32:795.

Shapiro AK et al: Pimozide treatment of tic and Tourette disorders. Pediatrics 1987;79:6.

Shults CW et al: Effects of coenzyme Q_{10} in early Parkinson disease: evidence of slowing of the functional decline. Arch Neurol 2002;59:1541.

Starr PA et al: Deep brain stimulation for movement disorders. Neurosurg Clin North Am 1998;9:381.

Tuite P, Ebbitt B: Dopamine agonists. Semin Neurol 2001;21:9.

Antipsychotic Agents & Lithium   29

William Z. Potter, MD, PhD, & Leo E. Hollister, MD*

I. ANTIPSYCHOTIC AGENTS

The terms **antipsychotic** and **neuroleptic** are used interchangeably to denote a group of drugs that have been used mainly for treating schizophrenia but are also effective in some other psychoses and agitated states.

History

Antipsychotic drugs have been used in western medicine for 50 years. Reserpine and chlorpromazine were the first drugs found to be useful in schizophrenia. Although chlorpromazine is still sometimes used for the treatment of psychoses, these forerunner drugs have been superseded by many newer agents. Their impact on psychiatry, however—especially on the treatment of schizophrenia—has been enormous: The number of patients requiring hospitalization in mental institutions has markedly decreased, and psychiatric thinking has shifted to a more biologic basis.

Nature of Psychosis & Schizophrenia

The term "psychosis" denotes a variety of mental disorders. Schizophrenia is a particular kind of psychosis characterized mainly by a clear sensorium but a marked thinking disturbance.

The pathogenesis of schizophrenia is unknown. Largely as a result of research stimulated by the discovery of antipsychotic drugs, a genetic predisposition has been proposed as a necessary but not always sufficient condition underlying psychotic disorder. This assumption has been supported by the observed familial incidence of schizophrenia. Completion of the first phase of the human genome project increases the likelihood of identifying multiple genes that contribute to the various clinical phenotypes subsumed under the broad diagnostic classification of schizophrenia. At least one gene—that which encodes for neuregulin 1—is associated with schizophrenia in Icelandic and northern European populations. In what way it actually contributes to schizophrenia and whether it applies to other populations have yet to be determined. The molecular basis for schizophrenia thus continues to elude definition, but a great deal of effort has been expended in attempting to link the disorder with abnormalities of amine neurotransmitter function, especially that of dopamine (see Box, The Dopamine Hypothesis). The defects of this hypothesis are significant, and it is now appreciated that the disorder is far more complex than originally supposed.

BASIC PHARMACOLOGY OF ANTIPSYCHOTIC AGENTS

Chemical Types

A number of chemical structures have been associated with antipsychotic properties. The drugs can be classified into several groups as shown in Figures 29–1 and 29–2.

A. PHENOTHIAZINE DERIVATIVES

Three subfamilies of phenothiazines, based primarily on the side chain of the molecule, were once the most widely used of the antipsychotics. Aliphatic derivatives (eg, **chlorpromazine**) and piperidine derivatives (eg, **thioridazine**) are the least potent. Piperazine derivatives are more potent in the sense that they are effective in lower doses. The piperazine derivatives are also more selective in their pharmacologic effects (Table 29–1).

B. THIOXANTHENE DERIVATIVES

This group of drugs is exemplified primarily by **thiothixene**. In general, these compounds are slightly less potent than their phenothiazine analogs.

C. BUTYROPHENONE DERIVATIVES

This group, of which **haloperidol** is the most widely used, has a very different structure from those of the two preceding groups. Diphenylbutylpiperidines are closely related compounds. These agents tend to be more potent and to have fewer autonomic effects.

D. MISCELLANEOUS STRUCTURES

The newer drugs, not all of which are available in the USA, have a variety of structures and include **pimozide,**

---

*Deceased

THE DOPAMINE HYPOTHESIS

The dopamine hypothesis for schizophrenia is the most fully developed of several hypotheses and is the basis for much of the rationale for drug therapy. Several lines of circumstantial evidence suggest that excessive dopaminergic activity plays a role in the disorder: (1) most antipsychotic drugs strongly block postsynaptic D_2 receptors in the central nervous system, especially in the mesolimbic-frontal system; (2) drugs that increase dopaminergic activity, such as levodopa (a precursor), amphetamines (releasers of dopamine), or apomorphine (a direct dopamine receptor agonist), either aggravate schizophrenia or produce psychosis de novo in some patients; (3) dopamine receptor density has been found, postmortem, to be increased in the brains of schizophrenics who have not been treated with antipsychotic drugs; (4) positron emission tomography (PET) has shown increased dopamine receptor density in both treated and untreated schizophrenics when compared with such scans of nonschizophrenic persons; and (5) successful treatment of schizophrenic patients has been reported to change the amount of homovanillic acid (HVA), a metabolite of dopamine, in the cerebrospinal fluid, plasma, and urine.

The dopamine hypothesis is far from complete, however. If an abnormality of dopamine physiology were completely responsible for the pathogenesis of schizophrenia, antipsychotic drugs would do a much better job of treating patients—but they are only partially effective for most and ineffective for some patients. Moreover, it appears that antagonists of the NMDA receptor such as phencyclidine, when administered to nonpsychotic subjects, produce much more "schizophrenia like" symptoms than do dopamine agonists. The recent cloning and characterization of multiple dopamine receptor types may permit more direct testing of the dopamine hypothesis if drugs can be developed that act selectively on each receptor type. The traditional antipsychotics bind D_2 50 times more avidly than D_1 or D_3 receptors. Until recently, the main thrust in drug development was to find agents that were more potent and more selective in blocking D_2 receptors. The fact that several of the atypical antipsychotic drugs have much less effect on D_2 receptors and yet are effective in schizophrenia has redirected attention to the role of other dopamine receptors and to nondopamine receptors, especially serotonin receptor subtypes that may mediate synergistic effects or protect against the extrapyramidal consequences of D_2 antagonism. As a result of these considerations, the direction of research has changed to a greater focus on compounds that may act on several transmitter-receptor systems. The great hope is to produce drugs with greater efficacy and fewer adverse effects, especially extrapyramidal toxicity.

---

molindone, loxapine, clozapine, olanzapine, quetiapine, risperidone, ziprasidone, and **aripiprazole** (Figure 29–2).

Pharmacokinetics

A. ABSORPTION AND DISTRIBUTION

Most antipsychotic drugs are readily but incompletely absorbed. Furthermore, many of these drugs undergo significant first-pass metabolism. Thus, oral doses of chlorpromazine and thioridazine have systemic availability from 25% to 35%, while haloperidol, which is less likely to be metabolized, has an average systemic availability of about 65%.

Most antipsychotics are highly lipid-soluble and protein-bound (92–99%). They tend to have large volumes of distribution (usually > 7 L/kg). Probably because these drugs are sequestered in lipid compartments of the body and have very high affinity for selected neurotransmitter receptors in the central nervous system, they generally have a much longer clinical duration of action than would be estimated from their plasma half-lives.

This is paralleled by prolonged occupancy of dopamine D_2 receptors in brain. Metabolites of chlorpromazine may be excreted in the urine weeks after the last dose of chronically administered drug. Similarly, full relapse may not occur until 6 weeks or more following discontinuation of many antipsychotic drugs.

B. METABOLISM

Most antipsychotics are almost completely metabolized by a variety of processes. Although some metabolites retain activity, eg, 7-hydroxychlorpromazine and reduced haloperidol, metabolites are not considered to be highly important to the action of these drugs. The sole exception is mesoridazine, the major metabolite of thioridazine, which is more potent than the parent compound and accounts for most of the effect. This compound has been marketed as a separate entity.

C. EXCRETION

Very little of these drugs is excreted unchanged, because they are almost completely metabolized to more polar substances.

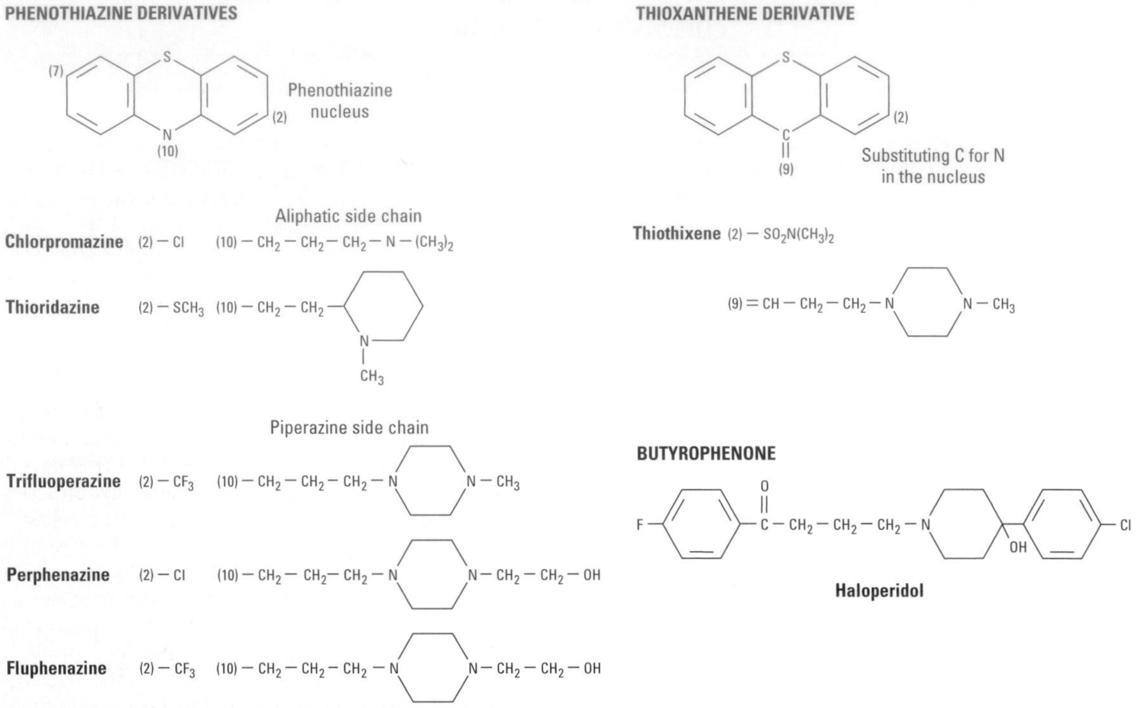

PHENOTHIAZINE DERIVATIVES

THIOXANTHENE DERIVATIVE

BUTYROPHENONE

Haloperidol

Figure 29–1. Structural formulas of some older antipsychotic drugs: phenothiazines, thioxanthenes, and butyrophenones. Only representative members of each type are shown.

Pharmacologic Effects

The first phenothiazine antipsychotic drugs, with chlorpromazine as the prototype, proved to have a wide variety of central nervous system, autonomic, and endocrine effects. These actions were traced to blocking effects at a wide range of receptors, including dopamine and α-adrenoceptor, muscarinic, H_1 histaminic, and serotonin (5-HT$_2$) receptors. Dopamine receptor effects quickly became the major focus of interest.

A. DOPAMINERGIC SYSTEMS

Five important dopaminergic systems or pathways are now recognized in the brain. The first pathway—the one most closely related to behavior—is the **mesolimbic-mesocortical** pathway, which projects from cell bodies near the substantia nigra to the limbic system and neocortex. The second system—the **nigrostriatal** pathway—consists of neurons that project from the substantia nigra to the caudate and putamen; it is involved in the coordination of voluntary movement. The third pathway—the **tuberoinfundibular** system—connects arcuate nuclei and periventricular neurons to the hypothalamus and posterior pituitary. Dopamine released by

these neurons physiologically inhibits prolactin secretion. The fourth dopaminergic system—the **medullary-periventricular** pathway—consists of neurons in the motor nucleus of the vagus whose projections are not well defined. This system may be involved in eating behavior. The fifth pathway—the **incertohypothalamic** pathway—forms connections from the medial zona incerta to the hypothalamus and the amygdala. It appears to regulate the anticipatory motivational phase of copulatory behavior in rats.

After dopamine was recognized as a neurotransmitter in 1959, investigators showed that its effects on electrical activity in central synapses and on production of cAMP by adenylyl cyclase could be blocked by most antipsychotic drugs. This evidence led to the conclusion in the early 1960s that these drugs should be considered **dopamine antagonists.** The antipsychotic action is now thought to be produced (at least in part) by their ability to block dopamine in the mesolimbic and mesofrontal systems. Furthermore, the antagonism of dopamine in the nigrostriatal system explains the unwanted effect of parkinsonism produced by these drugs. The hyperprolactinemia that follows treatment with antipsychotics is caused by blockade of dopamine's tonic inhibitory effect

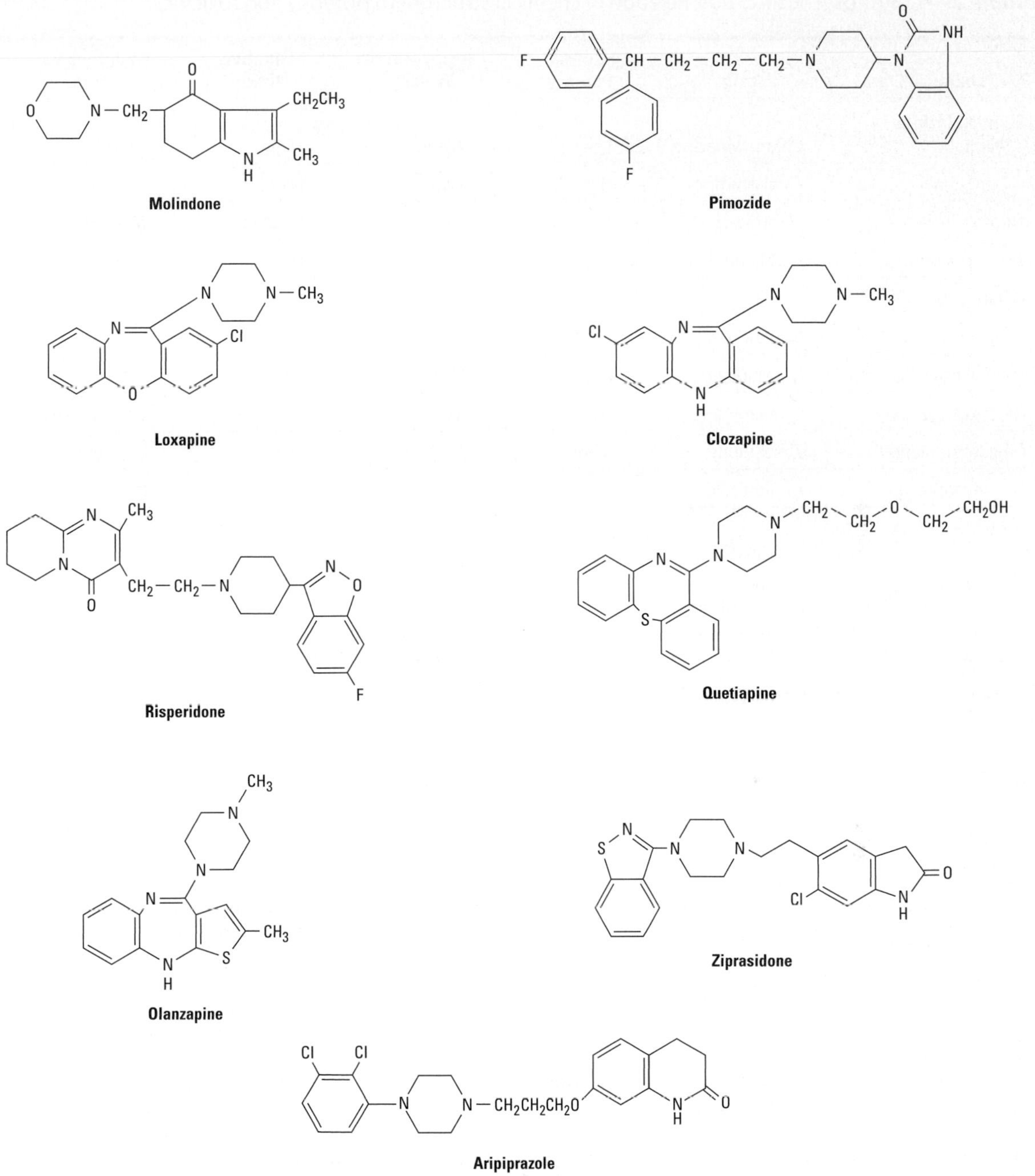

Molindone

Pimozide

Loxapine

Clozapine

Risperidone

Quetiapine

Olanzapine

Ziprasidone

Aripiprazole

Figure 29–2. Structural formulas of some newer antipsychotic drugs.

Table 29–1. Antipsychotic drugs: Relation of chemical structure to potency and toxicities.

Chemical Class	Drug	Clinical Potency	Extrapyramidal Toxicity	Sedative Action	Hypotensive Actions
Phenothiazines					
Aliphatic	Chlorpromazine	Low	Medium	High	High
Piperazine	Fluphenazine	High	High	Low	Very low
Thioxanthene	Thiothixene	High	Medium	Medium	Medium
Butyrophenone	Haloperidol	High	Very high	Low	Very low
Dibenzodiazepine	Clozapine	Medium	Very low	Low	Medium
Benzisoxazole	Risperidone	High	Low[1]	Low	Low
Thienobenzodiazepine	Olanzapine	High	Very low	Medium	Low
Dibenzothiazepine	Quetiapine	Low	Very low	Medium	Low to medium
Dihydroindolone	Ziprasidone	Medium	Very low	Low	Very low
Dihydrocarbostyril	Aripiprazole	High	Very low	Very low	Low

[1]At dosages below 8 mg/d.

on prolactin release from the pituitary. Thus, the same pharmacodynamic action may have distinct psychiatric, neurologic, and endocrinologic consequences.

B. DOPAMINE RECEPTORS AND THEIR EFFECTS

At present, five different dopamine receptors have been described, consisting of two separate families, the D_1-like and D_2-like receptor groups. The D_1 receptor is coded by a gene on chromosome 5, increases cAMP by activation of adenylyl cyclase, and is located mainly in the putamen, nucleus accumbens, and olfactory tubercle. The second member of this family, D_5, is coded by a gene on chromosome 4, also increases cAMP, and is found in the hippocampus and hypothalamus. The therapeutic potency of antipsychotic drugs does not correlate with their affinity for binding the D_1 receptor (Figure 29–3, top). The D_2 receptor is coded on chromosome 11, decreases cAMP (by inhibition of adenylyl cyclase), and inhibits calcium channels but opens potassium channels. It is found both pre- and postsynaptically on neurons in the caudate-putamen, nucleus accumbens, and olfactory tubercle. A second member of this family, the D_3 receptor, also coded by a gene on chromosome 11, is thought to decrease cAMP, and is located in the frontal cortex, medulla, and midbrain. D_4 receptors, the newest members of the D_2-like family, also decrease cAMP. All dopamine receptors have seven-transmembrane domains and are G protein-coupled.

The activation of D_2 receptors by a variety of direct or indirect agonists (eg, amphetamines, levodopa, apomorphine) causes increased motor activity and stereo-

typed behavior in rats, a model that has been extensively used for antipsychotic drug screening. When given to humans, the same drugs aggravate schizophrenia. The antipsychotic agents block D_2 receptors stereoselectively for the most part, and their binding affinity is very strongly correlated with clinical antipsychotic and extrapyramidal potency (Figure 29–3, bottom). Continuous treatment with antipsychotic drugs has been reported in some studies to produce a transient increase in levels of a dopamine metabolite, homovanillic acid (HVA), in the cerebrospinal fluid, plasma, and urine. After 1–3 weeks, HVA levels decrease to lower than normal levels, and this decrease persists. These changes may be explained as follows: The initial period of receptor blockade causes a compensatory increase in transmitter turnover, resulting in increased levels of HVA. With chronic therapy, feedback inhibition caused by the increased synaptic levels of dopamine results in decreased dopamine release and turnover. Some studies have failed to confirm these findings.

As noted above, these findings have been incorporated into the dopamine hypothesis of schizophrenia. However, many questions have not been satisfactorily answered, and many observations have not been fully confirmed. For example, dopamine receptors exist in both high- and low-affinity forms, and it is not known whether schizophrenia or the antipsychotic drugs alter the proportions of receptors in these two forms. With the introduction of aripiprazole, which in preclinical studies shows partial agonism at D_2 and 5-HT$_{1A}$ receptors, the relevance of the proportion of receptors in var-

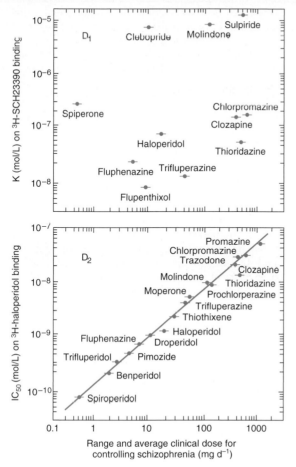

Figure 29–3. Correlations between the therapeutic potency of antipsychotic drugs and their affinity for binding to dopamine D_1 *(top)* or D_2 receptors *(bottom)*. Potency is indicated on the horizontal axes; it decreases to the right. Binding affinity for D_1 receptors was measured by displacing the selective D_1 ligand SCH 23390; affinity for D_2 receptors was similarly measured by displacing the selective D_2 ligand haloperidol. Binding affinity decreases upward. (Modified and reproduced, with permission, from Seeman P: Dopamine receptors and the dopamine hypothesis of schizophrenia. Synapse 1987;1:133.)

ious affinity states may prove especially important for understanding the degree of response to this agent.

Furthermore, the drug-induced progression of extrapyramidal changes—from diminished function (resembling parkinsonism) to increased activity (manifested by dyskinesias)—often occurs over a period of months to years. This time scale is much longer than that described for other drug-induced changes in receptor function. Of most importance, newer drugs—clozapine, olanzapine, quetiapine, and aripiprazole—are not very potent antagonists at the D_2 receptor, which suggests that additional actions are critical to their antipsychotic effects.

It has not been convincingly demonstrated that antagonism of any dopamine receptor other than the D_2 receptor plays any role in the action of antipsychotic drugs. Selective D_3 receptor antagonists may prove therapeutic but are not yet available. Specific D_1 receptor antagonists have been developed, and at least one is reputed to have failed in clinical trials. Attempts to assess the effects of D_4 antagonism have met with discouraging early anecdotal reports. Participation of glutamate, GABA, and acetylcholine receptors in the patho physiology of schizophrenia has also been proposed. Agents targeted at glutamatergic and cholinergic systems are just beginning to be evaluated in schizophrenia.

C. DIFFERENCES AMONG ANTIPSYCHOTIC DRUGS

Although all effective antipsychotic drugs block D_2 receptors, the degree of this blockade in relation to other actions on receptors varies considerably between drugs. Vast numbers of ligand-receptor binding experiments have been performed in an effort to discover a single receptor action that would best predict antipsychotic efficacy. For example, in vitro binding studies indicate that chlorpromazine and thioridazine block α_1 adrenoceptors more potently than D_2 receptors. They also block serotonin 5-HT$_2$ receptors relatively strongly. However, their affinity for D_1 receptors as measured by displacement of a selective D_1 ligand, SCH 23390, is relatively weak (Figure 29–3). Drugs such as perphenazine and haloperidol act mainly on D_2 receptors; they have some effect on 5-HT$_2$ and α_1 receptors but negligible effects on D_1 receptors. Pimozide acts almost exclusively on D_2 receptors. The atypical antipsychotic clozapine, which shows marked clinical differences from the others, binds more to D_4, 5-HT$_2$, α_1, and histamine H$_1$ receptors than to either D_2 or D_1 receptors. Risperidone is about equally potent in blocking D_2 and 5-HT$_2$ receptors. Olanzapine is somewhat more potent as an antagonist of 5-HT$_2$ receptors, with lesser and approximately equal potency at D_1, D_2, and α_1 receptors. Quetiapine is a lower-potency compound with relatively similar antagonism of 5-HT$_2$, D_2, α_1, and α_2 receptors. Like clozapine, both olanzapine and quetiapine are also potent inhibitors of H$_1$ histamine receptors, which is consistent with their sedative properties. The most recently marketed antipsychotic, aripiprazole, is reported to have partial agonist effects at D_2 and 5-HT$_{1A}$ receptors. A summary of the relative receptor-binding affinities of three key agents in such comparisons illustrates the difficulty in drawing simple conclusions from such experiments:

Chlorpromazine: $\alpha_1 = 5\text{-HT}_2 > D_2 > D_1$
Haloperidol: $D_2 > D_1 = D_4 > \alpha_1 > 5\text{-HT}_2$
Clozapine: $D_4 = \alpha_1 > 5\text{-HT}_2 > D_2 = D_1$

Current research is directed toward discovering atypical antipsychotic compounds that are either more selective for the mesolimbic system (to reduce their effects on the extrapyramidal system) or have effects on central neurotransmitter receptors—such as those for acetylcholine and excitatory amino acids—that have been proposed as new targets for antipsychotic action.

In contrast to the search for *efficacy,* such differences in the receptor effects of various antipsychotics do explain many of their *toxicities* (Tables 29–1 and 29–2). In particular, extrapyramidal toxicity appears to be associated with high D_2 potency.

D. PSYCHOLOGICAL EFFECTS

Most antipsychotic drugs cause unpleasant subjective effects in nonpsychotic individuals; the combination of sleepiness, restlessness, and autonomic effects creates experiences unlike those associated with more familiar sedatives or hypnotics. Nonpsychotic persons also experience impaired performance as judged by a number of psychomotor and psychometric tests. Psychotic individuals, however, may actually show improvement in their performance as the psychosis is alleviated.

E. NEUROPHYSIOLOGIC EFFECTS

Antipsychotic drugs produce shifts in the pattern of electroencephalographic frequencies, usually slowing them and increasing their synchronization. The slowing (hypersynchrony) is sometimes focal or unilateral, which may lead to erroneous diagnostic interpretations. Both the frequency and the amplitude changes induced by psychotropic drugs are readily apparent and can be quantitated by sophisticated electrophysiologic techniques.

F. ENDOCRINE EFFECTS

Older antipsychotic drugs produce striking adverse effects on the reproductive system. Amenorrhea-galactorrhea, false-positive pregnancy tests, and increased libido have been reported in women, whereas men have experienced decreased libido and gynecomastia. Some of these effects are secondary to blockade of dopamine's tonic inhibition of prolactin secretion; others may be due to increased peripheral conversion of androgens to estrogens. Absent or minimal increases of prolactin after some of the newer antipsychotics such as olanzapine, quetiapine, and aripiprazole may be a marker of diminished D_2 antagonism and hence reduced risks of extrapyramidal system dysfunction and tardive dyskinesia as well as endocrine dysfunction.

G. CARDIOVASCULAR EFFECTS

Orthostatic hypotension and high resting pulse rates frequently result from use of the "high-dose" (low potency) phenothiazines. Mean arterial pressure, peripheral resistance, and stroke volume are decreased, and heart rate is increased. These effects are predictable from the autonomic actions of these agents (Table 29–2). Abnormal ECGs have been recorded, especially with thioridazine. Changes include prolongation of QT interval and abnormal configurations of the ST segment and T waves, the latter being rounded, flattened, or notched. These changes are readily reversed by withdrawing the drug.

Table 29–2. Adverse pharmacologic effects of antipsychotic drugs.

Type	Manifestations	Mechanism
Autonomic nervous system	Loss of accommodation, dry mouth, difficulty urinating, constipation	Muscarinic cholinoceptor blockade
	Orthostatic hypotension, impotence, failure to ejaculate	Alpha adrenoceptor blockade
Central nervous system	Parkinson's syndrome, akathisia, dystonias	Dopamine receptor blockade
	Tardive dyskinesia	Supersensitivity of dopamine receptors
	Toxic-confusional state	Muscarinic blockade
Endocrine system	Amenorrhea-galactorrhea, infertility, impotence	Dopamine receptor blockade resulting in hyperprolactinemia
Other	Weight gain	Possibly combined H_1 and 5-HT_2 blockade

Among the newest antipsychotics, prolongation of the QT or QT$_c$ interval—with increased risk of dangerous arrhythmias—has been of such concern that the atypical drug sertindole was withdrawn shortly after being marketed. Ziprasidone carries a warning about risk of significant QT$_c$ prolongation.

H. ANIMAL SCREENING TESTS

Inhibition of conditioned (but not unconditioned) avoidance behavior is one of the most predictive tests of antipsychotic action. Another is the inhibition of amphetamine- or apomorphine-induced stereotyped behavior. This inhibition is undoubtedly related to the D$_2$ receptor-blocking action of the drugs, countering these two dopamine agonists. Other tests that may predict antipsychotic action are reduction of exploratory behavior without undue sedation, induction of a cataleptic state, inhibition of intracranial self-stimulation of reward areas, and prevention of apomorphine-induced vomiting. Most of these tests are difficult to relate to any model of clinical psychosis.

As mentioned earlier, the psychosis produced by phencyclidine (PCP) is a model for schizophrenia. As this drug is an antagonist of the NMDA glutamate receptor, attempts have been made to develop antipsychotics that work as NMDA agonists. Sigma opioid and cholecystokinin type b (CCK$_b$) antagonism have also been suggested as potential targets. Thus far, NMDA receptor-based models have pointed to use of agents that modulate glutamate release as potential antipsychotics.

CLINICAL PHARMACOLOGY OF ANTIPSYCHOTIC AGENTS

Indications

A. PSYCHIATRIC INDICATIONS

Schizophrenia is the primary indication for these drugs, which are presently the mainstay of treatment for this condition. Unfortunately, some patients do not respond at all and virtually none show a complete response.

Antipsychotics are also indicated for schizoaffective disorders, which share characteristics of both schizophrenia and affective disorders. The psychotic aspects of the illness require treatment with antipsychotic drugs, which may be used with other drugs such as antidepressants, lithium, or valproic acid. The manic episode in bipolar affective disorder often requires treatment with antipsychotic agents, though lithium or valproic acid supplemented with high-potency benzodiazepines (eg, lorazepam or clonazepam) may suffice in milder cases. Recent controlled trials support the efficacy of monotherapy with atypical antipsychotics in the acute phase (up to 4 weeks) of mania, and olanzapine has been approved for this indication.

As mania subsides, the antipsychotic drug may be withdrawn, although maintenance treatment with atypical antipsychotics has become more common. Nonmanic excited states may also be managed by antipsychotics, often in combination with benzodiazepines.

Other indications for the use of antipsychotics include Tourette's syndrome and the need to control disturbed behavior in patients with senile dementia of the Alzheimer type. The drugs may also be used with antidepressants to control agitation or psychosis in depressed patients. Such patients have been reported to develop tardive dyskinesia more readily, so they must be dosed sparingly with the older typical potent D$_2$ antagonists. Olanzapine, risperidone, quetiapine, and aripiprazole should prove to be better tolerated. It appears possible that some of the newer drugs such as olanzapine will show "antidepressant" efficacy in schizophrenia, as was reported for thioridazine decades ago. Antipsychotics are not indicated for the treatment of various withdrawal syndromes, eg, opioid withdrawal.

Antipsychotics in small doses have been promoted (wrongly) for the relief of anxiety associated with minor emotional disorders. The antianxiety sedatives (see Chapter 22) are far better in every respect, including safety and acceptability to patients. Ziprasidone in low doses may turn out to be an exception to this rule, since early studies suggest a favorable risk-benefit ratio in some types of anxiety.

B. NONPSYCHIATRIC INDICATIONS

Most older antipsychotic drugs, with the exception of thioridazine, have a strong antiemetic effect. This action is due to dopamine receptor blockade, both centrally (in the chemoreceptor trigger zone of the medulla) and peripherally (on receptors in the stomach). Some drugs, such as prochlorperazine and benzquinamide, are promoted solely as antiemetics. Phenothiazines with shorter side chains have considerable H$_1$ receptor-blocking action and have been used for relief of pruritus or, in the case of promethazine, as preoperative sedatives. The butyrophenone droperidol is used in combination with an opioid, fentanyl, in neuroleptanesthesia. The use of these drugs for anesthesia is described in Chapter 25.

Drug Choice

Choice among antipsychotic drugs is based mainly on differences in pharmacologic properties and an appreciation of side effects and possible differences in efficacy. Since use of the older drugs is still widespread, especially for patients treated in the public sector, knowledge of such agents as chlorpromazine and haloperidol remains relevant. Thus, one should be familiar with one member of each of the three subfamilies of phenothiazines, a member of the thioxanthine and butyrophenone group, and all of the newer compounds—clozapine, risperidone, olanzapine, quetiapine, ziprasidone, and aripiprazole. Each may have special benefits for selected patients. A representative group of antipsychotic drugs is presented in Table 29–3.

New antipsychotic drugs have been shown in some trials to be more effective than older ones for treating negative symptoms (emotional blunting, social withdrawal, lack of motivation). The floridly psychotic form of the illness accompanied by uncontrollable behavior probably responds equally well to all potent antipsychotics but is still frequently treated with older drugs

Table 29–3. Some representative antipsychotic drugs.

Drug Class	Drug	Advantages	Disadvantages
Phenothiazines			
Aliphatic	Chlorpromazine[1] (Thorazine)	Generic, inexpensive	Many adverse effects, especially autonomic
Piperidine	Thioridazine[2] (Mellaril)	Slight extrapyramidal syndrome; generic	800 mg/d limit; no parenteral form; cardiotoxicity
Piperazine	Fluphenazine[3] (Permitil, Prolixin)	Depot form also available (enanthate, decanoate)	(?) Increased tardive dyskinesia
Thioxanthene	Thiothixene (Navane)	Parenteral form also available; (?) decreased tardive dyskinesia	Uncertain
Butyrophenone	Haloperidol (Haldol)	Parenteral form also available; generic	Severe extrapyramidal syndrome
Dibenzoxazepine	Loxapine (Loxitane)	(?) No weight gain	Uncertain
Dibenzodiazepine	Clozapine (Clozaril)	May benefit treatment-resistant patients; little extrapyramidal toxicity	May cause agranulocytosis in up to 2% of patients
Benzisoxazole	Risperidone (Risperdal)	Broad efficacy; little or no extrapyramidal system dysfunction at low doses	Extrapyramidal system dysfunction, hypotension with higher doses
Thienobenzodiazepine	Olanzapine (Zyprexa)	Effective against negative as well as positive symptoms; little or no extrapyramidal system dysfunction	Weight gain
Dibenzothiazepine	Quetiapine (Seroquel)	Similar to risperidone; perhaps less weight gain	Dose must be adjusted if there is associated hypotension; short $t_{1/2}$ and twice-daily dosing
Dihydroindolone	Ziprasidone (Geodon)	Perhaps less weight gain than clozapine, parenteral form available	QT_c prolongation
Dihydrocarbostyril	Aripiprazole (Abilify)	Lower weight gain liability, long half-life, novel mechanism potential	Uncertain, novel toxicities possible

[1]Other aliphatic phenothiazines: promazine, triflupromazine.

[2]Other piperidine phenothiazines: mesoridazine.

[3]Other piperazine phenothiazines: perphenazine, prochlorperazine, trifluoperazine.

that offer intramuscular formulations for acute and chronic treatment. Moreover, the low cost of these drugs contributes to their widespread use despite their clear disadvantages in terms of extrapyramidal side effects and hyperprolactinemia. Superiority over haloperidol in terms of overall response (positive and negative symptoms) of clozapine, olanzapine, and risperidone has been demonstrated in controlled trials. More comparative studies with aripiprazole are needed to evaluate its relative efficacy. Moreover, the superior side effect profile of the newer agents and low (to absent) risk of tardive dyskinesia suggests that these should provide the first line of treatment.

It is not necessary for practitioners to know all of the drugs intimately, but they should be familiar with the effects—including the adverse effects—of one or two drugs in each class. The best guide for selecting a drug for an individual patient is the patient's past responses to drugs. Within the older group, the trend has been away from "low-potency" agents such as chlorpromazine and thioridazine to the "high-potency" drugs such as thiothixene, haloperidol, and fluphenazine. At present, use of clozapine is limited to those patients who have failed to respond to substantial doses of conventional antipsychotic drugs or those who have disabling tardive dyskinesia. The agranulocytosis and seizures associated with this drug prevent more widespread use. Risperidone's superior side effects profile (compared with haloperidol) at dosages of 6 mg/d or less and the lower risk of tardive dyskinesia have contributed to its very widespread use. Olanzapine may have even lower risk and has also achieved widespread use. Whether any of the other recently introduced antipsychotics can substitute for clozapine remains to be established.

Dosage

The range of effective dosages among various antipsychotics is quite broad. Therapeutic margins are substantial. Assuming that dosages are appropriate, antipsychotics, with the exception of clozapine and perhaps olanzapine, are of equal efficacy in broadly selected groups of patients. However, some patients who fail to respond to one drug may respond to another, and for this reason several drugs may have to be tried to find the one most effective for an individual patient. Quite possibly, this phenomenon might be due to the differing profiles of receptor actions of the various drugs. Patients who have become refractory to two or three antipsychotics given in substantial doses now become candidates for treatment with clozapine. This drug, in dosages up to 900 mg/d, salvages about 30–50% of patients previously refractory to 60 mg/d of haloperidol. In such cases, the increased risk of clozapine can well be justified. Risperidone does not appear to substitute for

clozapine, although reports are mixed. Whether olanzapine or quetiapine will show efficacy similar to that of clozapine remains to be determined. If this is shown to be the case, and if evidence of their safety is sustained, one of these newer agents could emerge as the preferred first-line antipsychotic.

Some dosage relationships between various antipsychotic drugs, as well as possible therapeutic ranges, are shown in Table 29–4.

Plasma Concentrations & Clinical Effects

Attempts to define a therapeutic range of plasma concentrations of antipsychotic agents are beset by many difficulties. Ranges of 2–20 ng/mL have been suggested for haloperidol, though such a wide range is not very helpful clinically. Clinical monitoring of plasma concentrations of these drugs, though technically feasible, is not warranted at this time.

Parenteral Preparations

Well-tolerated parenteral forms of the high-potency older drugs are available for rapid initiation of treatment as well as for maintenance treatment in noncompliant patients. Since the parenterally administered drugs may have much greater bioavailability than the oral forms, doses should be only a fraction of what might be given orally. Fluphenazine decanoate and haloperidol decanoate are suitable for long-term parenteral maintenance therapy in patients who cannot or will not take oral medication.

Dosage Schedules

Antipsychotics may be given in divided daily doses initially while an effective dosage level is being sought. They need not always be equally divided doses, even when given orally. After an effective daily dosage has been defined for an individual patient, doses can be given less frequently. Once-daily doses, usually given at night, are feasible for many patients during chronic maintenance treatment. Simplification of dosage schedules leads to better compliance. Maximum dose sizes of many drugs are being increased by manufacturers to meet the needs of once-daily dosing.

Maintenance Treatment

A very small minority of schizophrenic patients may recover from an acute episode and require no further drug therapy for prolonged periods. In most cases the choice is between "as needed" increased doses or addition of other drugs for exacerbations versus continual maintenance treatment with full therapeutic doses. The choice will depend on social factors such as the availability of family or friends familiar with the symptoms of early relapse and ready access to care.

Table 29–4. Dose relationships of antipsychotics.

	Minimum Effective Therapeutic Dose (mg)	Usual Range of Daily Doses (mg)
Chlorpromazine (Thorazine)	100	100–1000
Thioridazine (Mellaril)	100	100–800
Mesoridazine (Lidanar, Serentil)	50	50–400
Trifluoperazine (Stelazine)	5	5–60
Perphenazine (Trilafon)	10	8–64
Fluphenazine (Permitil, Prolixin)	2	2–60
Thiothixene (Navane)	2	2–120
Haloperidol (Haldol)	2	2–60
Loxapine (Loxitane)	10	20–160
Molindone (Lidone, Moban)	10	20–200
Clozapine (Clozaril)	50	300–600
Olanzapine (Zyprexa)	5	10–30
Quetiapine (Seroquel)	150	150–800
Risperidone (Risperdal)	4	4–16
Ziprasidone (Geodon)	40	80–160
Aripiprazole (Abilify)	10	10–30

Drug Combinations

Combining antipsychotic drugs confounds evaluation of the efficacy of the drugs being used. Addition of other classes of drugs, however, is widespread, with more emerging experimental data supporting such practices. Tricyclic antidepressants or, more often, selective serotonin reuptake inhibitors may be used with antipsychotics for clear symptoms of depression complicating schizophrenia. Lithium or valproic acid is sometimes added to antipsychotic agents with benefit to patients who do not respond to the latter drugs alone. It is uncertain whether such instances represent misdiagnosed cases of mania or schizoaffective disorder. Sedative drugs may be added for relief of anxiety or insomnia not controlled by antipsychotics.

The drugs most frequently combined with antipsychotics are antiparkinsonism agents (see below).

Adverse Reactions

Most of the unwanted effects of antipsychotics are extensions of their known pharmacologic actions (Tables 29–1 and 29–2), but a few are allergic and some are idiosyncratic.

A. BEHAVIORAL EFFECTS

The older typical antipsychotic drugs are unpleasant to take. Many patients stop taking these drugs because of the adverse effects, which may be mitigated by giving small doses during the day and the major portion at bedtime. A "pseudodepression" that may be due to drug-induced akinesia usually responds to treatment with antiparkinsonism drugs. Other "pseudodepressions" may be due to using higher doses than needed in a partially remitted patient, in which case decreasing the dose may relieve the symptoms. Toxic-confusional states may occur with very high doses of drugs that have prominent antimuscarinic actions.

B. NEUROLOGIC EFFECTS

Extrapyramidal reactions occurring early during treatment with older agents include typical **Parkinson's syndrome, akathisia** (uncontrollable restlessness), and **acute dystonic reactions** (spastic retrocollis or torticollis). Parkinsonism can be treated, when necessary, with conventional antiparkinsonism drugs of the antimuscarinic type or, in rare cases, with amantadine. Parkinsonism may be self-limiting, so that an attempt to withdraw antiparkinsonism drugs should be made every 3–4 months. Akathisia and dystonic reactions will also respond to such treatment, but many prefer to use a sedative antihistamine with anticholinergic properties, eg, diphenhydramine, which can be given either parenterally or orally.

Tardive dyskinesia, as the name implies, is a late-occurring syndrome of abnormal choreoathetoid movements. It is the most important unwanted effect of antipsychotic drugs. It has been proposed that it is caused by a relative cholinergic deficiency secondary to supersensitivity of dopamine receptors in the caudate-putamen. Older women treated for long periods are most susceptible to the disorder, though it can occur at any age and in either sex. The prevalence varies enormously, but tardive dyskinesia is estimated to have occurred in 20–40% of chronically treated patients prior to the introduction of the newer atypical antipsychotics. Early recognition is important, since advanced cases may be difficult to reverse. Many treatments have been proposed, but their evaluation is confounded by the fact that the course of the disorder is variable and sometimes self-limited. Most authorities agree that the first step would be to try to discontinue or reduce the dose of the current antipsychotic or switch to one of the newer atypical agents. A logical second step would be to eliminate all drugs with central anticholinergic action, particularly antiparkinsonism drugs and tricyclic antidepressants. These two steps are often enough to bring about improvement. If they fail, the addition of diazepam in doses as high as 30–40 mg/d may add to the improvement by enhancing GABAergic activity.

Seizures, while recognized as a complication of chlorpromazine treatment, were so rare with the high-potency older drugs as to merit little consideration. However, de novo seizures may occur in 2–5% of patients treated with clozapine.

C. Autonomic Nervous System Effects

Most patients are able to tolerate the antimuscarinic adverse effects of antipsychotic drugs. Those who are made too uncomfortable or who develop urinary retention or other severe symptoms can be switched to an agent without significant antimuscarinic action. Orthostatic hypotension or impaired ejaculation—common complications of therapy with chlorpromazine or mesoridazine—should be managed by switching to drugs with less marked adrenoceptor-blocking actions.

D. Metabolic and Endocrine Effects

Weight gain is very common, especially with clozapine and olanzapine, and requires monitoring of food intake, especially carbohydrates. Hyperglycemia may develop, but whether secondary to weight gain-associated insulin resistance or due to other potential mechanisms remains to be clarified. Hyperprolactinemia in women results in the amenorrhea-galactorrhea syndrome and infertility; in men, loss of libido, impotence, and infertility may result.

E. Toxic or Allergic Reactions

Agranulocytosis, cholestatic jaundice, and skin eruptions occur rarely with the high-potency antipsychotic drugs currently used.

In contrast to other antipsychotic agents, clozapine causes agranulocytosis in a small but significant number of patients—approximately 1–2% of those treated. This serious, potentially fatal effect can develop rapidly, usually between the sixth and eighteenth weeks of therapy. It is not known whether it represents an immune reaction, but it appears to be reversible upon discontinuance of the drug. *Because of the risk of agranulocytosis, patients receiving clozapine must have weekly blood counts for the first 6 months of treatment and every 3 weeks thereafter.*

F. Ocular Complications

Deposits in the anterior portions of the eye (cornea and lens) are a common complication of chlorpromazine therapy. They may accentuate the normal processes of aging of the lens. Thioridazine is the only antipsychotic drug that causes retinal deposits, which in advanced cases may resemble retinitis pigmentosa. The deposits are usually associated with "browning" of vision. The maximum daily dose of thioridazine has been limited to 800 mg/d to reduce the possibility of this complication.

G. Cardiac Toxicity

Thioridazine in doses exceeding 300 mg daily is almost always associated with minor abnormalities of T waves that are easily reversible. Overdoses of thioridazine are associated with major ventricular arrhythmias, cardiac conduction block, and sudden death; it is not certain whether thioridazine can cause these same disorders when used in therapeutic doses. In view of possible additive antimuscarinic and quinidine-like actions with various tricyclic antidepressants, thioridazine should be combined with the latter drugs only with great care. Among the atypical agents, ziprasidone carries the greatest risk of QT prolongation and therefore should not be combined with drugs that prolong the QT interval, including thioridazine, pimozide, and quinidine.

H. Use in Pregnancy; Dysmorphogenesis

Although the antipsychotic drugs appear to be relatively safe in pregnancy, a small increase in teratogenic risk could be missed. Questions about whether to use these drugs during pregnancy and whether to abort a pregnancy in which the fetus has already been exposed must be decided individually.

I. Neuroleptic Malignant Syndrome

This life-threatening disorder occurs in patients who are extremely sensitive to the extrapyramidal effects of antipsychotics. The initial symptom is marked muscle rigidity. If sweating is impaired, as it often is during treatment with anticholinergic drugs, fever may ensue, often reaching dangerous levels. The stress leukocytosis and high fever associated with this syndrome may erroneously suggest an infectious process. Autonomic instability, with altered blood pressure and pulse rate, is often present. Creatine kinase isozymes are usually elevated, reflecting muscle damage. This syndrome is believed to result from an excessively rapid blockade of postsynaptic dopamine receptors. A severe form of extrapyramidal syndrome follows. Early in the course, vigorous treatment of the extrapyramidal syndrome with antiparkinsonism drugs is worthwhile. Muscle relaxants, particularly diazepam, are often helpful. The use of other muscle relaxants, such as dantrolene, or dopamine agonists, such as bromocriptine, has been reported to be helpful. If fever is present, cooling by physical measures should be tried. Various minor forms of this syndrome are now recognized.

Drug Interactions

Antipsychotics produce more important pharmacodynamic than pharmacokinetic interactions because of their multiple effects. Additive effects may occur when these drugs are combined with others that have sedative effects, α-adrenoceptor-blocking action, anticholinergic effects, and—for thioridazine and ziprasidone—quinidine-like action.

A variety of pharmacokinetic interactions have been reported, but none are of major clinical significance.

Overdoses

Poisonings with antipsychotics are rarely fatal, with the exception of those due to mesoridazine and thioridazine. In general, drowsiness proceeds to coma, with an intervening period of agitation. Neuromuscular excitability may be increased and proceed to convulsions. Pupils are miotic, and deep tendon reflexes are decreased. Hypotension and hypothermia are the rule, though fever may be present later in the course. The lethal effects of mesoridazine and thioridazine are related to induction of ventricular tachyarrhythmias. Patients should be monitored in an intensive care setting for the usual vital signs, venous pressure, arterial blood gases, and electrolytes. Gastric lavage should be considered even if several hours have elapsed since the drug was taken, because gastrointestinal motility is often decreased and tablets may still be present in the stomach (Chapter 59). Activated charcoal effectively binds most of these drugs, following which a saline cathartic may be given. Hypotension often responds to fluid replacement. If a pressor agent is to be used, norepinephrine or dopamine is preferred to epinephrine, whose unopposed β-adrenoceptor-stimulant action in the presence of α blockade may cause vasodilation. Seizures may be treated with either diazepam or phenytoin, the latter being given with an initial loading dose. Management of overdoses of thioridazine and mesoridazine, which are complicated by cardiac arrhythmias, is similar to that for tricyclic antidepressants (see Chapter 30).

New Approaches

The atypical antipsychotics are at least as potent in inhibiting 5-HT$_2$ receptors as they are in inhibiting D$_2$ receptors. The newest, aripiprazole, appears to be a partial agonist of D$_2$ receptors—ie, it stimulates certain D$_2$ receptors while blocking others depending on their locations in the brain and the concentration of drug. Varying degrees of antagonism of α$_1$ and α$_2$ adrenoceptors are also seen with risperidone, clozapine, olanzapine, quetiapine, and aripiprazole. The clinical relevance of these actions remains to be ascertained.

Unconventional Drugs

The efficacy of propranolol as a treatment for schizophrenia remains uncertain after 30 years of study. Patients with marked agitation, hostility, and belligerence may be controlled by the addition of propranolol to a regimen of conventional antipsychotic drugs. High-dose treatment with benzodiazepines may control disturbed behavior, just as barbiturates did 35 years ago. Levodopa, thyrotropin-releasing hormone, endorphins, and apomorphine have been ineffective. Megavitamin therapy has been discredited scientifically, but adherents still persist.

Benefits & Limitations of Drug Treatment

As noted at the beginning of this chapter, these drugs have had a major impact on psychiatric treatment. First, they have shifted the care of patients from mental institutions to the community. For many patients, this shift has provided a better life under more humane circumstances and in many cases has made possible life without frequent use of physical restraints. For others, the tragedy of an aimless existence is now being played out in the streets of our communities rather than in mental institutions.

Second, these drugs have markedly shifted psychiatric thinking to a more biologic orientation. Partly because of research stimulated by the effects of these drugs on schizophrenia, we now know much more about central nervous system physiology and pharmacology than we did before the introduction of these agents. However, despite a great amount of research, schizophrenia remains a scientific mystery and a personal disaster for the patient. While most schizophrenic patients obtain some degree of benefit from these drugs—in some cases substantial benefit—none are made well by them.

II. LITHIUM & OTHER MOOD-STABILIZING DRUGS

Lithium carbonate is often referred to as an "antimanic" drug, but in many parts of the world it is considered a "mood-stabilizing" agent because of its primary action of preventing mood swings in patients with bipolar affective (manic-depressive) disorder. Discovery of its benefits was based on an incorrect hypothesis and extremely good fortune in choosing the correct dosage. Carbamazepine has also been recognized as effective in some groups of manic-depressive patients despite not being formally approved for such use. Valproate has recently been approved for the treatment of mania and is being evaluated as a mood stabilizer. Atypical antipsychotics, beginning with olanzapine, are being investigated and approved as antimanic agents and potential mood stabilizers.

Nature of Bipolar Affective Disorder

Bipolar affective (manic-depressive) disorder is a frequently diagnosed and very serious psychiatric disorder. Patients with cyclic attacks of mania have many symptoms of paranoid schizophrenia (grandiosity, bellicosity, paranoid thoughts, and overactivity). The gratifying response to lithium therapy of patients with bipolar disorder has made such diagnostic distinctions important.

The episodes of mood swings characteristic of this condition are generally unrelated to life events. The exact biologic disturbance has not been identified, but a preponderance of catecholamine-related activity is thought to be present. Drugs that increase this activity tend to exacerbate mania, whereas those that reduce activity of dopamine or norepinephrine relieve mania. Acetylcholine or glutamate may also be involved. The nature of the abrupt switch from mania to depression experienced by some patients is uncertain. Bipolar disorder has a strong familial component. Genetic studies have identified at least three possible linkages to different chromosomes.

BASIC PHARMACOLOGY OF LITHIUM

Pharmacokinetics

Lithium is a small monovalent cation. Its pharmacokinetics are summarized in Table 29–5.

Pharmacodynamics

Despite considerable investigation, the mode of action of lithium remains unclear. The major possibilities being investigated include (1) effects on electrolytes and ion transport; (2) effects on neurotransmitters and their release; and (3) effects on second messengers and intracellular enzymes that mediate transmitter action. The last of these three approaches appears to be the most promising.

A. EFFECTS ON ELECTROLYTES AND ION TRANSPORT

Lithium is closely related to sodium in its properties. It can substitute for sodium in generating action potentials and in Na^+-Na^+ exchange across the membrane. It inhibits the latter process, ie, Li^+-Na^+ exchange is gradually slowed after lithium is introduced into the body. At therapeutic concentrations (around 1 mmol/L), it does not significantly affect the Na^+/Ca^{2+} exchange process or the Na^+/K^+ ATPase sodium pump.

B. EFFECTS ON NEUROTRANSMITTERS

Lithium appears to enhance some of the actions of serotonin, though findings have been contradictory. Its effects on norepinephrine are variable. The drug may decrease

Table 29–5. Pharmacokinetics of lithium.

Absorption	Virtually complete within 6–8 hours; peak plasma levels in 30 minutes to 2 hours
Distribution	In total body water; slow entry into intracellular compartment. Initial volume of distribution is 0.5 L/kg, rising to 0.7–0.9 L/kg; some sequestration in bone. No protein binding.
Metabolism	None
Excretion	Virtually entirely in urine. Lithium clearance about 20% of creatinine. Plasma half-life about 20 hours.
Target plasma concentration	0.6–1.4 meq/L
Dosage	0.5 meq/kg/d in divided doses

norepinephrine and dopamine turnover, and these effects, if confirmed, might be relevant to its antimanic action. Lithium also appears to block the development of dopamine receptor supersensitivity that may accompany chronic therapy with antipsychotic agents. Finally, lithium may augment the synthesis of acetylcholine, perhaps by increasing choline uptake into nerve terminals. Some clinical studies have suggested that increasing cholinergic activity may mitigate mania. However, as noted below, a second-messenger effect of lithium may obviate any effect of increased acetylcholine release.

C. EFFECTS ON SECOND MESSENGERS

One of the best-defined effects of lithium is its action on inositol phosphates. Early studies of lithium demonstrated changes in brain inositol phosphate levels, but the significance of these changes was not appreciated until the second-messenger roles of inositol-1,4,5-trisphosphate (IP_3) and diacylglycerol (DAG) were discovered. As described in Chapter 2, IP_3 and DAG are important second messengers for both α-adrenergic and muscarinic transmission. Lithium inhibits several important enzymes in the normal recycling of membrane phosphoinositides, including conversion of IP_2 to IP_1 (inositol monophosphate) and the conversion of IP to inositol (Figure 29–4). This block leads to a depletion of phosphatidylinositol-4,5-bisphosphate (PIP_2), the membrane precursor of IP_3 and DAG. Over time, the effects of transmitters on the cell will diminish in pro-portion to the amount of activity in the PIP_2-dependent pathways. Before therapy, such activity might be greatly increased in mania; thus, lithium could cause a selective depression of the overactive circuits.

Studies of noradrenergic effects in isolated brain tissue indicate that lithium can inhibit norepinephrine-sensitive adenylyl cyclase. Such an effect could relate to both its antidepressant and its antimanic effects. The relationship of these effects to lithium's actions on IP_3 mechanisms is currently unknown.

Since lithium affects second-messenger systems involving both activation of adenylyl cyclase and phosphoinositol turnover, it is not surprising that G proteins are also found to be affected. Several studies suggest that lithium may uncouple receptors from their G proteins; indeed, two of lithium's most common side effects, polyuria and subclinical hypothyroidism, may be due to uncoupling of the vasopressin and TSH receptors from their G proteins.

The major current working hypothesis for lithium's therapeutic mechanism of action supposes that its effects on phosphoinositol turnover, leading to an early relative reduction of myoinositol in human brain, are part of an initiating cascade of intracellular changes. Effects on specific isoforms of protein kinase C may be most relevant. Alterations of protein kinase C-mediated signaling alter gene expression and the production of proteins implicated in long-term neuroplastic events that could underlie long-term mood stabilization.

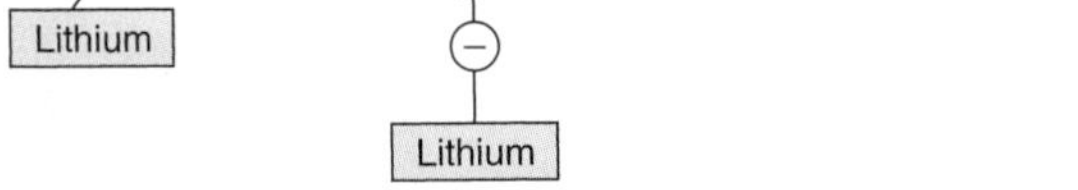

CLINICAL PHARMACOLOGY OF LITHIUM

Bipolar Affective Disorder

Until recently, lithium carbonate was the universally preferred treatment for bipolar disorder, especially in the manic phase. With the approval of valproate and olanzapine for this indication, a smaller fraction of bipolar patients now receive lithium. This trend is reinforced by the slow onset of action of lithium, which has often been supplemented with concurrent use of antipsychotic drugs or potent benzodiazepines in severely manic patients. The overall success rate for achieving remission from the manic phase of bipolar disorder has been reported to be 60–80%. However, among patients who require hospitalization, success rates are considerably lower. A similar situation applies to maintenance treatment, which is about 60% effective overall but less in severely ill patients. These considerations have led to increased use of combined treatment in severe cases. After mania is controlled, the antipsychotic drug may be stopped, then the benzodiazepine and lithium continued as maintenance therapy.

Figure 29–4. Effect of lithium on the IP_3 and DAG second-messenger system. The schematic diagram shows the synaptic membrane of a neuron. (PIP_2, phosphatidylinositol-4,5-bisphosphate; PLC, phospholipase-C; G, coupling protein; EFFECTS, activation of protein kinase C, mobilization of intracellular Ca^{2+}, etc.) Lithium, by inhibiting the recycling of inositol substrates, may cause depletion of the second-messenger source PIP_2 and therefore reduce the release of IP_3 and DAG. Lithium may also act by other mechanisms.

The depressive phase of manic-depressive disorder often requires concurrent use of an antidepressant drug (see Chapter 30). Tricyclic antidepressant agents have been linked to precipitation of mania, with more rapid cycling of mood swings, although most patients do not show this effect. Selective serotonin reuptake inhibitors are less likely to induce mania but may have limited efficacy. Bupropion has shown some promising effects but may induce mania—like tricyclic antidepressants—at higher doses. As shown in recent controlled trials, the anticonvulsant lamotrigine is effective for many patients with bipolar depression. For some patients, however, one of the older MAO inhibitors may be the antidepressant of choice.

Unlike antipsychotic or antidepressant drugs, which exert several actions on the central or autonomic nervous system, lithium ion at therapeutic concentrations is devoid of autonomic blocking effects and of activating or sedating effects, though it can produce nausea and tremor.

Another attribute of considerable interest has been the prophylactic use of lithium in preventing both mania and depression. It is indeed remarkable that a so-called functional psychosis can be controlled so easily by such a simple chemical as lithium carbonate.

Other Applications

Acute endogenous depression is not generally considered to be an indication for treatment with lithium. Alcohol and substance abuse have a high association with bipolar illness. However, recurrent endogenous depressions with a cyclic pattern are controlled by either lithium or imipramine, both of which are superior to a placebo.

Schizoaffective disorders are characterized by a mixture of schizophrenic symptoms and altered affect in the form of depression or excitement. Antipsychotic drugs alone or combined with lithium are used in the excited as well as in the maintenance phases; clozapine may be particularly effective. Various antidepressants are added if depression is present, but none has been adequately studied in this condition.

While lithium alone is rarely successful in treating schizophrenia, adding it to an antipsychotic may salvage an otherwise treatment-resistant patient. Carbamazepine may work equally well when added to an antipsychotic.

An interesting application of lithium that is relatively well supported by controlled studies is as an adjunct to tricyclic antidepressants and selective serotonin reuptake inhibitors in patients with unipolar depression who do not respond fully to monotherapy with the antidepressant. For this application, concentrations of lithium at the lower end of the recommended range for manic depressive illness appear to be adequate.

Monitoring Treatment

Clinicians have relied heavily on measurements of serum concentrations for assessing both the dosage required for satisfactory treatment of acute mania and the adequacy of maintenance treatment. These measurements are customarily taken 10–12 hours after the last dose, so all data in the literature pertaining to these concentrations reflect this interval.

An initial determination of serum lithium concentration should be obtained about 5 days after the start of treatment, at which time steady-state conditions should have been attained for the dosage chosen. If the clinical response suggests a change in dosage, simple arithmetic (new dose equals present dose times desired blood level divided by present blood level) should produce the desired level. The serum concentration attained with the adjusted dosage can be checked in another 5 days. Once the desired concentration has been achieved, levels can be measured at increasing intervals unless the schedule is influenced by intercurrent illness or the introduction of a new drug into the treatment program.

Maintenance Treatment

The decision to use lithium as *prophylactic* treatment depends on many factors: the frequency and severity of previous episodes, a crescendo pattern of appearance, and the degree to which the patient is willing to follow a program of indefinite maintenance therapy. If the present attack was the patient's first or if the patient is unreliable, one might prefer to terminate treatment after the attack has subsided. Patients who have one or more episodes of illness per year are candidates for maintenance treatment. While some patients can be maintained with serum levels as low as 0.6 meq/L, the best results in groups of patients have been obtained with higher levels, such as 0.9 meq/L.

Drug Interactions

Renal clearance of lithium is reduced about 25% by diuretics (eg, thiazides), and doses may need to be reduced by a similar amount. A similar reduction in lithium clearance has been noted with several of the newer nonsteroidal anti-inflammatory drugs that block synthesis of prostaglandins. This interaction has not been reported for either aspirin or acetaminophen. All neuroleptics tested to date, with the possible exception of clozapine and the newer antipsychotics, may produce more severe extrapyramidal syndromes when combined with lithium.

Adverse Effects & Complications

Many adverse effects associated with lithium treatment occur at varying times after treatment is started. Some are harmless, but it is important to be alert to adverse effects that may signify impending serious toxic reactions.

A. NEUROLOGIC AND PSYCHIATRIC ADVERSE EFFECTS

Tremor is one of the most frequent adverse effects of lithium treatment, occurring at therapeutic dosage levels. Propranolol and atenolol, which have been reported to be effective in essential tremor, also alleviate lithium-induced tremor. Other reported neurologic abnormalities include choreoathetosis, motor hyperactivity, ataxia, dysarthria, and aphasia. Psychiatric disturbances at toxic concentrations are generally marked by mental confusion and withdrawal or bizarre motor movements. Appearance of any new neurologic or psychiatric symptoms or signs is a clear indication for temporarily stopping treatment with lithium and close monitoring of serum levels.

B. EFFECTS ON THYROID FUNCTION

Lithium probably decreases thyroid function in most patients exposed to the drug, but the effect is reversible or nonprogressive. Few patients develop frank thyroid enlargement, and fewer still show symptoms of hypothyroidism. Although initial thyroid testing followed by regular monitoring of thyroid function has been proposed, such procedures are not cost-effective. Obtaining a serum TSH concentration every 6–12 months, however, is prudent.

C. RENAL ADVERSE EFFECTS

Polydipsia and polyuria are frequent but reversible concomitants of lithium treatment, occurring at therapeutic serum concentrations. The principal physiologic lesion involved is loss of the ability of the collecting tubule to conserve water under the influence of antidiuretic hormone, resulting in excessive free water clearance (**nephrogenic diabetes insipidus**). Lithium-induced diabetes insipidus is resistant to vasopressin but responds to amiloride.

An extensive literature has accumulated concerning other forms of renal dysfunction during long-term lithium therapy, including **chronic interstitial nephritis** and **minimal change glomerulopathy** with nephrotic syndrome. Some instances of decreased glomerular filtration rate have been encountered but no instances of marked azotemia or renal failure.

Patients receiving lithium should avoid dehydration and the associated increased concentration of lithium in urine. Periodic tests of renal concentrating ability should be performed to detect changes.

D. EDEMA

Edema is a frequent adverse effect of lithium treatment and may be related to some effect of lithium on sodium retention. Although weight gain may be expected in patients who become edematous, water retention does not account for the weight gain observed in up to 30% of patients taking lithium.

E. CARDIAC ADVERSE EFFECTS

The bradycardia-tachycardia ("sick sinus") syndrome is a definite contraindication to the use of lithium because the ion further depresses the sinus node. T wave flattening is often observed on the ECG but is of questionable significance.

F. USE DURING PREGNANCY

Renal clearance of lithium increases during pregnancy and reverts to lower levels immediately after delivery. A patient whose serum lithium concentration is in a good therapeutic range during pregnancy may develop toxic levels following delivery. Special care in monitoring lithium levels is needed at these times. Lithium is transferred to nursing infants through breast milk, in which it has a concentration about one-third to one-half that of serum. Lithium toxicity in newborns is manifested by lethargy, cyanosis, poor suck and Moro reflexes, and perhaps hepatomegaly.

The issue of dysmorphogenesis is not settled. An earlier report suggested an increase in the frequency of cardiac anomalies, especially Ebstein's anomaly, in lithium babies, but the most recent data suggest that lithium carries a relatively low risk of teratogenic effects.

G. MISCELLANEOUS ADVERSE EFFECTS

Transient acneiform eruptions have been noted early in lithium treatment. Some of them subside with temporary discontinuance of treatment and do not recur with its resumption. Folliculitis is less dramatic and probably occurs more frequently. Leukocytosis is always present during lithium treatment, probably reflecting a direct effect on leukopoiesis rather than mobilization from the marginal pool. This "adverse effect" has now become a therapeutic effect in patients with low leukocyte counts.

Overdoses

Therapeutic overdoses are more common than those due to deliberate or accidental ingestion of the drug. Therapeutic overdoses are usually due to accumulation of lithium resulting from some change in the patient's status, such as diminished serum sodium, use of diuretics, or fluctuating renal function. Since the tissues will have already equilibrated with the blood, the plasma concentrations of lithium may not be excessively high in proportion to the degree of toxicity; any value over 2 meq/L must be considered as indicating likely toxicity. As lithium is a small ion, it is dialyzed readily. Both peritoneal dialysis and hemodialysis are effective, though the latter is preferred. Dialysis should be continued until the plasma concentration falls below the usual therapeutic range.

VALPROIC ACID

Valproic acid (valproate), discussed in detail elsewhere as an antiepileptic (see Chapter 24), has been demonstrated to have antimanic effects and is now being widely used for this indication in the USA. Overall, it shows efficacy equivalent to that of lithium during the early weeks of treatment. Importantly, valproic acid has been effective in some patients who have failed to respond to lithium. Moreover, its side effect profile is such that one can rapidly increase the dose over a few days to produce blood levels in the apparent therapeutic range, with nausea being the only limiting factor in some patients. The starting dose is 750 mg/d, increasing rapidly to the 1500–2000 mg range with a recommended maximum dose of 60 mg/kg/d.

Combinations of valproic acid with other psychotropic medications likely to be used in the management of either phase of bipolar illness are generally well tolerated. Valproic acid is becoming recognized as an appropriate first-line treatment for mania, though it is not clear that it will be as effective as lithium as a maintenance treatment in all subsets of patients. Many clinicians argue for combining valproic acid and lithium in patients who do not fully respond to either agent alone.

CARBAMAZEPINE

Carbamazepine has been considered to be a reasonable alternative to lithium when the latter is less than optimally efficacious. It may be used to treat acute mania and also for prophylactic therapy. Adverse effects (discussed in Chapter 24) are generally no greater and sometimes are less than those associated with lithium. Carbamazepine may be used alone or, in refractory patients, in combination with lithium or, rarely, valproate. The mode of action of carbamazepine is unclear, but it may reduce the sensitization of the brain to repeated episodes of mood swing. Such a mechanism might be similar to its anticonvulsant effect.

The use of carbamazepine as a mood stabilizer is similar to its use as an anticonvulsant (see Chapter 24). Dosage usually begins with 200 mg twice daily, with increases as needed. Maintenance dosage is similar to that used for treating epilepsy, ie, 800–1200 mg/d. Plasma concentrations between 3 and 14 mg/L are considered desirable, though no therapeutic range has been established. Although blood dyscrasias have figured prominently in the adverse effects of carbamazepine when it is used as an anticonvulsant, they have not been a major problem with its use as a mood stabilizer. Overdoses of the drug are a major emergency and should be managed in general like overdoses of tricyclic antidepressants.

PREPARATIONS AVAILABLE

ANTIPSYCHOTIC AGENTS
Aripiprazole (Abilify)
  Oral: 10, 15, 20, 30 mg tablets
Chlorpromazine (generic, Thorazine, others)
  Oral: 10, 25, 50, 100, 200 mg tablets; 10 mg/5 mL syrup; 30, 100 mg/mL concentrate
  Oral sustained-release: 30, 75, 150 mg capsules
  Rectal: 25, 100 mg suppositories
  Parenteral: 25 mg/mL for IM injection
Clozapine (generic, Clozaril)
  Oral: 25, 100 mg tablets
Fluphenazine (generic, Permitil, Prolixin)
  Oral: 1, 2.5, 5, 10 mg tablets; 2.5 mg/5 mL elixir; 5 mg/mL concentrate
  Parenteral: 2.5 mg/mL for IM injection
Fluphenazine esters (generic [decanoate only], Prolixin Enanthate, Prolixin Decanoate)
  Parenteral: 25 mg/mL

Haloperidol (generic, Haldol)
  Oral: 0.5, 1, 2, 5, 10, 20 mg tablets; 2 mg/mL concentrate
  Parenteral: 5 mg/mL for IM injection
Haloperidol ester (Haldol Decanoate)
  Parenteral: 50, 100 mg/mL for IM injection
Loxapine (Loxitane)
  Oral: 5, 10, 25, 50 mg capsules; 25 mg/mL concentrate
  Parenteral: 50 mg/mL for IM injection
Mesoridazine (Serentil)
  Oral: 10, 25, 50, 100 mg tablets; 25 mg/mL concentrate
  Parenteral: 25 mg/mL for IM injection
Molindone (Moban)
  Oral: 5, 10, 25, 50, 100 mg tablets; 20 mg/mL concentrate
Olanzapine (Zyprexa)
  Oral: 2.5, 5, 7.5, 10, 15, 20 mg tablets; 5, 10, 15, 20 mg orally disintegrating tablets.

Perphenazine (generic, Trilafon)
Oral: 2, 4, 8, 16 mg tablets; 16 mg/5 mL concentrate
Parenteral: 5 mg/mL for IM or IV injection
Pimozide (Orap)
Oral: 1, 2 mg tablets
Prochlorperazine (generic, Compazine)
Oral: 5, 10, mg tablets; 5 mg/5 mL syrup
Oral sustained-release: 10, 15 mg capsules
Rectal: 2.5, 5, 25 mg suppositories
Parenteral: 5 mg/mL for IM injection
Promazine (generic, Sparine)
Oral: 25, 50 mg tablets
Parenteral: 25, 50 mg/mL for IM injection
Quetiapine (Seroquel)
Oral: 25, 100, 200, 300 mg tablets
Risperidone (Risperdal)
Oral: 0.25, 0.5, 1, 2, 3, 4 mg tablets; 1 mg/mL oral solution
Thioridazine (generic, Mellaril, others)
Oral: 10, 15, 25, 50, 100, 150, 200 mg tablets; 30, 100 mg/mL concentrate; 25, 100 mg/5 mL suspension
Thiothixene (generic, Navane)
Oral: 1, 2, 5, 10, 20 mg capsules; 5 mg/mL concentrate

Trifluoperazine (generic, Stelazine)
Oral: 1, 2, 5, 10 mg tablets; 10 mg/mL concentrate
Parenteral: 2 mg/mL for IM injection
Triflupromazine (Vesprin)
Parenteral: 10, 20 mg/mL for IM injection
Ziprasidone (Geodon)
Oral: 20, 40, 60, 80 mg capsules
Parenteral: 20 mg/mL for IM injection

MOOD STABILIZERS

Carbamazepine (generic, Tegretol, others)
Oral: 200 mg tablets, 100 mg chewable tablets; 100 mg/5 mL oral suspension.
Oral extended-release: 100, 200, 400 mg tablets; 200, 300 mg capsules
Divalproex (Depakote)
Oral: 125, 250, 500 mg delayed-release tablets
Lithium carbonate (generic, Eskalith) (**Note:** 300 mg lithium carbonate = 8.12 meq Li$^+$.)
Oral: 150, 300, 600 mg capsules; 300 mg tablets; 8 meq/5 mL syrup
Oral sustained-release: 300, 450 mg tablets
Valproic acid (generic, Depakene)
Oral: 250 mg capsules; 250 mg/5 mL syrup

REFERENCES

ANTIPSYCHOTICS

Beasley CM et al: Olanzapine versus placebo and haloperidol acute phase results of the North American double-blind olanzapine trial. Neuropsychopharmacology 1996;14:111.

Bilder RM et al: Neurocognitive effects of clozapine, olanzapine, risperidone, and haloperidol in patients with chronic schizophrenia or schizoaffective disorder. Am J Psychiatry 2002;159:1018.

Braver TS, Barch DM, Cohen JD: Cognition and control in schizophrenia: a computational model of dopamine and prefrontal function. Biol Psychiatry 1999;46:312.

Breier A, Berg PH: The psychosis of schizophrenia: prevalence, response to atypical antipsychotics, and prediction of outcome. Biol Psychiatry 1999;46:361.

Carlsson A, Waters N, Carlsson ML: Neurotransmitter interactions in schizophrenia—therapeutic implications. Biol Psychiatry 1999;46:1388.

Carpenter WT et al: Deficit psychopathology and a paradigm shift in schizophrenia research. Biol Psychiatry 1999;46:352.

Dickey W: The neuroleptic malignant syndrome. Prog Neurobiol 1991;36:423.

Farde L et al: Central D_2-dopamine receptor occupancy in schizophrenic patients treated with antipsychotic drugs. Arch Gen Psychiatry 1987;45:71.

Freudenreich O, Goff DC: Antipsychotic combination therapy in schizophrenia. A review of efficacy and risks of current combinations. Acta Psychiatr Scand 2002;106:323.

Friedhoff AJ et al: Report on schizophrenia of the American College of Neuropsychopharmacology. The Ad Hoc Committee on Schizophrenia: Neuropsychopharmacology 1987;1:89.

Haddad PM, Anderson IM: Antipsychotic-related QT$_c$ prolongation, torsade de pointes and sudden death. Drugs 2002;62:1649.

Harrison P, Owen M: Genes for schizophrenia? Recent findings and their pathophysiological implications. Lancet 2003;361:417.

Hashimoto F, Sherma CB, Jeffery WH: Neuroleptic malignant syndrome and dopaminergic blockade. Arch Intern Med 1984;144:629.

Hollister LE, Csernansky JG: Antipsychotic drugs. In: *Clinical Pharmacology of Psychotherapeutic Drugs*, 3rd ed. Churchill Livingstone, 1990.

Hugenholtz GW et al: Short-acting parenteral antipsychotics drive choice for classical versus atypical agents. Eur J Clin Pharmacol 2003;58:757.

Jackson DM et al: Preclinical findings with new antipsychotic agents: What makes them atypical? Acta Psychiatr Scand 1994;89(Suppl 380):41.

Jacobsen E: The early history of psychotherapeutic drugs. Psychopharmacology 1986;89:138.

Jibson MD, Tandon R: New atypical antipsychotic medications. J Psychiatr Res 1998;32:215.

Kane JM et al: Clozapine for the treatment of treatment-resistant schizophrenia: Results of a US multicenter trial. Psychopharmacology 1989;99:560.

Kane JM: Pharmacologic treatment of schizophrenia. Biol Psychiatry 1999;46:1396.

Lehmann HE, Wilson WH, Deutsch M: Minimal maintenance medication: Effects of three dose schedules on relapse rates and symptoms in chronic schizophrenic outpatients. Compr Psychiatry 1983;24:293.

Marder SR, Meibach R: Risperidone in the treatment of patients with chronic schizophrenia. Am J Psychiatry 1994;151:825.

McElroy SL et al: Clozapine in the treatment of psychotic mood disorders, schizoaffective disorders, and schizophrenia. J Clin Psychiatry 1991;52:411.

McGavin JK, Goa KL: Aripiprazole. CNS Drugs 2002;779:786.

Meltzer HY: Treatment of schizophrenia and spectrum disorders: pharmacotherapy, psychosocial treatments, and neurotransmitter interactions. Biol Psychiatry 1999;46:1321.

Seeman P: Dopamine receptors and the dopamine hypothesis of schizophrenia. Synapse 1987;1:133.

Stefansson H et al: Neuregulin 1 and susceptibility to schizophrenia. Am J Hum Genet 2002;71:877.

Tarsy D, Baldessarini RJ: The pathophysiologic basis of tardive dyskinesia. Biol Psychiatry 1977;12:431.

Tauscher J et al: Significant dissociation of brain and plasma kinetics with antipsychotics. Mol Psychiatry 2002;7:317.

MOOD STABILIZERS

Amdisen A: History of lithium. (Letter.) Biol Psychiatry 1987;22:522.

Baraban JM, Worley PF, Snyder SH: Second messenger systems and psychoactive drug action: Focus on the phosphoinositide system and lithium. Am J Psychiatry 1989;146:1251.

Bowden CL et al: Efficacy of divalproex vs lithium, placebo in the treatment of mania. JAMA 1994;271:918.

Bowden CL: Valproate in mania. In: Manji HK, Bowden CL, Belmaker RH (editors). *Bipolar Medications: Mechanisms of Action.* American Psychiatric Press, 2000.

Bunney WE Jr, Garland-Bunney BL: Mechanisms of action of lithium in affective illness: Basic and clinical implications. In:

Meltzer HY (editor). *Psychopharmacology: The Third Generation of Progress.* Raven Press, 1987.

Cowan WM et al: The human genome project and its impact on psychiatry. Annu Rev Neurosci 2002;25:1.

Goodwin FK, Ghaemi SN: Bipolar disorder: state of the art. Dialogues Clin Neurosci 1999;1:41.

Goodwin FK, Jamison KR: *Manic-Depressive Illness.* Oxford Univ Press, 1990.

Hodgkinson S: Molecular genetic evidence for heterogeneity in manic depression. Nature 1987;325:805.

Jope RS: Anti-bipolar therapy: mechanism of action of lithium. Mol Psychiatry 1999;4:117.

Kimmel SE et al: Clozapine in treatment-refractory mood disorders. (Review.) J Clin Psychiatry 1994;55:91.

Manji HK, Chen G: PKC, MAP kinases and the bcl-2 family of proteins as long-term targets for mood stabilizers. Mol Psychiatry 2002;(7 Suppl 1):S46.

Manji HK, Lenox RH: Ziskind-Somerfeld Research Award. Protein kinase C signaling in the brain: molecular transduction of mood stabilization in the treatment of manic-depressive illness. Biol Psychiatry 1999;46:1328.

Manji HK, Potter WZ, Lenox RH: Signal transduction pathways. Molecular targets for lithium's actions. Arch Gen Psychiatry 1995;52:531.

McElroy SL et al: Valproate in the treatment of bipolar disorder: Literature review and clinical guidelines. J Clin Psychopharmacol 1992;12(Suppl):42S.

Prien RF, Galenberg AJ: Alternatives to lithium for preventive treatment of bipolar disorder. Am J Psychiatry 1989;146:840.

Prien RF, Potter WZ: NIMH workshop report on the treatment of bipolar disorder. Psychopharmacol Bull 1990;26:409.

Schou M: Lithium treatment at 52. J Affect Disord 2001;67:21.

Sklar P: Linkage analysis in psychiatric disorders: the emerging picture. Ann Rev Genomics Hum Genet 2002;3:371.

Tondo L, Jamison KR, Baldessarini RJ: Effect of lithium maintenance on suicidal behavior in major mood disorders. Ann N Y Acad Sci 1997;836:339.

Zimmerman U et al: Epidemiology, implications and mechanisms underlying drug-induced weight gain in psychiatric patients. J Psychiatr Res 2003;37:193.

Antidepressant Agents

30

William Z. Potter, MD, PhD, & Leo E. Hollister, MD

Major depression is one of the most common psychiatric disorders. At any given moment, about 5–6% of the population is depressed (point prevalence), and an estimated 10% of people may become depressed during their lives (lifetime prevalence). The symptoms of depression are often subtle and unrecognized both by patients and by physicians. Patients with vague complaints that resist explanation as manifestations of somatic disorders and those who might be simplistically described as "neurotic" should be suspected of being depressed.

Depression is a heterogeneous disorder that has been characterized and classified in a variety of ways. According to the American Psychiatric Association's fourth edition (1994) of the *Diagnostic and Statistical Manual of Mental Disorders (DSM-IV)*, several diagnoses of affective disorders are possible. Major depression and dysthymia (minor) are pure depressive syndromes, whereas bipolar disorder and cyclothymic disorder signify depression in association with mania. A simplified classification based on presumed origin is as follows: (1) "reactive" or "secondary" depression (most common), occurring in response to real stimuli such as grief, illness, etc; (2) "endogenous" depression, a genetically determined biochemical disorder manifested by inability to experience ordinary pleasure or to cope with ordinary life events; and (3) depression associated with bipolar affective (manic-depressive) disorder. Drugs discussed in this chapter are used chiefly in management of the second type. Table 30–1 indicates how the three types may be differentiated.

An intensive effort to formalize guidelines for the treatment of depression is provided by the cross-disciplinary publication of the Depression Guideline Panel (1993) and its update on newer pharmacotherapies (Mulrow et al, 1999). Pharmacologic treatment is emphasized, though a continuing role for electroconvulsive therapy for delusional or severe forms of life-threatening depression is noted. Despite intensive research, the mechanisms of action of various pharmacologic treatments are still not understood, though most are believed to involve effects on two monoamine neurotransmitters: serotonin and norepinephrine.

The Pathogenesis of Major Depression: The Amine Hypothesis

Soon after the introduction of reserpine in the early 1950s, it became apparent that the drug could induce depression in patients being treated for hypertension and schizophrenia as well as in normal subjects. Within the next few years, pharmacologic studies revealed that the principal mechanism of action of reserpine was to inhibit the storage of amine neurotransmitters such as serotonin and norepinephrine in the vesicles of presynaptic nerve endings. Reserpine induced depression and depleted stores of amine neurotransmitters; therefore, it was reasoned, depression must be associated with decreased functional amine-dependent synaptic transmission. This idea provided the basis for what became known as the amine hypothesis of depression. A major puzzle in applying this hypothesis was the fact that although the pharmacologic actions of both tricyclic and MAO inhibitor classes of antidepressants are prompt, the clinical effects require weeks to become manifest. Attempts have been made to explain this observation by invoking slow compensatory responses to the initial blockade of amine reuptake or MAO inhibition (see below).

While the amine hypothesis is undoubtedly too simplistic, it has provided the major experimental models for the discovery of new antidepressant drugs. As a result, all the currently available antidepressant drugs—except bupropion—are classified as having their primary actions on the metabolism, reuptake, or selective receptor antagonism of serotonin, norepinephrine, or both.

I. BASIC PHARMACOLOGY OF ANTIDEPRESSANTS

Chemistry

A variety of different chemical structures have been found to have antidepressant activity. With the possible exception of bupropion, however, the core antidepres-

Table 30–1. Differentiation of types of depression.

Type	Diagnostic Features	Comments
Reactive	Loss (adverse life events). Physical illness (myocardial infarct, cancer). Drugs (anti-hypertensives, alcohol, hormones). Other psychiatric disorders (senility).	More than 60% of all depressions. Core depressive syndrome: depression, anxiety, bodily complaints, tension, guilt. May respond spontaneously or to a variety of ministrations.
Major depressive (endogenous)	Precipitating life event not adequate for degree of depression. Autonomous (unresponsive to changes in life). May occur at any age (childhood to old age). Biologically determined (family history).	About 25% of all depressions. Core depressive syndrome plus "vital" signs: abnormal rhythms of sleep, motor activity, libido, appetite. Usually responds specifically to antidepressants or electroconvulsive therapy. Tends to recur throughout life.
Bipolar affective (manic-depressive)	Characterized by episodes of mania. Cyclic; mania alone, rare; depression alone, occasional; mania-depression, usual.	About 10–15% of all depressions. May be misdiagnosed as endogenous if hypomanic episodes are missed. Lithium carbonate stabilizes mood. Mania may require antipsychotic drugs as well; depression managed with antidepressants.

sant action of even the newest agents derives from mechanisms engaged by antidepressants introduced 4 decades ago.

A. TRICYCLIC ANTIDEPRESSANTS (TCAs) (FIGURE 30–1)

Tricyclic antidepressants—so called because of the characteristic three-ring nucleus—have been used clinically for four decades. They closely resemble the phenothiazines chemically and, to a lesser extent, pharmacologically. Like the latter drugs, they were first thought to be useful as antihistamines with sedative properties and later as antipsychotics. The discovery of their antidepressant properties was a fortuitous clinical observation. **Imipramine** and **amitriptyline** are the prototypical drugs of the class as mixed norepinephrine and serotonin uptake inhibitors though they also have several other properties.

B. HETEROCYCLICS; SECOND- AND THIRD-GENERATION DRUGS

Between 1980 and 1996, a number of heterocyclic agents denoted as second-generation and third-generation or heterocyclic antidepressants were introduced. Four of the agents classified as "second-generation" are available for clinical use in the USA and are shown in Figure 30–2. **Amoxapine** and **maprotiline** resemble the structure of the tricyclic agents, while **trazodone** and **bupropion** are distinctive. The heterocyclic agents are not notably different from the older agents in potency. Since 1990, **venlafaxine,** a chemically unique third-generation agent; **mirtazapine,** an analog of a widely used European antidepressant; and **nefazodone,** developed on the basis of trazodone, have been introduced. The

structures of these compounds are shown in Figure 30–3.

C. SELECTIVE SEROTONIN REUPTAKE INHIBITORS (SSRIs)

Among the major drawbacks of most first-generation antidepressants have been their many "irrelevant" pharmacologic actions, a trait inherited from the phenothiazine antipsychotic agents. As far as has been determined, the antimuscarinic, antihistaminic, and α adrenoceptor-blocking actions of tricyclic antidepressants contribute only to the toxicity of these agents. Since the introduction of **fluoxetine**—an effective and more selective antidepressant with minimal autonomic toxicity—four more selective serotonin reuptake inhibitors have been introduced as well as the active enantiomeric form of one, *(S)*-citalopram. All are structurally distinct from the tricyclic molecules (Figure 30–4).

D. MONOAMINE OXIDASE (MAO) INHIBITORS

MAO inhibitors may be classified as hydrazides, exemplified by the C–N–N moiety, as is the case with **phenelzine** and **isocarboxazid** (no longer marketed); or nonhydrazides, which lack such a moiety, as with **tranylcypromine** (Figure 30–5). Tranylcypromine closely resembles dextroamphetamine, which is itself a weak inhibitor of MAO. Tranylcypromine retains some of the sympathomimetic characteristics of the amphetamines. The hydrazides appear to combine irreversibly with the enzyme, while tranylcypromine has a prolonged duration of effect even though it is not bound irreversibly. These older MAO inhibitors are nonselective inhibitors of both MAO-A and MAO-B.

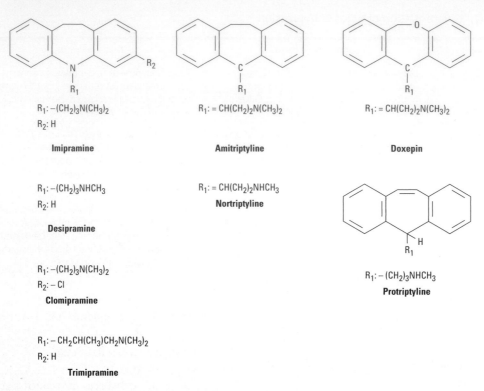

R₁: –(CH₂)₃N(CH₃)₂
R₂: H

Imipramine

R₁: = CH(CH₂)₂N(CH₃)₂

Amitriptyline

R₁: = CH(CH₂)₂N(CH₃)₂

Doxepin

R₁: –(CH₂)₃NHCH₃
R₂: H

Desipramine

R₁: = CH(CH₂)₂NHCH₃

Nortriptyline

R₁: –(CH₂)₃N(CH₃)₂
R₂: – Cl

Clomipramine

R₁: – (CH₂)₃NHCH₃

Protriptyline

R₁: – CH₂CH(CH₃)CH₂N(CH₃)₂
R₂: H

Trimipramine

Figure 30–1. Structural relationships between various tricyclic antidepressants (TCAs).

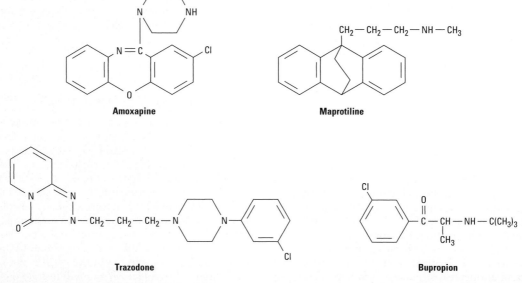

Amoxapine

Maprotiline

Trazodone

Bupropion

Figure 30–2. Second-generation antidepressants.

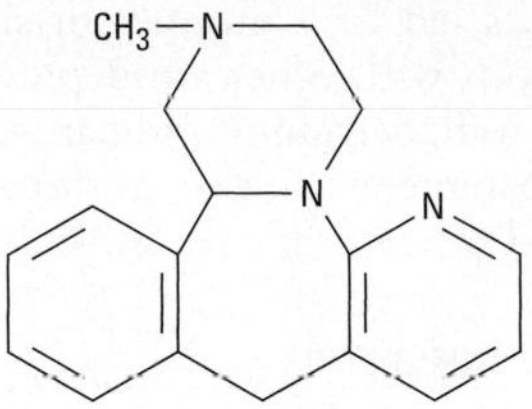

Mirtazapine

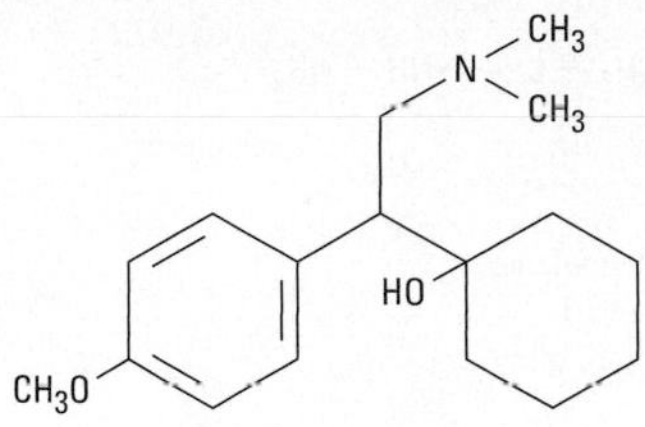

Venlafaxine

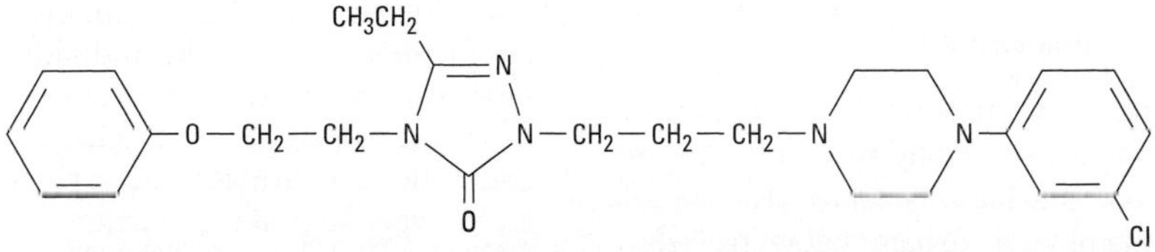

Nefazodone

Figure 30–3. Third-generation antidepressants.

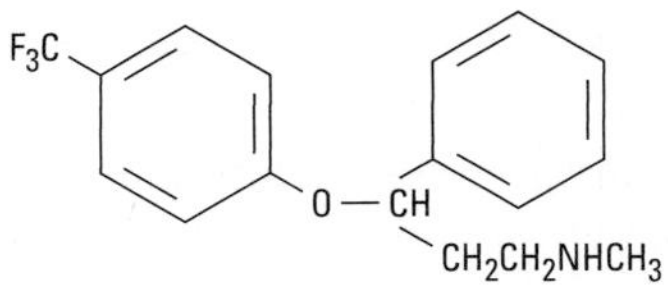

Fluoxetine

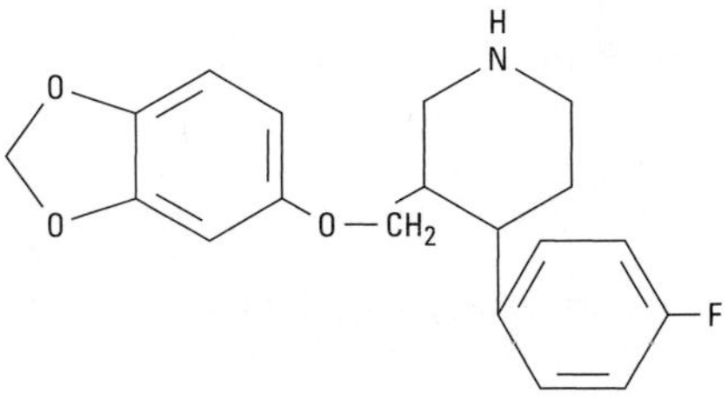

Paroxetine

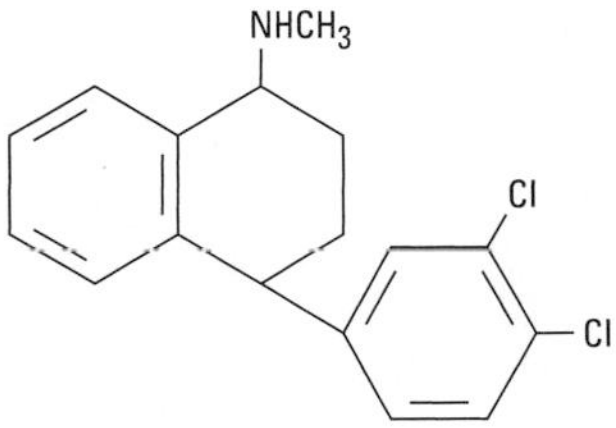

Sertraline

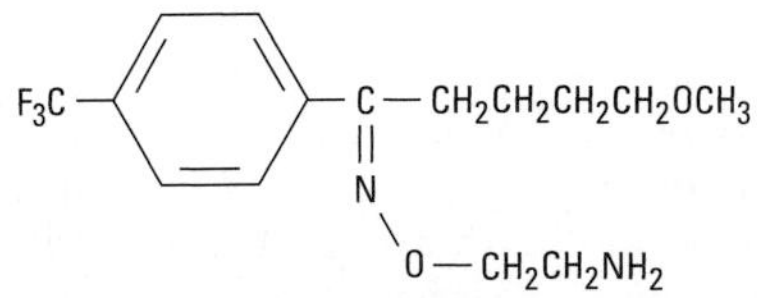

Fluvoxamine

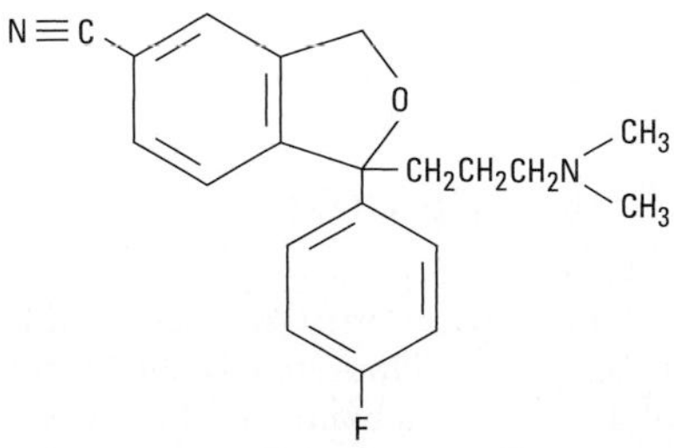

Citalopram

Figure 30–4. Selective serotonin reuptake inhibitors (SSRIs).

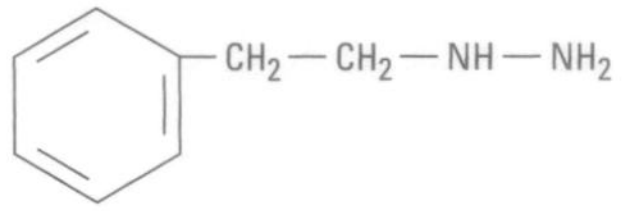

Figure 30–5. Some monoamine oxidase inhibitors. Phenelzine is the hydrazide of phenylethylamine (Figure 9–3), while tranylcypromine has a cyclopropyl amine side chain and closely resembles dextroamphetamine (see Figure 9–4). These agents are unselective and produce an extremely long-lasting inhibition of the enzyme.

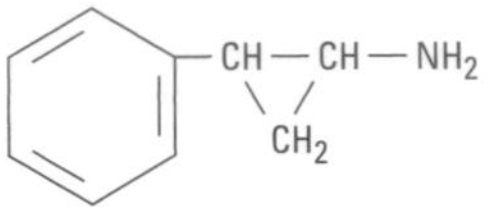

Pharmacokinetics

A. TRICYCLICS

Most tricyclics are incompletely absorbed and undergo significant first-pass metabolism. As a result of high protein binding and relatively high lipid solubility, volumes of distribution tend to be very large. Tricyclics are metabolized by two major routes: transformation of the tricyclic nucleus and alteration of the aliphatic side chain. Monodemethylation of tertiary amines leads to active metabolites such as desipramine and nortriptyline (which are themselves available as drugs; Figure 30–1). The pharmacokinetic parameters of various antidepressants are summarized in Table 30–2.

B. HETEROCYCLICS

The pharmacokinetics of these drugs are similar to those of the tricyclics (Table 30–2). Some may have active metabolites. Trazodone and venlafaxine have short plasma half-lives, which mandates divided doses during the day when beginning treatment, though once-a-day dosing may be possible later. Extended-release forms of bupropion and venlafaxine allow for once-a-day dosing in some patients from the outset.

C. SELECTIVE SEROTONIN REUPTAKE INHIBITORS (SSRIs)

The pharmacokinetic parameters of these drugs are summarized in Table 30–2. Fluoxetine is notable for the long half-life of its active metabolite, norfluoxetine (7–9 days at steady state). This long $t_{1/2}$ has allowed for the introduction of a formulation for once-weekly dosing. Fluoxetine inhibits various drug-metabolizing enzymes,

which has led to a number of significant drug-drug interactions with other antidepressants and with other drugs as well. Sertraline and paroxetine have pharmacokinetic parameters similar to those of tricyclics. Citalopram and fluvoxamine resemble fluoxetine.

D. MAO INHIBITORS

The monoamine oxidase inhibitors (MAOIs) are readily absorbed from the gastrointestinal tract. The hydrazide inhibitor phenelzine is acetylated in the liver and manifests differences in elimination depending on the acetylation phenotype of the individual (see Chapter 4). However, inhibition of MAO persists even after these drugs are no longer detectable in plasma. Therefore, conventional pharmacokinetic parameters (half-life, etc) are not very helpful in governing dosage. It is prudent to assume that the drug effect will persist for from 7 days (tranylcypromine) to 2 or 3 weeks (phenelzine) after discontinuance of the drug.

Pharmacodynamics

A. ACTION OF ANTIDEPRESSANTS ON BIOGENIC AMINE NEUROTRANSMITTERS

The amine hypothesis was buttressed by studies on the mechanism of action of various types of antidepressant drugs (Figure 30–6). Tricyclics block the amine (norepinephrine or serotonin) reuptake pumps, which terminate amine neurotransmission (see Table 30–3 and Chapter 6). Such an action presumably permits a longer sojourn of neurotransmitter at the receptor site. MAO inhibitors block a major degradative pathway for the amine neurotransmitters, which permits more amines to accumulate in presynaptic stores and more to be released. Some of the second-generation antidepressants have similar effects on amine neurotransmitters, while others have mild or minimal effects on reuptake or metabolism. In contrast, trazodone, nefazodone, and mirtazapine stand out as agents in which antagonism of subtypes of serotonin receptors (5-HT$_{2A}$ or 5-HT$_{2C}$) may be important in their action. Mirtazapine is unique in including antagonism of α_2 norepinephrine receptors as presumably contributing to its therapeutic effects. Bupropion has been found to alter the output of norepinephrine in humans following chronic administration through some as yet unidentified primary mechanism as well as occupying about 25% of dopamine uptake pumps in the brain as revealed by positron emission tomography. Since it has been shown that effective doses of SSRIs occupy 80% of serotonin uptake sites, the clinical relevance of 25% dopamine uptake occupancy is uncertain. Thus, even the newest antidepressants can still be categorized as working through serotonergic and noradrenergic effects with the possibility of a role for

Table 30–2. Pharmacokinetic parameters of various antidepressants.[1,2]

Drug	Bioavailability (percent)	Protein Binding (percent)	Plasma $t_{1/2}$ (hours)	Active Metabolites	Volume of Distribution (L/kg)	Therapeutic Plasma Concentrations (ng/mL)
Amitriptyline	31–61	82–96	31–46	Nortriptyline	5–10	80–200 total
Amoxapine	nd	nd	8	7-,8-Hydroxy	nd	nd
Bupropion	60–80	85	14–37	Hydroxy, threohydro, erythreohydro	20–30	25–100
Citalopram	51–93	70–80	23–75	Desmethyl	12–16	nd
Clomipramine	nd	nd	22–84	Desmethyl	7–20	240–700
Desipramine	60–70	73–90	14–62	Hydroxy	22–59	> 125
Doxepin	13–45	nd	8–24	Desmethyl	9–33	30–150
Escitalopram	80	56	27–59	5-Desmethyl	12	nd
Fluoxetine	70	94	24–96	Norfluoxetine	12–97	nd
Fluvoxamine	> 90	77	7–63	None	> 5	nd
Imipramine	29–77	76–95	9–24	Desipramine	15–30	> 180 total
Maprotiline	66–75	88	21–52	Desmethyl	15–28	200–300
Mirtazapine	nd	nd	20–40	Desmethyl	nd	nd
Nefazodone	15–23	98	2–4	Hydroxy, *m*-chlorophenyl piperazine	nd	nd
Nortriptyline	32–79	93–95	18–93	10-Hydroxy	21–57	50–150
Paroxetine	50	95	24	None	28–31	nd
Protriptyline	77–93	90–95	54–198	nd	19–57	70–170
Sertraline	nd	98	22–35	Desmethyl	20	nd
Trazodone	nd	nd	4–9	*m*-Chloro-phenyl-piperazine	nd	nd
Venlafaxine	nd	27–30	4–10	*O*-Desmethyl	nd	nd

[1]Range includes active metabolites.
[2]nd = no data found.

dopamine. A potential dopaminergic mechanism has often been invoked as relevant to the efficacy of MAOIs.

B. RECEPTOR AND POSTRECEPTOR EFFECTS

Considerable attention has been paid to the ultimate postsynaptic effects of increased neurotransmitters in the synapses. In tests of postsynaptic effects, cAMP concentrations have consistently *decreased* rather than increased, in spite of the presumably longer duration of action of the transmitters. In addition, the number of postsynaptic β-adrenoceptors has shown a measurable decrease that follows the same delayed time course as clinical improvement in patients. Thus, the initial increase in neurotransmitter seen with some antidepressants appears to produce, over time, a compensatory decrease in receptor activity, ie, down-regulation of receptors. Decreases in

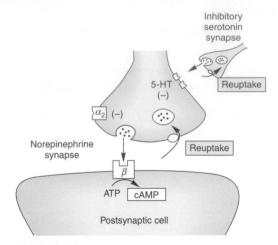

Figure 30–6. Schematic diagram showing some of the potential sites of action of antidepressant drugs. Chronic therapy with these drugs has been proved to reduce reuptake of norepinephrine or serotonin (or both), reduce the number of postsynaptic β receptors, and reduce the generation of cAMP. The MAO inhibitors act on MAO in the nerve terminals and cause the same effects on β receptors and cAMP generation.

norepinephrine-stimulated cAMP and in β-adrenoceptor binding have been conclusively shown for selective norepinephrine uptake inhibitors, those with mixed action on norepinephrine and serotonin, monoamine oxidase inhibitors, and even electroconvulsive therapy. Such changes do not consistently occur after the selective serotonin uptake inhibitors, α_2 receptor antagonists, and mixed serotonin antagonists.

It has also been emphasized that enhanced serotonergic transmission, albeit mediated through diverse mechanisms, might be a common (but not universal) long-term effect of antidepressants. This could occur, for instance, without increasing the concentration of neurotransmitter at the receptor site if there were an increase in serotonin receptor sensitivity. Thus, chronic treatment with tricyclic agents or electroconvulsive shock increases the electrophysiologic response to microiontophoretically applied serotonin in various areas of the rat brain. And selective receptor antagonism of either norepinephrine or serotonin receptors may lead to enhanced extracellular serotonin due to the complex manner in which these neurotransmitters are interregulated. One current hypothesis holds that enhanced stimulation or responsiveness of postsynaptic 5-HT$_{1A}$ receptors is particularly important in the action of antidepressants.

Most recently, long-term intracellular changes involving phosphorylation of various regulatory ele-

ments, including those within the nucleus, have been implicated as relevant to antidepressant action. It is possible that effects on certain neurotrophic factors—factors critical to sustained survival and function of neurons in the adult nervous system—may be central to the actions of antidepressants.

No clinical studies have directly tested the relevance of these findings from animals for norepinephrine and serotonin function in humans and their relationship to the mode of action of antidepressants. One of the most interesting approaches has been to reduce the amino acid precursor of serotonin, tryptophan, in the diet and, by implication, the amount of available neurotransmitter in the brain, since tryptophan availability can be rate-limiting in the formation of serotonin under certain experimental conditions. Using this approach, it was found that a tryptophan-depleted diet produces low plasma tryptophan and acutely reverses antidepressant responses to SSRIs but not to selective or mixed norepinephrine uptake inhibitors. Similarly, depletion of the norepinephrine amino acid precursor tyrosine can reverse antidepressant effects of the relatively selective norepinephrine reuptake inhibitor, desipramine. These findings indirectly support the hypothesis that enhanced serotonin throughput is necessary for the antidepressant action of serotonin but not norepinephrine uptake inhibitors. The same appears to be true of norepinephrine throughput and norepinephrine reuptake inhibitors. However, tryptophan depletion does not consistently worsen the condition of unmedicated depressed patients. Thus, there is no clear relationship between serotonin and depression or antidepressant mechanisms in general.

C. EFFECTS OF SPECIFIC ANTIDEPRESSANTS

1. Tricyclics—The first-generation antidepressants demonstrate varying degrees of selectivity for the reuptake pumps for norepinephrine and serotonin (Table 30–3). They also have numerous autonomic actions, as described below under Adverse Effects.

2. Second-generation agents—Amoxapine is a metabolite of the antipsychotic drug loxapine and retains some of its antipsychotic action and dopamine receptor antagonism. A combination of antidepressant and antipsychotic actions might make it a suitable drug for depression in psychotic patients. However, the dopamine antagonism may cause akathisia, parkinsonism, amenorrhea-galactorrhea syndrome, and perhaps tardive dyskinesia.

Maprotiline (a tetracyclic drug) is most like desipramine in terms of its potent norepinephrine uptake inhibition. Like the latter drug, it has fewer sedative and antimuscarinic actions than the older tricyclics.

Clinical experience with trazodone has indicated

Table 30–3. Pharmacologic differences among several antidepressants.[1]

Drug	Sedative Action	Antimus-carinic Action	Block of Amine Pump for:		
			Serotonin	Norepinephrine	Dopamine
Amitriptyline	+++	+++	+++	++	0
Amoxapine	++	++	+	++	+
Bupropion	0	0	+,0	+,0	+
Citalopram, escitalopram	0	0	+++	0	0
Clomipramine	+++	++	+++	+++	0
Desipramine	+	+	0	+++	0
Doxepin	+++	+++	++	+	0
Fluoxetine	+	+	+++	0,+	0,+
Fluvoxamine	0	0	+++	0	0
Imipramine	++	++	+++	++	0
Maprotiline	++	++	0	+++	0
Mirtazapine[2]	+++	0	0	0	0
Nefazodone	++	+++	+,0	0	0
Nortriptyline	++	++	+++	++	0
Paroxetine	+	0	+++	0	0
Protriptyline	0	++	?	+++	?
Sertraline	+	0	+++	0	0
Trazodone	+++	0	++	0	0
Venlafaxine	0	0	+++	++	0,+

[1]0 = none; + = slight; ++ = moderate; +++ = high; ? = uncertain.
[2]Significant α_2-adrenoceptor antagonism.

unpredictable efficacy for depression though it has proved very useful as a hypnotic, sometimes being combined with MAOIs, which disturb sleep.

3. Third-generation agents—Three antidepressants—nefazodone, venlafaxine, and mirtazapine—are all related to earlier agents in either structure or mechanism of action. Nefazodone is closely related to trazodone but is less sedating. It produces fewer adverse sexual effects than the SSRIs but is a potent inhibitor of CYP3A4. (Fluvoxamine causes the same inhibition of CYP3A4.)

Venlafaxine is a potent inhibitor of serotonin reuptake and a weaker inhibitor of norepinephrine transport such that at lower therapeutic doses it behaves like an SSRI. At high doses (more than 225 mg/d) it produces mild to moderate increases of heart rate and blood pressure attributable to norepinephrine reuptake inhibition. Doses in the range of 300 mg/d or greater may confer broader therapeutic effects than SSRIs, but a careful titration up to these doses is needed to control adverse effects.

Mirtazapine, a drug derived from mianserin—an antidepressant available outside the USA—is a potent antihistaminic with greater sedating effects than the other second- and third-generation antidepressants. Its use is also more likely to be associated with weight gain. The hypothesized mechanism of action of mirtazapine combines 5-HT$_2$ receptor and α-adrenoceptor antagonism and, if established in humans, would be unique among available drugs. Thus, mirtazapine may prove beneficial in patients who can tolerate its sedative effects and do not respond well to SSRIs or cannot tolerate the sexual or other adverse effects of the other antidepressants.

4. Selective serotonin reuptake inhibitors—Fluoxetine was the first SSRI to reach general clinical use. Paroxetine and sertraline differ mainly in having shorter half-lives and different potencies as inhibitors of specific P450 isoenzymes. While the SSRIs have not been shown to be more effective overall than prior drugs, they lack many of the toxicities of the tricyclic and heterocyclic antidepressants. Thus, patient acceptance has been high despite adverse effects such as nausea, decreased libido, and even decreased sexual function.

A dangerous pharmacodynamic interaction may occur when fluoxetine or one of the newer selective serotonin reuptake inhibitors is used in the presence of a monoamine oxidase inhibitor. The combination of increased stores of the monoamine plus inhibition of reuptake after release is thought to result in marked increases of serotonin in the synapses, leading to a **serotonin syndrome.** This sometimes fatal syndrome includes hyperthermia, muscle rigidity, myoclonus, and rapid changes in mental status and vital signs.

5. MAO inhibitors—MAO-A (isoform A) is the amine oxidase primarily responsible for norepinephrine, serotonin, and tyramine metabolism. MAO-B is more selective for dopamine. The irreversible inhibitors available in the USA are nonselective and block both forms of the enzyme. Irreversible block of MAO, characteristic of the older MAO inhibitors, allows significant accumulation of tyramine and loss of the first-pass metabolism that protects against tyramine in foods. As a result, the irreversible MAO inhibitors are subject to a very high risk of hypertensive reactions to tyramine ingested in food. From the evidence available to date, the reversible, short-acting MAO inhibitor moclobemide, which is available in several countries (but not the USA), appears to be relatively free of this interaction. (The selective MAO-B inhibitor selegiline loses selectivity at antidepressant dosage. Because its action is on the enzyme that metabolizes dopamine, it is most useful in the treatment of Parkinson's disease [Chapter 28].)

II. CLINICAL PHARMACOLOGY OF ANTIDEPRESSANTS

Clinical Indications

The major indication for these drugs is to treat depression, but a number of other uses have been established by clinical experience and controlled trials.

A. DEPRESSION

This indication has been kept broad deliberately, even though evidence from clinical studies strongly suggests that the drugs are specifically useful only in major depressive episodes. Major depressive episodes are diagnosed not so much by their severity as by their quality. Formerly, they were referred to as "endogenous," "vital," or "vegetative"—reflecting the characteristic disturbances of major body rhythms of sleep, hunger and appetite, sexual drive, and motor activity. The diagnosis of major depression may be uncertain in individual patients, so that on balance this condition is underdiagnosed and undertreated. The depressed phase of bipolar illness definitely requires pharmacologic treatment given the high rate of suicide in persons with this disorder. Standard antidepressants are usually added to lithium or another antimanic agent; SSRIs are less likely to induce mania than the older tricyclic agents. There are, however, few controlled studies on their relative efficacy or proper duration of use. Recent controlled studies provide evidence that the anticonvulsant lamotrigine may have special promise in bipolar depression.

B. PANIC DISORDER

Imipramine was first shown in 1962 to have a beneficial effect in the acute episodes of anxiety that have come to be known as panic attacks. Recent studies have shown it to be as effective as MAO inhibitors and benzodiazepines. It has also been demonstrated that SSRIs are effective in panic disorder. In some instances, benzodiazepines are preferred, as they are well tolerated and their clinical effects become evident promptly. Alternatively, if one wishes to avoid the physiologic dependence associated with chronic benzodiazepine use, SSRIs are acceptable for many patients though they require several weeks to produce full therapeutic effects.

C. OBSESSIVE-COMPULSIVE DISORDERS

The serotonin reuptake inhibitors have been shown to be uniquely effective for treating these disorders. Recent studies have focused on fluoxetine and other selective serotonin reuptake-inhibiting drugs, although clomipramine, a mixed serotonin and norepinephrine uptake inhibitor, may be more potent. Fluvoxamine is marketed exclusively for this disorder in the United States.

D. ENURESIS

Enuresis is an established indication for tricyclics. Proof of efficacy for this indication is substantial, but drug therapy is not the preferred approach. The beneficial effect of drug treatment lasts only as long as drug treatment is continued. Institutionalized elderly patients with incontinence are often treated with imipramine. Unfortunately, this age group is also the most sensitive to the anticholinergic hallucinogenic effects of the drug.

E. CHRONIC PAIN

Clinicians in pain clinics have found tricyclics to be especially useful for treating a variety of chronically painful states that often cannot be definitively diagnosed. Whether such painful states represent depressive equivalents or whether such patients become secondarily depressed after some initial pain-producing insult is not clear. It is even possible that the tricyclics work directly on pain pathways.

Controlled studies of higher doses of venlafaxine, which inhibit both norepinephrine and serotonin uptake, show efficacy in pain. **Duloxetine**, a mixed uptake inhibitor soon to be marketed, has similar effects. SSRIs, however, are not effective for chronic pain.

F. OTHER INDICATIONS

Certain antidepressants have been shown to be effective for eating disorders, especially bulimia (fluoxetine), and attention deficit hyperkinetic disorder (imipramine, desipramine). **Atomoxetine** was recently introduced for the treatment of attention deficit hyperactivity disorder (ADHD). This selective inhibitor of norepinephrine reuptake was shown to be as effective as a standard drug in this condition (methylphenidate; see Chapter 9) and possibly better tolerated. This drug should not be used concurrently with MAO inhibitors.

SSRIs show efficacy in social phobia, and combined serotonin and norepinephrine uptake inhibitors are effective in generalized anxiety disorder.

Drug Choice

Controlled comparisons of the available antidepressants have usually led to the conclusion that they are roughly equivalent drugs. Although this may be true for groups of patients, individual patients may for uncertain reasons fare better on one drug than on another. European studies show that patients depressed enough to be hospitalized respond better to classic tricyclics than to monotherapy with SSRIs. Meta-analyses of outpatient studies also show greater efficacy of tricyclics than SSRIs in patients who complete trials. The greater tolerability of the SSRIs, however, makes them the preferred agent for most patients. At high doses (> 225 mg), venlafaxine also shows greater efficacy than the SSRIs. Thus, finding the right drug and the right dose for the individual patient must be accomplished empirically. The past history of the patient's drug experience is the most valuable guide. At times such a history may lead to the exclusion of tricyclics, as in the case of patients who have responded well in the past to MAO inhibitors.

Tricyclics and the second- and third-generation agents differ mainly in the degree of sedation they produce (greatest with amitriptyline, doxepin, trazodone, and mirtazapine) and their antimuscarinic effects (greatest with amitriptyline and doxepin; Table 30–3). SSRIs are generally free of sedative effects and remarkably safe in overdose. Combined with the ease of once-a-day dosing, these qualities may explain why they have become the most widely prescribed antidepressants.

None of the newer antidepressants have been shown to be more effective overall than the tricyclics with which they have been compared. Solid evidence to support a claim of more rapid onset of action has been difficult to obtain. Amoxapine and maprotiline seem to have as many sedative and autonomic actions as most tricyclics; more recently introduced antidepressants such as bupropion and venlafaxine have fewer, although nefazodone and mirtazapine are very sedating. Amoxapine and maprotiline are at least as dangerous as the tricyclics when taken in overdoses; the other newer agents seem to be safer.

No special indications for particular types of depression have been found for the selective serotonin reuptake inhibitors or other newer antidepressants. The popularity of these drugs, despite their higher cost, is due principally to their greater acceptance by patients. A provocative clinical report that fluoxetine use increased suicidal or aggressive ideation was not supported by subsequent analyses of massive data bases. Suicidal thoughts are part of the depressive syndrome.

Clinical reports, prescription databases, and a few trials support the use of selective serotonin reuptake inhibitors in combination with the older tricyclics, especially desipramine; with bupropion; and, most recently, with mirtazapine in patients who do not show an adequate response to a single agent.

MAO inhibitors are helpful in patients described as having "atypical" depressions—usually patients with considerable attendant anxiety, phobic features, and hypochondriasis.

Few clinicians use lithium, an antimanic agent, as primary treatment for depression. However, some have found that lithium along with one of the other antidepressants may achieve a favorable response not obtained by the antidepressant alone. Another potential use of lithium is to prevent relapses of depression.

Dosages

The usual daily dose ranges of antidepressants are shown in Table 30–4. Doses are almost always determined empirically; the patient's acceptance of adverse effects is the usual limiting factor. Tolerance to some of the objectionable effects may develop, so that the usual pattern of treatment has been to start with small doses, increasing either to a predetermined daily dose, or to one that produces relief of depression, or to the maximum tolerated dose (except in the case of nortriptyline, which loses efficacy at plasma concentrations over 150 ng/mL).

Table 30–4. Usual daily doses of antidepressant drugs.

Drug	Dose (mg)
Tricyclics	
Amitriptyline	75–200
Clomipramine	75–300
Desipramine	75–200
Doxepin	75–300
Imipramine	75–200
Nortriptyline	75–150
Protriptyline	20–40
Trimipramine	75–200
Second- and third-generation agents	
Amoxapine	150–300
Bupropion	200–400
Maprotiline	75–300
Mirtazapine	15–60
Nefazodone	200–600
Trazodone	50–600
Venlafaxine	75–225
Monoamine oxidase inhibitors	
Phenelzine	45–75
Tranylcypromine	30–60
Selective serotonin reuptake inhibitors	
Citalopram	20–60
Escitalopram	10–30
Fluoxetine	10–60
Fluvoxamine	100–300
Paroxetine	20–50
Sertraline	50–200

MAO inhibitors, bupropion, fluoxetine, sertraline, paroxetine, citalopram, and venlafaxine are customarily given early in the day when initiating treatment, as they can be somewhat stimulating and may cause insomnia if given late. After a few weeks on the drug, however, any such effects should disappear and time of day administered is rarely important. Virtually all the other antidepressants have varying degrees of sedative effects and are best given near bedtime. Autonomic adverse effects also tend to be less troublesome if the dose is given late.

Maintenance Treatment

Whether or not to undertake long-term maintenance treatment of a depressed patient depends entirely on the natural history of the disorder. If the depressive episode was the patient's first and if it responded quickly and satisfactorily to drug therapy, it is rational to gradually withdraw treatment over a period of a few weeks after treating for 6–9 months. If relapse does not occur, drug treatment can be stopped until another episode occurs, which is unpredictable but highly probable. Pooled data from randomized trials covering 6–36 months reveal more than 50% reduction in relapses or recurrences if patients are maintained on an antidepressant. Thus, a patient who has had previous episodes of depression—especially if each succeeding one was more severe and more difficult to treat—is a candidate for maintenance therapy. Maintenance therapy requires the full dosage used to obtain the initial response. The duration of treatment varies, though many patients require maintenance treatment indefinitely.

Monitoring Plasma Concentrations

Routine monitoring of plasma concentrations of antidepressants, while technically feasible for most drugs, is of uncertain value (except for nortriptyline). However, studies suggest that at least 20% of patients become noncompliant at some time or other. Thus, a "poor response" in a patient for whom an adequate dosage of drug has been prescribed may be shown by measurement of the plasma drug concentration to be due merely to failure to take the drug.

Unresponsive Patients

One third or more of patients do not respond (defined as 50% or more improvement), and over half fail to achieve or maintain full remission on any single treatment. In evaluating a patient's resistance to treatment, one should consider the five D's: diagnosis, drug, dose, duration of treatment, and different treatment.

Diagnosis might be reassessed if the patient shows little response over a period of 2–3 weeks of adequate dosage or plasma concentrations. Whether or not the patient is bipolar, lithium might be added (see Chapter 29); if psychotic, treatment might be augmented with an antipsychotic. Combination of an SSRI with desipramine or bupropion appears relatively safe and effective for some patients. Similarly, mirtazapine can be effectively combined with SSRIs. There is no good pharmacologic rationale for combining venlafaxine with SSRIs since it is itself a potent serotonin reuptake inhibitor; rather, it might be considered for combination with bupropion or mirtazapine. Some clinicians believe that several weeks or months of treatment should be tried before giving up on a drug or combination. The morbidity of depression, however, is such that long delays in attaining relief are demoralizing.

A generally accepted strategy is to begin treatment with an SSRI in mild to moderate outpatient depression and then augment by adding a drug of a different class for more impaired patients. Otherwise, switch to a drug of different class. Most clinicians would prefer to move through various antidepressant drug classes in the search for the right drug rather than through various drugs within a class.

Dose and duration of treatment must be considered. Many treatment failures are due to inadequate dosage, which should be pushed to the limits of the patient's tolerance in refractory cases. The duration of treatment before giving up on a drug is a matter of clinical judgment.

Finally, some patients may need a completely different type of treatment, such as electroconvulsive therapy (ECT). ECT is often viewed as a treatment of last resort, but it should not be withheld from patients with this disorder who cannot be helped by drug therapy. For patients with psychotic depression, ECT may be a treatment of first choice.

Noncompliance is an important cause of lack of response to drugs. Patients should be warned also that noticeable improvement may be slow, perhaps taking 3 weeks or more. Inability to tolerate adverse effects and discouragement with treatment are two major causes for noncompliance and for failure of antidepressants to show efficacy.

Adverse Effects

Adverse effects of various antidepressants are summarized in Table 30–5. Most common unwanted effects are minor, but they may seriously affect patient compliance; the more seriously depressed the patient is, the more likely it is that unwanted effects will be tolerated. Most normal persons find that even moderate doses of many antidepressants cause disagreeable symptoms, especially the classic tertiary amine tricyclics: amitriptyline, imipramine, clomipramine, and doxepin. With the SSRIs, transient nausea is the most frequent complaint, and decreased libido and sexual dysfunction create the greatest concerns during maintenance treatment.

Drug Interactions

A. Pharmacodynamic Interactions

Many of the pharmacodynamic interactions of antidepressants with other drugs have already been discussed. Sedative effects may be additive with other sedatives, especially alcohol. Patients taking tricyclics should be warned that use of alcohol may lead to greater than expected impairment of driving ability. MAO inhibitors, by increasing stores of catecholamines, sensitize the patient to indirectly acting sympathomimetics such as tyramine, which is found in some fermented foods and beverages, and to sympathomimetic drugs such as diethylpropion, phenylpropanolamine, or botanicals containing ephedrine. Such sensitization can result in dangerous and—rarely—fatal hypertensive reactions. The serious interaction between MAO inhibitors and selective serotonin reuptake inhibitors has been mentioned; the serotonin syndrome is potentially lethal and must be avoided.

Table 30–5. Adverse effects of antidepressants.

Tricyclics	
	Sedation (sleepiness, additive effects with other sedative drugs)
	Sympathomimetic (tremor, insomnia)
	Antimuscarinic (blurred vision, constipation, urinary hesitancy, confusion)
	Cardiovascular (orthostatic hypotension, conduction defects, arrhythmias)
	Psychiatric (aggravation of psychosis, withdrawal syndrome)
	Neurologic (seizures)
	Metabolic-endocrine (weight gain, sexual disturbances)
Monoamine oxidase inhibitors	Sleep disturbances, weight gain, postural hypotension, sexual disturbances (phenelzine)
Amoxapine	Similar to the tricyclics with the addition of some effects associated with the antipsychotics (Chapter 29)
Maprotiline	Similar to tricyclics; seizures are dose-related
Mirtazapine	Somnolence, increased appetite, weight gain, dizziness
Trazodone, nefazadone	Drowsiness, dizziness, insomnia, nausea, agitation
Venlafaxine	Nausea, somnolence, sweating, dizziness, sexual disturbances, hypertension, anxiety
Bupropion	Dizziness, dry mouth, sweating, tremor, aggravation of psychosis, potential for seizures at high doses
Fluoxetine and other serotonin reuptake inhibitors	Gastrointestinal symptoms, decreased libido, sexual dysfunction, anxiety (acutely), insomnia, tremor

B. Pharmacokinetic Interactions

The most likely pharmacokinetic interactions are between the potent inhibitors of P450 2D6, paroxetine and fluoxetine, and those drugs highly dependent on this pathway for clearance (eg, desipramine, nortriptyline, flecainide; see also Chapter 4). Actual instances of clinically significant interactions are extremely rare, there being only a handful of case reports after cumulative exposure of more than 50 million patients to these SSRI drugs. Inhibition of P450 3A4 could possibly occur at high concentrations of nefazodone and fluvoxamine and block the metabolism of the many substrates of this isoform.

Overdoses

A. Tricyclics

Tricyclics are extremely dangerous when taken in overdose quantities, and depressed patients are more likely than others to be suicidal. Prescriptions should therefore be limited to amounts less than 1.25 g, or 50 dose units of 25 mg, on a "no refill" basis. If suicide is a serious possibility, the tablets should be entrusted to a family member. The drugs must be kept away from children. Both accidental and deliberate overdoses continue to occur and are serious medical emergencies. Major effects and management of overdosage are discussed in Chapter 59.

B. Second- and Third-Generation Drugs

Overdoses of amoxapine are characterized by severe neurotoxicity, with seizures that are difficult to control. Overdoses of maprotiline also have a tendency to cause seizures as well as cardiotoxicity. Overdoses of the other heterocyclic drugs appear to create only minor problems and can usually be managed with purely supportive measures. For example, in one recorded case even 11 g of nefazodone failed to cause serious injury.

C. MAO Inhibitors

Intoxication with MAO inhibitors is unusual. Agitation, delirium, and neuromuscular excitability are followed by obtunded consciousness, seizures, shock, and hyperthermia. Supportive treatment is usually all that is required, though sedative phenothiazines with α adrenoceptor-blocking action, such as chlorpromazine, may be useful.

D. Selective Serotonin Reuptake Inhibitors

A few deaths have occurred during overdosage of SSRIs when other drugs were also being taken. The likelihood of fatalities from SSRI overdoses is extremely low. In case of overdose, only supportive treatment can be offered, since the high volume of distribution, as with other antidepressants, rules out removal of drug by dialysis. As much as 2.6 g of sertraline has been taken with survival. Overdoses of paroxetine are relatively benign: Up to 850 mg has been taken with no evidence of cardiotoxicity.

 PREPARATIONS AVAILABLE

Tricyclics
  Amitriptyline (generic, Elavil, others)
    Oral: 10, 25, 50, 75, 100, 150 mg tablets
    Parenteral: 10 mg/mL for IM injection
  Clomipramine (generic, Anafranil; labeled only for obsessive-compulsive disorder)
    Oral: 25, 50, 75 mg capsules
  Desipramine (generic, Norpramin, Pertofrane)
    Oral: 10, 25, 50, 75, 100, 150 mg tablets
  Doxepin (generic, Sinequan, others)
    Oral: 10, 25, 50, 75, 100, 150 mg capsules; 10 mg/mL concentrate
  Imipramine (generic, Tofranil, others)
    Oral: 10, 25, 50 mg tablets (as hydrochloride); 75, 100, 125, 150 mg capsules (as pamoate)
    Parenteral: 25 mg/2 mL for IM injection
  Nortriptyline (generic, Aventyl, Pamelor)
    Oral: 10, 25, 50, 75 mg capsules; 10 mg/5 mL solution
  Protriptyline (generic, Vivactil)
    Oral: 5, 10 mg tablets

  Trimipramine (Surmontil)
    Oral: 25, 50, 100 mg capsules

Second- & Third-Generation Drugs
  Amoxapine (generic, Asendin)
    Oral: 25, 50, 100, 150 mg tablets
  Bupropion (generic, Wellbutrin)
    Oral: 75, 100 mg tablets; 100, 150 mg sustained-release tablets
  Maprotiline (generic, Ludiomil)
    Oral: 25, 50, 75 mg tablets
  Mirtazapine (Remeron)
    Oral: 15, 30, 45 mg tablets
  Nefazodone (Serzone)
    Oral: 50, 100, 150, 200, 250 mg tablets
  Trazodone (generic, Desyrel)
    Oral: 50, 100, 150, 300 mg tablets
  Venlafaxine (Effexor)
    Oral: 25, 37.5, 50, 75, 100 mg tablets; 37.5, 75, 150 mg extended-release tablets

SELECTIVE SEROTONIN REUPTAKE INHIBITORS

Citalopram (Celexa)
Oral: 20, 40 mg tablets
Escitalopram (Lexapro)
Oral: 5, 10, 20 mg tablets
Fluoxetine (generic, Prozac)
Oral: 10, 20 mg pulvules; 10 mg tablets; 20 mg/5 mL liquid
Oral delayed release (Prozac Weekly): 90 mg capsules
Fluvoxamine (Luvox, labeled only for obsessive-compulsive disorder)
Oral: 25, 50, 100 mg tablets

Paroxetine (Paxil)
Oral: 10, 20, 30, 40 mg tablets; 10 mg/5 mL suspension; 12.5, 25, 37.5 mg controlled-release tablets
Sertraline (Zoloft)
Oral: 25, 50, 100 mg tablets

MONOAMINE OXIDASE INHIBITORS

Phenelzine (Nardil)
Oral: 15 mg tablets
Tranylcypromine (Parnate)
Oral: 10 mg tablets

OTHER

Atomoxetine (Strattera)
Oral: 10, 18, 25, 40, 60 mg capsules

REFERENCES

American Psychiatric Association: *Diagnostic and Statistical Manual of Mental Disorders,* 4th ed. American Psychiatric Association, 1994.

American Psychiatric Association: APA practice guideline for major depressive disorder in adults. Am J Psychiatry 1993;150 (Suppl):1.

Anderson IM, Tomenson BM: Selective serotonin reuptake inhibitors versus tricyclic antidepressants: A meta-analysis of efficacy and tolerability. J Affect Disord 2000;58:19.

Blackwell B: Side effects of antidepressant drugs. In: *American Psychiatric Association Annual Review,* vol 6. Hales RE, Frances AJ (editors). American Psychiatric Association, 1987.

Bodkin IA et al: Combining serotonin reuptake inhibition and bupropion in partial responders to antidepressant monotherapy. J Clin Psychiatry 1997;58:137.

Briley M: New hope in the treatment of painful symptoms in depression. Curr Opin Investig Drugs 2003;4:42.

Burke WJ: Expert on Investigational Drugs. Ashley Publications: Abstract, 2002, vol. 11, no. 10, p. 1477.

Depression Guideline Panel: Depression in Primary Care: Volume 2. Treatment of Major Depression. Clinical Practice Guideline, Number 5. Rockville, MD: U.S. Department of Health and Human Services, Public Health Service, Agency for Health Care Policy and Research, AHCPR, Pub. No. 93-0551. April 1993.

Derby LE, Jick H, Dean AD: Antidepressant drugs and suicide. J Clin Psychopharmacol 1992;12:235.

Duman RS, Heninger G, Nestler E: A molecular and cellular theory of depression. Arch Gen Psychiatry 1997;54:597.

Ernst CL, Goldberg JF: Antidepressant properties of anticonvulsant drugs for bipolar disorder. J Clin Psychopharmacol 2003;23:182.

Fava M et al: Lithium and tricyclic augmentation of fluoxetine treatment for resistant major depression: A double-blind, controlled study. Am J Psychiatry 1994;151:1372.

Frommer DA et al: Tricyclic antidepressant overdose: A review. JAMA 1987;257:521.

Garver DL, Davis JM: Biogenic amine hypothesis of affective disorders. Life Sci 1979;24:383.

Geddes JR et al: Relapse prevention with antidepressant drug treatment in depressive disorders: a systematic review. Lancet 2003;361:653.

Griest JH et al: Efficacy and tolerability of serotonin transport inhibitors in obsessive-compulsive disorder. Arch Gen Psychiatry 1995;52:53.

Haddjeri N, Blier P, deMontigny C: Noradrenergic modulation of central serotonergic neurotransmission: acute and long-term actions of mirtazapine. Int Clin Psychopharmacol 1995;10(Suppl 4):11.

Harvey AT et al: Evidence of the dual mechanisms of action of venlafaxine. Arch Gen Psychiatry 2000;57:503.

Jick SS et al: Antidepressants and convulsions. J Clin Psychopharmacol 1992;12:241.

Lebowitz BD et al: Diagnosis and treatment of depression in late life. Consensus statement update. JAMA 1997;278:1186.

McGrath PJ et al: A double-blind crossover trial of imipramine and phenelzine for outpatients with treatment-refractory depression. Am J Psychiatry 1993; 150:118.

Merikangas KR et al: Workgroup Reports: NIMH Strategic Plan for Mood Disorders Research, Future of Genetics of Mood Disorders Research. Biol Psychiatry 2002;52:457.

Meyer JH et al: Occupancy of serotonin transporters by paroxetine and citalopram during treatment of depression: a [(11)C]DASB PET imaging study. Am J Psychiatry 2001;158:1843.

Mulrow CD et al: Treatment of Depression: Newer Pharmacotherapies. Evidence Report/Technology Assessment No. 7. (Prepared by the San Antonio Evidence-Based Practice Center based at The University of Texas Health Science Center at San Antonio under Contract 290-97-0012.) AHCPR Publication No, 99-E014. Rockville, MD: Agency for Health Care Policy and Research. February 1999.

Murphy DL: Neuropsychiatric disorders and the multiple human brain serotonin receptor subtypes and subsystems. Neuropsychopharmacology 1990;3:457.

Nelson JC: Treatment of refractory depression. Depress Anxiety 1997;5:165.

Nestler EJ et al: Preclinical models: status of basic research in depression. Biol Psychiatry 2002;52:503.

Potter WZ: Adrenoceptors and serotonin receptor function: Relevance to antidepressant mechanisms of action. J Clin Psychiatry 1996;57(Suppl 4):4.

Preskorn SH: Selection of an antidepressant: mirtazapine. J Clin Psychiatry 1997;58(Suppl 6):3.

Reimherr FW et al: Antidepressant efficacy of sertraline: A double blind placebo and amitriptyline-controlled multicenter comparison study in outpatients with major depression. J Clin Psychiatry 1990;51(Suppl 12B):18.

Rudorfer MV, Manji HK, Potter WZ: Comparative tolerability profiles of the newer versus older antidepressants. Drug Saf 1994;10:1846.

Rush JA, Ryan ND: Current and emerging therapeutics for depression. In: Davis KL et al (editors). *Neuropsychopharmacology: The Fifth Generation of Progress.* Lippincott Williams & Wilkins, 2002.

Sachs G: Treatment-resistant bipolar depression. Psychiatr Clin North Am 1996;19:215.

Schatzberg AF, Nemeroff CB (editors): *The American Psychiatric Press Textbook of Psychopharmacology.* American Psychiatric Press, 1995.

Schatzberg I et al: Molecular and cellular mechanisms in depression. In: Davis KL et al (editors). *Neuropsychopharmacology. The Fifth Generation of Progress.* Lippincott Williams & Wilkins, 2002.

Shen WW: Cytochrome P450 monooxygenases and interactions of psychotropic drugs: A five-year update. Int J Psychiatry Med 1995;25:277.

Stein DJ, Spadaccini E, Hollander E: Meta-analysis of pharmacotherapy trials for obsessive-compulsive disorder. Int Clin Psychopharmacol 1995;10:11.

Stahl SM et al: Comparative efficacy between venlafaxine and SSRIs: A pooled analysis of patients with depression. Biol Psychiatry 2002;52:1166.

Sternbach H: The serotonin syndrome. Am J Psychiatry 1991;148:705.

Thase ME, Rush AJ: Treatment-resistant depression. In: Bloom FE, Kupfer DJ (editors). *Psychopharmacology: The Fourth Generation of Progress.* Raven Press, 1995.

Weissman MM et al: Cross-national epidemiology of major depression and bipolar disorder. JAMA 1996;276:293.

Opioid Analgesics & Antagonists

31

Mark A. Schumacher, PhD, MD, Allan I. Basbaum, PhD, & Walter L. Way, MD

Morphine, the prototypical opioid agonist, has long been known to relieve severe pain with remarkable efficacy. The opium poppy is the source of crude opium from which Serturner in 1803 isolated the pure alkaloid morphine—named after Morpheus, the Greek god of dreams. It remains the standard against which all drugs that have strong analgesic action are compared. These drugs are collectively known as "opioid analgesics" and include not only the natural and semisynthetic alkaloid derivatives from opium but also include synthetic surrogates, other opioid-like drugs whose actions are blocked by the nonselective antagonist naloxone, plus several endogenous peptides that interact with the several subtypes of opioid receptors.

I. BASIC PHARMACOLOGY OF THE OPIOID ANALGESICS

Source

Incision of the poppy seed pod reveals a white substance that turns into a brown gum that is crude opium. Opium contains many alkaloids, the principle one being morphine which is present in a concentration of about 10%. Codeine is synthesized commercially from morphine.

Classification & Chemistry

Opioid drugs include full agonists, partial agonists, and antagonists (see Chapter 2 for definitions). Figure 31–1 shows the chemical structures of morphine, a natural opioid; codeine, a semisynthetic opioid; fentanyl, a pharmacologically similar synthetic; and naloxone, a nonselective opioid antagonist. Morphine is a full agonist at the μ (mu) opioid receptor, whereas codeine functions as a partial (or "weak") μ receptor agonist. As shown in Figure 31–1, simple substitution of an allyl group on the nitrogen of the full *agonist* morphine plus addition of a single hydroxyl group results in naloxone, a strong μ receptor *antagonist*. Some opioids, eg, nalbuphine, are capable of producing an agonist (or partial agonist) effect at one opioid receptor subtype and an antagonist effect at another. Not only can the activating properties of opioid analgesics be manipulated by pharmaceutical chemistry, certain opioid analgesics are modified in the liver resulting in compounds with greater analgesic action (see below, Pharmacokinetics, Metabolism).

Endogenous Opioid Peptides

Opioid alkaloids (eg, morphine) produce analgesia through actions at regions in the brain that contain peptides which have opioid-like pharmacologic properties. The general term currently used for these endogenous substances is **endogenous opioid peptides,** which replaces the previous term **endorphin.**

Three families of endogenous opioid peptides have been described in detail. The best-characterized of the opioid peptides possessing analgesic activity are the pentapeptides methionine-enkephalin (**met-enkephalin**) and leucine-enkephalin (**leu-enkephalin**). Leu- and met-enkephalin have slightly higher affinity for the δ (delta) than for the μ opioid receptor (Table 31–1). These endogenous opioid peptides are derived from three precursor proteins: prepro-opiomelanocortin (POMC), preproenkephalin (proenkephalin A), and preprodynorphin (proenkephalin B). POMC contains the met-enkephalin sequence, β-**endorphin,** and several nonopioid peptides, including adrenocorticotropic hormone (ACTH), β-lipotropin, and melanocyte-stimulating hormone. Preproenkephalin contains six copies of met-enkephalin and one copy of leu-enkephalin. Preprodynorphin yields several active opioid peptides that contain the leu-enkephalin sequence. These are **dynorphin A, dynorphin B,** and α and β neoendorphins. More recently, the endogenous peptides **endomorphin-1** and **endomorphin-2,** have been found to possess many of the properties of opioid peptides, notably analgesia and high affinity binding to the μ receptor. Current research is focused on whether endomorphins selectively activate μ receptor subtypes. Both the endogenous opioid precursor molecules and the endomorphins are present at central nervous system (CNS) sites that have been implicated in pain modulation. Evidence suggests

497

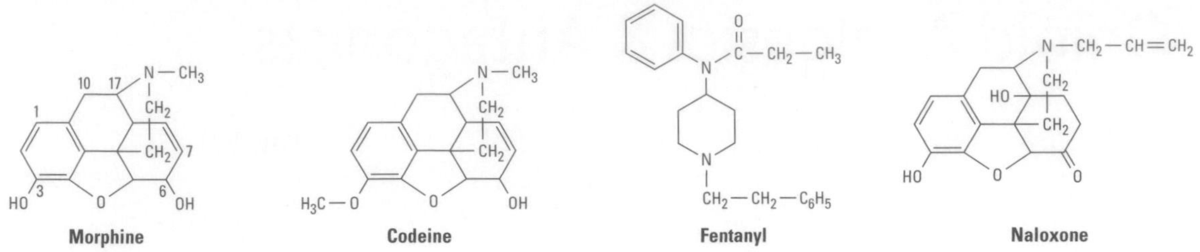

Figure 31–1. Chemical structures of three opioid analgesics and an antagonist.

that they can be released during stressful conditions such as pain or the anticipation of pain to diminish the sensation of noxious stimuli.

In contrast to the analgesic role of leu- and met-enkephalin, an analgesic action of dynorphin A—through its binding to κ (kappa) opioid receptors—remains controversial. Dynorphin A is also found in the dorsal horn of the spinal cord where it plays a critical role in the *sensitization* of nociceptive neurotransmision. Increased levels of dynorphin can be found in the dorsal horn following tissue injury and inflammation. This elevated dynorphin level is believed to increase pain and induce a state of long-lasting hyperalgesia. The pro-nociceptive action of dynorphin in the spinal cord appears to be independent of the opioid receptor system. Rather, dynorphin A can bind and activate the *N*-methyl-D-aspartate (NMDA) receptor complex, a site of action that is the focus of intense therapeutic development.

Recently, a novel receptor-ligand system homologous to the opioid peptides has been found. The principle receptor for this system is the G protein-coupled **orphanin opioid-receptor-like subtype 1 (ORL1)**. Its endogenous ligand has been termed **nociceptin** by one group of investigators and **orphanin FQ** by another group. This ligand-receptor sytem is currently known as the **N/OFQ** system. Nociceptin is structurally similar to dynorphin but acts only at the ORL1 receptor. Although widely expressed in the CNS and periphery, this system has a diverse pharmacology, capable of opposing classic μ receptor–mediated analgesia as well as modulating drug reward, reinforcement, learning, and memory processes.

Pharmacokinetics

Some of the pharmacologic properties of clinically important opioids are summarized in Table 31–2.

A. ABSORPTION

Most opioid analgesics are well absorbed when given by subcutaneous, intramuscular, and oral routes. However, because of the first-pass effect, the oral dose of the opioid (eg, morphine) may need to be much higher than the parenteral dose to elicit a therapeutic effect. Considerable interpatient variability exists in first-pass opioid metabolism, making prediction of an effective oral dose difficult. Certain analgesics such as codeine and oxycodone are effective orally because they have reduced first-pass metabolism, which is primarily due to a methyl group on their aromatic hydroxyl group. Nasal insufflation of certain opioids can result in rapid therapeutic blood levels by avoiding first-pass metabolism. Other

Table 31–1. Opioid receptor subtypes, endogenous opioid peptide affinity, and some of their functions.

Receptor Subtype	Functions	Endogenous Opioid Peptide Affinity
μ (mu)	Supraspinal and spinal analgesia; sedation; inhibition of respiration; slowed GI transit; modulation of hormone and neurotransmitter release	Endorphin > enkephalins > dynorphins
δ (delta)	Supraspinal and spinal analgesia; modulation of hormone and neurotransmitter release	Enkephalins > > endorphins and dynorphins
κ (kappa)	Supraspinal and spinal analgesia; psychotomimetic effects; slowed GI transit	Dynorphins >> endorphin and enkephalins

GI, gastrointestinal.

Table 31–2. Common opioid analgesics.

Generic Name	Trade Name	Approximate Dose (mg)	Oral:Parenteral Potency Ratio	Duration of Analgesia (hours)	Intrinsic Activity
Morphine[1]		10	Low	4–5	High
Hydromorphone	Dilaudid	1.5	Low	4–5	High
Oxymorphone	Numorphan	1.5	Low	3–4	High
Methadone	Dolophine	10	High	4–6	High
Meperidine	Demerol	60–100	Medium	2–4	High
Fentanyl	Sublimaze	0.1	Low	1–1.5	High
Sufentanil	Sufenta	0.02	Parenteral only	1–1.5	High
Alfentanil	Alfenta	Titrated	Parenteral only	0.25–0.75	High
Levorphanol	Levo-Dromoran	2–3	High	4–5	High
Codeine		30–60[4]	High	3–4	Low
Hydrocodone[2]		5–10	Medium	4–6	Moderate
Oxycodone[1,3]	Percodan	4.5[4]	Medium	3–4	Moderate
Propoxyphene	Darvon	60–120[3,4]	Oral only	4–5	Very low
Pentazocine	Talwin	30–50[4]	Medium	3–4	Moderate
Nalbuphine	Nubain	10	Parenteral only	3–6	High
Buprenorphine	Buprenex	0.3	Low	4–8	High
Butorphanol	Stadol	2	Parenteral only	3–4	High

[1]Available in sustained-release forms, morphine (MSContin); oxycodone (OxyContin).

[2]Available in tablets containing acetaminophen (Norco, Vicodin, Lortab, others).

[3]Available in tablets containing acetaminophen (Percocet); aspirin (Percodan).

[4]Analgesic efficacy at this dose not equivalent to 10 mg of morphine. See text for explanation.

routes of opioid administration include oral mucosal and the application of transdermal patches, which can provide delivery of potent analgesics over days.

B. DISTRIBUTION

The uptake of opioids by various organs and tissues is a function of both physiologic and chemical factors. Although all opioids bind to plasma proteins with varying affinity, the drugs rapidly leave the blood compartment and localize in highest concentrations in tissues that are highly perfused such as the brain, lungs, liver, kidneys, and spleen. Drug concentrations in skeletal muscle may be much lower, but this tissue serves as the main reservoir because of its greater bulk. Even though blood flow to fatty tissue is much lower than to the highly perfused tissues, accumulation can be very important particularly after frequent high-dose adminis-

tration or continuous infusion of highly lipophilic opioids that are slowly metabolized, eg, fentanyl.

C. METABOLISM

The opioids are converted in large part to polar metabolites (mostly glucuronides), which are then readily excreted by the kidneys. For example, morphine, which contains free hydroxyl groups, is primarily conjugated to morphine-3-glucuronide (M3G), a compound with neuroexcitatory properties. Moreover, approximately 10% of morphine is metabolized to morphine-6-glucuronide (M6G), an active metabolite with greater analgesic potency than morphine. Despite their limited ability to cross the blood-brain barrier, accumulation of these metabolites may produce unexpected side effects in patients with renal failure or when exceptionally large doses of morphine are administered. This can result in M3G-induced CNS excitation (seizures) or enhanced and prolonged opioid action produced by M6G. Similarly, hydromorphone is metabolized to hydromorphone-3-glucuronide (H3G), which has CNS excitatory properties. However, hydromorphone has not been shown to form the 6-glucuronide metabolite.

Esters (eg, heroin, remifentanil) are rapidly hydrolyzed by common tissue esterases. Heroin (diacetylmorphine) is hydrolyzed to monoacetylmorphine and finally to morphine, which is then conjugated with glucuronic acid.

Hepatic oxidative metabolism is the primary route of degradation of the phenylpiperidine opioids (fentanyl, alfentanil, sufentanil) and eventually leaves only small quantities of the parent compound unchanged for excretion. No active metabolites of fentanyl have been reported. The P450 isozyme CYP3A4 metabolizes fentanyl by N-dealkylation in the liver. CYP3A4 is also present in the mucosa of the small intestine and contributes to the first-pass metabolism of fentanyl when it is taken orally. Codeine, oxycodone, and hydrocodone undergo metabolism in the liver by P450 isozyme CYP2D6, resulting in the production of metabolites of greater potency. Genetic polymorphism of CYP2D6 has been documented and linked to the variation in analgesic response seen among patients. Nevertheless, these metabolites may be of minor consequence because the parent compounds (codeine, oxycodone, hydrocodone) are currently believed to be directly responsible for the majority of their analgesic actions.

Accumulation of a demethylated metabolite of meperidine, normeperidine, may occur in patients with decreased renal function or those receiving multiple high doses of the drug. In sufficiently high concentrations, normeperidine may cause seizures.

D. Excretion

Polar metabolites, including glucuronide conjugates of opioid analgesics, are excreted mainly in the urine. Small amounts of unchanged drug may also be found in the urine. Glucuronide conjugates are also found in the bile, but enterohepatic circulation represents only a small portion of the excretory process.

Pharmacodynamics

A. Mechanism of Action

Opioid agonists produce analgesia by binding to specific G protein-coupled receptors, located primarily in brain and spinal cord regions involved in the transmission and modulation of pain.

1. Receptor types—As noted above, three major classes of opioid receptors (μ, δ, and κ) have been identified in

various nervous system sites and in other tissues (Table 31–1). Each of the three major receptors has now been cloned. All are members of the G protein-coupled family of receptors and show significant amino acid sequence homologies. Multiple receptor subtypes have been proposed based on pharmacologic criteria, including μ_1, μ_2, δ_1, δ_2, κ_1, κ_2, and κ_3. However, genes encoding only one subtype from each of the μ, δ, and κ receptor families have been isolated and characterized thus far. One plausible explanation is that μ receptor subtypes arise from alternate splice variants of a common gene. Since an opioid drug may function with different potencies as an agonist, partial agonist, or antagonist at more than one receptor class or subtype, it is not surprising that these agents are capable of diverse pharmacologic effects.

2. Cellular actions—At the molecular level, opioid receptors form a family of proteins that physically couple to G proteins and through this interaction affect ion channel gating, modulate intracellular Ca^{2+} disposition, and alter protein phosphorylation (see Chapter 2). The opioids have two well-established direct actions on neurons: (1) they close voltage-gated Ca^{2+} channels on presynaptic nerve terminals and thereby reduce transmitter release and (2) they hyperpolarize and thus inhibit postsynaptic neurons by opening K^+ channels. Figure 31–2 schematically illustrates the presynaptic action at all three receptor types and the postsynaptic effect at μ receptors on nociceptive afferents in the spinal cord. The presynaptic action—depressed transmitter release—has been demonstrated for release of a large number of neurotransmitters including glutamate, the principle excitatory amino acid released from noci-

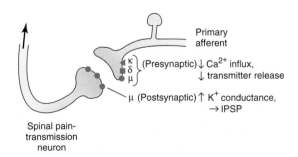

Figure 31–2. Spinal sites of opioid action. Mu (μ), delta (δ), and kappa (κ) agonists reduce transmitter release from presynaptic terminals of nociceptive primary afferents. Mu-agonists also hyperpolarize second-order pain transmission neurons by increasing K^+ conductance, evoking an inhibitory postsynaptic potential.

ceptive nerve terminals, as well as acetylcholine, norepinephrine, serotonin, and substance P.

3. Relation of physiologic effects to receptor type— The majority of currently available opioid analgesics act primarily at the μ opioid receptor. Analgesia, as well as the euphoriant, respiratory depressant, and physical dependence properties of morphine result principally from actions at μ receptors. In fact, the μ receptor was originally defined using the relative potencies for clinical analgesia of a series of opioid alkaloids. However, opioid analgesic effects are complex and include interaction with δ and κ receptors. This is supported by the study of genetic knockouts of the μ, δ, and κ genes in mice. Delta receptor agonists retain analgesic properties in μ receptor knockout mice. The development of δ receptor selective agonists could be clinically useful if their side-effect profiles (respiratory depression, risk of dependence) were more favorable than those found with current μ receptor agonists, such as morphine. Although morphine does act at κ and δ receptor sites, it is unclear to what extent this contributes to its analgesic action. The endogenous opioid peptides differ from most of the alkaloids in their affinity for the δ and κ receptors (Table 31–1). For example, leu-enkephalin has a high affinity for the δ receptor and dynorphin for the κ receptor.

In an effort to develop opioid analgesics with a reduced incidence of respiratory depression or propensity for addiction and dependence, compounds that show preference for κ opioid receptors have been developed. Butorphanol and nalbuphine have shown some clinical success as analgesics, but they can cause dysphoric reactions and have limited potency. Interestingly, butorphanol has also been shown to cause significantly greater analgesia in women than in men. The reason for this difference is not known.

4. Receptor distribution and neural mechanisms of analgesia— Opioid receptor binding sites have been localized autoradiographically using high-affinity radioligand binding with antibodies to unique peptide sequences in each receptor subtype. All three major receptors are present in high concentrations in the dorsal horn of the spinal cord (site **B**, Figure 31–3). Receptors are present both on spinal cord pain transmission neurons and on the primary afferents that relay the pain message to them (Figure 31–3, left side). Opioid agonists inhibit the release of excitatory transmitters from these primary afferents, and they directly inhibit the dorsal horn pain transmission neuron. Thus, opioids exert a powerful analgesic effect directly upon the spinal cord. This **spinal action** has been exploited clinically by direct application of opioid agonists to the spinal cord, which provides a regional analgesic effect while reducing the unwanted respiratory depression,

nausea and vomiting, and sedation that may occur from the **supraspinal actions** of systemically administered opioids.

Under most circumstances, opioids are given systemically and so act simultaneously at both spinal and supraspinal sites; interaction at these two sites tends to increase their overall analgesic efficacy. Different combinations of opioid receptors are found in the supraspinal regions implicated in pain transmission and modulation (Figure 31–3). Of particular importance are opioid binding sites in pain-modulating descending pathways (Figure 31–3, right), including the rostral ventral medulla, the locus ceruleus, and the midbrain periaqueductal gray area. At these sites as at others, opioids directly inhibit neurons, yet neurons that send processes to the spinal cord and inhibit pain transmission neurons are activated by the drugs. This activation has been shown to result from the inhibition of inhibitory neurons in several locations (Figure 31–4).

When pain-relieving opioid drugs are given systemically, they presumably act upon brain circuits normally regulated by endogenous opioid peptides. Part of the pain-relieving action of exogenous opioids involves the release of endogenous opioid peptides. An exogenous opioid agonist (eg, morphine) may act primarily and directly at the μ receptor, but this action may evoke the release of endogenous opioids that additionally act at δ and κ receptors. Thus, even a receptor-selective ligand can initiate a complex sequence of events involving multiple synapses, transmitters, and receptor types.

Animal and human clinical studies demonstrate that both endogenous and exogenous opioids can also produce opioid-mediated analgesia at sites *outside* the CNS. Pain associated with inflammation seems especially sensitive to these peripheral opioid actions. The identification of functional μ receptors on the peripheral terminals of sensory neurons supports this hypothesis. Furthermore, activation of peripheral μ receptors results in a decrease in sensory neuron activity and transmitter release. Peripheral administration of opioids, eg, into the knees of patients undergoing arthroscopic knee surgery, has shown some clinical benefit. If they can be developed, opioids selective for a peripheral site would be useful adjuncts in the treatment of inflammatory pain (see Box, Ion Channels & Novel Analgesics). Moreover, new peripherally acting dynorphins may provide a novel means to treat visceral pain.

5. Tolerance and physical dependence— With frequently repeated administration of therapeutic doses of morphine or its surrogates, there is a gradual loss in effectiveness, ie, tolerance. To reproduce the original response, a larger dose must be administered. Along with tolerance, physical dependence develops. Physical dependence is defined as the occurrence of a characteris-

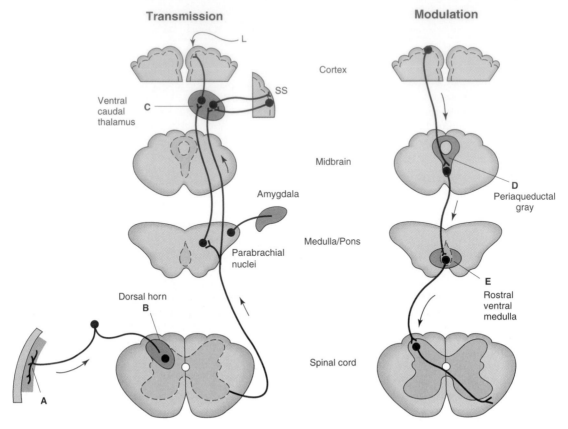

Transmission

Modulation

Cortex

Ventral caudal thalamus

Midbrain

Amygdala

Periaqueductal gray

Medulla/Pons

Parabrachial nuclei

Dorsal horn

Rostral ventral medulla

Spinal cord

Figure 31–3. Putative sites of action of opioid analgesics (darker color). On the left, sites of action on the pain transmission pathway from the periphery to the higher centers are shown. **A:** Direct action of opioids on inflamed peripheral tissues. **B:** Inhibition occurs in the spinal cord. **C:** Possible site of action in the thalamus. Different thalamic regions project to somatosensory (SS) or limbic (L) cortex. Parabrachial nuclei (medulla/pons) projects to the amygdala. On the right, actions of opioids on pain-modulating neurons in the midbrain **(D)** and medulla **(E)** indirectly control pain transmission pathways.

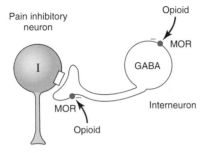

Pain inhibitory neuron

Opioid

MOR

GABA

Interneuron

MOR

Opioid

Figure 31–4. Brainstem local circuitry underlying μ opioid receptor (MOR)–mediated analgesia. The pain inhibitory neuron (*I*) is indirectly excited by opioids (exogenous or endogenous) that inhibit an inhibitory (GABAergic) interneuron *(GABA).*

tic withdrawal or **abstinence syndrome** when the drug is stopped or an antagonist is administered.

The mechanism of development of tolerance and physical dependence is poorly understood, but persistent activation of μ receptors such as occurs with the treatment of severe chronic pain appears to play a primary role in its induction and maintenance. Current concepts have shifted away from tolerance being driven by a simple up-regulation of the cyclic adenosine monophosphate (cAMP) system or a down-regulation and recycling of μ receptors from the cell surface to cryptic intracellular sites. Although these processes are associated with tolerance, they are not sufficient to explain it. Recent research suggests that the δ opioid receptor is an important component in the maintenance of tolerance. In addition, the concept of **receptor uncoupling** has gained prominence.

ION CHANNELS & NOVEL ANALGESICS

Even the most severe acute pain (that lasting hours to days) can usually be well controlled—with significant but tolerable adverse effects—with currently available analgesics, especially the opioids. Chronic pain (lasting weeks to months), however, is not very satisfactorily managed with opioids. It is now known that in chronic pain, presynaptic receptors on sensory nerve terminals in the periphery contribute to increased excitability of sensory nerve endings (peripheral sensitization). The hyperexcitable sensory neuron bombards the spinal cord, leading to increased excitability and synaptic alterations in the dorsal horn (central sensitization). Such changes appear to be important in chronic inflammatory and neuropathic pain states (Basbaum, 1999; Woolf, 2000).

In the effort to discover better analgesic drugs for chronic pain, renewed attention is being paid to synaptic transmission in nociception and sensory processing. Potentially important ion channels associated with these processes in the periphery include members of the transient receptor potential family as TRPV1 (capsaicin receptor) that is activated by heat and products of inflammation as well as P2X receptors (responsive to purines released from tissue damage). A special type of tetrodotoxin-resistant voltage-gated sodium channel (Nav1.8), also known as the PN3/SNS channel, is apparently uniquely associated with nociceptive neurons in dorsal root ganglia. Mexiletine, which is useful in some chronic pain

states, may act by blocking this channel. Certain blockers of voltage-gated N-type calcium channels have shown analgesic effects. A synthetic peptide related to the marine snail toxin ω-conotoxin, which selectively blocks these calcium channels, is in clinical trials as an analgesic. Gabapentin, an anticonvulsant analog of GABA (see Chapter 24), is an effective treatment for neuropathic (nerve injury) pain. It has recently been shown to block the pain and hyperalgesia associated with inflammation. Potential sites of action of gabapentin include the alpha-2-delta family of calcium channels.

N-methyl-D-aspartate (NMDA) receptors appear to play a very important role in central sensitization at both spinal and supraspinal levels. Although certain NMDA antagonists have demonstrated analgesic activity (eg, ketamine), it has been difficult to find agents with an acceptably low profile of side effects or neurotoxicity. GABA and acetylcholine (through nicotinic receptors) appear to control the central synaptic release of several transmitters involved in nociception. Nicotine itself and certain nicotine analogs cause analgesia. A nicotinic agonist found in certain frogs (epibatidine) has significant analgesic effect.

Although none of the studies described has yet yielded an approved analgesic drug, they have already provided a better understanding of nociception and analgesia.

Under this hypothesis, tolerance is due to a dysfunction of structural interactions between the μ receptor and G-proteins, second messenger systems, and their target ion channels. Moreover, a particular ion channel complex, the NMDA receptor, has been shown to play a critical role in tolerance development and maintenance because NMDA receptor antagonists such as ketamine can block tolerance development. The development of novel NMDA receptor antagonists or other strategies to recouple μ receptors to their target ion channels provides hope for achieving a clinically effective means to prevent or reverse opioid analgesic tolerance. In addition to the development of tolerance, persistent administration of opioid analgesics has been observed to *increase* the sensation of pain. Spinal dynorphin is a leading candidate for the mediation of opioid-induced pain and hyperalgesia.

B. ORGAN SYSTEM EFFECTS OF MORPHINE AND ITS SURROGATES

The actions described below for morphine, the prototypic opioid agonist, can also be observed with other opi-

oid agonists even though some variation between individual agents does occur. Agents with partial agonist or mixed receptor effects, when given to a patient who has not recently received an agonist agent, also produce analgesia but with minor additional variations in effects as noted below. Characteristics of specific members of these two groups are discussed below. When given to a subject who *has* received an agonist, the pure antagonists and the mixed agents have very different effects from those observed in a subject who *has not* received an agonist. This is discussed further at the end of this chapter.

1. Central nervous system effects—The principal effects of opioid analgesics with affinity for μ receptors are on the CNS; the more important ones include analgesia, euphoria, sedation, and respiratory depression. With repeated use, a high degree of tolerance occurs to all of these effects (Table 31–3).

a. Analgesia—Pain consists of both sensory and affective (emotional) components. Opioid analgesics are unique in that they can reduce both aspects of the pain experience, especially the affective aspect.

b. Euphoria—Typically, patients or intravenous drug users who receive intravenous morphine experience a pleasant floating sensation with lessened anxiety and distress. However, dysphoria, an unpleasant state characterized by restlessness and malaise, may sometimes occur.

c. Sedation—Drowsiness and clouding of mentation are frequent concomitants of opioid action. There is little or no amnesia. Sleep is induced by opiates more frequently in the elderly than in young, healthy individuals. Ordinarily, the patient can be easily aroused from this sleep. However, the combination of morphine with other central depressant drugs such as the sedative-hypnotics may result in very deep sleep. Marked sedation occurs more frequently with compounds closely related to the phenanthrene derivatives and less frequently with the synthetic agents such as meperidine and fentanyl. In standard analgesic doses, morphine (a phenanthrene) disrupts normal REM and non-REM sleep patterns. This disrupting effect is probably characteristic of all opioids. In contrast to humans, a number of species (cats, horses, cows, pigs) may manifest excitation rather than sedation when given opioids. These paradoxic effects are at least partially dose-dependent.

d. Respiratory depression—All of the opioid analgesics can produce significant respiratory depression by inhibiting brainstem respiratory mechanisms. Alveolar P_{CO_2} may increase, but the most reliable indicator of this depression is a depressed response to a carbon dioxide challenge. The respiratory depression is dose-related and is influenced significantly by the degree of sensory input occurring at the time. For example, it is possible to partially overcome opioid-induced respiratory depression by stimulation of various sorts. When strongly painful stimuli that have prevented the depressant action of a large dose of an opioid are relieved, respiratory depression may suddenly become marked. A small to moderate decrease in respiratory function, as measured by Pa_{CO_2} elevation, may be well-tolerated in the patient without prior respiratory impairment. However, in individuals with increased intracranial pressure, asthma, chronic obstructive pulmonary disease, or cor pulmonale, this decrease in respiratory function may not be tolerated.

e. Cough suppression—Suppression of the cough reflex is a well-recognized action of opioids. Codeine in particular has been used to advantage in persons suffering from pathologic cough and in patients in whom it is necessary to maintain ventilation via an endotracheal tube. However, cough suppression by opioids may allow accumulation of secretions and thus lead to airway obstruction and atelectasis.

f. Miosis—Constriction of the pupils is seen with virtually all opioid agonists. Miosis is a pharmacologic action to which little or no tolerance develops (Table 31–3); thus, it is valuable in the diagnosis of opioid overdose. Even in highly tolerant addicts, miosis will be seen. This action, which can be blocked by opioid antagonists, is mediated by parasympathetic pathways, which, in turn, can be blocked by atropine.

g. Truncal rigidity—An intensification of tone in the large trunk muscles has been noted with a number of opioids. It was originally believed that truncal rigidity involved a spinal cord action of these drugs, but there is now evidence that it results from an action at supraspinal levels. Truncal rigidity reduces thoracic compliance and thus interferes with ventilation. The effect is most apparent when high doses of the highly lipid-soluble opioids (eg, fentanyl, sufentanil, alfentanil) are rapidly administered intravenously. Truncal rigidity may be overcome by administration of an opioid antagonist, which of course will also antagonize the analgesic action of the opioid. Preventing truncal rigidity while preserving analgesia requires the concomitant use of neuromuscular blocking agents.

h. Nausea and vomiting—The opioid analgesics can activate the brainstem chemoreceptor trigger zone to produce nausea and vomiting. There may also be a vestibular component in this effect because ambulation seems to increase the incidence of nausea and vomiting.

2. Peripheral effects—

a. Cardiovascular system—Most opioids have no significant *direct* effects on the heart and no major effects on cardiac rhythm (except bradycardia). Meperidine is an exception to this generalization because its antimuscarinic action may result in tachycardia. Blood pressure is usually well maintained in subjects receiving opioids unless the cardiovascular system is stressed, in which case hypotension may occur. This hypotensive effect is probably due to peripheral arterial and venous

Table 31–3. Degrees of tolerance that may develop to some of the effects of the opioids.

High	Moderate	Minimal or None
Analgesia	Bradycardia	Miosis
Euphoria, dysphoria		Constipation
Mental clouding		Convulsions
Sedation		
Respiratory depression		
Antidiuresis		
Nausea and vomiting		
Cough suppression		

dilation, which has been attributed to a number of mechanisms including central depression of vasomotor-stabilizing mechanisms and release of histamine. No consistent effect on cardiac output is seen, and the electrocardiogram is not significantly affected. However, caution should be exercised in patients with decreased blood volume, since the above mechanisms make these patients quite susceptible to hypotension. Opioid analgesics affect cerebral circulation minimally except when PCO_2 rises as a consequence of respiratory depression. Increased PCO_2 leads to cerebral vasodilation associated with a decrease in cerebral vascular resistance, an increase in cerebral blood flow, and an increase in intracranial pressure.

b. Gastrointestinal tract—Constipation has long been recognized as an effect of opioids. Opioid receptors exist in high density in the gastrointestinal tract, and the constipating effects of the opioids are mediated through an action on the local enteric nervous system (see Chapter 6) as well as the CNS. In the stomach, motility (rhythmic contraction and relaxation) may decrease but tone (persistent contraction) may increase—particularly in the central portion; gastric secretion of hydrochloric acid is decreased. Small intestine resting tone is increased, with periodic spasms, but the amplitude of nonpropulsive contractions is markedly decreased. In the large intestine, propulsive peristaltic waves are diminished and tone is increased; this delays passage of the fecal mass and allows increased absorption of water, which leads to constipation. The large bowel actions are the basis for the use of opioids in management of diarrhea.

c. Biliary tract—The opioids constrict biliary smooth muscle, which may result in biliary colic. The sphincter of Oddi may constrict, resulting in reflux of biliary and pancreatic secretions and elevated plasma amylase and lipase levels.

d. Renal—Renal function is depressed by opioids. It is believed that in humans this is chiefly due to decreased renal plasma flow. Opioids can decrease systemic blood pressure and glomerular filtration rate. In addition, μ opioids have been found to have an antidiuretic effect in humans. Mechanisms may involve both the CNS and peripheral sites, but the relative contributions of each are unknown. Opioids also enhance renal tubular sodium reabsorption. The role of opioid-induced changes in antidiuretic hormone (ADH) release is controversial. Ureteral and bladder tone are increased by therapeutic doses of the opioid analgesics. Increased sphincter tone may precipitate urinary retention, especially in postoperative patients. Occasionally, ureteral colic caused by a renal calculus is made worse by opioid-induced increase in ureteral tone.

e. Uterus—The opioid analgesics may prolong labor. The mechanism for this action is unclear, but both peripheral and central effects of the opioids can reduce uterine tone.

f. Neuroendocrine—Opioid analgesics stimulate the release of ADH, prolactin, and somatotropin but inhibit the release of luteinizing hormone. These effects suggest that endogenous opioid peptides, through effects in the hypothalamus, play regulatory roles in these systems (Table 31–1).

g. Pruritus—Therapeutic doses of the opioid analgesics produce flushing and warming of the skin accompanied sometimes by sweating and itching; CNS effects and peripheral histamine release may be responsible for these reactions. Opioid-induced pruritus and occasionally urticaria appear more frequently when opioid analgesics are administered parenterally. In addition, when opioids such as morphine are administered to the neuraxis by the spinal or epidural route, their usefulness may be limited by intense pruritus over the lips and torso.

h. Miscellaneous—The opioids may modulate the actions of the immune system by effects on lymphocyte proliferation, antibody production, and chemotaxis. Natural killer cell cytolytic activity and lymphocyte proliferative responses to mitogens are usually inhibited by opioids. Although the mechanisms involved are complex, activation of central opioid receptors could mediate a significant component of the changes observed in peripheral immune function. In general, these effects are mediated by the sympathetic nervous system in the case of acute administration and by the hypothalamic-pituitary-adrenal system in the case of prolonged administration of opioids.

C. EFFECTS OF DRUGS WITH BOTH AGONIST AND ANTAGONIST ACTIONS

Buprenorphine is an opioid agonist that displays high binding affinity but low intrinsic activity at the μ receptor. Its slow rate of dissociation from the μ receptor has also made it an attractive alternative to methadone for the management of opioid withdrawal. It functions as an *antagonist* at the δ and κ receptors and for this reason is referred to as a "mixed agonist-antagonist." Although buprenorphine is used as an analgesic, it can antagonize the action of more potent μ agonists such as morphine. Buprenorphine also binds to ORL1, the orphanin receptor. Whether this property also participates in opposing μ receptor function is under study. Pentazocine and nalbuphine are other examples of opioid analgesics with mixed agonist-antagonist properties. Psychotomimetic effects, with hallucinations, nightmares, and anxiety, have been reported following use of drugs with mixed agonist-antagonist actions.

II. CLINICAL PHARMACOLOGY OF THE OPIOID ANALGESICS

Successful treatment of pain is a challenging task that begins with careful attempts to assess the source and magnitude of the pain. The amount of pain experienced by the patient is often described in terms of a numeric visual analog scale (VAS) with word descriptors ranging from no pain (0) to excruciating pain (10). A similar scale can be used with children and with patients who cannot speak; this scale depicts five faces ranging from smiling (no pain) to crying (maximum pain).

In severe pain, the administration of an opioid analgesic is usually considered a primary part of the overall management plan. Determining the route of administration (oral, parenteral, neuraxial), duration of drug action, ceiling effect (maximal intrinsic activity), duration of therapy, potential for unwanted side effects, and the patient's past experience with opioids should all be addressed. One of the principal errors made by physicians in this setting is a failure to adequately assess a patient's pain and to match its severity with an appropriate level of therapy. Just as important is the principle that following delivery of the therapeutic plan, its effectiveness must be reevaluated and the plan modified if necessary if the response was excessive or inadequate.

Use of opioid drugs in acute situations may be contrasted with their use in chronic pain management, where a multitude of other factors must be considered, including the development of tolerance to and physical dependence on to opioid analgesics.

Clinical Use of Opioid Analgesics

A. ANALGESIA

Severe, *constant* pain is usually relieved with opioid analgesics with high intrinsic activity (see Table 31–2); whereas sharp, intermittent pain does not appear to be as effectively controlled.

The pain associated with cancer and other terminal illnesses must be treated aggressively and often requires a multidisciplinary approach for effective management. Such conditions may require continuous use of potent opioid analgesics and will be associated with some degree of tolerance and dependence. However, this should not be used as a barrier to providing patients with the best possible care and quality of life. Research in the hospice movement has demonstrated that fixed-interval administration of opioid medication (ie, a regular dose at a scheduled time) is more effective in achieving pain relief than dosing on demand. New dosage forms of opioids that allow slower release of the drug are now available

(eg, sustained-release forms of morphine (MSContin) and oxycodone (OxyContin). Their purported advantage is a longer and more stable level of analgesia.

If disturbances of gastrointestinal function prevent the use of oral sustained-release morphine, the fentanyl transdermal system (fentanyl patch) can be used over long periods. Furthermore, buccal transmucosal fentanyl can be used for episodes of breakthrough pain (see Alternative Routes of Administration, below). Administration of strong opioids by nasal insufflation has been shown to be efficacious, and nasal preparations are now available in some countries. Approval of such formulations in the USA is growing. In addition, stimulant drugs such as the amphetamines have been shown to enhance the analgesic actions of the opioids and thus may be very useful adjuncts in the patient with chronic pain.

Opioid analgesics are often used during obstetric labor. Because opioids cross the placental barrier and reach the fetus, care must be taken to minimize neonatal depression. If this occurs, immediate injection of the antagonist naloxone will reverse the depression. The phenylpiperidine drugs (eg, meperidine) appear to produce less depression, particularly respiratory depression, in newborn infants than does morphine; this may justify their use in obstetric practice.

The acute, severe pain of renal and biliary colic often requires a strong agonist opioid for adequate relief. However, the drug-induced increase in smooth muscle tone may cause a paradoxical *increase* in pain secondary to increased spasm. An increase in the dose of opioid is usually successful in providing adequate analgesia.

B. ACUTE PULMONARY EDEMA

The relief produced by intravenous morphine in dyspnea from pulmonary edema associated with left ventricular failure is remarkable. The mechanism is not clear but probably involves reduced *perception* of shortness of breath and reduced patient anxiety as well as reduced cardiac preload (reduced venous tone) and afterload (decreased peripheral resistance). Morphine can be particularly useful when treating painful myocardial ischemia with pulmonary edema.

C. COUGH

Suppression of cough can be obtained at doses lower than those needed for analgesia. However, in recent years the use of opioid analgesics to allay cough has diminished largely because a number of effective synthetic compounds have been developed that are neither analgesic nor addictive. These agents are discussed below.

D. DIARRHEA

Diarrhea from almost any cause can be controlled with the opioid analgesics, but if diarrhea is associated with infection such use must not substitute for appropriate chemotherapy. Crude opium preparations (eg, paregoric) were used in the past to control diarrhea, but now synthetic surrogates with more selective gastrointestinal effects and few or no CNS effects, eg, diphenoxylate, are used. Several preparations are available specifically for this purpose.

E. APPLICATIONS IN ANESTHESIA

The opioids are frequently used as premedicant drugs before anesthesia and surgery because of their sedative, anxiolytic, and analgesic properties. The opioids are also used intraoperatively both as adjuncts to other anesthetic agents and, in high doses (eg, 0.02–0.075 mg/kg of fentanyl), as a primary component of the anesthetic regimen (see Chapter 25), most commonly in cardiovascular surgery and other types of high-risk surgery where a primary goal is to minimize cardiovascular depression. In such situations, mechanical respiratory assistance must be provided.

Because of their direct action on the superficial neurons of the spinal cord dorsal horn, opioids can also be used as regional analgesics, by administration into the epidural or subarachnoid spaces of the spinal column. A number of studies have demonstrated that long-lasting analgesia with minimal adverse effects can be achieved by epidural administration of 3–5 mg of morphine, followed by slow infusion through a catheter placed in the epidural space. It was initially assumed that the epidural application of opioids might selectively produce analgesia without impairment of motor, autonomic, or sensory functions other than pain. However, respiratory depression may occur after the drug is injected into the epidural space and may require reversal with naloxone. Other effects such as pruritus and nausea and vomiting are common after epidural and subarachnoid administration of opioids and may also be reversed with naloxone if necessary. Currently, the epidural route is favored because adverse effects are less common. Morphine is the most frequently used agent, but the use of low doses of local anesthetics in combination with fentanyl infused through a thoracic epidural catheter has also become an accepted method of pain control in patients recovering from major upper abdominal surgery. In rare cases, chronic pain management specialists may elect to surgically implant a programmable infusion pump connected to a spinal catheter for continuous infusion of opioids or other analgesic compounds.

F. ALTERNATIVE ROUTES OF ADMINISTRATION

Rectal suppositories of morphine and hydromorphone have long been used when oral and parenteral routes are undesirable. The **transdermal patch** provides stable blood levels of drug and better pain control while avoiding the need for repeated parenteral injections. Fentanyl has been the most successful opioid in transdermal application and finds great use in patients experiencing chronic pain. The **intranasal** route avoids repeated parenteral drug injections and the first-pass metabolism of orally administered drugs. Butorphanol is the only opioid currently available in the USA in a nasal formulation but more are expected. Another alternative to parenteral administration is the **buccal transmucosal** route, which uses a fentanyl citrate lozenge or a "lollipop" mounted on a stick.

Another type of pain control called **patient-controlled analgesia (PCA)** is now in widespread use. With PCA, the patient controls a parenteral (usually intravenous) infusion device by depressing a button to deliver a preprogrammed dose of the desired opioid analgesic. Claims of better pain control using less opioid are supported by well-designed clinical trials, making this approach very useful in postoperative pain control. However, health care personnel must be very familiar with the use of PCAs to avoid overdosage secondary to misuse or improper programming. There is a proven risk of respiratory depression with hypoxia that requires careful monitoring of vital signs and sedation level.

Toxicity & Undesired Effects

Direct toxic effects of the opioid analgesics that are extensions of their acute pharmacologic actions include respiratory depression, nausea, vomiting, and constipation (Table 31–4). In addition, tolerance and dependence, diagnosis and treatment of overdosage, as well as contraindications must be considered.

A. TOLERANCE AND DEPENDENCE

Drug dependence of the opioid type is marked by a relatively specific withdrawal or abstinence syndrome. Just as there are pharmacologic differences between the various opioids, there are also differences in psychologic dependence and the severity of withdrawal effects. For example, withdrawal from dependence upon a strong

Table 31–4. Adverse effects of the opioid analgesics.

Behavioral restlessness, tremulousness, hyperactivity (in dysphoric reactions)
Respiratory depression
Nausea and vomiting
Increased intracranial pressure
Postural hypotension accentuated by hypovolemia
Constipation
Urinary retention
Itching around nose, urticaria (more frequent with parenteral and spinal administration)

agonist is associated with more severe withdrawal signs and symptoms than withdrawal from a mild or moderate agonist. Administration of an opioid *antagonist* to an opioid-dependent person is followed by brief but severe withdrawal symptoms (see antagonist-precipitated withdrawal, below). The potential for physical and psychologic dependence of the partial agonist-antagonist opioids appear to be less than that of the agonist drugs.

1. Tolerance—Although development of tolerance begins with the first dose of an opioid, tolerance generally does not become clinically manifest until after 2–3 weeks of frequent exposure to ordinary therapeutic doses. Tolerance develops most readily when large doses are given at short intervals and is minimized by giving small amounts of drug with longer intervals between doses.

Depending on the compound and the effect measured, the degree of tolerance may be as great as 35-fold. Marked tolerance may develop to the analgesic, sedating, and respiratory depressant effects. It is possible to produce respiratory arrest in a nontolerant person with a dose of 60 mg of morphine, whereas in addicts maximally tolerant to opioids as much as 2000 mg of morphine taken over a 2- or 3-hour period may not produce significant respiratory depression. Tolerance also develops to the antidiuretic, emetic, and hypotensive effects but not to the miotic, convulsant, and constipating actions (Table 31–3).

Tolerance to the sedating and respiratory effects of the opioids dissipates within a few days after the drugs are discontinued. Tolerance to the emetic effects may persist for several months after withdrawal of the drug. The rates at which tolerance appears and disappears, as well as the degree of tolerance, may also differ considerably among the different opioid analgesics and among individuals using the same drug. For instance, tolerance to methadone develops more slowly and to a lesser degree than to morphine.

Tolerance develops also to analgesics with mixed receptor effects but to a lesser extent than to the agonists. Such effects as hallucinations, sedation, hypothermia, and respiratory depression are reduced after repeated administration of the mixed receptor drugs. However, tolerance to the latter agents does not generally include cross-tolerance to the agonist opioids. It is also important to note that tolerance does not develop to the antagonist actions of the mixed agents nor to those of the pure antagonists.

Cross-tolerance is an extremely important characteristic of the opioids, ie, patients tolerant to morphine show a reduction in analgesic response to other agonist opioids. This is particularly true of those agents with primarily μ receptor agonist activity. Morphine and its congeners exhibit cross-tolerance not only with respect to their analgesic actions but also to their euphoriant, sedative, and respiratory effects. However, the cross-tolerance existing among the μ receptor agonists can often be partial or incomplete. This clinical observation has led to the concept of "opioid rotation," which has been used in the treatment of cancer pain for many years. A patient who is experiencing decreasing effectiveness of one opioid analgesic regimen is "rotated" to a different opioid analgesic (eg, morphine to hydromorphone; hydromorphone to methadone) and typically experiences significantly improved analgesia at a reduced overall equivalent dosage. Another approach is to "recouple" opioid receptor function through the use of adjunctive nonopioid agents. NMDA receptor antagonists (eg, ketamine, dextromethorphan) have shown promise in preventing or reversing opioid-induced tolerance in animals and humans. Routine use of these agents awaits the outcome of well-controlled studies to determine their clinical effectiveness in reducing postoperative pain and morphine requirements.

2. Physical dependence—The development of physical dependence is an invariable accompaniment of tolerance to repeated administration of an opioid of the μ type. Failure to continue administering the drug results in a characteristic withdrawal or **abstinence syndrome** that reflects an exaggerated rebound from the acute pharmacologic effects of the opioid.

The signs and symptoms of withdrawal include rhinorrhea, lacrimation, yawning, chills, gooseflesh (piloerection), hyperventilation, hyperthermia, mydriasis, muscular aches, vomiting, diarrhea, anxiety, and hostility (see Chapter 32). The number and intensity of the signs and symptoms are largely dependent on the degree of physical dependence that has developed. Administration of an opioid at this time suppresses abstinence signs and symptoms almost immediately.

The time of onset, intensity, and duration of abstinence syndrome depend on the drug used and may be related to its biologic half-life. With morphine or heroin, withdrawal signs usually start within 6–10 hours after the last dose. Peak effects are seen at 36–48 hours, after which most of the signs and symptoms gradually subside. By 5 days, most of the effects have disappeared, but some may persist for months. In the case of meperidine, the withdrawal syndrome largely subsides within 24 hours, whereas with methadone several days are required to reach the peak of the abstinence syndrome, and it may last as long as 2 weeks. The slower subsidence of methadone effects is associated with a less intense immediate syndrome, and this is the basis for its use in the detoxification of heroin addicts. After the abstinence syndrome subsides, tolerance also disappears as evidenced by a restoration in sensitivity to the opioid agonist. However, despite the loss of physical dependence on the opioid, craving for it may persist for many months.

A transient, explosive abstinence syndrome—**antagonist-precipitated withdrawal**—can be induced in a subject physically dependent on opioids by administering naloxone or other antagonist. Within 3 minutes after injection of the antagonist, signs and symptoms similar to those seen after abrupt discontinuance appear, peaking in 10–20 minutes and largely subsiding after 1 hour. Even in the case of methadone, withdrawal of which results in a relatively mild abstinence syndrome, the antagonist-precipitated abstinence syndrome may be very severe.

In the case of agents with mixed effects, withdrawal signs and symptoms can be induced after repeated administration followed by abrupt discontinuance of pentazocine, cyclazocine, or nalorphine, but the syndrome appears to be somewhat different from that produced by morphine and other agonists. Anxiety, loss of appetite and body weight, tachycardia, chills, increase in body temperature, and abdominal cramps have been noted.

3. Psychologic dependence—The euphoria, indifference to stimuli, and sedation usually caused by the opioid analgesics, especially when injected intravenously, tend to promote their compulsive use. In addition, the addict experiences abdominal effects that have been likened to an intense sexual orgasm. These factors constitute the primary reasons for opioid abuse liability and are strongly reinforced by the development of physical dependence.

Obviously, the risk of causing dependence is an important consideration in the therapeutic use of these drugs. *Despite that risk, under no circumstances should adequate pain relief ever be withheld simply because an opioid exhibits potential for abuse or because legislative controls complicate the process of prescribing narcotics.* Furthermore, certain principles can be observed by the clinician to minimize problems presented by tolerance and dependence when using opioid analgesics:

Establish therapeutic goals before starting opioid therapy. This tends to limit the potential for physical dependence. The patient should be included in this process.

Once a therapeutic dose is established, attempt to limit dosage to this level. This goal is facilitated by use of a written treatment contract which specifically prohibits early refills and having multiple prescribing physicians.

Instead of opioid analgesics—especially in chronic management—consider using other types of analgesics or compounds exhibiting less pronounced withdrawal symptoms on discontinuance.

Frequently evaluate continuing analgesic therapy and the patient's need for opioids.

B. Diagnosis and Treatment of Opioid Overdosage

Intravenous injection of naloxone dramatically reverses coma due to opioid overdose but not that due to other CNS depressants. Use of the antagonist should not, of course, delay the institution of other therapeutic measures, especially respiratory support.

See also following Antagonists section and Chapter 59.

C. Contraindications and Cautions in Therapy

1. Use of pure agonists with weak partial agonists—When a weak partial agonist such as pentazocine is given to a patient also receiving a full agonist (eg, morphine), there is a risk of diminishing analgesia or even inducing a state of withdrawal; combining full agonist with partial agonist opioids should be avoided.

2. Use in patients with head injuries—Carbon dioxide retention caused by respiratory depression results in cerebral vasodilation. In patients with elevated intracranial pressure, this may lead to lethal alterations in brain function.

3. Use during pregnancy—In pregnant women who are chronically using opioids, the fetus may become physically dependent in utero and manifest withdrawal symptoms in the early postpartum period. A daily dose as small as 6 mg of heroin (or equivalent) taken by the mother will result in a mild withdrawal syndrome in the infant, and twice that much may result in severe signs and symptoms, including irritability, shrill crying, diarrhea, or even seizures. Recognition of the problem is aided by a careful history and physical examination. When withdrawal symptoms are judged to be relatively mild, treatment is aimed at control of these symptoms with such drugs as diazepam; with more severe withdrawal, camphorated tincture of opium (paregoric; 0.4 mg of morphine/mL) in an oral dose of 0.12–0.24 mL/kg is used. Oral doses of methadone (0.1–0.5 mg/kg) have also been used.

4. Use in patients with impaired pulmonary function—In patients with borderline respiratory reserve, the depressant properties of the opioid analgesics may lead to acute respiratory failure.

5. Use in patients with impaired hepatic or renal function—Because morphine and its congeners are metabolized primarily in the liver, their use in patients in prehepatic coma may be questioned. Half-life is prolonged in patients with impaired renal function, and morphine and its active glucuronide metabolite, may accumulate; dosage can often be reduced in such patients.

6. Use in patients with endocrine disease—Patients with adrenal insufficiency (Addison's disease) and those with hypothyroidism (myxedema) may have prolonged and exaggerated responses to opioids.

Drug Interactions

Because seriously ill or hospitalized patients may require a large number of drugs, there is always a possibility of drug interactions when the opioid analgesics are administered. Table 31–5 lists some of these drug interactions and the reasons for not combining the named drugs with opioids.

SPECIFIC AGENTS

The following section describes the most important widely used opioid analgesics, along with features peculiar to specific agents. Data about doses approximately equivalent to 10 mg of intramuscular morphine, oral versus parenteral efficacy, duration of analgesia, and intrinsic activity (maximum efficacy) are presented in Table 31–2.

STRONG AGONISTS

1. Phenanthrenes

Morphine, **hydromorphone,** and **oxymorphone** are strong agonists useful in treating severe pain. These prototypic agents have been described in detail above. **Heroin** (diamorphine, diacetylmorphine) is potent and fast-acting, but its use is prohibited in the USA and Canada. In recent years, there has been considerable agitation to revive its use. However, double-blind studies have not supported the claim that heroin is more effec-

Table 31–5. Opioid drug interactions.

Drug Group	Interaction With Opioids
Sedative-hypnotics	Increased central nervous system depression, particularly respiratory depression.
Antipsychotic tranquilizers	Increased sedation. Variable effects on respiratory depression. Accentuation of cardiovascular effects (antimuscarinic and α-blocking actions).
MAO inhibitors	Relative contraindication to all opioid analgesics because of the high incidence of hyperpyrexic coma; hypertension has also been reported.

MAO, monoamine oxidase.

tive than morphine in relieving severe chronic pain, at least when given by the intramuscular route.

2. Phenylheptylamines

Methadone has undergone a dramatic revival as a potent and clinically useful analgesic. It can be administered by the oral, intravenous, subcutaneous, and rectal routes. It is well absorbed from the gastrointestinal tract and its bioavailability far exceeds that of oral morphine. Methadone is not only a potent μ receptor agonist but its racemic mixture of d- and l-methadone isomers can block both NMDA receptors and monoaminergic reuptake. These nonopioid receptor properties may help explain its ability to relieve difficult-to-treat pain (neuropathic, cancer pain), especially when a previous trial of morphine has failed. In this regard, when analgesic tolerance or intolerable side effects have developed with the use of increasing doses of morphine or hydromorphone, "opioid rotation" to methadone has provided superior analgesia at 10–20% of the morphine-equivalent daily dose. In contrast to its use in suppressing symptoms of opioid withdrawal, use of methadone as an analgesic typically requires administration at intervals of at least every 8 hours. However, given methadone's highly variable pharmacokinetics and long half-life (25–52 hours), initial administration should be closely monitored to avoid potentially harmful side effects, such as respiratory depression.

Methadone is widely known for its use in the treatment of opioid abuse. Tolerance and physical dependence develop more slowly with methadone than with morphine. The withdrawal signs and symptoms occurring after abrupt discontinuance of methadone are milder, although more prolonged, than those of morphine. These properties make methadone a useful drug for detoxification and for maintenance of the chronic relapsing heroin addict.

For detoxification of a heroin-dependent addict, low doses of methadone (5–10 mg orally) are given two or three times daily for 2 or 3 days. Upon discontinuing methadone, the addict experiences a mild but endurable withdrawal syndrome.

For maintenance therapy of the opioid recidivist, tolerance to 50–100 mg/d of oral methadone may be deliberately produced; in this state, the addict experiences cross-tolerance to heroin that prevents most of the addiction-reinforcing effects of heroin. One rationale of maintenance programs is that blocking the reinforcement obtained from abuse of illicit opioids removes the drive to obtain them, thereby reducing criminal activity and making the addict more amenable to psychiatric and rehabilitative therapy. The pharmacologic basis for the use of methadone in maintenance programs is sound and the sociologic basis is rational, but some methadone programs fail because nonpharmacologic management is inadequate.

The concurrent administration of methadone to heroin addicts known to be recidivists has been questioned due to the increased risk of overdose death secondary to respiratory arrest. Buprenorphine, a partial μ receptor agonist with long-acting properties, has been found to be effective in opioid detoxification and maintenance programs and is presumably associated with a lower risk of such overdose fatalities.

3. Phenylpiperidines

Meperidine and **fentanyl** are the most widely used agents in this family of synthetic opioids. Meperidine has significant antimuscarinic effects, which may be a contraindication if tachycardia would be a problem. It is also reported to have a negative inotropic action on the heart. The potential for producing seizures secondary to accumulation of normeperidine in patients receiving high doses of meperidine or with renal compromise must be considered. The fentanyl subgroup now includes **sufentanil, alfentanil,** and **remifentanil** in addition to the parent compound, fentanyl. These opioids differ mainly in their potency and biodisposition. Sufentanil is five to seven times more potent than fentanyl. Alfentanil is considerably less potent than fentanyl, acts more rapidly, and has a markedly shorter duration of action. Remifentanil is metabolized very rapidly by blood and nonspecific tissue esterases, making its pharmacokinetic and pharmacodynamic half-lives extremely short.

4. Morphinans

Levorphanol is a synthetic opioid analgesic closely resembling morphine in its action.

MILD TO MODERATE AGONISTS

1. Phenanthrenes

Codeine (Figure 31–1), **oxycodone, dihydrocodeine,** and **hydrocodone** are all somewhat less efficacious than morphine (they are partial agonists) or have adverse effects that limit the maximum tolerated dose when one attempts to achieve analgesia comparable to that of morphine. These compounds are rarely used alone but are combined in formulations containing aspirin or acetaminophen and other drugs.

2. Phenylheptylamines

Propoxyphene is chemically related to methadone but has low analgesic activity. Various studies have reported its potency at levels ranging from no better than placebo to half as potent as codeine, ie, 120 mg propoxyphene = 60 mg codeine. Its true potency probably lies somewhere between these extremes, and its analgesic effect is additive to that of an optimal dose of aspirin. However, its low efficacy makes it unsuitable, even in combination with aspirin, for severe pain. Although propoxyphene has a low abuse liability, the increasing incidence of deaths associated with its misuse has caused it to be scheduled as a controlled substance with low potential for abuse.

3. Phenylpiperidines

Diphenoxylate and its metabolite, **difenoxin,** are not used for analgesia but for the treatment of diarrhea. They are scheduled for minimal control (difenoxin is schedule IV, diphenoxylate schedule V; see inside front cover) because the likelihood of their abuse is remote. The poor solubility of the compounds limits their use for parenteral injection. As antidiarrheal drugs, they are used in combination with atropine. The atropine is added in a concentration too low to have a significant antidiarrheal effect but is presumed to further reduce the likelihood of abuse.

Loperamide is a phenylpiperidine derivative used to control diarrhea. Its potential for abuse is considered very low because of its limited access to the brain. It is therefore available without a prescription.

The usual dose with all of these antidiarrheal agents is two tablets to start and then one tablet after each diarrheal stool.

OPIOIDS WITH MIXED RECEPTOR ACTIONS

Care should be taken not to administer any partial agonist or drug with mixed opioid receptor actions to patients receiving pure agonist drugs because of the unpredictability of both drugs' effects: reduction of analgesia or precipitation of an explosive abstinence syndrome may result.

1. Phenanthrenes

Nalbuphine is a strong κ receptor *agonist* and a μ receptor *antagonist;* it is given parenterally. At higher doses there seems to be a definite ceiling—not noted with morphine—to the respiratory depressant effect. Unfortunately, when respiratory depression does occur, it may be relatively resistant to naloxone reversal.

Buprenorphine is a potent and long-acting phenanthrene derivative that is a partial μ receptor agonist. Its long duration of action is due to its slow dissociation from μ receptors. This property renders its effects resistant to naloxone reversal. Its clinical applications are much like those of nalbuphine. In addition, studies continue to suggest that buprenorphine is as effective as methadone in the detoxification and maintenance of heroin abusers.

2. Morphinans

Butorphanol produces analgesia equivalent to nalbuphine and buprenorphine but appears to produce more sedation at equianalgesic doses. Butorphanol is considered to be predominantly a κ agonist. However, it may also act as a partial agonist or antagonist at the μ receptor.

3. Benzomorphans

Pentazocine is a κ agonist with weak μ antagonist or partial agonist properties. It is the oldest mixed agent available. It may be used orally or parenterally. However, because of its irritant properties, the injection of pentazocine subcutaneously is not recommended.

Dezocine is a compound structurally related to pentazocine. It has its highest affinity for μ receptors and less interaction with κ receptors. Although it is said to be equivalent in efficacy to morphine, its use is associated with the same problems observed with all opioids that have mixed receptor actions.

MISCELLANEOUS

Tramadol is a central-acting analgesic whose mechanism of action is predominantly based on enhanced serotonergic neurotransmission. As such, its analgesic effectiveness can be blocked by coadministration of the serotonin (5-HT$_3$) receptor antagonist ondansetron. Tramadol also inhibits norepinephrine transporter function and is a weak μ receptor agonist, since it is only partially antagonized by naloxone. The recommended dosage is 50–100 mg orally four times daily. Toxicity includes association with seizures; the drug is relatively contraindicated in patients with a history of epilepsy and for use with other drugs that lower the seizure threshold. Other side effects include nausea and dizziness, but these symptoms typically abate following several days of therapy. Surprisingly, no clinically relevant effects on respiration or the cardiovascular system have thus far been reported. Given the fact that the analgesic action of tramadol is largely independent of μ receptor action, this agent may be useful in atypical pain such as chronic neuropathic pain.

ANTITUSSIVES

As noted above, the opioid analgesics are among the most effective drugs available for the suppression of cough. This effect is often achieved at doses below those

necessary to produce analgesia. The receptors involved in the antitussive effect appear to differ from those associated with the other actions of opioids. For example, the antitussive effect is also produced by stereoisomers of opioid molecules that are devoid of analgesic effects and addiction liability (see below).

The physiologic mechanism of cough is complex, and little is known about the specific mechanism of action of the opioid antitussive drugs. It is likely that both central and peripheral effects play a role.

The opioid derivatives most commonly used as antitussives are dextromethorphan, codeine, levopropoxyphene, and noscapine (levopropoxyphene and noscapine are not available in the USA). While these agents (other than codeine) are largely free of the adverse effects associated with the opioids, they should be used with caution in patients taking monoamine oxide (MAO) inhibitors (see Table 31–5). Antitussive preparations usually also contain expectorants to thin and liquefy respiratory secretions.

Dextromethorphan is the dextrorotatory stereoisomer of a methylated derivative of levorphanol. It is purported to be free of addictive properties and produces less constipation than codeine. The usual antitussive dose is 15–30 mg three or four times daily. It is available in many over-the-counter products. Dextromethorphan has also been found to enhance the analgesic action of morphine and presumably other μ receptor agonists.

Codeine, as noted above, has a useful antitussive action at doses lower than those required for analgesia. Thus, 15 mg is usually sufficient to relieve cough.

Levopropoxyphene is the stereoisomer of the weak opioid agonist dextropropoxyphene. It is devoid of opioid effects, although sedation has been described as a side effect. The usual antitussive dose is 50–100 mg every 4 hours.

THE OPIOID ANTAGONISTS

The pure opioid antagonist drugs **naloxone** (Figure 31–1), **naltrexone,** and **nalmefene** are morphine derivatives with bulkier substituents at the N$_{17}$ position. These agents have a relatively high affinity for μ opioid binding sites. They have lower affinity for the other receptors but can also reverse agonists at δ and κ sites.

Pharmacokinetics

Naloxone has poor efficacy when given by the oral route and a short duration of action (1–2 hours) when given by injection. Metabolic disposition is chiefly by glucuronide conjugation like that of the agonist opioids with free hydroxyl groups. Naltrexone is well absorbed after oral administration but may undergo rapid first-pass metabolism. It has a half-life of 10 hours, and a single oral dose of 100 mg will block the effects of injected heroin for up to 48 hours. Nalmefene, the newest of these agents, is a derivative of naltrexone but is available only for intravenous administration. Like naloxone, nalmefene is used for opioid overdose but has a longer half-life (8–10 hours).

Pharmacodynamics

When given in the absence of an agonist drug, these antagonists are almost inert at doses that produce marked antagonism of agonist effects.

When given intravenously to a morphine-treated subject, the antagonist will completely and dramatically reverse the opioid effects within 1–3 minutes. In individuals who are acutely depressed by an overdose of an opioid, the antagonist will effectively normalize respiration, level of consciousness, pupil size, bowel activity, and awareness of pain. In dependent subjects who appear normal while taking opioids, naloxone or naltrexone will almost instantaneously precipitate an abstinence syndrome, as described previously.

There is no tolerance to the antagonistic action of these agents, nor does withdrawal after chronic administration precipitate an abstinence syndrome.

Clinical Use

Naloxone is a pure antagonist and is preferred over older weak agonist-antagonist agents that had been used primarily as antagonists, eg, nalorphine and levallorphan.

The major application of naloxone is in the treatment of acute opioid overdose (see also Chapter 59). *It is very important that the relatively short duration of action of* *naloxone be borne in mind, because a severely depressed patient may recover after a single dose of naloxone and appear normal, only to relapse into coma after 1–2 hours.*

The usual initial dose of naloxone is 0.1–0.4 mg intravenously for life-threatening respiratory and CNS depression. Treatment is with the same drug, 0.4–0.8 mg given intravenously, and repeated whenever necessary. In using naloxone in the severely opioid-depressed newborn, it is important to start with doses of 5–10 μg/kg and to consider a second dose of up to a total of 25 μg/kg if no response is noted.

Low-dose naloxone (0.04 mg) has an increasing role in the treatment of adverse effects that are commonly associated with the use of intravenous or epidural opioids. Careful titration of the naloxone dosage can often eliminate the itching, nausea, and vomiting while sparing the analgesia. Oral naloxone, and more recently developed nonabsorbable analogs of naloxone, have been shown to be efficacious in the treatment of opioid-induced ileus or constipation. The principal mechanism behind this selective therapeutic effect is believed to be local inhibition of μ receptors in the gut with minimal systemic absorption.

Because of its long duration of action, naltrexone has been proposed as a maintenance drug for addicts in treatment programs. A single dose given on alternate days blocks virtually all of the effects of a dose of heroin. It might be predicted that this approach to rehabilitation would not be popular with a large percentage of drug users unless they are motivated to become drug-free. There is evidence that naltrexone decreases craving for alcohol in chronic alcoholics, and it has been approved by the US Food and Drug Administration for this purpose (see Chapter 23).

PREPARATIONS AVAILABLE[1]

ANALGESIC OPIOIDS
  Alfentanil (Alfenta)
    Parenteral: 0.5 mg/mL for injection
  Buprenorphine (Buprenex, others)
    Oral: 2, 8 mg sublingual tablets
    Parenteral: 0.3 mg/mL for injection
  Butorphanol (generic, Stadol)
    Parenteral: 1, 2 mg/mL for injection
    Nasal (generic, Stadol NS): 10 mg/mL nasal spray
  Codeine (sulfate or phosphate) (generic)
    Oral: 15, 30, 60 mg tablets, 15 mg/5 mL solution
    Parenteral: 30, 60 mg/mL for injection
  Dezocine (Dalgan)
    Parenteral: 5, 10, 15 mg/mL for injection

Fentanyl
  Parenteral (generic, Sublimaze): 50 mg/mL for injection
  Fentanyl Transdermal System (Duragesic): 25, 50, 75, 100 μg/h delivery
  Fentanyl Oralet: 100, 200, 300, 400 μg oral lozenge
  Fentanyl Actiq: 200, 400, 600, 800, 1200, 1600 μg lozenge on a stick
Hydromorphone (generic, Dilaudid)
  Oral: 1, 2, 3, 4, 8 mg tablets; 5 mg/mL liquid
  Parenteral: 1, 2, 4, 10 mg/mL for injection
  Rectal: 3 mg suppositories

[1]Antidiarrheal opioid preparations are listed in Chapter 63.

Levomethadyl acetate (Orlaam)
Oral: 10 mg/mL solution. *Note:* Approved only for the treatment of narcotic addiction.
Levorphanol (generic, Levo-Dromoran)
Oral: 2 mg tablets
Parenteral: 2 mg/mL for injection
Meperidine (generic, Demerol)
Oral: 50, 100 mg tablets; 50 mg/5 mL syrup
Parenteral: 25, 50, 75, 100 mg per dose for injection
Methadone (generic, Dolophine)
Oral: 5, 10 mg tablets; 40 mg dispersible tablets; 1, 2, 10 mg/mL solutions
Parenteral: 10 mg/mL for injection
Morphine sulfate (generic, others)
Oral: 10, 15, 30 mg tablets; 15, 30 mg capsules; 10, 20, 100 mg/5 mL solution
Oral sustained-release tablets (MS-Contin, others): 15, 30, 60, 100, 200 mg tablets);
Oral sustained-release capsules (Kadian): 20, 50, 100 mg capsules
Parenteral: 0.5, 1, 2, 4, 5, 8, 10, 15, 25, 50 mg/mL for injection
Rectal: 5, 10, 20, 30 mg suppositories
Nalbuphine (generic, Nubain)
Parenteral: 10, 20 mg/mL for injection
Oxycodone (generic)
Oral: 5 mg tablets, capsules; 1, 20 mg/mL solutions
Oral sustained-release (OxyContin): 10, 20, 40, 80, 100 mg tablets
Oxymorphone (Numorphan)
Parenteral: 1, 1.5 mg/mL for injection
Rectal: 5 mg suppositories
Pentazocine (Talwin)
Oral: See combinations.
Parenteral: 30 mg/mL for injection
Propoxyphene (generic, Darvon Pulvules, others)
Oral: 65 mg capsules, 100 mg tablets. *Note:* This product is not recommended.
Remifentanil (Ultiva)
Parenteral: 3, 5, 10 mg powder for reconstitution for injection
Sufentanil (generic, Sufenta)
Parenteral: 50 μg/mL for injection
Tramadol (Ultram)
Oral: 50 mg tablets

ANALGESIC COMBINATIONS[2]
Codeine/acetaminophen (generic, Tylenol w/ Codeine, others)
Oral: 15, 30, 60 mg codeine plus 300 or 325 mg acetaminophen tablets or capsules; 12 mg codeine plus 120 mg acetaminophen tablets
Codeine/aspirin (generic, Empirin Compound, others)
Oral: 30, 60 mg codeine plus 325 mg aspirin tablets
Hydrocodone/acetaminophen (generic, Norco, Vicodin, Lortab, others)
Oral: 2.5, 5, 7.5, 10 mg hydrocodone plus 500 or 650 mg acetaminophen tablets
Hydrocodone/ibuprofen (Vicoprofen)
Oral: 7.5 mg hydrocodone plus 200 mg ibuprofen
Oxycodone/acetaminophen (generic, Percocet, Tylox, others). *Note:* High-dose acetaminophen has potential for hepatic toxicity with repeated use.
Oral: 5 mg oxycodone plus 325 or 500 mg acetaminophen tablets
Oxycodone/aspirin (generic, Percodan)
Oral: 4.9 mg oxycodone plus 325 mg aspirin
Propoxyphene/aspirin or acetaminophen (Darvon Compound-65, others). *Note:* This product is not recommended.
Oral: 65 mg propoxyphene plus 389 mg aspirin plus 32.4 mg caffeine; 50, 65, 100 mg propoxyphene plus 325 or 650 mg acetaminophen.

OPIOID ANTAGONISTS
Nalmefene (Revex)
Parenteral: 0.1, 1 mg/mL for injection
Naloxone (Narcan, various)
Parenteral: 0.4, 1 mg/mL; 0.02 mg/mL (for neonatal use) for injection
Naltrexone (ReVia, Depade)
Oral: 50 mg tablets

ANTITUSSIVES
Codeine (generic, others)
Oral: 15, 30, 60 mg tablets; constituent of many proprietary syrups[2]
Dextromethorphan (generic, Benylin DM, Delsym, others)
Oral: 2.5, 5, 7.5, 15 mg lozenges; 3.5, 5, 7.5, 10, 15 mg/5 mL syrup; 30 mg sustained-action liquid; constituent of many proprietary syrups[1]

---

[2] Dozens of combination products are available; only a few of the most commonly prescribed ones are listed here. Codeine combination products available in several strengths are usually denoted No. 2 (15 mg codeine), No. 3 (30 mg codeine), and No. 4 (60 mg codeine). Prescribers should be aware of the possible danger of renal damage with acetaminophen, aspirin, and nonsteroidal anti-inflammatory drugs contained in these analgesic combinations.

REFERENCES

Akil H et al: Endogenous opioids: overview and current issues. Drug Alcohol Depend 1998;51:127.

Arcioni R et al: Ondansetron inhibits the analgesic effects of tramadol: a possible 5-HT(3) spinal receptor involvement in acute pain in humans. Anesth Analg 2002;94:1553.

Basbaum AI, Woolf CJ: Pain. Curr Biol 1999;9:R429.

Basbaum AI, Jessel T: The Perception of Pain. In Kandel ER et al (editors): *Principles of Neural Science*, 4th ed, McGraw-Hill, 2000.

Benedetti C, Bonica JJ (editors): Recent advances in intraspinal pain therapy. Acta Anaesthesiol Scand 1987;31(Suppl 85):1.

Benedetti C, Premuda L: The history of opium and its derivatives. In: Benedetti C et al (editors). *Advances in Pain Research and Therapy*, vol 14. Raven Press, 1990.

Bolan EA, Tallarida RJ, Pasternak GW: Synergy between mu opioid ligands: evidence for functional interactions among mu opioid receptor subtypes. J Pharmacol Exp Ther 2002;303:557.

Bonci A, Williams JT: Increased probability of GABA release during withdrawal from morphine. J Neurosci 1997;17:796.

Braga PC: Centrally acting opioid drugs. In: Braga PC, Allegra L (editors). *Cough.* Raven Press, 1989.

Crain SM, Shen K-F: Opioids can evoke direct receptor-mediated excitatory effects on sensory neurons. Trends Pharmacol Sci 1990;11:77.

Davis MP, Walsh D: Methadone for relief of cancer pain: a review of pharmacokinetics, pharmacodynamics, drug interactions and protocols of administration. Support Care Cancer 2001;9:73.

De Kock M, Lavand'homme P, Waterloos H: "Balanced analgesia" in the perioperative period: is there a place for ketamine? Pain 2001;92:373.

Eilers HM et al: The reversal of fentanyl-induced tolerance by administration of "small-dose" ketamine. Anesth Analg 2001;93:213.

Evans CJ et al: Cloning of a delta opioid receptor by functional expression. Science 1992;258:1952.

Ferner RE, Daniels AM: Office-based treatment of opioid-dependent patients. N Engl J Med 2003;348:81.

Ferrante FM: Principles of opioid pharmacotherapy: Practical implications of basic mechanisms. J Pain Symptom Manage 1996;11:265.

Fields HL, Basbaum AI: Central nervous system mechanisms of pain modulation. In: Wall PD, Melzack R (editors). *Textbook of Pain.* Churchill Livingstone, 1999.

Fields HL, Heinricher MM, Mason P: Neurotransmitters in nociceptive modulatory circuits. Annu Rev Neurosci 1991;14:219.

Foley KM: Misconceptions and controversies regarding the use of opioids in cancer pain. Anticancer Drugs 1995;6(Suppl 3):4.

Galamba JM et al: Continuous subcutaneous infusion of opioids in cancer patients. Ugeskr Laeger 1995;157:4126.

Gear RW et al: Kappa opioids produce significantly greater analgesia in women than in men. Nature Med 1996;2:1248.

Goldman D, Barr CS: Restoring the addicted brain. N Engl J Med 2002;347:843.

Hill HF, Mather LE: Patient-controlled analgesia. Pharmacokinetic and therapeutic considerations. Clin Pharmacokinet 1993;24:124.

Irwin RS, Curley FJ, Bennett FM: Appropriate use of antitussives and protussives: A practical review. Drugs 1993;46:80.

Julius D, Basbaum AI: Molecular mechanisms of nociception. Nature 2001;413:203.

Kaiko RF et al: Pharmacokinetic-pharmacodynamic relationships of controlled release oxycodone. Clin Pharmacol Ther 1996;59:52.

Kapusta D: Opioid mechanisms controlling renal function. Clin Exp Pharmacol Physiol 1995;22:891.

Kieffer BL: Opioids: first lessons from knockout mice. Trends Pharmacol Sci 1999;20:19.

Kirkwood LC et al: Characterization of the human cytochrome P450 enzymes involved in the metabolism of dihydrocodeine. Br J Clin Pharmacol 1997;44:549.

Kovelowski CJ et al: Supraspinal cholecystokinin may drive tonic descending facilitation mechanisms to maintain neuropathic pain in the rat. Pain 2000;87:265.

Kromer W: Endogenous and exogenous opioids in the control of gastrointestinal motility and secretion. Pharmacol Rev 1988;40:121.

Kuhar MJ, Pasternak GW (editors): *Analgesics: Neurochemical, Behavioral, and Clinical Perspectives.* Raven Press, 1984.

Labroo RB et al: Fentanyl metabolism by human hepatic and intestinal cytochrome P450 3A4: implications for interindividual variability in disposition, efficacy, and drug interactions. Drug Metab Dispos 1997;25:1072.

Laughlin TM, Larson AA, Wilcox GL: Mechanisms of induction of persistent nociception by dynorphin. J Pharmacol Exp Ther 2001;299:6.

Liu JG, Anand KJ: Protein kinases modulate the cellular adaptations associated with opioid tolerance and dependence. Brain Res Brain Res Rev 2001;38:1.

Marais E, Klugbauer N, Hofmann F: Calcium channel alpha(2)delta subunits-structure and Gabapentin binding. Mol Pharmacol 2001;59:1243.

Marubio LM et al: Reduced antinociception in mice lacking neuronal nicotinic receptor subunits Nature. 1999;398:805.

McGaraughty S, Heinricher MM: Microinjection of morphine into various amygdaloid nuclei differentially affects nociceptive responsiveness and RVM neuronal activity. Pain 2002;96:153.

Mellon RD et al: Evidence for central opioid receptors in the immunomodulatory effects of morphine: Review of potential mechanisms of action. J Neuroimmunology 1998;83:19.

Mercadante S: Opioid rotation for cancer pain: rationale and clinical aspects. Cancer 1999;86:1856.

Meunier J, Mouledous L, Topham CM: The nociceptin (ORL1) receptor: molecular cloning and functional architecture. Peptides 2000;21:893.

Mitchell JM, Basbaum AI, Fields HL: A locus and mechanism of action for associative morphine tolerance. Nat Neurosci 2000;3:47.

Pan YX et al: Generation of the mu opioid receptor (MOR-1) protein by three new splice variants of the Oprm gene. Proc Natl Acad Sci U S A 2001;98:14084.

Parris WC et al: The use of controlled-release oxycodone for the treatment of chronic cancer pain: a randomized, double-blind study. J Pain Symptom Manage 1998;16:205.

Paul D et al: Pharmacological characterization of morphine 6-β glucuronide, a very potent morphine metabolite. J Pharmacol Exp Ther 1989;251:477.

Pechnik RN: Effect of opioids on the hypothalamo-pituitary-adrenal axis. Annu Rev Pharmacol Toxicol 1993;32:353.

Perneger TV et al: Risk of kidney failure associated with use of acetaminophen, aspirin, and nonsteroidal anti-inflammatory drugs. N Engl J Med 1994;331:1675.

Quock RM et al: The delta-opioid receptor: molecular pharmacology, signal transduction, and the determination of drug efficacy. Pharmacol Rev 1999;51:503.

Rasmussen K et al: Opiate withdrawal from the rat locus coeruleus [sic]: Behavioral, electrophysiologic, and biochemical correlates. J Neurosci 1990;10:2308.

Rouveix B: Opiates and immune function. Therapie 1992;47:503.

Self DW, Nestler E: Molecular mechanisms of drug reinforcement and addiction. Annu Rev Neurosci 1995;18:463.

Shir Y et al: Methadone is safe for treating hospitalized patients with severe pain. Can J Anaesth 2001;48:1109.

Sindrup SH, Jensen TS: Efficacy of pharmacological treatments of neuropathic pain: an update and effect related to mechanism of drug action. Pain 1999;83:389.

Smith MT: Neuroexcitatory effects of morphine and hydromorphone: evidence implicating the 3-glucuronide metabolites. Clin Exp Pharmacol Physiol 2000;27:524.

Smith NT et al: Seizures during opioid anesthetic induction: Are they opioid-induced rigidity? Anesthesiology 1989;71:852.

Stein C: The control of pain in peripheral tissue by opioids. N Engl J Med 1995;332:1685.

Thirlwell MP et al: Pharmacokinetics and clinical efficacy of oral morphine solution and controlled-release morphine tablets in cancer patients. Cancer 1989;63:2275.

Tzschentke TM: Behavioral pharmacology of buprenorphine, with a focus on preclinical models of reward and addiction. Psychopharmacology (Berl) 2002;161:1.

Vanderah TW et al: Mechanisms of opioid-induced pain and antinociceptive tolerance: descending facilitation and spinal dynorphin. Pain 2001;92:5.

Von Dossow V et al: Thoracic epidural anesthesia combined with general anesthesia: the preferred anesthetic technique for thoracic surgery. Anesth Analg 2001;92:848.

Wang Z et al: Pronociceptive actions of dynorphin maintain chronic neuropathic pain. J Neurosci 2001;21:1779.

Way EL: Opioid tolerance and physical dependence and their relationship. In: Herz A et al (editors). *Handbook of Experimental Pharmacology*. Vol 104: II. Opioids. Springer, 1993.

Weinbroum AA et al: Dextromethorphan for the reduction of immediate and late postoperative pain and morphine consumption in orthopedic oncology patients: a randomized, placebo-controlled, double-blind study. Cancer 2002; 95:1164.

Williams JT, Christie MJ, Manzoni O: Cellular and synaptic adaptations mediating opioid dependence. Physiol Rev 2001;81:299.

Woolf CJ, Salter MW: Neuronal plasticity: increasing the gain in pain. Science 2000;288:1765.

Yaster M, Deshpande JK: Management of pediatric pain with opioid analgesics. J Pediatr 1988;113:421.

Yeadon M, Kitchen I: Opioids and respiration. Prog Neurobiol 1989;33:1.

Yuan CS et al: Methylnaltrexone for reversal of constipation due to chronic methadone use: a randomized controlled trial. JAMA 2000;283:367.

Zadina JE: A potent and selective endogenous agonist for the mu-opiate receptor. Nature 1997;386:499.

Zhao GM et al: Profound spinal tolerance after repeated exposure to a highly selective mu-opioid peptide agonist: role of delta-opioid receptors. J Pharmacol Exp Ther 2002;302:188.

Zubieta JK et al: Regional mu opioid receptor regulation of sensory and affective dimensions of pain. Science 2001;293:311.

Drugs of Abuse

Thomas R. Kosten, MD

The term "drug abuse" is unfortunate because it connotes social disapproval and may have different meanings to different people. One must also distinguish drug abuse from drug misuse. Abuse of a drug might be construed as any use of a drug for nonmedical purposes, usually for altering consciousness but also for body-building. To misuse a drug might be to take it for the wrong indication, in the wrong dosage, or for too long a period, to mention only a few obvious examples. In the context of drug abuse, the drug itself is of less importance than the pattern of use. For example, taking 50 mg of diazepam to heighten the effect of a daily dose of methadone is an abuse of diazepam. On the other hand, taking the same excessive daily dose of the drug but only for its anxiolytic effect is misusing diazepam.

Dependence is a biologic phenomenon often associated with "drug abuse." **Psychologic dependence** is manifested by compulsive drug-seeking behavior in which the individual uses the drug repetitively for personal satisfaction, often in the face of known risks to health. Cigarette smoking is an example. Deprivation of the agent for a short period of time typically results in a strong desire or *craving* for it. **Physiologic dependence** is present when withdrawal of the drug produces symptoms and signs that are frequently the opposite of those sought by the user. It has been suggested that the body adjusts to a new level of homeostasis during the period of drug use and reacts in opposite fashion when the new equilibrium is disturbed. Alcohol withdrawal syndrome is perhaps the best-known example, but milder degrees of withdrawal may be observed in people who drink a lot of coffee every day. Psychologic dependence almost always precedes physiologic dependence but does not inevitably lead to it. **Addiction** is usually taken to mean a state of physiologic and psychologic dependence, but the word is too imprecise for scientific usage.

Tolerance signifies a decreased response to the effects of the drug, necessitating ever larger doses to achieve the same effect. Tolerance is closely associated with the phenomenon of physiologic dependence. It is largely due to compensatory responses that mitigate the drug's pharmacodynamic action. **Metabolic tolerance** due to increased disposition of the drug after chronic use is occasionally reported. **Behavioral tolerance,** an ability to compensate for the drug's effects, is another possible mechanism of tolerance. **Functional tolerance,** which may be the most common type, is due to compensatory changes in receptors, effector enzymes, or membrane actions of the drug.

A number of experimental techniques have been devised to predict the ability of a drug to produce dependence and to assess its likelihood for abuse. Most of these techniques employ self-administration of the drug by animals. The rates of reinforcement can be altered so as to make the animal work harder for each dose of drug, providing a semiquantitative measure as well. Comparisons are made against a standard drug in the class, eg, morphine among the opioids. Withdrawal of dependent animals from drugs assesses the nature of the withdrawal syndrome and can be used to test drugs that might cross-substitute for the standard drug. Most agents with significant potential for psychologic or physiologic dependence can be readily detected by these techniques. The actual abuse liability, however, is difficult to predict, since many variables enter into the decision to abuse drugs.

Cultural Considerations

Each society accepts certain drugs as licit and condemns others as illicit. In the USA and most of Western Europe, the "national drugs" are caffeine, nicotine, and alcohol. In the Middle East, cannabis may be added to the list of licit drugs, whereas alcohol is forbidden. Among certain Native American tribes, peyote, a hallucinogen, may be used licitly for religious purposes. In the Andes of South America, cocaine is used to allay hunger and enhance the ability to perform arduous work at high altitudes. Thus, which drugs are licit or illicit or—to use other terminology—"used" or "abused" is a social judgment. A major social cost of relegating any substance to the illicit category is the criminal activity that often results, since purveyors of the substance are lured into illegal traffic by the opportunity to make large profits, while dependent users may resort to robbery, prostitution, and other types of antisocial behavior to support their habits. A major social and medical cost associated with *parenteral* abuse of drugs is the high incidence of transmission of HIV and hepatitis virus through the sharing of needles.

Current attitudes in the USA to drugs of this type are reflected in the Schedule of Controlled Drugs (see inside front cover). This schedule is quite similar to those published by international control bodies. Such schedules affect principally ethical and law-abiding manufacturers and prescribers of the drugs and have little deterrent effect on illicit manufacturers or suppliers. Such schedules have been circumvented by the synthesis of "designer" drugs that make small modifications of the chemical structures of drugs with little or no change in their pharmacodynamic actions. Thus, schedules must constantly be revised to include these attempts to produce compounds not currently listed.

Because of the high social cost of drug abuse, many countries attempt to interdict their entry across borders. While surveys may indicate that the use of drugs such as cocaine and marijuana is increasing or decreasing, it is difficult to attribute such changes to law enforcement policies. Little progress has been made in decreasing the demand for illicit drugs. Some persons have argued that the only reasonable solution to the problem is legalization of the drugs. Such proposals are obviously highly controversial.

Any use of mind-altering drugs is based on a complicated interplay between three factors: the user, the setting in which the drug is taken, and the drug. Thus, the personality of the user and the setting may have a strong influence on what the user experiences. Nonetheless, it is usually possible to identify a pharmacologic "core" of drug effects that will be experienced by almost anyone under almost any circumstances if the dosage is adequate.

Neurobiology of Abused Drugs

During the last 20 years, substantial progress has been made in elucidating the neurobiology of abused drugs and their effects not only on neurotransmitter receptors and reuptake carriers but also on the cascade of second, third, and fourth intracellular messenger systems (Nestler, 2001). Many abused drugs act through G protein-linked receptors such as the opioid, cannabinoid, and dopamine receptors. These G proteins frequently are coupled to the cyclic adenosine monophosphate (cAMP) second messenger system, and through phosphorylation of various intracellular proteins a cascade of changes occurs in the cytoplasm and nucleus. Immediate early genes such as c-*fos* and c-*jun* are activated followed by regulation of other genes with more sustained effects on protein transcription that may lead to the observed down-regulation of receptor numbers and up-

regulation of second messenger systems. These effects on DNA are also reflective of genetic risk factors for drug dependence; it is estimated that up to 50% of the risk for dependence is due to polygenic inheritance. Extensive studies are underway for alcohol, opioids, and stimulants including nicotine in order to identify specific genes associated with this risk.

For each of the classes of abused drugs a complex molecular biology has been described, including specific neuroanatomic substrates linked to different neurotransmitters during acute intoxication and during withdrawal after dependence is established. Acute reinforcing effects of abused drugs are clearly a function of specific receptor binding but are also related to the *rate of change* in synaptic levels of dopamine, a key neurotransmitter involved in reinforcement in the nucleus accumbens. The chronic effects of abused drugs include tolerance and sensitization as well as the neurobiologic substrates for withdrawal symptoms. Much has been learned about these neurobiologic substrates for withdrawal in opioid dependence, including the activation of adrenergic brain systems such as the locus ceruleus during withdrawal. The latter findings have important treatment implications, such as the use of clonidine for opioid withdrawal.

Other drug classes, such as the benzodiazepines, have specific receptors on chloride channels associated with the neurotransmitter γ-aminobutyric acid (GABA), while other abused drugs, such as phencyclidine, bind to sites on excitatory amino acid receptor-channel complexes. The functions of other receptors that bind abused drugs such as opioid and cannabinoid receptors also have been clarified with the identification of endogenous ligands for these receptors, such as β-endorphin for the μ opioid receptor and anandamide for the cannabinoid receptor. These binding sites appear to be critical for the acute effects of these abused drugs, and substantial progress has been made in understanding the neurotransmitter basis for reinforcement of most abused drugs including recent work with the inhalant toluene (Riegel and French, 2002). The dopamine neurons connecting the ventral tegmental area to the nucleus accumbens have been considered the major reinforcement pathway for a wide range of abused drugs, but their role in reinforcement has been most clearly established for cocaine and amphetamine and less clearly for other drugs, particularly inhalants and several hallucinogens.

The neurobiologic findings in animal models have been increasingly confirmed in human studies. These human studies include pharmacologic challenges with neuroendocrine and behavioral outcomes, assessments of endogenous ligands in cerebrospinal fluid from drug-dependent patients, and neuroimaging studies, particularly neuroreceptor imaging. Available radioligands have permitted examination in humans of dopamine receptors and transporters, opioid receptors, and functional brain activity based on blood flow or glucose utilization. These receptor-neuroimaging studies have demonstrated that chronic abuse of drugs which can produce tolerance, dependence, and sensitization may have associated effects on receptor numbers (eg, dopamine D_2 receptors decrease in cocaine abusers) and on transporter numbers (eg, dopamine transporters increase in cocaine abusers). Blood flow and glucose utilization studies have shown that acute drug use is associated with substantial reductions in cerebral metabolic activity and that the rate of change is a correlate of the reinforcing effects of abused drugs.

In the following sections, we review current knowledge about the molecular neurobiology of each class of abused drugs and their clinical pharmacology.

OPIOIDS

History

The nepenthe (Gk "free from sorrow") mentioned in the *Odyssey* probably contained opium. Opium smoking was widely practiced in China and the Near East until recently. Isolation of active opium alkaloids and the introduction of the hypodermic needle, allowing parenteral use of morphine, increased opioid use in the West. The first of several "epidemics" of opioid use in the USA followed the Civil War. About 4% of adults in the USA used opiates regularly during the postbellum period. By the 1900s, the number had dropped to about 1 in 400 people in the USA, but the problem was still considered serious enough to justify passage of the Harrison Narcotic Act just before World War I. A new epidemic of opioid use started around 1964 and has continued unabated ever since. While fear of AIDS has reduced intravenous use of heroin, recent increases in its purity have led to markedly increased intranasal use. Present estimates are that the number of opioid-dependent people in the USA has stabilized at around 750,000.

Chemistry & Pharmacology

The most commonly abused drugs in this group are heroin, morphine, oxycodone, and—among health professionals—meperidine. The chemistry and general pharmacology of these agents are presented in Chapter 31.

Tolerance to the mental effects of opioids develops with long-term use. The need for ever-increasing amounts of drugs to sustain the desired euphoriant effects—as well as to avoid the discomfort of withdrawal—has the expected consequence of strongly reinforcing dependence once it has started. The role of endogenous opioid peptides in opioid dependence is uncertain.

Clinical Aspects

Intravenous administration is routine not only because it is the most efficient route but also because it produces a bolus of high concentration of drug that reaches the brain to produce a "rush," followed by euphoria, a feeling of tranquility, and sleepiness ("the nod"). Heroin produces effects that last 3–5 hours, and several doses a day are required to forestall manifestations of withdrawal in dependent persons. Symptoms of opioid withdrawal begin 8–10 hours after the last dose. Many of these symptoms resemble those of increased activity of the autonomic nervous system. Lacrimation, rhinorrhea, yawning, and sweating appear first. Restless sleep followed by weakness, chills, gooseflesh ("cold turkey"), nausea and vomiting, muscle aches, and involuntary movements ("kicking the habit"), hyperpnea, hyperthermia, and hypertension occur in later stages of the withdrawal syndrome. The acute course of withdrawal may last 7–10 days. A secondary phase of protracted abstinence lasts for 26–30 weeks and is characterized by hypotension, bradycardia, hypothermia, mydriasis, and decreased responsiveness of the respiratory center to carbon dioxide.

Heroin users in particular tend to be polydrug users, also using alcohol, sedatives, cannabinoids, and stimulants. None of these other drugs serve as substitutes for opioids, but they have desired additive effects. One needs to be sure that the person undergoing a withdrawal reaction is not also withdrawing from alcohol or other sedatives, which might be more dangerous and more difficult to manage.

Besides the ever-present risk of fatal overdose, hepatitis B and AIDS are among the many potential complications of sharing contaminated hypodermic syringes. Bacterial infections lead to septic complications such as meningitis, osteomyelitis, and abscesses in various organs. Attempts to illicitly manufacture meperidine have resulted in the highly specific neurotoxin 1-methyl-4-phenyl-1,2,3,6-tetrahydropyridine (MPTP), which produces parkinsonism in users (see Chapter 28).

Treatment

Treatment of acute overdoses of opioids can be lifesaving and is described in Chapters 31 and 59. In long-term treatment of opioid-dependent persons, pharmacologic and psychosocial approaches are often combined. Chronic users tend to prefer pharmacologic approaches; those with shorter histories of drug abuse are more amenable to detoxification and psychosocial interventions.

Pharmacologic treatment is most often used for detoxification. The principles of detoxification are the same for all drugs: to substitute a longer-acting, orally active, pharmacologically equivalent drug for the abused drug, stabilize the patient on that drug, and then gradually withdraw the substituted drug. **Methadone** is admirably suited for such use in opioid-dependent persons. **Clonidine**, a centrally acting sympatholytic agent, has also been used for detoxification. By reducing central sympathetic outflow, clonidine mitigates many of the signs of sympathetic overactivity. Clonidine has no narcotic action and is not addictive. Lofexidine, a clonidine analog with less hypotensive effect, is being developed for use.

While it is easy to detoxify patients, the recidivism rate (return to abuse of the agent) is high. Methadone maintenance therapy, which substitutes a long-acting orally active opioid for heroin, has been effective in some settings. A single dose can be given each day. Methadone saturates the opioid receptors and prevents the desired sudden onset of central nervous system effects normally produced by intravenous administration of additional opiates. An even longer-acting methadone analog, L-acetylmethadol, allows three times a week rather than daily dosing and reduced abuse potential, but its association with sudden cardiac death due to prolonged QT arrhythmias has made its use uncommon. Another candidate drug for use in this setting is buprenorphine, a partial opioid agonist, that can be given once daily or even less often at sublingual doses of 4–32 mg daily depending on the patient. The lower doses are useful for detoxification from heroin, while the higher doses are for longer maintenance treatment. Treatment in an office-based primary care setting is a potential advantage of this agent over methadone (Kosten, 2002).

Use of a narcotic antagonist is a rational alternative to the above agonist-based therapies because blocking the action of self-administered opioids should eventually extinguish the habit, but this therapy is poorly accepted by patients. Naltrexone, a long-acting orally active pure opioid antagonist, can be given three times a week at doses of 100–150 mg and a depot form for monthly administration is being developed. Because it is an antagonist, the patient must first be detoxified from opioid dependence before starting naltrexone.

Psychosocial approaches include drug-free residential communities, which use peer group pressures, emphasizing confrontation and discussion.

BARBITURATES, OTHER SEDATIVE-HYPNOTICS, & GHB

History

Ethanol is the sedative-hypnotic with the longest history of both use and abuse; it is discussed in Chapter 23.

Barbiturates were introduced in 1903; they have been largely replaced in medical practice by newer agents, especially **benzodiazepines** in the 1960s (see Chapter 22). Short-acting members of the sedative-hypnotic group are widely abused and the most recent addition to this abused group is **gamma-hydroxybutyric acid (GHB)**.

Chemistry & Pharmacology

The chemical relationships among this class of drugs are reviewed in Chapter 22. Depending on the dose, these drugs produce sedation, hypnosis, anesthesia, coma, and death. Both barbiturates and benzodiazepines can be classified pharmacokinetically into short- and long-acting compounds; GHB is relatively short-acting. Most abuse involves short-acting drugs, eg, secobarbital or pentobarbital sodium, and not long-acting ones, eg, phenobarbital. Drugs with half-lives in the range of 8–24 hours produce a rapidly evolving, severe withdrawal syndrome; those with longer half-lives, eg, 48–96 hours, produce a withdrawal syndrome that is slower in onset and less severe but longer in duration. Drugs with half-lives longer than 96 hours usually have a built-in tapering-off action that reduces the possibility of withdrawal reactions.

Clinical Aspects

Although statistics on alcoholism are extensive, no one knows how many persons are dependent on prescription sedatives. However, physiologic dependence has been relatively rare and usually occurs following long-term treatment with doses of 40 mg/d or more of diazepam or its equivalent. These abusers often are codependent on other drugs such as opioids, alcohol, or stimulants. "Therapeutic dose dependence" at doses of 15–30 mg/d of diazepam may be characterized by weight loss, changes in perception, paresthesias, and headache.

Finally, very rapid onset benzodiazepines have been widely reported as a means of "date rape," by using a small tasteless dose of the drug to make the victim incapable of protecting herself (or himself). This produces intoxication but not dependence. The drug most commonly used in this situation has been **flunitrazepam** (Rohypnol, "roofies," not available in the USA) and more recently GHB. The amnesia-producing effects of the benzodiazepines (see Chapter 22) make the victim unable to describe the events after she or he has recovered.

As these drugs are usually taken orally and the tablets or capsules are consistent in drug content, inadvertent fatal overdoses of single agents are rare. Tolerance may develop to the sedative effect but not to the respiratory depressant effect. Thus, if these drugs are used with other respiratory depressants, eg, large amounts of alcohol or opioids, fatalities can occur.

The withdrawal syndrome from sedatives is almost identical to that from alcohol and includes anxiety, tremors, twitches, and nausea and vomiting. In the case of long-acting drugs, symptoms may not appear for 2–3 days, and initial symptoms may suggest a recrudescence of those originally treated (nervousness, anxiety). Only by the fourth or fifth day can one be sure that a withdrawal reaction is under way. Convulsions are a late manifestation when they do occur—often not until the eighth or ninth day. Following this, the syndrome subsides. Severe cases are associated with delirium, hallucinations, and other psychosis-like manifestations.

Treatment

If short-acting drugs have been abused, chlordiazepoxide or phenobarbital is substituted as the pharmacologically equivalent agent. If long-acting drugs have been used, the same drug may be continued. The patient is stabilized on whatever dose is required to cause signs and symptoms to abate, and the drug is then gradually withdrawn. The rate of decrement may be 15–25% of the daily dose early in treatment, with later decrements of 5–10%. Complete detoxification can usually be achieved in less than 2 weeks.

No specific treatment programs have been developed for prescription sedative abusers. The problem is so often complicated by abuse of other drugs that it may be more expeditious to enroll the patient in a program designed for alcoholics or opiate-dependent persons. Patients with psychiatric disorders that can be defined, especially those with depression, may be treated with drug therapy specific for the underlying disorder.

STIMULANTS

History

In this section, caffeine is discussed only briefly and the focus is on other stimulants that produce psychiatric disorders. **Caffeine** can lead to a withdrawal syndrome characterized by lethargy, irritability, and headache, but withdrawal appears to occur in less than 3% of regular coffee drinkers. Moreover, the morbidity associated with caffeine overdose, which can include disturbing effects on sleep and heart rhythm, is much less than the morbidity associated with other stimulants.

Nicotine is one of the most widely used licit drugs because it is heavily promoted and produces powerful psychologic and physical dependence. About 28% of adults in the USA still smoke cigarettes because they have become dependent on nicotine. The use of smokeless tobacco products (eg, snuff, chewing tobacco) has increased in adolescents. Deaths directly attributable to smoking account for 20% of all deaths and 30% of cancer deaths in the USA. It is estimated that about 90% of cases of chronic obstructive pulmonary disease in the USA are due to smoking. **Cocaine** is a plant product that has been used for at least 1200 years in the custom of chewing coca leaves by natives of the South American Andes. In contrast, **amphetamine** was synthesized in the late 1920s and has a large number of analogs including **methylphenidate** (Ritalin) and **methylenedioxymethamphetamine** (MDMA, "ecstasy"). A closely related natural alkaloid, **cathinone,** is found in **khat,** a plant that produces effects indistinguishable from those of the amphetamines.

Chemistry & Pharmacology

Despite their similar behavioral effects, caffeine, nicotine, cocaine, and amphetamine have very different structures and sites of action in the brain. Caffeine, a methylxanthine compound, appears to exert its central actions (and perhaps some of its peripheral ones as well) by blocking adenosine receptors. Because caffeine does not act on the dopaminergic brain structures related to reward and addiction, its abuse and dependence potential are quite small. As noted in the above section Neurobiology of Abused Drugs, dopamine is very important in the reward system of the brain; its increase probably accounts for the high dependence potential of cocaine. Cocaine binds to the dopamine reuptake transporter in the central nervous system, effectively inhibiting reuptake of dopamine as well as norepinephrine. Amphetamines probably act mainly by increasing release of catecholaminergic neurotransmitters, including dopamine, by reversal of the vesicular transporter. A useful model of the action of these two drugs in the reward centers of the CNS is shown in Figure 32–1. Cocaine reduces reuptake of dopamine into the neuron by inhibiting the dopamine reuptake transporter. Amphetamine causes the intracellular release of dopamine within the terminal and reverses the transporter direction so that dopamine is released into the synapse by reverse transport rather than ordinary exocytosis. In addition, amphetamine inhibits intracellular MAO metabolism of dopamine. Note that both drugs result in an increase in the concentration of dopamine in the synapse.

Clinical Aspects

One common pattern of amphetamine or cocaine abuse is called a "run." Repeated smoked or intravenous injections are self-administered to obtain a "rush"—an orgasm-like reaction—followed by a feeling of mental alertness and marked euphoria. When free base cocaine is smoked, entry through the lungs is almost as fast as by intravenous injection, so that effects are more accentuated than when the drug is snorted (Figure 32–2). Because the plasma half-life of cocaine is short, effects following a single dose persist only for an hour or so and repeated dosing may occur every 30 minutes. Because tolerance develops quickly, abusers may take monumental doses compared with those used medically, eg, as anorexiants. Total daily amphetamine doses as high as 4000 mg have been reported. After several days of such spree use, subjects may enter a paranoid schizophrenia-like state. Typically, delusions that bugs are crawling under their skin develop, which leads to scratching and characteristic discrete excoriations. Finally, the spree is terminated by exhaustion from lack of sleep and lack of food, followed by a withdrawal syndrome. A typical pattern of withdrawal includes a ravenous appetite, exhaustion, and mental depression. This syndrome may last for several days after the drug is withdrawn.

Besides the paranoid psychosis associated with chronic use of amphetamines, a specific lesion associated with chronic amphetamine use is necrotizing arteritis, which may involve many small and medium-sized arteries and lead to fatal brain hemorrhage or renal failure. Overdoses

of amphetamines are rarely fatal; they can usually be managed by sedating the patient with benzodiazepines.

Overdoses of cocaine are often rapidly fatal, victims dying within minutes from arrhythmias, seizures, or respiratory depression. Those who survive for 3 hours usually recover fully. Intravenous administration of diazepam, propranolol, or calcium channel-blocking drugs may be the best treatment. The local anesthetic action of cocaine contributes to the production of seizures. The powerful vasoconstrictive action of cocaine has led to a significant number of patients with severe acute hypertensive episodes resulting in myocardial infarcts and strokes. This vasoconstrictive effect may also contribute to the multiple brain perfusion defects that have been described using single photon emission computed tomography (SPECT) blood flow imaging in cocaine abusers (Kosten, 1998). Finally, an epidemic of "cocaine babies" born to mothers who are using cocaine heavily has posed a major new challenge to health care facilities in the inner cities (Mayes, 1999). There are clear-cut deleterious effects on the pregnancy, with increased fetal morbidity and mortality as well as early childhood impairment in learning and attention.

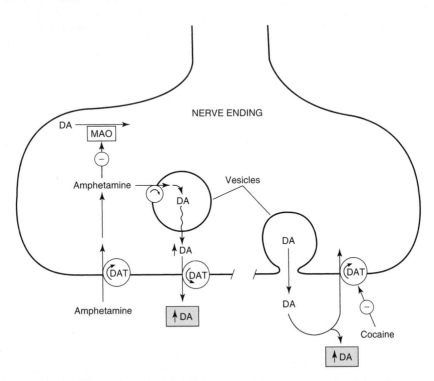

Figure 32–1. A model for the action of cocaine and amphetamine at a dopaminergic synapse in the central nervous system. Cocaine (right side) blocks the dopamine reuptake transporter (DAT). Amphetamine (left side) has several effects. It enters the nerve ending via reverse transport by the DAT and displaces dopamine (DA) from vesicles by altering their pH. It also inhibits dopamine metabolism by MAO in the nerve ending. The increased intraneuronal dopamine causes reversal of the DAT and dopamine floods into the synapse.

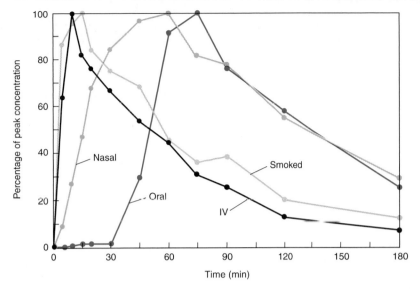

Figure 32–2. Comparison of blood concentrations achieved when cocaine is administered by different routes. Time to peak is nearly as fast by smoking as by intravenous injection. (Modified and reproduced, with permission, from Jones RT: The pharmacology of cocaine smoking in humans. In: *Research Findings on Smoking of Abused Substances. National Institute on Drug Abuse Research Monograph 99.* Chiang CN, Hawks RL [editors]. US Government Printing Office, 1990.)

Treatment

Subjects with residual emotional disorders, either schizophreniform psychosis or mental depression, may require treatment with antipsychotic or antidepressant drugs during weaning from stimulants. Dopamine agonists have been suggested to mitigate withdrawal from cocaine, reduce craving during abstinence, and facilitate abstinence, but neither these nor other agents have shown reliable efficacy. Depression occurs in up to 40% of stimulant-dependent patients, and antidepressants may be helpful for relapse prevention.

Nicotine dependence may respond to replacement therapy with either nicotine gum or transdermal patches, and detoxification from nicotine dependence has been described using clonidine. Bupropion, an antidepressant, also shows efficacy for smoking cessation. The nicotinic receptor blocker mecamylamine, which has good central nervous system access, has been used with limited efficacy. Overall, success rates for smoking abstinence at 1 year are about 20%, with even less success for depressed smokers.

HALLUCINOGENS

History

Almost every society has found some bark, skin, leaf, vine, berry, fungus, or weed that contains "hallucino-genic" materials, but neither hallucinations nor psychotic states are typically induced by these drugs. The more recent "club drugs" including MDMA have also been considered to be like hallucinogens, but club drugs are better considered as related to either stimulants (MDMA) or sedatives (GHB).

Chemistry & Pharmacology

The LSD-like group of drugs includes **lysergic acid diethylamide (LSD), mescaline, psilocybin,** and their related compounds. LSD is a synthetic agent related to the ergot alkaloids (see Chapter 16), while mescaline, a phenethylamine derivative, and psilocybin, an indol-ethylamine derivative, are found in nature. Representative structures are shown in Figure 32–3. These drugs also have chemical resemblances to three major neurotransmitters: norepinephrine, dopamine, and serotonin. LSD interacts with several serotonin (5-HT) receptor subtypes in the brain. The drug displays agonist activity at 5-HT$_{1A}$ and 5-HT$_{1C}$ receptors. These actions may be more relevant to LSD's hallucinogenic action than its 5-HT$_2$ receptor antagonism, because a number of other drugs with good antagonist effects at central 5-HT$_2$ receptors are not hallucinogenic.

Phencyclidine (PCP, "angel dust," many other names) is a synthetic phenylcyclohexylamine derivative originally used as a veterinary anesthetic. Ketamine, an

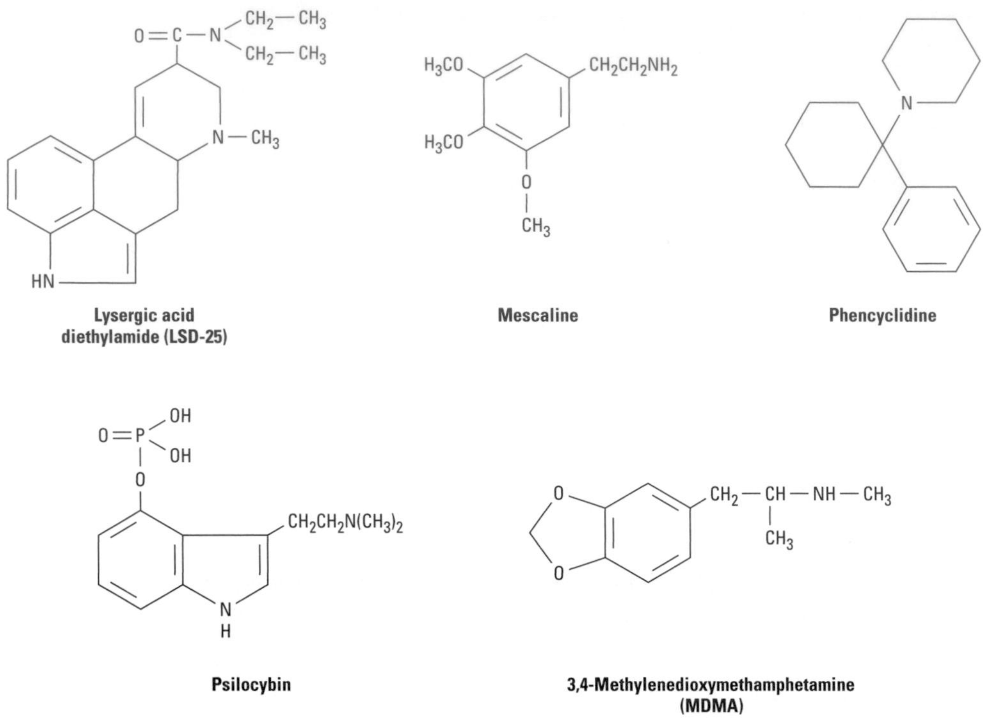

Figure 32–3. Chemical structures of lysergic acid diethylamide (LSD), mescaline, phencyclidine, psilocybin, and the amphetamine analog MDMA.

analog, replaced phencyclidine as an anesthetic for use in humans (see Chapter 25). It too produces some emergent hallucinogenic effects. Since the 1970s, PCP and more recently ketamine have become widely accepted by drug abusers as desirable hallucinogenic agents. Phencyclidine may be smoked (by mixing the powder with tobacco), "snorted," taken orally, or injected intravenously.

Receptors for PCP have been identified in the brain, and PCP acts as an antagonist on the N-methyl-D-aspartate (NMDA) subtype of glutamate receptors. The drug is unique among hallucinogens in that animals will self-administer it.

The deliriant hallucinogens, exemplified by scopolamine (see Chapter 8) and some synthetic centrally acting cholinoceptor-blocking agents, are different chemically as well as pharmacologically from the LSD group. Their effects seem to be entirely explainable by blockade of central muscarinic receptors. Similar mental effects may be seen during therapeutic or deliberate overdoses of commonly used medications with antimuscarinic action, such as anticholinergic antiparkinsonism drugs, tricyclic antidepressants, and antispasmodics. Occasional instances of abuse of these therapeutic agents have occurred.

Clinical Effects

LSD produces a series of somatic, perceptual, and psychological effects that overlap each other. Dizziness, weakness, tremors, nausea, and paresthesias are prominent somatic symptoms. Blurring of vision, distortions of perspective, organized visual illusions or "hallucinations," less discriminant hearing, and a change in sense of time are common perceptual abnormalities. Impaired memory, difficulty in thinking, poor judgment, and altered mood are prominent psychological effects. Physiologically, LSD produces signs of central stimulation and overactivity of the sympathetic nervous system, manifested by dilated pupils, increased heart rate, mild elevation of blood pressure, tremor, and alertness. Virtually identical effects are produced by mescaline and psilocybin when they are given in equivalent doses. The onset of effects is fairly rapid, but the duration varies with the dose and is usually measured in hours. Phenomena may vary considerably from one user to another owing to such factors as the personality and expectations of the user and the circumstances under which the drug is taken, but the above effects occur in almost everyone. Waxing and waning of effects is typical.

Usual doses of LSD in humans are approximately 1–2 µg/kg, making it one of the most potent pharmacologic agents known. The drug is equally effective parenterally or orally and consequently is almost always taken by mouth. Psilocybin is usually taken in doses of 250 µg/kg and mescaline in doses of 5–6 mg/kg. Despite these differences in potency, the effects are virtually indistinguishable.

PCP and ketamine produce detachment, disorientation, distortions of body image, and loss of proprioception. Somatic symptoms and signs include numbness, nystagmus, sweating, rapid heart rate, and hypertension. Overdosage has been fatal, as contrasted with the absence of known human fatalities directly caused by drugs of the LSD group.

Scopolamine and other antimuscarinic drugs produce delirium with fluctuating levels of awareness, disorientation, marked difficulty in thinking, marked loss of memory, and bizarre delusions. Most subjects, at least under experimental conditions, find these drugs to be unpleasant and have little desire to repeat the experience.

Use of these hallucinogens has not been associated with dependence or physiologic withdrawal symptoms. This is probably because tolerance develops rapidly, so that closely spaced dosing would be necessary to cause dependence; such frequent dosing is unusual.

Treatment

Common adverse psychologic consequences of hallucinogenic drugs include panic reactions ("bad trips") and acute psychotic reactions with PCP. Treatment includes benzodiazepines for sedation and constant monitoring by a nondrugged companion for several hours. Acidification of the urine (see Chapter 59) may hasten PCP excretion.

Overdoses of the antimuscarinic agents can be treated with infusions of physostigmine, but supportive care is usually preferred.

MARIJUANA

History

Use of **cannabis** has been recorded for thousands of years, and about 200–300 million people use it currently, including 30–40 million persons in the USA. Recent surveys suggest its use is starting at an earlier age (sixth to eighth grade, 11–13 years). Because of proposed medical uses, it has been legalized in several states, although federal law prohibits its distribution for any purpose. Much cannabis is now grown indoors using genetically altered strains with 10-fold higher levels of Δ^9-**tetrahydrocannabinol** (**THC**) (see below).

Chemistry & Pharmacology

With the exception of THC and its analogs, no other cannabinoids have definite psychoactivity, and the content of THC varies considerably among plants. Special genetic plant lines may produce as much as 4–6% THC content.

Δ^9-Tetrahydrocannabinol (THC)

The preferred route of administration in Western countries is by smoking. The high lipid solubility of the drug leads to extensive sequestration in the lipid compartments of the body, and metabolites may be excreted for as long as a week after a single dose.

A G protein-coupled cannabinoid receptor (CB1) is most numerous in the outflow nuclei of the basal ganglia, the substantia nigra, pars reticulata, globus pallidus, hippocampus, and brainstem. Positron emission tomographic (PET) studies have revealed increases in metabolism following THC in the same areas in which receptors are localized, suggesting that these receptors are closely involved in the clinical actions of the drug.

THC has a variety of pharmacologic effects that resemble those of amphetamines, LSD, alcohol, sedatives, atropine, and morphine. Important opioid interactions include reduction in opioid dependence in CB1 knockout mice lacking the CB1 receptor.

Clinical Effects

The expert smoker of marijuana is usually aware of a drug effect after two or three inhalations. As smoking continues, the effects increase, reaching a maximum about 20 minutes after the smoke has been finished. Most effects of the drug usually have vanished after 3 hours, by which time plasma concentrations are low. Peak effects after oral administration may be delayed until 3–4 hours after drug ingestion but may last for 6–8 hours.

The early stage is one of being "high" and is characterized by euphoria, uncontrollable laughter, alteration of time sense, depersonalization, and sharpened vision. Later, the user becomes relaxed and experiences introspective and dream-like states if not actual sleep. Thinking or concentrating becomes difficult, though by force of will the subject can attend.

Two characteristic physiologic signs of cannabis intoxication are increased pulse rate and reddening of the conjunctiva. The latter correlates well with the presence of detectable plasma concentrations. Pupil size is not changed. The blood pressure may fall, especially in the upright position. An antiemetic effect may be present. Muscle weakness, tremors, unsteadiness, and increased deep tendon reflexes may also be noted. Virtually any psychologic test shows impairment if the doses are large enough and the test difficult enough. No distinctive biochemical changes have been found in humans.

Tolerance has been demonstrated in virtually every animal species that has been tested. It is apparent in humans only among heavy long-term users of the drug. Different degrees of tolerance develop for different effects of the drug, with tolerance for the tachycardic effect developing fairly rapidly. A mild withdrawal syndrome has been noted following chronic use at very high doses.

Three epidemiologic studies in developing countries have failed to find definite evidence of impairment among heavy users of cannabis, but field studies may lack sensitivity. Experimental studies in which subjects have smoked heavily for varying periods have shown a lower serum testosterone level in men and airway narrowing. Reports of effects on immune mechanisms, chromosomes, and cell metabolism are often contradictory. Effects on the fetus are still uncertain.

Heavy smokers of marijuana may be subject to some of the same problems of chronic bronchitis, airway obstruction, and squamous cell metaplasia as smokers of tobacco cigarettes. Angina pectoris may be aggravated by the speeding of the heart rate, orthostatic hypotension, and increased carboxyhemoglobin. Driving ability is likely to be impaired but is not easily demonstrated with usual testing. "Amotivational syndrome," in which promising young people with obvious social advantages lose interest in school and career and enter the drug culture, is a real phenomenon, but one cannot be sure whether drug use is the cause of the problem or simply a matter of personal choice. Acute panic reactions, toxic delirium, paranoid states, and frank psychoses are rare. Brain damage has not been confirmed in humans, although some suggestion of ultrastructural damage has been found in animals.

Therapeutic THC is called **dronabinol** (Marinol) and has been marketed with approval by the Food and Drug Administration to reduce nausea and vomiting in patients undergoing cancer chemotherapy and to stimulate appetite in AIDS patients. It has also been shown to reduce intraocular pressure in glaucoma. **Levonantradol,** an analog, may be useful as an analgesic.

Few abusers seek treatment, but recent studies have suggested that behavioral treatments can stop abuse and improve cognitive functioning.

INHALANTS

Chemistry

Four types of inhalants are abused: (1) anesthetic gases; (2) industrial solvents, including a variety of hydrocarbons, such as toluene; (3) aerosol propellants, such as various fluorocarbons; and (4) organic nitrites, such as amyl or butyl nitrite. The mode of action of the inhalant anesthetics has been discussed in Chapter 25.

Clinical Aspects

Anesthetic gases such as **nitrous oxide** produce difficulty in concentrating, dreaminess, euphoria, numbness and tingling, unsteadiness, and visual and auditory disturbances. Nitrous oxide is usually taken as 35% N_2O mixed with oxygen; administration of 100% nitrous oxide may cause asphyxia and death. **Ether** and **chloroform** are readily available, and after an initial period of exhilaration, the person often loses consciousness.

Industrial solvents include **gasoline,** and various toxins such as **toluene, benzene,** and **trichloroethylene.** The clinical effects of industrial solvent inhalation are short, lasting only 5–15 minutes. Rags or "toques" are soaked in the solvent and the fumes inhaled. **Aerosol propellants** are usually inhaled from a plastic bag. Euphoria and a relaxed "drunk" feeling are followed by disorientation, slow passage of time, and possibly hallucinations.

Organic nitrites (**amyl nitrite** and **isobutyl nitrite**) cause dizziness, giddiness, rapid heart rate, lowered blood pressure, "speeding," and flushing of the skin. These effects last only a few minutes and can readily be repeated. The main effect of the drug on sexual performance is probably to enhance or prolong erection through the release of nitric oxide in the corpora cavernosa (see Chapter 19).

Toxicity from chronic use of inhalants can be severe. Industrial solvents have produced liver, kidney, peripheral nerve, and possibly brain damage in animals, bone marrow suppression, and pulmonary disease. In human neuroimaging studies using magnetic resonance imaging, demyelination of white matter has been described in chronic abusers. Fluorocarbon inhalation has resulted in sudden deaths, due either to ventricular arrhythmias or to asphyxiation. Nitrites have been rather safe but might pose hazards (especially arrhythmias) for persons with preexisting cardiovascular problems. Finally, recent data have indicated that nitrate inhalants may reduce lymphocyte counts and natural killer cell activity, thereby acting as a cofactor for AIDS progression.

STEROIDS

History

Anabolic steroids were first used in competitive sports during the 1940s, and by the late 1980s, use was widespread in adolescents with distribution points in gymnasiums and physical fitness centers. However, the first urine testing for anabolic steroids did not occur until 1976 at the Olympic Games because of the fairly difficult assay methods needed for detection. These drugs are discussed in Chapter 40.

Clinical Use & Effects

Oral and injectable formulations of different steroids are often "stacked," ie, used simultaneously. Because detection of these different steroids is difficult and expensive, the history from the patient rather than urine toxicology is more generally useful for detecting anabolic steroid abuse. Anabolic steroids were added to Schedule III of the Controlled Substances Act in 1990.

Anabolic steroids are typically abused in a cyclic fashion, with a cycle of 4–18 weeks on steroids and 1 month to 1 year off. Abuse of other psychoactive drugs may occur in up to a third of these patients, but this is low compared with other substance abusers because of concerns about health and appearance by steroid abusers. The primary effects sought by abusers are increased muscle mass and strength, not euphoria. In the context of an adequate diet and sufficient physical activity, a significant increase in muscle mass and strength can be produced by these steroids.

Among the behavioral manifestations of heavy use are increases in aggression, changes in libido and sexual functions, and mood changes with occasional psychotic features. In studies comparing doses of 40–240 mg/d of methyltestosterone in a double-blind inpatient trial, irritability, mood swings, violent feelings, and hostility were greater during the high-dose period than at baseline. This clear ability of androgenic steroids to provoke aggression and irritability has aroused concerns about violence toward family members by abusers. In two prospective controlled trials using blinded administration, mood disturbances were reported in more than 50% of bodybuilders using anabolic steroids. Both increases and decreases in libido have been reported in studies comparing anabolic steroid abusers with nonusing athletes. Cognitive impairment, including distractibility, forgetfulness, and confusion, has also been demonstrated in controlled trials. A withdrawal syndrome has been described, with common symptoms being fatigue, depressed mood, and a craving for steroids.

Clinical findings may include hypertrophied muscles, acne, oily skin, hirsutism in females, gynecomastia in males, and needle punctures. Edema and jaundice may develop in heavy users. Common laboratory abnormalities include elevated hemoglobin and hematocrit measurements, elevated low-density lipoprotein cholesterol and depressed high-density lipoprotein cholesterol levels. Liver function test results may be elevated, and luteinizing hormone levels are usually depressed.

Treatment

Controlled trials of psychosocial treatments for anabolic steroid dependence have not been reported, and these individuals rarely present to substance abuse treatment programs. Patients may come to the attention of mental health professionals as a result of excessive aggression, sexual dysfunction, or mood disturbances. Peer counseling by former bodybuilders and group support may be of particular value for these users. Nutritional counseling and consultation with a fitness expert may also be helpful. Since gymnasiums are a frequent site for acquisition of steroids, abusers need to avoid these places until recovery is firmly established.

REFERENCES

GENERAL

Everitt BJ, Dickinson A, Robbins TW: The neuropsychological basis of addictive behaviour. Brain Res Brain Res Rev 2001; 36:129.

Gottschalk PC, Jacobsen LK, Kosten TR: Current concepts in pharmacotherapy of substance abuse. Curr Psychiatry Rep 1999; 1:172.

Melichar JK, Daglish MR, Nutt DJ: Addiction and withdrawal–current views. Curr Opin Pharmacol 2001;1:84.

Musto DF: *The American Disease: Origins of Narcotic Control,* 3rd ed. Oxford Univ Press, 1999.

Nestler EJ: Molecular basis of long-term plasticity underlying addiction. Nat Rev Neurosci 2001;2:119.

Van Etten ML, Anthony JC: Comparative epidemiology of initial drug opportunities and transitions to first use: Marijuana, cocaine, hallucinogens and heroin. Drug Alcohol Depend 1999;54:117.

Walker A, Rosenberg M, Balaban-Gil K: Neurodevelopmental and neurobehavioral sequelae of selected substances of abuse and psychiatric medications in utero. Child Adolesc Psychiatr Clin N Am 1999;8:845.

Weiss F et al: Compulsive drug-seeking behavior and relapse. Neuroadaptation, stress, and conditioning factors. Ann N Y Acad Sci 2001;937:1.

Websites: www.health.org and www.drugabuse.gov

OPIOIDS

Dole VP: Implications of methadone maintenance treatment for theories of narcotic addiction. JAMA 1988;260:3025.

Gonzalez G, Oliveto A, Kosten TR: Treatment of heroin (Diamorphine) addiction: Current approaches and future prospects. Drugs 2002;62:1331.

O'Connor PG, Kosten TR: Rapid and ultrarapid opioid detoxification techniques. JAMA 1998;279:229.

Websites: Kosten TR. Office based treatment of opiate dependent patients with buprenorphine. Web-based training course for American Psychiatric Association 2002: http://www.psych.org/cme/apacme/courses/opiate/introduction.cfm.

SEDATIVES & GHB

Lader MH: Limitations on the use of benzodiazepines in anxiety and insomnia: Are they justified? Eur Neuropsychopharmacol 1999;9 (Suppl 6):S399.

Longo LP, Johnson B: Addiction: Part I. Benzodiazepines—side effects, abuse risk, and alternatives. Am Fam Physician 2000;61:2121.

Okun MS et al: GHB: An important pharmacologic and clinical update. J Pharm Pharm Sci 2001;4:167.

STIMULANTS

Balfour D, Le Houezec J: Advances in neuroscience and pharmacology of nicotine. 3rd SRNT Europe Conference, Nicotine Tob Res 2002;4:229.

Davidson C et al: Methamphetamine neurotoxicity: Necrotic and apoptotic mechanisms and relevance to human abuse and treatment. Brain Res Brain Res Rev 2001;36:1.

Feinstein AR et al: Do caffeine-containing analgesics promote dependence? A review and evaluation. Clin Pharmacol Ther 2000;68:457.

Gainetdinov RR, Sotnikova TD, Caron MG: Monoamine transporter pharmacology and mutant mice. Trends Pharmacol Sci 2002;23:367.

Hughes JR et al: Recent advances in the pharmacotherapy of smoking. JAMA 1999;281:72.

Kosten TR: Pharmacotherapy of cerebral ischemia in cocaine dependence. Drug Alcohol Depend 1998;49:133.

Kosten TR et al: Human therapeutic cocaine vaccine: Safety and immunogenicity. Vaccine 2002;20:1196.

Kosten TR, George TP, Kosten TA: The potential of dopamine agonists in drug addiction. Exp Opin Investig Drugs 2002;11:491.

Mayes LC: Developing brain and in utero cocaine exposure: Effects on neural ontogeny. Devel Psychopathol 1999;11:685.

Nehlig A: Are we dependent upon coffee and caffeine? A review on human and animal data. Neurosci Biobehav Rev 1999;23:563.

Reneman L et al: Cortical serotonin transporter density and verbal memory in individuals who stopped using 3,4-methylenedioxymethamphetamine (MDMA or "ecstasy"): Preliminary findings. Arch Gen Psychiatry 2001;58:901.

Srisurapanont M et al: Treatment for amphetamine dependence and abuse. Cochrane Database System Review 2001;(4):CD003022.

HALLUCINOGENS

Curran HV, Monaghan L: In and out of the K-hole: A comparison of the acute and residual effects of ketamine in frequent and infrequent ketamine users. Addiction 2001;96:749.

Halpern JH, Pope HG Jr: Hallucinogens on the Internet: A vast new source of underground drug information. Am J Psychiatry 2001;158:481.

Koesters SC, Rogers PD, Rajasingham CR: MDMA ("ecstasy") and other "club drugs." The new epidemic. Pediatr Clin North Am 2002;49:415.

Web site: www.clubdrugs.org

MARIJUANA

Ashton CH: Pharmacology and effects of cannabis: A brief review. Br J Psychiatry 2001;178:101.

Budney AJ et al: Marijuana abstinence effects in marijuana smokers maintained in their home environment. Arch Gen Psychiatry 2001;58:917.

Gruber AJ, Pope HG Jr: Marijuana use among adolescents. Pediatr Clin North Am 2002;49:389.

Joy JE, Watson SJ Jr, Benson JA (editors): *Marijuana and Medicine: Assessing the Science Base.* National Academy Press; 1999.

Maldonado R, Rodríguez de Fonseca F: Cannabinoid addiction: Behavioral models and neural correlates. J Neurosci 2002;22:3326.

Pope HG Jr et al: Neuropsychological performance in long-term cannabis users. Arch Gen Psychiatry 2001;58:909.

INHALANTS

Neumark YD, Delva J, Anthony JC: The epidemiology of adolescent inhalant drug involvement. Arch Pediatr Adolesc Med 1998;152:781.

Riegel AC, French ED: Abused inhalants and central reward pathways: Electrophysiological and behavioral studies in the rat. Ann N Y Acad Sci 2002;965:281.

Rosenberg NL et al: Neuropsychologic impairment and MRI abnormalities associated with chronic solvent abuse. J Toxicol Clin Toxicol 2002;40:21.

Soderberg LS: Immunomodulation by nitrite inhalants may predispose abusers to AIDS and Kaposi's sarcoma. J Neuroimmunol 1998;83:157.

STEROIDS

Bagatell CJ, Bremner WJ: Androgens in men—uses and abuses. N Engl J Med 1996;334:707.

Bahrke MS et al: Risk factors associated with anabolic-androgenic steroid use among adolescents. Sports Med 2000;29:397.

Pope HG, Kouri EM, Husons MD: Effects of supraphysiological doses of testosterone on mood and aggression in normal men. Arch Gen Psychiatry 2000;57:133.

Zorpette G: Andro angst. Scientific American 1998;279:22.

Web site: www.steroidabuse.org

SECTION VI
Drugs Used to Treat Diseases of the Blood, Inflammation, & Gout

Agents Used in Anemias; Hematopoietic Growth Factors

33

Susan B. Masters, PhD

Hematopoiesis, the production from undifferentiated stem cells of circulating erythrocytes, platelets, and leukocytes, is a remarkable process that produces over 200 billion new cells per day in the normal person and even greater numbers of blood cells in people with conditions that cause loss or destruction of blood cells. The hematopoietic machinery resides primarily in the bone marrow in adults and requires a constant supply of three essential nutrients—**iron, vitamin B_{12}, and folic acid**— as well as the presence of **hematopoietic growth factors,** proteins that regulate the proliferation and differentiation of hematopoietic cells. Inadequate supplies of either the essential nutrients or the growth factors result in deficiency of functional blood cells. **Anemia,** a deficiency in oxygen-carrying erythrocytes, is the most common and easily treated of these conditions, but **thrombocytopenia** and **neutropenia** are not rare and in some forms are amenable to drug therapy. In this chapter, we first consider treatment of anemia due to deficiency of iron, vitamin B_{12}, or folic acid and then turn to the medical use of hematopoietic growth factors to combat anemia, thrombocytopenia, and neutropenia.

AGENTS USED IN ANEMIAS

IRON

Basic Pharmacology

Iron deficiency is the most common cause of chronic anemia—anemia that develops over time. Like other forms of chronic anemia, iron deficiency anemia leads to pallor, fatigue, dizziness, exertional dyspnea, and other generalized symptoms of tissue ischemia. The cardiovascular adaptations to chronic anemia—tachycardia, increased cardiac output, vasodilation—can worsen the condition of patients with underlying cardiovascular disease.

Iron forms the nucleus of the iron-porphyrin heme ring, which together with globin chains forms hemoglobin. Hemoglobin reversibly binds oxygen and provides the critical mechanism for oxygen delivery from the lungs to other tissues. In the absence of adequate iron, small erythrocytes with insufficient hemoglobin are formed, giving rise to microcytic hypochromic anemia.

Pharmacokinetics

The body has an elaborate system for maintaining the supply of the iron required for hematopoiesis. It involves specialized transport and storage proteins whose concentrations are regulated by the body's demand for hemoglobin synthesis and adequate iron stores (Table 33–1). The vast majority of the iron used to support hematopoiesis is reclaimed from catalysis of the hemoglobin in old erythrocytes. Normally, only a small amount of iron is lost from the body each day, so dietary requirements are small and easily fulfilled by the iron available in a wide variety of foods. However, in special populations with either increased iron requirements (eg, growing children, pregnant women) or increased losses of iron (eg, menstruating women), iron requirements can exceed normal dietary supplies and iron deficiency can develop.

A. ABSORPTION

Iron is normally absorbed in the duodenum and proximal jejunum, though the more distal small intestine can absorb iron if necessary. The average diet in the USA contains 10–15 mg of elemental iron daily. A normal individual without iron deficiency absorbs 5–10% of this iron, or about 0.5–1 mg daily. Iron absorption increases in response to low iron stores or increased iron requirements. Total iron absorption increases to 1–2 mg/d in normal menstruating women and may be as high as 3–4 mg/d in pregnant women. Infants and adolescents also have increased iron requirements during rapid growth periods.

Iron is available in a wide variety of foods but is especially abundant in meat. The iron in meat protein can be efficiently absorbed, since heme iron in meat hemoglobin and myoglobin can be absorbed intact without first having to be broken down into elemental iron. Iron in other foods, especially vegetables and grains, is often tightly bound to phytates or other complexing agents and may be much less available for absorption. Nonheme iron in foods and iron in inorganic iron salts and complexes must be reduced to ferrous (Fe^{2+}) iron before it can be absorbed by the intestinal mucosal cells. Such absorption is decreased by the presence of chelators or complexing agents in the intestinal lumen and is increased in the presence of hydrochloric acid and vitamin C.

Iron crosses the intestinal mucosal cell by active transport. The rate of iron uptake is regulated by mucosal cell iron stores such that more iron is transported when stores are low. Together with iron split from absorbed heme, the newly absorbed iron can be made available for immediate transport from the mucosal cell to the plasma via transferrin or can be stored in the mucosal cell as ferritin, a water-soluble complex consisting of a core crystal of ferric hydroxide covered by a shell of a specialized storage protein called apoferritin. In general, when total body iron stores are high and iron requirements by the body are low, newly absorbed iron is diverted into ferritin in the intestinal mucosal cells rather than being transported to other sites. When iron stores are low or iron requirements are high, however, newly absorbed iron is immediately transported from the mucosal cells to the bone marrow for the production of hemoglobin.

B. TRANSPORT

Iron is transported in the plasma bound to **transferrin**, a β-globulin that specifically binds ferric iron. The transferrin-ferric iron complex enters maturing erythroid cells by a specific receptor mechanism. Transferrin receptors—integral membrane glycoproteins present in large numbers on proliferating erythroid cells—bind the transferrin-iron complex and internalize the iron, releasing it within the cell. The transferrin and transferrin receptor are then recycled, providing an efficient mechanism for incorporating iron into hemoglobin in developing red blood cells.

Increased erythropoiesis is associated with an increase in the number of transferrin receptors on developing erythroid cells. Iron store depletion and iron deficiency anemia are associated with an increased concentration of serum transferrin.

C. STORAGE

Iron binds avidly to a protein, **apoferritin**, and forms the complex **ferritin.** Iron is stored, primarily as ferritin, in intestinal mucosal cells and in macrophages in the liver, spleen, and bone. Apoferritin synthesis is regulated by the levels of free iron. When these levels are low, apo-

Table 33–1. Iron distribution in normal adults.[1,2]

	Iron Content (mg)	
	Men	**Women**
Hemoglobin	3050	1700
Myoglobin	430	300
Enzymes	10	8
Transport (transferrin)	8	6
Storage (ferritin and other forms)	750	300
Total	4248	2314

[1]Adapted, with permission, from Brown EB: Iron deficiency anemia. In: *Cecil Textbook of Medicine,* 16th ed. Wyngaarden JB, Smith LH (editors). Saunders, 1982.

[2]Values are based on data from various sources and assume that "normal" men weigh 80 kg and have a hemoglobin of 16 g/dL and that "normal" women weigh 55 kg and have a hemoglobin of 14 g/dL.

ferritin synthesis is inhibited and the balance of iron binding shifts toward transferrin. When free iron levels are high, more apoferritin is produced in an effort to safely sequester more iron and protect organs from the toxic effects of excess free iron.

Ferritin is also detectable in plasma. Since the ferritin present in plasma is in equilibrium with storage ferritin in reticuloendothelial tissues, the plasma (or serum) ferritin level can be used to estimate total body iron stores.

D. ELIMINATION

There is no mechanism for excretion of iron. Small amounts are lost by exfoliation of intestinal mucosal cells into the stool, and trace amounts are excreted in bile, urine, and sweat. These losses account for no more than 1 mg of iron per day. Because the body's ability to increase excretion of iron is so limited, regulation of iron balance must be achieved by changing intestinal absorption and storage of iron, in response to the body's needs.

Clinical Pharmacology

A. INDICATIONS FOR THE USE OF IRON

The only clinical indication for the use of iron preparations is the treatment or prevention of iron deficiency anemia. Iron deficiency is commonly seen in populations with increased iron requirements. These include infants, especially premature infants; children during rapid growth periods; and pregnant and lactating women. Iron deficiency also occurs frequently after gastrectomy and in patients with severe small bowel disease that results in generalized malabsorption. Iron deficiency in these gastrointestinal conditions is due to inadequate iron absorption.

The most common cause of iron deficiency in adults is blood loss. Menstruating women lose about 30 mg of iron with each menstrual period; women with heavy menstrual bleeding may lose much more. Thus, many premenopausal women have low iron stores or even iron deficiency. In men and postmenopausal women, the most common site of blood loss is the gastrointestinal tract. Patients with unexplained iron deficiency anemia should be evaluated for occult gastrointestinal bleeding.

As iron deficiency develops, storage iron decreases and then disappears; next, serum ferritin decreases; and then serum iron decreases and iron-binding capacity increases, resulting in a decrease in iron-binding (transferrin) saturation. Thereafter, anemia begins to develop. Red cell indices (mean corpuscular volume [MCV]: normal = 80–100 fL; mean corpuscular hemoglobin concentration [MCHC]: normal = 32–36 g/dL) are usually low normal when iron deficiency anemia is mild, but cells become progressively more microcytic (low MCV) and hypochromic (low MCHC) as anemia becomes more severe. By the time iron deficiency is diagnosed, serum iron is usually less than 40 µg/dL; total iron-binding capacity (TIBC) is greater than 400 µg/dL; iron-binding saturation is less than 10%; and serum ferritin is less than 10 µg/L. These laboratory measurements can be used to confirm a diagnosis of iron deficiency anemia in patients who present with signs and symptoms of microcytic anemia.

B. TREATMENT

The treatment of iron deficiency anemia consists of administration of oral or parenteral iron preparations. Oral iron corrects the anemia just as rapidly and completely as parenteral iron in most cases if iron absorption from the gastrointestinal tract is normal.

1. Oral iron therapy—A wide variety of oral iron preparations are available. Since ferrous iron is most efficiently absorbed, only ferrous salts should be used. Ferrous sulfate, ferrous gluconate, and ferrous fumarate are all effective and inexpensive and are recommended for the treatment of most patients.

Different iron salts provide different amounts of elemental iron, as shown in Table 33–2. In an iron-deficient individual, about 50–100 mg of iron can be incorporated into hemoglobin daily, and about 25% of oral iron given as ferrous salt can be absorbed. Therefore, 200–400 mg of elemental iron should be given daily to correct iron deficiency most rapidly. Patients unable to tolerate such large doses of iron can be given lower daily doses of iron, which results in slower but still complete correction of iron deficiency. Treatment with oral iron should be continued for 3–6 months. This will correct the anemia and replenish iron stores.

Common adverse effects of oral iron therapy include nausea, epigastric discomfort, abdominal cramps, constipation, and diarrhea. These effects are usually dose-

Table 33–2. Some commonly used oral iron preparations.

Preparation	Tablet Size	Elemental Iron per Tablet	Usual Adult Dosage (Tablets per Day)
Ferrous sulfate, hydrated	325 mg	65 mg	3–4
Ferrous sulfate, desiccated	200 mg	65 mg	3–4
Ferrous gluconate	325 mg	36 mg	3–4
Ferrous fumarate	200 mg	66 mg	3–4
Ferrous fumarate	325 mg	106 mg	2–3

related and can often be overcome by lowering the daily dose of iron or by taking the tablets immediately after or with meals. Some patients have less severe gastrointestinal adverse effects with one iron salt than another and benefit from changing preparations. Patients taking oral iron develop black stools; this itself has no clinical significance but may obscure the diagnosis of continued gastrointestinal blood loss.

2. Parenteral iron therapy—Parenteral therapy should be reserved for patients with documented iron deficiency unable to tolerate or absorb oral iron and patients with extensive chronic blood loss who cannot be maintained with oral iron alone. This includes patients with various postgastrectomy conditions and previous small bowel resection, inflammatory bowel disease involving the proximal small bowel, and malabsorption syndromes.

Iron dextran is a stable complex of ferric hydroxide and low-molecular-weight dextran containing 50 mg of elemental iron per milliliter of solution. **Iron-sucrose complex** and **iron sodium gluconate complex** are newer, alternative preparations. These agents can be given either by deep intramuscular injection or by intravenous infusion. Adverse effects of parenteral iron therapy include local pain and tissue staining (brown discoloration of the tissues overlying the injection site), headache, light-headedness, fever, arthralgias, nausea and vomiting, back pain, flushing, urticaria, bronchospasm, and, rarely, anaphylaxis and death.

Most adults with iron deficiency anemia require 1–2 g of replacement iron, or 20–40 mL of iron dextran. Most physicians prefer to give the entire dose in a single intravenous infusion in several hundred milliliters of normal saline over 1–2 hours. Intravenous administration eliminates the local pain and tissue staining that often occur with the intramuscular route and allows delivery of the entire dose of iron necessary to correct the iron deficiency at one time. There is no clear evidence that any of the adverse effects, including anaphylaxis, are more likely to occur with intravenous than with intramuscular administration.

Owing to the risk of a hypersensitivity reaction, a small test dose of iron dextran should always be given before full intramuscular or intravenous doses are given. Patients with a strong history of allergy and patients who have previously received parenteral iron are more likely to have hypersensitivity reactions following treatment with parenteral iron dextran.

Clinical Toxicity

A. ACUTE IRON TOXICITY

Acute iron toxicity is seen almost exclusively in young children who have ingested a number of iron tablets. Although adults are able to tolerate large doses of oral iron without serious consequences, as few as ten tablets of any of the commonly available oral iron preparations can be lethal in young children. Patients taking oral iron preparations should be instructed to store tablets in child-proof containers out of the reach of children.

Large amounts of oral iron cause necrotizing gastroenteritis, with vomiting, abdominal pain, and bloody diarrhea followed by shock, lethargy, and dyspnea. Subsequently, improvement is often noted, but this may be followed by severe metabolic acidosis, coma, and death. Urgent treatment of acute iron toxicity is necessary, especially in young children. Activated charcoal, a highly effective adsorbent for most toxins, *does not* bind iron and thus is ineffective. Whole bowel irrigation (see Chapter 59) should be performed to flush out unabsorbed pills. **Deferoxamine,** a potent iron-chelating compound, can be given systemically to bind iron that has already been absorbed and to promote its excretion in urine and feces. Appropriate supportive therapy for gastrointestinal bleeding, metabolic acidosis, and shock must also be provided.

B. CHRONIC IRON TOXICITY

Chronic iron toxicity (iron overload), also known as **hemochromatosis,** results when excess iron is deposited in the heart, liver, pancreas, and other organs. It can lead to organ failure and death. It most commonly occurs in patients with inherited hemochromatosis, a disorder characterized by excessive iron absorption, and in patients who receive many red cell transfusions over a long period of time.

Chronic iron overload in the absence of anemia is most efficiently treated by intermittent phlebotomy. One unit of blood can be removed every week or so until all of the excess iron is removed. Iron chelation therapy using parenteral deferoxamine is much less efficient as well as more complicated, expensive, and hazardous, but it can be useful for severe iron overload that cannot be managed by phlebotomy.

VITAMIN B$_{12}$

Vitamin B$_{12}$ serves as a cofactor for several essential biochemical reactions in humans. Deficiency of vitamin B$_{12}$ leads to anemia, gastrointestinal symptoms, and neurologic abnormalities. While deficiency of vitamin B$_{12}$ due to an inadequate supply in the diet is unusual, deficiency of B$_{12}$ in adults—especially older adults—due to abnormal absorption of dietary vitamin B$_{12}$ is a relatively common and easily treated disorder.

Chemistry

Vitamin B$_{12}$ consists of a porphyrin-like ring with a central cobalt atom attached to a nucleotide. Various organic groups may be covalently bound to the cobalt atom, forming different cobalamins. Deoxyadenosyl-cobalamin and methylcobalamin are the active forms of the vitamin in humans. **Cyanocobalamin** and **hydroxo-cobalamin** (both available for therapeutic use) and other cobalamins found in food sources are converted to the above active forms. The ultimate source of vitamin B_{12} is from microbial synthesis; the vitamin is not synthesized by animals or plants. The chief dietary source of vitamin B_{12} is microbially derived vitamin B_{12} in meat (especially liver), eggs, and dairy products. Vitamin B_{12} is sometimes called **extrinsic factor** to differentiate it from **intrinsic factor,** a protein normally secreted by the stomach.

Pharmacokinetics

The average diet in the USA contains 5–30 μg of vitamin B_{12} daily, 1–5 μg of which is usually absorbed. The vitamin is avidly stored, primarily in the liver, with an average adult having a total vitamin B_{12} storage pool of 3000–5000 μg. Only trace amounts of vitamin B_{12} are normally lost in urine and stool. Since the normal daily requirements of vitamin B_{12} are only about 2 μg, it would take about 5 years for all of the stored vitamin B_{12} to be exhausted and for megaloblastic anemia to develop if B_{12} absorption stopped. Vitamin B_{12} in physiologic amounts is absorbed only after it complexes with **intrinsic factor,** a glycoprotein secreted by the parietal cells of the gastric mucosa. Intrinsic factor combines with the vitamin B_{12} that is liberated from dietary sources in the stomach and duodenum, and the intrinsic factor-vitamin B_{12} complex is subsequently absorbed in the distal ileum by a highly specific receptor-mediated transport system. Vitamin B_{12} deficiency in humans most often results from malabsorption of vitamin B_{12}, due either to lack of intrinsic factor or to loss or malfunction of the specific absorptive mechanism in the distal ileum. Nutritional deficiency is rare but may be seen in strict vegetarians after many years without meat, eggs, or dairy products.

Once absorbed, vitamin B_{12} is transported to the various cells of the body bound to a plasma glycoprotein, transcobalamin II. Excess vitamin B_{12} is transported to the liver for storage. Significant amounts of vitamin B_{12} are excreted in the urine only when very large amounts are given parenterally, overcoming the binding capacities of the transcobalamins (50–100 μg).

Pharmacodynamics

Two essential enzymatic reactions in humans require vitamin B_{12} (Figure 33–1). In one, methylcobalamin serves as an intermediate in the transfer of a methyl group from N^5-methyltetrahydrofolate to methionine

A. Methyl transfer

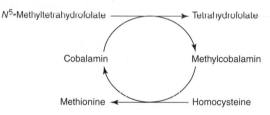

B. Isomerization of L-Methylmalonyl-CoA

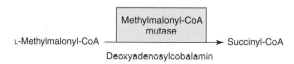

Figure 33–1. Enzymatic reactions that use vitamin B_{12}. See text for details.

(Figure 33–1A; Figure 33–2, reaction 1). In the absence of vitamin B_{12}, conversion of the major dietary and storage folate, N^5-methyltetrahydrofolate, to tetrahydrofolate, the precursor of folate cofactors, cannot occur. As a result, a deficiency of folate cofactors necessary for several biochemical reactions involving the transfer of one-carbon groups develops. In particular, the depletion of tetrahydrofolate prevents synthesis of adequate supplies of the deoxythymidylate (dTMP) and purines required for DNA synthesis in rapidly dividing cells as shown in Figure 33–3, reaction 2. The accumulation of folate as N^5-methyltetrahydrofolate and the associated depletion of tetrahydrofolate cofactors in vitamin B_{12} deficiency have been referred to as the "methylfolate trap." This is the biochemical step whereby vitamin B_{12} and folic acid metabolism are linked and explains why the megaloblastic anemia of vitamin B_{12} deficiency can be partially corrected by ingestion of relatively large amounts of folic acid. Folic acid can be reduced to dihydrofolate by the enzyme dihydrofolate reductase (Figure 33–2, reaction 3) and thus serve as a source of the tetrahydrofolate required for synthesis of the purines and dTMP that are needed for DNA synthesis.

The other enzymatic reaction that requires vitamin B_{12} is isomerization of methylmalonyl-CoA to succinyl-CoA by the enzyme methylmalonyl-CoA mutase (Figure 33–1B). In vitamin B_{12} deficiency, this conversion cannot take place, and the substrate, methylmalonyl-CoA, accumulates. In the past, it was thought that abnormal accumulation of methylmalonyl-CoA causes the neurologic manifestations of vitamin B_{12} deficiency. However, newer evidence instead implicates the disruption of the methionine synthesis pathway as the cause of neurologic problems. Whatever the biochemical expla-

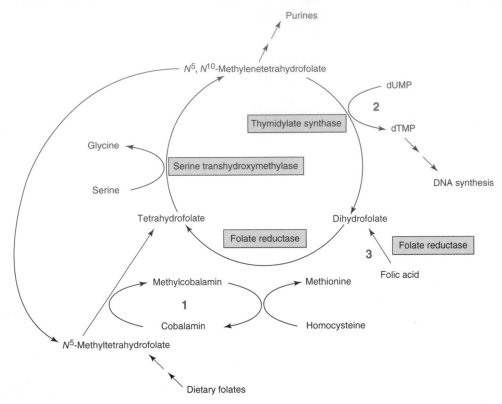

Figure 33–2. Enzymatic reactions that use folates. Section 1 shows the vitamin B_{12}-dependent reaction that allows most dietary folates to enter the tetrahydrofolate cofactor pool and becomes the "folate trap" in vitamin B_{12} deficiency. Section 2 shows the dTMP cycle. Section 3 shows the pathway by which folate enters the tetrahydrofolate cofactor pool. Double arrows indicate pathways with more than one intermediate step.

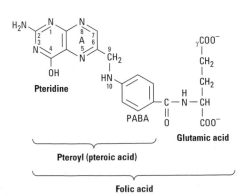

Figure 33–3. The structure and numbering of atoms of folic acid. (Reproduced, with permission, from Murray RK et al: *Harper's Biochemistry,* 24th ed. McGraw-Hill, 1996)

nation for neurologic damage, the important point is that administration of folic acid in the setting of vitamin B_{12} deficiency will not prevent *neurologic* manifestations even though it will largely correct the *anemia* caused by the vitamin B_{12} deficiency.

Clinical Pharmacology

Vitamin B_{12} is used to treat or prevent deficiency. There is no evidence that vitamin B_{12} injections have any benefit in persons who do not have vitamin B_{12} deficiency. The most characteristic clinical manifestation of vitamin B_{12} deficiency is megaloblastic anemia. The typical clinical findings in megaloblastic anemia are macrocytic anemia (MCV usually > 120 fL), often with associated mild or moderate leukopenia or thrombocytopenia (or both), and a characteristic hypercellular bone marrow with megaloblastic maturation of erythroid and other precursor cells. Vitamin B_{12} deficiency also causes a neurologic syndrome that usually begins with paresthesias and weakness in peripheral nerves and progresses to spasticity, ataxia, and other central nervous system dysfunctions. A characteristic pathologic feature of the neurologic syndrome is degeneration of myelin sheaths followed by disruption of axons in the dorsal and lateral horns of the spinal cord and in peripheral nerves. Correction of vitamin B_{12} deficiency arrests the progression of neurologic disease, but it may not fully reverse neurologic symptoms that have been present for several months. Although most patients with neurologic abnormalities caused by vitamin B_{12} deficiency have full-blown megaloblastic anemias when first seen, occasional patients have few if any hematologic abnormalities.

Once a diagnosis of megaloblastic anemia is made, it must be determined whether vitamin B_{12} or folic acid deficiency is the cause. (Other causes of megaloblastic anemia are very rare.) This can usually be accomplished by measuring serum levels of the vitamins. The Schilling test, which measures absorption and urinary excretion of radioactively labeled vitamin B_{12}, can be used to further define the mechanism of vitamin B_{12} malabsorption when this is found to be the cause of the megaloblastic anemia.

The most common causes of vitamin B_{12} deficiency are pernicious anemia, partial or total gastrectomy, and diseases that affect the distal ileum, such as malabsorption syndromes, inflammatory bowel disease, or small bowel resection.

Pernicious anemia results from defective secretion of intrinsic factor by the gastric mucosal cells. Patients with pernicious anemia have gastric atrophy and fail to secrete intrinsic factor (as well as hydrochloric acid). The Schilling test shows diminished absorption of radioactively labeled vitamin B_{12}, which is corrected when hog intrinsic factor is administered with radioactive B_{12}, since the vitamin can then be normally absorbed.

Vitamin B_{12} deficiency also occurs when the region of the distal ileum that absorbs the vitamin B_{12}-intrinsic factor complex is damaged, as when the ileum is involved with inflammatory bowel disease, or when the ileum is surgically resected. In these situations, radioactively labeled vitamin B_{12} is not absorbed in the Schilling test, even when intrinsic factor is added. Other rare causes of vitamin B_{12} deficiency include bacterial overgrowth of the small bowel, chronic pancreatitis, and thyroid disease. Rare cases of vitamin B_{12} deficiency in children have been found to be secondary to congenital deficiency of intrinsic factor and congenital selective vitamin B_{12} malabsorption due to defects of the receptor sites in the distal ileum.

Since almost all cases of vitamin B_{12} deficiency are caused by malabsorption of the vitamin, parenteral injections of vitamin B_{12} are required for therapy. For patients with potentially reversible diseases, the underlying disease should be treated after initial treatment with parenteral vitamin B_{12}. Most patients, however, do not have curable deficiency syndromes and require lifelong treatment with vitamin B_{12} injections.

Vitamin B_{12} for parenteral injection is available as cyanocobalamin or hydroxocobalamin. Hydroxocobalamin is preferred because it is more highly protein-bound and therefore remains longer in the circulation. Initial therapy should consist of 100–1000 μg of vitamin B_{12} intramuscularly daily or every other day for 1–2 weeks to replenish body stores. Maintenance therapy consists of 100–1000 μg intramuscularly once a month for life. If neurologic abnormalities are present, maintenance therapy injections should be given every 1–2 weeks for 6 months before switching to monthly injections. Oral vitamin B_{12}-intrinsic factor mixtures and liver extracts should not be used to treat vitamin B_{12} deficiency; however, oral doses of 1000 μg of vitamin B_{12} daily are usually sufficient to treat patients with pernicious anemia who refuse or cannot tolerate the injections.

FOLIC ACID

Reduced forms of folic acid are required for essential biochemical reactions that provide precursors for the synthesis of amino acids, purines, and DNA. Folate deficiency is not uncommon, even though the deficiency is easily corrected by administration of folic acid. The consequences of folate deficiency go beyond the problem of anemia because folate deficiency is implicated as a cause of congenital malformations in newborns and may play a role in vascular disease (see Box, Folic Acid Supplementation: A Public Health Dilemma).

Chemistry

Folic acid (pteroylglutamic acid) is a compound composed of a heterocycle, *p*-aminobenzoic acid, and glutamic acid (Figure 33–3). Various numbers of glutamic acid moieties may be attached to the pteroyl portion of the molecule, resulting in monoglutamates, triglutamates, or polyglutamates. Folic acid can undergo reduction, catalyzed by the enzyme dihydrofolate reductase ("folate reductase"), to give dihydrofolic acid (Figure 33–2, reaction 3). Tetrahydrofolate can subsequently be transformed to folate cofactors possessing one-carbon units attached to the 5-nitrogen, to the 10-nitrogen, or to both positions (Figure 33–2). The folate cofactors are interconvertible by various enzymatic reactions and serve the important biochemical function of donating one-carbon units at various levels of oxidation. In most of these, tetrahydrofolate is regenerated and becomes available for reutilization.

FOLIC ACID SUPPLEMENTATION: A PUBLIC HEALTH DILEMMA

By January 1998, all products made from enriched grains in the USA were required to be supplemented with folic acid. This FDA ruling was issued to reduce the incidence of congenital neural tube defects. Scientific studies show a strong correlation between maternal folic acid deficiency and the incidence of neural tube defects such as spinal bifida and anencephaly. The FDA requirement for folic acid supplementation is a public health measure aimed at the significant number of women in the USA who do not receive prenatal care and are not aware of the importance of adequate folic acid ingestion for preventing birth defects in their babies. Pregnant women have increased requirements for folic acid; at least 400 μg/d is recommended. It is estimated that the level of folic acid fortification now required in enriched grain products provides an additional 80–100 μg of folic acid per day to the diet of women of childbearing age and 70–120 μg/d to the diet of middle-aged and older adults.

There may be an added benefit for adults. N^5-methyltetrahydrofolate is required for the conversion of homocysteine to methionine (Figure 33–1; Figure 33–2, reaction 1). Impaired synthesis of N^5-methyltetrahydrofolate results in elevated serum concentrations of homocysteine. Data from several sources suggest a positive correlation between elevated serum homocysteine and occlusive vascular diseases such as ischemic heart disease and stroke. Clinical data suggest that the folate supplementation program has improved the folate status and reduced the prevalence of hyperhomocysteinemia in a population of middle-

aged and older adults who did not use vitamin supplements. It is possible, though as yet unproved, that the increased ingestion of folic acid will also reduce the risk of vascular disease in this population.

While these two potential benefits of supplemental folic acid are compelling, the decision to require folic acid in grains was—and still is—controversial. As described in the text, ingestion of folic acid can partially or totally correct the anemia caused by vitamin B_{12} deficiency. However, folic acid supplementation *will not* prevent the potentially irreversible neurologic damage caused by vitamin B_{12} deficiency. People with pernicious anemia and other forms of vitamin B_{12} deficiency are usually identified because of signs and symptoms of anemia, which tend to occur before neurologic symptoms. The opponents of folic acid supplementation are concerned that increased folic acid intake in the general population will mask vitamin B_{12} deficiency and increase the prevalence of neurologic disease in our elderly population. To put this in perspective, approximately 4000 pregnancies, including 2500 live births, in the USA each year are affected by neural tube defects. In contrast, it is estimated that over 10% of the elderly population in the USA, or several million people, are at risk of the neuropsychiatric complications of vitamin B_{12} deficiency (Rothenberg, 1999). In acknowledgment of this controversy, the FDA kept its requirements for folic acid supplementation at a somewhat low level. They also recommend that all adults should keep their ingestion of folic acid below 1 mg/d.

Pharmacokinetics

The average diet in the USA contains 500–700 μg of folates daily, 50–200 μg of which is usually absorbed, depending on metabolic requirements (pregnant women may absorb as much as 300–400 μg of folic acid daily). Various forms of folic acid are present in a wide variety of plant and animal tissues; the richest sources are yeast, liver, kidney, and green vegetables. Normally, 5–20 mg of folates are stored in the liver and other tissues. Folates are excreted in the urine and stool and are also destroyed by catabolism, so serum levels fall within a few days when intake is diminished. Since body stores of folates are relatively low and daily requirements high, folic acid deficiency and megaloblastic anemia can develop within 1–6 months after the intake of folic acid stops, depending on the patient's nutritional status and the rate of folate utilization.

Unaltered folic acid is readily and completely absorbed in the proximal jejunum. Dietary folates, however, consist primarily of polyglutamate forms of N^5-methyltetrahydrofolate. Before absorption, all but one of the glutamyl residues of the polyglutamates must be hydrolyzed by the enzyme α-1-glutamyl transferase ("conjugase") within the brush border of the intestinal mucosa. The monoglutamate N^5-methyltetrahydrofolate is subsequently transported into the bloodstream by both active and passive transport and is then widely distributed throughout the body. Inside cells, N^5-methyltetrahydrofolate is converted to tetrahydrofolate by the demethylation reaction that requires vitamin B_{12} (Figure 33–2, reaction 1).

Pharmacodynamics

Tetrahydrofolate cofactors participate in one-carbon transfer reactions. As described above in the section on vitamin B_{12}, one of these essential reactions produces the dTMP needed for DNA synthesis. In this reaction, the enzyme thymidylate synthase catalyzes the transfer of the one-carbon unit of N^5,N^{10}-methylenetetrahydrofolate to deoxyuridine monophosphate (dUMP) to form dTMP (Figure 33–2, reaction 2). Unlike all of the other enzymatic reactions that utilize folate cofactors, in this reaction the cofactor is oxidized to dihydrofolate, and for each mole of dTMP produced, one mole of tetrahydrofolate is consumed. In rapidly proliferating tissues, considerable amounts of tetrahydrofolate can be consumed in this reaction, and continued DNA synthesis requires continued regeneration of tetrahydrofolate by reduction of dihydrofolate, catalyzed by the enzyme dihydrofolate reductase. The tetrahydrofolate thus produced can then reform the cofactor N^5,N^{10}-methylenetetrahydrofolate by the action of serine transhydroxymethylase and thus allow for the continued synthesis of dTMP. The combined catalytic activities of dTMP synthase, dihydrofolate reductase, and serine transhydroxymethylase are often referred to as the dTMP synthesis cycle. Enzymes in the dTMP cycle are the targets of two anticancer drugs; methotrexate inhibits dihydrofolate reductase, and a metabolite of 5-fluorouracil inhibits thymidylate synthase (see Chapter 55).

Cofactors of tetrahydrofolate participate in several other essential reactions. As described above, N^5-methylenetetrahydrofolate is required for the vitamin B_{12}-dependent reaction that generates methionine from homocysteine (Figure 33–1A; Figure 33–2, reaction 1). In addition, tetrahydrofolate cofactors donate one-carbon units during the de novo synthesis of essential purines. In these reactions, tetrahydrofolate is regenerated and can reenter the tetrahydrofolate cofactor pool.

Clinical Pharmacology

Folate deficiency results in a megaloblastic anemia that is microscopically indistinguishable from the anemia caused by vitamin B_{12} deficiency (see above). However, folate deficiency does not cause the characteristic neurologic syndrome seen in vitamin B_{12} deficiency. In patients with megaloblastic anemia, folate status is assessed with assays for serum folate or for red blood cell folate. Red blood cell folate levels are often of greater diagnostic value than serum levels, since serum folate levels tend to be quite labile and do not necessarily reflect tissue levels.

Folic acid deficiency, unlike vitamin B_{12} deficiency, is often caused by inadequate dietary intake of folates. Alcoholics and patients with liver disease develop folic acid deficiency because of poor diet and diminished hepatic storage of folates. There is also evidence that alcohol and liver disease interfere with absorption and metabolism of folates. Pregnant women and patients with hemolytic anemia have increased folate requirements and may become folic acid-deficient, especially if their diets are marginal. Evidence implicates maternal folic acid deficiency in the occurrence of fetal neural tube defects, eg, spina bifida. (See Box, Folic Acid Supplementation: A Public Health Dilemma.) Patients with malabsorption syndromes also frequently develop folic acid deficiency. Folic acid deficiency is occasionally associated with cancer, leukemia, myeloproliferative disorders, certain chronic skin disorders, and other chronic debilitating diseases. Patients who require renal dialysis also develop folic acid deficiency, because folates are removed from the plasma each time the patient is dialyzed.

Folic acid deficiency can be caused by drugs that interfere with folate absorption or metabolism. Phenytoin, some other anticonvulsants, oral contraceptives, and isoniazid can cause folic acid deficiency by interfering with folic acid absorption. Other drugs such as methotrexate and, to a lesser extent, trimethoprim and pyrimethamine, inhibit dihydrofolate reductase and may result in a deficiency of folate cofactors and ultimately in megaloblastic anemia.

Parenteral administration of folic acid is rarely necessary, since oral folic acid is well absorbed even in patients with malabsorption syndromes. A dose of 1 mg of folic acid orally daily is sufficient to reverse megaloblastic anemia, restore normal serum folate levels, and replenish body stores of folates in almost all patients. Therapy should be continued until the underlying cause of the deficiency is removed or corrected. Therapy may be required indefinitely for patients with malabsorption or dietary inadequacy. Folic acid supplementation to prevent folic acid deficiency should be considered in high-risk patients, including pregnant women, alcoholics, and patients with hemolytic anemia, liver disease, certain skin diseases, and patients on renal dialysis.

HEMATOPOIETIC GROWTH FACTORS

The hematopoietic growth factors are glycoprotein hormones that regulate the proliferation and differentiation of hematopoietic progenitor cells in the bone marrow. The first growth factors to be identified were called colony-stimulating factors because they could stimulate the growth of colonies of various bone marrow progenitor cells in vitro. In the past decade, many of these growth factors have been purified and cloned, and their effects on hematopoiesis have been extensively studied. Quantities of these growth factors sufficient for clinical use are produced by recombinant DNA technology.

Of the known hematopoietic growth factors, **erythropoietin (epoetin alfa)**, **granulocyte colony-stimu-**

lating factor (**G-CSF**), **granulocyte-macrophage colony-stimulating factor** (**GM-CSF**), and **interleukin 11** are currently in clinical use. Thrombopoietin is undergoing clinical trials and will probably become available soon. Other potentially useful hematopoietic factors are still in development.

The hematopoietic growth factors have complex effects on the function of a wide variety of cell types, including nonhematologic cells. Their utility in other areas of medicine, particularly as potential anticancer and anti-inflammatory drugs, is being investigated.

ERYTHROPOIETIN

Chemistry & Pharmacokinetics

Erythropoietin, a 34-39 kDA glycoprotein, was the first human hematopoietic growth factor to be isolated. It was originally purified from the urine of patients with severe anemia. Recombinant human erythropoietin (rHuEpo, epoetin alfa) is produced in a mammalian cell expression system using recombinant DNA technology. After intravenous administration, erythropoietin has a serum half-life of 4–13 hours in patients with chronic renal failure. It is not cleared by dialysis. It is measured in international units (IU). Darbopoetin alfa is a glycosylated form of erythropoietin and differs from it functionally only in having a twofold to threefold longer half-life.

Pharmacodynamics

Erythropoietin stimulates erythroid proliferation and differentiation by interacting with specific erythropoietin receptors on red cell progenitors. It also induces release of reticulocytes from the bone marrow. Endogenous erythropoietin is produced by the kidney in response to tissue hypoxia. When anemia occurs, more erythropoietin is produced by the kidney, signaling the bone marrow to produce more red blood cells. This results in correction of the anemia provided that bone marrow response is not impaired by red cell nutritional deficiency (especially iron deficiency), primary bone marrow disorders (see below), or bone marrow suppression from drugs or chronic diseases.

Normally there is an inverse relationship between the hematocrit or hemoglobin level and the serum erythropoietin level. Nonanemic individuals have serum erythropoietin levels of less than 20 IU/L. As the hematocrit and hemoglobin levels fall and anemia becomes more severe, the serum erythropoietin level rises exponentially. Patients with moderately severe anemias usually have erythropoietin levels in the 100–500 IU/L range, and patients with severe anemias may have levels of thousands of IU/L. The most important exception to this inverse relationship is in the anemia of chronic renal failure. In patients with renal disease, erythropoietin levels are usually low because the kidneys cannot produce the growth factor. These patients are the most likely to respond to treatment with exogenous erythropoietin. In most primary bone marrow disorders (aplastic anemia, leukemias, myeloproliferative and myelodysplastic disorders, etc) and most nutritional and secondary anemias, endogenous erythropoietin levels are high, so there is less likelihood of a response to exogenous erythropoietin (but see below).

Clinical Pharmacology

The availability of erythropoietin has had a significant positive impact for patients with chronic renal failure. Erythropoietin consistently improves the hematocrit and hemoglobin level and usually eliminates the need for transfusions in these patients. An increase in reticulocyte count is usually observed in about 10 days and an increase in hematocrit and hemoglobin levels in 2–6 weeks. Most patients can maintain a hematocrit of about 35% with erythropoietin doses of 50–150 IU/kg intravenously or subcutaneously three times a week. Failure to respond to erythropoietin is most commonly due to concurrent iron deficiency, which can be corrected by giving oral iron. Folate supplementation may also be necessary in some patients.

In selected patients, erythropoietin may also be useful for the treatment of anemia due to primary bone marrow disorders and secondary anemias. This includes patients with aplastic anemia and other bone marrow failure states, myeloproliferative and myelodysplastic disorders, multiple myeloma and perhaps other chronic bone marrow malignancies, and the anemias associated with chronic inflammation, AIDS, and cancer. Patients with these disorders who have disproportionately low serum erythropoietin levels for their degree of anemia are most likely to respond to treatment with this growth factor. Patients with endogenous erythropoietin levels of less than 100 IU/L have the best chance of response, though patients with erythropoietin levels between 100 and 500 IU/L respond occasionally. These patients generally require higher erythropoietin doses (150–300 IU/kg three times a week) to achieve a response, and responses are often incomplete.

Erythropoietin has been used successfully to offset the anemia produced by zidovudine treatment in patients with HIV infection and in the treatment of the anemia of prematurity. It can also be used to accelerate erythropoiesis after phlebotomies, when blood is being collected for autologous transfusion for elective surgery, or for treatment of iron overload (hemochromatosis).

Erythropoietin is one of the drugs banned by the International Olympic Committee. The use of erythropoietin by athletes is based on their hope that increased red blood cell concentration will increase oxygen delivery and improve performance.

Toxicity

The most common adverse effects of erythropoietin are associated with a rapid increase in hematocrit and hemoglobin and include hypertension and thrombotic complications. These difficulties can be minimized by raising the hematocrit and hemoglobin slowly and by adequately monitoring and treating hypertension. Allergic reactions have been infrequent and mild.

MYELOID GROWTH FACTORS

Chemistry & Pharmacokinetics

G-CSF and **GM-CSF**, the two myeloid growth factors currently available for clinical use, were originally purified from cultured human cell lines. Recombinant human G-CSF (**rHuG-CSF; filgrastim**) is produced in a bacterial expression system using recombinant DNA technology. It is a nonglycosylated peptide of 175 amino acids, with a molecular weight of 18 kDa. Recombinant human GM-CSF (**rHuGM-CSF; sargramostim**) is produced in a yeast expression system using recombinant DNA technology. It is a partially glycosylated peptide of 127 amino acids, with three molecular species with molecular weights of 15,500, 15,800, and 19,500. These preparations have serum half-lives of 2–7 hours after intravenous or subcutaneous administration. **Pegfilgrastim**, a covalent conjugation product of filgrastim and a form of polyethylene glycol, has a much longer serum half-life than recombinant G-CSF, and so it can be injected once per myelosuppressive chemotherapy cycle instead of daily for several days.

Pharmacodynamics

The myeloid growth factors stimulate proliferation and differentiation by interacting with specific receptors found on various myeloid progenitor cells. These receptors are members of the superfamily of receptors that transduce signals by association with cytoplasmic tyrosine kinases in the JAK/STAT pathway (see Chapter 2). G-CSF stimulates proliferation and differentiation of progenitors already committed to the neutrophil lineage. It also activates the phagocytic activity of mature neutrophils and prolongs their survival in the circulation. G-CSF also has a remarkable ability to mobilize hematopoietic stem cells, ie, to increase their concentration in peripheral blood. This biologic effect underlies a major advance in transplantation—the use of peripheral blood stem cells (PBSCs) instead of bone marrow stem cells for autologous and allogeneic hematopoietic stem cell transplantation (see below).

GM-CSF has broader biologic actions than G-CSF. It is a multipotential hematopoietic growth factor that stimulates proliferation and differentiation of early and late granulocytic progenitor cells as well as erythroid and megakaryocyte progenitors. Like G-CSF, GM-CSF also stimulates the function of mature neutrophils. GM-CSF acts together with interleukin-2 to stimulate T cell proliferation and appears to be a locally active factor at the site of inflammation. GM-CSF mobilizes peripheral blood stem cells, but it is significantly less efficacious than G-CSF in this regard.

Clinical Pharmacology

Neutropenia, a common adverse effect of the cytotoxic drugs used to treat cancer, puts patients at high risk of serious infection. Unlike the treatment of anemia and thrombocytopenia, transfusion of neutropenic patients with granulocytes collected from donors is performed rarely and with limited success. The introduction of G-CSF in 1991 represented a milestone in the treatment of chemotherapy-induced neutropenia. This growth factor dramatically accelerates the rate of neutrophil recovery after dose-intensive myelosuppressive chemotherapy (Figure 33–4). It reduces the duration of neutropenia

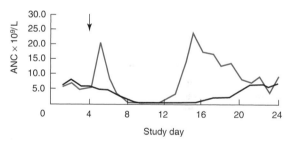

Figure 33–4. Effects of G-CSF (color) or placebo (black line) on absolute neutrophil count (ANC) after cytotoxic chemotherapy for lung cancer. Doses of chemotherapeutic drugs were administered on days 1 and 3. G-CSF or placebo injections were started on day 4 and continued daily through day 12 or 16. The first peak in ANC reflects the recruitment of mature cells by G-CSF. The second peak reflects a marked increase in new neutrophil production by the bone marrow under stimulation by G-CSF. Treated patients in this study had fewer days of neutropenia, days of antibiotic treatment, and days of hospitalization. They also had a lower incidence of infections. (Normal ANC is 2.2–8.6 × 10⁹/L.) (Modified and reproduced, with permission, from Crawford et al: Reduction by granulocyte colony-stimulating factor of fever and neutropenia induced by chemotherapy in patients with small-cell lung cancer. N Engl J Med 1991;325:164.)

and usually raises the nadir, the lowest neutrophil count seen following a cycle of chemotherapy.

While the ability of G-CSF to increase neutrophil counts after myelosuppressive chemotherapy is nearly universal, its impact upon clinical outcomes is more variable. Some clinical trials have shown that G-CSF reduces episodes of febrile neutropenia, requirements for broad-spectrum antibiotics, and days of hospitalization; however, other trials failed to find these favorable outcomes. To date, no clinical trial has shown improved survival in cancer patients treated with G-CSF. Clinical guidelines for the use of G-CSF after cytotoxic chemotherapy have been published (Ozer et al, 2001). These guidelines recommend reserving G-CSF for patients with a prior episode of febrile neutropenia after cytotoxic chemotherapy, patients receiving dose-intensive chemotherapy, patients at high risk of febrile neutropenia, and patients who are unlikely to survive an episode of febrile neutropenia. Pegfilgrastim is an alternative to G-CSF for prevention of chemotherapy-induced febrile neutropenia. Pegfilgrastim can be administered less frequently, and it may shorten the period of severe neutropenia slightly more than G-CSF.

Like G-CSF and pegfilgrastim, GM-CSF also reduces the duration of neutropenia after cytotoxic chemotherapy. It has been more difficult to show that GM-CSF reduces the incidence of febrile neutropenia, probably because GM-CSF itself can induce fever. In the treatment of chemotherapy-induced neutropenia, G-CSF, 5 μg/kg/d, or GM-CSF, 250 μg/m²/d, is usually started within 24–72 hours after completing chemotherapy and is continued until the absolute neutrophil count is > 10,000 cells/μL. Pegfilgrastim is given as a single dose instead of as daily injections.

The utility and safety of the myeloid growth factors in the postchemotherapy supportive care of patients with acute myeloid leukemia (AML) has been the subject of a number of clinical trials. Since leukemic cells arise from progenitors whose proliferation and differentiation are normally regulated by hematopoietic growth factors, including GM-CSF and G-CSF, there was concern that myeloid growth factors could stimulate leukemic cell growth and increase the rate of relapse. The results of randomized clinical trials suggest that both G-CSF and GM-CSF are safe following induction and consolidation treatment of myeloid and lymphoblastic leukemia. There has been no evidence that these growth factors reduce the rate of remission or increase relapse rate. On the contrary, the growth factors accelerate neutrophil recovery and reduce infection rates and days of hospitalization. Both G-CSF and GM-CSF have FDA approval for treatment of patients with AML.

G-CSF and GM-CSF have also been shown to be effective in treating the neutropenia associated with congenital neutropenia, cyclic neutropenia, myelodysplasia, and aplastic anemia. Many patients with these disorders respond with a prompt and sometimes dramatic increase in neutrophil count. In some cases this results in a decrease in the frequency of infections. Since G-CSF and GM-CSF do not stimulate the formation of erythrocytes or platelets, they are sometimes used in combination with other growth factors for treatment of pancytopenia.

The myeloid growth factors play an important role in autologous stem cell transplantation for patients undergoing high-dose chemotherapy. High-dose chemotherapy with autologous stem cell support is increasingly being used to treat patients with tumors that are resistant to standard doses of chemotherapeutic drugs. The high-dose regimens produce extreme myelosuppression; the myelosuppression is then counteracted by reinfusion of the patient's own hematopoietic stem cells (which are collected prior to chemotherapy). The administration of G-CSF or GM-CSF early after autologous stem cell transplantation has been shown to reduce the time to engraftment and to recovery from neutropenia in patients receiving stem cells obtained either from bone marrow or from peripheral blood. These effects are seen in patients being treated for lymphoma or for solid tumors. G-CSF and GM-CSF are also used to support patients who have received allogeneic bone marrow transplantation for treatment of hematologic malignancies or bone marrow failure states. In this setting, the growth factors speed the recovery from neutropenia without increasing the incidence of acute graft-versus-host disease.

Probably the most important role of the myeloid growth factors in transplantation is for mobilization of peripheral blood stem cells (PBSCs). Stem cells collected from peripheral blood have nearly replaced bone marrow as the hematopoietic preparation used for autologous transplantation. The cells can be collected in an outpatient setting with a procedure that avoids much of the risk and discomfort of bone marrow collection, including the need for general anesthesia. In addition, there is evidence that PBSC transplantation results in more rapid engraftment of all hematopoietic cell lineages and in reduced rates of graft failure or delayed platelet recovery. The use of PBSCs for allogeneic transplantation is also being investigated. In allogeneic transplantation, donors are treated with G-CSF in order to mobilize their PBSCs prior to leukapheresis, the procedure that separates the fraction containing stem cells from the other components in blood.

G-CSF is the cytokine most commonly used for PBSC mobilization because of its increased efficacy and reduced toxicity compared with GM-CSF. To mobilize stem cells, patients or donors are given 5–10 μg/kg/d subcutaneously for 4 days. On the fifth day, they undergo leukapheresis. The success of PBSC transplantation depends upon transfusion of adequate numbers of stem cells. CD34, an antigen present on early progenitor cells and absent from later, committed, cells, is used as a marker for the requisite stem cells. The goal is to reinfuse at least 5×10^6 CD34 cells/kg; this number of CD34 cells usually results in prompt and durable engraftment of all cell lineages. It can take several separate leukaphereses to collect enough CD34 cells, especially from older patients and patients who have been exposed to radiotherapy or chemotherapy.

Toxicity

Although the two growth factors have similar effects on neutrophil counts, G-CSF is used more frequently because it is better tolerated. G-CSF can cause bone pain, which clears when the drug is discontinued. GM-CSF can cause more severe side effects, particularly at higher doses. These include fevers, malaise, arthralgias, myalgias, and a capillary leak syndrome characterized by peripheral edema and pleural or pericardial effusions. Allergic reactions may occur but are infrequent. Splenic rupture is a rare but serious complication of the use of G-CSF for PBSC.

MEGAKARYOCYTE GROWTH FACTORS

Chemistry & Pharmacokinetics

Interleukin-11 (IL-11) is a 65–85 kDa protein produced by fibroblasts and stromal cells in the bone marrow. **Oprelvekin,** the recombinant form of interleukin-11 approved for clinical use, is produced by expression in *E coli*. The half-life of IL-11 is 7–8 hours when the drug is injected subcutaneously.

Thrombopoietin, a 65–85 kDa glycosylated protein, is constitutively expressed by a variety of organs and cell types. Hepatocytes appear to be the major source of human thrombopoietin, and patients with cirrhosis and thrombocytopenia have low serum thrombopoietin levels. Recombinant thrombopoietin is produced by expression in human cells; the recombinant product contains two intramolecular disulfide bonds and a number of carbohydrate side chains.

Pharmacodynamics

Interleukin-11 acts through a specific cell surface cytokine receptor to stimulate the growth of multiple lymphoid and myeloid cells. It acts synergistically with other growth factors to stimulate the growth of primitive megakaryocytic progenitors and, most importantly, increases the number of peripheral platelets and neutrophils.

Acting through its own cytokine receptor, thrombopoietin also independently stimulates the growth of primitive megakaryocytic progenitors. In addition, it stimulates mature megakaryocytes and even activates mature platelets to respond to aggregation-inducing stimuli. The critical in vivo role of thrombopoietin has been demonstrated in genetically engineered knockout mice who lack either thrombopoietin or its receptor. These mice have marked thrombocytopenia but do not display anemia or leukopenia.

Clinical Pharmacology

Patients with thrombocytopenia have a high risk of hemorrhage. While platelet transfusion is commonly used to treat thrombocytopenia, this procedure can cause adverse reactions in the recipient; furthermore, a significant number of patients fail to exhibit the expected increase in platelet count.

Interleukin-11 is the first growth factor to gain FDA approval for treatment of thrombocytopenia. It is approved for the secondary prevention of thrombocytopenia in patients receiving cytotoxic chemotherapy for treatment of nonmyeloid cancers. Clinical trials show that it reduces the number of platelet transfusions required by patients who experienced severe thrombocytopenia after a previous cycle of chemotherapy. Although IL-11 has broad stimulatory effects on hematopoietic cell lineages in vitro, it does not appear to have significant effects on the leukopenia or neutropenia caused by myelosuppressive chemotherapy. Interleukin-11 is given by subcutaneous injection at a dose of 50 μg/kg/d. It is started 6–24 hours after completion of chemotherapy and continued for 14–21 days or until the platelet count passes the nadir and rises to > 50,000 cells/μL.

Recombinant thrombopoietin is still an investigational agent. The primary focus of current clinical trials is for the treatment of chemotherapy-induced thrombocytopenia and thrombocytopenia accompanying hematologic stem cell transplantation. Other trials are looking into the possibility of administering thrombopoietin to normal donors in order to increase the number of cells recovered by platelet apheresis. Approval of the latter application will require that thrombopoietin be shown to have an excellent short- and long-term safety profile.

Toxicity

The most common side effects of interleukin-11 are fatigue, headache, dizziness, and cardiovascular effects. The cardiovascular effects include anemia (due to hemodilution), dyspnea (due to fluid accumulation in the lungs), and transient atrial arrhythmias. Hypokalemia has also been seen in some patients. All of these adverse effects appear to be reversible. In the limited clinical trial data available thus far, recombinant thrombopoietin appears to be well tolerated.

PREPARATIONS AVAILABLE

Darbopoetin alfa (Aranesp)
Parenteral: 25, 40, 60, 100, 150, 200, 300, 500 μg/mL for IV or SC injection

Deferoxamine (Desferal)
Parenteral: 500 mg vials for IM, SC, or IV injection

Epoetin alfa (erythropoietin, Epo) (Epogen, Procrit)
Parenteral: 2000, 3000, 4000, 10,000, 20,000 IU/mL vials for IV or SC injection

Filgrastim (G-CSF) (Neupogen)
Parenteral: 300 μg vials for IV or SC injection

Folic acid (folacin, pteroylglutamic acid) (generic)
Oral: 0.4, 0.8, 1 mg tablets
Parenteral: 5 mg/mL for injection

Iron (generic)
Oral: See Table 33–2.
Parenteral (Iron dextran) (InFeD, DexFerrum): 50 mg elemental iron/mL
Parenteral (Sodium ferric gluconate complex) (Ferrlecit): 12.5 mg elemental iron/mL

Parenteral (Iron sucrose)(Venofer): 20 mg elemental iron/mL

Oprelvekin (interleukin-11) (Neumega)
Parenteral: 5 mg vials for SC injection

Pegfilgrastim (Neulasta)
Parenteral: 10 mg/mL solution in single-dose syringe

Sargramostim (GM-CSF) (Leukine)
Parenteral: 250, 500 μg vials for IV infusion

Vitamin B$_{12}$ (generic cyanocobalamin or hydroxocobalamin)
Oral (cyanocobalamin): 100, 500, 1000 μg tablets, 100, 250, 500 μg lozenges
Nasal (Nascobal): 5000 μg/mL (500 μg/spray)
Parenteral (cyanocobalamin): 100, 1000 μg/mL for IM or SC injection
Parenteral (hydroxocobalamin): 1000 μg/mL for IM injection only

REFERENCES

American Society of Clinical Oncology Practice Guidelines Website, http://www.asco.org/ac/1,1003,12-002130,00.asp

Crawford J et al: Reduction by granulocyte colony-stimulating factor of fever and neutropenia induced by chemotherapy in patients with small-cell lung cancer. N Engl J Med 1991;325:164.

Du X, Williams DA: Interleukin-11: review of molecular, cell biology and clinical use. Blood 1997;89:3897.

Fetscher S, Mertelsmann R: Supportive care in hematological malignancies: hematopoietic growth factors, infections, transfusion therapy. Curr Opin Hematol 1999;6:262.

Fisher JW: Erythropoietin: physiology and pharmacology update. Exp Biol Med 2003;228:1.

Gazitt Y: Comparison between granulocyte colony-stimulating factor and granulocyte-macrophage colony stimulating factor in the mobilization of peripheral blood stem cells. Curr Opin Hematol 2002;9:190.

Green R, Miller JW: Folate deficiency beyond megaloblastic anemia: hyperhomocysteinemia and other manifestations of dysfunctional folate status. Semin Hematol 1999;36:47.

Harker LA: Physiology and clinical applications of platelet growth factors. Curr Opin Hematol 1999;6:127.

Jacques PF et al: The effects of folic acid fortification on plasma folate and total homocysteine concentrations. N Engl J Med 1999;340:1449.

Kuter DJ, Begley CG: Recombinant human thrombopoietin: basic biology and evaluation of clinical studies. Blood 2002;100:3457.

Ozer H et al: 2000 update of recommendations for the use of hematopoietic colony-stimulating factors: evidence-based, clinical practice guidelines. American Society of Clinical Oncology Growth Factors Expert Panel. J Clin Oncol 2001;19:1583.

Rothenberg SP: Increasing the dietary intake of folate: pros and cons. Semin Hematol 1999;36:65.

Selhub J: Homocysteine metabolism. Annu Rev Nutr 1999;19:217.

Shpall EJ: The utilization of cytokines in stem cell mobilization strategies. Bone Marrow Transplant 1999;23(Suppl 2):S13.

Wickramasinghe SN: The wide spectrum and unresolved issues of megaloblastic anemia. Semin Hematol 1999;36:3.

Zittoun J, Zittoun R: Modern clinical testing strategies in cobalamin and folate deficiency. Semin Hematol 1999;36:35.

Drugs Used in Disorders of Coagulation

34

Julie Hambleton, MD

Excessive bleeding and thrombosis may represent altered states of hemostasis. Impaired hemostasis results in spontaneous bleeding; stimulated hemostasis results in thrombus formation. The drugs used to arrest abnormal bleeding and to inhibit thrombosis are the subjects of this chapter.

MECHANISMS OF BLOOD COAGULATION

Thrombogenesis

Hemostasis is the spontaneous arrest of bleeding from a damaged blood vessel. The normal vascular endothelial cell is not thrombogenic, and circulating blood platelets and clotting factors do not normally adhere to it to an appreciable extent. The immediate hemostatic response of a damaged vessel is **vasospasm**. Within seconds, platelets stick to the exposed collagen of the damaged endothelium (**platelet adhesion**) and to each other (**platelet aggregation**). Platelets then lose their individual membranes and form a gelatinous mass during **viscous metamorphosis**. This **platelet plug** quickly arrests bleeding but must be reinforced by fibrin for long-term effectiveness. Fibrin reinforcement results from local stimuli to blood coagulation: the exposed collagen of damaged vessels and the membranes and released contents of platelets (Figure 34–1). The local production of thrombin not only releases platelet **adenosine diphosphate (ADP)**, a powerful inducer of platelet aggregation, but also stimulates the synthesis of prostaglandins from the arachidonic acid of platelet membranes. These powerful substances are composed of two groups of eicosanoids (Chapter 18) that have opposite effects on thrombogenesis. **Thromboxane A_2 (TXA_2)** is synthesized within platelets and induces thrombogenesis and vasoconstriction. **Prostacyclin (PGI_2)** is synthesized within vessel walls and inhibits thrombogenesis. **Serotonin (5-HT)** is also released from the platelets, stimulating further aggregation and vasoconstriction.

The platelet is central to normal hemostasis and to all thromboembolic disease. A **white thrombus** forms initially in high-pressure arteries by adherence of circulating platelets to areas of abnormal endothelium as described above. The growing thrombus of aggregated platelets reduces arterial flow. This localized stasis triggers fibrin formation, and a red thrombus forms around the nidal white thrombus.

A **red thrombus** can form around a white thrombus as mentioned above or de novo in low-pressure veins, initially by adherence of platelets (as in arteries) but followed promptly by the process of blood coagulation so that the bulk of the thrombus forms a long tail consisting of a fibrin network in which red cells are enmeshed. These tails become detached easily and travel as emboli to the pulmonary arteries. Such emboli often arise from a deep venous thrombosis (DVT)—a thrombus in the veins of the legs or pelvis. Although all thrombi are mixed, the platelet nidus dominates the arterial thrombus and the fibrin tail the venous thrombus. Arterial thrombi cause serious disease by producing local occlusive ischemia; venous thrombi, by giving rise to distant embolization.

Blood Coagulation

Blood coagulates by the transformation of soluble fibrinogen into insoluble fibrin. Several circulating proteins interact in a cascading series of limited proteolytic reactions. At each step, a clotting factor zymogen (eg, factor VII) undergoes limited proteolysis and becomes an active protease (eg, factor VIIa). Thus, each protease factor activates the next clotting factor until finally a solid fibrin clot is formed. Fibrinogen (factor I), the soluble precursor of fibrin, is the substrate for the enzyme thrombin (factor IIa). This protease is formed during coagulation by activation of its zymogen, prothrombin (factor II). Prothrombin is bound by calcium to a platelet phospholipid (PL) surface, where activated factor X (Xa), in the presence of factor Va, converts it into circulating thrombin. Several of the blood clotting factors are targets for drug therapy (Table 34–1).

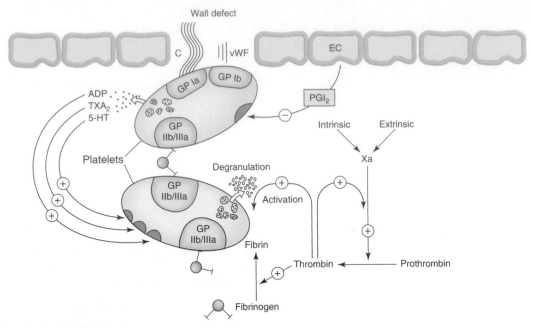

Figure 34–1. Thrombus formation at the site of the damaged vascular wall (EC, endothelial cell) and the role of platelets and clotting factors. Platelet membrane receptors include the glycoprotein (GP) Ia receptor, binding to collagen (C); GP Ib receptor binding, von Willebrand factor (vWF), and GP IIb/IIIa, which binds fibrinogen and other macromolecules. Antiplatelet prostacyclin (PGI$_2$) is released from the endothelium. Aggregating substances released from the degranulating platelet include ADP, TXA$_2$, and 5-HT. Production of factor Xa is detailed in Figure 34–2. (Redrawn and reproduced, with permission, from Simoons ML, Decker JW: New directions in anticoagulant and antiplatelet treatment. [Editorial.] Br Heart J 1995;74:337.)

The main initiator of blood coagulation is the tissue factor (TF)/factor VIIa pathway. The exposure of TF on damaged endothelium binds and activates circulating factor VII (Figure 34–2). This complex, in turn, activates factors X and IX, with the eventual generation of thrombin. Thrombin, in turn, activates upstream proteins, primarily factors V, VIII, and XI, resulting in further thrombin generation. Additionally, thrombin is a potent activator of platelets, converts fibrinogen to fibrin, and activates factor XIII, resulting in an insoluble, cross-linked fibrin molecule.

The TF/factor VII/factor X process is inhibited and regulated by tissue factor pathway inhibitor (TFPI). Oral anticoagulant drugs inhibit the hepatic synthesis of several clotting factors. Heparin inhibits the activity of several of these activated clotting factors by enhancing the anticoagulant activity of **antithrombin,** which inactivates the serine proteases IIa, IXa, Xa, XIa, and XIIa. The endogenous anticoagulants protein C and protein S diminish amplification in the blood clotting cascade by proteolysis of factors Va and VIIIa.

Regulation of Coagulation & Fibrinolysis

Blood coagulation and thrombus formation must be confined to the smallest possible area to achieve local hemostasis in response to bleeding from trauma or surgery without causing disseminated coagulation or impaired blood flow. Two major systems regulate and delineate these processes: **fibrin inhibition** and **fibrinolysis.**

Plasma contains protease inhibitors that rapidly inactivate the coagulation proteins as they escape from the site of vessel injury. The most important proteins of this system are α_1-antiprotease, α_2-macroglobulin, α_2-antiplasmin, and antithrombin. If this system is overwhelmed, generalized intravascular clotting may occur. This process is called **disseminated intravascular coagulation (DIC)** and may follow massive tissue injury, cell lysis in malignant neoplastic disease, obstetric emergencies such as abruptio placentae, or bacterial sepsis.

The central process of fibrinolysis is conversion of inactive plasminogen to the proteolytic enzyme **plasmin.** Injured cells release activators of plasminogen.

Table 34–1. Blood clotting factors and drugs that affect them.[1]

Component or Factor	Common Synonym	Target for the Action of:
I	Fibrinogen	
II	Prothrombin	Heparin (IIa); warfarin (synthesis)
III	Tissue thromboplastin	
IV	Calcium	
V	Proaccelerin	
VII	Proconvertin	Warfarin (synthesis)
VIII	Antihemophilic factor (AHF)	
IX	Christmas factor, plasma thromboplastin component (PTC)	Warfarin (synthesis)
X	Stuart-Prower factor	Heparin (Xa); warfarin (synthesis)
XI	Plasma thromboplastin antecedent (PTA)	
XII	Hageman factor	
XIII	Fibrin-stabilizing factor	
Proteins C and S		Warfarin (synthesis)
Plasminogen		Thrombolytic enzymes, aminocaproic acid

[1]See Figure 34–2 and text for additional details.

Plasmin remodels the thrombus and limits the extension of thrombosis by proteolytic digestion of fibrin.

Regulation of the fibrinolytic system is useful in therapeutics. Increased fibrinolysis is effective therapy for thrombotic disease. **Tissue plasminogen activator (t-PA), urokinase,** and **streptokinase** all activate the fibrinolytic system (Figure 34–3). Conversely, decreased fibrinolysis protects clots from lysis and reduces the bleeding of hemostatic failure. **Aminocaproic acid** is a clinically useful inhibitor of fibrinolysis. Heparin and the oral anticoagulant drugs do not affect the fibrinolytic mechanism.

I. BASIC PHARMACOLOGY OF THE ANTICOAGULANT DRUGS

INDIRECT THROMBIN INHIBITORS

The indirect thrombin inhibitors are so named because their antithrombotic effect is exerted by their interaction with antithrombin. **Unfractionated heparin (UFH), low-molecular-weight heparin (LMWH),** and the synthetic pentasaccharide **fondaparinux** bind to antithrombin and enhance its inactivation of factor Xa. UFH and to a lesser extent LMWH also enhance antithrombin's inactivation of thrombin (IIa).

HEPARIN

Chemistry & Mechanism of Action

Heparin is a heterogeneous mixture of sulfated mucopolysaccharides. It binds to endothelial cell surfaces and a variety of plasma proteins. As noted above, its biologic activity is dependent upon the plasma protease inhibitor **antithrombin.** Antithrombin inhibits clotting factor proteases, especially thrombin (IIa), IXa, and Xa, by forming equimolar stable complexes with them. In the absence of heparin, these reactions are slow; in the presence of heparin, they are accelerated 1000-fold. Only about a third of the molecules in commercial heparin preparations have an accelerating effect because the remainder lack the unique pentasaccharide sequence needed for high-affinity binding to antithrombin (Figure 34–4). The active heparin molecules bind tightly to antithrombin and cause a conformational change in this inhibitor. The conformational change of antithrombin exposes its active site for more rapid interaction with the proteases (the activated clotting factors). Heparin cat-

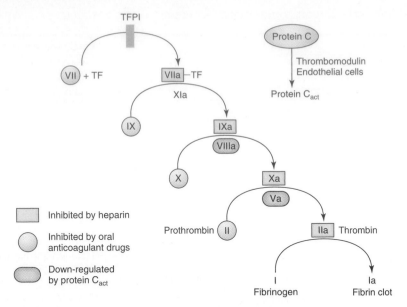

Figure 34–2. A model of blood coagulation. With tissue factor (TF), factor VII forms an activated complex (VIIa-TF) that catalyzes the activation of factor IX to factor IXa. Activated factor XIa also catalyzes this reaction. Tissue factor pathway inhibitor (TFPI) inhibits the catalytic action of the VIIa-TF complex. The cascade proceeds as shown, resulting ultimately in the conversion of fibrinogen to fibrin, an essential component of a functional clot. The two major anticoagulant drugs, heparin and warfarin (an oral anticoagulant), have very different actions. Heparin, acting in the blood, directly activates anticlotting factors, specifically antithrombin, which inactivates the factors enclosed in rectangles. Warfarin, acting in the liver, inhibits the synthesis of the factors enclosed in circles. Proteins C and S exert anticlotting effects by inactivating activated factors Va and VIIIa.

alyzes the antithrombin-protease reaction without being consumed. Once the antithrombin-protease complex is formed, heparin is released intact for renewed binding to more antithrombin.

The antithrombin binding region of commercial unfractionated heparin consists of repeating sulfated disaccharide units composed of D-glucosamine-L-iduronic acid and D-glucosamine-D-glucuronic acid (Figure 34–4). High-molecular-weight (HMW) fractions of heparin with high affinity for antithrombin markedly inhibit blood coagulation by inhibiting all three factors, especially thrombin and factor Xa. Unfractionated heparin has a MW range of 5000–30,000. In contrast, the shorter-chain low-molecular-weight (LMW) fractions of heparin inhibit activated factor X but have less effect on thrombin (and on coagulation in general) than the HMW species. Nevertheless, numerous studies have demonstrated that LMW heparins such as **enoxaparin, dalteparin,** and **tinzaparin** are effective in several thromboembolic conditions. In fact, these LMW heparins—in comparison with UFH—have equal efficacy, increased bioavailability from the subcutaneous site of injection, and less frequent dosing requirements (once or twice daily is sufficient).

Because commercial heparin consists of a family of molecules of different molecular weights, the correlation between the concentration of a given heparin preparation and its effect on coagulation often is poor. Therefore, UFH is standardized by bioassay. Heparin sodium USP must contain at least 120 USP units per milligram. Heparin is generally used as the sodium salt, but calcium heparin is equally effective. Lithium heparin is used in vitro as an anticoagulant for blood samples. Commercial heparin is extracted from porcine intestinal mucosa and bovine lung. Enoxaparin is obtained from the same sources as regular heparin, but doses are specified in milligrams. Dalteparin, tinzaparin and danaparoid (an LMW heparanoid containing heparan sulfate, dermatan sulfate, and chondroitin sulfate that is no longer available in the United States), on the other hand, are specified in anti-factor Xa units.

Toxicity

The major adverse effect of heparin is bleeding. This risk can be decreased by scrupulous patient selection, careful control of dosage, and close monitoring of the activated partial thromboplastin time (aPTT) in those

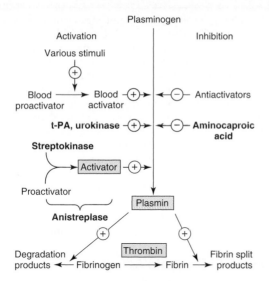

Figure 34–3. Schematic representation of the fibrinolytic system. Plasmin is the active fibrinolytic enzyme. Several clinically useful activators are shown on the left in bold. Anistreplase is a combination of streptokinase and the proactivator plasminogen. Aminocaproic acid (right) inhibits the activation of plasminogen to plasmin and is useful in some bleeding disorders.

patients receiving unfractionated heparin. Levels for UFH may also be determined by protamine titration (therapeutic levels 0.2–0.4 unit/mL) or anti-Xa units (therapeutic levels 0.3–0.7 unit/mL). Weight-based dosing of the LMW heparins results in predictable pharmacokinetics and plasma levels in patients with normal renal function. Therefore, LMW heparin levels are not generally measured except in the setting of renal insufficiency, obesity, and pregnancy. LMW heparin levels are determined by anti-Xa units. Peak therapeutic levels are 0.5–1 unit/mL for twice daily dosing, determined 4

hours after administration, and approximately 1.5 units/mL for once daily dosing. Elderly women and patients with renal failure are more prone to hemorrhage. Heparin is of animal origin and should be used cautiously in patients with allergy. Increased loss of hair and reversible alopecia have been reported. Long-term heparin therapy is associated with osteoporosis and spontaneous fractures. Heparin accelerates the clearing of postprandial lipemia by causing the release of lipoprotein lipase from tissues, and long-term use is associated with mineralocorticoid deficiency.

Heparin causes transient thrombocytopenia in 25% or more of patients and severe thrombocytopenia in 5%. Mild platelet reduction within the first 5 days of therapy may result from heparin-induced aggregation that is postulated to be benign and transient in character. A smaller subset of patients may develop an antibody-mediated thrombocytopenia that is associated with paradoxical thrombosis. In these instances, the heparin-induced antibody is directed against the heparin-platelet factor 4 complex. These antigen-antibody complexes bind to Fc receptors on adjacent platelets, causing aggregation and thromboembolism. The following points should be considered in all patients receiving heparin: Platelet counts should be performed frequently; thrombocytopenia should be considered to be heparin-induced; any new thrombus can be the result of heparin; and thromboembolic disease thought to be heparin-induced should be treated by discontinuance of heparin and administration of an alternative drug, such as a direct thrombin inhibitor (see below). Administration of warfarin alone is contraindicated since it may exacerbate the prothrombotic state associated with heparin-induced thrombocytopenia.

Contraindications

Heparin is contraindicated in patients who are hypersensitive to the drug, are actively bleeding, or have hemophilia, significant thrombocytopenia, purpura,

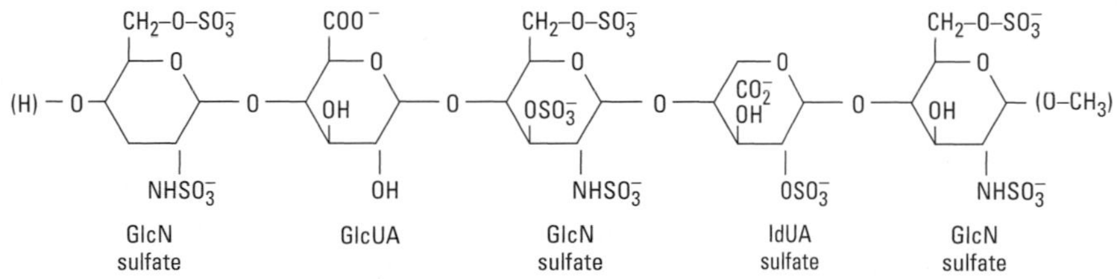

Figure 34–4. Subunit structure of heparin. The small polymer section shown illustrates the repeating disaccharide units typical of heparin. The sequence shows the critical pentasaccharide portion required for binding to antithrombin. In addition to those shown, other saccharides occur. Heparin is a strongly acidic molecule because of its high content of anionic sulfate and carboxylic acid groups. GlcN, glucosamine; IdUA, iduronic acid; GlcUA, glucuronic acid. The same five residues with the terminal groups shown in parentheses, constitute fondaparinux.

severe hypertension, intracranial hemorrhage, infective endocarditis, active tuberculosis, ulcerative lesions of the gastrointestinal tract, threatened abortion, visceral carcinoma, or advanced hepatic or renal disease. Heparin should be avoided in those patients who have recently had surgery of the brain, spinal cord, or eye and in patients who are undergoing lumbar puncture or regional anesthetic block. Despite the apparent lack of placental transfer, heparin should be used in pregnant women only when clearly indicated.

Administration & Dosage

The indications for the use of heparin are described in the section on clinical pharmacology. A plasma concentration of heparin of 0.2–0.4 unit/mL (by protamine titration) or 0.3–0.7 unit/mL (anti-Xa units) usually prevents pulmonary emboli in patients with established venous thrombosis. This concentration of heparin will prolong the activated partial thromboplastin time (aPTT) to 2–2.5 times that of the control value. This degree of anticoagulant effect should be maintained throughout the course of *continuous* intravenous heparin therapy. When *intermittent* heparin administration is used, the aPTT should be measured 6 hours after the administered dose to maintain prolongation of the aPTT to 2–2.5 times that of the control value.

Continuous intravenous administration of heparin is accomplished via an infusion pump. After an initial bolus injection of 80-100 units/kg, a continuous infusion of about 15-22 units/kg/h is required to maintain the aPTT at 2–2.5 times control. Patients with acute pulmonary emboli often require larger doses than these during the first few days because of binding to a variety of acute phase proteins, such as factor VIII and von Willebrand factor, and increased heparin clearance. Subcutaneous administration of heparin, as in low-dose prophylaxis, is achieved with 5000 units every 8–12 hours. Because of the danger of hematoma formation at the injection site, heparin must never be administered intramuscularly.

Prophylactic enoxaparin is given subcutaneously in a dosage of 30 mg twice daily or 40 mg once daily. Full-dose enoxaparin therapy is 1 mg/kg subcutaneously every 12 hours. This corresponds to a therapeutic anti-factor Xa level of 0.5–1 unit/mL. Selected patients may be treated with enoxaparin 1.5 mg/kg once a day, with a target anti-Xa level of 1.5 units/mL. The prophylactic dose of dalteparin is 5000 units subcutaneously once a day; therapeutic dosing is 200 units/kg once a day for venous disease or 120 units/kg every 12 hours for acute coronary syndrome. The use of LMW heparins is discouraged or contraindicated in patients with renal insufficiency or body weight greater than 150 kg.

The synthetic pentasaccharide molecule fondaparinux (Figure 34–4) avidly binds antithrombin with high spe-cific activity, resulting in efficient inactivation of factor Xa. Fondaparinux has a long half-life of 15 hours, allowing for once-daily dosing by subcutaneous administration. A series of phase 3 studies in orthopedic patients comparing fondaparinux 2.5 mg subcutaneously daily beginning 6 hours postoperatively versus enoxaparin either 40 mg daily or 30 mg twice daily found fondaparinux to be superior in preventing development of asymptomatic deep venous thrombosis. A phase 3 study evaluating the use of fondaparinux coupled with warfarin compared with LMWH plus warfarin in the treatment of acute venous thromboembolic disease found these two treatment approaches equivalent. Increased bleeding with fondaparinux is seen in patients administered the drug sooner than 6 hours postoperatively, in those who weigh less than 50 kg, and in those with renal insufficiency.

Reversal of Heparin Action

Excessive anticoagulant action of heparin is treated by discontinuance of the drug. If bleeding occurs, administration of a specific antagonist such as protamine sulfate is indicated. Protamine is a highly basic peptide that combines with heparin as an ion pair to form a stable complex devoid of anticoagulant activity. For every 100 units of heparin remaining in the patient, administer 1 mg of protamine sulfate intravenously; the rate of infusion should not exceed 50 mg in any 10-minute period. Excess protamine must be avoided; it also has an anticoagulant effect. Neutralization of LMW heparin by protamine is incomplete. Limited experience suggests that 1 mg of protamine sulfate may be used to partially neutralize 1 mg of enoxaparin. Protamine will not reverse the activity of fondaparinux. Excess danaparoid can be removed by plasmapheresis.

DIRECT THROMBIN INHIBITORS

The direct thrombin inhibitors (DTI) are a relatively new class of agents that exert their anticoagulant effect by directly binding to the active site of thrombin, thereby inhibiting thrombin's downstream effects. The DTIs bind thrombin without additional binding proteins, such as antithrombin, and they do not bind to other plasma proteins, such as platelet factor 4. **Hirudin** and **bivalirudin** are bivalent DTIs in that they bind at both the catalytic or active site of thrombin as well as at a substrate recognition site. **Argatroban** and **melagatran** are small molecules that bind only at the thrombin active site.

HIRUDIN

For a number of years, surgeons have used medicinal leeches (*Hirudo medicinalis*) to prevent thrombosis in the fine vessels of reattached digits. Hirudin is a specific, irreversible thrombin inhibitor from the leech that is now available in recombinant form as **lepirudin.** Its action is independent of antithrombin, which means it can reach and inactivate fibrin-bound thrombin in thrombi. Lepirudin has little effect on platelets or the bleeding time. Like heparin, it must be administered parenterally and is monitored by the aPTT. Lepirudin is FDA-approved for use in patients with thrombosis related to heparin-induced thrombocytopenia. This drug has a short half-life, but it accumulates in renal insufficiency and no antidote exists. Up to 40% of patients on long-term infusions develop an antibody directed against the thrombin-lepirudin complex. These antigen-antibody complexes are not cleared by the kidney and may result in an enhanced anticoagulant effect.

Bivalirudin, another bivalent inhibitor of thrombin, is administered intravenously, with a rapid onset and offset of action. The drug has a short half-life with clearance that is 20% renal and the remainder metabolic. Bivalirudin inhibits platelet activation and been FDA-approved for use in percutaneous coronary angioplasty.

Argatroban is a small molecule thrombin inhibitor that is FDA approved for use in patients with heparin-induced thrombocytopenia (HIT) with or without thrombosis and coronary angioplasty in patients with HIT. It, too, has a short half-life, is given by continuous intravenous infusion, and monitoring is done by aPTT. Its clearance is not affected by renal disease but is dependent on liver function. The drug requires dose reduction in patients with liver disease. Patients on argatroban will demonstrate elevated INRs because of test interference, rendering the transition to warfarin difficult.

Melagatran is the fourth parenteral drug in this class. It and its oral prodrug, ximelagatran, are under intensive study. Attractive features of ximelagatran include predictable pharmacokinetics and bioavailability—allowing for fixed dosing and predictable anticoagulant response; no need for routine coagulation monitoring; lack of interaction with P450-interacting drugs; rapid onset and offset of action—allowing for immediate anticoagulation and thus no need for overlap with additional anticoagulant drugs. A published phase 3 trial in patients status post major orthopedic surgery found ximelagatran equivalent to warfarin in preventing postoperative DVT. Clinical trials in patients with acute DVT and chronic atrial fibrillation are on-going.

WARFARIN & THE COUMARIN ANTICOAGULANTS

Chemistry & Pharmacokinetics

The clinical use of the coumarin anticoagulants can be traced to the discovery of an anticoagulant substance formed in spoiled sweet clover silage. It produced a deficiency of plasma prothrombin and consequent hemorrhagic disease in cattle. The toxic agent was identified as bishydroxycoumarin and synthesized as dicumarol. This drug and its congeners, most notably warfarin (Figure 34–5), are widely used as rodenticides in addition to their application as antithrombotic agents in humans. Warfarin is the most reliable member of this group, and the other coumarin anticoagulants are almost never used in the USA.

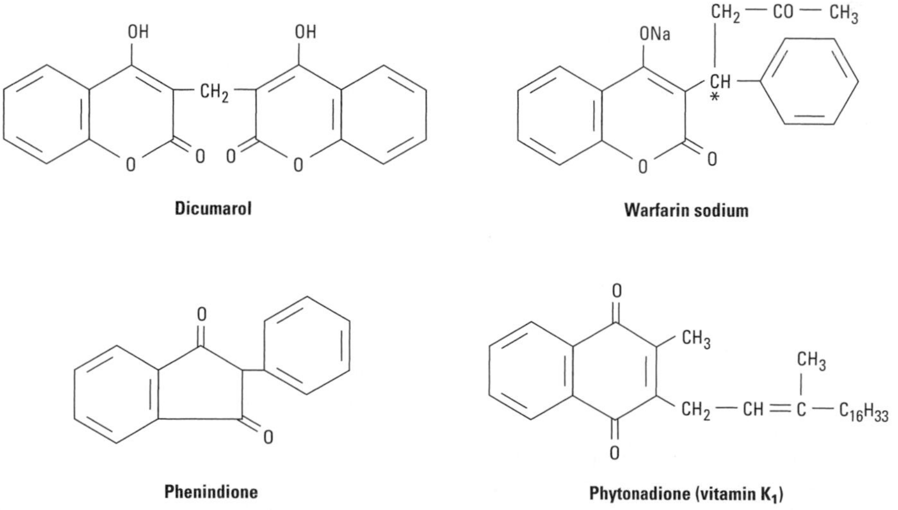

Dicumarol

Warfarin sodium

Phenindione

Phytonadione (vitamin K₁)

Figure 34–5. Structural formulas of several oral anticoagulant drugs and of vitamin K. The carbon atom of warfarin shown at the asterisk is an asymmetric center.

Warfarin is generally administered as the sodium salt and has 100% bioavailability. Over 99% of racemic warfarin is bound to plasma albumin, which may contribute to its small volume of distribution (the albumin space), its long half-life in plasma (36 hours), and the lack of urinary excretion of unchanged drug. Warfarin used clinically is a racemic mixture composed of equal amounts of two enantiomorphs. The levorotatory *S*-warfarin is four times more potent than the dextrorotatory *R*-warfarin. This observation is useful in understanding the stereoselective nature of several drug interactions involving warfarin.

Mechanism of Action

Coumarin anticoagulants block the γ-carboxylation of several glutamate residues in prothrombin and factors VII, IX, and X as well as the endogenous anticoagulant proteins C and S (Figure 34–2). The blockade results in incomplete molecules that are biologically inactive in coagulation. This protein carboxylation is physiologically coupled with the oxidative deactivation of vitamin K. The anticoagulant prevents reductive metabolism of the inactive vitamin K epoxide back to its active hydroquinone form (Figure 34–6). Mutational change of the responsible enzyme, vitamin K epoxide reductase, can give rise to genetic resistance to warfarin in humans and especially in rats.

There is an 8- to 12-hour delay in the action of warfarin. Its anticoagulant effect results from a balance between partially inhibited synthesis and unaltered degradation of the four vitamin K-dependent clotting factors. The resulting inhibition of coagulation is dependent on their degradation rate in the circulation. These half-lives are 6, 24, 40, and 60 hours for factors VII, IX, X, and II, respectively. Larger initial doses of warfarin—up to about 0.75 mg/kg—hasten the onset of the anticoagulant effect. Beyond this dosage, the speed of onset is independent of the dose size. The only effect of a larger loading dose is to prolong the time that the plasma concentration of drug remains above that required for suppression of clotting factor synthesis. The only difference among oral anticoagulants in producing and maintaining hypoprothrombinemia is the half-life of each drug.

Toxicity

Warfarin crosses the placenta readily and can cause a hemorrhagic disorder in the fetus. Furthermore, fetal proteins with γ-carboxyglutamate residues found in bone and blood may be affected by warfarin; the drug can cause a serious birth defect characterized by abnormal bone formation. Thus, warfarin should never be administered during pregnancy. Cutaneous necrosis with reduced activity of protein C sometimes occurs

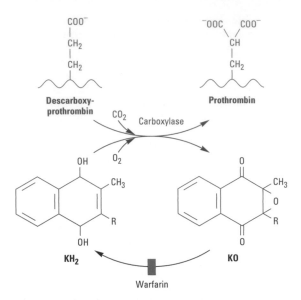

Figure 34–6. Vitamin K cycle—metabolic interconversions of vitamin K associated with the synthesis of vitamin K-dependent clotting factors. Vitamin K$_1$ or K$_2$ is activated by reduction to the hydroquinone form (KH$_2$). Stepwise oxidation to vitamin K epoxide (KO) is coupled to prothrombin carboxylation by the enzyme carboxylase. The reactivation of vitamin K epoxide is the warfarin-sensitive step (warfarin). The R on the vitamin K molecule represents a 20-carbon phytyl side chain in vitamin K$_1$ and a 30- to 65-carbon polyprenyl side chain in vitamin K$_2$.

during the first weeks of therapy. Rarely, the same process causes frank infarction of breast, fatty tissues, intestine, and extremities. The pathologic lesion associated with the hemorrhagic infarction is venous thrombosis, suggesting that it is caused by warfarin-induced depression of protein C synthesis.

Administration & Dosage

Treatment with warfarin should be initiated with standard doses of 5–10 mg rather than the large loading doses formerly used. The initial adjustment of the prothrombin time takes about 1 week, which usually results in a maintenance dose of 5–7 mg/d. The prothrombin time should be increased to a level representing a reduction of prothrombin activity to 25% of normal and maintained there for long-term therapy. When the activity is less than 20%, the warfarin dosage should be reduced or omitted until the activity rises above 20%.

The therapeutic range for oral anticoagulant therapy is now defined in terms of an international normalized ratio (INR). The INR is the prothrombin time ratio (test/control) obtained if the more sensitive international reference thromboplastin made from human brain is used rather than the less sensitive rabbit brain thromboplastin used in North America. Randomized prospective studies with the INR system have resulted in use of lower doses of anticoagulant drug and less bleeding, yet the efficacy is equal to that of the regimens with higher doses. These less intensive and lower dose regimens are efficacious for many therapeutic indications. Analysis of several clinical trials in patients with artificial heart valves has led to the recommendation that dosage be adjusted to achieve an INR of 2.5–3.5.

Drug Interactions

The oral anticoagulants often interact with other drugs and with disease states. These interactions can be broadly divided into **pharmacokinetic** and **pharmacodynamic** effects (Table 34–2). Pharmacokinetic mechanisms for drug interaction with oral anticoagulants are mainly **enzyme induction, enzyme inhibition,** and **reduced plasma protein binding.** Pharmacodynamic mechanisms for interactions with warfarin are **synergism** (impaired hemostasis, reduced clotting factor synthesis, as in hepatic disease), **competitive antagonism** (vitamin K), and an **altered physiologic control loop for vitamin K** (hereditary resistance to oral anticoagulants).

The most serious interactions with warfarin are those that increase the anticoagulant effect and the risk of bleeding. The most dangerous of these interactions are the pharmacokinetic interactions with the pyrazolones phenylbutazone and sulfinpyrazone. These drugs not only augment the hypoprothrombinemia but also inhibit platelet function and may induce peptic ulcer disease (see

Chapter 36). The mechanisms for their hypoprothrombinemic interaction are a stereoselective inhibition of oxidative metabolic transformation of S-warfarin (the more potent isomer) and displacement of albumin-bound warfarin, increasing the free fraction. For this and other reasons, neither phenylbutazone nor sulfinpyrazone is in common use in the USA. Metronidazole, fluconazole, and trimethoprim-sulfamethoxazole also stereoselectively inhibit the metabolic transformation of S-warfarin, whereas amiodarone, disulfiram, and cimetidine inhibit metabolism of both enantiomorphs of warfarin. Aspirin, hepatic disease, and hyperthyroidism augment warfarin pharmacodynamically—aspirin by its effect on platelet function and the latter two by increasing the turnover rate of clotting factors. The third-generation cephalosporins eliminate the bacteria in the intestinal tract that produce vitamin K and, like warfarin, also directly inhibit vitamin K epoxide reductase. Heparin directly prolongs the prothrombin time by inhibiting the activity of several clotting factors.

Barbiturates and rifampin cause a marked *decrease* of the anticoagulant effect by induction of the hepatic enzymes that transform racemic warfarin. Cholestyramine binds warfarin in the intestine and reduces its absorption and bioavailability.

Pharmacodynamic reductions of anticoagulant effect occur with vitamin K (increased synthesis of clotting factors), the diuretics chlorthalidone and spironolactone (clotting factor concentration), hereditary resistance (mutation of vitamin K reactivation cycle molecules), and hypothyroidism (decreased turnover rate of clotting factors).

Drugs with *no* significant effect on anticoagulant therapy include ethanol, phenothiazines, benzodiazepines, acetaminophen, opioids, indomethacin, and most antibiotics.

Table 34–2. Pharmacokinetic and pharmacodynamic drug and body interactions with oral anticoagulants.

Increased Prothrombin Time		Decreased Prothrombin Time	
Pharmacokinetic	**Pharmacodynamic**	**Pharmacokinetic**	**Pharmacodynamic**
Amiodarone	**Drugs**	Barbiturates	**Drugs**
Cimetidine	Aspirin (high doses)	Cholestyramine	Diuretics
Disulfiram	Cephalosporins, third-	Rifampin	Vitamin K
Metronidazole[1]	generation		**Body factors**
Fluconazole[1]	Heparin		Hereditary resistance
Phenylbutazone[1]	**Body factors**		Hypothyroidism
Sulfinpyrazone[1]	Hepatic disease		
Trimethoprim-sulfamethoxazole	Hyperthyroidism		

[1]Stereoselectively inhibits the oxidative metabolism of the (S)-warfarin enantiomorph of racemic warfarin.

Reversal of Action

Excessive anticoagulant effect and bleeding from warfarin can be reversed by stopping the drug and administering vitamin K_1 (phytonadione), fresh-frozen plasma, prothrombin complex concentrates (PCC) such as Bebulin and Proplex T, and recombinant factor VIIa (rFVIIa). The disappearance of excessive effect is not correlated with plasma warfarin concentrations but rather with reestablishment of normal activity of the clotting factors. A modest excess of anticoagulant effect without bleeding may require no more than cessation of the drug. The warfarin effect can be rapidly reversed in the setting of severe bleeding with the administration of a prothrombin complex or recombinant factor VIIa coupled with intravenous vitamin K.

Analogs & Variants

Vitamin K antagonists other than warfarin are seldom used, because they have less favorable pharmacologic properties or greater toxicity. **Dicumarol** is incompletely absorbed and frequently causes gastrointestinal symptoms. **Phenprocoumon** has a long half-life of 6 days—a disadvantage should toxicity occur. The indanedione group, which includes phenindione and diphenadione, has potentially serious adverse effects in the kidney and liver and is of little clinical use.

II. BASIC PHARMACOLOGY OF THE FIBRINOLYTIC DRUGS

Fibrinolytic drugs rapidly lyse thrombi by catalyzing the formation of the serine protease **plasmin** from its precursor zymogen, plasminogen (Figure 34–3). These drugs (**streptokinase, alteplase, anistreplase, tissue plasminogen activator, reteplase, tenecteplase,** and **urokinase**) create a generalized lytic state when administered intravenously. Thus, both protective hemostatic thrombi and target thromboemboli are broken down. The Box, Thrombolytic Drugs for Acute Myocardial Infarction describes the use of these drugs in one major application.

Pharmacology

Streptokinase is a protein (but not an enzyme in itself) synthesized by streptococci that combines with the proactivator plasminogen. This enzymatic complex catalyzes the conversion of inactive plasminogen to active plasmin. **Urokinase** is a human enzyme synthesized by the kidney that directly converts plasminogen to active plasmin. Plasmin itself cannot be used because naturally occurring inhibitors in plasma prevent its effects. However, the absence of inhibitors for urokinase and the streptokinase-proactivator complex permit their use clinically. Plasmin formed inside a thrombus by these activators is protected from plasma antiplasmins, which allows it to lyse the thrombus from within.

Anistreplase (anisoylated plasminogen streptokinase activator complex; APSAC) consists of a complex of purified human plasminogen and bacterial streptokinase that has been acylated to protect the enzyme's active site. When administered, the acyl group spontaneously hydrolyzes, freeing the activated streptokinase-proactivator complex. This product (recently discontinued in the USA) allows for rapid intravenous injection, greater clot selectivity (ie, more activity on plasminogen associated with clots than on free plasminogen in the blood), and more thrombolytic activity.

Plasminogen can also be activated endogenously by **tissue plasminogen activators** (t-PA). These activators preferentially activate plasminogen that is bound to fibrin, which (in theory) confines fibrinolysis to the formed thrombus and avoids systemic activation. Human t-PA is manufactured as alteplase by means of recombinant DNA technology.

Reteplase is another recombinant human t-PA from which several amino acid sequences have been deleted. Reteplase is less expensive to produce than t-PA. Because it lacks the major fibrin-binding domain, reteplase is less fibrin-specific than t-PA. **Tenecteplase** is a mutant form of t-PA that has a longer half-life, and it can be given as an intravenous bolus. Tenecteplase is slightly more fibrin-specific than t-PA.

Indications & Dosage

Use of fibrinolytic drugs by the intravenous route is indicated in cases of **multiple pulmonary emboli** that are not massive enough to require surgical management. Intravenous fibrinolytic drugs are also indicated in cases of **central deep venous thrombosis** such as the superior vena caval syndrome and ascending thrombophlebitis of the iliofemoral vein. They have also been used intra-arterially, especially for peripheral vascular disease.

Thrombolytic therapy in the management of **acute myocardial infarction** requires careful patient selection, the use of a specific thrombolytic agent, and the benefit of adjuvant therapy. Considerable controversy surrounds the question of greater safety or efficacy of t-PA compared with the other thrombolytic agents (see the accompanying Box, Thrombolytic Drugs for Acute Myocardial Infarction).

Streptokinase is administered by intravenous infusion of a loading dose of 250,000 units, followed by 100,000 units/h for 24–72 hours. Patients with antistreptococcal antibodies can develop fever, allergic reactions, and therapeutic resistance. Urokinase requires a loading dose of 300,000 units given over 10 minutes and a maintenance dose of 300,000 units/h for 12 hours. Alteplase (t-PA) is given by intravenous infusion of 60 mg over the first hour and then 40 mg at a rate of 20 mg/h. Reteplase is given as two intravenous bolus injections of 10 units each, separated by 30 minutes. Tenecteplase is given as a single intravenous bolus of 0.5 mg/kg. Anistreplase is given as a single intravenous injection of 30 units over 3–5 minutes. A single course of fibrinolytic drugs is expensive: hundreds of dollars for streptokinase and thousands for urokinase and t-PA.

Recombinant tissue plasminogen activator has increasingly been used for patients presenting with acute stroke symptoms. A recent outcomes study demon-strated an advantage with respect to neurologic disabil-ity at 1 year in those patients with acute ischemic stroke who received intravenous t-PA within 3 hours after onset of symptoms.

III. BASIC PHARMACOLOGY OF ANTIPLATELET AGENTS

Platelet function is regulated by three categories of sub-stances. The first group consists of agents generated out-side the platelet that interact with platelet membrane receptors, eg, catecholamines, collagen, thrombin, and

---

THROMBOLYTIC DRUGS FOR ACUTE MYOCARDIAL INFARCTION

Background: The paradigm shift in 1980 on the cau-sation of acute myocardial infarction to acute coro-nary occlusion by a thrombus created the rationale for thrombolytic therapy of this common lethal dis-ease. At that time—and for the first time—intra-venous thrombolytic therapy for acute myocardial infarction in the European Cooperative Study Group trial was found to reduce mortality significantly. Later studies, with thousands of patients in each trial, pro-vided enough statistical power for the 20% reduction in mortality to be considered statistically significant. Although the standard of care in areas with adequate facilities and experience in percutaneous coronary intervention (PCI) now favors catheterization and placement of a stent, thrombolytic therapy is still very important where PCI is not readily available.

Patients: The selection of patients for throm-bolytic therapy is critical. The diagnosis of acute myocardial infarction is made clinically and is con-firmed by electrocardiography. Patients with ST seg-ment elevation and bundle branch block on electro-cardiography do best; those with ST segment depression or a normal ECG do less well; and those with non-Q-wave acute myocardial infarction may even be harmed. All trials to date show the greatest benefit for thrombolytic therapy when it is given early, within 6 hours after symptomatic onset of acute myocardial infarction.

Clinical trials: One of the trials (ISIS-3) showed that streptokinase plus aspirin performed as well as recombinant tissue-type plasminogen activator (rt-PA) or complex formulations of streptokinase such as anistreplase (APSAC). The GUSTO trial showed a small advantage for the much more expensive t-PA over streptokinase, but with a significantly higher risk of hemorrhagic stroke. Nine clinical trials—each con-taining over 1000 patients with suspected acute myocardial infarction—reported 11.6% mortality at 35 days in the control group and 9.5% in the treat-ment group, an 18% reduction in mortality.

Adjunctive drugs: The best results occur with thrombolytic drugs supplemented by other drugs. β-Blocker drugs reduced myocardial ischemia and infarct size, prevented arrhythmias, decreased rein-farction, and improved survival in ISIS-1 and GISSI-1. Aspirin alone and with streptokinase reduced mor-tality in ISIS-2. Nitroglycerin, given early in acute myocardial infarction for pain relief, had no beneficial effect on mortality in GISSI-3 and ISIS-4. Oral antico-agulants are best used in patients with depressed left ventricular function or systemic embolization. Heparin was a necessary adjunct for t-PA in GUSTO but was less useful with streptokinase plus aspirin because of the increased risk of bleeding. ACE inhibitors reduced infarct expansion and arrhyth-mias and improved survival in GISSI-3. Direct throm-bin inhibitors like hirudin and bivalirudin are under-going clinical trials to better determine their efficacy in conjunction with thrombolytic therapy (TIMI-9B, GUSTO-2A, OASIS, HERO).

Summary: Thrombolytic drugs reduce the mor-tality of acute myocardial infarction. The early and appropriate use of any thrombolytic drug probably transcends individual advantages. Adjunctive drugs like aspirin, β-blockers, and ACE inhibitors reduce mortality even further. The principles of manage-ment are outlined in part 7 of the American Heart Association Guidelines, 2000.

prostacyclin. The second category contains agents generated within the platelet that interact with membrane receptors, eg, ADP, prostaglandin D_2, prostaglandin E_2, and serotonin. The third group comprises agents generated within the platelet that act within the platelet, eg, prostaglandin endoperoxides and thromboxane A_2, the cyclic nucleotides cAMP and cGMP, and calcium ion. From this list of agents, several targets for platelet inhibitory drugs have been identified (Figure 34–1): inhibition of prostaglandin metabolism (aspirin), inhibition of ADP-induced platelet aggregation (clopidogrel, ticlopidine), and blockade of GP IIb/IIIa receptors on platelets (abciximab, tirofiban, and eptifibatide). Dipyridamole and cilostazol are additional antiplatelet drugs.

ASPIRIN

The prostaglandin **thromboxane A_2** is an arachidonate product that causes platelets to change shape, to release their granules, and to aggregate (see Chapter 18). Drugs that antagonize this pathway interfere with platelet aggregation in vitro and prolong the bleeding time in vivo. **Aspirin** is the prototype of this class of drugs. Drugs that modulate the intraplatelet concentration of cAMP do not prolong the bleeding time. However, dietary therapy can be useful in the prophylaxis of thrombosis. Ingestion of the unsaturated fatty acid **eicosapentaenoic acid,** which is high in cold water fish, generates prostaglandin I_3, an effective antiaggregating substance like prostacyclin, and thromboxane A_3, which is much less active than TXA_2 (Chapter 18).

As described in Chapter 18, aspirin inhibits the synthesis of thromboxane A_2 by irreversible acetylation of the enzyme cyclooxygenase. Other salicylates and nonsteroidal anti-inflammatory drugs also inhibit cyclooxygenase but have a shorter duration of inhibitory action because they cannot acetylate cyclooxygenase, ie, their action is reversible.

The FDA has approved the use of 325 mg/d for *primary* prophylaxis of myocardial infarction but urges caution in this use of aspirin by the general population except when prescribed as an adjunct to risk factor management by smoking cessation and lowering of blood cholesterol and blood pressure. Meta-analysis of many published trials of aspirin and other antiplatelet agents confirms the value of this intervention in the *secondary* prevention of vascular events among patients with a history of vascular events.

CLOPIDOGREL & TICLOPIDINE

Clopidogrel and ticlopidine reduce platelet aggregation by inhibiting the ADP pathway of platelets. These drugs are thienopyridine derivatives that achieve their antiplatelet effects by irreversibly blocking the ADP receptor on platelets. Unlike aspirin, these drugs have no effect on prostaglandin metabolism. Randomized clinical trials with both drugs report efficacy in the prevention of vascular events among patients with transient ischemic attacks, completed strokes, and unstable angina pectoris. Use of clopidogrel or ticlopidine to prevent thrombosis is now considered standard practice in patients undergoing placement of a coronary stent.

Adverse effects of ticlopidine include nausea, dyspepsia, and diarrhea in up to 20% of patients, hemorrhage in 5%, and, most seriously, leukopenia in 1%. The leukopenia is detected by regular monitoring of the white blood cell count during the first 3 months of treatment. Development of thrombotic thrombocytopenic purpura (TTP) has also been associated with the ingestion of ticlopidine. The dosage of ticlopidine is 250 mg twice daily. It is particularly useful in patients who cannot tolerate aspirin. Doses of ticlopidine less than 500 mg/d may be efficacious with fewer adverse effects.

Clopidogrel has fewer adverse effects than ticlopidine and is rarely associated with neutropenia. Thrombotic thrombocytopenic purpura associated with clopidogrel has recently been reported. Because of its superior side effect profile and dosing requirements, clopidogrel is preferred over ticlopidine. The antithrombotic effects of clopidogrel are dose-dependent; within 5 hours after an oral loading dose of 300 mg, 80% of platelet activity will be inhibited. The maintenance dose of clopidogrel is 75 mg/d, which achieves maximum platelet inhibition. The duration of the antiplatelet effect is 7–10 days.

BLOCKADE OF PLATELET GP IIB/IIIA RECEPTORS

The glycoprotein IIb/IIIa inhibitors are used in patients with acute coronary syndromes. These drugs target the platelet IIb/IIIa receptor complex (Figure 34–1). The IIb/IIIa complex functions as a receptor mainly for fibrinogen and vitronectin but also for fibronectin and von Willebrand factor. Activation of this receptor complex is the "final common pathway" for platelet aggregation. There are approximately 50,000 copies of this complex on the platelet surface. Persons lacking this receptor have a bleeding disorder called Glanzmann's thrombasthenia.

Abciximab, a humanized monoclonal antibody directed against the IIb/IIIa complex including the vibronectin receptor, was the first agent approved in this class of drugs. It has been approved for use in percutaneous coronary intervention and in acute coronary syndromes. **Eptifibatide** is an analog of the sequence at the extreme carboxyl terminal of the delta chain of fibrinogen, which mediates the binding of fibrinogen to the receptor. **Tirofiban** is a smaller molecule with similar properties. Eptifibatide and tirofiban inhibit ligand binding to the IIb/IIIa receptor by their occupancy of the receptor but do not block the vibronectin receptor.

The three agents described above are administered parenterally. Oral formulations of IIb/IIIa antagonists have been developed and are in various stages of development. Thus far, however, lack of efficacy and significant thrombocytopenia have prevented progress with the oral analogs.

ADDITIONAL ANTIPLATELET-DIRECTED DRUGS

Dipyridamole is a vasodilator that inhibits platelet function by inhibiting adenosine uptake and cyclic GMP phosphodiesterase activity. Dipyridamole by itself has little or no beneficial effect. Therefore, therapeutic use of this agent is primarily in combination with aspirin to prevent cerebrovascular ischemia. It may also be used in combination with warfarin for primary prophylaxis of thromboemboli in patients with prosthetic heart valves. A combination of dipyridamole complexed with 25 mg of aspirin is now available for secondary prophylaxis of cerebrovascular disease.

Cilostazol is a newer phosphodiesterase inhibitor that promotes vasodilation and inhibition of platelet aggregation. Cilostazol is used primarily to treat intermittent claudication.

IV. CLINICAL PHARMACOLOGY OF DRUGS USED TO PREVENT CLOTTING

VENOUS THROMBOSIS

Risk Factors

A. INHERITED DISORDERS

The inherited disorders characterized by an tendency to form thrombi (thrombophilia) derive from either quantitative or qualitative abnormalities of the natural anticoagulant system. Deficiencies in the natural anticoagulants antithrombin, protein C, and protein S account for approximately 15% of selected patients with juvenile or recurrent thrombosis and 5–10% of unselected cases

of acute venous thrombosis. Additional causes of thrombophilia include the factor V Leiden mutation, hyperhomocystinemia, and the prothrombin 20210 mutation that together account for the greater number of hypercoagulable patients.

B. ACQUIRED DISEASE

The increased risk of thromboembolism associated with arrhythmia, primarily atrial fibrillation, and the placement of mechanical heart valves has long been recognized. Similarly, prolonged bed rest, high-risk surgical procedures, and the presence of cancer are clearly associated with an increased incidence of deep venous thrombosis and embolism.

Antithrombotic Management

A. PREVENTION

Primary prevention of venous thrombosis reduces the incidence of and mortality rate from pulmonary emboli. Heparin and warfarin may be used to prevent venous thrombosis. Subcutaneous administration of low-dose unfractionated heparin, low-molecular-weight heparin, or fondaparinux provides effective prophylaxis. Warfarin is also effective but requires laboratory monitoring of the prothrombin time.

B. TREATMENT OF ESTABLISHED DISEASE

Treatment for established venous thrombosis is initiated with unfractionated or low-molecular-weight heparin for the first 5–7 days, with an overlap with warfarin. Once therapeutic effects of warfarin have been established, therapy with warfarin is continued for a minimum of 3–6 months. Patients with recurrent disease or identifiable, nonreversible risk factors may be treated indefinitely. Small thrombi confined to the calf veins may be managed without anticoagulants if there is documentation over time that the thrombus is not extending.

Warfarin readily crosses the placenta. It can cause hemorrhage at any time during pregnancy as well as developmental defects when administered during the first trimester. Therefore, venous thromboembolic disease in pregnant women is generally treated with heparin, best administered by subcutaneous injection.

ARTERIAL THROMBOSIS

Activation of platelets is considered an essential process for arterial thrombosis. Thus, treatment with platelet-inhibiting drugs such as aspirin and ticlopidine or clopidogrel is indicated in patients with transient ischemic attacks and strokes or unstable angina and acute myocardial infarction. In angina and infarction, these drugs are often used in conjunction with β-blockers, calcium channel blockers, and fibrinolytic drugs.

V. DRUGS USED IN BLEEDING DISORDERS

VITAMIN K

Vitamin K confers biologic activity upon prothrombin and factors VII, IX, and X by participating in their postribosomal modification. Vitamin K is a fat-soluble substance found primarily in leafy green vegetables. The dietary requirement is low, because the vitamin is additionally synthesized by bacteria that colonize the human intestine. Two natural forms exist: vitamins K_1 and K_2. Vitamin K_1 (phytonadione; Figure 34–5) is found in food. Vitamin K_2 (menaquinone) is found in human tissues and is synthesized by intestinal bacteria.

Vitamins K_1 and K_2 require bile salts for absorption from the intestinal tract. Vitamin K_1 is available clinically in 5 mg tablets and 50 mg ampules. Onset of effect is delayed for 6 hours but the effect is complete by 24 hours when treating depression of prothrombin activity by excess warfarin or vitamin K deficiency. Intravenous administration of vitamin K_1 should be slow, because rapid infusion can produce dyspnea, chest and back pain, and even death. Vitamin K repletion is best achieved with intravenous or oral administration, because its bioavailability after subcutaneous administration is erratic. Vitamin K_1 is currently administered to all newborns to prevent the hemorrhagic disease of vitamin K deficiency, which is especially common in premature infants. The water-soluble salt of vitamin K_3 (menadione) should never be used in therapeutics. It is particularly ineffective in the treatment of warfarin overdosage. Vitamin K deficiency frequently occurs in hospitalized patients in intensive care units because of poor diet, parenteral nutrition, recent surgery, multiple antibiotic therapy, and uremia. Severe hepatic failure results in diminished protein synthesis and a hemorrhagic diathesis that is unresponsive to vitamin K.

PLASMA FRACTIONS

Sources & Preparations

Deficiencies in plasma coagulation factors can cause bleeding (Table 34–3). Spontaneous bleeding occurs when factor activity is less than 5–10% of normal. Factor VIII deficiency (classic hemophilia, or hemophilia A) and factor IX deficiency (Christmas disease, or hemophilia B) account for most of the heritable coagulation defects. Concentrated plasma fractions are available for the treatment of these deficiencies. Administration of plasma-derived, heat- or detergent-treated factor concentrates and recombinant factor concentrates are the standard treatments for bleeding associated with hemophilia. Lyophilized factor VIII concentrates are prepared from large pools of plasma. Transmission of viral diseases such as hepatitis B and C and AIDS is reduced or eliminated by pasteurization and by extraction of plasma with solvents and detergents. The best use of these therapeutic materials requires diagnostic specificity of the deficient factor and quantitation of its activity in plasma. Intermediate purity factor VIII concentrates (as opposed to recombinant or high-purity concentrates) contain significant amounts of von Willebrand factor. Humate-P is a factor VIII concentrate that is approved by the FDA for the treatment of bleeding associated with von Willebrand disease.

Clinical Uses

An uncomplicated hemorrhage into a joint should be treated with sufficient factor VIII or factor IX replacement to maintain a level of at least 30–50% of the normal concentration for 24 hours. Soft tissue hematomas require a minimum of 100% activity for 7 days. Hematuria requires at least 10% activity for 3 days. Surgery and major trauma require a minimum of 100% activity for 10 days. The initial loading dose for factor VIII is 50 units/kg of body weight to achieve 100% activity of factor VIII from a baseline of $\leq$ 1%, assuming a normal hemoglobin. Each unit of factor VIII per kilogram of body weight raises its activity in plasma 2%. Replacement should be administered every 12 hours. Factor IX therapy requires twice the dose of factor VIII, but with an administration of about every 24 hours because of its longer half-life. Recombinant factor IX has only 80% recovery compared to plasma-derived factor IX products. Therefore, dosing with recombinant factor IX requires 120% of the dose used with the plasma-derived product.

Desmopressin acetate (arginine vasopressin) increases the factor VIII activity of patients with mild hemophilia A or von Willebrand disease. It can be used in preparation for minor surgery such as tooth extraction without any requirement for infusion of clotting factors if the patient has a documented adequate response. High-dose intranasal desmopressin (see Chapter 17) is available and has been shown to be efficacious and well tolerated by patients.

Freeze-dried concentrates of plasma containing prothrombin, factors IX and X, and varied amounts of factor VII (Proplex, etc) are commercially available for treating deficiencies of these factors (Table 34–3). Each unit of factor IX per kilogram of body weight raises its activity in plasma 1.5%. Heparin is often added to inhibit coagulation factors activated by the manufacturing process. However, addition of heparin does not eliminate all thromboembolic events.

Table 34–3. Therapeutic products for the treatment of coagulation disorders.

Factor	Deficiency State	Hemostatic Levels	Half-Life of Infused Factor	Replacement Source
I	Hypofibrinogenemia	1 g/dL	4 days	Cryoprecipitate FFP
II	Prothrombin deficiency	30–40%	3 days	Prothrombin complex concentrates (intermediate purity factor IX concentrates)
V	Factor V deficiency	20%	1 day	FFP
VII	Factor VII deficiency	30%	4-6 hours	FFP Prothrombin complex concentrates (Intermediate purity factor IX concentrates) rFVIIa
VIII	Hemophilia A	30–50% 100% for major bleeding or trauma	12 hours	Recombinant factor VIII products Plasma-derived high purity concentrates [1]Cryoprecipitate Some patients with mild deficiency will respond to DDAVP
IX	Hemophilia B Christmas disease	30–50% 100% for major bleeding or trauma	24 hours	Recombinant F IX products Plasma-derived high purity concentrates
X	Stuart-Prower defect	25%	36 hours	FFP Prothrombin complex concentrates
XI	Hemophilia C	30–50%	3 days	FFP
XII	Hageman defect	Not required		Treatment not necessary
Von Willebrand	Von Willebrand disease	30%	Approximately 10 hours	Intermediate purity factor VIII concentrates that contain von Willebrand factor Some patients respond to DDAVP [1]Cryoprecipitate
XIII	Factor XIII deficiency	5%	6 days	FFP Cryoprecipitate

FFP, fresh frozen plasma.

Antithrombin and activated protein C concentrates are available for the appropriate indications that include thrombosis in the setting of antithrombin deficiency and sepsis respectively.

[1]Cryoprecipate should be used to treat bleeding in the setting of factor VIII deficiency and von Willebrand disease only in an emergency in which pathogen-inactivated products are not available.

Some preparations of factor IX concentrate contain *activated* clotting factors, which has led to their use in treating patients with inhibitors or antibodies to factor VIII or factor IX. Two products are available expressly for this purpose: **Autoplex** (with factor VIII correctional activity) and **Feiba** (with factor VIII inhibitor bypassing activity). These products are not uniformly successful in arresting hemorrhage, and the factor IX inhibitor titers often rise after treatment with them. Acquired inhibitors of coagulation factors may also be treated with porcine factor VIII (for factor VIII inhibitors) and recombinant activated factor VII. Recombinant activated factor VII (**NovoSeven**) is being increasingly used to treat coagulopathy associated with liver disease and major blood loss in trauma and surgery. These recombinant and plasma-derived factor concentrates are very expensive, and the indications for them are very precise. Therefore, close consultation with a hematologist knowledgeable in this area is essential.

Cryoprecipitate is a plasma protein fraction obtainable from whole blood. It is used to treat deficiencies or qualitative abnormalities of fibrinogen, such as that which occurs with disseminated intravascular coagulation and liver disease. A single unit of cryoprecipitate contains 300 mg of fibrinogen.

Cryoprecipitate may also be used for patients with factor VIII deficiency and von Willebrand disease if desmopressin is not indicated and a pathogen-inactivated recombinant or plasma-derived product is not available. The concentration of factor VIII and von Willebrand factor in cryoprecipitate is not as great as that found in the concentrated plasma fractions. Moreover, cryoprecipitate is not treated in any manner to decrease the risk of viral exposure. For infusion, the frozen cryoprecipitate unit is thawed and dissolved in a small volume of sterile citrate-saline solution and pooled with other units. Rh-negative women with potential for childbearing should receive only Rh-negative cryoprecipitate because of possible contamination of the product with Rh-positive blood cells.

FIBRINOLYTIC INHIBITORS: AMINOCAPROIC ACID

Aminocaproic acid (EACA), which is chemically similar to the amino acid lysine, is a synthetic inhibitor of fibrinolysis. It competitively inhibits plasminogen activation (Figure 34–3). It is rapidly absorbed orally and is cleared from the body by the kidney. The usual oral dosage of EACA is 6 g four times a day. When the drug is administered intravenously, a 5 g loading dose should be infused over 30 minutes to avoid hypotension. **Tranex-** amic acid is an analog of aminocaproic acid and has the same properties. It is administered orally with a 15 mg/kg loading dose followed by 30 mg/kg every 6 hours, but the drug is not currently available in the United States.

Clinical uses of aminocaproic acid are as adjunctive therapy in hemophilia, as therapy for bleeding from fibrinolytic therapy, and as prophylaxis for rebleeding from intracranial aneurysms. Treatment success has also been reported in patients with postsurgical gastrointestinal bleeding and postprostatectomy bleeding and bladder hemorrhage secondary to radiation- and drug-induced cystitis. Adverse effects of the drug include intravascular thrombosis from inhibition of plasminogen activator, hypotension, myopathy, abdominal discomfort, diarrhea, and nasal stuffiness. The drug should not be used in patients with disseminated intravascular coagulation or genitourinary bleeding of the upper tract, eg, kidney and ureters, because of the potential for excessive clotting.

SERINE PROTEASE INHIBITORS: APROTININ

Aprotinin is a serine protease inhibitor ("serpin") that inhibits fibrinolysis by free plasmin and may have other antihemorrhagic effects as well. It also inhibits the plasmin-streptokinase complex in patients who have received that thrombolytic agent. Aprotinin will reduce bleeding—by as much as 50%—from many types of surgery, especially that involving extracorporeal circulation for open heart procedures and liver transplantation. It is currently approved for use in patients undergoing coronary artery bypass grafting who are at high risk of excessive blood loss. In placebo-controlled trials, adverse effects of aprotinin were little different from those reported in patients in the placebo group. In larger studies, a possible association with anaphylaxis has been reported in < 0.5% of cases. Therefore, a small test dose is recommended before the full therapeutic dose is given.

PREPARATIONS AVAILABLE

Abciximab (ReoPro)
 Parenteral: 2 mg/mL for IV injection
Alteplase recombinant [t-PA] (Activase*)
 Parenteral: 50, 100 mg lyophilized powder to reconstitute for IV injection
Aminocaproic acid (generic, Amicar)
 Oral: 500 mg tablets; 250 mg/mL syrup
 Parenteral: 250 mg/mL for IV injection

Anisindione (Miradon)
 Oral: 50 mg tablets
Antihemophilic factor [factor VIII, AHF] (Alphanate, Bioclate*, Helixate*, Hemofil M, Koate-HP, Kogenate*, Monoclate, Recombinate,* others)
 Parenteral: in vials

FIBRINOLYTIC DRUGS

Davydov L et al: Tenecteplase: A review. Clinical Therapeutics 2001;23:982.

Thrombolytic therapy with streptokinase in acute ischemic stroke. The Multicenter Acute Stroke Trial–Europe Study Group. N Engl J Med 1996;335:145.

Weitz J, Hirsh J: New antithrombotic agents. Chest 1998;(5 Suppl)114:715S.

ANTITHROMBOTIC DRUGS

American Heart Association: Guidelines 2000 for cardiopulmonary resuscitation and emergency cardiovascular care. Part 7. Circulation 2000;102:I-172.

Chew DP, Bhatt DL: Optimizing glycoprotein IIb/IIIa inhibition: lessons from recent randomized controlled trials. Internal Medicine J 2002;32:338.

Hurlen M et al: Warfarin, aspirin, or both after myocardial infarction. N Engl J Med 2002;347:969.

BLEEDING DISORDERS

Mannucci PM, Tuddenham EGD: The hemophilias—from royal genes to gene therapy. N Engl J Med 2001;344:1773.

Mannucci PM: How I treat patients with von Willebrand disease. Blood 2001;97:1915.

Mannucci PM: Hemostatic drugs. N Engl J Med 1998;339:245.

Anti-inhibitor coagulant complex (Autoplex T, Feiba VH Immuno)
Parenteral: in vials

Antithrombin III (Thrombate III)
Parenteral: 500, 1000 IU powder to reconstitute for IV injection

Aprotinin (Trasylol)
Parenteral: 10,000 units/mL in 100 and 200 mL vials

Argatroban
Parenteral: 100 mg/ml in 2.5 mL vials

Bivalirudin (Angiomax)
Parenteral: 250 mg per vial

Cilostazol (Pletal)
Oral: 50, 100 mg tablets

Clopidogrel (Plavix)
Oral: 75 mg tablets

Coagulation factor VIIa recombinant (Novo-Seven*)
Parenteral: 1.2, 4.8 mg powder/vial for IV injection

Dalteparin (Fragmin)
Parenteral: 2500, 5000, 10,000 anti-factor Xa units/0.2 mL for SC injection only

Danaparoid (Orgaran)
Parenteral: 750 anti-Xa units/vial

Dipyridamole (Persantine)
Oral: 25, 50, 75 mg tablets
Oral combination product (Aggrenox): 200 mg extended-release dipyridamole plus 25 mg aspirin

Enoxaparin (low-molecular-weight heparin, Lovenox)
Parenteral: pre-filled, multiple-dose syringes for SC injection only

Eptifibatide (Integrilin)
Parenteral: 0.75, 2 mg/mL for IV infusion

Factor VIIa: see Coagulation factor VIIa recombinant

Factor VIII: see Antihemophilic factor

Factor IX complex, human (AlphaNine SD, Bebulin VH, BeneFix*, Konyne 80, Mononine, Profilnine SD, Proplex T, Proplex SX-T)
Parenteral: in vials

Fondaparinux (Arixtra)
Parenteral: 2.5 mg in 0.5 mL single-dose prefilled syringes

Heparin sodium (generic, Liquaemin)
Parenteral: 1000, 2000, 2500, 5000, 10,000, 20,000, 40,000 units/mL for injection

Lepirudin (Refludan*)
Parenteral: 50 mg powder for IV injection

Phytonadione [K_1] (generic, Mephyton, AquaMephyton)
Oral: 5 mg tablets
Parenteral: 2, 10 mg/mL aqueous colloidal solution or suspension for injection

Protamine (generic)
Parenteral: 10 mg/mL for injection

Reteplase (Retavase*)
Parenteral: 10.8 IU powder for injection

Streptokinase (Streptase)
Parenteral: 250,000, 750,000, 1,500,000 IU per vial powders to reconstitute for injection

Tenecteplase (TNKase)
Parenteral: 50 mg powder for injection

Ticlopidine (Ticlid)
Oral: 250 mg tablets

Tinzaparin (Innohep)
Parenteral: 20,000 anti-Xa units/mL for subcutaneous injection only

Tirofiban (Aggrastat)
Parenteral: 50, 250 µg/mL for IV infusion

Tranexamic acid (Cyklokapron)
Oral: 500 mg tablets
Parenteral: 100 mg/mL for IV infusion

Urokinase (Abbokinase)
Parenteral: 250,000 IU per vial for systemic use

Warfarin (generic, Coumadin)
Oral: 1, 2, 2.5, 3, 4, 5, 6, 7.5, 10 mg tablets

---

* Recombinant product.

REFERENCES

BLOOD COAGULATION

Dahlback B: Blood coagulation. Lancet 2000;355:1627.

Morrissey JH: Tissue factor: an enzyme cofactor and a true receptor. Thromb Haemost 2001;86:66.

Rosenberg RD, Aird WC: Vascular-bed-specific hemostasis and hypercoagulable states. N Engl J Med 1999;340:1555.

ANTICOAGULANT DRUGS

Dalen JE, Hirsh J, Guyatt GH (editors): Sixth ACCP Consensus Conference on Antithrombotic Therapy. Chest 2001;119(Suppl):1.

Ridker PM et al: Long-term, low-intensity warfarin therapy for the prevention of recurrent venous thromboembolism. N Engl J Med 2003;348:15.

Weitz JI, Bates, SM: Beyond heparin and aspirin: New treatments for unstable angina and non-Q-wave myocardial infarction. Arch Intern Med 2000;160:749.

Agents Used in Hyperlipidemia

35

Mary J. Malloy, MD, & John P. Kane, MD, PhD

The lipids of human plasma are transported in macromolecular complexes termed **lipoproteins.** A number of metabolic disorders that involve elevations in levels of any of the lipoprotein species are thus termed **hyperlipoproteinemias** or **hyperlipidemias.** The term **hyperlipemia** denotes increased levels of triglycerides in plasma.

The two major clinical sequelae of the hyperlipoproteinemias are acute pancreatitis and atherosclerosis. The former occurs in patients with marked hyperlipemia. Control of triglycerides can prevent recurrent attacks of this life-threatening disease.

Atherosclerosis is the leading cause of death for both sexes in the USA and other Western countries. Lipoproteins that contain **apolipoprotein (apo) B100** convey lipids into the artery wall. These are the **low-density (LDL), intermediate-density (IDL), very low density (VLDL),** and **lipoprotein(a) (Lp[a]) lipoproteins.**

The characteristic cellular components in atherosclerotic plaques are foam cells, which are transformed macrophages and smooth muscle cells filled with **cholesteryl esters.** This is the result of endocytosis of chemically modified lipoproteins via at least four species of **scavenger receptors.** Chemical modification of lipoproteins by free radicals creates ligands for scavenger receptors. The atheroma grows with the accumulation of foam cells, collagen, fibrin, and frequently calcium. Whereas lesions can slowly occlude coronary vessels, clinical symptoms are more frequently precipitated by rupture of unstable plaques, leading to activation of platelets and formation of occlusive thrombi. These acute events are thought to reflect inflammatory activities of macrophages.

Although treatment of hyperlipidemia can cause slow physical regression of plaques, the well-documented reduction in acute coronary events that follows vigorous treatment is attributable chiefly to mitigation of the inflammatory activity of macrophages and is evident within 2–3 months after starting therapy.

High-density lipoproteins (HDL) exert several

ACRONYMS	
ACAT	Acyl-CoA:cholesterol acyl-transferase
Apo	Apolipoprotein
CETP	Cholesteryl ester transfer protein
HDL	High-density lipoproteins
HMG-CoA	3-Hydroxy-3-methylglutaryl-coenzyme A
IDL	Intermediate-density lipoproteins
LCAT	Lecithin:cholesterol acyltransferase
LDL	Low-density lipoproteins
Lp(a)	Lipoprotein(a)
LPL	Lipoprotein lipase
PPAR-α	Peroxisome proliferator-activated receptor-alpha
VLDL	Very low density lipoproteins

antiatherogenic effects. They participate in pathways that retrieve cholesterol from the artery wall and inhibit the oxidation of atherogenic lipoproteins. Low levels of HDL (hypoalphalipoproteinemia) are an independent risk factor for coronary disease. The use of drugs that increase levels of HDL is indicated in patients with hypoalphalipoproteinemia.

Cigarette smoking is a major risk factor for coronary disease. It is associated with reduced levels of HDL, impairment of cholesterol retrieval, cytotoxic effects on the endothelium, increased oxidation of lipoproteins, and stimulation of thrombogenesis.

Normal coronary arteries can dilate in response to ischemia, increasing delivery of oxygen to the myocardium. This is mediated by nitric oxide, which acts upon smooth muscle cells of the arterial media. This function is impaired by atherogenic lipoproteins in several phenotypes of hyperlipidemia, aggravating ischemic manifestations of atherosclerosis. Reducing levels of atherogenic lipoproteins and inhibition of their oxidation helps restore endothelial function.

Because atherogenesis is multifactorial, therapy should be directed toward all the modifiable risk factors. Atherosclerosis is a dynamic process. Quantitative angiographic measurements in clinical trials have demonstrated that net regression of plaques can occur during aggressive lipid-lowering therapy. Large primary and secondary prevention trials have shown significant reduction in mortality from new coronary events and in all-cause mortality. Therefore, the timely diagnosis and treatment of lipoprotein disorders can be expected to decrease morbidity and mortality due to coronary disease.

Many of the hyperlipidemic states are associated with the development of xanthomas. These lesions, which are produced by deposition of lipid in tendons or skin, may be painful or cosmetically unacceptable to the patient. Because xanthomas regress with lipid-lowering therapy, this provides another indication for treatment.

PATHOPHYSIOLOGY OF HYPERLIPOPROTEINEMIA

NORMAL LIPOPROTEIN METABOLISM

Structure

Lipoproteins are particles with hydrophobic core regions containing cholesteryl esters and triglycerides. Unesterified cholesterol, phospholipids, and apoproteins surround the core. Certain lipoproteins contain very high-molecular-weight B proteins that exist in two forms: **B48,** which is formed in the intestine and found in chylomicrons and their remnants; and **B100,** synthesized in liver and found in **VLDL, VLDL remnants** (intermediate-density lipoproteins; **IDL**), **LDL** (formed from VLDL), and the **Lp(a) lipoproteins.**

Synthesis & Catabolism

A. CHYLOMICRONS

Chylomicrons are formed in the intestine and carry **triglycerides** of dietary origin, **unesterified cholesterol,** and **cholesteryl esters.** They transit the thoracic duct to the bloodstream.

Triglycerides are removed from chylomicrons in extrahepatic tissues through a pathway shared with VLDL that involves hydrolysis by the **lipoprotein lipase**

(LPL) system. A progressive decrease in particle diameter occurs as triglycerides in the core are depleted. Surface lipids and small apoproteins are transferred to HDL. The resultant chylomicron remnants are taken up by receptor-mediated endocytosis into hepatocytes.

B. VERY LOW DENSITY LIPOPROTEINS (VLDL)

VLDL are secreted by the liver and provide a means for export of triglycerides to peripheral tissues (Figure 35–1). VLDL triglycerides are hydrolyzed by LPL, yielding free fatty acids for storage in adipose tissue and for oxidation in tissues such as cardiac and skeletal muscle. Depletion of triglycerides produces remnants (IDL). Some IDL are endocytosed directly by liver. The remainder are converted to LDL by further removal of triglycerides mediated by hepatic lipase. This process explains the clinical phenomenon of the "beta shift," the increase of LDL (beta-lipoprotein) in serum as a hypertriglyceridemic state subsides. Increased levels of LDL can also result from increased secretion of its precursor VLDL as well as from decreased LDL catabolism.

C. LOW-DENSITY LIPOPROTEINS (LDL)

A major pathway by which LDL are catabolized in hepatocytes and other cells involves receptor-mediated endocytosis. Cholesteryl esters from the LDL core are hydrolyzed, yielding free cholesterol for the synthesis of cell membranes. Cells also obtain cholesterol by de novo synthesis via a pathway involving the formation of mevalonic acid by HMG-CoA reductase. Production of this enzyme and of LDL receptors is transcriptionally regulated by the content of cholesterol in the cell. Normally, about 70% of LDL is removed from plasma by hepatocytes. Even more cholesterol is delivered to the liver via remnants of VLDL and chylomicrons. Thus, the liver plays a major role in the cholesterol economy. Unlike other cells, hepatocytes are capable of eliminating cholesterol by secretion of cholesterol in bile and by conversion of cholesterol to bile acids.

D. LP(A) LIPOPROTEIN

Lp(a) lipoprotein is formed from LDL and the Lp(a) protein linked by a disulfide bridge. Lp(a) protein is highly homologous with plasminogen but is not activated by tissue plasminogen activator. It occurs in a number of isoforms of different molecular weights. Levels of Lp(a) in serum vary from nil to over 200 mg/dL and are determined chiefly by genetic factors. Lp(a) can be found in atherosclerotic plaques and may also contribute to coronary disease by inhibiting thrombolysis. Levels are elevated in nephrosis.

E. HIGH-DENSITY LIPOPROTEINS (HDL)

The apoproteins of HDL are secreted by the liver and intestine. Much of the lipid comes from the surface

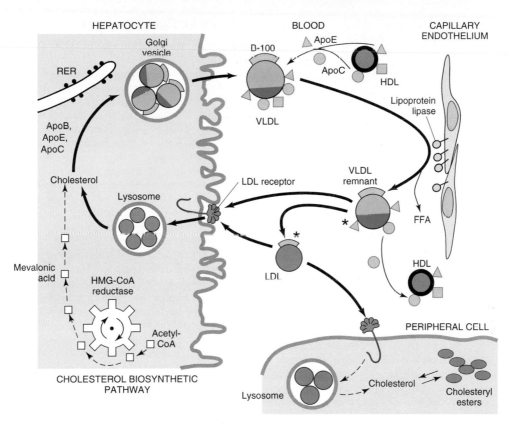

Figure 35–1. Metabolism of lipoproteins of hepatic origin. The heavy arrows show the primary pathways. Nascent VLDL are secreted via the Golgi apparatus. They acquire additional C lipoproteins and apo E from HDL. VLDL are converted to VLDL remnants (IDL) by lipolysis via lipoprotein lipase in the vessels of peripheral tissues. In the process, C apolipoproteins and a portion of the apo E are given back to HDL. Some of the VLDL remnants are converted to LDL by further loss of triglycerides and loss of apo E. A major pathway for LDL degradation involves the endocytosis of LDL by LDL receptors in the liver and the peripheral tissues, for which apo B100 is the ligand. (Dark color denotes cholesteryl esters; light color, triglycerides; the asterisk denotes a functional ligand for LDL receptors; triangles indicate apolipoprotein E; circles and squares represent C apolipoproteins; RER denotes rough endoplasmic reticulum.) (Modified and redrawn, with permission, from Kane J, Malloy M: Disorders of lipoproteins. In: Rosenberg RN et al (editors). *The Molecular and Genetic Basis of Neurological Disease*. Butterworth-Heinemann, 1993.)

monolayers of chylomicrons and VLDL during lipolysis. HDL also acquire cholesterol from peripheral tissues in a pathway that protects the cholesterol homeostasis of cells. In this process, free cholesterol is transported from the cell membrane by a transporter protein, ABCA1, acquired by a small particle termed prebeta-1 HDL, and then esterified by lecithin:cholesterol acyltransferase (LCAT), leading to the formation of larger HDL species. The cholesteryl esters are transferred to VLDL, IDL, LDL, and chylomicron remnants with the aid of cholesteryl ester transfer protein (CETP). Much of the cholesteryl ester thus transferred is ultimately delivered to the liver by endocytosis of the acceptor lipoproteins.

HDL can also deliver cholesteryl esters directly to the liver via a docking receptor (scavenger receptor, SR-BI) that does not endocytose the lipoproteins.

LIPOPROTEIN DISORDERS

Lipoprotein disorders are detected by measuring lipids in serum after a 10-hour fast. Risk of atherosclerotic heart disease increases with concentrations of the atherogenic lipoproteins, is inversely related to levels of

HDL, and is modified by other risk factors (Table 35–1). Evidence from clinical trials suggests that LDL cholesterol levels of 60–70 mg/dL may be optimal for patients with coronary disease. Ideally, triglyceride levels should be below 150 mg/dL. Differentiation requires identification of the lipoproteins involved (Table 35–2). Diagnosis of a primary lipoprotein disorder usually requires further clinical and genetic data as well as ruling out secondary hyperlipidemias (Table 35–3).

Phenotypes of abnormal lipoprotein distribution are described in this section. Drugs mentioned for use in these conditions are described in the following section on basic and clinical pharmacology.

THE PRIMARY HYPERTRIGLYCERIDEMIAS

Hypertriglyceridemia is linked epidemiologically with increased risk of coronary disease. VLDL and its remnants have been found in atherosclerotic plaques. In some kindreds, hypertriglyceridemia may be the only evident risk factor. These patients tend to have cholesterol-rich VLDL of small particle diameter. Hypertriglyceridemic patients with coronary disease or a family history of premature coronary disease should be treated aggressively. In others, treatment decisions should be based on the aggregate of risk factors. Because clearance of triglycerides by the LPL system is saturated at about 800 mg/dL of triglycerides, patients with higher levels should be treated to prevent acute pancreatitis.

Table 35–1. National Cholesterol Education Program: Adult Treatment Guidelines (2001).

	Desirable	Borderline to High[1]	High
Total cholesterol	< 200 (5.2)[2]	200–239[2] (5.2–6.2)	> 240 (6.2)[2]
LDL cholesterol	< 130 (3.4)[3]	130–159 (3.4–4.1)	> 160 (4.1)
HDL cholesterol Men Women	> 40 (1.04) > 50 (1.30)		> 60 (1.55)
Triglycerides	< 150 (1.7)	150–199 (1.7–2.3)	> 200 (2.3)

[1] Consider as high if coronary disease or more than 2 risk factors are present
[2] mg/dL (mmol/L)
[3] Optimal level is < 100 (2.6)

Primary Chylomicronemia

Chylomicrons are not present in the serum of normal individuals who have fasted 10 hours. The recessive traits of lipoprotein lipase deficiency and cofactor deficiency are usually associated with severe lipemia (2000–2500 mg/dL triglycerides when the patient is consuming a typical American diet). These disorders might not be diagnosed until an attack of acute pancreatitis occurs. Patients may have eruptive xanthomas, hepatosplenomegaly, hypersplenism, and lipid-laden foam cells in bone marrow, liver, and spleen. The lipemia is aggravated by estrogens because they stimulate VLDL production, and pregnancy may cause marked increases in triglycerides despite strict dietary control. Although these patients have a predominant chylomicronemia, they may also have moderately elevated VLDL, presenting with a pattern of mixed lipemia (fasting chylomicronemia and elevated VLDL). LPL deficiency is diagnosed by assay of lipolytic activity after intravenous injection of heparin; cofactor deficiency is diagnosed by isoelectric focusing of the VLDL proteins. A presumptive diagnosis of these disorders is made by demonstrating a pronounced decrease in levels of triglycerides a few days after sharp restriction of oral fat intake. Marked restriction of the total fat content in the diet provides effective long-term treatment. Niacin or a fibrate may be of some benefit.

Familial Hypertriglyceridemia

A. SEVERE (USUALLY MIXED LIPEMIA)

A pattern of mixed lipemia usually results from impaired removal of triglyceride-rich lipoproteins. Factors that increase VLDL production aggravate the lipemia because VLDL and chylomicrons are competing substrates for LPL. The primary mixed lipemias probably represent a variety of modes of inheritance. Most patients have the centripetal pattern of obesity with insulin resistance. Other factors that lead to an increased rate of secretion of VLDL also worsen the lipemia. Eruptive xanthomas, lipemia retinalis, epigastric pain, and pancreatitis are variably present depending on the severity of the lipemia. Treatment is primarily dietary, with restriction of total fat, avoidance of alcohol and exogenous estrogens, and weight reduction. Some patients may require treatment with a fibrate or niacin.

B. MODERATE (ENDOGENOUS LIPEMIA)

Primary increases of VLDL probably reflect a number of genetic determinants and are worsened by factors that increase the rate of VLDL secretion from liver, ie, obesity, alcohol, diabetes, and estrogens. A major indication for treatment is the presence of atherosclerosis in the patient or the patient's family. Treatment includes

Table 35–2. The primary hyperlipoproteinemias and their drug treatment.

Disorder	Manifestations	Single Drug[1]	Drug Combination
Primary chylomicronemia (familial lipoprotein lipase or cofactor deficiency)	Chylomicrons, VLDL increased	Dietary management (niacin, fibrate)	Niacin plus fibrate
Familial hypertriglyceridemia Severe	VLDL, chylomicrons increased	Niacin, fibrate	Niacin plus fibrate
Moderate	VLDL increased; chylomicrons may be increased	Niacin, fibrate	
Familial combined hyperlipoproteinemia	VLDL increased	Niacin, fibrate	
	LDL increased	Niacin, reductase inhibitor, ezetimibe	Two or three of the individual drugs
	VLDL, LDL increased	Niacin, reductase inhibitor	Niacin plus resin or reductase inhibitor or ezetimibe
Familial dysbetalipoproteinemia	VLDL remnants, chylomicron remnants increased	Fibrate, niacin	Fibrate plus niacin, or niacin plus reductase inhibitor
Familial hypercholesterolemia Heterozygous	LDL increased	Reductase inhibitor, resin, niacin, ezetimibe	Two or three of the individual drugs
Homozygous	LDL increased	Niacin, atorvastatin, ezetimibe, rosuvastatin	Niacin plus reductase inhibitor plus ezetimibe
Familial ligand-defective apoB	LDL increased	Niacin, reductase inhibitor, ezetimibe	Niacin plus reductase inhibitor or ezetimibe
Lp(a) hyperlipoproteinemia	Lp(a) increased	Niacin	

[1]Single-drug therapy should be evaluated before drug combinations are used.

weight reduction, restriction of all types of dietary fat, and avoidance of alcohol. Fibrates or niacin usually produce further reduction in triglyceride levels if dietary measures are not sufficient. Marine omega fatty acids may also be of value.

Familial Combined Hyperlipoproteinemia

In kindreds with this disorder, individuals may have elevated levels of VLDL, LDL, or both, and the pattern may change with time. Familial combined hyperlipoproteinemia involves an approximate doubling in VLDL secretion. It seems to be transmitted as a semi-dominant trait. Triglycerides can be increased by the factors noted above. Elevations of cholesterol and triglycerides are generally moderate, and xanthomas are usually absent. Drug treatment is warranted because the risk of coronary atherosclerosis is increased and diet

alone does not normalize lipid levels. A reductase inhibitor or ezetimibe in combination with niacin is usually required to treat these patients.

Familial Dysbetalipoproteinemia

In this disorder, remnants of chylomicrons and VLDL accumulate. Levels of LDL are usually decreased. Because remnants are rich in cholesteryl esters, the level of cholesterol may be as high as that of triglycerides. Diagnosis is confirmed by the absence of the E3 and E4 isoforms of apo E. Patients often develop tuberous or tuberoeruptive xanthomas, or characteristic planar xanthomas of the palmar creases. They tend to be obese, and some have impaired glucose tolerance. These factors, as well as hypothyroidism, can aggravate the lipemia. Coronary and peripheral atherosclerosis occur with increased frequency. Weight loss, together with decreased fat, cho-

Table 35–3. Secondary causes of hyperlipoproteinemia.

Hypertriglyceridemia	Hypercholesterolemia
Diabetes mellitus	Hypothyroidism
Alcohol ingestion	Early nephrosis
Severe nephrosis	Resolving lipemia
Estrogens	Immunoglobulin-lipoprotein complex disorders
Uremia	Anorexia nervosa
Corticosteroid excess	Cholestasis
Myxedema	Hypopituitarism
Glycogen storage disease	Corticosteroid excess
Hypopituitarism	
Acromegaly	
Immunoglobulin-lipoprotein complex disorders	
Lipodystrophy	
Isotretinoin	
Protease inhibitors	

lesterol, and alcohol consumption, may be sufficient treatment, but a fibrate or niacin is needed in most cases. These agents can be given together in more resistant cases, or a reductase inhibitor may be added.

THE PRIMARY HYPERCHOLESTEROLEMIAS

Familial Hypercholesterolemia

Familial hypercholesterolemia is an autosomal dominant trait. Although levels of LDL tend to increase throughout childhood, the diagnosis can often be made on the basis of elevated umbilical cord blood cholesterol. In most heterozygotes, cholesterol levels commonly range from 260 to 500 mg/dL. Triglycerides are usually normal, tendinous xanthomatosis is often present, and arcus corneae and xanthelasma may appear in the third decade. Coronary atherosclerosis tends to occur prematurely. Homozygous familial hypercholesterolemia, which can lead to coronary disease in childhood, is characterized by levels of cholesterol often exceeding 1000 mg/dL and early tuberous and tendinous xanthomatosis. These patients may also develop elevated plaque-like xanthomas of the aortic valve, digital webs, buttocks, and extremities.

Defects of LDL receptors underlie this disorder. Some individuals have combined heterozygosity for alleles producing nonfunctional and kinetically impaired receptors. Levels of LDL in compliant heterozygous patients can be normalized with combined drug regimens (Figure 35–2). Those whose receptors retain even minimal function may partially respond to resins or

reductase inhibitors. Niacin and atorvastatin may benefit patients with no receptor function.

Familial Ligand-Defective Apolipoprotein B

Defects in the ligand domain of apo B100 (the region that binds to the LDL receptor) impair the endocytosis of LDL, leading to hypercholesterolemia of moderate severity. Tendon xanthomas may occur. These disorders are as prevalent as familial hypercholesterolemia. Response to reductase inhibitors is variable. Up-regulation of LDL receptors in liver increases endocytosis of LDL precursors but does not increase uptake of ligand-defective LDL particles. Niacin often has beneficial effects by reducing VLDL production.

Familial Combined Hyperlipoproteinemia (FCH)

As described above, some persons in kindreds with this disorder have only an elevation in LDL. Serum cholesterol is usually less than 350 mg/dL. Premature coronary disease is common. Dietary and drug treatment, usually with niacin or a reductase inhibitor, is indicated. It is fre-

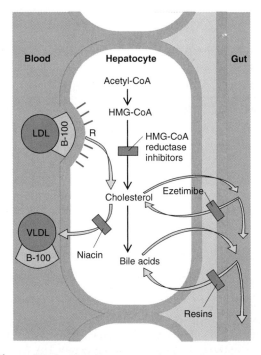

Figure 35–2. Sites of action of HMG-CoA reductase inhibitors, niacin, ezetimibe, and resins used in treating hyperlipidemias. LDL receptors (R) are increased by treatment with resins and HMG-CoA reductase inhibitors.

quently necessary to add niacin to normalize LDL or to reduce triglycerides if treatment is initiated with a resin.

Lp(a) Hyperlipoproteinemia

This familial disorder, which is associated with increased atherogenesis, is determined chiefly by alleles that dictate increased production of the Lp(a) lipoprotein. Niacin reduces levels of Lp(a) in many patients.

Other Disorders

Deficiency of cholesterol 7α-hydroxylase can cause elevated LDL in the heterozygous state. Homozygotes can also have elevated triglycerides, resistance to reductase inhibitors, and premature gallstones. Autosomal recessive hypercholesterolemia is due to mutations in a protein that assists in endocytosis of LDL. Niacin and ezetimibe may be useful in these disorders.

HDL Deficiency

Certain rare genetic disorders are associated with extremely low levels of HDL in serum. These include Tangier disease and disorders of LCAT. Familial hypoalphalipoproteinemia is a more common disorder in which levels of HDL cholesterol are usually below 35 mg/dL, with apparent codominant transmission. These patients tend to have premature atherosclerosis, and the low HDL may be the only identified risk factor. Treatment should include special attention to avoidance of other risk factors. Niacin increases HDL cholesterol in many of these patients. Reductase inhibitors and fibric acid derivatives exert lesser effects.

In the presence of hypertriglyceridemia, HDL cholesterol is low because of exchange of cholesteryl esters from HDL into triglyceride-rich lipoproteins. This may contribute to the atherogenic effect of hypertriglyceridemia. In most, treatment of the hypertriglyceridemia will result in normalization of HDL.

SECONDARY HYPERLIPOPROTEINEMIA

Before primary disorders can be diagnosed, secondary causes of the phenotype must be considered. The more common conditions are summarized in Table 35–3. The lipoprotein abnormality usually resolves if the underlying disorder can be treated successfully.

DIETARY MANAGEMENT OF HYPERLIPOPROTEINEMIA

Dietary measures are always initiated first and may obviate the need for drugs. Exceptions are patients with familial hypercholesterolemia or familial combined hyperlipidemia in whom diet and drug therapy should be started simultaneously. Cholesterol, saturated fats, and trans fats are the principal factors that influence LDL levels, whereas total fat and calorie restriction is important in management of triglycerides.

Lipoprotein levels are also affected—but to a lesser extent—by other dietary factors. Increases in VLDL occur when carbohydrate intake is increased but tend to normalize after several months. Sucrose and other simple sugars raise VLDL levels in hypertriglyceridemic patients. Some forms of dietary fiber reduce LDL modestly. Alcohol can cause significant hypertriglyceridemia by increasing hepatic secretion of VLDL. Synthesis and secretion of VLDL are increased by excess calories. Caloric restriction, especially in obese subjects, reduces VLDL and often LDL as well. During weight loss, LDL and VLDL levels may be much lower than can be maintained during neutral caloric balance. The conclusion that diet suffices for management can only be arrived at after weight has stabilized for at least 1 month.

Most patients with elevated LDL can be managed with a diet restricted in cholesterol and saturated fat but with sufficient calories to achieve and maintain ideal body weight. Total fat calories should be 20–25%, with saturated fats less than 8% and cholesterol less than 200 mg/d. Reductions in serum cholesterol range from 10% to 20% on this regimen. Use of complex carbohydrates and fiber is recommended, and monounsaturated fats should predominate within the fat allowance. Weight reduction and caloric restriction are especially important for patients with elevated VLDL and IDL. Those with hypertriglyceridemia should avoid alcohol.

The effect of dietary fats on hypertriglyceridemia is dependent upon the disposition of double bonds in the fatty acid. Omega-3 fatty acids found in fish oils—but not those from plant sources—can induce profound lowering of triglycerides in some patients with endogenous or mixed lipemia. In contrast, the omega-6 fatty acids present in vegetable oils may cause triglycerides to increase.

Patients with primary chylomicronemia and some with mixed lipemia must consume a diet severely restricted in total fat—10–15 g/d, of which 5 g should be vegetable oils rich in essential fatty acids. Supplementation of fat-soluble vitamins should be given.

Supplementation with the antioxidant vitamins ascorbic acid (250 mg) and mixed natural tocopherols (50 IU on alternate days) may be beneficial. Higher doses may vitiate the impact of lipid lowering therapy. Other naturally occurring antioxidants such as resveratrol, β-catechin, selenium, and various carotenoids found in a variety of fruits and vegetables may provide additional antioxidant defense. Homocysteine, which initiates proatherogenic changes in endothelium, can be reduced in many patients by restriction of total protein intake to the amount required for amino acid replacement. Daily supplementation with up to 2 mg of folic acid plus other B vitamins is also recommended.

BASIC & CLINICAL PHARMACOLOGY OF DRUGS USED IN HYPERLIPIDEMIA

The decision to use drug therapy is based on the specific metabolic defect and its potential for causing atherosclerosis or pancreatitis. Suggested regimens for the principal lipoprotein disorders are presented in Table 35–2. Diet should be continued for achievement of the full potential of the drug regimen. Drugs should be avoided in pregnant and lactating women and those likely to become pregnant. All drugs that alter plasma lipoprotein concentrations may require adjustment of doses of warfarin and indandione anticoagulants. Children with heterozygous familial hypercholesterolemia may be treated with a resin or reductase inhibitor, usually after 7 or 8 years of age, when myelination of the central nervous system is essentially complete. The decision to treat a child should be based on the level of LDL, other risk factors, the family history, and the child's age. Drugs are rarely indicated before age 18.

COMPETITIVE INHIBITORS OF HMG-COA REDUCTASE (REDUCTASE INHIBITORS; "STATINS")

These compounds are structural analogs of HMG-CoA (3-hydroxy-3-methylglutaryl-coenzyme A). (Figure 35–3). **Lovastatin, atorvastatin, fluvastatin, pravastatin, simvastatin,** and **rosuvastatin** belong to this class. They are most effective in reducing LDL. Other effects include decreased oxidative stress and vascular inflammation with increased stability of atherosclerotic lesions. It has become standard practice to initiate reductase inhibitor therapy immediately after myocardial infarction, irrespective of lipid levels.

Chemistry & Pharmacokinetics

Lovastatin and simvastatin are inactive lactone prodrugs that are hydrolyzed in the gastrointestinal tract to the active β-hydroxyl derivatives, whereas pravastatin has an open, active lactone ring. Atorvastatin, fluvastatin, and rosuvastatin are fluorine-containing congeners that are active as given. Absorption of the ingested doses of the reductase inhibitors varies from 40% to 75% with the exception of fluvastatin, which is almost completely absorbed. All have high first-pass extraction by the liver. Most of the absorbed dose is excreted in the bile; about 5–20% is excreted in the urine. Plasma half-lives of these drugs range from 1 hour to 3 hours except for atorvastatin, which has a half-life of 14 hours, and rosuvastatin, 19 hours.

Mechanism of Action

HMG-CoA reductase mediates the first committed step in sterol biosynthesis. The active forms of the reductase inhibitors are structural analogs of the HMG-CoA intermediate (Figure 35–3) that is formed by HMG-CoA reductase in the synthesis of mevalonate. These analogs cause partial inhibition of the enzyme and thus may impair the synthesis of isoprenoids such as ubiquinone and dolichol and the prenylation of proteins. It is not known whether this has biologic significance. However, the reductase inhibitors clearly induce an increase in high-affinity LDL receptors. This effect increases both the fractional catabolic rate of LDL and the liver's extraction of LDL precursors (VLDL remnants), thus reducing plasma LDL (Figure 35–2). Because of marked first-pass hepatic extraction, the major effect is on liver. Preferential activity in liver of some congeners appears to be attributable to tissue-specific differences in uptake. Limited reduction of LDL levels in patients who lack functional LDL receptors indicates that decreases in de novo cholesterologenesis also contribute to cholesterol reduction. Modest decreases in plasma triglycerides and small increases in HDL also occur.

Therapeutic Uses & Dosage

Reductase inhibitors are useful alone or with resins, niacin, or ezetimibe in reducing levels of LDL. Women who are pregnant, lactating, or likely to become pregnant should not be given these agents. Use in children is restricted to those with homozygous familial hypercholesterolemia and selected patients with heterozygous familial hypercholesterolemia.

Because cholesterol biosynthesis occurs predominantly at night, reductase inhibitors—except atorvastatin and rosuvastatin—should be given in the evening if a single daily dose is used. Absorption generally (with the exception of pravastatin) is enhanced by taking the dose with food. Daily doses of lovastatin vary from 10 mg to 80 mg. Pravastatin is nearly as potent on a mass basis as lovastatin up to the maximum recommended daily dose, 80 mg. Simvastatin is twice as potent and is

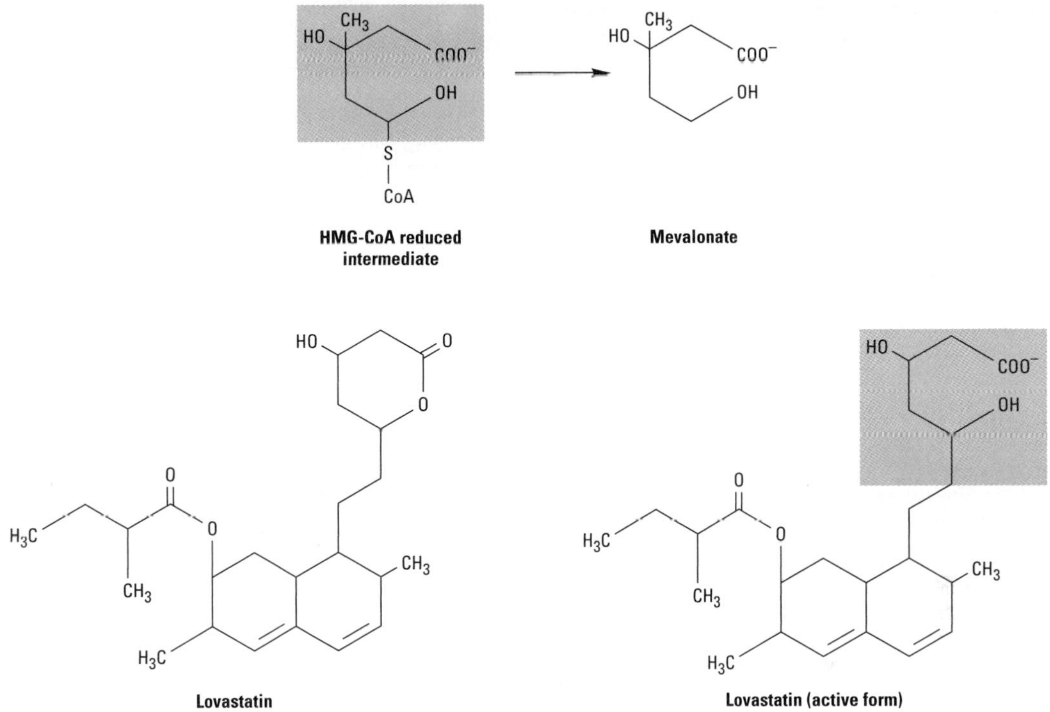

Figure 35–3. Inhibition of HMG-CoA reductase. **Top:** The HMG-CoA intermediate that is the immediate precursor of mevalonate, a critical compound in the synthesis of cholesterol. **Bottom:** The structure of lovastatin and its active form, showing the similarity to the normal HMG-CoA intermediate (shaded areas).

given in doses of 5–80 mg daily. Fluvastatin appears to be about half as potent as lovastatin on a mass basis and is given in doses of 10–80 mg daily. Atorvastatin is given in doses of 10–80 mg/d, and rosuvastatin, the most efficacious agent for severe hypercholesterolemia, at 10–40 mg/d. The dose-response curves of pravastatin and especially of fluvastatin tend to level off in the upper part of the dosage range in patients with moderate to severe hypercholesterolemia. Those of lovastatin, simvastatin, and atorvastatin are more nearly linear.

Toxicity

Elevations of serum aminotransferase activity (up to three times the normal level) occur in some patients. These increases are often intermittent and usually not associated with other evidence of hepatic toxicity. Therapy may be continued in such patients in the absence of symptoms if aminotransferase levels are measured frequently. In about 2% of patients, some of whom have underlying liver disease or a history of alcohol abuse,

aminotransferase levels may exceed three times the normal limit. This effect, which can occur at any time, portends more severe hepatic toxicity. These patients may present with malaise, anorexia, and precipitous decreases in LDL. Medication should be discontinued immediately in these patients and in asymptomatic patients whose aminotransferase activity is persistently elevated to more than three times the upper limit of normal. These agents should be used with caution and in reduced dosage in patients with hepatic parenchymal disease. In general, aminotransferase activity should be measured at baseline, at 1–2 months, and then every 6 months (if stable).

Minor increases in creatine kinase activity in plasma are observed in some patients receiving reductase inhibitors, frequently associated with heavy physical activity. Rarely, patients may have marked elevations in kinase activity, often accompanied by generalized pain or weakness in skeletal muscles. If the drug is not discontinued, rhabdomyolysis may cause myoglobinuria, which may lead to renal shutdown. Myopathy may occur with monotherapy, but there is an increased incidence in patients receiving a reductase inhibitor concurrently with certain other drugs. The catabolism of lovastatin, simvastatin, and atorvastatin proceeds chiefly through cytochrome P450 3A4, whereas that of fluvastatin and rosuvastatin is mediated by CYP2C9. Pravastatin is catabolized through other pathways, including sulfation. The 3A4-dependent reductase inhibitors tend to accumulate in plasma in the presence of drugs that inhibit or compete for the 3A4 cytochrome. These include the macrolide antibiotics, cyclosporine, ketoconazole and its congeners, HIV protease inhibitors, tacrolimus, nefazodone, fibrates, and others (see Chapter 4). Concomitant use of reductase inhibitors with amiodarone or verapamil also causes an increased risk of myopathy. Conversely, drugs such as phenytoin, griseofulvin, barbiturates, rifampin, and thiazolidinediones increase expression of CYP3A4 and can reduce the plasma concentrations of the 3A4-dependent reductase inhibitors. Inhibitors of CYP2C9 such as ketoconazole and its congeners, metronidazole, sulfinpyrazone, amiodarone, and cimetidine may increase plasma levels of fluvastatin and rosuvastatin. Pravastatin appears to be the drug of choice for use with verapamil, the ketoconazole group of antifungal agents, macrolides, and cyclosporine. Plasma levels of lovastatin, simvastatin, and atorvastatin may be elevated in patients ingesting more than 1 liter of grapefruit juice daily.

Creatine kinase activity should be measured frequently in patients receiving potentially interacting drug combinations. In all patients, creatine kinase levels should be measured before treatment and then every 6–12 months (depending on the dose). If significant muscle pain, tenderness, or weakness appears, creatine kinase activity should be measured immediately and the drug discontinued if activity is elevated over baseline. The myopathy usually reverses promptly upon cessation of therapy. If the association is unclear, the patient can be rechallenged under close surveillance. Myopathy in the absence of elevated creatine kinase activity has been reported. Rarely, hypersensitivity syndromes have been reported that include a lupus-like disorder and peripheral neuropathy.

These drugs should be temporarily discontinued in the event of serious illness, trauma, or major surgery.

NIACIN (NICOTINIC ACID)

Niacin (but not niacinamide) decreases VLDL and LDL levels—and Lp(a) in most patients. It often increases HDL levels significantly.

Chemistry & Pharmacokinetics

Niacin (vitamin B_3) is converted in the body to the amide, which is incorporated into niacinamide adenine dinucleotide (NAD). It is excreted in the urine unmodified and as several metabolites.

Mechanism of Action

Niacin inhibits VLDL secretion, in turn decreasing production of LDL (Figure 35–2). Increased clearance of VLDL via the LPL pathway contributes to triglyceride reduction. Niacin has no effect on bile acid production. Excretion of neutral sterols in the stool is increased acutely as cholesterol is mobilized from tissue pools and a new steady state is reached. The catabolic rate for HDL is decreased. Fibrinogen levels are reduced, and levels of tissue plasminogen activator appear to increase. Niacin inhibits the intracellular lipase of adipose tissue via receptor-mediated signaling, possibly reducing VLDL production by decreasing the flux of free fatty acids to liver. Sustained inhibition of lipolysis has not been established, however.

Therapeutic Uses & Dosage

In combination with a resin or reductase inhibitor, niacin normalizes LDL in most patients with heterozygous familial hypercholesterolemia and other forms of hypercholesterolemia. These combinations are also indicated in some cases of nephrosis. In severe mixed lipemia that is incompletely responsive to diet, niacin often produces marked reduction of triglycerides, an effect enhanced by marine omega-3 fatty acids. It is useful in patients with combined hyperlipoproteinemia and in those with familial dysbetalipoproteinemia. Niacin reduces levels of Lp(a) in many subjects. It is clearly the most effective agent for increasing levels of HDL.

For treatment of heterozygous familial hypercholesterolemia, most patients require 2–6 g of niacin daily; more than this should not be given. For other types of hypercholesterolemia and for hypertriglyceridemia, 1.5–3.5 g daily is often sufficient. The drug should be given in divided doses with meals, starting with 100 mg two or three times daily and increasing gradually.

Toxicity

Most persons experience a harmless cutaneous vasodilation and sensation of warmth after each dose when the drug is started or the dose is increased. Taking 0.3 g of aspirin one half hour beforehand blunts this prostaglandin-mediated effect. Ibuprofen, once daily, also mitigates the flush. Tachyphylaxis to flushing usually occurs within a few days at doses above 1.5–3 g daily. Care providers should warn patients to expect the flush and explain that it is a harmless side effect. Pruritus, rashes, dry skin or mucous membranes, and acanthosis nigricans have been reported. The latter contraindicates use of niacin because of its association with insulin resistance. Some patients experience nausea and abdominal discomfort. Many can continue the drug at reduced dosage, with inhibitors of gastric acid secretion, or use of antacids not containing aluminum. Niacin should be avoided in patients with severe peptic disease.

Reversible elevations in aminotransferases up to twice normal may occur, usually not associated with liver toxicity. However, liver function should be monitored regularly. Rarely, true hepatotoxicity may occur and is an indication for discontinuing the drug. The association of severe hepatic dysfunction, including acute necrosis, with the use of sustained-release preparations of niacin has been reported. Experience to date with one of these, given at bedtime in doses of 2 g or less, suggests that acute liver failure may be avoided. Carbohydrate tolerance may be moderately impaired, but this is also reversible. In some patients with latent diabetes, however, this effect may be incompletely reversible. Niacin may be given to diabetics who are receiving insulin and to some receiving oral agents if insulin resistance is not increased. Hyperuricemia occurs in some patients and occasionally precipitates gout. Allopurinol can be given with niacin if needed. Rarely, niacin is associated with arrhythmias, mostly atrial, and a reversible toxic amblyopia. Patients should be instructed to report blurring of distance vision. Niacin may potentiate the action of antihypertensive agents, requiring adjustment of their dosages. Dryness of mucous membranes is occasionally reported.

FIBRIC ACID DERIVATIVES

Gemfibrozil and **fenofibrate** decrease levels of VLDL and, in some patients, LDL as well. Another fibrate, **bezafibrate,** is not yet available in the USA.

Chemistry & Pharmacokinetics

Gemfibrozil is absorbed quantitatively from the intestine and is tightly bound to plasma proteins. It undergoes enterohepatic circulation and readily passes the placenta. The plasma half-life is 1.5 hours. Seventy percent is eliminated through the kidneys, mostly unmodified. The liver modifies some of the drug to hydroxymethyl, carboxyl, or quinol derivatives. Fenofibrate is a methylethyl ester that is hydrolyzed completely in the intestine. Its plasma half-life is 20 hours. Sixty percent is excreted in the urine as the glucuronide, and about 25% in feces.

Gemfibrozil

Fenofibrate

Mechanism of Action

These agents function primarily as ligands for the nuclear transcription receptor, peroxisome proliferator-activated receptor-alpha (PPAR-α). They increase lipolysis of lipoprotein triglyceride via LPL. Intracellular lipolysis in adipose tissue is decreased. Levels of VLDL decrease, in part as a result of decreased secretion by the liver. Only modest reductions of LDL occur in most patients. In others, especially those with combined hyperlipidemia, LDL often increases as triglycerides are reduced. HDL cholesterol increases moderately. Part of this apparent increase is a consequence of decreasing triglycerides in plasma, with reduction in exchange of triglycerides into HDL in place of cholesteryl esters. Some increase in HDL protein has been reported.

Therapeutic Uses & Dosage

These drugs are useful in hypertriglyceridemias in which VLDL predominate and in dysbetalipoproteinemia. They also may be of benefit in treating the hypertriglyceridemia that results from treatment with viral protease inhibitors. The usual dose of gemfibrozil is 600 mg orally once or twice daily. The dosage of fenofibrate is one to three 54 mg tablets (or a single 160 mg tablet) daily. Absorption of both drugs is improved when they are taken with food.

Toxicity

Rare adverse effects include rashes, gastrointestinal symptoms, myopathy, arrhythmias, hypokalemia, and high blood levels of aminotransferases or alkaline phosphatase. A few patients show decreases in white blood count or hematocrit. Both agents potentiate the action of coumarin and indanedione anticoagulants, and doses of these agents should be adjusted. Rhabdomyolysis has occurred rarely. Risk of myopathy increases when fibrates are given with reductase inhibitors. These drugs should be avoided in patients with hepatic or renal dysfunction. There appears to be a modest increase in the risk of cholesterol gallstones, reflecting an increase in the cholesterol content of bile. Therefore, fibrates should be used with caution in patients with biliary tract disease or in those at high risk such as women, obese patients, and Native Americans.

BILE ACID-BINDING RESINS

Colestipol, cholestyramine, and **colesevelam** are useful only for isolated increases in LDL. In patients who also have hypertriglyceridemia, VLDL levels may be further increased during treatment with resins.

Chemistry & Pharmacokinetics

These agents are large polymeric cationic exchange resins that are insoluble in water. They bind bile acids in the intestinal lumen and prevent their reabsorption. The resin itself is not absorbed.

Mechanism of Action

The bile acids, metabolites of cholesterol, are normally efficiently reabsorbed in the jejunum and ileum (Figure 35–2). Excretion is increased up to tenfold when resins are given, resulting in enhanced conversion of cholesterol to bile acids in liver via 7α-hydroxylation, normally controlled by negative feedback by bile acids. Increased uptake of LDL and IDL from plasma results from up-regulation of LDL receptors, particularly in liver. Therefore, the resins are without effect in patients with homozygous familial hypercholesterolemia who have no functioning receptors but may be useful in patients with receptor-defective combined heterozygous states.

Therapeutic Uses & Dosage

The resins are used in treatment of patients with primary hypercholesterolemia, producing approximately 20% reduction in LDL cholesterol in maximal dosage. If resins are used to treat LDL elevations in persons with combined hyperlipidemia, they may cause an increase in VLDL requiring the addition of a second agent such as niacin. Resins are also used in combination with other drugs to achieve further hypocholesterolemic effect (see below). They may be helpful in relieving pruritus in patients who have cholestasis and bile salt accumulation. Because they bind digitalis glycosides, the resins may be useful in digitalis toxicity.

Colestipol and cholestyramine are available as granular preparations. Colestipol is also available in 1 g tablets that must be swallowed whole. The maximum dose is 16 g daily. A gradual increase of dosage of granules from 4 or 5 g/d to 20 g/d is recommended. Total dosages of 30–32 g/d may be needed for maximum effect. The usual dosage for a child is 10–20 g/d. Granular resins are mixed with juice or water and allowed to hydrate for 1 minute. Colesevelam is available in 625 mg tablets. The maximum dose is six tablets daily. Resins should be taken in two or three doses with meals, and they lack effect when taken between meals.

Toxicity

Common complaints are constipation and bloating, usually relieved by increasing dietary fiber or mixing psyllium seed with the resin. Resins should be avoided in patients with diverticulitis. Heartburn and diarrhea are occasionally reported. In patients who have preexisting bowel disease or cholestasis, steatorrhea may occur. Malabsorption of vitamin K occurs rarely, leading to hypoprothrombinemia. Prothrombin time should be measured frequently in patients who are taking resins and anticoagulants. Malabsorption of folic acid has been reported rarely. Increased formation of gallstones, particularly in obese persons, was an anticipated adverse effect but has rarely occurred in practice. An occasional problem is dry flaking skin, relieved by application of lanolin.

Absorption of certain drugs, including those with neutral or cationic charge as well as anions, may be impaired by the resins. These include digitalis glycosides, thiazides, warfarin, tetracycline, thyroxine, iron salts, pravastatin, fluvastatin, folic acid, phenylbutazone, aspirin, and ascorbic acid. Any additional medication (except niacin) should be given 1 hour before or at least 2 hours after the resin to ensure adequate absorption. Colesevelam does not bind digoxin, warfarin, or reductase inhibitors.

INHIBITORS OF INTESTINAL STEROL ABSORPTION

Ezetimibe is the first member of a new group of drugs that inhibit intestinal absorption of phytosterols and cholesterol. Its primary clinical effect is reduction of LDL levels.

Chemistry & Pharmacokinetics

Ezetimibe is readily absorbed and conjugated in the intestine to an active glucuronide, reaching peak blood levels in 12–14 hours. It undergoes enterohepatic circulation. Its half-life is 22 hours. Approximately 80% of the drug is excreted in feces. Plasma ezetimibe concentrations are substantially increased when it is administered with fibrates and reduced when it is given with cholestyramine. Other resins may also decrease its absorption. There are no significant interactions with warfarin or digoxin.

Ezetimibe

Mechanism of Action

Ezetimibe is a selective inhibitor of intestinal absorption of cholesterol and phytosterols. It is effective even in the absence of dietary cholesterol because it inhibits reabsorption of cholesterol excreted in the bile.

Therapeutic Uses & Dosage

The effect on cholesterol absorption is constant over the dosage range of 5–20 mg/d. Therefore, a single daily dose of 10 mg is used. Average reduction in LDL cholesterol with ezetimibe alone in patients with primary hypercholesterolemia is about 18%, with minimal increases in HDL cholesterol. It is also effective in patients with phytosterolemia. Ezetimibe is apparently synergistic with reductase inhibitors, producing decrements as great as 25% in LDL cholesterol beyond that achieved with the reductase inhibitor alone.

Toxicity

Ezetimibe does not appear to be a substrate for cytochrome P450 enzymes. Preliminary data reveal a low incidence of reversible impaired hepatic function with a small increase in incidence when given with a reductase inhibitor. Liver function tests should be done before starting the drug and then at intervals of 2–4 months.

TREATMENT WITH DRUG COMBINATIONS

Combined drug therapy is useful (1) when VLDL levels are significantly increased during treatment of hypercholesterolemia with a resin; (2) when LDL and VLDL levels are both elevated initially; (3) when LDL or VLDL levels are not normalized with a single agent, or (4) when elevated levels of Lp(a) or HDL deficiency coexist with other hyperlipidemias.

1. Fibric Acid Derivatives & Bile Acid-Binding Resins

This combination is sometimes useful in treating patients with familial combined hyperlipidemia who are intolerant of niacin. However, it may increase the risk of cholelithiasis.

2. HMG-CoA Reductase Inhibitors & Bile Acid-Binding Resins

This highly synergistic combination is useful for treatment of familial hypercholesterolemia but may not control levels of VLDL in some patients with familial combined hyperlipoproteinemia. Pravastatin, atorvastatin, and fluvastatin should be given at least 1 hour before or 4 hours after the resin to ensure their absorption.

3. Niacin & Bile Acid-Binding Resins

This combination effectively controls VLDL levels during resin therapy of familial combined hyperlipoproteinemia or other disorders involving both increased VLDL and LDL levels. When VLDL and LDL levels are both initially increased, doses of niacin as low as 1–3 g/d may be sufficient in combination with a resin. The niacin-resin combination is effective for treating heterozygous familial hypercholesterolemia. Niacin also significantly elevates levels of HDL cholesterol and frequently decreases levels of Lp(a).

Quantitative evidence of reversal of coronary disease was demonstrated with this regimen in three major clinical trials. Effects on lipoprotein levels are sustained, and no additional adverse effects have developed other than those encountered when the drugs are used singly. The drugs may be taken together, because niacin does not bind to the resins. LDL levels in patients with heterozygous familial hypercholesterolemia are usually normalized with daily doses of up to 6.5 g of niacin with 24–30 g of resin.

4. Niacin & Reductase Inhibitors

This regimen is more effective than either agent alone in treating familial hypercholesterolemia. Experience indicates that it is the most efficacious and practical combination for treatment of familial combined hyperlipoproteinemia.

5. Reductase Inhibitors & Ezetimibe

This combination is synergistic in treating primary hypercholesterolemia and has some use in the treatment of homozygous familial hypercholesterolemia.

6. Ternary Combination of Resins, Niacin, & Reductase Inhibitors

These agents act in a complementary fashion to normalize cholesterol in patients with severe disorders involving elevated LDL. The effects are sustained, and little compound toxicity has been observed. Effective doses of the individual drugs may be lower than when each is used alone—eg, as little as 1–2 g of niacin may substantially increase the effects of the other agents.

PREPARATIONS AVAILABLE

Atorvastatin (Lipitor)
  Oral: 10, 20, 40, 80 mg tablets
Cholestyramine (generic, Questran, Questran Light)
  Oral: 4 g packets anhydrous granules cholestyramine resin; 210 g (Questran Light), 378 g (Questran) cans
Colesevelam (Welchol)
  Oral: 625 mg tablets
Colestipol (Colestid)
  Oral: 5 g packets granules; 300, 500 g bottles; 1 g tablets
Ezetimibe (Zetia)
  Oral: 10 mg tablets
Fenofibrate (Tricor)
  Oral: 54, 160 mg tablets

Fluvastatin (Lescol)
  Oral: 20, 40 mg capsules; extended release (Lescol XL): 80 mg capsules
Gemfibrozil (generic, Lopid)
  Oral: 600 mg tablets
Lovastatin (generic, Mevacor)
  Oral: 10, 20, 40, 80 mg tablets; extended release tablets (Altocar) 10, 20, 40, 60 mg
Niacin, nicotinic acid, vitamin B$_3$ (generic, others)
  Oral: 100, 250, 500, 1000 mg tablets
Pravastatin (Pravachol)
  Oral: 10, 20, 40, 80 mg tablets
Rosuvastatin (Crestor)
  Oral: 5, 10, 20, 40 mg tablets
Simvastatin (Zocor)
  Oral: 5, 10, 20, 40, 80 mg tablets

REFERENCES

ATHEROSCLEROSIS: MECHANISMS & EPIDEMIOLOGY

Libby P: Current concepts of the pathogenesis of the acute coronary syndromes. Circulation 2001;104:365.

Libby P, Ridker PM, Maseri A: Inflammation and atherosclerosis. Circulation 2002;105:1135.

Malloy MJ, Kane JP: A risk factor for atherosclerosis: triglyceride-rich lipoproteins. Adv Intern Med 2001;47:111.

Seman LJ, McNamara JR, Schaefer EJ: Lipoprotein(a), homocysteine, and remnant-like particles: emerging risk factors. Curr Opin Cardiol 1999;14:186.

Steinberg D et al: Beyond cholesterol: Modifications of low density lipoprotein that increase its atherogenicity. N Engl J Med 1989;320:915.

ATHEROSCLEROSIS: REGRESSION

Brown BG et al: Regression of coronary artery disease as a result of intensive lipid-lowering therapy in men with high levels of apolipoprotein B. N Engl J Med 1990;323:1289.

Brown BG et al: Simvastatin and niacin, antioxidant vitamins, or the combination for the prevention of coronary disease. N Engl J Med 2001;345:1583.

Kane JP et al: Regression of coronary atherosclerosis during treatment of familial hypercholesterolemia with combined drug regimens. JAMA 1990;264:3007.

OUTCOME STUDIES

Rubins HB et al: Gemfibrozil for the secondary prevention of coronary heart disease in men with low levels of high-density lipoprotein cholesterol. Veterans Affairs High-Density Lipoprotein Cholesterol Intervention Trial Study Group. N Engl J Med 1999;341:410.

Scandinavian Simvastatin Survival Study: Randomized trial of cholesterol lowering in 4444 patients with coronary heart disease: The Scandinavian Simvastatin Survival Study (4S). Lancet 1994;345:1383.

Sacks FM et al: The effect of pravastatin on coronary events after myocardial infarction in patients with average cholesterol levels. Cholesterol and Recurrent Events Investigators. N Engl J Med 1996;335:1001.

Schwartz GG et al: Effects of atorvastatin on early recurrent ischemic events in acute coronary syndromes: the MIRACL study: a randomized controlled trial. JAMA 2001;285:1711.

Shepherd J et al: Prevention of coronary heart disease with pravastatin in men with hypercholesterolemia. N Engl J Med 1995;338:1301.

DIETARY TREATMENT

Albert CM et al: Blood levels of long-chain n-3 fatty acids and the risk of sudden death. N Engl J Med 2002;345:1113.

Kromhout D et al: Prevention of coronary heart disease by diet and lifestyle. Circulation 2002;105:893.

DRUG TREATMENT

Executive Summary of the Third Report of the National Cholesterol Education Program (NCEP): Expert Panel on Detection, Evaluation, and Treatment of High Blood Cholesterol in Adults (Adult Treatment Panel III). JAMA 2001;285:2486.

Knopp RH: Drug treatment of lipid disorders. N Engl J Med 1999;341:498.

Malloy MJ et al: Complementarity of colestipol, niacin, and lovastatin in treatment of severe familial hypercholesterolemia. Ann Intern Med 1987;107:616.

Stein EA: Managing dyslipidemia in the high-risk patient. Am J Cardiol 2002;89(5A):50C.

Nonsteroidal Anti-Inflammatory Drugs, Disease-Modifying Antirheumatic Drugs, Nonopioid Analgesics, & Drugs Used in Gout

36

William Wagner, MD, Puja Khanna, MD, & Daniel E. Furst, MD

THE IMMUNE RESPONSE

The immune response occurs when immunologically competent cells are activated in response to foreign organisms or antigenic substances liberated during the acute or chronic inflammatory response. The outcome of the immune response for the host may be beneficial, as when it causes invading organisms to be phagocytosed or neutralized. On the other hand, the outcome may be deleterious if it leads to chronic inflammation without resolution of the underlying injurious process (see Chapter 56). Chronic inflammation involves the release of a number of mediators that are not prominent in the acute response. One of the most important conditions involving these mediators is rheumatoid arthritis, in which chronic inflammation results in pain and destruction of bone and cartilage that can lead to severe disability and in which systemic changes occur that can result in shortening of life.

The cell damage associated with inflammation acts on cell membranes to cause leukocytes to release lysosomal enzymes; arachidonic acid is then liberated from precursor compounds, and various eicosanoids are synthesized. As discussed in Chapter 18, the cyclooxygenase pathway of arachidonate metabolism produces prostaglandins, which have a variety of effects on blood vessels, on nerve endings, and on cells involved in inflammation. The discovery of cyclooxygenase (COX) isoforms (COX-1 and COX-2) led to the concepts that the constitutive COX-1 isoform tends to be homeostatic in function, while COX-2 is induced during inflammation and tends to facilitate the inflammatory response. On this basis, highly selective COX-2 inhibitors have been developed and marketed on the assumption that such selective inhibitors would be safer than nonselective COX-1 inhibitors but without loss of efficacy. The lipoxygenase pathway of arachidonate metabolism yields leukotrienes, which have a powerful chemotactic effect on eosinophils, neutrophils, and macrophages and promote bronchoconstriction and alterations in vascular permeability.

Kinins, neuropeptides, and histamine are also released at the site of tissue injury, as are complement components, cytokines, and other products of leukocytes and platelets. Stimulation of the neutrophil membranes produces oxygen-derived free radicals. Superoxide anion is formed by the reduction of molecular oxygen, which may stimulate the production of other reactive molecules such as hydrogen peroxide and hydroxyl radicals. The interaction of these substances with arachidonic acid results in the generation of chemotactic substances, thus perpetuating the inflammatory process.

THERAPEUTIC STRATEGIES

The treatment of patients with inflammation involves two primary goals: first, the relief of pain, which is often the presenting symptom and the major continuing complaint of the patient; and second, the slowing or—in theory—arrest of the tissue-damaging process. In rheumatoid arthritis, response to therapy can be quantitated by means of the American College of Rheumatology scoring system values ACR20, ACR50, and ACR70, which denote the percentage of patients showing an improvement of 20%, 50%, or 70% in a global assessment of signs and symptoms.

Reduction of inflammation with **nonsteroidal anti-inflammatory drugs** (NSAIDs) often results in relief of pain for significant periods. Furthermore, most of the nonopioid analgesics (aspirin, etc) also have anti-inflammatory effects, so they are appropriate for the treatment of both acute and chronic inflammatory conditions.

The **glucocorticoids** also have powerful anti-inflammatory effects and when first introduced were considered to be the ultimate answer to the treatment of inflammatory arthritis. Unfortunately, the toxicity associated with chronic corticosteroid therapy limits their use except in the control of acute flare-ups of joint disease. Therefore, the nonsteroidal anti-inflammatory drugs have assumed a major role in the long-term treatment of arthritis.

Another important group of agents are characterized as **slow-acting antirheumatic drugs (SAARDs)** or **disease-modifying antirheumatic drugs (DMARDs)**. They may slow the bone damage associated with rheumatoid arthritis and are thought to affect more basic inflammatory mechanisms than do the NSAIDs. Unfortunately, they may also be more toxic than the nonsteroidal anti-inflammatory agents.

I. NONSTEROIDAL ANTI-INFLAMMATORY DRUGS

Salicylates and other similar agents used to treat rheumatic disease share the capacity to suppress the signs and symptoms of inflammation. These drugs also exert antipyretic and analgesic effects, but it is their anti-inflammatory properties that make them most useful in the management of disorders in which pain is related to the intensity of the inflammatory process.

Although all NSAIDs are not FDA-approved for the whole range of rheumatic diseases, all are probably effective in rheumatoid arthritis, seronegative spondyloarthropathies (eg, psoriatic arthritis and arthritis associated with inflammatory bowel disease), osteoarthritis, localized musculoskeletal syndromes (eg, sprains and strains, low back pain), and gout (except tolmetin, which appears to be ineffective in gout). Since aspirin, the original NSAID, has a number of adverse effects, many other NSAIDs have been developed in attempts to improve upon aspirin's efficacy and decrease its toxicity.

Chemistry & Pharmacokinetics

The NSAIDs are grouped in several chemical classes, some of which are shown in Figure 36–1. This chemical diversity yields a broad range of pharmacokinetic characteristics (Table 36–1). Although there are many differences in the kinetics of NSAIDs, they have some general properties in common. All but one of the NSAIDs are weak organic acids as given; the exception, nabumetone, is a ketone prodrug that is metabolized to the acidic active drug. Most of these drugs are well absorbed, and food does not substantially change their bioavailability. Most of the NSAIDs are highly metabolized, some by phase I followed by phase II mechanisms and others by direct glucuronidation (phase II) alone. Metabolism of most NSAIDs proceeds, in part, by way of the CYP3A or CYP2C families of P450 enzymes in the liver. While renal excretion is the most important route for final elimination, nearly all undergo varying degrees of biliary excretion and reabsorption (enterohepatic circulation). In fact, the degree of lower gastrointestinal tract irritation correlates with the amount of enterohepatic circulation. Most of the NSAIDs are highly protein-bound ($\geq$ 98%), usually to albumin. Some of the NSAIDs (eg, ibuprofen) are racemic mixtures, while one, naproxen, is provided as a single enantiomer and a few have no chiral center (eg, diclofenac).

All NSAIDs can be found in synovial fluid after repeated dosing. Drugs with short half-lives remain in the joints longer than would be predicted from their half-lives, while drugs with longer half-lives disappear from the synovial fluid at a rate proportionate to their half-lives.

Pharmacodynamics

The anti-inflammatory activity of the NSAIDs is mediated chiefly through inhibition of biosynthesis of prostaglandins. Various NSAIDs have additional possible mechanisms of action, including inhibition of chemotaxis, down-regulation of interleukin-1 production, decreased production of free radicals and superoxide, and interference with calcium-mediated intracellular events. Aspirin irreversibly acetylates and blocks platelet cyclooxygenase, while most non-COX-selective NSAIDs are reversible inhibitors. Selectivity for COX-1 versus COX-2 is variable and incomplete for the older members, but highly selective COX-2 inhibitors (celecoxib, rofecoxib, and valdecoxib) are now available and other highly selective coxibs are being developed. The highly selective COX-2 inhibitors do not affect platelet function at their usual doses. In testing using human whole blood, aspirin, indomethacin, piroxicam, and sulindac were somewhat more effective in inhibiting COX-1; ibuprofen and meclofenamate inhibited the two isozymes about equally. The efficacy of COX-2-selective drugs equals that of the older NSAIDs, while gastrointestinal safety may be improved. On the other hand, highly selective COX-2 inhibitors may increase the incidence of edema and hypertension.

The NSAIDs decrease the sensitivity of vessels to bradykinin and histamine, affect lymphokine production from T lymphocytes, and reverse vasodilation. To varying degrees, all newer NSAIDs are analgesic, anti-inflammatory, and antipyretic, and all (except the COX-2-selective agents and the nonacetylated salicylates) inhibit platelet aggregation. NSAIDs are all gastric irritants as well, though as a group the newer agents tend to

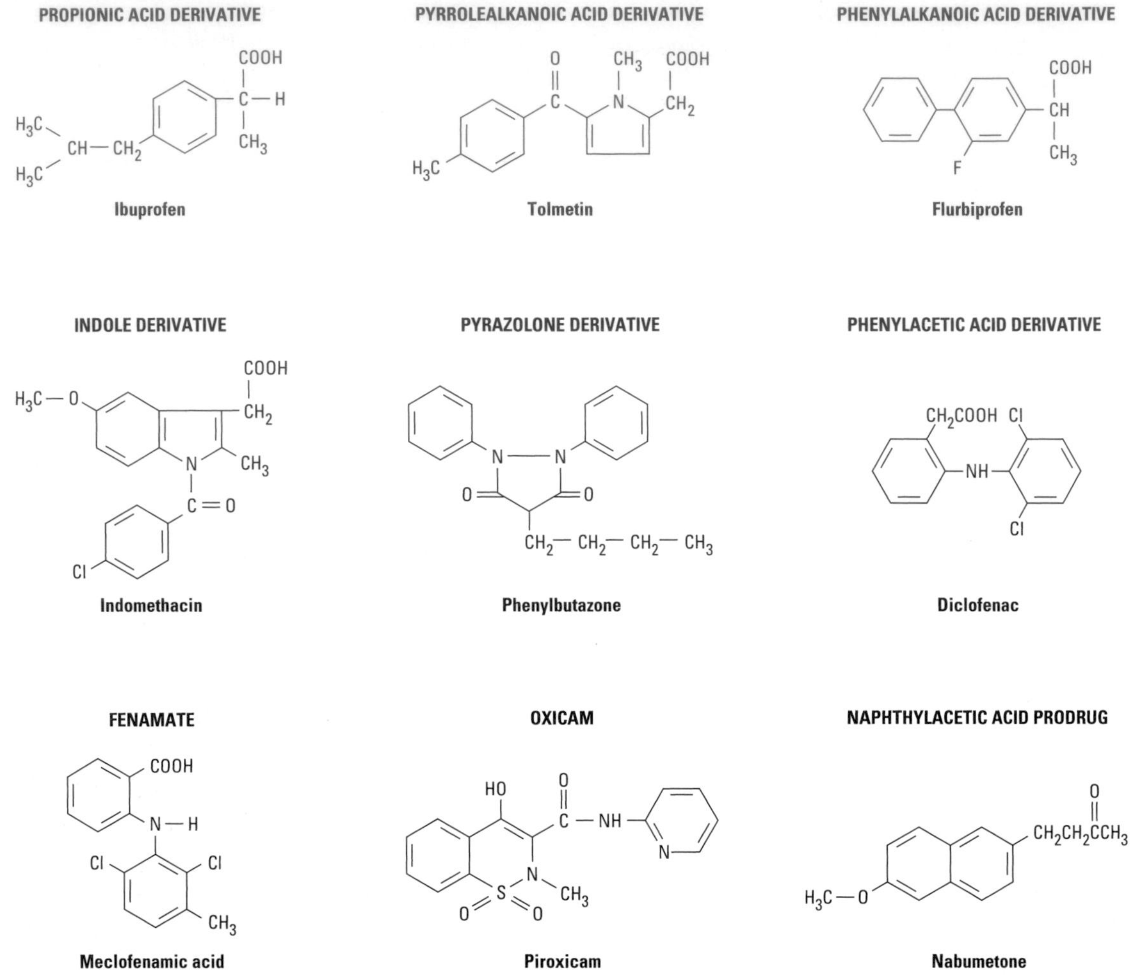

PROPIONIC ACID DERIVATIVE

PYRROLEALKANOIC ACID DERIVATIVE

PHENYLALKANOIC ACID DERIVATIVE

Ibuprofen

Tolmetin

Flurbiprofen

INDOLE DERIVATIVE

PYRAZOLONE DERIVATIVE

PHENYLACETIC ACID DERIVATIVE

Indomethacin

Phenylbutazone

Diclofenac

FENAMATE

OXICAM

NAPHTHYLACETIC ACID PRODRUG

Meclofenamic acid

Piroxicam

Nabumetone

Figure 36–1. Chemical structures of some NSAIDs.

cause less gastric irritation than aspirin. Nephrotoxicity has been observed for all of the drugs for which extensive experience has been reported, and hepatotoxicity can also occur with any NSAID.

Although these drugs effectively inhibit inflammation, there is no evidence that—in contrast to drugs such as methotrexate and gold—they alter the course of an arthritic disorder.

1. Aspirin

Aspirin's long use and availability without prescription diminishes its glamour compared to that of the newer NSAIDs. Aspirin is now rarely used as an anti-inflammatory medication; it has been replaced by ibuprofen and naproxen, since they are effective, are also available over the counter, and have good to excellent safety records.

Pharmacokinetics

Salicylic acid is a simple organic acid with a pK_a of 3.0. Aspirin (acetylsalicylic acid; ASA) has a pK_a of 3.5 (see Table 1–1). Sodium salicylate and aspirin (Figure 36–2) are equally effective anti-inflammatory drugs, though aspirin may be more effective as an analgesic. The salicylates are rapidly absorbed from the stomach and upper small intestine, yielding a peak plasma salicylate level within 1–2 hours. Aspirin is absorbed as such and is rapidly hydrolyzed (serum half-life 15 minutes) to acetic acid and salicylate by esterases in tissue and blood. Salicylate is bound to albumin, but the binding is saturable

Table 36–1. Properties of aspirin and some nonsteroidal anti-inflammatory drugs.

Drug	Half-life (hours)	Urinary Excretion of Unchanged Drug	Recommended Anti-inflammatory Dosage
Aspirin	0.25	< 2%	1200–1500 mg tid
Salicylate[1]	2–19	2–30%	See footnote 2
Apazone	15	62%	600 mg bid
Celecoxib	11	27%[3]	100–200 mg bid
Diclofenac	1.1	< 1%	50–75 mg qid
Diflunisal	13	3–9%	500 mg bid
Etodolac	6.5	< 1%	200–300 mg qid
Fenoprofen	2.5	30%	600 mg qid
Flurbiprofen	3.8	< 1%	300 mg tid
Ibuprofen	2	< 1%	600 mg qid
Indomethacin	4–5	16%	50–70 mg tid
Ketoprofen	1.8	< 1%	70 mg tid
Ketorolac	4–10	58%	10 mg qid[4]
Meclofenamate	3	2–4%	100 mg qid
Meloxicam	20	Data not found	7.5–15 mg qd
Nabumetone[5]	26	1%	1000–2000 mg qd[6]
Naproxen	14	< 1%	375 mg bid
Oxaprozin	58	1–4%	1200–1800 mg qd[6]
Piroxicam	57	4–10%	20 mg qd[6]
Rofecoxib	17	72%[3]	12.5–50 mg qd
Sulindac	8	7%	200 mg bid
Tolmetin	1	7%	400 mg qid
Valdecoxib	8–11	90[3]	10 mg qd

[1]Major anti-inflammatory metabolite of aspirin.
[2]Salicylate is usually given in the form of aspirin.
[3]Total urinary excretion including metabolites.
[4]Recommended for treatment of acute (eg, surgical) pain only.
[5]Nabumetone is a prodrug; the half-life and urinary excretion are for its active metabolite.
[6]A single daily dose is sufficient because of the long half-life.

so that the unbound fraction increases as total concentration increases. Ingested salicylate and that generated by the hydrolysis of aspirin may be excreted unchanged, but the metabolic pathways for salicylate disposition become saturated when the total body load of salicylate exceeds 600 mg. Beyond this amount, increases in salicylate dosage increase salicylate concentration disproportionately. As doses of aspirin increase, salicylate elimination half-life increases from 3–5 hours (for 600 mg/d dosage) to 12–16 hours (dosage > 3.6 g/d). Alkalinization of the urine increases the rate of excretion of free salicylate and its water-soluble conjugates.

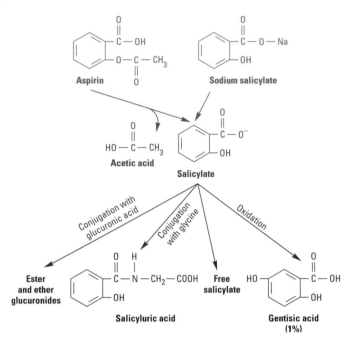

Figure 36–2. Structure and metabolism of the salicylates. (Modified and reproduced, with permission, from Meyers FH, Jawetz E, Goldfien A: *Review of Medical Pharmacology,* 7th ed. McGraw-Hill, 1980.)

Mechanisms of Action

A. ANTI-INFLAMMATORY EFFECTS

Aspirin is a nonselective inhibitor of both COX isoforms (Figure 36–3), but salicylate is much less effective in inhibiting either isoform. Nonacetylated salicylates may work as oxygen radical scavengers. Aspirin irreversibly inhibits COX and inhibits platelet aggregation, while nonacetylated salicylates do not.

Aspirin also interferes with the chemical mediators of the kallikrein system (see Chapter 17), thus inhibiting granulocyte adherence to damaged vasculature, stabilizing lysosomes, and inhibiting the chemotaxis of polymorphonuclear leukocytes and macrophages.

B. ANALGESIC EFFECTS

Aspirin is most effective in reducing pain of mild to moderate intensity through its effects on inflammation and because it probably inhibits pain stimuli at a subcortical site.

C. ANTIPYRETIC EFFECTS

Aspirin reduces elevated temperature, whereas normal body temperature is only slightly affected. Aspirin's antipyretic effect is probably mediated by both COX inhibition in the central nervous system and inhibition of IL-1 (which is released from macrophages during episodes of inflammation).

D. ANTIPLATELET EFFECTS

Single low doses of aspirin (81 mg daily) produce a slightly prolonged bleeding time, which doubles if administration is continued for a week (see Chapter 34). The change is due to irreversible inhibition of platelet COX, so that aspirin's antiplatelet effect lasts 8–10 days (the life of the platelet).

Clinical Uses

A. ANALGESIA, ANTIPYRESIS, AND ANTI-INFLAMMATORY EFFECTS

Aspirin is employed for mild to moderate pain of varied origin but is not effective for severe visceral pain. Aspirin and other NSAIDs have been combined with opioid analgesics for treatment of cancer pain, where their anti-inflammatory effects act synergistically with the opioids to enhance analgesia. High-dose salicylates are effective for treatment of rheumatic fever, rheumatoid arthritis, and other inflammatory joint conditions.

B. OTHER EFFECTS

Aspirin decreases the incidence of transient ischemic attacks, unstable angina, coronary artery thrombosis with myocardial infarction, and thrombosis after coronary artery bypass grafting (see Chapter 34).

Epidemiologic studies suggest that long-term use of

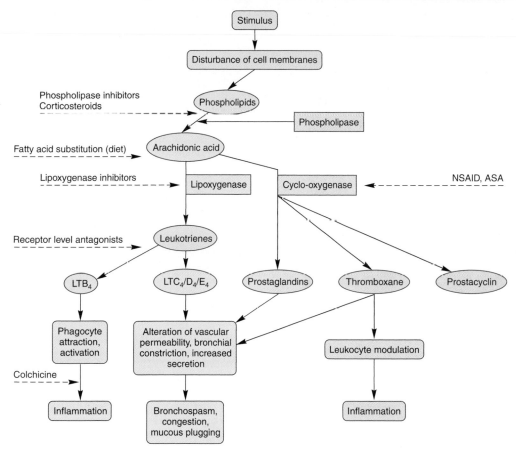

Figure 36–3. Scheme for mediators derived from arachidonic acid and sites of drug action (dashed arrows).

aspirin at low dosage is associated with a lower incidence of colon cancer, possibly related to its COX-inhibiting effects.

Dosage

The optimal analgesic or antipyretic dose of aspirin is less than the 0.6–0.65 g oral dose commonly used. Larger doses may prolong the effect. The usual dose may be repeated every 4 hours. The anti-inflammatory dose for children is 50–75 mg/kg/d in divided doses and the average starting anti-inflammatory dose for adults is 45 mg/kg/d in divided doses (Table 36–1). The relationship of salicylate blood levels to therapeutic effect and toxicity is illustrated in Figure 36–4.

Adverse Effects

At the usual dosage, aspirin's main adverse effects are gastric upset (intolerance) and gastric and duodenal ulcers,

while hepatotoxicity, asthma, rashes, and renal toxicity occur less frequently. Upper gastrointestinal bleeding associated with aspirin use is usually related to erosive gastritis. A 3 mL increase in fecal blood loss is routinely associated with aspirin administration; the blood loss is greater for higher doses. On the other hand, some mucosal adaptation occurs in many patients, so that blood loss declines back to baseline over 4–6 weeks; ulcers have been shown to heal while aspirin was taken concomitantly.

With higher doses, patients may experience "salicylism"—vomiting, tinnitus, decreased hearing, and vertigo—reversible by reducing the dosage. Still larger doses of salicylates cause hyperpnea through a direct effect on the medulla. At toxic salicylate levels, respiratory alkalosis followed by metabolic acidosis (salicylate accumulation), respiratory depression, and even cardiotoxicity and glucose intolerance can occur (Figure 36–4). Two grams or less of aspirin daily usually increases serum uric acid levels, whereas doses exceeding 4 g daily decrease urate

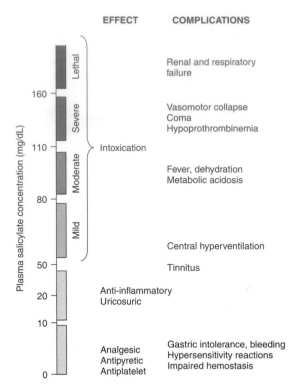

Figure 36–4. Approximate relationships of plasma salicylate levels to pharmacodynamics and complications. (Modified and reproduced, with permission, from Hollander J, McCarty D Jr: *Arthritis and Allied Conditions.* Lea & Febiger, 1972.)

levels (see Drugs Used in Gout, below). Like other NSAIDs, aspirin can cause elevation of liver enzymes (a frequent but mild effect), hepatitis (rare), decreased renal function, bleeding, rashes, and asthma.

The antiplatelet action of aspirin contraindicates its use by patients with hemophilia. Although previously not recommended during pregnancy, aspirin may be valuable in treating preeclampsia-eclampsia.

When overdosing occurs, gastric lavage is advised and an alkaline, high urine output state should be maintained (see Chapter 59). Hyperthermia and electrolyte abnormalities should be treated. In severe toxic reactions, ventilatory assistance may be required. Sodium bicarbonate infusions may be employed to alkalinize the urine, which will increase the amount of salicylate excreted.

NONACETYLATED SALICYLATES

These drugs include magnesium choline salicylate, sodium salicylate, and salicylsalicylate. All nonacetylated salicylates are effective anti-inflammatory drugs, though they may be less effective analgesics than aspirin. Because they are much less effective than aspirin as cyclooxygenase inhibitors, they may be preferable when cyclooxygenase inhibition is undesirable, such as in patients with asthma, those with bleeding tendencies, and even (under close supervision) those with renal dysfunction.

The nonacetylated salicylates are administered in the same dosage as aspirin and can be monitored using serum salicylate measurements.

COX-2 SELECTIVE INHIBITORS

COX-2 selective inhibitors, or coxibs, were developed in an attempt to inhibit prostacyclin synthesis by the COX-2 isoenzyme induced at sites of inflammation without affecting the action of the constitutively active "housekeeping" COX-1 isoenzyme found in the gastrointestinal tract, kidneys, and platelets. Coxibs selectively bind to and block the active site of the COX-2 enzyme much more effectively than that of COX-1. COX-2 inhibitors have analgesic, antipyretic, and anti-inflammatory effects similar to those of nonselective NSAIDs but with fewer gastrointestinal side effects. Likewise, COX-2 inhibitors have been shown to have no impact on platelet aggregation, which is mediated by the COX-1 isoenzyme. As a result, COX-2 inhibitors do not offer the cardioprotective effects of traditional nonselective NSAIDs, which has resulted in some patients taking low-dose aspirin in addition to a coxib regimen to maintain this effect. Unfortunately, because COX-2 is constitutively active within the kidney, recommended doses of COX-2 inhibitors cause renal toxicities similar to those associated with traditional NSAIDs. They are not recommended for patients with severe renal insufficiency. Furthermore, some clinical data have suggested a higher incidence of cardiovascular thrombotic events associated with COX-2 inhibitors such as rofecoxib, but this issue has not yet been settled. Data from animal studies have also pointed to the role of the COX-2 enzyme in bone repair, resulting in a recommendation for short-term use of different drugs in postoperative patients and those undergoing bone repair. COX-2 inhibitors have been recommended mainly for treatment of osteoarthritis and rheumatoid arthritis, but other indications include primary familial adenomatous polyposis, dysmenorrhea, acute gouty arthritis, acute musculoskeletal pain, and perhaps ankylosing spondylitis.

1. Celecoxib

Celecoxib is a highly selective COX-2 inhibitor—about 10–20 times more selective for COX-2 than for COX-1.

Pharmacokinetic and dosage considerations are given in Table 36–1.

Colooooxib

Celecoxib is as effective as other NSAIDs in rheumatoid arthritis and osteoarthritis, and in trials it has caused fewer endoscopic ulcers than most other NSAIDs. Because it is a sulfonamide, celecoxib may cause rashes. It does not affect platelet aggregation. It interacts occasionally with warfarin—as would be expected of a drug metabolized via CYP2C9.

The coxibs continue to be investigated to determine whether their effect on prostacyclin production could lead to a prothrombotic state. The frequency of other adverse effects approximates that of other NSAIDs. Celecoxib causes no more edema or renal effects than other members of the NSAID group, but edema and hypertension have been documented.

2. Etoricoxib

Etoricoxib, a bipyridine derivative, is a second-generation COX-2-selective inhibitor with the highest selectivity ratio of any coxib for inhibition of COX-2 relative to COX-1. It is extensively metabolized by hepatic P450 enzymes followed by renal excretion and has an elimination half-life of 22 hours. Etoricoxib is approved in the United Kingdom for acute treatment of the signs and symptoms of osteoarthritis (60 mg once daily) and rheumatoid arthritis (90 mg once daily), for treatment of acute gouty arthritis (120 mg once daily), and for relief of acute musculoskeletal pain (60 mg once daily). Approval in the United States is pending. Clinical data have demonstrated that 90 mg of etoricoxib once daily has superior efficacy compared with 500 mg of naproxen twice daily for treatment of patients with rheumatoid arthritis over 12 weeks. Other studies have shown etoricoxib to have similar efficacy to traditional NSAIDs for treatment of osteoarthritis, acute gouty arthritis, and primary dysmenorrhea and a gastrointestinal safety profile similar to that of other coxibs. Since etoricoxib has structural similarities to diclofenac, it is appropriate to monitor hepatic function carefully in patients using this drug.

3. Meloxicam

Meloxicam is an enolcarboxamide related to piroxicam that has been shown to preferentially inhibit COX-2 over COX-1, particularly at its lowest therapeutic dose of 7.5 mg/d. It is not as selective as the other coxibs. The drug is popular in Europe and many other countries for most rheumatic diseases and has recently been approved for treatment of osteoarthritis in the USA. Its efficacy in this condition and rheumatoid arthritis is comparable to that of other NSAIDs. It is associated with fewer clinical gastrointestinal symptoms and complications than piroxicam, diclofenac, and naproxen. Similarly, while meloxicam is known to inhibit synthesis of thromboxane A_2, it appears that even at supratherapeutic doses its blockade of thromboxane A_2 does not reach levels that result in decreased in vivo platelet function. Other toxicities are similar to those of other NSAIDs.

4. Rofecoxib

Rofecoxib, a furanose derivative, is a potent, selective COX-2 inhibitor (Table 36–1). In the USA, rofecoxib is approved for osteoarthritis and rheumatoid arthritis, and it also appears to be analgesic and antipyretic—in common with other NSAIDs. This drug does not inhibit platelet aggregation and appears to have little effect on gastric mucosal prostaglandins or lower gastrointestinal tract permeability. At high doses it is associated with occasional edema and hypertension. Other toxicities are similar to those of other coxibs.

Rofecoxib

5. Valdecoxib

Valdecoxib, a diaryl-substituted isoxazole, is a new highly selective COX-2 inhibitor. Pharmacokinetic characteristics and dosage in arthritis are set forth in Table 36–1. In primary dysmenorrhea, dosage is 20 mg twice daily, and the drug is as effective as nonselective

NSAIDs for this indication. Gastrointestinal and other toxicities are similar to those of the other coxibs. Valdecoxib has no effect on platelet aggregation or bleeding time. Serious reactions have been reported in sulfonamide-sensitive individuals.

Valdecoxib

NONSELECTIVE COX INHIBITORS

1. Diclofenac

Diclofenac is a phenylacetic acid derivative that is relatively nonselective as a cyclooxygenase inhibitor. Pharmacokinetic and dosage characteristics are set forth in Table 36–1.

Adverse effects occur in approximately 20% of patients and include gastrointestinal distress, occult gastrointestinal bleeding, and gastric ulceration, though ulceration may occur less frequently than with some other NSAIDs. A preparation combining diclofenac and misoprostol decreases upper gastrointestinal ulceration but may result in diarrhea. Another combination of diclofenac and omeprazole was also effective with respect to the prevention of recurrent bleeding, but renal adverse effects were common in high-risk patients. Diclofenac at a dosage of 150 mg/d appears to impair renal blood flow and glomerular filtration rate. Elevation of serum aminotransferases may occur more commonly with this drug than with other NSAIDs.

A 0.1% ophthalmic preparation is recommended for prevention of postoperative ophthalmic inflammation and can be used after intraocular lens implantation and strabismus surgery. A topical gel containing 3% diclofenac is effective for solar keratoses. Diclofenac in rectal suppository form can be considered a drug of choice for preemptive analgesia and postoperative nausea. In Europe, diclofenac is also available as an oral mouthwash and for intramuscular administration.

2. Diflunisal

Although diflunisal is derived from salicylic acid, it is not metabolized to salicylic acid or salicylate. It undergoes an enterohepatic cycle with reabsorption of its glucuronide metabolite followed by cleavage of the glucuronide to again release the active moiety. Diflunisal is subject to capacity-limited metabolism, with serum half-lives at various dosages approximating that of salicylates (Table 36–1). It is claimed to be particularly effective for cancer pain with bone metastases and for pain control in dental (third molar) surgery. A 2% diflunisal oral ointment is a clinically useful analgesic for painful oral lesions.

Because its clearance depends on renal function as well as hepatic metabolism, diflunisal's dosage should be limited in patients with significant renal impairment. Its adverse event profile is similar to those of other NSAIDs; pseudoporphyria has also been reported.

3. Etodolac

Etodolac is a racemic acetic acid derivative with an intermediate half-life (Table 36–1). It is slightly more COX-2-selective than most other NSAIDs, with a COX-2:COX-1 activity ratio of about 10. Unlike many other racemic NSAIDs, etodolac does not undergo chiral inversion in the body. Etodolac produces good postoperative pain relief after coronary artery bypass operations, although transient impairment of renal function has been reported. There are no data to suggest that etodolac differs significantly from other NSAIDs except in its pharmacokinetic parameters, though it has been claimed to cause less gastric toxicity in terms of ulcer disease than other nonselective NSAIDs.

4. Fenoprofen

Fenoprofen, a propionic acid derivative, is the NSAID most closely associated with the toxic effect of interstitial nephritis. This rare toxicity may be associated with a local T cell response in renal tissue.

Other adverse effects of fenoprofen include nausea, dyspepsia, peripheral edema, rash, pruritus, central nervous system and cardiovascular effects, tinnitus, and drug interactions. However, the latter effects are less common than with aspirin.

5. Flurbiprofen

Flurbiprofen is a propionic acid derivative with a possibly more complex mechanism of action than other NSAIDs. Its *(S)(−)* enantiomer inhibits COX nonselectively, but it has been shown in rat tissue to also affect TNF-α and nitric oxide synthesis. Hepatic metabolism is extensive; its *(R)(+)* and *(S)(−)* enantiomers are metabolized differently, and it does not undergo chiral conversion. It does demonstrate enterohepatic circulation.

The efficacy of flurbiprofen at dosages of 200–400 mg/d is comparable to that of aspirin and other

NSAIDs in clinical trials for patients with rheumatoid arthritis, ankylosing spondylitis, gout, and osteoarthritis. It is also available in a topical ophthalmic formulation for inhibition of intraoperative miosis. Flurbiprofen intravenously has been found to be effective for perioperative analgesia in minor ear, neck, and nose surgery and in lozenge form for sore throat.

Although its adverse effect profile is similar to that of other NSAIDs in most ways, flurbiprofen is also associated rarely with cogwheel rigidity, ataxia, tremor, and myoclonus.

6. Ibuprofen

Ibuprofen is a simple derivative of phenylpropionic acid. In doses of about 2400 mg daily, ibuprofen is equivalent to 4 g of aspirin in anti-inflammatory effect. Pharmacokinetic characteristics are given in table 36–1.

Oral ibuprofen is often prescribed in lower doses (< 2400 mg/d), at which it has analgesic but not anti-inflammatory efficacy. It is available over the counter in low-dose forms under several trade names. A topical cream preparation appears to be absorbed into fascia and muscle; an (S)(−) formulation has been tested. Ibuprofen cream was more effective than placebo cream for the treatment of primary knee osteoarthritis. A liquid gel preparation of ibuprofen 400 mg provided faster relief and superior overall efficacy in postsurgical dental pain. In comparison with indomethacin, ibuprofen decreases urine output less and also causes less fluid retention than indomethacin. Ibuprofen has been shown to be effective in closing patent ductus arteriosus in preterm infants, with much the same efficacy and safety as indomethacin. Oral ibuprofen is as effective as intravenous administration in this condition.

Gastrointestinal irritation and bleeding occur, though less frequently than with aspirin. The use of ibuprofen concomitantly with aspirin may *decrease* the total anti-inflammatory effect. The drug is relatively contraindicated in individuals with nasal polyps, angioedema, and bronchospastic reactivity to aspirin. In addition to the gastrointestinal symptoms (which can be modified by ingestion with meals), rash, pruritus, tinnitus, dizziness, headache, aseptic meningitis (particularly in patients with systemic lupus erythematosus), and fluid retention have been reported. Interaction with anticoagulants is uncommon.

The concomitant administration of ibuprofen antagonizes the irreversible platelet inhibition induced by aspirin. Thus, treatment with ibuprofen in patients with increased cardiovascular risk may limit the cardioprotective effects of aspirin. Rare hematologic effects include agranulocytosis and aplastic anemia. Effects on the kidney (as with all NSAIDs) include acute renal failure, interstitial nephritis, and nephrotic syndrome, but these occur very rarely. Finally, hepatitis has been reported.

7. Indomethacin

Indomethacin, introduced in 1963, is an indole derivative (Figure 36–1). It is a potent nonselective COX inhibitor and may also inhibit phospholipase A and C, reduce neutrophil migration, and decrease T cell and B cell proliferation. Probenecid prolongs indomethacin's half-life by inhibiting both renal and biliary clearance.

Clinical Uses

Indomethacin enjoys the usual indications for use in rheumatic conditions and is particularly popular for gout and ankylosing spondylitis. In addition, it has been used to treat patent ductus arteriosus. Indomethacin has been tried in numerous small or uncontrolled trials for many conditions, including Sweet's syndrome, juvenile rheumatoid arthritis, pleurisy, nephrotic syndrome, diabetes insipidus, urticarial vasculitis, postepisiotomy pain, and prophylaxis of heterotopic ossification in arthroplasty, and many others. An ophthalmic preparation seems to be efficacious for conjunctival inflammation (alone and in combination with gentamicin) to reduce pain after traumatic corneal abrasion. Gingival inflammation is reduced after administration of indomethacin oral rinse. Epidural injections produce a degree of pain relief similar to that achieved with methylprednisolone in postlaminectomy syndrome.

Adverse Effects

At higher dosages, at least a third of patients have reactions to indomethacin requiring discontinuance. The gastrointestinal effects may include abdominal pain, diarrhea, gastrointestinal hemorrhage, and pancreatitis. Headache is experienced by 15–25% of patients and may be associated with dizziness, confusion, and depression. Rarely, psychosis with hallucinations has been reported. Hepatic abnormalities are rare. Serious hematologic reactions have been noted, including thrombocytopenia and aplastic anemia. Hyperkalemia has been reported and is related to inhibition of the synthesis of prostaglandins in the kidney. Renal papillary necrosis has also been observed. Bolus injections decrease organ blood flow and impair urinary output, although continuous infusion does not. A number of interactions with other drugs have been reported (see Appendix II). As is true for other potent cyclooxygenase inhibitors also, use of indomethacin should be avoided in patients with nasal polyps or angioedema, in whom asthma may be precipitated.

8. Ketoprofen

Ketoprofen is a propionic acid derivative that inhibits both cyclooxygenase (nonselectively) and lipoxygenase.

Its pharmacokinetic characteristics are given in Table 36–1. Concurrent administration of probenecid elevates ketoprofen levels and prolongs its plasma half-life.

The effectiveness of ketoprofen at dosages of 100–300 mg/d is equivalent to that of other NSAIDs in the treatment of rheumatoid arthritis, osteoarthritis, gout, dysmenorrhea, and other painful conditions. In spite of its dual effect on prostaglandins and leukotrienes, ketoprofen is not superior to other NSAIDs. Its major adverse effects are on the gastrointestinal tract and the central nervous system.

9. Ketorolac

Ketorolac is an NSAID promoted for systemic use mainly as an analgesic, not as an anti-inflammatory drug (though it has typical NSAID properties). Pharmacokinetics are presented in Table 36–1. The drug does appear to have significant analgesic efficacy and has been used successfully to replace morphine in some situations involving mild to moderate postsurgical pain. It is most often given intramuscularly or intravenously, but an oral dose formulation is available. When used with an opioid, it may decrease the opioid requirement by 25–50%. An ophthalmic preparation is available for anti-inflammatory applications. Toxicities are similar to those of other NSAIDs, although renal toxicity may be more common with chronic use.

10. Meclofenamate & Mefenamic Acid

Meclofenamate and mefenamic acid (Table 36–1) inhibit both COX and phospholipase A_2. Meclofenamate appears to have adverse effects similar to those of other NSAIDs, though diarrhea and abdominal pain may be more common; it has no advantages over other NSAIDs. This drug enhances the effect of oral anticoagulants. Meclofenamate is contraindicated in pregnancy; its efficacy and safety have not been established for young children.

Mefenamic acid is probably less effective than aspirin as an anti-inflammatory agent and is clearly more toxic. It should not be used for longer than 1 week and should not be given to children.

11. Nabumetone

Nabumetone is the only nonacid NSAID in current use; it is converted to the active acetic acid derivative in the body. It is given as a ketone prodrug that resembles naproxen in structure (Figure 36–1). Its half-life of more than 24 hours (Table 36–1) permits once-daily dosing, and the drug does not appear to undergo enterohepatic circulation. Renal impairment results in a doubling of its half-life and a 30% increase in area under the curve. Its properties are very similar to those of other NSAIDs, though it may be less damaging to the stomach than some other NSAIDs when given at a dosage of 1000 mg/d. Unfortunately, higher doses (eg, 1500–2000 mg/d) are often needed, and this is a very expensive NSAID. Like naproxen, nabumetone has been reported to cause pseudoporphyria and photosensitivity in some patients. Other adverse effects mirror those of other NSAIDs.

12. Naproxen

Naproxen is a naphthylpropionic acid derivative. It is the only NSAID presently marketed as a single enantiomer, and it is a nonselective COX inhibitor. Naproxen's free fraction is 41% higher in women than in men, though albumin binding is very high in both sexes (Table 36–1). Naproxen is effective for the usual rheumatologic indications and is available both in a slow-release formulation and as an oral suspension. A topical preparation and an ophthalmic solution are also available.

The incidence of upper gastrointestinal bleeding in OTC use is low but still double that of OTC ibuprofen (perhaps due to a dose effect). Rare cases of allergic pneumonitis, leukocytoclastic vasculitis, and pseudoporphyria as well as the more common NSAID-associated adverse effects have been noted.

13. Oxaprozin

Oxaprozin is another propionic acid derivative NSAID. As noted in Table 36–1, its major difference from the other members of this subgroup is a very long half-life (50–60 hours), though oxaprozin does not undergo enterohepatic circulation. Because of its long half-life, oxaprozin can be given once a day, and dosage adjustments should be made at intervals no shorter than 5 days. The drug appears to have the same benefits and risks that are associated with other NSAIDs. It is mildly uricosuric, making it potentially more useful in gout than some other NSAIDs.

14. Phenylbutazone

Phenylbutazone, a pyrazolone derivative, rapidly gained favor after its introduction in 1949 for the treatment of rheumatic syndromes, but its toxicities—particularly the hematologic effects (including aplastic anemia)—have resulted in its withdrawal from the North American and most European markets. It is rarely used today.

15. Piroxicam

Piroxicam, an oxicam (Figure 36–1), is a nonselective COX inhibitor but at high concentrations also inhibits polymorphonuclear leukocyte migration, decreases oxygen radical production, and inhibits lymphocyte function. Its long half-life (Table 36–1) permits once-daily dosing.

Piroxicam can be used for the usual rheumatic indications. Toxicity includes gastrointestinal symptoms (20% of patients), dizziness, tinnitus, headache, and rash. When piroxicam is used in dosages higher than 20 mg/d, an increased incidence of peptic ulcer and bleeding is encountered. Epidemiologic studies suggest that this risk is as much as 9.5 times higher with piroxicam than with other NSAIDs.

16. Sulindac

Sulindac is a sulfoxide prodrug. It is reversibly metabolized to the active sulfide metabolite, which is excreted in bile and then reabsorbed from the intestine. The enterohepatic cycling prolongs the duration of action to 12–16 hours.

The indications and adverse reactions of sulindac are similar to those of other NSAIDs. In addition to its rheumatic disease indications, sulindac suppresses familial intestinal polyposis; it may inhibit the development of colon, breast, and prostate cancer in humans. It appears to inhibit the occurrence of gastrointestinal cancer in rats. The latter effect may be caused by the sulfone rather than the sulfide.

Because the sulfide may be reoxidized to the inactive prodrug in the kidney, sulindac may inhibit renal COX less than other NSAIDs, though reversible renal failure and nephrotic syndrome have been observed with this drug. Among the more severe reactions, Stevens-Johnson epidermal necrolysis syndrome, thrombocytopenia, agranulocytosis, and nephrotic syndrome have all been observed. Like diclofenac, sulindac may have some propensity to cause elevation of serum aminotransferases; it is also sometimes associated with cholestatic liver damage, which disappears or becomes quiescent when the drug is stopped.

17. Tenoxicam

Tenoxicam is an oxicam similar to piroxicam and shares its nonselective COX inhibition, long half-life (72 hours), efficacy, and toxicity profile. It is available abroad but not in the USA.

18. Tiaprofen

Tiaprofen is a racemic propionic acid derivative but does not undergo stereoconversion. It has a short serum half-life (1–2 hours) with an increase to 2–4 hours in the elderly. This drug inhibits renal uric acid reabsorption and thus decreases serum uric acid slightly. It is available for oral and intramuscular administration. Its efficacy and adverse event profiles mirror those of other NSAIDs, but tiaprofen is not available in the USA.

19. Tolmetin

Tolmetin is a nonselective COX inhibitor. Its short half-life means that it must be given frequently, and it is therefore not often used. It is similar to other NSAIDs in efficacy except in gout, in which it is ineffective (for unknown reasons). Its toxicity profile is also similar to those of other NSAIDs, with the rare additional problem of allergic IgM-related thrombocytopenic purpura.

20. Azapropazone & Carprofen

These drugs are available in many other countries but are not sold in the USA. Azapropazone (apazone), a pyrazolone derivative, is structurally related to phenylbutazone but appears less likely to cause agranulocytosis. Its half-life of 12–16 hours may be doubled in patients with decreased renal function. Carprofen is a propionic acid derivative with a half-life of 10–16 hours. The indications and adverse effects of azapropazone and carprofen are similar to those of other NSAIDs.

CLINICAL PHARMACOLOGY OF THE NSAIDs

All NSAIDs, including aspirin, are about equally efficacious with a few exceptions—tolmetin seems not to be effective for gout, and aspirin is less effective than other NSAIDs (eg, indomethacin) for ankylosing spondylitis. Thus, NSAIDs tend to be differentiated on the basis of toxicity and cost-effectiveness. For example, the gastrointestinal and renal side effects of ketorolac limit its use. Fries et al (1993), using a toxicity index, estimated that indomethacin, tolmetin, and meclofenamate were associated with the greatest toxicity, while salsalate, aspirin, and ibuprofen were least toxic. The selective COX-2 inhibitors were not included in this analysis.

For patients with renal insufficiency, nonacetylated salicylates may be best. Fenoprofen is less used because of its rare association with interstitial nephritis. Diclofenac and sulindac are associated with more liver function test abnormalities than other NSAIDs. The relatively expensive and selective COX-2 inhibitors are probably safest for patients at high risk for gastrointestinal bleeding. These drugs or a nonselective NSAID plus omeprazole or misoprostol may be appropriate in those patients at highest risk for gastrointestinal bleeding; in this subpopulation of patients, they are cost-effective despite their high acquisition costs.

The choice of an NSAID thus requires a balance of efficacy, cost-effectiveness, safety, and numerous personal factors (eg, other drugs also being used, concurrent illness, compliance, medical insurance coverage), so that there is no "best" NSAID for all patients. There may, however, be one or two best NSAIDs for a specific person.

II. DISEASE-MODIFYING ANTIRHEUMATIC DRUGS (DMARDs)

Careful clinical and epidemiologic studies have shown that rheumatoid arthritis is an immunologic disease that causes significant systemic effects which shorten life in addition to the joint disease that reduces mobility and quality of life. NSAIDs offer mainly symptomatic relief; they reduce inflammation and the pain it causes and often preserve function, but they have little effect on the progression of bone and cartilage destruction. Interest has therefore centered on finding treatments that might arrest—or at least slow—this progression by modifying the disease itself. The effects of disease-modifying therapies may take 6 weeks to 6 months to become evident, ie, they are slow-acting compared with NSAIDs. These therapies include methotrexate, azathioprine, penicillamine, hydroxychloroquine and chloroquine, organic gold compounds, sulfasalazine, leflunomide, tumor necrosis factor (TNF)-blocking agents, and immunoadsorption apheresis. Considerable controversy surrounds the long-term efficacy of many of these therapies.

METHOTREXATE

Methotrexate is now considered the first DMARD of choice in the treatment of rheumatoid arthritis and is used in up to 60% of patients. It is active in this condition at much lower doses than those needed in cancer chemotherapy (see Chapter 55).

Mechanism of Action

Methotrexate's principal mechanism of action at the low doses used in the rheumatic diseases probably relates to inhibition of aminoimidazolecarboxamide (AICAR) transformylase and thymidylate synthetase, with secondary effects on polymorphonuclear chemotaxis. While there is some effect on dihydrofolate reductase—and this effects lymphocyte and macrophage function—it is more likely its effect on AICAR transformylase that accounts for the major portion of its action in autoimmune disease.

Pharmacokinetics

The drug is approximately 70% absorbed after oral administration (see Chapter 55). It is metabolized to a less active hydroxylated metabolite, and both the parent compound and the metabolite are polyglutamated within cells, where they stay for prolonged periods. Methotrexate's serum half-life is usually only 6–9 hours, although it may be as long as 24 hours in some individuals. Methotrexate's concentration is increased in the presence of hydroxychloroquine. This drug is excreted principally in the urine, but up to 30% may be excreted in bile.

Indications

Although the most common methotrexate dosing regimens for the treatment of rheumatoid arthritis are 15 or 17.5 mg weekly, there is an increased effect up to 30 or 35 mg weekly. The drug decreases the rate of appearance of new erosions. Evidence supports its use in juvenile chronic arthritis, and it has been used in psoriasis, psoriatic arthritis, polymyositis, dermatomyositis, Wegener's granulomatosis, giant cell arteritis, subacute lupus erythematosus, and vasculitis.

Adverse Effects

Nausea and mucosal ulcers are the most common toxicities. Progressive dose-related hepatotoxicity in the form of enzyme elevation occurs frequently, but cirrhosis is rare (< 1%). Liver toxicity is not related to methotrexate concentrations, and liver biopsy follow-up is only recommended every 5 years. A rare "hypersensitivity" lung reaction with acute shortness of breath is documented, as are pseudolymphomatous reactions. The incidence of gastrointestinal and liver function test abnormalities can be reduced by the use of leucovorin 24 hours after each weekly dose or by the use of daily folic acid. This drug is contraindicated in pregnancy.

CHLORAMBUCIL

Mechanism of Action & Pharmacokinetics

Chlorambucil, probably through its metabolite phenylacetic acid mustard, cross-links DNA, thereby preventing cell replication. Its bioavailability is about 70% and it is completely metabolized, with excretion completed within 24 hours.

Indications

One controlled, double-blind trial plus anecdotal evidence attest to the efficacy of chlorambucil in rheumatoid arthritis. Chlorambucil has also been used in Behçet's disease, systemic lupus erythematosus, vasculitis, and other autoimmune disorders.

Adverse Effects

The most common toxicity is dose-related bone marrow suppression. Infertility with azoospermia and amenorrhea also occurs. The risk of neoplasia is increased, with the relative risk of leukemia increased about tenfold compared with the general population, especially after more than 3 years of use.

CYCLOPHOSPHAMIDE

Mechanism of Action

Cyclophosphamide's major active metabolite is phosphoramide mustard, which cross-links DNA to prevent cell replication. It suppresses T cell and B cell function by 30–40%; the T cell suppression correlates with clinical response in the rheumatic diseases.

Pharmacokinetics

See Chapter 55.

Indications

Cyclophosphamide is active against rheumatoid arthritis when given orally at dosages of 2 mg/kg/d but not when given intravenously. It is used regularly to treat systemic lupus erythematosus, vasculitis, Wegener's granulomatosis, and other severe rheumatic diseases.

Adverse Effects

Cyclophosphamide causes significant dose-related infertility in both men and women as well as bone marrow suppression, alopecia, hemorrhagic cystitis, and, rarely, bladder carcinoma (see Chapter 55).

CYCLOSPORINE

Mechanism of Action

Through regulation of gene transcription, cyclosporine inhibits IL-1 and IL-2 receptor production and secondarily inhibits macrophage-T cell interaction and T cell responsiveness (see Chapter 56). T cell-dependent B cell function is also affected.

Pharmacokinetics

Cyclosporine absorption is incomplete and somewhat erratic, although a new microemulsion formulation improves its consistency and provides 20 to 30% bioavailability. Grapefruit juice increases cyclosporine bioavailability up to 62%. Cyclosporine is metabolized by CYP3A and consequently is subject to a large number of drug interactions (see Chapter 56 and Appendix II).

Indications

Cyclosporine is approved for use in rheumatoid arthritis and retards the appearance of new bony erosions. Its usual dosage is 3–5 mg/kg/d divided into two doses. Anecdotal reports suggest that it may be useful in systemic lupus erythematosus, polymyositis and dermatomyositis, Wegener's granulomatosis, and juvenile chronic arthritis.

Adverse Effects

Cyclosporine has significant nephrotoxicity, and its toxicity can be increased by drug interactions with diltiazem, potassium-sparing diuretics, and other drugs inhibiting CYP3A. Serum creatinine should be closely monitored. Other toxicities include hypertension, hyperkalemia, hepatotoxicity, gingival hyperplasia, and hirsutism.

AZATHIOPRINE

Mechanism of Action

Azathioprine acts through its major metabolite, 6-thioguanine. 6-Thioguanine suppresses inosinic acid synthesis, B cell and T cell function, immunoglobulin production, and IL-2 secretion (see Chapter 56).

Pharmacokinetics

The metabolism of azathioprine is bimodal, with rapid metabolizers clearing the drug four times more rapidly than slow metabolizers. Production of 6-thioguanine is dependent on thiopurine methyltransferase (TPMT), and patients with low or absent TPMT activity (0.3% of the population) are at particularly high risk of myelosuppression by excess concentrations of the parent drug if dosage is not adjusted.

Indications

Azathioprine is approved for use in rheumatoid arthritis and is used at a dosage of 2 mg/kg/d. Controlled trials show efficacy in psoriatic arthritis, reactive arthritis, polymyositis, systemic lupus erythematosus, and Behçet's disease

Adverse Effects

Azathioprine's toxicity includes bone marrow suppression, gastrointestinal disturbances, and some increase in infection risk. As noted in Chapter 56, lymphomas may be increased with azathioprine use. Rarely, fever, rash, and hepatotoxicity signal acute allergic reactions.

MYCOPHENOLATE MOFETIL

Mechanism of Action

Mycophenolate mofetil (MMF) is converted to mycophenolic acid, the active form of the drug. The active product inhibits cytosine monophosphate dehydrogenase and secondarily, inhibits T cell lymphocyte proliferation; downstream, it interferes with leukocyte adhesion to endothelial cells through inhibition of E-selectin, P-selectin, and intercellular adhesion molecule 1.

Pharmacokinetics

See Chapter 56.

Indications

MMF has been shown to be effective for the treatment of renal disease due to systemic lupus erythematosus and may be useful in vasculitis and Wegener's granulomatosis. While occasionally used at a dosage of 2 g/d to treat rheumatoid arthritis, there are few controlled data regarding its efficacy in this disease.

Adverse Effects

Comparisons with azathioprine in the renal transplantation literature show that MMF and azathioprine have similar gastrointestinal, hematopoietic, and hepatic toxicity profiles, with a possibly decreased incidence of fungal infections among patients treated with MMF. Hepatic toxicities are infrequent but must be monitored.

CHLOROQUINE & HYDROXYCHLOROQUINE

Mechanism of Action

Chloroquine and hydroxychloroquine are used mainly in malaria (see Chapter 53). The mechanism of the anti-inflammatory action of these drugs in rheumatic diseases is unclear. The following mechanisms have been proposed: suppression of T lymphocyte responses to mitogens, decreased leukocyte chemotaxis, stabilization of lysosomal enzymes, inhibition of DNA and RNA synthesis, and the trapping of free radicals.

Pharmacokinetics

Antimalarials are rapidly absorbed but only 50% protein-bound in the plasma. They are very extensively tissue-bound, particularly in melanin-containing tissues such as the eyes. The drugs are deaminated in the liver and have blood elimination half-lives of up to 45 days.

Indications

Antimalarials are approved for rheumatoid arthritis, but they are not considered very efficacious DMARDs. Dose-response and serum concentration-response relationships have been documented for hydroxychloroquine. While antimalarials improve symptoms, there is

no evidence that these compounds alter bony damage in rheumatoid arthritis at their usual dosages (up to 6.4 mg/kg/d hydroxychloroquine or 200 mg/d chloroquine). It usually takes 3–6 months to obtain a response. Antimalarials are often used for the treatment of the skin manifestations, serositis, and joint pains of systemic lupus erythematosus, and they have been used in Sjögren's syndrome.

Adverse Effects

Although ocular toxicity may occur at dosages greater than 250 mg/d chloroquine and greater than 6.4 mg/kg/d hydroxychloroquine, it rarely occurs at lower doses. Nevertheless, ophthalmologic monitoring every 6–12 months is advised. Other toxicities include dyspepsia, nausea, vomiting, abdominal pain, rashes, and nightmares. These drugs appear to be relatively safe in pregnancy.

GOLD

Gold compounds were first proved to be effective in a large double-blind trial in 1960. Because of their toxicity, they are used infrequently today. Their intramuscular formulations (**aurothiomalate** and **aurothioglucose**) contain 50% elemental gold. The oral formulation (**auranofin**) contains 29% elemental gold.

Mechanism of Action

Gold alters the morphology and functional capabilities of human macrophages—possibly its major mode of action. As a result, monocyte chemotactic factor-1, interleukin-8, interleukin-1β production, and vascular endothelial growth factor are all inhibited. Intramuscular gold compounds also alter lysosomal enzyme activity, reduce histamine release from mast cells, inactivate the first component of complement, and suppress the phagocytic activities of polymorphonuclear leukocytes. Auranofin also inhibits release of prostaglandin E_2 and leukotriene B_4.

Pharmacokinetics

These compounds have high bioavailability after intramuscular administration and tend to concentrate in synovial membranes, liver, kidney, spleen, lymph nodes, and bone marrow. One month after an intramuscular injection, 75–80% of the drug is eliminated from the serum, but intramuscular gold's total body half-life is approximately 1 year. Auranofin is only about 25% bioavailable. Gold compounds are excreted approximately 66% in the urine and 33% via the feces. There has generally been no correlation found between serum gold concentration and either efficacy or toxicity.

Indications

Gold is effective for active rheumatoid arthritis and has been shown to slow radiologic progression of the disease. It has also been used in Sjögren's syndrome and juvenile rheumatoid arthritis, while use in psoriatic arthritis is controversial. In Japan, gold is used to treat asthma. The oral form of gold is effective in rheumatoid arthritis, but it appears less effective than the intramuscular formulation and is generally felt to have only modest effects.

Clinical Use

Intramuscular gold is given as a test dose of 5–25 mg and then as 50 mg intramuscular doses weekly for 20 weeks. Continued treatment, with maintained response, frequently allows lengthening of the dosing interval to 2, 3, or 4 weeks. Oral gold is generally given as 6 mg doses daily.

Adverse Effects

Pruritic skin rashes occur in 15–20% of patients, sometimes associated with eosinophilia. Stomatitis and a metallic taste in the mouth are common. Hematologic abnormalities, including thrombocytopenia, leukopenia, and even pancytopenia occur in 1–10% of patients. Aplastic anemia, while very rare, may be fatal. Eight to 10 percent of patients develop proteinuria that may progress to nephrotic syndrome. Other rare toxicities include enterocolitis, cholestatic jaundice, peripheral neuropathy, and pulmonary infiltrates. Corneal deposition of gold occurs but has little clinical import. Nitritoid reactions (sweating, flushing, and headaches) can occur, especially with gold thiomalate, and are presumably due to the vehicle rather than the gold salts. Adverse effects cause 30–40% of patients to discontinue gold therapy within a year.

PENICILLAMINE

Penicillamine, a metabolite of penicillin, is an analog of amino acid cystine. The D isomer has been used in rheumatoid arthritis. Penicillamine is rarely used today because of toxicity.

$$HS-\underset{\underset{CH_3}{|}}{\overset{\overset{CH_3}{|}}{C}}-\underset{\underset{NH_2}{|}}{\overset{\overset{H}{|}}{C}}-COOH$$

Penicillamine

SULFASALAZINE

Mechanism of Action

Sulfasalazine is metabolized to sulfapyridine and 5-aminosalicylic acid, and it is thought that the sulfapyridine is probably the active moiety when treating rheumatoid arthritis (unlike inflammatory bowel disease; see Chapter 63). Some authorities believe that the parent compound, sulfasalazine, also has an effect. In treated arthritis patients, IgA and IgM rheumatoid factor production are decreased. Suppression of T cell responses to concanavalin and inhibition of in vitro B cell proliferation have also been documented. It is not clear how these findings relate to the clinical efficacy of sulfasalazine in rheumatoid arthritis.

Pharmacokinetics

Only 10–20% of orally administered sulfasalazine is absorbed, although a fraction undergoes enterohepatic recirculation into the bowel, where sulfasalazine is reduced by intestinal bacteria to liberate sulfapyridine and 5-aminosalicylic acid. Sulfapyridine is well absorbed while 5-aminosalicylic acid remains unabsorbed. Some sulfasalazine is excreted unchanged in the urine whereas sulfapyridine is excreted after hepatic acetylation and hydroxylation. Sulfasalazine's half-life is 6–17 hours.

Indications

Sulfasalazine is effective in rheumatoid arthritis and reduces the rate of appearance of new joint damage. It has been used in juvenile chronic arthritis and ankylosing spondylitis and its associated uveitis. The usual regimen is 2–3 g/d.

Adverse Effects

Approximately 30% of patients using sulfasalazine discontinue the drug because of toxicity. Common adverse effects include nausea, vomiting, headache, and rash. Hemolytic anemia and methemoglobinemia also occur, but rarely. Neutropenia occurs in 1.4–4.4% of patients, while thrombocytopenia is very rare. Pulmonary toxicity and positive double-stranded DNA are occasionally seen, but drug-induced lupus is rare. Reversible infertility occurs in men, but sulfasalazine does not affect fertility in women. The drug does not appear to be teratogenic.

TNF-α BLOCKING AGENTS

Cytokines play a central role in the immune response (see Chapter 56) and in rheumatoid arthritis. Although a wide range of cytokines are expressed in the joints of rheumatoid arthritis patients, TNF-α appears to be at the heart of the inflammatory process.

TNF-α effects cellular function via activation of specific membrane-bound TNF receptors ($TNFR_1$, $TNFR_2$). Administered soluble TNF receptors, by combining with soluble TNF-α, can inhibit the effects of the endogenous cytokine. Monoclonal anti-TNF antibodies can, in theory, cross-link TNF receptors on the cell surface and inhibit T cell and macrophage function. Three drugs interfering with TNF-α have been approved for the treatment of rheumatoid arthritis.

1. Adalimumab

Mechanism of Action

Adalimumab is a recombinant human anti-TNF monoclonal antibody. This compound complexes with soluble TNF-α and prevents its interaction with p55 and p75 cell surface receptors. This results in down-regulation of macrophage and T cell function.

Pharmacokinetics

Adalimumab is given subcutaneously and has a half-life of 9–14 days. Its clearance is decreased by approximately 30% in the presence of methotrexate, and the formation of human antimonoclonal antibody is decreased from 12% to 4% when methotrexate is given at the same time.

Indications

The compound is indicated for the treatment of rheumatoid arthritis and decreases the rate of formation of new erosions. It is effective both as monotherapy and in combination with methotrexate. The usual dose is 40 mg every other week, though increased responses may be evident at higher dosages. Adalimumab is presently being tested in psoriasis, psoriatic arthritis, ankylosing spondylitis, and juvenile chronic arthritis.

Adverse Effects

In common with the other TNF-α blocking agents, the risk of macrophage-dependent infection (including tuberculosis and other opportunistic infections) must be considered when using adalimumab, and screening for latent tuberculosis or active tuberculosis is recommended before starting adalimumab or other TNF-α blocking agents. There is no evidence of an increased incidence of solid malignancies when adalimumab is used. It is not clear if the incidence of lymphomas is increased by adalimumab. A low incidence of newly formed double-stranded (ds) DNA antibodies and antinuclear antibodies (ANAs) has been documented when using adalimumab, but clinical lupus is extremely rare. Rare leukopenias and vasculitis, apparently associated with adalimumab, have been documented.

2. Infliximab

Mechanism of Action

Infliximab is a chimeric (25% mouse, 75% human) monoclonal antibody that binds with high affinity to soluble and possibly membrane-bound TNF-α. Its mechanism of action probably is the same as that of adalimumab.

Pharmacokinetics

Infliximab is given as an intravenous infusion at doses ranging from 3 mg/kg to 10 mg/kg, although the usual dose is 3–5 mg/kg. While most studies used an every-8-week regimen, a number of patients require dosing every 6–7 weeks. There is a relationship between serum concentration and effect, though individual clearances vary markedly. The terminal half-life is 9–12 days without accumulation after repeated dosing at the recommended interval of 8 weeks. After intermittent therapy, infliximab elicits up to a 62% incidence of human antichimeric antibodies. Concurrent therapy with methotrexate markedly decreases the prevalence of human antichimeric antibodies.

Indications

Infliximab is effective in rheumatoid arthritis and ulcerative colitis and is being used in other diseases, including psoriasis, psoriatic arthritis, juvenile chronic arthritis, Wegener's granulomatosis, giant cell arteritis, and sarcoidosis. In rheumatoid arthritis, a regimen of infliximab plus methotrexate decreases the rate of formation of new erosions more than methotrexate alone over 52–104 weeks. While it is recommended that methotrexate be used in conjunction with infliximab, a number of other DMARDs, including antimalarials, azathioprine, and cyclosporine, can be used as background therapy for this drug.

Adverse Effects

Upper respiratory tract infections, nausea, headache, sinusitis, rash, and cough are common when using infliximab, although their incidence does not appear to be very different from that of methotrexate. As a potent macrophage inhibitor, infliximab can be associated with activation of latent tuberculosis, and screening for latent tuberculosis is recommended prior to starting this therapy. Other opportunistic infections have been documented, although rarely. There is no evidence for an increased incidence of solid malignancies or lymphoma, but as with adalimumab, lymphomas should be looked for. It is not clear whether there is an increased incidence of demyelinating syndromes associated with infliximab. Rare cases of leukopenia and vasculitis have been documented. The incidence of positive ANA and double-stranded DNA is increased, although clinical lupus erythematosus remains an extremely rare occurrence and the presence of ANA and dsDNA does not contraindicate the use of infliximab. Infusion site reactions occur in approximately 3–11% of patients, and the combined use of antihistamines and H_2 blocking agents apparently prevents some of these reactions.

3. *Etanercept*

Mechanism of Action

Etanercept is a recombinant fusion protein consisting of two soluble TNF p75 receptor moieties linked to the Fc portion of human IgG1; it binds TNF-α molecules and also inhibits lymphotoxin-α.

Pharmacokinetics

Etanercept is given subcutaneously in a dosage of 25 mg twice weekly. The drug is slowly absorbed, with peak concentration 72 hours after drug administration. Etanercept has a mean serum elimination half-life of 4.5 days. Fifty milligrams given once weekly gives the same area under the curve and minimum serum concentrations as 25 mg twice weekly.

Indications

Etanercept is approved for the treatment of rheumatoid arthritis, juvenile chronic arthritis, and psoriatic arthritis and ankylosing spondylitis. It is used both as monotherapy and with methotrexate background; over 70% of patients taking etanercept are also using methotrexate. Etanercept decreases the rate of formation of new erosions relative to methotrexate alone. While etanercept is ineffective for treatment of ulcerative colitis, it is being used in many rheumatic syndromes such as scleroderma, Wegener's granulomatosis, giant cell arteritis, and sarcoidosis.

Adverse Effects

The incidence of activation of latent tuberculosis in patients treated with etanercept may be lower than that caused by other TNF blocking agents, but this difference is not statistically significant and it is appropriate to screen patients for latent or active tuberculosis prior to starting this medication. Similarly, opportunistic infections can occur when using etanercept. The incidence of solid malignancies is not increased, but as with other TNF-blocking agents one must be alert for lymphomas (although their incidence may not be increased compared with other DMARDs or active rheumatoid arthritis itself). While positive ANAs and double-stranded DNAs may be found in patients receiving this drug, these findings do not contraindicate continued use if clinical lupus symptoms do not occur. Injection site reactions occur in 20–40% of patients, although they rarely result in discontinuation of therapy. Although antietanercept antibodies appear sporadically in up to 16% of patients, the presence of the antibodies does not appear to interfere with efficacy or to presage toxicity.

LEFLUNOMIDE

Mechanism of Action

Leflunomide undergoes rapid conversion, both in the intestine and in the plasma, to its active metabolite, A77-1726. This metabolite inhibits dihydroorotate dehydrogenase, leading to a decrease in ribonucleotide synthesis and the arrest of stimulated cells in the G1 phase of cell growth. Consequently, leflunomide inhibits T cell proliferation and production of autoantibodies by B cells. Secondary effects include increases of interleukin-10 receptor mRNA, decreased interleukin-8 receptor type A mRNA, and decreased TNF-α-dependent NFκB activation.

Pharmacokinetics

Leflunomide is completely absorbed and has a mean plasma half-life of 19 days. A77-1726 is subject to enterohepatic recirculation and is efficiently reabsorbed. Cholestyramine can enhance leflunomide excretion and increases total clearance by approximately 50%.

Indications

Leflunomide is as effective as methotrexate in rheumatoid arthritis, including inhibition of bony damage. In one study, combined treatment with methotrexate and leflunomide resulted in a 46.2% ACR20 response compared with 19.5% in patients receiving methotrexate alone.

Adverse Effects

Diarrhea or loose bowels occur in approximately 25% of patients given leflunomide, although only about 3–5% discontinue drug because of this effect. Elevation in liver enzymes also occurs. Both effects can be reduced by decreasing the dose of leflunomide. Other adverse effects associated with leflunomide are mild alopecia, weight gain, and increased blood pressure. Leukopenia and thrombocytopenia occur rarely. This drug is contraindicated in pregnancy.

COMBINATION THERAPY WITH DMARDs

In a 1998 study, approximately half of North American rheumatologists treated moderately aggressive rheumatoid arthritis with combination therapy. Combinations of DMARDs can be designed rationally on the basis of complementary mechanisms of action, nonoverlapping pharmacokinetics, and nonoverlapping toxicity.

When added to methotrexate background therapy, cyclosporine, chloroquine, leflunomide, infliximab, adalimumab, and etanercept have all shown improved efficacy. In contrast, azathioprine, auranofin, or sulfasalazine plus methotrexate results in no additional therapeutic benefit. Other combinations have occasionally been used, including the combination of intramuscular gold with hydroxychloroquine. A triple-therapy regimen (methotrexate, sulfasalazine, and hydroxychloroquine) was recently tested and compared with methotrexate plus sulfasalazine or methotrexate plus hydroxychloroquine. Seventy-eight percent of the triple therapy group achieved an ACR20 response at 2 years, compared with 60% of those treated with methotrexate plus hydroxychloroquine and 49% of those treated with methotrexate plus sulfasalazine.

While it might be anticipated that combination therapy might result in more toxicity, this is often not the case. Combination therapy for patients not responding adequately to monotherapy is becoming the rule in the treatment of rheumatoid arthritis.

IMMUNOABSORPTION APHERESIS

Extracorporeal immunoabsorption of plasma over columns containing an inert silica matrix and covalently attached highly purified staphylococcal protein A (Prosorba column) involves apheresis of about 1200 mL plasma weekly for 3 months.

Mechanism of Action

Although this treatment has been available for idiopathic thrombocytopenic purpura for several years, its mechanism of action is not understood. Removal of IgG and IgG-containing immune complexes does not explain its effects in rheumatoid arthritis. The most recent hypothesis for this treatment's mechanism of action is down-regulation of B cell function through the release of small amounts of staphylococcal protein A complexed with immunoglobulins.

Indications

This treatment has generally been used in patients who have failed numerous other therapies, so its low efficacy in rheumatoid arthritis is better than it appears. The study establishing efficacy in rheumatoid arthritis showed a 41.7% ACR20 response among Prosorba-treated patients compared with 15.6% in the sham-treated group. Further testing is clearly indicated.

Adverse Effects

Common adverse events include joint pain, joint swelling, and hypotension. Central intravenous line usage may be associated with pulmonary emboli and sepsis. Other events, such as nausea, rash, pruritus, flushing, and fever occurred in 1–6% of treatments in both sham and treatment groups in the double-blind trial. Rare leukocytoclastic vasculitis has been documented.

GLUCOCORTICOID DRUGS

The general pharmacology of corticosteroids, including mechanism of action, pharmacokinetics, and other applications, is discussed in Chapter 39.

Indications

Corticosteroids have been used in 60–70% of rheumatoid arthritis patients. Their effects are prompt and dramatic, and they are capable of slowing the appearance of new bone erosions. Corticosteroids may be administered for certain serious extra-articular manifestations such as pericarditis or eye involvement or during periods of exacerbation. When prednisone is required for long-term therapy, the dosage should not exceed 7.5 mg daily, and gradual reduction of the dose should be encouraged. Alternate-day corticosteroid therapy is usually unsuccessful in rheumatoid arthritis.

Other rheumatic diseases in which the corticosteroids' potent anti-inflammatory effects may be useful include vasculitis, systemic lupus erythematosus, Wegener's granulomatosis, psoriatic arthritis, giant cell arteritis, sarcoidosis, and even gout.

Intra-articular corticosteroids are often helpful to alleviate painful symptoms and, when successful, are preferable to increasing the dosage of systemic medication.

Adverse Effects

Prolonged use of these drugs leads to serious and disabling toxic effects as described in Chapter 39. There is controversy over whether many of these side effects occur at doses below 7.5 mg prednisone equivalent daily, although many experts believe that even 5 mg/d can cause these effects in susceptible individuals.

DIETARY MANIPULATION OF INFLAMMATION

Arachidonic acid is an eicosatetraenoic acid that is metabolized by the cyclooxygenase and lipoxygenase pathways, yielding several mediators (see Chapter 18). These mediators have potent effects on many systems, including the immune system. It has been demonstrated that dietary manipulation which substitutes unsaturated fatty acids (such as eicosapentaenoic acid, found in marine fish) causes the alternative fatty acids to be metabolized, changing the final prostaglandin and leukotriene products of the process. The products of eicosapentaenoic acid metabolism are less potent than the corresponding mediators derived from arachidonic acid (sometimes by several orders of magnitude), and they diminish the activities of the eicosatetraenoic mediators by competing with them for shared target-cell receptors.

The results of clinical studies suggest that therapy with dietary eicosapentaenoic acid decreases both morning stiffness and the number of tender joints in patients with rheumatoid arthritis and erythema associated with psoriasis. The efficacy of dietary eicosapentaenoic acid approximates that of the NSAIDs. These preliminary results and the near absence of significant adverse effects suggest that dietary alteration or supplementation to provide 1–4 g/d of eicosapentaenoic acid may be a beneficial addition to conventional treatment of rheumatoid arthritis.

III. OTHER ANALGESICS

Acetaminophen is one of the most important drugs used for the treatment of mild to moderate pain when an anti-inflammatory effect is not necessary. Phenacetin, a prodrug that is metabolized to acetaminophen, is more toxic than its active metabolite and has no rational indications.

ACETAMINOPHEN

Acetaminophen is the active metabolite of phenacetin and is responsible for its analgesic effect. It is a weak COX-1 and COX-2 inhibitor in peripheral tissues and possesses no significant anti-inflammatory effects. Recent evidence suggests that acetaminophen may inhibit a third enzyme, COX-3, in the central nervous system. COX-3 appears to be a splice variant product of the COX-1 gene.

N-Acetyl-*p*-aminophenol
(acetaminophen)

Pharmacokinetics

Acetaminophen is administered orally. Absorption is related to the rate of gastric emptying, and peak blood concentrations are usually reached in 30–60 minutes. Acetaminophen is slightly bound to plasma proteins and is partially metabolized by hepatic microsomal enzymes and converted to acetaminophen sulfate and glucuronide, which are pharmacologically inactive (Figure 4–4). Less than 5% is excreted unchanged. A minor but highly active metabolite (*N*-acetyl-*p*-benzoquinone) is important in large doses because of its toxicity to both liver and kidney. The half-life of acetaminophen is 2–3 hours and is relatively unaffected by renal function. With toxic doses or liver disease, the half-life may be increased twofold or more.

Indications

Although equivalent to aspirin as an effective analgesic and antipyretic agent, acetaminophen differs in that it lacks anti-inflammatory properties. It does not affect uric acid levels and lacks platelet-inhibiting properties. The drug is useful in mild to moderate pain such as headache, myalgia, postpartum pain, and other circumstances in which aspirin is an effective analgesic. Acetaminophen alone is inadequate therapy for inflammatory conditions such as rheumatoid arthritis, though it may be used as an analgesic adjunct to anti-inflammatory therapy. For mild analgesia, acetaminophen is the preferred drug in patients allergic to aspirin or when salicylates are poorly tolerated. It is preferable to aspirin in patients with hemophilia or a history of peptic ulcer and in those in whom bronchospasm is precipitated by aspirin. Unlike aspirin, acetaminophen does not antagonize the effects of uricosuric agents; it may be used concomitantly with probenecid in the treatment of gout. It is preferred to aspirin in children with viral infections.

Adverse Effects

In therapeutic doses, a mild increase in hepatic enzymes may occasionally occur in the absence of jaundice; this is reversible when the drug is withdrawn. With larger doses, dizziness, excitement, and disorientation are seen. Ingestion of 15 g of acetaminophen may be fatal, death being caused by severe hepatotoxicity with centrilobular necrosis, sometimes associated with acute renal tubular necrosis (see Chapters 4 and 59). Early symptoms of hepatic damage include nausea, vomiting, diarrhea, and abdominal pain. Recent data also implicate acetaminophen in rare cases of renal damage without hepatic damage. This damage has occurred even after usual doses of acetaminophen. Therapy is much less satisfactory than for aspirin overdose. In addition to supportive therapy, the measure that has proved most useful is the provision of sulfhydryl groups in the form of acetylcysteine to neutralize the toxic metabolites (see Chapter 59).

Hemolytic anemia and methemoglobinemia, reported with the use of phenacetin, are rarely noted with acetaminophen. Interstitial nephritis and papillary necrosis—serious complications of phenacetin—although anticipated with widespread chronic use of acetaminophen, have not occurred. Gastrointestinal bleeding does not occur. Caution should be exercised in patients with liver disease.

Dosage

Acute pain and fever may be effectively treated with 325–500 mg four times daily and proportionately less for children. Steady state conditions are attained within a day.

PHENACETIN

Phenacetin is no longer prescribed in the USA and has been removed from many over-the-counter analgesic combinations. However, it is still present in a number of proprietary analgesics in this country and is in common use in many other parts of the world. The association between the excessive use of analgesic combinations—especially those that contain phenacetin—and the development of renal failure has been recognized for almost 30 years.

IV. DRUGS USED IN GOUT

Gout is a familial metabolic disease characterized by recurrent episodes of acute arthritis due to deposits of monosodium urate in joints and cartilage. Formation of uric acid calculi in the kidneys may also occur. Gout is usually associated with high serum levels of uric acid, a poorly soluble substance that is the major end product of purine metabolism. In most mammals, uricase converts uric acid to the more soluble allantoin; this enzyme is absent in humans.

The treatment of gout is aimed at relieving the acute gouty attack and preventing recurrent gouty episodes and urate lithiasis. Therapy for an attack of acute gouty arthritis is based on our current understanding of the pathophysiologic events that occur in this disease (Figure 36–5). Urate crystals are initially phagocytosed by synoviocytes, which then release prostaglandins, lysosomal enzymes, and interleukin-1. Attracted by these chemotactic mediators, polymorphonuclear leukocytes migrate into the joint space and amplify the ongoing inflammatory process. In the later phases of the attack, increased numbers of mononuclear phagocytes (macrophages) appear, ingest the urate crystals, and release more inflammatory mediators. This sequence of events suggests that the most effective agents for the management of acute urate crystal-induced inflammation are those that suppress different phases of leukocyte activation.

Before starting chronic therapy for gout, patients in whom hyperuricemia is associated with gout and urate lithiasis must be clearly distinguished from those who have only hyperuricemia. In an asymptomatic person with hyperuricemia, the efficacy of long-term drug treatment is unproved. In some individuals, uric acid levels may be elevated up to 2 SD above the mean for a lifetime without adverse consequences.

COLCHICINE

Colchicine is an alkaloid isolated from the autumn crocus, *Colchicum autumnale*. Its structure is shown in Figure 36–6.

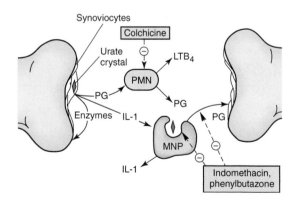

Figure 36–5. Pathophysiologic events in a gouty joint. Synoviocytes phagocytose urate crystals and then secrete inflammatory mediators, which attract and activate polymorphonuclear leukocytes (PMN) and mononuclear phagocytes (MNP) (macrophages). Drugs active in gout inhibit crystal phagocytosis and polymorphonuclear leukocyte and macrophage release of inflammatory mediators. (PG, prostaglandin; IL-1, interleukin-1; LTB$_4$, leukotriene B$_4$.)

Pharmacokinetics

Colchicine is absorbed readily after oral administration and reaches peak plasma levels within 2 hours. Metabolites of the drug are excreted in the intestinal tract and urine.

Pharmacodynamics

Colchicine dramatically relieves the pain and inflammation of gouty arthritis in 12–24 hours without altering the metabolism or excretion of urates and without other analgesic effects. Colchicine produces its anti-inflammatory effects by binding to the intracellular protein tubulin, thereby preventing its polymerization into microtubules and leading to the inhibition of leukocyte migration and phagocytosis. It also inhibits the formation of leukotriene B_4. Several of colchicine's adverse effects are produced by its inhibition of tubulin polymerization and cell mitosis.

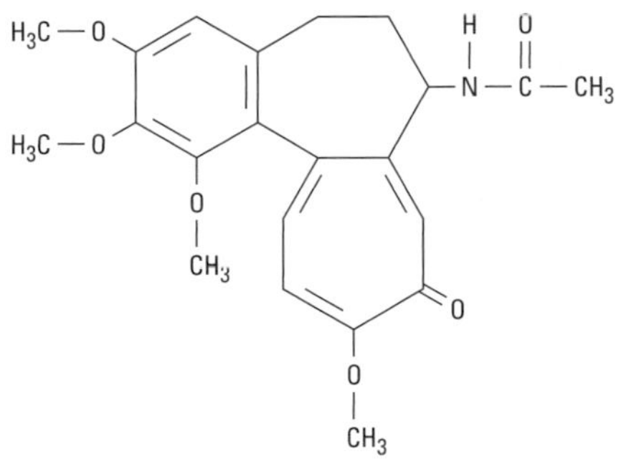

Colchicine

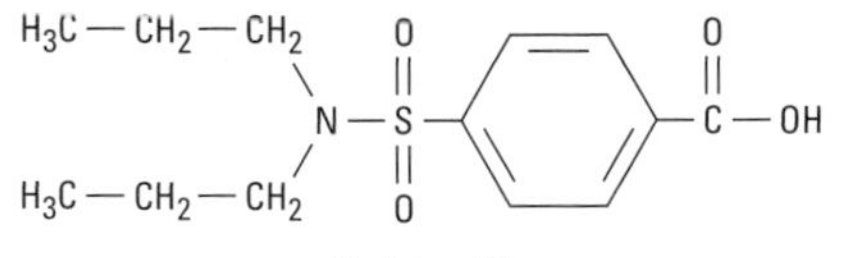

Probenecid

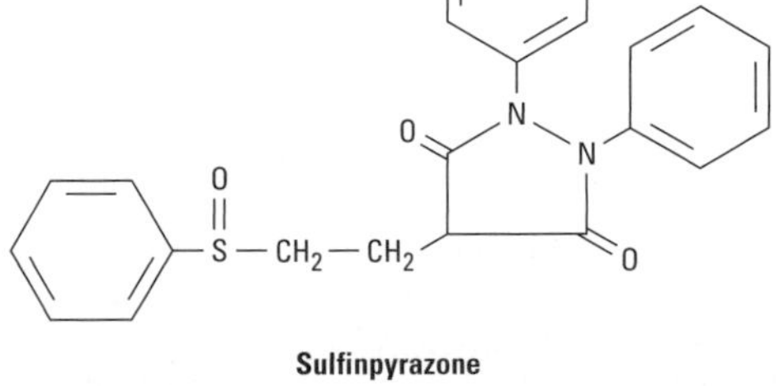

Sulfinpyrazone

Figure 36–6. Colchicine and uricosuric drugs.

Indications

Colchicine was the traditional drug used for alleviating the inflammation of acute gouty arthritis. Although colchicine is more specific in gout than the NSAIDs, other agents (eg, indomethacin and other NSAIDs [except aspirin]) have replaced it in the treatment of acute gout because of the troublesome diarrhea associated with colchicine therapy. Colchicine is now used for the prophylaxis of recurrent episodes of gouty arthritis, is effective in preventing attacks of acute Mediterranean fever, and may have a mild beneficial effect in sarcoid arthritis and in hepatic cirrhosis.

Adverse Effects

Colchicine often causes diarrhea and may occasionally cause nausea, vomiting, and abdominal pain. Colchicine may rarely cause hair loss and bone marrow depression as well as peripheral neuritis and myopathy.

Acute intoxication after ingestion of large (nontherapeutic) doses of the alkaloid is characterized by burning throat pain, bloody diarrhea, shock, hematuria, and oliguria. Fatal ascending central nervous system depression has been reported. Treatment is supportive.

Dosage

The prophylactic dose of colchicine is 0.6 mg one to three times daily. For terminating an attack of gout, the traditional initial dose of colchicine is usually 0.6 or 1.2 mg, followed by 0.6 mg every 2 hours until pain is relieved or nausea and diarrhea appear. The total dose can be given intravenously if necessary, but it should be remembered that as little as 8 mg in 24 hours may be fatal.

NSAIDs IN GOUT

In addition to inhibiting prostaglandin synthase, indomethacin and other NSAIDs also inhibit urate crystal phagocytosis. Indomethacin is commonly used as initial treatment of gout as the replacement for colchicine. Three or four doses of 50 mg every 6 hours are given; when a response occurs, the dosage is reduced to 25 mg three or four times daily for about 5 days.

All other NSAIDs except aspirin, salicylates, and tolmetin have been successfully used to treat acute gouty episodes. Oxaprozin, which lowers serum uric acid, is theoretically a good NSAID though it should not be given to patients with uric acid stones because it increases uric acid excretion in the urine. These agents appear to be as effective and safe as the older drugs.

URICOSURIC AGENTS

Probenecid and sulfinpyrazone are uricosuric drugs employed to decrease the body pool of urate in patients

with tophaceous gout or in those with increasingly frequent gouty attacks. In a patient who excretes large
amounts of uric acid, the uricosuric agents should be
avoided so as not to precipitate the formation of uric
acid calculi.

Chemistry

Uricosuric drugs are organic acids (Figure 36–6) and, as
such, act at the anionic transport sites of the renal
tubule (see Chapter 15). Sulfinpyrazone is a metabolite
of an analog of phenylbutazone.

Pharmacokinetics

Probenecid is completely reabsorbed by the renal tubules
and is metabolized very slowly. Sulfinpyrazone or its
active hydroxylated derivative is rapidly excreted by the
kidneys. Even so, the duration of its effect after oral
administration is almost as long as that of probenecid.

Pharmacodynamics

Uric acid is freely filtered at the glomerulus. Like many
other weak acids, it is also both reabsorbed and secreted
in the middle segment of the proximal tubule. Uricosuric drugs—probenecid, sulfinpyrazone, and large
doses of aspirin—affect these active transport sites so
that net reabsorption of uric acid in the proximal tubule
is decreased. Because aspirin in small (analgesic or
antipyretic) doses causes net retention of uric acid by
inhibiting the secretory transporter, it should not be
used for analgesia in patients with gout. The secretion of
other weak acids (eg, penicillin) is also reduced by uricosuric agents. Probenecid was originally developed to
prolong penicillin blood levels.

As the urinary excretion of uric acid increases, the
size of the urate pool decreases, although the plasma
concentration may not be greatly reduced. In patients
who respond favorably, tophaceous deposits of urate are
reabsorbed, with relief of arthritis and remineralization
of bone. With the ensuing increase in uric acid excretion, a predisposition to the formation of renal stones is
augmented rather than decreased; therefore, the urine
volume should be maintained at a high level, and at least
early in treatment the urine pH should be kept above
6.0 by the administration of alkali.

Indications

Uricosuric therapy should be initiated if several acute
attacks of gouty arthritis have occurred, when evidence
of tophi appears, or when plasma levels of uric acid in
patients with gout are so high that tissue damage is
almost inevitable. Therapy should not be started until
2–3 weeks after an acute attack.

Adverse Effects

Adverse effects do not provide a basis for preferring one
or the other of the uricosuric agents. Both of these
organic acids cause gastrointestinal irritation, but sulfinpyrazone is more active in this regard. Probenecid is
more likely to cause allergic dermatitis, but a rash may
appear after the use of either compound. Nephrotic syndrome has resulted from the use of probenecid. Both
sulfinpyrazone and probenecid may rarely cause aplastic
anemia.

Contraindications & Cautions

It is essential to maintain a large urine volume to minimize the possibility of stone formation.

Dosage

Probenecid is usually started at a dosage of 0.5 g orally
daily in divided doses, progressing to 1 g daily after 1
week. Sulfinpyrazone is started at a dosage of 200 mg
orally daily, progressing to 400–800 mg daily. It should
be given in divided doses with food to reduce adverse
gastrointestinal effects.

ALLOPURINOL

An alternative to increasing uric acid excretion in the
treatment of gout is to reduce its synthesis by inhibiting
xanthine oxidase with allopurinol.

Chemistry

The structure of allopurinol, an isomer of hypoxanthine, is shown in Figure 36–7.

Pharmacokinetics

Allopurinol is approximately 80% absorbed after oral
administration. Like uric acid, allopurinol is itself
metabolized by xanthine oxidase. The resulting compound, alloxanthine, retains the capacity to inhibit xanthine oxidase and has a long enough duration of action
so that allopurinol need be given only once a day.

Pharmacodynamics

Dietary purines are not an important source of uric
acid. The quantitatively important amounts of purine
are formed from amino acids, formate, and carbon dioxide in the body. Those purine ribonucleotides not incorporated into nucleic acids and those derived from the
degradation of nucleic acids are converted to xanthine
or hypoxanthine and oxidized to uric acid (Figure
36–7). When this last step is inhibited by allopurinol,
there is a fall in the plasma urate level and a decrease in

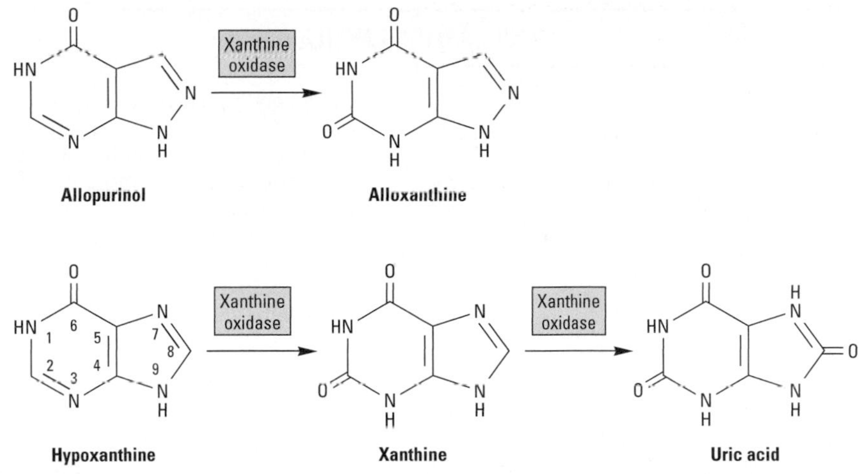

Figure 36–7. Inhibition of uric acid synthesis by allopurinol. (Modified and reproduced, with permission, from Meyers FH, Jawetz E, Goldfien A: *Review of Medical Pharmacology,* 7th ed. McGraw-Hill, 1980.)

the size of the urate pool with a concurrent rise in the more soluble xanthine and hypoxanthine.

Indications

Treatment of gout with allopurinol, as with uricosuric agents, is begun with the expectation that it will be continued for years if not for life. Although allopurinol is often the first urate-lowering drug used, its most rational indications are as follows: (1) in chronic tophaceous gout, in which reabsorption of tophi is more rapid than with uricosuric agents; (2) in patients with gout whose 24-hour urinary uric acid on purine-free diet exceeds 600–700 mg; (3) when probenecid or sulfinpyrazone cannot be used because of adverse effects or allergic reactions, or when they are providing less than optimal therapeutic effect; (4) for recurrent renal stones; (5) in patients with renal functional impairment; or (6) when serum urate levels are grossly elevated. One should attempt to lower serum urate levels to less than 6.5 mg/dL. Aside from gout, allopurinol is used as an antiprotozoal agent (see Chapter 52) and is indicated to prevent the massive uricosuria following therapy of blood dyscrasias that could otherwise lead to renal calculi.

Adverse Effects

Acute attacks of gouty arthritis occur early in treatment with allopurinol, when urate crystals are being withdrawn from the tissues and plasma levels are below normal. To prevent acute attacks, colchicine or indomethacin should be given during the initial period of therapy with allopurinol unless allopurinol is being used in combination with probenecid or sulfinpyrazone. Gastrointestinal intolerance, including nausea, vomiting, and diarrhea, may occur. Peripheral neuritis and necrotizing vasculitis, depression of bone marrow elements, and, rarely, aplastic anemia may also occur. Hepatic toxicity and interstitial nephritis have been reported. An allergic skin reaction characterized by pruritic maculopapular lesions occurs in 3% of patients. Isolated cases of exfoliative dermatitis have been reported. In very rare cases, allopurinol has become bound to the lens, resulting in cataracts.

Interactions & Cautions

When chemotherapeutic mercaptopurines are being given concomitantly with allopurinol, their dosage must be reduced by about 75%. Allopurinol may also increase the effect of cyclophosphamide. Allopurinol inhibits the metabolism of probenecid and oral anticoagulants and may increase hepatic iron concentration. Safety in children and during pregnancy has not been established.

Dosage

The initial dosage of allopurinol is 100 mg/d. It may be titrated to 300 mg/d depending on the serum uric acid response.

Colchicine or an NSAID should be given during the first weeks of allopurinol therapy to prevent the gouty arthritis episodes that sometimes occur.

PREPARATIONS AVAILABLE

NSAIDs

Aspirin, acetylsalicylic acid (generic, Easprin, others)
Oral (regular, enteric-coated, buffered): 81, 165, 325, 500, 650, 800, 975 mg tablets; 81, 650, 800 mg timed- or extended-release tablets
Rectal: 120, 200, 300, 600 mg suppositories

Celecoxib (Celebrex)
Oral: 100, 200 mg capsules

Choline salicylate (Arthropan)
Oral: 870 mg/5 mL liquid

Diclofenac (generic, Cataflam, Voltaren)
Oral: 50 mg tablets; 25, 50, 75 mg delayed-release tablets; 100 mg extended-release tablets
Ophthalmic: 0.1% solution

Diflunisal (generic, Dolobid)
Oral: 250, 500 mg tablets

Etodolac (generic, Lodine)
Oral: 200, 300 mg capsules; 400, 500 mg tablets; 400, 500, 600 mg extended-release tablets

Fenoprofen (generic, Nalfon)
Oral: 200, 300 mg capsules; 600 mg tablets

Flurbiprofen (generic, Ansaid)
Oral: 50, 100 mg tablets
Ophthalmic (generic, Ocufen): 0.03% solution

Ibuprofen (generic, Motrin, Rufen, Advil [OTC], Nuprin [OTC], others)
Oral: 100, 200, 400, 600, 800 mg tablets; 50, 100 mg chewable tablets; 200 mg capsules; 100 mg/2.5 mL suspension, 100 mg/5 mL suspension; 40 mg/mL drops

Indomethacin (generic, Indocin, others)
Oral: 25, 50 mg capsules; 75 mg sustained-release capsules; 25 mg/5 mL suspension
Rectal: 50 mg suppositories

Ketoprofen (generic, Orudis, others)
Oral: 12.5 mg tablets; 25, 50, 75 mg capsules; 100, 150, 200 mg extended-release capsules

Ketorolac tromethamine (generic, Toradol)
Oral: 10 mg tablets
Parenteral: 15, 30 mg/mL for IM injection
Ophthalmic: 0.5% solution

Magnesium salicylate (Doan's Pills, Magan, Mobidin)
Oral: 545, 600 mg tablets; 467, 500, 580 mg caplets

Meclofenamate sodium (generic)
Oral: 50, 100 mg capsules

Mefenamic acid (Ponstel)
Oral: 250 mg capsules

Meloxicam (Mobic)
Oral: 7.5 mg tablets

Nabumetone (Relafen)
Oral: 500, 750 mg tablets

Naproxen (generic, Naprosyn, Anaprox, Aleve [otc])
Oral: 200, 250, 375, 500 mg tablets; 375, 550 mg sustained-release tablets; 375, 500 mg delayed-release tablets; 125 mg/5 mL suspension

Oxaprozin (Daypro)
Oral: 600 mg tablets

Piroxicam (generic, Feldene)
Oral: 10, 20 mg capsules

Rofecoxib (Vioxx)
Oral: 12.5, 25, 50 mg tablets; 12.5, 25 mg/5 mL suspension

Salsalate, salicylsalicylic acid (generic, Disalcid)
Oral: 500, 750 mg tablets; 500 mg capsules

Sodium salicylate (generic)
Oral: 325, 650 mg enteric-coated tablets

Sodium thiosalicylate (generic, Rexolate)
Parenteral: 50 mg/mL for IM injection

Sulindac (generic, Clinoril)
Oral: 150, 200 mg tablets

Suprofen (Profenal)
Topical: 1% ophthalmic solution

Tolmetin (Tolectin, generic [400 mg only])
Oral: 200, 600 mg tablets; 400 mg capsules

Valdecoxib (Bextra)
Oral: 10, 20 mg tablets

DISEASE-MODIFYING ANTIRHEUMATIC DRUGS

Anakinra (Kineret)
Parenteral: 100 mg solution for SC injection

Adalimumab (Humira)
Parenteral: 40 mg/0.8 mL for SC injection

Auranofin (Ridaura)
Oral: 3 mg capsules

Aurothioglucose (Solganal)
Parenteral: 50 mg/mL suspension for injection

Etanercept (Enbrel)
Parenteral: 25 mg powder for subcutaneous injection

Gold sodium thiomalate (generic, Aurolate)
Parenteral: 50 mg/mL for injection

Hydroxychloroquine (Plaquenil)
Oral: 200 mg tablets

Infliximab (Remicade)
Parenteral: 100 mg powder for IV infusion

Leflunomide (Arava)
Oral: 10, 20, 100 mg tablets

Methotrexate (generic, Rheumatrex)
Oral: 2.5 mg tablets

Penicillamine (Cuprimine, Depen)
Oral: 125, 250 mg capsules; 250 mg tablets

Sulfasalazine (Azulfidine)
Oral: 500 mg tablets; 500 mg delayed-release tablets

ACETAMINOPHEN

Acetaminophen (generic, Tylenol, Tempra, Panadol, Acephen, others)
Oral: 160, 325, 500, 650 mg tablets; 80 mg chewable tablets; 160, 500, 650 mg caplets; 325, 500 mg capsules; 80, 120, 160 mg/5 mL elixir; 500 mg/15 mL elixir; 100 mg/mL solution
Rectal: 80, 120, 125, 300, 325, 650 mg suppositories

DRUGS USED IN GOUT

Allopurinol (generic, Zyloprim, others)
Oral: 100, 300 mg tablets
Colchicine (generic)
Oral: 0.5 and 0.6 mg tablets
Parenteral: 0.5 mg/mL for injection
Probenecid (generic)
Oral: 500 mg tablets
Sulfinpyrazone (generic, Anturane)
Oral: 100 mg tablets; 200 mg capsules

REFERENCES

GENERAL

Harris ED Jr: Rheumatoid arthritis. Pathophysiology and implications for therapy. N Engl J Med 1990;322:1277.

Hellman DB, Stone JH: Arthritis and musculoskeletal disorders. In: Tierney LM Jr, McPhee ST, Papadakis MA (editors). *Current Medical Diagnosis & Treatment 2004*. McGraw-Hill, 2004.

Singh G et al: Toxicity profiles of disease modifying antirheumatic drugs in rheumatoid arthritis. J Rheumatol 1991;18:188.

Vane J, Botting R: Inflammation and the mechanism of action of anti-inflammatory drugs. FASEB J 1987;1:89.

Walson PD, Mortensen ME: Pharmacokinetics of common analgesics, anti-inflammatories and antipyretics in children. Clin Pharmacokinet 1989;17(Suppl 1):116.

Williams KM, Day RO, Briet SN: Biochemical actions and clinical pharmacology of anti-inflammatory drugs. Adv Drug Res 1993;24:121.

NSAIDs

Alberti MM et al: Combined indomethacin/gentamicin eyedrops to reduce pain after traumatic corneal abrasion. Eur J Ophthalmol 2001;11:233.

Barthel T et al: Prophylaxis of heterotopic ossification after total hip arthroplasty: a prospective randomized study comparing indomethacin and meloxicam. Acta Orthop Scand 2002;73:611.

Baudouin C et al: Efficacy of indomethacin 0.1% and fluorometholone 0.1% on conjunctival inflammation following chronic application of antiglaucomatous drugs. Graefes Arch Clin Exp Ophthalmol 2002;240:929.

Bensen W et al: Efficacy and safety of valdecoxib in treating the signs and symptoms of rheumatoid arthritis: a randomized, controlled comparison with placebo and naproxen. Rheumatology (Oxford) 2002;41:1008.

Bombardier C: An evidence-based evaluation of the gastrointestinal safety of coxibs. Am J Cardiol 2002;89(Suppl 6A):3D.

Bombardier C et al: Comparison of upper gastrointestinal toxicity of rofecoxib and naproxen in patients with rheumatoid arthritis. VIGOR Study Group. N Engl J Med 2000;343:1520.

Bonney SL et al: Renal safety of two analgesics used over the counter: ibuprofen and aspirin. Clin Pharmacol Ther 1986;40:373.

Brix AE: Renal papillary necrosis. Toxicol Pathol 2002;30:672.

Catella-Lawson F et al: Cyclooxygenase inhibitors and the antiplatelet effects of aspirin. N Engl J Med 2001;345:1809.

Chan FK et al: Celecoxib versus diclofenac and omeprazole in reducing the risk of recurrent ulcer bleeding in patients with arthritis. N Engl J Med 2002;347:2104.

Christmann V et al: Changes in cerebral, renal and mesenteric blood flow velocity during continuous and bolus infusion of indomethacin. Acta Paediatr 2002;91:440.

Cochrane DJ, Jarvis B, Keating GM: Etoricoxib. Drugs 2002;62:2637.

Comfort MB et al: A study of the comparative efficacy of three common analgesics in the control of pain after third molar surgery under local anaesthesia. Aust Dent J 2002;47:327.

Daniels SE et al: Valdecoxib, a cyclooxygenase-2-specific inhibitor, is effective in treating primary dysmenorrhea. Obstet Gynecol 2002;100:350.

Deeks JJ, Smith LA, Bradley MD: Efficacy, tolerability, and upper gastrointestinal safety of celecoxib for treatment of osteoarthritis and rheumatoid arthritis: systematic review of randomised controlled trials. BMJ 2002;325:619.

Furst DE et al: Dose response and safety study of meloxicam up to 22.5 mg daily in rheumatoid arthritis: a 12 week multicenter, double blind, dose response study versus placebo and diclofenac. J Rheumatol 2002;29:436.

Hanna MH et al: Comparative study of analgesic efficacy and morphine-sparing effect of intramuscular dexketoprofen trometamol with ketoprofen or placebo after major orthopaedic surgery. Br J Clin Pharmacol 2003;55:126.

Hurwitz ES et al: Public Health Service Study of Reye's syndrome and medications. Report of the main study. JAMA 1987;257:1905.

Immer FF et al: Pain treatment with a COX-2 inhibitor after coronary artery bypass operation: a randomized trial Ann Thorac Surg 2003;75:490.

Kivitz A et al: Randomized placebo-controlled trial comparing efficacy and safety of valdecoxib with naproxen in patients with osteoarthritis. J Fam Pract 2002;51:530.

Knijff-Dutmer EA et al: Platelet function is inhibited by non-selective non-steroidal anti-inflammatory drugs but not by cyclooxygenase-2-selective inhibitors in patients with rheumatoid arthritis. Rheumatology (Oxford) 2002;41:458.

Lago P et al: Safety and efficacy of ibuprofen versus indomethacin in preterm infants treated for patent ductus arteriosus: a randomized controlled trial. Eur J Pediatr 2002;161:202.

Laine L et al: Serious lower gastrointestinal clinical events with non-selective NSAID or coxib use. Gastroenterology 2003;124:288.

Lau H et al: Prospective randomized trial of preemptive analgesics following ambulatory inguinal hernia repair: intravenous ketorolac versus diclofenac suppository. Aust N Z J Surg 2002;72:704.

Laurell CG, Zetterstrom C: Effects of dexamethasone, diclofenac, or placebo on the inflammatory response after cataract surgery. Br J Ophthalmol 2002;86:1380.

Lesko SM et al: Asthma morbidity after short-term use of ibuprofen in children. Pediatrics 2002;109:E20.

Makarowski W et al: Efficacy and safety of the COX-2 specific inhibitor valdecoxib in the management of osteoarthritis of the hip: a randomized, double-blind, placebo-controlled comparison with naproxen. Osteoarthritis Cartilage 2002;10:290.

Matsumoto AK et al: A randomized, controlled, clinical trial of etoricoxib in the treatment of rheumatoid arthritis. J Rheumatol 2002;29:1623.

Meade EA, Smith WL, DeWitt DL: Differential inhibition of prostaglandin endoperoxide synthase (cyclooxygenase) isozymes by aspirin and other nonsteroidal anti-inflammatory drugs. J Biol Chem 1993;268:6610.

Mitchell JA et al: Selectivity of nonsteroidal antiinflammatory drugs as inhibitors of constitutive and inducible cyclooxygenase. Proc Natl Acad Sci U S A 1994;90:11693.

Moran EM: Epidemiological and clinical aspects of nonsteroidal anti-inflammatory drugs and cancer risks. J Environ Pathol Toxicol Oncol 2002;21:193.

Niccoli L, Bellino S, Cantini F: Renal tolerability of three commonly employed non-steroidal anti-inflammatory drugs in elderly patients with osteoarthritis. Clin Exp Rheumatol 2002;20:201.

Norton ME et al: Neonatal complications after the administration of indomethacin for preterm labor. N Engl J Med 1993;329:1602.

Olson NZ et al: Onset of analgesia for liquigel ibuprofen 400 mg, acetaminophen 1000 mg, ketoprofen 25 mg, and placebo in the treatment of postoperative dental pain. J Clin Pharmacol 2001;41:1238.

Papa V et al: Topical naproxen sodium for inhibition of miosis during cataract surgery. Prospective, randomized clinical trials. Eye 2002;16:292.

Paulus HE, Furst DE: Aspirin and other non-steroidal anti-inflammatory drugs. In: McCarty DJ (editor). *Arthritis and Allied Conditions,* 10th ed. Lea & Febiger, 1985.

Ray WA et al: COX-2 selective non-steroidal anti-inflammatory drugs and risk of serious coronary heart disease. Lancet 2002;360:1071.

Reicin AS et al: Comparison of cardiovascular thrombotic events in patients with osteoarthritis treated with rofecoxib versus non-selective nonsteroidal anti-inflammatory drugs (ibuprofen, diclofenac, and nabumetone). Am J Cardiol 2002;89:204.

Riendeau D et al: Etoricoxib (MK-0663): preclinical profile and comparison with other agents that selectively inhibit cyclooxygenase-2. J Pharmacol Exp Ther 2001;296:558.

Roda A et al: Bioavailability of a new ketoprofen formulation for once-daily oral administration. Int J Pharm 2002;241:165.

Rovensky J et al: Treatment of knee osteoarthritis with a topical non-steroidal anti-inflammatory drug. Results of a randomized, double-blind, placebo-controlled study on the efficacy and safety of a 5% ibuprofen cream. Drugs Exp Clin Res 2001;27:209.

Schachtel BP et al: Demonstration of dose response of flurbiprofen lozenges with the sore throat pain model. Clin Pharmacol Ther 2002;71:375.

Seckin B et al: Effects of indomethacin suppository and lidocaine pomade for the relief of post-episiotomy pain. Int J Gynaecol Obstet 2002;78:159.

Thun MJ, Namboodiri MM, Heath CW Jr: Aspirin use and reduced risk of fatal colon cancer. N Engl J Med 1991;325:1593.

DISEASE-MODIFYING ANTIRHEUMATIC DRUGS & GLUCOCORTICOIDS

Arend WP, Dayer J-M: Cytokines and cytokine inhibitors or antagonists in rheumatoid arthritis. Arthritis Rheum 1990;33:305.

Arnold M, Schreiber L, Brooks P: Immunosuppressive drugs and corticosteroids in the treatment of rheumatoid arthritis. Drugs 1988;36:340.

Balint JP Jr: Immune modulation associated with extracorporeal immunoadsorption treatments utilizing protein A/silica columns. Artif Organs 1996;20:906.

Burke GW et al: Removal of preformed cytotoxic antibody using PROSORBA (Staph Protein-A-Silica) column without immunosuppression. Transplant Proc 1997;29:2249.

Caldwell J, Gendreau RM, Furst D: A pilot study using a staph protein A column (Prosorba) to treat refractory rheumatoid arthritis. J Rheumatol 1999;26:1657.

Carette S et al: A double blind placebo-controlled study of auranofin in patients with psoriatic arthritis. Arthritis Rheum 1989;32:158.

Charles P et al: Regulation of cytokines, cytokine inhibitors, and acute-phase proteins following anti-TNF-α therapy in rheumatoid arthritis. J Immunol 1999;163:1521.

Clements PJ: Alkylating agents. In: Dixon J, Furst DE (editors). *Second Line Agents in the Treatment of Rheumatic Diseases.* Marcel Dekker, 1991.

Clements PJ: Cytotoxic immunosuppressive drugs. In: Paulus HE, Furst DE, Dromgoole SH (editors). *Drugs For Rheumatic Diseases.* Marcel Dekker, 1991.

Felson DT et al: The Prosorba column for treatment of refractory rheumatoid arthritis: a randomized, double-blind, sham-controlled trial. Arthritis Rheum 1999;42:2153.

Fennelly DW et al: A phase II trial of extracorporeal plasma immunoadsorption of patient plasma with PROSORBA columns for treating metastatic breast cancer. Cancer 1995;75:2099.

Fox DA, McCune WJ: Immunologic and clinical effects of cytotoxic drugs used in the treatment of rheumatoid arthritis and systemic lupus erythematosus. Concepts Immunopathol 1989;7:20.

Fries JF et al: The relative toxicity of disease-modifying antirheumatic drugs. Arthritis Rheum 1993;36:297.

Furst DE: Rational use of disease-modifying antirheumatic drugs. Drugs 1990;39:19.

Garrison L, McDonnell ND: Etanercept: therapeutic use in patients with rheumatoid arthritis. Ann Rheum Dis 1999;58(Suppl I):I165.

Harriman G, Harper LK, Schaible TF: Summary of clinical trials in rheumatoid arthritis using infliximab, an anti-TNFα treatment. Ann Rheum Dis 1999;58:161.

Jarvis B, Faulds D: Etanercept: a review of its use in rheumatoid arthritis. Drugs 1999;57:945.

Jones RE, Moreland LW: Tumor necrosis factor inhibitors for rheumatoid arthritis. Bull Rheum Dis 1999;48:14.

Kowal A, Carstens JH Jr, Schnitzer TJ: Cyclosporine in rheumatoid arthritis. In: Furst DE, Weinblatt ME (editors). *Immunomodulators in the Rheumatic Diseases*. Marcel Dekker, 1990.

Kremer JM, Phelps CT: Long-term prospective study of the use of methotrexate in the treatment of rheumatoid arthritis. Update after a mean of 90 months. Arthritis Metab 1992;35:138.

Maini RN et al: Antitumour necrosis factor specific antibody (infliximab) treatment provides insights into the pathophysiology of rheumatoid arthritis. Ann Rheum Dis 1999;58:156.

Maini RN et al: Therapeutic efficacy of multiple intravenous infusions of anti-tumor necrosis factor α monoclonal antibody combined with low-dose weekly methotrexate in rheumatoid arthritis. Arthritis Rheum 1998;41:1552.

Moreland LW et al: Etanercept therapy in rheumatoid arthritis. A randomized, controlled trial. Ann Intern Med 1999;130:478.

Shiroky JB et al: Low-dose methotrexate with leucovorin (folinic acid) in the management of rheumatoid arthritis. Results of a multicenter randomized, double-blind, placebo-controlled trial. Arthritis Rheum 1993;36:795.

Snyder HW Jr, Balint JP Jr, Jones FR: Modulation of immunity in patients with autoimmune disease and cancer treated by extracorporeal immunoadsorption with PROSORBA columns. Semin Hematol 1989;26:31.

van der Hyde D et al: Sulphasalazine versus hydroxychloroquine in rheumatoid arthritis: 3 year followup. Lancet 1990;335:539.

van der Poll T et al: Effect of a recombinant dimeric tumor necrosis factor receptor on inflammatory responses to intravenous endotoxin in normal humans. Blood 1997;89:3727.

Wallis WJ et al: Biologic agents and immunotherapy in rheumatoid arthritis. Progress and perspective. Rheum Dis Clin North Am 1998;24:537.

Wiesenhutter CW, Irish BL, Bertram JH: Treatment of patients with refractory rheumatoid arthritis with extracorporeal protein A immunoadsorption columns: a pilot trial. J Rheumatol 1994;21:804.

EICOSAPENTAENOIC ACID

Kremer JM et al: Effects of manipulation of dietary fatty acids on clinical manifestations of rheumatoid arthritis. Lancet 1985;1:184.

Maurice PDL et al: Effects of dietary supplementation with eicosapentaenoic acid in patients with psoriasis. In: Samuelsson B, Paoletti R, Ramwell P (editors). *Advances in Prostaglandin, Thromboxane, and Leukotriene Research*. Raven Press, 1987.

OTHER ANALGESICS

Black M: Acetaminophen hepatotoxicity. Annu Rev Med 1984;35:577.

Chandrasekharan NV et al: COX-3, a cyclooxygenase-1 variant inhibited by acetaminophen and other analgesic/antipyretic drugs: Cloning, structure, and expression. Proc Natl Acad Sci U S A 2002;99:13926.

Linden CH, Rumack BH: Acetaminophen overdose. Emerg Med Clin North Am 1984;2:103.

Styrt B, Sugarman B: Antipyresis and fever. Arch Intern Med 1990;150:1589.

DRUGS USED IN GOUT

Emmerson BT: The management of gout. N Engl J Med 1996;334:445.

Famey JP: Colchicine in therapy: State of the art and new perspectives for an old drug. Clin Exp Rheum 1988;6:305.

Star VL, Hochberg MC: Prevention and management of gout. Drugs 1993;45:212.

Terkeltaub RA: Gout and mechanisms of crystal-induced inflammation. Curr Opinion Rheumatol 1993;5:510.

SECTION VII
Endocrine Drugs

Hypothalamic & Pituitary Hormones

37

Paul A. Fitzgerald, MD

The control of metabolism, growth, and reproduction is mediated by a combination of neural and endocrine systems located in the hypothalamus and pituitary gland. The pituitary weighs about 0.6 g and rests in the bony sella turcica under a layer of dura mater and is bordered by the cavernous sinuses. It consists of an anterior lobe (adenohypophysis) and a posterior lobe (neurohypophysis). The pituitary is connected to the overlying hypothalamus by a stalk of neurosecretory fibers and blood vessels, including a portal venous system that drains the hypothalamus and perfuses the anterior pituitary. The portal venous system carries small regulatory peptide hormones (Table 37–1) from the hypothalamus to the anterior pituitary.

The posterior lobe hormones are synthesized in the hypothalamus and transported via the neurosecretory fibers in the stalk of the pituitary to the posterior lobe, from which they are released into the circulation.

Hypothalamic and pituitary hormones (and their synthetic analogs) have pharmacologic applications in three areas: (1) as replacement therapy for hormone deficiency states; (2) as drug therapy and (3) as diagnostic tools for performing stimulation tests.

ACRONYMS

ACTH	Adrenocorticotropic hormone
CRH	Corticotropin-releasing hormone
FSH	Follicle-stimulating hormone
GHBP	Growth hormone-binding protein
GHRH	Growth hormone-releasing hormone
GnRH	Gonadotropin-releasing hormone
GRH	Growth hormone-releasing hormone
IGF-I, -II	Insulin-like growth factor -I, -II
LH	Luteinizing hormone
LHRH	Luteinizing hormone-releasing hormone
β-LPH	β-Lipotropin
PRL	Prolactin
rbGH	Recombinant bovine growth hormone
rhGH	Recombinant human growth hormone
rhTSH	Recombinant human thyroid-stimulating hormone
SRIH	Somatotropin release-inhibiting hormone (somatostatin)
TRH	Thyrotropin-releasing hormone
TSH	Thyroid-stimulating hormone (thyrotropin)

HYPOTHALAMIC & ANTERIOR PITUITARY HORMONES

Hypothalamic regulatory hormones include growth hormone-releasing hormone (GHRH); a growth hormone-inhibiting hormone (somatostatin); thyrotropin-releasing hormone (TRH); corticotropin-releasing hormone (CRH); gonadotropin-releasing hormone (GnRH), also called luteinizing hormone-releasing hormone (LHRH); and prolactin-inhibiting hormone (dopamine).

Anterior pituitary hormones include growth hormone (GH), thyrotropin (TSH), follicle-stimulating hormone (FSH), luteinizing hormone (LH), prolactin (PRL), and adrenocorticotropin (ACTH). Another peptide, β-lipotropin (β-LPH), is derived from the same prohormone, pro-opiomelanocortin, as ACTH. β-LPH is secreted from the pituitary (along with ACTH), and is a precursor of the opioid peptide β-endorphin (see Chapter 31).

MECHANISMS OF HORMONE ACTION

The hypothalamic and pituitary hormones are all peptides that exert their effects by binding to target cell surface membrane receptors with high specificity and affinity.

GHRH, Somatostatin, TRH, TSH, CRH, ACTH, GnRH, FSH, LH, & Dopamine

The receptors for these hormones are typical seven-transmembrane-domain serpentine peptides (see Chapter 2). Each hormone acts as a ligand within a receptor pocket, inducing conformational activating changes in the receptor. The conformational changes in the receptor's intracellular third loop and carboxyl terminal tail activate an adjacent intracellular G protein. The G_{14} protein is associated with the receptors for GnRH and TRH, G_i with the dopamine receptor, and G_s protein with the receptors for the other hormones listed above.

A. GHRH, CRH, GnRH, TSH, ACTH, FSH, LH, and Dopamine

The G protein-GTP complexes related to receptors for these hormones activate adenylyl cyclase, which synthesizes the second messenger cAMP. Cyclic AMP activates protein kinases, which phosphorylate certain intracellular proteins (eg, enzymes), thus producing the hormonal effect. Conversely, dopamine binding to lactotroph receptors causes conformational changes in its G_i protein that reduce the activity of adenylyl cyclase and inhibit the secretion of prolactin.

B. Somatostatin

The α-GTP complexes related to somatostatin receptors exert effects on potassium channels, thereby inhibiting GH secretion.

C. Thyrotropin-Releasing Hormone

The G protein complexes related to thyrotrophs' TRH receptors affect phosphoinositide-specific phospholipase C, which increases intracellular cytoplasmic free calcium, thereby stimulating TSH secretion.

Growth Hormone & Prolactin

The receptors for both GH and PRL consist of similar single peptides. The two types of receptors have extra-

Table 37–1. Links between hypothalamic, pituitary, and target gland hormones.

Hypothalamic Hormone	Pituitary Hormone	Target Organ	Target Organ Hormone
Growth hormone-releasing hormone (GHRH) (+) Somatotropin release-inhibiting hormone (SRIH, somatostatin) (–)	Growth hormone (somatotropin, GH)	Liver	Insulin-like growth factors (IGF, somatomedins)
Corticotropin-releasing hormone (CRH) (+)	Adrenocorticotropin (ACTH)	Adrenal cortex	Glucocorticoids, mineralocorticoids, androgens
Thyrotropin-releasing hormone (TRH) (+)	Thyroid-stimulating hormone (TSH)	Thyroid	Thyroxine, triiodothyronine
Gonadotropin-releasing hormone (GnRH)	Follicle-stimulating hormone (FSH) Luteinizing hormone (LH)	Gonads	Estrogen, progesterone, testosterone
Dopamine (–)	Prolactin (PRL)	Breast	—

(+), stimulant; (–), inhibitor.

cellular amino terminal hormone-binding domains. Both receptors pass through the cell membrane, where an intracellular carboxyl terminal sequence activates a tyrosine kinase, JAK2, causing phosphorylation on tyrosines of intracellular proteins and gene regulation. Fragments of GH receptors circulate in plasma (GH binding protein, GHBP), binding about 50% of the circulating growth hormone.

GROWTH HORMONE-RELEASING HORMONE (GHRH) & GROWTH HORMONE-RELEASING PEPTIDES (GHRPS)

Growth hormone-releasing hormone is a peptide hormone found in the hypothalamus that stimulates synthesis and release of growth hormone (GH) from the pituitary. It is sometimes abbreviated GRH and was originally named growth hormone-releasing factor (GRF). It was first isolated from rare pancreatic tumors that caused acromegaly by stimulating excessive GH secretion by pituitary somatotroph cells (an unusual cause—almost all cases of acromegaly are caused by pituitary tumors). In the hypothalamus, cells in the arcuate nuclei secrete GHRH into the hypophysial-pituitary portal venous system.

Chemistry & Pharmacokinetics

A. STRUCTURE

Naturally occurring GHRH has been isolated as both 40 and 44 amino acid peptides ($GHRH_{40}$, $GHRH_{44}$), which are derived from precursor molecules of 107 and 108 amino acids. GHRH bears distinct structural homologies to certain gastrointestinal peptide hormones such as gastrin, gastric inhibitory peptide, secretin, and vasoactive intestinal polypeptide. Full biologic activity of GHRH lies in the 1–29 amino terminal segment.

Growth hormone-releasing peptides comprise several groups of small synthetic peptide analogs of GHRH that can stimulate GH secretion. **Sermorelin** is the commercially available acetate salt of a synthetic 29-amino-acid peptide that is the amino terminal segment of GHRH. It has also been called GRH_{1-29} and $GHRH_{1-29}$. Sermorelin is similar to native GHRH in its ability to stimulate GH secretion. Similar peptides (GHRP-2, GHRP-6, and **hexarelin**, an analog of GHRP-6) also have clinical activity.

B. ABSORPTION, METABOLISM, AND EXCRETION

GHRH is not currently available commercially; in research use it may be administered intravenously, subcutaneously, or intranasally, and the relative potencies (defined as incremental growth hormone release) by

these three routes are 300, 10, and 1, respectively. Intravenous GHRH (1 μg/kg) has a distribution half-life of 4 minutes and an elimination half-life of 53 minutes. Subcutaneous GHRH has a similar elimination half-life but a distribution half-life of about 10 minutes. Peak serum levels of GHRH (1 μg/kg) are 37 times higher after intravenous administration compared with subcutaneous injection. Sermorelin, 2 μg/kg subcutaneously, reaches peak serum concentrations in 5–20 minutes; its bioavailability is 6%. The half-life of sermorelin is about 12 minutes after either subcutaneous or intravenous injection.

Clinical Pharmacology

A. DIAGNOSTIC USES

GHRH is not currently available commercially. GHRH or GHRPs such as sermorelin may be given intravenously to test pituitary GH secretory capacity as part of the clinical evaluation of childhood short stature. It is used after GH deficiency has already been established by clinical criteria, including testing with conventional stimuli for GH secretion, ie, exercise, insulin-induced hypoglycemia, intravenous arginine, oral carbidopa/levodopa, and oral clonidine. In such children, a normal GH response to GHRH indicates that GH deficiency is due to hypothalamic dysfunction. A subnormal response is not diagnostic. A rise in the serum growth hormone level demonstrates the somatotrophs' ability to produce GH and predicts a favorable response to GHRH therapy.

The response of GH to GHRH can be blunted by prior treatment with octreotide, glucocorticoids, and cyclooxygenase inhibitors such as aspirin or indomethacin. GH response to GHRH is also blunted in hypothyroidism, in obesity, and in adults over 40 years of age. Exogenous growth hormone therapy should be discontinued for at least a week prior to GHRH testing.

B. THERAPEUTIC USES

Synthetic human growth hormone is now usually used for treatment of growth hormone deficiency (see below).

Sermorelin is commercially available (see above). It and other GHRH analogs, given subcutaneously, can also stimulate GH (and thereby growth) in certain GH-deficient children with short stature. Sermorelin is given only to children who have had a positive growth hormone response to the diagnostic test and who have a bone age of less than 7.5 years (girls) or 8 years (boys). A physician experienced in its use must carefully monitor treatment. If successful in promoting growth, treatment is continued until the desired height is reached or the epiphyses have fused, whichever comes first. Children who have an inadequate response are evaluated for hypothyroidism and considered for growth hormone therapy.

Dosage

A. DIAGNOSTIC USE

Sermorelin may be used as a diagnostic test for pituitary GH reserve according to the following protocol: After an overnight fast, the patient has blood drawn for GH at −15 and 0 minutes; sermorelin 1 μg/kg is injected intravenously, followed by a 3 mL normal saline flush of the infusion line. Blood for GH is then drawn at 15, 30, 45, and 60 minutes following the injection. Serum GH levels must reach a peak of over 2 ng/mL to be considered a positive response.

B. THERAPEUTIC USE

Sermorelin is usually given subcutaneously at a dosage of 0.03 mg/kg body weight once daily at bedtime. Alternative regimens include GHRH, 2–5 μg/kg subcutaneously every 6–12 hours. GHRP-2 has been administered intranasally in doses of 5–20 μg/kg. Hexarelin has clinical activity in doses of 20 μg/kg intranasally.

Toxicity

Intravenous GHRH usually causes acute but transient adverse effects lasting several minutes. These effects include flushing, injection site pain and erythema, nausea, headache, metallic taste, pallor, and chest tightness.

Chronic subcutaneous GHRH therapy causes injection site reactions (pain, swelling, erythema) in about 20% of patients. Other reported adverse reactions have included headaches, flushing, dysphagia, dizziness, hyperactivity, somnolence, and urticaria.

GHRH analogs are not known to cause or stimulate malignancies, and long-term carcinogenic potential has not been studied. It is recommended that GHRH treatment be terminated if a malignancy is detected. GHRH treatment is not recommended for patients with GH deficiency due to an intracranial neoplasm.

SOMATOSTATIN (GROWTH HORMONE-INHIBITING HORMONE, SOMATO-TROPIN RELEASE-INHIBITING HORMONE)

Somatostatin, a 14-amino-acid peptide, is found in the hypothalamus and other parts of the central nervous system. It has been sequenced (Figure 37–1) and synthesized. It inhibits growth hormone release in normal individuals. Somatostatin has also been identified in the pancreas and other sites in the gastrointestinal tract. It has been shown to inhibit the release of glucagon, insulin, and gastrin.

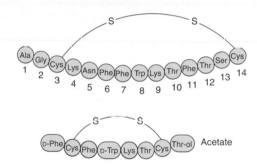

Figure 37–1. **Above:** Amino acid sequence of somatostatin. **Below:** Sequence of the synthetic analog, octreotide (SMS 201-995).

Exogenously administered somatostatin is rapidly cleared from the circulation, with an initial half-life of 1–3 minutes. The kidney appears to play an important role in its metabolism and excretion.

Peptides have been synthesized that partially separate the various properties of somatostatin. A 7-aminoheptanoic acid derivative containing only four of the 14 amino acids of somatostatin has been found to block the effect of somatostatin.

Clinical Pharmacology of Octreotide (Somatostatin Analog)

Somatostatin has limited therapeutic usefulness because of its short duration of action and its multiple effects on many secretory systems. Octreotide is 45 times more potent than somatostatin in inhibiting growth hormone release but only twice as potent in reducing insulin secretion. Because of this relatively reduced effect on pancreatic B cells, hyperglycemia rarely occurs during treatment. The greater potency of octreotide as compared with somatostatin is not due to differences in affinity for somatostatin receptors. Rather, it appears to be due to octreotide's much lower clearance and longer half-life. The plasma elimination half-life of octreotide is about 80 minutes, 30 times longer in humans than the half-life of somatostatin.

Octreotide, in doses of 50–200 μg given subcutaneously every 8 hours, reduces symptoms caused by a variety of hormone-secreting tumors: acromegaly; the carcinoid syndrome; gastrinoma; glucagonoma; nesidioblastosis; the watery diarrhea, hypokalemia, and achlorhydria (WDHA) syndrome; and "diabetic diarrhea." Somatostatin receptor scintigraphy, using radiolabeled octreotide, is useful in localizing neuroendocrine tumors having somatostatin receptors and helps predict the response to octreotide therapy. Octreotide is also useful for the acute control of bleeding from esophageal varices.

Octreotide acetate injectable suspension (octreotide long-acting release; Sandostatin LAR) is a slow-release formulation in which octreotide is incorporated into microspheres. It is instituted only after a brief course of shorter-acting octreotide has been demonstrated to be effective and tolerated. The microspheres must be carefully put into suspension and immediately injected into a gluteal muscle. Injections into alternate gluteal muscles are repeated at 4-week intervals in doses of 20–40 mg. Octreotide is extremely costly.

Adverse effects of therapy include nausea with or without vomiting, abdominal cramps, flatulence, and steatorrhea with bulky bowel movements. Biliary sludge and gallstones may occur after 6 months of use in 20–30% of patients. However, the yearly incidence of symptomatic gallstones is about 1%. Cardiac effects include sinus bradycardia (25%) and conduction disturbances (10%). Pain at the site of injection is common, especially with the long-acting octreotide suspension. Vitamin B_{12} deficiency may occur with long-term use of octreotide.

PEGVISOMANT (GROWTH HORMONE RECEPTOR ANTAGONIST)

Pegvisomant is a new GH receptor antagonist that is proving useful for the treatment of acromegaly. Pegvisomant is the polyethylene glycol (PEG) derivative of a mutant growth hormone (B2036) that has increased affinity for one site of the GH receptor but a reduced affinity at its second binding site. This allows dimerization of the receptor but blocks the conformational changes required for signal transduction. Pegvisomant has less GH receptor antagonism than does B2036, but pegylation reduces its clearance rate and improves its overall clinical effectiveness. When pegvisomant was administered to 160 acromegalic patients subcutaneously daily for 12 months or more, serum levels of IGF-I fell into the normal range in 97% while serum levels of GH rose during treatment; two patients experienced growth of their GH-secreting pituitary tumors, and two patients developed increases in liver enzymes.

GROWTH HORMONE (SOMATOTROPIN, GH)

Growth hormone is a peptide hormone produced by the anterior pituitary. It produces growth at open epiphyses via stimulation of insulin-like growth factor I (IGF-I, somatomedin C). It also causes lipolysis in adipose tissue and growth of skeletal muscle.

Chemistry & Pharmacokinetics

A. STRUCTURE

Human pituitary GH (**somatotropin**) is a 191-amino-acid peptide with two sulfhydryl bridges. Its structure closely resembles that of prolactin and the placental hormone human chorionic somatomammotropin. Pituitary-derived GH is no longer used (see below). Animal GH is not completely homologous to human GH and is ineffective in humans.

Recombinant human growth hormone (**rhGH**) is the growth hormone preparation in widespread use. It is synthesized by introducing plasmids containing the gene for human growth hormone into a strain of microorganisms that synthesize rhGH, which is purified for pharmacologic use. **Somatropin** has a 191-amino-acid sequence that is identical with human growth hormone. **Somatrem** has 192 amino acids consisting of the 191 amino acids of growth hormone plus an extra methionine residue at the amino terminal end. These preparations all appear to be equipotent.

B. ABSORPTION, METABOLISM, AND EXCRETION

Circulating endogenous growth hormone has a half-life of 20–25 minutes and is predominantly cleared by the liver. Human growth hormone can be administered subcutaneously, with peak levels occurring in 2–4 hours and active blood levels persisting for 36 hours.

Somatropin injectable suspension (Nutropin Depot) is a long-acting preparation of rhGH enclosed within biodegradable microspheres. These microspheres degrade slowly after subcutaneous injection such that the rhGH is released over about 1 month.

Pharmacodynamics

Recombinant human growth hormone is equipotent with native pituitary growth hormone. The metabolic consequence of a pharmacologic dose of growth hormone is an initial insulin-like effect with increased tissue uptake of both glucose and amino acids and decreased lipolysis. Within a few hours, there is a peripheral insulin-antagonistic effect with impaired glucose uptake and increased lipolysis.

Pharmacologic doses of growth hormone cause longitudinal growth indirectly via another class of peptide hormones, the somatomedins, or insulin-like growth factors (IGFs). Growth hormone stimulates synthesis of somatomedins IGF-I and IGF-II (predominantly in growth plate cartilage and the liver); somatomedins promote uptake of sulfate into cartilage and are probably the actual mediators of the cellular processes associated with bone growth. This growth can be traced back to the molecular level, where increased incorporation of thymidine into DNA and uridine into RNA occurs (indicating cellular proliferation) along with increased conversion of proline to hydroxyproline (indicating cartilage synthesis).

Growth hormone deficiency leads to inadequate somatomedin production and short stature. Rarely, short stature may be caused by IGF-I deficiency despite high growth hormone levels (Laron dwarfism) or a lack of a pubertal surge of IGF-I (pygmies).

Clinical Pharmacology

A. Growth Hormone Deficiency

Genetic GH deficiency may present in the newborn with hypoglycemic seizures. Acquired GH deficiency is caused by damage to the pituitary or hypothalamus. In childhood, GH deficiency presents as short stature and adiposity. Criteria for diagnosis of growth hormone deficiency usually include (1) a growth rate below 4 cm per year and (2) the absence of a serum growth hormone response to two growth hormone secretagogues. The prevalence of congenital growth hormone deficiency is approximately 1:4000 live births.

Therapy with rhGH permits many children with short stature to achieve normal adult height.

Adults with GH deficiency tend to have generalized obesity, reduced muscle mass, asthenia, and reduced cardiac output. Adult-onset GH deficiency is usually found in the presence of other pituitary hormone deficiencies, and is usually due to damage to the hypothalamus or pituitary caused by tumor, infection, surgery, or radiation therapy.

The precise testing required to diagnose GH deficiency is controversial. Treatment of GH-deficient adults can cause increased lean body mass and bone density, decreased fat mass, increased exercise tolerance, and an improved sense of well-being. Adverse effects often include arthralgias and fluid retention.

B. Growth Hormone-Responsive States

Some non-growth hormone-deficient short children with a delayed bone age and a slow growth rate achieve increased growth with short-term growth hormone therapy. Selected "normal variant short stature" children can be offered a trial of growth hormone following a baseline period of measurement to confirm a subnormal growth rate. During the first 6 months of treatment, the height velocity must increase by 2 cm per year for treatment to continue. Girls with Turner's syndrome frequently respond to high-dose growth hormone therapy with increased growth velocity and increased height as adults.

In 1993, the FDA approved the use of recombinant bovine growth hormone (rbGH) in dairy cattle to increase milk production. Although milk and meat from rbGH-treated cows appears to be safe, these cows have a higher frequency of mastitis, which could increase antibiotic use and result in greater antibiotic residues in milk and meat.

C. Experimental Uses

Therapy with rhGH appears to be effective for infants with intrauterine growth retardation. Children with growth retardation following renal transplantation also appear to respond to rhGH therapy. Hypophosphatemia due to hyperphosphaturia (eg, X-linked hypophosphatemic vitamin D-resistant rickets) has been improved by adding rhGH to the treatment regimen.

Serum levels of growth hormone normally decline with aging. Elderly men treated with rhGH for 6 months had an increase in muscle mass and bone density and a drop of 13% in fat mass, but functional abilities remained unchanged. Available data do not support the use of rhGH to reverse the manifestations of normal aging.

Dosage

The therapeutic dosage of recombinant human growth hormone must be individualized. It is usually given in the evening by subcutaneous injection in the thighs, rotating the sites of injections. One milligram of standard rhGH preparations is equivalent to 3 units.

A. Children

Treatment is begun with 0.025 mg/kg daily and may be increased to a maximum of 0.045 mg/kg daily. Somatropin injectable suspension (Nutropin Depot) is a long-acting preparation of rhGH that is administered subcutaneously in doses of 1.5 mg/kg monthly or 0.75 mg/kg twice monthly. Children must be observed closely for slowing of growth velocity, which could indicate a need to increase the dosage or the possibility of epiphysial fusion or intercurrent problems such as hypothyroidism or malnutrition. Children with Turner's syndrome or chronic renal insufficiency require somewhat higher doses. The injection should be given at least 3 hours after dialysis to reduce the risk of hematoma formation due to residual heparin effect.

B. Adults

The required dosage for adults is lower than that for children. Treatment is begun at about 0.2 mg three times weekly and titrated upward gradually at intervals of 2–4 weeks to a maximum of 0.025 mg/kg/d (adults under age 35) or 0.0125 mg/kg/d (adults over age 35) given three to seven times weekly according to clinical response. Somatropin injectable suspension is administered subcutaneously to adult men in doses of 0.2–0.4 mg/kg every 2 weeks; it is administered to adult women taking oral estrogen in doses of 0.4–0.6 mg/kg every 2 weeks. Women usually require higher dosages than men, perhaps because of concomitant use of oral estrogens. Clinical response and adverse effects best determine the final therapeutic dosage. Serum IGF-I levels (age- and sex-adjusted) can also be used.

Toxicity & Contraindications

Before 1985, GH was obtained from human cadaver pituitary glands. A small number of individuals who received cadaver-derived pooled growth hormone preparations developed Creutzfeldt-Jakob disease, a fatal neurodegenerative disease that presented many years after GH treatment. (This disease is caused by prions, infectious proteins containing no DNA or RNA, which escaped the usual purification processes.) Distribution of pituitary-derived GH ceased in 1985. Recombinant human growth hormone carries no such risk.

Children generally tolerate GH treatment well. A rarely reported side effect is intracranial hypertension, which may present with vision changes, headache, nausea, or vomiting. Some children develop scoliosis during rapid growth. Patients with Turner's syndrome have an increased risk of otitis media while taking GH. Hypothyroidism is commonly discovered during GH treatment, so periodic assessment of thyroid function is indicated. Pancreatitis, gynecomastia, and nevus growth have occurred in patients receiving GH. Adults tend to have more adverse effects from GH therapy. Peripheral edema, myalgias, and arthralgias (especially in the hands and wrists) occur commonly but remit with dosage reduction. Carpal tunnel syndrome can occur. GH treatment increases the activity of cytochrome P450 isoforms, which could reduce the serum levels of drugs metabolized by that enzyme system (see Chapter 4). There has been no increased incidence of malignancy among patients receiving GH therapy, but GH treatment is contraindicated in a patient with a known malignancy. Proliferative retinopathy may rarely occur. GH treatment of critically ill patients appears to increase mortality.

Side effects of the long-acting somatropin injectable suspension have included injection-site nodules that persist for 5–7 days (96%), edema, arthralgias, transient fatigue (24%), mild-moderate nausea (24%), and headache (36%).

THYROTROPIN-RELEASING HORMONE (PROTIRELIN, TRH)

Thyrotropin-releasing hormone, or protirelin, is a tripeptide hormone found in the paraventricular nuclei of the hypothalamus as well as in other parts of the brain. TRH is secreted into the portal venous system and stimulates the pituitary to produce thyroid-stimulating hormone (TSH, thyrotropin), which in turn stimulates the thyroid to produce thyroxine (T_4) and triiodothyronine (T_3). TRH stimulation of thyrotropin is blocked by thyroxine and potentiated by lack of thyroxine.

Chemistry & Pharmacokinetics

TRH is (pyro)Glu-His-Pro-NH_2. It is administered intravenously over 1 minute. Rapid plasma inactivation occurs, with a half-life of 4–5 minutes.

Pharmacodynamics

Peak serum thyrotropin levels occur 20–30 seconds after intravenous TRH injection in healthy individuals. In hyperthyroidism, the serum thyrotropin level is suppressed. In primary hypothyroidism, thyrotropin levels are high and the thyrotropin response to TRH may be accentuated. In secondary (pituitary) hypothyroidism, serum thyrotropin levels are "inappropriately" normal or low (using a sensitive TSH assay); TSH often fails to rise after TRH administration. In tertiary (hypothalamic) hypothyroidism, the baseline serum thyrotropin level may be normal or low and the thyrotropin response to TRH may be normal or blunted.

TRH infusion leads to stimulation of prolactin release by the pituitary in healthy individuals but has no effect on cells producing growth hormone or ACTH. In certain types of pituitary tumors, however, the neoplastic cells may respond abnormally to TRH by releasing growth hormone (in acromegaly), by releasing ACTH (in Cushing's disease), or by failing to release prolactin (in most prolactinomas). Infusion of TRH or TRH analogs has been reported to improve the outcome of partial spinal cord injuries.

Clinical Pharmacology

TRH testing (see above) is now rarely used to diagnose hyperthyroidism or hypothyroidism, having been supplanted by sensitive assays for serum thyrotropin (see below).

Dosage

The dose of protirelin for diagnostic use is 500 μg for adults and 7 μg/kg for children aged 6 years or older but not to exceed the adult dose. A baseline thyrotropin level should be obtained, followed by three further determinations at 15, 30, and 60 minutes postinfusion. The test is performed with the patient supine while blood pressure is monitored.

Toxicity

Most patients given intravenous TRH note adverse effects lasting for a few minutes: an urge to urinate, a metallic taste, nausea, flushing, or light-headedness. Transient hypertension or hypotension may occur, and marked blood pressure fluctuations have been reported in a few patients.

THYROID-STIMULATING HORMONE (THYROTROPIN, TSH) & THYROTROPIN ALPHA (rhTSH)

Thyrotropin is an anterior pituitary hormone that stimulates the thyroid to produce and synthesize thyroxine (T_4), triiodothyronine (T_3), and thyroglobulin. Thyrotropin alpha is a commercially available analog of TSH that is used to help detection of metastatic differentiated thyroid carcinoma; it is also known as recombinant human TSH (rhTSH).

Chemistry & Pharmacokinetics

A. STRUCTURE

Thyrotropin is a glycoprotein consisting of two peptide (alpha and beta) subunits joined noncovalently. The TSH-alpha subunit in humans has 89 amino acids and is virtually identical to that of the alpha subunit of FSH, LH, and hCG. The TSH-beta subunit has 112 amino acids and confers thyroid specificity. Carbohydrate side chains glycosylate each subunit prior to secretion and are important for hormone action. Native TSH is actually secreted as a mixture of glycosylation variants, having both sialylated and sulfated forms.

Thyrotropin alpha is a purified synthetic analog of native pituitary TSH that is produced in a Chinese hamster ovary cell line cotransfected with recombinant plasmids containing DNA sequences that encode the alpha and beta subunits of TSH. Like native TSH, thyrotropin alpha is a heterodimeric glycoprotein containing an alpha subunit of 92 amino acids with two glycosylation sites and a beta subunit of 118 amino acids with one glycosylation site. These subunits are slightly longer than those of pituitary TSH but contain amino acid sequences identical to those of native TSH. Like pituitary TSH, synthetic thyrotropin alpha is a mixture of glycosylated variants, but with only sialylated forms.

B. ABSORPTION, METABOLISM, AND EXCRETION

Following an intramuscular injection of thyrotropin alpha (0.9 mg), the peak rhTSH concentration is reached in about 10 hours (range, 3–24 hours). The mean elimination half-life of thyrotropin alpha is 22 hours. Pituitary TSH is cleared by the kidneys and liver. Little unchanged thyrotropin is found in the urine.

Pharmacodynamics

Thyrotropin alpha has the biologic properties of pituitary TSH. It binds to TSH receptors on both normal thyroid and differentiated thyroid cancer cells. The TSH-activated receptor stimulates intracellular adenylyl cyclase activity. Increased cAMP production causes increased iodine uptake and increased production of thyroid hormones and thyroglobulin.

Clinical Pharmacology

A. DIAGNOSTIC USES

Patients with well-differentiated (papillary or follicular) thyroid carcinoma are treated with surgical resection of the cancer along with total or near-total thyroidectomy. Total thyroidectomy normally reduces the serum levels of thyroid hormones and thyroglobulin to undetectable levels. Postoperatively, these patients must take oral thyroid hormone in order to maintain clinical euthyroidism and to suppress pituitary TSH secretion, thereby preventing any stimulation of tumor growth by TSH. Since thyroid cancer can recur years after apparent cure, such patients should have follow-up TSH-stimulated whole-body ^{131}I scans and serum thyroglobulin determinations. However, the aggressiveness of follow-up surveillance must be individualized according to each patient's risk of recurrence. Traditionally, patients have had to endure prolonged withdrawal of thyroid hormone replacement for many weeks before these tests in order to allow their TSH levels to rise high enough to stimulate any remaining tumor cells to resume their uptake of ^{131}I and their secretion of thyroglobulin. The use of thyrotropin alpha can obviate the need for cessation of thyroid hormone replacement prior to the diagnostic whole-body ^{131}I scan and serum thyroglobulin determination.

B. THERAPEUTIC USES

Treatment of metastatic differentiated thyroid cancer requires the administration of large doses of [131]I (30–200 mCi) in the presence of persistently high serum levels of TSH (see Chapter 38). Patients must withdraw from thyroid hormone replacement in order to achieve this. For treatment purposes, thyrotropin alpha administration cannot substitute for thyroid hormone withdrawal.

Dosage

Thyrotropin alpha injections can stimulate uptake of ^{131}I by thyroid cancer or residual thyroid. The preparation is stored as a lyophilized powder that must be reconstituted before use. The dosage is 0.9 mg intragluteally (not intravenously) every 24 hours for two doses (eg, Monday and Tuesday). Twenty-four hours after the final thyrotropin injection (eg, Wednesday), ^{131}I is administered in a dosage of at least 4 mCi (a larger dose than in hypothyroid patients, since iodine clearance is faster in euthyroid patients). Then, 48 hours after the ^{131}I administration (eg, Friday), a serum thyroglobulin is drawn and a scan is obtained using a gamma camera, with neck, anterior whole body, and posterior whole-body imaging. If the scan shows probable metastases or if the serum thyroglobulin level (using a sensitive assay) is > 2.5 ng/mL, further evaluation and treatment are indicated.

Toxicity

Side effects of thyrotropin injections include nausea (11%), headache (7%), and asthenia (3%). Hyperthyroidism can occur in patients with significant metastases or residual normal thyroid. Thyrotropin has caused neurologic deterioration in 7% of patients with brain metastases.

CORTICOTROPIN-RELEASING HORMONE (CRH)

CRH is a hypothalamic hormone that stimulates release of ACTH and β-endorphin from the pituitary.

Chemistry & Pharmacokinetics

A. STRUCTURE

Human CRH is a 41-amino-acid peptide. An analog of human CRH is sheep (ovine) CRH, which also contains 41 amino acids. These molecules differ in seven amino acids.

B. ABSORPTION, METABOLISM, AND EXCRETION

CRH is administered intravenously. The first-phase half-lives of human and sheep CRH are 9 minutes and 18 minutes, respectively. The peptide is metabolized in various tissues, and less than 1% is excreted in the urine.

Pharmacodynamics

ACTH released by CRH stimulation of the pituitary subsequently stimulates the adrenal cortex to produce cortisol and androgens. Ovine CRH is more potent than human CRH.

Clinical Pharmacology

CRH is used only for diagnostic purposes. In Cushing's syndrome, CRH has been used to distinguish Cushing's disease from ectopic ACTH secretion. CRH generally elicits an increase in ACTH and cortisol secretion in Cushing's disease but usually not in the ectopic ACTH syndrome. However, exceptions occur frequently, making this test unreliable. A more reliable test depends on differential concentrations of ACTH. In patients with Cushing's disease, ACTH levels in blood drawn from the inferior petrosal sinuses draining the pituitary are more than 2.5 times higher than levels in simultaneously drawn peripheral venous blood. When tumors are associated with ectopic ACTH production, no such difference is observed. Concurrent administration of CRH (ovine) further improves the distinction between blood levels of ACTH when Cushing's disease is present.

Preparations & Dosage

Synthetic human and ovine CRH are available. Sheep CRH is used more frequently because of its longer half-life and slightly greater potency. CRH may be dissolved in water or dilute acid but not in saline. A dose of 1 mg/kg is used for diagnostic testing.

Toxicity

Intravenous bolus doses of 1 mg/kg produce transient facial flushing and, rarely, dyspnea.

ADRENOCORTICOTROPIN (CORTICOTROPIN, ACTH, ACTH$_{1-24}$)

Adrenocorticotropin is a peptide hormone produced in the anterior pituitary. Its primary endocrine function is to stimulate synthesis and release of cortisol by the adrenal cortex. Corticotropin can be used therapeutically, but a synthetic derivative is more commonly—and almost exclusively—used to assess adrenocortical responsiveness. A substandard adrenocortical response to exogenous corticotropin administration indicates adrenocortical insufficiency.

Chemistry & Pharmacokinetics

A. STRUCTURE

Human ACTH is a single peptide chain of 39 amino acids. The amino terminal portion containing amino acids 1–24 is necessary for full biologic activity. The remaining amino acids (25–39) confer species specificity. Synthetic human ACTH$_{1-24}$ is known as cosyntropin. The amino terminal amino acids 1–13 are identical to melanocyte-stimulating hormone (α-MSH), which has been found in animals but not in humans. In states of excessive pituitary ACTH secretion (Addison's disease or an ACTH-secreting pituitary tumor), hyperpigmentation—caused by the α-MSH activity intrinsic to ACTH—may be noted.

ACTH from animal sources is assayed biologically by measuring the depletion of adrenocortical ascorbic acid that follows subcutaneous administration of the ACTH.

B. ABSORPTION, METABOLISM, AND EXCRETION

Both porcine and synthetic corticotropin are given parenterally. Corticotropin cannot be administered orally because of gastrointestinal proteolysis.

The biologic half-lives of $ACTH_{1-39}$ and $ACTH_{1-24}$ are under 20 minutes. Tissue uptake occurs in the liver and kidneys. $ACTH_{1-39}$ is transformed into a biologically inactive substance, probably by modification of a side chain. ACTH is not excreted in the urine in significant amounts. The effects of long-acting repository forms of porcine corticotropin persist for up to 18 hours with a gelatin complex of the peptide and up to several days with a zinc hydroxide complex.

Pharmacodynamics

ACTH stimulates the adrenal cortex to produce glucocorticoids, mineralocorticoids, and androgens. ACTH increases the activity of cholesterol esterase, the enzyme that catalyzes the rate-limiting step of steroid hormone production: cholesterol $\rightarrow$ pregnenolone. ACTH also stimulates adrenal hypertrophy and hyperplasia. When given chronically in pharmacologic doses, corticotropin causes increased skin pigmentation.

Clinical Pharmacology

A. Diagnostic Uses

ACTH stimulation of the adrenals will fail to elicit an appropriate response in states of adrenal insufficiency. A rapid test for ruling out adrenal insufficiency employs cosyntropin (see below). Plasma cortisol levels are measured before and either 30 minutes or 60 minutes following an intramuscular or intravenous injection of 0.25 mg of cosyntropin. A normal plasma cortisol response is a stimulated peak level exceeding 20 µg/dL. A subnormal response indicates primary or secondary adrenocortical insufficiency that can be differentiated using endogenous plasma ACTH levels (which are increased in primary adrenal insufficiency and decreased in the secondary form). An incremental rise in plasma aldosterone generally occurs in secondary but not primary adrenal insufficiency after cosyntropin stimulation.

ACTH stimulation may distinguish three forms of "late-onset" (nonclassic) congenital adrenal hyperplasia from states of ovarian hyperandrogenism, all of which may be associated with hirsutism. In patients with deficiency of 21-hydroxylase, ACTH stimulation results in an incremental rise in plasma 17-hydroxyprogesterone, the substrate for the deficient enzyme. Patients with 11-hydroxylase deficiency manifest a rise in 11-deoxycortisol, while those with 3β-hydroxy-δ5 steroid dehydrogenase deficiency show an increase of 17-hydroxypregnenolone in response to ACTH stimulation.

B. Therapeutic Uses

Corticotropin therapy has been virtually abandoned since it has no therapeutic advantage over direct administration of glucocorticoids.

Dosage

Cosyntropin is the preferred preparation for diagnostic use. The standard diagnostic test dose of 0.25 mg is equivalent to 25 units of porcine corticotropin. ACTH is rarely indicated but is available for use in doses of 10–20 units four times daily. Repository ACTH, 40–80 units, may be administered every 24–72 hours.

Toxicity & Contraindications

The toxicity of therapeutic doses of ACTH resembles that of the glucocorticoids (see Chapter 39), with the added adverse effect of hyperandrogenism in women. The occasional development of antibodies to animal ACTH or to depot cosyntropin (a preparation not currently available in the USA) has produced anaphylactic reactions or refractoriness to ACTH therapy in a few individuals. Painful swelling occurs at the injection site more often with the zinc hydroxide depot preparation than with the gelatin preparation. Contraindications are similar to those of glucocorticoids. When immediate effects are desired, glucocorticoids are preferable.

There are virtually no adverse effects from diagnostic doses of cosyntropin.

GONADOTROPIN-RELEASING HORMONE (GNRH; LUTEINIZING HORMONE-RELEASING HORMONE [LHRH]; GONADORELIN HYDROCHLORIDE)

GnRH is produced in the arcuate nucleus of the hypothalamus. GnRH is secreted into the hypothalamic-pituitary venous plexus and binds to cell surface receptors of the anterior pituitary gonadotroph cells. Pulsatile GnRH secretion is required to stimulate the gonadotroph cell to produce and release luteinizing hormone (LH) and follicle stimulating hormone (FSH).

Divergent production of the two gonadotropins is controlled by the frequency of GnRH pulses. In women, increasing levels of estradiol at midcycle have a positive feedback upon the hypothalamus that increases GnRH secretion, resulting in a sudden increase in LH secretion. This LH-surge induces the ovulation of the dominant ovarian follicle, with subsequent luteinization in the ovary that secretes progesterone; this changes the uterine proliferative endometrium to a secretory endometrium that is receptive to a fertilized ovum.

Ironically, sustained non-pulsatile administration of GnRH or GnRH analogs *inhibits* the release of FSH and LH by the pituitary in both women and men, resulting in hypogonadism.

Chemistry & Pharmacokinetics

A. STRUCTURE

GnRH is a decapeptide found in all mammals. It is derived from a precursor (proGnRH) with 92 amino acids. Pharmaceutical GnRH is synthetic. Analogs (eg, leuprolide, nafarelin, buserelin, goserelin, and histrelin) with D-amino acids at position 6 and with ethylamide substituted for glycine at position 10 are more potent and longer-lasting than native GnRH.

5-O-Pro-His-Trp-Ser-Tyr-Gly-Leu-Arg-Pro-Gly-NH$_2$
GnRH (gonadorelin)

5-O-Pro-His-Trp-Ser-Tyr-D-Leu-Leu-Arg-Pro-NHCH$_2$CH$_3$
Leuprolide

5-O-Pro-His-Trp-Ser-Tyr-D-Nal-*Leu-Arg-Pro-Gly-NH$_2$
Nafarelin

5-O-Pro-His-Trp-Ser-Tyr-D-Ser(t-Bu)-Leu-Arg-Pro-NHNHCONH$_2$
Goserelin

5-O-Pro-His-Trp-Ser-Tyr-D-His(N^τ-PhCH$_2$)-Leu-Arg-Pro-NHCH$_2$CH$_3$
Histrelin

*D-Nal = D-3-(2-naphthyl)-alanine.

B. ABSORPTION, METABOLISM, AND EXCRETION

GnRH may be administered intravenously or subcutaneously. GnRH analogs may be administered subcutaneously, intramuscularly, or via nasal spray. The half-life of intravenous GnRH is 4 minutes, and the half-lives of subcutaneous and intranasal GnRH analogs are 3 hours. Degradation occurs in the hypothalamus and pituitary. GnRH analogs have increased affinity for GnRH receptors and reduced susceptibility to degradation.

Pharmacodynamics

GnRH binds to receptors on pituitary gonadotrophs. Pulsatile intravenous administration of GnRH every 1–4 hours stimulates FSH and LH secretion. As noted above, GnRH administered continuously or GnRH analogs administered in depot formulations inhibit gonadotropin release.

Clinical Pharmacology

A. DIAGNOSTIC USES

Delayed puberty in a hypogonadotropic adolescent may be due to a constitutional delay or to hypogonadotropic hypogonadism. The LH response (but not the FSH response) to GnRH can distinguish between these two conditions. Serum LH levels are measured before and then 15, 30, 45, 60, and 120 minutes after a 100 mg intravenous or subcutaneous bolus of GnRH. A peak LH response exceeding 15.6 mIU/mL is normal and suggests impending puberty, whereas an impaired LH response suggests hypogonadotropic hypogonadism due to either pituitary or hypothalamic disease (but may also be seen in constitutional delay of adolescence).

B. THERAPEUTIC USES

1. Stimulation—GnRH can stimulate pituitary function and is used to treat infertility caused by hypothalamic hypogonadotropic hypogonadism in both sexes. A portable battery-powered programmable pump and intravenous tubing allows pulsatile GnRH therapy every 90 minutes.

2. Suppression—Leuprolide, nafarelin, goserelin, and histrelin are GnRH analog agonists that induce hypogonadism when given continuously. Such GnRH agonists are used to treat prostate cancer, uterine fibroids, endometriosis, polycystic ovary syndrome, and precocious puberty. Many in vitro fertilization programs sequentially use a GnRH analog to suppress endogenous gonadotropin release, along with exogenous gonadotropins to achieve synchronous follicular development.

GnRH analog therapy for the purpose of producing pituitary suppression leads to a transient rise in sex hormone concentration during the first 2 weeks of treatment. This can be deleterious during treatment of prostate cancer, precocious puberty, and infertility.

Dosage: Gonadorelin (GnRH, Factrel)

Gonadorelin hydrochloride is available in a lyophilized powder that is reconstituted and injected either subcutaneously or intravenously.

A. DIAGNOSTIC USE

Gonadorelin has been used to test pituitary luteinizing hormone (LH) responsiveness. Administered as a 100 μg test dose, the average times to peak LH levels are 34 minutes (men) or 72 minutes (women) following subcutaneous gonadorelin and 27 minutes (men) or 36 minutes (women) following intravenous gonadorelin. There is considerable individual variation in response.

B. FEMALE INFERTILITY

Gonadorelin is administered intravenously, 5 μg every 90 minutes from a portable pump. The woman is followed carefully with serum estradiol levels, and an ovarian ultrasound examination is done weekly before refilling the GnRH pump. When an ovarian follicle reaches 14 mm in diameter, ovulation is induced with hCG,

5000 units subcutaneously, and the luteal phase is maintained with hCG, 1500 units every 3 days for 12 days.

C. Male Infertility

For male infertility caused by hypothalamic GnRH deficiency, gonadorelin treatment is begun only after preparatory hCG injections continued for up to 1 year in men with prepubertal hypogonadotropic hypogonadism. A portable pump infuses gonadorelin intravenously every 90 minutes. Serum testosterone levels and semen analyses must be done regularly. At least 3–6 months of bolus infusions are required before significant numbers of sperm are seen. The preferable alternative to intravenous gonadorelin treatment is subcutaneously administered gonadotropins.

Dosage: Leuprolide (GnRH Analog, Lupron)

Leuprolide is available in solution for daily subcutaneous injection and in slow-release depot preparations in which leuprolide is lyophilized in microspheres given by intramuscular injection.

A. Endometriosis and Uterine Fibroids

Women with endometriosis receive treatment courses of 6 months' duration. Concomitant low-dose hormone replacement therapy has been reported to diminish bone loss without significantly decreasing clinical effectiveness. Women with uterine fibroids that are symptomatic (menorrhagia, anemia, pain) receive treatment courses of 3 months, by which time women have amenorrhea or reduced menorrhagia; uterine fibroids are reduced in size an average of 37%. Intramuscular depot preparations containing 3.75 mg (monthly) or 11.5 mg (every 3 months) are used.

B. Prostate Cancer

Leuprolide is usually used in depot form, 7.5 mg intramuscularly monthly, 22.5 mg intramuscularly at 84-day intervals, or 30 mg intramuscularly at 4-month intervals.

C. Central Precocious Puberty

Leuprolide aqueous solution is started at a dosage of 0.05 mg/kg body weight injected subcutaneously daily. If the clinical response is inadequate, the dose can be increased by increments of 0.01 mg/kg body weight. Pediatric depot preparations are also available. The dose can be titrated upward according to the endocrine response.

Leuprolide is indicated for treatment of central precocious puberty (onset of secondary sex characteristics before 8 years in girls or 9 years in boys). Prior to use, central precocious puberty must be confirmed by a puberty gonadotropin response to GnRH and a bone age at least 1 year beyond chronologic age. Pretreatment

evaluation must also include sex steroid levels compatible with precocious puberty and not congenital adrenal hyperplasia; a βhCG level to exclude a chronic gonadotropin-secreting tumor; an MRI of the brain to exclude an intracranial tumor; and an ultrasound examination of the adrenals and ovaries or testes to exclude a steroid-secreting tumor.

Dosage: Nafarelin (GnRH Analog, Synarel) Nasal Solution

Nafarelin is available as Synarel, a nasal preparation. The head should be tilted back and 30 seconds allowed to elapse between each spray. Nafarelin is rapidly absorbed by the nasal mucosa. Maximum serum levels occur in 10–40 minutes. Rhinitis is a common side effect. Sneezing should be avoided after administration. Nasal decongestants must not be used for 2 hours following each dose.

A. Endometriosis

Treatment is begun between days 2 and 4 of the menstrual cycle. The initial dose is one spray (0.1 mL, 0.2 mg) into one nostril in the morning and another spray into the opposite nostril in the evening. Amenorrhea occurs in about 65%, 80%, and 90% of women at 2, 3, and 4 months of treatment, respectively. About 60% of women become symptom-free by the end of treatment, and of these, about 50% remain symptom-free 6 months after cessation of treatment. Withdrawal menstrual bleeding occurs commonly during the first 2 months of nafarelin therapy. If bleeding persists despite good patient compliance, the dosage may be increased to one spray into each nostril twice daily.

B. Central Precocious Puberty

The recommended initial daily dose of nafarelin for central precocious puberty is 1.6 mg/d. This is achieved with two unit dose sprays (each spray contains 0.1 mL, 0.2 mg) into each nostril twice daily. If adequate suppression of puberty is not achieved, the dose may be increased to 1.8 mg/d, given as 3 sprays (total) three times daily. Pretreatment evaluation and follow-up are the same as for leuprolide.

C. Uterine Fibroids

Nafarelin nasal spray has been used to shrink uterine fibroids and reduce menometrorrhagia, dysmenorrhea, and pelvic discomfort. Required doses range from 50 μg to 400 μg intranasally twice daily for 3–6 months.

Dosage: Goserelin (GnRH Analog, Zoladex) Implants

Goserelin acetate is available in the form of implantable cylinders, 1–1.5 mm in diameter, that are placed subcutaneously in the upper abdominal area. Goserelin is metabolized in the liver and excreted in the urine. Clearance is greater in women than in men. Stimulation of gonadotropins occurs in the first weeks of therapy, followed by suppression.

A. Endometriosis, Breast Cancer, and Dysfunctional Uterine Bleeding

Implants containing 3.6 mg of goserelin are injected subcutaneously every 28 days.

B. Prostate Cancer

Implants containing 10.8 mg goserelin are injected subcutaneously every 12 weeks.

Toxicity

GnRH (gonadorelin) may cause headache, light-headedness, nausea, and flushing. Local swelling often occurs at subcutaneous injection sites. Generalized hypersensitivity dermatitis has occurred after long-term subcutaneous administration. Rare acute hypersensitivity reactions include bronchospasm and anaphylaxis. Sudden pituitary apoplexy and blindness has been reported following administration of GnRH to a patient with a gonadotropin-secreting pituitary tumor.

GnRH analog (leuprolide, nafarelin, goserelin) treatment of women may cause hot flushes and sweats (89%) and headaches (29%). Depression, diminished libido, generalized pain, vaginal dryness, and breast atrophy may also occur. Ovarian cysts may develop within the first 2 months of therapy and generally resolve by 6 weeks, but may persist and require discontinuation of therapy. Osteoporosis may occur with prolonged use, so patients may be monitored with bone densitometry prior to repeated treatment courses. Cholesterol and triglyceride levels may rise. Contraindications include pregnancy and breast-feeding.

GnRH analog (leuprolide, goserelin) treatment in men causes serum testosterone levels to rise for about 1 week; this can precipitate pain in men with bone metastases. In men with vertebral metastases, initial growth of tumor can produce neurologic symptoms. It can also temporarily worsen symptoms of urinary obstruction. Within about 2 weeks, serum testosterone levels fall to the hypogonadal range. Other adverse effects in men include hot flushes and sweats (59%), edema (13%), gynecomastia, decreased libido, decreased hematocrit, and asthenia. For men with prostate cancer, GnRH agonists are often given together with an antiandrogen (see Chapter 40), which may exacerbate hypogonadal symptoms while reducing the risk of exacerbation of bone pain.

GnRH analog (leuprolide, nafarelin) treatment of children is generally well tolerated. However, temporary exacerbation of precocious puberty may occur during the first few weeks of therapy. Injection site reactions occur in about 5%. Nafarelin nasal spray may cause or aggravate sinusitis.

Dosage: Cetrorelix Acetate for Injection (GnRH Antagonist)

Cetrorelix is a synthetic decapeptide that reversibly binds to pituitary GnRH receptors without activating them. Cetrorelix thus inhibits the secretion of FSH and LH in a dose-dependent manner by competing with natural hypothalamic GnRH for pituitary cell surface receptors. At the doses used for in vitro fertilization, cetrorelix produces an immediate suppression of LH; this delays the LH surge and thus delays ovulation. At higher doses, cetrorelix also suppresses FSH secretion, thus inhibiting the secretion of estradiol from the ovaries.

Cetrorelix is absorbed rapidly following subcutaneous injection, with maximum plasma concentrations occurring 1–2 hours after administration. Following a subcutaneous dose of 3 mg, the duration of action is at least 4 days; daily administration of 0.25 mg maintains GnRH antagonism.

A. In Vitro Fertilization (IVF)

GnRH antagonists produce less ovarian hyperstimulation during IVF than do GnRH analogs. Cetrorelix suppresses endogenous FSH and LH while recombinant FSH (rFSH) is being given to prepare the ova for ovulation-induction by hCG administration. Ovarian stimulation is commenced with rFSH on the second or third day of the menstrual cycle. When serum estradiol rises to levels that indicate sufficient ovarian stimulation (requiring 5–9 days), cetrorelix is administered subcutaneously in order to prevent a natural LH that could cause premature spontaneous ovulation, obviating laparoscopic harvest of the ova. Cetrorelix may be administered subcutaneously in a dose of 3 mg, followed by 0.25 mg daily if hCG stimulation has not been given within the next 4 days. Alternatively, cetrorelix may be given subcutaneously in doses of 0.25 mg subcutaneously daily, beginning on the fifth or sixth day of FSH stimulation and continued daily until hCG is administered.

B. Endometriosis

Cetrorelix has been given in doses of 3 mg by subcutaneous injection of a depot preparation once weekly for 8 weeks.

C. Uterine Fibroids

Cetrorelix has been given in doses of 3 mg by subcutaneous injection every 4 days for 2–4 weeks prior to surgery. Therapy is commenced on the first day of the menstrual cycle.

FOLLICLE-STIMULATING HORMONE (FSH)

Follicle-stimulating hormone is a glycoprotein hormone consisting of two chains and, like LH, is produced by gonadotroph cells in the anterior pituitary. FSH and LH regulate gonadal function by increasing cAMP in the target gonadal tissue. FSH, like other pituitary glycoproteins, is composed of a common alpha subunit that promotes hormone action and a unique beta subunit that confers specificity. The principal function of FSH is to stimulate gametogenesis and follicular development in women and spermatogenesis in men. FSH acts on the immature follicular cells of the ovary and induces development of the mature follicle and oocyte. Both LH and FSH are needed for proper ovarian steroidogenesis. LH stimulates androgen production by these cells, and FSH stimulates androgen conversion into estrogens by the granulosa cells. In the testes, FSH acts on the Sertoli cells and stimulates their production of androgen-binding protein.

FSH has been commercially available since the 1960s. It was first extracted from the urine of postmenopausal women, which contains a substance with FSH-like properties (but with 4% of the potency) and an LH-like substance. This purified extract of FSH and LH, derived from the urine of postmenopausal women, remains available and is known as menotropins, or human menopausal gonadotropins (hMG). A purified preparation of human FSH, also extracted from the urine of postmenopausal women, contains virtually no LH and is know as urofollitropin, or urinary FSH (uFSH). In 1996, a synthetic modified form of FSH became available, known as follitropin alpha, or recombinant FSH (rFSH). Preparations of rFSH have batch-to-batch consistency and are free from possible urinary contaminants. The cost of rFSH is about three times that of hMG. It is controversial whether in vitro fertilization protocols using rFSH are significantly more successful than protocols using uFSH or hMG.

These preparations are used in states of infertility to stimulate ovarian follicle development in women and spermatogenesis in men. In both sexes, they must be used in conjunction with a luteinizing hormone, ie, human chorionic gonadotropin (hCG), to permit ovulation and implantation in women and testosterone production and full masculinization in men.

Pharmacokinetics

Over a 7- to 12-day course of daily hMG or urofollitropin administration (intended to mimic the follicular phase of the ovarian cycle in women with hypothalamic amenorrhea), FSH levels gradually rise to twice their baseline level. LH levels increase to 1.5 times their baseline with hMG, but they do not rise with urofollitropin.

Pharmacodynamics

Ovarian follicular growth and maturation will occur during hMG or FSH treatment of gonadotropin-deficient women. Ovulation requires administration of chorionic gonadotropin when adequate follicular maturation has occurred.

In men with gonadotropin deficiencies, pretreatment with chorionic gonadotropin produces external sexual maturation; addition of a subsequent course of hMG (or rFSH plus hCG) will stimulate spermatogenesis and lead to fertility.

Clinical Pharmacology

FSH or hMG are indicated for pituitary or hypothalamic hypogonadism with infertility. Anovulatory women with the following conditions may benefit from hMG: primary amenorrhea, secondary amenorrhea, polycystic ovary syndrome, and anovulatory cycles. Both hMG and FSH are used by in vitro fertilization programs for controlled ovarian hyperstimulation.

Over 50% of men with hypogonadotropic hypogonadism become fertile after hMG or hCG/FSH administration.

Dosage

An ampule of menotropins contains 75 IU or 150 IU of FSH and an equal amount of LH. One international unit of LH is approximately equivalent to 0.5 IU of hCG. An ampule of urofollitropin contains 75 IU of FSH and less than 1 IU of LH. Human menopausal gonadotropins, FSH, and hCG are administered intramuscularly.

A. WOMEN

In hypothalamic hypogonadism and for in vitro fertilization, one or two ampules are administered daily for 5–12 days until evidence of adequate follicular maturation is present. Serum estradiol levels should be measured and a cervical examination performed every 1 or 2 days. When appropriate follicular maturation has occurred, hMG or FSH is discontinued; the following day, hCG (5000–10,000 IU) is administered intramuscularly to induce ovulation.

B. MEN

Following pretreatment with 5000 IU of hCG three times weekly for up to 12 months to achieve masculinization and a normal serum testosterone level, menotropins is administered as one ampule (75 units) three times weekly in combination with hCG, 2000 IU twice weekly. At least 4 months of combined treatment are usually necessary before spermatozoa appear in the ejaculate. If there is no response, the menotropins dose may be doubled. When adding menotropins to hCG therapy, the dose of hCG must be reduced to keep serum testosterone in the high normal range and avoid hyperandrogenism.

Toxicity & Contraindications

Overstimulation of the ovary with hMG can lead to uncomplicated ovarian enlargement in approximately 20% of patients. This usually resolves spontaneously. A more serious complication, the "hyperstimulation syndrome," occurs in 0.5–4% of patients. It is characterized by hMG-induced ovarian enlargement, ascites, hydrothorax, and hypovolemia, sometimes to the point of shock. Hemoperitoneum (from a ruptured ovarian cyst), fever, or arterial thromboembolism can occur. The frequency of multiple births is approximately 20%. A reported 25% incidence of spontaneous abortions may be due to earlier diagnosis of pregnancy in treated than in untreated patients, with recognition of very early abortion. There may, however, be abnormal development and premature degeneration of corpus luteum in some treated patients. Gynecomastia occasionally occurs in men. An association between ovarian cancer and fertility drugs has been reported (Spirtas et al, 1993). However, it is not known which, if any, fertility drugs are causally related to cancer.

Human menopausal gonadotropin, uFSH or rFSH should be administered only by a physician experienced in treating infertility. Before treatment of women, a thorough gynecologic evaluation must be performed to rule out uterine, tubal, or ovarian diseases as well as pregnancy. In cases of irregular bleeding, uterine cancer should be ruled out.

LUTEINIZING HORMONE (LH) & HUMAN CHORIONIC GONADOTROPIN (hCG)

Luteinizing hormone is a glycoprotein hormone consisting of two chains and, like FSH, is produced by gonadotroph cells in the anterior pituitary. LH is primarily responsible for regulation of gonadal steroid hormone production. In men, LH acts on testicular Leydig cells to stimulate testosterone production. In the ovary, LH acts in concert with FSH to stimulate follicular development. LH acts on the mature follicle to induce ovulation, and it stimulates the corpus luteum in the luteal phase of the menstrual cycle to produce progesterone and androgens.

There is no LH preparation presently available for clinical use. **Human chorionic gonadotropin**—with an almost identical structure—is available and can be used as a luteinizing hormone substitute.

Human chorionic gonadotropin is a hormone produced by the human placenta and excreted into the urine, whence it can be extracted and purified. Human chorionic gonadotropin is a glycoprotein consisting of a 92-amino-acid alpha chain virtually identical to that of FSH, LH, and TSH and a beta chain of 145 amino acids that resembles that of LH except for the presence of a carboxyl terminal sequence of 30 amino acids not present in LH.

The function of hCG is to stimulate the ovarian corpus luteum to produce progesterone and maintain the placenta. It is very similar to LH in structure and is used to treat both men and women with LH deficiency.

Pharmacokinetics

Human chorionic gonadotropin is well absorbed after intramuscular administration and has a biologic half-life of 8 hours, compared with 30 minutes for LH. The difference may lie in the high sialic acid content of hCG compared with that of LH. It is apparently modified in the body prior to urinary excretion, because the half-life measured by immunoassay far exceeds that measured by bioassay.

Pharmacodynamics

Human chorionic gonadotropin stimulates production of gonadal steroid hormones. The interstitial and corpus luteal cells of the female produce progesterone, and the Leydig cells of the male produce testosterone. hCG can be used to mimic a midcycle LH surge and trigger ovulation in a hypogonadotropic woman.

Clinical Pharmacology

A. DIAGNOSTIC USES

In prepubertal boys with undescended gonads, hCG can be used to distinguish a truly retained (cryptorchid) testis from a retracted (pseudocryptorchid) one. Testicular descent during a course of hCG administration usually foretells permanent testicular descent at puberty, when circulating LH levels rise. Lack of descent usually means that orchiopexy will be necessary to preserve spermatogenesis.

Patients with constitutional delay in onset of puberty can be distinguished from those with hypogonadotropic hypogonadism using repeated hCG stimulation. Serum testosterone and estradiol levels rise in the former but not in the latter group.

B. THERAPEUTIC USES

As described above, hCG can be used in combination with hMG, uFSH, or rFSH to induce ovulation in women with hypogonadotropic hypogonadism or as part of an in vitro fertilization program. hCG stimulates testosterone secretion by the testes of men with hypogonadotropic hypogonadism. In such men, the increased intratesticular testosterone levels promote spermatogenesis, but FSH is often needed for fertility.

In patients with AIDS-related Kaposi's sarcoma, injection of hCG into the lesions has been reported to cause regression in a dose-related manner.

Dosage

The dosages for female and male infertility are described under hMG dosage. For prepubertal cryptorchidism, a dosage of 500–4000 units three times weekly for up to 6 weeks has been advocated.

Toxicity & Contraindications

Reported adverse effects include headache, depression, edema, precocious puberty, gynecomastia, or (rarely) production of antibodies to hCG. Human chorionic gonadotropin should be administered for infertility only by a physician with experience in this field. Androgen-dependent neoplasia and precocious puberty are contraindications to its use.

PROLACTIN

Prolactin is a 198-amino-acid peptide hormone produced in the anterior pituitary. Its structure resembles that of growth hormone. Prolactin is the principal hormone responsible for lactation. Milk production is stimulated by prolactin when appropriate circulating levels of estrogens, progestins, corticosteroids, and insulin are present. A deficiency of prolactin—which can occur in states of pituitary deficiency—is manifested by failure to lactate or by a luteal phase defect. In hypothalamic destruction, prolactin levels may be elevated as a result of impaired transport of prolactin-inhibiting hormone (dopamine) to the pituitary. Hyperprolactinemia can produce galactorrhea and hypogonadism and may be associated with symptoms of a pituitary mass. No preparation is available for use in prolactin-deficient patients. For patients with symptomatic hyperprolactinemia, inhibition of prolactin secretion can be achieved with cabergoline and other dopamine agonists.

DOPAMINE AGONISTS

Dopamine is released by the hypothalamus to inhibit prolactin release from the anterior pituitary. **Bromocriptine, cabergoline,** and **pergolide** are ergot derivatives with a very high affinity for dopamine D_2 receptors in the pituitary. **Quinagolide** is a nonergot drug with similar D_2 receptor affinity. These drugs lower circulating prolactin levels and shrink pituitary prolactin-secreting

tumors. The chemical structure and pharmacokinetic features of bromocriptine are presented in Chapter 16.

Dopamine agonists decrease pituitary prolactin secretion through a dopamine-mimetic action on the pituitary at two central nervous system loci: (1) they decrease dopamine turnover in the tuberoinfundibular neurons of the arcuate nucleus, generating increased hypothalamic dopamine; and (2) they act directly on pituitary dopamine receptors to inhibit prolactin release.

These agents, like L-dopa, stimulate pituitary growth hormone release in normal subjects and—paradoxically—suppress growth hormone release in acromegalics.

Pharmacokinetics

Cabergoline reaches peak plasma levels within 2–3 hours after a 1 mg oral dose. It has a half-life of 63–69 hours. Metabolites are excreted mostly in feces. Bromocriptine is metabolized more quickly.

All dopamine agonists may be administered orally. Additionally, bromocriptine and cabergoline are absorbed systemically after intravaginal insertion of tablets. Following intravaginal administration, serum levels peak more gradually.

Clinical Pharmacology

A. Prolactin-Secreting Adenomas

A dopamine agonist is the usual initial treatment for prolactinomas. Significant reduction in both tumor size and serum prolactin levels occurs in about 85% of those receiving these drugs for 6 months or longer.

B. Amenorrhea-Galactorrhea

Dopamine agonists are useful for treating problems induced by hyperprolactinemia: amenorrhea, galactorrhea, breast tenderness (mastodynia), infertility, and hypogonadism.

C. Physiologic Lactation

Dopamine agonists can prevent breast engorgement when breast feeding is not desired. Their use for this purpose has been discouraged because of toxicity (see below).

D. Acromegaly

A dopamine agonist alone or in combination with pituitary surgery, irradiation, or octreotide may be used to treat acromegaly. Acromegalic patients seldom respond adequately to bromocriptine unless the pituitary tumor secretes prolactin as well as growth hormone.

E. Parkinson's Disease and Restless Legs Syndrome

Cabergoline, bromocriptine, and pergolide have been used in Parkinson's disease to improve motor function and reduce levodopa requirements as discussed in Chapter 28. Cabergoline has also been effective in restless legs syndrome.

Preparations & Dosage

Cabergoline is initiated at 0.25 mg orally or vaginally twice weekly. It may be increased gradually according to serum prolactin determinations, up to a maximum of 1 mg twice weekly.

Bromocriptine is generally taken after the evening meal at the initial dose of 1.25 mg; the dose is then increased as tolerated. Most patients require 2.5–7.5 mg daily; acromegalics require higher doses, up to 20 mg/d. Bromocriptine tablets may be administered intravaginally to reduce nausea. Long-acting oral bromocriptine formulations (Parlodel SRO) and intramuscular formulations (Parlodel L.A.R.) are available outside the USA.

Quinagolide (CV 205-502, Norprolac) in doses of 0.15–0.6 mg/d orally, suppresses prolactin and shrinks most prolactinomas. It also decreases cyclic mastodynia. Quinagolide is sometimes better tolerated than ergot-derived dopamine agonists. It is not available in the USA.

Toxicity & Contraindications

Dopamine agonists may cause nausea, headache, light-headedness, orthostatic hypotension, and fatigue. Psychiatric manifestations occasionally occur even at lower doses and may take months to resolve. Erythromelalgia occurs rarely. High dosages of ergot-derived preparations may cause cold-induced peripheral digital vasospasm. Pulmonary infiltrates may occur with chronic high-dosage therapy. Cabergoline appears to cause nausea less often than bromocriptine. Vaginal administration of cabergoline or bromocriptine also tends to reduce nausea, but may cause vaginal irritation.

Dopamine agonist therapy during the early weeks of pregnancy has not been associated with an increased risk of spontaneous abortion or congenital malformations. Although there has been a longer experience with the safety of bromocriptine during early pregnancy, there is growing evidence that cabergoline is also safe to use in women with macroprolactinomas who must continue a dopamine agonist during pregnancy. In patients with small pituitary adenomas, dopamine agonist therapy is discontinued upon conception since there is usually no growth of microadenomas during pregnancy. Patients with very large adenomas require vigilance for tumor progression and often require a dopamine agonist throughout pregnancy. There have been rare reports of stroke or coronary thrombosis in postpartum women taking bromocriptine to suppress postpartum lactation.

If a woman who is receiving a dopamine agonist is late in having her menses, a pregnancy test is necessary; if she is amenorrheic, pregnancy tests should be performed regularly because ovulation may occur before menstruation resumes.

POSTERIOR PITUITARY HORMONES

Two posterior pituitary hormones are known: vasopressin and oxytocin. Their structures are very similar. Posterior pituitary hormones are synthesized in the hypothalamus and then transported to the posterior pituitary, where they are stored and then released into the circulation.

OXYTOCIN

Oxytocin is a peptide hormone secreted by the posterior pituitary that elicits milk ejection in lactating women. It may contribute to the initiation of labor. Oxytocin is released during sexual orgasm.

Chemistry & Pharmacokinetics

A. STRUCTURE (FIGURE 37–2.)

Oxytocin is a nine-amino-acid peptide composed of a six-amino-acid disulfide ring and a three-membered tail. Oxytocin and vasopressin differ from vasotocin—the only posterior pituitary hormone found in nonmammalian vertebrates—by only one amino acid residue each.

B. ABSORPTION, METABOLISM, AND EXCRETION

Oxytocin is usually administered intravenously for stimulation of labor. It is also available as a nasal spray to

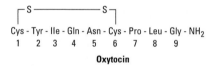

Figure 37–2. Posterior pituitary hormones. (Modified and reproduced, with permission, from Ganong WF: *Review of Medical Physiology,* 21st ed. McGraw-Hill, 2003.)

induce lactation postpartum. It is inactive if swallowed, because it is destroyed in the stomach and intestine. Oxytocin is not bound to plasma proteins and is catabolized by the kidneys and liver, with a circulating half-life of 5 minutes.

Pharmacodynamics

Oxytocin alters transmembrane ionic currents in myometrial smooth muscle cells to produce sustained uterine contraction. The sensitivity of the uterus to oxytocin increases during pregnancy. Oxytocin-induced myometrial contractions can be inhibited by β-adrenoceptor agonists, magnesium sulfate, or inhalation anesthetics. Oxytocin also causes contraction of myoepithelial cells surrounding mammary alveoli, which leads to milk ejection. Without oxytocin-induced contraction, normal lactation cannot occur. Oxytocin has weak antidiuretic and pressor activity.

Clinical Pharmacology

A. DIAGNOSTIC USES

Oxytocin infusion near term will produce uterine contractions that decrease the fetal blood supply. The fetal heart rate response to a standardized oxytocin challenge test provides information about placental circulatory reserve. An abnormal response suggests intrauterine growth retardation and may warrant immediate cesarean delivery.

B. THERAPEUTIC USES

Oxytocin is used to induce labor and augment dysfunctional labor for (1) conditions requiring early vaginal delivery (eg, Rh problems, maternal diabetes, or preeclampsia), (2) uterine inertia, and (3) incomplete abortion. Oxytocin can also be used for control of postpartum uterine hemorrhage. Impaired milk ejection may respond to nasal oxytocin. Synthetic peptide and nonpeptide oxytocin antagonists that can prevent premature labor are being investigated.

Dosage

Oxytocin is frequently given to induce and maintain labor after the cervix has ripened naturally or with the aid of misoprostol. For induction of labor, oxytocin should be administered intravenously via an infusion pump with appropriate fetal and maternal monitoring. An initial infusion rate of 1 mU/min is increased every 15–30 minutes until a physiologic contraction pattern is established. The maximum infusion rate is 20 mU/min. For postpartum uterine bleeding, 10–40 units is added to 1 L of 5% dextrose, and the infusion rate is titrated to control uterine atony. Alternatively, 10 units can be

given intramuscularly after delivery of the placenta. To induce milk let-down, one puff is sprayed into each nostril in the sitting position 2–3 minutes before nursing.

Toxicity & Contraindications

When oxytocin is used properly, serious toxicity is rare. Among the reported adverse reactions are maternal deaths due to hypertensive episodes, uterine rupture, water intoxication, and fetal deaths. Afibrinogenemia has also been reported.

Contraindications include fetal distress, prematurity, abnormal fetal presentation, cephalopelvic disproportion, and other predispositions for uterine rupture.

VASOPRESSIN (ANTIDIURETIC HORMONE, ADH)

Vasopressin is a peptide hormone released by the posterior pituitary in response to rising plasma tonicity or falling blood pressure. Vasopressin possesses antidiuretic and vasopressor properties. A deficiency of this hormone results in diabetes insipidus (see Chapters 15 and 17).

Chemistry & Pharmacokinetics

A. STRUCTURE

Vasopressin is a nonapeptide with a six-amino-acid ring and a three-amino-acid side chain. The residue at position 8 is arginine in humans and in most other mammals except pigs and related species, whose vasopressin contains lysine at position 8 (Figure 37–2).

B. ABSORPTION, METABOLISM, AND EXCRETION

Vasopressin is administered by intravenous, intramuscular, or intranasal routes; oral absorption is slight. The half-life of circulating ADH is approximately 20 minutes, with renal and hepatic catabolism via reduction of the disulfide bond and peptide cleavage. A small amount of vasopressin is excreted as such in the urine.

Pharmacodynamics

Vasopressin interacts with two types of receptors. V_1 receptors are found on vascular smooth muscle cells and mediate vasoconstriction (see Chapter 17). V_2 receptors are found on renal tubule cells and mediate antidiuresis through increased water permeability and water resorption in the collecting tubules. Extrarenal V_2-like receptors mediate release of coagulation factor VIII_c and von Willebrand factor.

Desmopressin acetate (DDAVP, 1-desamino-8-D-arginine vasopressin) is a long-acting synthetic analog of vasopressin with minimal V_1 activity and an antidiuretic-to-pressor ratio 4000 times that of vasopressin.

Clinical Pharmacology

Vasopressin and desmopressin are the alternative treatments of choice for pituitary diabetes insipidus. Bedtime desmopressin therapy ameliorates nocturnal enuresis by decreasing nocturnal urine production. Vasopressin infusion is effective in some cases of esophageal variceal bleeding and colonic diverticular bleeding.

Dosage

A. AQUEOUS VASOPRESSIN

Synthetic aqueous vasopressin is a short-acting preparation for intramuscular, subcutaneous, or intravenous administration. The dose is 5–10 units subcutaneously or intramuscularly every 3–6 hours for transient diabetes insipidus and 0.1–0.5 units/min intravenously for gastrointestinal bleeding.

B. DESMOPRESSIN ACETATE

This is the preferred treatment for most patients with central diabetes insipidus. Desmopressin may be administered intranasally, intravenously, subcutaneously, or orally. The typical nasal dosage is 10–40 μg (0.1–0.4 mL) daily in one to three divided doses. Nasal desmo-

pressin is available as a unit dose spray that delivers 0.1 mL per spray; it is also available with a calibrated nasal tube that can be made to deliver a more precise dose. Injectable desmopressin is approximately ten times more bioavailable than intranasal desmopressin. The dosage by injection is 1–4 μg (0.25–1 mL) daily every 12–24 hours as needed for polyuria, polydipsia, or hypernatremia.

For nocturnal enuresis, desmopressin, 10–20 μg (0.1–0.2 mL) intranasally at bedtime, is used.

Desmopressin is also available as an oral preparation. The usual dose is 0.1–0.2 mg every 12–24 hours.

Desmopressin is also used for the treatment of coagulopathy in hemophilia A and von Willebrand's disease (see Chapter 34).

Toxicity & Contraindications

Headache, nausea, abdominal cramps, agitation, and allergic reactions occur rarely. Therapy can result in hyponatremic convulsions.

Vasopressin (but not desmopressin) can cause vasoconstriction and should be used cautiously in patients with coronary artery disease. Nasal insufflation of desmopressin may be less effective when nasal congestion is present.

PREPARATIONS AVAILABLE

Bromocriptine (Parlodel)
 Oral: 2.5 mg tablets, 5 mg capsules
Cabergoline (Dostinex)
 Oral: 0.5 mg scored tablets
Cetrorelix (Cetrotide)
 Parenteral: 0.25, 3.0 mg/vial with diluent for subcutaneous injection
Chorionic gonadotropin [hCG] (generic, Profasi, A.P.L., Pregnyl, others)
 Parenteral: powder to reconstitute 500, 1000, 2000 units/mL for injection
Corticorelin ovine (Acthrel)
 Parenteral: 100 μg for IV injection
Corticotropin (H.P. Acthar Gel)
 Parenteral: 80 units/mL
Cosyntropin (Cortrosyn)
 Parenteral: 0.25 mg/vial with diluent for IV or IM injection
Desmopressin (DDAVP, Stimate)
 Nasal: 0.1, 1.5 mg/mL solution
 Nasal: 100 μg/mL spray pump and rhinal tube delivery system
 Parenteral: 4 μg/mL solution for injection
 Oral: 0.1, 0.2 mg tablets

Follitropin alfa (Gonal-F)
 Parenteral: 37.5, 150 IU powder for injection
Follitropin beta [FSH] (Follistim)
 Parenteral: 75 IU powder for injection
Ganirelix (Antagon)
 Parenteral: 500 μg/mL for injection
Gonadorelin acetate [GnRH] (Lutrepulse)
 Parenteral: powder to reconstitute for injection via Lutrepulse pump (0.8, 3.2 mg/vial)
Gonadorelin hydrochloride [GnRH] (Factrel)
 Parenteral: 100, 500 mg for injection
Goserelin acetate (Zoladex)
 Parenteral: 3.6, 10.8 mg subcutaneous implant
Histrelin (Supprelin)
 Parenteral: 120, 300, 600 mg for subcutaneous injection
Leuprolide (generic, Lupron)
 Parenteral: 5 mg/mL for subcutaneous injection
 Parenteral depot suspension (Lupron Depot, Depot-Ped, Depot-3, Depot-4): lyophilized micro-spheres to reconstitute for IM injection (3.75, 7.5, 11.25, 15, 22.5, 30 mg/vial)
 Parenteral implant: 72 mg

Menotropins [hMG] (Pergonal, Repronex)
Parenteral: 75 IU FSH and 75 IU LH activity, 150 IU FSH and 150 IU LH activity, each with diluent

Nafarelin (Synarel)
Nasal: 2 mg/mL (200 µg/spray)

Octreotide (Sandostatin)
Parenteral: 0.05, 0.1, 0.2, 0.5, 1.0 mg/mL for subcutaneous or IV administration
Parenteral depot injection (Sandostatin LAR Depot): 10, 20, 30 mg for IM injection only

Oxytocin (generic, Pitocin, Syntocinon)
Parenteral: 10 units/mL for injection
Nasal: 40 units/mL spray

Pergolide (Permax)
Oral: 0.05, 0.25, 1.0 mg tablets

Protirelin (Thypinone, Relefact TRH, Thyrel TRH)
Parenteral: 500 mg/mL for injection

Sermorelin (Geref)
Parenteral: 0.5, 1.0 mg for subcutaneous injection; 50 µg powder to reconstitute for intravenous injection

Somatrem (Protropin)
Parenteral: 5, 10 mg/vial with diluent for subcutaneous or IM injection

Somatropin (Genotropin, Humatrope, Nutropin, Nutropin AQ, Norditropin, Serostim, Saizen)
Parenteral: 0.2, 0.4, 0.6, 0.8, 1.0, 1.2, 1.4, 1.5, 1.6, 1.8, 2, 4, 5, 5.8, 6, 8, 10, 12, 13.5, 13.8, 15, 18, 22.5, 24 mg/vial with diluent for subcutaneous or IM injection

Thyrotropin alpha (Thyrogen)
Parenteral: 1.1 mg (> 4 IU)/vial with diluent for IM injection

Triptorelin (Trelstar)
Parenteral: 3.75, 11.25 mg for IM injection

Urofollitropin (Fertinex, Bravelle)
Parenteral: powder to reconstitute for injection, 75, 150 IU FSH activity per ampule

Vasopressin (generic, Pitressin)
Parenteral: 20 pressor units/mL for IM or subcutaneous administration

REFERENCES

HYPOTHALAMIC RELEASING & INHIBITING HORMONES

Agarwal SK: Comparative effects of GnRH agonist therapy. Review of clinical studies and their implications. J Reprod Med 1998;43(Suppl):293.

Bell GI, Reisine T: Molecular biology of somatostatin receptors. Trends Neurosci 1993;16:34.

Biller BM: Hyperprolactinemia. Int J Fertil Womens Med 1999;44:74.

Buchter D et al: Pulsatile GnRH or human chorionic gonadotropin/human menopausal gonadotropin as effective treatment for men with hypogonadotropic hypogonadism: a review of 42 cases. Eur J Endocrinol 1998;139:298.

Cannavo S et al: Cabergoline: a first-choice treatment in patients with previously untreated prolactin-secreting pituitary adenoma. J Endocrinol Invest 1999;22:354.

Catt KJ: Molecular mechanisms of hormone action: Control of target cell function by peptide and catecholamine hormones. In: Felig P, Baxter JD, Frohman LA (editors). *Endocrinology and Metabolism,* 3rd ed. McGraw-Hill, 1995.

Celio L et al: Premenopausal breast cancer patients treated with a gonadotropin-releasing hormone analog alone or in combination with an aromatase inhibitor: a comparative endocrine study. Anticancer Res 1999;19:2261.

de Jong D et al: High dose gonadotropin-releasing hormone antagonist (ganirelix) may prevent ovarian hyperstimulation syndrome caused by ovarian stimulation for in-vitro fertilization. Hum Reprod 1998;13:573.

Elias KA et al: In vitro characterization of four novel classes of growth hormone-releasing peptides. Endocrinology 1995; 136:5694.

Findling JW, Raff H: Newer diagnostic techniques and problems in Cushing's disease. Endocrinol Metab Clin North Am 1999;28:191.

Ghigo E et al: Diagnostic and therapeutic uses of growth hormone-releasing substances in adult and elderly subjects. Baillieres Clin Endocrinol Metab 1998;12:341.

Gill PS et al: The effects of preparations of human chorionic gonadotropin on AIDS-related Kaposi's sarcoma. N Engl J Med 1996;335:1261.

Gillis JC et al: Octreotide long-acting release (LAR). A review of its pharmacological properties and therapeutic use in the management of acromegaly. Drugs 1997;53:681.

Growth Hormone Antagonist for Proliferative Diabetic Retinopathy Study Group: The effect of a growth hormone receptor antagonist drug on proliferative diabetic retinopathy. Ophthalmology 2001;108:2266.

Homann CN et al: Sleep attacks in patients taking dopamine agonists: review. BMJ 2002;324:1483.

Klingmuller D et al: Hormonal responses to the new potent GnRH antagonist Cetrorelix. Acta Endocrinol 1993;128:15.

Lamberts SWJ et al: Octreotide. N Engl J Med 1996;334:246.

Locatelli V, Torsello A: Growth hormone secretagogues: focus on the growth hormone-releasing peptides. Pharmacol Res 1997;36:415.

Loewe C, Dragovic LJ: Acute coronary artery thrombosis in a postpartum woman receiving bromocriptine. Am J Forensic Med Pathol 1998;19:258.

Minaguchi H, Wong JM, Snabes MC: Clinical use of nafarelin in the treatment of leiomyomas. A review of the literature. J Reprod Med 2000;45:481.

Morange I et al: Prolactinomas resistant to bromocriptine: long-term efficacy of quinagolide and outcome of pregnancy. Eur J Endocrinol 1996;135:413.

Pitts LH et al: Treatment with thyrotropin-releasing hormone (TRH) in patients with traumatic spinal cord injuries. J Neurotrauma 1995;12:235.

Spencer CA et al: Thyrotropin (TSH)-releasing hormone stimulation test responses employing third and fourth generation TSH assays. J Clin Endocrinol Metab 1993;76:494.

Tang XT et al: Cellular mechanisms of growth inhibition of human epithelial ovarian cancer cell line by LH-releasing hormone antagonist cetrorelix. J Clin Endocrinol Metab 2002;87:3721.

Van Eijck CH et al: Somatostatin receptor imaging and therapy of pancreatic endocrine tumors. Ann Oncol 1999; 10(Suppl):177.

ANTERIOR PITUITARY HORMONES

Abdennebi L et al: Generating FSH antagonists and agonists through immunization against FSH receptor N-terminal decapeptides. J Mol Endocrinol 1999;22:151.

Abdu TA et al: Comparison of the low dose short synacthen test (1 mcg), the conventional dose short synacthen test (250 mcg), and the insulin tolerance test for assessment of the hypothalamo-pituitary-adrenal axis in patients with pituitary disease. J Clin Endocrinol Metab 1999;84:838.

Bevan JS et al: Primary medical therapy for acromegaly: an open, prospective, multicenter study of the effects of subcutaneous and intramuscular slow-release octreotide on growth hormone, insulin-like growth factor-I, and tumor size. J Clin Endocrinol Metab 2002;87:4554.

Bornstein SR, Chrousos GP: Adrenocorticotropin (ACTH)- and non-ACTH-mediated regulation of the adrenal cortex: neural and immune inputs. J Clin Endocrinol Metab 1999;84:1729.

Carter-Su C, Schwartz J, Smit LS: Molecular mechanism of growth hormone action. Annu Rev Physiol 1996;58:187.

Cook DM et al: The pharmacokinetic and pharmacodynamic characteristics of a long-acting growth hormone (GH) preparation (Nutropin Depot) in GH-deficient adults. J Clin Endocrinol Metab 2002;87:4508.

Daya S: Updated meta-analysis of recombinant follicle-stimulating hormone (FSH) versus urinary FSH for ovarian stimulation in assisted reproduction. Fertil Steril 2002;77:711.

Demling R: Growth hormone therapy in critically ill patients. N Engl J Med 1999;341:837.

Drake WM et al: Optimizing growth hormone replacement therapy by dose titration in hypopituitary adults. J Clin Endocrinol Metab 1998;83:3913.

Goffin V, Touraine P: Pegvisomant. Pharmacia. Curr Opin Investig Drugs 2002;3:752.

Ladenson PW: Strategies for thyrotropin use to monitor patients with treated thyroid carcinoma. Thyroid 1999;9:429.

Liu PY et al: Efficacy and safety of recombinant human follicle stimulating hormone (Gonal-F) with urinary human chorionic gonadotrophin for induction of spermatogenesis and fertility in gonadotrophin-deficient men. Hum Reprod 1999; 14:1540.

Papadakis MA et al: Growth hormone replacement in healthy older men improves body composition but not functional ability. Ann Intern Med 1996;124:708.

Prevost RR: Recombinant follicle-stimulating hormone: new biotechnology for infertility. Pharmacotherapy 1998;18:1001.

Ricci E et al: Pregnancy outcome after cabergoline treatment in early weeks of gestation. Reprod Toxicol 2002;16:791.

Rose MP: Follicle stimulating hormone international standards and reference preparations for the calibration of immunoassays and bioassays. Clin Chem Acta 1998;273:103.

Schultz PN et al. Quinagolide in the management of prolactinoma. Pituitary 2000;3:239.

Schmidt DN, Wallace K: How to diagnose hypopituitarism. Learning the features of secondary hormonal deficiencies. Postgrad Med 1998;104:77.

Spirtas R et al: Fertility drugs and ovarian cancer: Red alert or red herring? Fertil Steril 1993;59:291.

van der Lely AJ et al: Long-term treatment of acromegaly with pegvisomant, a growth hormone receptor antagonist. Lancet 2001;358:1754.

Van Wely M et al: Human menopausal gonadotropin versus recombinant follicle stimulation hormone for ovarian stimulation in assisted reproductive cycles (Cochrane Review). Cochrane Database Syst Rev 2003;(1):CD003973.

Weintraub BD, Szkudlinski MS: Development and in vitro characterization of human recombinant thyrotropin. Thyroid 1999;9:447.

Windisch PA et al: Recombinant human growth hormone for AIDS-associated wasting. Ann Pharmacother 1998;32:437.

Zward-van Rijkom JE, Broekmans FJ, Leufkens HG: From HMG through purified urinary FSH preparations to recombinant FSH: a substitution study. Hum Reprod 2002;17:857.

POSTERIOR PITUITARY HORMONES

Deitcher SR et al: Intranasal DDAVP induced increases in plasma von Willebrand factor alter the pharmacokinetics of high-purity factor VIII concentrates in severe haemophilia A patients. Haemophilia 1999;5:88.

Harman JH Jr, Kim A: Current trends in cervical ripening and labor induction. Am Fam Physician 1999;60:477.

Ray JG: DDAVP use during pregnancy: an analysis of its safety for mother and child. Obstet Gynecol Surv 1998;53:450.

Shindel A et al: Hyponatremia associated with desmopressin for the treatment of nocturnal polyuria. Urology 2002;60:344.

Thyroid & Antithyroid Drugs

Francis S. Greenspan, MD, & Betty J. Dong, PharmD

Because of its anatomic prominence, the thyroid was one of the first of the endocrine glands to be associated with the clinical conditions caused by its malfunction.

THYROID PHYSIOLOGY

The normal thyroid gland secretes sufficient amounts of the thyroid hormones—triiodothyronine (T_3) and tetraiodothyronine (T_4, thyroxine)—to normalize growth and development, body temperature, and energy levels. These hormones contain 59% and 65% (respectively) of iodine as an essential part of the molecule. Calcitonin, the second type of thyroid hormone, is important in the regulation of calcium metabolism and is discussed in Chapter 42.

Iodide Metabolism

The recommended daily adult iodide (I^-)* intake is 150 μg (200 μg during pregnancy).

Iodide, ingested from food, water, or medication, is rapidly absorbed and enters an extracellular fluid pool. The thyroid gland removes about 75 μg a day from this pool for hormone secretion, and the balance is excreted in the urine. If iodide intake is increased, the fractional iodine uptake by the thyroid is diminished.

Biosynthesis of Thyroid Hormones

Once taken up by the thyroid gland, iodide undergoes a series of enzymatic reactions that convert it into active thyroid hormone (Figure 38–1). The first step is the transport of iodide into the thyroid gland by an intrinsic follicle cell basement membrane protein called the sodium/iodide symporter (NIS). This can be inhibited by such anions as SCN^-, TcO_4^-, and ClO_4^-. Iodide is then oxidized by thyroidal peroxidase to iodine, in which form it rapidly iodinates tyrosine residues within the thyroglobulin molecule to form monoiodotyrosine (MIT) and diiodotyrosine (DIT). This process is called **iodide organification.** Thyroidal peroxidase is tran-

---

* In this chapter, the term "iodine" denotes all forms of the element; the term "iodide" denotes only the ionic form, I^-.

siently blocked by high levels of intrathyroidal iodide and blocked more persistently by thioamide drugs. Two molecules of DIT combine within the thyroglobulin molecule to form L-thyroxine (T_4). One molecule of MIT and one molecule of DIT combine to form T_3. In addition to thyroglobulin, other proteins within the gland may be iodinated, but these iodoproteins do not have hormonal activity. Thyroxine, T_3, MIT, and DIT are released from thyroglobulin by **exocytosis** and **proteolysis** of thyroglobulin at the apical colloid border. The MIT and DIT are deiodinated within the gland, and the iodine is reutilized. This process of proteolysis is also blocked by high levels of intrathyroidal iodide. The ratio of T_4 to T_3 within thyroglobulin is approximately 5:1, so that most of the hormone released is thyroxine. Most of the T_3 circulating in the blood is derived from peripheral metabolism of thyroxine (see below).

Transport of Thyroid Hormones

T_4 and T_3 in plasma are reversibly bound to protein, primarily thyroxine-binding globulin (TBG). Only about 0.04% of total T_4 and 0.4% of T_3 exist in the free form. Many physiologic and pathologic states and drugs affect T_4, T_3, and thyroid transport. However, the actual levels of free hormone generally remain normal, reflecting feedback control.

Peripheral Metabolism of Thyroid Hormones

The primary pathway for the peripheral metabolism of thyroxine is deiodination. Deiodination of T_4 may occur by monodeiodination of the outer ring, producing 3,5,3'-triiodothyronine (T_3), which is three to four times more potent than T_4. Alternatively, deiodination may occur in the inner ring, producing 3,3',5'-triiodothyronine (reverse T_3, or rT_3), which is metabolically inactive (Figure 38–2). Drugs such as ipodate, β-blockers, and corticosteroids, and severe illness or starvation inhibit the 5'-deiodinase necessary for the conversion of T_4 to T_3, resulting in low T_3 and high rT_3 levels in the serum. Normal levels of thyroid hormone in the serum are listed in Table 38–1. The low serum

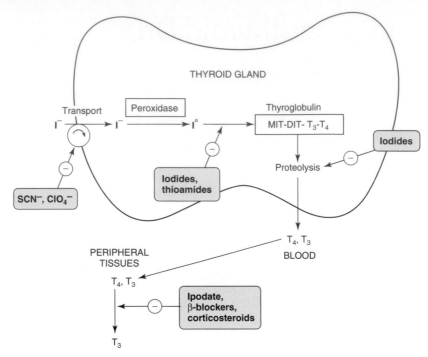

Figure 38–1. Biosynthesis of thyroid hormones. The sites of action of various drugs that interfere with thyroid hormone biosynthesis are shown.

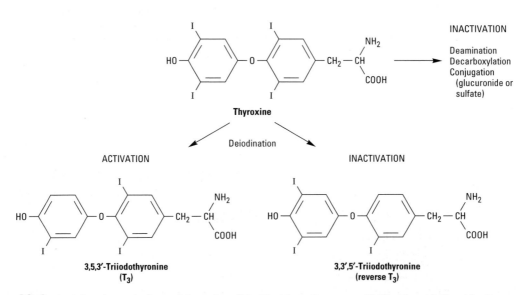

Figure 38–2. Peripheral metabolism of thyroxine. (Modified from Greenspan FS: The Thyroid Gland. In: Greenspan FS, Gardner D [editors]: *Basic & Clinical Endocrinology,* 6th ed. McGraw-Hill, 2001.)

Table 38–1. Summary of thyroid hormone kinetics.

Variable	T$_4$	T$_3$
Volume of distribution	10 L	40 L
Extrathyroidal pool	800 μg	54 μg
Daily production	75 μg	25 μg
Fractional turnover per day	10%	60%
Metabolic clearance per day	1.1 L	24 L
Half-life (biologic)	7 days	1 day
Serum levels		
Total	5–11 μg/dL (64–132 nmol/L)	95–190 ng/dL (1.5–2.9 nmol/L)
Free	0.7–1.86 ng/dL (9–24 pmol/L)	0.2–0.52 ng/dL (3–8 pmol/L)
Amount bound	99.96%	99.6%
Biologic potency	1	4
Oral absorption	80%	95%

levels of T$_3$ and rT$_3$ in normal individuals are due to the high metabolic clearances of these two compounds.

Control of Thyroid Function

The tests used to evaluate thyroid function are listed in Table 38–2.

A. Thyroid-Pituitary Relationships

Control of thyroid function via thyroid-pituitary feedback is also discussed in Chapter 37. Briefly, hypothalamic cells secrete thyrotropin-releasing hormone (TRH) (Figure 38–3). TRH is secreted into capillaries of the pituitary portal venous system, and in the pituitary gland, TRH stimulates the synthesis and release of thyroid-stimulating hormone (TSH). TSH in turn stimulates an adenylyl cyclase–mediated mechanism in the thyroid cell to increase the synthesis and release of T$_4$ and T$_3$. These thyroid hormones act in a negative feedback fashion in the pituitary to block the action of TRH and in the hypothalamus to inhibit the synthesis and secretion of TRH. Other hormones or drugs may also affect the release of TRH or TSH.

B. Autoregulation of the Thyroid Gland

The thyroid gland also regulates its uptake of iodide and thyroid hormone synthesis by intrathyroidal mechanisms that are independent of TSH. These mechanisms are primarily related to the level of iodine in the blood.

Large doses of iodine inhibit iodide organification (Figure 38–1). In certain disease states (eg, Hashimoto's thyroiditis), this can result in inhibition of thyroid hormone synthesis and hypothyroidism.

C. Abnormal Thyroid Stimulators

In Graves' disease (see below), lymphocytes secrete a TSH receptor-stimulating antibody (TSH-R Ab [stim]), also known as thyroid-stimulating immunoglobulin (TSI). This immunoglobulin binds to the TSH receptor and turns on the gland in the same fashion as TSH itself. The duration of its effect, however, is much longer than that of TSH. TSH receptors are also found in orbital fibrocytes, which may be stimulated by high levels of TSH-R Ab [stim].

I. BASIC PHARMACOLOGY OF THYROID & ANTITHYROID DRUGS

THYROID HORMONES

Chemistry

The structural formulas of thyroxine and triiodothyronine as well as reverse triiodothyronine (rT$_3$) are shown

Table 38–2. Normal values for thyroid function tests.

Name of Test	Normal Value[1]	Results in Hypothyroidism	Results in Hyperthyroidism
Total thyroxine by RIA (T$_4$ [RIA])	5–12 µg/dL (64–154 nmol/L)	Low	High
Total triiodothyronine by RIA (T$_3$ [RIA])	70–132 ng/dL (1.1–2.0 nmol/L)	Normal or low	High
Resin T$_3$ uptake (RT$_3$U)	25–35%	Low	High
Free thyroxine index (FT$_4$I)[1]	1.3–4.2	Low	High
Free T$_3$ index (FT$_3$I)	17.5–46	Normal or low	High
Free FT$_4$ (FT$_4$)	0.7–1.86 (9–24 pmol/L)	Low	High
Free T$_3$ (FT$_3$)	0.2–0.42 ng/dL (3–8 pmol/L)	Low	High
Thyrotropic hormone (TSH)	0.5–5.0 µIU/mL (0.5–5.0 mIU/L)	High[2]	Low
^{123}I uptake at 24 hours	5–35%	Low	High
Thyroglobulin autoantibodies (Tg-ab)	< 1 IU/mL	Often present	Usually present
Thyroid peroxidase antibodies (TPA)	< 1 IU/mL	Often present	Usually present
Isotope scan with ^{123}I or ^{99m}TcO$_4$	Normal pattern	Test not indicated	Diffusely enlarged gland
Fine-needle aspiration biopsy (FNA)	Normal pattern	Test not indicated	Test not indicated
Serum thyroglobulin	< 40 ng/mL	Test not indicated	Test not indicated
Serum calcitonin	Male:< 8 ng/L (< 2.3 pmol/L); female:< 4 ng/L (< 1.17 pmol/L)	Test not indicated	Test not indicated

[1]Results may vary with different laboratories.

[2]Exception is central hypothyroidism

in Figure 38–2. All of these naturally occurring molecules are levo (L) isomers. The synthetic dextro (D) isomer of thyroxine, dextrothyroxine, has approximately 4% of the biologic activity of the L isomer as evidenced by its lesser ability to suppress TSH secretion and correct hypothyroidism.

Pharmacokinetics

Thyroxine is absorbed best in the duodenum and ileum; absorption is modified by intraluminal factors such as food, drugs, and intestinal flora. Oral bioavailability of current preparations of L-thyroxine averages 80% (Table 38–1). In contrast, T$_3$ is almost completely absorbed (95%). T$_4$ and T$_3$ absorption appears not to be affected by mild hypothyroidism but may be impaired in severe myxedema with ileus. These factors are important in switching from oral to parenteral therapy. For parenteral use, the intravenous route is preferred for both hormones.

In patients with hyperthyroidism, the metabolic clearances of T$_4$ and T$_3$ are increased and the half-lives decreased; the opposite is true in patients with hypothyroidism. Drugs that induce hepatic microsomal enzymes (eg, rifampin, phenobarbital, carbamazepine, phenytoin) increase the metabolism of both T$_4$ and T$_3$ (Table 38–3). Despite this change in clearance, the normal hormone concentration is maintained in euthyroid patients as a result of compensatory hyperfunction of the thyroid. However, patients receiving T$_4$ replacement medication may require increased dosages to maintain clinical effectiveness. A similar compensation occurs if binding sites are altered. If TBG sites are increased by pregnancy, estrogens, or oral contraceptives, there is an initial shift of hormone from the free to the bound state and a decrease in its rate of elimination until the normal hormone concentration is restored. Thus, the concentration of total and bound hormone will increase, but the concentration of free hormone and the steady state

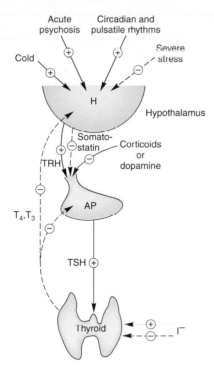

Figure 38–3. The hypothalamic-pituitary-thyroid axis. Acute psychosis or prolonged exposure to cold may activate the axis. Hypothalamic TRH stimulates pituitary TSH release, while somatostatin and dopamine inhibit it. TSH stimulates T_4 and T_3 synthesis and release from the thyroid, and they in turn inhibit both TRH and TSH synthesis and release. Small amounts of iodide are necessary for hormone production, but large amounts inhibit T_3 and T_4 production and release. (Solid arrows, stimulatory influence; dashed arrows, inhibitory influence. H, hypothalamus, HP, anterior pituitary.)

elimination will remain normal. The reverse occurs when thyroid binding sites are decreased.

Mechanism of Action

A model of thyroid hormone action is depicted in Figure 38–4, which shows the free forms of thyroid hormones, T_4 and T_3, dissociated from thyroid-binding proteins, entering the cell by diffusion or possibly by active transport. Within the cell, T_4 is converted to T_3 by 5'-deiodinase, and the T_3 enters the nucleus, where T_3 binds to a specific T_3 receptor protein, a member of the *c-erb* oncogene family, which also includes the steroid hormone receptors and receptors for vitamins A and D. The T_3 receptor exists in two forms, α and β. Differing concentrations of receptor forms in different

tissues may account for variations in T_3 effect on different tissues.

Most of the effects of thyroid on metabolic processes appear to be mediated by activation of nuclear receptors that lead to increased formation of RNA and subsequent protein synthesis, eg, increased formation of Na^+/K^+ ATPase. This is consistent with the observation that the action of thyroid is manifested in vivo with a time lag of hours or days after its administration.

Large numbers of thyroid hormone receptors are found in the most hormone-responsive tissues (pituitary, liver, kidney, heart, skeletal muscle, lung, and intestine), while few receptor sites occur in hormone-unresponsive tissues (spleen, testes). The brain, which lacks an anabolic response to T_3, contains an intermediate number of receptors. In congruence with their biologic potencies, the affinity of the receptor site for T_4 is about ten times lower than that for T_3. The number of nuclear receptors may be altered to preserve body homeostasis. For example, starvation lowers both circulating T_3 hormone and cellular T_3 receptors.

Effects of Thyroid Hormones

The thyroid hormones are responsible for optimal growth, development, function, and maintenance of all body tissues. Excess or inadequate amounts result in the signs and symptoms of thyrotoxicosis or hypothyroidism (Table 38–4). Since T_3 and T_4 are qualitatively similar, they may be considered as one hormone in the discussion that follows.

Thyroid hormone is critical for nervous, skeletal, and reproductive tissues. Its effects depend on protein synthesis as well as potentiation of the secretion and action of growth hormone. Thyroid deprivation in early life results in irreversible mental retardation and dwarfism—symptoms typical of congenital cretinism.

Effects on growth and calorigenesis are accompanied by a pervasive influence on metabolism of drugs as well as carbohydrates, fats, proteins, and vitamins. Many of these changes are dependent upon or modified by activity of other hormones. Conversely, the secretion and degradation rates of virtually all other hormones, including catecholamines, cortisol, estrogens, testosterone, and insulin, are affected by thyroid status.

Many of the manifestations of thyroid hyperactivity resemble sympathetic nervous system overactivity (especially in the cardiovascular system), although catecholamine levels are not increased. Changes in catecholamine-stimulated adenylyl cyclase activity as measured by cAMP are found with changes in thyroid activity. Possible explanations include increased numbers of β receptors or enhanced amplification of the β receptor signal. Other clinical symptoms reminiscent of excessive epinephrine activity (and partially alleviated by

Table 38–3. Drug effects and thyroid function.

Drug Effect	Drugs
Change in thyroid hormone synthesis	
Inhibition of TRH or TSH secretion without induction of hypothyroidism	Dopamine, levodopa, corticosteroids, somatostatin
Inhibition of thyroid hormone synthesis or release with the induction of hypothyroidism (or occasionally hyperthyroidism)	Iodides (including amiodarone), lithium, aminoglutethimide
Alteration of thyroid hormone transport and serum total T_3 and T_4 levels, but usually no modification of FT_4 or TSH	
Increased TBG	Estrogens, tamoxifen, heroin, methadone, mitotane
Decreased TBG	Androgens, glucocorticoids
Displacement of T_3 and T_4 from TBG with transient hyperthyroxinemia	Salicylates, fenclofenac, mefenamic acid, furosemide
Alteration of T_4 and T_3 metabolism with modified serum T_3 and T_4 levels but not FT_4 or TSH levels	
Induction of increased hepatic enzyme activity	Phenytoin, carbamazepine, phenobarbital, rifampin, rifabutin
Inhibition of 5'-deiodinase with decreased T_3, increased rT_3	Iopanoic acid, ipodate, amiodarone, β-blockers, corticosteroids, propylthiouracil
Other interactions	
Interference with T_4 absorption	Cholestyramine, colestipol, aluminum hydroxide, sucralfate, reloxifene, ferrous sulfate, some calcium preparations, bran
Induction of autoimmune thyroid disease with hypothyroidism or hyperthyroidism	Interferon-α, interleukin-2

adrenoceptor antagonists) include lid lag and retraction, tremor, excessive sweating, anxiety, and nervousness. The opposite constellation of symptoms is seen in hypothyroidism (Table 38–4).

Thyroid Preparations

See the Preparations Available section at the end of this chapter for a list of available preparations. These preparations may be synthetic (levothyroxine, liothyronine, liotrix) or of animal origin (desiccated thyroid).

Synthetic levothyroxine is the preparation of choice for thyroid replacement and suppression therapy because of its stability, content uniformity, low cost, lack of allergenic foreign protein, easy laboratory measurement of serum levels, and long half-life (7 days), which permits once-daily administration. In addition, T_4 is converted to T_3 intracellularly; thus, administration of T_4 produces both hormones. Generic levothyroxine preparations can be used because they provide comparable efficacy and are more cost-effective than branded preparations.

Although liothyronine is three to four times more potent than levothyroxine, it is not recommended for routine replacement therapy because of its shorter half-life (24 hours), which requires multiple daily doses; its higher cost; and the greater difficulty of monitoring its adequacy of replacement by conventional laboratory tests. Furthermore, because of its greater hormone activity and consequent greater risk of cardiotoxicity, T_3 should be avoided in patients with cardiac disease. It is best used for short-term suppression of TSH. Because oral administration of T_3 is unnecessary, use of the more expensive mixture of thyroxine and liothyronine (liotrix) instead of levothyroxine is never required.

The use of desiccated thyroid rather than synthetic preparations is never justified, since the disadvantages of protein antigenicity, product instability, variable hormone concentrations, and difficulty in laboratory monitoring far outweigh the advantage of low cost. Significant amounts of T_3 found in some thyroid extracts and liotrix may produce significant elevations in T_3 levels and toxicity. Equivalent doses are 100 mg (1.5 g) of desiccated thyroid, 100 μg of levothyroxine, and 37.5 μg of liothyronine.

The shelf life of synthetic hormone preparations is about 2 years, particularly if they are stored in dark bot-

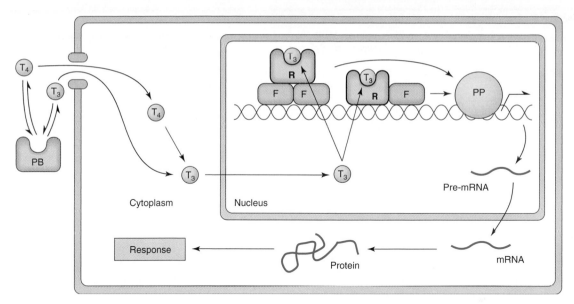

Figure 38–4. Regulation of transcription by thyroid hormones. T_3 and T_4 are triiodothyronine and thyroxine, respectively. PB, plasma binding protein; F, transcription factor; R, receptor; PP, proteins that bind at the proximal promoter. (Reproduced, with permission, from Baxter JD: General concepts of endocrinology. In: Greenspan FS, Baxter JD (editors). *Basic & Clinical Endocrinology*, 4th ed. Originally published by Appleton & Lange. Copyright © 1994 by The McGraw-Hill Companies, Inc.)

tles to minimize spontaneous deiodination. The shelf life of desiccated thyroid is not certainly known, but its potency is better preserved if it is kept dry.

ANTITHYROID AGENTS

Reduction of thyroid activity and hormone effects can be accomplished by agents that interfere with the production of thyroid hormones; by agents that modify the tissue response to thyroid hormones; or by glandular destruction with radiation or surgery. "Goitrogens" are agents that suppress secretion of T_3 and T_4 to subnormal levels and thereby increase TSH, which in turn produces glandular enlargement (goiter). The antithyroid compounds used clinically include the thioamides, iodides, and radioactive iodine.

1. Thioamides

The thioamides methimazole and propylthiouracil are major drugs for treatment of thyrotoxicosis. In the United Kingdom, carbimazole, which is converted to methimazole in vivo, is widely used. Methimazole is about ten times more potent than propylthiouracil.

The chemical structures of these compounds are shown in Figure 38–5. The thiocarbamide group is essential for antithyroid activity.

Pharmacokinetics

Propylthiouracil is rapidly absorbed, reaching peak serum levels after 1 hour. The bioavailability of 50–80% may be due to incomplete absorption or a large first-pass effect in the liver. The volume of distribution approximates total body water with accumulation in the thyroid gland. Most of an ingested dose of propylthiouracil is excreted by the kidney as the inactive glucuronide within 24 hours.

In contrast, methimazole is completely absorbed but at variable rates. It is readily accumulated by the thyroid gland and has a volume of distribution similar to that of propylthiouracil. Excretion is slower than with propylthiouracil; 65–70% of a dose is recovered in the urine in 48 hours.

The short plasma half-life of these agents (1.5 hours for propylthiouracil and 6 hours for methimazole) has little influence on the duration of the antithyroid action or the dosing interval because both agents are accumulated by the thyroid gland. For propylthiouracil, giving the drug every 6–8 hours is reasonable since a single 100 mg dose can inhibit 60% of iodine organification for 7 hours. Since a single 30 mg dose of methimazole exerts an antithyroid effect for longer than 24 hours, a single daily dose is effective in the management of mild to moderate hyperthyroidism.

Table 38–4. Manifestations of thyrotoxicosis and hypothyroidism.

System	Thyrotoxicosis	Hypothyroidism
Skin and appendages	Warm, moist skin; sweating; heat intolerance; fine, thin hair; Plummer's nails; pretibial dermopathy (Graves' disease)	Pale, cool, puffy skin; dry and brittle hair; brittle nails
Eyes, face	Retraction of upper lid with wide stare; periorbital edema; exophthalmos; diplopia (Graves' disease)	Drooping of eyelids; periorbital edema; loss of temporal aspects of eyebrows; puffy, nonpitting facies; large tongue
Cardiovascular system	Decreased peripheral vascular resistance, increased heart rate, stroke volume, cardiac output, pulse pressure; high-output heart failure; increased inotropic and chronotropic effects; arrhythmias; angina	Increased peripheral vascular resistance; decreased heart rate, stroke volume, cardiac output, pulse pressure; low-output heart failure; ECG: bradycardia, prolonged PR interval, flat T wave, low voltage; pericardial effusion
Respiratory system	Dyspnea; decreased vital capacity	Pleural effusions; hypoventilation and CO_2 retention
Gastrointestinal system	Increased appetite; increased frequency of bowel movements; hypoproteinemia	Decreased appetite; decreased frequency of bowel movements; ascites
Central nervous system	Nervousness; hyperkinesia; emotional lability	Lethargy; general slowing of mental processes; neuropathies
Musculoskeletal system	Weakness and muscle fatigue; increased deep tendon reflexes; hypercalcemia; osteoporosis	Stiffness and muscle fatigue; decreased deep tendon reflexes; increased alkaline phosphatase, LDH, AST
Renal system	Mild polyuria; increased renal blood flow; increased glomerular filtration rate	Impaired water excretion; decreased renal blood flow; decreased glomerular filtration rate
Hematopoietic system	Increased erythropoiesis; anemia[1]	Decreased erythropoiesis; anemia[1]
Reproductive system	Menstrual irregularities; decreased fertility; increased gonadal steroid metabolism	Hypermenorrhea; infertility; decreased libido; impotence; oligospermia; decreased gonadal steroid metabolism
Metabolic system	Increased basal metabolic rate; negative nitrogen balance; hyperglycemia; increased free fatty acids; decreased cholesterol and triglycerides; increased hormone degradation; increased requirements for fat- and water-soluble vitamins; increased drug metabolism	Decreased basal metabolic rate; slight positive nitrogen balance; delayed degradation of insulin, with increased sensitivity; increased cholesterol and triglycerides; decreased hormone degradation; decreased requirements for fat- and water-soluble vitamins; decreased drug metabolism

[1]The anemia of hyperthyroidism is usually normochromic and caused by increased red blood cell turnover. The anemia of hypothyroidism may be normochromic, hyperchromic, or hypochromic and may be due to decreased production rate, decreased iron absorption, decreased folic acid absorption, or to autoimmune pernicious anemia.

Both thioamides cross the placental barrier and are concentrated by the fetal thyroid, so that caution must be employed when using these drugs in pregnancy. Of the two, propylthiouracil is preferable in pregnancy because it is more strongly protein-bound and therefore crosses the placenta less readily. In addition, it is not secreted in sufficient quantity in breast milk to preclude breast-feeding.

Pharmacodynamics

The thioamides act by multiple mechanisms. The major action is to prevent hormone synthesis by inhibiting the thyroid peroxidase-catalyzed reactions and blocking iodine organification. In addition, they block coupling of the iodotyrosines. They do not block uptake of iodide by the gland. Propylthiouracil and (to a much lesser

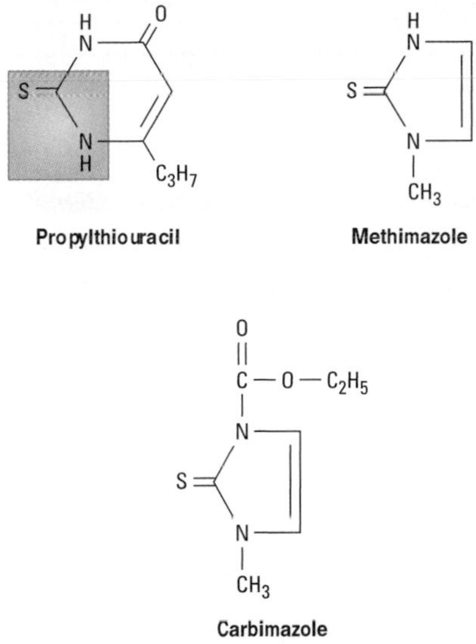

Figure 38–5. Structure of thioamides. The thiocarbamide moiety is shown in color.

extent) methimazole inhibit the peripheral deiodination of T_4 and T_3 (Figure 38–1). Since the synthesis rather than the release of hormones is affected, the onset of these agents is slow, often requiring 3–4 weeks before stores of T_4 are depleted.

Toxicity

Adverse reactions to the thioamides occur in 3–12% of treated patients. Most reactions occur early. The most common adverse effect is a maculopapular pruritic rash, at times accompanied by systemic signs such as fever. Rare adverse effects include an urticarial rash, vasculitis, arthralgia, a lupus-like reaction, cholestatic jaundice, hepatitis, lymphadenopathy, hypoprothrombinemia, exfoliative dermatitis, polyserositis, and acute arthralgia.

The most dangerous complication is agranulocytosis, an infrequent but potentially fatal adverse reaction. It occurs in 0.3–0.6% of patients taking thioamides, but the risk may be increased in older patients and in those receiving high-dose methimazole therapy (over 40 mg/d). The reaction is usually rapidly reversible when the drug is discontinued, but antibiotic therapy may be necessary for complicating infections. Colony-stimulating factors (eg, G-CSF; see Chapter 33) may hasten recovery of the granulocytes. The cross-sensitivity between propylthiouracil and methimazole is about 50%; therefore, switching drugs in patients with severe reactions is not recommended.

2. Anion Inhibitors

Monovalent anions such as perchlorate (ClO_4^-), pertechnetate (TcO_4^-), and thiocyanate (SCN^-) can block uptake of iodide by the gland through competitive inhibition of the iodide transport mechanism. Since these effects can be overcome by large doses of iodides, their effectiveness is somewhat unpredictable.

The major clinical use for potassium perchlorate is to block thyroidal reuptake of I^- in patients with iodide-induced hyperthyroidism (eg, amiodarone-induced hyperthyroidism). However, potassium perchlorate is rarely used clinically because it has been shown to cause aplastic anemia.

3. Iodides

Prior to the introduction of the thioamides in the 1940s, iodides were the major antithyroid agents; today they are rarely used as sole therapy.

Pharmacodynamics

Iodides have several actions on the thyroid. They inhibit organification and hormone release and decrease the size and vascularity of the hyperplastic gland. In susceptible individuals, iodides can induce hyperthyroidism (jodbasedow phenomenon) or precipitate hypothyroidism.

In pharmacologic doses (> 6 mg daily), the major action of iodides is to inhibit hormone release, possibly through inhibition of thyroglobulin proteolysis. Rapid improvement in thyrotoxic symptoms occurs within 2–7 days—hence the value of iodide therapy in thyroid storm. In addition, iodides decrease the vascularity, size, and fragility of a hyperplastic gland, making the drugs valuable as preoperative preparation for surgery.

Clinical Use of Iodide

Disadvantages of iodide therapy include an increase in intraglandular stores of iodine, which may delay onset of thioamide therapy or prevent use of radioactive iodine therapy for several weeks. Thus, iodides should be initiated after onset of thioamide therapy and avoided if treatment with radioactive iodine seems likely. Iodide should not be used alone, because the gland will escape from the iodide block in 2–8 weeks, and its withdrawal may produce severe exacerbation of thyrotoxicosis in an iodine-enriched gland. Chronic use of iodides in pregnancy should be avoided, since they cross the placenta and can cause fetal goiter. In radiation emergencies, the thyroid-blocking effects of potassium iodide can protect the gland from subsequent damage if administered before radiation exposure.

Toxicity

Adverse reactions to iodine (iodism) are uncommon and in most cases reversible upon discontinuance. They include acneiform rash (similar to that of bromism), swollen salivary glands, mucous membrane ulcerations, conjunctivitis, rhinorrhea, drug fever, metallic taste, bleeding disorders and, rarely, anaphylactoid reactions.

4. Iodinated Contrast Media

The iodinated contrast agents—ipodate and iopanoic acid by mouth, or diatrizoate intravenously—are valuable in the treatment of hyperthyroidism, although they are not labeled for this indication. These drugs rapidly inhibit the conversion of T_4 to T_3 in the liver, kidney, pituitary gland, and brain. This accounts for the dramatic improvement in both subjective and objective parameters. For example, a decrease in heart rate is seen after only 3 days of oral administration of 0.5–1 g/d. T_3 levels often return to normal during this time. The prolonged effect of suppressing T_4 as well as T_3 suggests that inhibition of hormone release due to the iodine released may be an additional mechanism of action. Fortunately, these agents are relatively nontoxic. They provide useful adjunctive therapy in the treatment of thyroid storm and offer valuable alternatives when iodides or thioamides are contraindicated. Surprisingly, these agents may not interfere with ^{131}I retention as much as iodides despite their large iodine content. Their toxicity is similar to that of the iodides, and their safety in pregnancy is undocumented.

5. Radioactive Iodine

[131]I is the only isotope used for treatment of thyrotoxicosis (others are used in diagnosis). Administered orally in solution as sodium ^{131}I, it is rapidly absorbed, concentrated by the thyroid, and incorporated into storage follicles. Its therapeutic effect depends on emission of β rays with an effective half-life of 5 days and a penetration range of 400–2000 μm. Within a few weeks after administration, destruction of the thyroid parenchyma is evidenced by epithelial swelling and necrosis, follicular disruption, edema, and leukocyte infiltration. Advantages of radioiodine include easy administration, effectiveness, low expense, and absence of pain. Fears of radiation-induced genetic damage, leukemia, and neoplasia have not been realized after more than 30 years of clinical experience with radioiodine. Radioactive iodine should not be administered to pregnant women or nursing mothers, since it crosses the placenta and is excreted in breast milk.

6. Adrenoceptor-Blocking Agents

Beta blockers without intrinsic sympathomimetic activity are effective therapeutic adjuncts in the management of thyrotoxicosis since many of these symptoms mimic those associated with sympathetic stimulation. Propranolol has been the β-blocker most widely studied and used in the therapy of thyrotoxicosis.

II. CLINICAL PHARMACOLOGY OF THYROID & ANTITHYROID DRUGS

HYPOTHYROIDISM

Hypothyroidism is a syndrome resulting from deficiency of thyroid hormones and is manifested largely by a reversible slowing down of all body functions (Table 38–4). In infants and children, there is striking retardation of growth and development that results in dwarfism and irreversible mental retardation.

The etiology and pathogenesis of hypothyroidism are outlined in Table 38–5. Hypothyroidism can occur with or without thyroid enlargement (goiter). The laboratory diagnosis of hypothyroidism in the adult is easily made by the combination of a low free thyroxine (or low free thyroxine index) and elevated serum TSH (Table 38–2).

The most common cause of hypothyroidism in the USA at this time is probably Hashimoto's thyroiditis, an immunologic disorder in genetically predisposed individuals. In this condition, there is evidence of humoral immunity in the presence of antithyroid antibodies and lymphocyte sensitization to thyroid antigens.

Management of Hypothyroidism

Except for hypothyroidism caused by drugs (Table 38–5), which can be treated by simply removing the depressant agent, the general strategy of replacement therapy is appropriate. The most satisfactory preparation is levothyroxine. Infants and children require more T_4 per kilogram of body weight than adults. The average dosage for an infant 1–6 months of age is 10–15 μg/kg/d, whereas the average dosage for an adult is about 1.7 μg/kg/d. There is some variability in the absorption of thyroxine, so this dosage may vary from patient to patient. Because of the long half-life of thyroxine, the dose can be given once daily. Children should be monitored for normal growth and development. Serum TSH and free thyroxine should be measured at regular intervals and maintained within the normal range. It takes 6–8 weeks after starting a given dose of thyroxine to reach steady state levels in the bloodstream. Thus, dosage changes should be made slowly.

Table 38–5. Etiology and pathogenesis of hypothyroidism.

Cause	Pathogenesis	Goiter	Degree of Hypothyroidism
Hashimoto's thyroiditis	Autoimmune destruction of thyroid	Present early, absent later	Mild to severe
Drug-induced[1]	Blocked hormone formation	Present	Mild to moderate
Dyshormonogenesis	Impaired synthesis of T_4 due to enzyme deficiency	Present	Mild to severe
Radiation, ^{131}I, x-ray, thyroidectomy	Destruction or removal of gland	Absent	Severe
Congenital (cretinism)	Athyreosis or ectopic thyroid, iodine deficiency; TSH receptor-blocking antibodies	Absent or present	Severe
Secondary (TSH deficit)	Pituitary or hypothalamic disease	Absent	Mild

[1]Iodides, lithium, fluoride, thioamides, aminosalicylic acid, phenylbutazone, amiodarone, etc.

In long-standing hypothyroidism, in older patients, and in patients with underlying cardiac disease, it is imperative to start treatment with reduced dosage. In such adult patients, levothyroxine is given in a dosage of 12.5–25 μg/d for 2 weeks, increasing the daily dose by 25 μg every 2 weeks until euthyroidism or drug toxicity is observed. In older patients, the heart is very sensitive to the level of circulating thyroxine, and if angina pectoris or cardiac arrhythmia develops, it is essential to stop or reduce the dose of thyroxine immediately. In younger patients or those with very mild disease, full replacement therapy may be started immediately.

The toxicity of thyroxine is directly related to the hormone level. In children, restlessness, insomnia, and accelerated bone maturation and growth may be signs of thyroxine toxicity. In adults, increased nervousness, heat intolerance, episodes of palpitation and tachycardia, or unexplained weight loss may be the presenting symptoms. If these symptoms are present, it is important to monitor serum TSH (Table 38–2), which will determine whether the symptoms are due to excess thyroxine blood levels. Chronic overtreatment with T_4, particularly in elderly patients, can increase the risk of atrial fibrillation and accelerated osteoporosis.

Special Problems in Management of Hypothyroidism

A. MYXEDEMA AND CORONARY ARTERY DISEASE

Since myxedema frequently occurs in older persons, it is often associated with underlying coronary artery disease. In this situation, the low levels of circulating thyroid hormone actually protect the heart against increasing demands that could result in angina pectoris or myocardial infarction. Correction of myxedema must be done cautiously to avoid provoking arrhythmia, angina, or acute myocardial infarction.

B. MYXEDEMA COMA

Myxedema coma is an end state of untreated hypothyroidism. It is associated with progressive weakness, stupor, hypothermia, hypoventilation, hypoglycemia, hyponatremia, water intoxication, shock, and death.

Management of myxedema coma is a medical emergency. The patient should be treated in the intensive care unit, since tracheal intubation and mechanical ventilation may be required. Associated illnesses such as infection or heart failure must be treated by appropriate therapy. It is important to give all preparations intravenously, because patients with myxedema coma absorb drugs poorly from other routes. Intravenous fluids should be administered with caution to avoid excessive water intake. These patients have large pools of empty T_3 and T_4 binding sites that must be filled before there is adequate free thyroxine to affect tissue metabolism. Accordingly, the treatment of choice in myxedema coma is to give a loading dose of levothyroxine intravenously—usually 300–400 μg initially, followed by 50 μg daily. Intravenous T_3 can also be used but may be more cardiotoxic and more difficult to monitor. Intravenous hydrocortisone is indicated if the patient has associated adrenal or pituitary insufficiency but is probably not necessary in most patients with primary myxedema. Opioids and sedatives must be used with extreme caution.

C. HYPOTHYROIDISM AND PREGNANCY

Hypothyroid women frequently have anovulatory cycles and are therefore relatively infertile until restoration of the euthyroid state. This has led to the widespread use of thyroid hormone for infertility, although there is no evidence for its usefulness in infertile euthyroid patients. In a pregnant hypothyroid patient receiving thyroxine, it is extremely important that the daily dose of thyroxine be adequate because early development of the fetal brain depends on maternal thyroxine. In many hypothyroid patients, a modest increase in the thyroxine dose (about 20–30%) is required to normalize the serum TSH level during pregnancy. Because of the elevated maternal TBG, the free thyroxine index (FT_4I) or free thyroxine (FT_4) and TSH (Table 38–2) must be used to monitor maternal thyroxine dosages.

HYPERTHYROIDISM

Hyperthyroidism (thyrotoxicosis) is the clinical syndrome that results when tissues are exposed to high levels of thyroid hormone (Table 38–4).

1. Graves' Disease

The most common form of hyperthyroidism is Graves' disease, or diffuse toxic goiter. The presenting signs and symptoms of Graves' disease are set forth in Table 38–4.

Pathophysiology

Graves' disease is considered to be an autoimmune disorder in which there is a genetic defect in suppressor T lymphocytes, and helper T lymphocytes stimulate B lymphocytes to synthesize antibodies to thyroidal antigens. The antibody described previously (TSH-R Ab [stim]) is directed against the TSH receptor site in the thyroid cell membrane and has the capacity to stimulate the thyroid cell. Spontaneous remission occurs but may require 1 to 15 years.

Laboratory Diagnosis

In most patients with hyperthyroidism, T_3, T_4, RT_3U, FT_4, and FT_4I will all be elevated and TSH is suppressed (Table 38–2). Radioiodine uptake is usually markedly elevated as well. Antithyroglobulin antibodies, thyroid peroxidase, and TSH-R Ab [stim] are often present.

Management of Graves' Disease

The three primary methods for controlling hyperthyroidism are antithyroid drug therapy, surgical thyroidectomy, and destruction of the gland with radioactive iodine.

A. ANTITHYROID DRUG THERAPY

Drug therapy is most useful in young patients with small glands and mild disease. Methimazole or propyl-thiouracil is administered until the disease undergoes spontaneous remission. This is the only therapy that leaves an intact thyroid gland, but it does require a long period of treatment and observation (1–2 years), and there is a 60–70% incidence of relapse.

Antithyroid drug therapy is usually begun with large divided doses, shifting to maintenance therapy with single daily doses when the patient becomes clinically euthyroid. However, mild to moderately severe thyrotoxicosis can often be controlled with methimazole given in a single morning dose of 30–40 mg; once-daily dosing may enhance adherence. Maintenance therapy requires 5–15 mg once daily. Alternatively, therapy is started with propylthiouracil, 100–150 mg every 6 or 8 hours, followed after 4–8 weeks by gradual reduction of the dose to the maintenance level of 50–150 mg once daily. In addition to inhibiting iodine organification, propylthiouracil also inhibits the conversion of T_4 to T_3, so it brings the level of activated thyroid hormone down more quickly than does methimazole. The best clinical guide to remission is reduction in the size of the goiter. Laboratory tests most useful in monitoring the course of therapy are serum T_3 by RIA, FT_4 or FT_4I, and serum TSH.

Reactivation of the autoimmune process may occur when the dosage of antithyroid drug is lowered during maintenance therapy and TSH begins to drive the gland. TSH release can be prevented by the daily administration of 50–150 μg of levothyroxine with 5–15 mg of methimazole or 50–150 mg of propylthiouracil for the second year of therapy. The relapse rate with this program is probably comparable to the rate with antithyroid therapy alone, but the risk of hypothyroidism and overtreatment is avoided.

Reactions to antithyroid drugs have been described above. A minor rash can often be controlled by antihistamine therapy. Because the more severe reaction of agranulocytosis is often heralded by sore throat or high fever, patients receiving antithyroid drugs must be instructed to discontinue the drug and seek immediate medical attention if these symptoms develop. White cell and differential counts and a throat culture are indicated in such cases, followed by appropriate antibiotic therapy.

B. THYROIDECTOMY

A near-total thyroidectomy is the treatment of choice for patients with very large glands or multinodular goiters. Patients are treated with antithyroid drugs until euthyroid (about 6 weeks). In addition, for 2 weeks prior to surgery, they receive saturated solution of potassium iodide, 5 drops twice daily, to diminish vascularity of the gland and simplify surgery. About 80–90% of patients will require thyroid supplementation following near-total thyroidectomy.

C. Radioactive Iodine

Radioiodine therapy utilizing ^{131}I is the preferred treatment for most patients over 21 years of age. In patients without heart disease, the therapeutic dose may be given immediately in a range of 80–120 µCi/g of estimated thyroid weight corrected for uptake. In patients with underlying heart disease or severe thyrotoxicosis and in elderly patients, it is desirable to treat with antithyroid drugs (preferably methimazole) until the patient is euthyroid. The medication is then stopped for 5–7 days before the appropriate dose of ^{131}I is administered. Iodides should be avoided to ensure maximal ^{131}I uptake. Six to 12 weeks following the administration of radioiodine, the gland will shrink in size and the patient will usually become euthyroid or hypothyroid. A second dose may be required in some patients. Hypothyroidism occurs in about 80% of patients following radioiodine therapy. Serum FT_4 and TSH levels should be monitored. When hypothyroidism develops, prompt replacement with oral levothyroxine, 50–150 µg daily, should be instituted.

D. Adjuncts to Antithyroid Therapy

During the acute phase of thyrotoxicosis, β-adrenoceptor-blocking agents without intrinsic sympathomimetic activity are extremely helpful. Propranolol, 20–40 mg orally every 6 hours, will control tachycardia, hypertension, and atrial fibrillation. Propranolol is gradually withdrawn as serum thyroxine levels return to normal. Diltiazem, 90–120 mg three or four times daily, can be used to control tachycardia in patients in whom β-blockers are contraindicated, eg, those with asthma. Other calcium channel blockers may not be as effective as diltiazem. Adequate nutrition and vitamin supplements are essential. Barbiturates accelerate T_4 breakdown (by hepatic enzyme induction) and may be helpful both as sedatives and to lower T_4 levels.

2. Toxic Uninodular Goiter & Toxic Multinodular Goiter

These forms of hyperthyroidism occur often in older women with nodular goiters. FT_4 is moderately elevated or occasionally normal, but T_3 by RIA is strikingly elevated. Single toxic adenomas can be managed with either surgical excision of the adenoma or with radioiodine therapy. Toxic multinodular goiter is usually associated with a large goiter and is best treated by preparation with methimazole or propylthiouracil followed by subtotal thyroidectomy.

3. Subacute Thyroiditis

During the acute phase of a viral infection of the thyroid gland, there is destruction of thyroid parenchyma with transient release of stored thyroid hormones. A similar state may occur in patients with Hashimoto's thyroiditis. These episodes of transient thyrotoxicosis have been termed "spontaneously resolving hyperthyroidism." Supportive therapy is usually all that is necessary, such as propranolol for tachycardia and aspirin or nonsteroidal anti-inflammatory drugs to control local pain and fever. Corticosteroids may be necessary in severe cases to control the inflammation.

4. Special Problems

Thyroid Storm

Thyroid storm, or thyrotoxic crisis, is sudden acute exacerbation of all of the symptoms of thyrotoxicosis, presenting as a life-threatening syndrome. Vigorous management is mandatory. Propranolol, 1–2 mg slowly intravenously or 40–80 mg orally every 6 hours, is helpful to control the severe cardiovascular manifestations. If propranolol is contraindicated by the presence of severe heart failure or asthma, hypertension and tachycardia may be controlled with diltiazem, 90–120 mg orally three or four times daily or 5–10 mg/h by intravenous infusion (asthmatic patients only). Release of thyroid hormones from the gland is retarded by the administration of saturated solution of potassium iodide, 10 drops orally daily, or iodinated contrast media (eg, sodium ipodate, 1 g orally daily). The latter medication will also block peripheral conversion of T_4 to T_3. Hormone synthesis is blocked by the administration of propylthiouracil, 250 mg orally every 6 hours. If the patient is unable to take propylthiouracil by mouth, a rectal formulation can be prepared and administered in a dosage of 400 mg every 6 hours as a retention enema. Methimazole may also be prepared for rectal administration in a dose of 60 mg daily. Hydrocortisone, 50 mg intravenously every 6 hours, will protect the patient against shock and will block the conversion of T_4 to T_3, rapidly bringing down the level of thyroactive material in the blood.

Supportive therapy is essential to control fever, heart failure, and any underlying disease process that may have precipitated the acute storm. In rare situations, where the above methods are not adequate to control the problem, plasmapheresis or peritoneal dialysis has been used to lower the levels of circulating thyroxine.

Ophthalmopathy

Although severe ophthalmopathy is rare, it is difficult to treat. Management requires effective treatment of the thyroid disease, usually by total surgical excision or ^{131}I ablation of the gland plus oral prednisone therapy (see below). In addition, local therapy may be necessary, eg, elevation of the head to diminish periorbital edema and artificial tears to relieve corneal drying. Smoking cessation should be advised to prevent progression of the ophthalmopathy. For the severe, acute inflammatory reaction, a short course of prednisone, 60–100 mg orally daily for about a week and then 60–100 mg every other day, tapering the dose over a period of 6–12 weeks, may be effective. If steroid therapy fails or is contraindicated, irradiation of the posterior orbit, using well-collimated high-energy x-ray therapy, will frequently result in marked improvement of the acute process. Threatened loss of vision is an indication for surgical decompression of the orbit. Eyelid or eye muscle surgery may be necessary to correct residual problems after the acute process has subsided.

Dermopathy

Dermopathy or pretibial myxedema will often respond to topical corticosteroids applied to the involved area and covered with an occlusive dressing.

Thyrotoxicosis During Pregnancy

Ideally, women in the childbearing period with severe disease should have definitive therapy with ^{131}I or subtotal thyroidectomy *prior* to pregnancy in order to avoid an acute exacerbation of the disease during pregnancy or following delivery. If thyrotoxicosis does develop during pregnancy, radioiodine is contraindicated because it crosses the placenta and may injure the fetal thyroid. In the first trimester, the patient can be prepared with propylthiouracil and a subtotal thyroidectomy performed safely during the mid trimester. It is essential to give the patient a thyroid supplement during the balance of the pregnancy. However, most patients are treated with propylthiouracil during the pregnancy, and the decision regarding long-term management can be made after delivery. The dosage of propylthiouracil must be kept to the minimum necessary for control of the disease (ie, < 300 mg daily), because it may affect the function of the fetal thyroid gland. Methimazole is a potential alternative, although there is concern about a possible risk of fetal scalp defects.

Neonatal Graves' Disease

Graves' disease may occur in the newborn infant, either due to passage of TSH-R Ab [stim] through the placenta, stimulating the thyroid gland of the neonate, or to genetic transmission of the trait to the fetus. Laboratory studies reveal an elevated free thyroxine, a markedly elevated T_3, and a low TSH—in contrast to the normal infant, in whom TSH is elevated at birth. TSH-R Ab [stim] is usually found in the serum of both the child and the mother.

If caused by maternal TSH-R Ab [stim], the disease is usually self-limited and subsides over a period of 4–12 weeks, coinciding with the fall in the infant's TSH-R Ab [stim] level. However, treatment is necessary because of the severe metabolic stress the infant experiences. Therapy includes propylthiouracil in a dose of 5–10 mg/kg/d in divided doses at 8-hour intervals; Lugol's solution (8 mg of iodide per drop), 1 drop every 8 hours; and propranolol, 2 mg/kg/d in divided doses. Careful supportive therapy is essential. If the infant is very ill, oral prednisone, 2 mg/kg/d in divided doses, will help block conversion of T_4 to T_3. These medications are gradually reduced as the clinical picture improves and can be discontinued by 6–12 weeks.

NONTOXIC GOITER

Nontoxic goiter is a syndrome of thyroid enlargement without excessive thyroid hormone production. Enlargement of the thyroid gland is usually due to TSH stimulation from inadequate thyroid hormone synthesis. The most common cause of nontoxic goiter worldwide is iodide deficiency, but in the USA, it is Hashimoto's thyroiditis. Less common causes include dietary goitrogens, dyshormonogenesis, and neoplasms (see below).

Goiter due to iodide deficiency is best managed by prophylactic administration of iodide. The optimal daily iodide intake is 150–200 μg. Iodized salt and iodate used as preservatives in flour and bread are excellent sources of iodine in the diet. In areas where it is difficult to introduce iodized salt or iodate preservatives, a solution of iodized poppyseed oil has been administered intramuscularly to provide a long-term source of inorganic iodine.

Goiter due to ingestion of goitrogens in the diet is managed by elimination of the goitrogen or by adding sufficient thyroxine to shut off TSH stimulation. Similarly, in Hashimoto's thyroiditis and dyshormonogenesis, adequate thyroxine therapy—150–200 μg/d orally—will suppress pituitary TSH and result in slow regression of the goiter as well as correction of hypothyroidism.

THYROID NEOPLASMS

Neoplasms of the thyroid gland may be benign (adenomas) or malignant. Some adenomas will regress following thyroxine therapy; those that do not should be rebiopsied or surgically removed. Management of thyroid carcinoma requires a total thyroidectomy, postoperative radioiodine therapy in selected instances, and lifetime replacement with levothyroxine. The evaluation for recurrence of some thyroid malignancies requires withdrawal of thyroxine replacement for 4–6 weeks—

accompanied by the development of hypothyroidism. Tumor recurrence is likely if there is a rise in serum thyroglobulin (ie, a tumor marker) or a positive ^{131}I scan when TSH is elevated. Alternatively, administration of recombinant human TSH (Thyrogen) can produce comparable TSH elevations without discontinuing thyroxine and avoiding hypothyroidism. Recombinant human TSH is administered intramuscularly once daily for 2 days. A rise in serum thyroglobulin or a positive ^{131}I scan will indicate a recurrence of the thyroid cancer.

PREPARATIONS AVAILABLE

THYROID AGENTS

Levothyroxine [T$_4$] (generic, Levoxyl, Levo-T, Synthroid, Unithroid)
Oral: 0.025, 0.05, 0.075, 0.088, 0.1, 0.112, 0.125, 0.137, 0.15, 0.175, 0.2, 0.3 mg tablets
Parenteral: 200, 500 μg per vial (100 μg/mL when reconstituted) for injection

Liothyronine [T$_3$] (generic, Cytomel, Triostat)
Oral: 5, 25, 50 μg tablets
Parenteral: 10 μg/mL

Liotrix [a 4:1 ratio of T$_4$:T$_3$] (Thyrolar)
Oral: tablets containing 12.5, 25, 30, 50, 60, 100, 120, 150, 180 μg T$_4$ and one fourth as much T$_3$

Thyroid desiccated [USP] (generic, Armour Thyroid, Thyroid Strong, Thyrar, S-P-T)
Oral: tablets containing 15, 30, 60, 90, 120, 180, 240, 300 mg; capsules (S-P-T) containing 120, 180, 300 mg

ANTITHYROID AGENTS

Diatrizoate sodium (Hypaque)
Parenteral: 25% (150 mg iodine/mL); 50% (300 mg iodine/mL) (unlabeled use)

Iodide (^{131}I) **sodium** (Iodotope, Sodium Iodide I 131 Therapeutic)
Oral: available as capsules and solution

Iopanoic acid (Telepaque)
Oral: 500 mg tablets (unlabeled use)

Ipodate sodium (Oragrafin Sodium, Bilivist)
Oral: 500 mg capsules (unlabeled use)

Methimazole (Tapazole)
Oral: 5, 10 mg tablets

Potassium iodide
Oral solution (generic, SSKI): 1 g/mL
Oral solution (Lugol's solution): 100 mg/mL potassium iodide plus 50 mg/mL iodine
Oral syrup (Pima): 325 mg/5 mL
Oral controlled action tablets (Iodo-Niacin): 135 mg potassium iodide plus 25 mg niacinamide hydroiodide
Oral potassium iodide tablets (generic, IOSAT, RAD-Block, Thyro-Block): 65, 130 mg

Propylthiouracil [PTU] (generic)
Oral: 50 mg tablets

Thyrotropin; recombinant human TSH (Thyrogen)
Parenteral: 0.9 mg per vial

REFERENCES

GENERAL

Greenspan FS: Thyroid gland. In: Greenspan FS, Gardner DG (editors). *Basic & Clinical Endocrinology,* 7th ed. McGraw-Hill, 2003.

American Thyroid Association (http://thyroid.org/)

GUIDELINES

Harris PE: The management of thyroid cancer in adults: a review of new guidelines. Clin Med 2002;2:144.

Ladenson PW et al: American Thyroid Association Guidelines for detection of thyroid dysfunction. Arch Intern Med 2000;160:1573.

US Department of Health and Human Services: Potassium iodide as a thyroid blocking agent in radiation emergencies. December 2001 (http://www.fda.gov/cder/guidance/index.htm)

HYPOTHYROIDISM

Bunevicius R et al: Effects of thyroxine as compared with thyroxine plus triiodothyronine in patients with hypothyroidism. N Engl J Med 1999;340:424.

Cooper DS: Clinical practice: subclinical hypothyroidism. N Engl J Med 2001;345:260.

Dong BJ et al: Bioequivalence of generic and brand-name levothyroxine products in the treatment of hypothyroidism. JAMA 1997;277:1205.

Gruters A et al: Long-term consequences of congenital hypothyroidism in the era of screening programs. Endocrinol Metab 2002;16:369.

Ringel MD: Management of hypothyroidism and hyperthyroidism in the intensive care unit. Crit Care Clinics 2001;17:59.

Smallridge RC, Ladenson PW: Hypothyroidism in pregnancy: consequences to neonatal health. J Clin Endocrinol Metab 2001;86:2349.

Wiersinga QM: Thyroid hormone replacement therapy. Horm Res 2001;56(Suppl 1):74.

HYPERTHYROIDISM

Atkins P et al: Drug therapy for hyperthyroidism in pregnancy: safety issues for mother and fetus. Drug Safety 2000;23:229.

Fontanilla JC et al: The use of oral radiographic contrast agents in the management of hyperthyroidism. Thyroid 2001;11:561.

Greenspan SL, Greenspan FS: The effects of thyroid hormone on skeletal integrity. Ann Intern Med 1999;130:750.

Nabil N, Miner DJ, Amatruda JM: Methimazole: An alternative route of administration. J Clin Endocrinol Metab 1982;54:180.

Toft AD: Clinical practice: subclinical hyperthyroidism. N Engl J Med 2001;345:512.

Walter RM, Bartle WR: Rectal administration of propylthiouracil in the treatment of Graves' disease. Am J Med 1990;88:69.

NONTOXIC GOITER, NODULES, & CANCER

Lawrence W Jr, Kaplan BJ: Diagnosis and management of patients with thyroid nodules. J Surg Oncol 2002;80:157.

Mazzaferri EL, Kloos RT: Clinical review 128: Current approaches to primary therapy for papillary and follicular thyroid cancer. J Clin Endocrinol Metab 2001;86:1447.

Meier CA: Thyroid nodules: pathogenesis, diagnosis and treatment. Baillieres Best Pract Res Clin Endocrinol Metab 2000;14:559.

THE EFFECTS OF DRUGS ON THYROID FUNCTION

Arafah BM: Increased need for thyroxine in women with hypothyroidism during estrogen therapy. N Engl J Med 2001;344:1743.

Dong BJ: How medications affect thyroid function. West J Med 2000;172:102.

Markou K et al: Iodine-induced hyperthyroidism. Thyroid 2001;11:501.

Martino E et al: The effects of amiodarone on the thyroid. Endocr Rev 2001;22:240.

Adrenocorticosteroids & Adrenocortical Antagonists

39

George P. Chrousos, MD

The natural adrenocortical hormones are steroid molecules produced and released by the adrenal cortex. Both natural and synthetic corticosteroids are used for diagnosis and treatment of disorders of adrenal function. They are also used—more often and in much larger doses—for treatment of a variety of inflammatory and immunologic disorders.

Secretion of adrenocortical steroids is controlled by the pituitary release of corticotropin (ACTH). Secretion of the salt-retaining hormone aldosterone is primarily under the influence of angiotensin. Corticotropin has some actions that do not depend upon its effect on adrenocortical secretion. However, its pharmacologic value as an anti-inflammatory agent and its use in testing adrenal function depend on its secretory action. Its pharmacology is discussed in Chapter 37 and will be reviewed only briefly here.

Inhibitors of the synthesis or antagonists of the action of the adrenocortical steroids are important in the treatment of several conditions. These agents are described at the end of this chapter.

ADRENOCORTICOSTEROIDS

The adrenal cortex releases a large number of steroids into the circulation. Some have minimal biologic activity and function primarily as precursors, and there are some for which no function has been established. The hormonal steroids may be classified as those having important effects on intermediary metabolism (glucocorticoids), those having principally salt-retaining activity (mineralocorticoids), and those having androgenic or estrogenic activity (see Chapter 40). In humans, the major glucocorticoid is cortisol and the most important mineralocorticoid is aldosterone. Quantitatively, dehydroepiandrosterone (DHEA) in its sulfated form (DHEAS) is the major adrenal androgen, since about 20 mg is secreted daily. However, DHEA and two other

adrenal androgens, androstenediol and androstenedione, are weak androgens or estrogens, mostly by peripheral conversion to testosterone and dehydrotestosterone or estradiol and estrone. Adrenal androgens constitute the major endogenous precursors of estrogen in women after menopause and in younger patients in whom ovarian function is deficient or absent.

THE NATURALLY OCCURRING GLUCOCORTICOIDS; CORTISOL (HYDROCORTISONE)

Pharmacokinetics

Cortisol (also called hydrocortisone, compound F) exerts a wide range of physiologic effects, including regulation of intermediary metabolism, cardiovascular function, growth, and immunity. Its synthesis and secretion are tightly regulated by the central nervous system, which is very sensitive to negative feedback by the circulating cortisol and exogenous (synthetic) glucocorticoids. Cortisol is synthesized from cholesterol (as shown in Figure 39–1). The mechanisms controlling its secretion are discussed in Chapter 37.

In the normal adult, in the absence of stress, 10–20 mg of cortisol is secreted daily. The rate of secretion follows a circadian rhythm governed by pulses of ACTH that peak in the early morning hours and after meals (Figure 39–2). In plasma, cortisol is bound to circulating proteins. Corticosteroid-binding globulin (CBG), an α_2-globulin synthesized by the liver, binds 90% of the circulating hormone under normal circumstances. The remainder is free (about 5–10%) or loosely bound to albumin (about 5%) and is available to exert its effect on target cells. When plasma cortisol levels exceed 20–30 μg/dL, CBG is saturated, and the concentration of free cortisol rises rapidly. CBG is increased in pregnancy and with estrogen administration and in hyperthyroidism. It is decreased by hypothyroidism, genetic defects in synthesis, and protein deficiency states. Albumin has a large capacity but low affinity for cortisol, and

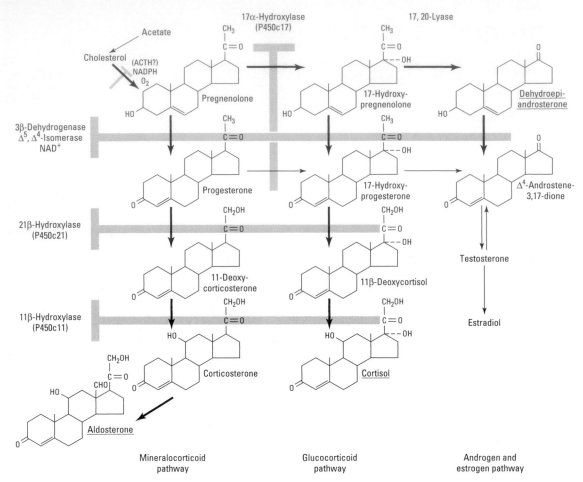

Figure 39–1. Outline of major pathways in adrenocortical hormone biosynthesis. The major secretory products are underlined. Pregnenolone is the major precursor of corticosterone and aldosterone, and 17-hydroxypregnenolone is the major precursor of cortisol. The enzymes and cofactors for the reactions progressing down each column are shown on the left and across columns at the top of the figure. When a particular enzyme is deficient, hormone production is blocked at the points indicated by the shaded bars. (Modified after Welikey et al; reproduced, with permission, from Ganong WF: *Review of Medical Physiology,* 17th ed. Originally published by Appleton & Lange. Copyright © 1995 by The McGraw-Hill Companies, Inc.)

for practical purposes albumin-bound cortisol should be considered free. Synthetic corticosteroids such as dexamethasone are largely bound to albumin rather than CBG.

The half-life of cortisol in the circulation is normally about 60–90 minutes; half-life may be increased when hydrocortisone (the pharmaceutical preparation of cortisol) is administered in large amounts or when stress, hypothyroidism, or liver disease is present. Only 1% of cortisol is excreted unchanged in the urine as free cortisol; about 20% of cortisol is converted to cortisone by

11-hydroxysteroid dehydrogenase in the kidney and other tissues with mineralocorticoid receptors (see below) before reaching the liver. Most cortisol is inactivated in the liver by reduction of the 4,5 double bond in the A ring and subsequent conversion to tetrahydrocortisol and tetrahydrocortisone by 3-hydroxysteroid dehydrogenase. (See Figure 39–4 for carbon numbering.) Some is converted to cortol and cortolone by reduction of the C_{20} ketone. There are small amounts of other metabolites. About one third of the cortisol produced daily is excreted in the urine as dihydroxy ketone

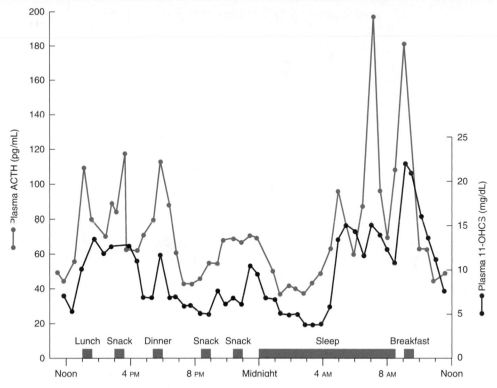

Figure 39–2. Fluctuations in plasma ACTH and glucocorticoids throughout the day in a normal girl (age 16). The ACTH was measured by immunoassay and the glucocorticoids as 11-oxysteroids *(11-OHCS)*. Note the greater ACTH and glucocorticoid rises in the morning, before awakening from sleep. (Reproduced, with permission, from Krieger DT et al: Characterization of the normal temporal pattern of plasma corticosteroid levels. J Clin Endocrinol Metab 1971;32:266.)

metabolites and is measured as 17-hydroxysteroids. Many cortisol metabolites are conjugated with glucuronic acid or sulfate at the C_3 and C_{21} hydroxyls, respectively, in the liver; they then reenter the circulation and are excreted in the urine.

In some species (eg, the rat), corticosterone is the major glucocorticoid. It is less firmly bound to protein and therefore metabolized more rapidly. The pathways of its degradation are similar to those of cortisol.

Pharmacodynamics

A. MECHANISM OF ACTION

Most of the known effects of the glucocorticoids are mediated by widely distributed glucocorticoid receptors. These proteins are members of the superfamily of nuclear receptors that includes steroid, sterol (vitamin D), thyroid, retinoic acid, and many other receptors with unknown or nonexistent ligands (orphan receptors). All these receptors interact with the promoters of—and regulate the transcription of—target genes

(Figure 39–3). In the absence of the hormonal ligand, glucocorticoid receptors are primarily cytoplasmic, in oligomeric complexes with heat shock proteins (Hsp). The most important of these are two molecules of Hsp90, though other proteins are certainly involved. Free hormone from the plasma and interstitial fluid enters the cell and binds to the receptor, inducing conformational changes that allow it to dissociate from the heat shock proteins. The ligand-bound receptor complex then is actively transported into the nucleus, where it interacts with DNA and nuclear proteins. As a homodimer, it binds to glucocorticoid receptor elements (GRE) in the promoters of responsive genes. The GRE is composed of two palindromic sequences that bind to the hormone receptor dimer.

In addition to binding to GREs, the ligand-bound receptor also forms complexes with and influences the function of other transcription factors, such as AP1 and NF-κB, which act on non-GRE-containing promoters, to contribute to the regulation of transcription of their responsive genes. These transcription factors have broad

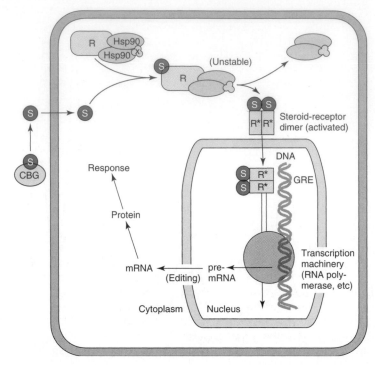

Figure 39–3. A model of the interaction of a steroid, S (eg, cortisol), and its receptor, R, and the subsequent events in a target cell. The steroid is present in the blood in bound form on the corticosteroid-binding globulin, CBG, but enters the cell as the free molecule. The intracellular receptor is bound to stabilizing proteins, including two molecules of heat shock protein 90 (Hsp90) and several others, denoted as "X" in the figure. This receptor complex is incapable of activating transcription. When the complex binds a molecule of cortisol, an unstable complex is created and the Hsp90 and associated molecules are released. The steroid-receptor complex is able to enter the nucleus, bind to the glucocorticoid response element (GRE) on the gene, and regulate transcription by RNA polymerase II and associated transcription factors. A variety of regulatory factors (not shown) may participate in facilitating (coactivators) or inhibiting (corepressors) the steroid response. The resulting mRNA is edited and exported to the cytoplasm for the production of protein that brings about the final hormone response.

actions on the regulation of growth factors, proinflammatory cytokines, etc, and to a great extent mediate the anti-growth, anti-inflammatory, and immunosuppressive effects of glucocorticoids. These factors represent new targets in the development of a new generation of glucocorticoid agonists or antagonists with response selectivity or tissue selectivity.

Two genes for the corticoid receptor have been identified, one encoding the classic glucocorticoid receptor and the other the mineralocorticoid receptor. Alternative splicing of human glucocorticoid receptor pre-mRNA generates two highly homologous isoforms, termed hGR alpha and hGR beta. hGR alpha is the classic ligand-activated glucocorticoid receptor which, in the hormone-bound state, modulates the expression of glucocorticoid-responsive genes. In contrast, hGR

beta does not bind glucocorticoids and is transcriptionally inactive. However, hGR beta is able to inhibit the effects of hormone-activated hGR alpha on glucocorticoid-responsive genes, playing the role of a physiologically relevant endogenous inhibitor of glucocorticoid action.

The glucocorticoid receptor is composed of about 800 amino acids and can be divided into three functional domains (Figure 2–6). The glucocorticoid-binding domain is located at the carboxyl terminal of the molecule and is the area where free glucocorticoids bind. The DNA-binding domain is located in the middle of the protein and contains nine cysteine residues. This region folds into a "two-finger" structure stabilized by zinc ions connected to cysteines to form two tetrahedrons. This part of the molecule binds to the GREs that regulate glucocorticoid action on glucocorticoid-regulated genes. The zinc-fingers represent the basic structure by which the DNA-binding domain recognizes specific nucleic acid sequences. The amino-terminal domain is highly antigenic. It is involved in the transactivational activity of the receptor and increases its specificity.

The interaction of glucocorticoid receptors with GREs or other transcription factors is facilitated or inhibited by several families of proteins called steroid receptor "coregulators" divided respectively into "coactivators" and "corepressors." They do this by serving as bridges between the receptors and other nuclear proteins and by expressing enzymatic activities such as histone acetylase or deacetylase that alter the conformation of nucleosomes and the transcribability of genes.

Between 10% and 20% of expressed genes in a cell are regulated by glucocorticoids. The number and affinity of receptors for the hormone, the complement of transcription factors and coregulators, and posttranscription events determine the relative specificity of these hormones' actions in various cells. The effects of glucocorticoids are mainly due to proteins synthesized from mRNA transcribed by their target genes.

Some of the effects of glucocorticoids can be attributed to their binding to aldosterone receptors (AR). Indeed, ARs bind aldosterone and cortisol with similar affinity. A mineralocorticoid effect of cortisol is avoided in some tissues by expression of 11β-hydroxysteroid dehydrogenase type 2, the enzyme responsible for biotransformation to its 11-keto derivative (cortisone), which has minimal affinity for aldosterone receptors.

Prompt effects such as initial feedback suppression of pituitary ACTH occur in minutes and are too rapid to be explained on the basis of gene transcription and protein synthesis. It is not known how these effects are mediated. Among the proposed mechanisms are direct effects on cell membrane receptors for the hormone or nongenomic effects of the classic hormone-bound glucocorticoid receptor. The putative membrane receptors might be entirely different from the known intracellular receptors.

B. Physiologic Effects

The glucocorticoids have widespread effects because they influence the function of most cells in the body. The major metabolic consequences of glucocorticoid secretion or administration are due to direct actions of these hormones in the cell. However, some important effects are the result of homeostatic responses by insulin and glucagon. Although many of the effects of glucocorticoids are dose-related and become magnified when large amounts are administered for therapeutic purposes, there are also other effects—called "permissive" effects—in the absence of which many normal functions become deficient. For example, the response of

vascular and bronchial smooth muscle to catecholamines is diminished in the absence of cortisol and restored by physiologic amounts of this glucocorticoid. Furthermore, the lipolytic responses of fat cells to catecholamines, ACTH, and growth hormone are attenuated in the absence of glucocorticoids.

C. Metabolic Effects

The glucocorticoids have important dose-related effects on carbohydrate, protein, and fat metabolism. The same effects are responsible for some of the serious adverse effects associated with their use in therapeutic doses. Glucocorticoids stimulate and are required for gluconeogenesis and glycogen synthesis in the fasting state. They stimulate phosphoenolpyruvate carboxykinase, glucose-6-phosphatase, and glycogen synthase and the release of amino acids in the course of muscle catabolism.

Glucocorticoids increase serum glucose levels and thus stimulate insulin release and inhibit the uptake of glucose by muscle cells, while they stimulate hormone-sensitive lipase and thus lipolysis. The increased insulin secretion stimulates lipogenesis and to a lesser degree inhibits lipolysis, leading to a net increase in fat deposition combined with increased release of fatty acids and glycerol into the circulation.

The net results of these actions are most apparent in the fasting state, when the supply of glucose from gluconeogenesis, the release of amino acids from muscle catabolism, the inhibition of peripheral glucose uptake, and the stimulation of lipolysis all contribute to maintenance of an adequate glucose supply to the brain.

D. Catabolic and Antianabolic Effects

Although glucocorticoids stimulate protein and RNA synthesis in the liver, they have catabolic and antianabolic effects in lymphoid and connective tissue, muscle, fat, and skin. Supraphysiologic amounts of glucocorticoids lead to decreased muscle mass and weakness and thinning of the skin. Catabolic and antianabolic effects on bone are the cause of osteoporosis in Cushing's syndrome and impose a major limitation in the long-term therapeutic use of glucocorticoids. In children, glucocorticoids reduce growth. This effect may be partially prevented by administration of growth hormone in high doses.

E. Anti-inflammatory and Immunosuppressive Effects

Glucocorticoids dramatically reduce the manifestations of inflammation. This is due to their profound effects on the concentration, distribution, and function of peripheral leukocytes and to their suppressive effects on the inflammatory cytokines and chemokines and on other lipid and glucolipid mediators of inflammation. Inflammation, regardless of its cause, is characterized by the extravasation and infiltration of leukocytes into the affected tissue. These events are mediated by a complex series of interactions of white cell adhesion molecules with those on endothelial cells and are inhibited by glucocorticoids. After a single dose of a short-acting glucocorticoid, the circulating concentration of neutrophils increases while the lymphocytes (T and B cells), monocytes, eosinophils, and basophils in the circulation decrease in number. The changes are maximal at 6 hours and are dissipated in 24 hours. The increase in neutrophils is due both to the increased influx into the blood from the bone marrow and decreased migration from the blood vessels, leading to a reduction in the number of cells at the site of inflammation. The reduction in circulating lymphocytes, monocytes, eosinophils, and basophils is primarily the result of their movement from the vascular bed to lymphoid tissue.

Glucocorticoids also inhibit the functions of tissue macrophages and other antigen-presenting cells. The ability of these cells to respond to antigens and mitogens is reduced. The effect on macrophages is particularly marked and limits their ability to phagocytose and kill microorganisms and to produce tumor necrosis factor-α, interleukin-1, metalloproteinases, and plasminogen activator. Both macrophages and lymphocytes produce less interleukin-12 and interferon-γ, important inducers of TH1 cell activity, and cellular immunity.

In addition to their effects on leukocyte function, glucocorticoids influence the inflammatory response by reducing the prostaglandin, leukotriene, and platelet-activating factor synthesis that results from activation of phospholipase A_2. Finally, glucocorticoids reduce expression of cyclooxygenase II, the inducible form of this enzyme, in inflammatory cells, thus reducing the amount of enzyme available to produce prostaglandins (Chapters 18 and 36).

Glucocorticoids cause vasoconstriction when applied directly to the skin, possibly by suppressing mast cell degranulation. They also decrease capillary permeability by reducing the amount of histamine released by basophils and mast cells.

The anti-inflammatory and immunosuppressive effects of glucocorticoids are largely due to the actions described above. In humans, complement activation is unaltered, but its effects are inhibited. Antibody production can be reduced by large doses of steroids, though it is unaffected by moderate dosages (eg, 20 mg/d of prednisone). The efficacy of glucocorticoids in the control of transplant rejection is augmented by their ability to reduce antigen expression from the grafted tissue, delay revascularization, and interfere with the sensitization of cytotoxic T lymphocytes and the generation of primary antibody-forming cells.

The anti-inflammatory and immunosuppressive effects of these agents are widely useful therapeutically but are also responsible for some of their most serious adverse effects (see below).

F. OTHER EFFECTS

Glucocorticoids have important effects on the nervous system. Adrenal insufficiency causes marked slowing of the alpha rhythm of the EEG and is associated with depression. Increased amounts of glucocorticoids often produce behavioral disturbances in humans: initially insomnia and euphoria and subsequently depression. Large doses of glucocorticoids may increase intracranial pressure (pseudotumor cerebri).

Glucocorticoids given chronically suppress the pituitary release of ACTH, GH, TSH, and LH.

Large doses of glucocorticoids have been associated with the development of peptic ulcer, possibly by suppressing the local immune response against *Helicobacter pylori*. They also promote fat redistribution in the body, with increase of visceral, facial, nuchal, and supraclavicular fat, and they appear to antagonize the effect of vitamin D on calcium absorption. The glucocorticoids also have important effects on the hematopoietic system. In addition to their effects on leukocytes described above, they increase the number of platelets and red blood cells.

In the absence of physiologic amounts of cortisol, renal function (particularly glomerular filtration) is impaired, vasopressin secretion is augmented, and there is an inability to excrete a water load normally.

Glucocorticoids have important effects on the development of the fetal lungs. Indeed, the structural and functional changes in the lungs near term, including the production of pulmonary surface-active material required for air breathing (surfactant), are stimulated by glucocorticoids.

SYNTHETIC CORTICOSTEROIDS

Glucocorticoids have become important agents for use in the treatment of many inflammatory, allergic, hematologic, and other disorders. This has stimulated the development of many synthetic steroids with anti-inflammatory and immunosuppressive activity.

Pharmacokinetics

A. SOURCE

Pharmaceutical steroids are usually synthesized from cholic acid (obtained from cattle) or steroid sapogenins, in particular diosgenin and hecopenin, found in plants of the Liliaceae and Dioscoreaceae families. Further modifications of these steroids have led to the marketing of a large group of synthetic steroids with special characteristics that are pharmacologically and therapeutically important (Table 39–1; Figure 39–4).

Table 39–1. Some commonly used natural and synthetic corticosteroids for general use.

Agent	Activity[1]			Equivalent Oral Dose (mg)	Forms Available
	Anti-inflammatory	Topical	Salt-Retaining		
Short- to medium-acting glucocorticoids					
Hydrocortisone (cortisol)	1	1	1	20	Oral, injectable, topical
Cortisone	0.8	0	0.8	25	Oral, injectable, topical
Prednisone	4	0	0.3	5	Oral
Prednisolone	5	4	0.3	5	Oral, injectable, topical
Methylprednisolone	5	5	0	4	Oral, injectable, topical
Meprednisone[2]	5		0	4	Oral, injectable
Intermediate-acting glucocorticoids					
Triamcinolone	5	5[3]	0	4	Oral, injectable, topical
Paramethasone[2]	10		0	2	Oral, injectable
Fluprednisolone	15	7	0	1.5	Oral
Long-acting glucocorticoids					
Betamethasone	25–40	10	0	0.6	Oral, injectable, topical
Dexamethasone	30	10	0	0.75	Oral, injectable, topical
Mineralocorticoids					
Fludrocortisone	10	10	250	2	Oral, injectable, topical
Desoxycorticosterone acetate	0	0	20		Injectable, pellets

[1]Potency relative to hydrocortisone.
[2]Outside USA.
[3]Acetonide: Up to 100.

B. DISPOSITION

The metabolism of the naturally occurring adrenal steroids has been discussed above. The synthetic corticosteroids (Table 39–1) are in most cases rapidly and completely absorbed when given by mouth. Although they are transported and metabolized in a fashion similar to that of the endogenous steroids, important differences exist.

Alterations in the glucocorticoid molecule influence its affinity for glucocorticoid and mineralocorticoid receptors as well as its protein-binding avidity, side chain stability, rate of reduction, and metabolic products. Halogenation at the 9 position, unsaturation of the Δ1–2 bond of the A ring, and methylation at the 2 or 16 position prolong the half-life by more than 50%. The Δ1 compounds are excreted in the free form. In some cases, the agent given is a prodrug—eg, prednisone is rapidly converted to the active product prednisolone in the body.

Pharmacodynamics

The actions of the synthetic steroids are similar to those of cortisol (see above). They bind to the specific intracellular receptor proteins and produce the same effects but have different ratios of glucocorticoid to mineralocorticoid potency (Table 39–1).

Clinical Pharmacology

A. DIAGNOSIS AND TREATMENT OF DISTURBED ADRENAL FUNCTION

1. Adrenocortical insufficiency—

a. Chronic (Addison's disease)—Chronic adrenocortical insufficiency is characterized by weakness, fatigue, weight loss, hypotension, hyperpigmentation, and inability to maintain the blood glucose level during fasting. In such individuals, minor noxious, traumatic,

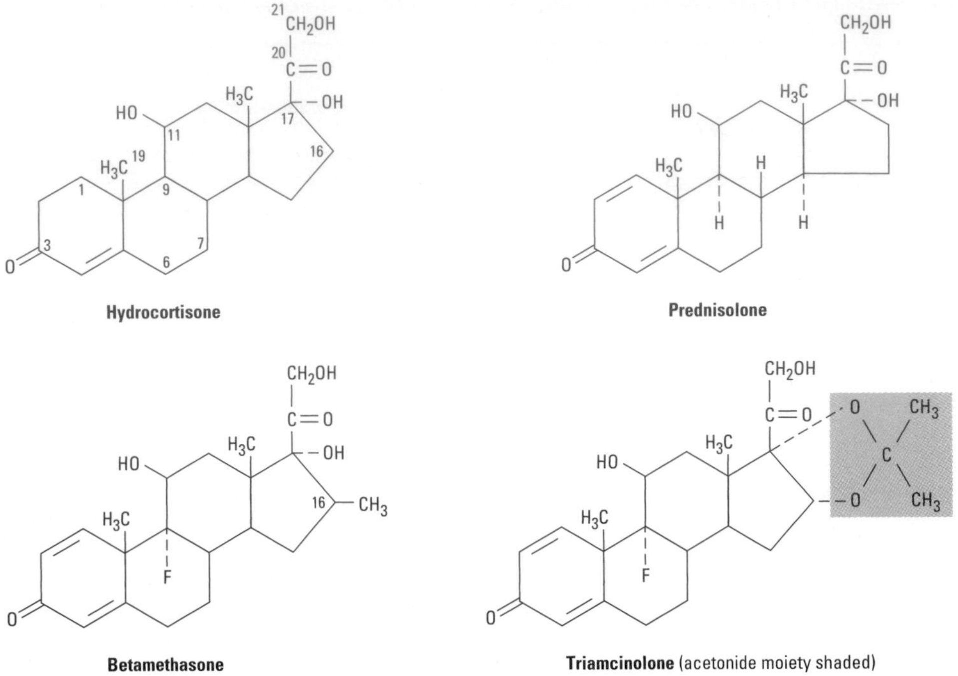

Figure 39–4. Chemical structures of several glucocorticoids. The acetonide-substituted derivatives (eg, triamcinolone acetonide) have increased surface activity and are useful in dermatology. Dexamethasone is identical to betamethasone except for the configuration of the methyl group at C_{16}: in betamethasone it is beta (projecting *up* from the plane of the rings); in dexamethasone it is alpha.

or infectious stimuli may produce acute adrenal insufficiency with circulatory shock and even death.

In primary adrenal insufficiency, about 20–30 mg of hydrocortisone must be given daily, with increased amounts during periods of stress. Although hydrocortisone has some mineralocorticoid activity, this must be supplemented by an appropriate amount of a salt-retaining hormone such as fludrocortisone. Synthetic glucocorticoids that are long-acting and devoid of salt-retaining activity should not be administered to these patients.

b. Acute—When acute adrenocortical insufficiency is suspected, treatment must be instituted immediately. Therapy consists of correction of fluid and electrolyte abnormalities and treatment of precipitating factors in addition to large amounts of parenteral hydrocortisone.

Hydrocortisone sodium succinate or phosphate in doses of 100 mg intravenously is given every 8 hours until the patient is stable. The dose is then gradually reduced, achieving maintenance dosage within 5 days. The administration of salt-retaining hormone is resumed when the total hydrocortisone dosage has been reduced to 50 mg/d.

2. Adrenocortical hypo- and hyperfunction—

a. Congenital adrenal hyperplasia—This group of disorders is characterized by specific defects in the synthesis of cortisol. In pregnancies at high risk for congenital adrenal hyperplasia, fetuses can be protected from genital abnormalities by administration of dexamethasone to the mother. The most common defect is a decrease in or lack of P450c21 (21β-hydroxylase) activity.*

As can be seen in Figure 39–1, this would lead to a reduction in cortisol synthesis and produce a compensatory increase in ACTH release. The gland becomes hyperplastic and produces abnormally large amounts of precursors such as 17-hydroxyprogesterone that can be diverted to the androgen pathway, leading to virilization. Metabolism of this compound in the liver leads to pregnanetriol, which is characteristically excreted into

---

* Names for the adrenal steroid synthetic enzymes include the following:
  P450c11 (11β-hydroxylase)
  P450c17 (17α-hydroxylase)
  P450c21 (21β-hydroxylase)

the urine in large amounts in this disorder and can be used to make the diagnosis and to monitor efficacy of glucocorticoid substitution. However, the most reliable method of detecting this disorder is the increased response of plasma 17-hydroxyprogesterone to ACTH stimulation.

If the defect is in 11-hydroxylation, large amounts of deoxycorticosterone are produced, and because this steroid has mineralocorticoid activity, hypertension with or without hypokalemic alkalosis ensues. When 17-hydroxylation is defective in the adrenals and gonads, hypogonadism is also present. However, increased amounts of 11-deoxycorticosterone (DOC; see page 653) are formed, and the signs and symptoms associated with mineralocorticoid excess—such as hypertension and hypokalemia—are also observed.

When first seen, the infant with congenital adrenal hyperplasia may be in acute adrenal crisis and should be treated as described above, using appropriate electrolyte solutions and an intravenous preparation of hydrocortisone in stress doses.

Once the patient is stabilized, oral hydrocortisone, 12–18 mg/m²/d in two unequally divided doses (two thirds in the morning, one third in late afternoon) is begun. The dosage is adjusted to allow normal growth and bone maturation and to prevent androgen excess. Alternate-day therapy with prednisone has also been used to achieve greater ACTH suppression without increasing growth inhibition. Fludrocortisone, 0.05–0.2 mg/d, should also be administered by mouth, with added salt to maintain normal blood pressure, plasma renin activity, and electrolytes.

b. Cushing's syndrome—Cushing's syndrome is usually the result of bilateral adrenal hyperplasia secondary to an ACTH-secreting pituitary adenoma (Cushing's disease) but occasionally is due to tumors or nodular hyperplasia of the adrenal gland or ectopic production of ACTH by other tumors. The manifestations are those associated with the chronic presence of excessive glucocorticoids. When glucocorticoid hypersecretion is marked and prolonged, a rounded, plethoric face and trunk obesity are striking in appearance. The manifestations of protein loss are often found and include muscle wasting, thinning, purple color striae and easy bruising of the skin, poor wound healing, and osteoporosis. Other serious disturbances include mental disorders, hypertension, and diabetes. This disorder is treated by surgical removal of the tumor producing ACTH or cortisol, irradiation of the pituitary tumor, or resection of one or both adrenals. These patients must receive large doses of cortisol during and following the surgical procedure. Doses of up to 300 mg of soluble hydrocortisone may be given as a continuous intravenous infusion on the day of surgery. The dose must be reduced slowly to normal replacement levels, since rapid reduction in dose may produce withdrawal symptoms, including fever and joint pain. If adrenalectomy has been performed, long-term maintenance is similar to that outlined above for adrenal insufficiency.

c. Aldosteronism—Primary aldosteronism usually results from the excessive production of aldosterone by an adrenal adenoma. However, it may also result from abnormal secretion by hyperplastic glands or from a malignant tumor. The clinical findings of hypertension, weakness, and tetany are related to the continued renal loss of potassium, which leads to hypokalemia, alkalosis, and elevation of serum sodium concentrations. This syndrome can also be produced in disorders of adrenal steroid biosynthesis by excessive secretion of deoxycorticosterone, corticosterone, or 18-hydroxycorticosterone—all compounds with inherent mineralocorticoid activity.

In contrast to patients with secondary aldosteronism (see below), these patients have low (suppressed) levels of plasma renin activity and angiotensin II. When treated with deoxycorticosterone acetate (20 mg/d intramuscularly for 3 days—no longer available in the USA) or fludrocortisone (0.2 mg twice daily orally for 3 days), they fail to retain sodium and their secretion of aldosterone is not significantly reduced. When the disorder is mild, it may escape detection when serum potassium levels are used for screening. However, it may be detected by an increased ratio of plasma aldosterone to renin. Patients are generally improved when treated with spironolactone, and the response to this agent is of diagnostic and therapeutic value.

3. Use of glucocorticoids for diagnostic purposes—It is sometimes necessary to suppress the production of ACTH in order to identify the source of a particular hormone or to establish whether its production is influenced by the secretion of ACTH. In these circumstances, it is advantageous to employ a very potent substance such as dexamethasone because the use of small quantities reduces the possibility of confusion in the interpretation of hormone assays in blood or urine. For example, if complete suppression is achieved by the use of 50 mg of cortisol, the urinary 17-hydroxycorticosteroids will be 15–18 mg/24 h, since one third of the dose given will be recovered in urine as 17-hydroxycorticosteroid. If an equivalent dose of 1.5 mg of dexamethasone is employed, the urinary excretion will be only 0.5 mg/24 h and blood levels will be low.

The **dexamethasone suppression test** is used for the diagnosis of Cushing's syndrome and has also been used in the differential diagnosis of depressive psychiatric states. As a screening test, dexamethasone, 1 mg, is given orally at 11 PM, and a plasma sample is obtained in the morning. In normal individuals, the morning cortisol concentration is usually less than 3 μg/dL, whereas in Cushing's syndrome the level is usually greater than 5 μg/dL. The results are not reliable in the presence of depression, anxiety, concurrent illness, and other stressful conditions or if the patient receives a medication that enhances the catabolism of dexamethasone in the liver. To distinguish between hypercortisolism due to anxiety, depression, and alcoholism (pseudo-Cushing syndrome) and bona fide Cushing's syndrome, a combined test is carried out, consisting of dexamethasone (0.5 mg orally every 6 hours for 2 days) followed by a standard corticotropin-releasing hormone (CRH) test (1 mg/kg given as a bolus intravenous infusion 2 hours after the last dose of dexamethasone).

In patients in whom the diagnosis of Cushing's syndrome has been established clinically and confirmed by a finding of elevated free cortisol in the urine, suppression with large doses of dexamethasone will help to distinguish patients with Cushing's disease from those with steroid-producing tumors of the adrenal cortex or with the ectopic ACTH syndrome. Dexamethasone is given in a dosage of 0.5 mg orally every 6 hours for 2 days, followed by 2 mg orally every 6 hours for 2 days, and the urine is then assayed for cortisol or its metabolites (Liddle's test); or dexamethasone is given as a single dose of 8 mg at 11 PM and the plasma cortisol is measured at 8 AM the following day. In patients with Cushing's disease, the suppressant effect of dexamethasone will usually produce a 50% reduction in hormone levels. In patients in whom suppression does not occur, the ACTH level will be low in the presence of a cortisol-producing adrenal tumor and elevated in patients with an ectopic ACTH-producing tumor.

B. Corticosteroids and Stimulation of Lung Maturation in the Fetus

Lung maturation in the fetus is regulated by the fetal secretion of cortisol. Treatment of the mother with large doses of glucocorticoid reduces the incidence of respiratory distress syndrome in infants delivered prematurely. When delivery is anticipated before 34 weeks of gestation, intramuscular betamethasone, 12 mg, followed by an additional dose of 12 mg 18–24 hours later, is commonly used. Betamethasone is chosen because maternal protein binding and placental metabolism of this corticosteroid is less than that of cortisol, allowing increased transfer across the placenta to the fetus.

C. Corticosteroids and Nonadrenal Disorders

The synthetic analogs of cortisol are useful in the treatment of a diverse group of diseases unrelated to any known disturbance of adrenal function (Table 39–2). The usefulness of corticosteroids in these disorders is a function of their ability to suppress inflammatory and immune responses, as described above. In disorders in which host response is the cause of the major manifestations of the disease, these agents are useful. In instances where the inflammatory or immune response is important in controlling the pathologic process, therapy with corticosteroids may be dangerous but justified to prevent irreparable damage from an inflammatory response—if used in conjunction with specific therapy for the disease process.

Since the corticosteroids are not usually curative, the pathologic process may progress while clinical manifestations are suppressed. Therefore, chronic therapy with these drugs should be undertaken with great care and only when the seriousness of the disorder warrants their use and less hazardous measures have been exhausted.

In general, attempts should be made to bring the disease process under control using medium- to intermediate-acting glucocorticoids such as prednisone and prednisolone (Table 39–1), as well as all ancillary measures possible to keep the dose low. Where possible, alternate-day therapy should be utilized (see below). Therapy should not be decreased or stopped abruptly. When prolonged therapy is anticipated, it is helpful to obtain chest x-rays and a tuberculin test, since glucocorticoid therapy can reactivate dormant disease. The presence of diabetes, peptic ulcer, osteoporosis, and psychologic disturbances should be taken into consideration, and cardiovascular function should be assessed.

Toxicity

The benefits obtained from use of the glucocorticoids vary considerably. Use of these drugs must be carefully weighed in each patient against their widespread effects on every part of the organism. The major undesirable effects of the glucocorticoids are the result of their hormonal actions (see above), which lead to the clinical picture of iatrogenic Cushing's syndrome (see below).

When the glucocorticoids are used for short periods (less than 2 weeks), it is unusual to see serious adverse effects even with moderately large doses. However, insomnia, behavioral changes (primarily hypomania), and acute peptic ulcers are occasionally observed even after only a few days of treatment. Acute pancreatitis is a rare but serious acute adverse effect of high-dose glucocorticoids.

A. Metabolic Effects

Most patients who are given daily doses of 100 mg of hydrocortisone or more (or the equivalent amount of synthetic steroid) for longer than 2 weeks undergo a series of changes that have been termed iatrogenic Cushing's syndrome. The rate of development is a function of the dose and the genetic background of the patient. In the face, rounding, puffiness, fat deposition, and plethora usually appear (moon facies). Similarly, fat

Table 39–2. Some therapeutic indications for the use of glucocorticoids in nonadrenal disorders.

Disorder	Examples
Allergic reactions	Angioneurotic edema, asthma, bee stings, contact dermatitis, drug reactions, allergic rhinitis, serum sickness, urticaria
Collagen-vascular disorders	Giant cell arteritis, lupus erythematosus, mixed connective tissue syndromes, polymyositis, polymyalgia rheumatica, rheumatoid arthritis, temporal arteritis
Eye diseases	Acute uveitis, allergic conjunctivitis, choroiditis, optic neuritis
Gastrointestinal diseases	Inflammatory bowel disease, nontropical sprue, subacute hepatic necrosis
Hematologic disorders	Acquired hemolytic anemia, acute allergic purpura, leukemia, autoimmune hemolytic anemia, idiopathic thrombocytopenic purpura, multiple myeloma
Systemic inflammation	Acute respiratory distress syndrome; (sustained therapy with moderate dosage accelerates recovery and decreases mortality)
Infections	Gram-negative septicemia; (occasionally helpful to suppress excessive inflammation)
Inflammatory conditions of bones and joints	Arthritis, bursitis, tenosynovitis
Neurologic disorders	Cerebral edema (large doses of dexamethasone are given to patients following brain surgery to minimize cerebral edema in the postoperative period), multiple sclerosis
Organ transplants	Prevention and treatment of rejection (immunosuppression)
Pulmonary diseases	Aspiration pneumonia, bronchial asthma, prevention of infant respiratory distress syndrome, sarcoidosis
Renal disorders	Nephrotic syndrome
Skin diseases	Atopic dermatitis, dermatoses, lichen simplex chronicus (localized neurodermatitis), mycosis fungoides, pemphigus, seborrheic dermatitis, xerosis
Thyroid diseases	Malignant exophthalmos, subacute thyroiditis
Miscellaneous	Hypercalcemia, mountain sickness

tends to be redistributed from the extremities to the trunk, the back of the neck, and the supraclavicular fossae. There is an increased growth of fine hair over the face, thighs and trunk. Steroid-induced punctate acne may appear, and insomnia and increased appetite are noted. In the treatment of dangerous or disabling disorders, these changes may not require cessation of therapy. However, the underlying metabolic changes accompanying them can be very serious by the time they become obvious. The continuing breakdown of protein and diversion of amino acids to glucose production increase the need for insulin and over a period of time result in weight gain; visceral fat deposition; myopathy and muscle wasting; thinning of the skin, with striae and bruising; hyperglycemia; and eventually the development of osteoporosis, diabetes, and aseptic necrosis of the hip. Wound healing is also impaired under these circumstances. When diabetes occurs, it is treated by diet and insulin. These patients are often resistant to insulin but rarely develop ketoacidosis. In general, patients treated with corticosteroids should be on high-protein and potassium-enriched diets.

B. OTHER COMPLICATIONS

Other serious side effects include peptic ulcers and their consequences. The clinical findings associated with certain disorders, particularly bacterial and mycotic infections, may be masked by the corticosteroids, and patients must be carefully watched to avoid serious mishap when large doses are used. The frequency of severe myopathy is greater in patients treated with long-acting glucocorticoids. The administration of such compounds has been associated with nausea, dizziness, and weight loss in some patients. It is treated by changing drugs, reducing dosage, and increasing potassium and protein intake.

Hypomania or acute psychosis may occur, particularly in patients receiving very large doses of corticosteroids. Long-term therapy with intermediate- and long-acting steroids is associated with depression and the development of posterior subcapsular cataracts. Psychiatric follow-up and periodic slit lamp examination is indicated in such patients. Increased intraocular pressure is common, and glaucoma may be induced. Benign intracranial hypertension also occurs. In dosages of 45 mg/m²/d or more of hydrocortisone or its equivalent, growth retardation occurs in children. Medium-, intermediate-, and long-acting glucocorticoids have greater growth-suppressing potency than the natural steroid at equivalent doses.

When given in greater than physiologic amounts, steroids such as cortisone and hydrocortisone, which have mineralocorticoid effects in addition to glucocorticoid effects, cause some sodium and fluid retention and loss of potassium. In patients with normal cardiovascular and renal function, this leads to a hypokalemic, hypochloremic alkalosis and eventually a rise in blood pressure. In patients with hypoproteinemia, renal disease, or liver disease, edema may also occur. In patients with heart disease, even small degrees of sodium retention may lead to heart failure. These effects can be minimized by using synthetic non-salt-retaining steroids, sodium restriction, and judicious amounts of potassium supplements.

C. ADRENAL SUPPRESSION

When corticosteroids are administered for more than 2 weeks, adrenal suppression may occur. If treatment extends over weeks to months, the patient should be given appropriate supplementary therapy at times of minor stress (twofold dose increases for 24–48 hours) or severe stress (up to tenfold dose increases for 48–72 hours) such as accidental trauma or major surgery. If corticosteroid dosage is to be reduced, it should be tapered slowly. If therapy is to be stopped, the reduction process should be quite slow when the dose reaches replacement levels. It may take 2–12 months for the hypothalamic-pituitary-adrenal axis to function acceptably, and cortisol levels may not return to normal for another 6–9 months. The glucocorticoid-induced suppression is not a pituitary problem, and treatment with ACTH does not reduce the time required for the return of normal function.

If the dose is reduced too rapidly in patients receiving glucocorticoids for a certain disorder, the symptoms of the disorder may reappear or increase in intensity. However, patients without an underlying disorder (eg, patients cured surgically of Cushing's disease) will also develop symptoms with rapid reductions in corticosteroid levels. These symptoms include anorexia, nausea or vomiting, weight loss, lethargy, headache, fever, joint or muscle pain, and postural hypotension. Although many of these symptoms may reflect true glucocorticoid deficiency, they may also occur in the presence of normal or even elevated plasma cortisol levels, suggesting glucocorticoid dependence.

Contraindications & Cautions

A. SPECIAL PRECAUTIONS

Patients receiving these drugs must be monitored carefully for the development of hyperglycemia, glycosuria, sodium retention with edema or hypertension, hypokalemia, peptic ulcer, osteoporosis, and hidden infections.

The dosage should be kept as low as possible, and intermittent administration (eg, alternate-day) should be employed when satisfactory therapeutic results can be obtained on this schedule. Even patients maintained on relatively low doses of corticosteroids may require supplementary therapy at times of stress, such as when surgical procedures are performed or intercurrent illness or accidents occur.

B. CONTRAINDICATIONS

These agents must be used with great caution in patients with peptic ulcer, heart disease or hypertension with heart failure, certain infectious illnesses such as varicella and tuberculosis, psychoses, diabetes, osteoporosis, or glaucoma.

Selection of Drug & Dosage Schedule

Since these preparations differ with respect to relative anti-inflammatory and mineralocorticoid effect, duration of action, cost, and dosage forms available (Table 39–1), these factors should be taken into account in selecting the drug to be used.

A. ACTH VERSUS ADRENOCORTICAL STEROIDS

In patients with normal adrenals, ACTH was used to induce the endogenous production of cortisol to obtain similar effects. However, except when the increase in androgens is desirable, the use of ACTH as a therapeutic agent has been abandoned. Instances in which ACTH was claimed to be more effective than glucocorticoids were probably due to the administration of smaller amounts of corticosteroids than were produced by the dosage of ACTH.

B. DOSAGE

In determining the dosage regimen to be used, the physician must consider the seriousness of the disease, the amount of drug likely to be required to obtain the desired effect, and the duration of therapy. In some diseases, the amount required for maintenance of the desired therapeutic effect is less than the dose needed to obtain the initial effect, and the lowest possible dosage for the needed effect should be determined by gradually lowering the dose until a small increase in signs or symptoms is noted.

When it is necessary to maintain continuously elevated plasma corticosteroid levels in order to suppress ACTH, a slowly absorbed parenteral preparation or small oral doses at frequent intervals are required. The opposite situation exists with respect to the use of corticosteroids in the treatment of inflammatory and allergic disorders. The same total quantity given in a few doses may be more effective than when given in many smaller doses or in a slowly absorbed parenteral form.

Severe autoimmune conditions involving vital organs must be treated aggressively, and undertreatment is as dangerous as overtreatment. In order to minimize the deposition of immune complexes and the influx of leukocytes and macrophages, 1 mg/kg/d of prednisone in divided doses is required initially. This dose is maintained until the serious manifestations respond. The dose can then be gradually reduced.

When large doses are required for prolonged periods of time, **alternate-day** administration of the compound may be tried after control is achieved. When used in this manner, very large amounts (eg, 100 mg of prednisone) can sometimes be administered with less marked adverse effects because there is a recovery period between each dose. The transition to an alternate-day schedule can be made after the disease process is under control. It should be done gradually and with additional supportive measures between doses. A typical schedule for a patient previously maintained on 50 mg of prednisone daily could be as follows:

Day 1:	50 mg	Day 7:	75 mg
2:	40 mg	8:	5 mg
3:	60 mg	9:	70 mg
4:	30 mg	10:	5 mg
5:	70 mg	11:	65 mg
6:	10 mg	12:	5 mg, etc

When selecting a drug for use in large doses, a medium- or intermediate-acting synthetic steroid with little mineralocorticoid effect is advisable. If possible, it should be given as a single morning dose.

C. SPECIAL DOSAGE FORMS

The use of local therapy, such as topical preparations for skin disease, ophthalmic forms for eye disease, intra-articular injections for joint disease, inhaled steroids for asthma, and hydrocortisone enemas for ulcerative colitis, provides a means of delivering large amounts of steroid to the diseased tissue with reduced systemic effects.

Beclomethasone dipropionate and several other glucocorticoids—primarily budesonide and flunisolide and mometasone furoate, administered as aerosols—have been found to be effective in the treatment of asthma (see Chapter 20). The switch from therapy with systemic glucocorticoids to aerosol therapy must be undertaken with caution, since manifestations of glucocorticoid deficiency will appear if adrenal function has been suppressed. In such patients, a slow, graded reduction of systemic therapy and monitoring of endogenous adrenal function should accompany the institution of aerosol administration.

Beclomethasone dipropionate, triamcinolone acetonide, budesonide, flunisolide, and mometasone furoate are available as nasal sprays for the topical treatment of allergic rhinitis. They are effective at doses (one or two sprays one, two, or three times daily) that in most patients result in plasma levels too low to influence adrenal function or have any other systemic effects.

Corticosteroids incorporated in ointments, creams, lotions, and sprays are used extensively in dermatology. These preparations are discussed in more detail in Chapter 62.

MINERALOCORTICOIDS (ALDOSTERONE, DEOXYCORTICOSTERONE, FLUDROCORTISONE)

The most important mineralocorticoid in humans is aldosterone. However, small amounts of deoxycorticosterone (DOC) are also formed and released. Although the amount is normally insignificant, DOC was of some importance therapeutically in the past. Its actions, effects, and metabolism are qualitatively similar to those described below for aldosterone.

Fludrocortisone, a synthetic corticosteroid, is the most commonly prescribed salt-retaining hormone.

1. Aldosterone

Aldosterone is synthesized mainly in the zona glomerulosa of the adrenal cortex. Its structure and synthesis are illustrated in Figure 39–1.

The rate of aldosterone secretion is subject to several influences. ACTH produces a moderate stimulation of its release, but this effect is not sustained for more than a few days in the normal individual. Although aldosterone is no less than one third as effective as cortisol in suppressing ACTH, the quantities of aldosterone produced by the adrenal cortex and its plasma concentrations are insufficient to participate in any significant feedback control of ACTH secretion.

In the absence of of ACTH, aldosterone secretion falls to about half the normal rate, indicating that other factors, eg, angiotensin, are able to maintain and perhaps regulate its secretion (see Chapter 17). Independent variations between cortisol and aldosterone secretion can also be demonstrated by means of lesions in the nervous system such as decerebration, which decreases the secretion of cortisol while increasing the secretion of aldosterone.

Physiologic & Pharmacologic Effects

Aldosterone and other steroids with mineralocorticoid properties promote the reabsorption of sodium from the distal convoluted and cortical collecting renal tubules, loosely coupled to the excretion of potassium and hydrogen ion. Sodium reabsorption in the sweat and salivary glands, gastrointestinal mucosa, and across cell membranes in general is also increased. Excessive levels of aldosterone produced by tumors or overdosage with synthetic mineralocorticoids lead to hypernatremia, hypokalemia, metabolic alkalosis, increased plasma volume, and hypertension.

Mineralocorticoids act by binding to the mineralocorticoid receptor in the cytoplasm of target cells, especially principal cells of the distal convoluted and collecting tubules of the kidney. The drug-receptor complex activates a series of events similar to those described above for the glucocorticoids and illustrated in Figure 39–3. It is of interest that this receptor has the same affinity for cortisol, which is present in much higher concentrations in the extracellular fluid. The specificity for mineralocorticoids at this site appears to be conferred, at least in part, by the presence of the enzyme 11β-hydroxysteroid dehydrogenase, which converts cortisol to cortisone. The latter has low affinity for the receptor and is inactive as a mineralocorticoid or glucocorticoid.

Metabolism

Aldosterone is secreted at the rate of 100–200 μg/d in normal individuals with a moderate dietary salt intake. The plasma level in men (resting supine) is about 0.007 μg/dL. The half-life of aldosterone injected in tracer quantities is 15–20 minutes, and it does not appear to be firmly bound to serum proteins.

The metabolism of aldosterone is similar to that of cortisol, about 50 μg/24 h appearing in the urine as conjugated tetrahydroaldosterone. Approximately 5–15 μg/24 h is excreted free or as the 3-oxo glucuronide.

2. Deoxycorticosterone (DOC)

DOC, which also serves as a precursor of aldosterone (Figure 39–1), is normally secreted in amounts of about 200 μg/d. Its half-life when injected into the human circulation is about 70 minutes. Preliminary estimates of its concentration in plasma are approximately 0.03 μg/dL. The control of its secretion differs from that of aldosterone in that the secretion of DOC is primarily under the control of ACTH. Although the response to ACTH is enhanced by dietary sodium restriction, a low-salt diet does not increase DOC secretion. The secretion of DOC may be markedly increased in abnormal conditions such as adrenocortical carcinoma and congenital adrenal hyperplasia with reduced P450c11 or P450c17 activity.

3. Fludrocortisone

This compound, a potent steroid with both glucocorticoid and mineralocorticoid activity, is the most widely used mineralocorticoid. Doses of 0.1 mg two to seven times weekly have potent salt-retaining activity and are used in the treatment of adrenocortical insufficiency associated with mineralocorticoid deficiency. These dosages are too small to have important anti-inflammatory or antigrowth effects.

ADRENAL ANDROGENS

The adrenal cortex secretes large amounts of dehydroepiandrosterone (DHEA) and smaller amounts of androstenedione and testosterone. Although these androgens are thought to contribute to the normal maturation process, they do not stimulate or support major androgen-dependent pubertal changes in humans. Recent studies suggest that DHEA and its sulfate (DHEAS) may have other important physiologic actions (see also Chapter 65). If that is correct, these results are probably due to the peripheral conversion of DHEA to more potent androgens or to estrogens and interaction with androgen and estrogen receptors, respectively. Additional effects may be exerted through an interaction with the $GABA_A$ and glutamate receptors in the brain or with a newly discovered nuclear receptor in several central and peripheral sites. The therapeutic use of DHEA in humans is being explored, but the substance has already been adopted with uncritical enthusiasm by members of the sports drug culture and the vitamin and food supplement culture. The results of a placebo-controlled trial of DHEA in patients with systemic lupus erythematosus were recently reported as well as those of a study of DHEA replacement in women with adrenal insufficiency. In both studies a beneficial effect was seen, with significant improvement of the disease in the former and a clearly added sense of well-being in the latter. The androgenic or estrogenic actions of DHEA could explain the effects of the compound in both situations.

ANTAGONISTS OF ADRENOCORTICAL AGENTS

SYNTHESIS INHIBITORS & GLUCOCORTICOID ANTAGONISTS

1. *Metyrapone*

Metyrapone (Figure 39–5) is a relatively selective inhibitor of steroid synthesis. It inhibits 11-hydroxylation, interfering with cortisol and corticosterone synthesis. In the presence of a normal pituitary gland, there is a compensatory increase in 11-deoxycortisol secretion. This response is a measure of the capacity of the anterior pituitary to produce ACTH and has been adapted for clinical use as a diagnostic test. Although the toxicity of metyrapone is much lower than that of mitotane (see below), the drug may produce transient dizziness and gastrointestinal disturbances. This agent has not been widely used for the treatment of Cushing's syndrome.

However, in doses of 0.25 g twice daily to 1 g four times daily, metyrapone can reduce cortisol production to normal levels in some patients with endogenous Cushing's syndrome. Thus, it may be useful in the management of severe manifestations of cortisol excess while the cause of this condition is being determined or in conjunction with radiation or surgical treatment. It is the only adrenal-inhibiting medication that can be administered to pregnant women with Cushing's syndrome. The major adverse effects observed are salt and water retention and hirsutism resulting from diversion of the 11-deoxycortisol precursor to DOC and androgen synthesis.

Metyrapone is commonly used in tests of adrenal function. The blood levels of 11-deoxycortisol and the urinary excretion of 17-hydroxycorticoids are measured before and after administration of the compound. Normally, there is a twofold or greater increase in the urinary 17-hydroxycorticoid excretion. A dose of 300–500 mg every 4 hours for six doses is often used, and urine collections are made on the day before and the day after treatment. In patients with Cushing's syndrome, a normal response to metyrapone indicates that the cortisol excess is not the

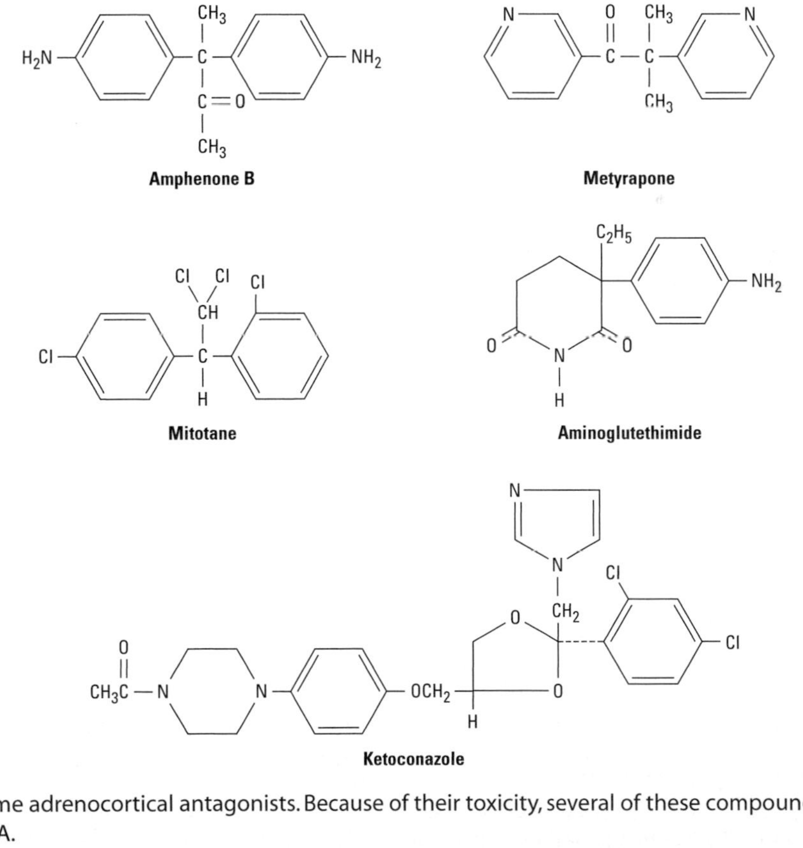

Figure 39–5. Some adrenocortical antagonists. Because of their toxicity, several of these compounds are no longer available in the USA.

result of a cortisol-secreting adrenal carcinoma or adenoma, since secretion by such tumors produces suppression of ACTH and atrophy of normal adrenal cortex.

Adrenal function may also be tested by administering metyrapone, 2–3 g orally at midnight, and measuring the level of ACTH or 11-deoxycortisol in blood drawn at 8 AM, or by comparing the excretion of 17-hydroxycorticosteroids in the urine during the 24-hour periods preceding and following administration of the drug. In patients with suspected or known lesions of the pituitary, this procedure is a means of estimating the ability of the gland to produce ACTH. The drug has been withdrawn from the market in the USA but is available on a compassionate basis.

2. Aminoglutethimide

Aminoglutethimide (Figure 39–5) blocks the conversion of cholesterol to pregnenolone and causes a reduction in the synthesis of all hormonally active steroids (Figure 39–1). It has been used in conjunction with dexamethasone or hydrocortisone to reduce or eliminate estrogen production in patients with carcinoma of the breast. In a dosage of 1 g/d it was well tolerated; however, with higher dosages, lethargy and skin rash was a common effect. The use of aminoglutethimide in breast cancer patients has now been supplanted by the use of tamoxifen, an estrogen antagonist or another class of drugs, the aromatase inhibitors (see Chapter 40). Aminoglutethimide can be used in conjunction with metyrapone or ketoconazole to reduce steroid secretion in patients with Cushing's syndrome due to adrenocortical cancer who do not respond to mitotane.

Aminoglutethimide also apparently increases the clearance of some steroids. It has been shown to enhance the metabolism of dexamethasone, reducing its half-life from 4–5 hours to 2 hours.

3. Ketoconazole

Ketoconazole, an antifungal imidazole derivative (see Chapter 48), is a potent and rather nonselective inhibitor of adrenal and gonadal steroid synthesis. This compound inhibits the cholesterol side chain cleavage, P450c17, C17,20-lyase, 3β-hydroxysteroid dehydrogenase, and P450c11 enzymes required for steroid hormone synthesis. The sensitivity of the P450 enzymes to this compound in mammalian tissues is much lower than that needed to treat fungal infections, so that its inhibitory effects on steroid biosynthesis are seen only at high doses.

Ketoconazole has been used for the treatment of patients with Cushing's syndrome due to several causes. Dosages of 200–1200 mg/d have produced a reduction in hormone levels and impressive clinical improvement. This drug has some hepatotoxicity and should be started at 200 mg/d and slowly increased by 200 mg/d every 2–3 days up to a total daily dose of 1000 mg.

4. Mifepristone (RU 486)

The search for a glucocorticoid receptor antagonist finally succeeded in the early 1980s with the development of the 11β-aminophenyl-substituted 19-norsteroid called RU 486, later named mifepristone. This compound has strong antiprogestin activity and initially was proposed as a contraceptive-contragestive agent. High doses of mifepristone exert antiglucocorticoid activity by blocking the glucocorticoid receptor, since mifepristone binds to it with high affinity, causing (1) some stabilization of the Hsp-glucocorticoid receptor complex and, thus, inhibition of the dissociation of the RU 486-bound glucocorticoid receptor from the Hsp chaperone proteins; and (2) alteration of the interaction of the glucocorticoid receptor with coregulators, favoring the formation of a transcriptionally inactive complex in the cell nucleus. The result is inhibition of glucocorticoid receptor activation.

The mean half-life of mifepristone is 20 hours. This is longer than that of many natural and synthetic glucocorticoid agonists (dexamethasone has a half-life of 4–5 hours). Less than 1% of the daily dose is excreted in the urine, suggesting a minor role of kidneys in the clearance of the compound. The long plasma half-life of mifepristone results from extensive and strong binding to plasma proteins. Less than 5% of the compound is found in the free form when plasma is analyzed by equilibrium dialysis. Mifepristone can bind to albumin and α_1-acid glycoprotein, but it has no affinity for CBG.

In humans, mifepristone causes generalized glucocorticoid resistance. Given orally to several patients with Cushing's syndrome due to ectopic ACTH production or adrenal carcinoma, it was able to reverse the cushingoid phenotype, to eliminate carbohydrate intolerance, normalize blood pressure, correct thyroid and gonadal hormone suppression, and ameliorate the psychologic sequelae of hypercortisolism in these patients. To date, the application of mifepristone can only be recommended for inoperable patients with ectopic ACTH secretion or adrenal carcinoma who have failed to respond to other therapeutic manipulations. Its pharmacology and use in women as a progesterone antagonist are discussed in Chapter 40.

5. Mitotane

Mitotane (Figure 39–5) has adrenolytic properties in dogs and to a lesser extent in humans. This drug is administered orally in divided doses up to 12 g daily. About one-third of patients with adrenal carcinoma show a reduction in tumor mass. In 80% of patients, the toxic effects are sufficiently severe to require dose reduction. These include diarrhea, nausea, vomiting, depression, somnolence, and skin rashes. The drug has been withdrawn from the market in the USA but is available on a compassionate basis.

6. Trilostane

Trilostane is a 3β-17 hydroxysteroid dehydrogenase inhibitor that interferes with the synthesis of adrenal and gonadal hormones and is comparable to aminoglutethimide. Its side effects are predominantly gastrointestinal; adverse effects occur in about 50% of patients with both agents. There is no cross-resistance or crossover of side effects between these compounds.

MINERALOCORTICOID ANTAGONISTS

In addition to agents that interfere with aldosterone synthesis (see above), there are steroids that compete with aldosterone for binding sites and decrease its effect peripherally. Progesterone is mildly active in this respect.

Spironolactone is a 7α acetylthiospironolactone. Its onset of action is slow, and the effects last for 2–3 days after the drug is discontinued. It is used in the treatment of primary aldosteronism in dosages of 50–100 mg/d. This agent reverses many of the manifestations of aldosteronism. It has been useful in establishing the diagnosis in some patients and in ameliorating the signs and symptoms when surgical removal of an adenoma is delayed. When used diagnostically for the detection of aldosteronism in hypokalemic patients with hypertension, dosages of 400–500 mg/d for 4–8 days—with an adequate intake of sodium and potassium—will restore potassium levels to or toward normal. This agent is also useful in preparing these patients for surgery. Dosages of 300–400 mg/d for 2 weeks are used for this purpose and may reduce the incidence of cardiac arrhythmias.

Spironolactone is also an androgen antagonist and as such is used in treatment of hirsutism in women. Dosages of 50–200 mg/d cause a reduction in the density, diameter, and rate of growth of facial hair in patients with idiopathic hirsutism or hirsutism secondary to androgen excess. The effect can usually be seen in 2 months and becomes maximal in about 6 months.

Spironolactone

The use of spironolactone as a diuretic is discussed in Chapter 15. The drug has benefits in heart failure greater than those predicted from its diuretic effects alone (see Chapter 13). Adverse effects reported for spironolactone include hyperkalemia, cardiac arrhythmia, menstrual abnormalities, gynecomastia, sedation, headache, gastrointestinal disturbances, and skin rashes.

Eplerenone, a new aldosterone antagonist, has been approved for the treatment of hypertension (see Chapter 11). This aldosterone receptor antagonist is somewhat more selective than spironolactone and has no reported effects on androgen receptors. The standard dosage in hypertension is 50–100 mg/d. The most common toxicity is hyperkalemia but this is usually mild.

Drospirenone, a progestin in a new oral contraceptive, also antagonizes the effects of aldosterone.

PREPARATIONS AVAILABLE[1]

GLUCOCORTICOIDS FOR ORAL & PARENTERAL USE
Betamethasone (Celestone)
  Oral: 0.6 mg tablets; 0.6 mg/5 mL syrup
Betamethasone sodium phosphate (Celestone Phosphate)
  Parenteral: 4 mg/mL for IV, IM, intralesional, or intra-articular injection

---

[1] Glucocorticoids for Aerosol Use: See Chapter 20.
Glucocorticoids for Dermatologic Use: See Chapter 62.
Glucocorticoids for Gastrointestinal Use: See Chapter 63.

Cortisone (generic, Cortone Acetate)
  Oral: 5, 10, 25 mg tablets
  Parenteral: 50 mg/mL solution
Dexamethasone (generic, Decadron, others)
  Oral: 0.25, 0.5, 0.75, 1, 1.5, 2, 4, 6 mg tablets; 0.5 mg/5 mL elixir; 0.5 mg/5 mL, 0.5 mg/0.5 mL solution
Dexamethasone acetate (generic, Decadron-LA, others)
  Parenteral: 8 mg/mL suspension for IM, intralesional, or intra-articular injection; 16 mg/mL suspension for intralesional injection

Dexamethasone sodium phosphate (generic, Decadron Phosphate, others)
Parenteral: 4, 10, 20 mg/mL for IV, IM, intralesional, or intra-articular injection; 24 mg/mL for IV use only

Hydrocortisone [cortisol] (generic, Cortef)
Oral: 5, 10, 20 mg tablets

Hydrocortisone acetate (generic)
Parenteral: 25, 50 mg/mL suspension for intralesional, soft tissue, or intra-articular injection

Hydrocortisone cypionate (Cortef)
Oral: 10 mg/5 mL suspension

Hydrocortisone sodium phosphate (Hydrocortone)
Parenteral: 50 mg/mL for IV, IM, or SC injection

Hydrocortisone sodium succinate (generic, Solu-Cortef)
Parenteral: 100, 250, 500, 1000 mg/vial for IV, IM injection

Methylprednisolone (generic, Medrol)
Oral: 2, 4, 8, 16, 24, 32 mg tablets

Methylprednisolone acetate (generic, Depo-Medrol)
Parenteral: 20, 40, 80 mg/mL for IM, intralesional, or intra-articular injection

Methylprednisolone sodium succinate (generic, Solu-Medrol)
Parenteral: 40, 125, 500, 1000, 2000 mg/vial for injection

Prednisolone (generic, Delta-Cortef, Prelone)
Oral: 5 mg tablets; 5, 15 mg/5 mL syrup

Prednisolone acetate (generic)
Parenteral: 25, 50 mg/mL for soft tissue or intra-articular injection

Prednisolone sodium phosphate (Hydeltrasol, others)
Oral: 5 mg/5 mL solution
Parenteral: 20 mg/mL for IV, IM, intra-articular, or intralesional injection

Prednisolone tebutate (generic)
Oral: 5 mg/5 mL liquid
Parenteral: 20 mg/mL for intra-articular or intralesional injection

Prednisone (generic, Meticorten)
Oral: 1, 2.5, 5, 10, 20, 50 mg tablets; 1, 5 mg/mL solution and syrup

Triamcinolone (generic, Aristocort, Kenacort)
Oral: 4, 8 mg tablets; 4 mg/5 mL syrup

Triamcinolone acetonide (generic, Kenalog)
Parenteral: 3, 10, 40 mg/mL for IM, intra-articular, or intralesional injection

Triamcinolone diacetate (generic)
Parenteral: 25, 40 mg/mL for IM, intra-articular, or intralesional injection

Triamcinolone hexacetonide (Aristospan)
Parenteral: 5, 20 mg/mL for intra-articular, intralesional, or sublesional injection

MINERALOCORTICOIDS

Fludrocortisone acetate (generic, Florinef Acetate)
Oral: 0.1 mg tablets

ADRENAL STEROID INHIBITORS

Aminoglutethimide (Cytadren)
Oral: 250 mg tablets

Ketoconazole (generic, Nizoral)
Oral: 200 mg tablets (unlabeled use)

Mitotane (Lysodren)
Oral: 500 mg tablets

REFERENCES

Bamberger CM et al: Glucocorticoid receptor-beta, a potential endogenous inhibitor of glucocorticoid action in humans. J Clin Invest 1995;95:2435.

Bamberger CM, Schulte HM, Chrousos GP: Molecular determinants of glucocorticoid receptor function and tissue sensitivity to glucocorticoids. Endocr Rev 1996;17:245.

Barnes PJ, Adcock I: Anti-inflammatory actions of steroids: Molecular mechanisms. Trends Pharmacol Sci 1993;14:436.

Baulieu EE: The steroid hormone antagonist RU486: Mechanism at the cellular level and clinical applications. Endocrinol Metab Clin North Am 1991;20:873.

Bentley AM et al: Prednisolone treatment in asthma: Reduction in the numbers of eosinophils, T cells, tryptase-only positive mast cells, and modulation of IL-4, IL-5, and interferon-gamma cytokine gene expression within the bronchial mucosa. Am J Resp Crit Care Med 1996;153:551.

Bikle DD et al: Elevated 1,25-dihydroxyvitamin D levels in patients with chronic obstructive pulmonary disease treated with prednisone. J Clin Endocrinol Metab 1993;76:456

Caelles C, Gonzalez-Sancho JM, Munoz A: Nuclear hormone receptor antagonism with AP-1 by inhibition of the JNK pathway. Genes Dev Dec 1997;11:3351.

Calandra T et al: MIF as a glucocorticoid-induced modulator of cytokine production. Nature 1995;376:68.

Chin R: Adrenal crisis. Crit Care Clin 1991;7:23.

Chrousos GP: The hypothalamic-pituitary-adrenal axis and immune-mediated inflammation. N Engl J Med 1995;332:1351.

Chrousos GP, Harris AG: Hypothalamic-pituitary-adrenal axis suppression and inhaled corticosteroid therapy. 1. General principles. Neuroimmunomodulation 1998;5:277.

Chrousos GP, Harris AG: Hypothalamic-pituitary-adrenal axis suppression and inhaled corticosteroid therapy. 2. Review of the literature. Neuroimmunomodulation 1998;5:288.

Chrousos GP: Secondary adrenal insufficiency. In: Lamberts SWJ (editor). *The Diagnosis and Treatment of Pituitary Insufficiency.* Bioscientifica, 1997.

Chrousos GP: Glucocorticoid therapy and withdrawal. Curr Pract Med 1999;1:291.

Chrousos GP et al: Molecular mechanisms of glucocorticoid resistance/hypersensitivity. Am J Resp Crit Care Med 1996;154(Suppl 2 Part 2):S39.

Cummings JJ, D'Eugenio DB, Gross SJ: A controlled trial of dexamethasone in preterm infants at high risk for bronchopulmonary dysplasia. N Engl J Med 1989;320:1505.

Dorr HG, Sippell WG: Prenatal dexamethasone treatment in pregnancies at risk for congenital adrenal hyperplasia due to 21-hydroxylase deficiency: Effect on midgestational amniotic fluid steroid levels. J Clin Endocrinol Metab 1993;76:117.

Elenkov IJ, Chrousos GP: Stress hormones, TH1/TH2 patterns, pro/anti-inflammatory cytokines and susceptibility to disease. Trends Endocrinol Metab 1999;10:359.

Engelhardt D, Weber MM: Therapy of Cushing's syndrome with steroid biosynthesis inhibitors. J Steroid Biochem Mol Biol 1994;49:261.

Franchimont D et al: Glucocorticoids and inflammation revisited: The state of the art. Neuroimmunomodulation 2002–03; 10:247.

Funder JW et al: Apparent mineralocorticoid excess, pseudohypoaldosteronism, and urinary electrolyte excretion: Toward a redefinition of mineralocorticoid action. FASEB J 1990;4:3234.

Graber AL et al: Natural history of pituitary-adrenal recovery following long-term suppression with corticosteroids. J Clin Endocrinol Metab 1965;25:11.

Hahn BH, Mazzaferri EL: Glucocorticoid-induced osteoporosis. Hosp Pract (Off Ed) Aug 1995;30:45.

Hammond GL: Molecular properties of corticosteroid binding globulin and the sex-steroid binding proteins. Endocr Rev 1990;11:65.

Henriques HF III, Lebovic D: Defining and focusing perioperative steroid supplementation. Am Surg 1995;61:809.

Hochberg Z, Pacak K, Chrousos GP: Endocrine withdrawal syndromes. Endocrine Rev 2003;24:523.

Hyams JS, Carey DE: Corticosteroids and growth. J Pediatr 1988;113:249.

James VHT (editor): *The Adrenal Gland,* 2nd ed. Raven Press, 1992.

Johnson TS et al: Prevention of acute mountain sickness by dexamethasone. N Engl J Med 1984;310:683.

Kalantaridou S, Chrousos GP: Clinical review 148: Monogenic disorders of puberty. J Clin Endocrinol Metab 2002;87:2481.

Koch CA, Pacak K, Chrousos GP: Endocrine tumors. In: Pizzo PA, Poplack DG (editors). *Principles and Practice of Pediatric Oncology,* 4th ed. Lippincott Williams & Wilkins, 2002.

Koch CA, Pacak K, Chrousos GP: The molecular pathogenesis of hereditary and sporadic adrenocortical and adrenomedullary tumors. J Clin Endocrinol Metab 2002;87:5367.

Koukouritaki E et al: Dexamethasone alters rapidly actin polymerization dynamics in human endometrial cells: Evidence for nongenomic actions involving cAMP turnover. J Cell Biochem 1996;62:251.

Lamberts SWJ, Koper JW, de Jong FH: The endocrine effects of long-term treatment with mifepristone (RU 486). J Clin Endocrinol Metab 1991;73:187.

Levine BD et al: Dexamethasone in the treatment of acute mountain sickness. N Engl J Med 1989;321:1707.

Luton J-P et al: Clinical features of adrenocortical carcinoma, prognostic factors, and the effect of mitotane therapy. N Engl J Med 1990;322:1190.

McKay LI, Cidlowski JA: Cross-talk between nuclear factor-κ B and the steroid hormone receptors: Mechanisms of mutual antagonism. Mol Endocrinol 1998;12:45.

Mao J, Regelson W, Kalimi M: Molecular mechanism of RU486 action: A review. Mol Cellular Biochem 1992;109:1.

Margioris A, Gravanis A, Chrousos G: Glucocorticoids and Mineralocorticoids. In: Brondy G et al (editors). *Human Pharmacology: Molecular to Clinical.* 2nd ed. Mosby, 1994.

Margioris AN, Chrousos GP: Adrenal disorders. In: Vinken PJ, Bruyn GW (editors). *Handbook of Clinical Neurology.* Part II, *Systemic Diseases.* Elsevier, 1998.

Meduri GV, Chrousos GP: Duration of glucocorticoid treatment and outcome in sepsis: Is the right drug used the wrong way? (Editorial.) Chest 1998;114:355.

Meduri GU et al: Prolonged methylprednisolone treatment suppresses systemic inflammation in patients with unresolving ARDS: evidence for inadequate endogenous glucocorticoid secretion and inflammation-induced immune cell resistance to glucocorticoids. Am J Resp Crit Care Med 2002;165:983.

Morales AJ et al: Effects of replacement dose of dehydroepiandrosterone in men and women of advancing age. J Clin Endocrinol Metab 1994;78:1360.

Muller M, Renkawitz R: The glucocorticoid receptor. Biochim Biophys Acta 1991;1088:171.

New ML: Prenatal diagnosis and treatment of congenital adrenal hyperplasia due to 21-hydroxylase deficiency. Development Pharmacol Therap 1990;15:200.

Ning YM, Sanchez ER: In vivo evidence for the generation of a glucocorticoid receptor-heat shock protein-90 complex incapable of binding hormone by the calmodulin antagonist phenoxybenzamine. Mol Endocrinol 1996;10:14.

Oelkers W et al: Effects of a new oral contraceptive containing an antimineralocorticoid progestin, drospirenone, on the renin-aldosterone system, body weight, blood pressure, glucose tolerance, and lipid metabolism. J Clin Endocrinol Metab 1995;80:1816.

Philips A et al: Antagonism between Nur77 and glucocorticoid receptor for control of transcription. Mol Cell Biol 1997;17:5952.

Ray A, Prefontaine KE: Physical association and functional antagonism between the p65 subunit of transcription factor NF-κ B and the glucocorticoid receptor. Proc Natl Acad Sci U S A 1994;91:752.

Rogatsky I, Logan SK, Garabedian MJ: Antagonism of glucocorticoid receptor transcriptional activation by the c-Jun N-terminal kinase. Proc Natl Acad Sci U S A 1998;95:2050.

Sambrook P et al: Prevention of corticosteroid osteoporosis. N Engl J Med 1993;329:1747.

Scheinman RI et al: Role of transcriptional activation of IκBα in mediation of immunosuppression by glucocorticoids. Science 1995;270:283.

Schobitz B, Reul JM, Holsboer F: The role of the hypothalamic-pituitary-adrenocortical system during inflammatory conditions. Crit Rev Neurobiol 1994;8:263.

Smith DF, Toft DO: Steroid receptors and their associated proteins. Mol Endocrinol 1993;4:7.

Sonino N et al: Ketoconazole treatment in Cushing's syndrome: Experience in 34 patients. Clin Endocrinol 1991;35:347.

Tabarin A et al: Use of ketoconazole in the treatment of Cushing's disease and ectopic ACTH syndrome. Clin Endocrinol 1991;34:63.

Tappy L et al: Mechanisms of dexamethasone-induced insulin resistance in healthy humans. J Clin Endocrinol Metab 1994;79:1063.

Tsigos C, Chrousos GP: Differential diagnosis and management of Cushing's syndrome. Annu Rev Med 1996;47:443.

Tsigos C, Kamilaris T, Chrousos GP: Adrenal diseases. In: Moore WT, Eastman R (editors). *Diagnostic Endocrinology*, 2nd ed. BC Decker, 1996.

Tyrell JB, Findling JW, Aron DC: Adrenal cortex. In: Greenspan FS, Gardner DG (editors). *Basic & Clinical Endocrinology*, 7th ed. McGraw-Hill, 2003.

Williams CJ et al: Multicentre cross-over study of aminoglutethimide and trilostane in advanced postmenopausal breast cancer. Clin Oncol 1995;7:87.

The Gonadal Hormones & Inhibitors

40

George P. Chrousos, MD

I. THE OVARY (ESTROGENS, PROGESTINS, OTHER OVARIAN HORMONES, ORAL CONTRACEPTIVES, INHIBITORS & ANTAGONISTS, & OVULATION-INDUCING AGENTS)

The ovary has important gametogenic functions that are integrated with its hormonal activity. In the human female, the gonad is relatively quiescent during childhood, the period of rapid growth and maturation. At puberty, the ovary begins a 30- to 40-year period of cyclic function called the **menstrual cycle** because of the regular episodes of bleeding that are its most obvious manifestation. It then fails to respond to gonadotropins secreted by the anterior pituitary gland, and the cessation of cyclic bleeding that occurs is called the **menopause.**

The mechanism responsible for the onset of ovarian function at the time of puberty is thought to be neural in origin, because the immature gonad can be stimulated by gonadotropins already present in the pituitary and because the pituitary is responsive to exogenous hypothalamic gonadotropin-releasing hormone. The maturation of centers in the brain may withdraw a childhood-related inhibitory effect upon hypothalamic arcuate nucleus neurons, allowing them to produce **gonadotropin-releasing hormone (GnRH)** in pulses with the appropriate amplitude, which stimulates the release of **follicle-stimulating hormone (FSH)** and **luteinizing hormone (LH)** (see Chapter 37). At first, small amounts of the latter two hormones are released during the night, and the limited quantities of ovarian estrogen secreted in response start to cause breast development. Subsequently, FSH and LH are secreted throughout the day and night, causing secretion of higher amounts of estrogen and leading to further breast

enlargement, alterations in fat distribution, and a growth spurt that culminates in epiphysial closure in the long bones. The beginning of ovarian function at puberty is called **gonadarche.**

A year or so after gonadarche, sufficient estrogen is produced to induce endometrial changes and periodic bleeding. After the first few irregular cycles, which may be anovulatory, normal cyclic function is established.

At the beginning of each cycle, a variable number of follicles (vesicular follicles), each containing an ovum, begin to enlarge in response to FSH. After 5 or 6 days, one follicle, called the dominant follicle, begins to develop more rapidly. The outer theca and inner granulosa cells of this follicle multiply and, under the influence of LH, synthesize and release estrogens at an increasing rate. The estrogens appear to inhibit FSH release and may lead to regression of the smaller, less mature follicles. The mature dominant ovarian follicle consists of an ovum surrounded by a fluid-filled antrum lined by granulosa and theca cells. The estrogen secretion reaches a peak just before midcycle, and the granulosa cells begin to secrete progesterone. These changes stimulate the brief surge in LH and FSH release that precedes and causes ovulation. When the follicle ruptures, the ovum is released into the abdominal cavity near the opening of the uterine tube.

Following the above events, the cavity of the ruptured follicle fills with blood (corpus hemorrhagicum), and the luteinized theca and granulosa cells proliferate and replace the blood to form the corpus luteum. The cells of this structure produce estrogens and progesterone for the remainder of the cycle, or longer if pregnancy occurs.

If pregnancy does not occur, the corpus luteum begins to degenerate and ceases hormone production, eventually becoming a corpus albicans. The endometrium, which proliferated during the follicular phase and developed its glandular function during the luteal phase, is shed in the process of menstruation. These events are summarized in Figure 40–1.

The ovary normally ceases its gametogenic and endocrine function with time. This change is accompanied by a cessation in uterine bleeding (menopause) and occurs at a mean age of 52 years in the USA. Although the ovary ceases to secrete estrogen, significant levels of estrogen persist in many women as a result of conversion of adrenal and ovarian steroids such as androstenedione to estrone and estradiol in adipose and possibly other nonendocrine tissues.

Disturbances in Ovarian Function

Disturbances of cyclic function are common even during the peak years of reproduction. A minority of these result from inflammatory or neoplastic processes that influence the functions of the uterus, ovaries, or pituitary. Many of the minor disturbances leading to periods of amenorrhea or anovulatory cycles are self-limited. They are often associated with emotional or physical stress and represent temporary alterations in the stress centers in the brain that control the secretion of gonadotropin-releasing hormone. Anovulatory cycles are also associated with eating disorders (bulimia, anorexia nervosa) and with severe exercise such as distance running and swimming. Among the more common organic causes of persistent ovulatory disturbances are pituitary prolactinomas and syndromes and tumors characterized by excessive ovarian or adrenal androgen production. Normal ovarian function can be modified by androgens produced by the adrenal cortex or tumors

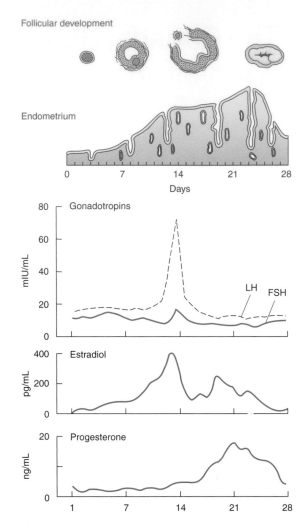

Figure 40–1. The menstrual cycle, showing plasma levels of pituitary and ovarian hormones and histologic changes.

arising from it. The ovary also gives rise to androgen-producing neoplasms such as arrhenoblastomas, as well as to estrogen-producing granulosa cell tumors.

THE ESTROGENS

Estrogenic activity is shared by a large number of chemical substances. In addition to the variety of steroidal estrogens derived from animal sources, numerous nonsteroidal estrogens have been synthesized. Many phenols are estrogenic, and estrogenic activity has been identified in such diverse forms of life as those found in ocean sediments. Estrogen-mimetic compounds (flavonoids) are found in many plants, including saw palmetto, and soybeans and other foods. Studies have shown that eating these plant products may produce slight estrogenic effects. Additionally, some compounds used in the manufacture of plastics (bisphenols, alkylphenols, phthalate phenols) have been found to be estrogenic. It has been proposed that these agents are associated with an increased breast cancer incidence in both women and men in the industrialized world.

Natural Estrogens

The major estrogens produced by women are estradiol (estradiol-17β, E₂), estrone (E₁), and estriol (E₃) (Figure 40–2). Estradiol is the major secretory product of the ovary. Although some estrone is produced in the ovary, most estrone and estriol are formed in the liver from estradiol or in peripheral tissues from androstenedione and other androgens. As noted above, during the first part of the menstrual cycle estrogens are produced in the ovarian follicle by the theca and granulosa cells. After ovulation, the estrogens as well as progesterone are synthesized by the luteinized granulosa and theca cells of the corpus luteum, and the pathways of biosynthesis are slightly different.

During pregnancy, a large amount of estrogen is synthesized by the fetoplacental unit—consisting of the fetal adrenal zone, secreting androgen precursor, and the placenta, which aromatizes it into estrogen. The estriol synthesized by the fetoplacental unit is released into the maternal circulation and excreted into the urine.

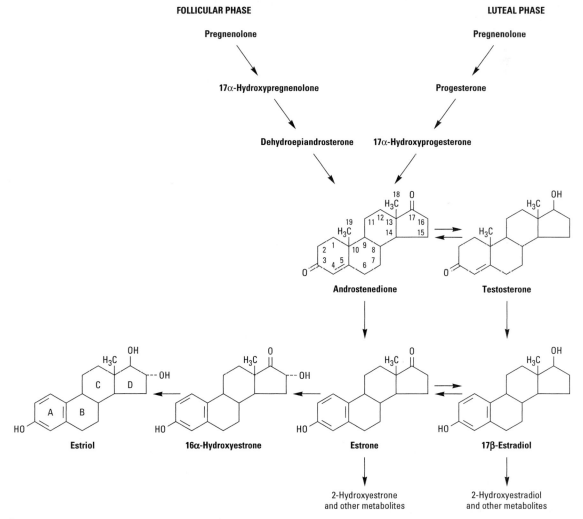

Figure 40–2. Biosynthesis and metabolism of estrogens.

Repeated assay of maternal urinary estriol excretion has been used in the assessment of fetal well-being.

One of the most prolific natural sources of estrogenic substances is the stallion, which liberates more of these hormones than the pregnant mare or pregnant woman. The equine estrogens—equilenin and equilin—and their congeners are unsaturated in the B as well as the A ring and are excreted in large quantities in urine, from which they can be recovered and used for medicinal purposes.

In normal women, estradiol is produced at a rate that varies during the menstrual cycle, resulting in plasma levels as low as 50 pg/mL in the early follicular phase to as high as 350–850 pg/mL at the time of the preovulatory peak (Figure 40–1).

Synthetic Estrogens

A variety of chemical alterations have been produced in the natural estrogens. The most important effect of these alterations has been to increase the oral effectiveness of the estrogens. Some structures are shown in Figure 40–3. Those with therapeutic use are listed in Table 40–1.

In addition to the steroidal estrogens, a variety of nonsteroidal compounds with estrogenic activity have been synthesized and used clinically. These include dienestrol, diethylstilbestrol, benzestrol, hexestrol, methestrol, methallenestril, and chlorotrianisene (Figure 40–3).

Pharmacokinetics

When released into the circulation, estradiol binds strongly to an α_2-globulin (sex hormone-binding globulin [SHBG]) and to albumin with lower affinity. Bound estrogen is relatively unavailable for diffusion into cells, so it is the free fraction that is physiologically active.

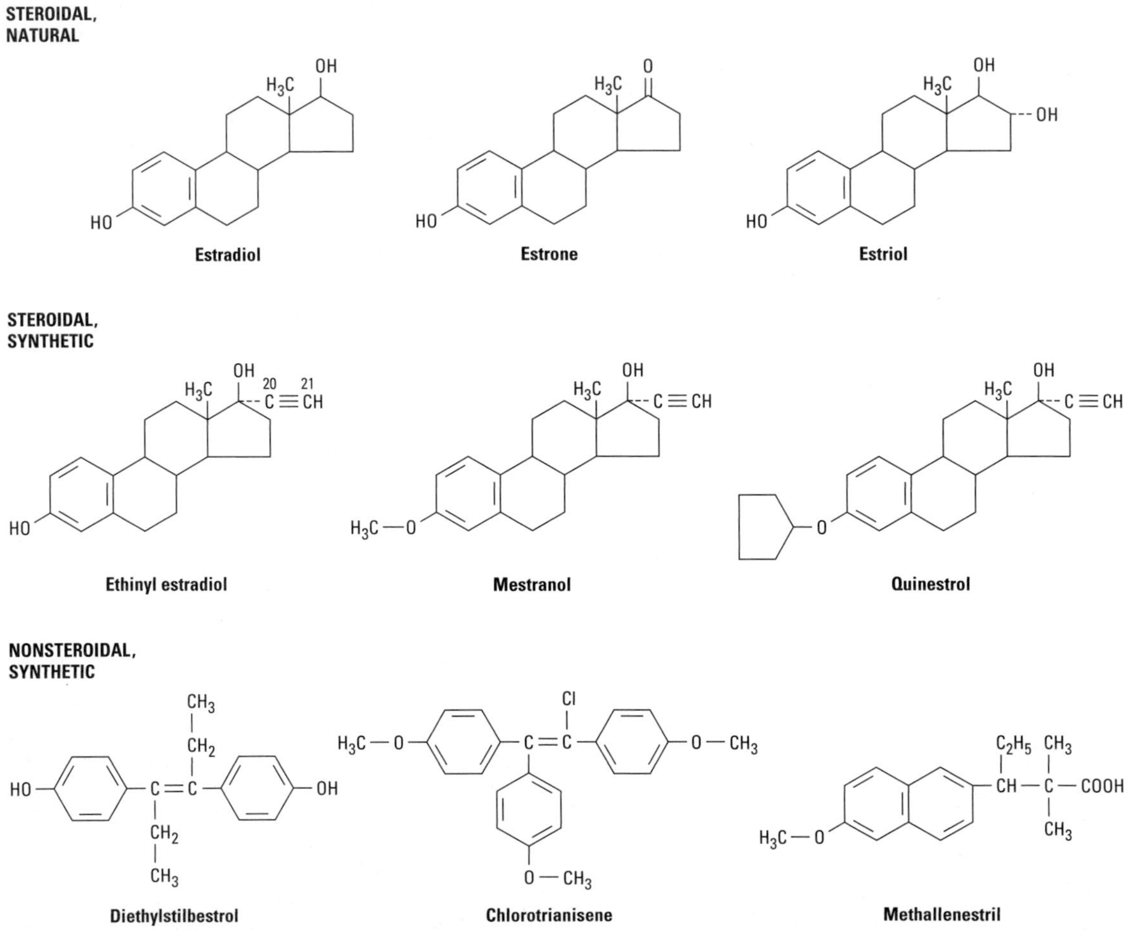

Figure 40–3. Compounds with estrogenic activity.

Table 40–1. Commonly used estrogens.

	Average Replacement Dosage
Ethinyl estradiol	0.005–0.02 mg/d
Micronized estradiol	1–2 mg/d
Estradiol cypionate	2–5 mg every 3–4 weeks
Estradiol valerate	2–20 mg every other week
Estropipate	1.25–2.5 mg/d
Conjugated, esterified, or mixed estrogenic substances:	
Oral	0.3–1.25 mg/d
Injectable	0.2–2 mg/d
Transdermal	Patch
Diethylstilbestrol	0.1–0.5 mg/d
Quinestrol	0.1–0.2 mg/week
Chlorotrianisene	12–25 mg/d
Methallenestril	3–9 mg/d

Estradiol is converted by the liver and other tissues to estrone and estriol (which have low affinity for the estrogen receptor) and their 2-hydroxylated derivatives and conjugated metabolites (which are too insoluble in lipid to cross the cell membrane readily) and excreted in the bile (Figure 40–2). However, the conjugates may be hydrolyzed in the intestine to active, reabsorbable compounds. Estrogens are also excreted in small amounts in the breast milk of nursing mothers.

Because significant amounts of estrogens and their active metabolites are excreted in the bile and reabsorbed from the intestine, the resulting enterohepatic circulation ensures that orally administered estrogens will have a high ratio of hepatic to peripheral effects. As noted below, the hepatic effects are thought to be responsible for some undesirable actions such as synthesis of increased clotting factors and plasma renin substrate. The hepatic effects of estrogen can be minimized by routes that avoid first-pass liver exposure, ie, vaginal, transdermal, or by injection.

Physiologic Effects

A. MECHANISM

Plasma estrogens in the blood and interstitial fluid are bound to sex hormone-binding globulin, from which they dissociate to enter the cell and bind to their receptor. Two genes code for two estrogen receptor isoforms, α and β, which are members of the superfamily of steroid, sterol, retinoic acid, and thyroid receptors. The estrogen receptors are found predominantly in the nucleus bound to heat shock proteins that stabilize them (Figure 39–3).

Binding of the hormone to its receptor alters its conformation and releases it from the stabilizing proteins (predominantly Hsp90). The receptor-hormone complex forms homodimers that bind to a specific sequence of nucleotides called estrogen response elements (EREs) in the promoters of various genes and regulate their transcription. The ERE is composed of two half-sites arranged as a palindrome separated by a small group of nucleotides called the spacer. The interaction of a receptor dimer with the ERE also involves a number of nuclear proteins, the coregulators, as well as components of the transcription machinery. The receptor may also bind to other transcription factors to influence the effects of these factors on their responsive genes.

The relative concentrations and types of receptors, receptor coregulators, and transcription factors confer the cell specificity of the hormone's actions. The genomic effects of estrogens are mainly due to proteins synthesized by translation of RNA transcribed from a responsive gene. Some of the effects of estrogens are indirect, mediated by the autocrine and paracrine actions of autacoids such as growth factors, lipids, glycolipids, and cytokines produced by the target cells in response to estrogen.

Rapid estrogen-induced effects such as granulosa cell Ca^{2+} uptake and increased uterine blood flow do not require gene activation. These appear to be mediated by nongenomic effects of the classic estrogen receptor-estrogen complex, influencing several intracellular signaling pathways.

B. FEMALE MATURATION

Estrogens are required for the normal sexual maturation and growth of the female. They stimulate the development of the vagina, uterus, and uterine tubes as well as the secondary sex characteristics. They stimulate stromal development and ductal growth in the breast and are responsible for the accelerated growth phase and the closing of the epiphyses of the long bones that occur at puberty. They contribute to the growth of axillary and pubic hair and alter the distribution of body fat to produce typical female body contours. Larger quantities also stimulate development of pigmentation in the skin, most prominent in the region of the nipples and areolae and in the genital region.

C. ENDOMETRIAL EFFECTS

In addition to its growth effects on uterine muscle, estrogen also plays an important role in the development of the endometrial lining. When estrogen production is properly coordinated with the production of progesterone during the normal human menstrual cycle, regular periodic bleeding and shedding of the endometrial lining occur. Continuous exposure to estrogens for prolonged periods leads to hyperplasia of the endometrium that is usually associated with abnormal bleeding patterns.

D. Metabolic and Cardiovascular Effects

Estrogens have a number of important metabolic and cardiovascular effects. They seem to be partially responsible for maintenance of the normal structure and function of the skin and blood vessels in women. Estrogens also decrease the rate of resorption of bone by promoting the apoptosis of osteoclasts and by antagonizing the osteoclastogenic and pro-osteoclastic effects of parathyroid hormone and interleukin-6. Estrogens also stimulate adipose tissue production of leptin and are in part responsible for the higher levels of this hormone in women than in men.

In addition to stimulating the synthesis of enzymes and growth factors leading to uterine and breast growth and differentiation, estrogens alter the production and activity of many other proteins in the body. Metabolic alterations in the liver are especially important, so that there is a higher circulating level of proteins such as transcortin (CBG), thyroxine-binding globulin (TBG), sex hormone-binding globulin (SHBG), transferrin, renin substrate, and fibrinogen. This leads to increased circulating levels of thyroxine, estrogen, testosterone, iron, copper, and other substances.

Alterations in the composition of the plasma lipids caused by estrogens are characterized by an increase in the high-density lipoproteins, a slight reduction in the low-density lipoproteins, and a reduction in plasma cholesterol levels. Plasma triglyceride levels are increased. Estrogens decrease hepatic oxidation of adipose tissue lipid to ketones and increase synthesis of triglycerides.

E. Effects on Blood Coagulation

Estrogens enhance the coagulability of blood. Many changes in factors influencing coagulation have been reported, including increased circulating levels of factors II, VII, IX, and X and decreased antithrombin III, partially as a result of the hepatic effects mentioned above. Increased plasminogen levels and decreased platelet adhesiveness have also been found (see Hormonal Contraception).

F. Other Effects

Estrogens induce the synthesis of progesterone receptors. They are responsible for estrous behavior in animals and may influence behavior and libido in humans. Administration of estrogens stimulates central components of the stress system, including the production of corticotropin-releasing hormone and the activity of the sympathetic system, and promotes a sense of well-being in women who are estrogen-deficient. They also facilitate the loss of intravascular fluid into the extracellular space, producing edema. The resulting decrease in plasma volume causes a compensatory retention of sodium and water by the kidney. Estrogens also modulate sympathetic nervous system control of smooth muscle function.

Clinical Uses*

A. Primary Hypogonadism

Estrogens have been used extensively for replacement therapy in estrogen-deficient patients. The estrogen deficiency may be due to primary failure of development of the ovaries, premature menopause, castration, or menopause.

Treatment of primary hypogonadism is usually begun at 11–13 years of age in order to stimulate the development of secondary sex characteristics and menses, to stimulate optimal growth, to prevent osteoporosis and to avoid the psychologic consequences of delayed puberty and estrogen deficiency. Treatment attempts to mimic the physiology of puberty. It is initiated with small doses of estrogen (0.3 mg conjugated estrogens or 5–10 µg ethinyl estradiol) on days 1–21 each month and is slowly increased to adult doses and maintained until the age of menopause (approximately 51 years of age). A progestin is added after the first uterine bleeding. When growth is completed, chronic therapy consists mainly of the administration of adult doses of both estrogens and progestins, as described below.

B. Postmenopausal Hormonal Therapy

In addition to the signs and symptoms that follow closely upon the cessation of normal ovarian function—such as loss of periods, vasomotor symptoms, sleep disturbances, and genital atrophy—there are longer-lasting changes that influence the health and well-being of postmenopausal women. These include an acceleration of bone loss, which in susceptible women may lead to vertebral, hip, and wrist fractures; and lipid changes, which may contribute to the acceleration of atherosclerotic cardiovascular disease noted in postmenopausal women. The effects of estrogens on bone have been extensively studied, and the effects of hormone withdrawal have been well-characterized. However, the role of estrogens and progestins in the cause and prevention of cardiovascular disease, which is responsible for 350,000 deaths per year, and breast cancer, which causes 35,000 deaths per year, is less well understood.

When normal ovulatory function ceases and the estrogen levels fall after menopause, oophorectomy, or premature ovarian failure, there is an accelerated rise in plasma cholesterol and LDL concentrations, while LDL receptors decline. HDL is not much affected, and levels remain higher than in men. VLDL and triglyceride levels are also relatively unaffected. Since cardiovascular

---

* The use of estrogens in contraception is discussed below.

disorders account for most deaths in this age group, the risk for these disorders constitutes a major consideration in deciding whether or not hormonal replacement therapy (HRT) is indicated and influences the selection of hormones to be administered. Estrogen replacement therapy has a beneficial effect on circulating lipids and lipoproteins, and this was earlier thought to be accompanied by a reduction in myocardial infarction by about 50% and of fatal strokes by as much as 40%. These findings, however, have been recently disputed by the results of a large controlled study from the Womens' Health Initative project showing no cardiovascular benefit from estrogen plus progestin replacement therapy in perimenopausal or postmenopausal patients. In fact, there may be a small increase in cardiovascular problems as well as breast cancer in women who received the replacement therapy. Interestingly, a small protective effect against colon cancer was observed. In other recent studies, a protective effect of estrogen replacement therapy against Alzheimer's disease was observed.

Progestins antagonize estrogen's effects on LDL and HDL to a variable extent. However, a large study has recently shown that the addition of a progestin to estrogen replacement therapy does not influence the cardiovascular risk.

Optimal management of the postmenopausal patient requires careful assessment of her symptoms as well as consideration of her age and the presence of (or risks for) cardiovascular disease, osteoporosis, breast cancer, and endometrial cancer. Bearing in mind the effects of the gonadal hormones on each of these disorders, the goals of therapy can then be defined and the risks of therapy assessed and discussed with the patient.

If the main indication for therapy is hot flushes and sleep disturbances, therapy with the lowest dose of estrogen required for symptomatic relief is recommended. Treatment may be required for only a limited period of time and the possible increased risk for breast cancer avoided. In women who have undergone hysterectomy, estrogens alone can be given 5 days per week or continuously, since progestins are not required to reduce the risk for endometrial hyperplasia and cancer. Hot flushes, sweating, insomnia, and atrophic vaginitis are generally relieved by estrogens; many patients experience some increased sense of well-being; and climacteric depression and other psychopathologic states are improved.

The role of estrogens in the prevention and treatment of osteoporosis has been carefully studied (see Chapter 42). The amount of bone present in the body is maximal in the young active adult in the third decade of life and begins to decline more rapidly in middle age in both men and women. The development of osteoporosis also depends on the amount of bone present at the start of this process, on vitamin D and calcium intake, and on the degree of physical activity. The risk of osteoporosis is highest in smokers who are thin, Caucasian, and inactive and have a low calcium intake and a strong family history of osteoporosis. Depression also is a major risk factor for development of osteoporosis in women.

Estrogens should be used in the smallest dosage consistent with relief of symptoms. In women who have not undergone hysterectomy, it is most convenient to prescribe estrogen on the first 21–25 days of each month. The recommended dosages of estrogen are 0.3–1.25 mg/d of conjugated estrogen or 0.01–0.02 mg/d of ethinyl estradiol. Dosages in the middle of these ranges have been shown to be maximally effective in preventing the decrease in bone density occurring at menopause. From this point of view, it is important to begin therapy as soon as possible after the menopause for maximum effect. In these patients and others not taking estrogen, calcium supplements that bring the total daily calcium intake up to 1500 mg are useful.

Patients at low risk of developing osteoporosis who manifest only mild atrophic vaginitis can be treated with topical preparations. The vaginal route of application is also useful in the treatment of urinary tract symptoms in these patients. It is important to realize, however, that although locally administered estrogens escape the first-pass effect (so that some undesirable hepatic effects are reduced), they are almost completely absorbed into the circulation, and these preparations should be given cyclically.

As noted below, the administration of estrogen is associated with an increased risk of endometrial carcinoma. The administration of a progestational agent with the estrogen prevents endometrial hyperplasia and markedly reduces the risk of this cancer. When estrogen is given for the first 25 days of the month and the progestin medroxyprogesterone (10 mg/d) is added during the last 10–14 days, the risk is only half of that in women not receiving hormone replacement therapy. On this regimen, some women will experience a return of symptoms during the period off estrogen administration. In these patients, the estrogen can be given continuously. If the progestin produces sedation or other undesirable effects, its dose can be reduced to 2.5–5 mg for the last 10 days of the cycle with a slight increase in the risk for endometrial hyperplasia. These regimens are usually accompanied by bleeding at the end of each cycle. Some women experience migraine headaches during the last few days of the cycle. The use of a continuous estrogen regimen will often prevent their occurrence. Women who object to the cyclic bleeding associated with sequential therapy can also consider continuous therapy. Daily therapy with 0.625 mg of conjugated equine estrogens and 2.5–5 mg of medroxyprogesterone will eliminate cyclic bleeding, control vasomotor symptoms, prevent genital atrophy, maintain bone density, and show a favorable lipid profile with a small decrease in LDL and an increase in HDL concentrations. These women have endometrial atrophy on biopsy. About half of these patients experience breakthrough bleeding during the first few months of therapy. Seventy to 80 percent become amenorrheic after the first 4 months, and most remain so. The main disadvantage of continuous therapy is the need for uterine biopsy when bleeding occurs after the first few months.

As noted above, estrogens may also be administered vaginally or transdermally. When estrogens are given by these routes, the liver is bypassed on the first circulation, and the ratio of the liver effects to peripheral effects is reduced.

In patients in whom estrogen replacement therapy is contraindicated, such as those with estrogen-sensitive tumors, relief of vasomotor symptoms may be obtained by the use of clonidine.

C. OTHER USES

Estrogens combined with progestins can be used to suppress ovulation in patients with intractable dysmenorrhea or when suppression of ovarian function is used in the treatment of hirsutism and amenorrhea due to excessive secretion of androgens by the ovary. Under these circumstances, greater suppression may be needed, and oral contraceptives containing 50 μg of estrogen or a combination of a low estrogen pill with GnRH suppression may be required.

Adverse Effects

Adverse effects of variable severity have been reported with the therapeutic use of estrogens. Many other effects reported in conjunction with hormonal contraceptives may be related to their estrogen content. These are discussed below.

A. UTERINE BLEEDING

Estrogen therapy is a major cause of postmenopausal uterine bleeding. Unfortunately, vaginal bleeding at this time of life may also be due to carcinoma of the endometrium. In order to avoid confusion, patients should be treated with the smallest amount of estrogen possible. It should be given cyclically so that bleeding, if it occurs, will be more likely to occur during the withdrawal period. As noted above, endometrial hyperplasia can be prevented by administration of a progestational agent with estrogen in each cycle.

B. CANCER

The relation of estrogen therapy to cancer continues to be the subject of active investigation. Although no adverse effect of short-term estrogen therapy on the incidence of breast cancer has been demonstrated, a small increase in the incidence of this tumor may occur with prolonged therapy. Although the risk factor is small (1.25), the impact may be great since this tumor occurs in 10% of women, and addition of progesterone does not confer a protective effect. Studies indicate that following unilateral excision of breast cancer, women receiving tamoxifen (an estrogen partial agonist, see below) show a 35% decrease in contralateral breast cancer compared with controls. These studies also demonstrate that tamoxifen is well tolerated by most patients, produces estrogen-like alterations in plasma lipid levels, and stabilizes bone mineral loss. Studies bearing on the possible efficacy of tamoxifen in postmenopausal women at high risk for breast cancer are under way. A recent study shows that postmenopausal hormone replacement therapy with estrogens plus progestins was associated with greater breast epithelial cell proliferation and breast epithelial cell density than estrogens alone or no replacement therapy. Furthermore, with estrogens plus progestins, breast proliferation was localized to the terminal duct-lobular unit of the breast, which is the main site of development of breast cancer. Thus, further studies are needed to conclusively assess the possible association between progestins and breast cancer risk.

Many studies show an increased risk of endometrial carcinoma in patients taking estrogens alone. The risk seems to vary with the dose and duration of treatment: 15 times as great in patients taking large doses of estrogen for 5 or more years, in contrast with two to four times greater in patients receiving lower doses for short periods. However, as noted above, the concomitant use of a progestin prevents this increased risk and may in fact reduce the incidence of endometrial cancer to less than that in the general population.

There have been a number of reports of adenocarcinoma of the vagina in young women whose mothers were treated with large doses of diethylstilbestrol early in pregnancy. These cancers are most common in young women (ages 14–44). The incidence is less than 1 per 1000 women exposed—too low to establish a cause-and-effect relationship with certainty. However, the risks for infertility, ectopic pregnancy, and premature delivery are also increased. It is now recognized that there is no indication for the use of diethylstilbestrol during pregnancy, and it should be avoided. It is not known whether other estrogens have a similar effect or whether the observed phenomena are peculiar to diethylstilbestrol. This agent should be used only for the treatment of cancer (eg, of the prostate) or as a "morning after" contraceptive (see below).

C. OTHER EFFECTS

Nausea and breast tenderness are common and can be minimized by using the smallest effective dose of estrogen. Hyperpigmentation also occurs. Estrogen therapy is associated with an increase in frequency of migraine headaches as well as cholestasis, gallbladder disease, and hypertension.

Contraindications

Estrogens should not be used in patients with estrogen-dependent neoplasms such as carcinoma of the endometrium or in those with — or at high risk for—carcinoma of the breast. They should be avoided in patients with undiagnosed genital bleeding, liver disease, or a history of thromboembolic disorder. In addition, the use of estrogens should be avoided by heavy smokers.

Preparations & Dosages

The dosages of commonly used natural and synthetic preparations are listed in Table 40–1. Although all of the estrogens produce almost the same hormonal effects, their potencies vary both between agents and depending on the route of administration. As noted above, estradiol is the most active endogenous estrogen, and it has the highest affinity for the estrogen receptor. However, its metabolites estrone and estriol have weak uterine effects.

For a given level of gonadotropin suppression, oral estrogen preparations have more effect on the circulating levels of CBG, SHBG, and a host of other liver proteins, including angiotensinogen, than do transdermal preparations. The oral route of administration allows greater concentrations of hormone to reach the liver, thus increasing the synthesis of these proteins. Transdermal preparations were developed to avoid this effect. When administered transdermally, 50–100 µg of estradiol has effects similar to those of 0.625–1.25 mg of conjugated oral estrogens on gonadotropin concentrations, endometrium, and vaginal epithelium. Furthermore, the transdermal estrogen preparations do not significantly increase the concentrations of renin substrate, CBG, and TBG and do not produce the characteristic changes in serum lipids. Combined oral preparations containing 0.625 mg of conjugated estrogens and 2.5 mg of medroxyprogesterone acetate are available for menopausal replacement therapy. Tablets containing 0.625 of conjugated estrogens and 5 mg of medroxyprogesterone acetate are available to be used in conjunction with conjugated estrogens in a sequential fashion. Estrogens alone are taken on days 1–14 and the combination on days 15–28.

THE PROGESTINS

Natural Progestins: Progesterone

Progesterone is the most important progestin in humans. In addition to having important hormonal effects, it serves as a precursor to the estrogens, androgens, and adrenocortical steroids. It is synthesized in the ovary, testis, and adrenal from circulating cholesterol. Large amounts are also synthesized and released by the placenta during pregnancy.

In the ovary, progesterone is produced primarily by the corpus luteum. Normal males appear to secrete 1–5 mg of progesterone daily, resulting in plasma levels of about 0.03 µg/dL. The level is only slightly higher in the female during the follicular phase of the cycle, when only a few milligrams per day of progesterone are secreted. During the luteal phase, plasma levels range from 0.5 µg/dL to more than 2 µg/dL (Figure 40–1). Plasma levels of progesterone are further elevated and reach their peak levels in the third trimester of pregnancy.

Synthetic Progestins

A variety of progestational compounds have been synthesized. Some are active when given by mouth. They are not a uniform group of compounds, and all of them differ from progesterone in one or more respects. Table 40–2 lists some of these compounds and their effects. In general, the 21-carbon compounds (hydroxyprogesterone, medroxyprogesterone, megestrol, and dimethisterone) are the most closely related, pharmacologically as well as chemically, to progesterone. A new group of third-generation synthetic progestins has been introduced, principally as components of oral contraceptives. These "19-nor, 13-ethyl" steroid compounds include desogestrel (Figure 40–4), gestodene, and norgestimate. They are claimed to have lower androgenic activity than older synthetic progestins.

Pharmacokinetics

Progesterone is rapidly absorbed following administration by any route. Its half-life in the plasma is approximately 5 minutes, and small amounts are stored temporarily in body fat. It is almost completely metabolized in one passage through the liver, and for that reason it is quite ineffective when the usual formulation is administered orally. However, high-dose oral micronized progesterone preparations have been developed that provide adequate progestational effect.

In the liver, progesterone is metabolized to pregnanediol and conjugated with glucuronic acid. It is excreted into the urine as pregnanediol glucuronide. The amount of pregnanediol in the urine has been used as an index of progesterone secretion. This measure has been very useful in spite of the fact that the proportion of secreted progesterone converted to this compound varies from day to day and from individual to individual. In addition to progesterone, 20α- and 20β-hydroxyproges-

Table 40–2. Activities of progestational agents.

	Route	Duration of Action	Activities[1]				
			Estro-genic	Andro-genic	Anties-trogenic	Antian-drogenic	Anabolic
Progesterone and derivatives							
Progesterone	IM	1 day	–	–	+	–	–
Hydroxyprogesterone caproate	IM	8–14 days	sl	sl	–	–	–
Medroxyprogesterone acetate	IM, PO	Tabs: 1–3 days; injection: 4–12 weeks	–	+	+	–	–
Megestrol acetate	PO	1–3 days	–	+	–	+	–
17-Ethinyl testosterone derivatives							
Dimethisterone	PO	1–3 days	–	–	sl	–	–
19-Nortestosterone derivatives							
Desogestrel	PO	1–3 days	–	–	–	–	–
Norethynodrel[2]	PO	1–3 days	+	–	–	–	–
Lynestrenol[3]	PO	1–3 days	+	+	–	–	+
Norethindrone[2]	PO	1–3 days	sl	+	+	–	+
Norethindrone acetate[2]	PO	1–3 days	sl	+	+	–	+
Ethynodiol diacetate[2]	PO	1–3 days	sl	+	+	–	–
L-Norgestrel[2]	PO	1–3 days	–	+	+	–	+

[1]**Interpretation:** + = active; – = inactive; sl = slightly active. Activities have been reported in various species using various end points and may not apply to humans.

[2]See Table 40–3.

[3]Not available in USA.

terone (20α- and 20β-hydroxy-4-pregnene-3-one) are also found. These compounds have about one fifth the progestational activity of progesterone in humans and other species. Little is known of their physiologic role, but 20α-hydroxyprogesterone is produced in large amounts in some species and may be of some importance biologically.

The usual routes of administration and durations of action of the synthetic progestins are listed in Table 40–2. Most of these agents are extensively metabolized to inactive products that are excreted mainly in the urine.

Physiologic Effects

A. MECHANISM

The mechanism of action of progesterone—described in more detail above—is similar to that of other steroid hormones. Progestins enter the cell and bind to proges-

terone receptors that are distributed between the nucleus and the cytoplasm. The ligand-receptor complex binds to a progesterone response element (PRE) to activate gene transcription. The response element for progesterone appears to be similar to the corticosteroid response element, and the specificity of the response depends upon which receptor is present in the cell as well as upon other cell-specific receptor coregulators and interacting transcription factors. The progesterone-receptor complex forms a dimer before binding to DNA. Like the estrogen receptor, it can form heterodimers as well as homodimers between two isoforms: A and B. These isoforms are produced by alternative splicing of the same gene.

B. EFFECTS OF PROGESTERONE

Progesterone has little effect on protein metabolism. It stimulates lipoprotein lipase activity and seems to favor fat deposition. The effects on carbohydrate metabolism

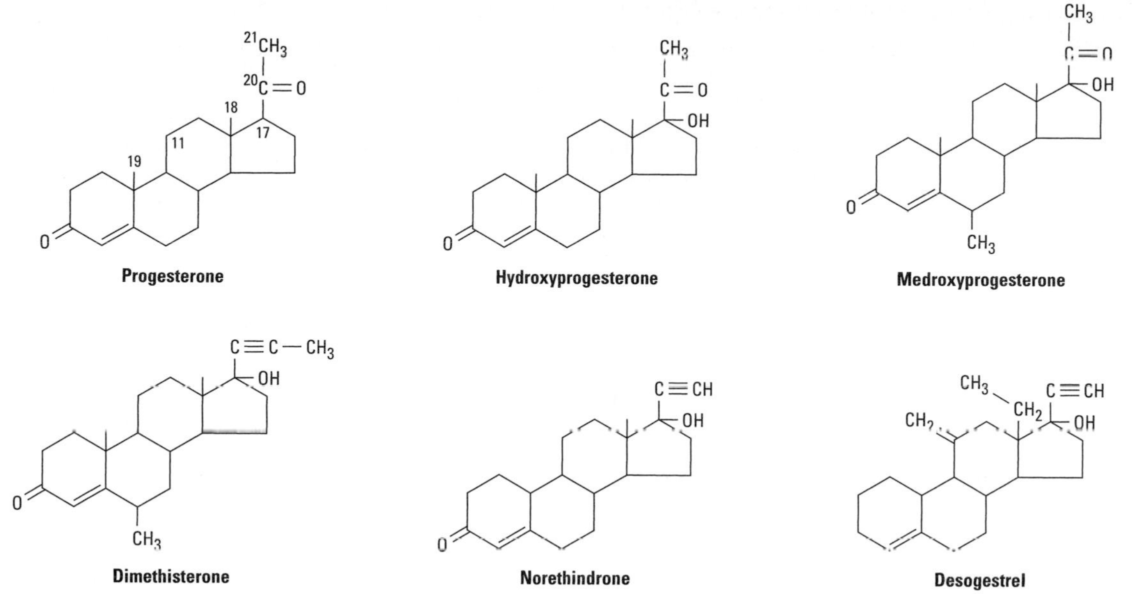

Figure 40–4. Progesterone and some progestational agents in clinical use. See Table 40–2.

are more marked. Progesterone increases basal insulin levels and the insulin response to glucose. There is usually no manifest change in carbohydrate tolerance. In the liver, progesterone promotes glycogen storage, possibly by facilitating the effect of insulin. Progesterone also promotes ketogenesis.

Progesterone can compete with aldosterone for the mineralocorticoid receptor of the renal tubule, causing a decrease in Na^+ reabsorption. This leads to an increased secretion of aldosterone by the adrenal cortex (eg, in pregnancy). Progesterone increases body temperature in humans. The mechanism of this effect is not known, but an alteration of the temperature-regulating centers in the hypothalamus has been suggested. Progesterone also alters the function of the respiratory centers. The ventilatory response to CO_2 is increased (synthetic progestins with an ethinyl group do not have respiratory effects). This leads to a measurable reduction in arterial and alveolar P_{CO_2} during pregnancy and in the luteal phase of the menstrual cycle. Progesterone and related steroids also have depressant and hypnotic effects on the brain.

Progesterone is responsible for the alveolobular development of the secretory apparatus in the breast. It also participates in the preovulatory LH surge and causes the maturation and secretory changes in the endometrium that are seen following ovulation (Figure 40–1).

Progesterone decreases the plasma levels of many amino acids and leads to increased urinary nitrogen excre-

tion. It induces changes in the structure and function of smooth endoplasmic reticulum in experimental animals.

Other effects of progesterone and its analogs are noted in the section on Hormonal Contraception.

C. SYNTHETIC PROGESTINS

The 21-carbon progesterone analogs antagonize aldosterone-induced sodium retention (see above). The remaining compounds ("19-nortestosterone" third-generation agents) produce a decidual change in the endometrial stroma, do not support pregnancy in test animals, are more effective gonadotropin inhibitors, and may have minimal estrogenic and androgenic or anabolic activity (Table 40–2, Figure 40–4). They are sometimes referred to as "impeded androgens." Progestins without androgenic activity include desogestrel, norgestimate, and gestodene. The first two of these compounds are dispensed in combination with ethinyl estradiol for oral contraception (Table 40–3) in the USA. Oral contraceptives containing the progestins cyproterone acetate (also an antiandrogen) in combination with ethinyl estradiol are investigational in the USA.

Clinical Uses of Progestins

A. THERAPEUTIC APPLICATIONS

The major uses of progestational hormones are for hormone replacement therapy (see above) and hormonal contraception (see below). In addition, they are useful in producing long-term ovarian suppression for other purposes. When used alone in large doses parenterally (eg, medroxyprogesterone acetate, 150 mg intramuscularly every 90 days), prolonged anovulation and amenorrhea result. This therapy has been employed in the treatment of dysmenorrhea, endometriosis, and bleeding disorders when estrogens are contraindicated, and for contraception. The major problem with this regimen is the prolonged time required in some patients for ovulatory function to return after cessation of therapy. It should not be used for patients planning a pregnancy in the near future. Similar regimens will relieve hot flushes in some menopausal women and can be used if estrogen therapy is contraindicated.

Medroxyprogesterone acetate, 10–20 mg orally twice weekly—or intramuscularly in doses of 100 mg/m^2 every 1–2 weeks—will prevent menstruation, but it will not arrest accelerated bone maturation in children with precocious puberty.

Progestins do not appear to have any place in the therapy of threatened or habitual abortion. Early reports of the usefulness of these agents resulted from the unwarranted assumption that after several abortions the likelihood of repeated abortions was over 90%. When progestational agents were administered to patients with previous abortions, a salvage rate of 80% was achieved. It is now recognized that similar patients abort only 20% of the time even when untreated. On the other hand, progesterone was experimentally given recently to delay premature labor with encouraging results.

Progesterone and medroxyprogesterone have been used in the treatment of women who have difficulty in conceiving and who demonstrate a slow rise in basal body temperature. There is no convincing evidence that this treatment is effective.

Preparations of progesterone and medroxyprogesterone have been used to treat premenstrual syndrome. Controlled studies have not confirmed the effectiveness of such therapy except when doses sufficient to suppress ovulation have been used.

B. DIAGNOSTIC USES

Progesterone can be used as a test of estrogen secretion. The administration of progesterone, 150 mg/d, or medroxyprogesterone, 10 mg/d, for 5–7 days, is followed by withdrawal bleeding in amenorrheic patients only when the endometrium has been stimulated by estrogens. A combination of estrogen and progestin can be given to test the responsiveness of the endometrium in patients with amenorrhea.

Contraindications, Cautions, & Adverse Effects

Studies of progestational compounds alone and with combination oral contraceptives indicate that the progestin in these agents may increase blood pressure in some patients. The more androgenic progestins also reduce plasma HDL levels in women. (See Hormonal Contraception, below.) Two recent studies suggest that combined progestin plus estrogen replacement therapy in postmenopausal women may increase breast cancer risk significantly compared with the risk in women taking estrogen alone. These findings require careful examination and if confirmed will lead to important changes in postmenopausal hormone replacement practice.

OTHER OVARIAN HORMONES

The normal ovary produces small amounts of **androgens,** including testosterone, androstenedione, and dehydroepiandrosterone. Of these, only testosterone has a significant amount of biologic activity, though androstenedione can be converted to testosterone or estrone in peripheral tissues. The normal woman produces less than 200 μg of testosterone in 24 hours, and about one third of this is probably formed in the ovary directly. The physiologic significance of these small amounts of androgens is not established, but they may be partly responsible for normal hair growth at puberty, for stimulation of female libido, and, possibly, for other important metabolic effects. Androgen production by the ovary may be markedly increased in some abnormal states, usually in association with hirsutism and amenorrhea as noted above.

The ovary also produces **inhibin** and **activin.** These peptides consist of several combinations of α and β subunits. The αβ dimer (inhibin) inhibits FSH secretion while the ββ dimer (activin) increases FSH secretion. Studies in primates indicate that inhibin has no direct effect on ovarian steroidogenesis but that activin modulates the response to LH and FSH. For example, simultaneous treatment with activin and human FSH enhances FSH stimulation of progesterone synthesis and aromatase activity in granulosa cells. When combined with LH, activin suppressed the LH-induced progesterone response by 50% but markedly enhanced basal and LH-stimulated aromatase activity. Activin may also act as a growth factor in other tissues. The physiologic roles of these modulators are not fully understood.

Relaxin is another peptide that can be extracted from the ovary. The three-dimensional structure of relaxin is related to that of growth-promoting peptides and is similar to that of insulin. Although the amino acid sequence differs from that of insulin, this hormone, like insulin, consists of two chains linked by disulfide bonds, cleaved from a prohormone. It is found in the ovary, placenta, uterus, and blood. Relaxin synthesis has been demonstrated in luteinized granulosa cells of the corpus luteum. It has been shown to increase glycogen synthesis and water uptake by the myometrium and decreases uterine contractility. In some species, it changes the mechanical properties of the cervix and pubic ligaments, facilitating delivery.

In women, relaxin has been measured by immunoassay. Levels were highest immediately after the LH surge and during menstruation. A physiologic role for this hormone has not been established.

Clinical trials with relaxin have been conducted in patients with dysmenorrhea. Relaxin has also been administered to patients in premature labor and during prolonged labor. When applied to the cervix of a woman at term, it facilitates dilation and shortens labor.

Several other nonsteroidal substances such as corticotropin-releasing hormone, follistatin, and prostaglandins are produced by the ovary. These probably have paracrine effects within the ovary.

HORMONAL CONTRACEPTION (ORAL, PARENTERAL, & IMPLANTED CONTRACEPTIVES)

A large number of oral contraceptives containing estrogens or progestins (or both) are now available for clinical use (Table 40–3). These preparations vary chemically and pharmacologically and have many properties in common as well as definite differences important for the correct selection of the right agent.

Two types of preparations are used for oral contraception: (1) combinations of estrogens and progestins and (2) continuous progestin therapy without concomitant administration of estrogens. The combination agents are further divided into monophasic forms (constant dosage of both components during the cycle) and biphasic or triphasic forms (dosage of one or both components is changed once or twice during the cycle). The preparations for oral use are all adequately absorbed, and in combination preparations the pharmacokinetics of neither drug is significantly altered by the other.

Only one implantable contraceptive preparation is available at present. Norgestrel, also utilized as the progestin component of some oral contraceptive preparations, is an effective suppressant of ovulation when it is released from subcutaneous implants. Intramuscular injection of large doses of medroxyprogesterone also provides contraceptive action of long duration.

Pharmacologic Effects

A. MECHANISM OF ACTION

The combinations of estrogens and progestins exert their contraceptive effect largely through selective inhibition of pituitary function that results in inhibition of ovulation. The combination agents also produce a change in

the cervical mucus, in the uterine endometrium, and in motility and secretion in the uterine tubes, all of which decrease the likelihood of conception and implantation. The continuous use of progestins alone does not always inhibit ovulation. The other factors mentioned, therefore, play a major role in the prevention of pregnancy when these agents are used.

B. EFFECTS ON THE OVARY

Chronic use of combination agents depresses ovarian function. Follicular development is minimal, and corpora lutea, larger follicles, stromal edema, and other morphologic features normally seen in ovulating women are absent. The ovaries usually become smaller even when enlarged before therapy.

The great majority of patients return to normal menstrual patterns when these drugs are discontinued. About 75% will ovulate in the first posttreatment cycle and 97% by the third posttreatment cycle. About 2% of patients remain amenorrheic for periods of up to several years after administration is stopped.

The cytologic findings on vaginal smears vary depending on the preparation used. However, with almost all of the combined drugs, a low maturation index is found because of the presence of progestational agents.

C. EFFECTS ON THE UTERUS

After prolonged use, the cervix may show some hypertrophy and polyp formation. There are also important effects on the cervical mucus, making it more like postovulation mucus, ie, thicker and less copious.

Agents containing both estrogens and progestins produce further morphologic and biochemical changes of the endometrial stroma under the influence of the progestin, which also stimulates glandular secretion throughout the luteal phase. The agents containing "19-nor" progestins—particularly those with the smaller amounts of estrogen—tend to produce more glandular atrophy and usually less bleeding.

D. EFFECTS ON THE BREAST

Stimulation of the breasts occurs in most patients receiving estrogen-containing agents. Some enlargement is generally noted. The administration of estrogens and combinations of estrogens and progestins tends to suppress lactation. When the doses are small, the effects on breast feeding are not appreciable. Studies of the transport of the oral contraceptives into breast milk suggest that only small amounts of these compounds cross into the milk, and they have not been considered to be of importance.

E. OTHER EFFECTS OF ORAL CONTRACEPTIVES

1. Effects on the central nervous system—The central nervous system effects of the oral contraceptives have

Table 40–3. Some oral and implantable contraceptive agents in use. The estrogen-containing compounds are arranged in order of increasing content of estrogen. (Ethinyl estradiol and mestranol have similar potencies.)

	Estrogen (mg)		Progestin (mg)	
Monophasic combination tablets				
Loestrin 21 1/20	Ethinyl estradiol	0.02	Norethindrone acetate	1.0
Desogen, Apri, Ortho-Cept	Ethinyl estradiol	0.03	Desogestrel	0.15
Brevicon, Modicon, Necon 0.5/35	Ethinyl estradiol	0.035	Norethindrone	0.5
Demulen 1/35	Ethinyl estradiol	0.035	Ethynodiol diacetate	1.0
Nelova 1/35 E, Ortho-Novum 1/35	Ethinyl estradiol	0.035	Norethindrone	1.0
Ovcon 35	Ethinyl estradiol	0.035	Norethindrone	0.4
Demulen 1/50	Ethinyl estradiol	0.05	Ethynodiol diacetate	1.0
Ovcon 50	Ethinyl estradiol	0.05	Norethindrone	1.0
Ovral-28	Ethinyl estradiol	0.05	D,L-Norgestrel	0.5
Norinyl 1/50, Ortho-Novum 1/50	Mestranol	0.05	Norethindrone	1.0
Biphasic combination tablets				
Jenest-28, Ortho-Novum 10/11, Necon 10/11, Nelova 10/11				
Days 1–10	Ethinyl estradiol	0.035	Norethindrone	0.5
Days 11–21	Ethinyl estradiol	0.035	Norethindrone	1.0
Triphasic combination tablets				
Triphasil, Tri-Levlen, Trivora				
Days 1–6	Ethinyl estradiol	0.03	L-Norgestrel	0.05
Days 7–11	Ethinyl estradiol	0.04	L-Norgestrel	0.075
Days 12–21	Ethinyl estradiol	0.03	L-Norgestrel	0.125
Ortho-Novum 7/7/7, Necon 7/7/7				
Days 1–7	Ethinyl estradiol	0.035	Norethindrone	0.5
Days 8–14	Ethinyl estradiol	0.035	Norethindrone	0.75
Days 15–21	Ethinyl estradiol	0.035	Norethindrone	1.0
Tri-Norinyl				
Days 1–7	Ethinyl estradiol	0.035	Norethindrone	0.5
Days 8–16	Ethinyl estradiol	0.035	Norethindrone	1.0
Days 17–21	Ethinyl estradiol	0.035	Norethindrone	0.5
Ortho-Tri-Cyclen				
Days 1–7	Ethinyl estradiol	0.035	Norgestimate	0.18
Days 8–14	Ethinyl estradiol	0.035	Norgestimate	0.215
Days 15–21	Ethinyl estradiol	0.035	Norgestimate	0.25
Daily progestin tablets				
Micronor, Nor-QD, Ortho Micronor, Nor-QD, Camila, Errin		...	Norethindrone	0.35
Ovrette		...	D,L-Norgestrel	0.075
Implantable progestin preparation				
Norplant System		...	L-Norgestrel (six tubes of 36 mg each)	

not been well studied in humans. A variety of effects of estrogen and progesterone have been noted in animals. Estrogens tend to increase excitability in the brain, whereas progesterone tends to decrease it. The thermogenic action of progesterone and some of the synthetic progestins is also thought to occur in the central nervous system.

It is very difficult to evaluate any behavioral or emotional effects of these compounds in humans. Although the incidence of pronounced changes in mood, affect, and behavior appears to be low, milder changes are commonly reported, and estrogens are being successfully employed in the therapy of premenstrual tension syndrome, postpartum depression, and climacteric depression.

2. Effects on endocrine function—The inhibition of pituitary gonadotropin secretion has been mentioned. Estrogens also alter adrenal structure and function. Estrogens given orally or at high doses increase the plasma concentration of the α_2-globulin that binds cortisol (corticosteroid-binding globulin). Plasma concentrations may be more than double the levels found in untreated individuals, and urinary excretion of free cortisol is elevated.

These preparations cause alterations in the renin-angiotensin-aldosterone system. Plasma renin activity has been found to increase, and there is an increase in aldosterone secretion.

Thyroxine-binding globulin is increased. As a result, total plasma thyroxine (T_4) levels are increased to those commonly seen during pregnancy. Since more of the thyroxine is bound, the free thyroxine level in these patients is normal. Estrogens also increase the plasma level of SHBG and decrease plasma levels of free androgens by increasing their binding; large amounts of estrogen may decrease androgens by gonadotropin suppression.

3. Effects on blood—Serious thromboembolic phenomena occurring in women taking oral contraceptives have given rise to a great many studies of the effects of these compounds on blood coagulation. A clear picture of such effects has not yet emerged. The oral contraceptives do not consistently alter bleeding or clotting times. The changes that have been observed are similar to those reported in pregnancy. There is an increase in factors VII, VIII, IX, and X and a decrease in antithrombin III. Increased amounts of coumarin anticoagulants may be required to prolong prothrombin time in patients taking oral contraceptives.

There is an increase in serum iron and total iron-binding capacity similar to that reported in patients with hepatitis.

Significant alterations in the cellular components of blood have not been reported with any consistency. A number of patients have been reported to develop folic acid deficiency anemias.

4. Effects on the liver—These hormones also have profound effects on the function of the liver. Some of these effects are deleterious and will be considered below in the section on adverse effects.

The effects on serum proteins result from the effects of the estrogens on the synthesis of the various α_2-globulins and fibrinogen. Serum haptoglobins that also arise from the liver are depressed rather than increased by estrogen.

Some of the effects on carbohydrate and lipid metabolism are probably influenced by changes in liver metabolism (see below).

Important alterations in hepatic drug excretion and metabolism also occur. Estrogens in the amounts seen during pregnancy or used in oral contraceptive agents delay the clearance of sulfobromophthalein and reduce the flow of bile. The proportion of cholic acid in bile acids is increased while the proportion of chenodeoxycholic acid is decreased. These changes may cause the observed increase in cholelithiasis associated with the use of these agents.

5. Effects on lipid metabolism—As noted above, estrogens increase serum triglycerides and free and esterified cholesterol. Phospholipids are also increased, as are high-density lipoproteins. Low-density lipoproteins usually decrease. Although the effects are marked with doses of 100 μg of mestranol or ethinyl estradiol, doses of 50 μg or less have minimal effects. The progestins (particularly the "19-nortestosterone" derivatives) tend to antagonize these effects of estrogen. Preparations containing small amounts of estrogen and a progestin may slightly decrease triglycerides and high-density lipoproteins.

6. Effects on carbohydrate metabolism—The administration of oral contraceptives produces alterations in carbohydrate metabolism similar to those observed in pregnancy. There is a reduction in the rate of absorption of carbohydrates from the gastrointestinal tract. Progesterone increases the basal insulin level and the rise in insulin induced by carbohydrate ingestion. Preparations with more potent progestins such as norgestrel may cause progressive decreases in carbohydrate tolerance over several years. However, the changes in glucose tolerance are reversible on discontinuing medication.

7. Effects on the cardiovascular system—These agents cause small increases in cardiac output associated with higher systolic and diastolic blood pressure and heart rate. The pressure returns to normal when treatment is terminated. Although the magnitude of the pressure change is small in most patients, it is marked in a few. It is important that blood pressure be followed in each patient. An increase in blood pressure has been reported to occur in few postmenopausal women treated with estrogens alone.

8. Effects on the skin—The oral contraceptives have been noted to increase pigmentation of the skin (chloasma). This effect seems to be enhanced in women with dark complexions and by exposure to ultraviolet light. Some of the androgen-like progestins might increase the production of sebum, causing acne in some patients. However, since ovarian androgen is suppressed, many patients note decreased sebum production, acne, and terminal hair growth. The sequential oral contraceptive preparations as well as estrogens alone often decrease sebum production.

Clinical Uses

The most important use of combined estrogens and progestins is for oral contraception. A large number of preparations are available for this specific purpose, some of which are listed in Table 40–3. They are specially packaged for ease of administration. In general, they are very effective; when these agents are taken according to directions, the risk of conception is extremely small. The pregnancy rate with combination agents is estimated to be about 0.5–1 per 100 woman years at risk. Contraceptive failure has been observed in some patients when one or more doses are missed, if phenytoin is also being used (which may increase catabolism of the compounds), or if antibiotics are taken that alter the enterohepatic cycle.

Progestins and estrogens are also useful in the treatment of endometriosis. When severe dysmenorrhea is the major symptom, the suppression of ovulation with estrogen alone may be followed by painless periods. However, in most patients this approach to therapy is inadequate. The long-term administration of large doses of progestins or combinations of progestins and estrogens prevents the periodic breakdown of the endometrial tissue and in some cases will lead to endometrial fibrosis and prevent the reactivation of implants for prolonged periods.

As is true with most hormonal preparations, many of the undesired effects are physiologic or pharmacologic actions that are objectionable only because they are not pertinent to the situation for which they are being used. Therefore, the product containing the smallest effective amounts of hormones should be selected for use.

Adverse Effects

The incidence of serious known toxicities associated with the use of these drugs is low. There are a number of reversible changes in intermediary metabolism. Minor adverse effects are frequent, but most are mild and many are transient. Continuing problems may respond to simple changes in pill formulation. Although it is not often necessary to discontinue medication for these reasons, as many as one third of all patients started on oral contraception discontinue use for reasons other than a desire to become pregnant.

A. MILD ADVERSE EFFECTS

1. Nausea, mastalgia, breakthrough bleeding, and edema are related to the amount of estrogen in the preparation. These effects can often be alleviated by a shift to a preparation containing smaller amounts of estrogen or to agents containing progestins with more androgenic effects.

2. Changes in serum proteins and other effects on endocrine function (see above) must be taken into account when thyroid, adrenal, or pituitary function is being evaluated. Increases in sedimentation rate are thought to be due to increased levels of fibrinogen.

3. Headache is mild and often transient. However, migraine is often made worse and has been reported to be associated with an increased frequency of cerebrovascular accidents. When this occurs or when migraine has its onset during therapy with these agents, treatment should be discontinued.

4. Withdrawal bleeding sometimes fails to occur—most often with combination preparations—and may cause confusion with regard to pregnancy. If this is disturbing to the patient, a different preparation may be tried or other methods of contraception used.

B. MODERATE ADVERSE EFFECTS

Any of the following may require discontinuance of oral contraceptives:

1. Breakthrough bleeding is the most common problem in using progestational agents alone for contraception. It occurs in as many as 25% of patients. It is more frequently encountered in patients taking low-dose preparations than in those taking combination pills with higher levels of progestin and estrogen. The biphasic and triphasic oral contraceptives (Table 40–3) decrease breakthrough bleeding without increasing the total hormone content.

2. Weight gain is more common with the combination agents containing androgen-like progestins. It can usually be controlled by shifting to preparations with less progestin effect or by dieting.

3. Increased skin pigmentation may occur, especially in dark-skinned women. It tends to increase with time, the incidence being about 5% at the end of the first year and about 40% after 8 years. It is thought to be exacerbated by vitamin B deficiency. It is often reversible upon discontinuance of medication but may disappear very slowly.

4. Acne may be exacerbated by agents containing androgen-like progestins (see Table 40–2), whereas agents containing large amounts of estrogen usually cause marked improvement in acne.

5. Hirsutism may also be aggravated by the "19-nortestosterone" derivatives, and combinations containing nonandrogenic progestins are preferred in these patients.

6. Ureteral dilation similar to that observed in pregnancy has been reported, and bacteriuria is more frequent.

7. Vaginal infections are more common and more difficult to treat in patients who are receiving oral contraceptives.

8. Amenorrhea occurs in some patients. Following cessation of administration of oral contraceptives, 95% of patients with normal menstrual histories resume normal periods and all but a few resume normal cycles during the next few months. However, some patients remain amenorrheic for several years. Many of these patients also have galactorrhea. Patients who have had menstrual irregularities before taking oral contraceptives are particularly susceptible to prolonged amenorrhea when the agents are discontinued. Prolactin levels should be measured in these patients, since many have prolactinomas.

C. SEVERE ADVERSE EFFECTS

1. Vascular disorders—Thromboembolism was one of the earliest of the serious unanticipated effects to be reported and has been the most thoroughly studied.

a. Venous thromboembolic disease—Superficial or deep thromboembolic disease in women not taking oral contraceptives occurs in about one patient per 1000 woman years. The overall incidence of these disorders in patients taking low-dose oral contraceptives is about threefold higher. The risk for this disorder is increased during the first month of contraceptive use and remains constant for several years or more. The risk returns to normal within a month when use is discontinued. The risk of venous thrombosis or pulmonary embolism is increased among women with predisposing conditions such as stasis, altered clotting factors such as antithrombin III, increased levels of homocysteine, or injury. Genetic disorders, including mutations in the genes governing the production of protein C (factor V Leiden), protein S, hepatic cofactor II, and others, markedly increase the risk of venous thromboembolism. The incidence of these disorders is too low for cost-effective screening by current methods, but prior episodes or a family history may be helpful in identifying patients with increased risk.

The incidence of venous thromboembolism is related to the estrogen but not the progestin content of oral contraceptives and is not related to age, parity, mild obesity, or cigarette smoking. Decreased venous blood flow, endothelial proliferation in veins and arteries, and increased coagulability of blood resulting from changes in platelet functions and fibrinolytic systems contribute to the increased incidence of thrombosis. The major plasma inhibitor of thrombin, antithrombin III, is substantially decreased during oral contraceptive use. This change occurs in the first month of treatment and lasts as long as treatment persists, reversing within a month thereafter.

b. Myocardial infarction—The use of oral contraceptives is associated with a slightly higher risk of myocardial infarction in women who are obese, have a history of preeclampsia or hypertension, or have hyperlipoproteinemia or diabetes. There is a much higher risk in women who smoke. The risk attributable to oral contraceptives in women 30–40 years of age who do not smoke is about 4 cases per 100,000 users per year, as compared with 185 cases per 100,000 among women 40–44 who smoke heavily. The association with myocardial infarction is thought to involve acceleration of atherogenesis because of decreased glucose tolerance, decreased levels of HDL, increased levels of LDL, and increased platelet aggregation. In addition, facilitation of coronary arterial spasm may also play a role in some of these patients. The progestational component of oral contraceptives decreases HDL cholesterol levels, in proportion to the androgenic activity of the progestin. The net effect, therefore, will depend on the specific composition of the pill used and the patient's susceptibility to the particular effects. Recent studies suggest that risk of infarction is not increased in past users who have discontinued oral contraceptives.

c. Cerebrovascular disease—The risk of strokes is concentrated in women over age 35. It is increased in current users of oral contraceptives but not in past users. However, subarachnoid hemorrhages have been found to be increased among both current and past users and may increase with time. The risk of thrombotic or hemorrhagic stroke attributable to oral contraceptives (based on older, higher-dose preparations) has been estimated to about 37 cases per 100,000 users per year.

In summary, available data indicate that oral contraceptives increase the risk of various cardiovascular disorders at all ages and among both smokers and nonsmokers. However, this risk appears to be concentrated in women 35 years of age or older who are heavy smokers. It is clear that these risk factors must be considered in each individual patient for whom oral contraceptives are being considered.

2. Gastrointestinal disorders—Many cases of cholestatic jaundice have been reported in patients taking progestin-containing drugs. The differences in incidence of these disorders from one population to another suggest that genetic factors may be involved. The jaundice caused by these agents is similar to that produced by other 17-alkyl-substituted steroids. It is most often observed in the first three cycles and is particularly common in women with a history of cholestatic jaundice during pregnancy. Jaundice and pruritus disappear 1–8 weeks after the drug is discontinued.

These agents have also been found to increase the incidence of symptomatic gallbladder disease, including cholecystitis and cholangitis. This is probably the result of the alterations responsible for jaundice and bile acid changes described above.

It also appears that the incidence of hepatic adenomas is increased in women taking oral contraceptives. Ischemic bowel disease secondary to thrombosis of the celiac and superior and inferior mesenteric arteries and veins has also been reported in women using these drugs.

3. Depression—Depression of sufficient degree to require cessation of therapy occurs in about 6% of patients treated with some preparations.

4. Cancer—The occurrence of malignant tumors in patients taking oral contraceptives has been studied extensively. It is now clear that these compounds *reduce* the risk of endometrial and ovarian cancer. The lifetime risk of breast cancer in the population as a whole does not seem to be affected by oral contraceptive use. Some studies have shown an increased risk in younger women, and it is possible that tumors that develop in younger women become clinically apparent sooner. The relation of risk of cervical cancer to oral contraceptive use is still controversial. It should be noted that a number of recent studies associate the use of oral contraceptives by women with cervical infection with the human papillomavirus to an increased risk of cervical cancer.

5. Other—In addition to the above effects, a number of other adverse reactions have been reported for which a causal relation has not been established. These include alopecia, erythema multiforme, erythema nodosum, and other skin disorders.

Contraindications & Cautions

These drugs are contraindicated in patients with thrombophlebitis, thromboembolic phenomena, and cardiovascular and cerebrovascular disorders or a past history of these conditions. They should not be used to treat vaginal bleeding when the cause is unknown. They should be avoided in patients with known or suspected tumor of the breast or other estrogen-dependent neoplasm. Since these preparations have caused aggravation of preexisting disorders, they should be avoided or used with caution in patients with liver disease, asthma, eczema, migraine, diabetes, hypertension, optic neuritis, retrobulbar neuritis, or convulsive disorders.

The oral contraceptives may produce edema, and for that reason they should be used with great caution in patients in heart failure or in whom edema is otherwise undesirable or dangerous.

Estrogens may increase the rate of growth of fibroids. Therefore, for women with these tumors, agents with the smallest amounts of estrogen and the most androgenic progestins should be selected. The use of progestational agents alone for contraception might be especially useful in such patients (see below).

These agents are contraindicated in adolescents in whom epiphysial closure has not yet been completed.

Women using oral contraceptives must be made aware of an important interaction that occurs with antimicrobial drugs. Because the normal gastrointestinal flora increases the enterohepatic cycling (and bioavailability) of estrogens, antimicrobial drugs that interfere with these organisms may reduce the efficacy of oral contraceptives. Additionally, coadministration with potent inducers of the hepatic microsomal metabolizing enzymes, such as rifampin, may increase liver catabolism of estrogens or progestins and diminish the efficacy of oral contraceptives.

Contraception With Progestins Alone

Small doses of progestins administered orally or by implantation under the skin can be used for contraception. They are particularly suited for use in patients for whom estrogen administration is undesirable. They are about as effective as intrauterine devices or combination pills containing 20–30 μg of ethinyl estradiol. There is a high incidence of abnormal bleeding.

Effective contraception can also be achieved by injecting 150 mg of depot medroxyprogesterone acetate (**DMPA**) every 3 months. After a 150 mg dose, ovulation is inhibited for at least 14 weeks. Almost all users experience episodes of unpredictable spotting and bleeding, particularly during the first year of use. Spotting and bleeding decrease with time, and amenorrhea is common. This preparation is not desirable for women planning a pregnancy soon after cessation of therapy because ovulation suppression can persist for as long as 18 months after the last injection. However, ovulation usually returns in a much shorter time. Long-term DMPA use reduces menstrual blood loss and is associated with a decreased risk of endometrial cancer. Suppression of endogenous estrogen secretion may be associated with a reversible reduction in bone density, and changes in plasma lipids are associated with an increased risk of atherosclerosis.

The progestin implant method utilizes the subcutaneous implantation of capsules containing a progestin (L-norgestrel). These capsules release one fifth to one third as much steroid as oral agents, are extremely effective, and last for 5–6 years. The low levels of hormone have little effect on lipoprotein and carbohydrate metabolism or blood pressure. The disadvantages include the need for surgical insertion and removal of capsules and some irregular bleeding rather than predictable menses. An association of intracranial hypertension with implanted norgestrel has been observed in a small number of women. Patients experiencing headache or visual disturbances should be checked for papilledema.

Contraception with progestins is useful in patients with hepatic disease, hypertension, psychosis or mental retardation, or prior thromboembolism. The side effects include headache, dizziness, bloating and weight gain of 1–2 kg, and a reversible reduction of glucose tolerance.

Postcoital Contraceptives

Pregnancy can be prevented following coitus by the administration of estrogens alone or in combination with progestins ("**morning after**" contraception). When treatment is begun within 72 hours, it is effective 99% of the time. Some effective schedules are shown in Table 40–4. The hormones are often administered with antiemetics, since 40% of the patients have nausea or vomiting. Other adverse effects include headache, dizziness, breast tenderness, and abdominal and leg cramps.

Mifepristone (RU 486), an antagonist at progesterone (and glucocorticoid) receptors, has a luteolytic effect and is effective as a postcoital contraceptive. When combined with a prostaglandin it is an effective abortifacient (see next page).

Beneficial Effects of Oral Contraceptives

It has become apparent that reduction in the dose of the constituents of oral contraceptives has markedly reduced mild and severe adverse effects, providing a relatively safe and convenient method of contraception for many young women. Treatment with oral contraceptives has now been shown to be associated with many benefits unrelated to contraception. These include a reduced risk of ovarian cysts, ovarian and endometrial cancer, and benign breast disease. There is a lower incidence of ectopic pregnancy. Iron deficiency and rheumatoid arthritis are less common, and premenstrual symptoms, dysmenorrhea, endometriosis, acne, and hirsutism may be ameliorated with their use.

ESTROGEN & PROGESTERONE INHIBITORS & ANTAGONISTS

TAMOXIFEN & RELATED PARTIAL AGONIST ESTROGENS

Tamoxifen is a competitive partial agonist inhibitor of estradiol at the estrogen receptor and is extensively used in the palliative treatment of advanced breast cancer in postmenopausal women. It is a nonsteroidal agent (see structure below) that is given orally. Peak plasma levels are reached in a few hours. Tamoxifen has an initial half-life of 7–14 hours in the circulation and is predominantly excreted by the liver. It is used in doses of 10–20 mg twice daily. Hot flushes and nausea and vomiting occur in 25% of patients, and many other minor adverse effects are observed. Studies of patients treated with tamoxifen as adjuvant therapy for early breast cancer have shown a 35% decrease in contralateral breast cancer. However, adjuvant therapy extended beyond 5 years in patients with breast cancer has shown no further improvement in outcome. **Toremifene** is a structurally similar compound with very similar properties, indications, and toxicities.

Table 40–4. Schedules for use of postcoital contraceptives.

Conjugated estrogens: 10 mg three times daily for 5 days

Ethinyl estradiol: 2.5 mg twice daily for 5 days

Diethylstilbestrol: 50 mg daily for 5 days

L-Norgestrel: 0.75 mg twice daily for 1 day (eg, Plan B[1])

Norgestrel, 0.5 mg, with ethinyl estradiol, 0.05 mg (eg, Ovral, Preven[1]): Four tablets (two immediately and two at 12 hours)

Mifepristone, 600 mg once with misoprostol 400 μg once

---

[1] Sold as emergency contraceptive kits.

Tamoxifen

Prevention of the expected loss of lumbar spine bone density and plasma lipid changes consistent with a reduction in the risk for atherosclerosis have also been reported in tamoxifen-treated patients following spontaneous or surgical menopause. However, this agonist activity also affects the uterus and increases the risk of endometrial cancer.

Raloxifene is another partial estrogen agonist-antagonist at some but not all target tissues. It has similar effects on lipids and bone but appears not to stimulate the endometrium or breast. Because of its apparent tissue selectivity it has been described as a **selective estrogen receptor modulator** (**SERM**), a term that could also be applied to tamoxifen and toremifene. Although subject to a high first-pass effect, raloxifene has a very large volume of distribution and a long half-life (> 24 hours), so it can be taken once a day. Raloxifene has been approved in the USA for the prevention of postmenopausal osteoporosis.

Clomiphene is an older partial agonist, a weak estrogen that also acts as a competitive inhibitor of endogenous estrogens. It has found use as an ovulation-inducing agent (see below).

MIFEPRISTONE

Mifepristone (RU 486) is a "19-norsteroid" that binds strongly to the progesterone receptor and inhibits the activity of progesterone. The drug has luteolytic properties in 80% of women when given in the midluteal period. The mechanism of this effect is unknown, but it may provide the basis for using mifepristone as a contraceptive (as opposed to an abortifacient). However, because the compound has a long half-life, large doses may prolong the follicular phase of the subsequent cycle and so make it difficult to use continuously for this purpose. A single dose of 600 mg is an effective emergency postcoital contraceptive, though it may result in delayed ovulation in the following cycle. As noted in Chapter 39, the drug also binds to and acts as an antagonist at the glucocorticoid receptor. Limited clinical studies suggest that mifepristone or other analogs with similar properties may be useful in the treatment of endometriosis, Cushing's syndrome, breast cancer, and possibly other neoplasms such as meningiomas that contain glucocorticoid or progesterone receptors.

Mifepristone

Mifepristone's major use thus far has been to terminate early pregnancies. Doses of 400–600 mg/d for 4 days or 800 mg/d for 2 days successfully terminated pregnancy in over 85% of the women studied. The major adverse effect was prolonged bleeding that on most occasions did not require treatment. The combination of a single oral dose of 600 mg of mifepristone and a vaginal pessary containing 1 mg of prostaglandin E_1 or oral misoprostol has been found to effectively terminate pregnancy in over 95% of patients treated during the first 7 weeks after conception. The adverse effects of the medications included vomiting, diarrhea, and abdominal or pelvic pain. As many as 5% of patients have vaginal bleeding requiring intervention. Because of these adverse effects, RU 486 is administered only by physicians at family planning centers. It is not in use in the United States at the time of this writing.

ZK 98734 (lilopristone) is a potent experimental progesterone inhibitor and abortifacient in doses of 25 mg twice daily. Like mifepristone, it also appears to have antiglucocorticoid activity.

DANAZOL

Danazol, an isoxazole derivative of ethisterone (17α-ethinyltestosterone) with weak progestational, androgenic, and glucocorticoid activities, is used to suppress ovarian function. Danazol inhibits the midcycle surge of LH and FSH and can prevent the compensatory increase in LH and FSH following castration in animals, but it does not significantly lower or suppress basal LH or FSH levels in normal women. Danazol binds to androgen, progesterone, and glucocorticoid receptors and can translocate the androgen receptor into the nucleus to initiate androgen-specific RNA synthesis. It does not bind to intracellular estrogen receptors, but it does bind to sex hormone-binding and corticosteroid-binding globulins. It inhibits P450scc (the cholesterol side chain-cleaving enzyme), 3β-hydroxysteroid dehydrogenase, 17α-hydroxysteroid dehydrogenase, P450c17 (17α-hydroxylase), P450c11 (11β-hydroxylase), and P450c21 (21β-hydroxylase). However, it does not inhibit aromatase, the enzyme required for estrogen synthesis. It increases the mean clearance of progesterone, probably by competing with the hormone for binding proteins, and may have similar effects on other active steroid hormones. Ethisterone, a major metabolite of danazol, has both progestational and mild androgenic effects.

Danazol is slowly metabolized in humans, having a half-life of over 15 hours. This results in stable circulating levels when the drug is administered twice daily. It is highly concentrated in the liver, adrenals, and kidneys and is excreted in both feces and urine.

Danazol has been employed as an inhibitor of gonadal function and has found its major use in the treatment of endometriosis. For this purpose, it can be given in a dosage of 600 mg/d. The dosage is reduced to 400 mg/d after 1 month and to 200 mg/d in 2 months. About 85% of patients show marked improvement in 3–12 months.

Danazol has also been used for the treatment of fibrocystic disease of the breast and hematologic or allergic disorders, including hemophilia, Christmas disease, idiopathic thrombocytopenic purpura, and angioneurotic edema.

The major adverse effects are weight gain, edema, decreased breast size, acne and oily skin, increased hair growth, deepening of the voice, headache, hot flushes, changes in libido, and muscle cramps. Although mild adverse effects are very common, it is seldom necessary to discontinue the drug because of them. Occasionally, because of its inherent glucocorticoid activity, danazol may cause adrenal suppression.

Danazol should be used with great caution in patients with hepatic dysfunction, since it has been reported to produce mild to moderate hepatocellular damage in some patients, as evidenced by enzyme changes. It is also contraindicated during pregnancy and breast feeding, as it may produce urogenital abnormalities in the offspring.

OTHER INHIBITORS

The prototypical steroidal inhibitor of aromatase (the enzyme required for estrogen synthesis) is **testolactone.** It is a weak inhibitor of the enzyme, and large quantities need to be administered to achieve clinical effect.

Anastrozole, a selective nonsteroidal inhibitor of aromatase, is effective in some women whose breast tumors have become resistant to tamoxifen. It is approved for use in such patients. **Letrozole** is similar. **Exemestane,** a steroid molecule, is an irreversible inhibitor of aromatase. Like anastrazole and letrozole, it is approved for use in women with advanced breast cancer (Chapter 55).

Several other aromatase inhibitors are undergoing clinical trials in patients with breast cancer. **Fadrozole** is a newer oral nonsteroidal (triazole) inhibitor of aromatase activity. These compounds appear to be as effective as tamoxifen. In addition to their use in breast cancer, aromatase inhibitors have been successfully employed as adjuncts to androgen antagonists in the treatment of precocious puberty and as primary treatment in the excessive aromatase syndrome.

Fulvestrant is a pure estrogen receptor antagonist that has been somewhat more effective than those with partial agonist effects and is effective in some patients who have become resistant to tamoxifen. ICI 164,384 inhibits dimerization of the occupied estrogen receptor and interferes with its binding to DNA. It has also been used experimentally in breast cancer patients who have become resistant to tamoxifen.

GnRH and its analogs (**nafarelin, buserelin,** etc) have become important in both stimulating and inhibiting ovarian function. They are discussed in Chapter 37.

OVULATION-INDUCING AGENTS

CLOMIPHENE

Clomiphene citrate, a partial estrogen agonist, is closely related to the estrogen chlorotrianisene (Figure 40–3). This compound is active when taken orally. Very little is known about its metabolism, but about half of the compound is excreted in the feces within 5 days after administration. It has been suggested that clomiphene is slowly excreted from an enterohepatic pool.

Pharmacologic Effects

A. MECHANISMS OF ACTION

Clomiphene is a partial agonist at estrogen receptors. The estrogenic agonist effects are best demonstrated in animals with marked gonadal deficiency. Clomiphene has also been shown to effectively inhibit the action of stronger estrogens. In humans it leads to an increase in the secretion of gonadotropins and estrogens by inhibiting estradiol's negative feedback effect on the gonadotropins.

B. EFFECTS

The pharmacologic importance of this compound rests on its ability to stimulate ovulation in women with oligomenorrhea or amenorrhea and ovulatory dysfunction. The majority of patients suffer from polycystic ovary syndrome, a common disorder affecting about 7% of women of reproductive age. The syndrome is characterized by gonadotropin-dependent ovarian hyperandrogenism associated with with oligo- or anovulation and infertility. The disorder is frequently accompanied by adrenal hyperandrogenism. Clomiphene has been suggested in order to block an inhibitory influence of estrogens on the hypothalamus, causing an ovulatory surge of gonadotropins and leading to ovulation.

Clinical Uses

Clomiphene is used for the treatment of disorders of ovulation in patients wishing to become pregnant. Usually, a single ovulation is induced by a single course of therapy, and the patient must be treated repeatedly until pregnancy is achieved, since normal ovulatory function does not usually resume. The compound is of no use in patients with ovarian or pituitary failure.

When clomiphene is administered in doses of 100 mg daily for 5 days, a rise in plasma LH and FSH is observed after several days. In patients who ovulate, the initial rise is followed by a second rise of gonadotropin levels just prior to ovulation.

Adverse Effects

The most common adverse effects in patients treated with this drug are hot flushes, which resemble those experienced by menopausal patients. They tend to be mild, and disappear when the drug is discontinued. There have been occasional reports of eye symptoms due to intensification and prolongation of afterimages. These are generally of short duration. Headache, constipation, allergic skin reactions, and reversible hair loss have been reported occasionally.

The effective use of clomiphene is associated with some stimulation of the ovaries and usually with ovarian enlargement. The degree of enlargement tends to be greater and its incidence higher in patients who have enlarged ovaries at the beginning of therapy.

A variety of other symptoms such as nausea and vomiting, increased nervous tension, depression, fatigue, breast soreness, weight gain, urinary frequency, and heavy menses have also been reported. However, these appear to result from the hormonal changes associated with an ovulatory menstrual cycle rather than from the medication. The incidence of multiple pregnancy is approximately 10%. Clomiphene has not been shown to have an adverse effect when inadvertently given to women who are already pregnant.

Contraindications & Cautions

Special precautions should be observed in patients with enlarged ovaries. These women are thought to be more sensitive to this drug and should receive small doses. Any patient who complains of abdominal symptoms should be examined carefully. Maximum ovarian enlargement occurs after the 5-day course has been completed, and many patients can be shown to have a palpable increase in ovarian size by the seventh to tenth days. Treatment with clomiphene for more than a year may be associated with an increased risk for low-grade ovarian cancer; however, the evidence for this effect is not conclusive.

Special precautions must also be taken in patients who have visual symptoms associated with clomiphene therapy, since these symptoms may make activities such as driving more hazardous.

Dosages

The recommended dosage of clomiphene citrate at the beginning of therapy is 50 mg/d for 5 days. If ovulation occurs, this same course may be repeated until pregnancy is achieved. If ovulation does not occur, the dosage is doubled to 100 mg/d for 5 days. If ovulation and menses occur, the next course can be started on the fifth day of the cycle. Experience to date suggests that patients who do not ovulate after three courses of 100 mg/d of clomiphene are not likely to respond to continued therapy. However, larger doses are effective in some individuals. Clomiphene is sometimes used in combination with gonadotropins, ie, a combination of LH and FSH.

About 80% of patients with anovulatory disorders or amenorrhea can be expected to respond by having ovulatory cycles. Approximately half of these patients become pregnant.

OTHER DRUGS USED IN OVULATORY DISORDERS

In addition to clomiphene, a variety of other hormonal and nonhormonal agents are used in treating anovulatory disorders. They are discussed in Chapter 37.

II. THE TESTIS (ANDROGENS & ANABOLIC STEROIDS, ANTIANDROGENS, & MALE CONTRACEPTION)

The testis, like the ovary, has both gametogenic and endocrine functions. The onset of gametogenic function of the testes is controlled largely by the secretion of FSH by the pituitary. High concentrations of testosterone locally are also required for continuing sperm production in the seminiferous tubules. The Sertoli cells in the seminiferous tubules may be the source of the estradiol produced in the testes via aromatization of locally produced testosterone. With LH stimulation, testosterone is produced by the interstitial or Leydig cells found in the spaces between the seminiferous tubules.

The Sertoli cells in the testis synthesize and secrete a variety of active proteins, including müllerian duct inhibitory factor, inhibin, and activin. As in the ovary, inhibin and activin appear to be the product of three genes that produce a common alpha subunit and two beta subunits, A and B. Activin is composed of the two beta subunits ($\beta_A\beta_B$). There are two inhibins (A and B), which contain the alpha subunit and one of the beta subunits. Activin stimulates pituitary FSH release and is structurally similar to transforming growth factor-β, which also increases FSH. The inhibins in conjunction with testosterone and dihydrotestosterone are responsible for the feedback inhibition of pituitary FSH secretion.

ANDROGENS & ANABOLIC STEROIDS

In humans, the most important androgen secreted by the testis is testosterone. The pathways of synthesis of testosterone in the testes are similar to those previously described for the adrenal and ovary (Figures 39–1 and 40–2).

In men, approximately 8 mg of testosterone is produced daily. About 95% is produced by the Leydig cells and only 5% by the adrenal. The testis also secretes small amounts of another potent androgen, dihydrotestosterone, as well as androstenedione and dehydroepiandrosterone, which are weak androgens. Pregnenolone and progesterone and their 17-hydroxylated derivatives are also released in small amounts. Plasma levels of testosterone in males are about 0.6 µg/dL after puberty and appear to decline after age 50. Testosterone is also present in the plasma of women in concentrations of approximately 0.03 µg/dL and is derived in approximately equal parts from the ovaries and adrenals and by the peripheral conversion of other hormones.

About 65% of circulating testosterone is bound to sex hormone-binding globulin. SHBG is increased in plasma by estrogen, by thyroid hormone, and in patients with cirrhosis of the liver. It is decreased by androgen and growth hormone and is lower in obese individuals. Most of the remaining testosterone is bound to albumin. Approximately 2% remains free and available to enter cells and bind to intracellular receptors.

Metabolism

In many target tissues, testosterone is converted to dihydrotestosterone by 5α-reductase. In these tissues, dihydrotestosterone is the major active androgen. The conversion of testosterone to estradiol by P450 aromatase also occurs in some tissues, including adipose tissue, liver, and the hypothalamus, where it may be of importance in regulating gonadal function.

The major pathway for the degradation of testosterone in humans occurs in the liver, with the reduction of the double bond and ketone in the A ring, as is seen in other steroids with a Δ^4-ketone configuration in the A ring. This leads to the production of inactive substances such as androsterone and etiocholanolone that are then conjugated and excreted in the urine.

Androstenedione, dehydroepiandrosterone (DHEA), and dehydroepiandrosterone sulfate (DHEAS) are also produced in significant amounts in humans, though largely in the adrenal rather than in the testes. They contribute slightly to the normal maturation process (adrenarche) supporting other androgen-dependent pubertal changes in the human, primarily development of pubic and axillary hair and bone maturation. As noted in Chapters 39 and 65, recent studies suggest that DHEA and DHEAS may have other central nervous system and metabolic effects and may prolong life in rabbits. In men they may improve the sense of well-being and inhibit atherosclerosis. In a recent placebo-controlled clinical trial in patients with systemic lupus erythematosus, DHEA demonstrated clear beneficial effects (see Adrenal Androgens, Chapter 39). Adrenal androgens are to a large extent metabolized in the same fashion as testosterone. Both steroids—but particularly androstenedione—can be converted by peripheral tissues to estrone in very small amounts (1–5%). The P450 aromatase enzyme responsible for this conversion is also found in the brain and is thought to play an important role in development.

Physiologic Effects

In the normal male, testosterone or its active metabolite 5α-dihydrotestosterone is responsible for the many changes that occur in puberty. In addition to the general growth-promoting properties of androgens on the body tissues, these hormones are responsible for penile and scrotal growth. Changes in the skin include the appearance of pubic, axillary, and beard hair. The sebaceous glands become more active, and the skin tends to become thicker and oilier. The larynx grows and the vocal cords become thicker, leading to a lower-pitched voice. Skeletal growth is stimulated and epiphysial closure accelerated. Other effects include growth of the prostate and seminal vesicles, darkening of the skin, and increased skin circulation. Androgens play an important role in stimulating and maintaining sexual function in men. Androgens increase lean body mass and stimulate body hair growth and sebum secretion. Metabolic effects include the reduction of hormone binding and other carrier proteins and increased liver synthesis of clotting factors, triglyceride lipase, α_1-antitrypsin, haptoglobin, and sialic acid. They also stimulate renal erythropoietin secretion and decrease high-density lipoprotein levels.

Synthetic Steroids With Androgenic & Anabolic Action

Testosterone, when administered by mouth, is rapidly absorbed. However, it is largely converted to inactive metabolites, and only about one sixth of the dose administered is available in active form. Testosterone can be administered parenterally, but it has a more prolonged absorption time and greater activity in the propionate, enanthate, undecanoate, or cypionate ester forms. These derivatives are hydrolyzed to release free testosterone at the site of injection. Testosterone derivatives alkylated at the 17 position, eg, methyltestosterone and fluoxymesterone, are active when given by mouth.

Testosterone and its derivatives have been used for their anabolic effects as well as for the treatment of testosterone deficiency. Although testosterone and other known active steroids can be isolated in pure form and measured by weight, biologic assays are still used in the investigation of new compounds. In some of these studies in animals, the anabolic effects of the compound as measured by trophic effects on muscles or the reduction of nitrogen excretion may be dissociated from the other androgenic effects. This has led to the marketing of compounds claimed to have anabolic activity associated with only weak androgenic effects. Unfortunately, this dissociation is less marked in humans than in the animals used for testing (Table 40–5), and all are potent androgens.

Pharmacologic Effects

A. MECHANISMS OF ACTION

Like other steroids, testosterone acts intracellularly in target cells. In skin, prostate, seminal vesicles, and epididymis, it is converted to 5α-dihydrotestosterone. In

Table 40–5. Androgens: Preparations available and relative androgenic:anabolic activity in animals.

	Androgenic: Anabolic Activity
Testosterone	1:1
Testosterone cypionate	1:1
Testosterone enanthate	1:1
Testosterone propionate	1:1
Methyltestosterone	1:1
Fluoxymesterone	1:2
Methandrostenolone (methandienone)	1:3
Oxymetholone	1:3
Ethylestrenol	1:4–1:8
Oxandrolone	1:3–1:13
Nandrolone phenpropionate	1:3–1:6
Nandrolone decanoate	1:2.5–1:4
Stanozolol	1:3–1:6
Dromostanolone propionate	1:3–1:4

these tissues, dihydrotestosterone is the dominant androgen. The distribution of this enzyme in the fetus is different and has important developmental implications.

Testosterone and dihydrotestosterone bind to the intracellular androgen receptor, initiating a series of events similar to those described above for estradiol and progesterone, leading to growth, differentiation, and synthesis of a variety of enzymes and other functional proteins.

B. EFFECTS

In the male at puberty, androgens cause development of the secondary sex characteristics (see above). In the adult male, large doses of testosterone—when given alone—or its derivatives suppress the secretion of gonadotropins and result in some atrophy of the interstitial tissue and the tubules of the testes. Since fairly large doses of androgens are required to suppress gonadotropic secretion, it has been postulated that inhibin, in combination with androgens, is responsible for the feedback control of secretion. In women, androgens are capable of producing changes similar to those observed in the prepubertal male. These include growth of facial and body hair, deepening of the voice, enlargement of the clitoris, frontal baldness, and prominent musculature. The natural androgens stimulate erythrocyte production.

The administration of androgens reduces the excretion of nitrogen into the urine, indicating an increase in protein synthesis or a decrease in protein breakdown within the body. This effect is much more pronounced in women and children than in normal men.

Clinical Uses

A. ANDROGEN REPLACEMENT THERAPY IN MEN

Androgens are used to replace or augment endogenous androgen secretion in hypogonadal men (Table 40–6). Even in the presence of pituitary deficiency, androgens are used rather than gonadotropin except when normal spermatogenesis is to be achieved. In patients with hypopituitarism, androgens are not added to the treatment regimen until puberty, at which time they are instituted in gradually increasing doses to achieve the growth spurt and the development of secondary sex characteristics. In these patients, therapy should be started with long-acting agents such as testosterone enanthate in doses of 50 mg intramuscularly, initially every 4, then every 3, and finally every 2 weeks, with each change taking place at 3-month intervals. The dose is then doubled to 100 mg every 2 weeks until maturation is complete. Finally, it is changed to the adult replacement dose of 200 mg at 2-week intervals. Testosterone propionate, though potent, has a short duration

Table 40–6. Androgen preparations for replacement therapy.

	Route of Administration	Dosage
Methyltestosterone	Oral Sublingual (buccal)	25–50 mg/d 5–10 mg/d
Fluoxymesterone	Oral	2–10 mg/d
Testosterone propionate	Sublingual (buccal) Intramuscular	5–20 mg/d 10–50 mg three times weekly
Testosterone enanthate	Intramuscular	See text
Testosterone cypionate	Intramuscular	See text
Testosterone	Transdermal	2.5–10 mg/d
	Topical gel (1%)	5–10 g gel/d

of action and is not practical for long-term use. Testosterone undecanoate can be given orally, administering large amounts of the steroid twice daily (eg, 40 mg/d); however, this is not recommended because oral testosterone administration has been associated with liver tumors. Testosterone can also be administered transdermally; skin patches or gels are available for scrotal or other skin area application. Two applications daily are usually required for replacement therapy. Implanted pellets and other longer-acting preparations are under study. The development of polycythemia or hypertension may require some reduction in dose.

B. Gynecologic Disorders

Androgens are used occasionally in the treatment of certain gynecologic disorders, but the undesirable effects in women are such that they must be used with great caution. Androgens have been used to reduce breast engorgement during the postpartum period, usually in conjunction with estrogens. The weak androgen danazol is used in the treatment of endometriosis (see above).

Androgens are sometimes given in combination with estrogens for replacement therapy in the postmenopausal period in an attempt to eliminate the endometrial bleeding that may occur when only estrogens are used and to enhance libido. They are also used for chemotherapy of breast tumors in premenopausal women.

C. Use as Protein Anabolic Agents

Androgens and anabolic steroids have been used in conjunction with dietary measures and exercises in an attempt to reverse protein loss after trauma, surgery, or prolonged immobilization and in patients with debilitating diseases.

D. Anemia

In the past, large doses of androgens were employed in the treatment of refractory anemias such as aplastic anemia, Fanconi's anemia, sickle cell anemia, myelofibrosis, and hemolytic anemias. Recombinant erythropoietin has largely replaced androgens for this purpose.

E. Osteoporosis

Androgens and anabolic agents have been used in the treatment of osteoporosis, either alone or in conjunction with estrogens. With the exception of substitution therapy in hypogonadism, bisphosphonates have largely replaced androgen use for this purpose.

F. Use as Growth Stimulators

These agents have been used to stimulate growth in boys with delayed puberty. If the drugs are used carefully, these children will probably achieve their expected adult height. If treatment is too vigorous, the patient may grow rapidly at first but will not achieve full final stature because of the accelerated epiphysial closure that occurs. It is difficult to control this type of therapy adequately even with frequent x-ray examination of the epiphyses, since the action of the hormones on epiphysial centers may continue for many months after therapy is discontinued.

G. Anabolic Steroid and Androgen Abuse in Sports

The use of anabolic steroids by athletes has received worldwide attention. Many athletes and their coaches believe that anabolic steroids—in doses 10–200 times larger than the daily normal production—increase strength and aggressiveness, thereby improving competitive performance. Although such effects have been demonstrated in women, many studies have failed to unequivocally demonstrate them in men. Placebo effects and the potential impact of minimal changes in championship competitions make evaluation of these studies very difficult. However, the adverse effects of these drugs clearly make their use inadvisable.

H. AGING

Androgen production falls with age in men and may contribute to the decline in muscle mass, strength, and libido. Preliminary studies of androgen replacement in aging males with low androgen levels show an increase in lean body mass and hematocrit and a decrease in bone turnover. Longer studies will be required to assess the usefulness of this therapy.

Adverse Effects

The adverse effects of these compounds are due largely to their masculinizing actions and are most noticeable in women and prepubertal children. In women, the administration of more than 200–300 mg of testosterone per month is usually associated with hirsutism, acne, amenorrhea, clitoral enlargement, and deepening of the voice. These effects may occur with even smaller doses in some women. Some of the androgenic steroids exert progestational activity leading to endometrial bleeding upon discontinuation. These hormones also alter serum lipids and could conceivably increase susceptibility to atherosclerotic disease in women. Except under the most unusual circumstances, androgens should not be used in infants. Recent studies in animals suggest that administration of androgens in early life may have profound effects on maturation of central nervous system centers governing sexual development, particularly in the female. Administration of these drugs to pregnant women may lead to masculinization or undermasculinization of the external genitalia in the female and male fetus, respectively. Although the above-mentioned effects may be less marked with the anabolic agents, they do occur.

Sodium retention and edema are not common but must be carefully watched for in patients with heart and kidney disease.

Most of the synthetic androgens and anabolic agents are 17-alkyl-substituted steroids. Administration of drugs with this structure is often associated with evidence of hepatic dysfunction, eg, increase in sulfobromophthalein retention and aspartate aminotransferase (AST) levels. Alkaline phosphatase values are also elevated. These changes usually occur early in the course of treatment, and the degree is proportionate to the dose. Bilirubin levels occasionally increase until clinical jaundice is apparent. The cholestatic jaundice is reversible upon cessation of therapy, and permanent changes do not occur. In older males, prostatic hyperplasia may develop, causing urinary retention.

Replacement therapy in men may cause acne, sleep apnea, erythrocytosis, gynecomastia, and azoospermia. Supraphysiologic doses of androgens produce azoospermia and decrease in testicular size, both of which may take months to recover after cessation of therapy. The alkylated androgens in high doses can produce peliosis hepatica, cholestasis, and hepatic failure. They lower plasma HDL_2 and may increase LDL. Hepatic adenomas and carcinomas have also been reported. Behavioral effects include psychologic dependence, increased aggressiveness, and psychotic symptoms.

Contraindications & Cautions

The use of androgenic steroids is contraindicated in pregnant women or women who may become pregnant during the course of therapy.

Androgens should not be administered to male patients with carcinoma of the prostate or breast. Until more is known about the effects of these hormones on the central nervous system in developing children, they should be avoided in infants and young children.

Special caution is required in giving these drugs to children to produce a growth spurt. In most patients, the use of somatotropin is more appropriate (Chapter 37).

Care should be exercised in the administration of these drugs to patients with renal or cardiac disease predisposed to edema. If sodium and water retention occurs, it will respond to diuretic therapy.

Methyltestosterone therapy is associated with creatinuria, but the significance of this finding is not known.

Caution: Several cases of hepatocellular carcinoma have been reported in patients with aplastic anemia treated with androgen anabolic therapy. Colony-stimulating factors (Chapter 33) should be used instead.

ANDROGEN SUPPRESSION & ANTIANDROGENS

ANDROGEN SUPPRESSION

The treatment of advanced prostatic carcinoma often requires orchiectomy or large doses of estrogens to reduce available endogenous androgen. The psychologic effects of the former and gynecomastia produced by the latter make these approaches undesirable. As noted in Chapter 37, the gonadotropin-releasing hormone analogs such as goserelin, nafarelin, buserelin, and

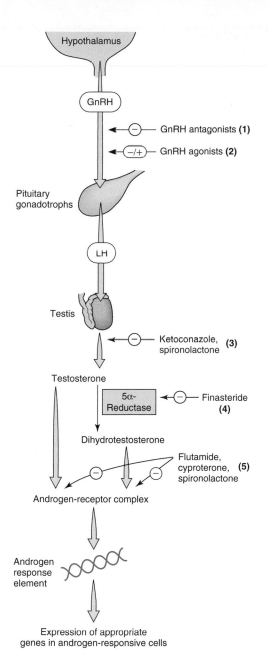

Figure 40–5. Control of androgen secretion and activity and some sites of action of antiandrogens. **(1)**, competitive inhibition of GnRH receptors; **(2)**, stimulation (+, pulsatile administration) or inhibition via desensitization of GnRH receptors (–, continuous administration); **(3)**, decreased synthesis of testosterone in the testis; **(4)**, decreased synthesis of dihydrotestosterone by inhibition of 5α-reductase; **(5)**, competition for binding to cytosol androgen receptors.

leuprolide acetate produce gonadal suppression when blood levels are continuous rather than pulsatile (see Chapter 37 and Figure 40–5). **Leuprolide acetate** is injected subcutaneously daily in doses of 1 mg (or depot leuprolide is given once every month or every 3 months) for the treatment of prostatic carcinoma. Goserelin is administered once every 4 weeks as a subcutaneous slow-release injection. Although testosterone levels fall to 10% of their initial values after a month with either of these drugs, they *increase* significantly in the beginning. This increase is usually associated with a flare of tumor activity and an increase in symptoms. The combination of a GnRH agonist and flutamide, an androgen antagonist (or equivalent, see below), can prevent the initial stimulation and provide a more effective inhibition of androgenic activity.

GnRH antagonists have also been under study, since they would have the advantage of eliminating the surge of androgen secretion seen at the beginning of GnRH analog therapy. Most of the compounds studied have the capacity to release histamine and are unsuitable for use. However, newer agents with less histamine-releasing activity are being studied.

ANTIANDROGENS

The potential usefulness of antiandrogens for the treatment of patients producing excessive amounts of testosterone has led to the search for effective drugs that can be used for this purpose. Several approaches to the problem, especially inhibition of synthesis and receptor antagonism, have met with some success.

Steroid Synthesis Inhibitors

Ketoconazole, used primarily for the treatment of fungal disease, is an inhibitor of adrenal and gonadal steroid synthesis, as described in Chapter 39. It does not affect ovarian aromatase, but it reduces human placental aromatase activity. It displaces estradiol and dihydrotestosterone from sex hormone-binding protein in vitro and increases the estradiol:testosterone ratio in plasma in vivo by a different mechanism. However, it does not appear to be clinically useful in women with increased androgens because of the toxicity associated with prolonged use of the 400–800 mg/d required. The drug has also been used experimentally to treat prostatic carcinoma, but the results have not been encouraging. Men treated with ketoconazole often develop reversible gynecomastia during therapy; this may be due to the demonstrated increase in the estradiol:testosterone ratio.

Conversion of Steroid Precursors to Androgens

Several compounds have been developed that inhibit the 17-hydroxylation of progesterone or pregnenolone, thereby preventing the action of the side chain-splitting enzyme and the further transformation of these steroid precursors to active androgens. A few of these compounds have been tested clinically but have been too toxic for prolonged use.

Since dihydrotestosterone—not testosterone—appears to be the essential androgen in the prostate, androgen effects in this and similar dihydrotestosterone-dependent tissues can be reduced by an inhibitor of 5α-reductase (Figure 40–5). **Finasteride**, a steroid-like inhibitor of this enzyme, is orally active and produces a reduction in dihydrotestosterone levels within 8 hours after administration that lasts for about 24 hours. The half-life is about 8 hours (longer in elderly individuals). Forty to 50 percent of the dose is metabolized; more than half is excreted in the feces. Finasteride has been reported to be moderately effective in reducing prostate size in men with benign prostatic hyperplasia and is approved for this use in the USA. The dosage is 5 mg/d. Its use in advanced prostatic carcinoma is under study. The drug is not approved for use in women or children, though it has been used successfully in the treatment of hirsutism in women and early male pattern baldness in men (1 mg/d).

Finasteride

Receptor Inhibitors

Cyproterone and **cyproterone acetate** are effective antiandrogens that inhibit the action of androgens at the target organ. The acetate form has a marked progestational effect that suppresses the feedback enhancement of LH and FSH, leading to a more effective antiandrogen effect. These compounds have been used in women for the treatment of hirsutism and in men to decrease excessive sexual drive and are being studied in other conditions in which the reduction of androgenic effects would be useful. Cyproterone acetate in a dosage of 2 mg/d administered concurrently with an estrogen is used in the treatment of hirsutism in women, doubling as a contraceptive pill; it has orphan drug status in the USA.

Flutamide, a substituted anilide, is a potent antiandrogen that has been used in the treatment of prostatic carcinoma. Though not a steroid, it behaves like a competitive antagonist at the androgen receptor. It is rapidly metabolized in humans. It frequently causes mild gynecomastia (probably by increasing testicular estrogen production) and occasionally causes mild reversible hepatic toxicity. Administration of this compound causes some improvement in most patients who have not had prior endocrine therapy. Preliminary studies indicate that flutamide is also useful in the management of excess androgen effect in women.

Flutamide

Bicalutamide and **nilutamide** are potent orally active antiandrogens that can be administered as a single daily dose and are used in patients with metastatic prostate carcinoma. Studies in patients with carcinoma of the prostate indicate that they are well tolerated. Bicalutamide is recommended for use in combination with a GnRH analog (to reduce tumor flare) and may have fewer gastrointestinal side effects than flutamide. A dosage of 150–200 mg/d (when used alone) is required to reduce prostate-specific antigen levels to those achieved by castration, but, in combination with a GnRH analog, 50 mg/d may be adequate. Nilutamide is approved for use following surgical castration in a dosage of 300 mg/d for 30 days followed by 150 mg/d.

Spironolactone, a competitive inhibitor of aldosterone (see Chapter 15), also competes with dihydrotestosterone for the androgen receptors in target tissues. It also reduces 17α-hydroxylase activity, lowering plasma levels of testosterone and androstenedione. It is used in dosages of 50–200 mg/d for the treatment of hirsutism in women and appears to be as effective as finasteride, flutamide, or cyproterone in this condition.

CHEMICAL CONTRACEPTION IN MEN

Although many studies have been conducted, an effective oral contraceptive for men has not yet been found. For example, various androgens, including testosterone and testosterone enanthate, in a dosage of 400 mg per month, produced azoospermia in less than half the men treated. Minor adverse reactions, including gynecomastia and acne, were encountered. Testosterone in combination with danazol was well tolerated but no more effective than testosterone alone. Androgens in combination with a progestin such as medroxyprogesterone acetate were no more effective. However, preliminary studies indicate that the intramuscular administration of 100 mg of testosterone enanthate weekly together with 500 mg of levonorgestrel daily orally can produce azoospermia in 94% of men.

Cyproterone acetate, a very potent progestin and antiandrogen, also produces oligospermia; however, it does not cause reliable contraception.

At present, pituitary hormones—and potent antagonist analogs of GnRH—are receiving increased attention. A GnRH antagonist in combination with testosterone has been shown to produce reversible azoospermia in nonhuman primates.

GOSSYPOL

Extensive trials of this cottonseed derivative have been conducted in China. This compound destroys elements of the seminiferous epithelium but does not alter the endocrine function of the testis in a major fashion.

Gossypol

In Chinese studies, large numbers of men were treated with 20 mg/d of gossypol or gossypol acetic acid for 2 months, followed by a maintenance dosage of 60 mg/wk. On this regimen, 99% of men developed sperm counts below 4 million/mL. Preliminary data indicate that recovery (return of normal sperm count) following discontinuance of gossypol administration is more apt to occur in men whose counts do not fall to extremely low levels and when administration is not continued for more than 2 years. Hypokalemia is the major adverse effect and may lead to transient paralysis. The drug has also been tried as an intravaginal spermicide contraceptive.

PREPARATIONS AVAILABLE[1]

ESTROGENS
Conjugated estrogens (Premarin)
Oral: 0.3, 0.625, 0.9, 1.25, 2.5 mg tablets
Parenteral: 25 mg/5 mL for IM, IV injection
Vaginal: 0.625 mg/g cream base
Dienestrol (Ortho Dienestrol, DV)
Vaginal: 10 mg/g cream
Diethylstilbestrol diphosphate (Stilphostrol)
Oral: 50 mg tablets
Parenteral: 50 mg/mL injection
Esterified estrogens (Menest, Estratab)
Oral: 0.3, 0.625, 1.25, 2.5 mg tablets
Estradiol cypionate in oil (generic, Depo-Estradiol Cypionate)
Parenteral: 5 mg/mL for IM injection
Estradiol (generic, Estrace)
Oral: 0.5, 1, 2 mg tablets
Vaginal: 0.1 mg/g cream
Estradiol transdermal (Estraderm, others)
Transdermal: patches with 0.025, 0.0375, 0.05, 0.075, 0.1 mg/d release rates
Estradiol valerate in oil (generic)
Parenteral: 10, 20, 40 mg/mL for IM injection

Estrone aqueous suspension (generic, Kestrone 5)
Parenteral: 5 mg/mL for injection
Estropipate (generic, Ogen)
Oral: 0.625, 1.25, 2.5, 5 mg tablets
Vaginal: 1.5 mg/g cream base
Ethinyl estradiol (Estinyl)
Oral: 0.02, 0.05, 0.5 mg tablets

PROGESTINS
Hydroxyprogesterone caproate (generic, Hylutin)
Parenteral: 125, 250 mg/mL for IM injection
Levonorgestrel (Norplant)
Kit for subcutaneous implant: 6 capsules of 36 mg each
Medroxyprogesterone acetate (generic, Provera)
Oral: 2.5, 5, 10 mg tablets
Parenteral (Depo-Provera): 150, 400 mg/mL for IM injection
Megestrol acetate (generic, Megace)
Oral: 20, 40 mg tablets; 40 mg/mL suspension
Norethindrone acetate (generic, Aygestin)
Oral: 5 mg tablets
Norgestrel (Ovrette) (See also Table 40–3)
Oral: 0.075 mg tablets

---

[1] Oral contraceptives are listed in Table 40–3.

Progesterone (generic)
Oral: 100 mg capsules
Topical: 8% vaginal gel
Parenteral: 50 mg/mL in oil for IM injection

ANDROGENS & ANABOLIC STEROIDS

Fluoxymesterone (generic, Halotestin)
Oral: 2, 5, 10 mg tablets
Methyltestosterone (generic)
Oral: 10, 25 mg tablets; 10 mg capsules; 10 mg buccal tablets
Parenteral: 200 mg/mL injection
Nandrolone decanoate (Deca-Durabolin, others)
Parenteral: 100, 200 mg/mL in oil for injection
Oxandrolone (Oxandrin)
Oral: 2.5 mg tablets
Oxymetholone (Androl-50)
Oral: 50 mg tablets
Stanozolol (Winstrol)
Oral: 2 mg tablets
Testolactone (Teslac)
Oral: 50 mg tablets
Testosterone aqueous (generic, others)
Parenteral: 25, 50, 100 mg/mL suspension for IM injection
Testosterone cypionate in oil (generic, others)
Parenteral: 100, 200 mg/mL for IM injection
Testosterone enanthate in oil (generic)
Parenteral: 200 mg/mL for IM injection
Testosterone propionate in oil (generic, Testex)
Parenteral: 100 mg/mL for IM injection
Testosterone transdermal system
Patch (Testoderm): 4, 5, 6 mg/24 h release rate
Patch (Androderm): 2.5, 5 mg/24 h release rate
Gel (Androgel): 25, 50 mg total
Testosterone pellets (Testopel)
Parenteral: 75 mg/pellet for parenteral injection (not IV)

ANTAGONISTS & INHIBITORS

(See Also Chapter 37)
Anastrozole (Arimidex)
Oral: 1 mg tablets
Bicalutamide (Casodex)
Oral: 50 mg tablets
Clomiphene (generic, Clomid, Serophene, Milophene)
Oral: 50 mg tablets
Danazol (generic, Danocrine)
Oral: 50, 100, 200 mg capsules
Dutasteride (Avodart)
Oral: 0.5 mg tablets
Exemestane (Aromasin)
Oral: 25 mg tablets
Finasteride
Oral: 1 mg tablets (Propecia); 5 mg tablets (Proscar)
Flutamide (Eulexin)
Oral: 125 mg capsules
Fulvestrant (Faslodex)
Parenteral: 50 mg/mL for IM injection
Letrozole (Femara)
Oral: 2.5 mg tablets
Mifepristone (Mifeprex)
Oral: 200 mg tablets
Nilutamide (Nilandron)
Oral: 50, 150 mg tablets
Raloxifene (Evista)
Oral: 60 mg tablets
Tamoxifen (generic, Nolvadex)
Oral: 10, 20 mg tablets
Toremifene (Fareston)
Oral: 60 mg tablets

REFERENCES

OVARIAN HORMONES

Adashi EY: Intraovarian peptides: Stimulators and inhibitors of follicular growth and differentiation. Endocrinol Metab Clin North Am 1992;21:1.

Ahokas A, Kaukoranta J, Aito M: Effect of oestradiol on postpartum depression. Psychopharmacology (Berl) 1999;146:108.

Bamberger CM, Schulte HM, Chrousos GP: Molecular determinants of glucocorticoid receptor function and tissue sensitivity. Endo Rev 1996;17:221.

Belchetz PE: Hormonal treatment of postmenopausal women. N Engl J Med 1994;330:1062.

Bhavnani BR, Cecutti A: Pharmacokinetics of 17β-dihydroequilin sulfate and 17β-dihydroequilin in normal postmenopausal women. J Clin Endocrinol Metab 1994;78:197.

Casper RF, Chapdelaine A: Estrogen and interrupted progestin: A new concept for hormone replacement therapy. Am J Obstet Gynecol 1993;168:1186.

Carranza-Lira S, Valentino-Figueroa ML: Estrogen therapy for depression in postmenopausal women. Int J Gynaecol Obstet 1999;65:35.

Chrousos GP, Torpy DJ, Gold PW: Interactions between the hypothalamic-pituitary-adrenal axis and the female reproductive system: Clinical implications. Ann Intern Med 1998;129:229.

Colditz GA et al: The use of estrogens and progestins and the risk of breast cancer in postmenopausal women. N Engl J Med 1995;332:1589.

Derksen RH: Dehydroepiandrosterone (DHEA) and systemic lupus erythematosus. Semin Arthritis Rheum 1998;27:335.

DiSaia PJ: Estrogen replacement therapy for the breast cancer survivor. J Soc Gynecol Invest 1996;3:57.

Draper MW et al: Antiestrogenic properties of raloxifene. Pharmacology 1995;50:209.

Edwards DP, Boonyaratanakornkit V: Rapid extranuclear signaling by the estrogen receptor (ER): MNAR couples ER and Src to the MAP Kinase signaling pathway. Mol Interventions 2002;3:12.

Giangrande PH, McDonnell DP: The A and B isoforms of the human progesterone receptor: Two functionally different transcription factors encoded by a single gene. Recent Prog Horm Res 1999;54:291.

Golditz GA, Egan KM, Stampfer MJ: Hormone replacement therapy and the risk of breast cancer: Results from epidemiologic studies. Am J Obstet Gynecol 1993;168:1473.

Grandien K, Berkenstam A, Gustafsson JA: The estrogen receptor gene: Promoter organization and expression. Int J Biochem Cell Biol 1997;29:1343.

Grodstein F et al: Postmenopausal estrogen and progestin use and the risk of cardiovascular disease. N Engl J Med 1996;335:453.

Hofseth L et al: Hormone replacement therapy with estrogens or estrogens plus medroxyprogesterone acetate is associated with increased epithelial proliferation in the normal postmenopausal breast. J Clin Endocrinol Metab 1999;84:4559.

Horrobin DF, Bennett CN: Depression and bipolar disorder: Relationships to impaired fatty acid and phospholipid metabolism and to diabetes, cardiovascular disease, immunological abnormalities, cancer, aging and osteoporosis. Possible candidate genes. Prostaglandins Leukot Essent Fatty Acids 1999;60:217.

Kalantaridou S, Chrousos GP: Monogenic disorders of puberty. J Clin Endocrinol Metab 2002;87:2481.

Lacey JV Jr et al: Oral contraceptives as risk factors for cervical adenocarcinomas and squamous cell carcinomas. Cancer Epidemiol Biomarkers Prev 1999;8:1079.

Latronico AC et al: Testicular and ovarian resistance to luteinizing hormone caused by homozygous inactivating mutations of the luteinizing hormone receptor gene. N Engl J Med 1996;334:507.

Manson JE et al: Estrogen plus progestin and the risk of coronary heart disease. N Engl J Med 2003;349:523.

Mastorakos G, Webster EL, Chrousos GP: Corticotropin-releasing hormone and its receptors in the ovary: Physiological implications. Ann New York Acad Sci 1993;687:20.

Merke DP et al: Future directions in the study and management of congenital adrenal hyperplasia due to 21-hydroxylase deficiency. Ann Intern Med 2002;136:320.

Morales AJ et al: Effects of replacement dose of dehydroepiandrosterone in men and women of advancing age. J Clin Endocrinol Metab 1994;78:1360.

Nabulsi AA et al: Association of hormone-replacement therapy with various cardiovascular risk factors in postmenopausal women. N Engl J Med 1993;328:1069.

Perez P et al: The estrogenicity of bisphenol A-related diphenylalkanes with various substituents at the central carbon and the hydroxy groups. Environ Health Perspect 1998;106:167.

Rittmaster RS: Medical treatment of androgen-dependent hirsutism. J Clin Endocrinol Metab 1995;80:2559.

Rossouw JE et al: Risks and benefits of estrogen plus progestin in healthy postmenopausal women: principal results from the Women's Health Initiative randomized controlled trial. JAMA 2002;288:321.

Sonnenscheim C, Soto AM: An updated review of environmental estrogen and androgen mimics and antagonists. J Steroid Biochem Mol Biol 1998;65:143.

Tesarik J, Mendoza C: Nongenomic effects of 17β-estradiol on maturing oocytes: Relationship to oocyte developmental potential. J Clin Endocrinol Metab 1995;80:1438.

Stock SM, Sande EM, Bremme KA: Leptin levels vary significantly during the menstrual cycle, pregnancy, and in vitro fertilization treatment: Possible relation to estradiol. Fertil Steril 1999;72:657.

Stratakis CA et al: The aromatase excess syndrome is associated with feminization of both sexes and autosomal dominant transmission of aberrant P450 aromatase gene transcription. J Clin Endocrinol Metab 1998;83:1348.

Westerveld HT et al: 17β-Estradiol improves postprandial lipid metabolism in postmenopausal women. J Clin Endocrinol Metab 1995;80:249.

Women's Health Initiative Investigators: Risk and benefits of estrogen plus progestin in healthy postmenopausal women. Principal results from the Women's Health Initiative randomized controlled trial. JAMA 2002;288:321.

Zandi PP et al: Hormone replacement therapy and incidence of Alzheimer's disease in older women. JAMA 2002;288:2123.

ORAL CONTRACEPTIVES

Azziz R: Leuprolide and estrogen versus oral contraceptive pills for the treatment of hirsutism: A prospective randomized study. J Clin Endocrinol Metab 1995;80:3406.

Baird DT, Glasier AF: Hormonal contraception. N Engl J Med 1993;328:1543.

Darncy PD: The androgenicity of progestins. Am J Med 1995;98:104S.

Fotherby K, Caldwell AD: New progestogens in oral contraception. Contraception 1994;49:1.

Grimes DA, Mishell DR Jr, Speroff L (editors): Contraceptive choices for women with medical problems. Am J Obstet Gynecol 1993;168(No 6 Part 2):1979.

Herbst AL, Berek JS: Impact of contraception on gynecologic cancers. Am J Obstet Gynecol 1993;168:1980.

Mishell DR Jr: Noncontraceptive health benefits of oral contraceptives. Am J Obstet Gynecol 1982;142:809.

Oelkers W et al: Effects of a new oral contraceptive containing an antimineralocorticoid progestogen, drospirenone, on the renin-aldosterone system, body weight, blood pressure, glucose tolerance, and lipid metabolism. J Clin Endocrinol Metab 1995;80:1816.

Polaneczky M et al: The use of levonorgestrel implants (Norplant) for contraception in adolescent mothers. N Engl J Med 1994;331:1201.

Weisberg E: Interactions between oral contraceptives and antifungals/antibacterials. Is contraceptive failure the result? Clin Pharmacokinet 1999;36:309.

ANDROGENS

Bagatell CJ, Bremner WJ: Androgens in men—uses and abuses. N Engl J Med 1996;334:707.

Bagatell CJ et al: Effects of endogenous testosterone and estradiol on sexual behavior in normal young men. J Clin Endocrinol Metab 1993;78:711.

Bebb RA et al: Combined administration of levonorgestrel and testosterone induces more rapid and effective suppression of spermatogenesis than testosterone alone: A promising male contraceptive approach. J Clin Endocrinol Metab 1996;81:757.

Bhasin S: Androgen treatment of hypogonadal men. J Clin Endocrinol Metab 1993;74:1221.

Butler GE et al: Oral testosterone undecanoate in the management of delayed puberty in boys: Pharmacokinetics and effects on sexual maturation and growth. J Clin Endocrinol Metab 1992;75:37.

Cunningham GR, Cordero E, Thornby JI: Testosterone replacement with transdermal therapeutic systems: Physiologic serum testosterone and elevated dihydrotestosterone levels. JAMA 1989;261:2525.

Kopera H: The history of anabolic steroids and a review of clinical experience with anabolic steroids. Acta Endocrinol 1985;271(Suppl):11.

Malarkey WB et al: Endocrine effects in female weight lifters who self administer testosterone and anabolic steroids. Am J Obstet Gynecol 1991;165:1385.

Meikle W et al: Enhanced transdermal delivery of testosterone across nonscrotal skin produces physiologic concentrations of testosterone and its metabolites in hypogonadal men. J Clin Endocrinol Metab 1992;74:623.

Mooradian AD, Morley JD, Korenman SG: Biological action of androgens. Endocr Rev 1987;8:1.

Tenover JS: Effects of testosterone supplementation in the aging male. J Clin Endocrinol Metab 1992;75:1092.

Wilson JD: Androgen abuse by athletes. Endocr Rev 1988;9:181.

Young NR et al: Body composition and muscle strength in healthy men receiving T enanthate for contraception. J Clin Endocrinol Metab 1993;77:1028.

INHIBITORS

Bagdade JD et al: Effects of tamoxifen treatment on plasma lipids and lipoprotein lipid concentration. J Clin Endocrinol Metab 1990;70:1132.

Baulieu E-E: Contragestion and other clinical applications of RU 486, an antiprogesterone at the receptor. Science 1989;245:1351.

Dallob AL et al: The effect of finasteride, a 5α-reductase inhibitor, on scalp skin testosterone and dihydrotestosterone concentrations in patients with male pattern baldness. J Clin Endocrinol Metab 1994;79:703.

Flack MR et al: Oral gossypol in the treatment of metastatic adrenal cancer. J Clin Endocrinol Metab 1993;76:1019.

Fruzzetti F et al: Effects of finasteride, a 5α-reductase inhibitor, on circulating androgen and gonadotropin secretion in hirsute women. J Clin Endocrinol Metab 1994;79:811.

Glasier A et al: Mifepristone (RU 486) compared with high-dose estrogen and progestogen for emergency postcoital contraception. N Engl J Med 1992;327:1041.

Grey AB et al: The effect of the anti-estrogen tamoxifen on cardiovascular risk factors in normal postmenopausal women. J Clin Endocrinol Metab 1995;80:8192.

Hill NCW, Ferguson J, MacKenzie IZ: The efficacy of oral mifepristone (RU 38,486) with a prostaglandin E$_1$ analog vaginal pessary for the termination of early pregnancy: Complications and patient acceptability. Am J Obstet Gynecol 1990:162:414.

Lipton A et al: Letrozole (CGS 20267). A phase I study of a new potent oral aromatase inhibitor of breast cancer. Cancer 1995;75:2132.

Love RR et al: Effects of tamoxifen on bone mineral density in postmenopausal women with breast cancer. N Engl J Med 1992;326:852.

McConnell JD et al: Finasteride, an inhibitor of 5α-reductase, suppresses prostatic dihydrotestosterone in men with benign prostatic hyperplasia. J Clin Endocrinol Metab 1992;74:505.

Miller AA et al: Fadrozole hydrochloride in postmenopausal patients with metastatic breast carcinoma. Cancer 1996;78:789.

Moghetti P et al: Clinical and hormonal effects of the 5α-reductase inhibitor finasteride in idiopathic hirsutism. J Clin Endocrinol Metab 1994;79:1115.

Peyron R et al: Early termination of pregnancy with mifepristone (RU 486) and the orally active prostaglandin misoprostol. N Engl J Med 1993; 328:1509.

Price VH: Treatment of hair loss. N Engl J Med 1999;341:964.

Porat O: Effects of gossypol on the motility of mammalian sperm. Mol Reprod Devel 1990;25:400.

Rabinovici J et al: Endocrine effects and pharmacokinetic characteristics of a potent new gonadotropin-releasing hormone antagonist (Ganirelix) with minimal histamine-releasing properties: Studies in postmenopausal women. J Clin Endocrinol Metab 1992;75:1220.

Rittmaster RS: Finasteride. (Drug Therapy.) N Engl J Med 1993;330:120.

Sawaya ME, Hordinsky MK: The antiandrogens: When and how they should be used. Dermatol Ther 1993;11:65.

Sciarra F: Anti-estrogens and aromatase inhibitors: Tamoxifen and testolactone. J Endocrinol Invest 1988;11:755.

Silvestre L et al: Voluntary interruption of pregnancy with mifepristone (RU 486) and a prostaglandin analog: A large-scale French experience. N Engl J Med 1990;322:645.

Spitz IM, Bardin WC: Mifepristone (RU-486)—A modulator of progestin and glucocorticoid action. N Engl J Med 1993;329:404.

Zilembo N et al: Formestane: An effective first-line endocrine treatment for advanced breast cancer. J Cancer Res Clin Oncol 1995;121:378.

Pancreatic Hormones & Antidiabetic Drugs

41

Martha S. Nolte, MD, & John H. Karam, MD*

THE ENDOCRINE PANCREAS

The endocrine pancreas in the adult human consists of approximately 1 million islets of Langerhans interspersed throughout the pancreatic gland. Within the islets, at least four hormone-producing cells are present (Table 41–1). Their hormone products include **insulin,** the storage and anabolic hormone of the body; **islet amyloid polypeptide (IAPP, or amylin),** whose metabolic function remains undefined; **glucagon,** the hyperglycemic factor that mobilizes glycogen stores; **somatostatin,** a universal inhibitor of secretory cells; and **pancreatic peptide,** a small protein that facilitates digestive processes by a mechanism not yet clarified.

The elevated blood glucose associated with diabetes mellitus results from absent or inadequate pancreatic insulin secretion, with or without concurrent impairment of insulin action. The disease states underlying the diagnosis of diabetes mellitus are now classified into four categories: type 1, "insulin-dependent diabetes," type 2, "noninsulin-dependent diabetes," type 3, "other," and type 4, "gestational diabetes mellitus" (Expert Committee 2002, Mayfield, 1998).

Type 1 Diabetes Mellitus

The hallmark of type 1 diabetes is selective B cell destruction and severe or absolute insulin deficiency. Administration of insulin is essential in patients with type 1 diabetes. Type 1 diabetes is further subdivided into immune and idiopathic causes. The immune form is the most common form of type 1 diabetes. In the USA, this form is diagnosed in approximately 1,500,000 individuals. Although most patients are younger than 30 years of age at the time of diagnosis, the onset can occur at any age. Type 1 diabetes is found in all ethnic groups, but the highest incidence is in people from northern Europe and from Sardinia. Susceptibility appears to involve a multifactorial genetic linkage but only 15–20% of patients have a positive family history.

Type 2 Diabetes Mellitus

Type 2 diabetes is characterized by tissue resistance to the action of insulin combined with a relative deficiency in insulin secretion. A given individual may have more resistance or more B cell deficiency, and the abnormalities may be mild or severe. Although insulin is produced by the B cells in these patients, it is inadequate to overcome the resistance, and the blood glucose rises. The impaired insulin action also affects fat metabolism, resulting in increased free fatty acid flux and triglyceride levels, and reciprocally low high-density lipoprotein (HDL) levels.

Individuals with type 2 diabetes may not require insulin to survive, but 30% or more will benefit from insulin therapy to control the blood glucose. It is likely that 10–20% of individuals in whom type 2 diabetes was initially diagnosed actually have both type 1 and type 2, or have a slowly progressing type 1, and ultimately will require full insulin replacement. Although persons with type 2 diabetes ordinarily will not develop ketosis, ketoacidosis may occur as the result of stress such as infection or use of medication that enhances resistance, eg, corticosteroids. Dehydration in untreated and poorly controlled individuals with type 2 diabetes can lead to a life-threatening condition called "nonketotic hyperosmolar coma". In this condition, the blood glucose may rise to 6–20 times the normal range and an altered mental state develops or the person loses consciousness. Urgent medical care and rehydration is required.

Type 3 Diabetes Mellitus

The type 3 designation refers to multiple **other** specific causes of an elevated blood glucose: nonpancreatic diseases, drug therapy, etc. For a complete, detailed list the

* Deceased.

693

Table 41–1. Pancreatic islet cells and their secretory products.

Cell Types	Approximate Percent of Islet Mass	Secretory Products
A cell (alpha)	20	Glucagon, proglucagon
B cell (beta)	75	Insulin, C-peptide, proinsulin, islet amyloid polypeptide (IAPP)
D cell (delta)	3–5	Somatostatin
F cell (PP cell)[1]	< 2	Pancreatic polypeptide (PP)

[1]Within pancreatic polypeptide-rich lobules of adult islets, located only in the posterior portion of the head of the human pancreas, glucagon cells are scarce (< 0.5%) and F cells make up as much as 80% of the cells.

reader is referred to Expert Committee, 2002 or Mayfield, 1998.

Type 4 Diabetes Mellitus

Gestational Diabetes (GDM) is defined as any abnormality in glucose levels noted for the first time during pregnancy. Gestational diabetes is diagnosed in approximately 4% of all pregnancies in the USA. During pregnancy, the placenta and placental hormones create an insulin resistance that is most pronounced in the last trimester. Risk assessment for diabetes is suggested starting at the first prenatal visit. High risk individuals should be screened immediately. Screening may be deferred in lower risk women until the 24th to 28th week of gestation.

INSULIN

Chemistry

Insulin is a small protein with a molecular weight in humans of 5808. It contains 51 amino acids arranged in two chains (A and B) linked by disulfide bridges; there are species differences in the amino acids of both chains. Proinsulin, a long single-chain protein molecule, is processed within the Golgi apparatus and packaged into granules, where it is hydrolyzed into insulin and a residual connecting segment called C-peptide by removal of four amino acids (shown in dashed circles in Figure 41–1).

Insulin and C-peptide are secreted in equimolar amounts in response to all insulin secretagogues; a small quantity of unprocessed or partially hydrolyzed proinsulin is released as well. While proinsulin may have some mild hypoglycemic action, C-peptide has no known physiologic function. Granules within the B cells store the insulin in the form of crystals consisting of two atoms of zinc and six molecules of insulin. The entire human pancreas contains up to 8 mg of insulin, representing approximately 200 biologic units. Originally, the unit was defined on the basis of the hypoglycemic activity of insulin in rabbits. With improved purification techniques, the unit is presently defined on the basis of weight, and present insulin standards used for assay purposes contain 28 units per milligram.

Insulin Secretion

Insulin is released from pancreatic B cells at a low basal rate and at a much higher stimulated rate in response to a variety of stimuli, especially glucose. Other stimulants such as other sugars (eg, mannose), certain amino acids (eg, leucine, arginine), and vagal activity are recognized. One mechanism of stimulated insulin release is diagrammed in Figure 41–2. As shown in the figure, hyperglycemia results in increased intracellular ATP levels, which close the ATP-dependent potassium channels. Decreased outward potassium efflux results in depolarization of the B cell and opening of voltage-gated calcium channels. The resulting increased intracellular calcium triggers secretion of the hormone. As noted below, the insulin secretagogue drug group (sulfonylureas, meglitinides, and D-phenylalanine) exploits parts of this mechanism.

Insulin Degradation

The liver and kidney are the two main organs that remove insulin from the circulation. The liver normally clears the blood of approximately 60% of the insulin released from the pancreas by virtue of its location as the terminal site of portal vein blood flow, with the kidney removing 35–40% of the endogenous hormone. However, in insulin-treated diabetics receiving subcutaneous insulin injections, this ratio is reversed, with as much as 60% of exogenous insulin being cleared by the kidney and the liver removing no more than 30–40%. The half-life of circulating insulin is 3–5 minutes.

Measurement of Circulating Insulin

The radioimmunoassay of insulin permits detection of insulin in picomolar quantities. The assay is based on antibodies developed in guinea pigs against bovine or pork insulin. Because of the similarities between these

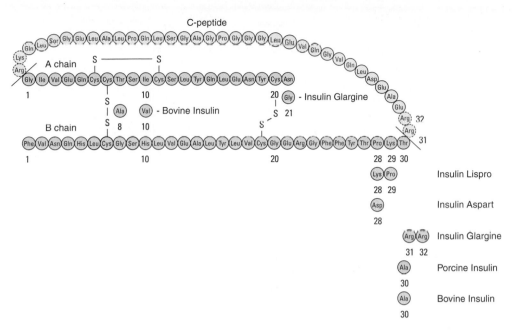

Figure 41–1. Structure of human proinsulin and commercially available insulin analogs. Insulin is shown as the shaded (darker color) peptide chains, A and B. Species differences in the A and B chains and amino acid modifications for insulin aspart, lispro, and glargine are noted.

two insulins and human insulin, the assay successfully measures the human hormone as well.

With this assay, basal insulin values of 5–15 μU/mL (30–90 pmol/L) are found in normal humans, with a peak rise to 60–90 μU/mL (360–540 pmol/L) during meals. Similar assays for measuring all of the known hormones of the endocrine pancreas (including C-peptide and proinsulin) have been developed.

The Insulin Receptor

Once insulin has entered the circulation, it is bound by specialized receptors that are found on the membranes of most tissues. The biologic responses promoted by these insulin-receptor complexes have been identified in the primary target tissues, ie, liver, muscle, and adipose tissue. The receptors bind insulin with high specificity and affinity in the picomolar range. The full insulin receptor consists of two covalently linked heterodimers, each containing an α subunit, which is entirely extracellular and constitutes the recognition site, and a β subunit that spans the membrane (Figure 41–3). The β subunit contains a tyrosine kinase. The binding of an insulin molecule to the α subunits at the outside surface of the cell activates the receptor and through a confor-

mational change brings the catalytic loops of the opposing cytoplasmic β subunits into closer proximity thereby facilitating phosphorylation of tyrosine residues and tyrosine kinase activity.

The first proteins to be phosphorylated by the activated receptor tyrosine kinases are the docking proteins, insulin receptor substrate-1 and -2 (IRS-1, IRS-2). After tyrosine phosphorylation at several critical sites, IRS-1 and IRS-2 bind to and activate other kinases—most importantly phosphatidylinositol-3-kinase—that produce further phosphorylations or to an adaptor protein such as growth factor receptor-binding protein 2 that translates the insulin signal to a guanine nucleotide-releasing factor that ultimately activates the GTP binding protein ras, and the mitogen activated protein kinase (MAPK) system. The particular IRS-phosphorylated tyrosine kinases have binding specificity with downstream molecules based on their surrounding 4–5 amino acid sequences or motifs that recognize specific Src homology 2 (SH2) domains on the other protein. This network of phosphorylations within the cell represents insulin's second message and results in multiple effects including translocation of glucose transporters (especially GLUT-4, Table 41–2) to the cell membrane with a resultant increase in glucose uptake; glycogen

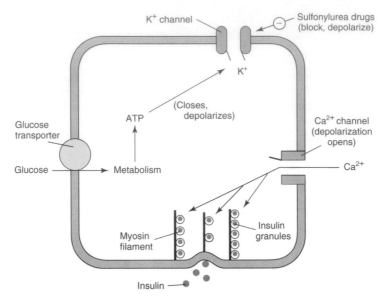

Figure 41–2. One model of control of insulin release from the pancreatic B cell by glucose and by sulfonylurea drugs. In the resting cell with normal (low) ATP levels, potassium diffuses down its concentration gradient through ATP-gated potassium channels, maintaining the intracellular potential at a fully polarized, negative level. Insulin release is minimal. If glucose concentration rises, ATP production increases, potassium channels close, and depolarization of the cell results. As in muscle and nerve, voltage-gated calcium channels open in response to depolarization, allowing more calcium to enter the cell. Increased intracellular calcium results in increased insulin secretion. Insulin secretagogues close the ATP-dependent potassium channel, thereby depolarizing the membrane and causing increased insulin release by the same mechanism. (Modified and reproduced, with permission, from *Basic & Clinical Endocrinology,* 4th ed. Greenspan F, Baxter JD [editors]. Originally published by Appleton & Lange. Copyright © 1994 by The McGraw-Hill Companies, Inc.)

synthase activity and increased glycogen formation; multiple effects on protein synthesis, lipolysis, and lipogenesis; and activation of transcription factors that enhance DNA synthesis and cell growth and division.

Various hormonal agents (eg, glucocorticoids) lower the affinity of insulin receptors for insulin; growth hormone in excess increases this affinity slightly. Aberrant serine and threonine phosphorylation of the insulin receptor β subunits or IRS molecules may result in insulin resistance and functional receptor down-regulation.

Effects of Insulin on Its Targets

Insulin promotes the storage of fat as well as glucose (both sources of energy) within specialized target cells (Figure 41–4) and influences cell growth and the metabolic functions of a wide variety of tissues (Table 41–3).

Characteristics of Available Insulin Preparations

Commercial insulin preparations differ in a number of ways, including differences in the recombinant DNA production techniques, amino acid sequence, concen-

tration, solubility, and the time of onset and duration of their biologic action. In 2003, seventeen insulin formulations were available in the USA.

A. PRINCIPAL TYPES AND DURATION OF ACTION OF INSULIN PREPARATIONS

Four principal types of insulins are available: (1) rapid-acting, with very fast onset and short duration; (2) short-acting, with rapid onset of action; (3) intermediate-acting; and (4) long-acting, with slow onset of action (Figure 41–5, Table 41–4). Rapid-acting and short-acting insulins are dispensed as clear solutions at neutral pH and contain small amounts of zinc to improve their stability and shelf-life. All other commercial insulins have been modified to provide prolonged action and are, with the exception of insulin glargine, dispensed as turbid suspensions at neutral pH with either protamine in phosphate buffer (neutral protamine Hagedorn [NPH] insulin) or varying concentrations of zinc in acetate buffer (ultralente and lente insulins). Insulin glargine is the only soluble long-acting insulin. The goal of subcutaneous insulin therapy is to replace the normal basal (overnight, fasting, and between meal) as well as prandial

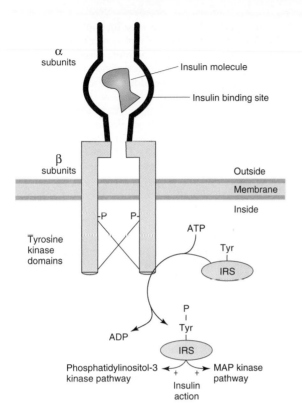

Figure 41–3. Schematic diagram of the insulin receptor heterodimer in the activated state. IRS, insulin receptor substrate; tyr, tyrosine; P, phosphate.

Table 41–2. Glucose transporters.

Transporter	Tissues	Glucose K_m (mmol/L)	Function
GLUT 1	All tissues, especially red cells, brain	1–2	Basal uptake of glucose; transport across the blood-brain barrier
GLUT 2	B cells of pancreas; liver, kidney; gut	15–20	Regulation of insulin release, other aspects of glucose homeostasis
GLUT 3	Brain, kidney, placenta, other tissues	< 1	Uptake into neurons, other tissues
GLUT 4	Muscle, adipose	≈ 5	Insulin-mediated uptake of glucose
GLUT 5	Gut, kidney	1–2	Absorption of fructose

(mealtime) insulin. Current regimens generally use intermediate- or long-acting insulins to provide basal or background coverage, and rapid-acting or short-acting insulin to meet the mealtime requirements. The latter insulins are given as supplemental doses to correct high blood sugars. Intensive therapy ("tight control") attempts to restore near-normal glucose patterns throughout the day while minimizing the risk of hypoglycemia. An exact reproduction of the normal glycemic profile is technically not possible because of the limitations inherent in subcutaneous administration of insulin. The most sophisticated insulin regimen delivers rapid-acting insulin through a continuous subcutaneous insulin infusion device; alternative intensive regimens referred to as multiple daily injections (MDI) use long-acting or intermediate-acting insulins with multiple boluses of rapid-acting or short-acting insulin. Conventional therapy presently consists of split-dose injections of mixtures of rapid- or short-acting and intermediate-acting insulins.

1. Rapid-acting insulin—Two rapid-acting insulin analogs are commercially available: **insulin lispro** and

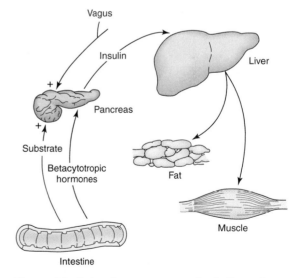

Figure 41–4. Insulin promotes synthesis (from circulating nutrients) and storage of glycogen, triglycerides, and protein in its major target tissues: liver, fat, and muscle. The release of insulin from the pancreas is stimulated by increased blood glucose, vagal nerve stimulation, and other factors (see text).

Table 41–3. Endocrine effects of insulin.

Effect on liver:
Reversal of catabolic features of insulin deficiency
  Inhibits glycogenolysis
  Inhibits conversion of fatty acids and amino acids to
    keto acids
  Inhibits conversion of amino acids to glucose
Anabolic action
  Promotes glucose storage as glycogen (induces
    glucokinase and glycogen synthase, inhibits
    phosphorylase)
  Increases triglyceride synthesis and very low density
    lipoprotein formation

Effect on muscle:
Increased protein synthesis
  Increases amino acid transport
  Increases ribosomal protein synthesis
Increased glycogen synthesis
  Increases glucose transport
  Induces glycogen synthase and inhibits phosphorylase

Effect on adipose tissue:
Increased triglyceride storage
  Lipoprotein lipase is induced and activated by insulin to
    hydrolyze triglycerides from lipoproteins
  Glucose transport into cell provides glycerol phosphate
    to permit esterification of fatty acids supplied by
    lipoprotein transport
  Intracellular lipase is inhibited by insulin

insulin aspart. The rapid-acting insulins permit more physiologic prandial insulin replacement because their rapid onset and early peak action more closely mimics normal endogenous prandial insulin secretion than does regular insulin, and they have the additional benefit of allowing insulin to be taken immediately before the meal without sacrificing glucose control. Their duration of action is rarely more than 3–5 hours, which decreases the risk of late postmeal hypoglycemia. They have the lowest variability of absorption of all available insulin formulations.

Insulin lispro, the first monomeric insulin analog to be marketed, is produced by recombinant technology wherein two amino acids near the carboxyl terminal of the B chain have been reversed in position: proline at position B28 has been moved to B29 and lysine at position B29 has been moved to B28 (Figure 41–1). Reversing these two amino acids does not interfere in any way with insulin lispro's binding to the insulin receptor, its circulating half-life, or with its immunogenicity, all of which are identical with those of human regular insulin. However, the advantage of this analog is its very low propensity—in contrast to human insulin—to self-associate in antiparallel fashion and form dimers. To enhance the shelf-life of insulin in vials, insulin lispro is stabilized into hexamers by a cresol preservative. When injected subcutaneously, the drug quickly dissociates into monomers and is rapidly absorbed with onset of action within 5–15 minutes, and reaching peak activity as early as 1 hour. The time to peak action is relatively constant, regardless of the dose. Its duration is seldom more than 3–5 hours.

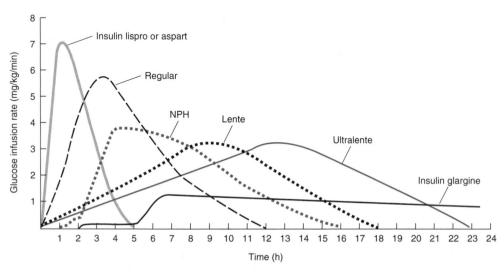

Figure 41–5. Extent and duration of action of various types of insulin as indicated by the glucose infusion rates (mg/kg/min) required to maintain a constant glucose concentration. The durations of action shown are typical of an average dose of 0.2–0.3 U/kg; with the exception of insulin lispro and insulin aspart, duration increases considerably when dosage is increased.

Table 41–4. Some insulin preparations available in the USA.[1,2]

Preparation	Species Source	Concentration
Rapid-acting insulins		
Insulin lispro, Humalog (Lilly)	Human analog	U100
Insulin Aspart, Novolog (Novo Nordisk)	Human analog	U100
Short-acting insulins		
Regular (Novo Nordisk)[3]	Human	U100
Regular Humulin (Lilly)	Human	U100, U500
Velosulin BR (Novo Nordisk)[4]	Human	U100
Intermediate-acting insulins		
Lente Humulin (Lilly)	Human	U100
Lente (Novo Nordisk)	Human	U100
NPH Humulin (Lilly)	Human	U100
NPH (Novo Nordisk)	Human	U100
Premixed insulins (% NPH, % regular)		
Novolin 70/30 (Novo Nordisk)	Human	U100
Humulin 70/30 and 50/50 (Lilly)	Human	U100
Premixed (% NP-analog, % rapid acting analog)	Human analog	U100
50/50 NPL, Lispro (Lilly)	Human analog	U100
75/25 NPL, Lispro (Lilly)	Human analog	U100
70/30 NPA, Aspart (NovoNordisk)	Human analog	U100
Long-acting insulins		
Ultralente Humulin U (Lilly)	Human	U100
Insulin glargine-lantus (Aventis/Hoechst Marion Roussel)	Human	U100

[1] Modified and reproduced, with permission, from Katzung BG (editor): *Drug Therapy,* 2nd ed. Originally published by Appleton & Lange. Copyright © 1991 by The McGraw-Hill Companies, Inc.

[2] All of these agents (except insulin lispro, insulin aspart, insulin glargine, and U500 regular Humulin) are available without a prescription. All insulins should be refrigerated and brought to room temperature just before injection.

[3] Novo Nordisk human insulins are termed Novolin R, L, and N.

[4] Velosulin contains phosphate buffer, which favors its use to prevent insulin aggregation in pump tubing but precludes its being mixed with lente insulin.

Insulin lispro has a low variability of absorption (5%) of all the commercial insulin preparations—compared with 25% for regular insulin and 25–50% or more for intermediate-acting and long-acting insulins. Although not specifically approved for use in continuous subcutaneous insulin infusion (CSII) pumps, when used in these devices or in intensive insulin regimens, insulin lispro is associated with significantly improved glycemic control compared with regular insulin, without increased incidence of hypoglycemia.

Insulin aspart is created by the substitution of the B28 proline with a negatively charged aspartic acid (Figure 41–1). This modification reduces the normal ProB28 and GlyB23 monomer-monomer interaction, thereby inhibiting insulin self-aggregation. Insulin aspart rapidly breaks into monomers after subcutaneous injection, displays an onset of action within 10–20 minutes, and exerts a peak effect within 1 hour, with an average duration of action of no longer than 3–5 hours. Its absorption and activity profile is similar to insulin lispro and more reproducible than regular insulin, but it has similar binding, activity, and mitogenicity characteristics to regular insulin and equivalent immunogenicity. Insulin aspart is approved for subcutaneous administration by injection as well as through CSII devices.

2. Short-acting insulin—Regular insulin is a short-acting soluble crystalline zinc insulin made by recombinant DNA techniques to produce a molecule identical to human insulin. Its effect appears within 30 minutes and peaks between 2 and 3 hours after subcutaneous injection and generally lasts 5–8 hours. In high concentrations, eg, in the vial, regular insulin molecules self-aggregate in antiparallel fashion to form dimers that stabilize around zinc ions to create insulin hexamers. The hexameric nature of regular insulin causes a delayed onset and prolongs the time to peak action. After subcutaneous injection, the insulin hexamers are too large and bulky to be transported across the vascular endothelium into the bloodstream. As the insulin depot is diluted by interstitial fluid and the concentration begins to fall, the hexamers break down into dimers and finally monomers. This results in three different rates of absorption of the injected insulin, with the final monomeric phase having the fastest uptake out of the injection site. As with all older insulin formulations, the duration of action as well as the time of onset and the intensity of peak action increase with the size of the dose. Clinically, this is a critical issue because the pharmacokinetics and pharmacodynamics of small doses of regular, NPH, lente, and ultralente, insulins differ greatly from those of large doses. Short-acting soluble insulin is the only type that should be administered intravenously as the dilution causes the hexameric insulin to immediately dissociate into monomers. It is particularly useful for intravenous therapy in the management of diabetic ketoacidosis and when the insulin requirement is changing rapidly, such as after surgery or during acute infections.

3. Intermediate-acting and long-acting insulins—

a. Lente insulin—Lente insulin is a mixture of 30% semilente (an amorphous precipitate of insulin with zinc ions in acetate buffer that has a relatively rapid onset of action) with 70% ultralente insulin (a poorly soluble crystal of zinc insulin that has a delayed onset and prolonged duration of action). These two components provide a combination of relatively rapid absorption with sustained long action, making lente insulin a useful therapeutic agent. As with regular insulin, the time of onset, time to peak, and duration of action are dose-dependent.

b. NPH (neutral protamine Hagedorn, or isophane) insulin—NPH insulin is an intermediate-acting insulin wherein absorption and the onset of action is delayed by combining appropriate amounts of insulin and protamine so that neither is present in an uncomplexed form ("isophane"). Protamine is a mixture of six major and some minor compounds of similar structure isolated from the sperm of rainbow trout. They appear to be basic, arginine-rich peptides with an average molecular weight of approximately 4400. To form an isophane complex (one in which neither component retains any free binding sites), approximately a 1:10 ratio by weight of protamine to insulin is required, representing approximately six molecules of insulin per molecule of protamine. After subcutaneous injection, proteolytic tissue enzymes degrade the protamine to permit absorption of insulin.

The onset and duration of action of NPH insulin are similar to those of lente insulin (Figure 41–5); it is usually mixed with regular, lispro, or aspart insulin and given two to four times daily for insulin replacement in patients with type 1 diabetes. The dose regulates the action profile, specifically, small doses have lower, earlier peaks and a short duration of action with the converse true for large doses.

c. Ultralente insulin—There has recently been a resurgence in the use of ultralente insulin, in combination with multiple injections of rapid-acting insulin, as a means of attempting optimal control in patients with type 1 diabetes. Human insulin (Humulin U [Lilly]) is the only ultralente insulin available in the USA. In contrast to the older animal insulin–based formulations, human ultralente has a shorter duration of action and more pronounced peak effect. To create a smoother background insulin profile and minimize the peak effect, it is recommended that the daily dose of human ultralente be split into two or more doses. This is especially needed in patients with type 1 diabetes to achieve basal insulin levels throughout the 24 hours that are more comparable to those achieved in normal subjects by basal endogenous secretion or by the overnight infusion rate programmed into insulin pumps.

d. Insulin glargine—Insulin glargine is a soluble, "peakless" (ie, having a broad plasma concentration plateau), ultra-long-acting insulin analog. This product was designed to provide reproducible, convenient, background insulin replacement. The attachment of two arginine molecules to the B chain carboxyl terminal and substitution of a glycine for asparagine at the A21 position created an analog that is soluble in solution but precipitates in the more neutral body pH after subcutaneous injection. Individual insulin molecules slowly dissolve away from the crystalline depot and provide a low, continuous level of circulating insulin. Insulin glargine has a slow onset of action (1–1.5 hours) and achieves a maximum effect after 4–5 hours. This maximum activity is maintained for 11–24 hours or longer. Glargine is usually given once daily, although some very insulin-sensitive individuals will benefit from split (twice a day) dosing. To maintain solubility, the formulation is unusually acidic (pH 4.0) and insulin glargine should not be mixed with other insulin. Separate syringes must be used to minimize the risk of contamination and subsequent loss of efficacy. The absorption pattern of insulin glargine appears to be independent of the anatomic site of injection, and this drug is associated with less immunogenicity than human insulin in animal studies. Glargine's interaction with the insulin receptor is similar to that of native insulin and shows no increase in mitogenic activity in vitro. It has sixfold to sevenfold greater binding than native insulin to the IGF1 receptor, but the clinical significance of this is unclear.

4. Mixtures of insulins—Since intermediate-acting insulins require several hours to reach adequate therapeutic levels, their use in type 1 diabetic patients requires supplements of lispro, aspart, or regular insulin before meals. For convenience, these are often mixed together in the same syringe before injection. When regular insulin is used, NPH is preferred to lente insulin as the intermediate-acting component in these mixtures because increased proportions of lente to regular insulin may retard the rapid action of admixed regular insulin, particularly if not injected immediately after mixing. This is due to precipitation of the regular insulin by excess zinc. Premixed formulations of 70%/30% NPH and regular and 50%/50% NPH and regular are available in the USA. Insulin lispro and aspart can be *acutely* mixed (ie, just before injection) with either NPH, lente, or ultralente insulin without affecting their rapid absorption. However, *premixed* preparations have thus far been unstable. To remedy this, intermediate insulins composed of isophane complexes of protamine with insulin lispro and insulin aspart have been developed. These intermediate insulins have been designated as "NPL" (neutral protamine lispro) and "NPA" (neutral protamine aspart) and have the same duration of action as NPH insulin. They have the advantage of permitting formulation as premixed combinations of NPL and insulin lispro, and NPA and insulin aspart and they have been shown to be safe and effective in clinical trials. The FDA has approved 50%/50% and 75%/30% NPL/insulin lispro and a 70%/30% NPA/insulin aspart premixed formulations. Additional ratios are available abroad. Insulin glargine must be given as a separate injection. It is not miscible acutely or in a premixed preparation with any other insulin formulation.

B. Species of Insulin

1. Beef and pork insulins—Historically, commercial insulin in the USA contained beef or pork insulin. Beef insulin differs by three amino acids from human insulin, whereas only a single amino acid distinguishes pork and human insulins (Figure 41–1). The beef hormone is slightly more antigenic than pork insulin in humans. Of the insulins manufactured from animal sources, only purified pork insulin is still available and it requires special ordering.

Human insulin, which is now less expensive than monospecies pork insulin and is also less immunogenic, has supplanted purified pork insulins.

2. Human insulins—Mass production of human insulin by recombinant DNA techniques is now carried out by inserting the human proinsulin gene into *Escherichia coli* or yeast and treating the extracted proinsulin to form the human insulin molecule.

Human insulin from *E coli* is available for clinical use as Humulin (Lilly) and dispensed as either regular, NPH, lente, or ultralente Humulin. Human insulin prepared biosynthetically in yeast is marketed by Novo Nordisk as human insulin injection in regular, lente, and NPH forms: Novolin R, Monotard Human Insulin (Novolin L), and Novolin N. The same company also produces a human insulin marketed as Velosulin (regular) that contains a phosphate buffer. This reduces aggregation of regular insulin molecules when used in infusion pumps. However, because of the tendency of phosphate to precipitate zinc ions, Velosulin should not be mixed with any of the lente insulins.

Human insulins appear to be as effective as—and considerably less immunogenic in diabetic patients than—beef-pork insulin mixtures and slightly less immunogenic than pork insulin.

C. Concentration

Currently, all insulins in the USA and Canada are available in a concentration of 100 U/mL (U100) and are dispensed in 10 mL vials. A limited supply of U500 regular human insulin is available for use in rare cases of severe insulin resistance in which larger doses of insulin are required.

Insulin Delivery Systems

The standard mode of insulin therapy is subcutaneous injection using conventional disposable needles and syringes. During the last 3 decades, much effort has gone into exploration of other means of administration.

A. Portable Pen Injectors

To facilitate multiple subcutaneous injections of insulin, particularly during intensive insulin therapy, portable pen-sized injectors have been developed. These contain cartridges of insulin and replaceable needles. Disposable insulin pens are also available for selected formulations. These include regular insulin, insulin lispro, insulin aspart, NPH insulin, and premixed 70%/30% and 50%/50% NPH/regular, 75% NPL/25% lispro, 50% NPL/50% lispro, and 70% NPA/30% aspart insulin. They have been well accepted by patients because they eliminate the need to carry syringes and bottles of insulin to the workplace and while traveling.

B. Continuous Subcutaneous Insulin Infusion Devices (CSII, Insulin Pumps)

Continuous subcutaneous insulin infusion devices are external open-loop pumps for insulin delivery. The devices have a user-programmable pump that delivers individualized basal and bolus insulin replacement doses based on blood glucose self-monitoring results. Normally, the 24-hour background basal rates are relatively constant from day to day, although temporarily altered rates can be superimposed to adjust for a short-term change in requirement. For example, the basal delivery rate might need to be decreased for several hours because of the increased insulin sensitivity associated with strenuous activity. In contrast, the bolus amounts frequently vary and are used to correct high blood glucose levels and to cover mealtime insulin requirements based on the carbohydrate content of the food and concurrent activity. The pump—which contains an insulin reservoir, the program chip, the keypad, and the display screen—is about the size of a pager. It is usually placed on a belt or in a pocket, and the insulin is infused through thin plastic tubing that is connected to the subcutaneously inserted infusion set. The abdomen is the favored site for the infusion set, although flanks and thighs are also used. The insulin reservoir, tubing, and infusion set need to be changed using sterile techniques every 2 or 3 days. CSII delivery is regarded as the most physiologic method of insulin replacement.

The use of these devices is encouraged for individuals who are unable to obtain target control while on multiple injection regimens and in circumstances where excellent glycemic control is desired, such as during pregnancy. Their optimal use requires responsible involvement and commitment by the patient. Velosulin (a regular insulin) and insulin aspart are the only insulins specifically approved for pump use. Although not formally approved for pump use, insulin lispro has been successfully delivered through CSII devices since it became commercially available. Insulins aspart and lispro are preferred pump insulins because their favorable pharmacokinetic attributes allow glycemic control without increasing the risk of hypoglycemia.

C. Inhaled Insulin

Clinical trials are in progress to evaluate the safety and efficacy of finely powdered and aerosolized insulin formulations delivered by inhalation. Insulin is readily absorbed into the bloodstream through alveolar walls, but the challenge has been to create particles that are small enough to pass through the bronchial tree without being trapped and still enter the alveoli in sufficient amounts to have a clinical effect. Insulin delivered by the inhaled route should have a rapid onset and a relatively short duration of action and could be used to cover mealtime insulin requirements or to correct high glucose levels, but not to provide background or basal insulin coverage. Safety concerns regarding pulmonary fibrosis or hypertension and excessive antibody formation may preclude or delay approval.

Treatment With Insulin

The current classification of diabetes mellitus identifies a group of patients who have virtually no insulin secretion and whose survival depends on administration of exogenous insulin. This insulin-dependent group (type 1) represents 5–10% of the diabetic population in the USA. Most type 2 diabetics do not require exogenous insulin for survival, but many need exogenous supplementation of their endogenous secretion to achieve optimum health. It is estimated that as many as 20% of type 2 diabetics in the USA (2–2.5 million people) are presently taking insulin.

Benefit of Glycemic Control in Diabetes Mellitus

The consensus of the American Diabetes Association is that intensive insulin therapy associated with comprehensive self-management training should become standard therapy in most type 1 patients after puberty (see Box, Benefits of Tight Glycemic Control in Type 1 Diabetes). Exceptions include patients with advanced renal disease and the elderly, since the risks of hypoglycemia outweigh the benefit of tight glycemic control in these groups. In children under the age of 7 years, the extreme susceptibility of the developing brain to damage from hypoglycemia contraindicates attempts at intensive glycemic control, particularly since diabetic complications do not seem to occur until some years after the onset of puberty. A similar conclusion regarding the benefits of tight control in type 2 diabetes was reached as the result of a large study in the United Kingdom.

Complications of Insulin Therapy

A. Hypoglycemia

1. Mechanisms and diagnosis—Hypoglycemic reactions are the most common complication of insulin therapy. They may result from a delay in taking a meal, inadequate carbohydrate consumed, unusual physical exertion, or a dose of insulin that is too large for immediate needs.

Rapid development of hypoglycemia in individuals with intact hypoglycemic awareness causes signs of autonomic hyperactivity, both sympathetic (tachycardia, palpitations, sweating, tremulousness) and

BENEFITS OF TIGHT GLYCEMIC CONTROL IN DIABETES

A long-term randomized prospective study involving 1441 type 1 patients in 29 medical centers reported in 1993 that "near normalization" of blood glucose resulted in a delay in onset and a major slowing of progression of microvascular and neuropathic complications of diabetes during follow-up periods of up to 10 years (Diabetes Control and Complications Trial [DCCT] Research Group, 1993).

In the intensively treated group a mean glycated hemoglobin of 7.2% (normal, < 6%) and a mean blood glucose of 155 mg/dL were achieved, while in the conventionally treated group, glycated hemoglobin averaged 8.9% with an average blood glucose of 225 mg/dL. Over the study period, which averaged 7 years, there was an approximately 60% reduction in risk in the tight control group compared with the standard control group with regard to diabetic retinopathy, nephropathy, and neuropathy.

The United Kingdom Prospective Diabetes Study (UKPDS) was a very large randomized prospective study carried out to study the effects of intensive glycemic control with several types of therapies and the effects of blood pressure control in type 2 diabetic patients. A total of 3867 newly diagnosed type 2 diabetic patients were studied over 10 years. A significant fraction of these were overweight and hypertensive. Patients were given dietary treatment alone or intensive therapy with insulin, chlorpropamide, glyburide, or glipizide. Metformin was an option for patients with inadequate response to other therapies. Tight control of blood pressure was added as a variable, with an angiotensin-converting enzyme inhibitor, β-blocker or, in some cases, a calcium channel blocker available for this purpose.

Tight control of diabetes, with reduction of HbA_{1c} from 9.1% to 7%, was shown to reduce the risk of microvascular complications overall compared with conventional therapy (mostly diet alone, which decreased HbA_{1c} to 7.9%). Cardiovascular complications were not noted for any particular therapy; metformin treatment alone reduced the risk of macrovascular disease (myocardial infarction, stroke).

Tight control of hypertension also had a surprisingly significant effect on microvascular disease (as well as more conventional hypertension-related sequela) in these diabetic patients. These studies show that tight glycemic control benefits both type 1 and type 2 patients.

---

parasympathetic (nausea, hunger) and may progress to convulsions and coma if untreated.

In individuals exposed to frequent hypoglycemic episodes during tight glycemic control, autonomic warning signals of hypoglycemia are less frequent or even absent. This dangerous acquired condition is termed "hypoglycemic unawareness." When patients lack the early warning signs of low blood glucose, they may not take corrective measures in time. In patients with persistent, untreated hypoglycemia, the manifestations of insulin excess may develop—confusion, weakness, bizarre behavior, coma, seizures—at which point they may not be able to procure or safely swallow glucose-containing foods. Hypoglycemic awareness may be restored by preventing frequent hypoglycemic episodes. An identification bracelet, necklace, or card in the wallet or purse, as well as some form of rapidly absorbed glucose, should be carried by every diabetic who is receiving hypoglycemic drug therapy.

2. Treatment of hypoglycemia—All of the manifestations of hypoglycemia are relieved by glucose administration. To expedite absorption, simple sugar or glucose should be given, preferably in a liquid form. To treat mild hypoglycemia in a patient who is conscious and able to swallow, orange juice, glucose gel, or any sugar-containing beverage or food may be given. If more severe hypoglycemia has produced unconsciousness or stupor, the treatment of choice is to give 20–50 mL of 50% glucose solution by intravenous infusion over a period of 2–3 minutes. If intravenous therapy is not available, 1 mg of glucagon injected either subcutaneously or intramuscularly will usually restore consciousness within 15 minutes to permit ingestion of sugar. If the patient is stuporous and glucagon is not available, small amounts of honey or syrup can be inserted into the buccal pouch. In general, however, oral feeding is contraindicated in unconscious patients. Emergency medical services should be called for all episodes of severely impaired consciousness.

B. IMMUNOPATHOLOGY OF INSULIN THERAPY

At least five molecular classes of insulin antibodies may be produced during the course of insulin therapy in diabetes: IgA, IgD, IgE, IgG, and IgM. There are two major types of immune disorders in these patients:

1. Insulin allergy—Insulin allergy, an immediate type hypersensitivity, is a rare condition in which local or systemic urticaria results from histamine release from tissue mast cells sensitized by anti-insulin IgE antibodies. In severe cases, anaphylaxis results. Because sensitivity is often to noninsulin protein contaminants, the highly purified and human insulins have markedly reduced the incidence of insulin allergy, especially local reactions.

2. Immune insulin resistance—A low titer of circulating IgG anti-insulin antibodies that neutralize the action of insulin to a negligable extent develops in most insulin-treated patients. Rarely, the titer of insulin antibodies will lead to insulin resistance and may be associated with other systemic autoimmune processes such as lupus erythematosus.

C. LIPODYSTROPHY AT INJECTION SITES

Injection of older insulin preparations sometimes led to atrophy of subcutaneous fatty tissue at the site of injection. This type of immune complication is almost never seen since the development of human insulin preparations of neutral pH. Injection of these newer preparations directly into the atrophic area often results in restoration of normal contours. Hypertrophy of subcutaneous fatty tissue remains a problem, even with the purified insulins, if injected repeatedly at the same site. However, this may be corrected by avoidance of that specific injection site or with liposuction.

ORAL ANTIDIABETIC AGENTS

Four categories of oral antidiabetic agents are now available in the USA: **insulin secretagogues** (sulfonylureas, meglitinides, D-phenylalanine derivatives), **biguanides, thiazolidinediones,** and α-**glucosidase inhibitors.** The sulfonylureas and biguanides have been available the longest and are the traditional initial treatment choice for type 2 diabetes. Novel classes of rapidly acting insulin secretagogues, the meglitinides and D-phenylalanine derivatives, are alternatives to the short-acting sulfonylurea, tolbutamide. The thiazolidinediones, under development since the early 1980s, are very effective agents that reduce insulin resistance. α-Glucosidase inhibitors have a relatively weak antidiabetic effect and significant adverse effects, and they are used primarily as adjunctive therapy in individuals who cannot achieve their glycemic goals with other medications.

INSULIN SECRETAGOGUES: SULFONYLUREAS

Mechanism of Action

The major action of sulfonylureas is to increase insulin release from the pancreas (Table 41–5). Two additional mechanisms of action have been proposed—a reduction of serum glucagon levels and closure of potassium chan-

Table 41–5. Regulation of insulin release in humans.[1]

Stimulants of insulin release
Glucose, mannose
Leucine
Vagal stimulation
Sulfonylureas

Amplifiers of glucose-induced insulin release
Enteric hormones:
Glucagon-like peptide 1(7–37)
Gastrin inhibitory peptide
Cholecystokinin
Secretin, gastrin
Neural amplifiers:
β-Adrenoceptor stimulation
Amino acids:
Arginine

Inhibitors of insulin release
Neural: α-Sympathomimetic effect of catecholamines
Humoral: Somatostatin
Drugs: Diazoxide, phenytoin, vinblastine, colchicine

[1]Modified and reproduced, with permission, from Greenspan FS, Strewler GJ (editors): *Basic & Clinical Endocrinology,* 5th ed. Originally published by Appleton & Lange. Copyright © 1997 by The McGraw-Hill Companies, Inc.

nels in extrapancreatic tissues. The latter is of unknown clinical significance.

A. INSULIN RELEASE FROM PANCREATIC B CELLS (FIGURE 41–2)

Sulfonylureas bind to a 140 kDa high-affinity sulfonylurea receptor that is associated with a B cell inward rectifier ATP-sensitive potassium channel. Binding of a sulfonylurea inhibits the efflux of potassium ions through the channel and results in depolarization. Depolarization, in turn, opens a voltage-gated calcium channel and results in calcium influx and the release of preformed insulin.

B. REDUCTION OF SERUM GLUCAGON CONCENTRATIONS

Chronic administration of sulfonylureas to type 2 diabetics reduces serum glucagon levels, which may contribute to the hypoglycemic effect of the drugs. The mechanism for this suppressive effect of sulfonylureas on glucagon levels is unclear but appears to involve indirect inhibition due to enhanced release of both insulin and somatostatin, which inhibit A cell secretion.

C. POTASSIUM CHANNEL CLOSURE IN EXTRAPANCREATIC TISSUES

Insulin secretagogues bind to sulfonylurea receptors in potassium channels in extrapancreatic tissues but the binding affinity varies among the drug classes and is much less avid than for the B cell receptors. The clinical significance of extrapancreatic binding is not known.

Efficacy & Safety of the Sulfonylureas

In 1970, the University Group Diabetes Program (UGDP) in the USA reported that the number of deaths due to cardiovascular disease in diabetic patients treated with tolbutamide was excessive compared with either insulin-treated patients or those receiving placebos. Due to design flaws, this study and its conclusions were not generally accepted. A study in the United Kingdom, the UKPDS, did not find an untoward cardiovascular effect of sulfonylurea usage in their large, long-term study.

The sulfonylureas continue to be widely prescribed and six are available in the USA (Table 41–6). They are conventionally divided into first-generation and second-generation agents, which differ primarily in their potency and adverse effects. The first-generation sulfonylureas are increasingly difficult to procure, and as the second-generation agents become generic and less expensive, the earlier compounds probably will be discontinued.

Table 41–6. Sulfonylureas.

Sulfonylurea	Chemical Structure	Daily Dose	Duration of Action (hours)
Tolbutamide (Orinase)		0.5–2 g in divided doses	6–12
Tolazamide (Tolinase)		0.1–1 g as single dose or in divided doses	10–14
Chlorpropamide (Diabinese)		0.1–0.5 g as single dose	Up to 60
Glyburide (glibenclamide[1]) (Diaβeta, Micronase, Glynase PresTab)		0.00125–0.02 g	10–24
Glipizide (glydiazinamide[1]) (Glucotrol, Glucotrol XL)		0.005–0.04g (0.02 g in Glucotrol XL)	10–24[2]
Glimepiride (Amaryl)		0.001–0.004 g	12–24

[1]Outside USA.
[2]Elimination half-life considerably shorter (see text).

1. First-Generation Sulfonylureas

Tolbutamide is well absorbed but rapidly metabolized in the liver. Its duration of effect is relatively short, with an elimination half-life of 4–5 hours, and it is best administered in divided doses. Because of its short half-life, it is the safest sulfonylurea for use in elderly diabetics. Prolonged hypoglycemia has been reported rarely, mostly in patients receiving certain drugs (eg, dicumarol, phenylbutazone, some sulfonamides) that inhibit the metabolism of tolbutamide.

Chlorpropamide has a half-life of 32 hours and is slowly metabolized in the liver to products that retain some biologic activity; approximately 20–30% is excreted unchanged in the urine. Chlorpropamide also interacts with the drugs mentioned above that depend on hepatic oxidative catabolism, and it is contraindicated in patients with hepatic or renal insufficiency. Dosages in excess of 500 mg daily increase the risk of jaundice. The average maintenance dosage is 250 mg daily, given as a single dose in the morning. Prolonged hypoglycemic reactions are more common in elderly patients, and the drug is contraindicated in this group. Other side effects include a hyperemic flush after alcohol ingestion in genetically predisposed patients and dilutional hyponatremia. Hematologic toxicity (transient leukopenia, thrombocytopenia) occurs in less than 1% of patients.

Tolazamide is comparable to chlorpropamide in potency but has a shorter duration of action. Tolazamide is more slowly absorbed than the other sulfonylureas, and its effect on blood glucose does not appear for several hours. Its half-life is about 7 hours. Tolazamide is metabolized to several compounds that retain hypoglycemic effects. If more than 500 mg/d is required, the dose should be divided and given twice daily. Dosages larger than 1000 mg daily do not further improve the degree of blood glucose control.

2. Second-Generation Sulfonylureas

The second-generation sulfonylureas are more frequently prescribed in the USA than the first-generation agents because they have fewer adverse effects and drug interactions. These potent sulfonylurea compounds—glyburide, glipizide, and glimepiride—should be used with caution in patients with cardiovascular disease or in elderly patients, in whom hypoglycemia would be especially dangerous.

Glyburide is metabolized in the liver into products with very low hypoglycemic activity. The usual starting dosage is 2.5 mg/d or less, and the average maintenance dosage is 5–10 mg/d given as a single morning dose; maintenance dosages higher than 20 mg/d are not recommended. A formulation of "micronized" glyburide (Glynase PresTab) is available in a variety of tablet sizes. However, there is some question as to its bioequivalence with nonmicronized formulations, and the FDA recommends careful monitoring to retitrate dosage when switching from standard glyburide doses or from other sulfonylurea drugs.

Glyburide has few adverse effects other than its potential for causing hypoglycemia. Flushing has rarely been reported after ethanol ingestion and the compound slightly enhances free water clearance. Glyburide is contraindicated in the presence of hepatic impairment and in patients with renal insufficiency.

Glipizide has the shortest half-life (2–4 hours) of the more potent agents. For maximum effect in reducing postprandial hyperglycemia, this agent should be ingested 30 minutes before breakfast, since absorption is delayed when the drug is taken with food. The recommended starting dosage is 5 mg/d, with up to 15 mg/d given as a single dose. When higher daily dosages are required, they should be divided and given before meals. The maximum total daily dosage recommended by the manufacturer is 40 mg/d, although some studies indicate that the maximum therapeutic effect is achieved by 15–20 mg of the drug. An extended-release preparation (Glucotrol XL) provides 24-hour action after a once-daily morning dose (maximum of 20 mg/d). However, this formulation appears to have sacrificed its lower propensity for severe hypoglycemia compared with longer-acting glyburide without showing any demonstrable therapeutic advantages over the latter (which can be obtained as a generic drug).

Because of its shorter half-life, glipizide is much less likely than glyburide to produce serious hypoglycemia. At least 90% of glipizide is metabolized in the liver to inactive products, and 10% is excreted unchanged in the urine. Glipizide therapy is therefore contraindicated in patients with significant hepatic or renal impairment, who would therefore be at high risk for hypoglycemia.

Glimepiride is approved for once-daily use as monotherapy or in combination with insulin. Glimepiride achieves blood glucose lowering with the lowest dose of any sulfonylurea compound. A single daily dose of 1 mg has been shown to be effective, and the recommended maximal daily dose is 8 mg. It has a long duration of effect with a half-life of 5 hours, allowing once-daily dosing and thereby improving compliance. It is completely metabolized by the liver to inactive products.

Secondary Failure & Tachyphylaxis to Sulfonylureas

Secondary failure, ie, failure to maintain a good response to sulfonylurea therapy over the long term—remains a disconcerting problem in the management of type 2 diabetes. A progressive decrease in B cell mass, reduction in physical activity, decline in lean body mass, or increase in ectopic fat deposition in chronic type 2 diabetes also may contribute to secondary failure.

INSULIN SECRETAGOGUES: MEGLITINIDES

The meglitinides are a relatively new class of insulin secretagogues. **Repaglinide,** the first member of the group, was approved for clinical use in 1998 (Table 41–7). These drugs modulate B cell insulin release by regulating potassium efflux through the potassium channels previously discussed. There is overlap with the sulfonylureas in their molecular sites of action since the meglitinides have two binding sites in common with the sulfonylureas and one unique binding site. Unlike the sulfonylureas, they have no direct effect on insulin exocytosis.

Repaglinide has a very fast onset of action, with a peak concentration and peak effect within approximately 1 hour after ingestion, but the duration of action is 5–8 hours. It is hepatically cleared by CYP3A4 with a plasma half-life of 1 hour. Because of its rapid onset, repaglinide is indicated for use in controlling postprandial glucose excursions. The drug should be taken just before each meal in doses of 0.25–4 mg (maximum, 16 mg/d); hypoglycemia is a risk if the meal is delayed or skipped or contains inadequate carbohydrate. This drug should be used cautiously in individuals with renal and hepatic impairment. Repaglinide is approved as monotherapy or in combination with biguanides. There

is no sulfur in its structure, so repaglinide may be used in type 2 diabetic individuals with sulfur or sulfonylurea allergy.

INSULIN SECRETAGOGUE: D-PHENYLALANINE DERIVATIVE

Nateglinide, a D-phenylalanine derivative, is the latest insulin secretagogue to become clinically available. Nateglinide stimulates very rapid and transient release of insulin from B cells through closure of the ATP-sensitive K^+ channel. It also partially restores initial insulin release in response to an intravenous glucose tolerance test. This may be a significant advantage of the drug because type 2 diabetes is associated with loss of this initial insulin response. The restoration of more normal insulin secretion may suppress glucagon release early in the meal and result in less endogenous or hepatic glucose production. Nateglinide may have a special role in the treatment of individuals with isolated postprandial hyperglycemia, but it has minimal effect on overnight or fasting glucose levels. It is efficacious when given alone or in combination with nonsecretagogue oral agents (such as metformin). In contrast to other insulin secretagogues, dose titration is not required.

Nateglinide is ingested just prior to meals. It is absorbed within 20 minutes after oral administration with a time to peak concentration of less than 1 hour and is hepatically metabolized by CYP2C9 and CYP3A4 with a half-life of 1.5 hours. The overall duration of action is less than 4 hours.

Table 41–7. Other insulin secretagogues.

Drug	Chemical Structure	Oral Dose	$t_{1/2}$	Duration of Action (hours)
Repaglinide (Prandin)		0.25–4 mg before meals	1 hour	4–5
Nateglinide (Starlix)		60–120 mg before meals	1 hour	4

Nateglinide amplifies the insulin secretory response to a glucose load but has a markedly diminished effect in the presence of normoglycemia. The incidence of hypoglycemia may be the lowest of all the secretagogues, and it has the advantage of being safe in individuals with very reduced renal function.

BIGUANIDES

The structure of metformin is shown below. Phenformin (an older biguanide) was discontinued in the USA because of its association with lactic acidosis and because there was no documentation of any long-term benefit from its use.

Metformin

Mechanisms of Action

A full explanation of the biguanides' mechanism of action remains elusive. Their blood glucose-lowering action does not depend on the presence of functioning pancreatic B cells. Patients with type 2 diabetes have considerably less fasting hyperglycemia as well as lower postprandial hyperglycemia after biguanides; however, hypoglycemia during biguanide therapy is essentially unknown. These agents are therefore more appropriately termed "euglycemic" agents. Currently proposed mechanisms of action include (1) direct stimulation of glycolysis in tissues, with increased glucose removal from blood; (2) reduced hepatic and renal gluconeogenesis; (3) slowing of glucose absorption from the gastrointestinal tract, with increased glucose to lactate conversion by enterocytes; and (4) reduction of plasma glucagon levels.

Metabolism & Excretion

Metformin has a half-life of 1.5–3 hours, is not bound to plasma proteins, is not metabolized, and is excreted by the kidneys as the active compound. As a consequence of metformin's blockade of gluconeogenesis, the drug may impair the hepatic metabolism of lactic acid. In patients with renal insufficiency, biguanides accumulate and thereby increase the risk of lactic acidosis, which appears to be a dose-related complication.

Clinical Use

Biguanides have been most often prescribed for patients whose hyperglycemia is due to ineffective insulin action, ie, insulin resistance syndrome. Because metformin is an insulin-sparing agent and does not increase weight or provoke hypoglycemia, it offers obvious advantages over insulin or sulfonylureas in treating hyperglycemia in such individuals. The UKPDS reported that metformin therapy decreases the risk of macrovascular as well as microvascular disease; this is in contrast to the other therapies, which only modified microvascular morbidity. Biguanides are also indicated for use in combination with insulin secretagogues or thiazolidinediones in type 2 diabetics in whom oral monotherapy is inadequate. Metformin is useful in the prevention of type 2 diabetes; the landmark Diabetes Prevention Program concluded that metformin is efficacious in preventing the new onset of type 2 diabetes in middle-aged, obese individuals with impaired glucose tolerance and fasting hyperglycemia. Interestingly, metformin did not prevent diabetes in older, leaner pre-diabetics.

The dosage of metformin is from 500 mg to a maximum of 2.55 g daily, with the lowest effective dose being recommended. A common schedule would be to begin with a single 500 mg tablet given with breakfast for several days. If this is tolerated without gastrointestinal discomfort and hyperglycemia persists, a second 500 mg tablet may be added with the evening meal. If further dose increases are required after 1 week, an additional 500 mg tablet can be added to be taken with the midday meal, or the larger (850 mg) tablet can be prescribed twice daily or even three times daily (the maximum recommended dosage) if needed. Dosage should always be divided, since ingestion of more than 1000 mg at any one time usually provokes significant gastrointestinal side effects.

Toxicities

The most frequent toxic effects of metformin are gastrointestinal (anorexia, nausea, vomiting, abdominal discomfort, diarrhea) and occur in up to 20% of patients. They are dose related, tend to occur at the onset of therapy, and are often transient. However, metformin may have to be discontinued in 3–5% of patients because of persistent diarrhea. Absorption of vitamin B_{12} appears to be reduced during long-term metformin therapy, and annual screening of serum vitamin B_{12} levels and red blood cell parameters has been encouraged by the manufacturer to determine the need for vitamin B_{12} injections. In the absence of hypoxia or renal or hepatic insufficiency, lactic acidosis is less common with metformin therapy than with phenformin therapy.

Biguanides are contraindicated in patients with renal disease, alcoholism, hepatic disease, or conditions predisposing to tissue anoxia (eg, chronic cardiopulmonary dysfunction), because of an increased risk of lactic acidosis induced by biguanide drugs in the presence of these diseases.

THIAZOLIDINEDIONES

Thiazolidinediones (Tzds) act to decrease insulin resistance. Their primary action is the nuclear regulation of genes involved in glucose and lipid metabolism and adipocyte differentiation. Tzds are ligands of **peroxisome proliferator-activated receptor-gamma (PPAR-γ)**, part of the steroid and thyroid superfamily of nuclear receptors. These PPAR receptors are found in muscle, fat, and liver. PPAR-γ receptors are complex and modulate the expression of the genes involved in lipid and glucose metabolism, insulin signal transduction, and adipocyte and other tissue differentiation. The available Tzds do not have identical clinical effects and new drug development will focus on defining PPAR effects and designing ligands that have selective action—much like the selective estrogen receptor ligands (see Chapter 40).

In addition to targeting adipocytes, myocytes, and hepatocytes, Tzds also have significant effects on vascular endothelium, the immune system, the ovaries, and tumor cells. Some of these responses may be independent of the PPAR-γ pathway.

In persons with diabetes, a major site of Tzd action is adipose tissue, where the drug promotes glucose uptake and utilization and modulates synthesis of lipid hormones or cytokines and other proteins involved in energy regulation. Tzds also regulate adipocyte apoptosis and differentiation. Numerous other effects have been documented in animal studies but applicability to human tissues has yet to be determined.

Two thiazolidinediones are currently available: pioglitazone and rosiglitazone (Table 41–8). Their distinct side chains create differences in therapeutic action, metabolism, metabolite profile, and adverse effects. A third compound, troglitazone, was withdrawn from the market because of hepatic toxicity thought to be related to its side chain.

Pioglitazone may have PPAR-α as well as PPAR-γ activity. It is absorbed within 2 hours of ingestion; although food may delay uptake, total bioavailability is not affected. Pioglitazone is metabolized by CYP2C8 and CYP3A4 to active metabolites. The bioavailability of numerous other drugs also degraded by these enzymes may be affected by pioglitazone therapy, including estrogen-containing oral contraceptives; additional methods of contraception are advised. Pioglitazone may be taken once daily; the usual starting dose is 15–30 mg. The triglyceride lowering effect is more significant than that observed with rosiglitazone. Pioglitazone is approved as a monotherapy and in combination with metformin, sulfonylureas, and insulin for the treatment of type 2 diabetes.

Rosiglitazone is rapidly absorbed and highly protein bound. It is metabolized in the liver to minimally active metabolites, predominantly by CYP2C8 and to a lesser extent by CYP2C9. It is administered once or twice daily; 4–8 mg is the usual total dose. Rosiglitazone shares the common Tzd adverse effects but does not seem to have any significant drug interactions. The drug is approved for use in type 2 diabetes as monotherapy or in combination with a biguanide or sulfonylurea.

Tzds are considered "euglycemics" and are efficacious in about 70% of new users. The overall response is similar to sulfonylurea and biguanide monotherapy. Individuals experiencing secondary failure to other oral agents should benefit from the addition (rather than substitution) of a Tzd. Because their mechanism of action involves gene regulation, the Tzds have a slow

Table 41–8. Thiazolidinediones.

Thiazolidinedione	Chemical Structure	Oral Dose
Pioglitazone (Actos)		15–45 mg once daily
Rosiglitazone (Avandia)		2–8 mg once daily

onset and offset of activity over weeks or even months. Combination therapy with sulfonylureas and insulin can lead to hypoglycemia and may require dosage adjustment. Long-term therapy is associated with a drop in triglyceride levels and a slight rise in HDL and low-density lipoprotein (LDL) cholesterol values. An adverse effect common to both Tzds is fluid retention, which presents as a mild anemia and peripheral edema especially when used in combination with insulin or insulin secretagogues. Many users have a dose-related weight gain (average 1–3 kg), which may be fluid-related. These agents should not be used during pregnancy, in the presence of significant liver disease, or if there is a concurrent diagnosis of heart failure. Anovulatory women may resume ovulation and should be counseled on the increased risk of pregnancy. Because of the hepatotoxicity observed with troglitazone, the FDA continues to require regular monitoring of liver function tests for the first year after initiation of Tzd therapy. To date, hepatotoxicity has not been associated with rosiglitazone or pioglitazone.

Thiazolidinediones have a theoretical benefit in the prevention of type 2 diabetes. One study reported that troglitazone therapy significantly decreased the recurrence of diabetes mellitus in high risk Hispanic women with a prior history of gestational diabetes. Other trials using clinically available Tzds are in progress.

ALPHA GLUCOSIDASE INHIBITORS

Only monosaccharides, such as glucose and fructose, can be transported out of the intestinal lumen and into the bloodstream. Complex starches, oligosaccharides, and disaccharides must be broken down into individual monosaccharides before being absorbed in the duodenum and upper jejunum. This digestion is facilitated by enteric enzymes, including pancreatic α-amylase, and

α-glucosidases that are attached to the brush border of the intestinal cells. **Acarbose** and **miglitol** (Table 41–9) are competitive inhibitors of the intestinal α-glucosidases and reduce the postprandial digestion and absorption of starch and disaccharides. Miglitol differs structurally from acarbose and is six times more potent in inhibiting sucrase. Although the binding affinity of the two compounds differs, acarbose and miglitol both target the α-glucosidases: sucrase, maltase, glycoamylase, dextranase. Miglitol alone has effects on isomaltase and on β-glucosidases, which split β-linked sugars such as lactose. Acarbose alone has a small effect on α-amylase. The consequence of enzyme inhibition is to minimize upper intestinal digestion and defer digestion (and thus absorption) of the ingested starch and disaccharides to the distal small intestine, thereby lowering postmeal glycemic excursions as much as 45–60 mg/dL and creating an insulin-sparing effect. Monotherapy with these drugs is associated with a modest drop (0.5–1%) in glycohemoglobin levels and a 20–25 mg/dL fall in fasting glucose levels. They are FDA-approved for use in individuals with type 2 diabetes as monotherapy and in combination with sulfonylureas, where the glycemic effect is additive. Both acarbose and miglitol are taken in doses of 25–100 mg just prior to ingesting the first portion of each meal; therapy should be initiated with the lowest dose and slowly titrated upward.

Prominent adverse effects include flatulence, diarrhea, and abdominal pain and result from the appearance of undigested carbohydrate in the colon that is then fermented into short-chain fatty acids, releasing gas. These side effects tend to diminish with ongoing use because chronic exposure to carbohydrate induces the expression of α-glucosidase in the jejunum and ileum, increasing distal small intestine glucose absorption and minimizing the passage of carbohydrate into the colon. Although not a problem with monotherapy or combination therapy with a biguanide, hypo-

Table 41–9. Alpha-glucosidase inhibitors.

Alpha-glucosidase Inhibitor	Chemical Structure	Oral Dose
Acarbose (Precose)		25–100 mg before meals
Miglitol (Glyset)		25–100 mg before meals

glycemia may occur with concurrent sulfonylurea treatment. Hypoglycemia should be treated with glucose (dextrose) and not sucrose, whose breakdown may be blocked. These drugs are contraindicated in patients with inflammatory bowel disease or any intestinal condition that could be worsened by gas and distention. Because both miglitol and acarbose are absorbed from the gut, these medications should not be prescribed in individuals with renal impairment. Acarbose has been associated with reversible hepatic enzyme elevation and should be used with caution in the presence of hepatic disease.

The STOP-NIDDM trial demonstrated that α-glucosidase therapy in prediabetic individuals successfully prevented a significant number of new cases of type 2 diabetes and helped restore β cell function. Diabetes prevention may become a further indication for this class of medications.

Combination Therapy With Oral Antidiabetic Agents & Insulin

A. COMBINATION THERAPY IN TYPE 2 DIABETES MELLITUS

Bedtime insulin has been suggested as an adjunct to oral antidiabetic therapy in patients with type 2 diabetes patients who have not responded to maximal oral therapy. Clinical practice has evolved to include sulfonylureas, meglitinides, D-phenylalanine derivatives, biguanides, thiazolidinediones, or α-glucosidase inhibitors given in conjunction with insulin.

Individuals unable to achieve glycemic control with bedtime insulin as described above generally require full insulin replacement and multiple daily injections of insulin. Insulin secretagogues are redundant when an individual is receiving multiple daily insulin injections, but cases of severe insulin resistance may benefit from the addition of one of the biguanides, thiazolidinediones, or α-glucosidase inhibitors. In some cases, multiple oral agents have been required together with insulin. When oral agents are added to the regimen of someone already taking insulin, the blood glucose should be closely monitored and the insulin dosage decreased as needed to avoid hypoglycemia.

B. COMBINATION THERAPY IN TYPE 1 DIABETES MELLITUS

There is no indication for combining insulin with insulin secretagogues (sulfonylureas, meglitinides, or D-phenylalanine derivatives) in individuals with type 1 diabetes. Type 1 diabetics with diets very high in starch may benefit from the addition of α-glucosidase inhibitors, but this is not typically practiced in the USA.

GLUCAGON

Chemistry & Metabolism

Glucagon is synthesized in the A cells of the pancreatic islets of Langerhans (see Table 41–1). Glucagon is a peptide—identical in all mammals—consisting of a single chain of 29 amino acids, with a molecular weight of 3485. Selective proteolytic cleavage converts a large precursor molecule of approximately 18,000 MW to glucagon. One of the precursor intermediates consists of a 69-amino-acid peptide called **glicentin**, which contains the glucagon sequence interposed between peptide extensions.

Glucagon is extensively degraded in the liver and kidney as well as in plasma, and at its tissue receptor sites. Because of its rapid inactivation by plasma, chilling of the collecting tubes and addition of inhibitors of proteolytic enzymes are necessary when samples of blood are collected for immunoassay of circulating glucagon. Its half-life in plasma is between 3 and 6 minutes, which is similar to that of insulin.

"Gut Glucagon"

Glicentin immunoreactivity has been found in cells of the small intestine as well as in pancreatic A cells and in effluents of perfused pancreas. The intestinal cells secrete **enteroglucagon**, a family of glucagon-like peptides, of which glicentin is a member, along with glucagon-like peptides 1 and 2 (GLP-1 and GLP-2). Unlike the pancreatic A cell, these intestinal cells lack the enzymes to convert glucagon precursors to true glucagon by removing the carboxyl terminal extension from the molecule.

The function of the enteroglucagons has not been clarified, although smaller peptides can bind hepatic glucagon receptors where they exert partial activity. A derivative of the 37-amino-acid form of GLP-1 that lacks the first six amino acids (GLP-1[7–37]) is a potent stimulant of insulin release. It represents the predominant form of GLP in the human intestine and has been termed "insulinotropin." It has been considered as a potential therapeutic agent in type 2 diabetes. However, it requires continuous subcutaneous infusion to produce a sustained lowering of both fasting and postprandial hyperglycemia in type 2 diabetic patients; therefore, its clinical usefulness is limited.

Pharmacologic Effects of Glucagon

A. METABOLIC EFFECTS

The first six amino acids at the amino terminal of the glucagon molecule bind to specific receptors on liver cells. This leads to a G_s protein-linked increase in adenylyl cyclase activity and the production of cAMP, which facilitates catabolism of stored glycogen and increases gluconeogenesis and ketogenesis. The immediate pharmacologic result of glucagon infusion is to raise blood glucose at the expense of stored hepatic glycogen. There is no effect on skeletal muscle glycogen, presumably because of the lack of glucagon receptors on skeletal muscle. Pharmacologic amounts of glucagon cause release of insulin from normal pancreatic B cells, catecholamines from pheochromocytoma, and calcitonin from medullary carcinoma cells.

B. Cardiac Effects

Glucagon has a potent inotropic and chronotropic effect on the heart, mediated by the cAMP mechanism described above. Thus, it produces an effect very similar to that of β-adrenoceptor agonists without requiring functioning β-receptors.

C. Effects on Smooth Muscle

Large doses of glucagon produce profound relaxation of the intestine. In contrast to the above effects of the peptide, this action on the intestine may be due to mechanisms other than adenylyl cyclase activation.

Clinical Uses

A. Severe Hypoglycemia

The major use of glucagon is for emergency treatment of severe hypoglycemic reactions in patients with type 1 diabetes when unconsciousness precludes oral feedings and use of intravenous glucose is not possible. Recombinant glucagon is currently available in 1 mg vials for parenteral use (Glucagon Emergency Kit). Nasal sprays have been developed for this purpose but have not yet received FDA approval.

B. Endocrine Diagnosis

Several tests use glucagon to diagnose endocrine disorders. In patients with type 1 diabetes mellitus, a standard test of pancreatic B cell secretory reserve utilizes 1 mg of glucagon administered as an intravenous bolus. Since insulin-treated patients develop circulating anti-insulin antibodies that interfere with radioimmunoassays of insulin, measurements of C-peptide are used to indicate B cell secretion.

C. Beta-Blocker Poisoning

Glucagon is sometimes useful for reversing the cardiac effects of an overdose of β-blocking agents because of its ability to increase cAMP production in the heart. However, it is not clinically useful in the treatment of cardiac failure.

D. Radiology of the Bowel

Glucagon has been used extensively in radiology as an aid to x-ray visualization of the bowel because of its ability to relax the intestine.

Adverse Reactions

Transient nausea and occasional vomiting can result from glucagon administration. These are generally mild, and glucagon is relatively free of severe adverse reactions.

ISLET AMYLOID POLYPEPTIDE (IAPP, AMYLIN)

IAPP is a 37-amino-acid peptide originally derived from islet amyloid deposits in pancreas material from patients with long-standing type 2 diabetes or insulinomas. It is produced by pancreatic B cells, packaged within B cell granules in a concentration 1–2% that of insulin, and secreted in response to B cell secretagogues. Approximately one molecule of IAPP is released for every ten molecules of insulin. A physiologic effect has not been established; however, pharmacologic doses inhibit the action of insulin to promote muscle uptake of glucose. IAPP appears to be a member of the superfamily of neuroregulatory peptides, with 46% homology with the calcitonin gene-related peptide CGRP (see Chapter 17). Whereas CGRP inhibits insulin secretion, this has not been demonstrated at physiologic concentrations of IAPP. Clinical trials have begun to evaluate IAPP and its analogs, eg, **pramlintide,** as adjuncts to insulin therapy in type 1 diabetic patients with recurrent episodes of severe insulin-induced hypoglycemia—episodes that are generally refractory to usual preventive measures.

REFERENCES

Aguilar-Bryan L et al: Cloning of the beta cell high-affinity sulfonylurea receptor: a regulator of insulin secretion. Science 1995;268:423.

Aviles-Santa L, Sinding J, Raskin P: Effects of metformin in patients with poorly controlled, insulin-treated type 2 diabetes mellitus. A randomized, double-blind, placebo-controlled trial. Ann Intern Med 1999;131:182.

Bailey CJ: New pharmacological approaches to glycemic control. Diabetes Rev 1999;7:94.

Bolli GB et al: Insulin analogues and their potential in the management of diabetes mellitus. Diabetologia 1999;42:1151.

PREPARATIONS AVAILABLE[1]

SULFONYLUREAS

Acetohexamide (Dymelor) (rarely used)
Oral: 250, 500 mg tablets

Chlorpropamide (generic, Diabinese)
Oral: 100, 250 mg tablets

Glimepiride (Amaryl)
Oral: 1, 2, 4 mg tablets

Glipizide (generic, Glucotrol, Glucotrol XL)
Oral: 5, 10 mg tablets; 5, 10 mg extended release tablets

Glyburide (generic, Diaβeta, Micronase, Glynase PresTab)
Oral: 1.25, 2.5, 5 mg tablets; 1.5, 3, 4.5, 6 mg Glynase PresTab, micronized tablets

Tolazamide (generic, Tolinase)
Oral: 100, 250, 500 mg tablets

Tolbutamide (generic, Orinase)
Oral: 500 mg tablets

MEGLITINIDE & RELATED DRUGS

Repaglinide (Prandin)
Oral: 0.5, 1, 2 mg tablets

Nateglinide (Starlix)
Oral: 60, 120 mg tablets

BIGUANIDE & BIGUANIDE COMBINATIONS

Metformin (Glucophage, Glucophage XR)
Oral: 500, 850, 1000 mg tablets; extended-release (XR): 500 mg tablets

METFORMIN COMBINATIONS

Glipizide plus metformin (Metaglip)
Oral: 2.5/250, 2.5/500, 5/500 mg tablets

Glyburide plus metformin (Glucovance)
Oral: 1.25/250, 2.5/500, 5/500 mg tablets

Rosiglitazone plus metformin (Avandamet)
Oral: 1/500, 2/500, 4/500 mg tablets

THIAZOLIDINEDIONE DERIVATIVES

Pioglitazone (Actos)
Oral: 15, 30, 45 mg tablets

Rosiglitazone (Avandia)
Oral: 2, 4, 8 mg tablets

ALPHA GLUCOSIDASE INHIBITORS

Acarbose (Precose)
Oral: 50, 100 mg tablets

Miglitol (Glyset)
Oral: 25, 50, 100 mg tablets

GLUCAGON

Glucagon (generic)
Parenteral: 1 mg lyophilized powder to reconstitute for injection

[1] See Table 41–4 for insulin preparations.

Brange J et al: Monomeric insulins and their experimental and clinical implications. Diabetes Care 1990;13:923.

Buchanan TA: Protection from type 2 diabetes persists in the TRIPOD cohort eight months after stopping troglitazone. Diabetes 2001;50(Suppl 2):A81.

Buse JB: Overview of current therapeutic options in type 2 diabetes. Rationale for combining oral agents with insulin therapy. Diabetes Care 1999;22(Suppl 3):C65.

Chan NN, Brain HPS, Feher MD: Metformin-associated lactic acidosis: a rare or very rare clinical entity. Diabet Med 1999;16:273.

Cherrington AD: Banting Lecture 1997. Control of glucose uptake and release by the liver in vivo. Diabetes 1999;48:1198.

Chiasson JL et al: Acarbose for prevention of type 2 diabetes mellitus: the STOP-NIDDM randomized trial. Lancet 2002;359:2072.

Cohen RD: Lactic acidosis: new perspectives on origins and treatment. Diabetes Rev 1994;2:86.

Cryer PE, Fisher JN, Shamoon H: Hypoglycemia. Diabetes Care 1994;17:734.

Cusi K, DeFronzo RA: Metformin: a review of its metabolic effects. Diabetes Rev 1998;6:89.

Day C: Thiazolidinediones: a new class of antidiabetic drugs. Diabet Med 1999;16:179.

DeFronzo RA et al: Efficacy of metformin in patients with non-insulin-dependent diabetes mellitus. N Engl J Med 1995;333:541.

DeFronzo RA: Pharmacologic therapy for type 2 diabetes mellitus. Ann Intern Med 1999;131:281.

Diabetes Control and Complications Trial Research Group: Epidemiology of severe hypoglycemia in the diabetes control and complications trial. Am J Med 1991;90:450.

Diabetes Control and Complications Trial Research Group: The effect of intensive treatment of diabetes on the development and progression of long-term complications in insulin-dependent diabetes mellitus. N Engl J Med 1993;329:977.

Diabetes Prevention Program Research Group: Reduction in the incidence of type 2 diabetes with lifestyle intervention or metformin. N Engl J Med 2002;346:393.

Dunn CJ et al: Nateglinide. Drugs 2000;60:607.

Dunn CJ, Peters DH: Metformin: a review of its pharmacological properties and therapeutic use in non-insulin-dependent diabetes mellitus. Drugs 1995;49:721.

Edwards CM et al: Glucagon-like peptide 1 has a physiological role in the control of postprandial glucose in humans: studies with the antagonist exendin 9-39. Diabetes 1999;48:86.

Eliasson L et al: PKC-dependent stimulation of exocytosis by sulfonylureas in pancreatic beta cells. Science 1996;271:813.

Emilien G, Maloteaux JM, Ponchon M: Pharmacological management of diabetes: recent progress and future perspective in daily drug treatment. Pharmacol Ther 1999;81:37.

Expert Committee on the Diagnosis and Classification of Diabetes Mellitus: Report of the expert committee on the diagnosis and classification of diabetes mellitus. Diabetes Care 2002;25(Suppl 1):S5.

Fehman H-C, Goke R, Goke B: Cell and molecular biology of the incretin hormones glucagon-like peptide I and glucose-dependent insulin-releasing polypeptide. Endocr Rev 1995;16:390.

Ferrannini E: Insulin resistance versus insulin deficiency in non-insulin-dependent diabetes mellitus: Problems and prospects. Endocr Rev 1998;19:477.

Gribble FM et al: Tissue specificity of sulfonylureas: Studies on cloned cardiac and beta cell K(ATP) channels. Diabetes 1998;47:1412.

Groop L et al: Comparison of pharmacokinetics, metabolic effects and mechanisms of action of glyburide and glipizide during long-term treatment. Diabetes Care 1987;10:671.

Heinemann L et al: Prandial glycemia after a carbohydrate-rich meal in type 1 diabetic patients. Using the rapid acting insulin analogue [Lys (B28), Pro (B29)] human insulin. Diabetic Med 1996;13:625.

Heinemann L et al: Time action profile of the long-acting insulin analog insulin glargine (HOE901) in comparison with those of NPH insulin and placebo. Diabetes Care 2000;23:644.

Howey DC et al: [Lys (B28), Pro (B29)]-human insulin: A rapidly absorbed analog of human insulin. Diabetes 1994;43:396.

Howlet HC, Bailey CJ: A risk-benefit assessment of metformin in type 2 diabetes mellitus. Drug Saf 1999;20:489.

Hunter SJ, Garvey WT: Insulin action and insulin resistance: Diseases involving defects in insulin receptors, signal transduction, and the glucose transport effector system. Am J Med 1998;105:331.

Kahn BB: Facilitative glucose transporters: Regulatory mechanisms and dysregulation in diabetes. J Clin Invest 1992;89:1367.

Kahn SE, Andrikopoulos S, Verchere CB: Islet amyloid: A long-recognized but underappreciated pathological feature of type 2 diabetes. Diabetes 1999;48:241.

Klonoff DC et al: Hypoglycemia following inadvertent and factitious sulfonylurea overdosages. Diabetes Care 1995;18:563.

Kumar U et al: Subtype-selective expression of the five somatostatin receptors (hSSTR1–5) in human pancreatic islet cells. Diabetes 1999;48:77.

Lalau JD et al: Role of metformin accumulation in metformin-associated lactic acidosis. Diabetes Care 1995;18:779.

Lalli C et al: Long term intensive treatment of type 1 diabetes with the short-acting insulin analog lispro in variable combination with NPH insulin at mealtime. Diabetes Care 1999;22:468.

Lebovitz HE: Alpha-glucosidase inhibitors as agents in the treatment of diabetes. Diabetes Rev 1998;6:132.

Lee WL, Zinman B: From insulin to insulin analogs: Progress in the treatment of type 1 diabetes. Diabetes Rev 1998;6:73.

Lefebvre PJ: Glucagon and its family revisited. Diabetes Care 1995;18:715.

Lepore M et al: Pharmacokinetics and pharmacodynamics of subcutaneous injection of long-acting human insulin analog glargine, NPH insulin and ultralente human insulin and continuous subcutaneous infusion of insulin lispro. Diabetes 2000;49:2142.

Levien TL: Nateglinide therapy for type 2 diabetes mellitus. Ann Pharmacother 2001;35:1426.

Maran A et al: Double blind clinical and laboratory study of hypoglycaemia with human and porcine insulin in diabetic patients reporting hypoglycaemia unawareness after transferring to human insulin. Br Med J 1993;306:167.

Marshak S et al: Impaired beta cell functions induced by chronic exposure of cultured human pancreatic islets to high glucose. Diabetes 1999;48:1230.

Mayfield J: Diagnosis and classification of diabetes mellitus: new criteria. Am Fam Physician 1998;58:1355.

McGarry D: Dysregulation of fatty acid metabolism in the etiology of type 2 diabetes. Diabetes 2002;51:7.

Meyer C, Doston JM, Gerich JE: Role of the human kidney in glucose counterregulation. Diabetes 1999;48:943.

Mori Y et al: Effect of troglitazone on body fat distribution in type 2 diabetic patients. Diabetes Care 1999;22:908.

Mudaliar S et al: New oral therapies for type 2 diabetes mellitus: The glitazones or insulin sensitizers. Annu Rev Med 2001;52:239.

Muhlhauser I, Koch J, Berger M: Pharmacokinetics and bioavailability of injected glucagon: differences between intramuscular, subcutaneous, and intravenous administration. Diabetes Care 1984;8:39.

Nyholm B et al: The amylin analog pramlintide improves glycemic control and reduces postprandial glucagon concentrations in patients with type 1 diabetes mellitus. Metabolism 1999;48:935.

Ottensmeyer FP et al: Mechanism of transmembrane signalling: insulin binding and the insulin receptor. Biochemistry 2000;39:12103.

Owens DR: Repaglinide: a new short-acting insulinotropic agent for the treatment of type 2 diabetes. Eur J Clin Invest 1999;29(Suppl 2):30.

Pampanelli S et al: Improved postprandial metabolic control after subcutaneous injection of a short-acting insulin analog (lispro) in IDDM of short duration with residual pancreatic beta-cell function. Diabetes Care 1995;18:1452.

Polonsky KS: The beta-cell in diabetes: from molecular genetics to clinical research. Diabetes 1995;44:705.

Rasmussen H et al: Physiology and pathophysiology of insulin secretion. Diabetes Care 1990;13:655.

Rassam AG et al: Optimal administration of lispro insulin in hyperglycemic type 1 diabetes. Diabetes Care 1999;22:133.

Reaven GM: Role of insulin resistance in human disease. Diabetes 1988;37:1595.

Renner R et al: Use of insulin lispro in continuous subcutaneous insulin infusion treatment. Results of a multicenter trial. German Humalog-CSII Study Group. Diabetes Care 1999;22:784.

Report of the Expert Committee on the Diagnosis and Classification of Diabetes Mellitus. Diabetes Care 1997;20:1183.

Resine T, Bell GI: Molecular biology of somatostatin receptors. Endocr Rev 1995;16:427.

Ritzel R et al: Pharmacokinetics, insulinotropic and glucagonostatic properties of GLP-1 (7-36 amide) after subcutaneous injection in healthy volunteers. Diabetologia 1995;38:720.

Rosak C et al: The effect of the timing and the administration of acarbose on postprandial hyperglycemia. Diabetic Med 1995;12:979.

Rosskamp RH, Park G: Long-acting insulin analogs. Diabetes Care 1999;22(Suppl 2):B109.

Saleh YM, Mudaliar SR, Henry RR: Metabolic and vascular effects of the thiazolidinedione, troglitazone. Diabetes Rev 1999;7:55.

Shank ML, DelPrato S, DeFronzo RA: Bedtime insulin/daytime glipizide: Effective therapy for sulfonylurea failures in NIDDM. Diabetes 1995;44:165.

Shepherd PR, Kahn BB: Glucose transporters and insulin action— implications for insulin resistance and diabetes mellitus. N Engl J Med 1999;341:248.

Stephens JM, Pilch PF: The metabolic regulation and vesicular transport of GLUT4, the major insulin responsive glucose transporter. Endocr Rev 1995;16:529.

Stumvoll M et al: Metabolic effects of metformin in non-insulin-dependent diabetes mellitus. N Engl J Med 1995;333:550.

Toft-Nielsen MB, Madsbad S, Holst JJ: Continuous subcutaneous infusion of glucagon-like peptide 1 lowers plasma glucose and reduces appetite in type 2 diabetic patients. Diabetes Care 1999;22:1137.

Torlone E et al: Pharmacokinetics, pharmacodynamics and glucose counterregulation following subcutaneous injection of the monomeric analogue [Lys (B28), Pro (B29)] in IDDM. Diabetologia 1994;37:713.

United Kingdom Prospective Diabetes Study (UKPDS) Group:

Effect of intensive blood-glucose control with metformin on complications in overweight patients with type 2 diabetes: UKPDS 34. Lancet 1998;352:854.

Efficacy of atenolol and captopril in reducing risk of macrovascular and microvascular complications in type 2 diabetes: UKPDS 39. BMJ 1998;317:713.

Glycemic control with diet, sulfonylurea, metformin, or insulin in patients with type 2 diabetes mellitus: Progressive requirement for multiple therapies: UKPDS 49. JAMA 1999;281:2005.

Intensive blood-glucose control with sulphonylureas or insulin compared with conventional treatment and risk of complications in patients with type 2 diabetes: UKPDS 33. Lancet 1998;352:837.

Tight blood pressure control and risk of macrovascular and microvascular complications in type 2 diabetes: UKPDS 38. BMJ 1998;317:703.

Virkamaki A, Kohjiro U, Kahn CR: Protein-protein interaction in insulin signaling and the molecular mechanisms of insulin resistance. J Clin Invest 1999;103:931.

Agents That Affect Bone Mineral Homeostasis

42

Daniel D. Bikle, MD, PhD

I. BASIC PHARMACOLOGY

Calcium and phosphate, the major mineral constituents of bone, are also two of the most important minerals for general cellular function. Accordingly, the body has evolved a complex set of mechanisms by which calcium and phosphate homeostasis are carefully maintained (Figure 42–1). Approximately 98% of the 1–2 kg of calcium and 85% of the 1 kg of phosphorus in the human adult are found in bone, the principal reservoir for these minerals. These functions are dynamic, with constant remodeling of bone and ready exchange of bone mineral with that in the extracellular fluid. Bone also serves as the principal structural support for the body and provides the space for hematopoiesis. Thus, abnormalities in bone mineral homeostasis can lead not only to a wide variety of cellular dysfunctions (eg, tetany, coma, muscle weakness) but also to disturbances in structural support of the body (eg, osteoporosis with fractures) and loss of hematopoietic capacity (eg, infantile osteopetrosis).

Calcium and phosphate enter the body from the intestine. The average American diet provides 600–1000 mg of calcium per day, of which approximately 100–250 mg is absorbed. This figure represents net absorption, since both absorption (principally in the duodenum and upper jejunum) and secretion (principally in the ileum) occur. The amount of phosphorus in the American diet is about the same as that of calcium. However, the efficiency of absorption (principally in the jejunum) is greater, ranging from 70% to 90% depending on intake. In the steady state, renal excretion of calcium and phosphate balances intestinal absorption. In general, over 98% of filtered calcium and 85% of filtered phosphate is reabsorbed by the kidney. The movement of calcium and phosphate across the intestinal and renal epithelia is closely regulated. Intrinsic disease of the intestine (eg, nontropical sprue) or kidney (eg, chronic renal failure) disrupts bone mineral homeostasis.

Two hormones serve as the principal regulators of calcium and phosphate homeostasis: the peptide parathyroid hormone (PTH) and the steroid vitamin D. Vitamin D is a prohormone rather than a true hormone, since it must be further metabolized to gain biologic activity. Other hormones—calcitonin, prolactin, growth hormone, insulin, thyroid hormone, glucocorticoids, and sex steroids—influence calcium and phosphate homeostasis under certain physiologic circumstances and can be considered secondary regulators. Deficiency or excess of these secondary regulators within a physiologic range does not produce the disturbance of calcium and phosphate homeostasis that is observed in situations of deficiency or excess of PTH and vitamin D. However, certain of these secondary regulators—especially calcitonin, glucocorticoids, and estrogens—are useful therapeutically and will be discussed in subsequent sections.

In addition to these hormonal regulators, calcium and phosphate themselves, other ions such as sodium and fluoride, and a variety of drugs (bisphosphonates, plicamycin, and diuretics) also alter calcium and phosphate homeostasis.

PRINCIPAL HORMONAL REGULATORS OF BONE MINERAL HOMEOSTASIS

PARATHYROID HORMONE

Parathyroid hormone (**PTH**) is a single-chain peptide hormone composed of 84 amino acids. It is produced in the parathyroid gland in a precursor form of 115 amino acids, the remaining 31 amino terminal amino acids being cleaved off prior to secretion. Within the gland is a calcium-sensitive protease capable of cleaving the intact hormone into fragments. Biologic activity resides in the amino terminal region such that synthetic 1–34 PTH is fully active. Loss of the first two amino terminal amino acids eliminates most biologic activity.

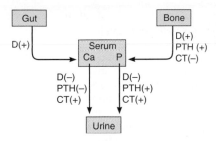

Figure 42–1. Some mechanisms contributing to bone mineral homeostasis. Calcium and phosphorus concentrations in the serum are controlled principally by two hormones, 1,25(OH)$_2$D$_3$ *(D)* and parathyroid hormone *(PTH)*, through their action on absorption from the gut and from bone and on excretion in the urine. Both hormones increase input of calcium and phosphorus from bone into the serum; vitamin D also increases absorption from the gut. Vitamin D decreases urinary excretion of both calcium and phosphorus, while PTH reduces calcium but increases phosphorus excretion. Calcitonin *(CT)* is a less critical hormone for calcium homeostasis, but in pharmacologic concentrations CT can reduce serum calcium and phosphorus by inhibiting bone resorption and stimulating their renal excretion. Feedback effects are not shown.

The metabolic clearance of intact PTH is rapid, with a half-time of disappearance measured in minutes. Most of the clearance occurs in the liver and kidney. The biologically inactive carboxyl terminal fragments produced during metabolism of the intact hormone have a much lower clearance, especially in renal failure. This accounts in part for the very high PTH values often observed in the past in patients with renal failure when measured by radioimmunoassays directed against the carboxyl terminal region of the molecule. However, most PTH assays currently in use measure the intact hormone by a double antibody method, so that this circumstance is less frequently encountered in clinical practice. PTH regulates calcium and phosphate flux across cellular membranes in bone and kidney, resulting in increased serum calcium and decreased serum phosphate. In bone, PTH increases the activity and number of osteoclasts, the cells responsible for bone resorption. However, this stimulation of osteoclasts is not a direct effect. Rather, PTH acts on the osteoblast (the bone-forming cell) to induce a membrane-bound protein called **RANK ligand.** This factor acts on osteoclasts and osteoclast precursors to increase both the numbers and the activity of osteoclasts. This action increases bone turnover or bone remodeling, a specific sequence of cellular events initiated by osteoclastic bone resorption and followed by osteoblastic bone formation. Although both bone resorption and bone formation are enhanced by PTH, the net effect of excess PTH is to increase bone resorption. PTH in low and intermittent doses may actually increase bone formation without first stimulating bone resorption. This has led to the recent approval of recombinant PTH 1-34(**teriparatide**) for the treatment of osteoporosis. In the kidney, PTH increases the ability of the nephron to reabsorb calcium and magnesium but reduces its ability to reabsorb phosphate, amino acids, bicarbonate, sodium, chloride, and sulfate. Another important action of PTH on the kidney is its stimulation of 1,25-dihydroxyvitamin D (1,25[OH]$_2$D) production.

VITAMIN D

Vitamin D is a secosteroid produced in the skin from 7-dehydrocholesterol under the influence of ultraviolet irradiation. Vitamin D is also found in certain foods and is used to supplement dairy products. Both the natural form (vitamin D$_3$, cholecalciferol) and the plant-derived form (vitamin D$_2$, ergocalciferol) are present in the diet. These forms differ in that ergocalciferol contains a double bond (C$_{22-23}$) and an additional methyl group in the side chain (Figure 42–2). In humans this difference apparently is of little physiologic consequence, and the following comments apply equally well to both forms of vitamin D.

Vitamin D is a prohormone that serves as precursor to a number of biologically active metabolites (Figure 42–2). Vitamin D is first hydroxylated in the liver to form 25-hydroxyvitamin D (25[OH]D). This metabolite is further converted in the kidney to a number of other forms, the best-studied of which are 1,25-dihydroxyvitamin D (1,25[OH]$_2$D) and 24,25-dihydroxyvitamin D (24,25[OH]$_2$D). Of the natural metabolites, only vitamin D, 25(OH)D (as **calcifediol**), and 1,25(OH)$_2$D (as **calcitriol**) are available for clinical use (see Table 42–1). Moreover, a number of analogs of 1,25(OH)$_2$ are being synthesized in an effort to extend the usefulness of this metabolite to a variety of nonclassic conditions. **Calcipotriene** (calcipotriol), for example, is currently being used to treat psoriasis, a hyperproliferative skin disorder. **Doxercalciferol** and **paricalcitol** have recently been approved for the treatment of secondary hyperparathyroidism in patients with renal failure. Other analogs are being investigated for the treatment of various malignancies. The regulation of vitamin D metabolism is complex, involving calcium, phosphate, and a variety of hormones, the most important of which is PTH, which stimulates the production of 1,25(OH)$_2$D by the kidney.

Vitamin D and its metabolites circulate in plasma tightly bound to a carrier protein, the vitamin D-binding protein. This α-globulin binds 25(OH)D and 24,25(OH)$_2$D with comparable high affinity and vitamin D and 1,25(OH)$_2$D with lower affinity. In normal subjects, the terminal half-life of injected calcifediol is 23 days, whereas in anephric subjects it is 42 days. The half-life of 24,25(OH)$_2$D is probably similar. Tracer studies with vitamin D have shown a rapid clearance from the blood. The liver appears to be the principal organ for clearance. Excess vitamin D is stored in adipose tissue. The metabolic clearance of calcitriol in humans indicates a rapid turnover, with a terminal half-life measured in hours. Several of the 1,25(OH)$_2$D analogs are bound poorly by the vitamin D-binding protein. As a result, their clearance is very rapid, with a terminal half-life measured in minutes. Such analogs have little of the hypercalcemic, hypercalciuric effects of

calcitriol, an important aspect of their use for the management of conditions such as psoriasis and hyperparathyroidism.

The mechanism of action of the vitamin D metabolites remains under active investigation. However, calcitriol is well established as the most potent agent with respect to stimulation of intestinal calcium and phosphate transport and bone resorption. Calcitriol appears to act on the intestine both by induction of new protein synthesis (eg, calcium-binding protein) and by modulation of calcium flux across the brush border and basolateral membranes by a means that does not require new protein synthesis. The molecular action of calcitriol on bone has received less attention. However, like PTH, calcitriol can induce RANK ligand in osteoblasts and proteins such as osteocalcin, which may regulate the

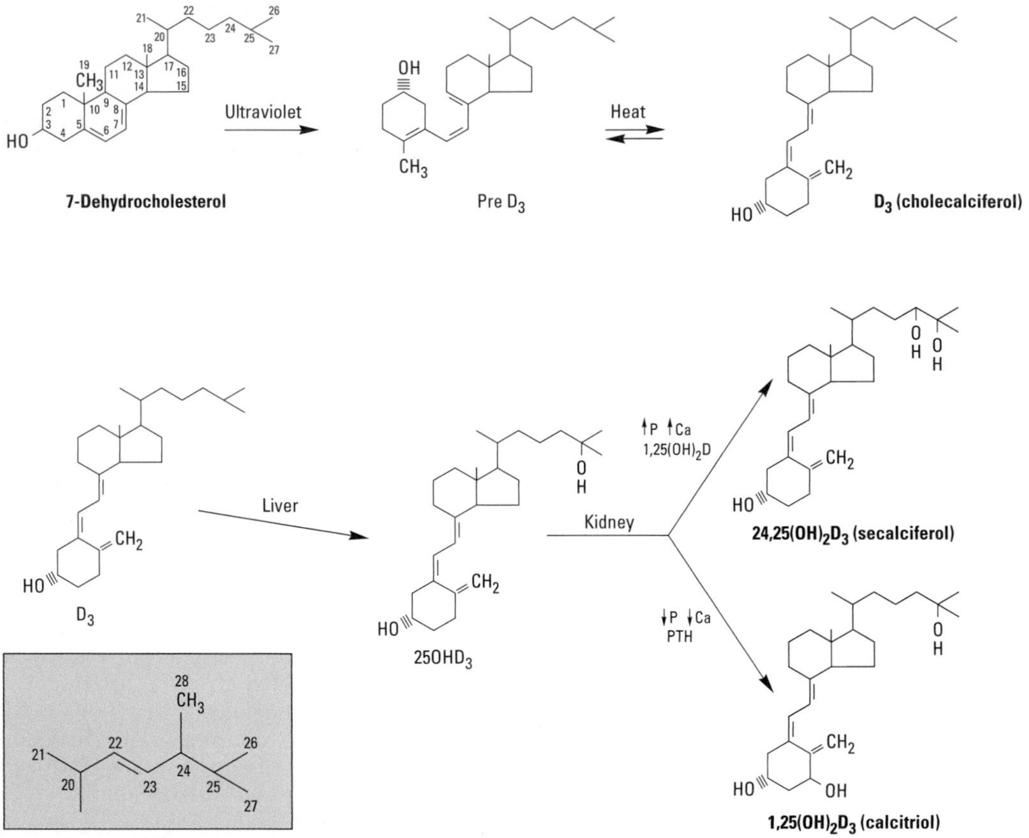

Figure 42–2. Conversion of 7-dehydrocholesterol to vitamin D$_3$ and metabolism of D$_3$ to 1,25(OH)$_2$D$_3$ and 24,25(OH)$_2$D$_3$. Control of the latter step is exerted primarily at the level of the kidney, where low serum phosphorus, low serum calcium, and high parathyroid hormone favor the production of 1,25(OH)$_2$D$_3$. The inset shows the side chain for ergosterol. Ergosterol undergoes similar transformation to vitamin D$_2$ (ergocalciferol), which, in turn, is metabolized to 25(OH)D$_2$, 1,25(OH)$_2$D$_2$, and 24,25(OH)$_2$D$_2$. In humans, corresponding D$_2$ and D$_3$ derivatives have equivalent effects and potency. They are therefore referred to in the text without a subscript.

mineralization process. The metabolites 25(OH)D and 24,25(OH)$_2$D are far less potent stimulators of intestinal calcium and phosphate transport or bone resorption. However, 25(OH)D appears to be more potent than 1,25(OH)$_2$D in stimulating renal reabsorption of calcium and phosphate and may be the major metabolite regulating calcium flux and contractility in muscle. Specific receptors for 1,25(OH)$_2$D exist in target tissues. However, the role and even the existence of receptors for 25(OH)D and 24,25(OH)$_2$D remain controversial.

The receptor for 1,25(OH)$_2$D exists in a wide variety of tissues—not just bone, gut, and kidney. In these "nonclassic" tissues, 1,25(OH)$_2$D exerts a number of actions including regulation of parathyroid hormone secretion from the parathyroid gland, insulin secretion from the pancreas, cytokine production by macrophages and T cells, and proliferation and differentiation of a large number of cells, including cancer cells. Thus, the clinical utility of 1,25(OH)$_2$D analogs is likely to expand.

INTERACTION OF PTH & VITAMIN D

A summary of the principal actions of PTH and vitamin D on the three main target tissues—intestine, kidney, and bone—is presented in Table 42–2. The net effect of PTH is to raise serum calcium and reduce serum phosphate; the net effect of vitamin D is to raise both. Regulation of calcium and phosphate homeostasis is achieved through a variety of feedback loops. Calcium is the principal regulator of PTH secretion. It binds to a novel ion recognition site that is part of a G_q protein–coupled receptor and links changes in intracellular free calcium concentration to changes in extracellular calcium. As serum calcium levels rise and bind to this receptor, intracellular calcium levels increase and inhibit PTH secretion. Phosphate regulates PTH secretion indirectly by forming complexes with calcium in the serum. Since it is the ionized concentration of calcium that is detected by the parathyroid gland, increases in serum phosphate levels reduce the ionized calcium and lead to enhanced PTH secretion. Such feedback regulation is appropriate to the net effect of PTH to raise serum calcium and reduce serum phosphate levels. Likewise, both calcium and phosphate at high levels reduce the amount of 1,25(OH)$_2$D produced by the kidney and increase the amount of 24,25(OH)$_2$D produced. Since 1,25(OH)$_2$D raises serum calcium and phosphate, whereas 24,25(OH)$_2$D has less effect, such feedback regulation is again appropriate. 1,25(OH)$_2$D itself directly inhibits PTH secretion (independently of its effect on serum calcium) by a direct action on PTH gene transcription. This provides yet another negative feedback loop, because PTH is a major stimulus for 1,25(OH)$_2$D production. This ability of 1,25(OH)$_2$D to inhibit PTH secretion directly is being exploited using calcitriol analogs that have less effect on serum calcium. Such drugs are proving useful in the management of secondary hyperparathyroidism accompanying renal failure and may be useful in selected cases of primary hyperparathyroidism.

SECONDARY HORMONAL REGULATORS OF BONE MINERAL HOMEOSTASIS

A number of hormones modulate the actions of PTH and vitamin D in regulating bone mineral homeostasis. Compared with that of PTH and vitamin D, the physiologic impact of such secondary regulation on bone mineral homeostasis is minor. However, in pharmacologic amounts, a number of these hormones have actions on the bone mineral homeostatic mechanisms that can be exploited therapeutically.

CALCITONIN

The calcitonin secreted by the parafollicular cells of the mammalian thyroid is a single-chain peptide hormone with 32 amino acids and a molecular weight of 3600. A disulfide bond between positions 1 and 7 is essential for biologic activity. Calcitonin is produced from a precursor with MW 15,000. The circulating forms of calcitonin are multiple, ranging in size from the monomer

Table 42–1. Vitamin D and its clinically available metabolites and analogs.

Chemical and Generic Names	Abbreviation
Vitamin D$_3$; cholecalciferol	D$_3$
Vitamin D$_2$; ergocalciferol	D$_2$
25-Hydroxyvitamin D$_3$; calcifediol	25(OH)D$_3$
1,25-Dihydroxyvitamin D$_3$; calcitriol	1,25(OH)$_2$D$_3$
24,25-Dihydroxyvitamin D$_3$; secalcifediol	24,25(OH)$_2$D$_3$
Dihydrotachysterol	DHT
Calcipotriene (calcipotriol)	None
1α-Hydroxyvitamin D$_2$; doxercalciferol	1α(OH)D$_2$
19-nor-1,25-Dihydroxyvitamin D$_2$; paricalcitol	19-nor-1,25(OH)D$_2$

Table 42–2. Actions of PTH and vitamin D on gut, bone, and kidney.

	PTH	Vitamin D
Intestine	Increased calcium and phosphate absorption (by increased 1,25 [OH]$_2$D production)	Increased calcium and phosphate absorption by 1,25(OH)$_2$D
Kidney	Decreased calcium excretion, increased phosphate excretion	Calcium and phosphate excretion may be decreased by 25(OH)D and 1,25(OH)$_2$D
Bone	Calcium and phosphate resorption increased by high doses. Low doses may increase bone formation.	Increased calcium and phosphate resorption by 1,25(OH)$_2$D; bone formation may be increased by 24,25(OH)$_2$D
Net effect on serum levels	Serum calcium increased, serum phosphate decreased	Serum calcium and phosphate both increased

(MW 3600) to forms with an apparent molecular weight of 60,000. Whether such heterogeneity includes precursor forms or covalently linked oligomers is not known. Because of its heterogeneity, calcitonin is standardized by bioassay in rats. Activity is compared to a standard maintained by the British Medical Research Council (MRC) and expressed as MRC units.

Human calcitonin monomer has a half-life of about 10 minutes with a metabolic clearance of 8–9 mL/kg/min. Salmon calcitonin has a longer half-life and a reduced metabolic clearance (3 mL/kg/min), making it more attractive as a therapeutic agent. Much of the clearance occurs in the kidney, although little intact calcitonin appears in the urine.

The principal effects of calcitonin are to lower serum calcium and phosphate by actions on bone and kidney. Calcitonin inhibits osteoclastic bone resorption. Although bone formation is not impaired at first after calcitonin administration, with time both formation and resorption of bone are reduced. Thus, the early hope that calcitonin would prove useful in restoring bone mass has not been realized. In the kidney, calcitonin reduces both calcium and phosphate reabsorption as well as reabsorption of other ions, including sodium, potassium, and magnesium. Tissues other than bone and kidney are also affected by calcitonin. Calcitonin in pharmacologic amounts decreases gastrin secretion and reduces gastric acid output while increasing secretion of sodium, potassium, chloride, and water in the gut. Pentagastrin is a potent stimulator of calcitonin secretion (as is hypercalcemia), suggesting a possible physiologic relationship between gastrin and calcitonin. In the adult human, no readily demonstrable problem develops in cases of calcitonin deficiency (thyroidectomy) or excess (medullary carcinoma of the thyroid). However, the ability of calcitonin to block bone resorption and lower serum calcium makes it a useful drug for the treatment of Paget's disease, hypercalcemia, and osteoporosis.

GLUCOCORTICOIDS

Glucocorticoid hormones alter bone mineral homeostasis by antagonizing vitamin D-stimulated intestinal calcium transport, by stimulating renal calcium excretion, and by blocking bone formation. Although these observations underscore the negative impact of glucocorticoids on bone mineral homeostasis, these hormones have proved useful in reversing the hypercalcemia associated with lymphomas and granulomatous diseases such as sarcoidosis (in which production of 1,25[OH]$_2$D is increased), or in cases of vitamin D intoxication. Prolonged administration of glucocorticoids is a common cause of osteoporosis in adults and stunted skeletal development in children.

ESTROGENS

Estrogens can prevent accelerated bone loss during the immediate postmenopausal period and at least transiently increase bone in the postmenopausal subject. The prevailing hypothesis advanced to explain these observations is that estrogens reduce the bone-resorbing action of PTH. Estrogen administration leads to an increased 1,25(OH)$_2$D level in blood, but estrogens have no direct effect on 1,25(OH)$_2$D production in vitro. The increased 1,25(OH)$_2$D levels in vivo following estrogen treatment may result from decreased serum calcium and phosphate and increased PTH. Estrogen receptors have been found in bone, suggesting that estrogen may have direct effects on bone remodeling. Recent case reports of men lacking the estrogen receptor or unable to produce estrogen because of aromatase deficiency noted marked osteopenia and failure to close epiphyses, further substantiating the role of estrogen in bone development, even in men. The principal therapeutic application for estrogen administration in disorders of bone mineral homeostasis is the treatment or prevention of postmenopausal osteoporosis. This application will increase as estrogen analogs lacking some of the deleterious effects of estrogen are developed (see Box, New Therapies for Osteoporosis).

NONHORMONAL AGENTS AFFECTING BONE MINERAL HOMEOSTASIS

BISPHOSPHONATES

The bisphosphonates are analogs of pyrophosphate in which the P–O–P bond has been replaced with a non-hydrolyzable P–C–P bond (Figure 42–3). **Etidronate, pamidronate,** and **alendronate** have now been joined by **risedronate, tiludronate,** and **zoledronate** for clinical use, and newer forms are likely to be available soon. The bisphosphonates owe at least part of their clinical usefulness and toxicity to their ability to retard formation and dissolution of hydroxyapatite crystals within and outside the skeletal system. However, the exact mechanism by which they selectively inhibit bone resorption is not clear.

The results from animal and clinical studies indicate that less than 10% of an oral dose of these drugs is absorbed. Food reduces absorption even further, necessitating their administration on an empty stomach. Because it causes gastric irritation, pamidronate is not available as an oral preparation. However, with the possible exception of etidronate, all currently available bisphosphonates have this complication. Nearly half of the absorbed drug accumulates in bone; the remainder is excreted unchanged in the urine. Decreased renal function, esophageal motility disorders, and peptic ulcer disease are the main contraindications to the use of these drugs. The portion bound to bone is retained for months, depending on the turnover of bone itself.

Etidronate and the other bisphosphonates exert a variety of effects on bone mineral homeostasis. Their physicochemical action of reducing hydroxyapatite formation and dissolution make them clinically useful. In particular, bisphosphonates are being evaluated for the treatment of hypercalcemia associated with malignancy, osteoporosis, and syndromes of ectopic calcification. Their usefulness in the management of Paget's disease is well established. Only alendronate and risedronate have been approved for the treatment of osteoporosis, but other bisphosphonates are being developed for this purpose. (See Box, New Therapies for Osteoporosis.) Contrary to expectations, alendronate appears to increase bone mineral density well beyond the 2-year period predicted for a drug whose effects are limited to blocking bone resorption. The bisphosphonates exert a variety of other cellular effects, including inhibition of $1,25(OH)_2D$ production, inhibition of intestinal cal-

cium transport, metabolic changes in bone cells such as inhibition of glycolysis, inhibition of cell growth, and changes in acid and alkaline phosphatase. Amino bisphosphonates such as alendronate have recently been found to block farnesyl pyrophosphate synthase, an enzyme in the mevalonate pathway that appears to be critical for osteoclast survival. Statins, which block mevalonate synthesis, stimulate bone formation at least in animal studies. Thus, the mevalonate pathway appears to be important in bone cell function and provides new targets for drug development. These effects vary depending on the bisphosphonate being studied (ie, only amino bisphosphonates have this property) and may account for some of the clinical differences observed in the effects of the various bisphosphonates on bone mineral homeostasis. However, with the exception of the induction of a mineralization defect by higher than approved doses of etidronate and gastric and esophageal irritation by pamidronate and by high doses of alendronate, these drugs have proved to be remarkably free of adverse effects. Esophageal irritation can be minimized by taking the drug with a full glass of water and remaining upright for 30 minutes.

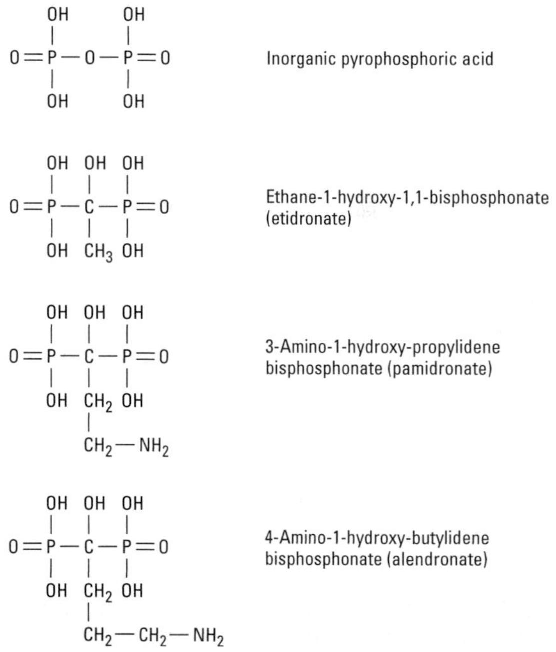

Figure 42–3. The structure of pyrophosphate and of the first three bisphosphonates—etidronate, pamidronate, and alendronate—that were approved for use in the USA.

PLICAMYCIN (MITHRAMYCIN)

Plicamycin is a cytotoxic antibiotic (see Chapter 55) that has been used clinically for two disorders of bone mineral metabolism: Paget's disease and hypercalcemia. The cytotoxic properties of the drug appear to involve its binding to DNA and interruption of DNA-directed RNA synthesis. The reasons for its usefulness in the treatment of Paget's disease and hypercalcemia are unclear but may relate to the need for protein synthesis to sustain bone resorption. The doses required to treat Paget's disease and hypercalcemia are about one tenth the amounts required to achieve cytotoxic effects.

THIAZIDES

The chemistry and pharmacology of this family of drugs are covered in Chapter 15. The principal application of thiazides in the treatment of bone mineral disorders is in reducing renal calcium excretion. Thiazides may increase the effectiveness of parathyroid hormone in stimulating reabsorption of calcium by the renal tubules or may act on calcium reabsorption secondarily by increasing sodium reabsorption in the proximal tubule. In the distal tubule, thiazides block sodium reabsorption at the luminal surface, increasing the calcium-sodium exchange at the basolateral membrane and thus enhancing calcium reabsorption into the blood at this site. Thiazides have proved to be quite useful in reducing the hypercalciuria and incidence of stone formation in subjects with idiopathic hypercalciuria. Part of their efficacy in reducing stone formation may lie in their ability to decrease urine oxalate excretion and increase urine magnesium and zinc levels (both of which inhibit calcium oxalate stone formation).

FLUORIDE

Fluoride is well established as effective for the prophylaxis of dental caries and has been under investigation for the treatment of osteoporosis. Both therapeutic applications originated from epidemiologic observations that subjects living in areas with naturally fluoridated water (1–2 ppm) had less dental caries and fewer vertebral compression fractures than subjects living in non-fluoridated water areas. Fluoride is accumulated by bones and teeth, where it may stabilize the hydroxyapatite crystal. Such a mechanism may explain the effectiveness of fluoride in increasing the resistance of teeth to dental caries, but it does not explain new bone growth.

Fluoride in drinking water appears to be most effective in preventing dental caries if consumed prior to the eruption of the permanent teeth. The optimum concentration in drinking water supplies is 0.5–1 ppm. Topical application is most effective if done just as the teeth erupt. There is little further benefit to giving fluoride after the permanent teeth are fully formed. Excess fluoride in drinking water leads to mottling of the enamel proportionate to the concentration above 1 ppm.

Because of the paucity of agents that stimulate new bone growth in patients with osteoporosis, the use of fluoride for this disorder has been examined (see Osteoporosis, below). Results of earlier studies indicated that fluoride alone without adequate calcium supplementation produced osteomalacia. More recent studies, in which calcium supplementation has been adequate, have demonstrated an improvement in calcium balance, an increase in bone mineral, and an increase in trabecular bone volume. However, studies of the ability of fluoride to reduce fractures reach opposite conclusions. Adverse effects observed—at the doses used for testing fluoride's effect on bone—include nausea and vomiting, gastrointestinal blood loss, arthralgias, and arthritis in a substantial proportion of patients. Such effects are usually responsive to reduction of the dose or giving fluoride with meals (or both). At present, fluoride is not approved by the Food and Drug Administration for use in osteoporosis.

II. CLINICAL PHARMACOLOGY

Disorders of bone mineral homeostasis generally present with abnormalities in serum or urine calcium levels (or both), often accompanied by abnormal serum phosphate levels. These abnormal mineral concentrations may themselves cause symptoms requiring immediate treatment (eg, coma in malignant hypercalcemia, tetany in hypocalcemia). More commonly, they serve as clues to an underlying disorder in hormonal regulators (eg, primary hyperparathyroidism), target tissue response (eg, chronic renal failure), or drug misuse (eg, vitamin D intoxication). In such cases, treatment of the underlying disorder is of prime importance.

Since bone and kidney play central roles in bone mineral homeostasis, conditions that alter bone mineral homeostasis usually affect either or both of these tissues secondarily. Effects on bone can result in osteoporosis (abnormal loss of bone; remaining bone histologically normal), osteomalacia (abnormal bone formation due to inadequate mineralization), or osteitis fibrosa (excessive bone resorption with fibrotic replacement of resorption cavities). Biochemical markers of skeletal involvement include changes in serum levels of the skeletal isoenzyme of alkaline phosphatase and osteocalcin (reflecting osteoblastic activity) and urine levels of hydroxyproline and pyridinoline cross-links (reflecting osteoclastic activity). The kidney becomes involved when the calcium-times-phosphate product in serum exceeds the point at which ectopic calcification occurs (nephrocalcinosis) or when the calcium-times-oxalate (or phosphate) product in urine exceeds saturation, leading to nephrolithiasis. Subtle early indicators of such renal involvement include polyuria, nocturia, and hyposthenuria. Radiologic evidence of nephrocalcinosis and stones is not generally observed until later. The degree of the ensuing renal failure is best followed by monitoring the decline in creatinine clearance.

ABNORMAL SERUM CALCIUM & PHOSPHATE LEVELS

HYPERCALCEMIA

Hypercalcemia causes central nervous system depression, including coma, and is potentially lethal. Its major causes (other than thiazide therapy) are hyperparathyroidism and cancer with or without bone metastases. Less common causes are hypervitaminosis D, sarcoidosis, thyrotoxicosis, milk-alkali syndrome, adrenal insufficiency, and immobilization. With the possible exception of hypervitaminosis D, these latter disorders seldom require emergency lowering of serum calcium. A number of approaches are used to manage the hypercalcemic crisis.

Saline Diuresis

In hypercalcemia of sufficient severity to produce symptoms, rapid reduction of serum calcium is required. The first steps include rehydration with saline and diuresis with furosemide. Most patients presenting with severe hypercalcemia have a substantial component of prerenal azotemia owing to dehydration, which prevents the kidney from compensating for the rise in serum calcium by excreting more calcium in the urine. Therefore, the initial infusion of 500—1000 mL/h of saline to reverse the dehydration and restore urine flow can by itself substantially lower serum calcium. The addition of a loop diuretic such as furosemide not only enhances urine flow but also inhibits calcium reabsorption in the ascending limb of the loop of Henle (see Chapter 15). Monitoring central venous pressure is important to forestall the development of heart failure and pulmonary edema in predisposed subjects. In many subjects, saline diuresis will suffice to reduce serum calcium levels to a point at which more definitive diagnosis and treatment of the underlying condition can be achieved. If this is not the case or if more prolonged medical treatment of hypercalcemia is required, the following agents are available (discussed in order of preference).

Bisphosphonates

Etidronate, 7.5 mg/kg in 250–500 mL saline, infused over several hours each day for 3 days, has proved quite useful in treating hypercalcemia of malignancy. More recently, pamidronate, 60–90 mg, infused over 2–4 hours, and zoledronate, 4 mg, infused over 15 minutes, have been approved for the same indication and appear to be more effective. This form of treatment is remarkably free of toxicity. The effects generally persist for weeks, but treatment can be repeated after a 7-day interval if necessary and if renal function is not impaired.

Calcitonin

Calcitonin has proved useful as ancillary treatment in a large number of patients. Calcitonin by itself seldom restores serum calcium to normal, and refractoriness frequently develops. However, its lack of toxicity permits frequent administration at high doses (200 MRC units or more). An effect on serum calcium is observed within 4–6 hours and lasts for 6–10 hours. Calcimar (salmon calcitonin) is available for parenteral and nasal administration.

Gallium Nitrate

Gallium nitrate is approved by the Food and Drug Administration for the management of hypercalcemia of malignancy and is undergoing trials for the treatment of advanced Paget's disease. This drug acts by inhibiting bone resorption. At a dosage of 200 mg/m² body surface area per day given as a continuous intravenous infusion in 5% dextrose for 5 days, gallium nitrate proved superior to calcitonin in reducing serum calcium in cancer patients. Because of potential nephrotoxicity, patients should be well-hydrated and have good renal output before starting the infusion.

Plicamycin (Mithramycin)

Because of its toxicity, plicamycin (mithramycin) is not the drug of first choice for the treatment of hypercalcemia. However, when other forms of therapy fail, 25–50 µg/kg given intravenously usually lowers serum calcium substantially within 24–48 hours. This effect can last for several days. This dose can be repeated as necessary. The most dangerous toxic effect is sudden thrombocytopenia followed by hemorrhage. Hepatic and renal toxicity can also occur. Hypocalcemia, nausea, and vomiting may limit therapy. Use of this drug must be accompanied by careful monitoring of platelet counts, liver and kidney function, and serum calcium levels.

Phosphate

Giving intravenous phosphate is probably the fastest and surest way to reduce serum calcium, but it is a hazardous procedure if not done properly. Intravenous phosphate should be used only after other methods of treatment (pamidronate, calcitonin, saline diuresis with furosemide, and plicamycin) have failed to control symptomatic hypercalcemia. Phosphate must be given slowly (50 mmol or 1.5 g elemental phosphorus over 6–8 hours) and the patient switched to oral phosphate (1–2 g/d elemental phosphorus, as one of the salts indicated below) as soon as symptoms of hypercalcemia have cleared. The risks of intravenous phosphate therapy include sudden hypocalcemia, ectopic calcification, acute renal failure, and hypotension. Oral phosphate can also lead to ectopic calcification and renal failure if serum calcium and phosphate levels are not carefully monitored, but the risk is less and the time of onset much longer. Phosphate is available in oral and intravenous forms as the sodium or potassium salt. Amounts required to provide 1 g of elemental phosphorus are as follows:

> **Intravenous:**
> In-Phos: 40 mL
> Hyper-Phos-K: 15 mL
> **Oral:**
> Fleet Phospho-Soda: 6.2 mL
> Neutra-Phos: 300 mL
> K-Phos-Neutral: 4 tablets

Glucocorticoids

Glucocorticoids have no clear role in the acute treatment of hypercalcemia. However, the chronic hypercalcemia of sarcoidosis, vitamin D intoxication, and certain cancers may respond within several days to glucocorticoid therapy. Prednisone in oral doses of 30–60 mg daily is generally used, though equivalent doses of other glucocorticoids are effective. The rationale for the use of glucocorticoids in these diseases differs, however. The hypercalcemia of sarcoidosis is secondary to increased production of $1,25(OH)_2D$, possibly by the sarcoid tissue itself. Glucocorticoid therapy directed at the reduction of sarcoid tissue results in restoration of normal serum calcium and $1,25(OH)_2D$ levels. The treatment of hypervitaminosis D with glucocorticoids probably does not alter vitamin D metabolism significantly but is thought to reduce vitamin D-mediated intestinal calcium transport. An action of glucocorticoids to reduce vitamin D-mediated bone resorption has not been excluded, however. The effect of glucocorticoids on the hypercalcemia of cancer is probably twofold. The malignancies responding best to gluco-corticoids (ie, multiple myeloma and related lympho-proliferative diseases) are sensitive to the lytic action of glucocorticoids, so part of the effect may be related to decreased tumor mass and activity. Glucocorticoids have also been shown to inhibit the secretion or effectiveness of cytokines elaborated by multiple myeloma and related cancers that stimulate osteoclastic bone resorption. Other causes of hypercalcemia—particularly primary hyperparathyroidism—do not respond to glucocorticoid therapy.

HYPOCALCEMIA

The main features of hypocalcemia are neuromuscular—tetany, paresthesias, laryngospasm, muscle cramps, and convulsions. The major causes of hypocalcemia in the adult are hypoparathyroidism, vitamin D deficiency, renal failure, and malabsorption. Neonatal hypocalcemia is a common disorder that usually resolves without therapy. The roles of PTH, vitamin D, and calcitonin in the neonatal syndrome are under active investigation. Large infusions of citrated blood can produce hypocalcemia by the formation of citrate-calcium complexes. Calcium and vitamin D (or its metabolites) form the mainstay of treatment of hypocalcemia.

Calcium

A number of calcium preparations are available for intravenous, intramuscular, and oral use. Calcium gluceptate (0.9 meq calcium/mL), calcium gluconate (0.45 meq calcium/mL), and calcium chloride (0.68–1.36 meq calcium/mL) are available for intravenous therapy. Calcium gluconate is the preferred form because it is less irritating to veins. Oral preparations include calcium carbonate (40% calcium), calcium lactate (13% calcium), calcium phosphate (25% calcium), and calcium citrate (21% calcium). Calcium carbonate is often the preparation of choice because of its high percentage of calcium, ready availability (eg, Tums), low cost, and antacid properties. In achlorhydric patients, calcium carbonate should be given with meals to increase absorption or the patient switched to calcium citrate, which is somewhat better absorbed. Combinations of vitamin D and calcium are available, but treatment must be tailored to the individual patient and individual disease, a flexibility lost by fixed-dosage combinations. Treatment of severe symptomatic hypocalcemia can be accomplished with slow infusion of 5–20 mL of 10% calcium gluconate. Rapid infusion can lead to cardiac arrhythmias. Less severe hypocalcemia is best treated with oral forms sufficient to provide approximately 400–800 mg of elemental calcium (1–2 g calcium carbonate) per day. Dosage must be adjusted to avoid hypercalcemia and hypercalciuria.

Vitamin D

When rapidity of action is required, $1,25(OH)_2D_3$ (calcitriol), 0.25–1 µg daily, is the vitamin D metabolite of choice, since it is capable of raising serum calcium within 24–48 hours. Calcitriol also raises serum phosphate, though this action is usually not observed early in treatment. The combined effects of calcitriol and all other vitamin D metabolites and analogs on both calcium and phosphate make careful monitoring of these mineral levels especially important to avoid ectopic calcification secondary to an abnormally high serum calcium × phosphate product. Since the choice of the appropriate vitamin D metabolite or analog for long-term treatment of hypocalcemia depends on the nature of the underlying disease, further discussion of vitamin D treatment will be found under the headings of the specific diseases.

HYPERPHOSPHATEMIA

Hyperphosphatemia is a frequent complication of renal failure but is also found in all types of hypoparathyroidism (idiopathic, surgical, and pseudo), vitamin D intoxication, and the rare syndrome of tumoral calcinosis. Emergency treatment of hyperphosphatemia is seldom necessary but can be achieved by dialysis or glucose and insulin infusions. In general, control of hyperphosphatemia involves restriction of dietary phosphate plus the use of phosphate binding gels such as sevelamer and of calcium supplements. Because of their potential to induce aluminum-associated bone disease, aluminum-containing antacids should be used sparingly and only when other measures fail to control the hyperphosphatemia.

HYPOPHOSPHATEMIA

A variety of conditions are associated with hypophosphatemia, including primary hyperparathyroidism, vitamin D deficiency, idiopathic hypercalciuria, vitamin D-resistant rickets, various other forms of renal phosphate wasting (eg, Fanconi's syndrome), overzealous use of phosphate binders, and parenteral nutrition with inadequate phosphate content. Acute hypophosphatemia may lead to a reduction in the intracellular levels of high-energy organic phosphates (eg, ATP), interfere with normal hemoglobin-to-tissue oxygen transfer by decreasing red cell 2,3-diphosphoglycerate levels, and lead to rhabdomyolysis. However, clinically significant acute effects of hypophosphatemia are seldom seen, and emergency treatment is generally not indicated. The long-term effects of hypophosphatemia include proximal muscle weakness and abnormal bone mineralization (osteomalacia). Therefore, hypophosphatemia should be avoided during other forms of therapy and treated in conditions such as hypophosphatemic rickets of which it is a cardinal feature. Oral forms of phosphate available for use are listed above in the section on hypercalcemia.

SPECIFIC DISORDERS INVOLVING THE BONE MINERAL-REGULATING HORMONES

PRIMARY HYPERPARATHYROIDISM

This rather common disease, if associated with symptoms and significant hypercalcemia, is best treated surgically. Oral phosphate and bisphosphonates have been tried but cannot be recommended. Asymptomatic patients with mild disease in general do not get worse and may be left untreated. The **calcimimetic agents,** a new class of drugs that act through the calcium receptor, are in clinical trials. If they prove efficacious, medical management of this disease will need to be reconsidered.

HYPOPARATHYROIDISM

In the absence of PTH (idiopathic or surgical hypoparathyroidism) or a normal target tissue response to PTH (pseudohypoparathyroidism), serum calcium falls and serum phosphate rises. In such patients, $1,25(OH)_2D$ levels are usually low, presumably reflecting the lack of stimulation by PTH of $1,25(OH)_2D$ production. The skeletons of patients with idiopathic or surgical hypoparathyroidism are normal except for a slow turnover rate. A number of patients with pseudohypoparathyroidism appear to have osteitis fibrosa, suggesting that the normal or high PTH levels found in such patients are capable of acting on bone but not on the kidney. The distinction between pseudohypoparathyroidism and idiopathic hypoparathyroidism is made on the basis of normal or high PTH levels but deficient renal response (ie, diminished excretion of cAMP or phosphate) in patients with pseudohypoparathyroidism.

The principal therapeutic concern is to restore normocalcemia and normophosphatemia. Under most circumstances, vitamin D (25,000–100,000 units three times per week) and dietary calcium supplements suffice. More rapid increments in serum calcium can be achieved with calcitriol, though it is not clear that this metabolite offers a substantial advantage over vitamin D itself for long-term therapy. Many patients treated with vitamin D develop episodes of hypercalcemia. This complication is more rapidly reversible with cessation of therapy using calcitriol rather than vitamin D. This would be of importance to the patient in whom such hypercalcemic crises are common. Dihydrotachysterol and 25(OH)D have not received much study as therapy for hypoparathyroidism, though both should be effective. Whether they offer advantages over vitamin D sufficient to justify their added expense remains to be seen.

NUTRITIONAL RICKETS

Vitamin D deficiency, once thought to be rare in this country, is being recognized more often, especially in the pediatric and geriatric populations on vegetarian diets and with reduced sunlight exposure. This problem can be avoided by daily intake of 400–800 units of vitamin D and treated by higher dosages (4000 units per day). No other metabolite is indicated. The diet should also contain adequate amounts of calcium and phosphate.

CHRONIC RENAL FAILURE

The major problems of chronic renal failure that impact on bone mineral homeostasis are the loss of $1,25(OH)_2D$ and $24,25(OH)_2D$ production, the retention of phosphate that reduces ionized calcium levels, and the secondary hyperparathyroidism that results. With the loss of $1,25(OH)_2D$ production, less calcium is absorbed from the intestine and less bone is resorbed under the influence of PTH. As a result hypocalcemia usually develops, furthering the development of hyperparathyroidism. The bones show a mixture of osteomalacia and osteitis fibrosa.

In contrast to the hypocalcemia that is more often associated with chronic renal failure, some patients may become hypercalcemic from two causes (in addition to overzealous treatment with calcium). The most common cause of hypercalcemia is the development of severe secondary (sometimes referred to as tertiary) hyperparathyroidism. In such cases, the PTH level in blood is very high. Serum alkaline phosphatase levels also tend to be high. Treatment often requires parathyroidectomy.

A less common circumstance leading to hypercalcemia is development of a form of osteomalacia characterized by a profound decrease in bone cell activity and loss of the calcium buffering action of bone. In the absence of kidney function, any calcium absorbed from the intestine accumulates in the blood. Therefore, such patients are very sensitive to the hypercalcemic action of $1,25(OH)_2D$. These individuals generally have a high serum calcium but nearly normal alkaline phosphatase and PTH levels. The bone in such patients generally has a high aluminum content, especially in the mineralization front, which may block normal bone mineralization. These patients do not respond favorably to parathyroidectomy. Deferoxamine, an agent used to chelate iron (see Chapter 58), also binds aluminum and is being used as therapy for this disorder.

Use of Vitamin D Preparations

The choice of vitamin D preparation to be used in the setting of chronic renal failure in the dialysis patient depends on the type and extent of bone disease and hyperparathyroidism. No consensus has been reached regarding the advisability of using any vitamin D metabolite in the predialysis patient. $1,25(OH)_2D_3$ (calcitriol) will rapidly correct hypocalcemia and at least partially reverse the secondary hyperparathyroidism and osteitis fibrosa. Many patients with muscle weakness and bone pain gain an improved sense of well-being.

Dihydrotachysterol, an analog of $1,25(OH)_2D$, is also available for clinical use, though it is used much less frequently than calcitriol. Dihydrotachysterol appears to be as effective as calcitriol, differing principally in its time course of action; calcitriol increases serum calcium in 1–2 days, whereas dihydrotachysterol requires 1–2 weeks. For an equipotent dose (0.2 mg dihydrotachysterol versus 0.5 µg calcitriol), dihydrotachysterol costs about one fourth as much as calcitriol. A disadvantage of dihydrotachysterol is the inability to measure it in serum. Neither dihydrotachysterol nor calcitriol corrects the osteomalacic component of renal osteodystrophy in the majority of patients, and neither should be used in patients with hypercalcemia, especially if the bone disease is primarily osteomalacic.

Calcifediol ($25[OH]D_3$) may also be used to advantage. Calcifediol is less effective than calcitriol in stimulating intestinal calcium transport, so that hypercalcemia is less of a problem with calcifediol. Like dihydrotachysterol, calcifediol requires several weeks to restore normocalcemia in hypocalcemic individuals with chronic renal failure. Presumably because of the reduced ability of the diseased kidney to metabolize calcifediol to more active metabolites, high doses (50–100 µg daily) must be given to achieve the supraphysiologic serum levels required for therapeutic effectiveness.

Vitamin D has been used in treating renal osteodystrophy. However, patients with a substantial degree of renal failure who are thus unable to convert vitamin D to its active metabolites usually are refractory to vitamin D. Its use is decreasing as more effective alternatives become available.

Two analogs of calcitriol, doxercalciferol and paricalcitol, are approved for the treatment of secondary hyperparathyroidism of chronic renal failure. Their principal advantage is that they are less likely than calcitriol to induce hypercalcemia. Their biggest impact will be in patients in whom the use of calcitriol may lead to unacceptably high serum calcium levels.

Regardless of the drug employed, careful attention to serum calcium and phosphate levels is required. Calcium supplements (dietary and in the dialysate) and phosphate restriction (dietary and with oral ingestion of phosphate binders) should be employed along with the use of vitamin D metabolites. Monitoring serum PTH and alkaline phosphatase levels is useful in determining whether therapy is correcting or preventing secondary hyperparathyroidism. Although not generally available, percutaneous bone biopsies for quantitative histomorphometry may help in choosing appropriate therapy and following the effectiveness of such therapy. Unlike the rapid changes in serum values, changes in bone morphology require months to years. Monitoring serum levels of the vitamin D metabolites is useful to determine compliance, absorption, and metabolism.

INTESTINAL OSTEODYSTROPHY

A number of gastrointestinal and hepatic diseases result in disordered calcium and phosphate homeostasis that ultimately leads to bone disease. The bones in such patients show a combination of osteoporosis and osteomalacia. Osteitis fibrosa does not occur (as it does in renal osteodystrophy). The common features that appear to be important in this group of diseases are malabsorption of calcium and vitamin D. Liver disease may, in addition, reduce the production of 25(OH)D from vitamin D, though the importance of this in all but patients with terminal liver failure remains in dispute. The malabsorption of vitamin D is probably not limited to exogenous vitamin D. The liver secretes into bile a substantial number of vitamin D metabolites and conjugates that are reabsorbed in (presumably) the distal jejunum and ileum. Interference with this process could deplete the body of endogenous vitamin D metabolites as well as limit absorption of dietary vitamin D.

In mild forms of malabsorption, vitamin D (25,000–50,000 units three times per week) should suffice to raise serum levels of 25(OH)D into the normal range. Many patients with severe disease do not respond to vitamin D. Clinical experience with the other metabolites is limited, but both calcitriol and calcifediol have been used successfully in doses similar to those recommended for treatment of renal osteodystrophy. Theoretically, calcifediol should be the drug of choice under these conditions, since no impairment of the renal metabolism of 25(OH)D to 1,25(OH)$_2$D and 24,25(OH)$_2$D exists in these patients. Both calcitriol and 24,25(OH)$_2$D may be of importance in reversing the bone disease. As in the other diseases discussed, treatment of intestinal osteodystrophy with vitamin D and its metabolites should be accompanied by appropriate dietary calcium supplementation and monitoring of serum calcium and phosphate levels.

OSTEOPOROSIS

Osteoporosis is defined as abnormal loss of bone predisposing to fractures. The estimated annual cost of fractures in older women and men in the USA was $13.8 billion (Incidence and costs, 1996). It is most common in postmenopausal women but also occurs in men. It may occur as a side effect of chronic administration of glucocorticoids or other drugs; as a manifestation of endocrine disease such as thyrotoxicosis or hyperparathyroidism; as a feature of malabsorption syndrome; as a consequence of alcohol abuse and cigarette smoking; or without obvious cause (idiopathic). The ability of some agents to reverse the bone loss of osteoporosis is shown in Figure 42–4. The postmenopausal form of osteoporosis may be accompanied by lower 1,25(OH)$_2$D levels and reduced intestinal calcium transport. This form of osteoporosis is due to estrogen deficiency and can be treated with estrogen (cycled with a progestin in women with a uterus to prevent endometrial carcinoma). However, concern that estrogen increases the risk of breast cancer and fails to reduce the development of heart disease has reduced enthusiasm for this form of therapy. Several estrogen-like drugs called SERMs (selective estrogen receptor modulators) have been developed that avoid the increased risk of breast and uterine cancer associated with estrogen while maintaining the benefit to bone. **Raloxifene** is such a drug approved for treatment of osteoporosis. Like tamoxifen, it appears to reduce the risk of breast cancer. Raloxifene protects against spine fractures but not hip fractures—unlike bisphosphonates and teriparatide, which protect against both. Raloxifene does not prevent hot flushes and imposes the same increased risk of thrombophlebitis as estrogen. To counter the reduced intestinal calcium transport associated with osteoporosis, vitamin D therapy is often employed in addition to dietary calcium supplementation. There is no clear evidence that pharmacologic doses of vitamin D are of much additional benefit beyond cyclic estrogens and calcium supplementation. However, in several large studies, vitamin D supplementation (400–800 IU/d) has been shown to be useful. In addition, calcitriol and its analog 1α(OH)D$_3$ have been shown to increase bone mass and reduce fractures in several recent studies. Use of these agents for osteoporosis is not FDA-approved, though they are used in other countries.

Despite early promise that **fluoride** might be useful in the prevention or treatment of postmenopausal osteoporosis, this form of therapy remains controversial. A new formulation of fluoride (slow release, lower dose) appears to avoid much of the toxicity of earlier formulations and may reduce fracture rates. This formulation is under consideration for approval by the FDA. **Teriparatide,** the recombinant form of PTH 1-34, has recently been approved for treatment of osteoporosis. Teriparatide is given in a dosage 20 μg subcutaneously daily. Like fluoride, teriparatide stimulates new bone formation, but unlike fluoride this new bone appears

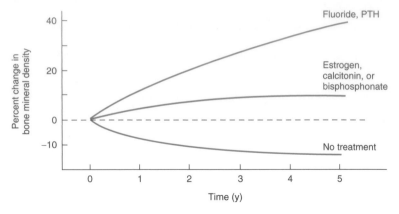

Figure 42–4. Typical changes in bone mineral density with time after the onset of menopause, with and without treatment. In the untreated condition, bone is lost during aging in both men and women. Fluoride and PTH promote new bone formation and can increase bone mineral density in subjects who respond to it throughout the period of treatment. In contrast, estrogen, calcitonin, and bisphosphonates block bone resorption. This leads to a transient increase in bone mineral density because bone formation is not initially decreased. However, with time, both bone formation and bone resorption are decreased and bone mineral density reaches a new plateau.

structurally normal and is associated with a substantial reduction in the incidence of fractures.

Calcitonin is approved for use in the treatment of postmenopausal osteoporosis. It has been shown to increase bone mass and reduce fractures, but only in the spine. It does not appear to be as effective as bisphosphonates or teriparatide.

Bisphosphonates are potent inhibitors of bone resorption. They increase bone density and reduce the risk of fractures in the hip, spine, and other locations. **Alendronate** and **risedronate** are approved for the treatment of osteoporosis, using either daily dosing schedules: alendronate 10 mg/d, risedronate 5 mg/d; or weekly schedules: alendronate 70 mg/wk, risedronate 35 mg/wk. These drugs are effective in men as well as women and for various causes of osteoporosis.

X-LINKED & AUTOSOMAL DOMINANT HYPOPHOSPHATEMIA

These disorders are manifested by the appearance of rickets and hypophosphatemia in children, though they may first present in adults. X-linked hypophosphatemia is caused by mutations in a gene encoding a protein called PHEX, which appears to be an endopeptidase. Mutations in the gene responsible for the autosomal dominant form target a newly discovered member of the fibroblast growth factor (FGF) family, FGF23. The current concept is that FGF23 blocks the renal uptake of phosphate and blocks $1,25(OH)_2D_3$ production. Normally PHEX cleaves and inactivates FGF23. Mutations in PHEX inactivate this enzyme, allowing FGF23 to accumulate. Similarly, mutations in FGF23 can prevent

cleavage by PHEX. In either case, intact and biologically active FGF23 accumulates, leading to phosphate wasting in the urine and hypophosphatemia.

Phosphate is critical to normal bone mineralization; when phosphate stores are deficient, a clinical and pathologic picture resembling vitamin D-deficient rickets develops. However, such children fail to respond to the usual doses of vitamin D employed in the treatment of nutritional rickets. A defect in $1,25(OH)_2D$ production by the kidney has also been noted, because the serum $1,25(OH)_2D$ levels tend to be low relative to the degree of hypophosphatemia observed. This combination of low serum phosphate and low or low-normal serum $1,25(OH)_2D$ provides the rationale for treating such patients with oral phosphate (1–3 g daily) and calcitriol (0.25–2 μg daily). Reports of such combination therapy are encouraging in this otherwise debilitating disease.

VITAMIN D-DEPENDENT RICKETS TYPES I & II

These distinctly different autosomal recessive diseases present as childhood rickets that does not respond to conventional doses of vitamin D. Type I vitamin D-dependent rickets is due to an isolated deficiency of $1,25(OH)_2D$ production caused by mutations in 25(OH)D-1α-hydroxylase. This condition can be treated with vitamin D (4000 units daily) or calcitriol (0.25–0.5 μg daily). Type II vitamin D-dependent rickets is caused by a target tissue defect in response to $1,25(OH)_2D$. Studies have shown a number of point mutations in the gene for the $1,25(OH)_2D$ receptor, which disrupt the functions of this receptor and lead to

NEW THERAPIES FOR OSTEOPOROSIS

Bone undergoes a continuous remodeling process involving bone resorption and formation. Any process that disrupts this balance by increasing resorption relative to formation results in osteoporosis. Inadequate sex hormone production is a major cause of osteoporosis in men and women. Estrogen replacement therapy at menopause is a well-established means of preventing osteoporosis in the female, but many women fear its adverse effects, particularly the increased risk of breast cancer from continued estrogen use (the well-demonstrated increased risk of endometrial cancer is prevented by cycling with a progestin), and do not like the persistence of menstrual bleeding that often accompanies this form of therapy. Medical enthusiasm for this treatment has waned with the demonstration that it does not protect against heart disease. Raloxifene is the first of the selective estrogen receptor modulators (SERMs; see Chapter 40) to be approved for the prevention of osteoporosis. Raloxifene shares some of the beneficial effects of estrogen on bone without increasing the risk of breast or endometrial cancer (it may actually reduce the risk of breast cancer). Although not as effective as estrogen in increasing bone density, raloxifene has been shown to reduce vertebral fractures.

Nonhormonal forms of therapy for osteoporosis with proved efficacy in reducing fracture risk have also been developed. Bisphosphonates such as alendronate and risedronate have been conclusively shown to increase bone density and reduce fractures over at least 5 years when used continuously at a dosage of 10 mg/d or 70 mg/wk for alendronate and 5 mg/d or 35 mg/wk for risedronate. Side-by-side trials between alendronate and calcitonin (another approved nonestrogen drug for osteoporosis) indicated greater efficacy for alendronate. Bisphosphonates are poorly absorbed and must be given on an empty stomach or infused intravenously. At the higher oral doses used in the treatment of Paget's disease, alendronate causes gastric irritation, but this is not a significant problem at the doses recommended for osteoporosis when patients are instructed to take the drug with a glass of water and remain upright. The most recently approved drug for osteoporosis is teriparatide, the recombinant form of PTH_{1-34}. Unlike other approved drugs for osteoporosis, teriparatide stimulates bone formation rather than inhibiting bone resorption. However, teriparatide must be given daily by subcutaneous injection. Its efficacy in preventing fractures appears to be at least as great as that of the bisphosphonates.

Thus, we now have several well-validated, efficacious forms of treatment for this common debilitating disease.

---

this syndrome. The serum levels of $1,25(OH)_2D$ are very high in type II but not in type I. Treatment with large doses of calcitriol has been claimed to be effective in restoring normocalcemia. Such patients are totally refractory to vitamin D. One recent report indicates a reversal of resistance to calcitriol when $24,25(OH)_2D$ was given. These diseases are rare.

NEPHROTIC SYNDROME

Patients with nephrotic syndrome can lose vitamin D metabolites in the urine, presumably by loss of the vitamin D-binding protein. Such patients may have very low 25(OH)D levels. Some of them develop bone disease. It is not yet clear what value vitamin D therapy has in such patients, since this complication of the nephrotic syndrome has only recently been recognized, and therapeutic trials with vitamin D (or any other vitamin D metabolite) have not yet been carried out. Since the problem is not related to vitamin D metabolism, one would not anticipate any advantage in using the more expensive vitamin D metabolites in place of vitamin D itself.

IDIOPATHIC HYPERCALCIURIA

This syndrome, characterized by hypercalciuria and nephrolithiasis with normal serum calcium and PTH levels, has been subdivided into three groups of patients: (1) hyperabsorbers, patients with increased intestinal absorption of calcium, resulting in high-normal serum calcium, low-normal PTH, and a secondary increase in urine calcium; (2) renal calcium leakers, patients with a primary decrease in renal reabsorption of filtered calcium, leading to low-normal serum calcium and high-normal serum PTH; and (3) renal phosphate leakers, patients with a primary decrease in renal reabsorption of phosphate, leading to stimulation of $1,25(OH)_2D$ production, increased intestinal calcium absorption, increased ionized serum calcium, low-normal PTH levels, and a secondary increase in urine calcium. There is some disagreement about this classification, and in many cases patients are not readily categorized. Many such patients present with mild hypophosphatemia, and oral phosphate has been used with some success to reduce stone formation. However, a clear role for phosphate in the treatment of this disorder has not been established. Therapy with hydrochlorothiazide, up to 50 mg twice daily, or chlorthalidone, 50–100 mg daily, is recommended, although equivalent doses of other thiazide diuretics work as well. Loop diuretics such as furosemide and ethacrynic acid should not be used, since they increase urinary calcium excretion. The major toxicity of thiazide diuretics, besides hypokalemia, hypomagnesemia, and hyperglycemia, is hypercalcemia. This is seldom more than a biochemical observation unless the patient has a disease such as hyperparathyroidism in which bone turnover is accelerated. Accordingly, one should screen patients for such disorders before starting thiazide therapy and monitor serum and urine calcium when therapy has begun.

An alternative to thiazides is allopurinol. Some studies indicate that hyperuricosuria is associated with idiopathic hypercalcemia and that a small nidus of urate crystals could lead to the calcium oxalate stone formation characteristic of idiopathic hypercalcemia. Allopurinol, 300 mg daily, may reduce stone formation by reducing uric acid excretion.

OTHER DISORDERS OF BONE MINERAL HOMEOSTASIS

PAGET'S DISEASE OF BONE

Paget's disease is a localized bone disease characterized by uncontrolled osteoclastic bone resorption with secondary increases in bone formation. This new bone is poorly organized, however. The cause of Paget's disease is obscure, though some studies suggest that a slow virus may be involved. The disease is fairly common, though symptomatic bone disease is less common. The biochemical parameters of elevated serum alkaline phosphatase and urinary hydroxyproline are useful for diagnosis. Along with the characteristic radiologic and bone scan findings, these biochemical determinations provide good markers by which to follow therapy. The goal of treatment is to reduce bone pain and stabilize or prevent other problems such as progressive deformity, hearing loss, high-output cardiac failure, and immobilization hypercalcemia. Calcitonin and bisphosphonates are the first-line agents for this disease. Treatment failures may respond to plicamycin. Calcitonin is administered subcutaneously or intramuscularly in doses of 50–100 MRC units every day or every other day. Nasal inhalation at 200–400 units per day is also effective. Higher or more frequent doses have been advocated when this initial regimen is ineffective. Improvement in bone pain and reduction in serum alkaline phosphatase and urine hydroxyproline levels require weeks to months. Often a patient who responds well initially will lose the response to calcitonin. This refractoriness is not correlated with the development of antibodies.

Sodium etidronate, alendronate, risedronate, and tiludronate are the bisphosphonates currently approved for clinical use in this condition in the USA. However, other bisphosphonates, including pamidronate, are being used in other countries. The recommended dosages of bisphosphonates are etidronate, 5 mg/kg/d; alendronate, 40 mg/d; risedronate, 30 mg/d; and tiludronate, 400 mg/d. Long-term (months to years) remission may be expected in patients who respond to these agents. Treatment should not exceed 6 months per course but can be repeated after 6 months if necessary. The principal toxicity of etidronate is the development of osteomalacia and an increased incidence of fractures when the dosage is raised substantially above 5 mg/kg/d. The newer bisphosphonates such as risedronate and alendronate do not share this side effect. Some patients treated with etidronate develop bone pain similar in nature to the bone pain of osteomalacia. This subsides after stopping the drug. The principal side effect of alendronate and the newer bisphosphonates is gastric irritation when used at these high doses. This is reversible on cessation of the drug.

The use of a potentially lethal cytotoxic drug such as plicamycin in a generally benign disorder such as Paget's disease is recommended only when other less toxic agents (calcitonin, alendronate) have failed and the symptoms are debilitating. Insufficient clinical data on long-term use of plicamycin are available to determine its usefulness for extended therapy. However, short courses involving 15–25 μg/kg/d intravenously for 5–10 days followed by 15 μg/kg intravenously each week have been used to control the disease.

ENTERIC OXALURIA

Patients with short bowel syndromes associated with fat malabsorption can present with renal stones composed of calcium and oxalate. Such patients characteristically have normal or low urine calcium levels but elevated urine oxalate levels. The reasons for the development of oxaluria in such patients are thought to be twofold: first, in the intestinal lumen, calcium (which is now bound to fat) fails to bind oxalate and no longer prevents its absorption; second, enteric flora, acting on the increased supply of nutrients reaching the colon, produce larger amounts of oxalate. Although one would ordinarily avoid treating a patient with calcium oxalate stones with calcium supplementation, this is precisely what is done in patients with enteric oxaluria. The increased intestinal calcium binds the excess oxalate and prevents its absorption. One to 2 g of calcium carbonate can be given daily in divided doses, with careful monitoring of urinary calcium and oxalate to be certain that urinary oxalate falls without a dangerous increase in urinary calcium.

PREPARATIONS AVAILABLE

VITAMIN D, METABOLITES, AND ANALOGS
Calcifediol (Calderol)
  Oral: 20, 50 µg capsules
Calcitriol
  Oral (Rocaltrol): 0.25, 0.5 µg capsules, 1 µg/mL solution
  Parenteral (Calcijex): 1 µg/mL for injection
Cholecalciferol [D₃] (vitamin D₃, Delta-D)
  Oral: 400, 1000 IU tablets
Dihydrotachysterol [DHT] (DHT, Hytakerol)
  Oral: 0.125 mg tablets, capsules; 0.2, 0.4 mg tablets; 0.2 mg/mL intensol solution
Doxercalciferol (Hectoral)
  Oral: 2.5 µg capsules
Ergocalciferol [D₂] (vitamin D₂, Calciferol, Drisdol)
  Oral: 50,000 IU capsules; 8000 IU/mL drops
  Parenteral: 500,000 IU/mL for injection
Paricalcitol (Zemplar)
  Parenteral: 5 µg/mL for injection

CALCIUM
Calcium acetate [25% calcium] (PhosLo)
  Oral: 668 mg (167 mg calcium) tablets; 333.5 mg (84.5 mg calcium), 667 mg (169 mg calcium) capsules
Calcium carbonate [40% calcium] (generic, Tums, Cal-Sup, Os-Cal 500, others)
  Oral: Numerous forms available containing 260–600 mg calcium per unit
Calcium chloride [27% calcium] (generic)
  Parenteral: 10% solution for IV injection only
Calcium citrate [21% calcium] (generic, Citracal)
  Oral: 950 mg (200 mg calcium), 2376 mg (500 mg calcium)
Calcium glubionate [6.5% calcium] (Calcionate, Calciquid)
  Oral: 1.8 g (115 mg calcium)/5 mL syrup
Calcium glucceptate [8% calcium] (Calcium Gluceptate)
  Parenteral: 1.1 g/5 mL solution for IM or IV injection
Calcium gluconate [9% calcium] (generic)
  Oral: 500 mg (45 mg calcium), 650 mg (58.5 mg calcium), 975 mg (87.75 mg calcium), 1 g (90 mg calcium) tablets
  Parenteral: 10% solution for IV or IM injection
Calcium lactate [13% calcium] (generic)
  Oral: 650 mg (84.5 mg calcium), 770 mg (100 mg calcium) tablets
Tricalcium phosphate [39% calcium] (Posture)
  Oral: 1565 mg (600 mg calcium) tablets (as phosphate)

PHOSPHATE AND PHOSPHATE BINDER
Phosphate
  Oral (Fleet Phospho-soda): solution containing 2.5 g phosphate/5 mL (816 mg phosphorus/5 mL; 751 mg sodium/5 mL)
  Oral (K-Phos-Neutral): tablets containing 250 mg phosphorus, 298 mg sodium
  Oral (Neutra-Phos): For reconstitution in 75 mL water, packet containing 250 mg phosphorus; 164 mg sodium; 278 mg potassium
  Oral (Neutra-Phos-K): For reconstitution in 75 mL water, packet containing 250 mg phosphorus; 556 mg potassium; 0 mg sodium
  Parenteral (potassium or sodium phosphate): 3 mmol/mL
Sevelamer (Renagel)
  Oral: 403 mg capsules

OTHER DRUGS
Alendronate (Fosamax)
  Oral: 5, 10, 35, 40, 70 mg tablets
Calcitonin-Salmon
  Nasal spray (Miacalcin): 200 IU/puff
  Parenteral (Calcimar, Miacalcin, Salmonine): 200 IU/mL for injection
Etidronate (Didronel)
  Oral: 200, 400 mg tablets
  Parenteral: 300 mg/6 mL for IV injection
Gallium nitrate (Ganite)
  Parenteral: 500 mg/20 mL vial
Pamidronate (generic, Aredia)
  Parenteral: 30, 60, 90 mg/vial
Plicamycin (mithramycin) (Mithracin)
  Parenteral: 2.5 mg per vial powder to reconstitute for injection
Risedronate (Actonel)
  Oral: 5, 30, 35 mg tablets
Sodium fluoride (generic)
  Oral: 0.55 mg (0.25 mg F), 1.1 mg (0.5 mg F), 2.2 mg (1.0 mg F) tablets; drops
Teriparatide (Forteo)
  Subcutaneous: 250 µg/mL from prefilled pen (3 mL)
Tiludronate (Skelid)
  Oral: 200 mg tablets
Zoledronic acid (Zometa)
  Parenteral: 4 mg/vial

REFERENCES

Austin LA, Heath HH III: Calcitonin: Physiology and pathophysiology. N Engl J Med 1981;304:269.

Berenson JR et al: American Society of Clinical Oncology clinical practice guidelines: The role of bisphosphonates in multiple myeloma. J Clin Oncol 2002;20:3719.

Bikle DD: Role of vitamin D, its metabolites, and analogs in the management of osteoporosis. Rheum Dis Clin North Am 1994;20:759.

Bikle DD: Vitamins D: New actions, new analogs, new therapeutic potential. Endocr Rev 1992;13:765.

Bilezikian JP: Management of acute hypercalcemia. N Engl J Med 1992;326:1196.

Chapuy MC et al: Vitamin D_3 and calcium to prevent hip fractures in elderly women. N Engl J Med 1992;327:1637.

Fisher JE, Rodan GA, Reszka AA: In vivo effects of bisphosphonates on the osteoclast mevalonate pathway. Endocrinology 2000;141:4793.

Hughes MR et al: Point mutations in the human vitamin D receptor gene associated with hypocalcemic rickets. Science 1988;242:1702.

HYP Consortium: A gene *(PEX)* with homologies to endopeptidases is mutated in patients with X-linked hypophosphatemic rickets. The HYP Consortium. Nat Genet 1995;11:130.

Incidence and costs to Medicare of fractures among Medicare beneficiaries ≥ 65 years—United States, July 1991–June 1992. MMWR Morb Mortal Wkly Rep 1996;45:877.

LaCroix AZ et al: Low-dose hydrochlorothiazide and preservation of bone mineral density in older adults. Ann Intern Med 2000;133:516.

Liberman et al: Effect of oral alendronate on bone mineral density and the incidence of fractures in postmenopausal osteoporosis. N Engl J Med 1995;333:1437.

Malluche HH et al: The use of deferoxamine in the management of aluminum accumulation in bone in patients with renal failure. N Engl J Med 1984;311:140.

Manolagas SC: Birth and death of bone cells: basic regulatory mechanisms and implications for the pathogenesis and treatment of osteoporosis. Endocr Rev 2000;21:115.

McClung MR et al: Effect of risedronate on the risk of hip fracture in elderly women. N Engl J Med 2001;344:333.

McIntyre CW et al: A prospective study of combination therapy for hyperphosphataemia with calcium-containing phosphate binders and sevelamer in hypercalcaemic haemodialysis patients. Nephrol Dial Transplant 2002;17:1643.

Mundy GR: Statins and their potential for osteoporosis. Bone 2001;29:495.

Neer RM et al: Effect of parathyroid hormone (1-34) on fractures and bone mineral density in postmenopausal women with osteoporosis. N Engl J Med 2001;344:1434.

Orwoll E et al: Alendronate for the treatment of osteoporosis in men. N Engl J Med 2000;343:604.

Osteoporosis prevention, diagnosis, and therapy. NIH Consensus Statement 2000;17:1.

Pak CYC et al: Safe and effective treatment of osteoporosis with intermittent slow release sodium fluoride: Augmentation of vertebral bone mass and inhibition of fracture. J Clin Endocrinol Metab 1989;68:150.

Prince RL et al: Prevention of postmenopausal osteoporosis: A comparative study of exercise, calcium supplementation, and hormone-replacement therapy. N Engl J Med 1991;325:1189.

Riggs BL et al: Effect of fluoride treatment on the fracture rate in postmenopausal women with osteoporosis. N Engl J Med 1990;322:802.

Rodan GA, Martin TJ: Therapeutic approaches to bone diseases. Science 2000;289:1508.

Strewler GJ: FGF23, hypophosphatemia, and rickets: has phosphatonin been found? Proc Natl Acad Sci U S A 2001;98:5945.

Suda T et al: Modulation of osteoclast differentiation and function by the new members of the tumor necrosis factor receptor and ligand families. Endocr Rev 1999;20:345.

Tohme JF et al: Diagnosis and treatment of hypocalcemic emergencies. The Endocrinologist 1996;6:10.

SECTION VIII.
Chemotherapeutic Drugs

INTRODUCTION TO ANTIMICROBIAL AGENTS

Antimicrobial agents are among the most dramatic examples of the advances of modern medicine. Many infectious diseases once considered incurable and lethal are now amenable to treatment with a few pills. The remarkably powerful and specific activity of antimicrobial drugs is due to their selectivity for targets that are either unique to microorganisms or much more important in them than in humans. Among these targets are bacterial and fungal cell wall-synthesizing enzymes (see Chapters 43 and 48), the bacterial ribosome (see Chapters 44 and 45), the enzymes required for nucleotide synthesis and DNA replication (see Chapter 46), and the machinery of viral replication (see Chapter 49). The special group of drugs used in mycobacterial infections is discussed in Chapter 47. The much older and less selective cytotoxic antiseptics and disinfectants are discussed in Chapter 50. The clinical uses of all of these agents are presented in Chapter 51.

Microorganisms can adapt to environmental pressures in a variety of effective ways, and their response to antibiotic pressure is no exception. An inevitable consequence of antimicrobial usage is the selection of resistant microorganisms. Overuse and inappropriate use of antibiotics has fueled a major increase in prevalence of multidrug-resistant pathogens, leading some to speculate that we are nearing the end of the antibiotic era. Unfortunately, as the need has grown in recent years, development of novel drugs has slowed. The most vulnerable molecular targets of antimicrobial drugs have been identified, and in many cases crystallized and characterized. Pending the identification of new targets and compounds, it seems likely that over the next decade we will have to rely on currently available families of drugs. In the face of continuing development of resistance, considerable effort will be required to maintain the effectiveness of these drug groups.

Beta-Lactam Antibiotics & Other Inhibitors of Cell Wall Synthesis

43

Henry F. Chambers, MD

BETA-LACTAM COMPOUNDS

PENICILLINS

The penicillins are classified as β-lactam drugs because of their unique four-membered lactam ring. They share features of chemistry, mechanism of action, pharmacologic and clinical effects, and immunologic characteristics with cephalosporins, monobactams, carbapenems, and β-lactamase inhibitors, which also are β-lactam compounds.

Chemistry

All penicillins have the basic structure shown in Figure 43–1. A thiazolidine ring (A) is attached to a β-lactam ring (B) that carries a secondary amino group (RNH–). Substituents (R; examples shown in Figure 43–2) can be attached to the amino group. Structural integrity of the 6-aminopenicillanic acid nucleus is essential for the biologic activity of these compounds. If the β-lactam ring is enzymatically cleaved by bacterial β-lactamases, the resulting product, penicilloic acid, lacks antibacterial activity.

A. CLASSIFICATION

The attachment of different substituents to 6-aminopenicillanic acid determines the essential pharmacologic and antibacterial properties of the resulting molecules. Penicillins can be assigned to one of three groups (below). Within each of these groups are compounds that are relatively stable to gastric acid and suitable for oral administration, eg, penicillin V, dicloxacillin, and amoxicillin. The side chains of some representatives of each group are shown in Figure 43–2, with a few distinguishing characteristics.

1. Penicillins (eg, penicillin G)—These have the greatest activity against gram-positive organisms, gram-negative cocci, and non-β-lactamase-producing anaerobes.

However, they have little activity against gram-negative rods. They are susceptible to hydrolysis by β lactamases.

2. Antistaphylococcal penicillins (eg, nafcillin)—These penicillins are resistant to staphylococcal β lactamases. They are active against staphylococci and streptococci but inactive against enterococci, anaerobic bacteria, and gram-negative cocci and rods.

3. Extended-spectrum penicillins (ampicillin and the antipseudomonal penicillins)—These drugs retain the antibacterial spectrum of penicillin and have improved activity against gram-negative organisms, but they are destroyed by β lactamases.

B. PENICILLIN UNITS AND FORMULATIONS

The activity of penicillin G was originally defined in units. Crystalline sodium penicillin G contains approximately 1600 units/mg (1 unit = 0.6 μg; 1 million units of penicillin = 0.6 g). Semisynthetic penicillins are prescribed by weight rather than units. The **minimum inhibitory concentration (MIC)** of any penicillin (or other antimicrobial) is usually given in μg/mL. Most penicillins are dispensed as the sodium or potassium salt of the free acid. Potassium penicillin G contains about 1.7 meq of K^+ per million units of penicillin (2.8 meq/g). Nafcillin contains Na^+, 2.8 meq/g. Procaine salts and benzathine salts of penicillin G provide repository forms for intramuscular injection. In dry crystalline form, penicillin salts are stable for long periods (eg, for years at 4 °C). Solutions lose their activity rapidly (eg, 24 hours at 20 °C) and must be prepared fresh for administration.

Mechanism of Action

Penicillins, like all β-lactam antibiotics, inhibit bacterial growth by interfering with a specific step in bacterial cell wall synthesis. The cell wall is a rigid outer layer that is not found in animal cells. It completely surrounds the cytoplasmic membrane (Figure 43–3), maintaining the shape of the cell and preventing cell lysis from high osmotic pressure. The cell wall is composed of a com-

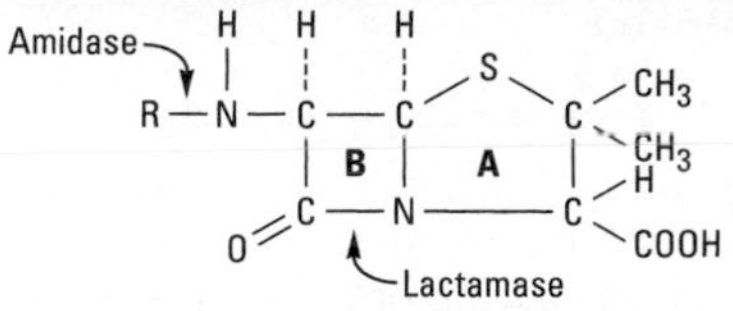

PENICILLIN

Substituted 6-aminopenicillanic acid

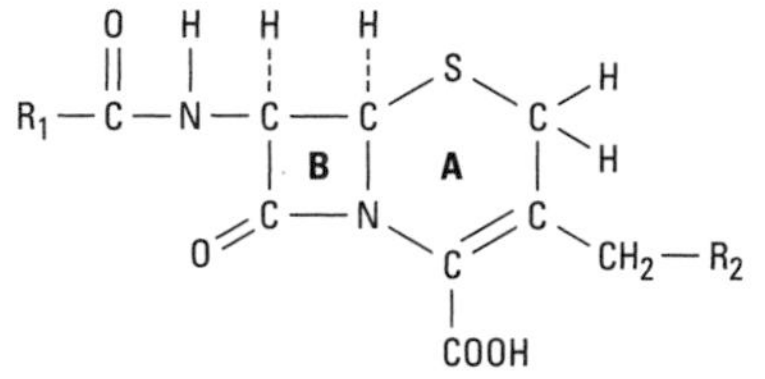

CEPHALOSPORIN

Substituted 7-aminocephalosporanic acid

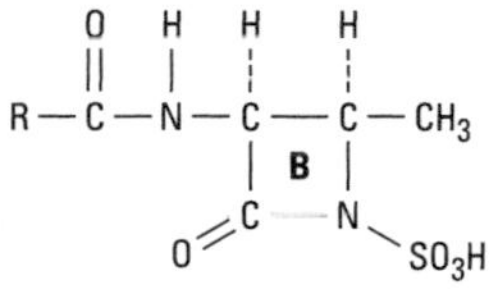

MONOBACTAM

Substituted 3-amino-4-methylmonobactamic acid (aztreonam)

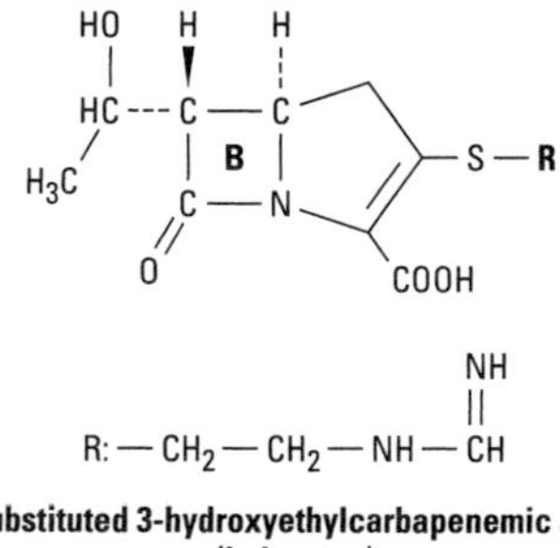

CARBAPENEM

Substituted 3-hydroxyethylcarbapenemic acid (imipenem)

Figure 43–1. Core structures of four β-lactam antibiotic families. The ring marked B in each structure is the β-lactam ring. The penicillins are susceptible to bacterial metabolism and inactivation by amidases and lactamases at the points shown. Note that the carbapenems have a different stereochemical configuration in the lactam ring that apparently imparts resistance to β lactamases. Substituents for the penicillin and cephalosporin families are shown in Figures 43–2 and 43–6, respectively.

plex cross-linked polymer, peptidoglycan (murein, mucopeptide), consisting of polysaccharides and polypeptides. The polysaccharide contains alternating amino sugars, *N*-acetylglucosamine and *N*-acetylmuramic acid (Figure 43–4). A five-amino-acid peptide is linked to the *N*-acetylmuramic acid sugar. This peptide terminates in D-alanyl-D-alanine. Penicillin-binding proteins (PBPs) catalyze the transpeptidase reaction that removes the terminal alanine to form a crosslink with a nearby peptide, which gives cell wall its structural rigidity. β-Lactam antibiotics are structural analogs of the natural D-Ala-D-Ala substrate and they are covalently bound by PBPs at the active site. After a β-lactam antibiotic has attached to the PBP, the transpeptidation reaction is inhibited (Figure 43–5), peptidoglycan synthesis is blocked, and the cell dies. The exact mechanism responsible for cell death is not completely understood, but autolysins, bacterial enzymes that remodel and break down cell wall, are involved. Penicillins and cephalosporins are bactericidal only if cells are actively growing and synthesizing cell wall.

Resistance

Resistance to penicillins and other β lactams is due to one of four general mechanisms: (1) inactivation of antibiotic by β lactamase, (2) modification of target PBPs, (3) impaired penetration of drug to target PBPs, and (4) the presence of an efflux pump. β-Lactamase production is the most common mechanism of resistance. More than 300 different β lactamases have been identified. Some, such as those produced by *Staphylococcus aureus,* haemophilus species, and *E coli,* are relatively narrow in substrate specificity and will hydrolyze penicillins but not cephalosporins. Other β lactamases, such as those produced by *Pseudomonas aeruginosa* and enterobacter species, are much broader in spectrum and will hydrolyze both cephalosporins and penicillins. Carbapenems, which are highly resistant to hydrolysis by penicillinases and cephalosporinases, are hydrolyzed by a metallo-β lactamase.

Alteration in target PBPs is responsible for methicillin resistance in staphylococci and penicillin resistance in pneumococci and enterococci. These resistant organisms produce PBPs that have low affinity for binding β-lactam antibiotics, and as a result they are not inhibited except at relatively high drug concentrations, which may exceed what is clinically achievable.

Resistance caused by impaired penetration of antibiotic to target PBPs, which occurs only in gram-negative species, is due to impermeability of an outer cell wall membrane that is present in gram-negative but not in gram-positive bacteria. β-Lactam antibiotics cross the outer membrane and enter gram-negative organisms via outer membrane protein channels (porins). Absence of the proper channel or down-regulation of its production can prevent or greatly reduce drug entry into the cell. Impaired penetration alone is usually not sufficient to confer resistance, because enough antibiotic eventually enters the cell to inhibit growth. However, this barrier can become important in the presence of a β lactamase, which hydrolyzes antibiotic as it slowly enters the cell. Gram-negative organisms also may produce an efflux pump, which consists of cytoplasmic and periplasmic protein components, that efficiently transport some β-lactam antibiotics from the periplasm back across the outer membrane (eg, extrusion of nafcillin by *Salmonella typhimurium*).

Pharmacokinetics

Absorption of orally administered drug differs greatly for different penicillins, depending in part on their acid stability and protein binding. Methicillin is acid-labile and gastrointestinal absorption of nafcillin is erratic, so neither is suitable for oral administration. Dicloxacillin, ampicillin, and amoxicillin are acid-stable and relatively

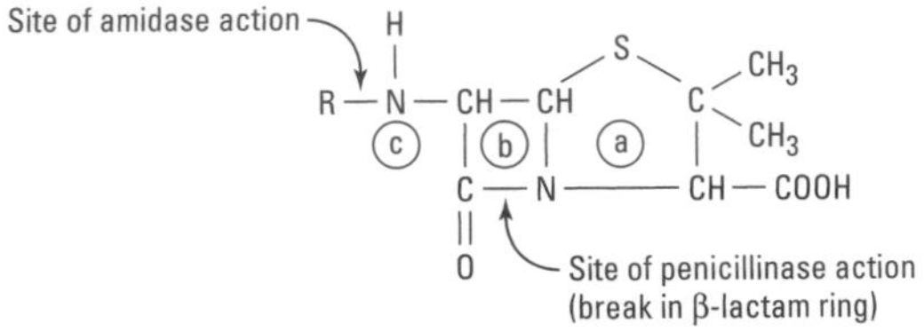

6-Aminopenicillanic acid

The following structures can each be substituted at the R to produce a new penicillin.

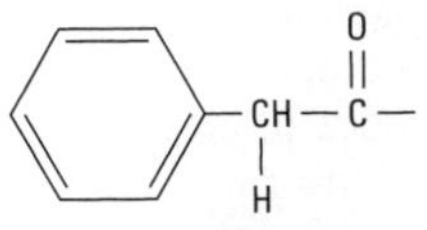

Penicillin G (benzylpenicillin):
High activity against gram-positive bacteria. Low activity against gram-negative bacteria. Acid-labile. Destroyed by β-lactamase. 60% protein-bound.

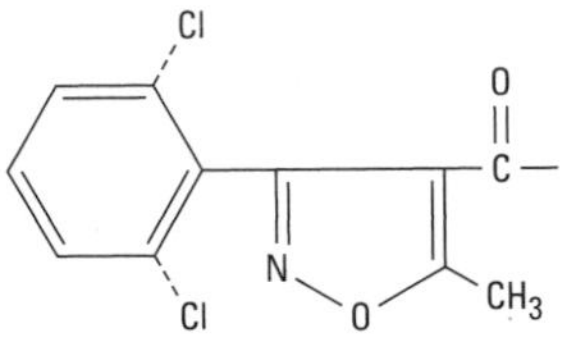

Oxacillin (no Cl atoms); cloxacillin (one Cl in structure); dicloxacillin (2 Cls in structure); flucloxacillin (one Cl and one F in structure) (isoxazolyl penicillins):
Similar to methicillin in β-lactamase resistance, but acid-stable. Can be taken orally. Highly protein-bound (95–98%).

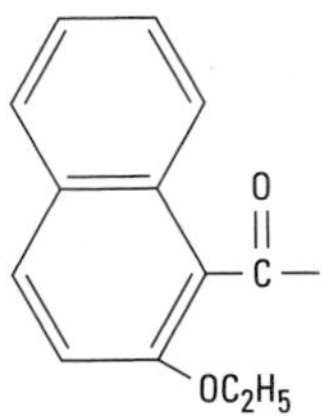

Nafcillin (ethoxynaphthamidopenicillin):
Similar to isoxazolyl penicillins. Less strongly protein-bound (90%). Resistant to staphylococcal β-lactamase.

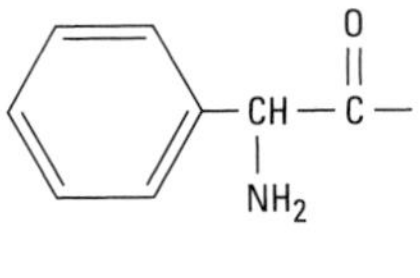

Ampicillin (alpha-aminobenzylpenicillin):
Similar to Penicillin G (destroyed by β-lactamase) but acid-stable and more active against gram-negative bacteria. Carbenicillin has –COONa instead of NH₂ group.

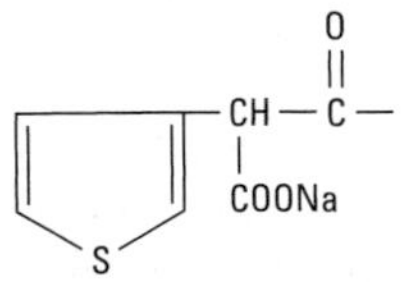

Ticarcillin:
Similar to carbenicillin but gives higher blood levels. Piperacillin, azlocillin, and mezlocillin resemble ticarcillin in action against gram-negative aerobes.

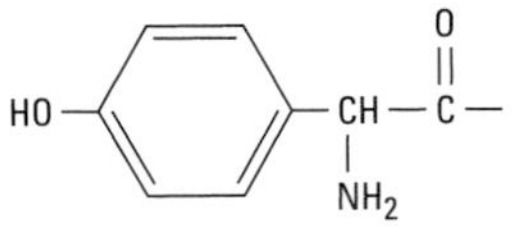

Amoxicillin:
Similar to ampicillin but better absorbed, gives higher blood levels.

Figure 43–2. Side chains of some penicillins (R groups of Figure 43–1).

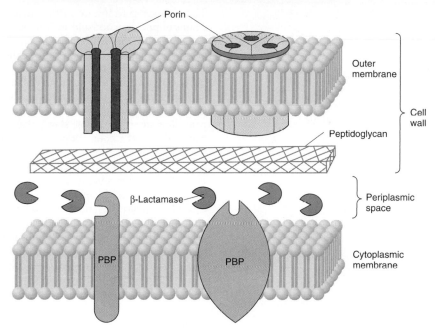

Figure 43–3. A highly simplified diagram of the cell envelope of a gram-negative bacterium. The outer membrane, a lipid bilayer, is present in gram-negative but not gram-positive organisms. It is penetrated by porins, proteins that form channels providing hydrophilic access to the cytoplasmic membrane. The peptidoglycan layer is unique to bacteria and is much thicker in gram-positive organisms than in gram-negative ones. Together, the outer membrane and the peptidoglycan layer constitute the cell wall. Penicillin-binding proteins (PBPs) are membrane proteins that cross-link peptidoglycan. β-lactamases, if present, reside in the periplasmic space or on the outer surface of the cytoplasmic membrane, where they may destroy β-lactam antibiotics that penetrate the outer membrane.

well absorbed, producing serum concentrations in the range of 4–8 μg/mL following a 500 mg oral dose. Absorption of most oral penicillins (amoxicillin being an exception) is impaired by food, and the drugs should be administered at least 1–2 hours before or after a meal.

After parenteral administration, absorption of most penicillins is complete and rapid. Administration by the intravenous route is preferred because of irritation and local pain produced by the intramuscular injection of large doses. Serum concentrations 30 minutes after an intravenous injection of 1 g of a penicillin (equivalent to approximately 1.6 million units of penicillin G) are 20–50 μg/mL. Only a fraction of the total drug in serum is present as free drug, the concentration of which is determined by protein binding. Highly protein-bound penicillins (eg, nafcillin) produce lower levels of free drug in serum than less protein-bound penicillins (eg, penicillin G, ampicillin). Protein binding becomes clinically relevant when the protein-bound fraction is approximately 95% or more. Penicillins are widely distributed in body fluids and tissues with the exceptions noted below. They are polar molecules, and

the concentration within cells is less than that in extracellular fluids.

Benzathine and procaine penicillins are formulated to delay absorption, resulting in prolonged blood and tissue concentrations. After a single intramuscular injection of 1.2 million units of benzathine penicillin, serum levels in excess of 0.02 μg/mL are maintained for 10 days and levels in excess of 0.003 μg/mL for 3 weeks. The latter is sufficient to protect against β-hemolytic streptococcal infection and the former to treat an established infection with these organisms. A 600,000 unit dose of procaine penicillin yields peak concentrations of 1–2 μg/mL and clinically useful concentrations for 12–24 hours after a single intramuscular injection.

Penicillin concentrations in most tissues are equal to those in serum. Penicillin is also excreted into sputum and milk to levels 3–15% of those present in the serum. Penetration into the eye, the prostate, and the central nervous system is poor. However, with active inflammation of the meninges, as in bacterial meningitis, penicillin concentrations of 1–5 μg/mL can be achieved with a daily parenteral dose of 18–24 million units.

These concentrations are sufficient to kill susceptible strains of pneumococci and meningococci.

Penicillin is rapidly excreted by the kidneys into the urine; small amounts are excreted by other routes. About 10% of renal excretion is by glomerular filtration and 90% by tubular secretion. The normal half-life of penicillin G is approximately 30 minutes; in renal failure, it may be as long as 10 hours. Ampicillin and the extended-spectrum penicillins are secreted more slowly than penicillin G and have half-lives of 1 hour. For penicillins that are cleared by the kidney, the dose must be adjusted according to renal function, with approximately one fourth to one third the normal dose being administered if creatinine clearance is 10 mL/min or less (Table 43–1). Nafcillin is primarily cleared by biliary excretion, and oxacillin, dicloxacillin, and cloxacillin are eliminated by both the kidney and biliary excretion—thus, no dosage adjustment is required for these drugs in renal failure. Because clearance of penicillins is less efficient in the newborn, doses adjusted for weight alone will result in higher systemic concentrations for longer periods than in the adult.

Clinical Uses

Oral penicillins, except for amoxicillin, should not be given at mealtimes (instead, give 1–2 hours before or after) to minimize binding to food proteins and acid inactivation. Blood levels of all penicillins can be raised by simultaneous administration of probenecid, 0.5 g (10 mg/kg in children) every 6 hours orally, which impairs tubular secretion of weak acids such as β-lactam compounds.

A. PENICILLIN

Penicillin G is the drug of choice for infections caused by streptococci, meningococci, enterococci, penicillin-susceptible pneumococci, non-β-lactamase-producing staphylococci, *Treponema pallidum* and many other

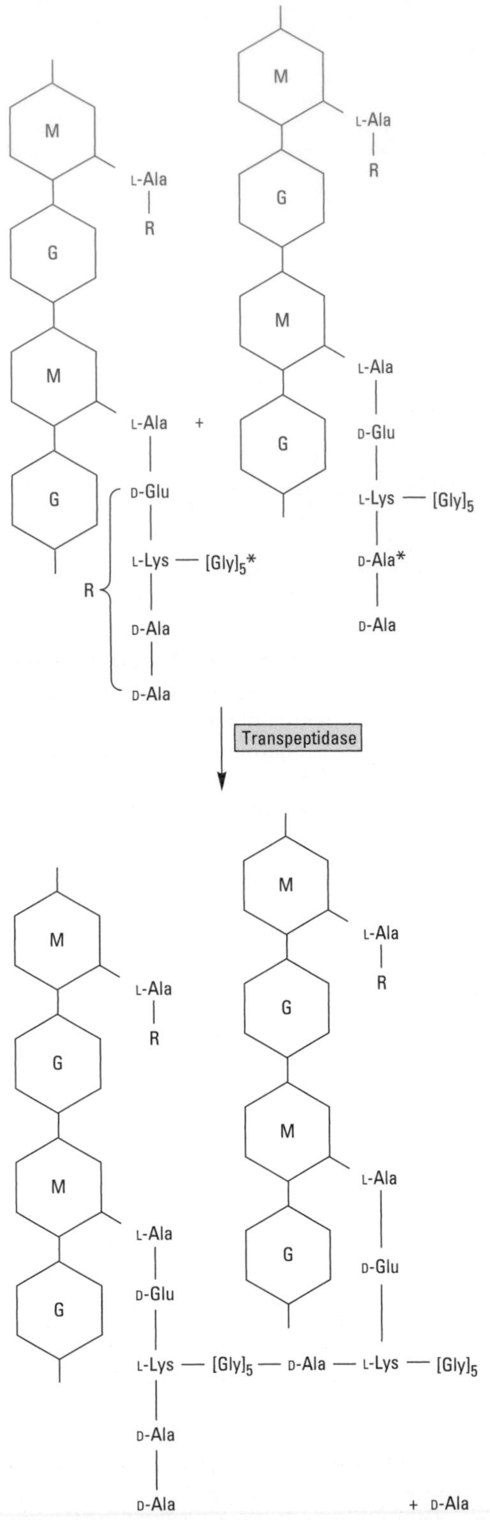

Figure 43–4. The transpeptidation reaction in *Staphylococcus aureus* that is inhibited by β-lactam antibiotics. The cell wall of gram-positive bacteria is made up of long peptidoglycan polymer chains consisting of the alternating aminohexoses N-acetylglucosamine (**G**) and N-acetylmuramic acid (**M**) with pentapeptide side chains linked (in *S aureus*) by pentaglycine bridges. The exact composition of the side chains varies among species. The diagram illustrates small segments of two such polymer chains and their amino acid side chains. These linear polymers must be cross-linked by transpeptidation of the side chains at the points indicated by the asterisk to achieve the strength necessary for cell viability.

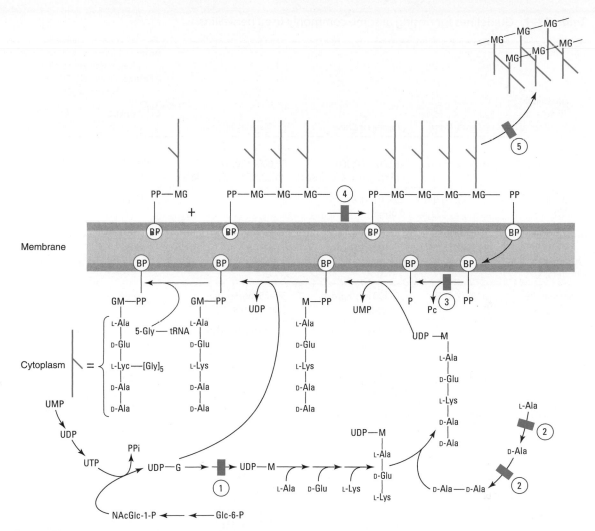

Figure 43–5. The biosynthesis of cell wall peptidoglycan, showing the sites of action of five antibiotics (shaded bars; 1 = fosfomycin, 2 = cycloserine, 3 = bacitracin, 4 = vancomycin, 5 = β-lactam antibiotics). Bactoprenol (BP) is the lipid membrane carrier that transports building blocks across the cytoplasmic membrane; M = *N*-acetylmuramic acid; Glc = glucose; NAcGlc or G = *N*-acetylglucosamine.

spirochetes, clostridium species, actinomyces, and other gram-positive rods and non-β-lactamase-producing gram-negative anaerobic organisms. Depending upon the organism, the site, and the severity of infection, effective doses range between 4 and 24 million units per day administered intravenously in four to six divided doses. Administration of high-dose penicillin G as a continuous intravenous infusion, although infrequently used, is also acceptable. Penicillin G when administered at doses of 18–24 million units is inhibitory for enterococci, but the simultaneous admin-

istration of an aminoglycoside is necessary to achieve a bactericidal effect, which is required when treating enterococcal endocarditis.

Penicillin V, the oral form of penicillin, is indicated only in minor infections because of its relatively poor bioavailability, the need for dosing four times a day, and its narrow antibacterial spectrum. Amoxicillin (see below) is often used instead.

Benzathine penicillin and procaine penicillin G for intramuscular injection yield low but prolonged drug levels. A single injection of benzathine penicillin, 1.2

Table 43–1. Guidelines for dosing of some commonly used penicillins.

Antibiotic (Route of Administration)	Adult Dose	Pediatric Dose[1]	Neonatal Dose[2]	Adjusted Dose as a Percentage of Normal Dose for Renal Failure Based on Creatinine Clearance (Cl_{cr})	
				Cl_{cr} Approx 50 mL/min	Cl_{cr} Approx 10 mL/min
Penicillins					
Penicillin G (IV)	1–4 mU q4–6h	25,000–400,000 units/kg/d in 4–6 doses	75,000–150,000 units/kg/d in 2 or 3 doses	50–75%	25%
Penicillin VK (PO)	0.25–0.5 g qid	25–50 mg/kg/d in 4 doses		None	None
Antistaphylococcal penicillins					
Cloxacillin, dicloxacillin (PO)	0.25–0.5 g qid	25–50 mg/kg/d in 4 doses		None	None
Nafcillin (IV)	1–2 g q4–6h	50–100 mg/kg/d in 4–6 doses	50–75 mg/kg/d in 2 or 3 doses	None	None
Oxacillin (IV)	1–2 g q4–6h	50–100 mg/kg/d in 4–6 doses	50–75 mg/kg/d in 2 or 3 doses	None	None
Extended-spectrum penicillins					
Amoxicillin (PO)	0.25–0.5 g tid	20–40 mg/kg/d in 3 doses		66%	33%
Amoxicillin/ potassium clavulanate (PO)	500/125– 875/125 mg bid–tid	20–40 mg/kg/d in 3 doses		66%	33%
Piperacillin (IV)	3–4 g q4–6h	300 mg/kg/d in 4–6 doses	150 mg/kg/d in 2 doses	50–75%	25–33%
Ticarcillin (IV)	3 g q4–6h	200–300 mg/kg/d in 4–6 doses	150–200 mg/kg/d in 2 or 3 doses	50–75%	25–33%

[1]The total dose should not exceed the adult dose.

[2]The dose shown is during the first week of life. The daily dose should be increased by approximately 33–50% after the first week of life. The lower dosage range should be used for neonates weighing less than 2 kg. After the first month of life, pediatric doses may be used.

million units intramuscularly, is satisfactory for treatment of β-hemolytic streptococcal pharyngitis. A similar injection given intramuscularly once every 3–4 weeks provides satisfactory prophylaxis against reinfection with β-hemolytic streptococci. Penicillin G benzathine, 2.4 million units intramuscularly once a week for 1–3 weeks, is effective in the treatment of syphilis, though its use for treatment of neurosyphilis is controversial. Procaine penicillin G, which in the past was used for treating uncomplicated pneumococcal pneumonia or gonorrhea, is rarely used nowadays because many strains are penicillin-resistant.

B. PENICILLINS RESISTANT TO STAPHYLOCOCCAL BETA LACTAMASE (METHICILLIN, NAFCILLIN, AND ISOXAZOLYL PENICILLINS)

These semisynthetic penicillins are indicated for infection by β-lactamase-producing staphylococci, although penicillin-susceptible strains of streptococci and pneumococci are also susceptible. Enterococci and methicillin-resistant strains of staphylococci are resistant.

An isoxazolyl penicillin such as oxacillin, cloxacillin, or dicloxacillin, 0.25–0.5 g orally every 4–6 hours (15–25 mg/kg/d for children), is suitable for treatment of mild localized staphylococcal infections. All of these drugs are relatively acid-stable and reasonably well absorbed from the gut. Food interferes with absorption, and the drugs must be administered 1 hour before or after meals.

For serious systemic staphylococcal infections, oxacillin or nafcillin, 8–12 g/d, is given by intermittent intravenous infusion of 1–2 g every 4–6 hours (50–100 mg/kg/d for children). Methicillin is no longer used because of its nephrotoxicity.

C. Extended-Spectrum Penicillins (Aminopenicillins, Carboxypenicillins, and Ureidopenicillins)

These drugs, which in general retain the spectrum of activity of penicillin G, differ in having greater activity against gram-negative bacteria due to their enhanced ability to penetrate the gram-negative outer membrane. Like penicillin G, they are inactivated by β-lactamases.

The aminopenicillins, ampicillin and amoxicillin, have the same spectrum and activity, but amoxicillin is better absorbed from the gut. A dosage of 250–500 mg of amoxicillin three times daily is equivalent to the same amount of ampicillin given four times daily. These drugs are given orally to treat urinary tract infections, sinusitis, otitis, and lower respiratory tract infections. Ampicillin and amoxicillin are the most active of the oral β-lactam antibiotics against penicillin-resistant pneumococci and are the preferred β-lactam antibiotics for treating infections suspected to be caused by these resistant strains. Ampicillin (but not amoxicillin) is effective for shigellosis but should not be used to treat uncomplicated salmonella gastroenteritis, as it may prolong the carrier state.

Ampicillin, at dosages of 4–12 g/d intravenously, is useful for treating serious infections caused by penicillin-susceptible organisms, including anaerobes, enterococci, *Listeria monocytogenes,* and susceptible strains of gram-negative cocci and bacilli such as *E coli, H influenzae,* and salmonella species. Many strains of gram-negative species produce β lactamases and are therefore resistant to ampicillin, precluding its use for empirical therapy of urinary tract infections, meningitis, and typhoid fever. Ampicillin is not active against klebsiella, enterobacter, *Pseudomonas aeruginosa,* citrobacter, serratia, indole-positive proteus species, and other gram-negative aerobes that are commonly encountered in hospital-acquired infections.

Carbenicillin, the first antipseudomonal carboxypenicillin, has become obsolete as a parenteral agent with the advent of more active, better tolerated agents. A derivative, carbenicillin indanyl sodium, is acid-stable and can be given orally in urinary tract infections. Ticarcillin, a carboxypenicillin that is similar to carbenicillin in activity but effective in lower doses, extends the ampicillin spectrum of activity (except that it is less active against enterococci) to include *Pseudomonas aeruginosa* and enterobacter species. The ureidopenicillins, piperacillin, mezlocillin, and azlocillin, resemble ticarcillin except that they are also active against selected gram-negative bacilli, such as *Klebsiella pneumoniae.* Because of the propensity of *P aeruginosa* to develop resistance during single drug therapy, an antipseudomonal penicillin generally is used in combination with an aminoglycoside for pseudomonal infections.

Ampicillin, amoxicillin, ticarcillin, and piperacillin are also available in combination with one of several β-lactamase inhibitors: clavulanic acid, sulbactam, or tazobactam. The addition of a β-lactamase inhibitor extends the activity of these penicillins to include β-lactamase-producing strains of *S aureus* as well as some β-lactamase-producing gram-negative bacteria (see below).

Adverse Reactions

The penicillins are remarkably nontoxic. Most of the serious adverse effects are due to hypersensitivity. All penicillins are cross-sensitizing and cross-reacting. The responsible antigenic determinants are degradation products of penicillins, particularly penicilloic acid and products of alkaline hydrolysis bound to host protein. A history of a penicillin reaction is not reliable; about 5–8% of people claim such a history, but only 5–10% of these will have an allergic reaction when given penicillin. Fewer than 1% of persons who previously received penicillin without incident will have an allergic reaction when given penicillin. Because of the potential for anaphylaxis, however, penicillin should be administered with caution or a substitute drug given if there is a history of penicillin allergy. The incidence of allergic reactions in small children is negligible.

Allergic reactions include anaphylactic shock (very rare—0.05% of recipients); serum sickness type reactions (now rare—urticaria, fever, joint swelling, angioneurotic edema, intense pruritus, and respiratory embarrassment occurring 7–12 days after exposure); and a variety of skin rashes. Oral lesions, fever, interstitial nephritis (an autoimmune reaction to a penicillin-protein complex), eosinophilia, hemolytic anemia and other hematologic disturbances, and vasculitis may also occur. Most patients allergic to penicillins can be treated with alternative drugs. However, if necessary (eg, treatment of enterococcal endocarditis or neurosyphilis in a highly penicillin-allergic patient), desensitization can be accomplished with gradually increasing doses of penicillin.

In patients with renal failure, penicillin in high doses can cause seizures. Nafcillin is associated with neutropenia; oxacillin can cause hepatitis; and methicillin causes interstitial nephritis. Large doses of penicillins given orally may lead to gastrointestinal upset, particularly nausea, vomiting, and diarrhea. Ampicillin has been associated with pseudomembranous colitis. Secondary infections such as vaginal candidiasis may occur. Ampicillin and amoxicillin can cause skin rashes that are not allergic in nature.

Problems Relating to the Use & Misuse of the Penicillins

Penicillins have been among the most misused antibiotics. As a result, 90% of all staphylococcal strains both in the hospital and in the community are β-lactamase producers, and the prevalence of methicillin-resistant strains of *S aureus* continues to increase. β-Lactamase-producing strains of *H influenzae* and *N gonorrhoeae* are now common. The prevalence of penicillin-resistant pneumococci exceeds 20% in some regions of the United States. Broad-spectrum penicillins also eradicate normal flora, thereby predisposing the patient to colonization and superinfection with opportunistic, drug-resistant species present within the hospital environment (proteus, pseudomonas, enterobacter, serratia, staphylococci, yeasts, etc).

CEPHALOSPORINS & CEPHAMYCINS

Cephalosporins and cephamycins are similar to penicillins chemically, in mechanism of action, and in toxicity. Cephalosporins are more stable than penicillins to many bacterial β-lactamases and therefore usually have a broader spectrum of activity. Cephalosporins are not active against enterococci and *Listeria monocytogenes*.

Chemistry

The nucleus of the cephalosporins, 7-aminocephalosporanic acid (Figure 43–6), bears a close resemblance to 6-aminopenicillanic acid (Figure 43–1). The intrinsic antimicrobial activity of natural cephalosporins is low, but the attachment of various R_1 and R_2 groups has yielded drugs of good therapeutic activity and low toxicity (Figure 43–6). The cephalosporins have molecular weights of 400–450. They are soluble in water and relatively stable to pH and temperature changes. Cephalosporins can be classified into four major groups or generations, depending mainly on the spectrum of antimicrobial activity. As a general rule, first-generation compounds have better activity against gram-positive organisms and the later compounds exhibit improved

activity against gram-negative aerobic organisms.

FIRST-GENERATION CEPHALOSPORINS

This group includes cefadroxil, cefazolin, cephalexin, cephalothin, cephapirin, and cephradine. These drugs are very active against gram-positive cocci, including pneumococci, streptococci, and staphylococci. Cephalosporins are not active against methicillin-resistant strains of staphylococci. *Escherichia coli, Klebsiella pneumoniae,* and *Proteus mirabilis* are often sensitive, but activity against *P aeruginosa,* indole-positive proteus, enterobacter, *Serratia marcescens,* citrobacter, and acinetobacter is poor. Anaerobic cocci (eg, peptococcus, peptostreptococcus) are usually sensitive, but *B fragilis* is not.

Pharmacokinetics & Dosage

A. ORAL

Cephalexin, cephradine, and cefadroxil are absorbed from the gut to a variable extent. After oral doses of 500 mg, serum levels are 15–20 μg/mL. Urine concentration is usually very high, but in most tissues levels are variable and generally lower than in serum. Cephalexin and cephradine are given orally in dosages of 0.25–0.5 g four times daily (15–30 mg/kg/d) and cefadroxil in dosages of 0.5–1 g twice daily. Excretion is mainly by glomerular filtration and tubular secretion into the urine. Drugs that block tubular secretion, eg, probenecid, may increase serum levels substantially. In patients with impaired renal function, dosage must be reduced (Table 43–2).

B. PARENTERAL

Cefazolin is the only first-generation parenteral cephalosporin still in general use. After an intravenous infusion of 1 g, the peak level of cefazolin is 90–120 μg/mL. The usual intravenous dosage of cefazolin for adults is 0.5–2 g intravenously every 8 hours. Cefazolin can also be administered intramuscularly. Excretion is via the kidney, and dose adjustments must be made for impaired renal function.

Clinical Uses

Although the first-generation cephalosporins have a broad spectrum of activity and are relatively nontoxic, they are rarely the drug of choice for any infection. Oral drugs may be used for the treatment of urinary tract infections, for minor staphylococcal lesions, or for minor polymicrobial infections such as cellulitis or soft tissue abscess. However, oral cephalosporins should not be relied upon in serious systemic infections.

Cefazolin penetrates well into most tissues. It is the

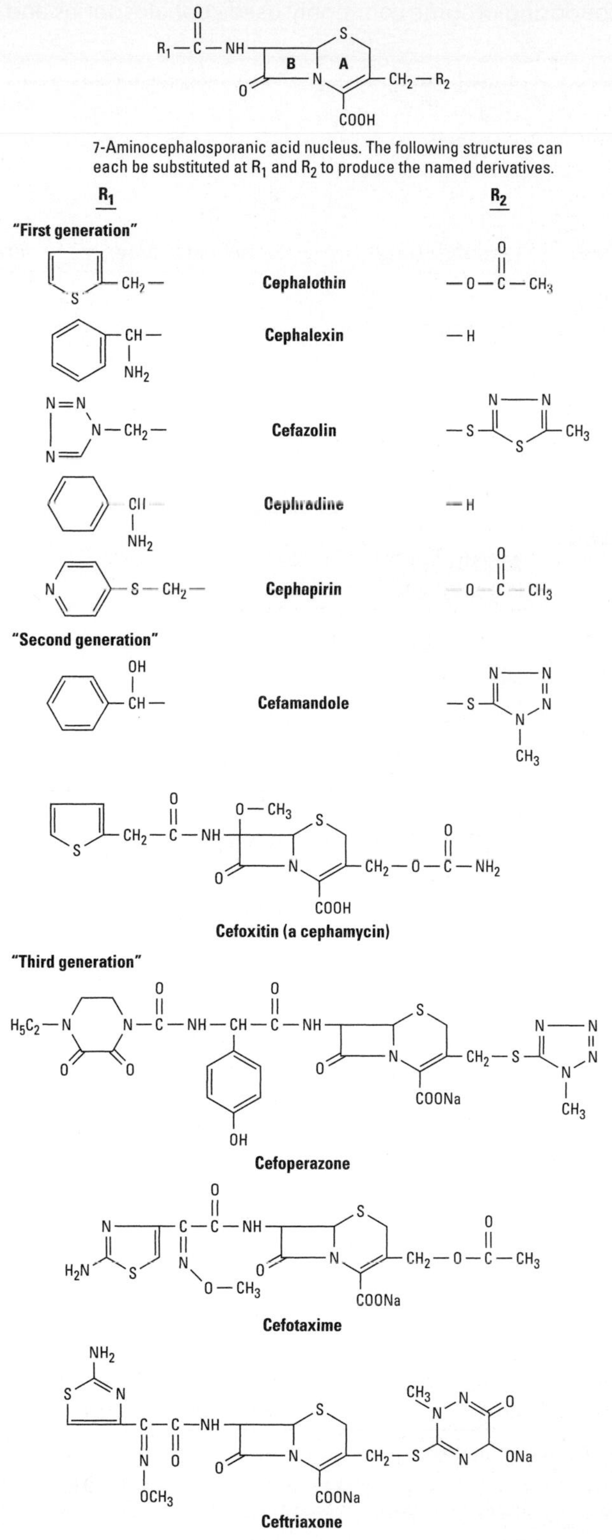

Figure 43–6. Structures of some cephalosporins. R_1 and R_2 structures are substituents on the 7-aminocephalosporanic acid nucleus pictured at the top. Other structures (cefoxitin and below) are complete in themselves.

Table 43–2. Guidelines for dosing of some commonly used cephalosporins and other cell-wall inhibitor antibiotics.

Antibiotic (Route of Administration)	Adult Dose	Pediatric Dose[1]	Neonatal Dose[2]	Adjusted Dose as a Percentage of Normal Dose for Renal Failure Based on Creatinine Clearance (Cl_{cr})	
				Cl_{cr} Approx 50 mL/min	Cl_{cr} Approx 10 mL/min
First-generation cephalosporins					
Cefadroxil (PO)	0.5–1 g qd–bid	30 mg/kg/d in 2 doses		50%	25%
Cephalexin, cephradine (PO)	0.25–0.5 g qid	25–50 mg/kg/d in 4 doses		50%	25%
Cefazolin (IV)	0.5–2 g q8h	25–100 mg/kg/d in 3 or 4 doses		50%	25%
Second-generation cephalosporins					
Cefoxitin (IV)	1–2 g q6–8h	75–150 mg/kg/d in 3 or 4 doses		50–75%	25%
Cefotetan (IV)	1–2 g q12h			50%	25%
Cefuroxime (IV)	0.75–1.5 g q8h	50–100 mg/kg/d in 3 or 4 doses		66%	25–33%
Cefuroxime axetil (PO)	0.25–0.5 g bid	0.125–0.25 g bid		None	25%
Third- and fourth-generation cephalosporins					
Cefotaxime (IV)	1–2 g q6–12h	50–200 mg/kg/d in 4–6 doses	100 mg/kg/d in 2 doses	50%	25%
Ceftazidime (IV)	1–2 g q8–12h	75–150 mg/kg/d in 3 doses	100–150 mg/kg/d in 2 or 3 doses	50%	25%
Ceftriaxone (IV)	1–4 g q24h	50–100 mg/kg/d in 1or 2 doses	50 mg/kg/d once a day	None	None
Cefepime (IV)	0.5–2 g q12h	75–120 mg/kg/d in 2 or 3 divided doses		50%	25%
Carbapenems					
Ertapenem (IM or IV)	1 g			100%[3]	50%
Imipenem (IV)	0.25–0.5 g q6–8h			75%	50%
Meropenem (IV)	1 g q8h (2 g q8h for meningitis)	60–120 mg/kg/d in 3 doses (maximum of 2 g q8h)		66%	50%
Glycopeptides					
Vancomycin (IV)	30 mg/kg/d in 2–3 doses	40 mg/kg/d in 3 or 4 doses	15 mg/kg load, then 20 mg/kg/d in 2 doses	40%	10%

[1]The total dose should not exceed the adult dose.

[2]The dose shown is during the first week of life. The daily dose should be increased by approximately 33–50% after the first week of life. The lower dosage range should be used for neonates weighing less than 2 kg. After the first month of life, pediatric doses may be used.

[3]50% of dose for $CL_{cr} < 30$ mL/min.

drug of choice for surgical prophylaxis. Second- and third-generation cephalosporins offer no advantage for surgical prophylaxis for most procedures, are far more expensive, and generally should not be used for that purpose. Cefazolin may be a choice in infections for which it is the least toxic drug (eg, *K pneumoniae*) and in persons with staphylococcal or streptococcal infections who have a history of a mild penicillin hypersensitivity reaction but not anaphylaxis. Cefazolin does not penetrate the central nervous system and cannot be used to treat meningitis. Cefazolin is an alternative to an antistaphylococcal penicillin for patients who are allergic to penicillin.

SECOND-GENERATION CEPHALOSPORINS

Members of this group include cefaclor, cefamandole, cefonicid, cefuroxime, cefprozil, loracarbef, and ceforanide and the structurally related cephamycins cefoxitin, cefmetazole, cefotetan, which have activity against anaerobes. This is a heterogeneous group of drugs with marked individual differences in activity, pharmacokinetics, and toxicity. In general, they are active against organisms affected by first-generation drugs, but in addition they have extended gram-negative coverage. Klebsiellae (including those resistant to cephalothin) are usually sensitive. Cefamandole, cefuroxime, cefonicid, ceforanide, and cefaclor are active against *H influenzae* but not against serratia or *B fragilis*. In contrast, cefoxitin, cefmetazole, and cefotetan are active against *B fragilis* and some serratia strains but are less active against *H influenzae*. All second-generation cephalosporins are less active against gram-positive bacteria than the first-generation drugs. As with first-generation agents, none are active against enterococci or *P aeruginosa*. Second-generation cephalosporins may exhibit in vitro activity against enterobacter species, but they should not be used to treat infections caused by these organisms because resistant mutants that constitutively express a chromosomal β-lactamase that hydrolyzes these compounds (as well as third-generation cephalosporins) are readily selected.

Pharmacokinetics & Dosage

A. ORAL

Cefaclor, cefuroxime axetil, cefprozil, and loracarbef can be given orally. The usual dosage for adults is 10–15 mg/kg/d in two to four divided doses; children should be given 20–40 mg/kg/d up to a maximum of 1 g/d. Except for cefuroxime axetil, these drugs are not predictably active against penicillin-resistant pneumococci and should be used cautiously, if at all, to treat suspected or proved pneumococcal infections. Cefaclor is more susceptible to β-lactamase hydrolysis compared with the other agents, and its utility is correspondingly diminished.

B. PARENTERAL

After a 1 g intravenous infusion, serum levels are 75–125 µg/mL for most second-generation cephalosporins, but they reach 200–250 µg/mL for cefonicid. There are marked differences among drugs in half-life, protein binding, and interval between doses. Cefonicid is highly protein-bound, a feature that has been implicated as a cause of treatment failures with serious staphylococcal infections. For cefoxitin (50–200 mg/kg/d), the interval is 6–8 hours. Cefotetan is administered every 12 hours; cefonicid or ceforanide, every 12–24 hours; and cefprozil, every 24 hours. In general, intramuscular injection is too painful to be used. In renal failure, dosage adjustments are required (Table 43–2).

Clinical Uses

The oral second-generation cephalosporins are active against β-lactamase-producing *H influenzae* or *Branhamella catarrhalis* and have been primarily used to treat sinusitis, otitis, or lower respiratory tract infections, in which these organisms have an important role. Because of their activity against anaerobes (including *B fragilis*), cefoxitin, cefotetan, or cefmetazole can be useful in such mixed anaerobic infections as peritonitis or diverticulitis. Cefuroxime is used to treat community-acquired pneumonia, particularly in cases where β-lactamase-producing *H influenzae* or *Klebsiella pneumoniae* is a consideration, but this drug has few other uses. Cefuroxime is the only second-generation drug that crosses the blood-brain barrier, but it is less effective in treatment of meningitis than ceftriaxone or cefotaxime and should not be used.

THIRD-GENERATION CEPHALOSPORINS

Third-generation agents include cefoperazone, cefotaxime, ceftazidime, ceftizoxime, ceftriaxone, cefixime, cefpodoxime proxetil, cefditoren pivoxil, ceftibuten, and moxalactam.

Antimicrobial Activity

The major features of these drugs (except cefoperazone) are their expanded gram-negative coverage and the ability of some to cross the blood-brain barrier. In addition to the gram-negative bacteria inhibited by other cephalosporins, third-generation drugs are active against citrobacter, *Serratia marcescens,* and providencia (though resistance can emerge during treatment of infections caused by these species due to selection of mutants that constitutively produce cephalosporinase). They are also effective against β-lactamase-producing strains of haemophilus and neisseria. Ceftazidime and cefoperazone are the two third-generation cephalosporins with useful activity against *P aeruginosa*. Like the second-generation drugs, third-generation cephalosporins are hydrolyzable by constitutively produced enterobacter chromosomal β-lactamase, and they are not reliably active against enterobacter species. Like enterobacter species, serratia, providencia, and citrobacter also produce a chromosomally encoded cephalosporinase that when constitutively expressed confers resistance to third-generation cephalosporins. Only ceftizoxime and moxalactam have good activity against *B fragilis*. Cefixime, ceftibuten, and cefpodoxime proxetil are oral agents possessing similar activity except that cefixime and ceftibuten are much less active against pneumococci (and completely inactive against penicillin-resistant strains) and have poor activity against *S aureus*.

Pharmacokinetics & Dosage

After intravenous infusion of 1 g of these drugs, serum levels are 60–140 μg/mL. They penetrate body fluids and tissues well and—with the exception of cefoperazone, cefixime, cefditoren pivoxil, ceftibuten, and cefpodoxime proxetil—achieve levels in the cerebrospinal fluid sufficient to inhibit most pathogens, including gram-negative rods, except perhaps pseudomonas.

The half-lives of these drugs and the necessary dosing intervals vary greatly: Ceftriaxone (half-life 7–8 hours) can be injected once every 24 hours at a dosage of 15–50 mg/kg/d. A single daily 1 g dose is sufficient for most serious infections, with 4 g once daily recommended for treatment of meningitis. Cefoperazone (half-life 2 hours) can be injected every 8–12 hours in a dosage of 25–100 mg/kg/d. The remaining drugs in the group (half-life 1–1.7 hours) can be injected every 6–8 hours in dosages between 2 and 12 g/d, depending on the severity of infection. Cefixime can be given orally (200 mg twice daily or 400 mg once daily) for respiratory or urinary tract infections. The dosage in adults for cefpodoxime proxetil and cefditoren pivoxil is 200–400 mg twice daily and for ceftibuten 400 mg once daily. The excretion of cefoperazone and ceftriaxone is mainly through the biliary tract, and no dosage adjustment is required in renal insufficiency. The others are excreted by the kidney and therefore require dosage adjustment in renal insufficiency.

Clinical Uses

Third-generation cephalosporins are used to treat a wide variety of serious infections caused by organisms that are resistant to most other drugs. Ceftriaxone (as a single 125 mg injection) and cefixime (as a single 400 mg oral dose) are first-line drugs for treatment of gonorrhea now that many strains of *N gonorrhoeae* are resistant to penicillin. Unfortunately, these drugs also are widely misused to treat infections that prove to be caused by strains that are susceptible to narrower spectrum agents. They should not be used to treat enterobacter infections even if the clinical isolate appears susceptible in vitro, because of emergence of resistance. Because of their penetration of the central nervous system, third-generation cephalosporins can be used to treat meningitis, including meningitis caused by pneumococci, meningococci, *H influenzae,* and susceptible enteric gram-negative rods, but not by *Listeria monocytogenes*. They should be used in combination with an aminoglycoside for treatment of meningitis caused by *P aeruginosa*. Ceftriaxone and cefotaxime are the most active cephalosporins against penicillin-resistant strains of pneumococci and are recommended for empirical therapy of serious infections that may be caused by these strains. Meningitis caused by highly penicillin-resistant strains of pneumococci (ie, those susceptible only to penicillin MICs > 1 μg/mL) may not respond even to these agents, and addition of vancomycin is recommended. Other potential indications include empirical therapy of sepsis of unknown cause in both the immunocompetent and the immunocompromised patient and treatment of infections for which a cephalosporin is the least toxic drug available. In neutropenic, febrile immunocompromised patients, third-generation cephalosporins are often used in combination with an aminoglycoside, but the necessity for including the aminoglycoside in the initial empirical regimen is controversial.

FOURTH-GENERATION CEPHALOSPORINS

Cefepime is an example of a so-called fourth-generation cephalosporin. It is more resistant to hydrolysis by chromosomal β lactamases (eg, those produced by enterobacter) and some extended-spectrum β lactamases that inactivate many of the third-generation cephalosporins. It has good activity against *P aeruginosa,* Enterobacteriaceae, *S aureus,* and *S pneumoniae*. It is highly active against haemophilus and neisseria. In animal models of meningitis, it penetrates well into cerebrospinal fluid. It is cleared by the kidneys and has a half-life of 2 hours, and its pharmacokinetic properties are very similar to those of ceftazidime. Unlike ceftazidime, however, cefepime has good activity against most penicillin-resistant strains of streptococci, and it may be useful in treatment of enterobacter infections.

Otherwise, its clinical role is similar to that of third-generation cephalosporins.

ADVERSE EFFECTS OF CEPHALOSPORINS

Allergy

Cephalosporins are sensitizing and may elicit a variety of hypersensitivity reactions that are identical to those of penicillins, including anaphylaxis, fever, skin rashes, nephritis, granulocytopenia, and hemolytic anemia. However, the chemical nucleus of cephalosporins is sufficiently different from that of penicillins so that some individuals with a history of penicillin allergy may tolerate cephalosporins. The frequency of cross-allergenicity between the two groups of drugs is uncertain but probably is around 5–10%. However, patients with a history of anaphylaxis to penicillins should not receive cephalosporins.

Toxicity

Local irritation can produce severe pain after intramuscular injection and thrombophlebitis after intravenous injection. Renal toxicity, including interstitial nephritis and even tubular necrosis, has been demonstrated and has caused the withdrawal of cephaloridine from clinical use.

Cephalosporins that contain a methylthiotetrazole group (eg, cefamandole, cefmetazole, cefotetan, cefoperazone) frequently cause hypoprothrombinemia and bleeding disorders. Administration of vitamin K_1, 10 mg twice weekly, can prevent this. Drugs with the methylthiotetrazole ring can also cause severe disulfiram-like reactions; consequently, alcohol and alcohol-containing medications must be avoided.

Superinfection

Many second- and particularly third-generation cephalosporins are ineffective against gram-positive organisms, especially methicillin-resistant staphylococci and enterococci. During treatment with such drugs,

these resistant organisms, as well as fungi, often proliferate and may induce superinfection.

OTHER BETA LACTAM DRUGS

MONOBACTAMS

These are drugs with a monocyclic β-lactam ring (Figure 43–1). They are relatively resistant to β lactamases and active against gram-negative rods (including pseudomonas and serratia). They have no activity against gram-positive bacteria or anaerobes. Aztreonam is the only monobactam available in the USA. It resembles aminoglycosides in its spectrum of activity. Aztreonam is given intravenously every 8 hours in a dose of 1–2 g, providing peak serum levels of 100 μg/mL. The half-life is 1–2 hours and is greatly prolonged in renal failure.

Penicillin-allergic patients tolerate aztreonam without reaction. Occasional skin rashes and elevations of serum aminotransferases occur during administration of aztreonam, but major toxicity has not yet been reported. The clinical usefulness of aztreonam has not been fully defined.

BETA-LACTAMASE INHIBITORS (CLAVULANIC ACID, SULBACTAM, & TAZOBACTAM)

These substances resemble β-lactam molecules (Figure 43–7) but themselves have very weak antibacterial action. They are potent inhibitors of many but not all bacterial β lactamases and can protect hydrolyzable penicillins from inactivation by these enzymes. β-Lactamase inhibitors are most active against Ambler class A β lactamases (plasmid-encoded transposable element [TEM] β-lactamases in particular) such as those produced by staphylococci, *H influenzae*, *N gonorrhoeae*, salmonella, shigella, *E coli*, and *K pneumoniae*. They are not good inhibitors of class C β-lactamases, which typically are chromosomally encoded and inducible, pro-

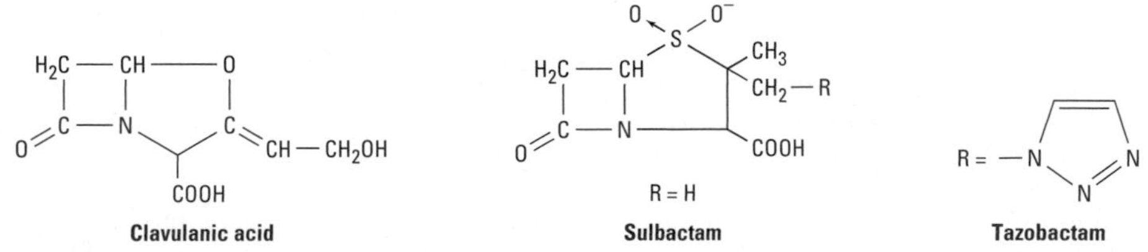

Figure 43–7. Structures of β-lactamase inhibitors.

duced by enterobacter, citrobacter, serratia, and pseudomonas, but they do inhibit chromosomal β lactamases of legionella, bacteroides, and branhamella.

The three inhibitors differ slightly with respect to pharmacology, stability, potency, and activity, but these differences are of little therapeutic significance. β-Lactamase inhibitors are available only in fixed combinations with specific penicillins. The antibacterial spectrum of the combination is determined by the companion penicillin, not the β-lactamase inhibitor. (The fixed combinations available in the USA are listed in the Preparations Available section.) An inhibitor will extend the spectrum of a penicillin provided that the inactivity of the penicillin is due to destruction by β lactamase and that the inhibitor is active against the β lactamase that is produced. Thus, ampicillin-sulbactam is active against β-lactamase-producing *S aureus* and *H influenzae* but not serratia, which produces a β lactamase that is not inhibited by sulbactam. Similarly, if a strain of *P aeruginosa* is resistant to piperacillin, it will also be resistant to piperacillin-tazobactam, since tazobactam does not inhibit the chromosomal β lactamase.

The indications for penicillin-β-lactamase inhibitor combinations are empirical therapy for infections caused by a wide range of potential pathogens in both immunocompromised and immunocompetent patients and treatment of mixed aerobic and anaerobic infections, such as intra-abdominal infections. Doses are the same as those used for the single agents except that the recommended dosage of piperacillin in the piperacillin-tazobactam combination is 3 g every 6 hours. This is less than the recommended 3–4 g every 4–6 hours for piperacillin alone, raising concerns about the use of the combination for treatment of suspected pseudomonal infection. Adjustments for renal insufficiency are made based on the penicillin component.

CARBAPENEMS

The carbapenems are structurally related to β-lactam antibiotics (Figure 43–1). Ertapenem, imipenem, and meropenem are licensed for use in the USA. Imipenem has a wide spectrum with good activity against many gram-negative rods, including *Pseudomonas aeruginosa,* gram-positive organisms, and anaerobes. It is resistant to most β lactamases but not metallo-β lactamases. *Enterococcus faecium,* methicillin-resistant strains of staphylococci, *Clostridium difficile, Burkholderia cepacia,* and *Stenotrophomonas maltophilia* are resistant. Imipenem is inactivated by dehydropeptidases in renal tubules, resulting in low urinary concentrations. Consequently, it is administered together with an inhibitor of renal dehydropeptidase, cilastatin, for clinical use. Meropenem is similar to imipenem but has slightly

greater activity against gram-negative aerobes and slightly less activity against gram-positives. It is not significantly degraded by renal dehydropeptidase and does not require an inhibitor. Ertapenem is less active than meropenem or imipenem against *Pseudomonas aeruginosa* and acinetobacter species. It is not degraded by renal dehydropeptidase.

Carbapenems penetrate body tissues and fluids well, including the cerebrospinal fluid. All are cleared renally, and the dose must be reduced in patients with renal insufficiency. The usual dose of imipenem is 0.25–0.5 g given intravenously every 6–8 hours (half-life 1 hour). The usual adult dose of meropenem is 1 g intravenously every 8 hours. Ertapenem has the longest half-life (4 hours) and is administered as a once-daily dose of 1 g intravenously or intramuscularly. Intramuscular ertapenem is irritating, and for that reason the drug is formulated with 1% lidocaine for administration by this route.

A carbapenem is indicated for infections caused by susceptible organisms that are resistant to other available drugs and for treatment of mixed aerobic and anaerobic infections. Carbapenems are active against many highly penicillin-resistant strains of pneumococci. A carbapenem is the β-lactam antibiotic of choice for treatment of enterobacter infections, since it is resistant to destruction by the β lactamase produced by these organisms. Strains of *Pseudomonas aeruginosa* may rapidly develop resistance to imipenem or meropenem, so simultaneous use of an aminoglycoside is recommended for infections caused by those organisms. Ertapenem is insufficiently active against *P aeruginosa* and should not be used to treat infections caused by that organism. Imipenem or meropenem with or without an aminoglycoside may be effective treatment for febrile neutropenic patients.

The most common adverse effects of carbapenems—which tend to be more common with imipenem—are nausea, vomiting, diarrhea, skin rashes, and reactions at the infusion sites. Excessive levels of imipenem in patients with renal failure may lead to seizures. Meropenem and ertapenem are less likely to cause seizures than imipenem. Patients allergic to penicillins may be allergic to carbapenems as well.

OTHER INHIBITORS OF CELL WALL SYNTHESIS

VANCOMYCIN

Vancomycin is an antibiotic produced by *Streptococcus orientalis.* With the single exception of flavobacterium, it is active only against gram-positive bacteria, particularly staphylococci. Vancomycin is a glycopeptide of molecular weight 1500. It is water-soluble and quite stable.

Mechanisms of Action & Basis of Resistance

Vancomycin inhibits cell wall synthesis by binding firmly to the D-Ala-D-Ala terminus of nascent peptidoglycan pentapeptide (Figure 43–5). This inhibits the transglycosylase, preventing further elongation of peptidoglycan and cross-linking. The peptidoglycan is thus weakened and the cell becomes susceptible to lysis. The cell membrane is also damaged, which contributes to the antibacterial effect.

Resistance to vancomycin in enterococci is due to modification of the D-Ala-D-Ala binding site of the peptidoglycan building block in which the terminal D-Ala is replaced by D-lactate. This results in the loss of a critical hydrogen bond that facilitates high-affinity binding of vancomycin to its target and loss of activity. This mechanism is also present in vancomycin-resistant S aureus strains (MIC ≥ 32 μg/mL), which have acquired the enterococcal resistance determinants. The mechanism for reduced vancomycin susceptibility of vancomycin-intermediate strains (MICs = 8–16 μg/mL) is not known.

Antibacterial Activity

Vancomycin is bactericidal for gram-positive bacteria in concentrations of 0.5–10 μg/mL. Most pathogenic staphylococci, including those producing β lactamase and those resistant to nafcillin and methicillin, are killed by 4 μg/mL or less. Vancomycin kills staphylococci relatively slowly and only if cells are actively dividing; the rate is less than that of the penicillins both in vitro and in vivo. Vancomycin is synergistic with gentamicin and streptomycin against E faecium and E faecalis strains that do not exhibit high levels of aminoglycoside resistance.

Pharmacokinetics

Vancomycin is poorly absorbed from the intestinal tract and is administered orally only for the treatment of antibiotic-associated enterocolitis caused by Clostridium difficile. Parenteral doses must be administered intravenously. A 1 hour intravenous infusion of 1 g produces blood levels of 15–30 μg/mL for 1–2 hours. The drug is widely distributed in the body. Cerebrospinal fluid levels 7–30% of simultaneous serum concentrations are achieved if there is meningeal inflammation. Ninety percent of the drug is excreted by glomerular filtration. In the presence of renal insufficiency, striking accumulation may occur (Table 43–2). In functionally anephric patients, the half-life of vancomycin is 6–10 days. The drug is not removed by hemodialysis.

Clinical Uses

The main indication for parenteral vancomycin is sepsis or endocarditis caused by methicillin-resistant staphylococci. However, vancomycin is not as effective as an antistaphylococcal penicillin for treatment of serious infections such as endocarditis caused by methicillin-susceptible strains. Vancomycin in combination with gentamicin is an alternative regimen for treatment of enterococcal endocarditis in a patient with serious penicillin allergy. Vancomycin (in combination with cefotaxime, ceftriaxone, or rifampin) is also recommended for treatment of meningitis suspected or known to be caused by a highly penicillin-resistant strain of pneumococcus (ie, MIC > 1 μg/mL). The recommended dosage is 30 mg/kg/d in two or three divided doses. A typical dosing regimen for most infections in adults with normal renal function is 1 g every 12 hours. The dosage in children is 40 mg/kg/d in three or four divided doses. Clearance of vancomycin is directly proportionate to creatinine clearance, and the dose is reduced accordingly in patients with renal insufficiency (see Moellering et al, 1981, for guidelines). For functionally anephric adult patients, a 1 g dose administered once a week is usually sufficient. Patients receiving a prolonged course of therapy should have serum concentrations checked. Recommended peak serum concentrations are 20–50 μg/mL, and trough concentrations are 5–15 μg/mL.

Oral vancomycin, 0.125–0.25 g every 6 hours, is used to treat antibiotic-associated enterocolitis caused by Clostridium difficile. However, because of the emergence of vancomycin-resistant enterococci and the strong selective pressure of oral vancomycin for these resistant organisms, metronidazole is strongly preferred as initial therapy and vancomycin should be reserved for treatment of refractory cases.

Adverse Reactions

Adverse reactions are encountered in about 10% of cases. Most reactions are minor. Vancomycin is irritating to tissue, resulting in phlebitis at the site of injection. Chills and fever may occur. Ototoxicity is rare and nephrotoxicity uncommon with current preparations. However, administration with another ototoxic or nephrotoxic drug, such as an aminoglycoside, increases the risk of these toxicities. Ototoxicity can be minimized by maintaining peak serum concentrations below 60 μg/mL. Among the more common reactions is the so-called "red man" or "red neck" syndrome. This infusion-related flushing is caused by release of histamine. It can be largely prevented by prolonging the infusion period to 1–2 hours or increasing the dosing interval.

TEICOPLANIN

Teicoplanin is a glycopeptide antibiotic that is very similar to vancomycin in mechanism of action and antibacterial spectrum. Unlike vancomycin, it can be given intramuscularly as well as intravenously. Teicoplanin has a long half-life (45–70 hours), permitting once-daily dosing. This drug is available in Europe but has not been approved for use in the United States.

FOSFOMYCIN

Fosfomycin trometamol, a stable salt of fosfomycin (**phosphonomycin**), inhibits a very early stage of bacterial cell wall synthesis (Figure 43–5). An analog of phosphoenolpyruvate, it is structurally unrelated to any other antimicrobial agent. It inhibits the cytoplasmic enzyme enolpyruvate transferase by covalently binding to the cysteine residue of the active site and blocking the addition of phosphoenolpyruvate to UDP-*N*-acetylglucosamine. This reaction is the first step in the formation of UDP-*N*-acetylmuramic acid, the precursor of *N*-acetylmuramic acid, which is found only in bacterial cell walls. The drug is transported into the bacterial cell by glycerophosphate or glucose 6-phosphate transport systems. Resistance is due to inadequate transport of drug into the cell.

Fosfomycin is active against both gram-positive and gram-negative organisms at concentrations ≤ 125 μg/mL. Susceptibility tests should be performed in growth medium supplemented with glucose 6-phosphate to minimize false-positive indications of resistance. In vitro synergism occurs when fosfomycin is combined with β-lactam antibiotics, aminoglycosides, or fluoroquinolones.

Fosfomycin trometamol is available in both oral and parenteral formulations, though only the oral preparation is approved for use in the United States. Oral bioavailability is approximately 40%. Peak serum concentrations are 10 μg/mL and 30 μg/mL following a 2 g or 4 g oral dose, respectively. The half-life is approximately 4 hours. The active drug is excreted by the kidney, with urinary concentrations exceeding MICs for most urinary tract pathogens.

Fosfomycin is approved for use as a single 3 g dose for treatment of uncomplicated lower urinary tract infections in women. The drug appears to be safe for use in pregnancy.

BACITRACIN

Bacitracin is a cyclic peptide mixture first obtained from the Tracy strain of *Bacillus subtilis* in 1943. It is active against gram-positive microorganisms. Bacitracin inhibits cell wall formation by interfering with dephosphorylation in cycling of the lipid carrier that transfers peptidoglycan subunits to the growing cell wall (Figure 43–5). There is no cross-resistance between bacitracin and other antimicrobial drugs.

Bacitracin is markedly nephrotoxic if administered systemically, producing proteinuria, hematuria, and nitrogen retention. Hypersensitivity reactions (eg, skin rashes) are rare. Because of its marked toxicity when used systemically, it is limited to topical use. Bacitracin is poorly absorbed. Topical application results in local antibacterial activity without significant systemic toxicity. The small amounts of bacitracin that are absorbed are excreted by glomerular filtration.

Bacitracin, 500 units/g in an ointment base (often combined with polymyxin or neomycin), is useful for the suppression of mixed bacterial flora in surface lesions of the skin, in wounds, or on mucous membranes. Solutions of bacitracin containing 100–200 units/mL in saline can be employed for irrigation of joints, wounds, or the pleural cavity.

CYCLOSERINE

Cycloserine is an antibiotic produced by *Streptomyces orchidaceus*. It is water-soluble and very unstable at acid pH. Cycloserine inhibits many gram-positive and gram-negative organisms, but it is used almost exclusively to treat tuberculosis caused by strains of *M tuberculosis* resistant to first-line agents. Cycloserine is a structural analog of D-alanine and inhibits the incorporation of D-alanine into peptidoglycan pentapeptide by inhibiting alanine racemase, which converts L-alanine to D-alanine, and D-alanyl-D-alanine ligase (Figure 43–5). After ingestion of 0.25 g of cycloserine blood levels reach 20–30 μg/mL—sufficient to inhibit many strains of mycobacteria and gram-negative bacteria. The drug is widely distributed in tissues. Most of the drug is excreted in active form into the urine. The dosage for treating tuberculosis is 0.5 to 1 g/d in two or three divided doses.

Cycloserine causes serious dose-related central nervous system toxicity with headaches, tremors, acute psychosis, and convulsions. If oral dosages are maintained below 0.75 g/d, such effects can usually be avoided.

PREPARATIONS AVAILABLE

PENICILLINS

Amoxicillin (generic, Amoxil, others)
Oral: 125, 200, 250, 400 mg chewable tablets; 500, 875 mg tablets; 250, 500 mg capsules; powder to reconstitute for 50, 125, 200, 250, 400 mg/mL solution

Amoxicillin/potassium clavulanate (generic, Augmentin)*
Oral: 250, 500, 875 mg tablets; 125, 200, 250, 400 mg chewable tablets; 1000 mg extended release tablet powder to reconstitute for 125, 200, 250 mg/5 mL suspension

Ampicillin (generic)
Oral: 250, 500 mg capsules; powder to reconstitute for 125, 250 mg suspensions
Parenteral: powder to reconstitute for injection (125, 250, 500 mg, 1, 2 g per vial)

Ampicillin/sulbactam sodium (generic, Unasyn)†
Parenteral: 1, 2 g ampicillin powder to reconstitute for IV or IM injection

Carbenicillin (Geocillin)
Oral: 382 mg tablets

Dicloxacillin (generic)
Oral: 250, 500 mg capsules

Mezlocillin (Mezlin)
Parenteral: powder to reconstitute for injection (in 1, 2, 3, 4 g vials)

Nafcillin (generic)
Oral: 250 mg capsules
Parenteral: 1, 2 g per IV piggyback units

Oxacillin (generic)
Oral: 250, 500 mg capsules; powder to reconstitute for 250 mg/5 mL solution
Parenteral: powder to reconstitute for injection (0.5, 1, 2, 10 g per vial)
Penicillin G (generic, Pentids, Pfizerpen)
Oral: 0.2, 0.25, 0.4, 0.5, 0.8 million unit tablets; powder to reconstitute 400,000 units/5mL suspension
Parenteral: powder to reconstitute for injection (1, 2, 3, 5, 10, 20 million units)

Penicillin G benzathine (Permapen, Bicillin)
Parenteral: 0.6, 1.2, 2.4 million units per dose

Penicillin G procaine (generic)
Parenteral: 0.6, 1.2 million units/mL for IM injection only

Penicillin V (generic, V-Cillin, Pen-Vee K, others)
Oral: 250, 500 mg tablets; powder to reconstitute for 125, 250 mg/5 mL solution

Piperacillin (Pipracil)
Parenteral: powder to reconstitute for injection (2, 3, 4 g per vial)

Piperacillin and tazobactam sodium (Zosyn)‡
Parenteral: 2, 3, 4 g powder to reconstitute for IV injection

Ticarcillin (Ticar)
Parenteral: powder to reconstitute for injection (1, 3, 6 g per vial)

Ticarcillin/clavulanate potassium (Timentin)§
Parenteral: 3 g powder to reconstitute for injection

CEPHALOSPORINS & OTHER BETA-LACTAM DRUGS

Narrow Spectrum (First-Generation) Cephalosporins

Cefadroxil (generic, Duricef)
Oral: 500 mg capsules; 1 g tablets; 125, 250, 500 mg/5 mL suspension

Cefazolin (generic, Ancef, Kefzol)
Parenteral: powder to reconstitute for injection (0.25, 0.5, 1 g per vial or IV piggyback unit)

Cephalexin (generic, Keflex, others)
Oral: 250, 500 mg capsules and tablets; 1 g tablets; 125, 250 mg/5 mL suspension

Cephalothin (generic, Keflin)¶
Parenteral: powder to reconstitute for injection and solution for injection (1 g per vial or infusion pack)

Cephapirin (Cefadyl)
Parenteral: powder to reconstitute for injection (1 g per vial or IV piggyback unit)

Cephradine (generic, Velosef)
Oral: 250, 500 mg capsules; 125, 250 mg/5 mL suspension
Parenteral: powder to reconstitute for injection (0.25, 0.5, 1, 2 g per vial)

Intermediate Spectrum (Second-Generation) Cephalosporins

Cefaclor (generic, Ceclor)
Oral: 250, 500 mg capsules; 375, 500 mg extended-release tablets; powder to reconstitute for 125, 187, 250, 375 mg/5 mL suspension

Cefamandole (Mandol)
Parenteral: 1, 2 g (in vials) for IM, IV injection

---

* Clavulanate content varies with the formulation; see package insert.
† Sulbactam content is half the ampicillin content.

‡ Tazobactam content is 12.5% of the piperacillin content.
§ Clavulanate content 0.1 g.
¶Not available in the USA.

Cefmetazole (Zefazone)
Parenteral: 1, 2 g powder for IV injection
Cefonicid (Monocid)
Parenteral: powder to reconstitute for injection (1, 10 g per vial)
Cefotetan (Cefotan)
Parenteral: powder to reconstitute for injection (1, 2, 10 g per vial)
Cefoxitin (Mefoxin)
Parenteral: powder to reconstitute for injection (1, 2, 10 g per vial)
Cefprozil (Cefzil)
Oral: 250, 500 mg tablets; powder to reconstitute 125, 250 mg/5mL suspension
Cefuroxime (generic, Ceftin, Kefurox, Zinacef)
Oral: 125, 250, 500 mg tablets; 125, 250 mg/5 mL suspension
Parenteral: powder to reconstitute for injection (0.75, 1.5, 7.5 g per vial or infusion pack)
Loracarbef (Lorabid)
Oral: 200, 400 mg capsules; powder for 100, 200 mg/5 mL suspension

Broad-Spectrum (Third- & Fourth-Generation) Cephalosporins
Cefdinir (Omnicef)
Oral: 300 mg capsules; 125 mg/5 mL suspension
Cefditoren (Spectracef)
Oral: 200 mg tablets
Cefepime (Maxipime)
Parenteral: powder for injection 0.5, 1, 2 g
Cefixime (Suprax)
Oral: 200, 400 mg tablets; powder for oral suspension, 100 mg/5 mL
Cefoperazone (Cefobid)
Parenteral: powder to reconstitute for injection (1, 2 g per vial, 10 g bulk)
Cefotaxime (Claforan)
Parenteral: powder to reconstitute for injection (0.5, 1, 2 g per vial)

Cefpodoxime proxetil (Vantin)
Oral: 100, 200 mg tablets; 50, 100 mg granules for suspension in 5 mL
Ceftazidime (generic, Fortaz, Tazidime)
Parenteral: powder to reconstitute for injection (0.5, 1, 2 g per vial)
Ceftibuten (Cedax)
Oral: 400 mg capsules; 90, 180 mg/5 mL powder for oral suspension
Ceftizoxime (Cefizox)
Parenteral: powder to reconstitute for injection and solution for injection (0.5, 1, 2 g per vial)
Ceftriaxone (Rocephin)
Parenteral: powder to reconstitute for injection (0.25, 0.5, 1, 2, 10 g per vial)

Carbapenems & Monobactam
Aztreonam (Azactam)
Parenteral: powder to reconstitute for injection (0.5, 1, 2 g)
Ertapenem (Invanz)
Parenteral: 1 g powder to reconstitute for intravenous (0.9% NaCl diluent) or intramuscular (1% lidocaine diluent) injection
Imipenem/cilastatin (Primaxin)
Parenteral: powder to reconstitute for injection (250, 500, 750 mg imipenem per vial)
Meropenem (Merrem IV)
Parenteral: powder for injection (0.5, 1 g per vial)

OTHER DRUGS DISCUSSED IN THIS CHAPTER
Cycloserine (Seromycin Pulvules)
Oral: 250 mg capsules
Fosfomycin (Monurol)
Oral: 3 g packet
Vancomycin (generic, Vancocin, Vancoled)
Oral: 125, 250 mg Pulvules; powder to reconstitute for 250 mg/5 mL, 500 mg/6 mL solution
Parenteral: 0.5, 1, 5, 10 g powder to reconstitute for IV injection

REFERENCES

Balbisi EA: Cefditoren, a new aminothiazolyl cephalosporin. Pharmacology 2002;22:1278.

Centers for Disease Control and Prevention: Vancomycin resistant *Staphylococcus aureus*—Pennsylvania, 2002. JAMA 2002;288:2116.

Chow JW et al: *Enterobacter* bacteremia: Clinical features and emergence of antibiotic resistance during therapy. Ann Intern Med 1991;115:585.

Eliopoulous GM, Moellering RC Jr: Azlocillin, mezlocillin, and piperacillin: New broad-spectrum penicillins. Ann Intern Med 1982;97:755.

Ertapenem (Invanz)—a new parenteral carbapenem. Med Lett Drugs Ther 2002;44:25.

Friedland IR, McCracken Jr GH: Management of infections caused by antibiotic-resistant *Streptococcus pneumoniae*. N Engl J Med 1994;331:377.

Fulton B, Perry CM: Cefpodoxime proxetil: A review of its use in the management of bacterial infections in pediatric patients. Paediatr Drugs 2001;3:137.

Ghuysen JM: Serine beta-lactamases and penicillin-binding proteins. Ann Rev Microbiol 1991;45:37.

Handsfield HH et al: A comparison of single-dose cefixime with ceftriaxone as treatment for uncomplicated gonorrhea. N Engl J Med 1991;325:1337.

Hiramatsu K et al: Methicillin resistant *Staphylococcus aureus* clinical strain with reduced vancomycin susceptibility. J Antimicrob Chemother 1997;40:135.

Livermore DM et al: In vitro activities of ertapenem (MK-0826) against recent clinical bacteria collected in Europe and Australia. Antimicrob Agents Chemother 2001;45:1860.

McHenry MC, Gavan TL: Vancomycin. Pediatr Clin North Am 1983;30:31.

Moellering RC et al: Vancomycin therapy in patients with impaired renal function: A nomogram for dosage. Ann Intern Med 1981;94:343.

Majumdar AK et al: Pharmacokinetics of ertapenem in healthy young volunteers. Antimicrob Agents Chemother 2002;46:3506.

Neu HC: Antistaphylococcal penicillins. Med Clin North Am 1982;66:51.

Neu HC: Carbenicillin and ticarcillin. Med Clin North Am 1982;66:61.

Nikaido H: Prevention of drug access to bacterial targets: Role of permeability barriers and active efflux. Science 1994;264:382.

Remington JS (editor): Carbapenems: A new class of antibiotics. (Symposium.) Am J Med 1985;78(Suppl 6A):1.

Sanders CC: Novel resistance selected by the new expanded-spectrum cephalosporins: A concern. J Infect Dis 1983;147:585.

Sieradzki K et al: The development of vancomycin resistance in a patient with methicillin-resistant *Staphylococcus aureus* infection. N Engl J Med 1999;340:517.

Smith TL et al: Emergence of vancomycin resistance in *Staphylococcus aureus*. Glycopeptide-Intermediate *Staphylococcus aureus* Working Group. N Engl J Med 1999;340:493.

Spratt BG: Resistance to antibiotics mediated by target alterations. Science 1994;264:389.

Sykes RB, Bonner DP: Discovery and development of the monobactams. Rev Infect Dis 1985;7(Suppl 4):S579.

Teasley DG et al: Trial of metronidazole vs. vancomycin for *Clostridium difficile:* Associated diarrhea and colitis. Lancet 1983;2:1043.

Walsh CT: Vancomycin resistance: Decoding the molecular logic. Science 1993;261:308.

Wilson WR et al: Antibiotic treatment of adults with infective endocarditis due to streptococci, enterococci, staphylococci, and HACEK microorganisms. JAMA 1995;274:1706.

Chloramphenicol, Tetracyclines, Macrolides, Clindamycin, & Streptogramins

44

Henry F. Chambers, MD

The drugs described in this chapter all share the property of inhibiting bacterial protein synthesis by binding to and interfering with their ribosomes.

CHLORAMPHENICOL

Crystalline chloramphenicol is a neutral, stable compound with the following structure:

Chloramphenicol

It is soluble in alcohol but poorly soluble in water. Chloramphenicol succinate, which is used for parenteral administration, is highly water-soluble. It is hydrolyzed in vivo with liberation of free chloramphenicol.

Antimicrobial Activity

Chloramphenicol is a potent inhibitor of microbial protein synthesis. It binds reversibly to the 50S subunit of the bacterial ribosome (Figure 44–1). It inhibits the peptidyl transferase step of protein synthesis. Chloramphenicol is a bacteriostatic broad-spectrum antibiotic that is active against both aerobic and anaerobic gram-positive and gram-negative organisms. It is active also against rickettsiae but not chlamydiae. Most gram-positive bacteria are inhibited at concentrations of 1–10

μg/mL, and many gram-negative bacteria are inhibited by concentrations of 0.2–5 μg/mL. *Haemophilus influenzae, Neisseria meningitidis,* and some strains of bacteroides are highly susceptible, and for them chloramphenicol may be bactericidal.

Low-level resistance may emerge from large populations of chloramphenicol-susceptible cells by selection of mutants that are less permeable to the drug. Clinically significant resistance is due to production of chloramphenicol acetyltransferase, a plasmid-encoded enzyme that inactivates the drug.

Pharmacokinetics

The usual dosage of chloramphenicol is 50–100 mg/kg/d. After oral administration, crystalline chloramphenicol is rapidly and completely absorbed. A 1 g oral dose produces blood levels between 10 and 15 μg/mL. Chloramphenicol palmitate is a prodrug that is hydrolyzed in the intestine to yield free chloramphenicol. The parenteral formulation, chloramphenicol succinate, yields free chloramphenicol by hydrolysis, giving blood levels somewhat lower than those achieved with orally administered drug. After absorption, chloramphenicol is widely distributed to virtually all tissues and body fluids, including the central nervous system and cerebrospinal fluid such that the concentration of chloramphenicol in brain tissue may be equal to that in serum. The drug penetrates cell membranes readily. Most of the drug is inactivated either by conjugation with glucuronic acid (principally in the liver) or by reduction to inactive aryl amines. Excretion of active chloramphenicol (about 10% of the total dose administered) and of inactive degradation products (about 90%

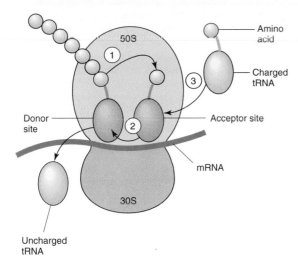

Figure 44–1. Steps in bacterial protein synthesis and targets of (1) chloramphenicol; (2) macrolides, clindamycin, and type B streptogramins; and (3) tetracyclines. The 70S ribosomal mRNA complex is shown with its 50S and 30S subunits. The peptidyl tRNA at the donor site donates the growing peptide chain to the aminoacyl tRNA at the acceptor site in a reaction catalyzed by peptidyl transferase. The tRNA, discharged of its peptide, is released from the donor site to make way for translocation of the newly formed peptidyl tRNA. The acceptor site is then free to be occupied by the next "charged" aminoacyl tRNA.

of the total) occurs by way of the urine. A small amount of active drug is excreted into bile or feces. The systemic dosage of chloramphenicol need not be altered in renal insufficiency, but it must be reduced markedly in hepatic failure. Newborns less than a week old and premature infants also clear chloramphenicol less well, and the dosage should be reduced to 25 mg/kg/d.

Clinical Uses

Because of potential toxicity, bacterial resistance, and the availability of other effective drugs (eg, cephalosporins), chloramphenicol is all but obsolete as a systemic drug. It may be considered for treatment of serious rickettsial infections, such as typhus or Rocky Mountain spotted fever, in children for whom tetracyclines are contraindicated, ie, those under 8 years of age. It is an alternative to a β-lactam antibiotic for treatment of meningococcal meningitis occurring in patients who have major hypersensitivity reactions to penicillin or bacterial meningitis caused by penicillin-resistant strains

of pneumococci. The dosage is 50–100 mg/kg/d in four divided doses.

Chloramphenicol is occasionally used topically in the treatment of eye infections because of its wide antibacterial spectrum and its penetration of ocular tissues and the aqueous humor. It is ineffective for chlamydial infections.

Adverse Reactions

A. GASTROINTESTINAL DISTURBANCES

Adults occasionally develop nausea, vomiting, and diarrhea. This is rare in children. Oral or vaginal candidiasis may occur as a result of alteration of normal microbial flora.

B. BONE MARROW DISTURBANCES

Chloramphenicol commonly causes a dose-related reversible suppression of red cell production at dosages exceeding 50 mg/kg/d after 1–2 weeks. Aplastic anemia is a rare consequence of chloramphenicol administration by any route. It is an idiosyncratic reaction unrelated to dose, though it occurs more frequently with prolonged use. It tends to be irreversible and can be fatal. Aplastic anemia probably develops in one of every 24,000–40,000 patients who have taken chloramphenicol.

C. TOXICITY FOR NEWBORN INFANTS

Newborn infants lack an effective glucuronic acid conjugation mechanism for the degradation and detoxification of chloramphenicol. Consequently, when infants are given dosages above 50 mg/kg/d, the drug may accumulate, resulting in the **gray baby syndrome,** with vomiting, flaccidity, hypothermia, gray color, shock, and collapse. To avoid this toxic effect, chloramphenicol should be used with caution in infants and the dosage limited to 50 mg/kg/d or less (during the first week of life) in full-term infants and 25 mg/kg/d in premature infants.

D. INTERACTION WITH OTHER DRUGS

Chloramphenicol inhibits hepatic microsomal enzymes that metabolize several drugs. Half-lives are prolonged, and the serum concentrations of phenytoin, tolbutamide, chlorpropamide, and warfarin are increased. Like other bacteriostatic inhibitors of microbial protein synthesis, chloramphenicol can antagonize bactericidal drugs such as penicillins or aminoglycosides.

TETRACYCLINES

All of the tetracyclines have the basic structure shown below:

	R$_7$	R$_6$	R$_5$	Renal Clearance (mL/min)
Chlortetracycline	— Cl	— CH$_3$	— H	35
Oxytetracycline	— H	— CH$_3$	— OH	90
Tetracycline	— H	— CH3	— H	65
Demeclocycline	— Cl	— H	— H	35
Methacycline	— H	═CH$_2$*	— OH	31
Doxycycline	— H	— CH$_3$*	— OH	16
Minocycline	— N(CH$_3$)$_2$	— H	— H	10

*There is no — OH at position 6 on methacycline and doxycycline.

Free tetracyclines are crystalline amphoteric substances of low solubility. They are available as hydrochlorides, which are more soluble. Such solutions are acid and, with the exception of chlortetracycline, fairly stable. Tetracyclines chelate divalent metal ions, which can interfere with their absorption and activity.

Antimicrobial Activity

Tetracyclines are broad-spectrum bacteriostatic antibiotics that inhibit protein synthesis. They are active against many gram-positive and gram-negative bacteria, including anaerobes, rickettsiae, chlamydiae, mycoplasmas, and L forms; and against some protozoa, eg, amebas. The antibacterial activities of most tetracyclines are similar except that tetracycline-resistant strains may remain susceptible to doxycycline or minocycline, drugs that are less rapidly transported by the pump that is responsible for resistance (see below). Differences in clinical efficacy are minor and attributable largely to features of absorption, distribution, and excretion of individual drugs.

Tetracyclines enter microorganisms in part by passive diffusion and in part by an energy-dependent process of active transport. Susceptible cells concentrate the drug intracellularly. Once inside the cell, tetracyclines bind reversibly to the 30S subunit of the bacterial ribosome, blocking the binding of aminoacyl-tRNA to the acceptor site on the mRNA-ribosome complex (Figure 44–1). This prevents addition of amino acids to the growing peptide.

Resistance

Three mechanisms of resistance to tetracycline have been described: (1) decreased intracellular accumulation due to either impaired influx or increased efflux by an active transport protein pump; (2) ribosome protection due to production of proteins that interfere with tetra-

cycline binding to the ribosome; and (3) enzymatic inactivation of tetracyclines. The most important of these is production of an efflux pump. The pump protein is encoded on a plasmid and may be transmitted by transduction or by conjugation. Because these plasmids commonly encode resistance genes for other drugs, eg, aminoglycosides, sulfonamides, and chloramphenicol, tetracycline resistance is a marker for resistance to multiple drugs.

Pharmacokinetics

Tetracyclines mainly differ in their absorption after oral administration and their elimination. Absorption after oral administration is approximately 30% for chlortetracycline; 60–70% for tetracycline, oxytetracycline, demeclocycline, and methacycline; and 95–100% for doxycycline and minocycline. A portion of an orally administered dose of tetracycline remains in the gut lumen, modifies intestinal flora, and is excreted in the feces. Absorption occurs mainly in the upper small intestine and is impaired by food (except doxycycline and minocycline); by divalent cations (Ca^{2+}, Mg^{2+}, Fe^{2+}) or Al^{3+}; by dairy products and antacids, which contain multivalent cations; and by alkaline pH. Specially buffered tetracycline solutions are formulated for intravenous administration.

Tetracyclines are 40–80% bound by serum proteins. Oral dosages of 500 mg every 6 hours of tetracycline hydrochloride or oxytetracycline produce peak blood levels of 4–6 μg/mL. Peak levels of 2–4 μg/mL are achieved with a 200 mg dose of doxycycline or minocycline. Intravenously injected tetracyclines give somewhat higher levels only temporarily. Tetracyclines are distributed widely to tissues and body fluids except for cerebrospinal fluid, where concentrations are 10–25% of those in serum. Minocycline reaches very high concentrations in tears and saliva, which makes it useful for eradication of the meningococcal carrier state. Tetracyclines cross the placenta to reach the fetus and are also excreted in milk. As a result of chelation with calcium, tetracyclines are bound to—and damage—growing bones and teeth. Carbamazepine, phenytoin, barbiturates, and chronic alcohol ingestion may shorten the half-life of doxycycline 50% by induction of hepatic enzymes that metabolize the drug.

Tetracyclines are excreted mainly in bile and urine. Concentrations in bile exceed those in serum tenfold. Some of the drug excreted in bile is reabsorbed from the intestine (enterohepatic circulation) and contributes to maintenance of serum levels. Ten to 50 percent of various tetracyclines is excreted into the urine, mainly by glomerular filtration. Ten to 40 percent of the drug in the body is excreted in feces. Doxycycline, in contrast to other tetracyclines, is eliminated by nonrenal mechanisms, does not accumulate significantly in renal failure, and requires no dosage adjustment, making it the tetracycline of choice for use in the setting of renal insufficiency.

Tetracyclines are classified as short-acting (chlortetracycline, tetracycline, oxytetracycline), intermediate-acting (demeclocycline and methacycline), or long-acting (doxycycline and minocycline) based on serum half-lives of 6–8 hours, 12 hours, and 16–18 hours, respectively. The almost complete absorption and slow excretion of doxycycline and minocycline allow for once-daily dosing.

Clinical Uses

A tetracycline is the drug of choice in infections with *Mycoplasma pneumoniae,* chlamydiae, rickettsiae, and some spirochetes. They are used in combination regimens to treat gastric and duodenal ulcer disease caused by *Helicobacter pylori.* They may be employed in various gram-positive and gram-negative bacterial infections, including vibrio infections, provided the organism is not resistant. In cholera, tetracyclines rapidly stop the shedding of vibrios, but tetracycline resistance has appeared during epidemics. Tetracyclines remain effective in most chlamydial infections, including sexually transmitted diseases. Tetracyclines are no longer recommended for treatment of gonococcal disease because of resistance. A tetracycline—usually in combination with an aminoglycoside—is indicated for plague, tularemia, and brucellosis. Tetracyclines are sometimes employed in the treatment of protozoal infections, eg, those due to *Entamoeba histolytica* or *Plasmodium falciparum.* Other uses include treatment of acne, exacerbations of bronchitis, community-acquired pneumonia, Lyme disease, relapsing fever, leptospirosis, and some nontuberculous mycobacterial infections (eg, *Mycobacterium marinum*). Tetracyclines formerly were used for a variety of common infections, including bacterial gastroenteritis, pneumonia (other than mycoplasmal or chlamydial pneumonia), and urinary tract infections. However, many strains of bacteria causing these infections now are resistant, and other agents have largely supplanted tetracyclines.

Minocycline, 200 mg orally daily for 5 days, can eradicate the meningococcal carrier state, but because of side-effects and resistance of many meningococcal strains, rifampin is preferred. Demeclocycline inhibits the action of ADH in the renal tubule and has been used in the treatment of inappropriate secretion of ADH or similar peptides by certain tumors (see Chapter 15).

A. ORAL DOSAGE

The oral dosage for rapidly excreted tetracyclines, equivalent to tetracycline hydrochloride, is 0.25–0.5 g four times daily for adults and 20–40 mg/kg/d for children (8 years of age and older). For severe systemic infections, the higher dosage is indicated, at least for the first few days. The daily dose is 600 mg for demeclocycline or methacycline, 100 mg once or twice a day for doxycycline, and 100 mg twice a day for minocycline. Doxycycline is the tetracycline of choice because it can be given as a once-daily dose and its absorption is not significantly affected by food. All tetracyclines chelate with metals, and none should be administered with milk, antacids, or ferrous sulfate. To avoid deposition in growing bones or teeth, tetracyclines should be avoided for pregnant women and for children under 8 years of age.

B. PARENTERAL DOSAGE

Several tetracyclines are available for intravenous injection in doses of 0.1–0.5 g every 6–12 hours (similar to oral doses), depending on the agent. Intramuscular injection is not recommended because of pain and inflammation at the injection site. Doxycycline is the preferred agent, at a dosage of 100 mg every 12–24 hours.

Adverse Reactions

Hypersensitivity reactions (drug fever, skin rashes) to tetracyclines are uncommon. Most adverse effects are due to direct toxicity of the drug or to alteration of microbial flora.

A. GASTROINTESTINAL ADVERSE EFFECTS

Nausea, vomiting, and diarrhea are the most common reasons for discontinuing tetracycline medication. These effects are attributable to direct local irritation of the intestinal tract. Nausea, anorexia, and diarrhea can usually be controlled by administering the drug with food or carboxymethylcellulose, reducing drug dosage, or discontinuing the drug.

Tetracyclines modify the normal flora, with suppression of susceptible coliform organisms and overgrowth of pseudomonas, proteus, staphylococci, resistant coliforms, clostridia, and candida. This can result in intestinal functional disturbances, anal pruritus, vaginal or oral candidiasis, or enterocolitis with shock and death. Pseudomembranous enterocolitis associated with *Clostridium difficile* should be treated with metronidazole.

B. BONY STRUCTURES AND TEETH

Tetracyclines are readily bound to calcium deposited in newly formed bone or teeth in young children. When the drug is given during pregnancy, it can be deposited in the fetal teeth, leading to fluorescence, discoloration, and enamel dysplasia; it can also be deposited in bone, where it may cause deformity or growth inhibition. If the drug is given for long periods to children under 8 years of age, similar changes can result.

C. Liver Toxicity

Tetracyclines can probably impair hepatic function, especially during pregnancy, in patients with preexisting hepatic insufficiency and when high doses are given intravenously. Hepatic necrosis has been reported with daily doses of 4 g or more intravenously.

D. Kidney Toxicity

Renal tubular acidosis and other renal injury resulting in nitrogen retention have been attributed to the administration of outdated tetracycline preparations. Tetracyclines given along with diuretics may produce nitrogen retention. Tetracyclines other than doxycycline may accumulate to toxic levels in patients with impaired kidney function.

E. Local Tissue Toxicity

Intravenous injection can lead to venous thrombosis. Intramuscular injection produces painful local irritation and should be avoided.

F. Photosensitization

Systemic tetracycline administration, especially of demeclocycline, can induce sensitivity to sunlight or ultraviolet light, particularly in fair-skinned persons.

G. Vestibular Reactions

Dizziness, vertigo, nausea, and vomiting have been particularly noted with doxycycline at doses above 100 mg. With dosages of 200–400 mg/d of minocycline, 35–70% of patients will have these reactions.

Medical & Social Implications of Overuse

Tetracyclines have been extensively used in animal feeds to enhance growth. This practice has contributed to the spread of tetracycline resistance among enteric bacteria and of plasmids that encode tetracycline resistance genes.

MACROLIDES

The macrolides are a group of closely related compounds characterized by a macrocyclic lactone ring (usually containing 14 or 16 atoms) to which deoxy sugars are attached. The prototype drug, erythromycin, which consists of two sugar moieties attached to a 14-atom lactone ring, was obtained in 1952 from *Streptomyces erythreus.* Clarithromycin and azithromycin are semisynthetic derivatives of erythromycin.

Erythromycin ($R_1 = CH_3$, $R_2 = H$)
Clarithromycin (R_1, $R_2 = CH_3$)

ERYTHROMYCIN

Chemistry

The general structure of erythromycin is shown above with the macrolide ring and the sugars desosamine and cladinose. It is poorly soluble in water (0.1%) but dissolves readily in organic solvents. Solutions are fairly stable at 4 °C but lose activity rapidly at 20 °C and at acid pH. Erythromycins are usually dispensed as various esters and salts.

Antimicrobial Activity

Erythromycin is effective against gram-positive organisms, especially pneumococci, streptococci, staphylococci, and corynebacteria, in plasma concentrations of 0.02–2 µg/mL. Mycoplasma, legionella, *Chlamydia trachomatis, C psittaci, C pneumoniae,* helicobacter, listeria, and certain mycobacteria *(Mycobacterium kansasii, Mycobacterium scrofulaceum)* are also susceptible. Gram-negative organisms such as neisseria species, *Bordetella pertussis, Bartonella henselae,* and *B quintana* (etiologic agents of cat-scratch disease and bacillary angiomatosis), some rickettsia species, *Treponema pallidum,* and campylobacter species are susceptible. *Haemophilus influenzae* is somewhat less susceptible.

The antibacterial action of erythromycin may be inhibitory or bactericidal, particularly at higher concentrations, for susceptible organisms. Activity is enhanced at alkaline pH. Inhibition of protein synthesis occurs via binding to the 50S ribosomal RNA. Protein synthesis is inhibited because aminoacyl translocation reactions and the formation of initiation complexes are blocked (Figure 44–1).

Resistance

Resistance to erythromycin is usually plasmid-encoded. Three mechanisms have been identified: (1) reduced permeability of the cell membrane or active efflux; (2) production (by Enterobacteriaceae) of esterases that hydrolyze macrolides; and (3) modification of the ribosomal binding site (so-called ribosomal protection) by chromosomal mutation or by a macrolide-inducible or constitutive methylase. Efflux and methylase production account for the vast majority of cases of resistance in gram-positive organisms. Cross-resistance is complete between erythromycin and the other macrolides. Constitutive methylase production also confers resistance to structurally unrelated but mechanistically similar compounds such as clindamycin and streptogramin B (so called macrolide-lincosamide-streptogramin, or MLS-type B, resistance), which share the same ribosomal binding site. Because nonmacrolides are poor inducers of the methylase, strains expressing an inducible methylase will appear susceptible in vitro. However, constitutive mutants that are resistant can be selected out and emerge during therapy with clindamycin.

Pharmacokinetics

Erythromycin base is destroyed by stomach acid and must be administered with enteric coating. Food interferes with absorption. Stearates and esters are fairly acid-resistant and somewhat better absorbed. The lauryl salt of the propionyl ester of erythromycin (erythromycin estolate) is the best-absorbed oral preparation. Oral dosage of 2 g/d results in serum erythromycin base and ester concentrations of approximately 2 μg/mL. However, only the base is microbiologically active, and its concentration tends to be similar regardless of the formulation. A 500 mg intravenous dose of erythromycin lactobionate produces serum concentrations of 10 μg/mL 1 hour after dosing. The serum half-life is approximately 1.5 h normally and 5 hours in patients with anuria. Adjustment for renal failure is not necessary. Erythromycin is not removed by dialysis. Large amounts of an administered dose are excreted in the bile and lost in feces, and only 5% is excreted in the urine. Absorbed drug is distributed widely except to the brain and cerebrospinal fluid. Erythromycin is taken up by polymorphonuclear leukocytes and macrophages. It traverses the placenta and reaches the fetus.

Clinical Uses

An erythromycin is the drug of choice in corynebacterial infections (diphtheria, corynebacterial sepsis, erythrasma); in respiratory, neonatal, ocular, or genital chlamydial infections; and in treatment of community-acquired pneumonia because its spectrum of activity includes the pneumococcus, mycoplasma, and legionella. Erythromycin is also useful as a penicillin substitute in penicillin-allergic individuals with infections caused by staphylococci (assuming that the isolate is susceptible), streptococci, or pneumococci. Emergence of erythromycin resistance in strains of group A streptococci and pneumococci (penicillin-resistant pneumococci in particular) has made macrolides less attractive as first-line agents for treatment of pharyngitis, skin and soft tissue infections, and pneumonia. Erythromycin has been recommended as prophylaxis against endocarditis during dental procedures in individuals with valvular heart disease, though clindamycin, which is better tolerated, has largely replaced it. Although erythromycin estolate is the best-absorbed salt, it imposes the greatest risk of adverse reactions. Therefore, the stearate or succinate salt may be preferred.

The oral dosage of erythromycin base, stearate, or estolate is 0.25–0.5 g every 6 hours (for children, 40 mg/kg/d). The dosage of erythromycin ethylsuccinate is 0.4–0.6 g every 6 hours. Oral erythromycin base (1 g) is sometimes combined with oral neomycin or kanamycin for preoperative preparation of the colon. The intravenous dosage of erythromycin glucepate or lactobionate is 0.5–1.0 g every 6 hours for adults and 20–40 mg/kg/d for children. The higher dosage is recommended when treating pneumonia caused by legionella species.

Adverse Reactions

A. GASTROINTESTINAL EFFECTS

Anorexia, nausea, vomiting, and diarrhea occasionally accompany oral administration. Gastrointestinal intolerance, which is due to a direct stimulation of gut motility, is the most frequent reason for discontinuing erythromycin and substituting another antibiotic.

B. LIVER TOXICITY

Erythromycins, particularly the estolate, can produce acute cholestatic hepatitis (fever, jaundice, impaired liver function), probably as a hypersensitivity reaction. Most patients recover from this, but hepatitis recurs if the drug is readministered. Other allergic reactions include fever, eosinophilia, and rashes.

C. DRUG INTERACTIONS

Erythromycin metabolites can inhibit cytochrome P450 enzymes and thus increase the serum concentrations of numerous drugs, including theophylline, oral anticoagulants, cyclosporine, and methylprednisolone. Erythromycin increases serum concentrations of oral digoxin by increasing its bioavailability.

CLARITHROMYCIN

Clarithromycin is derived from erythromycin by addition of a methyl group and has improved acid stability and oral absorption compared with erythromycin. Its mechanism of action is the same as that of erythromycin. Clarithromycin and erythromycin are virtually identical with respect to antibacterial activity except that clarithromycin is more active against *Mycobacterium avium* complex (see Chapter 47). Clarithromycin also has activity against *M leprae* and *Toxoplasma gondii.* Erythromycin-resistant streptococci and staphylococci are also resistant to clarithromycin.

A 500 mg dose produces serum concentrations of 2–3 μg/mL. The longer half-life of clarithromycin (6 hours) compared with erythromycin permits twice-daily dosing. The recommended dosage is 250–500 mg twice daily. Clarithromycin penetrates most tissues well, with concentrations equal to or exceeding serum concentrations.

Clarithromycin is metabolized in the liver. The major metabolite is 14-hydroxyclarithromycin, which also has antibacterial activity. A portion of active drug and this major metabolite is eliminated in the urine, and dosage reduction (eg, a 500 mg loading dose, then 250 mg once or twice daily) is recommended for patients with creatinine clearances less than 30 mL/min. Clarithromycin has drug interactions similar to those described for erythromycin.

The advantages of clarithromycin compared with erythromycin are lower frequency of gastrointestinal intolerance and less frequent dosing. Except for the specific organisms noted above, the two drugs are otherwise therapeutically very similar, and the choice of one over the other usually turns on issues of cost (clarithromycin being much more expensive) and tolerability.

AZITHROMYCIN

Azithromycin, a 15-atom lactone macrolide ring compound, is derived from erythromycin by addition of a methylated nitrogen into the lactone ring of erythromycin. Its spectrum of activity and clinical uses are virtually identical to those of clarithromycin. Azithromycin is active against *M avium* complex and *T gondii.* Azithromycin is slightly less active than erythromycin and clarithromycin against staphylococci and streptococci and slightly more active against *H influenzae.* Azithromycin is highly active against chlamydia.

Azithromycin differs from erythromycin and clarithromycin mainly in pharmacokinetic properties. A 500 mg dose of azithromycin produces relatively low serum concentrations of approximately 0.4 μg/mL. However, azithromycin penetrates into most tissues (except cerebrospinal fluid) and phagocytic cells extremely well, with tissue concentrations exceeding serum concentrations by 10- to 100-fold. The drug is slowly released from tissues (tissue half-life of 2–4 days) to produce an elimination half-life approaching 3 days. These unique properties permit once-daily dosing and shortening of the duration of treatment in many cases. For example, a single 1 g dose of azithromycin is as effective as a 7-day course of doxycycline for chlamydial cervicitis and urethritis. Community-acquired pneumonia can be treated with azithromycin given as a 500 mg loading dose, followed by a 250 mg single daily dose for the next 4 days.

Azithromycin is rapidly absorbed and well tolerated orally. It should be administered 1 hour before or 2 hours after meals. Aluminum and magnesium antacids do not alter bioavailability but delay absorption and reduce peak serum concentrations. Because it has a 15-member (not 14-member) lactone ring, azithromycin does not inactivate cytochrome P450 enzymes and therefore is free of the drug interactions that occur with erythromycin and clarithromycin.

KETOLIDES

Ketolides are semisynthetic 14-membered-ring macrolides, differing from erythromycin by substitution of a 3-keto group for the neutral sugar L-cladinose. **Telithromycin** is approved for clinical use. It is active in vitro against *S pyogenes, S pneumoniae, S aureus, H influenzae, Moraxella catarrhalis,* mycoplasmas, legionella species, chlamydia species, *Helicobacter pylori, N gonorrhoeae, Bacteroides fragilis, T gondii,* and nontuberculosis mycobacteria. Many macrolide-resistant strains are susceptible to ketolides because the structural modification of these compounds renders them poor substrates for efflux-pump mediated resistance and they bind to ribosomes of some bacterial species with higher affinity than macrolides.

Oral bioavailability is 57%, and tissue and intracellular penetration is generally good. Telithromycin is metabolized in the liver and eliminated by a combination of biliary and urinary routes of excretion. It is administered as a once-daily dose of 800 mg, which results in peak serum concentrations of approximately 2 μg/mL. Telithromycin is indicated for treatment of respiratory tract infections, including community-acquired bacterial pneumonia, acute exacerbations of chronic bronchitis, sinusitis, and streptococcal pharyngitis. Telithromycin is a reversible inhibitor of the CYP3A4 enzyme system.

CLINDAMYCIN

Clindamycin is a chlorine-substituted derivative of **lincomycin,** an antibiotic that is elaborated by *Streptomyces* *lincolnensis.* Lincomycin, although structurally distinct, resembles erythromycin in activity, but it is toxic and no longer used.

Clindamycin

Antibacterial Activity

Streptococci, staphylococci, and pneumococci are inhibited by clindamycin, 0.5–5 μg/mL. Enterococci and gram-negative aerobic organisms are resistant (in contrast to their susceptibility to erythromycin). Bacteroides species and other anaerobes, both gram-positive and gram-negative, are usually susceptible. *Clostridium difficile,* an important cause of pseudomembranous colitis, is resistant. Clindamycin, like erythromycin, inhibits protein synthesis by interfering with the formation of initiation complexes and with aminoacyl translocation reactions. The binding site for clindamycin on the 50S subunit of the bacterial ribosome is identical with that for erythromycin. Resistance to clindamycin, which generally confers cross-resistance to other macrolides, is due to (1) mutation of the ribosomal receptor site; (2) modification of the receptor by a constitutively expressed methylase (see section on erythromycin resistance, above); and (3) enzymatic inactivation of clindamycin. Gram-negative aerobic species are intrinsically resistant because of poor permeability of the outer membrane.

Pharmacokinetics

Oral dosages of clindamycin, 0.15–0.3 g every 6 hours (10–20 mg/kg/d for children), yield serum levels of 2–3 μg/mL. When administered intravenously, 600 mg of clindamycin every 8 hours gives levels of 5–15 μg/mL. The drug is about 90% protein-bound. Excretion is mainly via the liver, bile, and urine. Clindamycin penetrates well into most tissues, with brain and cerebrospinal fluid being important exceptions. It penetrates well into abscesses and is actively taken up and concentrated by phagocytic cells. Clindamycin is metabolized by the liver, and both active drug and active metabolites are excreted in bile. The half-life is about 2.5 hours in normal individuals, increasing to 6 hours in patients with anuria. No dosage adjustment is required for renal failure.

Clinical Uses

Clindamycin is indicated for treatment of severe anaerobic infection caused by bacteroides and other anaerobes that often participate in mixed infections. Clindamycin, sometimes in combination with an aminoglycoside or cephalosporin, is used to treat penetrating wounds of the abdomen and the gut; infections originating in the female genital tract, eg, septic abortion and pelvic abscesses; or aspiration pneumonia. Clindamycin is now recommended instead of erythromycin for prophylaxis of endocarditis in patients with valvular heart disease who are undergoing certain dental procedures. Clindamycin plus primaquine is an effective alternative to trimethoprim-sulfamethoxazole for moderate to moderately severe *Pneumocystis carinii* pneumonia in AIDS patients. It is also used in combination with pyrimethamine for AIDS-related toxoplasmosis of the brain.

Adverse Effects

Common adverse effects are diarrhea, nausea, and skin rashes. Impaired liver function (with or without jaundice) and neutropenia sometimes occur. Severe diarrhea and enterocolitis have followed clindamycin administration. Antibiotic-associated colitis that has followed administration of clindamycin and other drugs is caused by toxigenic *C difficile.* This potentially fatal complication must be recognized promptly and treated with metronidazole, 500 mg orally or intravenously three times a day (the preferred therapy), or vancomycin, 125 mg orally four times a day (less desirable given the increasing prevalence of vancomycin-resistant enterococci). Relapse may occur. Variations in the local prevalence of *C difficile* may account for the great differences in incidence of antibiotic-associated colitis. For unknown reasons, neonates given clindamycin may become colonized with toxigenic *C difficile* but do not develop colitis.

STREPTOGRAMINS

Quinupristin-dalfopristin is a combination of two streptogramins—quinupristin, a streptogramin B, and dalfopristin, a streptogramin A—in a 30:70 ratio. It is rapidly bactericidal for most organisms except *Enterococcus faecium,* which is killed slowly. It has a prolonged postantibiotic effect (up to 10 hours for *S aureus*) that may account for its prolonged antibacterial activity despite relatively short half-lives of the parent drugs.

Quinupristin-dalfopristin is active against gram-positive cocci, including multidrug-resistant strains of streptococci, penicillin-resistant strains of *S pneumoniae*, methicillin-susceptible and -resistant strains of staphylococci, and *E faecium* (but not *E faecalis*). Minimum inhibitory concentrations are 1 μg/mL or less. Resistance is due to modification of the quinupristin binding site (MLS-B type), enzymatic inactivation of dalfopristin, or efflux. Quinupristin is not an inducer of MLS-B resistance, but strains constitutively expressing the methylase may be inhibited but not killed by quinupristin-dalfopristin.

Quinupristin-dalfopristin is administered intravenously at a dosage of 7.5 mg/kg every 8–12 hours. Peak serum concentrations following an infusion of 7.5 mg/kg over 60 minutes are 3 μg/mL for quinupristin and 7 μg/mL for dalfopristin. Quinupristin and dalfopristin are rapidly metabolized, with half-lives of 0.85 and 0.7 hours, respectively. Elimination of approximately 75% of the parent compounds and their metabolites is by the fecal route. Renal elimination accounts for less than 20%. Dose adjustment is not necessary for renal failure, peritoneal dialysis, or hemodialysis. Patients with hepatic insufficiency may not tolerate the drug at usual doses, however, because of increased area under the concentration curve of both parent drugs and metabolites. This may necessitate a dose reduction to 7.5 mg/kg every 12 hours or 5 mg/kg every 8 hours in some patients. Quinupristin and dalfopristin are not metabolized by cytochrome P450 enzymes but significantly inhibit CYP 3A4, which metabolizes warfarin, diazepam, astemizole, terfenadine, cisapride, nonnucleoside reverse transcriptase inhibitors, and cyclosporine, among others. Dosage reduction of cyclosporine may be necessary.

Quinupristin-dalfopristin is approved for treatment of infections caused by vancomycin-resistant strains of *E faecium* but not *E faecalis*, which is intrinsically resistant, probably because of an efflux-type resistance mechanism. Quinupristin-dalfopristin also is likely to be approved for treatment of bacteremia or respiratory tract infections caused by methicillin-resistant staphylococci, streptococci, and penicillin-susceptible and penicillin-resistant strains of *S pneumoniae*. The principal toxicities are infusion-related events, such as pain at the infusion site, and an arthralgia-myalgia syndrome.

OXAZOLIDINONES

Linezolid is a member of the oxazolidinones, a new class of synthetic antimicrobials. It is active against gram-positive organisms including staphylococci, streptococci, enterococci, gram-positive anaerobic cocci, and gram-positive rods such as corynebacteria and *Listeria monocytogenes*. It is primarily a bacteriostatic agent except for streptococci for which it is bactericidal. There is modest in vitro activity against *Mycobacterium tuberculosis*.

Linezolid inhibits protein synthesis by preventing formation of the ribosome complex that initiates protein synthesis. Its unique binding site, located on 23S ribosomal RNA of the 50S subunit, results in no cross-resistance with other drug classes. Resistance is caused by mutation of the linezolid binding site on 23S ribosomal RNA.

The principal toxicity of linezolid is hematologic—reversible and generally mild. Thrombocytopenia is the most common manifestation (seen in approximately 3% of treatment courses), particularly when the drug is administered for longer than 2 weeks. Neutropenia may also occur, most commonly in patients with a predisposition to or underlying bone marrow suppression. Linezolid is 100% bioavailable after oral administration and has a half-life of 4–6 hours. It is metabolized by oxidative metabolism, yielding two inactive metabolites. It is neither an inducer nor an inhibitor of cytochrome P450 enzymes. Peak serum concentrations average 18 μg/mL following a 600 mg oral dose. The recommended dose for most indications is 600 mg twice daily, either orally or intravenously. It is approved for vancomycin-resistant *E faecium* infections; nosocomial pneumonia; community-acquired pneumonia; and skin infections, complicated or uncomplicated. It should be reserved for treatment of infections caused by multiply drug-resistant gram-positive bacteria.

REFERENCES

Bain KT, Wittbrodt ET: Linezolid for the treatment of resistant gram-positive cocci. Ann Pharmacother 2001;35:566.

Chant C, Ryba MJ: Quinupristin/dalfopristin (RP 59500): a new streptogramin antibiotic. Ann Pharmacother 1995;29:1022.

Chopra I, Hawkey PM, Hinton M: Tetracyclines, molecular and clinical aspects. J Antimicrob Chemother 1992;29:245.

Clarithromycin and azithromycin. Med Lett Drugs Ther 1992; 34:45.

Falages ME, Gorbach SL: Clindamycin and metronidazole. Med Clin North Am 1995;79:845.

Gee T et al: Pharmacokinetics and tissue penetration of linezolid following multiple oral doses. Antimicrob Agents Chemother 2001;45:1843.

Jacoby GA: Prevalence and resistance mechanisms of common bacterial respiratory pathogens. Clin Infect Dis 1993;18:951.

Jamjian C, Biedenbach DJ, Jones RN: In vitro evaluation of a novel ketolide antimicrobial agent, RU-64004. Antimicrob Agents Chemother 1997;41:454.

PREPARATIONS AVAILABLE

CHLORAMPHENICOL
Chloramphenicol (generic, Chloromycetin)
Oral: 250 mg capsules; 150 mg/5 mL suspension
Parenteral: 100 mg powder to reconstitute for injection

TETRACYCLINES
Demeclocycline (Declomycin)
Oral: 150, 300 mg tablets; 150 mg capsules
Doxycycline (generic, Vibramycin, others)
Oral: 50, 100 mg tablets and capsules; powder to reconstitute for 25 mg/5 mL suspension; 50 mg/5 mL syrup
Parenteral: 100, 200 mg powder to reconstitute for injection
Methacycline (Rondomycin)
Oral: 150, 300 mg capsules
Minocycline (Minocin)
Oral: 50, 100 mg tablets and capsules; 50 mg/5 mL suspension
Parenteral: 100 mg powder to reconstitute for injection
Oxytetracycline (generic, Terramycin)
Oral: 250 mg capsules
Parenteral: 50, 125 mg/mL for IM injection
Tetracycline (generic, Achromycin V, others)
Oral: 100, 250, 500 mg capsules; 250, 500 mg tablets; 125 mg/5 mL suspension
Parenteral: 100, 250 mg powder to reconstitute for IM injection; 250, 500 mg powder to reconstitute for IV injection

MACROLIDES
Azithromycin (Zithromax)
Oral: 250 mg capsules; powder for 100, 200 mg/5 mL oral suspension
Clarithromycin (Biaxin)
Oral: 250, 500 mg tablets, 500 mg extended release tablets; granules for 125, 250 mg/5 mL oral suspension

Erythromycin (generic, Ilotycin, Ilosone, E-Mycin, Erythrocin, others)
Oral (base): 250, 333, 500 mg enteric-coated tablets
Oral (base) delayed-release: 333 mg tablets, 250 capsules
Oral (estolate): 500 mg tablets; 250 mg capsules; 125, 250 mg/5 mL suspension
Oral (ethylsuccinate): 200, 400 mg film-coated tablets; 200, 400 mg/5 mL suspension
Oral (stearate): 250, 500 mg film-coated tablets
Parenteral: lactobionate, 0.5, 1 g powder to reconstitute for IV injection

KETOLIDES
Telithromycin (Proteck)
Oral: 800 mg tablets

LINCOMYCINS
Clindamycin (generic, Cleocin)
Oral: 75, 150, 300 mg capsules; 75 mg/5 mL granules to reconstitute for solution
Parenteral: 150 mg/mL in 2, 4, 6, 60 mL vials for injection

STREPTOGRAMINS
Quinupristin and dalfopristin (Synercid)
Parenteral: 30:70 formulation in 500 mg vial for reconstitution for IV injection

OXAZOLIDINONES
Linezolid (Zyvox)
Oral: 400, 600 mg tablets; 100 mg powder for solution
Parenteral: 2 mg/mL for IV infusion

Johnson CA et al: Pharmacokinetics of quinupristin-dalfopristin in continuous ambulatory peritoneal dialysis patients. Antimicrob Agents Chemother 1999;43:152.

Kanatani MS, Guglielmo BJ: The new macrolides azithromycin and clarithromycin. West J Med 1994;160:31.

Kang SL, Rybak MJ: Pharmacodynamics of RP 59500 alone and in combination with vancomycin against *Staphylococcus aureus* in an in vitro-infected fibrin clot model. Antimicrob Agents Chemother 1995;39:1505.

Malathum K et al: In vitro activities of two ketolides, HMR 3647 and HMR 3004, against gram-positive bacteria. Antimicrob Agents Chemother 1999;43:930.

Periti P et al: Pharmacokinetic drug interactions of macrolides. Clin Pharmacokinet 1992;23:106.

Schlossberg D: Azithromycin and clarithromycin. Med Clin North Am 1995;79:803.

Speer BS, Shoemaker MB, Salyers AA: Bacterial resistance to tetracycline: Mechanism, transfer, and clinical significance. Clin Microbiol Rev 1992;5:387.

Zhanel GG et al: The ketolides: a critical review. Drugs 2002;62:1771.

Aminoglycosides & Spectinomycin

Henry F. Chambers, MD

The drugs described in this chapter are, like those described in Chapter 44, protein synthesis inhibitors that interfere with ribosomal function. These agents are useful mainly against aerobic gram-negative microorganisms.

AMINOGLYCOSIDES

Aminoglycosides are a group of bactericidal antibiotics originally obtained from various streptomyces species and sharing chemical, antimicrobial, pharmacologic, and toxic characteristics. The group includes **streptomycin, neomycin, kanamycin, amikacin, gentamicin, tobramycin, sisomicin, netilmicin,** and others.

Aminoglycosides are used most widely against gram-negative enteric bacteria, especially in bacteremia and sepsis, in combination with vancomycin or a penicillin for endocarditis, and for treatment of tuberculosis. Streptomycin is the oldest and best-studied of the aminoglycosides. Gentamicin, tobramycin, and amikacin are the most widely employed aminoglycosides at present. Neomycin and kanamycin are now largely limited to topical or oral use.

General Properties of Aminoglycosides

A. Physical and Chemical Properties

Aminoglycosides have a hexose ring, either streptidine (in streptomycin) or 2-deoxystreptamine (other aminoglycosides), to which various amino sugars are attached by glycosidic linkages (Figures 45–1 and 45–2). They are water-soluble, stable in solution, and more active at alkaline than at acid pH. Aminoglycosides frequently exhibit synergism with β-lactams or vancomycin in vitro. In combination they eradicate organisms more rapidly than would be predicted from the activity of either single agent. However, at high concentrations aminoglycosides may complex with β-lactam drugs,

resulting in loss of activity, and they should not be mixed together for administration.

B. Mechanism of Action

The mode of action of streptomycin has been studied far more closely than that of other aminoglycosides, but probably all act similarly. Aminoglycosides are irreversible inhibitors of protein synthesis, but the precise mechanism for bactericidal activity is not known. The initial event is passive diffusion via porin channels across the outer membrane. Drug is then actively transported across the cell membrane into the cytoplasm by an oxygen-dependent process. The transmembrane electrochemical gradient supplies the energy for this process and transport is coupled to a proton pump. Low extracellular pH and anaerobic conditions inhibit transport by reducing the gradient. Transport may be enhanced by cell wall-active drugs, such as penicillin or vancomycin; this enhancement may be the basis of the synergism.

Once an aminoglycoside has entered the cell, it binds to specific 30S-subunit ribosomal proteins (S12 in the case of streptomycin). Protein synthesis is inhibited by aminoglycosides in at least three ways (Figure 45–3): (1) They interfere with the initiation complex of peptide formation; (2) they induce misreading of mRNA, which causes incorporation of incorrect amino acids into the peptide, resulting in a nonfunctional or toxic protein; and (3) they cause a breakup of polysomes into nonfunctional monosomes. These activities occur more or less simultaneously, and the overall effect is irreversible and lethal for the cell.

C. Mechanisms of Resistance

Three principal mechanisms have been established: (1) The microorganism produces a transferase enzyme or enzymes that inactivate the aminoglycoside by adenylylation, acetylation, or phosphorylation. This is the principal type of resistance encountered clinically. Specific transferase enzymes are discussed below. (2) Impaired entry of aminoglycoside into the cell. This may be genotypic, ie, resulting from mutation or deletion of a porin

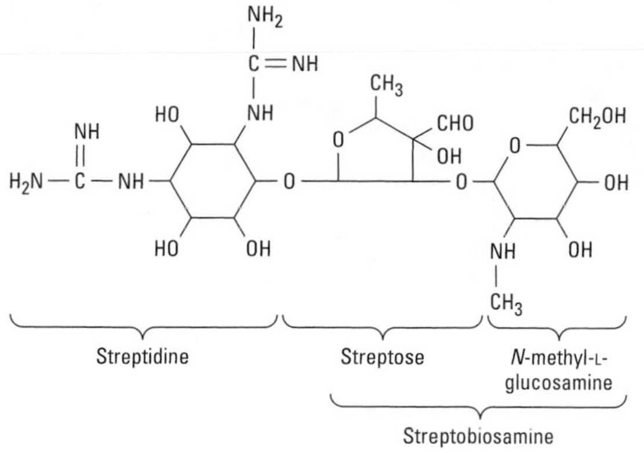

Figure 45–1. Structure of streptomycin.

protein or proteins involved in transport and maintenance of the electrochemical gradient; or phenotypic, eg, resulting from growth conditions under which the oxygen-dependent transport process described above is not functional. (3) The receptor protein on the 30S ribosomal subunit may be deleted or altered as a result of a mutation.

D. PHARMACOKINETICS AND ONCE-DAILY DOSING

Aminoglycosides are absorbed very poorly from the intact gastrointestinal tract; virtually the entire oral dose is excreted in feces after oral administration. However, the drugs may be absorbed if ulcerations are present. After intramuscular injection, aminoglycosides are well absorbed, giving peak concentrations in blood within 30–90 minutes. Aminoglycosides are usually administered intravenously as a 30–60 minute infusion; after a brief distribution phase this results in serum concentrations that are identical to those following intramuscular injection.

Traditionally, aminoglycosides have been administered in two or three equally divided daily doses for patients with normal renal function. However, once-daily aminoglycoside dosing may be preferred in certain

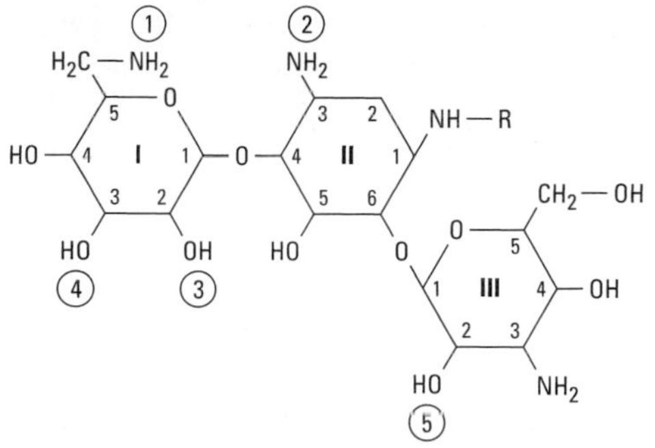

Figure 45–2. Structures of several important aminoglycoside antibiotics. Ring II is 2-deoxystreptamine. The resemblance between kanamycin and amikacin and between gentamicin, netilmicin, and tobramycin can be seen. The circled numerals on the kanamycin molecule indicate points of attack of plasmid-mediated bacterial transferase enzymes that can inactivate this drug. ①, ②, and ③, acetyltransferase; ④, phosphotransferase; ⑤, adenylyltransferase.) Amikacin is resistant to degradation at ②, ③, ④, and ⑤.

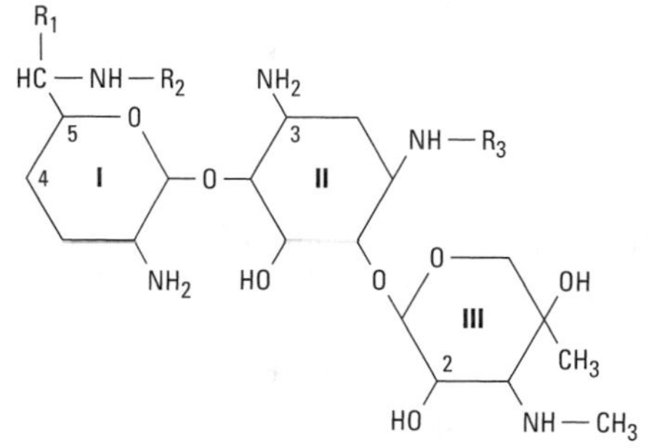

Kanamycin R = H

Amikacin $R = C - CH - CH_2 - CH_2 - NH_2$

Gentamicin, netilmicin

	Ring I			Ring II
	R_1	R_2	C4–C5 bond	R_3
Gentamicin C_1	CH_3	CH_3	Single	H
Gentamicin C_2	CH_3	H	Single	H
Gentamicin C_{1a}	H	H	Single	H
Netilmicin	H	H	Double	C_2H_5

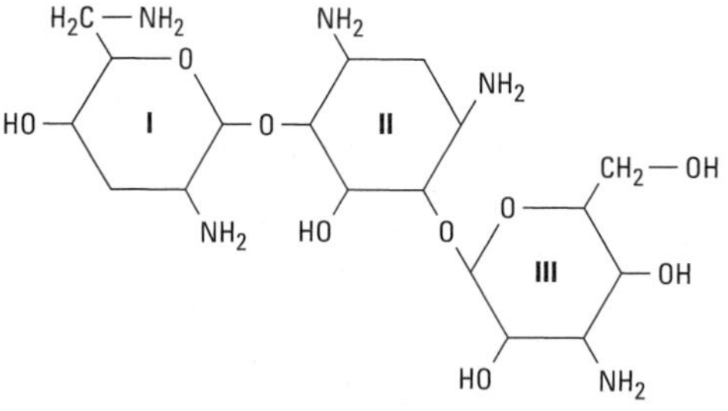

Tobramycin

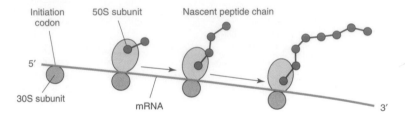

Normal bacterial cell

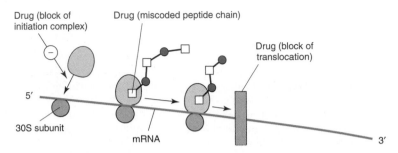

Aminoglycoside-treated bacterial cell

Figure 45–3. Putative mechanisms of action of the aminoglycosides. Normal protein synthesis is shown in the top panel. At least three different aminoglycoside effects have been described, as shown in the bottom panel: block of formation of the initiation complex; miscoding of amino acids in the emerging peptide chain due to misreading of the mRNA; and block of translocation on mRNA. Block of movement of the ribose may occur after the formation of a single initiation complex, resulting in an mRNA chain with only a single ribosome on it, a so-called monosome. (Reproduced, with permission, from Trevor AT, Katzung BG, Masters SB: *Pharmacology: Examination & Board Review,* 6th ed. McGraw-Hill, 2002.)

clinical situations. Aminoglycosides have **concentration-dependent killing**—ie, increasing concentrations kill an increasing proportion of bacteria and at a more rapid rate; and they have a significant **postantibiotic effect,** such that the antibacterial activity persists beyond the time during which measurable drug is present. The postantibiotic effect of aminoglycosides can reach several hours (see Chapter 51). Because of these properties, a given total amount of aminoglycoside may have better efficacy when administered as a single large dose than when administered as multiple smaller doses.

In contrast to the antimicrobial effect, aminoglycoside toxicity in the patient is both time- and concentration-dependent. Toxicity is unlikely to occur until a certain threshold concentration is achieved, but once that concentration is achieved the time above this threshold becomes critical. This threshold is imprecisely defined, but a trough concentration above 2 µg/mL is predictive of toxicity. At clinically relevant doses, the time above this threshold will be greater with multiple smaller doses of drug than with a single large dose.

Numerous clinical studies demonstrate that a single daily dose of aminoglycoside is just as effective—and no more (and often less) toxic—than multiple smaller doses. Therefore, many authorities now recommend that aminoglycosides be administered as a single daily dose in many clinical situations with the following exceptions: The efficacy of once-daily aminoglycoside dosing in combination therapy of enterococcal, streptococcal, and staphylococcal endocarditis remains to be defined; and the standard low-dose, thrice-daily administration is still recommended. The role of once-daily dosing in pregnancy and in pediatric patients is also not defined.

Once-daily dosing has potential practical advantages. For example, determination of serum concentrations is probably unnecessary unless aminoglycoside is given for more than 3 days. Less nursing time is required to give a drug once a day instead of three times a day. And once-a-day dosing lends itself to outpatient therapy.

Use of once-daily dosing does not eliminate responsibility for careful monitoring and dosage adjustment to minimize toxicity. Selection of the appropriate dose is particularly critical if renal insufficiency is present. Aminoglycosides are cleared by the kidney, and excretion is directly proportionate to creatinine clearance. Rapidly changing renal function, which may occur with acute renal failure in the patient with septic shock, must be anticipated to avoid overdose. Provided these pitfalls are avoided, once-daily aminoglycoside dosing is safe and effective. If the creatinine clearance is 100 mL/min, gentamicin is given as a 5 mg/kg dose (15 mg/kg for amikacin) over 30–60 minutes. If the creatinine clearance is 80 mL/min, the dose is 4 mg/kg (12 mg/kg for amikacin); and if creatinine clearance is 50 mL/min, the dose is 3 mg/kg (9 mg/kg for amikacin). If the creatinine clearance is less than 50 mL/min, a 2 mg/kg gentamicin loading dose is given and subsequent doses are adjusted as would normally be done. Serum concentrations need not be routinely checked until the second or third day of therapy depending on the stability of renal function and the anticipated duration of therapy. It is probably unnecessary to check peak concentrations, as they will be high. The goal is to administer drug so that concentrations of less than 1 µg/mL are present between 18 and 24 hours after dosing. This provides a sufficient period of time for washout of drug to occur before the next dose is given. This is most easily determined either by measuring serum concentrations in samples obtained 2 hours and 12 hours after dosing and then adjusting the dose based on the actual clearance of drug—or by measuring the concentration in a sample obtained 8 hours after a dose. If the 8-hour concentration is between 1.5 µg and 6 µg/mL, the target trough will be achieved at 18 hours.

Aminoglycosides are highly polar compounds that do not enter cells readily. They are largely excluded from the central nervous system and the eye. In the presence of active inflammation, however, cerebrospinal fluid levels reach 20% of plasma levels, and in neonatal meningitis the levels may be higher. Intrathecal or intraventricular injection is required for high levels in cerebrospinal fluid. Even after parenteral administration, concentrations of aminoglycosides are not high in most tissues except the renal cortex. Concentration in most secretions is also modest; in the bile, it may reach 30% of the blood level. Diffusion into pleural or synovial fluid may result in concentrations 50–90% of that of plasma with prolonged therapy.

The normal half-life of aminoglycosides in serum is 2–3 hours, increasing to 24–48 hours in patients with significant impairment of renal function. Aminoglycosides are only partially and irregularly removed by hemodialysis—eg, 40–60% for gentamicin—and even less effectively by peritoneal dialysis.

Dosage adjustments must be made to avoid accumulation of drug and toxicity in patients with renal insufficiency. Either the dose of drug is kept constant and the interval between doses is increased, or the interval is kept constant and the dose is reduced. Nomograms and formulas have been constructed relating serum creatinine levels to adjustments in treatment regimens. The simplest formula divides the dose (calculated on the basis of normal renal function) by the serum creatinine value (mg/dL). Thus, a 60 kg patient with normal renal function might receive 300 mg/d of gentamicin (maximum daily dose of 5 mg/kg), whereas a 60 kg patient with a serum creatinine of 3 mg/dL would receive 100 mg/d. However, this approach fails to take into account the age and gender of the patient, both of which significantly affect creatinine clearance without necessarily being reflected as a change in serum creatinine. Since aminoglycoside clearance is directly proportionate to the creatinine clearance, a better method for determining the aminoglycoside dose is to estimate creatinine clearance using the Cockcroft-Gault formula described in Chapter 61.

The daily dose of aminoglycoside is calculated by multiplying the maximum daily dose by the ratio of estimated creatinine clearance to normal creatinine clearance, ie, 120 mL/min, which is a typical value for a 70 kg young adult male. For a 60-year-old female weighing 60 kg with a serum creatinine of 3 mg/dL the corrected dosage of gentamicin would be approximately 50 mg/d, half the dose calculated by the simplest formula. There is considerable individual variation in aminoglycoside serum levels among patients with similar estimated creatinine clearance values. Therefore, it is mandatory, especially when using higher dosages for more than a few days or when renal function is rapidly changing, to measure serum drug levels in order to avoid severe toxicity. For a traditional twice- or thrice-daily dosing regimen, peak serum concentrations should be determined from a blood sample obtained 30–60 minutes after a dose and trough concentrations from a sample obtained just prior to the next dose.

E. Adverse Effects

All aminoglycosides are ototoxic and nephrotoxic. Ototoxicity and nephrotoxicity are more likely to be encountered when therapy is continued for more than 5 days, at higher doses, in the elderly, and in the setting of renal insufficiency. Concurrent use with loop diuretics (eg, furosemide, ethacrynic acid) or other nephrotoxic antimicrobial agents (eg, vancomycin or amphotericin) can potentiate nephrotoxicity and should be avoided if possible. Ototoxicity can manifest itself either as auditory damage, resulting in tinnitus and high-frequency hearing loss initially; or as vestibular damage, evident by vertigo, ataxia, and loss of balance. Nephrotoxicity results in rising serum creatinine levels or reduced creatinine clearance, though the earliest indication often is an increase in trough serum aminoglycoside concentrations. Neomycin, kanamycin, and amikacin are the most ototoxic agents. Streptomycin and gentamicin are the most vestibulotoxic. Neomycin, tobramycin, and gentamicin are the most nephrotoxic.

In very high doses, aminoglycosides can produce a curare-like effect with neuromuscular blockade that results in respiratory paralysis. This paralysis is usually reversible by calcium gluconate (given promptly) or neostigmine. Hypersensitivity occurs infrequently.

F. CLINICAL USES

Aminoglycosides are mostly used against gram-negative enteric bacteria, especially when the isolate may be drug-resistant and when there is suspicion of sepsis. They are almost always used in combination with a β-lactam antibiotic in order to extend coverage to include potential gram-positive pathogens and to take advantage of the synergism between these two classes of drugs. Penicillin aminoglycoside combinations also are used to achieve bactericidal activity in treatment of enterococcal endocarditis and to shorten duration of therapy for viridans streptococcal and staphylococcal endocarditis. Which aminoglycoside and what dose should be used depend upon the infection being treated and susceptibility of the isolate.

STREPTOMYCIN

Streptomycin (Figure 45–1) was isolated from a strain of *Streptomyces griseus*. The antimicrobial activity of streptomycin is typical of that of other aminoglycosides, as are the mechanisms of resistance. Resistance has emerged in most species, severely limiting the current usefulness of streptomycin, with the exceptions listed below. Ribosomal resistance to streptomycin develops readily, limiting its role as a single agent.

Clinical Uses

A. MYCOBACTERIAL INFECTIONS

Streptomycin is mainly used as a second-line agent for treatment of tuberculosis. The dosage is 0.5–1 g/d (7.5–15 mg/kg/d for children), which is given intramuscularly or intravenously. It should be used only in combination with other agents to prevent emergence of resistance. See Chapter 47 for additional information regarding its use in mycobacterial infections.

B. NONTUBERCULOUS INFECTIONS

In plague, tularemia, and sometimes brucellosis, streptomycin, 1 g/d (15 mg/kg/d for children), is given intramuscularly in combination with an oral tetracycline.

Penicillin plus streptomycin is effective for enterococcal endocarditis and 2-week therapy of viridans streptococcal endocarditis. Gentamicin has largely replaced streptomycin for these indications. Strepto-

mycin remains a useful agent for treating enterococcal infections, however, because approximately 15% of enterococcal isolates that are resistant to gentamicin (and therefore to netilmicin, tobramycin, and amikacin) will be susceptible to streptomycin.

Adverse Reactions

Fever, skin rashes, and other allergic manifestations may result from hypersensitivity to streptomycin. This occurs most frequently upon prolonged contact with the drug, either in patients who receive a prolonged course of treatment (eg, for tuberculosis) or in medical personnel who handle the drug. Desensitization is occasionally successful.

Pain at the injection site is common but usually not severe. The most serious toxic effect is disturbance of vestibular function—vertigo and loss of balance. The frequency and severity of this disturbance are proportionate to the age of the patient, the blood levels of the drug, and the duration of administration. Vestibular dysfunction may follow a few weeks of unusually high blood levels (eg, in individuals with impaired renal function) or months of relatively low blood levels. Vestibular toxicity tends to be irreversible. Streptomycin given during pregnancy can cause deafness in the newborn and therefore is relatively contraindicated.

GENTAMICIN

Gentamicin is an aminoglycoside (Figure 45–2) isolated from *Micromonospora purpurea*. It is effective against both gram-positive and gram-negative organisms, and many of its properties resemble those of other aminoglycosides. **Sisomicin** is very similar to the C_{1a} component of gentamicin.

Antimicrobial Activity

Gentamicin sulfate, 2–10 μg/mL, inhibits in vitro many strains of staphylococci and coliforms and other gram-negative bacteria. It is active alone, but also as a synergistic companion with β-lactam antibiotics, against pseudomonas, proteus, enterobacter, klebsiella, serratia, stenotrophomonas, and other gram-negative rods that may be resistant to multiple other antibiotics. Like all aminoglycosides, it has no activity against anaerobes.

Resistance

Streptococci and enterococci are relatively resistant to gentamicin owing to failure of the drug to penetrate into the cell. However, gentamicin in combination with vancomycin or a penicillin produces a potent bactericidal effect, which in part is due to enhanced uptake of drug that occurs with inhibition of cell wall synthesis.

Resistance to gentamicin rapidly emerges in staphylococci due to selection of permeability mutants. Ribosomal resistance is rare. Among gram-negative bacteria, resistance is most commonly due to plasmid-encoded aminoglycoside modifying enzymes. Gram-negative bacteria that are gentamicin-resistant usually will be susceptible to amikacin, which is much more resistant to modifying enzyme activity. The enterococcal enzyme that modifies gentamicin is a bifunctional enzyme that also inactivates amikacin, netilmicin, and tobramycin, but not streptomycin; the latter is modified by a different enzyme. This is why some gentamicin-resistant enterococci are susceptible to streptomycin.

Clinical Uses

A. INTRAMUSCULAR OR INTRAVENOUS ADMINISTRATION

At present, gentamicin is employed mainly in severe infections (eg, sepsis and pneumonia) caused by gram-negative bacteria that are likely to be resistant to other drugs, especially pseudomonas, enterobacter, serratia, proteus, acinetobacter, and klebsiella. Patients with these infections are often immunocompromised, and the combined action of the aminoglycoside with a cephalosporin or a penicillin may be life-saving. In such situations, 5–6 mg/kg/d of gentamicin is traditionally given intravenously in three equal doses. However, as noted above, studies indicate that once-daily administration is just as effective for some organisms and less toxic. Gentamicin is also used concurrently with penicillin G for bactericidal activity in endocarditis due to viridans streptococci or enterococci and in combination with nafcillin in selected cases of staphylococcal endocarditis. Gentamicin should not be used as a single agent to treat staphylococcal infections because resistance develops rapidly. Neither gentamicin nor any other aminoglycoside should be used for single-agent therapy of pneumonia because penetration of infected lung tissue is poor and local conditions of low pH and low oxygen tension contribute to poor activity.

Serum gentamicin concentrations and renal function should be monitored if gentamicin is administered for more than a few days or if renal function is changing (eg, in sepsis, which often is complicated by acute renal failure). For patients receiving every-8-hours dosing, target peak concentrations are 5–10 μg/mL and trough concentrations should be less than 1–2 μg/mL. Trough concentrations above 2 μg/mL indicate accumulation of drug and are associated with toxicity; in this case, the dose should be lowered or the interval extended to achieve the target range.

B. TOPICAL ADMINISTRATION

Creams, ointments, or solutions containing 0.1–0.3% gentamicin sulfate have been used for the treatment of infected burns, wounds, or skin lesions and the prevention of intravenous catheter infections. Topical gentamicin is partly inactivated by purulent exudates. Ten milligrams can be injected subconjunctivally for treatment of ocular infections.

C. INTRATHECAL ADMINISTRATION

Meningitis caused by gram-negative bacteria has been treated by the intrathecal injection of gentamicin sulfate, 1–10 mg/d. However, neither intrathecal nor intraventricular gentamicin was beneficial in neonates with meningitis, and intraventricular gentamicin was toxic, raising questions about the utility of this form of therapy. Moreover, the availability of third-generation cephalosporins for gram-negative meningitis has rendered this therapy obsolete in most cases.

Adverse Reactions

Nephrotoxicity is reversible and usually mild. It occurs in 5–25% of patients receiving the drug for longer than 3–5 days. Such toxicity requires, at the very least, adjustment of the dosing regimen and should prompt reconsideration of the necessity of using the drug, particularly if there is a less toxic alternative agent. Measurement of gentamicin serum levels is essential. Ototoxicity, which tends to be irreversible, manifests itself mainly as vestibular dysfunction, perhaps due to destruction of hair cells by prolonged elevated drug levels. Loss of hearing can also occur. The incidence of ototoxicity is 1–5% for patients receiving the drug for more than 5 days. Hypersensitivity reactions to gentamicin are uncommon.

TOBRAMYCIN

This aminoglycoside (Figure 45–2) has an antibacterial spectrum similar to that of gentamicin. While there is some cross-resistance between gentamicin and tobramycin, it is unpredictable in individual strains. Separate laboratory susceptibility tests are therefore necessary.

The pharmacokinetic properties of tobramycin are virtually identical to those of gentamicin. The daily dose of tobramycin is 5–6 mg/kg intramuscularly or intravenously, divided into three equal amounts and given every 8 hours. Monitoring blood levels in renal insufficiency is an essential guide to proper dosing.

Tobramycin has almost the same antibacterial spectrum as gentamicin with a few exceptions. Gentamicin is slightly more active against serratia, whereas tobramycin is slightly more active against pseudomonas; *Enterococcus faecalis* is susceptible to both gentamicin and tobramycin, but *E faecium* is resistant to tobramycin. Gentamicin and tobramycin are otherwise completely interchangeable clinically. Gentamicin is much less expensive, however, and is preferred for this reason.

Like other aminoglycosides, tobramycin is ototoxic and nephrotoxic. Nephrotoxicity of tobramycin may be slightly less than that of gentamicin, but the difference is clinically inconsequential.

AMIKACIN

Amikacin is a semisynthetic derivative of kanamycin; it is less toxic than the parent molecule (Figure 45–2). It is resistant to many enzymes that inactivate gentamicin and tobramycin, and it therefore can be employed against some microorganisms resistant to the latter drugs. Many gram-negative enteric bacteria, including many strains of proteus, pseudomonas, enterobacter, and serratia, are inhibited by 1–20 μg/mL amikacin in vitro. After the injection of 500 mg of amikacin every 12 hours (15 mg/kg/d) intramuscularly, peak levels in serum are 10–30 μg/mL.

Strains of multidrug-resistant *Mycobacterium tuberculosis,* including streptomycin-resistant strains, are usually susceptible to amikacin. Kanamycin-resistant strains may be cross-resistant to amikacin. The dosage of amikacin for tuberculosis is 7.5–15 mg/kg/d as a once-daily or two to three times weekly injection, always in combination with other drugs to which the isolate is susceptible.

Like all aminoglycosides, amikacin is nephrotoxic and ototoxic (particularly for the auditory portion of the eighth nerve). Serum concentrations should be monitored. Target peak serum concentrations for an every-12-hours dosing regimen are 20–40 μg/mL, and troughs should be maintained at less than 2 μg/mL.

NETILMICIN

This aminoglycoside became available in the USA in 1983. It shares many characteristics with gentamicin and tobramycin. However, the addition of an ethyl group to the 1-amino position of the 2-deoxystreptamine ring (ring II, Figure 45–2) sterically protects the netilmicin molecule from enzymatic degradation at the 3-amino (ring II) and 2-hydroxyl (ring III) positions. Consequently, netilmicin may not be inactivated by many gentamicin-resistant and tobramycin-resistant bacteria.

The dosage (5–7 mg/kg/d) and the routes of administration are the same as for gentamicin. It is completely therapeutically interchangeable with gentamicin or tobramycin and has similar toxicities.

NEOMYCIN & KANAMYCIN

These drugs are closely related. **Paromomycin** is also a member of this group. All have similar properties.

Antimicrobial Activity & Resistance

Drugs of the neomycin group are active against gram-positive and gram-negative bacteria and some mycobacteria. Pseudomonas and streptococci are generally resistant. Mechanisms of antibacterial action and resistance are the same as with other aminoglycosides. The widespread use of these drugs in bowel preparation for elective surgery has resulted in the selection of resistant organisms and some outbreaks of enterocolitis in hospitals. There is complete cross-resistance between kanamycin and neomycin.

Pharmacokinetics

Drugs of the neomycin group are not significantly absorbed from the gastrointestinal tract. After oral administration, the intestinal flora is suppressed or modified and the drug is excreted in the feces. Excretion of any absorbed drug is mainly through glomerular filtration into the urine.

Clinical Uses

Neomycin is too toxic for parenteral use. With the advent of more potent and less toxic aminoglycosides, parenteral administration of kanamycin has also been abandoned. Neomycin and kanamycin are now limited to topical and oral use.

A. TOPICAL ADMINISTRATION

Solutions containing 1–5 mg/mL are used on infected surfaces or injected into joints, the pleural cavity, tissue spaces, or abscess cavities where infection is present. The total amount of drug given in this fashion must be limited to 15 mg/kg/d because at higher doses enough drug may be absorbed to produce systemic toxicity. Whether topical application for active infection adds anything to appropriate systemic therapy is questionable. Ointments, often formulated as a neomycin-polymyxin-bacitracin combination, are sometimes applied to infected skin lesions or in the nares for suppression of staphylococci; they are largely ineffective.

B. ORAL ADMINISTRATION

In preparation for elective bowel surgery, 1 g of neomycin is given orally every 6–8 hours for 1–2 days, often combined with 1 g of erythromycin base. This reduces the aerobic bowel flora with little effect on anaerobes. In hepatic coma, the coliform flora can be suppressed for prolonged periods by giving 1 g every 6–8 hours together with reduced protein intake, thus reducing ammonia intoxication. Use of neomycin for hepatic coma has been almost entirely supplanted by lactulose, which is much less toxic. Paromomycin, 1 g every 6 hours orally for 2 weeks, has been effective in intestinal amebiasis.

Adverse Reactions

All members of the neomycin group have significant nephrotoxicity and ototoxicity. Auditory function is affected more than vestibular. Deafness has occurred, especially in adults with impaired renal function and prolonged elevation of drug levels.

The sudden absorption of postoperatively instilled kanamycin from the peritoneal cavity (3–5 g) has resulted in curare-like neuromuscular blockade and respiratory arrest. Calcium gluconate and neostigmine can act as antidotes.

While hypersensitivity is not common, prolonged application of neomycin-containing ointments to skin and eyes has resulted in severe allergic reactions.

SPECTINOMYCIN

Spectinomycin is an aminocyclitol antibiotic that is structurally related to aminoglycosides. It lacks amino sugars and glycosidic bonds.

Spectinomycin

While active in vitro against many gram-positive and gram-negative organisms, spectinomycin is used almost solely as an alternative treatment for gonorrhea in patients who are allergic to penicillin or whose gonococci are resistant to other drugs. The vast majority of gonococcal isolates are inhibited by 6 μg/mL of spectinomycin. Strains of gonococci may be resistant to spectinomycin, but there is no cross-resistance with other drugs used in gonorrhea. Spectinomycin is rapidly absorbed after intramuscular injection. A single dose of 40 mg/kg up to a maximum of 2 g is given. There is pain at the injection site and occasionally fever and nausea. Nephrotoxicity and anemia have been observed rarely.

PREPARATIONS AVAILABLE

Amikacin (generic, Amikin)
  Parenteral: 50, 250 mg (in vials) for IM, IV injection
Gentamicin (generic, Garamycin)
  Parenteral: 10, 40 mg/mL vials for IM, IV injection
Kanamycin (Kantrex)
  Oral: 500 mg capsules
  Parenteral: 500, 1000 mg for IM, IV injection; 75 mg for pediatric injection
Neomycin (generic, Mycifradin)
  Oral: 500 mg tablets; 125 mg/5 mL solution
Netilmicin (Netromycin)
  Parenteral: 100 mg/mL for IM, IV injection

Paromomycin (Humatin)
  Oral: 250 mg capsules
Spectinomycin (Trobicin)
  Parenteral: 2 g powder to reconstitute for IM injection
Streptomycin (generic)
  Parenteral: 400 mg/mL for IM injection
Tobramycin (generic, Nebcin)
  Parenteral: 10, 40 mg/mL for IM, IV injection; powder to reconstitute for injection

---

REFERENCES

Busse H-J, Wöstmann C, Bakker EP: The bactericidal action of streptomycin: Membrane permeabilization caused by the insertion of mistranslated proteins into the cytoplasmic membrane of *Escherichia coli* and subsequent caging of the antibiotic inside the cells due to degradation of these proteins. J Gen Microbiol 1992;138:551.

Edson RS, Terrell CL: The aminoglycosides: Streptomycin, kanamycin, gentamicin, tobramycin, amikacin, netilmicin, and sisomicin. Mayo Clin Proc 1987;62:916.

Gilbert DN: Mini-review: Once-daily aminoglycoside therapy. Antimicrob Agents Chemother 1991;35:399.

Hughes WT et al: Guidelines for the use of antimicrobial agents in neutropenic patients with unexplained fever. J Infect Dis 1990;161:381.

Krogstad DJ et al: Plasmid-mediated resistance to antibiotic synergism in enterococci. J Clin Invest 1978;61:1645.

McCormack JP, Jewesson PJ: A critical reevaluation of the "therapeutic range" of aminoglycosides. Clin Infect Dis 1992;14:320.

Nicolau DP et al: Experience with a once-daily aminoglycoside program administered to 2,184 adult patients. Antimicrob Agents Chemother 1995;39:650.

Nicolau DP et al: Once-daily aminoglycoside dosing: impact on requests and costs for therapeutic drug monitoring. Ther Drug Monit 1996;18:263.

Noone M et al: Prospective study of amikacin vs netilmicin in the treatment of severe infections in hospitalized patients. Am J Med 1989;86:809.

Prins JM et al: Once versus thrice daily gentamicin in patients with serious infections. Lancet 1993;341:335.

Smith CR et al: Double blind comparison of the nephrotoxicity and auditory toxicity of gentamicin and tobramycin. N Engl J Med 1980;302:1106.

Spera RV Jr, Farber BF: Multiply-resistant *Enterococcus faecium*. The nosocomial pathogen of the 1990s. JAMA 1992;268:2563.

Swan SK, Bennett WM: Drug dosing guide lines in patients with renal failure. West J Med 1992;156:633.

Wilson WR et al: Antibiotic treatment of adults with infective endocarditis due to streptococci, enterococci, staphylococci, and HACEK microorganisms. JAMA 1995;274:1706.

Sulfonamides, Trimethoprim, & Quinolones

Henry F. Chambers, MD

I. ANTIFOLATE DRUGS

SULFONAMIDES

Chemistry

The basic formula of the sulfonamides and their structural similarity to *p*-aminobenzoic acid (PABA) are shown in Figure 46–1. Sulfonamides with varying physical, chemical, pharmacologic, and antibacterial properties are produced by attaching substituents to the amido group ($-SO_2-NH-R$) or the amino group ($-NH_2$) of the sulfanilamide nucleus. Sulfonamides tend to be much more soluble at alkaline than at acid pH. Most can be prepared as sodium salts, which are used for intravenous administration.

Antimicrobial Activity

Susceptible microorganisms require extracellular PABA in order to form dihydrofolic acid (Figure 46–2), an essential step in the production of purines and the synthesis of nucleic acids. Sulfonamides are structural analogs of PABA that competitively inhibit dihydropteroate synthase. They inhibit growth by reversibly blocking folic acid synthesis. Sulfonamides inhibit both gram-positive and gram-negative bacteria, nocardia, *Chlamydia trachomatis,* and some protozoa. Some enteric bacteria, such as *E coli,* klebsiella, salmonella, shigella, and enterobacter, are inhibited. Interestingly, rickettsiae are not inhibited by sulfonamides but are actually stimulated in their growth.

Resistance

Mammalian cells (and some bacteria) lack the enzymes required for folate synthesis and depend upon exogenous sources of folate; therefore, they are not susceptible to sulfonamides. Sulfonamide resistance may occur as a result of mutations that cause overproduction of PABA, cause production of a folic acid-synthesizing enzyme that has low affinity for sulfonamides, or cause a loss of permeability to the sulfonamide. Dihydropteroate synthase with low sulfonamide affinity is often encoded on a plasmid that is transmissible and can disseminate rapidly and widely. Sulfonamide-resistant cells may be present in susceptible bacterial populations and can emerge under selective pressure.

Pharmacokinetics

Sulfonamides can be divided into three major groups: (1) oral, absorbable; (2) oral, nonabsorbable; and (3) topical. Sodium salts of sulfonamides in 5% dextrose in water can be given intravenously, but except for sulfamethoxazole-trimethoprim combinations, these are rarely used. The oral, absorbable sulfonamides can be classified as short-, medium-, or long-acting on the basis of their half-lives (Table 46–1). They are absorbed from the stomach and small intestine and distributed widely to tissues and body fluids (including the central nervous system and cerebrospinal fluid), placenta, and fetus. Absorbed sulfonamides become bound to serum proteins to an extent varying from 20% to over 90%. Therapeutic concentrations are in the range of 40–100 µg/mL of blood. Peak blood levels generally occur 2–6 hours after oral administration.

A portion of absorbed drug is acetylated or glucuronidated in the liver. Sulfonamides and inactivated metabolites are then excreted into the urine, mainly by glomerular filtration. In significant renal failure, the dosage of sulfonamide must be reduced.

Clinical Uses

Sulfonamides are infrequently used as single agents. Formerly drugs of choice for infections such as *Pneumocystis jiroveci* (formerly *P carinii*) pneumonia, toxoplasmosis, nocardiosis, and occasionally other bacterial infections, they have been largely supplanted by the fixed drug combination of trimethoprim-sulfamethoxazole. Many

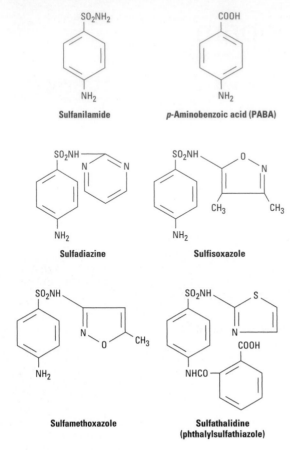

Figure 46–1. Structures of some sulfonamides and *p*-aminobenzoic acid.

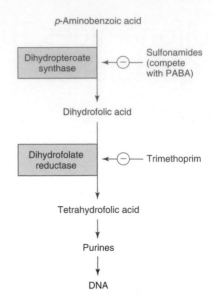

Figure 46–2. Actions of sulfonamides and trimethoprim.

synergistic because these drugs block sequential steps in the folate synthetic pathway blockade (Figure 46–2). The dosage of sulfadiazine is 1 g four times daily, with pyrimethamine given as a 75 mg loading dose followed by a 25 mg once-daily dose. Folinic acid, 10 mg orally

strains of formerly susceptible species, including meningococci, pneumococci, streptococci, staphylococci, and gonococci, are now resistant. Nevertheless, sulfonamides can be useful for treatment of urinary tract infections due to susceptible organisms and in other special clinical situations discussed below.

A. ORAL ABSORBABLE AGENTS

Sulfisoxazole and sulfamethoxazole are short- to medium-acting agents that are used almost exclusively to treat urinary tract infections. The usual adult dosage is 1 g of sulfisoxazole four times daily or 1 g of sulfamethoxazole two or three times daily.

Sulfadiazine achieves therapeutic concentrations in cerebrospinal fluid and in combination with pyrimethamine is first-line therapy for treatment of acute toxoplasmosis. Pyrimethamine, an antiprotozoal agent, is a potent inhibitor of dihydrofolate reductase. The combination of sulfadiazine and pyrimethamine is

Table 46–1. Pharmacokinetic properties of some sulfonamides and trimethoprim.

Drug	Half-Life	Oral Absorption
Sulfonamides		
Sulfacytine	Short	Prompt (peak levels in 1–4 hours)
Sulfisoxazole	Short (6 hours)	Prompt
Sulfamethizole	Short (9 hours)	Prompt
Sulfadiazine	Intermediate (10–17 hours)	Slow (peak levels in 4–8 hours)
Sulfamethoxazole	Intermediate (10–12 hours)	Slow
Sulfapyridine	No data	Slow
Sulfadoxine	Long (7–9 days)	Intermediate
Pyrimidines		
Trimethoprim	Intermediate (11 hours)	Prompt

each day, should also be administered to minimize bone marrow suppression.

Sulfadoxine is the only long-acting sulfonamide currently available in the United States. Urinary excretion—especially of the free form—is very slow, resulting in prolonged drug levels in serum. Sulfadoxine is available only as Fansidar, a combination formulation with pyrimethamine, which is used as a second-line agent in treatment for malaria (Chapter 53).

B. ORAL NONABSORBABLE AGENTS

Sulfasalazine (salicylazosulfapyridine) is widely used in ulcerative colitis, enteritis, and other inflammatory bowel disease (see Chapter 63).

C. TOPICAL AGENTS

Sodium sulfacetamide ophthalmic solution or ointment is effective treatment for bacterial conjunctivitis and as adjunctive therapy for trachoma. Mafenide acetate is used topically to prevent bacterial colonization and infection of burn wounds. Mafenide is absorbed from burn sites, and systemic levels are produced. The drug and its primary metabolite also inhibit carbonic anhydrase and can cause metabolic acidosis, a side effect that limits its usefulness. Silver sulfadiazine is a much less toxic topical sulfonamide and is preferred to mafenide for prevention of infection of burn wounds.

Adverse Reactions

All sulfonamides and their derivatives, including carbonic anhydrase inhibitors, thiazides, furosemide, bumetanide, torsemide, diazoxide, and the sulfonylurea hypoglycemic agents, are cross-allergenic. The most common adverse effects are fever, skin rashes, exfoliative dermatitis, photosensitivity, urticaria, nausea, vomiting, diarrhea, and difficulties referable to the urinary tract (see below). Stevens-Johnson syndrome, although relatively uncommon (ie, less than 1% of treatment courses), is a particularly serious and potentially fatal type of skin and mucous membrane eruption associated with sulfonamide use. Other unwanted effects include stomatitis, conjunctivitis, arthritis, hematopoietic disturbances (see below), hepatitis, and, rarely, polyarteritis nodosa and psychosis.

A. URINARY TRACT DISTURBANCES

Sulfonamides may precipitate in urine, especially at neutral or acid pH, producing crystalluria, hematuria, or even obstruction. This is rarely a problem with the more soluble sulfonamides (eg, sulfisoxazole). Sulfadiazine when given in large doses, particularly if fluid intake is poor, can cause crystalluria. Crystalluria is treated by administration of sodium bicarbonate to alkalinize the urine and fluids to maintain adequate hydration. Sulfonamides have also been implicated in various types of nephrosis and in allergic nephritis.

B. HEMATOPOIETIC DISTURBANCES

Sulfonamides can cause hemolytic or aplastic anemia, granulocytopenia, thrombocytopenia, or leukemoid reactions. Sulfonamides may provoke hemolytic reactions in patients whose red cells are deficient in glucose-6-phosphate dehydrogenase. Sulfonamides taken near the end of pregnancy increase the risk of kernicterus in newborns.

TRIMETHOPRIM & TRIMETHOPRIM-SULFAMETHOXAZOLE MIXTURES

Trimethoprim, a trimethoxybenzylpyrimidine, inhibits bacterial dihydrofolic acid reductase about 50,000 times more efficiently than the same enzyme of mammalian cells. Pyrimethamine, another benzylpyrimidine, inhibits the activity of dihydrofolic acid reductase of protozoa more than that of mammalian cells. Dihydrofolic acid reductases convert dihydrofolic acid to tetrahydrofolic acid, a step leading to the synthesis of purines and ultimately to DNA. Trimethoprim or pyrimethamine, given together with sulfonamides, produces sequential blocking in this metabolic sequence, resulting in marked enhancement (synergism) of the activity of both drugs (Figure 46–2). The combination often is bactericidal, compared to the bacteriostatic activity of a sulfonamide alone.

Trimethoprim

Pyrimethamine

Resistance

Resistance to trimethoprim can result from reduced cell permeability, overproduction of dihydrofolate reductase, or production of an altered reductase with reduced drug binding. Resistance can emerge by mutation, though more commonly it is due to plasmid-encoded trimethoprim-resistant dihydrofolate reductases. These resistant enzymes may be located within transposons on conjugative plasmids that exhibit a broad host range, accounting for rapid and widespread dissemination of trimethoprim resistance among numerous bacterial species.

Pharmacokinetics

Trimethoprim is usually given orally, alone or in combination with sulfamethoxazole, the latter chosen because it has a similar half-life. Trimethoprim-sulfamethoxazole can also be given intravenously. Trimethoprim is absorbed efficiently from the gut and distributed widely in body fluids and tissues, including cerebrospinal fluid. Because trimethoprim is more lipid-soluble than sulfamethoxazole, it has a larger volume of distribution than the latter drug. Therefore, when 1 part of trimethoprim is given with 5 parts of sulfamethoxazole (the ratio in the formulation), the peak plasma concentrations are in the ratio of 1:20, which is optimal for the combined effects of these drugs in vitro. About 65–70% of each participant drug is protein-bound, and 30–50% of the sulfonamide and 50–60% of the trimethoprim (or their respective metabolites) are excreted in the urine within 24 hours. The dose should be reduced by half for patients with creatinine clearances of 15 to 30 mL/min.

Trimethoprim (a weak base of pK_a 7.2) concentrates in prostatic fluid and in vaginal fluid, which are more acid than plasma. Therefore, it has more antibacterial activity in prostatic and vaginal fluids than many other antimicrobial drugs.

Clinical Uses

A. Oral Trimethoprim

Trimethoprim can be given alone (100 mg twice daily) in acute urinary tract infections. Most community-acquired organisms tend to be susceptible to the high concentrations that are found in the urine (200–600 µg/mL).

B. Oral Trimethoprim-Sulfamethoxazole

A combination of trimethoprim-sulfamethoxazole is effective treatment for *P jiroveci* pneumonia, shigellosis, systemic salmonella infections (caused by ampicillin- or chloramphenicol-resistant organisms), complicated urinary tract infections, prostatitis, some nontuberculous mycobacterial infections, and many others. It is active against many respiratory tract pathogens, including the pneumococcus, haemophilus species, *Moraxella catarrhalis,* and *Klebsiella pneumoniae* (but not *Mycoplasma pneumoniae*), making it a potentially useful alternative to β-lactam drugs for treatment of upper respiratory tract infections and community-acquired bacterial pneumonia. However, the increasing prevalence of strains of *E coli* (up to 30% or more) and pneumococci (particularly penicillin-resistant strains, but also some penicillin-susceptible strains) that are resistant to trimethoprim-sulfamethoxazole must be considered before using this combination for empirical therapy of upper urinary tract infections or pneumonia.

Two double-strength tablets (trimethoprim 160 mg plus sulfamethoxazole 800 mg) given every 12 hours is effective treatment for urinary tract infections and prostatitis. One half of the regular size (single-strength) tablet given three times weekly for many months may serve as prophylaxis in recurrent urinary tract infections of some women. Two double-strength tablets every 12 hours is effective treatment for infections caused by susceptible strains of shigella and salmonella. The dosage for children treated for shigellosis, urinary tract infection, or otitis media is 8 mg/kg trimethoprim and 40 mg/kg sulfamethoxazole every 12 hours.

Infections with *P jiroveci* and some other pathogens can be treated orally with high doses of the combination (dosed on the basis of the trimethoprim component at 15–20 mg/kg) or can be prevented in immunosuppressed patients by one double-strength tablet daily or three times weekly.

C. Intravenous Trimethoprim-Sulfamethoxazole

A solution of the mixture containing 80 mg trimethoprim plus 400 mg sulfamethoxazole per 5 mL diluted in 125 mL of 5% dextrose in water can be administered by intravenous infusion over 60–90 minutes. It is the agent of choice for moderately severe to severe pneumocystis pneumonia. It may be used for gram-negative bacterial sepsis, including that caused by some multidrug-resistant species such as enterobacter and serratia; shigellosis; typhoid fever; or urinary tract infection caused by a susceptible organism when the patient is unable to take the drug by mouth. The dosage is 10–20 mg/kg/d of the trimethoprim component.

D. Oral Pyrimethamine With Sulfonamide

Pyrimethamine and sulfadiazine have been used for treatment of leishmaniasis and toxoplasmosis. In falciparum malaria, the combination of pyrimethamine with sulfadoxine (Fansidar) has been employed (see Chapter 53).

Adverse Effects

Trimethoprim produces the predictable adverse effects of an antifolate drug, especially megaloblastic anemia, leukopenia, and granulocytopenia. This can be prevented by the simultaneous administration of folinic acid, 6–8 mg/d. Use of folinic acid to prevent hematologic toxicity resulting from trimethoprim-sulfamethoxazole during treatment of pneumocystis pneumonia in AIDS patients is associated with increased morbidity and treatment failures and is not recommended. In addition, the combination trimethoprim-sulfamethoxazole may cause all of the untoward reactions associated with sulfonamides. Nausea and vomiting, drug fever, vasculitis, renal damage, and central nervous system disturbances occasionally occur also. Patients with AIDS and pneumocystis pneumonia have a particularly high frequency of untoward reactions to trimethoprim-sulfamethoxazole, especially fever, rashes, leukopenia, diarrhea, elevations of hepatic aminotransferases, hyperkalemia, and hyponatremia.

II. DNA GYRASE INHIBITORS

FLUOROQUINOLONES

The important quinolones are synthetic fluorinated analogs of nalidixic acid. They are active against a variety of gram-positive and gram-negative bacteria. Quinolones block bacterial DNA synthesis by inhibiting bacterial topoisomerase II (DNA gyrase) and topoisomerase IV. Inhibition of DNA gyrase prevents the relaxation of positively supercoiled DNA that is required for normal transcription and replication. Inhibition of topoisomerase IV interferes with separation of replicated chromosomal DNA into the respective daughter cells during cell division.

Earlier quinolones (nalidixic acid, oxolinic acid, cinoxacin) did not achieve systemic antibacterial levels. These agents were useful only for treatment of lower urinary tract infections (see below); nalidixic acid and cinoxacin are still available. Fluorinated derivatives (ciprofloxacin, levofloxacin, and others; Figure 46–3 and Table 46–2) have greatly improved antibacterial activity compared with nalidixic acid and achieve bactericidal levels in blood and tissues.

Antibacterial Activity

Fluoroquinolones were originally developed because of their excellent activity against gram-negative aerobic bacteria; they had limited activity against gram-positive organisms. Several newer agents have improved activity against gram-positive cocci. This relative activity against gram-negative versus gram-positive species is useful for classification of these agents. Norfloxacin is the least active of the fluoroquinolones against both gram-negative and gram-positive organisms, with MICs fourfold to eightfold higher than those of ciprofloxacin, the prototype drug. Ciprofloxacin, enoxacin, lomefloxacin, levofloxacin,

ofloxacin, and pefloxacin comprise a second group of similar agents possessing excellent gram-negative activity and moderate to good activity against gram-positive bacteria. Minimum inhibitory concentrations (MICs) for gram-negative cocci and bacilli, including Enterobacteriaceae, pseudomonas, neisseria, haemophilus, and campylobacter, are 1–2 μg/mL and often less. Methicillin-susceptible strains of *S aureus* are generally susceptible to these fluoroquinolones, but methicillin-resistant strains of staphylococci are often resistant. Streptococci and enterococci tend to be less susceptible than staphylococci, and efficacy in infections caused by these organisms is limited. Ciprofloxacin is the most active agent of this group against gram-negatives, *P aeruginosa* in particular. Levofloxacin, the L-isomer of ofloxacin and twice as potent, has superior activity against gram-positive organisms, including *S pneumoniae*.

Gatifloxacin, moxifloxacin, sparfloxacin, and trovafloxacin comprise a third group of fluoroquinolones with improved activity against gram-positive organisms, particularly *S pneumoniae* and to some extent staphylococci. Although MICs of these agents for staphylococci are lower than those of ciprofloxacin (and the other compounds mentioned in the paragraph above) and may fall within the susceptible range, it is not known whether the enhanced activity is sufficient to permit use of these agents for treatment of infections caused by ciprofloxacin-resistant strains. None of these agents are as active as ciprofloxacin against gram-negative organisms. Fluoroquinolones also are active against agents of atypical pneumonia (eg, mycoplasmas and chlamydiae) and against intracellular pathogens such as legionella species and some mycobacteria, including *Mycobacterium tuberculosis* and *M avium* complex. Moxifloxacin and trovafloxacin, in addition to enhanced gram-positive activity, also have good activity—which other fluoroquinolones lack—against anaerobic bacteria.

Resistance

During fluoroquinolone therapy, resistant organisms emerge with a frequency of about one in 10^7–10^9, especially among staphylococci, pseudomonas, and serratia. Resistance is due to one or more point mutations in the quinolone binding region of the target enzyme or to a change in the permeability of the organism. DNA gyrase is the primary target in *E coli,* with single-step mutants exhibiting amino acid substitution in the A subunit of gyrase. Topoisomerase IV is a secondary target in *E coli* that is altered in mutants expressing higher levels of resistance. In staphylococci and streptococci, the situation is reversed: topoisomerase IV is usually the primary target, and gyrase is the secondary target. Resistance to one fluoroquinolone, particularly if of high level, generally confers cross-resistance to all other mem-

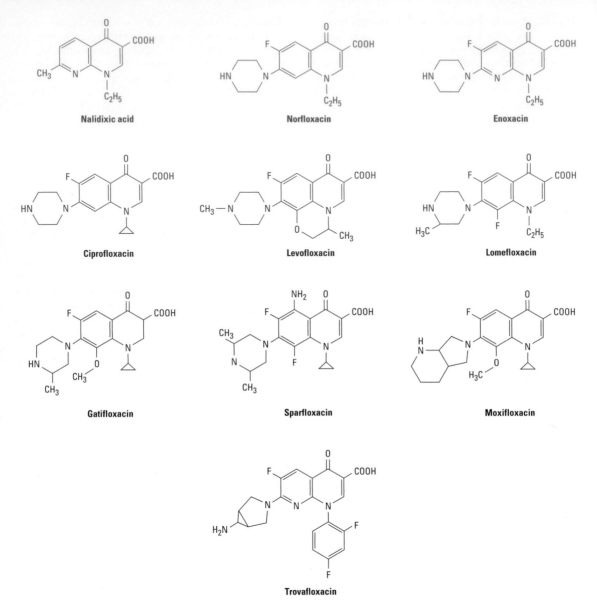

Figure 46–3. Structures of nalidixic acid and some fluoroquinolones.

bers of this class. With the increasing use of fluoro-quinolones for a variety of infections, including respiratory tract infections, fluoroquinolone resistance has emerged among strains of *Streptococcus pneumoniae*.

Pharmacokinetics

After oral administration, the fluoroquinolones are well absorbed (bioavailability of 80–95%) and distributed widely in body fluids and tissues (Table 46–2). Serum half-lives range from 3 hours (norfloxacin and cipro-floxacin) up to 10 (pefloxacin and fleroxacin) or longer (sparfloxacin). The relatively long half-lives of le-vofloxacin, moxifloxacin, sparfloxacin, and trovafloxacin permit once-daily dosing. The pharmacokinetics of ofloxacin and levofloxacin are identical. Oral absorption is impaired by divalent cations, including those in antacids. Serum concentrations of intravenously admin-

Table 46–2. Pharmacokinetic properties of fluoroquinolones.

Drug	Half-Life (h)	Oral Bioavailability (%)	Peak Serum Concentration (μg/mL)	Oral Dose (mg)	Primary Route of Excretion
Ciprofloxacin	3–5	70	2.4	500	Renal
Clinafloxacin	6	nd	2.5	200	Renal
Enoxacin	3–6	90	2.0	400	Renal
Gatifloxacin	8	98	3.4	400	Renal
Levofloxacin	5–7	95	5.7	500	Renal
Lomefloxacin	8	95	2.8	400	Renal
Moxifloxacin	9–10	> 85	3.1	400	Nonrenal
Norfloxacin	3.5–5	80	1.5	400	Renal
Ofloxacin	5–7	95	2.9	400	Renal
Sparfloxacin	18	92			50% renal, 50% fecal
Trovafloxacin	11	88	2.2	200	Nonrenal

istered drug are similar to those of orally administered drug. Alatrovafloxacin is the inactive, prodrug form of trovafloxacin for parenteral administration. It is rapidly converted to the active compound. Concentrations in prostate, kidney, neutrophils, and macrophages exceed serum concentrations. Most fluoroquinolones are eliminated by renal mechanisms, either tubular secretion or glomerular filtration (Table 46–2). Dose adjustment is required for patients with creatinine clearances less than 50 mL/min, the exact adjustment depending upon the degree of renal impairment and the specific fluoroquinolone being used. Dose adjustment for renal failure is not necessary for trovafloxacin or moxifloxacin. Nonrenally cleared fluoroquinolones are contraindicated in patients with hepatic failure.

Clinical Uses

Fluoroquinolones are effective in urinary tract infections even when caused by multidrug-resistant bacteria, eg, pseudomonas. Norfloxacin 400 mg, ciprofloxacin 500 mg, and ofloxacin 400 mg given orally twice daily are all effective. These agents are also effective for bacterial diarrhea caused by shigella, salmonella, toxigenic *E coli*, or campylobacter. Fluoroquinolones (except norfloxacin, which does not achieve adequate systemic concentrations) have been employed in infections of soft tissues, bones, and joints and in intra-abdominal and respiratory tract infections, including those caused by multidrug-resistant organisms such as pseudomonas and enterobacter.

Ciprofloxacin and ofloxacin are effective for gonococcal infection, including disseminated disease, and ofloxacin is effective for chlamydial urethritis or cervicitis. Ciprofloxacin is a second-line agent for legionellosis. Ciprofloxacin or levofloxacin is occasionally used for treatment of tuberculosis and atypical mycobacterial infections. They may be suitable for eradication of meningococci from carriers or for prophylaxis of infection in neutropenic patients.

Owing to their marginal activity against the pneumococcus, fluoroquinolones have not been routinely recommended for empirical treatment of pneumonia and other upper respiratory tract infections. However, levofloxacin, gatifloxacin, and moxifloxacin, with their enhanced gram-positive activity and activity against atypical pneumonia agents (eg, chlamydia, mycoplasma, and legionella), are likely to be effective and used increasingly for treatment of upper and lower respiratory tract infections.

Adverse Effects

Fluoroquinolones are extremely well tolerated. The most common effects are nausea, vomiting, and diarrhea. Occasionally, headache, dizziness, insomnia, skin rash, or abnormal liver function tests develop. Trovafloxacin has been associated with acute hepatitis and hepatic failure, which has led to its restricted indications. Photosensitivity has been reported with lomefloxacin and pefloxacin. Grepafloxacin was withdrawn by the manufacturer shortly after approval because of QT_c interval prolongation and its tendency to cause cardiac arrhythmias. QT_c prolongation may also occur with other fluoroquinolones—particularly sparfloxacin but also gatifloxacin, levofloxacin, and moxifloxacin. Ideally, these agents should be avoided or used with caution in patients with known QT_c interval prolongation or uncorrected hypokalemia; in those receiving class IA (eg, quinidine or procainamide) or class III antiarrhythmic agents (sotalol, ibutilide, amiodarone); and in patients who are receiving other agents known to increase the QT_c interval (eg, erythromycin, tricyclic antidepressants). Gatifloxacin has been associated with hyperglycemia in diabetic patients and with hypoglycemia in patients also receiving oral hypoglycemic agents.

Fluoroquinolones may damage growing cartilage and cause an arthropathy. Thus, they are not routinely recommended for use in patients under 18 years of age. However, the arthropathy is reversible, and there is a growing consensus that fluoroquinolones may be used in children in some cases (eg, for treatment of pseudomonal infections in patients with cystic fibrosis). Tendinitis, a

---

PREPARATIONS AVAILABLE

GENERAL-PURPOSE SULFONAMIDES

Sulfadiazine (generic)
Oral: 500 mg tablets
Sulfamethizole (Thiosulfil Forte)
Oral: 500 mg tablets
Sulfamethoxazole (generic, Gantanol, others)
Oral: 500 mg tablets; 500 mg/5 mL suspension
Sulfanilamide (AVC)
Vaginal cream: 15%
Sulfisoxazole (generic, Gantrisin)
Oral: 500 mg tablets; 500 mg/5 mL syrup
Ophthalmic: 4% solution

SULFONAMIDES FOR SPECIAL APPLICATIONS

Mafenide (Sulfamylon)
Topical: 85 mg/g cream; 5% solution
Silver sulfadiazine (generic, Silvadene)
Topical: 10 mg/g cream
Sulfacetamide sodium (generic)
Ophthalmic: 1, 10, 15, 30% solutions; 10% ointment

TRIMETHOPRIM

Trimethoprim (generic, Proloprim, Trimpex)
Oral: 100, 200 mg tablets
Trimethoprim-sulfamethoxazole [co-trimoxazole, TMP-SMZ] (generic, Bactrim, Septra, others)
Oral: 80 mg trimethoprim + 400 mg sulfamethoxazole per single-strength tablet; 160 mg trimethoprim + 800 mg sulfamethoxazole per double-strength tablet; 40 mg trimethoprim + 200 mg sulfamethoxazole per 5 mL suspension
Parenteral: 80 mg trimethoprim + 400 mg sulfamethoxazole per 5 mL for infusion (in 5 mL ampules and 5, 10, 20, 30, 50 mL vials)

QUINOLONES & FLUOROQUINOLONES

Cinoxacin (generic, Cinobac)
Oral: 250, 500 mg capsules

Ciprofloxacin (Cipro, Cipro I.V.)
Oral: 250, 500, 750 mg tablets; 50, 100 mg/mL suspension
Parenteral: 2, 10 mg/mL for IV infusion
Ophthalmic (Ciloxan): 3 mg/mL solution; 3.3 mg/g ointment
Enoxacin (Penetrex)
Oral: 200, 400 mg tablets
Gatifloxacin (Tequin)
Oral: 200, 400 mg tablets
Parenteral: 200, 400 mg for IV injection
Levofloxacin (Levaquin)
Oral: 250, 500, 750 mg for injection
Parenteral: 250, 500 mg for IV injection
Ophthalmic (Quixin): 5 mg/mL solution
Lomefloxacin (Maxaquin)
Oral: 400 mg tablets
Moxifloxacin (Avelox, Avelox I.V.)
Oral: 400 mg tablets
Parenteral: 400 mg in IV bag
Nalidixic acid (NegGram)
Oral: 250, 500, 1000 mg caplets; 250 mg/5 mL suspension
Norfloxacin (Noroxin)
Oral: 400 mg tablets
Ofloxacin (Floxin)
Oral: 200, 300, 400 mg tablets
Parenteral: 200 mg in 50 mL 5% D/W for IV administration; 20, 40 mg/mL for IV injection
Ophthalmic (Ocuflox): 3 mg/mL solution
Sparfloxacin (Zagam)
Oral: 200 mg tablets
Trovafloxacin (Trovan)
Oral: 100, 200 mg tablets
Intravenous: formulated as alatrovafloxacin 200 mg and 300 mg vials for IV infusion

rare complication that has been reported in adults, is potentially more serious because of the risk of tendon rupture. They should be avoided during pregnancy in the absence of specific data documenting their safety.

NALIDIXIC ACID & CINOXACIN

Nalidixic acid, the first antibacterial quinolone (Figure 46–3), was introduced in 1963. It is not fluorinated and is excreted too rapidly to be useful for systemic infections. Oxolinic acid and cinoxacin are similar in structure and function to nalidixic acid. Their mechanism of action is the same as that of the fluoroquinolones. These agents were useful only for the treatment of urinary tract infections and are rarely used now, having been made obsolete by the more efficacious fluorinated quinolones.

REFERENCES

Adrian PV, Klugman KP: Mutations in the dihydrofolate reductase gene of trimethoprim-resistant isolates of *Streptococcus pneumoniae.* Antimicrob Agents Chemother 1997;41:2406.

Bertino J Jr, Fish D: The safety profile of the fluoroquinolones. Clin Ther 2000;22:798.

Blondeau JM: Expanded activity and utility of the new fluoroquinolones: A review. Clin Ther 1999;21:3.

Davidson R et al: Resistance to levofloxacin and failure of treatment of pneumococcal pneumonia. N Engl J Med 2002;346:747.

Ferrero L, Cameron B, Crouzet J: Analysis of *gyrA* and *grlA* mutations in stepwise-selected ciprofloxacin-resistant mutants of *Staphylococcus aureus.* Antimicrob Agents Chemother 1995;39:1554.

Frothingham R: Rates of torsades de pointes associated with ciprofloxacin, ofloxacin, levofloxacin, gatifloxacin, and moxifloxacin. Pharmacotherapy 2001;21:1468.

Heikkila E et al: Analysis of localization of the type I trimethoprim resistance gene from *Escherichia coli* isolated in Finland. Antimicrob Agents Chemother 1991;35:1562.

Jones ME et al: Comparative activities of clinafloxacin, grepafloxacin, levofloxacin, moxifloxacin, ofloxacin, sparfloxacin, and trovafloxacin and nonquinolones linezolid, quinupristin-dalfopristin, gentamicin, and vancomycin against clinical isolates of ciprofloxacin-resistant and -susceptible *Staphylococcus aureus* strains. Antimicrob Agents Chemother 1999;43:421.

Pan XS, Fisher M: Cloning and characteristics of the *parC* and *parE* genes of *Streptococcus pneumoniae* encoding DNA topoisomerase IV: Role in fluoroquinolone resistance. J Bacteriol 1996;178:4060.

Radanst JM et al: Interaction of fluoroquinolones with other drugs: Mechanisms, variability, clinical significance, and management. Clin Infect Dis 1992;14:272.

Suh B, Lorber B: Quinolones. Med Clin North Am 1995;79:869.

Antimycobacterial Drugs

47

Henry F. Chambers, MD

Most antibiotics are more effective against rapidly growing organisms than against slowly growing ones. Because mycobacteria are very slowly growing organisms, they are relatively resistant to antibiotics. Mycobacterial cells can also be dormant and thus completely resistant to many drugs—or killed only very slowly by the few drugs that are active. The lipid-rich mycobacterial cell wall is impermeable to many agents. A substantial proportion of mycobacterial organisms are intracellular, residing within macrophages, and inaccessible to drugs that penetrate poorly. Finally, mycobacteria are notorious for their ability to develop resistance to any single drug. Combinations of drugs are required to overcome these obstacles and to prevent emergence of resistance during the course of therapy. The response of mycobacterial infections to chemotherapy is slow, and treatment must be administered for months to years depending on which drugs are used. The various drugs used to treat tuberculosis, which is caused by *Mycobacterium tuberculosis* and the closely related *M bovis,* atypical mycobacterial infections, and leprosy, which is caused by *M leprae,* are described in this chapter.

DRUGS USED IN TUBERCULOSIS

Isoniazid (INH), **rifampin, pyrazinamide, ethambutol,** and **streptomycin** are the five first-line agents for treatment of tuberculosis (Table 47–1). Isoniazid and rifampin are the two most active drugs. An isoniazid-rifampin combination administered for 9 months will cure 95–98% of cases of tuberculosis caused by susceptible strains. The addition of pyrazinamide to an isoniazid-rifampin combination for the first 2 months allows the total duration of therapy to be reduced to 6 months without loss of efficacy (Table 47–2). In practice, therapy is initiated with a four-drug regimen of isoniazid, rifampin, pyrazinamide, and either ethambutol or streptomycin until susceptibility of the clinical isolate has been determined. Neither ethambutol nor streptomycin adds substantially to the overall activity of the regimen (ie, the duration of treatment cannot be further reduced

if either drug is used), but they do provide additional coverage should the isolate prove to be resistant to isoniazid, rifampin, or both. Unfortunately, such resistance occurs in up to 10% of cases in the United States. Most patients with tuberculosis can be treated entirely as outpatients, with hospitalization being required only for those who are seriously ill or who require diagnostic evaluation.

ISONIAZID (INH)

Isoniazid is the most active drug for the treatment of tuberculosis caused by susceptible strains. It is a small (MW 137), simple molecule freely soluble in water. The structural similarity to pyridoxine is shown below.

Isoniazid

Pyridoxine

In vitro, isoniazid inhibits most tubercle bacilli in a concentration of 0.2 μg/mL or less and is bactericidal for actively growing tubercle bacilli. Isoniazid is less effective against atypical mycobacterial species. Isoniazid is able to penetrate into phagocytic cells and thus is active against both extracellular and intracellular organisms.

Mechanism of Action & Basis of Resistance

Isoniazid inhibits synthesis of mycolic acids, which are essential components of mycobacterial cell walls. Isoni-

Table 47–1. Antimicrobials used in the treatment of tuberculosis.

Drug	Typical Adult Dosage[1]
First-line agents (in approximate order of preference)	
Isoniazid	300 mg/d
Rifampin	600 mg/d
Pyrazinamide	25 mg/kg/d
Ethambutol	15–25 mg/kg/d
Streptomycin	15 mg/kg/d
Second-line agents	
Amikacin	15 mg/kg/d
Aminosalicylic acid	8–12 g/d
Capreomycin	15 mg/kg/d
Ciprofloxacin	1500 mg/d, divided
Clofazimine	200 mg/d
Cycloserine	500–1000 mg/d, divided
Ethionamide	500–750 mg/d
Levofloxacin	500 mg/d
Rifabutin	300 mg/d[2]
Rifapentine	600 mg once or twice weekly

[1]Assuming normal renal function.

[2]150 mg/d if used concurrently with a protease inhibitor.

azid is a prodrug that is activated by KatG, the mycobacterial catalase-peroxidase. The activated form of isoniazid exerts its lethal effect by forming a covalent complex with an acyl carrier protein (AcpM) and KasA, a beta-ketoacyl carrier protein synthetase, which blocks mycolic acid synthesis. Resistance to isoniazid has been associated with mutations resulting in overexpression of *inhA*, which encodes an NADH-dependent acyl carrier protein reductase; mutation or deletion of *katG*; promoter mutations resulting in overexpression of *ahpC*, a putative virulence gene involved in protection of the cell from oxidative stress; and mutations in *kasA*. Overproducers of *inhA* express low-level isoniazid resistance and cross-resistance to ethionamide. *KatG* mutants express high-level isoniazid resistance and are usually not cross-resistant to ethionamide.

Resistant mutants occur in susceptible mycobacterial populations with a frequency of about 1 bacillus in 10^6. Since tuberculous lesions often contain more than 10^8 tubercle bacilli, resistant mutants are readily selected out if isoniazid is given as the sole drug. However, addition of a second independently acting drug, to which resistance also emerges at a frequency of 1 in 10^6 to 1 in 10^8, is effective. The odds that a bacillus is resistant to both drugs are approximately 1 in $10^6 \times 10^6$, or 1 in 10^{12}, which is several orders of magnitude more than the number of infecting organisms. Single-drug therapy with isoniazid and failure to use isoniazid plus at least one other drug to which the infecting strain is susceptible (which is tantamount to single-drug therapy) has led to the 10–20% prevalence of isoniazid resistance in clinical isolates from the Caribbean and Southeast Asia. Currently, about 8–10% of primary clinical isolates in the United States are isoniazid-resistant.

Pharmacokinetics

Isoniazid is readily absorbed from the gastrointestinal tract. The administration of a 300-mg oral dose (5 mg/kg in children) results in peak plasma concentrations of 3–5 µg/mL within 1–2 hours. Isoniazid diffuses readily into all body fluids and tissues. The concentration in the central nervous system and cerebrospinal fluid ranges between 20% and 100% of simultaneous serum concentrations.

Metabolism of isoniazid, especially acetylation by liver N-acetyltransferase, is genetically determined (see Chapter 4). The average concentration of isoniazid in the plasma of rapid acetylators is about one third to one half of that in slow acetylators and average half-lives are less than 1 hour and 3 hours, respectively. Rapid acetylators were once thought to be more prone to hepatotoxicity, but this has not been proved. More rapid clearance of isoniazid by rapid acetylators is of no therapeutic consequence when appropriate doses are administered daily, but subtherapeutic concentrations may occur if drug is administered as a once-weekly dose.

Isoniazid metabolites and a small amount of unchanged drug are excreted mainly in the urine. The

Table 47–2. Recommended duration of therapy for tuberculosis.

Regimen (in Approximate Order of Preference)	Duration in Months
Isoniazid, rifampin, pyrazinamide	6
Isoniazid, rifampin	9
Rifampin, ethambutol, pyrazinamide	6
Rifampin, ethambutol	12
Isoniazid, ethambutol	18
All others	≥ 24

dose need not be adjusted in renal failure, but one third to one half of the normal dose is recommended in severe hepatic insufficiency.

Clinical Uses

The usual dosage of isoniazid is 5 mg/kg/d, with a typical adult dose being 300 mg given once daily. Up to 10 mg/kg/d may be used for serious infections or if malabsorption is a problem. A 15 mg/kg dose, or 900 mg, may be used in a twice-weekly dosing regimen in combination with a second antituberculous agent (eg, rifampin 600 mg). Pyridoxine, 25–50 mg/d is recommended for those with conditions predisposing to neuropathy, an adverse effect of isoniazid. Isoniazid is usually given by mouth but can be given parenterally in the same dosage.

Isoniazid as a single agent is also indicated for treatment of latent tuberculosis, which is usually determined by a positive tuberculin skin test. Isoniazid is routinely recommended for individuals who are at greatest risk for developing active disease after being infected such as very young children, persons who test positive within 2 years after a documented negative skin test (ie, recent converters), and immunocompromised individuals, especially HIV-infected and AIDS patients. Isoniazid is also indicated for prevention of tuberculosis in close contacts of active cases of pulmonary tuberculosis. The dosage is 300 mg/d (5 mg/kg/d) or 900 mg twice weekly for 9 months.

Adverse Reactions

The incidence and severity of untoward reactions to isoniazid are related to dosage and duration of administration.

A. Allergic Reactions

Fever and skin rashes are occasionally seen. Drug-induced systemic lupus erythematosus has been reported.

B. Direct Toxicity

Isoniazid-induced hepatitis is the most frequent major toxic effect. This is distinct from the minor increases in liver aminotransferases (up to three or four times normal) seen in 10–20% of patients, who usually are asymptomatic. Such increases do not require cessation of the drug. Clinical hepatitis with loss of appetite, nausea, vomiting, jaundice, and right upper quadrant pain occurs in 1% of isoniazid recipients and can be fatal, particularly if the drug is not discontinued promptly. There is histologic evidence of hepatocellular damage and necrosis. The risk of hepatitis depends on age. It occurs rarely under age 20, in 0.3% of those aged 21–35, 1.2% of those aged 36–50, and 2.3% for those aged 50 and above. The risk of hepatitis is greater in alcoholics and possibly during pregnancy and the postpartum period. Development of isoniazid hepatitis contraindicates further use of the drug.

Peripheral neuropathy is observed in 10–20% of patients given dosages greater than 5 mg/kg/d but is infrequently seen with the standard 300 mg adult dose. It is more likely to occur in slow acetylators and patients with predisposing conditions such as malnutrition, alcoholism, diabetes, AIDS, and uremia. Neuropathy is due to a relative pyridoxine deficiency. Isoniazid promotes excretion of pyridoxine, and this toxicity is readily reversed by administration of pyridoxine in a dosage as low as 10 mg/d. Central nervous system toxicity, which is less common, includes memory loss, psychosis, and seizures. These may also respond to pyridoxine.

Miscellaneous other reactions include hematologic abnormalities, provocation of pyridoxine deficiency anemia, tinnitus, and gastrointestinal discomfort. Isoniazid can reduce the metabolism of phenytoin, increasing its blood level and toxicity.

RIFAMPIN

Rifampin is a large (MW 823), complex semisynthetic derivative of rifamycin, an antibiotic produced by *Streptomyces mediterranei.* It is active in vitro against gram-positive and gram-negative cocci, some enteric bacteria, mycobacteria, and chlamydia. Susceptible organisms are inhibited by less than 1 μg/mL, but resistant mutants are present in all microbial populations at a frequency of approximately 1:10^6. Administration of rifampin as a single drug selects for these highly resistant organisms. There is no cross-resistance to other classes of antimicrobial drugs, but there is cross-resistance to other rifamycin derivatives, eg, rifabutin.

Antimycobacterial Activity, Resistance, & Pharmacokinetics

Rifampin binds strongly to the β subunit of bacterial DNA-dependent RNA polymerase and thereby inhibits RNA synthesis. Resistance results from one of several possible point mutations in *rpoB,* the gene for the beta subunit of RNA polymerase. These mutations prevent binding of rifampin to RNA polymerase. Human RNA polymerase does not bind rifampin and is not inhibited by it. Rifampin is bactericidal for mycobacteria. It readily penetrates most tissues and into phagocytic cells. It can kill organisms that are poorly accessible to many other drugs, such as intracellular organisms and those sequestered in abscesses and lung cavities.

Rifampin is well absorbed after oral administration and excreted mainly through the liver into bile. It then undergoes enterohepatic recirculation, with the bulk excreted as a deacylated metabolite in feces and a small amount in the urine. Dosage adjustment for renal insufficiency is not necessary. Usual doses result in serum levels of 5–7 μg/mL. Rifampin is distributed widely in body fluids and tissues. Rifampin is relatively highly protein-bound, but adequate cerebrospinal fluid concentrations are achieved only in the presence of meningeal inflammation.

Clinical Uses

A. MYCOBACTERIAL INFECTIONS

Rifampin, usually 600 mg/d (10 mg/kg/d) orally, is administered together with isoniazid, ethambutol, or another antituberculous drug in order to prevent emergence of drug-resistant mycobacteria. In some short-course therapies, 600 mg of rifampin is given twice weekly. Rifampin 600 mg daily or twice weekly for 6 months also is effective in some atypical mycobacterial infections and in leprosy when used together with a sulfone. Rifampin is an alternative to isoniazid prophylaxis for patients who are unable to take isoniazid or who have had close contact with a case of active tuberculosis caused by an isoniazid-resistant, rifampin-susceptible strain.

B. OTHER INDICATIONS

Rifampin is used in a variety of other clinical situations. An oral dosage of 600 mg twice daily for 2 days can eliminate meningococcal carriage. Rifampin, 20 mg/kg/d for 4 days, is used as prophylaxis in contacts of children with *Haemophilus influenzae* type b disease. Rifampin combined with a second agent is used to eradicate staphylococcal carriage. Rifampin combination therapy is also indicated for treatment of serious staphylococcal infections such as osteomyelitis and prosthetic valve endocarditis. Rifampin has been recommended also for use in combination with ceftriaxone or vancomycin in treatment of meningitis caused by highly penicillin-resistant strains of pneumococci.

Adverse Reactions

Rifampin imparts a harmless orange color to urine, sweat, tears, and contact lenses (soft lenses may be permanently stained). Occasional adverse effects include rashes, thrombocytopenia, and nephritis. It may cause cholestatic jaundice and occasionally hepatitis. Rifampin commonly causes light chain proteinuria. If administered less often than twice weekly, rifampin causes a flu-like syndrome characterized by fever, chills, myalgias, anemia, thrombocytopenia, and sometimes is associated with acute tubular necrosis. Rifampin strongly induces most cytochrome P450 isoforms (CYP1A2, CYP2C9, CYP2C19, CYP2D6, and CYP3A4), which increases the elimination of numerous other drugs including methadone, anticoagulants, some anticonvulsants, protease inhibitors, and contraceptives. Likewise, administration of rifampin with ketoconazole, cyclosporine, or chloramphenicol results in significantly lower serum levels of these drugs. Ketoconazole in turn may reduce rifampin serum concentrations by interfering with absorption.

ETHAMBUTOL

Ethambutol is a synthetic, water-soluble, heat-stable compound, the dextro- isomer of the structure shown below, dispensed as the dihydrochloride salt.

Ethambutol

Susceptible strains of *M tuberculosis* and other mycobacteria are inhibited in vitro by ethambutol, 1–5 μg/mL. Ethambutol is an inhibitor of mycobacterial arabinosyl transferases, which are encoded by the *embCAB* operon. Arabinosyl transferases are involved in the polymerization reaction of arabinoglycan, an essential component of the mycobacterial cell wall. Resistance to ethambutol is due to mutations resulting in overexpression of *emb* gene products or within the *embB* structural gene.

Ethambutol is well absorbed from the gut. Following ingestion of 25 mg/kg, a blood level peak of 2–5 μg/mL is reached in 2–4 hours. About 20% of the drug is excreted in feces and 50% in urine in unchanged form. Ethambutol accumulates in renal failure, and the dose should be reduced by half if creatinine clearance is less than 10 mL/min. Ethambutol crosses the blood-brain barrier only if the meninges are inflamed. Concentrations in cerebrospinal fluid are highly variable, ranging from 4% to 64% of serum levels in the setting of meningeal inflammation.

As with all antituberculous drugs, resistance to ethambutol emerges rapidly when the drug is used alone. Therefore, ethambutol is always given in combination with other antituberculous drugs.

Clinical Use

Ethambutol hydrochloride, 15–25 mg/kg, is usually given as a single daily dose in combination with isoniazid or rifampin. The higher dose is recommended for treatment of tuberculous meningitis. The dose of ethambutol is 50 mg/kg when a twice-weekly dosing schedule is used.

Adverse Reactions

Hypersensitivity to ethambutol is rare. The most common serious adverse event is retrobulbar neuritis causing loss of visual acuity and red-green color blindness. This dose-related side effect is more likely to occur at a dosage of 25 mg/kg/d continued for several months. With dosages of 15 mg/kg/d or less, visual disturbances are very rare. Periodic visual acuity testing is desirable if the 25 mg/kg/d dosage is used. Ethambutol is relatively contraindicated in children too young to permit assessment of visual acuity and red-green color discrimination.

PYRAZINAMIDE

Pyrazinamide (PZA) is a relative of nicotinamide, stable, slightly soluble in water, and quite inexpensive. At neutral pH, it is inactive in vitro, but at pH 5.5 it inhibits tubercle bacilli and some other mycobacteria at concentrations of approximately 20 μg/mL. Drug is taken up by macrophages and exerts its activity against intracellular organisms residing within this acidic environment.

Pyrazinamide is converted to pyrazinoic acid, the active form of the drug, by mycobacterial pyrazinamidase, which is encoded by *pncA*. The drug target and mechanism of action are unknown. Resistance is due to mutations in *pncA* that impair conversion of pyrazinamide to its active form. Impaired uptake of pyrazinamide may also contribute to resistance.

Pyrazinamide (PZA)

Clinical Use

Serum concentrations of 30–50 μg/mL at 1–2 hours after oral administration are achieved with dosages of 25 mg/kg/d. Pyrazinamide is well absorbed from the gastrointestinal tract and widely distributed in body tissues, including inflamed meninges. The half-life is 8–11 hours. A 50–70 mg/kg dose is used for twice-weekly or thrice-weekly treatment regimens. Pyrazinamide is an important front-line drug used in conjunction with isoniazid and rifampin in short-course (ie, 6-month) regimens as a "sterilizing" agent active against residual intracellular organisms that may cause relapse. Tubercle bacilli develop resistance to pyrazinamide fairly readily, but there is no cross-resistance with isoniazid or other antimycobacterial drugs.

Adverse Reactions

Major adverse effects of pyrazinamide include hepatotoxicity (in 1–5% of patients), nausea, vomiting, drug fever, and hyperuricemia. The latter occurs uniformly and is not a reason to halt therapy. Hyperuricemia may provoke acute gouty arthritis.

STREPTOMYCIN

The mechanism of action and other pharmacologic features of streptomycin have been discussed in Chapter 45. Most tubercle bacilli are inhibited by streptomycin, 1–10 μg/mL, in vitro. Nontuberculosis species of mycobacteria other than *Mycobacterium avium* complex (MAC) and *Mycobacterium kansasii* are resistant. All large populations of tubercle bacilli contain some streptomycin-resistant mutants. On average, 1 in 10^8 tubercle bacilli can be expected to be resistant to streptomycin at levels of 10–100 μg/mL. Resistance is due to a point mutation in either the *rpsL* gene encoding the S12 ribosomal protein gene or *rrs,* encoding 16S ribosomal rRNA, that alters the ribosomal binding site.

Streptomycin penetrates into cells poorly, and consequently it is active mainly against extracellular tubercle bacilli. Additional drugs are needed to eliminate intracellular organisms, which constitute a significant proportion of the total mycobacterial burden. Streptomycin crosses the blood-brain barrier and achieves therapeutic concentrations with inflamed meninges.

Clinical Use in Tuberculosis

Streptomycin sulfate remains an important drug in the treatment of tuberculosis. It is employed when an injectable drug is needed or desirable, principally in individuals with severe, possibly life-threatening forms of tuberculosis, eg, meningitis and disseminated disease, and in treatment of infections resistant to other drugs. The usual dosage is 15 mg/kg/d intramuscularly or intravenously daily for adults (20–40 mg/kg/d, not to exceed 1–1.5 g, for children) for several weeks, followed by 1–1.5 g two or three times weekly for several months. Serum concentrations of approximately 40 μg/mL are achieved 30–60 minutes after intramuscular injection of a 15 mg/kg dose. Other drugs are always given simultaneously to prevent emergence of resistance.

Adverse Reactions

Streptomycin is ototoxic and nephrotoxic. Vertigo and hearing loss are the most common side effects and may be permanent. Toxicity is dose-related, and the risk is increased in the elderly. As with all aminoglycosides, the dose must be adjusted according to renal function (see Chapter 45). Toxicity can be reduced by limiting therapy to no more than 6 months whenever possible.

ALTERNATIVE SECOND-LINE DRUGS FOR TUBERCULOSIS

The alternative drugs listed below are usually considered only (1) in the case of resistance to the drugs of first choice (which occurs with increasing frequency); (2) in case of failure of clinical response to conventional therapy; and (3) when expert guidance is available to deal with the toxic effects. For many of the second-line drugs listed below, the dosage, emergence of resistance, and long-term toxicity have not been fully established.

Ethionamide

Ethionamide is chemically related to isoniazid and also blocks the synthesis of mycolic acids. It is poorly water soluble and available only in oral form. It is metabolized by the liver.

Ethionamide

Most tubercle bacilli are inhibited in vitro by ethionamide, 2.5 μg/mL, or less. Some other species of mycobacteria also are inhibited by ethionamide, 10 μg/mL. Serum concentrations in plasma and tissues of approximately 20 μg/mL are achieved by a dosage of 1 g/d. Cerebrospinal fluid concentrations are equal to those in serum. A 1 g/d dosage, although effective in the treatment of tuberculosis, is poorly tolerated because of the intense gastric irritation and neurologic symptoms that commonly occur. Ethionamide is also hepatotoxic. Neurologic symptoms may be alleviated by pyridoxine.

Ethionamide is administered at an initial dosage of 250 mg once daily, which is increased in 250 mg increments to the recommended dosage of 1 g/d (or 15 mg/kg/d) if possible. The 1 g/d dosage, although theoretically desirable, is seldom tolerated, and one often must settle for a total daily dose of 500–750 mg.

Resistance to ethionamide as a single agent develops rapidly in vitro and in vivo. There can be low-level cross-resistance between isoniazid and ethionamide.

Capreomycin

Capreomycin is a peptide protein synthesis inhibitor antibiotic obtained from *Streptomyces capreolus*. Daily injection of 1 g intramuscularly results in blood levels of 10 μg/mL or more. Such concentrations in vitro are inhibitory for many mycobacteria, including multidrug-resistant strains of *M tuberculosis*.

Capreomycin (15 mg/kg/d) is an important injectable agent for treatment of drug-resistant tuberculosis. Strains of *M tuberculosis* that are resistant to streptomycin or amikacin (eg, the multidrug-resistant W strain) usually are susceptible to capreomycin. Resistance to capreomycin, when it occurs, may be due to an *rrs* mutation.

Capreomycin is nephrotoxic and ototoxic. Tinnitus, deafness, and vestibular disturbances occur. The injection causes significant local pain, and sterile abscesses may occur.

Dosing of capreomycin is the same as streptomycin. Toxicity is reduced if 1 g is given two or three times weekly after an initial response has been achieved with a daily dosing schedule.

Cycloserine

Cycloserine is an inhibitor of cell wall synthesis and is discussed in Chapter 43. Concentrations of 15–20 μg/mL inhibit many strains of *M tuberculosis*. The dosage of cycloserine in tuberculosis is 0.5–1 g/d in two divided doses. Cycloserine is cleared renally, and the dose should be reduced by half if creatinine clearance is less than 50 mL/min.

The most serious toxic effects are peripheral neuropathy and central nervous system dysfunction, including depression and psychotic reactions. Pyridoxine 150 mg/d should be given with cycloserine as this ameliorates neurologic toxicity. Adverse effects, which are most common during the first 2 weeks of therapy, occur in 25% or more of patients, especially at higher doses. Side effects can be minimized by monitoring peak serum concentrations. The peak concentration is reached 2–4 hours after dosing. The recommended range of peak concentrations is 20–40 μg/mL.

Aminosalicylic Acid (PAS)

Aminosalicylic acid is a folate synthesis antagonist that is active almost exclusively against *M tuberculosis*. It is structurally similar to *p*-aminobenzoic aid (PABA) and to the sulfonamides (see Chapter 46).

Aminosalicylic acid (PAS)

Tubercle bacilli are usually inhibited in vitro by aminosalicylic acid, 1–5 μg/mL. Aminosalicylic acid is readily absorbed from the gastrointestinal tract. Serum levels are 50 μg/mL or more after a 4 g oral dose. The dosage is 8–12 g/d orally for adults and 300 mg/kg/d for children. The drug is widely distributed in tissues and body fluids except the cerebrospinal fluid. Aminosalicylic acid is rapidly excreted in the urine, in part as active aminosalicylic acid and in part as the acetylated compound and other metabolic products. Very high concentrations of aminosalicylic acid are reached in the urine, which can result in crystalluria.

Aminosalicylic acid, formerly a first-line agent for treatment of tuberculosis, is used infrequently now because other oral drugs are better-tolerated. Gastrointestinal symptoms often accompany full doses of aminosalicylic acid. Anorexia, nausea, diarrhea, and epigastric pain and burning may be diminished by giving aminosalicylic acid with meals and with antacids. Peptic ulceration and hemorrhage may occur. Hypersensitivity reactions manifested by fever, joint pains, skin rashes, hepatosplenomegaly, hepatitis, adenopathy, and granulocytopenia, often occur after 3–8 weeks of aminosalicylic acid therapy, making it necessary to stop aminosalicylic acid administration temporarily or permanently.

Kanamycin & Amikacin

The aminoglycoside antibiotics are discussed in Chapter 45. Kanamycin has been used for treatment of tuberculosis caused by streptomycin-resistant strains, but the availability of less toxic alternatives (eg, capreomycin and amikacin) have rendered it obsolete.

The role of amikacin in treatment of tuberculosis has increased with the increasing incidence and prevalence of multidrug-resistant tuberculosis. Prevalence of amikacin-resistant strains is low (less than 5%), and most multidrug-resistant strains remain amikacin-susceptible. *M tuberculosis* is inhibited at concentrations of 1 μg/mL or less. Amikacin is also active against atypical mycobacteria. There is no cross-resistance between streptomycin and amikacin, but kanamycin resistance often indicates resistance to amikacin as well. Serum concentrations of 30–50 μg/mL are achieved 30–60 minutes after a 15 mg/kg intravenous infusion. Amikacin is indicated for treatment of tuberculosis suspected or known to be caused by streptomycin-resistant or multidrug-resistant strains. Amikacin must be used in combination with at least one and preferably two or three other drugs to which the isolate is susceptible for treatment of drug-resistant cases. The recommended dosage is 15 mg/kg/d intramuscularly or intravenously daily for 5 days a week for the first 2 months of therapy and then 1–1.5 g two or three times weekly to complete a 6-month course.

Ciprofloxacin & Levofloxacin

These drugs are discussed in Chapter 46. In addition to their activity against many gram-positive and gram-negative bacteria, ciprofloxacin and levofloxacin inhibit strains of *M tuberculosis* at concentrations less than 2 μg/mL. They are also active against atypical mycobacteria. Ofloxacin was used in the past, but levofloxacin is preferred because it is the L-isomer of ofloxacin (a racemic mixture of D- and L-stereoisomers), the active antibacterial component of ofloxacin, and it can be administered once daily. Levofloxacin tends to be slightly more active in vitro than ciprofloxacin against *M tuberculosis;* ciprofloxacin is slightly more active against atypical mycobacteria. Serum concentrations of 2–4 μg/mL and 4–8 μg/mL are achieved with standard oral doses of ciprofloxacin and levofloxacin, respectively.

Fluoroquinolones are an important recent addition to the drugs available for tuberculosis, especially for strains that are resistant to first-line agents. Resistance, which may result from any one of several single point mutations in the gyrase A subunit, develops rapidly if a fluoroquinolone is used as a single agent; thus, the drug must be used in combination with two or more other active agents. The standard dosage of ciprofloxacin is 750 mg orally twice a day. That of levofloxacin is 500–750 mg as a single daily dose.

Rifabutin (Ansamycin)

This antibiotic is derived from rifamycin and is related to rifampin. It has significant activity against *M tuberculosis, M avium-intracellulare* and *M fortuitum* (see below). Its activity is similar to that of rifampin, and cross-resistance with rifampin is virtually complete. Some rifampin-resistant strains may appear susceptible to rifabutin in vitro, but a clinical response is unlikely because the molecular basis of resistance, *rpoB* mutation, is the same. Rifabutin is both substrate and inducer of cytochrome P450 enzymes. Because it is a less potent inducer, rifabutin is indicated in place of rifampin for treatment of tuberculosis in HIV-infected patients who are receiving concurrent antiretroviral therapy with a protease inhibitor or nonnucleoside reverse transcriptase inhibitor (eg, efavirenz)—drugs which also are cytochrome P450 substrates. The usual dose of rifabutin is 300 mg/d unless the patient is receiving a protease inhibitor, in which case the dose should be reduced to 150 mg/d. If efavirenz (also a P450 inducer) is used, the recommended dose of rifabutin is 450 mg/d. (See Havlir 1999, and Centers 1998, for details.)

Rifabutin is effective in prevention and treatment of disseminated atypical mycobacterial infection in AIDS patients with CD4 counts below 50/μL. It is also effective for preventive therapy of tuberculosis, either alone in a 6-month regimen or with pyrazinamide in a 2-month regimen.

Rifapentine

Rifapentine is an analog of rifampin. It is active against both *M tuberculosis* and *M avium*. As with all rifamycins, it is a bacterial RNA polymerase inhibitor, and cross-resistance between rifampin and rifapentine is complete. Like rifampin, rifapentine is a potent inducer of cytochrome P450 enzymes, and it has the same drug interaction profile. Toxicity is similar to that of rifampin. Rifapentine and its microbiologically active metabolite, 25-desacetylrifapentine, have an elimination half-life of 13 hours. Rifapentine is indicated for treatment of tuberculosis caused by rifampin-susceptible strains. The dose is 600 mg once or twice weekly. Whether rifapentine is as effective as rifampin has not been established, and rifampin therefore remains the rifamycin of choice for treatment of tuberculosis.

DRUGS ACTIVE AGAINST ATYPICAL MYCOBACTERIA

About 10% of mycobacterial infections seen in clinical practice in the USA are caused not by *M tuberculosis* or *M leprae* but by nontuberculous or so-called "atypical" mycobacteria. These organisms have distinctive laboratory characteristics, occur in the environment, and are not communicable from person to person. Disease caused by these organisms is often less severe than tuberculosis. As a general rule, these mycobacterial species are less susceptible than *M tuberculosis* to antituberculous drugs. On the other hand, agents such as erythromycin, sulfonamides, or tetracycline, which are not effective against *M tuberculosis,* may be effective against atypical strains. Emergence of resistance during therapy is also a problem with these mycobacterial species, and active infection should be treated with combinations of drugs. *M kansasii* is susceptible to rifampin and ethambutol but relatively resistant to isoniazid and completely resistant to pyrazinamide. A three-drug combination of isoniazid, rifampin, and ethambutol is the conventional treatment for *M kansasii* infection. A few representative pathogens, with the clinical presentation and the drugs to which they are often susceptible, are given in Table 47–3.

M avium complex (MAC), which includes both *M avium* and *M intracellulare,* is an important and common cause of disseminated disease in late stages of AIDS (CD4 counts < 50/μL). *Mycobacterium avium* complex is much less susceptible than *M tuberculosis* to most antituberculous drugs. Combinations of agents are required to suppress the disease. Disseminated MAC is incurable and therapy is life-long if CD4 counts are below 200/μL. The need for multidrug therapy frequently leads to side effects that can be difficult to man-

Table 47–3. Clinical features and treatment options for infections with atypical mycobacteria.

Species	Clinical Features	Treatment Options
M kansasii	Resembles tuberculosis	Ciprofloxacin, clarithromycin, ethambutol, isoniazid, rifampin, trimethoprim-sulfamethoxazole
M marinum	Granulomatous cutaneous disease	Amikacin, clarithromycin, ethambutol, doxycycline, minocycline, rifampin, trimethoprim-sulfamethoxazole
M scrofulaceum	Cervical adenitis in children	Amikacin, erythromycin (or other macrolide), rifampin, streptomycin. (Surgical excision is often curative and the treatment of choice.)
M avium complex	Pulmonary disease in patients with chronic lung disease; disseminated infection in AIDS	Amikacin, azithromycin, clarithromycin, ciprofloxacin, ethambutol, ethionamide, rifabutin
M chelonae	Abscess, sinus tract, ulcer; bone, joint, tendon infection	Amikacin, doxycycline, imipenem, macrolides, tobramycin
M fortuitum	Abscess, sinus tract, ulcer; bone, joint, tendon infection	Amikacin, cefoxitin, ciprofloxacin, doxycycline, ofloxacin, trimethoprim-sulfamethoxazole
M ulcerans	Skin ulcers	Isoniazid, streptomycin, rifampin, minocycline. (Surgical excision may be effective.)

age. Azithromycin, 500 mg once daily, or clarithromycin, 500 mg twice daily, plus ethambutol, 15 mg/kg/d, is an effective and well-tolerated regimen for treatment of disseminated disease. Some authorities recommend use of a third agent, such as ciprofloxacin 750 mg twice daily or rifabutin, 300 mg once daily. Other agents that may be useful are listed in Table 47–3. Rifabutin in a single daily dose of 300 mg has been shown to reduce the incidence of *M avium* complex bacteremia in AIDS patients with CD4 < 200/μL but may not offer a survival advantage. Clarithromycin also effectively prevents MAC bacteremia in AIDS patients, but if breakthrough bacteremia occurs, the isolate often is resistant to both clarithromycin and azithromycin, precluding the use of the most effective drugs for treatment.

DRUGS USED IN LEPROSY

Mycobacterium leprae has never been grown in vitro, but animal models, such as growth in injected mouse footpads, have permitted laboratory evaluation of drugs. Only those drugs that have the widest clinical use are presented here. Because of increasing reports of dapsone resistance, treatment of leprosy with combinations of the drugs listed below is recommended.

DAPSONE & OTHER SULFONES

Several drugs closely related to the sulfonamides have been used effectively in the long-term treatment of leprosy. The most widely used is dapsone (diaminodiphenylsulfone). Like the sulfonamides, it inhibits folate synthesis. Resistance can emerge in large populations of *M leprae,* eg, in lepromatous leprosy, if very low doses are given. Therefore, the combination of dapsone, rifampin, and clofazimine is recommended for initial therapy. Dapsone may also be used to prevent and treat *Pneumocystis jiroveci* pneumonia in AIDS.

Dapsone

Sulfones are well absorbed from the gut and widely distributed throughout body fluids and tissues. Dapsone's half-life is 1–2 days, and drug tends to be retained in skin, muscle, liver, and kidney. Skin heavily infected with *M leprae* may contain several times as much of the drug as normal skin. Sulfones are excreted into bile and reabsorbed in the intestine. Excretion into urine is variable, and most excreted drug is acetylated. In renal failure, the dose may have to be adjusted. The usual adult dosage in leprosy is 100 mg daily. For children, the dose is proportionately less depending on weight.

Dapsone is usually well tolerated. Many patients develop some hemolysis, particularly if they have glucose-6-phosphate dehydrogenase deficiency. Methemoglobinemia is common, but usually is not a problem clinically. Gastrointestinal intolerance, fever, pruritus, and various rashes occur. During dapsone therapy of lepromatous leprosy, erythema nodosum leprosum often develops. It is sometimes difficult to distinguish reactions to dapsone from manifestations of the underlying illness. Erythema nodosum leprosum may be suppressed by **corticosteroids** or by **thalidomide.**

RIFAMPIN

This drug (see above) in a dosage of 600 mg daily can be strikingly effective in lepromatous leprosy. Because of the probable risk of emergence of rifampin-resistant *M leprae,* the drug is given in combination with dapsone or another antileprosy drug. A single monthly dose of 600 mg may be beneficial in combination therapy.

CLOFAZIMINE

Clofazimine is a phenazine dye that can be used as an alternative to dapsone. Its mechanism of action is unknown but may involve DNA binding.

Absorption of clofazimine from the gut is variable, and a major portion of the drug is excreted in feces. Clofazimine is stored widely in reticuloendothelial tissues and skin, and its crystals can be seen inside phagocytic reticuloendothelial cells. It is slowly released, so that the serum half-life may be 2 months.

Clofazimine is given for sulfone-resistant leprosy or when patients are intolerant to sulfone. A common dosage is 100 mg/d orally. The most prominent untoward effect is skin discoloration ranging from red-brown to nearly black. Gastrointestinal intolerance occurs occasionally.

PREPARATIONS AVAILABLE

DRUGS USED IN TUBERCULOSIS
Aminosalicylate sodium (Paser)
Oral: 4 g delayed release granules
Capreomycin (Capastat Sulfate)
Parenteral: 1 g powder to reconstitute for injection
Cycloserine (Seromycin Pulvules)
Oral: 250 mg capsules
Ethambutol (Myambutol)
Oral: 100, 400 mg tablets
Ethionamide (Trecator-SC)
Oral: 250 mg tablets
Isoniazid (generic)
Oral: 50, 100, 300 mg tablets; syrup, 50 mg/5 mL
Parenteral: 100 mg/mL for injection
Pyrazinamide (generic)
Oral: 500 mg tablets

Rifabutin (Mycobutin)
Oral: 150 mg capsules
Rifampin (generic, Rifadin, Rimactane)
Oral: 150, 300 mg capsules
Parenteral: 600 mg powder for IV injection
Rifapentine (Priftin)
Oral: 150 mg tablets
Streptomycin (generic)
Parenteral: 1 g lyophilized for IM injection

DRUGS USED IN LEPROSY
Clofazimine (Lamprene)
Oral: 50 mg capsules
Dapsone (generic)
Oral: 25, 100 mg tablets

REFERENCES

Bannerjee A et al: *inhA*, a gene encoding a target for isoniazid and ethionamide in *Mycobacterium tuberculosis*. Science 1994; 263:227.

Bass JB et al: Treatment of tuberculosis and tuberculosis infection in adults and children. Am J Crit Care Med 1994;149:1359.

Centers for Disease Control and Prevention. Prevention and treatment of tuberculosis in patients infected with human immunodeficiency virus: Principles of therapy and revised recommendations. MMWR Morb Mortal Wkly Rep 1998;47 (RR-20):1.

Diagnosis and treatment of disease caused by nontuberculous mycobacteria. Am J Respir Crit Care Med 1997;156(2 Part 2):S1.

Ellard GA: Chemotherapy of leprosy. Br Med Bull 1988;44:775.

Goble M et al: Treatment of 171 patients with pulmonary tuberculosis resistant to isoniazid and rifampin. N Engl J Med 1993;328:527.

Havlir DV, Barnes PF: Tuberculosis in patients with human immunodeficiency virus infection. N Engl J Med 1999; 340:367.

Horsburgh CR: *Mycobacterium avium* complex in AIDS. N Engl J Med 1991;324:1332.

Iseman MD: Treatment of multidrug-resistant tuberculosis. N Engl J Med 1993;329:784.

Jacobs RF et al: Intensive short course chemotherapy for tuberculous meningitis. Ped Infect Dis J 1992;11:194.

Jasmer RM, Nahid P, Hopewell PC: Latent tuberculosis infection. N Engl J Med 2002;347:1860.

Mdluli K et al: Inhibition of a *Mycobacterium tuberculosis* beta-ketoacyl ACP synthase by isoniazid. Science 1998;280:1607.

Morris S et al: Molecular mechanisms of multiple drug resistance in clinical isolates of *Mycobacterium tuberculosis*. J Infect Dis 1995;171:954.

Rapp RP et al: New macrolide antibiotics: Usefulness in infections caused by mycobacteria other than *Mycobacterium tuberculosis*. Ann Pharmacother 1994;28:1255.

Rifapentine—a long acting rifamycin for tuberculosis. Med Lett Drugs Ther 1999;41:21.

Sauret J et al: Treatment of pulmonary disease caused by *Mycobacterium kansasii*: Results of 18 versus 12 months chemotherapy. Tuber Lung Dis 1995;76:104.

Scorpio A, Zhang Y: Mutations in *pncA*, a gene encoding pyrazinamidase/nicotinamidase, cause resistance to the antituberculous drug pyrazinamide in tubercle bacillus. Nat Med 1996;2:662.

Sherman DR et al: Compensatory *ahpC* gene expression in isoniazid-resistant *Mycobacterium tuberculosis*. Science 1996; 272:1641.

Targeted tuberculin testing and treatment of latent tuberculosis infection. Am J Respir Crit Care Med 2000;161(4 Part 2):S221.

Telenti A et al: The *emb* operon, a gene cluster of *Mycobacterium tuberculosis* involved in resistance to ethambutol. Nat Med 1997;3:567.

Zhang Y et al: The catalase-peroxidase gene and isoniazid resistance of *Mycobacterium tuberculosis*. Nature 1992;358:591.

Antifungal Agents

48

Don Sheppard, MD, & Harry W. Lampiris, MD

Human fungal infections have increased dramatically in incidence and severity in recent years, due mainly to advances in surgery, cancer treatment, and critical care accompanied by increases in the use of broad-spectrum antimicrobials and the HIV epidemic. These changes have resulted in increased numbers of patients at risk for fungal infections.

Pharmacotherapy of fungal disease has been revolutionized by the introduction of the relatively nontoxic oral azole drugs and the echinocandins. Combination therapy is being reconsidered, and new formulations of old agents are becoming available. Unfortunately, the appearance of azole-resistant organisms, as well as the rise in the number of patients at risk for mycotic infections, has created new challenges

The antifungal drugs presently available fall into several categories: systemic drugs (oral or parenteral) for systemic infections, oral drugs for mucocutaneous infections, and topical drugs for mucocutaneous infections.

SYSTEMIC ANTIFUNGAL DRUGS FOR SYSTEMIC INFECTIONS

AMPHOTERICIN B

Amphotericin A and B are antifungal antibiotics produced by *Streptomyces nodosus*. Amphotericin A is not in clinical use.

Chemistry

Amphotericin B is an amphoteric polyene macrolide (polyene = containing many double bonds; macrolide = containing a large lactone ring of 12 or more atoms). It is nearly insoluble in water, and is therefore prepared as a colloidal suspension of amphotericin B and sodium desoxycholate for intravenous injection. Several new formulations have been developed in which amphotericin B is packaged in a lipid-associated delivery system (see Table 48–1 and Box, Liposomal Amphotericin B).

Pharmacokinetics

Amphotericin B is poorly absorbed from the gastrointestinal tract. Oral amphotericin B is thus effective only on fungi within the lumen of the tract and cannot be used for treatment of systemic disease. The intravenous injection of 0.6 mg/kg/d of amphotericin B results in average blood levels of 0.3–1 µg/mL; the drug is more than 90% bound by serum proteins. While it is mostly metabolized, some amphotericin B is excreted slowly in the urine over a period of several days. The serum $t_{1/2}$ is approximately 15 days. Hepatic impairment, renal impairment, and dialysis have little impact on drug concentrations and therefore no dose adjustment is required. The drug is widely distributed in most tissues, but only 2–3% of the blood level is reached in cerebrospinal fluid, thus occasionally necessitating intrathecal therapy for certain types of fungal meningitis.

Amphotericin B

792

LIPOSOMAL AMPHOTERICIN B

Therapy with amphotericin B is often limited by toxicity, especially drug-induced renal impairment. This has led to the development of lipid drug formulations on the assumption that lipid-packaged drug will bind to the mammalian membrane less readily, permitting the use of effective doses of the drug with lower toxicity. Liposomal amphotericin preparations package the active drug in lipid delivery vehicles, in contrast to the colloidal suspensions currently in use. Amphotericin binds to the lipids in these vehicles with an affinity between that for fungal ergosterol and that for human cholesterol. The lipid vehicle then serves as an amphotericin reservoir, reducing nonspecific binding to human cell membranes. This preferential binding allows for a reduction of toxicity without sacrificing efficacy and permits use of larger doses. Furthermore, some fungi contain lipases that may liberate free amphotericin B directly at the site of infection.

Three such formulations are now available and have differing pharmacologic properties as summarized in Table 48–1. While clinical trials have demonstrated different renal and infusion-related toxicities for these preparations compared with regular amphotericin B, there are no trials comparing the different formulations with each other. Limited studies have suggested at best a moderate improvement in the clinical efficacy of the lipid formulations compared to conventional amphotericin B. Because the lipid preparations are much more expensive, their use is usually restricted to patients intolerant to, or not responding to, conventional amphotericin treatment.

Mechanism of Action

Amphotericin B is selective in its fungicidal effect because it exploits the difference in lipid composition of fungal and mammalian cell membranes. **Ergosterol,** a cell membrane sterol, is found in the cell membrane of fungi, whereas the predominant sterol of bacteria and human cells is **cholesterol.** Amphotericin B binds to ergosterol and alters the permeability of the cell by forming amphotericin B-associated pores in the cell membrane. As suggested by its chemistry, amphotericin B combines avidly with lipids (ergosterol) along the double bond-rich side of its structure and associates with water molecules along the hydroxyl-rich side. This amphipathic characteristic facilitates pore formation by multiple amphotericin molecules, with the lipophilic portions around the outside of the pore and the hydrophilic regions lining the inside. The pore allows the leakage of intracellular ions and macromolecules, eventually leading to cell death. Some binding to human membrane sterols does occur, probably accounting for the drug's prominent toxicity.

Resistance to amphotericin B occurs if ergosterol binding is impaired, either by decreasing the membrane concentration of ergosterol or by modifying the sterol target molecule to reduce its affinity for the drug.

Adverse Effects

The toxicity of amphotericin B can be divided into two broad categories: immediate reactions, related to the infusion of the drug, and those occurring more slowly.

Table 48–1. Properties of conventional amphotericin B and some lipid formulations.[1]

Drug	Physical Form	Dosing (mg/kg/d)	C_{max}	Clearance	Nephro-toxicity	Infusional Toxicity	Daily Cost
Conventional formulation							
Fungizone	Micelles	1	--	--	--	--	24
Lipid formulations							
AmBisome	Spheres	3–5	↑	↓	↓	↓	1300
Amphotec	Disks	5	↓	↑	↓	↑(?)	660
Abelcet	Ribbons	5	↓	↑	↓	↓(?)	570

[1]Changes in C_{max} (peak plasma concentration), clearance, nephrotoxicity, and infusional toxicity are relative to conventional amphotericin B.

A. Infusion-Related Toxicity

These reactions are nearly universal and consist of fever, chills, muscle spasms, vomiting, headache, and hypotension. They can be ameliorated by slowing the infusion rate or decreasing the daily dose. Premedication with antipyretics, antihistamines, meperidine, or corticosteroids can be helpful. When starting therapy, many clinicians administer a test dose of 1 mg intravenously to gauge the severity of the reaction. This can serve as a guide to an initial dosing regimen and premedication strategy.

B. Slower Toxicity

Renal damage is the most significant toxic reaction. Renal impairment occurs in nearly all patients treated with clinically significant doses of amphotericin. The degree of azotemia is variable and often stabilizes during therapy, but can be serious enough to necessitate dialysis. A reversible component is associated with decreased renal perfusion and represents a form of prerenal renal failure. An irreversible component results from renal tubular injury and subsequent dysfunction. The irreversible form of amphotericin nephrotoxicity usually occurs in the setting of prolonged administration (> 4 g cumulative dose). Renal toxicity commonly presents with renal tubular acidosis and severe potassium and magnesium wasting. There is some evidence that the prerenal component can be attenuated with sodium loading, and it is common practice to administer normal saline infusions with the daily doses of amphotericin B.

Abnormalities of liver function tests are occasionally seen, as is a varying degree of anemia due to reduced erythropoietin production by damaged renal tubular cells. After intrathecal therapy with amphotericin, seizures and a chemical arachnoiditis may develop, often with serious neurologic sequelae.

Antifungal Activity

Amphotericin B remains the antifungal agent with the broadest spectrum of action. It has activity against the clinically significant yeasts, including *Candida albicans* and *Cryptococcus neoformans;* the organisms causing endemic mycoses, including *Histoplasma capsulatum, Blastomyces dermatitidis,* and *Coccidioides immitis;* and the pathogenic molds, such as *Aspergillus fumigatus* and mucor. Some fungal organisms such as *Candida lusitaniae* and *Pseudallescheria boydii* display intrinsic amphotericin B resistance.

Clinical Use

Owing to its broad spectrum of activity and fungicidal action, amphotericin B remains the drug of choice for nearly all life-threatening mycotic infections. It is often used as the initial induction regimen for serious fungal infections and is then replaced by one of the newer azole drugs (described below) for chronic therapy or prevention of relapse. Such induction therapy is especially important for immunosuppressed patients and those with severe fungal pneumonia, cryptococcal meningitis with altered mental status, or sepsis syndrome due to fungal infection. Once a clinical response has been elicited, these patients will then often continue maintenance therapy with an azole; therapy may be lifelong in patients at high risk for disease relapse. Amphotericin has also been used as empiric therapy for selected patients in whom the risks of leaving a systemic fungal infection untreated are high. The most common such patient is the cancer patient with neutropenia who remains febrile on broad-spectrum antibiotics.

For treatment of systemic fungal disease, amphotericin B is given by slow intravenous infusion at a dosage of 0.5–1 mg/kg/d. It is usually continued to a defined total dose (eg, 1–2 g), rather than a defined time span, as used with other antimicrobial drugs.

Intrathecal therapy for fungal meningitis is poorly tolerated and fraught with difficulties related to maintaining cerebrospinal fluid access. Thus, intrathecal therapy with amphotericin B is being increasingly supplanted by other therapies but remains an option in cases of fungal central nervous system infections that have not responded to other agents.

Local administration of amphotericin B has been used with success. Mycotic corneal ulcers and keratitis can be cured with topical drops as well as by direct subconjunctival injection. Fungal arthritis has been treated with adjunctive local injection directly into the joint. Candiduria responds to bladder irrigation with amphotericin B, and this route has been shown to produce no significant systemic toxicity.

FLUCYTOSINE

Flucytosine (5-FC) was discovered in 1957 during a search for novel antineoplastic agents. While devoid of anticancer properties, it became apparent that it was a potent antifungal agent. Flucytosine is a water-soluble pyrimidine analog related to the chemotherapeutic agent fluorouracil (5-FU). Its spectrum of action is much narrower than that of amphotericin B.

Flucytosine

Pharmacokinetics

Flucytosine is currently available in North America only in an oral formulation. The dosage is 100–150 mg/kg/d in patients with normal renal function. It is well (> 90%) absorbed, with serum concentrations peaking 1–2 hours after an oral dose. It is poorly protein-bound and penetrates well into all body fluid compartments, including the cerebrospinal fluid. It is eliminated by glomerular filtration with a half-life of 3–4 hours and is removed by hemodialysis. Levels rise rapidly with renal impairment and can lead to toxicity. Toxicity is more likely to occur in AIDS patients and in the presence of renal insufficiency. Peak serum concentrations should be measured periodically in patients with renal insufficiency and maintained between 50 and 100 µg/mL.

Mechanism of Action

Flucytosine is taken up by fungal cells via the enzyme cytosine permease. It is converted intracellularly first to 5-FU and then to 5-fluorodeoxyuridine monophosphate (F-dUMP) and fluorouridine triphosphate (FUTP), which inhibit DNA and RNA synthesis, respectively. Human cells are unable to convert the parent drug to its active metabolites.

Synergy with amphotericin B has been demonstrated in vitro and in vivo. It may be related to enhanced penetration of the flucytosine through amphotericin-damaged fungal cell membranes. In vitro synergy with azole drugs has also been seen, although the mechanism is unclear.

Resistance is thought to be mediated through altered metabolism of flucytosine, and, while uncommon in primary isolates, it develops rapidly in the course of flucytosine monotherapy.

Adverse Effects

The adverse effects of flucytosine result from metabolism (possibly by intestinal flora) to the toxic antineoplastic compound fluorouracil. Bone marrow toxicity with anemia, leukopenia, and thrombocytopenia are the most common adverse effects, with derangement of liver enzymes occurring less frequently. A form of toxic enterocolitis can occur. There seems to be a narrow therapeutic window, with an increased risk of toxicity at higher drug levels and resistance developing rapidly at subtherapeutic concentrations. The use of drug concentration measurements may be helpful in reducing the incidence of toxic reactions, especially when flucytosine is combined with nephrotoxic agents such as amphotericin B.

Clinical Use

The spectrum of activity of flucytosine is restricted to *Cryptococcus neoformans,* some candida species, and the dematiaceous molds that cause chromoblastomycosis. Flucytosine is not used as a single agent because of its demonstrated synergy with other agents and to avoid the development of secondary resistance. Clinical use at present is confined to combination therapy, either with amphotericin B for cryptococcal meningitis or with itraconazole for chromoblastomycosis.

AZOLES

Azoles are synthetic compounds that can be classified as either imidazoles or triazoles according to the number of nitrogen atoms in the five-membered azole ring as indicated below. The imidazoles consist of ketoconazole, miconazole, and clotrimazole (Figure 48–1). The latter two drugs are now used only in topical therapy. The triazoles include itraconazole, fluconazole, and voriconazole.

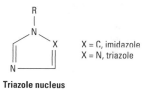

X = C, imidazole
X = N, triazole

Triazole nucleus

Pharmacology

The pharmacology of each of the azoles is unique and accounts for some of the variations in clinical use. Table 48–2 summarizes the differences among four of the azoles.

Mechanism of Action

The antifungal activity of azole drugs results from the reduction of ergosterol synthesis by inhibition of fungal cytochrome P450 enzymes. The specificity of azole drugs results from their greater affinity for fungal than for human cytochrome P450 enzymes. Imidazoles exhibit a lesser degree of specificity than the triazoles, accounting for their higher incidence of drug interactions and side effects.

Resistance to azoles occurs via multiple mechanisms. Once rare, increasing numbers of resistant strains are being reported, suggesting that increasing use of these agents for prophylaxis and therapy may be selecting for clinical drug resistance in certain settings.

Clinical Use

The spectrum of action of these medications is quite broad, ranging from many candida species, *Cryptococcus neoformans,* the endemic mycoses (blastomycosis, coccidioidomycosis, histoplasmosis), the dermatophytes,

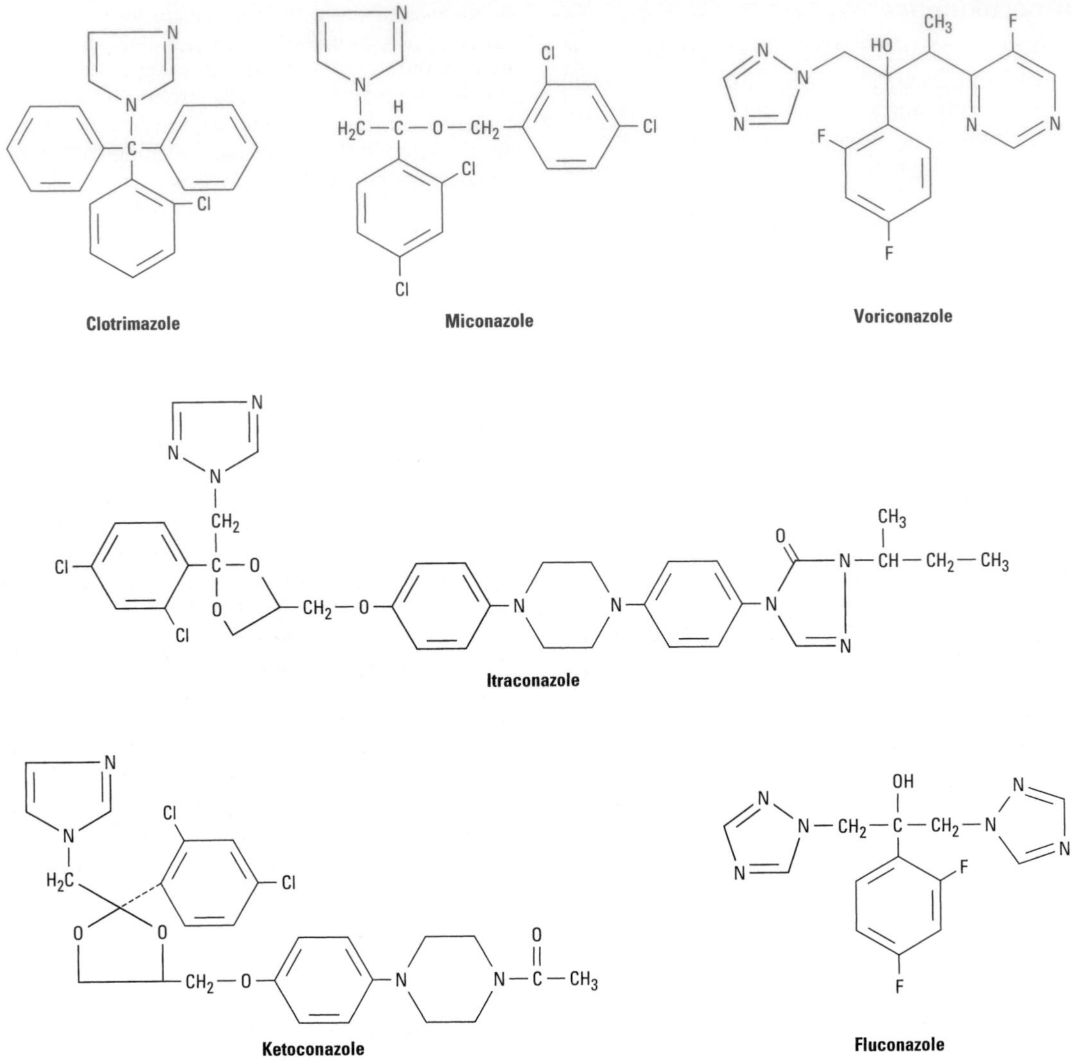

Figure 48–1. Structural formulas of some antifungal azoles.

and, in the case of itraconazole and voriconazole, even aspergillus infections. They are also useful in the treatment of intrinsically amphotericin-resistant organisms such as *Pseudallescheria boydii*.

Adverse Effects

As a group, the azoles are relatively nontoxic. The most common adverse reaction is relatively minor gastrointestinal upset. All azoles have been reported to cause abnormalities in liver enzymes and, very rarely, clinical hepatitis. Adverse effects specific to individual agents are discussed below.

Drug Interactions

All azole drugs affect the mammalian cytochrome P450 system of enzymes to some extent, and consequently they are prone to drug interactions. The most significant reactions are indicated below.

1. Ketoconazole

Ketoconazole was the first oral azole introduced into clinical use. It is distinguished from triazoles by its greater propensity to inhibit mammalian cytochrome P450 enzymes, ie, it is less selective for fungal P450 than

Table 48–2. Pharmacologic properties of four systemic azole drugs.

	Water Solubility	Absorption	CSF:Serum Concentration Ratio	$t_{1/2}$ (hours)	Elimination	Formulations
Ketoconazole	Low	Variable	< 0.1	7–10	Hepatic	Oral
Itraconazole	Low	Variable	< 0.01	24–42	Hepatic	Oral, IV
Fluconazole	High	High	> 0.7	22–31	Renal	Oral, IV
Voriconazole	High	High	...	6	Hepatic	Oral, IV

are the newer azoles. As a result, systemic ketoconazole has fallen out of clinical use in the USA and will not be discussed in any detail here. Its dermatologic use is discussed in Chapter 62.

2. Itraconazole

Itraconazole is available in oral and intravenous formulations and is used at a dosage of 100–400 mg/d. Drug absorption is increased by food and by low gastric pH. Like other lipid-soluble azoles, it interacts with hepatic microsomal enzymes, though to a lesser degree than ketoconazole. An important drug interaction is reduced bioavailability of itraconazole when taken with rifamycins (rifampin, rifabutin, rifapentine). It does not affect mammalian steroid synthesis, and its effects on the metabolism of other hepatically cleared medications are much less than those of ketoconazole. While itraconazole displays potent antifungal activity, effectiveness can be limited by reduced bioavailability. Newer formulations, including an oral liquid and an intravenous preparation, have utilized cyclodextran as a carrier molecule to enhance solubility and bioavailability. Like ketoconazole, it penetrates poorly into the cerebrospinal fluid. Itraconazole is the azole of choice for treatment of disease due to the dimorphic fungi histoplasma, blastomyces, and sporothrix. While itraconazole has activity against aspergillus species, this agent has been replaced by voriconazole as the azole of choice for aspergillosis. Itraconazole is used extensively in the treatment of dermatophytoses and onychomycosis.

3. Fluconazole

Fluconazole displays a high degree of water solubility and good cerebrospinal fluid penetration. Unlike ketoconazole and itraconazole, its oral bioavailability is high. Drug interactions are also less common because fluconazole has the least effect of all the azoles on hepatic microsomal enzymes. Because of fewer hepatic enzyme interactions and better gastrointestinal tolerance, flu-

conazole has the widest therapeutic index of the azoles, permitting more aggressive dosing in a variety of fungal infections. The drug is available in oral and intravenous formulations and is used at a dosage of 100–800 mg/d.

Fluconazole is the azole of choice in the treatment and secondary prophylaxis of cryptococcal meningitis. Intravenous fluconazole has been shown to be equivalent to amphotericin B in treatment of candidemia in ICU patients with normal white blood cell counts. Fluconazole is the agent most commonly used for the treatment of mucocutaneous candidiasis. Activity against the dimorphic fungi is limited to coccidioidal disease, and in particular for meningitis, where high doses of fluconazole often obviate the need for intrathecal amphotericin B. Fluconazole displays no activity against aspergillus or other filamentous fungi.

Prophylactic use of fluconazole has been demonstrated to reduce fungal disease in bone marrow transplant recipients and AIDS patients, but the emergence of fluconazole-resistant fungi has raised concerns about this indication.

4. Voriconazole

Voriconazole is the newest triazole to be licensed in the USA. It is available in intravenous and oral formulations. The recommended dosage is 400 mg/d. The drug is well absorbed orally, with a bioavailability exceeding 90%, and exhibits less protein binding than itraconazole. Metabolism is predominantly hepatic, but the propensity for inhibition of mammalian P450 appears to be low. Observed toxicities include rash, elevated hepatic enzymes, and transient visual disturbances. Visual disturbances are common, occurring in up to 30% of patients receiving voriconazole, and include blurring and changes in color vision or brightness. These visual changes usually occur immediately after a dose of voriconazole and resolve within 30 minutes.

Voriconazole is similar to itraconazole in its spectrum of action, having excellent activity against candida species (including fluconazole-resistant species such as

C krusei) and the dimorphic fungi. Voriconazole is less toxic than amphotericin B and may be more effective in the treatment of invasive aspergillosis.

ECHINOCANDINS

Echinocandins are the newest class of antifungal agent to be developed. They are large cyclic peptides linked to a long-chain fatty acid. **Caspofungin** is the only licensed agent in this category of antifungals, although several related agents are under active investigation.

Pharmacology

Caspofungin is available only in an intravenous form. The drug is administered as a single loading dose of 70 mg, followed by a daily dose of 50 mg. Caspofungin is water-soluble and highly protein-bound. The half-life is 9–11 hours, and the metabolites are excreted by the kidneys and gastrointestinal tract. Dosage adjustments are required only in the presence of severe hepatic insufficiency.

Mechanism of Action

Caspofungin acts at the level of the fungal cell wall by inhibiting the synthesis of $\beta(1-3)$ glucan. This results in disruption of the fungal cell wall and cell death.

Adverse Effects

Caspofungin is extremely well tolerated, with minor gastrointestinal side effects and flushing reported infrequently. Elevated liver enzymes have been noted in several patients receiving caspofungin in combination with cyclosporine, and this combination should be avoided.

Clinical Use

Caspofungin is currently licensed only for salvage therapy in patients with invasive aspergillosis who have failed to respond to amphotericin B. Clinical studies indicate that caspofungin is active also against candida species in the setting of mucocutaneous candidiasis and candidal bloodstream infections.

SYSTEMIC ANTIFUNGAL DRUGS FOR MUCOCUTANEOUS INFECTIONS

GRISEOFULVIN

Griseofulvin is a very insoluble fungistatic drug derived from a species of penicillium. Its only use is in the systemic treatment of dermatophytosis (Chapter 62). It is administered in a microcrystalline form at a dosage of 1 g/d. Absorption is improved when it is given with fatty foods. Griseofulvin's mechanism of action at the cellular level is unclear, but it is deposited in newly forming skin where it binds to keratin, protecting the skin from new infection. Since its action is to prevent infection of these new skin structures, it must be administered for 2–6 weeks for skin and hair infections to allow the replacement of infected keratin by the resistant structures. Nail infections may require therapy for months to allow regrowth of the new protected nail and is often followed by relapse. Adverse effects include an allergic syndrome much like serum sickness, hepatitis, and drug interactions with warfarin and phenobarbital. Griseofulvin has been largely replaced by newer antifungal medications such as itraconazole and terbinafine.

TERBINAFINE

Terbinafine is a synthetic allylamine that is available in an oral formulation and is used at a dosage of 250 mg/d. It is used in the treatment of dermatophytoses, especially onychomycosis (see Chapter 62). Like griseofulvin, it is a keratophilic medication, but unlike griseofulvin, it is fungicidal. Like the azole drugs, it interferes with ergosterol biosynthesis, but rather than interacting with the P450 system, terbinafine inhibits the fungal enzyme squalene epoxidase. This leads to the accumulation of the sterol squalene, which is toxic to the organism. One tablet given daily for 12 weeks achieves a cure rate of up to 90% for onychomycosis and is more effective than griseofulvin or itraconazole. Adverse effects are rare, consisting primarily of gastrointestinal upset and headache. Terbinafine does not seem to affect the P450 system and has demonstrated no significant drug interactions to date.

TOPICAL ANTIFUNGAL THERAPY

NYSTATIN

Nystatin is a polyene macrolide much like amphotericin B. It is too toxic for parenteral administration and is only used topically. It is currently available in creams, ointments, suppositories, and other forms for application to skin and mucous membranes. Nystatin is not absorbed to a significant degree from skin, mucous membranes, or the gastrointestinal tract. As a result, it has little toxicity, though oral use is often limited by the unpleasant taste.

Nystatin is active against most candida species and is most commonly used for suppression of local candidal infections. Some common indications include oropharyngeal thrush, vaginal candidiasis, and intertriginous candidal infections.

TOPICAL AZOLES

The two azoles most commonly used topically are clotrimazole and miconazole; several others are available (see Preparations Available, below). Both are available over-the-counter and are often used for vulvovaginal candidiasis. Oral clotrimazole troches are available for treatment of oral thrush and are a pleasant-tasting alternative to nystatin. In cream form, both agents are useful for dermatophytic infections, including tinea corporis, tinea pedis, and tinea cruris. Absorption is negligible, and adverse effects are rare.

Topical and shampoo forms of ketoconazole are also available and useful in the treatment of seborrheic dermatitis and pityriasis versicolor. Several other azoles are available for topical use (see Preparations Available).

TOPICAL ALLYLAMINES

Terbinafine and naftifine are allylamines available as topical creams (see Chapter 62). Both are effective for treatment of tinea cruris and tinea corporis. These are prescription drugs in the USA.

PREPARATIONS AVAILABLE

Amphotericin B
 Parenteral:
 Conventional formulation (Amphotericin B, Fungizone): 50 mg powder for injection
 Lipid formulations:
 (Abelcet): 100 mg/20 mL suspension for injection
 (AmBisome): 50 mg powder for injection
 (Amphotec): 50, 100 mg powder for injection
 Topical: 3% cream, lotion, ointment
Butaconazole (Femstat, Mycelex-3)
 Topical: 2% vaginal cream
Butenafine (Mentax)
 Topical: 1% cream
Caspofungin (Cancidas)
 Parenteral: 50, 70 mg powder for injection
Clotrimazole (Lotrimin, others)
 Topical: 1% cream, solution, lotion; 100, 200 mg vaginal suppositories
Econazole (Spectazole)
 Topical: 1% cream
Fluconazole (Diflucan)
 Oral: 50, 100, 150, 200 mg tablets; powder for 10, 40 mg/mL suspension
 Parenteral: 2 mg/mL in 100 and 200 mL vials
Flucytosine (Ancobon)
 Oral: 250, 500 mg capsules
Griseofulvin (Grifulvin, Grisactin, Fulvicin P/G)
 Oral microsize: 125, 250 mg capsules; 250 mg tablets, 125 mg/5 mL suspension
 Oral ultramicrosize:* 125, 165, 250, 330 mg tablets

Itraconazole (Sporanox)
 Oral: 100 mg capsules; 10 mg/mL solution
 Parenteral: 10 mg/mL for IV infusion
Ketoconazole (generic, Nizoral)
 Oral: 200 mg tablets
 Topical: 2% cream, shampoo
Miconazole (Micatin, others)
 Topical: 2% cream, powder, spray; 100, 200 mg vaginal suppositories
Naftifine (Naftin)
 Topical: 1% cream, gel
Natamycin (Natacyn)
 Topical: 5% ophthalmic suspension
Nystatin (generic, Mycostatin)
 Oral: 500,000 unit tablets
 Topical: 100,000 units/g cream, ointment, powder; 100,000 units vaginal tablets
Oxiconazole (Oxistat)
 Topical: 1% cream, lotion
Sulconazole (Exelderm)
 Topical: 1% cream, lotion
Terbinafine (Lamisil)
 Oral: 250 mg tablets
 Topical: 1% cream, gel
Terconazole (Terazol 3, Terazol 7)
 Topical: 0.4%, 0.8% vaginal cream; 80 mg vaginal suppositories
Tioconazole (Vagistat-1)
 Topical: 6.5% vaginal ointment
Tolnaftate (generic, Aftate, Tinactin)
 Topical: 1% cream, gel, solution, aerosol powder
Voriconazole (Vfend)
 Oral: 50, 200 mg tablets
 Parenteral: 200 mg vials, reconstituted to a 5 mg/mL solution

---

* Ultramicrosize formulations of griseofulvin are approximately 1.5 times more potent, milligram for milligram, than the microsize preparations.

REFERENCES

Brautigam M, Nolting S, Schopf RE: Randomized, double-blind comparison of terbinafine and itraconazole for treatment of tinea infection. Br Med J 1995;311:919.

Diekema DJ et al: Activities of caspofungin, itraconazole, posaconazole, ravuconazole, voriconazole, and amphotericin B against 448 recent clinical isolates of filamentous fungi. J Clin Microbiol 2003;41:3623.

Francis P, Walsh TJ: Evolving role of flucytosine in immunocompromised patients: New insights into safety, pharmacokinetics, and antifungal therapy. Clin Infect Dis 1992;15:1003.

Gallis HA, Drew RH, Pickard WW: Amphotericin B: 30 years of clinical experience. Rev Infect Dis 1990;12:308.

Groll A, Piscitelli SC, Walsh TJ: Clinical pharmacology of systemic antifungal agents: A comprehensive review of agents in clinical use, current investigational compounds, and putative targets for antifungal drug development. Adv Pharmacol 1998; 44:343.

Herbrecht R et al: Voriconazole versus amphotericin B for primary therapy of invasive aspergillosis. N Engl J Med 2002;347:408.

Rezabek GH, Friedman AD: Superficial fungal infections of the skin: Diagnosis and current treatment recommendations. Drugs 1992;43:674.

Saag MS, Dismukes WE: Azole antifungal agents: Emphasis on new triazoles. Antimicrob Agents Chemother 1988;32:1.

Sarosi GA, Davies SF: Therapy for fungal infections. Mayo Clin Proc 1994;69:1111.

Sheehan DJ, Hitchcock CA, Sibley CM: Current and emerging azole antifungal agents. Clin Microbiol Rev 1999;12:40.

Viviani MA: Flucytosine—what is its future? J Antimicrob Chemother 1995;35:241.

Wiederhold NP, Lewis RE: The echinocandin antifungals: An overview of the pharmacology, spectrum and clinical efficacy. Expert Opin Investig Drugs 2003;12:1313.

Wong-Beringer A, Jacobs RA, Guglielmo BJ: Lipid formulations of amphotericin B. Clinical efficacy and toxicities. Clin Infect Dis 1998;27:603.

Antiviral Agents

Sharon Safrin, MD

Viruses are obligate intracellular parasites; their replication depends primarily on synthetic processes of the host cell. Consequently, to be effective, antiviral agents must either block viral entry into or exit from the cell or be active inside the host cell. As a corollary, nonselective inhibitors of virus replication may interfere with host cell function and produce toxicity. The search for chemicals that inhibit virus-specific functions is currently one of the most active areas of pharmacologic investigation.

Research in antiviral chemotherapy began in the early 1950s, when the search for anticancer drugs generated several new compounds capable of inhibiting viral DNA synthesis. The two first-generation antivirals, 5-iododeoxyuridine and trifluorothymidine, had poor specificity (ie, they inhibited host cellular as well as viral DNA) that rendered them too toxic for systemic use. However, both are effective when used topically for the treatment of herpes keratitis.

Recent research has focused on the identification of agents with greater selectivity, in vivo stability, and lack of toxicity. Selective antiretroviral agents that inhibit a critical HIV-1 enzyme such as reverse transcriptase or the protease required for final packaging of the virus particle have become available. In many viral infections, replication of the virus peaks at or before the manifestation of clinical symptoms. Optimal clinical efficacy in many viral illnesses therefore depends either on early initiation of therapy (eg, acyclovir for treatment of varicella or zoster infection) or on prevention of infection (eg, chemoprophylaxis against influenza A using a neuraminidase inhibitor or amantadine. Alternatively, potent inhibition of viral replication may be of clinical benefit in chronic illnesses such as HIV infection or viral hepatitis.

Viral replication consists of several steps: (1) adsorption to and penetration into susceptible host cells; (2) uncoating of viral nucleic acid; (3) synthesis of early regulatory proteins, eg, nucleic acid polymerases; (4) synthesis of RNA or DNA; (5) synthesis of late, structural proteins; (6) assembly (maturation) of viral particles; and (7) release from the cell. Antiviral agents can potentially target any of these steps (Figure 49–1).

ACRONYMS & OTHER NAMES

3TC	Lamivudine
ara-A	Vidarabine
AZT	Zidovudine (previously azidothymidine)
CMV	Cytomegalovirus
CYP	Cytochrome P450
d4T	Stavudine
ddC	Zalcitabine
ddI	Didanosine
EBV	Epstein-Barr virus
HAART	Highly active antiretroviral therapy
HBV	Hepatitis B virus
HCV	Hepatitis C virus
HHV-6, -8	Human herpesvirus-6, -8
HIV	Human immunodeficiency virus
HSV-1, -2	Herpes simplex virus-1, -2
IDU, IDUR	Idoxuridine
IFN	Interferon
NNRTI	Nonnucleoside reverse transcriptase inhibitor
NRTI	Nucleoside reverse transcriptase inhibitor
PI	Protease inhibitor
RSV	Respiratory syncytial virus
VZV	Varicella-zoster virus

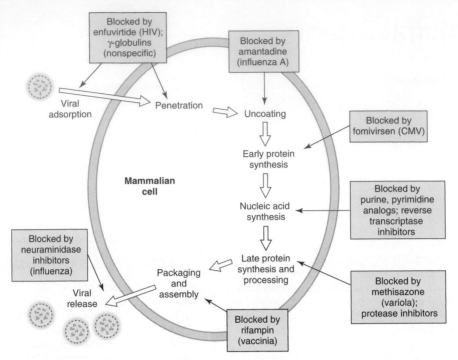

Figure 49–1. The major sites of antiviral drug action. (Modified and reproduced, with permission, from Trevor AT, Katzung BG, Masters SM: *Pharmacology: Examination & Board Review,* 6th ed. McGraw-Hill, 2002.)

I. AGENTS TO TREAT HERPES SIMPLEX VIRUS (HSV) & VARICELLA ZOSTER VIRUS (VZV) INFECTIONS

Three oral agents are licensed for the treatment of HSV and VZV infections: acyclovir, valacyclovir, and famciclovir. They have similar mechanisms of action and similar indications for clinical use; all are well tolerated. Acyclovir, licensed first, has been the most extensively studied; in addition, it is the only anti-HSV agent available for intravenous use in the United States. Neither valacyclovir nor famciclovir have been fully evaluated in pediatric patients; thus, they are not indicated for the treatment of varicella infection.

ACYCLOVIR

Acyclovir (Figure 49–2) is an acyclic guanosine derivative with clinical activity against HSV-1, HSV-2, and VZV. In vitro activity against Epstein-Barr virus,

cytomegalovirus, and human herpesvirus-6 is present but comparatively weaker.

Mechanism of Action

Acyclovir requires three phosphorylation steps for activation. It is converted first to the monophosphate derivative by the virus-specified thymidine kinase and then to the di- and triphosphate compounds by the host's cellular enzymes (Figure 49–3). Because it requires the viral kinase for initial phosphorylation, acyclovir is selectively activated and accumulates only in infected cells. Acyclovir triphosphate inhibits viral DNA synthesis by two mechanisms: competitive inhibition with deoxyGTP for the viral DNA polymerase, resulting in binding to the DNA template as an irreversible complex; and chain termination following incorporation into the viral DNA.

Pharmacokinetics

The bioavailability of oral acyclovir is 15–20% and is unaffected by food. Peak serum concentrations of approximately 1 μg/mL after a 200 mg oral dose and 1.5–2 μg/mL after an 800 mg dose are reached 1.5–2

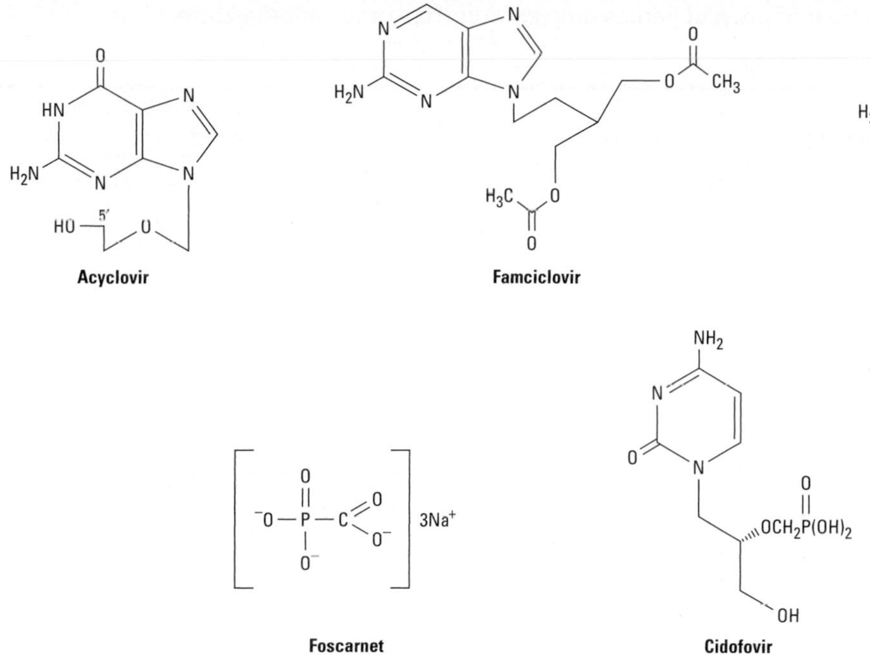

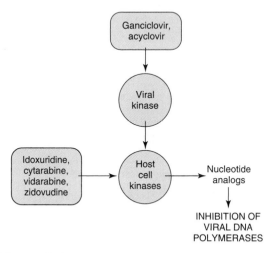

Figure 49–2. Chemical structures of some representative antiherpes agents.

Figure 49–3. Antiviral actions of purine and pyrimidine analogs. Acyclovir and ganciclovir (top) are phosphorylated first by viral kinase to the monophosphate. This intermediate and the drugs shown on the left are then phosphorylated by host cell kinases to the nucleotide analogs that inhibit viral replication. (Modified and reproduced, with permission, from Trevor AT, Katzung BG, Masters SM: *Pharmacology: Examination & Board Review,* 6th ed. McGraw-Hill, 2002.)

hours after dosing. Peak serum concentrations are 10 μg/mL and 20 μg/mL after intravenous infusions (over 1 hour) of 5 mg/kg and 10 mg/kg, respectively. Topical formulations produce local concentrations that may exceed 10 μg/mL in herpetic lesions, but systemic concentrations are undetectable.

Acyclovir is cleared primarily by glomerular filtration and tubular secretion. The half-life is approximately 3 hours in patients with normal renal function and 20 hours in patients with anuria. Acyclovir is readily cleared by hemodialysis but not by peritoneal dialysis.

Acyclovir diffuses into most tissues and body fluids to produce concentrations that are 50–100% of those in serum. Cerebrospinal fluid concentrations are 50% of serum values.

Clinical Uses (Table 49–1)

Oral acyclovir has multiple uses. In primary genital herpes, oral acyclovir shortens by approximately 5 days the duration of symptoms, the time of viral shedding, and the time to resolution of lesions; in recurrent genital herpes, the time course is shortened by 1–2 days. Treatment of primary genital herpes does not alter the frequency or severity of recurrent outbreaks. Long-term chronic suppression of genital herpes with oral acyclovir decreases the frequency both of symptomatic recurrences and of

Table 49–1. Agents to treat or prevent herpes simplex virus (HSV) and varicella-zoster virus (VZV) infections.

Agent	Route of Administration	Use	Recommended Adult Dosage and Regimen
Acyclovir[1]	Oral	First episode genital herpes	400 mg tid or 200 mg five times daily
		Recurrent genital herpes	400 mg tid or 200 mg five times daily or 800 mg bid
		Genital herpes suppression	400 mg bid
		Herpes proctitis	400 mg five times daily
		Mucocutaneous herpes in the immunocompromised host	400 mg five times daily
		Varicella	20 mg/kg (maximum 800 mg) four times daily
		Zoster	800 mg five times daily
	Intravenous	Severe HSV infection	5 mg/kg q8h
		Herpes encephalitis	10–15 mg/kg q8h
		Neonatal HSV infection	20 mg/kg q8h
		Varicella or zoster in the immunosuppressed host	10 mg/kg q8h
Famciclovir[1]	Oral	First episode genital herpes	250 mg tid
		Recurrent genital herpes	125 mg bid
		Genital herpes suppression	250 mg bid
		Zoster	500 mg tid
Valacyclovir[1]	Oral	First episode genital herpes	1 g bid
		Recurrent genital herpes	500 mg bid
		Genital herpes suppression	500 mg daily or twice daily
		Zoster	1 g tid
Foscarnet[1]	Intravenous	Acyclovir-resistant HSV and VZV infections	40 mg/kg q8-12h
Penciclovir	Topical	Recurrent herpes labialis	Thin film covering lesion every 2 hours
Trifluridine	Topical	Herpes keratitis	1 drop every 2 hours
		Acyclovir-resistant HSV infection	Thin film covering lesion five times daily

[1]Dosage must be reduced in patients with renal insufficiency.

asymptomatic viral shedding in patients with frequent recurrences, thus decreasing sexual transmission. However, outbreaks may resume upon discontinuation of suppressive acyclovir. In recurrent herpes labialis, oral acyclovir reduces the mean duration of pain but not the time to healing. Oral acyclovir decreases the total number of lesions and duration of varicella (if begun within 24 hours after the onset of rash) and cutaneous zoster (if begun within 72 hours). However, because VZV is less susceptible to acyclovir than HSV, higher doses are required (Table 49–1). A meta-analysis suggested that acyclovir was superior to placebo in reducing the duration of "zoster-associated pain," a continuous variable combining acute and chronic pain. When given prophylactically to patients undergoing organ transplantation, oral acyclovir (200 mg every 8 hours or 800 mg every 12 hours) or intravenous acyclovir (5 mg/kg every 8 hours) prevents reactivation of HSV infection. The benefit of acyclovir for prevention of CMV infections in transplant patients is controversial.

Intravenous acyclovir is the treatment of choice for herpes simplex encephalitis, neonatal HSV infection, and serious HSV or VZV infections (Table 49–1). In immunocompromised patients with zoster, intravenous acyclovir reduces the incidence of cutaneous and visceral dissemination.

Topical acyclovir is much less effective than oral therapy for primary HSV infection. It is of no benefit in treating recurrences.

Resistance

Resistance to acyclovir can develop in HSV or VZV through alteration in either the viral thymidine kinase or the DNA polymerase. Infections that are clinically resistant to acyclovir have been reported in immunocompromised hosts. Most clinical isolates are resistant on the basis of deficient thymidine kinase activity and thus are cross-resistant to valacyclovir, famciclovir, and ganciclovir. Agents such as foscarnet, cidofovir, and trifluridine do not require activation by viral thymidine kinase and thus have preserved activity against the most prevalent acyclovir-resistant strains.

Adverse Reactions

Acyclovir is generally well tolerated. Nausea, diarrhea, and headache have occasionally been reported. Intravenous infusion may be associated with reversible renal dysfunction due to crystalline nephropathy or neurologic toxicity (eg, tremors, delirium, seizures); however, these are uncommon with adequate hydration and avoidance of rapid infusion rates. Chronic daily suppressive use of acyclovir for more than 10 years has not been associated with untoward effects. High doses of acyclovir cause testicular atrophy in rats, but there has been no evidence of teratogenicity to date in a cumulative registry and no effect on sperm production was demonstrated in a placebo-controlled trial of patients receiving daily chronic acyclovir.

VALACYCLOVIR

Valacyclovir is the L-valyl ester of acyclovir. It is rapidly converted to acyclovir after oral administration, resulting in serum levels three to five times greater than those achieved with oral acyclovir and approximating those resulting from intravenous acyclovir administration. Oral bioavailability is about 48%. As with acyclovir, uses of valacyclovir include treatment of first atacks or recurrences of genital herpes, suppression of frequently recur-

rent genital herpes, treatment of herpes zoster infection, and, recently, as a 1-day treatment for orolabial herpes (Table 49–1). Valacyclovir has also been shown to be effective in preventing cytomegalovirus disease after organ transplantation when compared with placebo. In general, comparative studies have shown similar or slightly improved efficacy of valacyclovir versus acyclovir for all indications; furthermore, valacyclovir therapy was associated with a shorter duration of zoster-associated pain than acyclovir in one study, as well as a lower frequency of postherpetic neuralgia. Once-daily dosing of valacyclovir (500 mg) as chronic suppression in persons with recurrent genital herpes has recently been shown to markedly decrease the risk of sexual transmission. Valacyclovir is generally well tolerated, although nausea, diarrhea, and headache may occur. AIDS patients receiving high-dosage valacyclovir chronically (ie, 8 g/d) had an increased incidence of gastrointestinal intolerance as well as thrombotic microangiopathies such as thrombotic thrombocytopenic purpura and hemolytic-uremic syndrome. In transplant patients receiving valacyclovir (8 g/d), non-dose-limiting confusion and hallucinations were the most frequent side effects.

FAMCICLOVIR

Famciclovir is the diacetyl ester prodrug of 6-deoxypenciclovir, an acyclic guanosine analog (Figure 49–2). After oral administration, famciclovir is rapidly converted by first-pass metabolism to penciclovir, which shares many features with acyclovir. It is active in vitro against HSV-1, HSV-2, VZV, EBV, and HBV. Activation by phosphorylation is catalyzed by the virus-specified thymidine kinase in infected cells, followed by competitive inhibition of the viral DNA polymerase to block DNA synthesis. Unlike acyclovir, penciclovir does not cause chain termination. Penciclovir triphosphate has lower affinity for the viral DNA polymerase than acyclovir triphosphate, but it achieves higher intracellular concentrations and has a more prolonged intracellular effect in experimental systems. The most commonly encountered clinical mutants of HSV are thymidine kinase-deficient and are cross-resistant to acyclovir and famciclovir.

Pharmacokinetics

The bioavailability of penciclovir from orally administered famciclovir is 70%; less than 20% is plasma protein-bound. A peak serum concentration of 2 μg/mL is achieved following a 250 mg oral dose. Penciclovir triphosphate has an intracellular half-life of 10 hours in HSV-1-infected cells, 20 hours in HSV-2-infected cells, and 7 hours in VZV-infected cells in vitro. Penciclovir is excreted primarily in the urine.

Clinical Uses (Table 49–1)

Oral famciclovir is effective for the treatment of first and recurrent genital herpes attacks and for chronic daily suppression. It is also used to treat acute herpes zoster (shingles). In controlled trials in immunocompetent patients with zoster, famciclovir was similar to acyclovir in rates of cutaneous healing but was associated with a shorter duration of postherpetic neuralgia. Comparison of famciclovir to valacyclovir for treatment of herpes zoster in immunocompetent patients showed similar rates of cutaneous healing and pain resolution. However, neither drug decreased the incidence of postherpetic neuralgia.

Adverse Reactions

Oral famciclovir is generally well tolerated, although headache, diarrhea, and nausea may occur. As with acyclovir, testicular toxicity has been demonstrated in animals receiving repeated doses. However, men receiving daily famciclovir (250 mg every 12 hours) had no changes in sperm morphology or motility. The incidence of mammary adenocarcinoma was also increased in female rats receiving famciclovir for 2 years.

PENCICLOVIR

The guanosine analog penciclovir is the active metabolite of famciclovir (see above). Topical application of 1% penciclovir cream is effective for the treatment of recurrent herpes labialis in immunocompetent adults (Table 49–1). When therapy was initiated within 1 hour after the onset of signs or symptoms and continued every 2 hours during waking hours for 4 days, treatment with topical penciclovir resulted in a shortening of the mean duration of lesions, lesion pain, and virus shedding by approximately one-half day compared with placebo. Side effects are uncommon.

TRIFLURIDINE

Trifluridine (trifluorothymidine) is a fluorinated pyrimidine nucleoside that inhibits viral DNA synthesis. The compound has in vitro activity against HSV-1, HSV-2, vaccinia, and some adenoviruses. It is phosphorylated intracellularly to its active form by cellular enzymes, then competes with thymidine triphosphate for incorporation by the viral DNA polymerase. Incorporation of trifluridine triphosphate into both viral and cellular DNA prevents its systemic use. Application of a 1% solution is effective in treating primary keratoconjunctivitis and recurrent epithelial keratitis due to HSV-1 and HSV-2. Topical application of trifluridine solution, alone or in combination with interferon alfa, has been used successfully in the treatment of acyclovir-resistant HSV infections.

II. AGENTS TO TREAT CYTOMEGALOVIRUS (CMV) INFECTIONS

GANCICLOVIR

Ganciclovir is an acyclic guanosine analog (Figure 49–2) that requires triphosphorylation for activation prior to inhibiting the viral DNA polymerase. Initial phosphorylation is catalyzed by the virus-specified protein kinase phosphotransferase UL97 in CMV-infected cells. The activated compound competitively inhibits viral DNA polymerase and causes termination of viral DNA elongation. Ganciclovir has in vitro activity against CMV, HSV, VZV, EBV, and HHV-8. Its activity against CMV is up to 100 times greater than that of acyclovir.

Pharmacokinetics

Ganciclovir may be administered intravenously, orally, or via intraocular implant.

A 5 mg/kg dose of ganciclovir administered intravenously over 1 hour produces serum concentrations averaging 6–10 μg/mL, with trough levels of approximately 1 μg/mL. Cerebrospinal fluid concentrations are approximately 50% of those in serum. Intravitreal concentrations following intravenous administration average 1 μg/mL. The half-life is 2–4 hours with normal renal function. Clearance of the drug is linearly related to creatinine clearance. Ganciclovir is readily cleared by hemodialysis. The bioavailability of oral ganciclovir is poor (6–9% when taken with food).

In patients with an intraocular implant, ganclovir is released into the vitreous cavity at a rate of approximately 1.4 μg/h.

Clinical Uses (Table 49–2)

Intravenous ganciclovir has been shown to delay progression of CMV retinitis in patients with AIDS when compared with no treatment. Dual therapy with foscarnet and ganciclovir has been shown to be more effective in delaying progression of retinitis than either drug administered alone (see Foscarnet, below), although side effects are compounded. Intravenous ganciclovir is also used to treat CMV colitis and esophagitis. Intravenous ganciclovir, followed by either oral ganciclovir or high-dose oral acyclovir, reduces the risk of CMV infection in transplant recipients. Use of intravenous ganciclovir to treat CMV pneumonitis in immunocompromised patients may be beneficial, particularly in combination with intravenous cytomegalovirus immunoglobulin.

Table 49–2. Agents to treat cytomegalovirus (CMV) infection.

Agent	Route of Administration	Use	Recommended Adult Dosage
Cidofovir[1]	Intravenous	CMV retinitis treatment (induction or maintenance)	Induction: 5 mg/kg every 7 days Maintenance: 5 mg/kg every 14 davs
Fomivirsen	Intravitreal injection	CMV retinitis treatment (induction or maintenance)	Induction: 330 µg every14 days Maintenance: 330 µg every 4 weeks
Foscarnet[1]	Intravenous	CMV retinitis treatment (induction or maintenance)	Induction: 60 mg/kg q8h or 90 mg/kg q12h Maintenance: 90–120 mg/kg/d
Ganciclovir[1]	Intravenous	CMV retinitis treatment (induction or maintenance)	Induction: 5 mg/kg q12h Maintenance: 5 mg/kg/d or 6 mg/kg five times per week
	Oral	CMV prophylaxis	1 g tid
		CMV retinitis treatment (maintenance only)	1 g tid
	Intraocular implant	CMV retinitis treatment	4.5 mg every 6–8 months
Valganciclovir[1]	Oral	CMV retinitis treatment (induction or maintenance)	Induction: 900 mg bid Maintenance: 900 mg qd The drug should be taken with food.
	Oral	CMV prophylaxis	900 mg qd

[1]Dosage must be reduced in patients with renal insufficiency.

Oral ganciclovir is indicated for prevention of end-organ CMV disease in AIDS patients and as maintenance therapy of CMV retinitis following induction. Although less effective than intravenous ganciclovir, the risk of myelosuppression and of catheter-related complications is diminished.

Ganciclovir may also be administered intraocularly to treat CMV retinitis, either by direct intravitreal administration or via an intraocular implant. The implant, which achieves high and prolonged intraocular levels of ganciclovir, has been shown to delay progression of retinitis to a greater degree than systemic therapy with ganciclovir. Surgical replacement is required at intervals of 5–8 months. Owing to the lack of systemic protection against end-organ CMV disease (eg, colitis, esophagitis, ventriculitis) in patients treated with the ganciclovir implant alone—as well as the absence of protection against contralateral retinal CMV infection—concurrent therapy with a systemic anti-CMV agent is recommended. A recent study showed that the combination of either intravenous or oral ganciclovir and the ganciclovir intraocular implant in AIDS patients with CMV retinitis resulted in a decreased incidence of Kaposi's sarcoma over 6 months compared with those treated with the implant alone.

Resistance

Sporadic cases of ganciclovir-resistant CMV infection have been reported since the introduction of ganciclovir in the late 1980s; clinical manifestations may include progressive disease or prolonged viremia. Until recently, the majority of resistant cases were in patients with AIDS receiving prolonged therapy with ganciclovir. However, with the advent of more widespread use of oral ganciclovir, often in combination with more intensive immunosuppressive therapies, an increased frequency of ganciclovir-resistant CMV infection has been noted in organ transplant recipients. The most common mechanisms of resistance are mutations in UL97, resulting in decreased levels of the triphosphorylated (ie, active) form of ganciclovir; mutations in UL54, which result in a mutant DNA polymerase, occur less frequently. Isolates with mutations in UL97 are not cross-resistant with cidofovir or foscarnet, while mutations in UL54 may confer cross-resistance to cidofovir (and, less frequently, foscarnet). Performance of antiviral susceptibility testing is recommended in patients in whom resistance is suspected clinically, as is the substitution of alternative therapies (eg, foscarnet), and concomitant reduction in immunosuppressive therapies, if possible.

The addition of CMV hyperimmune globulin may also be considered.

Adverse Reactions & Drug Interactions

The most common side effect of systemic ganciclovir treatment (more common with intravenous than with oral administration) is myelosuppression, particularly neutropenia (20–40% of patients). Myelosuppression may be additive in patients receiving ganciclovir in combination with zidovudine, azathioprine, or mycophenolate mofetil. Central nervous system toxicity (headache, changes in mental status, seizures) has been rarely reported. Other potential adverse effects include fever, rash, abnormal liver function, and retinal detachment in patients with CMV retinitis. The drug is mitogenic in mammalian cells and carcinogenic and embryotoxic at high doses in animals and causes aspermatogenesis; the clinical significance of these preclinical data is unclear.

The primary potential adverse effects associated with the intraocular implant are vitreous hemorrhage and retinal detachment.

Levels of ganciclovir may rise in patients taking concurrent probenecid. Concurrent use of ganciclovir with didanosine may result in increased levels of didanosine.

VALGANCICLOVIR

Mechanism of Action

Valganciclovir is a monovalyl ester prodrug that is rapidly hydrolyzed to the active compound ganciclovir (see above) by intestinal and hepatic esterases when administered orally.

Pharmacokinetics

Valganciclovir is well absorbed and rapidly metabolized in the intestinal wall and liver to ganciclovir. The absolute bioavailability of oral valganciclovir is 60%, and steady state AUC increases by 30% with a high-fat meal. The $AUC_{0-24\ hr}$ resulting from valganciclovir (900 mg once daily) is similar to those noted after 5 mg/kg/d of intravenous ganciclovir. As with ganciclovir, the major route of elimination is renal, through glomerular filtration and active tubular secretion. Plasma concentrations of valganciclovir are reduced by approximately 50% by hemodialysis.

Clinical Uses (Table 49–2)

Valganciclovir is indicated for the treatment of CMV retinitis in patients with AIDS. A randomized, open-label study demonstrated similar efficacy of oral valganciclovir and intravenous ganciclovir for induction therapy. Although clinical data assessing maintenance therapy

with valganciclovir are not yet available, the pharmacokinetic profile would suggest similarity with intravenous ganciclovir. Potential side effects and drug interactions are those associated with ganciclovir (see above).

CIDOFOVIR

Cidofovir is a cytosine nucleotide analog with in vitro activity against CMV, HSV-1, HSV-2, VZV, EBV, HHV-6, HHV-8, adenovirus, poxviruses, polyomaviruses, and human papillomavirus. In contrast to ganciclovir, phosphorylation of cidofovir to the active diphosphate is independent of viral enzymes. After phosphorylation, cidofovir acts both as a potent inhibitor of and as an alternative substrate for viral DNA polymerase, competitively inhibiting DNA synthesis and becoming incorporated into the viral DNA chain. Isolates with resistance to cidofovir have been selected in vitro; these isolates tend to be cross-resistant with ganciclovir but retain susceptibility to foscarnet. Clinically significant resistance to cidofovir has not been reported to date.

Pharmacokinetics

Although the terminal half-life of cidofovir is about 2.6 hours, the active metabolite, cidofovir diphosphate, has a prolonged intracellular half-life of 17–65 hours, thus allowing widely spaced administration. A separate metabolite, cidofovir phosphocholine, has a half-life of at least 87 hours and may serve as an intracellular reservoir of active drug. Peak serum concentrations when administered with probenecid (see below) are about 19 μg/mL. Cerebrospinal fluid penetration is poor after intravenous administration. Elimination involves active renal tubular secretion. High-flux hemodialysis has been shown to reduce the serum levels of cidofovir by approximately 75%.

Clinical Uses

Intravenous cidofovir is effective for the treatment of CMV retinitis. Intravenous cidofovir must be administered with probenecid (2 g at 3 hours prior to the infusion and 1 g at 2 and 8 hours after), which blocks active tubular secretion and decreases nephrotoxicity. Cidofovir dosage must be adjusted for alterations in the calculated creatinine clearance or the presence of urine protein prior to each infusion, and aggressive adjunctive hydration is required. Initiation of cidofovir therapy is contraindicated in patients with existing renal insufficiency. Direct intravitreal administration of cidofovir is not recommended due to ocular toxicity.

Other potential uses of cidofovir that are currently under investigation include treatment of the polyomavirus-associated progressive multifocal leukoencephalopathy syndrome in patients with AIDS, postexposure prophylaxis against smallpox, and topical treatment of molluscum contagiosum. Topical cidofovir is not currently available in a standardized preparation.

Adverse Reactions

The primary adverse effect of intravenous cidofovir is a dose-dependent nephrotoxicity. Concurrent administration of other potentially nephrotoxic agents (eg, amphotericin B, aminoglycosides, nonsteroidal anti-inflammatory drugs, pentamidine, foscarnet) should be avoided. Prior administration of foscarnet may increase the risk of nephrotoxicity. Other potential side effects include uveitis, decreased intraocular pressure, and probenecid-related hypersensitivity reactions. Neutropenia and metabolic acidosis are rare. The drug caused mammary adenocarcinomas in rats and is embryotoxic.

FOSCARNET

Foscarnet (phosphonoformic acid) is an inorganic pyrophosphate compound (Figure 49–2) that inhibits viral DNA polymerase, RNA polymerase, and HIV reverse transcriptase directly, without requiring activation by phosphorylation. It has in vitro activity against HSV, VZV, CMV, EBV, HHV-6, HHV-8, and HIV. Resistance to foscarnet in HSV and CMV isolates is due to point mutations in the DNA polymerase gene and is typically associated with prolonged or repeated exposure to the drug. Mutations in the HIV-1 reverse transcriptase gene have also been described. Although foscarnet-resistant CMV isolates are typically cross-resistant to ganciclovir, activity is usually maintained against ganciclovir- and cidofovir-resistant isolates of CMV.

Pharmacokinetics

The drug is available in an intravenous formulation only; poor oral bioavailability and gastrointestinal intolerance preclude oral use. Peak serum concentrations averaging 80–100 μg/mL are achieved following an infusion of 60 mg/kg. Cerebrospinal fluid concentrations are 43–67% of steady state serum concentrations. Although the mean plasma half-life is 4.5–6.8 hours, up to 30% of the drug may be deposited in bone, with a half-life of several months. The clinical repercussions of this are unknown.

Clearance of foscarnet is primarily by the kidney and is directly proportionate to creatinine clearance. Serum drug concentrations are reduced by approximately 50% following a 3-hour hemodialysis.

Clinical Uses (Table 49–2)

Foscarnet is effective treatment for CMV retinitis, with an efficacy approximately equal to that of ganciclovir.

Foscarnet is also used for treatment of CMV colitis, CMV esophagitis, acyclovir-resistant HSV infection, and acyclovir-resistant VZV infection. The dose of foscarnet must be titrated according to the patient's calculated creatinine clearance prior to each infusion. Use of an infusion pump to control the rate of infusion is important to avoid toxicity, and relatively large volumes of fluid are required because of the drug's poor solubility. The combination of ganciclovir and foscarnet is synergistic in vitro against CMV and has been shown to be superior to either agent as monotherapy in delaying progression of retinitis. Foscarnet has been administered intravitreally for the treatment of CMV retinitis in patients with AIDS, but data regarding efficacy and safety are lacking.

As with ganciclovir, a decrease in the incidence of Kaposi's sarcoma has been observed in patients who have received foscarnet. However, treatment of patients with Kaposi's sarcoma using antiherpes agents has not been successful.

Adverse Reactions

Potential adverse effects of foscarnet include renal insufficiency, hypo- or hypercalcemia, and hypo- or hyperphosphatemia. Saline preloading helps to prevent nephrotoxicity, as does avoidance of concomitant administration of drugs with nephrotoxic potential (eg, amphotericin B, pentamidine, aminoglycosides). The risk of severe hypocalcemia is increased with concomitant use of pentamidine. Penile ulcerations associated with foscarnet therapy may be due to high levels of ionized drug in the urine. Nausea, vomiting, anemia, and fatigue have been reported; the risk of anemia may be additive in patients receiving concurrent zidovudine. Central nervous system toxicities include headache, hallucinations, and seizures. The drug caused chromosomal damage in preclinical studies.

FOMIVIRSEN

Fomivirsen is an oligonucleotide that inhibits human CMV through an antisense mechanism. Binding of fomivirsen to target mRNA results in inhibition of immediate early region 2 protein synthesis, thus inhibiting virus replication. Although resistant isolates have been induced under selection pressure in vitro, clinical resistance has not been observed to date. Cross-resistance between fomivirsen and other anti-CMV agents (ganciclovir, cidofovir, foscarnet) would not be expected. Fomivirsen is injected intravitreally for the treatment of CMV retinitis in patients with AIDS and is indicated for patients who are intolerant of or unresponsive to alternative therapies. The drug is slowly cleared from vitreous with a half-life of approximately 55 hours in humans and is subsequently cleared from the retina. Measurable concentrations of drug are not detected in the systemic circulation following intravitreal administration. Immediate therapy of CMV retinitis with fomivirsen was more effective in delaying progression than deferred treatment in a recent clinical trial. Concurrent systemic anti-CMV therapy is recommended to protect against extraocular and contralateral retinal CMV disease. Potential side effects include iritis and vitreitis as well as increased intraocular pressure and changes in vision. An interval of at least 2–4 weeks is recommended between cidofovir administration and use of fomivirsen because of the risk of ocular inflammation.

III. ANTIRETROVIRAL AGENTS

A large and increasing number of antiretroviral agents are currently available for treatment of HIV-1-infected patients (Table 49–3). When to initiate therapy is controversial, but it is clear that monotherapy with any one agent should be avoided because of the need for maximal potency to durably inhibit virus replication and to avoid premature development of resistance. A combination of agents (highly active antiretroviral therapy; HAART) is usually effective in reducing plasma HIV RNA levels and in gradually increasing CD4 cell counts, particularly in antiretroviral-naive patients. Also important in selection of agents is optimization of adherence, tolerability, and convenience. Given that many patients will ultimately experience at least one treatment failure, close monitoring of viral load and CD4 cell counts is critical to trigger appropriate changes in therapy. The judicious use of drug resistance testing should be considered in selecting an alternative regimen for a patient who is not responding to therapy.

NUCLEOSIDE REVERSE TRANSCRIPTASE INHIBITORS (NRTIs)

The NRTIs act by competitive inhibition of HIV-1 reverse transcriptase and can also be incorporated into the growing viral DNA chain to cause termination. Each requires intracytoplasmic activation as a result of phosphorylation by cellular enzymes to the triphosphate form. Most have activity against HIV-2 as well as HIV-1.

Lactic acidemia and severe hepatomegaly with steatosis have been reported with the use of NRTI agents, alone or in combination with other antiretroviral drugs. Obesity, prolonged nucleoside exposure, and risk factors for liver disease have been described as factors that increase risk for lactic acidemia; however, cases have also been reported in patients with no known risk factors. NRTI treatment should be suspended in the setting of rapidly rising aminotransferase levels, progressive hepatomegaly, or metabolic or lactic acidosis of unknown cause. Given their similar mechanism of action, it is probable that these cautions should be applied to treatment with nucleotide inhibitors as well (see page 816).

ZIDOVUDINE

Zidovudine (azidothymidine; AZT) is a deoxythymidine analog (Figure 49–4) that is well absorbed from the gut and distributed to most body tissues and fluids, including the cerebrospinal fluid, where drug levels are 60–65% of those in serum. Plasma protein binding is approximately 35%. The serum half-life averages 1 hour, and the intracellular half-life of the phosphorylated compound is 3.3 hours. Zidovudine is eliminated primarily by renal excretion following glucuronidation in the liver. Clearance of zidovudine is reduced by approximately 50% in uremic patients, and toxicity may increase in patients with advanced hepatic insufficiency.

As the first licensed antiretroviral agent, zidovudine has been well studied. Zidovudine has been shown to decrease the rate of clinical disease progression and prolong survival in HIV-infected individuals. Efficacy has also been demonstrated in the treatment of HIV-associated dementia and thrombocytopenia. In pregnancy, a regimen of oral zidovudine beginning between 14 and 34 weeks of gestation (100 mg five times a day), intravenous zidovudine during labor (2 mg/kg over 1 hour, then 1 mg/kg/h by continuous infusion), and zidovudine syrup to the neonate from birth through 6 weeks of age (2 mg/kg every 6 hours) has been shown to reduce the rate of vertical (mother-to-newborn) transmission of HIV by up to 23%.

As with other NRTI agents, resistance may limit clinical efficacy. High-level zidovudine resistance is generally seen in strains with three or more of the five most common mutations: M41L, D67N, K70R, T215F, and K219Q. However, the emergence of certain mutations that confer decreased susceptibility to one drug (eg, L74V in the case of didanosine and M184V in the case of lamivudine) seems to enhance susceptibility in previously zidovudine-resistant strains. Withdrawal of zidovudine exposure may permit the reversion of zidovudine-resistant HIV-1 isolates to the susceptible wild-type phenotype.

The most common adverse effect of zidovudine is myelosuppression, resulting in anemia or neutropenia. Gastrointestinal intolerance, headaches, and insomnia

Table 49–3. Currently available antiretroviral agents.

Agent	Class of Agent[1]	Recommended Adult Dosage (oral unless otherwise indicated)	Administration Recommendation	Common Side Effects	Comments
Abacavir	NRTI	300 mg bid		Rash, hypersensitivity reaction, nausea	Do not rechallenge after hypersensitivity reaction
Amprenavir	PI	1200 mg bid	Separate dosing from didanosine or antacids by 1 hour. Avoid high-fat meals.	Rash, diarrhea, nausea	See footnote 2 for concurrent drug contraindications. Oral solution contraindicated in young children and pregnant women.
Delavirdine	NNRTI	400 mg tid	Separate dosing from didanosine or antacids by 1 hour.	Rash, liver function abnormalities	Teratogenic; see footnote 2 for concurrent drug contraindications
Didanosine[3]	NRTI	150–200 mg bid, depending on weight. Enteric-coated: 250–400 mg qd, depending on weight	30 minutes before or 2 hours after meals	Peripheral neuropathy, pancreatitis, diarrhea, hyperuricemia	Contains antacid; avoid alcohol; avoid concurrent neuropathic drugs (eg, didanosine, zalcitabine, isoniazid)
Efavirenz	NNRTI	600 mg qd	Not to be taken with a fatty meal	Dizziness, insomnia, rash, transaminitis	Embryotoxic; see footnote 2 for concurrent drug contraindications
Enfuvirtide	Fusion inhibitor	90 mg bid subcutaneously	Reconstitute for subcutaneous administration	Local injection site reactions	Refrigeration required
Indinavir	PI	800 mg tid	With water or other liquids, 1 hour before or 2 hours after a meal. Drink at least 48 oz of liquid daily. Separate dosing with didanosine by 1 hour.	Nephrolithiasis, nausea, liver function abnormalities	Store in original container, which contains dessicant; see footnote 2 for concurrent drug contraindications
Lamivudine[3]	NRTI	150 mg bid or 300 mg qd, depending on weight		Nausea, headache, fatigue	Active against HBV as well as HIV -1
Lopinavir/-ritonavir	PI/PI	400 mg/l00 mg bid	With food. Separate dosing with didanosine by 1 hour.	Diarrhea, abdominal pain, nausea	The oral solution contains alcohol; store capsules and solution in refrigerator; see footnote 2 for concurrent drug contraindications.
Nelfinavir	PI	750 mg tid or 1250 mg bid	With food	Diarrhea, nausea, flatulence	See footnote 2 for concurrent drug contraindications
Nevirapine	NNRTI	200 mg bid		Rash, hepatitis, nausea, headache	Dose-escalate from 200 mg qd over 14 days to decrease frequency of rash. Avoid concurrent use with ketoconazole, methadone, and oral contraceptives.

(continued)

Table 49–3. Currently available antiretroviral agents (*continued*).

Agent	Class of Agent[1]	Recommended Adult Dosage (oral unless otherwise indicated)	Administration Recommendation	Common Side Effects	Comments
Ritonavir	PI	600 mg bid	With food. Separate dosing with didanosine by 2 hours.	Nausea, diarrhea, paresthesias, hepatitis	Dose-escalate over 5–10 days to improve tolerance. In combination with saquinavir (400 mg bid), use 400 mg bid ritonavir. Refrigerate capsules but not oral solution. See footnote 2 for concurrent drug contraindications; avoid concurrent oral contraceptives.
Saquinavir hard gel	PI	600 mg tid or- 400 mg bid with ritonavir 400 mg bid	Within 2 hours of a full meal	Nausea, diarrhea, rhinitis	Refrigeration recommended; see footnote 2 for concurrent drug contraindications.
Saquinavir soft gel	PI	1200 mg tid or 1800 mg bid or- 1600 mg qd with ritonavir 100 mg qd	Within 2 hours of a full meal	Nausea, diarrhea, abdominal pain, dyspepsia	Refrigeration recommended; see footnote 2 for concurrent drug contraindications.
Stavudine[3]	NRTI	30–40 mg bid, depending on weight		Peripheral neuropathy, stomatitis	Avoid concurrent neuropathic drugs (eg, didanosine, zalcitabine, isoniazid); avoid concurrent use with zidovudine
Tenofovir[4]	Nucleotide inhibitor	300 mg qd	With a meal. Separate dosing with didanosine by 1–2 hours	Nausea, vomiting, diarrhea, flatulence	
Zalcitabine[3]	NRTI	0.75 mg tid	Avoid administration with antacids or food	Peripheral neuropathy; oral ulcerations	Avoid concurrent neuropathic drugs (eg, didanosine, stavudine, isoniazid
Zidovudine[3]	NRTI	200 mg tid or 300 mg bid		Anemia, neutropenia, nausea, insomnia	Avoid concurrent myelosuppressive drugs (eg, ganciclovir, ribavirin)

[1]NRTI, nucleoside reverse transcriptase inhibitor; NNRTI, nonnucleoside reverse transcriptase inhibitor; PI, protease inhibitor.

[2]The following drugs are contraindicated as concurrent medications: astemizole, terfenadine, dihydroergotamine, cisapride, pimozide, midazolam, triazolam, flecainide, propafenone, rifampin, lovastatin, simvastatin, St. John's wort.

[3]Requires dose reduction in renal insufficiency.

[4]Should not be administered to patients with renal insufficiency.

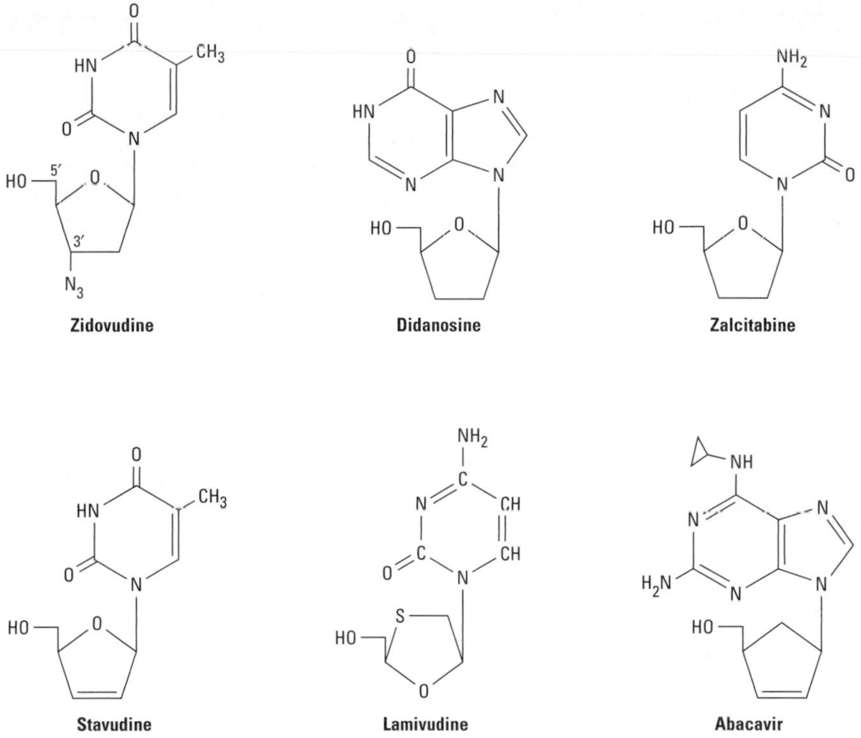

Figure 49–4. Chemical structures of some reverse transcriptase inhibitors.

may occur but tend to resolve during therapy. Less frequent side effects include thrombocytopenia, hyperpigmentation of the nails, and myopathy. Very high doses can cause anxiety, confusion, and tremulousness. Zidovudine causes vaginal neoplasms in mice; however, no human cases of genital neoplasms have been reported to date. Increased serum levels of zidovudine may occur with concomitant administration of probenecid, phenytoin, methadone, fluconazole, atovaquone, valproic acid, and lamivudine, either through inhibition of first-pass metabolism or through decreased clearance. Zidovudine may decrease phenytoin levels, and this warrants monitoring of serum phenytoin levels in epileptic patients taking both agents. Hematologic toxicity may be increased during coadministration of other myelosuppressive drugs such as ganciclovir, ribavirin, and cytotoxic agents. (See Box, Treatment of HIV-Infected Individuals: Importance of Pharmacokinetic Knowledge.)

DIDANOSINE

Didanosine (ddI) is a synthetic analog of deoxyadenosine (Figure 49–4). At acid pH, hydrolysis of the glycosidic bond between the sugar and the base moieties of ddI will inactivate the compound. Didanosine's AUC is reduced by 55% if it is ingested within 2 hours after a meal. Peak serum concentrations average 1 μg/mL after a 300 mg dose. Cerebrospinal fluid concentrations of the drug are approximately 20% of serum concentrations. Plasma protein binding is low (< 5%). The elimination half-life is 0.6–1.5 hours, but the intracellular half-life of the activated compound is as long as 12–24 hours. The drug is eliminated by glomerular filtration and tubular secretion. Dosage reduction is therefore required for low creatinine clearance, after hemodialysis or during continuous ambulatory peritoneal dialysis, and for low body weight (Table 49–3).

The original formulation, a buffered powder, has been replaced by chewable and dispersible buffered tablets with greater bioavailability (30–40%); a new enteric-coated formulation further improves patient convenience and tolerability. Since the chewable tablets contain both phenylalanine (36.5 mg) and sodium (1380 mg), caution should be exercised in patients with phenylketonuria and those taking sodium-restricted diets. Didanosine should be taken on an empty stomach and, because of the buffered formulation, should be administered at least 2 hours after administration of

---

TREATMENT OF HIV-INFECTED INDIVIDUALS: IMPORTANCE OF PHARMACOKINETIC KNOWLEDGE

In addition to knowledge about the clinical efficacy, adverse effect profile, and likelihood of emergence of resistance, the physician caring for an HIV-infected patient must be well versed in basic pharmacokinetics as well. Such patients are frequently taking multiple medications, including combinations of antiretroviral agents, prophylaxis or treatment for opportunistic infections, and opioid pain medications or methadone for maintenance therapy.

For example, an HIV-infected patient receiving ganciclovir for treatment of cytomegalovirus retinitis may be unable to tolerate concomitant therapies with the potential for additive myelosuppression, including zidovudine, ribavirin, or the interferons. Addition of colony-stimulating factor therapy for cytopenias or substitution of a different, nonmyelodepressant drug for ganciclovir may ultimately be necessary. In a patient taking didanosine (ddI), the ingestion of many other antiretroviral agents that may comprise their combination regimen, including delavirdine, indinavir, amprenavir, and tenofovir, must be separated by 2 or more hours in order to avoid interference with their absorption. Prescription of abacavir may be complicated by the fact that alcohol decreases the AUC of abacavir by 41%; the patient should be made aware of this potentially harmful interaction. The NNRTI agents and protease inhibitors for treatment of HIV infection are all metabolized by the cytochrome P450 enzyme system, primarily the 3A4 isoform. Many are also either inducers or inhibitors of CYP3A4 as well. Their myriad potential drug-drug interactions necessitate great caution during the treatment of AIDS patients. For example, an increased incidence of rifabutin-associated uveitis due to increased levels when given in combination with ritonavir is an important consideration when considering the addition of an agent for the prophylaxis or treatment against *Mycobacterium avium* complex (MAC) infection in a patient already on an effective HAART regimen. Similarly, the addition of clarithromycin for prophylaxis against MAC could potentially increase serum levels of delavirdine, ritonavir, and indinavir; conversely, levels of clarithromycin increase in the presence of indinavir and ritonavir but decrease with efavirenz. Most recently, however, these interactions have been used to advantage in the form of dual protease inhibitor regimens, based upon resultant increased plasma concentrations (C_{max}, C_{min}, and AUC) of the substrate (eg, saquinavir) when coadministered with an inducer (eg, ritonavir). Improved drug exposure, increased antiviral potency, more convenient dosing, and improved tolerability due to the use of lower doses are some of the benefits, thus improving patient adherence to the regimen. A newly licensed coformulation of lopinavir with ritonavir takes advantage of this phenomenon, known as "protease inhibitor boosting." Thus, a thorough working knowledge of potential drug-drug interactions is essential in the care of patients.

---

drugs requiring acidity for optimal absorption (eg, ketoconazole, itraconazole, dapsone).

Resistance to didanosine, due typically to mutation at codon 74 (L74V), may partially restore susceptibility to zidovudine but may confer cross-resistance to abacavir, zalcitabine, and lamivudine. High-level resistance (> 100-fold decreased susceptibility) has not been reported to date.

The major clinical toxicity associated with didanosine therapy is dose-dependent pancreatitis. Other risk factors for pancreatitis (eg, alcoholism, hypertriglyceridemia) are relative contraindications to administration of didanosine, and other drugs with the potential to cause pancreatitis should be avoided. Other reported adverse effects include painful peripheral distal neuropathy, diarrhea, hepatitis, esophageal ulceration, cardiomyopathy, and central nervous system toxicity (headache, irritability, insomnia). Asymptomatic hyperuricemia may precipitate attacks of gout in susceptible individuals. Reports of retinal changes and optic neuritis in patients receiving didanosine—particularly in adults receiving high doses and in children—indicate the utility of periodic retinal examinations.

Fluoroquinolones and tetracyclines should be administered at least 2 hours before or after didanosine in order to avoid decreased antibiotic plasma concentrations due to chelation. Coadministration with ganciclovir results in an increased AUC of didanosine and a decreased AUC of ganciclovir, while coadministration with methadone results in decreased didanosine serum levels.

LAMIVUDINE

Lamivudine (3TC) is a cytosine analog (Figure 49–4) with in vitro activity against HIV-1 that is synergistic with a variety of antiretroviral nucleoside analogs—including zidovudine and stavudine—against both zidovudine-sensitive and zidovudine-resistant HIV-1 strains. Activity against HBV is described below (see antihepatitis agents, page 821).

Oral bioavailability exceeds 80% and is not food-dependent. Peak serum levels after standard doses are 1.5 ± 0.5 μg/mL, and protein binding is less than 36%. In children, the mean CSF:plasma ratio of lamivudine was 0.2. Mean elimination half-life is 2.5 hours, while the intracellular half-life of the active 5′-triphosphate metabolite in HIV-1-infected cell lines is 10.5–15.5 hours. The majority of lamivudine is eliminated unchanged in the urine, and the dose should be reduced in patients with renal insufficiency or low body weight (Table 49–3). No supplemental doses are required after routine hemodialysis.

Lamivudine therapy rapidly selects—both in vitro and in vivo—for M184V-resistant mutants of HIV, which show high-level resistance to lamivudine and a reduction in susceptibility to abacavir, didanosine, and zalcitabine. Thus, lamivudine, like other antiretroviral agents, is best used in combination therapies that are fully suppressive of viral replication to reduce the generation of resistant mutants. The M184V mutation may restore phenotypic susceptibility to zidovudine, indicating that these two drugs in combination regimens may be particularly beneficial. However, HIV-1 strains resistant to both lamivudine and zidovudine have been isolated.

Potential side effects are headache, insomnia, fatigue, and gastrointestinal discomfort, though these are typically mild. Lamivudine's AUC increases when it is coadministered with trimethoprim-sulfamethoxazole. Peak levels of zidovudine increase when the drug is administered with lamivudine, though this effect is not felt to have clinical significance.

ZALCITABINE

Zalcitabine (ddC) is a cytosine analog (Figure 49–4) that has synergistic anti-HIV-1 activity with a variety of antiretroviral agents against both zidovudine-sensitive and zidovudine-resistant strains of HIV-1.

Zalcitabine has a relatively long intracellular half-life of 10 hours (despite its elimination half-life of 2 hours) and high oral bioavailability (> 80%). However, plasma levels decrease by 25–39% when the drug is administered with food or antacids. Plasma protein binding is low (< 4%). Cerebrospinal fluid concentrations are approximately 20% of those in the plasma.

Although a variety of mutations associated with in vitro resistance to zalcitabine have been described (eg, T69D, K65R, M186V), phenotypic resistance appears to be rare, particularly in combination regimens.

Zalcitabine therapy is associated with a dose-dependent peripheral neuropathy that can be treatment-limiting in 10–20% of patients but appears to be slowly reversible if treatment is stopped promptly. The potential for causing peripheral neuropathy constitutes a relative contraindication to use with other drugs that may cause neuropathy, including stavudine, didanosine, and isoniazid. Decreased renal clearance caused by amphotericin B, foscarnet, and aminoglycosides may increase the risk of zalcitabine neuropathy. The other major reported toxicity is oral and esophageal ulcerations. Pancreatitis occurs less frequently than with didanosine administration, but coadministration of other drugs that cause pancreatitis may increase the frequency of this adverse effect. Headache, nausea, rash, and arthralgias may occur but tend to be mild or resolve during therapy. Cardiomyopathy has rarely been reported. Zalcitabine causes thymic lymphomas in rodents, but no clinical correlates have been observed in humans.

Potential drug interactions include an increased AUC of zalcitabine when administered in combination with probenecid or cimetidine and decreased bioavailability when zalcitabine is coadministered with antacids or metoclopramide. Lamivudine inhibits the phosphorylation of zalcitabine in vitro, potentially interfering with its efficacy.

STAVUDINE

The thymidine analog stavudine (D4T) (Figure 49–4) has high oral bioavailability (86%) that is not food-dependent. The plasma half-life is 1.22 hours; the intracellular half-life is 3.5 hours; and mean cerebrospinal fluid concentrations are 55% of those of plasma. Plasma protein binding is negligible. Excretion is by active tubular secretion and glomerular filtration. The dosage of stavudine should be reduced in patients with renal insufficiency, in those receiving hemodialysis, and for low body weight (Table 49–3).

V75T and I50T mutations are associated with decreased in vitro susceptibility to stavudine; the former also confers decreased susceptibility to didanosine and zalcitabine. Clinically significant resistance to stavudine has been rare.

The major dose-limiting toxicity is a dose-related peripheral sensory neuropathy. The frequency of neuropathy may be increased when stavudine is administered with other neuropathy-inducing drugs such as zalcitabine and didanosine. Symptoms typically resolve completely upon discontinuation of stavudine; in such cases, a reduced dosage may be cautiously restarted. Potential adverse effects other than neuropathy include pancreatitis, arthralgias, and elevation in serum aminotransferases. Since zidovudine may reduce the phosphorylation of stavudine, these two drugs should generally not be used together.

ABACAVIR

In contrast to earlier NRTIs, abacavir is a guanosine analog. It is well absorbed following oral administration (83%), is unaffected by food, and is about 50% bound to plasma proteins. In single-dose studies, the elimination half-life was 1.5 hours. Cerebrospinal fluid levels are approximately one-third those of plasma. The drug is metabolized by alcohol dehydrogenase and glucuronosyltransferase to inactive metabolites that are eliminated primarily in the urine.

High-level resistance to abacavir appears to require at least two or three concomitant mutations (eg, M184V, L74V), and for that reason it tends to develop slowly. Although cross-resistance to lamivudine, didanosine, and zalcitabine has been noted in vitro in recombinant strains with abacavir-associated mutations, the clinical significance is unknown.

Hypersensitivity reactions, occasionally fatal, have been reported in 2–5% of patients receiving abacavir. Symptoms, which generally occur within the first 6 weeks of therapy, involve multiple organ systems and include fever, malaise, and gastrointestinal complaints. Skin rash may or may not be present. Laboratory abnormalities such as mildly elevated serum aminotransferase or creatine kinase levels are not specific for this reaction. Although the syndrome tends to resolve quickly with discontinuation of medication, rechallenge with abacavir following discontinuation results in return of symptoms within hours and may be fatal. Other adverse events may include rash, nausea and vomiting, diarrhea, headache, and fatigue. Adverse effects that appear to be infrequent include pancreatitis, hyperglycemia, and hypertriglyceridemia. Clinically significant adverse drug interactions have not been reported to date, though coadministration of alcohol and abacavir may result in an increase in abacavir's AUC.

NUCLEOTIDE INHIBITORS

TENOFOVIR

Tenofovir disoproxilfumarate is a prodrug that is converted in vivo to tenofovir, an acyclic nucleoside phosphonate (nucleotide) analog of adenosine. Like the NRTIs, tenofovir competitively inhibits HIV reverse transcriptase and causes chain termination after incorporation into DNA.

The oral bioavailability of tenofovir from tenofovir disopoxilfumarate, a water-soluble diester prodrug of the active ingredient tenofovir, in fasted patients is approximately 25%. Oral bioavailability is increased if the drug is ingested following a high-fat meal (increased AUC by about 40%); therefore, taking the drug along with a meal is recommended. Maximum serum concentrations are achieved in about 1 hour after taking the medication. Elimination occurs by a combination of glomerular filtration and active tubular secretion. However, only 70–80% of the dose is recovered in the urine, allowing for the possibility of hepatic metabolism as

well as alteration in hepatic insufficiency; the latter has not been studied.

Tenofovir is indicated for use in combination with other antiretroviral agents. Initial studies demonstrated potent HIV-1 suppression in treatment-experienced adults with evidence of viral replication despite ongoing antiretroviral therapy; similar benefit in antiretroviral-naive patients has yet to be demonstrated. The once-daily dosing regimen of tenofovir lends added convenience.

Varying degrees of cross-resistance to tenofovir by preexisting zidovudine-associated mutations (eg, M41L, L210W) may occur and diminish virologic response; these appear to depend on the number of specific mutations present. Presence of the 65R mutation also reduces virologic response. However, virologic response to tenofovir is not diminished in the lamivudine-abacavir-associated M184V mutation. Cross-resistance with protease inhibitor agents is unlikely.

Gastrointestinal complaints (eg, nausea, diarrhea, vomiting, and flatulence) are the most common side effects but rarely require discontinuation of therapy. Preclinical studies in several animal species have demonstrated bone toxicity (eg, osteomalacia); however, to date there has been no evidence of bone toxicity in humans. Tenofovir may compete with other drugs that are actively secreted by the kidneys, such as cidofovir, acyclovir, and ganciclovir. Tenofovir is not metabolized by the cytochrome P450 system, so drug interactions with agents metabolized by this system are unlikely. As with the NRTIs, lactic acidosis and hepatomegaly with steatosis should be watched for.

NONNUCLEOSIDE REVERSE TRANSCRIPTASE INHIBITORS (NNRTIs)

The NNRTIs bind directly to a site on the HIV-1 reverse transcriptase, resulting in blockade of RNA- and DNA-dependent DNA polymerase activities. The binding site is near to but distinct from that of the NRTIs. Unlike the latter group of agents, the NNRTIs neither compete with nucleoside triphosphates nor require phosphorylation to be active. Resistance to an NNRTI is generally rapid with monotherapy and is associated with the K103N mutation as well as the less critical Y181C/I mutation; cross-resistance among this class of agents, although observed in vitro, is of unknown clinical significance. There is no cross-resistance between the NNRTIs and the NRTIs or the protease inhibitors.

A syndrome of drug hypersensitivity has been described in patients receiving NNRTIs as well as in those receiving amprenavir or abacavir. Serious rashes, including Stevens-Johnson syndrome, have occurred.

NEVIRAPINE

The oral bioavailability of nevirapine is excellent (> 90%) and is not food-dependent. The drug is highly lipophilic, approximately 60% protein-bound, and achieves cerebrospinal fluid levels that are 45% of those in plasma. It is extensively metabolized by the CYP3A isoform to hydroxylated metabolites and then excreted, primarily in the urine.

Nevirapine is typically used as a component of a combination antiretroviral regimen. In addition, a single dose of nevirapine (200 mg) has recently been shown to be effective in the prevention of transmission of HIV from mother to newborn when administered to women at the onset of labor and followed by a 2-mg/kg oral dose given to the neonate within 3 days after delivery.

Severe and life-threatening skin rashes have occurred during nevirapine therapy, including Stevens-Johnson syndrome and toxic epidermal necrolysis. Nevirapine therapy should be immediately discontinued in patients with severe rash and in those with rash accompanied by constitutional symptoms. Rash occurs in approximately 17% of patients, most typically in the first 4–8 weeks of therapy, and is dose-limiting in about 7% of patients. When initiating therapy, gradual dose escalation over 14 days is recommended to decrease the frequency of rash. Fulminant hepatitis may occur in association with rash and fever, typically within the first 6 weeks of initiation of therapy, or may occur without a concomitant rash. Therefore, serial monitoring of liver function tests is strongly recommended. Other frequently reported adverse effects associated with nevirapine therapy are fever, nausea, headache, and somnolence.

Nevirapine is both a substrate and a moderate inducer of CYP3A metabolism, thus resulting in a 1.5-fold to twofold increase in oral clearance of itself and a corresponding decrease in the terminal phase half-life with repeated dosing—as well as decreased levels of indinavir and saquinavir if administered concurrently (see Table 49–4). Owing to an increase in nevirapine and a decrease in ketoconazole levels during coadministration, these two agents should not be given together. Nevirapine levels may increase during coadministration with inhibitors of CYP3A metabolism, such as cimetidine and the macrolide agents, and decrease in the presence of CYP3A inducers such as rifabutin and rifampin (see Table 4–2). Such agents should be coadministered cautiously and only if good alternatives are lacking.

DELAVIRDINE

Delavirdine has an oral bioavailability of about 85%, but this is reduced by antacids. It is extensively bound (about 98%) to plasma proteins. Cerebrospinal fluid levels average only 0.4% of the corresponding plasma concentrations, representing about 20% of the fraction not bound to plasma proteins. Caution should be used when administering delavirdine to patients with hepatic insufficiency because clinical experience in this situation is limited.

Table 49–4. Drug interactions pertaining to two-drug antiretroviral combinations.

Agent	Drugs That Will Increase Its Serum Levels	Drugs That Will Decrease Its Serum Levels
Amprenavir	Abacavir, delavirdine, indinavir, lopinavir, ritonavir, zidovudine	Didanosine, efavirenz, nevirapine, saquinavir
Delavirdine	Saquinavir	Didanosine, nelfinavir
Didanosine	Tenofovir	Delavirdine
Efavirenz	Ritonavir	
Indinavir	Delavirdine, lopinavir, nelfinavir, zidovudine	Amprenavir, delavirdine, efavirenz, nevirapine, ritonavir
Lamivudine	Nelfinavir	
Lopinavir	Delavirdine, ritonavir	
Nelfinavir	Delavirdine, efavirenz, ritonavir, saquinavir	
Ritonavir	Delavirdine, efavirenz	Didanosine, indinavir, zidovudine
Saquinavir	Delavirdine, lopinavir, nelfinavir, ritonavir	Efavirenz, nevirapine
Stavudine	Indinavir	
Zidovudine	Amprenavir, indinavir, lamivudine	Nelfinavir

Skin rash occurs in about 18% of patients receiving delavirdine; it typically occurs during the first month of therapy and does not preclude rechallenge. However, severe rash such as erythema multiforme and Stevens-Johnson syndrome have rarely been reported. Other adverse effects may include headache, fatigue, nausea, diarrhea, and increased serum aminotransferase levels. Delavirdine has been shown to be teratogenic in rats, causing ventricular septal defects and other malformations at exposures not unlike those achieved in humans. Thus, pregnancy should be avoided when taking delavirdine.

Delavirdine is extensively metabolized to inactive metabolites by the CYP3A and CYP2D6 enzymes. However, it also inhibits CYP3A and thus inhibits its own metabolism. In addition to its interactions with other antiretroviral agents (see Table 49–4), delavirdine will result in increased levels of numerous agents (Table 49–3). Dose reduction of indinavir and saquinavir should be considered if they are administered concurrently with delavirdine. Delavirdine plasma concentrations are reduced in the presence of antacids, phenytoin, phenobarbital, carbamazepine, rifabutin, and rifampin; concentrations are increased during coadministration with clarithromycin, fluoxetine, dexamethasone, and ketoconazole.

EFAVIRENZ

Efavirenz can be given once daily because of its long half-life (40–55 hours). It is moderately well absorbed following oral administration (45%), and bioavailability is increased to about 65% following a high-fat meal. Peak plasma concentrations are seen 3–5 hours after administration of daily doses; steady state plasma concentrations are reached in 6–10 days. Efavirenz is principally metabolized by CYP3A4 and CYP2B6 to inactive hydroxylated metabolites; the remainder is eliminated in the feces as unchanged drug. It is highly bound to albumin (> 99%). Cerebrospinal fluid levels range from 0.3% to 1.2% of plasma levels; these are approximately three times higher than the free fraction of efavirenz in the plasma. Because there is limited experience to date, caution is advised with use in patients with hepatic impairment.

The principal adverse effects of efavirenz involve the central nervous system (dizziness, drowsiness, insomnia, headache, confusion, amnesia, agitation, delusions, depression, nightmares, euphoria); these may occur in up to 50% of patients. They tend to occur during the first days of therapy and may resolve while medication is continued; administration at bedtime may be helpful. However, psychiatric symptoms may be severe. Skin rash has also been reported early in therapy in up to 28% of patients, is usually mild to moderate, and typically resolves despite continuation. Other potential adverse reactions include nausea and vomiting, diarrhea, crystalluria, elevated liver enzymes, and an increase in total serum cholesterol by 10–20%. High rates of fetal abnormalities occurred in pregnant monkeys exposed to efavirenz in doses roughly equivalent to the human dosage of 600 mg/d. Therefore, pregnancy should be avoided in women receiving efavirenz.

Efavirenz is a substrate, an inhibitor, and a moderate inducer of CYP3A4, thus inducing its own metabolism and interacting with the metabolism of many other drugs. Decreased plasma concentrations would be expected if efavirenz is administered concurrently with agents that induce CYP3A4 activity, including phenobarbital, rifampin, and rifabutin. The AUC of ethinyl estradiol is increased if coadminstered with efavirenz, and levels of clarithromycin are decreased. Efavirenz may reduce plasma methadone levels by 50% and thus should not be concurrently used. Coadministration of efavirenz with drugs that are highly dependent on CYP3A for clearance is contraindicated (see Table 4–2). Interactions with other antiretroviral agents are summarized in Table 49–4. The dose of indinavir should be increased if coadministered with efavirenz. Coadministration of efavirenz with saquinavir is to be avoided because of decreases in saquinavir plasma concentrations.

PROTEASE INHIBITORS

During the later stages of the HIV growth cycle, the Gag and Gag-Pol gene products are translated into polyproteins and then become immature budding particles. Protease is responsible for cleaving these precursor molecules to produce the final structural proteins of the mature virion core. By preventing cleavage of the Gag-Pol polyprotein, protease inhibitors result in the production of immature, noninfectious viral particles. Unfortunately, specific genotypic alterations that confer phenotypic resistance is fairly common with these agents, thus contraindicating monotherapy. The issue of cross-resistance among agents in this class of drugs is complex and requires further investigation; it appears to require a minimum of four substitutions in the gene.

A syndrome of redistribution and accumulation of body fat that includes central obesity, dorsocervical fat enlargement (buffalo hump), peripheral and facial wasting, breast enlargement, and a cushingoid appearance has been observed in patients receiving antiretroviral therapy. Although controversial, these abnormalities appear to be particularly associated with the use of protease inhibitors. Concurrent increases in triglyceride and LDL levels, along with glucose intolerance and insulin resistance, have been noted as well. The cause is not yet known.

Protease inhibitors have also been associated with increased spontaneous bleeding in patients with hemophilia A or B.

All of the antiretroviral protease inhibitors are substrates of the CYP3A4 isoenzyme. As such, there is a potential for drug-drug interactions. In addition, however, certain of the protease inhibitors are CYP3A4 inhibitors as well (eg, amprenavir, indinavir, lopinavir, nelfinavir, ritonavir, and saquinavir), thus having the potential to cause decreased clearance and increased plasma concentrations of other substrate drugs. For this reason, the CYP3A4 inhibitors should not be administered concurrently with agents that are heavily metabolized by CYP3A (see Table 4–2). Ritonavir also functions as a CYP3A4 inducer, such that potential drug-drug interactions may be clinically beneficial (see below).

SAQUINAVIR

In its original formulation as a hard gel capsule (saquinavir-H; Invirase), oral saquinavir was poorly bioavailable (about 4% in the fed state). It was therefore largely replaced in clinical use by a soft gel capsule formulation (saquinavir-S; Fortovase), in which absorption was increased approximately threefold. However, reformulation of saquinavir-H for once-daily dosing in combination with low-dose ritonavir (see below) has both improved antiviral efficacy and decreased the gastrointestinal side effects typically associated with saquinavir-S. Moreover, coadministration of saquinavir-H with ritonavir results in blood levels of saquinavir similar to those associated with saquinavir-S, thus capitalizing on the pharmacokinetic interaction of the two agents.

Both formulations of saquinavir should be taken within 2 hours after a fatty meal for enhanced absorption. Saquinavir has a large volume of distribution but is 98% protein-bound; penetration into the cerebrospinal fluid is negligible. The elimination half-life is 12 hours. Excretion is primarily in the feces. Reported adverse effects include gastrointestinal discomfort (nausea, diarrhea, abdominal discomfort, dyspepsia; these are more common with Fortovase) and rhinitis. Although refrigeration is recommended for storage, the capsules are stable at room temperature for up to 3 months.

Saquinavir is subject to extensive first-pass metabolism by CYP3A4, and functions as a CYP3A4 inhibitor as well as a substrate; thus, it should be used with the same precautions regarding drug-drug interactions as the other protease inhibitors. Coadministration with the CYP3A4 inhibitor ritonavir has been adopted by clinicians because inhibition of first-pass metabolism of saquinavir by ritonavir can result in higher—and thus more efficacious—levels of saquinavir (see Tables 49–3 and 49–4). Liver function tests should be monitored if saquinavir is coadministered with delavirdine.

The most common critical mutations are L90M and G48V, conferring an approximately tenfold decrease in susceptibility.

RITONAVIR

Ritonavir is an inhibitor of HIV-1 and HIV-2 proteases with high bioavailability (about 75%) that increases when the drug is given with food. Metabolism to an active metabolite occurs via the CYP3A and CYP2D6 isoforms; excretion is primarily in the feces. Caution is advised when administering the drug to persons with impaired hepatic function. Capsules (but not the oral solution) should be refrigerated for storage.

Resistance is associated with mutations at positions 84, 82, 71, 63, and 46, of which the I84V mutation appears to be the most critical.

The most common adverse effects of ritonavir are gastrointestinal disturbances, paresthesias (circumoral and peripheral), elevated serum aminotransferase levels, altered taste, and hypertriglyceridemia. Nausea, vomiting, and abdominal pain typically occur during the first few weeks of therapy, and patients should be told to expect them. Slow dose escalation over 4–5 days is recommended to decrease the frequency of dose-limiting side effects. Liver adenomas and carcinomas have been induced in male mice receiving ritonavir; no similar effects have been observed to date in humans.

Ease of administration is limited by ritonavir's numerous drug interactions. Ritonavir is both a substrate and an inhibitor of CYP3A4; as such, coadministration with agents heavily metabolized by CYP3A must be approached with the same precautions discussed above. In addition, since ritonavir is an inhibitor of the CYP3A4 isoenzyme, concurrent administration with other PIs results in increased plasma levels of the latter drugs; these interactions have been exploited to permit more convenient dosing (see Tables 49–3 and 49–4).

LOPINAVIR/RITONAVIR

Several studies have shown enhanced efficacy or improved tolerability of two protease inhibitors administered together. Lopinavir 100/ritonavir 400 is a licensed combination in which subtherapeutic doses of ritonavir inhibit the CYP3A-mediated metabolism of lopinavir, thereby resulting in increased exposure to lopinavir. Trough levels of lopinavir are greater than the median HIV-1 wild type 50% inhibitory concentration, thus maintaining potent viral suppression as well as providing a pharmacologic barrier to the emergence of resistance. In addition to improved patient compliance because of the reduced pill burden with twice-daily dosing, lopinavir/ritonavir is generally well tolerated.

Absorption is enhanced with food. Lopinavir is 98–99% protein-bound and is extensively metabolized by the CYP3A isozyme of the hepatic cytochrome P450 system, which is inhibited by ritonavir. Serum levels of lopinavir may be increased in patients with hepatic impairment.

The most common adverse effects are diarrhea, abdominal pain, nausea, vomiting, and asthenia. Potential drug-drug interactions are extensive (see Ritonavir and Table 49–4). Drugs that are highly dependent on CYP3A or CYP2D6 for clearance and for which elevated plasma concentrations may be serious or clinically significant—including those listed in Table 49–4 as well as those listed in Table 4–2—should not be given with lopinavir/ritonavir. Coadministration with rifampin, carbamazepine, phenobarbital, phenytoin, dexamethasone, or St. John's wort (*Hypericum perforatum*) may reduce levels of lopinavir.

INDINAVIR

Indinavir must be consumed on an empty stomach for maximal absorption. Oral bioavailability is about 65%, and the drug is about 60% protein-bound. Indinavir has the highest cerebrospinal fluid penetration of the existing protease inhibitors—up to 76% of serum levels. Excretion is primarily fecal. An increase in AUC by 60% and in half-life from 1.8 to 2.8 hours in the setting of hepatic insufficiency necessitates dose reduction.

Resistance may be associated with multiple mutations, and the number of codon alterations (typically substitutions) present tends to predict the level of phenotypic resistance. Mutations at positions at 46 or 82 seem to predict phenotypic resistance most consistently. Resistance to indinavir is associated with a loss of susceptibility to ritonavir; however, susceptibility to other protease inhibitors in indinavir-resistant isolates is less predictable.

The most common adverse effects are indirect hyperbilirubinemia and nephrolithiasis due to crystallization of the drug. Nephrolithiasis can occur within days after initiating therapy, with an estimated incidence of 3–15%, and may be associated with renal failure. Consumption of at least 48 oz of water daily is important to maintain adequate hydration and prevent nephrolithiasis. Thrombocytopenia, elevations of serum aminotransferase levels, nausea, diarrhea, and irritability have also been reported. There have also been rare cases of acute hemolytic anemia. In rats, high doses of indinavir are associated with development of thyroid adenomas.

Since indinavir is a substrate as well as an inhibitor of CYP3A4, numerous and complex drug interactions can occur as described above. Indinavir levels decrease with concurrent use of rifabutin, fluconazole, St. John's wort, and rifampin. Caution is advised with other 3A4 inducers also, including phenobarbital, phenytoin, carbamazepine, and dexamethasone. Dose reduction of indinavir should be considered if coadministered with delavirdine, ketoconazole, or itraconazole, while an increase in the dose of indinavir is indicated if the drug is coadministered with efavirenz or rifabutin.

NELFINAVIR

Nelfinavir has higher absorption in the fed state (increased AUC by two- to threefold), is extensively protein-bound (> 98%), undergoes metabolism by CYP3A, and is excreted primarily in the feces. The plasma half-life in humans is 3.5–5 hours. The D30N mutation appears to be particularly closely linked with phenotypic resistance in isolates obtained from clinical trials.

The most frequent adverse effects associated with nelfinavir are diarrhea and flatulence. Diarrhea can be dose-limiting but often responds to antidiarrheal medications. Like the other protease inhibitors, nelfinavir is an inhibitor of the CYP3A system, and multiple drug interactions may occur as described above. Interactions with antiretroviral agents are summarized in Table 49–4; others may be found in Table 4–2.

AMPRENAVIR

Amprenavir is rapidly absorbed from the gastrointestinal tract and can be taken with or without food. However, high-fat meals may decrease absorption and thus should be avoided. The plasma half-life is relatively long (7–10.6 hours). Protein binding is about 90%. Amprenavir is metabolized in the liver by CYP3A4; it is contraindicated in the setting of hepatic insufficiency.

The key in vitro resistance mutation to amprenavir appears to be I50V. Evidence to date suggests that cross-resistance to other members of the protease inhibitor class of drugs may be less prevalent with amprenavir than with previously available compounds.

The most common adverse effects of amprenavir have been nausea, diarrhea, vomiting, perioral paresthesias, depression, and rash. Up to 3% of patients in clinical trials to date have had rashes (including Stevens-Johnson syndrome) severe enough to warrant drug discontinuation.

Amprenavir is both a substrate and an inhibitor of CYP3A4 and is contraindicated with numerous other drugs (see Tables 49–3 and 4–2). The oral solution, which contains propylene glycol, is contraindicated in young children, pregnant women, and in those using metronidazole or disulfiram.

FUSION INHIBITORS

ENFUVIRTIDE

Enfuvirtide (formerly called T-20) is a newly approved antiretroviral agent of a novel class, ie, a fusion inhibitor that blocks entry into the cell. Enfuvirtide, a synthetic 36-amino-acid peptide, binds to the gp41 subunit of the viral envelope glycoprotein, preventing the conformational changes required for the fusion of the viral and cellular membranes.

Resistance to enfuvirtide can occur, and the frequency and mechanisms of this phenomenon are currently being investigated. However, enfuvirtide completely lacks cross-resistance to the other currently approved antiretroviral drug classes.

The drug is administered subcutaneously in combination with other antiretroviral agents in treatment-experienced patients with persistent HIV-1 replication despite ongoing therapy. Protein binding is high (92%), and metabolism appears to be by proteolytic hydrolysis without involvement of the cytochrome p450 system. Elimination half-life is 3.8 hours, and time to peak concentration is 8 hours.

The most common side effects associated with enfuvirtide therapy are local injection site reactions. Hypersensitivity reactions may occur, are of varying severity, and may recur on rechallenge. Eosinophilia has also been noted. No interactions have been identified that would require alteration of other antiretroviral drugs.

INVESTIGATIONAL ANTIRETROVIRAL AGENTS

New therapies are being sought offering the advantages of once-daily dosing, smaller pill size, lower incidences of adverse effects, new viral targets, and activity against virus that is resistant to other agents. Agents under evaluation or reformulation for once-daily dosing include stavudine and nevirapine. The NRTI agents amdoxovir and emtricitabine, the NNRTI agents DPC-083 and TMC-125, and the protease inhibitors atazanavir, tipranavir, and fosamprenavir (the prodrug of amprenavir) are among the new agents currently in development. In addition, new drug classes such as entry inhibitors and integrase inhibitors are under clinical investigation.

IV. ANTI-HEPATITIS AGENTS

Agents effective against hepatitis B virus (HBV) and hepatitis C virus (HCV) are now available (see Table 49–5). Although treatment is suppressive rather than curative, the high prevalence of these infections worldwide, with their concomitant morbidity and mortality, reflect a critical need for improved therapeutics.

LAMIVUDINE

The pharmacokinetics and safety profile of lamivudine are described above (see page 814). The more prolonged intracellular half-life in HBV cell lines (17–19 hours) than in HIV-infected cell lines (see above) allows for lower doses, administered less frequently, for hepatitis. Lamivudine can be safely administered to patients with decompensated liver disease.

Lamivudine achieves almost universal HBV DNA suppression, with decreases in viral replication by about 3-4 log copies in most patients. Response to lamivudine is more rapid than to interferon (see below), with HBV DNA levels decreasing by approximately 97% after 2 weeks of therapy and 98% by 1 year. However, evidence of viral replication recurs in over 80% upon discontinuation of therapy. Seroconversion of HBeAg antigen from positive to negative occurs in only about 20% of patients; yet in patients who do achieve seroconversion with lamivudine, the response is typically sustained. Progression to liver fibrosis is less frequent in patients treated with lamivudine compared with placebo. The height of the pretreatment serum ALT level may be the best predictor of HBeAg seroconversion.

Chronic therapy with lamivudine in patients with hepatitis may ultimately be limited by the emergence of lamivudine-resistant HBV isolates with YMDD mutation. Emergence of this mutation, which typically occurs within 8–9 months of therapy, is associated with reappearance of detectable levels of HBV DNA. The estimated rate of YMDD mutation is about 20% per year.

In the doses used for HBV infection, lamivudine has an excellent safety profile. No evidence of mitochondrial toxicity has been reported.

ADEFOVIR

Although initially and abortively developed for treatment of HIV infection, adefovir has been recently approved, at lower and less toxic doses, for treatment of HBV infection. Like tenofovir (see Antiretroviral Agents), adefovir is a nucleotide analog. As an analog of adenosine monophosphate, adefovir is phosphorylated by cellular kinases to the active disphosphate metabolite; it then competitively inhibits HBV DNA polymerase and results in chain termination after incorporation into the viral DNA.

Oral bioavailability is about 59% and is unaffected by meals. Peak serum levels occur at a median of 1.75

Table 49–5. Drugs used to treat viral hepatitis.

Agent	Indication	Recommended Adult Dosage	Route of Administration
Hepatitis B			
Lamivudine[1]	Chronic hepatitis B	100 mg once daily	Oral
Adefovir[1]	Chronic hepatitis B	10 mg once daily	Oral
Interferon alfa-2b	Chronic hepatitis B	5 million units once daily or– 10 million units three times weekly	Subcutaneous or intramuscular
Hepatitis C			
Interferon alfa-2b	Acute hepatitis C	5 million units once daily for 3 weeks, then 5 million units three times weekly	Subcutaneous or intramuscular
Interferon alfa-2a	Chronic hepatitis C[2]	3 million units three times weekly	Subcutaneous or intramuscular
Interferon alfa-2b	Chronic hepatitis C[2]	3 million units three times weekly	Subcutaneous or intramuscular
Interferon alfacon-1	Chronic hepatitis C[2]	9 μg three times weekly (consider 15 μg three times weekly if patient relapses or is unresponsive)	Subcutaneous
Pegylated interferon alfa-2a	Chronic hepatitis C[2]	180 μg once weekly	Subcutaneous
Pegylated interferon alfa-2b	Chronic hepatitis C[2]	40–150 μg once weekly, according to weight	Subcutaneous

[1]Dosage must be reduced in patients with renal insufficiency.

[2]For all agents, combination therapy with oral ribavirin is recommended if tolerated (dosage, 1000–1200 mg/d according to weight).

hours after dosing, and the terminal elimination half-life is approximately 7.5 hours. Protein binding is less than 4%. Adefovir is renally excreted by a combination of glomerular filtration and active tubular secretion. Dosing interval should be modified in patients with impaired renal function. Approximately 35% of the adefovir dose is removed during a 4-hour hemodialysis.

Recent placebo-controlled trials showed that adefovir resulted in significant suppression of HBV replication and improvement in liver histology and fibrosis at 1 year. However, as with lamivudine, serum HBV DNA reappeared following cessation of therapy.

Adefovir maintains activity against lamivudine-resistant strains of HBV, and no resistance to adefovir was detected in patients who had received continuous treatment for up to 1 year.

Adefovir is associated with a dose-dependent nephrotoxicity. The risk is low for treatment durations of up to 1 year at its recommended dosage for HBV but may rise in patients with preexisting renal dysfunction or in those treated for longer durations. Also, as with the antiretroviral nucleoside analogs (see Nucleoside Reverse Transcriptase Inhibitors), lactic acidosis and

severe hepatomegaly with steatosis may occur. When coadministered with ibuprofen, the AUC of adefovir is increased by about 23%, apparently due to higher oral bioavailabilty.

INTERFERON ALFA

Interferons are endogenous proteins that exert complex antiviral, immunomodulatory, and antiproliferative activities through cellular metabolic processes involving synthesis of both RNA and protein (see Chapter 56). They appear to function by binding to specific membrane receptors on the cell surface and initiating a series of intracellular events that include enzyme induction, suppression of cell proliferation, immunomodulatory activities, and inhibition of virus replication. They are classified according to the cell type from which they were derived, and each of the three immunologically distinct major classes of human interferons has unique physicochemical characteristics and different producer cells, inducers, and biologic effects.

Interferon alfa preparations are available for treatment of both HBV and HCV virus infections. Interferon alfa-2b is the only preparation licensed for treatment of HBV infection and for acute hepatitis C. Interferon alfa-2b leads to loss of HBeAg, normalization of serum aminotransferases, and sustained histologic improvement in approximately one-third of patients with chronic hepatitis B, thus reducing the risk of progressive liver disease.

In acute hepatitis C, the rate of clearance of the virus without therapy is estimated to be 15–30%. No therapy has yet been proved effective in the treatment of acute hepatitis C; however, a recent study suggested that interferon alfa-2b, in doses higher than those used for treatment of chronic hepatitis C (see Table 49–5), resulted in a sustained rate of clearance of 98%.

Several interferon alfa preparations are available for the treatment of patients with chronic hepatitis C infection, including interferon alfa-2a, interferon alfa-2b, interferon alfacon-2, pegylated interferon alfa-2a, and pegylated interferon alfa-2b, as described below. Factors associated with a favorable response to therapy include HCV genotype 2 or 3, absence of cirrhosis on liver biopsy, and low pretreatment HCV RNA levels. For all agents, combination therapy with oral ribavirin in patients with chronic hepatitis C is more effective than monotherapy with either interferon or ribavirin alone, increasing the percentage of previously untreated patients with a sustained virologic response from approximately 16% to approximately 40%. Therefore, monotherapy is recommended only in patients who cannot tolerate ribavirin. The time to maximal response may range from 24 weeks to 48 weeks of therapy.

Interferon alfa-2a and interferon alfa-2b may be administered subcutaneously or intramuscularly, while interferon alfacon-1 is administered subcutaneously (see Table 49–5). Maximum serum concentrations occur approximately 4 hours after intramuscular administration and approximately 7 hours after subcutaneous administration; elimination half-life is 2–5 hours for interferon alfa-2a and 2b, depending on the route of administration. The half-life of interferon alfacon-1 in patients with chronic hepatitis C ranged from 6 hours to 10 hours. Alfa interferons are filtered at the glomeruli and undergo rapid proteolytic degradation during tubular reabsorption, such that detection in the systemic circulation is negligible. Liver metabolism and subsequent biliary excretion are considered minor pathways.

Typical side effects are constitutional in nature, including a flu-like syndrome within 6 hours after dosing in more than 30% of patients that tends to resolve upon continued administration. Other potential adverse effects include thrombocytopenia, granulocytopenia, elevation in serum aminotransferase levels, induction of autoantibodies, nausea, fatigue, headache, arthralgias, rash, alopecia, anorexia, hypotension, and edema. Severe neuropsychiatric side effects may occur.

Absolute contraindications to therapy are psychosis, severe depression, neutropenia, thrombocytopenia, symptomatic heart disease, decompensated cirrhosis, uncontrolled seizures, and a history of organ transplantation (other than liver). Alfa interferons are abortifacient in primates and should not be administered in pregnancy.

PEGYLATED INTERFERON ALFA

Pegylated interferon alfa-2a (peginterferon alfa-2a) and pegylated interferon alfa-2b (peginterferon alfa-2b) have recently been introduced for the treatment of patients with chronic hepatitis C infection. In these agents, a linear or branched polyethylene glycol (PEG) moiety is attached to interferon by a covalent bond. Reduced clearance and sustained absorption results in an increased half-life and steadier drug concentrations, allowing for less frequent dosing.

In comparison with the nonpegylated interferon alfa compounds, the pegylated products have substantially longer terminal half-lives and slower clearance. Maximum serum concentrations occur between 15 hours and 44 hours after dosing and are sustained for up to 48–72 hours. For pegylated interferon alfa-2a, maximum serum concentrations occur at 72–96 hours after dosing and are sustained for up to 168 hours. In patients with chronic hepatitis C, the mean terminal half-life was 80 hours for pegylated interferon alfa-2a (versus 5.1 hours for interferon alfa-2a) and was about 40 hours for pegylated interferon alfa-2b (versus 2–3 hours for interferon alfa-2b). Renal elimination accounts for about 30% of clearance, and clearance is reduced by approximately half in subjects with impaired renal function. Although dose reduction in renal insufficiency is not specifically recommended, caution is advised in this setting.

Efficacy appears to be superior to therapy with nonpegylated interferons in controlled clinical trials, particularly as regards the proportion of patients with sustained virologic responses. As with the nonpegylated interferon alfa agents, combination therapy of the pegylated interferon alfa compounds with ribavirin is more effective than monotherapy.

Adverse events are similar to those of the interferon alfa agents described above. The PEG molecule is a nontoxic polymer that is readily excreted in the urine.

RIBAVIRIN

Ribavirin is a guanosine analog that is phosphorylated intracellularly by host cell enzymes. Although its mechanism of action has not been fully elucidated, it appears to interfere with the synthesis of guanosine triphosphate, to inhibit capping of viral messenger RNA, and to inhibit the viral RNA-dependent RNA polymerase of certain viruses. Ribavirin triphosphate inhibits the replication of DNA and RNA viruses, including influenza A and B, parainfluenza, respiratory syncytial virus, paramyxoviruses, HCV, and HIV-1.

The absolute oral bioavailability of ribavirin is about 64%, increases with high-fat meals, and decreases with coadministration of antacids. Since elimination is mostly through the urine, clearance is decreased in patients with creatinine clearances less than 30 mL/min.

Ribavirin capsules in combination with subcutaneous interferon alfa-2b are effective for the treatment of chronic hepatitis C infection in patients with compensated liver disease (see Antihepatitis Agents, above). Monotherapy with ribavirin alone is not effective.

Approximately 10–20% of patients experience a dose-dependent hemolytic anemia that may be dose-limiting. Other side effects are depression, fatigue, irritability, rash, cough, insomnia, nausea, and pruritus. Absolute contraindications to ribavirin therapy include anemia, end-stage renal failure, severe heart disease, and pregnancy. Ribavirin is both teratogenic in animals and mutagenic in mammalian cells.

INVESTIGATIONAL AGENTS

The nucleoside analogs entecavir and clevudine, the nucleotide analog emtricitabine, and the immunologic modulators theradigm-HBV and thymosin alpha-1 are new agents under evaluation for the treatment of HBV infection.

V. ANTI-INFLUENZA AGENTS

AMANTADINE & RIMANTADINE

Amantadine (1-aminoadamantane hydrochloride) and its α-methyl derivative, rimantadine, are cyclic amines that inhibit uncoating of the viral RNA of influenza A within infected host cells, thus preventing its replication. Rimantadine is four to ten times more active than amantadine in vitro. Steady state peak plasma levels in healthy young adults average 0.5—0.8 μg/mL for amantadine; elderly persons require only one half of the weight-adjusted dose for young adults to achieve equivalent trough plasma levels of 0.3 μg/mL. While amantadine is excreted unmetabolized in the urine, rimantadine undergoes extensive metabolism by hydroxylation, conjugation, and glucuronidation before urinary excretion. Dose reductions are required for both agents in the elderly, in renal insufficiency, and for rimantadine in patients with marked hepatic insufficiency. No supplemental doses of either agent are required after hemodial-

ysis. Plasma half-life is 12–18 hours for amantadine and 24–36 hours for rimantadine.

Both amantadine and rimantadine, in doses of 100 mg twice daily or 200 mg once daily, are approximately 70–90% protective in the prevention of clinical illness by influenza A. The effectiveness of postexposure prophylaxis is inconsistent. When begun within 1–2 days after the onset of clinical symptoms of influenza, both drugs reduce the duration of fever and systemic complaints by 1–2 days.

The primary target for both agents is the M2 protein within the viral membrane; this target incurs both specificity against influenza A (since influenza B contains a different protein in its membrane) and a mutation-prone site, causing the rapid development of resistance in up to 50% of treated individuals. Transmission of resistant virus to household contacts has been documented. Cross-resistance to zanamivir and oseltamivir does not occur.

The most common adverse effects are gastrointestinal intolerance and central nervous system complaints (eg, nervousness, difficulty in concentrating, lightheadedness); the latter are less frequent with rimantadine than with amantadine. The central nervous system toxicity of amantadine may be increased with concomitant antihistamines, anticholinergic drugs, hydrochlorothiazide, and trimethoprim-sulfamethoxazole. Serious neurotoxic reactions, occasionally fatal, may occur in association with high amantadine plasma concentrations (1–5 μg/mL). Acute amantadine overdose is associated with anticholinergic effects. Amantadine is teratogenic and embrytoxic in rodents, and birth defects have been reported after exposure during pregnancy.

ZANAMIVIR & OSELTAMIVIR

Neuraminidase is an essential viral glycoprotein for virus replication and release. The neuraminidase inhibitors zanamivir and oseltamivir have recently been approved for the treatment of acute uncomplicated influenza infection. When a 5-day course of therapy is initiated within 36–48 hours after the onset of symptoms, use of either agent shortens the severity and duration of illness and may decrease the incidence of respiratory complications in children and adults. Unlike amantadine and rimantidine, zanamivir and oseltamivir have activity against both influenza A and influenza B. Zanamivir is administered via oral inhaler. The compound displays poor oral bioavailability, limited plasma protein binding, rapid renal clearance, and absence of significant metabolism. Nasal and throat discomfort may occur—as well as bronchospasm in patients with reactive airway disease.

Oseltamivir is an orally administered prodrug that is activated in the gut and liver. Dosage is 75 mg twice daily. The half-life of oseltamivir is 6–10 hours, and excretion is primarily in the urine. In addition to treatment of influenza, prophylaxis once daily may be effective in preventing influenza. Potential side effects include nausea and vomiting, which may be decreased by administration with food.

Decreased susceptibility to zanamivir and oseltamivir in vitro is associated with mutations in viral neuraminidase or hemagglutinin. A resistant virus was recovered from an immunocompromised patient who had received zanamivir for 2 weeks. However, the incidence and clinical significance of resistance are not yet known.

VI. OTHER ANTIVIRAL AGENTS

INTERFERONS

Interferons have been studied for numerous clinical indications. In addition to HBV and HCV infections (see Antihepatitis Agents, above), intralesional injection of interferon alfa-2b or alfa-n3 may be used for treatment of condylomata acuminata.

RIBAVIRIN

In addition to oral administration for hepatitis C infection in combination with interferon alfa (see above), aerosolized ribavirin is administered by nebulizer (20 mg/mL for 12–18 hours per day for 3–7 days) to children and infants with severe respiratory syncytial virus (RSV) bronchiolitis or pneumonia, reducing the severity and duration of illness. Aerosolized ribavirin has also been used to treat influenza A and B infection but has not gained widespread use. Aerosolized ribavirin is generally well tolerated but may cause conjunctival or bronchial irritation. Health care workers should be protected against extended inhalation exposure.

Intravenous ribavirin decreases mortality in Lassa fever and other viral hemorrhagic fevers if started early. Clinical benefit has been reported in cases of severe measles pneumonitis, and continuous infusion of ribavirin decreased virus shedding in several patients with severe lower respiratory tract influenza or parainfluenza infections. Peak plasma concentrations are approximately tenfold higher than with oral administration and occur earlier (ie, at 0.5 hours after dosing). At steady state, cerebrospinal fluid levels are about 70% of those in plasma.

PALIVIZUMAB

Palivizumab is a humanized monoclonal antibody directed against the F glycoprotein on the surface of RSV. It was recently approved for the prevention of RSV infection in high-risk infants and children such as premature infants and those with bronchopulmonary dysplasia. A placebo-controlled trial utilizing once-monthly intramuscular injections (15 mg/kg) for 5 months beginning at the start of the RSV season demonstrated a 55% reduction in the risk of hospitalization for RSV in treated patients. The major observed adverse effect has been elevation in serum aminotransferase levels.

IMIQUIMOD

Imiquimod is an immune response modifier shown to be effective in the topical treatment of external genital and perianal warts (ie, condyloma acuminatum; see Chapter 62). The mechanism of action against these human papillomavirus (HPV)-induced lesions is unknown. The 5% cream is to be applied three times weekly. Local skin reactions are the most common side effect.

PREPARATIONS AVAILABLE

Abacavir (Ziagen)
 Oral: 300 mg tablets; 20 mg/mL solution
 Oral (Trizir): 300 mg tablets in combination with 150 mg lamivudine and 300 mg zidovudine
Acyclovir (generic, Zovirax)
 Oral: 200 mg capsules; 400, 800 mg tablets; 200 mg/5 mL suspension
 Parenteral: 50 mg/mL; powder to reconstitute for injection (500, 1000 mg/vial)
 Topical: 5% ointment
Adefovir (Hepsera)
 Oral: 10 mg tablets

Amantadine (generic, Symmetrel)
 Oral: 100 mg capsules, tablets; 50 mg/5 mL syrup
Amprenavir (Agenerase)
 Oral: 50, 150 mg capsules; 15 mg/mL solution
Cidofovir (Vistide)
 Parenteral: 375 mg/vial (75 mg/mL) for IV injection
Delavirdine (Rescriptor)
 Oral: 100, 200 mg tablets
Didanosine (dideoxyinosine, ddl)
 Oral (Videx): 25, 50, 100, 150, 200 mg tablets; 100, 167, 250 mg powder for oral solution; 2, 4 g powder for pediatric solution

Oral (Videx-EC): 125, 200, 250, 400 mg delayed release capsules

Efavirenz (Sustiva)
Oral: 50, 100, 200 mg capsules; 600 mg tablets

Enfuvirtide (Fuzeon)
Parenteral: 90 mg/mL for injection

Famciclovir (Famvir)
Oral: 125, 250, 500 mg tablets

Fomivirsen (Vitravene)
Intravitreal: 6.6 mg/mL for injection

Foscarnet (Foscavir)
Parenteral: 24 mg/mL for IV injection

Ganciclovir (Cytovene)
Oral: 250, 500 mg capsules
Parenteral: 500 mg/vial for IV injection
Intraocular implant (Vitrasert): 4.5 mg ganciclovir/implant

Idoxuridine (Herplex)
Ophthalmic: 0.1% solution

Imiquimod (Aldera)
Topical: 5% cream

Indinavir (Crixivan)
Oral: 100, 200, 333, 400 mg capsules

Interferon alfa-2a (Roferon-A)
Parenteral: 3, 6, 9, 36 million IU vials

Interferon alfa-2b (Intron-A)
Parenteral: 3, 5, 10, 18, 25, and 50 million IU vials

Interferon alfa-2b (Rebetron)
Parenteral: 3 million IU vials (supplied with oral ribavirin, 200 mg capsules)

Interferon alfa-n3 (Alferon N)
Parenteral: 5 million IU/vial

Interferon alfacon-1 (Infergen)
Parenteral: 9 and 15 μg vials

Lamivudine (Epivir)
Oral (Epivir): 150, 300 mg tablets; 10 mg/mL oral solution
Oral (Epivir-HBV): 100 mg tablets; 5 mg/mL solution
Oral (Combivir): 150 mg tablets in combination with 300 mg zidovudine
Oral (Trizir): 300 mg tablets in combination with 150 mg lamivudine and 300 mg zidovudine

Lopinavir/ritonavir (Kaletra)
Oral: 133.3 mg/33.3 mg capsules; 400 mg/100 mg per 5 mL solution

Nelfinavir (Viracept)
Oral: 250 mg tablets; 50 mg/g powder

Nevirapine (Viramune)
Oral: 200 mg tablets; 50 mg/5 mL suspension

Oseltamivir (Tamiflu)
Oral: 75 mg capsules; powder to reconstitute as suspension (12 mg/mL)

Palivizumab (Synagis)
Parenteral: 50, 100 mg/vial

Peginterferon alfa-2a (pegylated interferon-alfa 2a, Pegasys)
Parenteral: 180 μg/mL

Peginterferon alfa-2b (pegylated interferon-alfa 2b, PEG-Intron)
Parenteral: powder to reconstitute as 100, 160, 240, 300 μg/mL injection

Penciclovir (Denavir)
Topical: 1% cream

Ribavirin
Aerosol (Virazole): powder to reconstitute for aerosol; 6 gm/100 mL vial
Oral (Rebetol): 200 mg capsules
Oral (Rebetron): 200 mg in combination with 3 million units interferon alfa-2b (Intron-A)

Rimantadine (Flumadine)
Oral: 100 mg tablets; 50 mg/5 mL syrup

Ritonavir (Norvir)
Oral: 100 mg capsules; 80 mg/mL oral solution

Saquinavir
Oral (Invirase): 200 mg hard gel capsules
Oral (Fortovase): 200 mg soft gel capsules

Stavudine (Zerit)
Oral: 15, 20, 30, 40 mg capsules; powder for 1 mg/mL oral solution

Tenofovir (Viread)
Oral: 300 mg tablets

Trifluridine (Viroptic)
Topical: 1% ophthalmic solution

Valacyclovir (Valtrex)
Oral: 500, 1000 mg tablets

Valganciclovir (Valcyte)
Oral: 450 mg capsules

Zalcitabine (dideoxycytidine, ddC) (Hivid)
Oral: 0.375, 0.75 mg tablets

Zanamivir (Relenza)
Inhalational: 5 mg/rotadisk

Zidovudine (azidothymidine, AZT) (Retrovir)
Oral: 100 mg capsules, 300 mg tablets, 50 mg/5 mL syrup
Oral (Combivir): 300 mg tablets in combination with 150 mg lamivudine
Oral (Trizir): 300 mg tablets in combination with 150 mg lamivudine and 300 mg zidovudine
Parenteral: 10 mg/mL

REFERENCES

Baker DE: Pegylated interferons. Rev Gastroenterol Disord 2001;1:87.

Cocohoba JM, McNicholl IR: Valganciclovir: an advance in cytomegalovirus therapeutics. Ann Pharmacother 2001; 36:2075.

Drugs for non-HIV viral infections. Med Lett Drugs Ther 2002;44:9.

Geary RS, Henry SP, Grillone LR: Fomivirsen: Clinical pharmacology and potential drug interactions. Clin Pharmacokinet 2002; 41:255.

Johnson MA et al: Clinical pharmacokinetics of lamivudine. Clin Pharmacokinet 1999;36:41.

Kimberlin DW et al: Safety and efficacy of high-dose intravenous acyclovir in the management of neonatal herpes simplex virus infections. Pediatrics 2001;108:230.

Lauer GM, Walker BD: Hepatitis C infection. N Engl J Med 2001;345:41.

Malik AH, Lee WM: Chronic hepatitis B virus infection: treatment strategies for the next millenium. Ann Intern Med 2000; 132:723.

Martin DF et al: A controlled trial of valganciclovir as induction therapy for cytomegalovirus retinitis. N Engl J Med 2002; 346:1119.

Martin DF et al: Oral ganciclovir for patients with cytomegalovirus retinitis treated with a ganciclovir implant. N Engl J Med 1999;340:1063.

Piscitelli SC, Gallicano KD: Interactions among drugs for HIV and opportunistic infections. N Engl J Med 2001;344:984

Qazi NA et al: Lopinavir/ritonavir (ABT-378/r). Expert Opin Pharmacother 2002;3:315.

Recommendations for use of antiretroviral drugs in pregnant HIV-1-infected women for maternal health and interventions to reduce perinatal HIV-1 transmission in the United States. Med Lett Drugs Ther 2002;51(RR-18):1.

Sexually Transmitted Diseases Treatment Guidelines—2002. Med Lett Drugs Ther 2002;51(RR-6):1.

Whitley RJ: Herpes simplex virus infection. Semin Pediatr Infect Dis 2002;13:6.

Yeni PG et al: Antiretroviral treatment for adult HIV infection in 2002. Updated recommendations of the International AIDS Society—USA Panel. JAMA 2002;288:222.

RELEVANT WEB SITES

www.aidsinfo.nih.gov
www.cdc.gov
www.hivinsite.com

Miscellaneous Antimicrobial Agents; Disinfectants, Antiseptics, & Sterilants

50

Henry F. Chambers, MD

METRONIDAZOLE, MUPIROCIN, POLYMYXINS, & URINARY ANTISEPTICS

METRONIDAZOLE

Metronidazole is a nitroimidazole antiprotozoal drug (see Chapter 53) that also has potent antibacterial activity against anaerobes, including bacteroides and clostridium species. It is well absorbed after oral administration, widely distributed in tissues, and reaches serum levels of 4–6 μg/mL after a 250 mg oral dose. Metronidazole can also be given intravenously or by rectal suppository. The drug penetrates well into the cerebrospinal fluid, reaching levels similar to those in serum. Metronidazole is metabolized in the liver and may accumulate in hepatic insufficiency.

Metronidazole is indicated for treatment of anaerobic or mixed intra-abdominal infections, vaginitis (trichomonas, bacterial vaginosis), antibiotic-associated enterocolitis, and brain abscess. The typical dosage is 500 mg three times daily orally or intravenously (30 mg/kg/d). Vaginitis may respond to a single 2 g dose. A vaginal gel is available for topical use.

Adverse effects include nausea, diarrhea, stomatitis, and peripheral neuropathy with prolonged use. Metronidazole has a disulfiram-like effect, and patients should be instructed to avoid alcohol. Although teratogenic in some animals, metronidazole has not been associated with this effect in humans.

Other properties of metronidazole are discussed in Chapter 53.

MUPIROCIN

Mupirocin (pseudomonic acid) is a natural product produced by *Pseudomonas fluorescens*. It is rapidly inactivated after absorption, and systemic levels are undetectable. It is available as an ointment for topical application.

Mupirocin is active against gram-positive cocci, and its use is directed against *S aureus*, both methicillin-susceptible and methicillin-resistant strains. Mupirocin inhibits and kills staphylococci by inhibiting isoleucyl tRNA synthetase. Low-level resistance, defined as a minimum inhibitory concentration (MIC) of up to 100 μg/mL, is due to point mutation in the gene of the target enzyme. Low-level resistance has been observed after prolonged use, but local concentrations achieved with topical application are well above this MIC, and this level of resistance does not lead to clinical failure. High-level resistance, with MICs exceeding 1000 μg/mL, is due to the presence of a second isoleucyl tRNA synthetase gene, which is plasmid-encoded. High-level resistance results in complete loss of activity. Strains with high-level resistance have caused nosocomial (hospital) outbreaks of staphylococcal infection and colonization.

Mupirocin is indicated for topical treatment of minor skin infections, such as impetigo. Topical application over large infected areas, such as decubitus ulcers or open surgical wounds, has been identified as an important factor leading to emergence of mupirocin-resistant strains and is not recommended. Mupirocin is also indicated for intranasal application for elimination of methicillin-resistant *S aureus* carriage by patients or health care workers.

POLYMYXINS

The polymyxins are a group of basic peptides active against gram-negative bacteria. Polymyxins act like cationic detergents. They attach to and disrupt bacterial cell membranes. They also bind and inactivate endotoxin. Gram-positive organisms, proteus, and neisseria are resistant. Only polymyxin B is available in the USA.

Owing to their significant toxicity with systemic administration, polymyxins are now restricted to topical use. Ointments containing polymyxin B, 0.5 mg/g, in mixtures with bacitracin or neomycin (or both) are commonly applied to infected superficial skin lesions.

URINARY ANTISEPTICS

Urinary antiseptics are oral agents that exert antibacterial activity in the urine but have little or no systemic antibacterial effect. Their usefulness is limited to lower urinary tract infections. Prolonged suppression of bacteriuria by means of urinary antiseptics may be desirable in chronic urinary tract infections where eradication of infection by short-term systemic therapy has not been possible.

1. Nitrofurantoin

Nitrofurantoin is bacteriostatic and bactericidal for many gram-positive and gram-negative bacteria. *P aeruginosa* and many strains of proteus are resistant, but in nitrofurantoin-susceptible populations resistant mutants are rare. Clinical drug resistance emerges slowly. There is no cross-resistance between nitrofurantoin and other antimicrobial agents.

Nitrofurantoin is well absorbed after ingestion. It is metabolized and excreted so rapidly that no systemic antibacterial action is achieved. The drug is excreted into the urine by both glomerular filtration and tubular secretion. With average daily doses, concentrations of 200 μg/mL are reached in urine. In renal failure, urine levels are insufficient for antibacterial action, but high blood levels may cause toxicity.

The average daily dose for urinary tract infection in adults is 100 mg orally taken four times daily with food or milk. Nitrofurantoin is contraindicated in patients with severe renal insufficiency. Oral nitrofurantoin can be given for months for the suppression of chronic urinary tract infection. It is desirable to keep urinary pH below 5.5, which greatly enhances drug activity. A single daily dose of nitrofurantoin, 100 mg, can prevent recurrent urinary tract infections in some women.

Anorexia, nausea, and vomiting are the principal side effects of nitrofurantoin. Neuropathies and hemolytic anemia occur in glucose-6-phosphate dehydrogenase deficiency. Nitrofurantoin antagonizes the action of nalidixic acid. Rashes, pulmonary infiltration, and other hypersensitivity reactions have been reported.

2. Methenamine Mandelate & Methenamine Hippurate

Methenamine mandelate is the salt of mandelic acid and methenamine and possesses properties of both of these urinary antiseptics. Methenamine hippurate is the salt of hippuric acid and methenamine. Below pH 5.5, methenamine releases formaldehyde, which is antibacterial. Mandelic acid or hippuric acid taken orally is excreted unchanged in the urine, in which these drugs are bactericidal for some gram-negative bacteria when pH is less than 5.5.

Methenamine mandelate, 1 g four times daily, or methenamine hippurate, 1 g twice daily by mouth (children, 50 mg/kg/d or 30 mg/kg/d, respectively), is used only as a urinary antiseptic. Acidifying agents (eg, ascorbic acid, 4–12 g/d) may be given to lower urinary pH below 5.5. Sulfonamides should not be given at the same time because they may form an insoluble compound with the formaldehyde released by methenamine. Persons taking methenamine mandelate may exhibit falsely elevated tests for catecholamine metabolites.

The action of methenamine mandelate or hippurate is nonspecific against many different microorganisms and consists of the simultaneous effects of formaldehyde and acidity. Microorganisms such as proteus that make a strongly alkaline urine through release of ammonia from urea are usually resistant.

DISINFECTANTS, ANTISEPTICS, & STERILANTS

Disinfectants are strong chemical agents that inhibit or kill microorganisms (Table 50–1). **Antiseptics** are disinfecting agents with sufficiently low toxicity for host cells that they can be used directly on skin, mucous membranes, or wounds. **Sterilants** kill both vegetative cells and spores when applied to materials for appropriate times and temperatures. Some of the terms used in this context are defined in Table 50–2.

The process of disinfection prevents infection by reducing the number of potentially infective organisms either by killing, removing, or diluting them. Disinfection can be accomplished by application of chemical agents or use of physical agents such as ionizing irradiation, dry or moist heat, or superheated steam (auto-

Table 50–1. Activities of disinfectants.

	Bacteria				Viruses		Other		
	Gram-positive	Gram-negative	Acid-fast	Spores	Lipo-philic	Hydro-philic	Fungi	Amebic Cysts	Prions
Alcohols (isopropanol, ethanol)	HS	HS	S	R	S	V	—	—	R
Aldehydes (glutaraldehyde, formaldehyde)	HS	HS	MS	S (slow)	S	MS	S	—	R
Chlorhexidine gluconate	HS	MS	R	R	V	R	—	—	R
Sodium hypochlorite, chlorine dioxide	HS	HS	MS	S (pH 7.6)	S	S (at high conc)	MS	S	MS (at high conc)
Hexachlorophene	S (slow)	R	R	R	R	R	R	R	R
Povidone, iodine	HS	HS	S	S (at high conc)	S	R	S	S	R
Phenols, quaternary ammonium compounds	HS	HS	±	R	S	R	—	—	R
Strong oxidizing agents, cresols	HS	MS to R	R	R	S	R	R	R	R

Key: HS, highly susceptible; S, susceptible; MS, moderately susceptible; R, resistant; V, variable; —, no data.

clave, 120 °C) to kill microorganisms. Often a combination of agents is used, eg, water and moderate heat over time (pasteurization); ethylene oxide and moist heat (a sterilant); or addition of disinfectant to a detergent. Prevention of infection also can be achieved by washing, which dilutes the potentially infectious organism, or by establishing a barrier, eg, gloves, condom, or respirator, which prevents the pathogen from entry into the host.

Handwashing is the most important means of preventing transmission of infectious agents from person to person or from regions of high microbial load, eg, mouth, nose, or gut, to potential sites of infection. Regular handwashing is best done without disinfectants to minimize drying, irritation, and sensitization of the skin. Soap and warm water efficiently and effectively remove bacteria. Skin disinfectants along with detergent and water are usually used preoperatively as a surgical scrub for surgeons' hands and the patient's surgical incision.

Evaluation of effectiveness of antiseptics, disinfectants, and sterilants, although seemingly simple in principle, is very complex. Factors in any evaluation include the intrinsic resistance of the microorganism, the num-

ber of the microorganisms present, mixed populations of organisms, amount of organic material present (eg blood, feces, tissue), concentration and stability of disinfectant or sterilant, time and temperature of exposure, pH, and hydration and binding of the agent to surfaces. Specific, standardized assays of activity are defined for each use. Toxicity for humans also must be evaluated. The Environmental Protection Agency (EPA) regulates disinfectants and sterilants and the Food and Drug Administration regulates antiseptics.

Users of antiseptics, disinfectants, and sterilants need to consider their short-term and long-term toxicity since they may have general biocidal activity and may accumulate in the environment or in the body of the patient or caregiver using the agent. Disinfectants and antiseptics may also become contaminated by resistant microorganisms—eg, spores, *Pseudomonas aeruginosa*, or *Serratia marcescens*—and actually transmit infection. Most topical antiseptics interfere with wound healing to some degree. Simple cleansing with soap and water is less damaging than antiseptics to wounds. Topical antibiotics with a narrow spectrum of action and low toxicity (eg, bacitracin and mupirocin) can be used for

Table 50–2. Commonly used terms related to chemical and physical killing of microorganisms.

Antisepsis	Application of an agent to living tissue for the purpose of preventing infection
Decontamination	Destruction or marked reduction in number or activity of microorganisms
Disinfection	Chemical or physical treatment that destroys most vegetative microbes or viruses, but not spores, in or on inanimate surfaces
Sanitization	Reduction of microbial load on an inanimate surface to a level considered acceptable for public health purposes
Sterilization	A process intended to kill or remove all types of microorganisms, including spores, and usually including viruses with an acceptable low probability of survival
Pasteurization	A process that kills nonsporulating microorganisms by hot water or steam at 65–100 °C

temporary control of bacterial growth and are generally preferred to antiseptics. Methenamine mandelate releases formaldehyde in a low antibacterial concentration at acid pH and can be an effective urinary antiseptic for long-term control of urinary tract infections.

Some of the chemical classes of antiseptics, disinfectants, and sterilants are described briefly below. The reader is referred to the general references for descriptions of physical disinfection and sterilization methods.

ALCOHOLS

The two alcohols most frequently used for antisepsis and disinfection are ethanol and isopropyl alcohol (isopropanol). They are rapidly active, killing vegetative bacteria, *M tuberculosis,* and many fungi and inactivating lipophilic viruses. The optimum bactericidal concentration is 60–90% by volume in water. They probably act by denaturation of proteins. They are not used as sterilants because they are not sporicidal, do not penetrate protein-containing organic material, may not be active against hydrophilic viruses, and lack residual action because they evaporate completely. The alcohols are useful in situations where sinks with running water are not available for washing with soap and water. Their skin-drying effect can be partially alleviated by addition of emollients to the formulation.

Alcohols are flammable and must be stored in cool, well-ventilated areas. Alcohols must be allowed to evaporate before use of cautery, electrosurgery, or laser surgery. They may be damaging if applied directly to corneal tissue. Therefore, instruments such as tonometers that have been disinfected in alcohol should be rinsed with sterile water or the alcohol allowed to evaporate before they are used.

CHLORHEXIDINE

Chlorhexidine is a cationic biguanide with very low water solubility. Water-soluble chlorhexidine digluconate is used in water-based formulations as an antiseptic. It is active against vegetative bacteria and mycobacteria and has moderate activity against fungi and viruses. It strongly adsorbs to bacterial membranes, causing leakage of small molecules and precipitation of cytoplasmic proteins. It is active at pH 5.5–7.0. Chlorhexidine gluconate is slower in its action than alcohols, but because of its persistence it has residual activity when used repeatedly, producing bactericidal action equivalent to alcohols. It is most effective against gram-positive cocci and less active against gram-positive and gram-negative rods. Spore germination is inhibited by chlorhexidine. Chlorhexidine digluconate is resistant to inhibition by blood and organic materials. However, anionic and nonionic agents in moisturizers, neutral soaps, and surfactants may neutralize its action. Chlorhexidine digluconate formulations of 4% concentration have slightly greater antibacterial activity than newer 2% formulations. Chlorhexidine 0.5% in 70% alcohol formulations are available in some countries. Chlorhexidine has a very low skin-sensitizing or irritating capacity. Oral toxicity is low because chlorhexidine is poorly absorbed from the alimentary tract. Chlorhexidine must not be used during surgery on the middle ear because it causes sensorineural deafness. Similar neural toxicity may be encountered during neurosurgery.

HALOGENS

1. Iodine

Iodine in a 1:20,000 solution is bactericidal in 1 minute and kills spores in 15 minutes. Tincture of iodine USP contains 2% iodine and 2.4% sodium iodide in alcohol. It is the most active antiseptic for intact skin. It is not commonly used because of serious hypersensitivity reactions that may occur and because of its staining of clothing and dressings.

2. Iodophors

Iodophors are complexes of iodine with a surface-active agent such as **polyvinyl pyrrolidone (PVP; povidone-iodine)**. Iodophors retain the activity of iodine. They kill vegetative bacteria, mycobacteria, fungi, and lipid-containing viruses. They may be sporicidal upon prolonged exposure. Iodophors can be used as antiseptics or disinfectants, the latter containing more free iodine. The amount of free iodine is low, but it is released as the solution is diluted. An iodophor solution must be diluted according to the manufacturer's directions in order to obtain full activity.

Iodophors are less irritating and less likely to produce skin hypersensitivity than tincture of iodine. They act as rapidly as chlorhexidine and have a broader spectrum of action, including sporicidal action, but they lack the persistent action of chlorhexidine.

3. Chlorine

Chlorine is a strong oxidizing agent and universal disinfectant that is most commonly provided as a 5.25% **sodium hypochlorite** solution, a typical formulation for **household bleach.** As formulations may vary, the exact concentration should be verified on the label. A 1:10 dilution of household bleach provides 5000 ppm of available chlorine. The Centers for Disease Control and Prevention recommends this concentration for disinfection of blood spills. Less than 5 ppm kills vegetative bacteria, whereas up to 5000 ppm is necessary to kill spores. A concentration of 1000–10,000 ppm is tuberculocidal. One hundred ppm kills vegetative fungal cells in 1 hour, but fungal spores require 500 ppm. Viruses are inactivated by 200–500 ppm. Dilutions of 5.25% sodium hypochlorite made up in pH 7.5–8.0 tap water retain their activity for months when kept in tightly closed, opaque containers. Frequent opening and closing of the container reduces the activity markedly.

Because chlorine is inactivated by blood, serum, feces, and protein-containing materials, surfaces should be cleaned before chlorine disinfectant is applied. Undissociated hypochlorous acid (HOCl) is the active biocidal agent. When pH is increased, the less active hypochlorite ion, OCl⁻, is formed. When hypochlorite solutions contact formaldehyde, the carcinogen *bis*-chloromethyl is formed. Rapid evolution of irritating chlorine gas occurs when hypochlorite solutions are mixed with acid and urine. Solutions are corrosive to aluminum, silver, and stainless steel.

Alternative chlorine-releasing compounds include **chlorine dioxide** and **chloramine T.** These agents retain chlorine longer and have a prolonged bactericidal action.

PHENOLICS

Phenol itself (perhaps the oldest of the surgical antiseptics) is no longer used even as a disinfectant because of its corrosive effect on tissues, its toxicity upon absorp-

tion, and its carcinogenic effect. These adverse actions are diminished by forming derivatives in which a functional group replaces a hydrogen atom in the aromatic ring. The phenolic agents most commonly used are *o*-**phenylphenol,** *o*-**benzyl-***p***-chlorophenol,** and *p*-**tertiary amylphenol.** Mixtures of phenolic derivatives are often used. Some of these are derived from coal tar distillates, eg, cresols and xylenols. Skin absorption and skin irritation still occur with these derivatives, and appropriate care is necessary in their use. Detergents are often added to formulations to clean and remove organic material that may decrease the activity of a phenolic compound.

Phenolic compounds disrupt cell walls and membranes, precipitate proteins, and inactivate enzymes. They are bactericidal (including mycobacteria), fungicidal, and capable of inactivating lipophilic viruses. They are not sporicidal. Dilution and time of exposure recommendations of the manufacturer must be followed.

Phenolic disinfectants are used for hard surface decontamination in hospitals and laboratories, eg, floors, beds, and counter or bench tops. They are not recommended for use in nurseries and especially bassinets, where their use has been associated with hyperbilirubinemia. Use of **hexachlorophene** as a skin disinfectant has caused cerebral edema and convulsions in premature infants and occasionally in adults.

QUATERNARY AMMONIUM COMPOUNDS

The quaternary ammonium compounds ("quats") are cationic surface-active detergents. The active cation has at least one long water-repellent hydrocarbon chain, which causes the molecules to concentrate as an oriented layer on the surface of solutions and colloidal or suspended particles. The charged nitrogen portion of the cation has high affinity for water and prevents separation out of solution. The bactericidal action of quaternary compounds has been attributed to inactivation of energy-producing enzymes, denaturation of proteins, and disruption of the cell membrane. These agents are bacteriostatic, fungistatic, sporistatic, and also inhibit algae. They are bactericidal for gram-positive bacteria and moderately active against gram-negative bacteria. Lipophilic viruses are inactivated. They are not tuberculocidal or sporicidal, and they do not inactivate hydrophilic viruses. Quaternary ammonium compounds bind to the surface of colloidal protein in blood, serum, and milk and to fibers present in cotton, mops, cloths, and paper towels used to apply them, which can cause inactivation of the agent by removing it from solution. They are inactivated by anionic detergents (soaps), by many nonionic detergents, and by calcium, magnesium, ferric, and aluminum ions.

Quaternary compounds are used for sanitation of

noncritical surfaces (floors, bench tops, etc). Their low toxicity has led to their use as sanitizers in food production facilities. CDC recommends that quaternary ammonium compounds such as **benzalkonium chloride** *not* be used as antiseptics because several outbreaks of infections have occurred that were due to growth of pseudomonas and other gram-negative bacteria in quaternary ammonium antiseptic solutions.

ALDEHYDES

Formaldehyde and **glutaraldehyde** are used for disinfection or sterilization of instruments such as fiberoptic endoscopes, respiratory therapy equipment, hemodialyzers, and dental handpieces that can not withstand exposure to the high temperatures of steam sterilization. They are not corrosive for metal, plastic, or rubber. These agents have a broad spectrum of activity against microorganisms and viruses. They act by alkylation of chemical groups in proteins and nucleic acids. Failures of disinfection or sterilization can occur as a result of dilution below the known effective concentration, the presence of organic material, and the failure of liquid to penetrate into small channels in the instruments. Automatic circulating baths are available that increase penetration of aldehyde solution into the instrument while decreasing exposure of the operator to irritating fumes.

Formaldehyde is available as a 40% w/v solution in water (100% **formalin**). An 8% formaldehyde solution in water has a broad spectrum of activity against bacteria, fungi, and viruses. Sporicidal activity may take as long as 18 hours. Its rapidity of action is increased by solution in 70% isopropanol. Formaldehyde solutions are used for high-level disinfection of hemodialyzers, preparation of vaccines, and preservation and embalming of tissues. The 4% formaldehyde (10% formalin) solutions used for fixation of tissues and embalming may not be mycobactericidal.

Glutaraldehyde is a dialdehyde (1,5-pentanedial). Solutions of 2% w/v glutaraldehyde are most commonly used. The solution must be alkalinized to pH 7.4–8.5 for activation. Activated solutions are bactericidal, sporicidal, fungicidal, and virucidal for both lipophilic and hydrophilic viruses. Glutaraldehyde has greater sporicidal activity than formaldehyde, but its tuberculocidal activity may be less. Lethal action against mycobacteria and spores may require prolonged exposure. Once activated, solutions have a shelf life of 14 days, after which polymerization reduces activity. Other means of activation and stabilization can increase the shelf life. Since glutaraldehyde solutions are frequently reused, the most common reason for loss of activity is dilution and exposure to organic material. Test strips to measure residual activity are recommended.

Formaldehyde has a characteristic pungent odor and is highly irritating to respiratory mucous membranes and eyes at concentrations of 2–5 ppm. OSHA has declared that formaldehyde is a potential carcinogen and has established an employee exposure standard that limits the 8-hour time-weighted average (TWA) exposure to 0.75 ppm. Protection of health care workers from exposure to glutaraldehyde concentrations greater than 0.2 ppm is advisable. Increased air exchange, enclosure in hoods with exhausts, tight-fitting lids on exposure devices, and use of protective personal equipment such as goggles, respirators, and gloves may be necessary to achieve these exposure limits.

PEROXYGEN COMPOUNDS

The peroxygen compounds, **hydrogen peroxide** and **peracetic acid,** have high killing activity and a broad spectrum against bacteria, spores, viruses, and fungi when used in appropriate concentration. They have the advantage that their decomposition products are not toxic and do not injure the environment. They are powerful oxidizers that are used primarily as disinfectants and sterilants.

Hydrogen peroxide is a very effective disinfectant when used for inanimate objects or materials with low organic content such as water. Organisms with the enzymes catalase and peroxidase rapidly degrade hydrogen peroxide. The innocuous degradation products are oxygen and water. Concentrated solutions containing 90% w/v H_2O_2 are prepared electrochemically. When diluted in high-quality deionized water to 6% and 3% and put into clean containers, they remain stable. Hydrogen peroxide has been proposed for disinfection of respirators, acrylic resin implants, plastic eating utensils, soft contact lenses, and cartons intended to contain milk or juice products. Concentrations of 10–25% hydrogen peroxide are sporicidal. Vapor phase hydrogen peroxide (VPHP) is a cold gaseous sterilant that has the potential to replace the toxic or carcinogenic gases ethylene oxide and formaldehyde. VPHP does not require a pressurized chamber and is active at temperatures as low as 4 °C and concentrations as low as 4 mg/L. It is incompatible with liquids and cellulose products. It penetrates the surface of some plastics.

Peracetic acid (CH_3COOOH) is prepared commercially from 90% hydrogen peroxide, acetic acid, and sulfuric acid as a catalyst. It is explosive in the pure form. It is usually used in dilute solution and transported in containers with vented caps to prevent increased pressure as oxygen is released. Peracetic acid is more active than hydrogen peroxide as a bactericidal and sporicidal agent. Concentrations of 250–500 ppm are effective against a broad range of bacteria in 5 minutes at pH 7.0 at 20 °C. Bacterial spores are inactivated by 500–30,000 ppm peracetic acid. Only slightly increased concentrations are necessary in the presence of organic matter. Viruses require variable exposures. Enteroviruses require 2000 ppm for 15–30 minutes for inactivation.

An automated machine has been developed for sterilization of medical, surgical, and dental instruments. It uses buffered peracetic acid liquid of 0.1–0.5% concentration. Peracetic acid sterilization systems have been adopted for hemodialyzers. The food processing and beverage industries use peracetic acid extensively because the breakdown products in high dilution do not produce objectionable odor, taste, or toxicity. Since rinsing is not necessary in this use, time and money are saved.

Peracetic acid is a potent tumor promoter but a weak carcinogen. It is not mutagenic in the Ames test.

HEAVY METALS

Heavy metals, principally mercury and silver, are now rarely used as disinfectants. Mercury is an environmental hazard, and some pathogenic bacteria have developed plasmid-mediated resistance to mercurials. Hypersensitivity to thimerosal is common, possibly in as high as 40% of the population. These compounds are absorbed from solution by rubber and plastic closures. Nevertheless, **thimerosal** 0.001–0.004% is still used as a preservative of vaccines, antitoxins, and immune sera.

Inorganic silver salts are strongly bactericidal. **Silver nitrate**, 1:1000, has been most commonly used, particularly as a preventive for gonococcal ophthalmitis in newborns. Antibiotic ointments have replaced silver nitrate for this indication. **Silver sulfadiazine** slowly releases silver and is used to suppress bacterial growth in burn wounds (see Chapter 46).

STERILANTS

For many years, pressurized **steam (autoclaving)** at 120 °C for 30 minutes has been the basic method for sterilizing instruments and decontaminating materials. When autoclaving is not possible, as is the case with lensed instruments and materials containing plastic and rubber, **ethylene oxide**—diluted with either fluorocarbon or carbon dioxide to diminish explosive hazard—was used at 440–1200 mg/L at 45–60 °C with 30–60% relative humidity. The higher concentrations have been used to increase penetration.

Ethylene oxide is classified as a mutagen and carcinogen. The OSHA permissible exposure limit (PEL) for ethylene oxide is 1 ppm calculated as a time-weighted average. Alternative sterilants now being used increasingly include vapor phase hydrogen peroxide, peracetic acid, ozone, gas plasma, chlorine dioxide, formaldehyde, and propylene oxide. Each of these sterilants has potential advantages and problems. Automated peracetic acid systems are being used increasingly for high-

level decontamination and sterilization of endoscopes and hemodialyzers because of their effectiveness, automated features, and the low toxicity of the residual products of sterilization.

PRESERVATIVES

Disinfectants are used as preservatives to prevent the overgrowth of bacteria and fungi in pharmaceutical products, laboratory sera and reagents, cosmetic products, and contact lenses. Multi-use vials of medication that may be reentered through a rubber diaphragm, and eye and nose drops, require preservatives. Preservatives should not be irritant or toxic to tissues to which they will be applied, must be effective in preventing growth of microorganisms likely to contaminate them, and must have sufficient solubility and stability to remain active.

Commonly used preservative agents include organic acids such as **benzoic acid** and salts, the **parabens,** (alkyl esters of *p*-hydroxybenzoic acid), sorbic acid and salts, phenolic compounds, quaternary ammonium compounds, alcohols, and mercurials such as thimerosal in 0.001–0.004% concentration.

REFERENCES

MISCELLANEOUS ANTIMICROBIAL AGENTS

Bartlett JG: Anti-anaerobic antibacterial agents. Lancet 1982;2:478.

Cunha BA: Nitrofurantoin—An update. Obstet Gynecol Surv 1989;44:399.

Edwards DI: Nitroimidazole drugs—action and resistance mechanisms. (Two parts.) J Antimicrob Chemother 1993;31:9, 201.

Hamilton-Miller JM, Brumfitt W: Methenamine and its salts as urinary antiseptics. Invest Urol 1977;14:287.

Larson E: Guidelines for use of topical antimicrobial agents. Am J Infect Dis Control 1988;16:233.

Ronald AR, Harding KM: Urinary infection prophylaxis in women. Ann Intern Med 1981;94:268.

Scully BE: Metronidazole. Med Clin North Am 1988;72:623.

Teasley DG et al: Trial of metronidazole vs vancomycin for *Clostridium difficile:* Associated diarrhea and colitis. Lancet 1983; 2:1043.

DISINFECTANTS, ANTISEPTICS, & STERILANTS

Ascenzi JM (editor): *Handbook of Disinfectants and Antiseptics.* Marcel Dekker, 1996.

Best M et al: Efficacies of selected disinfectants against *Mycobacterium tuberculosis.* J Clin Microbiol 1990;28:2234.

Bischoff WE et al: Handwashing compliance by health care workers: The impact of introducing an accessible, alcohol-based hand antiseptic. Arch Intern Med 2000;160:1017.

Block SS (editor): *Disinfection, Sterilization and Preservation,* 5th ed. Lippincott Williams & Wilkins, 2001.

PREPARATIONS AVAILABLE

MISCELLANEOUS ANTIMICROBIAL DRUGS

Methenamine hippurate (Hiprex, Urex)
Oral: 1.0 g tablets

Methenamine mandelate (generic)
Oral: 0.5, 1 g tablets; 0.5 g/5 mL suspension

Metronidazole (generic, Flagyl)
Oral: 250, 500 mg tablets; 375 mg capsules; 750 mg extended-release tablets
Parenteral: 5 mg/mL; 500 mg for injection

Mupirocin (Bactroban)
Topical: 2% ointment, cream

Nitrofurantoin (Macrodantin, generic)
Oral: 25, 50, 100 mg capsules

Polymyxin B (Polymyxin B Sulfate)
Parenteral: 500,000 units per vial for injection
Ophthalmic: 500,000 units per vial

DISINFECTANTS, ANTISEPTICS, & STERILANTS

Benzalkonium (generic, Zephiran)
Topical: 17% concentrate; 50% solution; 1:750 solution

Benzoyl peroxide (generic)
Topical: 2.5%, 5%, 10% liquid; 5%, 5.5%, 10% lotion; 5%, 10% cream; 2.5%, 4%, 5%, 6%, 10%, 20% gel

Chlorhexidine gluconate (Hibiclens, Hibistat, others)

Topical: 2, 4% cleanser, sponge; 0.5% rinse in 70% alcohol
Oral rinse (Peridex, Periogard): 0.12%

Glutaraldehyde (Cidex)
Instruments: 2, 3.2% solution

Hexachlorophene (pHisoHex)
Topical: 3% liquid; 0.23% foam

Iodine aqueous (generic, Lugol's Solution)
Topical: 2–5% in water with 2.4% sodium iodide or 10% potassium iodide

Iodine tincture (generic)
Topical: 2% iodine or 2.4% sodium iodide in 47% alcohol, in 15, 30, 120 mL and in larger quantities

Nitrofurazone (generic, Furacin)
Topical: 0.2% solution, ointment, and cream

Oxychlorosene sodium (Clorpactin)
Topical: 2 g powder for solution for irrigation, instillation, or rinse

Povidone-iodine (generic, Betadine)
Topical: available in many forms, including aerosol, ointment, antiseptic gauze pads, skin cleanser (liquid or foam), solution, and swab-sticks

Silver nitrate (generic)
Topical: 10, 25, 50% solution

Thimerosal (generic, Mersol)
Topical: 1:1000 tincture and solution

Doebbing BN et al: Comparative efficacy of alternative handwashing agents in reducing infections in intensive care units. N Engl J Med 1992;327:88.

Gardner JF, Peel MM: *Introduction to Sterilization, Disinfection and Infection Control,* 3rd ed. Churchill Livingston, 1997.

Kaye ET, Kaye KM: Topical antibacterial agents. Infect Dis Clin North Am 1995;9:547.

Lewis DL, Arens M: Resistance of microorganisms to disinfection in dental and medical devices. Nat Med 1995;1:956.

Maki DG et al: Prospective randomized trial of povidone-iodine, alcohol and chlorhexidine for prevention of infection associated with central venous and arterial catheters. Lancet 1991;338:339.

Russell AD: Bacterial spores and chemical sporicidal agents. Clin Microbiol Rev 1990;3:99.

Rutala WA et al: Disinfection practices for endoscopes and other semicritical items. Infect Control Hosp Epidemiol 1991; 12:282.

Rutula WA: Guidelines for selection and use of disinfectants. Am J Infect Control 1990;18:99.

Widmer AF, Frei R: Decontamination, disinfection, and sterilization. In: Murray PR et al (editors). *Manual of Clinical Microbiology,* 7th ed. American Society for Microbiology, 1999.

Clinical Use of Antimicrobial Agents

Harry W. Lampiris, MD, & Daniel S. Maddix, PharmD

The development of antimicrobial drugs represents one of the most important advances in therapeutics, both in the control or cure of serious infections and in the prevention and treatment of infectious complications of other therapeutic modalities such as cancer chemotherapy and surgery. However, there is overwhelming evidence that antimicrobial agents are vastly overprescribed in outpatient settings in the United States, and the availability of antimicrobial agents without prescription in many developing countries has—by facilitating the development of resistance—already severely limited therapeutic options in the treatment of life-threatening infections. Therefore, the clinician should first determine whether antimicrobial therapy is warranted for a given patient. The specific questions one should ask include the following:

1. Is an antimicrobial agent indicated on the basis of clinical findings? Or is it prudent to wait until such clinical findings become apparent?
2. Have appropriate clinical specimens been obtained to establish a microbiologic diagnosis?
3. What are the likely etiologic agents for the patient's illness?
4. What measures should be taken to protect individuals exposed to the index case to prevent secondary cases, and what measures should be implemented to prevent further exposure?
5. Is there clinical evidence (eg, from clinical trials) that antimicrobial therapy will confer clinical benefit for the patient?

Once a specific cause is identified based upon specific microbiologic tests, the following further questions should be considered:

1. If a specific microbial pathogen is identified, can a narrower-spectrum agent be substituted for the initial empirical drug?
2. Is one agent or a combination of agents necessary?
3. What is the optimal dose, route of administration, and duration of therapy?

4. What specific tests (eg, susceptibility testing) should be undertaken to identify patients who will not respond to treatment?
5. What adjunctive measures can be undertaken to eradicate the infection? For example, is surgery feasible for removal of devitalized tissue or foreign bodies—or drainage of an abscess—into which antimicrobial agents may be unable to penetrate? Is it possible to decrease the dosage of immunosuppressive therapy in patients who have undergone organ transplantation or to give immunomodulatory drugs or antitoxins to patients with preexisting immune deficiency?

EMPIRICAL ANTIMICROBIAL THERAPY

Antimicrobial agents are frequently used before the pathogen responsible for a particular illness or the susceptibility to a particular antimicrobial agent is known. This use of antimicrobial agents is called empirical (or presumptive) therapy and is based upon experience with a particular clinical entity. The usual justification for empirical therapy is the hope that early intervention will improve the outcome, and in the best case this has been established by placebo-controlled, double-blind prospective clinical trials. For example, treatment of febrile episodes in neutropenic cancer patients with empirical antimicrobial therapy has been demonstrated to have impressive morbidity and mortality benefits even though the specific bacterial agent responsible for fever is determined for only a minority of such episodes. Conversely, there are many clinical situations in which empirical therapy may not be useful or may actually be harmful. For example, neutropenic patients with fever and pulmonary infiltrates may have a wide variety of causes for their clinical illness, including viruses, bacteria, mycobacteria, fungi, protozoa, and noninfectious disorders. In this setting, it may be more prudent to obtain specimens by sputum culture or via bronchoalveolar lavage early in order to offer narrow-spectrum therapy based upon culture results.

Lastly, there are many clinical entities, such as certain episodes of community-acquired pneumonia, in which it is difficult to identify a specific pathogen. In such cases, a clinical response to empirical therapy may be an important clue to the likely pathogen.

Approach to Empirical Therapy

Initiation of empirical therapy should follow a specific and systematic approach.

A. FORMULATE A CLINICAL DIAGNOSIS OF MICROBIAL INFECTION

Using all available data, the clinician should conclude that there is anatomic evidence of infection (eg, pneumonia, cellulitis, sinusitis).

B. OBTAIN SPECIMENS FOR LABORATORY EXAMINATION

Examination of stained specimens by microscopy or simple examination of an uncentrifuged sample of urine for white blood cells and bacteria may provide important etiologic clues in a very short time.

C. FORMULATE A MICROBIOLOGIC DIAGNOSIS

The history, physical examination, and immediately available laboratory results (eg, Gram's stain of urine or sputum) may provide highly specific information. For example, in a young man with urethritis and a Gram-stained smear from the urethral meatus demonstrating intracellular gram-negative diplococci, the most likely pathogen is *Neisseria gonorrhoeae*. In the latter instance, however, the clinician should be aware that a significant number of patients with gonococcal urethritis have uninformative Gram stains for the organism and that a significant number of patients with gonococcal urethritis harbor concurrent chlamydial infection that is not demonstrated on the Gram-stained smear.

D. DETERMINE THE NECESSITY FOR EMPIRICAL THERAPY

This is an important clinical decision based partly upon experience and partly upon data from clinical trials. Empirical therapy is indicated when there is a significant risk of serious morbidity if therapy is withheld until a specific pathogen is detected by the clinical laboratory.

In other settings, empirical therapy may be indicated for public health reasons rather than for demonstrated superior outcome of therapy in a specific patient. For example, urethritis in a young sexually active man usually requires treatment for *N gonorrhoeae* and *Chlamydia trachomatis* despite the absence of microbiologic confirmation at the time of diagnosis. Because there is a high risk of noncompliance with follow-up visits in this patient population, empirical therapy is warranted to ensure cure of the infection at the first visit in order to prevent further transmission.

E. INSTITUTE TREATMENT

Selection of empirical therapy may be based upon the microbiologic diagnosis or a clinical diagnosis without available microbiologic clues. If no microbiologic information is available, the antimicrobial spectrum of the agent or agents chosen must necessarily be broader, taking into account the most likely pathogens responsible for the patient's illness.

Choice of Antimicrobial Agent

Selection from among several drugs depends upon **host factors** which include the following: (1) concomitant disease states (eg, AIDS, severe chronic liver disease); (2) prior adverse drug effects; (3) impaired elimination or detoxification of the drug (this may be genetically predetermined but more frequently is associated with impaired renal or hepatic function due to underlying disease); (4) age of the patient; and (5) pregnancy status.

Pharmacologic factors include (1) the kinetics of absorption, distribution, and elimination; (2) the ability of the drug to be delivered to the site of infection; (3) the potential toxicity of an agent; and (4) pharmacokinetic or pharmacodynamic interactions with other drugs.

Knowledge of the susceptibility of an organism to a specific agent in a hospital or community setting is important in the selection of empirical therapy. Pharmacokinetic differences among agents with similar antimicrobial spectrums may be exploited to reduce the frequency of dosing (eg, ceftriaxone may be conveniently given every 24 hours). Lastly, increasing consideration is being given to the cost of antimicrobial therapy, especially when multiple agents with comparable efficacy and toxicity are available for a specific infection.

Brief guides to empirical therapy based upon presumptive microbial diagnosis and site of infection are given in Tables 51–1 and 51–2.

ANTIMICROBIAL THERAPY OF INFECTIONS WITH KNOWN ETIOLOGY

INTERPRETATION OF CULTURE RESULTS

Properly obtained and processed specimens for culture frequently yield reliable information about the cause of infection. The lack of a confirmatory microbiologic diagnosis may be due to the following:

Table 51–1. Empiric antimicrobial therapy based on microbiologic etiology.

Suspected or Proved Disease or Pathogen	Drugs of First Choice	Alternative Drugs
Gram-negative cocci (aerobic)		
Moraxella (Branhamella) catarrhalis	TMP-SMZ,[1] cephalosporin (second- or third-generation)	Erythromycin, quinolone, clarithromycin, azithromycin
Neisseria gonorrhoeae[2]	Ceftriaxone, cefixime	Spectinomycin, quinolone
Neisseria meningitidis	Penicillin G	Chloramphenicol, cephalosporin (third-generation)[3]
Gram-negative rods (aerobic)		
E coli, klebsiella, proteus	Cephalosporin (first- or second-generation), TMP-SMZ	Quinolone, aminoglycoside
Enterobacter, citrobacter, serratia	TMP-SMZ, quinolone, imipenem	Antipseudomonal penicillin,[4] aminoglycoside[5], cefepime
Shigella	Quinolone	TMP-SMZ, ampicillin, cefixime, ceftriaxone
Salmonella	TMP-SMZ, quinolone, cephalosporin (third-generation)	Chloramphenicol, ampicillin
Campylobacter jejuni	Erythromycin	Tetracycline, quinolone
Brucella species	Doxycycline + rifampin or aminoglycoside[5]	Chloramphenicol + aminoglycoside or TMP-SMZ
Helicobacter pylori	Bismuth + metronidazole + tetracycline or amoxicillin	Proton pump inhibitor + amoxicillin and clarithromycin
Vibrio species	Tetracycline	Quinolone, TMP-SMZ
Pseudomonas aeruginosa	Antipseudomonal penicillin + aminoglycoside[5]	Antipseudomonal penicillin + quinolone; cefepime, ceftazidime, imipenem, or aztreonam ± aminoglycoside
Burkholderia cepacia (formerly *Pseudomonas cepacia*)	TMP-SMZ	Ceftazidime, chloramphenicol
Stenotrophomonas maltophilia (formerly *Xanthomonas maltophilia*)	TMP-SMZ	Minocycline, ticarcillin-clavulanate, quinolone
Legionella species	Azithromycin + rifampin or quinolone + rifampin	Clarithromycin, erythromycin, doxycycline
Gram-positive cocci (aerobic)		
Streptococcus pneumoniae, penicillin-susceptible (MIC ≤ 2)	Penicillin[6]	Doxycycline, ceftriaxone, cefuroxime, erythromycin, imipenem, meropenem, linezolid
penicillin-resistant (MIC ≥ 4)	Ceftriaxone, vancomycin	Carbapenems, linezolid
Streptococcus pyogenes (group A)	Penicillin, clindamycin	Erythromycin, cephalosporin (first-generation)
Streptococcus agalactiae (group B)	Penicillin (+ aminoglycoside?[5])	Vancomycin
Viridans streptococci	Penicillin	Cephalosporin (first- or third-generation), vancomycin

Table 51–1. Empiric antimicrobial therapy based on microbiologic etiology (*continued*).

Suspected or Proved Disease or Pathogen	Drugs of First Choice	Alternative Drugs
Staphylococcus aureus Beta-lactamase-negative	Penicillin	Cephalosporin (first-generation), vancomycin
Beta-lactamase-positive	Penicillinase-resistant penicillin[7]	As above
Methicillin-resistant	Vancomycin	TMP-SMZ, minocycline, linezolid, quinupristin-dalfopristin
Enterococcus species[8]	Penicillin ± aminoglycoside[5]	Vancomycin ± aminoglycoside
Gram-positive rods (aerobic) Bacillus species (non *anthracis*)	Vancomycin	Imipenem, quinolone, clindamycin
Listeria species	Ampicillin (± aminoglycoside[5])	TMP-SMZ
Nocardia species	Sulfadiazine, TMP-SMZ	Minocycline, imipenem, amikacin
Anaerobic bacteria Gram-positive (clostridia, peptococcus, actinomyces, peptostreptococcus)	Penicillin, clindamycin	Vancomycin, imipenem, chloramphenicol
Clostridium difficile	Metronidazole	Vancomycin, bacitracin
Bacteroides fragilis	Metronidazole, clindamycin	Chloramphenicol, imipenem, beta-lactam–beta-lactamase-inhibitor combinations
Fusobacterium, prevotella, porphyromonas	Metronidazole, clindamycin, penicillin	As for *B fragilis*
Mycobacteria *Mycobacterium tuberculosis*	Isoniazid + rifampin + ethambutol + pyrazinamide	Streptomycin, quinolone, amikacin, ethionamide, cycloserine, PAS
Mycobacterium leprae Multibacillary Paucibacillary	Dapsone + rifampin + clofazimine Dapsone + rifampin	
Mycoplasma pneumoniae	Tetracycline, erythromycin	Azithromycin, clarithromycin, quinolone
Chlamydia *trachomatis*	Tetracycline, azithromycin	Clindamycin, ofloxacin
pneumoniae	Tetracycline, erythromycin	Clarithromycin, azithromycin
psittaci	Tetracycline	Chloramphenicol
Spirochetes *Borrelia recurrentis*	Doxycycline	Erythromycin, chloramphenicol, penicillin
Borrelia burgdorferi Early Late	Doxycycline, amoxicillin, ceftriaxone	Cefuroxime axetil, penicillin
Leptospira species	Penicillin	Tetracycline
Treponema species	Penicillin	Tetracycline, azithromycin, ceftriaxone

(*continued*)

Table 51–1. Empiric antimicrobial therapy based on microbiologic etiology *(continued).*

Suspected or Proved Disease or Pathogen	Drugs of First Choice	Alternative Drugs
Fungi		
Aspergillus species	Amphotericin B, voriconazole	Itraconazole, caspofungin
Blastomyces species	Amphotericin B	Itraconazole, ketoconazole[9]
Candida species, torulopsis species	Amphotericin B, caspofungin	Fluconazole, itraconazole
Cryptococcus	Amphotericin B ± flucytosine (5-FC)	Fluconazole
Coccidioides immitis	Amphotericin B	Fluconazole, itraconazole, ketoconazole
Histoplasma capsulatum	Amphotericin B	Itraconazole
Mucoraceae (rhizopus, absidia)	Amphotericin B	
Sporothrix schenkii	Amphotericin B	Itraconazole

[1]Trimethoprim-sulfamethoxazole (TMP-SMZ) is a mixture of one part trimethoprim plus five parts sulfamethoxazole.

[2]Quinolones are not recommended for empiric therapy of gonococcal infections acquired in Southeast Asia, Hawaii, and the Pacific Coast of the United States. Azithromycin 2 g is an alternative agent for the treatment of gonococcal urethritis and cervicitis.

[3]First-generation cephalosporins: Cephalothin, cephapirin, or cefazolin for parenteral administration; cephalexin or cephradine for oral administration. Second-generation cephalosporins: Cefuroxime, cefamandole, cefonicid for parenteral administration; cefaclor, cefuroxime axetil, cefprozil, ceftibuten for oral administration. Third-generation cephalosporins: Cefoperazone, cefotaxime, ceftizoxime, ceftriaxone for parenteral administration; cefixime, cefpodoxime for oral administration.

[4]Antipseudomonal penicillin: Carbenicillin, ticarcillin, azlocillin, mezlocillin, piperacillin.

[5]Generally, streptomycin and gentamicin are used to treat infections with gram-positive organisms, whereas gentamicin, tobramycin, and amikacin are used to treat infections with gram-negatives.

[6]See footnote 3 in Table 51–2 for guidelines on the treatment of penicillin-resistant pneumococcal meningitis.

[7]Parenteral nafcillin, oxacillin; or methicillin; oral dicloxacillin, cloxacillin, or oxacillin.

[8]There is no regimen that is reliably bactericidal for vancomycin-resistant enterococcus. Regimens that have been reported to be efficacious include single-drug therapy with chloramphenicol, tetracycline, nitrofurantoin (for urinary tract infection); potential regimens for bacteremia include ampicillin + vancomycin and ampicillin + ciprofloxacin + gentamicin.

[9]Ketoconazole does not penetrate the central nervous system and is unsatisfactory for meningitis.

(1) Sample error, eg, obtaining cultures after antimicrobial agents have been administered.

(2) Noncultivable or slow-growing organisms, (*Histoplasma capsulatum,* bartonella species), where cultures are often discarded before sufficient growth has occurred for detection.

(3) Requesting *bacterial* cultures when infection is due to other organisms.

(4) Not recognizing the need for special media or isolation techniques (eg, charcoal yeast extract agar for isolation of legionella species, shell-vial tissue culture system for rapid isolation of CMV).

Even in the setting of a classic infectious disease for which isolation techniques have been established for decades (eg, pneumococcal pneumonia, pulmonary tuberculosis, streptococcal pharyngitis), the sensitivity of the culture technique may be inadequate to identify all cases of the disease.

GUIDING ANTIMICROBIAL THERAPY OF ESTABLISHED INFECTIONS

Susceptibility Testing

Testing bacterial pathogens in vitro for their susceptibility to antimicrobial agents is extremely valuable in confirming susceptibility, ideally to a narrow-spectrum nontoxic antimicrobial drug. Tests measure the concentration of drug required to inhibit growth of the organism (minimal inhibitory concentration [MIC]) or to kill

Table 51–2. Empiric antimicrobial therapy based on site of infection.

Presumed Site of Infection	Common Pathogens	Drugs of First Choice	Alternative Drugs
Bacterial endocarditis			
Acute	*Staphylococcus aureus*	Penicillinase-resistant penicillin[1] + gentamicin	Vancomycin + gentamicin
Subacute	Viridans streptococci, enterococci	Penicillin + gentamicin	Vancomycin + gentamicin
Septic arthritis			
Child	*H influenzae, S aureus,* β-hemolytic streptococci	Ceftriaxone	Ampicillin-sulbactam
Adult, nongonococcal	*S aureus,* Enterobacteriaceae	Cefazolin	Vancomycin, quinolone
Acute otitis media, sinusitis	*H influenzae, S pneumoniae, M catarrhalis*	Amoxicillin	Amoxicillin-clavulanate, cefuroxime axetil, TMP-SMZ
Cellulitis	*S aureus,* group A streptococcus	Penicillinase-resistant penicillin, cephalosporin (first-generation)[2]	Vancomycin
Meningitis			
Neonate	Group B streptococcus, *E coli,* listeria	Ampicillin + cephalosporin (third-generation)	Ampicillin + aminoglycoside, chloramphenicol
Child	*H influenzae,* pneumococcus, meningococcus	Ceftriaxone or cefotaxime ± vancomycin[3]	Chloramphenicol
Adult	Pneumococcus, meningococcus	Ceftriaxone, cefotaxime	Vancomycin + ceftriaxone or cefotaxime[3]
Peritonitis due to ruptured viscus	Coliforms, *B fragilis*	Metronidazole + cephalosporin (third-generation), piperacillin-tazobactam	Imipenem
Pneumonia			
Neonate	As in neonatal meningitis		
Child	Pneumococcus, *S aureus, H influenzae*	Ceftriaxone, cefuroxime, cefotaxime	Ampicillin-sulbactam
Adult (community-acquired)	Pneumococcus, mycoplasma, legionella, *H influenzae, S aureus, C pneumonia,* coliforms	**Outpatient:** Erythromycin, amoxicillin, doxycycline **Inpatient:** Macrolide[4] + cefotaxime, ceftriaxone	**Outpatient:** Azithromycin, clarithromycin, quinolone **Inpatient:** Macrolide + piperacillin-tazobactam, ticarcillin-clavulanate, or cefuroxime; quinolone
Septicemia	Any	Vancomycin + aminoglycoside + cephalosporin (third-generation) or piperacillin + tazobactam	
Septicemia with granulocytopenia	Any	Antipseudomonal penicillin + aminoglycoside; ceftazidime; cefepime; consider addition of amphotericin B if fever persists beyond 5 days of empiric therapy	

[1]See footnote 7, Table 51–1.
[2]See footnote 3, Table 51–1.
[3]When meningitis with penicillin-resistant pneumococcus is suspected, empiric therapy with this regimen is recommended.
[4]Erythromycin, clarithromycin, or azithromycin (an azalide) may be used.

the organism (minimal bactericidal concentration [MBC]). The results of these tests can then be correlated with known drug concentrations in various body compartments. Only MICs are routinely measured in most infections, whereas in infections in which bactericidal therapy is required for eradication of infection (eg, meningitis, endocarditis, sepsis in the granulocytopenic host), MBC measurements occasionally may be useful.

Specialized Assay Methods

A. BETA-LACTAMASE ASSAY

For some bacteria (eg, haemophilus species), the susceptibility patterns of strains are similar except for the production of β lactamase. In these cases, extensive susceptibility testing may not be required and a direct test for β-lactamase utilizing a chromogenic β-lactam substrate (nitrocephin disk) may be substituted.

B. SYNERGY STUDIES

These in vitro tests attempt to measure synergistic, additive, indifferent, or antagonistic drug interactions. In general, these tests have not been standardized and have not correlated well with clinical outcome. (See section on combination chemotherapy for details.)

MONITORING THERAPEUTIC RESPONSE: DURATION OF THERAPY

The therapeutic response may be monitored microbiologically or clinically. Cultures of specimens taken from infected sites should eventually become sterile or demonstrate eradication of the pathogen and are useful for documenting recurrence or relapse. Follow-up cultures may also be useful for detecting superinfections or the development of resistance. Clinically, the patient's systemic manifestations of infection (malaise, fever, leukocytosis) should abate and the clinical findings should improve (eg, as shown by clearing of radiographic infiltrates or lessening hypoxemia in pneumonia).

The duration of therapy required for cure depends on the pathogen, the site of infection, and host factors (immunocompromised patients generally require longer courses of treatment). Precise data on duration of therapy exist for some infections (eg, streptococcal pharyngitis, syphilis, gonorrhea, tuberculosis, cryptococcal meningitis in non-AIDS patients). In many other situations, duration of therapy is determined empirically. For serious infections, continuing therapy for 7–10 days after the patient has become afebrile is a good rule of thumb. For recurrent infections (eg, sinusitis, urinary tract infections), longer courses of antimicrobial therapy are frequently necessary for eradication.

Clinical Failure of Antimicrobial Therapy

When the patient has an inadequate clinical or microbiologic response to antimicrobial therapy selected by in vitro susceptibility testing, systematic investigation should be undertaken to determine the cause of failure. Errors in susceptibility testing are rare, but the original results should be confirmed by repeat testing. Drug dosing and absorption should be scrutinized and tested directly using serum measurements, pill counting, or directly observed therapy.

The clinical data should be reviewed to determine whether the patient's immune function is adequate and, if not, what can be done to maximize it. For example, are adequate numbers of granulocytes present and are HIV infection, malnutrition, or underlying malignancy present? The presence of abscesses or foreign bodies should also be considered. Lastly, culture and susceptibility testing should be repeated to determine if superinfection has occurred with another organism or if the original pathogen has developed drug resistance.

ANTIMICROBIAL PHARMACODYNAMICS

The time course of drug concentration is closely related to the antimicrobial effect at the site of infection and to any toxic effects. Pharmacodynamic factors include pathogen susceptibility testing, drug bactericidal versus bacteriostatic activity, and drug synergism, antagonism, and postantibiotic effects. Together with pharmacokinetics, pharmacodynamic information permits the selection of optimal antimicrobial dosage regimens.

Bacteriostatic Versus Bactericidal Activity

Antibacterial agents may be classified as bacteriostatic or bactericidal (Table 51–3). For agents that are primarily bacteriostatic, inhibitory drug concentrations are much

Table 51–3. Bacteriostatic and bactericidal antibacterial agents.

Bactericidal agents	Bacteriostatic agents
Aminoglycosides	Chloramphenicol
Bacitracin	Clindamycin
Beta-lactam antibiotics	Ethambutol
Isoniazid	Macrolides
Metronidazole	Nitrofurantoin
Polymyxins	Novobiocin
Pyrazinamide	Oxazolidinones
Quinolones	Sulfonamides
Quinupristin-dalfopristin	Tetracyclines
Rifampin	Trimethoprim
Vancomycin	

lower than bactericidal drug concentrations. In general, cell wall-active agents are bactericidal, and drugs that inhibit protein synthesis are bacteriostatic.

The classification of antibacterial agents as bactericidal or bacteriostatic has limitations. Some agents that are considered to be bacteriostatic may be bactericidal against selected organisms. On the other hand, enterococci are inhibited but not killed by vancomycin, penicillin, or ampicillin used as single agents.

Bacteriostatic and bactericidal agents are equivalent for the treatment of most infectious diseases in immunocompetent hosts. Bactericidal agents should be selected over bacteriostatic ones in circumstances in which local or systemic host defenses are impaired. Bactericidal agents are required for treatment of endocarditis and other endovascular infections, meningitis, and infections in neutropenic cancer patients.

Bactericidal agents can be divided into two groups: agents that exhibit **concentration-dependent killing** (eg, aminoglycosides and quinolones) and agents that exhibit **time-dependent killing** (eg, β-lactams and vancomycin). For drugs whose killing action is concentration-dependent, the rate and extent of killing increase with increasing drug concentrations. Concentration-dependent killing is one of the pharmacodynamic factors responsible for the efficacy of once-daily dosing of aminoglycosides.

For drugs whose killing action is time-dependent, bactericidal activity continues as long as serum concentrations are greater than the MBC. Drug concentrations of time-dependent killing agents that lack a postantibiotic effect should be maintained above the MIC for the entire interval between doses.

Postantibiotic Effect

Persistent suppression of bacterial growth after limited exposure to an antimicrobial agent is known as the postantibiotic effect (PAE). The PAE can be expressed mathematically as follows:

$$PAE = T - C$$

where T is the time required for the viable count in the test (in vitro) culture to increase tenfold above the count observed immediately before drug removal and C is the time required for the count in an untreated culture to increase tenfold above the count observed immediately after completion of the same procedure used on the test culture. The PAE reflects the time required for bacteria to return to logarithmic growth.

Proposed mechanisms include (1) recovery after reversible nonlethal damage to cell structures; (2) persistence of the drug at a binding site or within the periplasmic space; and (3) the need to synthesize new enzymes before growth can resume. Most antimicrobials possess significant in vitro PAEs (≥ 1.5 hours) against suscepti-

ble gram-positive cocci (Table 51–4). Antimicrobials with significant PAEs against susceptible gram-negative bacilli are limited to carbapenems and agents that inhibit protein or DNA synthesis.

In vivo PAEs are usually much longer than in vitro PAEs. This is thought to be due to **postantibiotic leukocyte enhancement** (**PALE**) and exposure of bacteria to subinhibitory antibiotic concentrations. The efficacy of once-daily dosing regimens is in part due to the PAE. Aminoglycosides and quinolones possess concentration-dependent PAEs; thus, high doses of aminoglycosides given once daily result in enhanced bactericidal activity and extended PAEs. This combination of pharmacodynamic effects allows aminoglycoside serum concentrations that are below the MICs of target organisms to remain effective for extended periods of time.

PHARMACOKINETIC CONSIDERATIONS

Route of Administration

Many antimicrobial agents have similar pharmacokinetic properties when given orally or parenterally (ie, tetracyclines, trimethoprim-sulfamethoxazole, quinolones, chloramphenicol, metronidazole, clindamycin, rifampin, and fluconazole). In most cases, oral therapy with these drugs is equally effective, less costly, and results in fewer complications than parenteral therapy.

The intravenous route is preferred in the following situations: (1) for critically ill patients; (2) for patients with bacterial meningitis or endocarditis; (3) for patients with nausea, vomiting, gastrectomy, or diseases

Table 51–4. Antibacterial agents with in vitro postantibiotic effects ≥ 1.5 hours.

Against gram-positive cocci	Against gram-negative bacilli
Aminoglycosides	Aminoglycosides
Carbapenems	Carbapenems
Cephalosporins	Chloramphenicol
Chloramphenicol	Quinolones
Clindamycin	Rifampin
Macrolides	Tetracyclines
Oxazolidinones	
Penicillins	
Quinolones	
Quinupristin-dalfopristin	
Rifampin	
Sulfonamides	
Tetracyclines	
Trimethoprim	
Vancomycin	

that may impair oral absorption; and (4) when giving antimicrobials that are poorly absorbed following oral administration.

Conditions That Alter Antimicrobial Pharmacokinetics

Various diseases and physiologic states alter the pharmacokinetics of antimicrobial agents. Impairment of renal or hepatic function may result in decreased elimination. Table 51–5 lists drugs that require dosage reduction in patients with renal or hepatic insufficiency. Failure to reduce antimicrobial agent dosage in such patients may cause toxic side effects. Conversely, patients with burns, cystic fibrosis, or trauma may have increased dosage requirements for selected agents. The pharmacokinetics of antimicrobials are also altered in the elderly, in neonates, and in pregnancy.

Drug Concentrations in Body Fluids

Most antimicrobial agents are well distributed to most body tissues and fluids. Penetration into the cerebrospinal fluid is an exception. Most do not penetrate uninflamed meninges to an appreciable extent. In the presence of meningitis, however, the cerebrospinal fluid concentrations of many antimicrobials increase (Table 51–6).

Monitoring Serum Concentrations of Antimicrobial Agents

For most antimicrobial agents, the relationship between dose and therapeutic outcome is well established, and serum concentration monitoring is unnecessary for these drugs. To justify routine serum concentration monitoring, it should be established (1) that a direct relationship exists between drug concentrations and efficacy or toxicity; (2) that substantial interpatient variability exists in serum concentrations on standard doses; (3) that a small difference exists between therapeutic and toxic serum concentrations; (4) that the clinical efficacy or toxicity of the drug is delayed or difficult to measure; and (5) that an accurate assay is available.

In clinical practice, serum concentration monitoring is routinely performed on patients receiving aminoglycosides. Despite the lack of supporting evidence for its utility or need, serum vancomycin concentration monitoring is also widespread. Flucytosine serum concentration monitoring has been shown to reduce toxicity when doses are adjusted to maintain peak concentrations below 100 μg/mL.

MANAGEMENT OF ANTIMICROBIAL DRUG TOXICITY

Owing to the large number of antimicrobials available, it is usually possible to select an effective alternative in patients who develop serious drug toxicity (Table 51–1). However, for some infections there are no effective alternatives to the drug of choice. For example, in patients with neurosyphilis who have a history of anaphylaxis to penicillin, it is necessary to perform skin testing and desensitization to penicillin. It is important to obtain a clear history of drug allergy and other adverse drug reac-

Table 51–5. Antimicrobial agents that require dosage adjustment or are contraindicated in patients with renal or hepatic impairment.

Dosage Adjustment Needed in Renal Impairment	Contraindicated in Renal Impairment	Dosage Adjustment Needed in Hepatic Impairment
Acyclovir, adefovir, amantadine, aminoglycosides, aztreonam, cephalosporins,[1] clarithromycin, cycloserine, didanosine, ethambutol, famciclovir, fluconazole, flucytosine, foscarnet, ganciclovir, imipenem, lamivudine, meropenem, penicillins,[3] quinolones,[4] rimantadine, stavudine, terbinafine, trimethoprim-sulfamethoxazole, valacyclovir, vancomycin, zalcitabine, zidovudine	Cidofovir, itraconazole (IV), methenamine, nalidixic acid, nitrofurantoin, ribavirin, sulfonamides (long-acting), tetracyclines[2]	Amprenavir, caspofungin, chloramphenicol, clindamycin, erythromycin, indinavir, metronidazole, rimantadine, voriconazole

[1]Except cefoperazone and ceftriaxone.
[2]Except doxycycline and possibly minocycline.
[3]Except antistaphylococcal penicillins (eg, nafcillin and dicloxacillin).
[4]Except trovafloxacin and moxifloxacin.

Table 51–6. Cerebrospinal fluid (CSF) penetration of selected antimicrobials.

Antimicrobial Agent	CSF Concentration (Uninflamed Meninges) as Percent of Serum Concentration	CSF Concentration (Inflamed Meninges) as Percent of Serum Concentration
Ampicillin	2–3	2–100
Aztreonam	2	5
Cefotaxime	22.5	27–36
Ceftazidime	0.7	20–40
Ceftriaxone	0.8–1.6	16
Cefuroxime	20	17–88
Ciprofloxacin	6–27	26–37
Imipenem	3.1	11–41
Meropenem	0–7	1–52
Nafcillin	2–15	5–27
Penicillin G	1–2	8–18
Sulfamethoxazole	40	12–47
Trimethoprim	< 41	12–69
Vancomycin	0	1–53

tions. A patient with a documented antimicrobial allergy should carry a card with the name of the drug and a description of the reaction. Cross-reactivity between penicillins and cephalosporins is less than 10%. Cephalosporins may be administered to patients with penicillin-induced maculopapular rashes but should be avoided in patients with a history of penicillin-induced immediate hypersensitivity reactions. The cross-reactivity between penicillins and imipenem may exceed 50%. On the other hand, aztreonam does not cross-react with penicillins and can be safely administered to patients with a history of penicillin-induced anaphylaxis. For mild reactions, it may be possible to continue therapy with use of adjunctive agents or dosage reduction.

Adverse reactions to antimicrobials occur with increased frequency in several groups, including neonates, geriatric patients, renal failure patients, and AIDS patients. Dosage adjustment of the drugs listed in Table 51–5 is essential for the prevention of adverse effects in patients with renal failure. In addition, several agents are contraindicated in patients with renal impairment because of increased rates of serious toxicity (Table 51–5). See the preceding chapters for discussions of specific drugs.

Polypharmacy also predisposes to drug interactions. Although the mechanism is not known, AIDS patients have an unusually high incidence of toxicity to a number of drugs, including clindamycin, aminopenicillins, and sulfonamides. Many of these reactions, including rash and fever, may respond to dosage reduction or treatment with corticosteroids and antihistamines. Other examples are discussed in the preceding chapters and in Appendix II.

ANTIMICROBIAL DRUG COMBINATIONS

RATIONALE FOR COMBINATION ANTIMICROBIAL THERAPY

Most infections should be treated with a single antimicrobial agent. Although indications for combination therapy exist, antimicrobial combinations are often overused in clinical practice. The unnecessary use of antimicrobial combinations increases toxicity and costs and may occasionally result in reduced efficacy due to antagonism of one drug by another. Antimicrobial combinations should be selected for one or more of the following reasons:

(1) To provide broad-spectrum empirical therapy in seriously ill patients.

(2) To treat polymicrobial infections such as intra-abdominal abscesses. The antimicrobial combination chosen should cover the most common known or suspected pathogens but need not cover all possible pathogens. The availability of antimicrobials with excellent polymicrobial coverage (eg, β-lactamase inhibitor combinations or imipenem) may reduce the need for combination therapy in the setting of polymicrobial infections.

(3) To decrease the emergence of resistant strains. The value of combination therapy in this setting has been clearly demonstrated for tuberculosis.

(4) To decrease dose-related toxicity by using reduced doses of one or more components of the drug regimen. The use of flucytosine in combination with amphotericin B for the treatment of cryptococcal meningitis in non-HIV-infected patients allows for a reduction in amphotericin B dosage with decreased amphotericin B-induced nephrotoxicity.

(5) To obtain enhanced inhibition or killing. This use of antimicrobial combinations is discussed in the paragraphs that follow.

SYNERGISM & ANTAGONISM

When the inhibitory or killing effects of two or more antimicrobials used together are significantly greater than expected from their effects when used individually, synergism is said to result. Synergism is marked by a fourfold or greater reduction in the MIC or MBC of each drug when used in combination versus when used alone.

The interaction between two antimicrobial agents can be expressed by the fractional inhibitory concentration (FIC) index:

$$FIC_{index} = FIC_A + FIC_B$$

$$FIC_A = \frac{MIC\ of\ drug\ A\ in\ combination}{MIC\ of\ drug\ A\ alone}$$

$$FIC_B = \frac{MIC\ of\ drug\ B\ in\ combination}{MIC\ of\ drug\ B\ alone}$$

The fractional *bactericidal* concentration (FBC) index can be determined by substituting MBCs for MICs in the above equations. Synergism for combinations of two drugs requires an FIC or FBC index of ≤ 0.5. Antagonism occurs when the combined inhibitory or killing effects of two or more antimicrobials are significantly less than expected when the drugs are used individually. Antibiotic antagonism is marked by an FIC or FBC index of 4 or more.

Mechanisms of Synergistic Action

The need for synergistic combinations of antimicrobials has been clearly established for the treatment of enterococcal endocarditis. Bactericidal activity is essential for the optimal management of bacterial endocarditis. Penicillin or ampicillin in combination with gentamicin or streptomycin is superior to monotherapy with a penicillin or vancomycin. When tested alone, penicillins and vancomycin are only bacteriostatic against susceptible enterococcal isolates. When these agents are combined with an aminoglycoside, however, bactericidal activity results. The addition of gentamicin or streptomycin to penicillin allows for a reduction in the duration of therapy for selected patients with viridans streptococcal endocarditis. There is some evidence that synergistic combinations of antimicrobials may be of benefit in the treatment of gram-negative bacillary infections in febrile neutropenic cancer patients and in systemic infections caused by *Pseudomonas aeruginosa*.

Other synergistic antimicrobial combinations have been shown to be more effective than monotherapy with individual components. Trimethoprim-sulfamethoxazole has been successfully used for the treatment of bacterial infections and *Pneumocystis jiroveci (carinii)* pneumonia.* Beta-lactamase inhibitors restore the activity of intrinsically active but hydrolyzable β-lactams against organisms such as *S aureus* and *Bacteroides fragilis*. Three major mechanisms of antimicrobial synergism have been established:

1. Blockade of Sequential Steps in a Metabolic Sequence: Trimethoprim-sulfamethoxazole is the best-known example of this mechanism of synergy (see Chapter 46). Blockade of the two sequential steps in the folic acid pathway by trimethoprim-sulfamethoxazole results in a much more complete inhibition of growth than achieved by either component alone.

2. Inhibition of Enzymatic Inactivation: Enzymatic inactivation of β-lactam antibiotics is a major mechanism of antibiotic resistance. Inhibition of β-lactamase by β-lactamase inhibitor drugs (eg, sulbactam) results in synergism.

3. Enhancement of Antimicrobial Agent Uptake: Penicillins and other cell wall-active agents can increase the uptake of aminoglycosides by a number of bacteria, including staphylococci, enterococci, streptococci, and *P aeruginosa*. It is thought that enterococci are intrinsically resistant to aminoglycosides because of permeability barriers. Similarly, amphotericin B is thought to enhance the uptake of flucytosine by fungi.

Mechanisms of Antagonistic Action

There are few clinically relevant examples of antimicrobial antagonism. The most striking example was

---

Pneumocystis jiroveci is a fungal organism found in humans (*P carinii* infects animals) that responds to antiprotozoal drugs. See Chapter 53.

reported in a study of patients with pneumococcal meningitis. Patients who were treated with the combination of penicillin and chlortetracycline had a mortality rate of 79% versus a mortality rate of 21% in patients who received penicillin monotherapy (illustrating the first mechanism set forth below).

The use of an antagonistic antimicrobial combination does not preclude other potential beneficial interactions. For example, rifampin may antagonize the action of antistaphylococcal penicillins or vancomycin against staphylococci. However, the aforementioned antimicrobials may prevent the emergence of resistance to rifampin.

Two major mechanisms of antimicrobial antagonism have been established:

1. Inhibition of Cidal Activity by Static Agents: Bacteriostatic agents such as tetracyclines and chloramphenicol can antagonize the action of bactericidal cell wall-active agents because cell wall-active agents require that the bacteria be actively growing and dividing.

2. Induction of Enzymatic Inactivation: Some gram-negative bacilli, including enterobacter species, *P aeruginosa, Serratia marcescens,* and *Citrobacter freundii,* possess inducible β-lactamases. Beta-lactam antibiotics such as imipenem, cefoxitin, and ampicillin are potent inducers of β-lactamase production. If an inducing agent is combined with an intrinsically active but hydrolyzable β-lactam such as piperacillin, antagonism may result.

ANTIMICROBIAL PROPHYLAXIS

Antimicrobial agents are effective in preventing infections in many settings. Antimicrobial prophylaxis should be used in circumstances in which efficacy has been demonstrated and benefits outweigh the risks of prophylaxis. Antimicrobial prophylaxis may be divided into surgical prophylaxis and nonsurgical prophylaxis.

Surgical Prophylaxis

Surgical wound infections are a major category of nosocomial infections. The estimated annual cost of surgical wound infections in the United States is $1.5 billion.

The National Research Council (NRC) Wound Classification Criteria have served as the basis for recommending antimicrobial prophylaxis. The NRC criteria consist of four classes (see Box, National Research Council (NRC) Wound Classification Criteria).

The Study of the Efficacy of Nosocomial Infection Control (SENIC) identified four independent risk factors for postoperative wound infections: operations on the abdomen, operations lasting more than 2 hours, contaminated or dirty wound classification, and the presence of at least three medical diagnoses. Patients with at least two SENIC risk factors who undergo clean surgical procedures are at increased risk of developing surgical wound infections and should receive antimicrobial prophylaxis.

Surgical procedures that necessitate the use of antimicrobial prophylaxis include contaminated and clean-contaminated operations, selected operations in which postoperative infection may be catastrophic such as open heart surgery, clean procedures that involve placement of prosthetic materials, and any procedure in an immunocompromised host. The operation should carry a significant risk of postoperative site infection or cause significant bacterial contamination.

General principles of antimicrobial surgical prophylaxis include the following:

(1) The antibiotic should be active against common surgical wound pathogens; unnecessarily broad coverage should be avoided.

NATIONAL RESEARCH COUNCIL (NRC) WOUND CLASSIFICATION CRITERIA

Clean: Elective, primarily closed procedure; respiratory, gastrointestinal, biliary, genitourinary, or oropharyngeal tract not entered; no acute inflammation and no break in technique; expected infection rate ≤ 2%.

Clean contaminated: Urgent or emergency case that is otherwise clean; elective, controlled opening of respiratory, gastrointestinal, biliary, or oropharyngeal tract; minimal spillage or minor break in technique; expected infection rate ≤ 10%.

Contaminated: Acute nonpurulent inflammation present; major technique break or major spill from hollow organ; penetrating trauma less than 4 hours old; chronic open wounds to be grafted or covered; expected infection rate about 20%.

Dirty: Purulence or abscess present; preoperative perforation of respiratory, gastrointestinal, biliary, or oropharyngeal tract; penetrating trauma more than 4 hours old; expected infection rate about 40%.

(2) The antibiotic should have proved efficacy in clinical trials.

(3) The antibiotic must achieve concentrations greater than the MIC of suspected pathogens, and these concentrations must be present at the time of incision.

(4) The shortest possible course—ideally a single dose—of the most effective and least toxic antibiotic should be used.

(5) The newer broad-spectrum antibiotics should be reserved for therapy of resistant infections.

(6) If all other factors are equal, the least expensive agent should be used.

The proper selection and administration of antimicrobial prophylaxis is of utmost importance. Common indications for surgical prophylaxis are shown in Table 51–7. Cefazolin is the prophylactic agent of choice for head and neck, gastroduodenal, biliary tract, gynecologic, and clean procedures. Local wound infection patterns should be considered when selecting antimicrobial prophylaxis. The selection of vancomycin over cefazolin may be necessary in hospitals with high rates of methicillin-resistant *S aureus* or *Staphylococcus epidermidis* infections. The antibiotic should be present in adequate concentrations at the operative site prior to incision and throughout the procedure; initial dosing is dependent on the volume of distribution, peak levels, clearance, protein binding, and bioavailability. Parenteral agents should be administered during the interval beginning 60 minutes before incision; administration up to the time of incision is preferred. In cesarean section, the

Table 51–7. Recommendations for surgical antimicrobial prophylaxis.

Type of Operation	Common Pathogens	Drug of Choice
Cardiac (with median sternotomy)	Staphylococci, enteric gram-negative rods	Cefazolin
Noncardiac, thoracic	Staphylococci, streptococci, enteric gram-negative rods	Cefazolin
Vascular (abdominal and lower extremity)	Staphylococci, enteric gram-negative rods	Cefazolin
Neurosurgical (craniotomy)	Staphylococci	Cefazolin
Orthopedic (with hardware insertion)	Staphylococci	Cefazolin
Head and neck (with entry into the oropharynx)	*S aureus*, oral flora	Cefazolin
Gastroduodenal (high-risk patients[1])	*S aureus*, oral flora, enteric gram-negative rods	Cefazolin
Biliary tract (high-risk patients[2])	*S aureus*, enterococci, enteric gram-negative rods	Cefazolin
Colorectal (elective surgery)	Enteric gram-negative rods, anaerobes	Oral erythromycin plus neomycin[3]
Colorectal (emergency surgery or obstruction)	Enteric gram-negative rods, anaerobes	Cefoxitin, cefotetan, or cefmetazole
Appendectomy	Enteric gram-negative rods, anaerobes	Cefoxitin, ceftizoxime, cefotetan, or cefmetazole
Hysterectomy	Enteric gram-negative rods, anaerobes, enterococci, group B streptococci	Cefazolin
Cesarean section	Enteric gram-negative rods, anaerobes, enterococci, group B streptococci	Cefazolin[4]

[1]Gastric procedures for cancer, ulcer, bleeding, or obstruction; morbid obesity; suppression of gastric acid secretion.

[2]Age > 60, acute cholecystitis, prior biliary tract surgery, common duct stones, jaundice, or diabetes mellitus.

[3]In conjunction with mechanical bowel preparation.

[4]Administer immediately following cord clamping.

antibiotic is administered after umbilical cord clamping. If short-acting agents such as cefoxitin are used, doses should be repeated if the procedure exceeds 3–4 hours in duration. Single-dose prophylaxis is effective for most procedures and results in decreased toxicity and antimicrobial resistance.

Improper administration of antimicrobial prophylaxis leads to excessive surgical wound infection rates. Common errors in antibiotic prophylaxis include selection of the wrong antibiotic, administering the first dose too early or too late, failure to repeat doses during prolonged procedures, excessive duration of prophylaxis, and inappropriate use of broad-spectrum antibiotics.

Nonsurgical Prophylaxis

Nonsurgical prophylaxis includes the administration of antimicrobials to prevent colonization or asymptomatic infection as well as the administration of drugs following colonization by or inoculation of pathogens but before the development of disease. Nonsurgical prophylaxis is indicated in individuals who are at high risk for temporary exposure to selected virulent pathogens and in patients who are at increased risk for developing infection because of underlying disease (eg, immunocompromised hosts). Prophylaxis is most effective when directed against organisms that are predictably susceptible to antimicrobial agents. Common indications for nonsurgical prophylaxis are listed in Table 51–8.

Table 51–8. Recommendations for nonsurgical antimicrobial prophylaxis.

Infection to Be Prevented	Indication	Drug of Choice	Efficacy
Anthrax	Suspected exposure	Ciprofloxacin or doxycycline	Proposed effective
Cholera	Close contacts of a case	Tetracycline	Proposed effective
Diphtheria	Unimmunized contacts	Penicillin or erythromycin	Proposed effective
Endocarditis	Dental, oral, or upper respiratory tract procedures[1] in at-risk patients[2]	Amoxicillin or clindamycin	Proposed effective
	Genitourinary or gastrointestinal procedures[3] in at-risk patients[2]	Ampicillin or vancomycin and gentamicin	Proposed effective
Genital herpes simplex	Recurrent infection (≥ 4 episodes per year)	Acyclovir	Excellent
Influenza B	Unvaccinated geriatric patients, immunocompromised hosts, and healthcare workers during outbreaks	Oseltamivir	Good
Perinatal herpes simplex type 2 infection	Mothers with primary HSV or frequent recurrent genital HSV	Acyclovir	Proposed effective
Group B streptococcal (GBS) infection	Mothers with cervical or vaginal GBS colonization and their newborns with one or more of the following: (a) onset of labor or membrane rupture before 37 weeks' gestation, (b) prolonged rupture of membranes (> 12 hours), (c) maternal intrapartum fever, (d) history of GBS bacteriuria during pregnancy, (e) mothers who have given birth to infants who had early GBS disease or with a history of streptococcal bacteriuria during pregnancy	Ampicillin or penicillin	Excellent
Haemophilus influenzae type B infection	Close contacts of a case in incompletely immunized children (< 48 months old)	Rifampin	Excellent

(continued)

Table 51–8. Recommendations for nonsurgical antimicrobial prophylaxis (*continued*).

Infection to Be Prevented	Indication	Drug of Choice	Efficacy
HIV infection	Health care workers exposed to blood after needle-stick injury	Zidovudine and lamivudine ± indinavir or nelfinavir	Good
	Pregnant HIV-infected women who are at ≥ 14 weeks of gestation Newborns of HIV-infected women for the first 6 weeks of life, beginning 8–12 hours after birth	Zidovudine	Excellent
Influenza A	Unvaccinated geriatric patients, immunocompromised hosts, and health care workers during outbreaks	Amantadine	Good
Malaria	Travelers to areas endemic for chloroquine-susceptible disease	Chloroquine	Excellent
	Travelers to areas endemic for chloroquine-resistant disease	Mefloquine	Excellent
Meningococcal infection	Close contacts of a case	Rifampin	Excellent
Mycobacterium avium complex	HIV-infected patients with CD4 count < 75/μL	Azithromycin or clarithromycin	Excellent
Otitis media	Recurrent infection	Amoxicillin	Good
Pertussis	Close contacts of a case	Erythromycin	Excellent
Plague	Close contacts of a case	Tetracycline	Proposed effective
Pneumococcemia	Children with sickle cell disease or asplenia	Penicillin	Excellent
Pneumocystis jiroveci pneumonia (PCP)	High-risk patients (eg AIDS, leukemia, transplant)	Trimethoprim-sulfamethoxazole	Excellent
Rheumatic fever	History of rheumatic fever or known rheumatic heart disease	Benzathine penicillin	Excellent
Toxoplasmosis	HIV-infected patients with IgG antibody to *Toxoplasma* and CD4 count < 100/μL	Trimethoprim-sulfamethoxazole	Good
Tuberculosis	Persons with positive tuberculin skin tests and one or more of the following: (a) HIV infection, (b) close contacts with newly diagnosed disease, (c) recent skin test conversion, (d) medical conditions that increase the risk of developing tuberculosis, (e) age < 35	Isoniazid, rifampin or pyrazinamide	Excellent
Urinary tract infections (UTI)	Recurrent infection	Trimethoprim-sulfamethoxazole	Excellent

[1]Prophylaxis is recommended for the following: dental procedures known to induce gingival or mucosal bleeding, tonsillectomy or adenoidectomy, surgical procedures that involve respiratory mucosa, and rigid bronchoscopy.

[2]Risk factors include the following: prosthetic heart valves, previous bacterial endocarditis, congenital cardiac malformations, rheumatic and other acquired valvular dysfunction, and mitral valve prolapse with valvular regurgitation.

[3]Prophylaxis is recommended for the following: surgical procedures that involve intestinal mucosa, sclerotherapy for esophageal varices, esophageal or urethral dilation, biliary tract surgery, cystoscopy, urethral catheterization or urinary tract surgery in the presence of urinary tract infection, prostatic surgery, incision and drainage of infected tissue, vaginal hysterectomy, and vaginal delivery in the presence of infection.

REFERENCES

Antimicrobial prophylaxis in surgery. Med Lett Drugs Ther 2001;43:92.

ASHP Therapeutic Guidelines for Nonsurgical Antimicrobial Prophylaxis. American Society of Health-System Pharmacists. Am J Health Syst Pharm 1999;56:1201.

Bartlett JG et al: Practice guidelines for the management of community-acquired pneumonia in adults. Infectious Diseases Society of America. Clin Infect Dis 2000;31:347.

Blumberg HM et al: American Thoracic Society/Centers for Disease Control and Prevention/Infectious Diseases Society of America: treatment of tuberculosis. Am J Respir Crit Care Med 2003;167:603.

Bochner BS et al: Anaphylaxis. N Engl J Med 1991;324:1785.

Classen DC et al: The timing of prophylactic administration of antibiotics and the risk of surgical-wound infection. N Engl J Med 1992;326:281.

Craig WA: Pharmacokinetic/pharmacodynamic parameters: rationale for antibacterial dosing of mice and men. Clin Infect Dis 1998;26:1.

Craven DE et al: Nosocomial pneumonia: emerging concepts in diagnosis, management and prophylaxis. Curr Opin Crit Care 2002;8:421.

Dajani AS et al: Prevention of bacterial endocarditis. Recommendations by the American Heart Association. JAMA 1997; 277:1794.

Dellinger EP et al: Quality standard for antimicrobial prophylaxis in surgical procedures. Infect Control Hosp Epidemiol 1994;15:182.

Gonzales R et al: Principles of appropriate antibiotic use for treatment of acute respiratory tract infections in adults: background, specific aims, and methods. Ann Intern Med 2001;134:479.

Jones RN, Pfaller MA: Bacterial resistance: a worldwide problem. Diagn Microbiol Infect Dis 1998;31:379.

Kaye D: Antibacterial therapy: Pharmacodynamics, pharmacology, newer agents. Infect Dis Clin North Am 2000;14:265.

Mangram AJ et al: Guideline for prevention of surgical site infection, 1999. Hospital Infection Control Practices Advisory Committee. Infect Control Hosp Epidemiol 1999;20:250.

Martone WJ, Nichols RL: Recognition, prevention, surveillance, and management of surgical site infections: introduction to the problem and symposium overview. Clin Infect Dis 2001;33(Suppl 2):S67.

National Nosocomial Infections Surveillance (NNIS) System Report. Data Summary from January 1992–June 2001, issued August 2001. Am J Infect Control 2001;29:404.

Osmon DR: Antimicrobial prophylaxis in adults. Mayo Clin Proc 2000;75:98.

Sexually transmitted diseases treatment guidelines 2002. Centers for Disease Control and Prevention. MMWR Morb Mortal Wkly Rep 2002;51(RR-6):1.

USPHS/IDSA guidelines for preventing opportunistic infections among HIV-infected persons—2002. MMWR Morb Mortal Wkly Rep 2002;51(RR-8):1.

Wilson WR et al: Antibiotic treatment of adults with infective endocarditis due to streptococci, enterococci, staphylococci and HACEK microorganisms. JAMA 1995;274:1706.

Basic Principles of Antiparasitic Chemotherapy

Ching Chung Wang, PhD, & Alice Lee Wang, PhD

In its general scientific sense, the term "parasite" includes all of the known infectious agents such as viruses, bacteria, fungi, protozoa, and helminths. In this and the two following chapters, the term is used in a restricted sense to denote the protozoa and helminths. It has been estimated that 3 billion (3×10^9) humans suffer from parasitic infections, plus a much greater number of domestic and wild animals. Although these diseases constitute the most widespread human health problem in the world today, they have for various reasons also been the most neglected.

In theory, the parasitic infections should be relatively easy to treat because the etiologic agents are known in almost all cases. Furthermore, recent advances in cell culture techniques have made possible in vitro cultivation of many of the important parasites. These advances have not only laid to rest the traditional view that parasites somehow depend on a living host for their existence but have also enabled us to study parasites by methods similar to those employed in investigations of bacteria, including biochemistry, molecular biology, and immunologic pharmacology. However, many problems remain to be solved before more effective chemotherapeutic agents will be discovered and made available for all of the parasitic diseases.

Targets of Chemotherapy

A rational approach to antiparasitic chemotherapy requires comparative biochemical and physiologic investigations of host and parasite to discover differences in essential processes that will permit selective inhibition in the parasite and not in the host. One might expect that the parasite would have many deficiencies in its metabolism associated with its parasitic nature. This is true of many parasites—the oversimplified metabolic pathways are usually indispensable for survival of the parasite and thus represent points of vulnerability. However, oversimplified metabolic pathways are not the only opportunity for attack. Although the parasite lives in a metabolically luxurious environment and may become "lazy," the environment is not entirely friendly and the parasite

must have defense mechanisms in order to survive—ie, to defend itself against immunologic attack, proteolytic digestion, etc, by the host. In some instances, necessary nutrients are not supplied to the parasite from the host, though the latter can obtain the same nutrients from the diet. In this situation, the parasite will have acquired the synthetic activity needed for its survival. Finally, the great evolutionary distance between host and parasite has in some cases resulted in sufficient differences among individual enzymes or functional pathways to allow selective inhibition of the parasite. Thus, there can be three major types of potential targets for chemotherapy of parasitic diseases: (1) unique essential enzymes found only in the parasite; (2) similar enzymes found in both host and parasite but indispensable only for the parasite; and (3) common biochemical functions found in both parasite and host but with different pharmacologic properties. Examples of specific targets and drugs that act on them are summarized in Table 52–1. This chapter discusses antiparasitic mechanisms based upon these examples and provides background information for the drugs described in Chapters 53 and 54.

ESSENTIAL ENZYMES FOUND ONLY IN PARASITES

These enzymes would appear to be the cleanest targets for chemotherapy. Like enzymes involved in the synthesis of bacterial cell walls (see Chapter 43), inhibition of these enzymes should have no effect on the host. Unfortunately, only a few of these enzymes have been discovered among the parasitic protozoa. Furthermore, their usefulness as chemotherapeutic targets is sometimes limited because of the development of drug resistance. Examples of important target enzymes in this category are discussed in the following pages.

Enzymes for Dihydropteroate Synthesis

Intracellular protozoa of the phylum Apicomplexa such as plasmodium, toxoplasma, and eimeria have long

Table 52–1. Identified targets for chemotherapy in parasites.

Targets	Parasites	Inhibitors
Unique essential enzymes		
Enzymes for dihydropteroate synthesis	Apicomplexa	Sulfones and sulfonamides
Glycolipid synthesis	African trypanosomes	None
Pyruvate:ferrodoxin oxidoreductase	Anaerobic protozoa	Nitroimidazoles
Pyruvate phosphate dikinase	Anaerobic protozoa	None
Nucleoside phosphotransferase	Flagellated protozoa	Allopurinol riboside and formycin B
Trypanothione reductase and peroxidase	Kinetoplastida	Nifurtimox
Indispensable enzymes		
Lanosterol C-14α demethylase	Leishmania and *Trypanosoma cruzi*	Azoles
Purine phosphoribosyl transferase	Protozoa	Allopurinol
Purine nucleoside kinase	*Trichomonas vaginalis* and *Entamoeba histolytica*	None
Ornithine decarboxylase	African trypanosomes	α-Difluoromethylornithine
(S)-Adenosylmethionine decarboxylase	African trypanosomes	Diamidines
Glycolytic enzymes	Kinetoplastida	Glycerol plus salicylhydroxamic acid and suramin
Common indispensable biochemical functions with different pharmacologic properties		
Dihydrofolate reductase-thymidylate synthase bifunctional enzyme	Apicomplexa and Kinetoplastida	Pyrimethamine
Thiamin transporter	Coccidia	Amprolium
Mitochondrial electron transporter	Apicomplexa	4-Hydroxyquinolines and 2-hydroxynaphthoquinones
Microtubules	Helminth	Benzimidazoles
Nervous synaptic transmission	Helminth and ectoparasite	Levamisole, piperazine, milbemycins, and avermectins

been known to respond to sulfonamides and sulfones. This has led to the assumption that Apicomplexa must synthesize their own folate in order to survive. The reaction of 2-amino-4-hydroxy-6-hydroxymethyl-dihydropteridine diphosphate with *p*-aminobenzoate to form 7,8-dihydropteroate has been demonstrated in cell-free extracts of the human malaria parasite *Plasmodium falciparum*. 2-Amino-4-hydroxy-6-hydroxymethyl-dihydropteridine pyrophosphokinase and 7,8-dihydropteroate synthase have also been identified. Sulfathiazole, sulfaguanidine, and sulfanilamide act as competitive inhibitors of *p*-aminobenzoate. It has not been possible to demonstrate dihydrofolate synthase activity in the parasites, which raises the possibility that 7,8-dihydropteroate may have substituted for dihydro-

folate in malaria parasites. Similar lack of recognition of folate as substrate was also observed in the dihydrofolate reductase of *Eimeria tenella,* a parasite of chickens.

However, lack of utilization of exogenous folate may not fully explain the apparently indispensable nature of the synthesis of 7,8-dihydropteroate in plasmodium, toxoplasma, and eimeria. It is known that most of the folate molecules in mammalian cells are linked with polyglutamates in the cytoplasm and are transported across cell membranes with difficulty. It may compound the problem of obtaining 7,8-dihydropteroate or dihydrofolate for the parasite and makes all of the enzymes involved in their synthesis attractive targets for anti-Apicocomplexa chemotherapy.

The gene encoding 7,8-dihydropteroate synthase

was cloned from *P falciparum* and found to encode a bifunctional enzyme that includes the pyrophosphokinase at the amino terminal of the protein. Discrepancies were observed in the sequences of 7,8-dihydropteroate synthase portion of the genes from sulfadoxine-sensitive versus sulfadoxine-resistant *P falciparum,* thus confirming that this enzyme is the target for the antimalarial sulfonamide drugs.

The sulfones and sulfonamides synergize with the inhibitors of dihydrofolate reductase, and the combinations have been effective in controlling malaria, toxoplasmosis, and coccidiosis. Fansidar, a combination of sulfadoxine and pyrimethamine, has been successful in controlling some strains of chloroquine-resistant *Plasmodium falciparum* malaria (see Chapter 53). However, reports of Fansidar resistance have increased in recent years. New inhibitors effective against the sulfonamide-resistant 7,8-dihydropteroate synthase are needed.

The pharmacologic properties of parasite 7,8-dihydropteroate synthases may differ from those of the bacterial enzymes. For instance, metachloridine and 2-ethoxy-*p*-aminobenzoate are both ineffective against sulfonamide-sensitive bacteria, but the former has antimalarial activity and the latter is effective against infection by the chicken parasite *Eimeria acervulina;* both activities can be reversed by *p*-aminobenzoate.

Pyruvate:Ferredoxin Oxidoreductase

Certain anaerobic protozoal parasites lack mitochondria and mitochondrial activities for generating ATP and disposing of electrons. They possess, instead, ferredoxin-like or flavodoxin-like low-redox-potential electron transport proteins. In trichomonad flagellates and rumen ciliates, the process takes place in a membrane-limited organelle called the hydrogenosome. By the actions of pyruvate:ferredoxin oxidoreductase (PFOR) and hydrogenase in the hydrogenosome, H_2 is produced by these organisms under anaerobic conditions as the major means of electron disposition. Although entamoeba species and *Giardia lamblia* have no hydrogenosome, a ferredoxin has been isolated from *Entamoeba histolytica,* and the genes encoding ferredoxin and pyruvate:ferredoxin oxidoreductase have been isolated from *E histolytica* and *G lamblia.*

Pyruvate:ferredoxin oxidoreductase has no counterpart in mammalian systems. In contrast to the mammalian pyruvate dehydrogenase complex, pyruvate:ferredoxin oxidoreductase is incapable of reducing pyridine nucleotides because of its low redox potential (approximately −400 mV). However, this low potential can also transfer electrons from pyruvate to the nitro groups of metronidazole and other 5-nitroimidazole derivatives to form cytotoxic reduced products that bind to DNA and proteins. This is apparently why anaerobic protozoal species are highly susceptible to drugs such as metronidazole. Despite the recent development of drug resistance in some *Trichomonas vaginalis* strains and the possibility of carcinogenic properties (see Chapter 53), metronidazole remains the drug of choice for controlling anaerobic protozoal parasite infections. Nitazoxanide, an agent recently approved for use against *G lamblia* and *Cryptosporidium parvum,* apparently acts through an active metabolite, tizoxanide, which inhibits the pyruvate:ferredoxin oxidoreductase pathway.

Though pyruvate:ferredoxin oxidoreductase activates the prodrug metronidazole, it may not perform an essential function in the anaerobic parasites. The enzyme activity was significantly lower in metronidazole-resistant *G lamblia.* Some aerobic metronidazole-resistant *T vaginalis* strains have no detectable pyruvate:ferredoxin oxidoreductase activity but are viable. A knockdown of expression of this enzyme in *G lamblia* by ribozyme-antisense chimeric RNA resulted in facilitated cell growth under aerobic condition and metronidazole resistance.

Pyruvate Phosphate Dikinase

Glycolysis provides the main source of ATP in *Trypanosoma brucei, E histolytica,* and *G lamblia,* which possess pyruvate kinase as well as a pyruvate phosphate dikinase for converting phosphoenolpyruvate (PEP) to pyruvate and generating ATP. Pyruvate phosphate dikinase is not a homolog of pyruvate kinase but is closely related to PEP synthase from bacteria. The enzyme catalyzes conversion of PEP to pyruvate accompanied by the synthesis of ATP from AMP and pyrophosphate. Genes encoding the enzyme have been isolated from *E histolytica* and *G lamblia* and have demonstrated considerable structural divergences. No specific inhibitor of this enzyme has yet been identified.

Nucleoside Phosphotransferases

All the protozoal parasites studied thus far are deficient in de novo synthesis of purine nucleotides. The various purine salvage pathways in these parasites are thus essential for their survival and growth. Among the leishmania species, a unique salvage enzyme has been identified—purine nucleoside phosphotransferase—that can transfer the phosphate group from a variety of monophosphate esters, including *p*-nitrophenylphosphate, to the 5' position of purine nucleosides. This enzyme also phosphorylates purine nucleoside analogs such as allopurinol riboside, formycin B, 9-deazainosine, and thiopurinol riboside, converting them to the corresponding nucleotides. These nucleotides are either further converted to triphosphates and eventually incorporated into nucleic acid of leishmania or become inhibitors of other essential enzymes in purine metabolism. Consequently, allopurinol riboside, formycin B, 9-deazainosine, and thiopurinol riboside all act as antileishmanial agents both in vitro and in vivo. Allopurinol riboside is particularly interesting because it is remarkably nontoxic to the mammalian host.

The mechanism of action of these purine nucleoside analogs is thus not by blocking purine salvage in leishmania because there are many other major purine salvage enzymes in the organism that remain unaffected. The nucleoside transferase is a minor enzyme, but it recognizes a number of false substrates and converts them to products toxic to leishmania. This approach of identifying "subversive substrates" for a purine salvage enzyme as potential antiparasitic targets does not depend on the lack of de novo purine nucleotide synthesis in these parasites. It could be applied—in any parasite—to any enzyme that happens to recognize a subversive substrate.

Trichomonad flagellates appear to be deficient in de novo synthesis of both purines and pyrimidines. Their salvage thus becomes indispensable for these parasites. In *T vaginalis,* for instance, the supply route for thymidine 5′-monophosphate (TMP) is provided by a single salvage pathway that converts exogenous thymidine to TMP by the action of a thymidine phosphotransferase. The enzyme activity is not affected by thymidine kinase inhibitors such as acyclovir but is inhibitable by guanosine or 5-fluorodeoxyuridine; both compounds also inhibit the in vitro growth of the parasites. This enzyme is an attractive target for chemotherapeutic treatment of the anaerobic protozoal parasites.

Purine Nucleoside Kinase

Exogenous adenosine is the precursor of the entire purine nucleotide pool in *T vaginalis* through its partial conversion to inosine and the action of purine nucleoside kinase, a unique enzyme in the organism, which converts adenosine and inosine to the corresponding nucleotides. It performs a critical role in *T vaginalis* purine salvage and has a unique substrate specificity suitable as a target of chemotherapy.

Trypanothione Synthase, Reductase, & Peroxidase

Protozoa with kinetoplasts are unusual in that a considerable proportion of their intracellular spermidine and glutathione is found in the unique conjugate N^1-N^8-(glutathionyl)spermidine, which has been assigned the name trypanothione. Trypanothione synthase, reductase, and peroxidase activities have been detected in these parasites. A knockout of the gene encoding trypanothione reductase from the African trypanosome

Trypanosoma brucei resulted in apparent cessation of growth of the organism. Nifurtimox, a nitrofuran derivative effective in treating Chagas' disease (caused by *Trypanosoma cruzi*), has been found to be a potent inhibitor of trypanothione reductase, and other inhibitors are under study. No extensive studies of trypanothione synthetase or peroxidase have been performed. The antitrypanosomal trivalent arsenicals are taken up by the African trypanosome *Trypanosoma brucei* and complex with trypanothione, forming a product that is also an effective inhibitor of trypanothione reductase.

Glycolipid Synthetic Enzymes

The variant surface glycoprotein on the plasma membranes of bloodstream African trypanosomes provides the organisms with the means of evading host immune responses. The glycoprotein is anchored to the cell surface by a glycosyl phosphatidylinositol that contains myristate as its only fatty acid component. Thus, the introduction of a subversive substrate to replace myristate from the glycolipid anchor could result in loss of the variant surface glycoprotein, which might suppress development of trypanosomes in mammalian blood. A myristate analog, 10-(propoxy)decanoic acid, was found incorporated into the glycolipid and also active against *T brucei* in in vitro tests. However, further validation of this approach to antitrypanosomal chemotherapy must await results of in vivo tests.

Shikimate Pathway Enzymes

The availability of *P falciparum* genome database led to the identification of shikimate pathway enzymes in this organism. The pathway is known to exist in bacteria, fungi, algae, and plants but not in mammals. A herbicide, glyphosate, known to inhibit the enzyme 5′-enolpyruvylshikimate 3-phosphate synthase, was found to inhibit growth of *P falciparum.* However, it is not known if the in vitro antimalarial action of glyphosate is by inhibiting this enzyme. Furthermore, the shikimate pathway leads to biosynthesis of aromatic amino acids. Since *P falciparum* grows on digested hemoglobin, it is not clear if biosynthesis of aromatic amino acids plays an essential role in this organism.

Isoretinoid Biosynthetic Enzymes

A mevalonate-independent isoprenoid biosynthetic pathway occurring only among bacteria, algae, and plants was also identified in *P falciparum* and *T gondii.* **Fosmidomycin,** known to inhibit 1-deoxy-D-xylulose-5-phosphate isomerase in this pathway, was found to also inhibit in vitro growth of *P falciparum* and to cure *P vinckei* infection in mice. However, the same questions about whether the pathway plays an indispensable role in this parasitic organism and whether fosmidomycin inhibits the parasites by inhibiting the particular enzyme remain to be answered.

ENZYMES INDISPENSABLE ONLY IN PARASITES

Because of the many metabolic deficiencies among parasites resulting from the unique environments in which parasites live in their hosts, there are enzymes whose functions may be essential for the survival of the parasites, but the same enzymes are not indispensable to the host—ie, the host may be able to survive the complete loss of these enzyme functions by achieving the same result through alternative pathways. This discrepancy opens up opportunities for antiparasitic chemotherapy, though insufficiently selective inhibition of parasite enzymes remains an important safety concern.

Lanosterol C-14α Demethylase

T cruzi and leishmania contain ergosterol as the principal sterol in plasma membranes. The **azole antifungal agents** (eg, ketoconazole, miconazole, itraconazole), which are known to act by inhibiting the cytochrome P450-dependent C-14α demethylation of lanosterol in the ergosterol biosynthetic pathway, also inhibit growth of *T cruzi* and leishmania by blocking C-14α demethylation of lanosterol in these parasites. Recently, an antifungal bistriazole, D0870, demonstrated encouraging in vivo anti-*T cruzi* activity in mouse infection models. It is thus likely that lanosterol C-14α demethylase plays an essential role in ergosterol synthesis and therefore qualifies as a target for chemotherapy against *T cruzi* and leishmania.

The same C-14α demethylation of lanosterol is also required for cholesterol synthesis in mammals. As rather nonselective inhibitors of lanosterol C-14α demethylases, the azoles may exert a variety of endocrine side effects by inhibiting this enzyme in the adrenal glands and gonads while remaining acceptable as systemic antifungal agents. Because of its excessive toxicity, D0870 was not developed as an antifungal or antiparasitic agent. However, since human and yeast lanosterol C-14α demethylases share only 38–42% sequence identities, there may be a good chance of designing inhibitors that are more selective against the fungal or parasitic enzymes.

Purine Phosphoribosyl Transferases

The absence of de novo purine nucleotide synthesis in protozoal parasites as well as in the trematode *Schistosoma mansoni* is reflected in the relative importance of purine phosphoribosyl transferases in many parasite species.

G lamblia has an exceedingly simple scheme of purine salvage. It possesses only two pivotal enzymes: the adenine and guanine phosphoribosyl transferases, which convert exogenous adenine and guanine to the corresponding nucleotides. There is no salvage of hypoxanthine, xanthine, or any purine nucleosides and no interconversion between adenine and guanine nucleotides in the parasite. Functions of the two phosphoribosyl transferases are thus both essential for the survival and development of *G lamblia* (Figure 52–1). The guanine phosphoribosyl transferase is an interesting enzyme because it does not recognize hypoxanthine, xanthine, or adenine as substrate. This substrate specificity distinguishes the giardia enzyme from the mammalian enzyme, which uses hypoxanthine, and the bacterial one, which uses xanthine as substrate. Design of a highly specific inhibitor of this enzyme is thus possible. The crystal structures of both guanine and adenine phosphoribosyltransferases from *G lamblia* have been solved recently, which should provide good opportunities for specific inhibitor design.

T foetus depends primarily on a single enzyme, hypoxanthine-guanine-xanthine phosphoribosyltransferase, for replenishing the needed purine nucleotides. The three-dimensional structure of this enzyme was recently solved. It bears significant distinctions in both structure and function when compared with the mammalian enzyme, thus providing an excellent opportunity for specific inhibitor design.

Other protozoan parasites such as *Toxoplasma gondii* and *P falciparum* have also been found to contain a unique hypoxanthine-guanine-xanthine phosphoribosyltransferase. Detailed crystal structures of the two enzymes have been solved recently. However, there is an adenosine kinase-mediated purine salvage pathway in *T gondii* that can apparently bypass the inhibition of phosphoribosyltransferase, making this organism less vulnerable. On the other hand, the genome database of *P falciparum* suggests that the phosphoribosyltransferase is the only purine salvage enzyme in this organism. More biochemical and pharmacologic evidence will be needed for verifying it as a bona fide target for chemotherapy.

Ornithine Decarboxylase

Polyamines, which are found in almost all organisms, are required for cell proliferation. Ornithine decarboxylase, the key enzyme that controls formation of the polyamine putrescine from ornithine, has been identified in all protozoan parasites examined except *T cruzi*. **Eflornithine** (alpha-difluoromethylornithine; DFMO), a suicide inhibitor of ornithine decarboxylases, has good in vitro activity against virtually all protozoan parasites

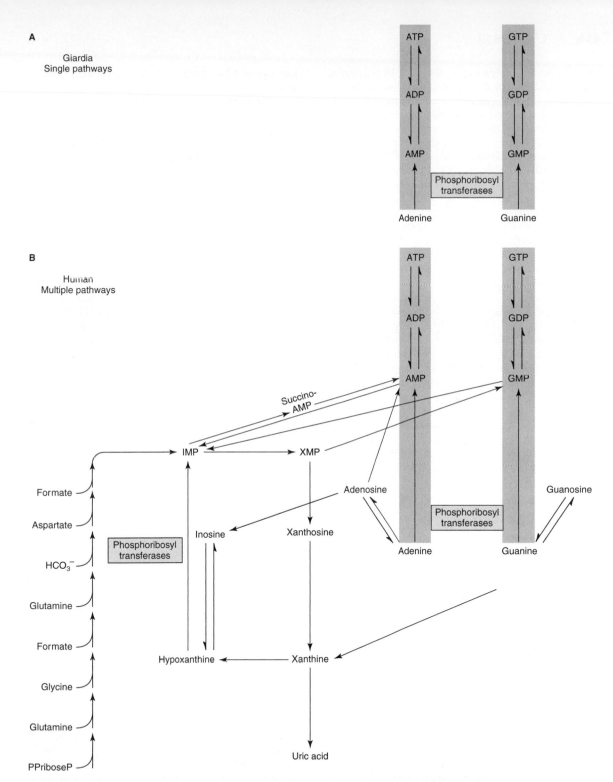

Figure 52–1. Purine metabolism in *Giardia lamblia* **(A)** and in humans **(B)**. *G lamblia* lacks enzymes both for de novo synthesis of essential purine nucleotides and for interconversion of these purine nucleotides. (AMP, GMP, IMP, XMP, etc, adenosine monophosphate, guanosine monophosphate, inosine monophosphate, xanthosine monophosphate, etc.)

propagated in culture media deficient in polyamine. However, when this drug is tested in vivo, it demonstrates activity only against African trypanosomes. This is attributable to the fact that mammalian blood, where the African trypanosomes reside, contains little polyamine. The parasite must therefore synthesize its own polyamine. Thus, inhibition of the parasite ornithine decarboxylase by eflornithine depletes the parasite of polyamines, causing it to enter a dormant state in which it can eventually be eliminated by the host's immune system. In contrast, parasites located inside or on the surface of mammalian cells are surrounded by high concentrations of polyamines. This may explain why *T cruzi* can proliferate without any endogenous ornithine decarboxylase.

Mammalian ornithine decarboxylase is characterized by its striking inducibility and very short half-life. Ornithine decarboxylase in African trypanosomes is much more stable. The relatively short half-life of eflornithine allows replacement of irreversibly inhibited mammalian enzyme by rapid turnover, whereas the more stable parasite enzyme remains inhibited. This difference may explain the therapeutic antitrypanosomal action of eflornithine and its lack of toxic effect on the mammalian host. Eflornithine is highly effective against *T gambiense* but much less so against *T rhodesiense*. This difference may be explained by the finding that *T rhodesiense* ornithine decarboxylase, like the mammalian enzyme, has a much shorter half-life than that of *T gambiense*.

(S)-Adenosylmethionine Decarboxylase

This is the second enzyme required for synthesis of the polyamine spermidine from putrescine and spermine from spermidine. It has recently been identified in African as well as American trypanosomes and is apparently essential for proliferation of the former in the mammalian bloodstream. This enzyme is effectively inhibited by a variety of diamidine derivatives, including berenil and pentamidine. These agents belong to a family of chemical compounds known to have specific activity against African trypanosomes, without any effect on other kinetoplastids such as leishmania and *T cruzi*.

Glycolytic Enzymes

In the bloodstream form of African trypanosomes such as *Trypanosoma brucei brucei*, the single mitochondrion lacks both cytochrome and functional Krebs cycle enzymes. The organism is entirely dependent on glycolysis for its production of ATP. Under aerobic conditions, one glucose molecule can generate only two molecules of ATP, with two pyruvate molecules excreted

into the host bloodstream as the end product. This low energy yield makes it necessary to have glycolysis in *T b brucei* proceed at an extremely high rate to enable the trypanosome to divide every 7 hours. The high glycolytic rate, 50 times that of the mammalian host, is made possible not only by the abundant glucose supply in the host's blood but also by the clustering of most of the glycolytic enzymes of the parasite in membrane-bound microbody organelles called glycosomes (Figure 52–2). Since lactate dehydrogenase is absent from the parasite, the regeneration of NAD from NADH in the glycosome during glycolysis depends on a dihydroxyacetone phosphate:glycerol 3-phosphate shuttle plus a glycerol-3-phosphate oxidase. Thus, under anaerobic conditions, glycerol 3-phosphate cannot be oxidized back to dihydroxyacetone phosphate and accumulates inside the glycosome. This accumulation, together with the accumulation of ADP due to depletion of NAD, eventually drives the reversed glycerol kinase-catalyzed reaction in the glycosome to generate glycerol and ATP. Thus, under anaerobic conditions, *T b brucei* generates only one ATP molecule from each glucose molecule and excretes equimolar pyruvate and glycerol as end products.

This delicate and indispensable glycolytic system appears to be an attractive target for antitrypanosomal chemotherapy. It has been shown that glycerol-3-phosphate oxidase can be inhibited in the parasite with **salicylhydroxamic acid (SHAM)** to bring *T b brucei* into an anaerobic condition. Glycolysis can then be stopped by inhibiting the reversed glycerol kinase-catalyzed reaction with added **glycerol**. This SHAM plus glycerol combination can lyse the African trypanosome bloodstream forms in vitro within minutes and is very effective in suppressing parasitemia in infected animals.

The systems involved in glycosome biogenesis may also be targets for antitrypanosomal therapy. The drug **suramin** contains six negatively charged sulfonyl groups and has a molecular weight of 1429. These sulfonyl groups may facilitate binding of the drug to some of the basic amino acids known to be present in several essential glycosomal enzymes. This would result in immobilization of the enzymes before transport into the glycosome, with a resultant crippling of glycosomal function.

Most of the crystal structures of the glycolytic enzymes in the glycosome of *T brucei* have been solved. The geometry of the active site in glycosomal glyceraldehyde-3-phosphate dehydrogenase was used for structure-based inhibitor design and resulted in the synthesis of N-6-(1-naphthalenemethyl)-2'-(3-methoxybenzimido) adenosine. It has an IC$_{50}$ of 2 μmol/L on the *T brucei* enzyme and an ED$_{50}$ of 30 μmol/L on in vitro cultured *T brucei* bloodstream cells. It has similarly potent activity against the same enzymes in *L mexicana* and *T cruzi* but has no effect on human enzyme or

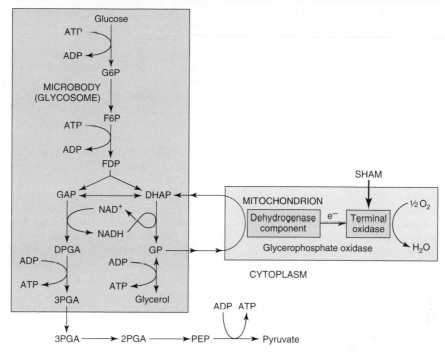

Figure 52–2. Glycolytic pathway in long, slender bloodstream forms of *Trypanosoma brucei brucei*. The principal site of inhibition by trypanocidal drugs in vivo is indicated by SHAM and the bold arrow. (SHAM, salicylhydroxamic acid; G6P, glucose 6-phosphate; F6P, fructose 6-phosphate; FDP, fructose 1,6-diphosphate; GAP, glyceraldehyde 3-phosphate; DHAP, dihydroxyacetone phosphate; GP, *sn*-glycerol 3-phosphate; DPGA, 1,3-diphosphoglycerate; 3PGA and 2PGA, 3- and 2-phosphoglycerate; PEP, phosphoenolpyruvate.) (Modified and reproduced, with permission, from Fairlamb A: Biochemistry of trypanosomiasis and rational approaches to chemotherapy. Trends Biochem Sci 1982;7:249.)

mammalian cells up to its maximal solubility. This approach may thus lead to more effective agents against Kinetoplastida.

INDISPENSABLE BIOCHEMICAL FUNCTIONS FOUND IN BOTH PARASITE & HOST BUT WITH DIFFERENT PHARMACOLOGIC PROPERTIES

In the parasite, these functions have differentiated sufficiently to become probable targets for antiparasitic chemotherapy, not because of the parasitic nature of the organism or its unique environment but, more likely, because of the long evolutionary distances separating the parasite and the host. It is thus difficult to discover these targets through studying metabolic deficiency or special nutritional requirements of the parasite. They have usually been found by investigating the modes of action of some well-established antiparasitic agents discovered by screening methods in the past. More

recently, comparison of genome databases between the host and the parasite has become practical. The target may not be a single well-defined enzyme but may include transporters, receptors, cellular structural components, or other specific functions essential for survival of the parasite.

Dihydrofolate Reductase-Thymidylate Synthase Bifunctional Enzyme

Dihydrofolate reductase (DHFR), a classic target in antimicrobial and anticancer chemotherapy, has been shown to be a useful therapeutic target in plasmodium, toxoplasma, and eimeria species. **Pyrimethamine** is the prototypical DHFR inhibitor, exerting inhibitory effects in all three groups. However, pyrimethamine resistance in *P falciparum* has become widespread in recent years. This is largely attributable to specific point mutations in *P falciparum* DHFR that have rendered the enzyme less susceptible to the inhibitor.

A highly unusual feature of DHFR in Apicomplexa and Kinetoplastida is its association with thymidylate synthase in the same protein. DHFR activity is always located at the amino terminal portion, while the thymidylate synthase activity resides in the carboxyl terminal. The two enzyme functions do not appear to be interdependent; eg, the DHFR portion of the *P falciparum* enzyme molecule was found to function normally in the absence of the thymidylate synthase portion. It is likely that since the protozoan parasites do not perform de novo synthesis of purine nucleotides, the primary function of the tetrahydrofolate produced by DHFR is to provide 5,10-methylenetetrahydrofolate only for the thymidylate synthase-catalyzed reaction. Physical association of the two enzymes may improve efficiency of TMP synthesis. If an effective means of disrupting the coordination between the two activities can be developed, this bifunctional protein may qualify as a target for antiparasitic therapy.

Thiamin Transporter

Carbohydrate metabolism provides the main energy source in coccidia. Diets deficient in thiamin, riboflavin, or nicotinic acid—all cofactors in carbohydrate metabolism—result in suppression of parasitic infestation of chickens by *E tenella* and *E acervulina*. A thiamin analog, **amprolium**—1-[(4-amino-2-propyl-5-pyrimidinyl)-methyl]-2-picolinium chloride—has long been used as an effective anticoccidial agent in chickens and cattle with relatively low host toxicity. The antiparasitic activity of amprolium is reversible by thiamin and is recognized to involve inhibition of thiamin transport in the parasite. Unfortunately, amprolium has a rather narrow spectrum of antiparasitic activity; it has poor activity against toxoplasmosis, a closely related parasitic infection.

Mitochondrial Electron Transporter

Mitochondria of *E tenella* appear to lack cytochrome c and to contain cytochrome o—a cytochrome oxidase commonly found in the bacterial respiratory chain—as the terminal oxidase. Certain 4-hydroxyquinoline derivatives such as buquinolate, decoquinate, and methyl benzoquate that have long been known to be relatively nontoxic and effective anticoccidial agents have been found to act on the parasites by inhibiting mitochondrial respiration. Direct investigation on isolated intact *E tenella* mitochondria indicated that the 4-hydroxyquinolines have no effect on NADH oxidase or succinoxidase activity but that they are extremely potent inhibitors of NADH- or succinate-induced mitochondrial respiration. On the other hand, the ascorbate-induced *E tenella* mitochondrial respiration was totally insusceptible to these 4-hydroxyquinolines. The block

by the anticoccidial agents thus may be located between the oxidases and cytochrome b in the electron transport chain. A certain component at this location must be essential for mediating the electron transport and would appear to be highly sensitive to the 4-hydroxyquinolines. This component must be a very specific chemotherapeutic target in eimeria species, since the 4-hydroxyquinolines have no effect on chicken liver and mammalian mitochondrial respiration and no activity against any parasites other than eimeria.

Many 2-hydroxynaphthoquinones have demonstrated therapeutic activities against Apicomplexa. **Parvaquinone** and **buparvaquinone** have been developed for the treatment of theileriosis in cattle and other domestic animals. **Atovaquone** is an antimalarial drug and is also used in the treatment of *Pneumocystis jiroveci* and *P carinii* infections. The 2-hydroxynaphthoquinones are analogs of ubiquinone. The primary site of action of atovaquone in *Plasmodium* is the cytochrome bc_1 complex, where an apparent drug-binding site is present in cytochrome b. In plasmodium, ubiquinone also plays an important role as an electron acceptor for dihydroorotate oxidase. Consequently, pyrimidine biosynthesis in plasmodium is also inhibited by atovaquone. This chemical compound has also been found to be active against *T gondii* cysts in the brains of infected mice.

A major problem in the use of the antiparasitic 4-hydroxyquinolones and 2-hydroxynaphthoquinones is resistance that can develop with extraordinarily high frequency. It may be attributable to their mitochondrial site of action, which is known to have a high frequency of mutation.

Microtubules

Microtubules are an important part of the cytoskeleton and the mitotic spindle and consist of α- and β-tubulin subunit proteins. Recent comparisons of α- and β-tubulins from several species of parasitic nematodes indicated the presence of multiple isoforms with varying isoelectric points. This variation is interesting not only in pointing out the evolutionary relations among eukaryotic cells but useful also in classifying the tubulins in parasites as potential targets for antiparasitic chemotherapy. A group of benzimidazole derivatives have long been established as highly effective anthelmintics. **Mebendazole** was among the first such anthelmintics found to act primarily by blocking transport of secretory granules and movement of other subcellular organelles in the parasitic nematode *Ascaris lumbricoides*. This inhibition coincides with the disappearance of cytoplasmic microtubules from the intestinal cells of the worm. The microtubular systems of the host cells are unaffected by the treatment. Mebendazole and **fenbendazole**, another anthelmintic benzimidazole, have also been shown to compete with colchicine binding to *A lumbricoides* embryonic tubulins with 250–400 times higher potencies than the binding competition to bovine brain tubulins. These differential binding affinities may explain the selective toxicity of benzimidazoles toward parasitic nematodes.

Synaptic Transmission

Invertebrate nervous systems in helminths and arthropods differ from those of vertebrates in important ways. The motoneurons in invertebrates, for example, are unmyelinated and are thus more susceptible to disturbances of nerve membranes than are the myelinated somatic motor fibers of vertebrates. Muscle fibers in arthropods are innervated by excitatory synapses, in which L-glutamic acid is the neurotransmitter, and by inhibitory nerves, which have γ-aminobutyric acid (GABA) as transmitter. Cholinergic nerves are concentrated in the central nervous system of arthropods. In nematodes, free-living species, eg, *Caenorhabditis elegans,* and gastrointestinal parasitic species, eg, *A lumbricoides,* appear to have identical neuronal systems and synaptic transmission. Cholinergic excitatory and glutamate inhibitory synapses are found in the ventral central cords, and GABAergic inhibitory synapses are identified at the neuromuscular junctions of the worms. The mammalian hosts, on the other hand, have mainly nicotinic receptors at the neuromuscular junctions (see Chapter 6), and the GABA synapses and $GABA_A$ receptors are primarily confined within the central nervous system protected by the blood-brain barrier (Chapter 21).

Neurotoxicant anthelmintics must be administered systemically to mammalian hosts to reach the parasitic nematodes. Therefore, if absorbed, they must be nontoxic to the nervous system of the host. Furthermore, they must penetrate the thick cuticle of the nematodes in order to be effective. It is therefore difficult to find a useful anthelmintic that acts on the nervous system of these parasites. Nevertheless, the majority of presently available anthelmintics do act on the nerves of nematodes. They can be classified into three groups: (1) those acting as ganglionic nicotinic acetylcholine agonists; (2) those acting directly or indirectly as GABA agonists; and (3) those acting on the chloride ion channel. The first category includes **levamisole, pyrantel pamoate, oxantel pamoate,** and **bephenium.** The acetylcholine receptors at the neuromuscular junctions of nematodes are of the ganglionic nicotinic type; these agonists are quite effective in causing muscular contraction of the worms. Experimentally, the ganglionic nicotinic antagonist mecamylamine can reverse the action of these anthelmintics.

The second category consists of only one drug, **piperazine,** an older agent that apparently acts as a GABA agonist at the neuromuscular junction and causes flaccid paralysis of the nematode.

The third category consists of a family of natural compounds, the **milbemycins** and **avermectins.** They act on the ventral cord interneuron and on the motoneuron junction of arthropods to cause paralysis by facilitating the opening of the chloride ion channel. Therefore, both the milbemycins and the avermectins are potent anthelmintics, insecticides, and antiectoparasitic agents with no cross-resistance problems with agents acting on the cholinergic systems. Picrotoxin, a specific blocker of the chloride ion channel, can reverse all of the physiologic effects of these drugs (see Chapter 21).

Ivermectin, a simple derivative of the mixture of avermectin B_{1a} and avermectin B_{1b}, is highly effective as an anthelmintic in domestic animals. It is also effective in controlling onchocerciasis by eliminating the microfilariae. It is currently in wide clinical use in West Africa. Avermectins have little effect on the mammalian central nervous system because they do not cross the blood-brain barrier readily. However, when isolated mammalian brain synaptosomes and synaptic membranes are used as models for investigation, specific high-affinity binding sites for the avermectins can be identified in GABAergic nerves. This drug binding stimulates GABA release from the presynaptic end of the GABA nerve and enhances the postsynaptic GABA binding. Avermectins also stimulate benzodiazepine binding to its receptor and enhance diazepam muscle relaxant activity in vivo. There is little doubt that milbemycins and avermectins act on chloride channels associated with GABA receptors and amplify GABA functions in the mammalian central nervous system. In the free-living nematode, *C elegans,* however, avermectin was found to interact with glutamate-gated chloride ion channels. The complementary DNA encoding an avermectin-sensitive, glutamate-gated chloride channel was recently identified and isolated. This channel may be an attractive target for future studies of antinematode chemotherapy.

Little is known about the nervous systems of cestodes and trematodes except that they probably differ from those of nematodes, since milbemycins and avermectins have no effect on them. However, a highly effective antischistosomal and antitapeworm agent, **praziquantel** (see Chapter 54), is known to enhance Ca^{2+} influx and induce muscular contraction in those parasites, though it exerts no action on nematodes or insects. Some benzodiazepine derivatives have activities similar to those of praziquantel; these activities are unrelated to the anxiolytic activities in the mammalian central nervous system. The nerves and muscles in schistosomes and tapeworms are thus interesting subjects for future chemotherapeutic studies.

Drugs Whose Mechanisms Have Not Yet Been Conclusively Identified

In spite of considerable progress in defining the mechanisms of action of the drugs described above, there are still wide gaps in our understanding of a number of other important antiparasitic agents. These include the compounds presented in Table 52–2. From the biochemical activities that have been identified for them, it appears that many are capable of binding DNA, and some can uncouple oxidative phosphorylation in mammals. These types of activity, which are toxic to the host but could also be involved in the antiparasitic action, may have been preferentially detectable in random screens routinely used for antiparasitic agents in the past.

Table 52–2. Some major antiparasitic agents with undefined mechanisms of action.

Antiparasitic Agents	Possibly Relevant Biochemical Activities
Antiamebiasis agents	
Diloxanide furoate	Unknown
Emetine	Inhibitor of eukaryote protein synthesis
Halogenated hydroxyquinolines	Unknown
Paromomycin	Inhibitor of prokaryote protein synthesis
Antifascioliasis agents	
Bithionol	Oxidative phosphorylation uncoupler
Rafoxanide	Oxidative phosphorylation uncoupler
Antifilariasis agent	
Diethylcarbamazine	Inhibitor of lipoxygenase
Antileishmaniasis agents	
Amphotericin B	Voltage-dependent channel maker in cell membrane
Pentavalent antimonials	Unknown
Antimalarials	
Chloroquine	DNA binding, lysosomal neutralization, and hematoporphyrin binding
Primaquine	Its quinoline quinone metabolite is an oxidant
Quinacrine	DNA binding and flavoenzyme inhibition
Quinine	DNA binding and membrane binding
Antischistosomal agents	
Praziquantel	Opening of Ca^{2+} channels
Hycanthone	DNA binding
Metrifonate	Acetylcholinesterase inhibition
Niridazole	Metabolites binding to DNA
Oxamniquine	DNA binding
Trivalent antimonials	Inhibition of phosphofructokinase
Antitapeworm agent	
Niclosamide	Oxidative phosphorylation uncoupler
Antitrypanosomiasis agent	
Melarsen oxide	Inhibitor of trypanothione reductase

REFERENCES

Aronov AM et al: Rational design of selective submicromolar inhibitors of *Tritrichomonas foetus* hypoxanthine-guanine-xanthine phosphoribosyltransferase. Biochemistry 2000;39:4684.

Aronov AM et al: Structure-based design of submicromolar, biologically active inhibitors of trypanosomatid glyceraldehyde-3-phosphate dehydrogenase. Proc Natl Acad Sci U S A 1999; 96:4273.

Aronov AM et al: Virtual screening of combinatorial libraries across a gene family, in search of inhibitors of *Giardia lamblia* guanine phosphoribosyltransferase. Antimicrob Agents Chemother 2001;45:2571.

Dan M, Wang AL, Wang CC: Inhibition of pyruvate-ferredoxin oxidoreductase gene expression in *Giardia lamblia* by virus-mediated hammerhead ribozyme. Mol Microbiol 2000; 36:447.

Donald RGK et al: Insertional tagging, cloning and expression of the *Toxoplasma gondii* hypoxanthine-xanthine-guanine phosphoribosyltransferase gene: Use as a selectable marker for stable transformation. J Biol Chem 1996;271:14010.

Fritz LC, Wang CC, Gorio A: Avermectin B_{1a} irreversibly blocks post-synaptic potentials at the lobster neuromuscular junction by reducing muscle membrane resistance. Proc Natl Acad Sci U S A 1979;76:2062.

Kinch LN et al: Cloning and kinetic characterization of the *Trypanosoma cruzi* S-adenosylmethionine decarboxylase. Mol Biochem Parasitol 1999;101:1.

Munagala N, Wang CC: The pivotal role of guanine phosophoribosyltransferase in purine salvage by *Giardia lamblia*. Mol Microbiol 2002;44:1073.

Munagala N, Wang CC: The purine nucleoside phosphorylase from *Trichomonas vaginalis* is a homologue of the bacterial enzyme. Biochemistry 2002;277:39973.

Nevalainen L, Hrdý I, Müller M: Sequence of a *Giardia lamblia* gene coding for the glycolytic enzyme, pyruvate phosphate dikinase. Mol Biochem Parasitol 1996;77:217.

Roberts CW et al: Shikimate pathway in apicomplexan parasites. Nature 1999;397:219.

Roberts F et al: Evidence for the shikimic pathway in apicomplexan parasites. Nature 1998;393:801

Rodriguez MA et al: Cloning and characterization of the *Entamoeba histolytica* pyruvate:ferredoxin oxidoreductase gene. Mol Biochem Parasitol 1996;78:273.

Sarver AE, Wang CC: The adenine phosphoribosyltransferase from *Giardia lamblia* has a unique reaction mechanism and unusual substrate binding properties. J Biol Chem 2002;277:39973.

Shi W et al: Closed-site complexers of adenine phosphoribosyltransferase from *Giardia lamblia* reveal a mechanism of ribosyl migration. J Biol Chem 2002;277:39981.

Sommer JM, Ma H, Wang CC: Cloning, expression, and characterization of an unusual guanine phosphoribosyltransferase from *Giardia lamblia*. Mol Biochem Parasitol 1996;78:185.

Somoza JR et al: The crystal structure of the hypoxanthine-guanine-xanthine phosphoribosyltransferase from the protozoan parasite *Tritrichomonas foetus*. Biochemistry 1996;35:7032.

Somoza JR et al: Rational design of antimicrobials: Blocking purine salvage in a parasitic protozoan. Biochemistry 1998;37:5344.

Stromstedt M, Rozman D, Waterman MR: The ubiquitously expressed human CYP51 encodes lanosterol 14α-demethylase, a cytochrome P450 whose expression is regulated by oxysterols. Arch Biochem Biophys 1996;329:73.

Townson SM, Upcroft JA, Upcroft P: Characterization and purification of pyruvate:ferredoxin oxidoreductase from *Giardia duodenalis*. Mol Biochem Parasitol 1996;79:183.

Urbina JA et al: Cure of short- and long-term experimental Chagas' disease using D0870. Science 1996;273:969.

Vial HJ: Isoprenoid biosynthesis and drug targeting in the Apicomplexa. Parasitol Today 2000;16:140.

Wiesner JH et al: Inhibitors of the nonmevalonate pathway of isoprenoid biosynthesis as antimalarial drugs. Science 1999;285:1573.

Antiprotozoal Drugs

Philip J. Rosenthal, MD

TREATMENT OF MALARIA

Four species of plasmodium cause human malaria: *Plasmodium falciparum, P vivax, P malariae,* and *P ovale.* Although all may cause significant illness, *P falciparum* is responsible for nearly all serious complications and deaths. Drug resistance is an important therapeutic problem, most notably with *P falciparum.*

PARASITE LIFE CYCLE

An anopheline mosquito inoculates plasmodium sporozoites to initiate human infection. Circulating sporozoites rapidly invade liver cells, and exoerythrocytic stage tissue schizonts mature in the liver. Merozoites are subsequently released from the liver and invade erythrocytes. Only erythrocytic parasites cause clinical illness. Repeated cycles of infection can lead to the infection of many erythrocytes and serious disease. Sexual stage gametocytes also develop in erythrocytes before being taken up by mosquitoes, where they develop into infective sporozoites.

In *P falciparum* and *P malariae* infection, only one cycle of liver cell invasion and multiplication occurs, and liver infection ceases spontaneously in less than 4 weeks. Thus, treatment that eliminates erythrocytic parasites will cure these infections. In *P vivax* and *P ovale* infections, a dormant hepatic stage, the hypnozoite, is not eradicated by most drugs, and subsequent relapses can therefore occur after therapy directed against erythrocytic parasites. Eradication of both erythrocytic and hepatic parasites is required to cure these infections.

DRUG CLASSIFICATION

Several classes of antimalarial drugs are available (Table 53–1; Figure 53–1). Drugs that eliminate developing or dormant liver forms are called **tissue schizonticides;** those that act on erythrocytic parasites are **blood schizonticides;** and those that kill sexual stages and prevent transmission to mosquitoes are **gametocides.** No one available agent can reliably effect a **radical cure,** ie, eliminate both hepatic and erythrocytic stages. Few available agents are **causal prophylactic drugs,** ie, capable of preventing erythrocytic infection. However, all effective chemoprophylactic agents kill erythrocytic parasites before they grow sufficiently in number to cause clinical disease.

CHEMOPROPHYLAXIS & TREATMENT

When patients are counseled on the prevention of malaria, it is imperative to emphasize measures to prevent mosquito bites (insect repellents, insecticides, and bed nets), since parasites are increasingly resistant to multiple drugs and no chemoprophylactic regimen is fully protective. Current recommendations from the Centers for Disease Control and Prevention (CDC) include the use of chloroquine for chemoprophylaxis in the few areas infested by only chloroquine-sensitive malaria parasites (principally the Caribbean and Central America west of the Panama Canal), mefloquine or Malarone for most other malarious areas, and doxycycline for areas with a very high prevalence of multidrug-resistant falciparum malaria (principally border areas of Thailand) (Table 53–2). CDC recommendations should be checked regularly (Phone: 877-FYI-TRIP; Internet: www.cdc.gov/travel/), as these may change in response to changing resistance patterns and increasing experience with new drugs. In some circumstances, it may be appropriate for travelers to carry supplies of drugs with them in case they develop a febrile illness when medical attention is unavailable. Regimens for self-treatment should generally include either quinine or artemisinin derivatives, which, though not available in the USA, are widely available in other countries. Most authorities do not recommend routine terminal chemoprophylaxis with primaquine to eradicate dormant hepatic stages of *P vivax* and *P ovale* after travel, but this may be appropriate in some circumstances, especially for travelers with major exposure to these parasites.

Treatment of malaria that presents in the USA is straightforward (Table 53–3). Nonfalciparum infections and falciparum malaria from areas without known resistance should be treated with chloroquine. Vivax and ovale malaria should subsequently be treated with primaquine to eradicate liver forms. However, for *P vivax,* chloroquine-resistance is increasingly reported and pri-

Table 53–1. Major antimalarial drugs.

Drug	Class	Use
Chloroquine	4-Aminoquinoline	Treatment and chemoprophylaxis of infection with sensitive parasites
Amodiaquine[1]	4-Aminoquinoline	Treatment of infection with some chloroquine-resistant *P falciparum* strains
Quinine	Quinoline methanol	Oral treatment of infections with chloroquine-resistant *P falciparum*
Quinidine	Quinoline methanol	Intravenous therapy of severe infections with *P falciparum*
Mefloquine	Quinoline methanol	Chemoprophylaxis and treatment of infections with *P falciparum*
Primaquine	8-Aminoquinoline	Radical cure and terminal prophylaxis of infections with *P vivax* and *P ovale*
Sulfadoxine-pyrimethamine (Fansidar)	Folate antagonist combination	Treatment of infections with some chloroquine-resistant *P falciparum*
Proguanil[1]	Folate antagonist	Chemoprophylaxis (with chloroquine)
Doxycycline	Tetracycline	Treatment (with quinine) of infections with *P falciparum;* chemoprophylaxis
Halofantrine[1]	Phenanthrene methanol	Treatment of infections with some chloroquine-resistant *P falciparum*
Lumefantrine[1]	Amyl alcohol	Treatment of *P falciparum* malaria in fixed combination with artemether (Coartem)
Artemisinins[1]	Sesquiterpene lactone endoperoxides	Treatment of infection with multidrug-resistant *P falciparum*
Atovaquone-proguanil (Malarone)	Quinone-folate antagonist combination	Treatment and chemoprophylaxis of *P falciparum* infection

[1]Not available in the USA.

maquine may fail to eradicate liver stages. Falciparum malaria from most areas is best treated with oral quinine or intravenous quinidine, in either case plus doxycycline or, for children, clindamycin. Other agents that are generally effective against resistant falciparum malaria include mefloquine and halofantrine, both of which have toxicity concerns at treatment dosages, and the artemisinin derivatives artesunate and artemether (alone or in combination, as discussed below).

CHLOROQUINE

Chloroquine has been the drug of choice for both treatment and chemoprophylaxis of malaria since the 1940s, but its utility against *P falciparum* has been seriously compromised by drug resistance. It remains the drug of choice for the treatment of sensitive *P falciparum* and other species of human malaria parasites.

Chemistry & Pharmacokinetics

Chloroquine is a synthetic 4-aminoquinoline (Figure 53–1) formulated as the phosphate salt for oral use. It is rapidly and almost completely absorbed from the gas-

trointestinal tract, reaches maximum plasma concentrations in about 3 hours, and is rapidly distributed to the tissues. It has a very large apparent volume of distribution of 100–1000 L/kg and is slowly released from tissues and metabolized. Chloroquine is principally excreted in the urine with an initial half-life of 3–5 days but a much longer terminal elimination half-life of 1–2 months.

Antimalarial Action & Resistance

A. ANTIMALARIAL ACTION

When not limited by resistance, chloroquine is a highly effective blood schizonticide. It is also moderately effective against gametocytes of *P vivax, P ovale,* and *P malariae* but not against those of *P falciparum.* Chloroquine is not active against liver stage parasites.

B. MECHANISM OF ACTION

The mechanism of action remains controversial. Chloroquine probably acts by concentrating in parasite food vacuoles, preventing the polymerization of the hemoglobin breakdown product, heme, into hemozoin,

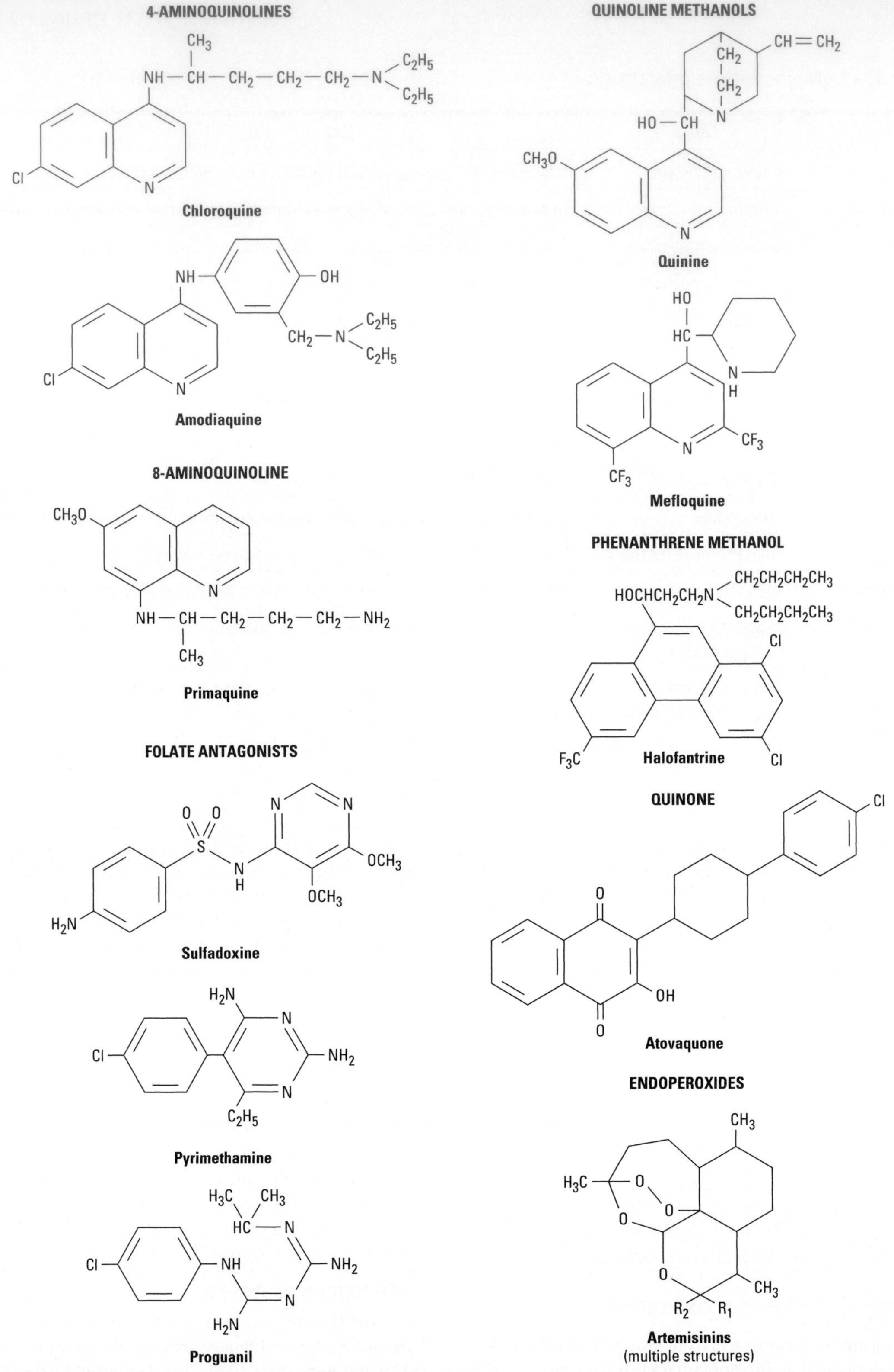

Figure 53–1. Structural formulas of antimalarial drugs.

Table 53–2. Drugs for the prevention of malaria in travelers.[1]

Drug	Use[2]	Adult Dosage[3]
Chloroquine	Areas without resistant *P falciparum*	500 mg weekly
Mefloquine	Areas with chloroquine-resistant *P falciparum*	250 mg weekly
Doxycycline	Areas with multidrug-resistant *P falciparum*	100 mg daily
Malarone	Areas with chloroquine-resistant *P falciparum*	1 tablet (250 mg atovaquone/100 mg proguanil) daily
Primaquine[4]	Terminal prophylaxis of *P vivax* and *P ovale* infections	26.3 mg (15 mg base) daily for 14 days after travel

[1]Recommendations may change, as resistance to all available drugs is increasing. See text for additional information on toxicities and cautions. For additional details and pediatric dosing, see CDC guidelines (phone: 877-FYI-TRIP; http://www.cdc.gov). Travelers to remote areas should consider carrying effective therapy (see text) for use if they develop a febrile illness and cannot reach medical attention quickly.

[2]Areas without known chloroquine-resistant *P falciparum* are Central America west of the Panama Canal, Haiti, Dominican Republic, Egypt, and most malarious countries of the Middle East. Mefloquine or Malarone are currently recommended for other malarious areas except for border areas of Thailand, where doxycycline is recommended.

[3]For drugs other than primaquine, begin 1–2 weeks before departure (except 2 days before for doxycycline and Malarone) and continue for 4 weeks after leaving the endemic area (except 1 week for Malarone). All dosages refer to salts.

[4]Screen for G6PD deficiency before using primaquine.

and thus eliciting parasite toxicity due to the buildup of free heme.

C. RESISTANCE

Resistance to chloroquine is now very common among strains of *P falciparum* and uncommon but increasing for *P vivax*. In *P falciparum,* mutations in a putative transporter, PfCRT, have been correlated with resistance. Chloroquine resistance can be reversed by certain agents, including verapamil, desipramine, and chlorpheniramine, but the clinical value of resistance-reversing drugs is not established.

Clinical Uses

A. TREATMENT

Chloroquine is the drug of choice for the treatment of nonfalciparum and sensitive falciparum malaria. It rapidly terminates fever (in 24–48 hours) and clears parasitemia (in 48–72 hours) caused by sensitive parasites. It is also still used to treat falciparum malaria in many areas with widespread resistance, in particular most of Africa, owing to its safety and low cost and the fact that many partially immune individuals respond to treatment even when infecting parasites are partially resistant to chloroquine. However, other agents are preferred to treat potentially resistant falciparum malaria, especially in nonimmune individuals. Chloroquine does not eliminate dormant liver forms of *P vivax* and *P ovale,* and for

that reason primaquine must be added for the radical cure of these species.

B. CHEMOPROPHYLAXIS

Chloroquine is the preferred chemoprophylactic agent in malarious regions without resistant falciparum malaria. Eradication of *P vivax* and *P ovale* requires a course of primaquine to clear hepatic stages.

C. AMEBIC LIVER ABSCESS

Chloroquine reaches high liver concentrations and may be used for amebic abscesses that fail initial therapy with metronidazole (see below).

Adverse Effects

Chloroquine is usually very well tolerated, even with prolonged use. Pruritus is common, primarily in Africans. Nausea, vomiting, abdominal pain, headache, anorexia, malaise, blurring of vision, and urticaria are uncommon. Dosing after meals may reduce some adverse effects. Rare reactions include hemolysis in glucose 6-phosphate dehydrogenase (G6PD)-deficient persons, impaired hearing, confusion, psychosis, seizures, agranulocytosis, exfoliative dermatitis, alopecia, bleaching of hair, hypotension, and electrocardiographic changes (QRS widening, T wave abnormalities). The long-term administration of high doses of chloroquine for rheumatologic diseases (Chapter 36) can result in

Table 53–3. Treatment of malaria.

Clinical Setting	Drug Therapy[1]	Alternative Drugs
Chloroquine-sensitive *P falciparum* and *P malariae* infections	Chloroquine phosphate, 1 g then 500 mg in 6 hours, followed by 500 mg daily for 2 days *or–* Chloroquine phosphate, 1 g at 0 and 24 hours, then 0.5 g at 48 hours	
P vivax and *P ovale* infections	Chloroquine (as above), then (if G6PD normal) primaquine, 26.3 mg daily for 14 days	
Uncomplicated infections with chloroquine-resistant *P falciparum*	Quinine sulfate, 650 mg 3 times daily for 3–7 days *plus one of the following–* Doxycycline, 100 mg twice daily for 7 days *or–* Clindamycin, 600 mg twice daily for 7 days *or–* Fansidar, three tablets once	Mefloquine, 15 mg/kg once or 750 mg, then 500 mg in 6–8 hours *or–* Malarone, 4 tablets (total of 1 g atovaquone, 400 mg proguanil) daily for 3 days *or–* Artesunate or artemether single daily doses of 4 mg/kg on day 0, 2 mg/kg on days 2 and 3, 1 mg/kg on days 4–7 *or–* Halofantrine, 500 mg every 6 hours for 3 doses; repeat in 1 week
Severe or complicated infections with *P falciparum*[3]	Quinidine gluconate,[2,3] 10 mg/kg IV over 1–2 hours, then 0.02 mg/kg IV/min *or–* 15 mg/kg IV over 4 hours, then 7.5 mg/kg IV over 4 hours every 8 hours.	Artesunate,[3] 2.4 mg/kg IV or IM, then 1.2 mg/kg every 12 hours for 1 day, then every day *or–* Artemether,[3] 3.2 mg/kg IM, then 1.6 mg/kg/d IM

[1]All dosages are oral and refer to salts unless otherwise indicated. See text for additional information on all agents, including toxicities and cautions. See CDC guidelines (phone: 877-FYI-TRIP; http://www.cdc.gov) for additional information and pediatric dosing.

[2]Cardiac monitoring should be in place during intravenous administration of quinidine.

[3]With all parenteral regimens, change to an oral regimen as soon as the patient can tolerate it.

irreversible ototoxicity, retinopathy, myopathy, and peripheral neuropathy. These abnormalities are rarely if ever seen with standard-dose weekly chemoprophylaxis, even when given for prolonged periods. Large intramuscular injections or rapid intravenous infusions of chloroquine hydrochloride can result in severe hypotension and respiratory and cardiac arrest. Parenteral administration of chloroquine is best avoided, but if other drugs are not available for parenteral use, it should be infused slowly.

Contraindications & Cautions

Chloroquine is contraindicated in patients with psoriasis or porphyria, in whom it may precipitate acute attacks of these diseases. It should generally not be used in those with retinal or visual field abnormalities or myopathy. Chloroquine should be used with caution in patients with a history of liver disease or neurologic or hematologic disorders. The antidiarrheal agent kaolin and calcium- and magnesium-containing antacids interfere with the absorption of chloroquine and should not be coadministered with the drug. Chloroquine is considered safe in pregnancy and for young children.

AMODIAQUINE

Amodiaquine is closely related to chloroquine, and it probably shares mechanisms of action and resistance with that drug. Amodiaquine has been widely used to treat malaria because of its low cost, limited toxicity, and, in some areas, effectiveness against chloroquine-resistant strains of *P falciparum*. Important toxicities of amodiaquine, including agranulocytosis, aplastic anemia, and hepatotoxicity, have limited use of the drug in recent years. However, recent reevaluation has shown that serious toxicity from amodiaquine is rare, and some authorities now advocate its use as a replacement for chloroquine (especially in combination regimens) in areas with high rates of resistance but limited resources. Chemoprophylaxis with amodiaquine is best avoided because of its apparent increased toxicity with long-term use.

QUININE & QUINIDINE

Quinine and quinidine remain first-line therapies for falciparum malaria—especially severe disease—though toxicity concerns complicate therapy. Resistance to quinine is uncommon but increasing.

Chemistry & Pharmacokinetics

Quinine is derived from the bark of the cinchona tree, a traditional remedy for intermittent fevers from South America. The alkaloid quinine was purified from the bark in 1820, and it has been used in the treatment and prevention of malaria since that time. Quinidine, the dextrorotatory stereoisomer of quinine, is at least as effective as parenteral quinine in the treatment of severe falciparum malaria. After oral administration, quinine is rapidly absorbed, reaches peak plasma levels in 1–3 hours, and is widely distributed in body tissues. The use of a loading dose in severe malaria allows the achievement of peak levels within a few hours. The pharmacokinetics of quinine varies among populations. Individuals with malaria develop higher plasma levels of the drug than healthy controls, but toxicity is not increased, apparently because of increased protein binding. The half-life of quinine also is higher in those with severe malaria (18 hours) than in healthy controls (11 hours). Quinidine has a shorter half life than quinine, mostly as a result of decreased protein binding. Quinine is primarily metabolized in the liver and excreted in the urine.

Antimalarial Action & Resistance

A. ANTIMALARIAL ACTION

Quinine is a rapidly acting, highly effective blood schizonticide against the four species of human malaria parasites. The drug is gametocidal against *P vivax* and *P ovale* but not *P falciparum*. It is not active against liver stage parasites. The mechanism of action of quinine is unknown.

B. RESISTANCE

Increasing in vitro resistance of parasites from a number of areas suggests that quinine resistance will be an increasing problem. Resistance to quinine is already common in some areas of Southeast Asia, especially border areas of Thailand, where the drug may fail if used alone to treat falciparum malaria. However, quinine still provides at least a partial therapeutic effect in most patients.

Clinical Uses

A. PARENTERAL TREATMENT OF SEVERE FALCIPARUM MALARIA

Quinine dihydrochloride or quinidine gluconate is the treatment of choice for severe falciparum malaria. Quinine can be administered slowly intravenously or, in a dilute solution, intramuscularly, but parenteral preparations of this drug are not available in the USA. Quinidine is now the standard therapy in the USA for the parenteral treatment of severe falciparum malaria. The drug can be administered in divided doses or by continuous intravenous infusion; treatment should begin with a loading dose to rapidly achieve effective plasma concentrations. Because of its cardiac toxicity and the relative unpredictability of its pharmacokinetics, intravenous quinidine should be administered with cardiac monitoring. Therapy should be changed to oral quinine as soon as the patient has improved and can tolerate oral medications.

B. ORAL TREATMENT OF FALCIPARUM MALARIA

Quinine sulfate is appropriate first-line therapy for uncomplicated falciparum malaria except when the infection was transmitted in an area without documented chloroquine-resistant malaria. Quinine is commonly used with a second drug (most often doxycycline) to shorten quinine's duration of use (usually to 3 days) and limit toxicity. Quinine is less effective than chloroquine against other human malarias and is more toxic, and it is therefore not used to treat infections with these parasites.

C. MALARIAL CHEMOPROPHYLAXIS

Quinine is not generally used in chemoprophylaxis owing to its toxicity, although a daily dose of 325 mg is effective.

D. BABESIOSIS

Quinine is first-line therapy, in combination with clindamycin, for the treatment of infection with *Babesia microti* or other human babesial infections.

Adverse Effects

Therapeutic dosages of quinine and quinidine commonly cause tinnitus, headache, nausea, dizziness, flushing, and visual disturbances, a constellation of symptoms termed **cinchonism.** Mild symptoms of cinchonism do not warrant the discontinuation of therapy. More severe findings, often after prolonged therapy, include more marked visual and auditory abnormalities, vomiting, diarrhea, and abdominal pain. Hypersensitivity reactions include skin rashes, urticaria, angioedema, and bronchospasm. Hematologic abnormalities include hemolysis (especially with G6PD deficiency), leukopenia, agranulocytosis, and thrombocytopenia. Therapeutic doses may cause hypoglycemia through stimulation of insulin release; this is a particular problem in severe infections and in pregnant patients, who have increased sensitivity to insulin. Quinine can stimulate uterine contractions, especially in the third trimester. However, this effect is mild, and quinine and quinidine remain the drugs of choice for severe falciparum malaria even during pregnancy. Intravenous infusions of the drugs may cause thrombophlebitis.

Severe hypotension can follow too-rapid intravenous infusions of quinine or quinidine. Electrocardiographic abnormalities (QT prolongation) are fairly common with intravenous quinidine, but dangerous arrhythmias are uncommon when the drug is administered appropriately in a monitored setting.

Blackwater fever is a rare severe illness that includes marked hemolysis and hemoglobinuria in the setting of quinine therapy for malaria. It appears to be due to a hypersensitivity reaction to the drug, though its pathogenesis is uncertain.

Contraindications & Cautions

Quinine (or quinidine) should be discontinued if signs of severe cinchonism, hemolysis, or hypersensitivity occur. It should be avoided if possible in those with underlying visual or auditory problems. It must be used with great caution in those with underlying cardiac abnormalities. Quinine should not be given concurrently with mefloquine and should be used with caution in a patient with malaria who has previously received mefloquine chemoprophylaxis. Absorption may be blocked by aluminum-containing antacids. Quinine can raise plasma levels of warfarin and digoxin. Dosage must be reduced in renal insufficiency.

MEFLOQUINE

Mefloquine is effective therapy for many chloroquine-resistant strains of *P falciparum* and against other species. Although toxicity is a concern, mefloquine is the recommended chemoprophylactic drug for use in most malaria-endemic regions with chloroquine-resistant strains.

Chemistry & Pharmacokinetics

Mefloquine hydrochloride is a synthetic 4-quinoline methanol that is chemically related to quinine. It can only be given orally because severe local irritation occurs with parenteral use. It is well absorbed, and peak plasma concentrations are reached in about 18 hours. Mefloquine is highly protein-bound, extensively distributed in tissues, and eliminated slowly, allowing a single-dose treatment regimen. The terminal elimination half-life is about 20 days, allowing weekly dosing for chemoprophylaxis. With weekly dosing, steady state drug levels are reached over a number of weeks; this interval can be shortened to 4 days by beginning a course with three consecutive daily doses of 250 mg, though this is not standard practice. Mefloquine and acid metabolites of the drug are slowly excreted, mainly in the feces. The drug can be detected in the blood for months after the completion of therapy.

Antimalarial Action & Resistance

A. ANTIMALARIAL ACTION

Mefloquine has strong blood schizonticidal activity against *P falciparum* and *P vivax,* but it is not active against hepatic stages or gametocytes. The mechanism of action of mefloquine is unknown.

B. RESISTANCE

Sporadic resistance to mefloquine has been reported from many areas. At present, resistance appears to be uncommon except in regions of Southeast Asia with high rates of multidrug resistance (especially border areas of Thailand). Mefloquine resistance appears to be associated with resistance to quinine and halofantrine but not with resistance to chloroquine.

Clinical Uses

A. CHEMOPROPHYLAXIS

Mefloquine is effective in prophylaxis against most strains of *P falciparum* and probably all other human malarial species as well. Mefloquine is recommended by the CDC for chemoprophylaxis in all malarious areas except for those with no chloroquine resistance (where chloroquine is preferred) and some rural areas of Southeast Asia with a high prevalence of mefloquine resistance. As with chloroquine, eradication of *P vivax* and *P ovale* requires a course of primaquine.

B. TREATMENT

Mefloquine is effective in treating most falciparum malaria. The drug is not appropriate for treating individuals with severe or complicated malaria since quinine and quinidine are more rapidly active and drug resistance is less likely with those agents.

Adverse Effects

Adverse effects with weekly dosing with mefloquine for chemoprophylaxis include nausea, vomiting, dizziness, sleep and behavioral disturbances, epigastric pain, diarrhea, abdominal pain, headache, rash, and dizziness. Neuropsychiatric toxicities have received a good deal of publicity, but despite frequent anecdotal reports of seizures and psychosis, a number of controlled studies have found the frequency of serious adverse effects from mefloquine to be no higher than that with other common antimalarial chemoprophylactic regimens. Leukocytosis, thrombocytopenia, and aminotransferase elevations have been reported.

The adverse effects listed above are more common with the higher dosages required for treatment. These effects may be lessened by splitting administration of the drug into two doses separated by 6–8 hours. The incidence of neuropsychiatric symptoms appears to be about ten times more common than with chemoprophylactic dosing, with widely varying frequencies of up to about 50% being reported. Serious neuropsychiatric toxicities (depression, confusion, acute psychosis, or seizures) have been reported in less than one in 1000 treatments, but some authorities believe that these toxicities are actually more common. Mefloquine can also alter cardiac conduction, and arrhythmias and bradycardia have been reported.

Contraindications & Cautions

Mefloquine is contraindicated if there is a history of epilepsy, psychiatric disorders, arrhythmia, cardiac conduction defects, or sensitivity to related drugs. It should not be coadministered with quinine, quinidine, or halofantrine, and caution is required if quinine or quinidine is used to treat malaria after mefloquine chemoprophylaxis. Theoretical risks of mefloquine use must be balanced with the risk of contracting falciparum malaria. The CDC no longer advises against mefloquine use in patients receiving β-adrenoceptor antagonists. Mefloquine is also now considered safe in young children. Available data suggest that mefloquine use is safe throughout pregnancy, though experience in the first trimester is limited. An older recommendation to avoid mefloquine use in those requiring fine motor skills (eg, airline pilots) is controversial. Mefloquine chemoprophylaxis should be discontinued if significant neuropsychiatric symptoms develop.

PRIMAQUINE

Primaquine is the drug of choice for the eradication of dormant liver forms of *P vivax* and *P ovale*.

Chemistry & Pharmacokinetics

Primaquine phosphate is a synthetic 8-aminoquinoline. The drug is well absorbed orally, reaching peak plasma levels in 1–2 hours. The plasma half-life is 3–8 hours. Primaquine is widely distributed to the tissues, but only a small amount is bound there. It is rapidly metabolized and excreted in the urine. Its three major metabolites appear to have less antimalarial activity but more potential for inducing hemolysis than the parent compound.

Antimalarial Action & Resistance

A. ANTIMALARIAL ACTION

Primaquine is active against hepatic stages of all human malaria parasites. It is the only available agent active against the dormant hypnozoite stages of *P vivax* and *P ovale*. Primaquine is also gametocidal against the four human malaria species. Primaquine acts against erythrocytic stage parasites, but this activity is too weak to play an important role. The mechanism of antimalarial action is unknown.

B. RESISTANCE

Some strains of *P vivax* in New Guinea, Southeast Asia, and perhaps Central and South America are relatively resistant to primaquine. Liver forms of these strains may not be eradicated by a single standard treatment with primaquine and may require repeated therapy with increased doses (eg, 30 mg base daily for 14 days) for radical cure.

Clinical Uses

A. THERAPY (RADICAL CURE) OF ACUTE VIVAX AND OVALE MALARIA

Standard therapy for these infections includes chloroquine to eradicate erythrocytic forms and primaquine to eradicate liver hypnozoites and prevent a subsequent relapse. Chloroquine is given acutely, and therapy with primaquine is withheld until the G6PD status of the patient is known. If the G6PD level is normal, a 14-day course of primaquine is given.

B. TERMINAL PROPHYLAXIS OF VIVAX AND OVALE MALARIA

Standard chemoprophylaxis does not prevent a relapse of vivax or ovale malaria, as the hypnozoite forms of these parasites are not eradicated by chloroquine or other available agents. To markedly diminish the likelihood of relapse, some authorities advocate the use of primaquine after the completion of travel to an endemic area.

C. CHEMOPROPHYLAXIS OF MALARIA

Primaquine has been studied as a daily chemoprophylactic agent. Daily treatment with 0.5 mg/kg of base provided good levels of protection against falciparum and vivax malaria. However, potential toxicities of long-term use remain a concern, and primaquine is not routinely recommended for this purpose.

D. GAMETOCIDAL ACTION

A single dose of primaquine (45 mg base) can be used as a control measure to render *P falciparum* gametocytes noninfective to mosquitoes. This therapy is of no clinical benefit to the patient but will disrupt transmission.

E. PNEUMOCYSTIS JIROVECI INFECTION

The combination of clindamycin and primaquine is an alternative regimen for the treatment of pneumocystosis, particularly mild to moderate disease. This regimen offers improved tolerance compared with high-dose trimethoprim-sulfamethoxazole or pentamidine, though its efficacy against severe pneumocystis pneumonia is not well studied. (See also page 873.)

Adverse Effects

Primaquine in recommended doses is generally well tolerated. It infrequently causes nausea, epigastric pain, abdominal cramps, and headache, and these symptoms are more common with higher dosages and when the drug is taken on an empty stomach. More serious but rare adverse effects include leukopenia, agranulocytosis, leukocytosis, and cardiac arrhythmias. Standard doses of primaquine may cause hemolysis or methemoglobinemia (manifested by cyanosis), especially in persons with G6PD deficiency or other hereditary metabolic defects.

Contraindications & Cautions

Primaquine should be avoided in patients with a history of granulocytopenia or methemoglobinemia, in those receiving potentially myelosuppressive drugs (eg, quinidine), and in those with disorders that commonly include myelosuppression. It is never given parenterally because it may induce marked hypotension.

Patients should be tested for G6PD deficiency before primaquine is prescribed. When a patient is deficient in G6PD, treatment strategies may consist of withholding therapy and treating subsequent relapses, if they occur, with chloroquine; treating patients with standard dosing, paying close attention to their hematologic status; or treating with weekly primaquine (45 mg base) for 8 weeks. G6PD-deficient individuals of Mediterranean and Asian ancestry are most likely to have severe deficiency, while those of African ancestry usually have a milder biochemical defect. This difference can be taken into consideration in choosing a treatment strategy. In any event, primaquine should be discontinued if there is evidence of hemolysis or anemia. Primaquine should be avoided in pregnancy because the fetus is relatively G6PD-deficient and thus at risk of hemolysis.

INHIBITORS OF FOLATE SYNTHESIS

Inhibitors of enzymes involved in folate metabolism are used, generally in combination regimens, for the treatment and prevention of malaria.

Chemistry & Pharmacokinetics

Pyrimethamine is a 2,4-diaminopyrimidine related to trimethoprim (see Chapter 46). Proguanil is a biguanide derivative (Figure 53–1). Both drugs are slowly but adequately absorbed from the gastrointestinal tract. Pyrimethamine reaches peak plasma levels 2–6 hours after an oral dose, is bound to plasma proteins, and has an elimination half-life of about 3.5 days. Proguanil reaches peak plasma levels about 5 hours after an oral dose and has an elimination half-life of about 16 hours. Therefore, proguanil must be administered daily for chemoprophylaxis, whereas pyrimethamine can be given once a week. Pyrimethamine is extensively metabolized before excretion. Proguanil is a prodrug; only its triazine metabolite, cycloguanil, is active. Fansidar, a fixed combination of the sulfonamide sulfadoxine (500 mg per tablet) and pyrimethamine (25 mg per tablet), is well absorbed. Its components display peak plasma levels within 2–8 hours and are excreted mainly by the kidneys. Average half-lives are about 170 hours for sulfadoxine and 90 hours for pyrimethamine.

Antimalarial Action & Resistance

A. ANTIMALARIAL ACTION

Pyrimethamine and proguanil act slowly against erythrocytic forms of susceptible strains of all four human malaria species. Proguanil also has some activity against hepatic forms. Neither drug is adequately gametocidal or effective against the persistent liver stages of *P vivax* or *P ovale*. Sulfonamides and sulfones are weakly active against erythrocytic schizonts but not against liver stages or gametocytes. They are not used alone as antimalarials but are effective in combination with other agents.

B. MECHANISM OF ACTION

Pyrimethamine and proguanil selectively inhibit plasmodial dihydrofolate reductase, a key enzyme in the pathway for synthesis of folate. Sulfonamides and sulfones inhibit another enzyme in the folate pathway, dihydropteroate synthase. As described in Chapter 46 and shown in Figure 46–2, combinations of inhibitors of these two enzymes provide synergistic activity.

C. RESISTANCE

In many areas, resistance to folate antagonists and sulfonamides is common for *P falciparum* and less common for *P vivax*. Resistance is due primarily to mutations in dihydrofolate reductase and dihydropteroate synthase. Because different mutations may mediate resistance to different agents, cross-resistance is not uniformly seen.

Clinical Uses

A. CHEMOPROPHYLAXIS

Chemoprophylaxis with single folate antagonists is no longer recommended because of frequent resistance, but a number of agents are used in combination regimens. The combination of chloroquine (500 mg weekly) and proguanil (200 mg daily) is used widely as an alternative to mefloquine. This combination has lower efficacy—but also probably less toxicity—than mefloquine. It is anticipated that the efficacy of the combination will continue to decrease as resistance to both chloroquine and proguanil increases. Fansidar and Maloprim (the latter is a combination of pyrimethamine and the sulfone dapsone) are both effective against sensitive parasites with weekly dosing, but they are no longer recommended because of resistance and toxicity.

B. TREATMENT OF CHLOROQUINE-RESISTANT FALCIPARUM MALARIA

Fansidar is commonly used to treat uncomplicated falciparum malaria. At present it is first-line therapy for this indication in some tropical countries and is considered the appropriate therapy after chloroquine treatment failure in most of Africa. Advantages of Fansidar in the developing world are relatively low rates of drug resistance and toxicity, ease of administration (a single oral dose), and low cost. However, rates of resistance are increasing. Fansidar is a less optimal regimen than quinine when both drugs are available, especially for nonimmune individuals. It should not be used for severe malaria, as it is slower-acting than other available agents. Fansidar can also be used as an adjunct to quinine therapy to shorten the course of quinine and limit toxicity. Fansidar is not reliably effective in vivax malaria, and its usefulness against *P ovale* and *P malariae* has not been adequately studied. A new antifolate-sulfone combination, chlorproguanil-dapsone, may soon be available for the treatment of uncomplicated falciparum malaria in Africa. Chlorproguanil-dapsone is highly effective in regions with fairly high levels of resistance to Fansidar, and its shorter half-life may prevent the selection of resistant parasites.

C. PRESUMPTIVE TREATMENT OF FALCIPARUM MALARIA

Fansidar is also used as presumptive therapy for travelers who develop fever while traveling in malaria-endemic regions and who are unable to obtain medical evaluation. Ideally, such patients obtain medical attention as soon as possible after the initiation of therapy to verify the diagnosis and develop an optimal treatment plan. This strategy is increasingly questionable as resistance to Fansidar increases. Alternative presumptive regimens are quinine and mefloquine, which are more toxic but less likely to fail due to drug resistance, or the artemisinin analogs artesunate and artemether, which are not available in the USA.

D. TOXOPLASMOSIS

Pyrimethamine, in combination with sulfadiazine, is first-line therapy for the treatment of toxoplasmosis, including acute infection, congenital infection, and disease in immunocompromised patients. For immunocompromised patients, high-dose therapy is required followed by chronic suppressive therapy. Folinic acid is included to limit myelosuppression. Toxicity from the combination is usually due primarily to sulfadiazine. The replacement of sulfadiazine with clindamycin provides an effective alternative regimen.

E. PNEUMOCYSTOSIS

Pneumocystis jiroveci is the cause of human pneumocystosis and is now recognized to be a fungus, but this organism is discussed in this chapter because it responds to antiprotozoal drugs, not antifungals. (The related species *P carinii* is now recognized to be the cause of animal infections.) First-line therapy of pneumocystosis is trimethoprim plus sulfamethoxazole (see also Chapter 46). Standard treatment includes high-dose intravenous (15–20 mg trimethoprim and 75–100 mg sulfamethoxazole per day in three or four divided doses) or oral (two double-strength tablets every 8 hours) therapy for 21 days. High-dose therapy entails significant toxicity, especially in patients with AIDS. Important toxicities include nausea, vomiting, fever, rash, leukopenia, hyponatremia, elevated hepatic enzymes, azotemia, anemia, and thrombocytopenia. Less common effects include severe skin reactions, mental status changes, pancreatitis, and hypocalcemia. Trimethoprim-sulfamethoxazole is also the standard chemoprophylactic drug for the prevention of *P jiroveci* infection in immunocompromised individuals. Dosing is one double-strength tablet daily or three times per week. The chemoprophylactic dosing schedule is much better tolerated than high-dose therapy in immunocompromised patients, but rash, fever, leukopenia, or hepatitis may necessitate changing to another drug.

Adverse Effects & Cautions

Most patients tolerate pyrimethamine and proguanil well. Gastrointestinal symptoms, skin rashes, and itching are rare. Mouth ulcers and alopecia have been described with proguanil. Fansidar is no longer recommended for chemoprophylaxis because of uncommon but severe cutaneous reactions, including erythema multiforme, Stevens-Johnson syndrome, and toxic epidermal necrolysis. Severe reactions appear to be much less common with single-dose therapy, and use of the drug is justified by the risks associated with falciparum malaria. Rare adverse effects with a single dose of Fansidar are those associated with other sulfonamides, including hematologic, gastrointestinal, central nervous system, dermatologic, and renal toxicity. Maloprim is no longer recommended for chemoprophylaxis because of unacceptably high rates of agranulocytosis. Folate antagonists should be used cautiously in the presence of renal or hepatic dysfunction. Although pyrimethamine is teratogenic in animals, Fansidar has been safely used in pregnancy for therapy and as an intermittent chemoprophylactic regimen to improve pregnancy outcomes. Proguanil is considered safe in pregnancy. With the use of any folate antagonist in pregnancy, folate supplements should be coadministered.

ANTIBIOTICS

A number of antibiotics in addition to the folate antagonists and sulfonamides are modestly active antimalarials. The mechanisms of action of these drugs are unclear. They may inhibit protein synthesis or other functions in two plasmodial prokaryote-like organelles, the mitochondrion and the apicoplast. None of the antibiotics should be used as single agents for the treatment of malaria because their action is much slower than those of standard antimalarials.

Tetracycline and doxycycline (see Chapter 44) are active against erythrocytic schizonts of all human malaria parasites. They are not active against liver stages. Doxycycline is commonly used in the treatment of falciparum malaria in conjunction with quinidine or quinine, allowing a shorter and better-tolerated course of quinine. Doxycycline has also become a standard chemoprophylactic drug for use in areas of Southeast Asia with high rates of resistance to other antimalarials, including mefloquine. Doxycycline side effects include infrequent gastrointestinal symptoms, candidal vaginitis, and photosensitivity. Its safety in long-term chemoprophylaxis has not been extensively evaluated.

Clindamycin (see Chapter 44) is slowly active against erythrocytic schizonts and can be used in conjunction with quinine or quinidine in those for whom doxycycline is not recommended, such as children and pregnant women. Azithromycin (see Chapter 44) also has antimalarial activity and is now under study as an alternative chemoprophylactic drug. Antimalarial activity of fluoroquinolones has been demonstrated, but efficacy for the therapy or chemoprophylaxis of malaria has been suboptimal.

Antibiotics also are active against other protozoans. Tetracycline and erythromycin are alternative therapies for the treatment of intestinal amebiasis. Clindamycin, in combination with other agents, is effective therapy for toxoplasmosis, pneumocystosis, and babesiosis. Spiramycin is a macrolide antibiotic that is used to treat primary toxoplasmosis acquired during pregnancy. Treatment lowers the risk of the development of congenital toxoplasmosis.

ATOVAQUONE

Atovaquone, a hydroxynaphthoquinone (Figure 53–1), was initially developed as an antimalarial but has been approved by the FDA for the treatment of mild to moderate *P jiroveci* pneumonia. The drug is only administered orally. Its bioavailability is low and erratic but absorption is increased by fatty food. The drug is heavily protein-bound and has a half-life of 2–3 days. Most of the drug is eliminated unchanged in the feces. The mechanism of action of atovaquone is uncertain. In plasmodia it appears to disrupt mitochondrial electron transport.

Atovaquone is an alternative therapy for *P jiroveci* infection, though its efficacy is lower than that of trimethoprim-sulfamethoxazole. Standard dosing is 750 mg taken with food three times daily for 21 days. Adverse effects include fever, rash, nausea, vomiting, diarrhea, headache, and insomnia. Serious adverse effects appear to be minimal, although experience with the drug remains limited. Atovaquone has also been effective in small numbers of immunocompromised patients with toxoplasmosis unresponsive to other agents, though its role in this disease is not yet defined.

Initial use of atovaquone to treat malaria led to disappointing results, with frequent failures apparently due to the selection of resistant parasites during therapy. In contrast, Malarone, a fixed combination of atovaquone (250 mg) and proguanil (100 mg), has been shown to be highly effective for both the treatment and chemoprophylaxis of falciparum malaria, and it is now approved for both indications in the USA. For chemoprophylaxis, Malarone must be taken daily (Table 53–2). It has an advantage over mefloquine and doxycycline in requiring shorter periods of treatment before and after the period at risk for malaria transmission, but it is more expensive than the other agents. It should be taken with food. Malarone is generally well tolerated. Adverse effects include abdominal pain, nausea, vomiting, diarrhea, headache, and rash, and these are more common with the higher dose required for treatment. Reversible elevations in liver enzymes have been reported. The safety of atovaquone in pregnancy is unknown. Plasma concentrations of atovaquone are decreased about 50% by coadministration of tetracycline or rifampin.

HALOFANTRINE & LUMEFANTRINE

Halofantrine hydrochloride, a phenanthrene-methanol related to quinine, is effective against erythrocytic (but not other) stages of all four human malaria species. Oral absorption is variable and is enhanced with food. Because of toxicity concerns, it should not be taken with meals. Plasma levels peak 16 hours after dosing, and the half-life is about 4 days. Excretion is mainly in the feces. The mechanism of action of halofantrine is unknown. The drug is not available in the USA (although it has been approved by the FDA), but it is widely available in malaria-endemic countries.

Halofantrine is rapidly effective against most chloroquine-resistant strains of *P falciparum,* but its use is limited by irregular absorption and cardiac toxicity. Cross-resistance with mefloquine may occur. As treatment for falciparum malaria, halofantrine is given orally in three 500-mg doses at 6-hour intervals, and this course is best repeated in 1 week for nonimmune individuals. Because of toxicity concerns and irregular absorption, halofantrine should not be used for chemoprophylaxis.

Halofantrine is generally well tolerated. The most common adverse effects are abdominal pain, diarrhea, vomiting, cough, rash, headache, pruritus, and elevated liver enzymes. Of greater concern, the drug alters cardiac conduction, with dose-related prolongation of QT and PR intervals. This effect is seen with standard doses and is worsened by prior mefloquine therapy. Rare instances of dangerous arrhythmias and some deaths have been reported. The drug is contraindicated in patients with cardiac conduction defects and should not be used in those who have recently taken mefloquine. The drug is embryotoxic in animal studies and is therefore contraindicated in pregnancy.

Lumefantrine, an aryl alcohol related to halofantrine, is available as a fixed-dose combination with artemether as Coartem in some countries. The half-life of lumefantrine, when used in combination, is 4.5 hours. As with halofantrine, oral absorption is highly variable and improved when the drug is taken with food. Coartem is highly effective for the treatment of falciparum malaria, but it is expensive and requires twice-daily dosing. Coartem does not appear to cause the cardiac toxicity seen with halofantrine.

ARTEMISININ & ITS DERIVATIVES

Artemisinin (**qinghaosu**) is a sesquiterpene lactone endoperoxide, the active component of an herbal medicine that has been used as an antipyretic in China for over 2000 years. Artemisinin is insoluble and can only be used orally. Analogs have been synthesized to increase solubility and improve antimalarial efficacy. The most important of these analogs are **artesunate** (water-soluble; useful for oral, intravenous, intramuscular, and rectal administration) and **artemether** (lipid-soluble; useful for oral, intramuscular, and rectal administration). Two other important analogs under study are arteether and

artelinic acid. Artemisinin and its analogs are rapidly absorbed, with peak plasma levels occurring in 1–2 hours and half-lives of 1–3 hours after oral administration. The compounds are rapidly metabolized to the active metabolite dihydroartemisinin. Drug levels appear to decrease after a number of days of therapy. None of the artemisinins are available in the USA, but artemether and artesunate are widely available in other countries.

Artemisinin and analogs are very rapidly acting blood schizonticides against all human malaria parasites. Artemisinin has no effect on hepatic stages. Artemisinin-resistant *P falciparum* has not yet been identified. The antimalarial activity of artemisinin probably results from the production of free radicals that follows the iron-catalyzed cleavage of the artemisinin endoperoxide bridge in the parasite food vacuole.

Artemisinins—in particular artesunate and artemether—are coming to play a key role in the treatment of multidrug-resistant *P falciparum* malaria. They are the only drugs reliably effective against quinine-resistant strains. The efficacy of the artemisinins is limited somewhat by their short plasma half-lives. Recrudescence rates are unacceptably high after short-course or even 7 days of therapy, and these drugs are generally best used in conjunction with another agent. Also because of their short-half lives, they are not useful in chemoprophylaxis. In a number of studies of severe malaria, artemether and artesunate were about as effective as quinine, though mortality from severe malaria remained high.

Artesunate is widely available—although quite expensive—for the treatment of uncomplicated and severe falciparum malaria. It is commonly used in combination with mefloquine to treat highly resistant falciparum malaria in Thailand. Artemether is available alone and as a fixed-dose combination with lumefantrine (see above). In the setting of multidrug resistance, many authorities now advocate combination therapy including an artemisinin as the optimal treatment for falciparum malaria, although concerns regarding high cost, recrudescence, and toxicity remain.

Artemisinins appear to be better tolerated than most antimalarials. The most commonly reported adverse effects have been nausea, vomiting, and diarrhea. Irreversible neurotoxicity has been seen in animals, but only after doses much higher than those used to treat malaria. Artemisinins should be avoided in pregnancy if possible because teratogenicity has been seen in animal studies.

TREATMENT OF AMEBIASIS

Amebiasis is infection with *Entamoeba histolytica.* This agent can cause asymptomatic intestinal infection, mild to moderate colitis, severe intestinal infection (dysentery), ameboma, liver abscess, and other extraintestinal infections. The choice of drugs for amebiasis depends on the clinical presentation (Figure 53–2; Table 53–4).

Treatment of Specific Forms of Amebiasis

A. ASYMPTOMATIC INTESTINAL INFECTION

Asymptomatic carriers generally are not treated in endemic areas but in nonendemic areas they are treated with a luminal amebicide. A tissue amebicidal drug is unnecessary. Standard luminal amebicides are diloxanide furoate, iodoquinol, and paromomycin. Each drug eradicates carriage in about 80–90% of patients

with a single course of treatment. Therapy with a luminal amebicide is also required in the treatment of all other forms of amebiasis.

B. AMEBIC COLITIS

Metronidazole plus a luminal amebicide is the treatment of choice for colitis and dysentery. Tetracyclines and erythromycin are alternative drugs for moderate colitis but are not effective against extraintestinal disease. Dehydroemetine or emetine can also be used, but these agents are best avoided (when possible) because of their toxicity.

C. EXTRAINTESTINAL INFECTIONS

The treatment of choice is metronidazole plus a luminal amebicide. A 10-day course of metronidazole cures over

Table 53–4. Treatment of amebiasis.[1]

Clinical Setting	Drugs of Choice and Adult Dosage	Alternative Drugs and Adult Dosage
Asymptomatic intestinal infection	Luminal agent: Diloxanide furoate,[2] 500 mg 3 times daily for 10 days or– Iodoquinol, 650 mg 3 times daily for 21 days or– Paromomycin, 10 mg/kg 3 times daily for 7 days	
Mild to moderate intestinal infection	Metronidazole, 750 mg 3 times daily (or 500 mg IV every 6 hours) for 10 days plus– Luminal agent (see above)	Luminal agent (see above) plus either– Tetracycline, 250 mg 3 times daily for 10 days or– Erythromycin, 500 mg 4 times daily for 10 days
Severe intestinal infection	Metronidazole, 750 mg 3 times daily (or 500 mg IV every 6 hours) for 10 days plus– Luminal agent (see above)	Luminal agent (see above) plus either– Tetracycline, 250 mg 3 times daily for 10 days or– Dehydroemetine[3] or emetine,[2] 1 mg/kg SC or IM for 3–5 days
Hepatic abscess, ameboma, and other extraintestinal disease	Metronidazole, 750 mg 3 times daily (or 500 mg IV every 6 hours) for 10 days plus– Luminal agent (see above)	Dehydroemetine[3] or emetine,[2] 1 mg/kg SC or IM for 8–10 days, followed by (liver abscess only) chloroquine, 500 mg twice daily for 2 days, then 500 mg daily for 21 days plus– Luminal agent (see above)

[1]Route is oral unless otherwise indicated. See text for additional details and cautions.
[2]Not available in the USA.
[3]Available in the USA only from the Drug Service, CDC, Atlanta (404-639-3670).

95% of uncomplicated liver abscesses. For unusual cases where initial therapy with metronidazole has failed, aspiration of the abscess and the addition of chloroquine to a repeat course of metronidazole should be considered. Dehydroemetine and emetine are toxic alternative drugs.

METRONIDAZOLE

Metronidazole, a nitroimidazole (Figure 53–2), is the drug of choice for the treatment of extraluminal amebiasis. It kills trophozoites but not cysts of *E histolytica* and effectively eradicates intestinal and extraintestinal tissue infections.

Chemistry & Pharmacokinetics

Oral metronidazole is readily absorbed and permeates all tissues by simple diffusion. Intracellular concentrations rapidly approach extracellular levels. Peak plasma concentrations are reached in 1–3 hours. Protein binding is low (< 20%), and the half-life of the unchanged drug is 7.5 hours. The drug and its metabolites are excreted mainly in the urine. Plasma clearance of metronidazole is decreased in patients with impaired liver function.

Mechanism of Action

The nitro group of metronidazole is chemically reduced in anaerobic bacteria and sensitive protozoans. Reactive reduction products appear to be responsible for antimicrobial activity.

Clinical Uses

A. AMEBIASIS

Metronidazole is the drug of choice for the treatment of all tissue infections with *E histolytica*. It is not reliably

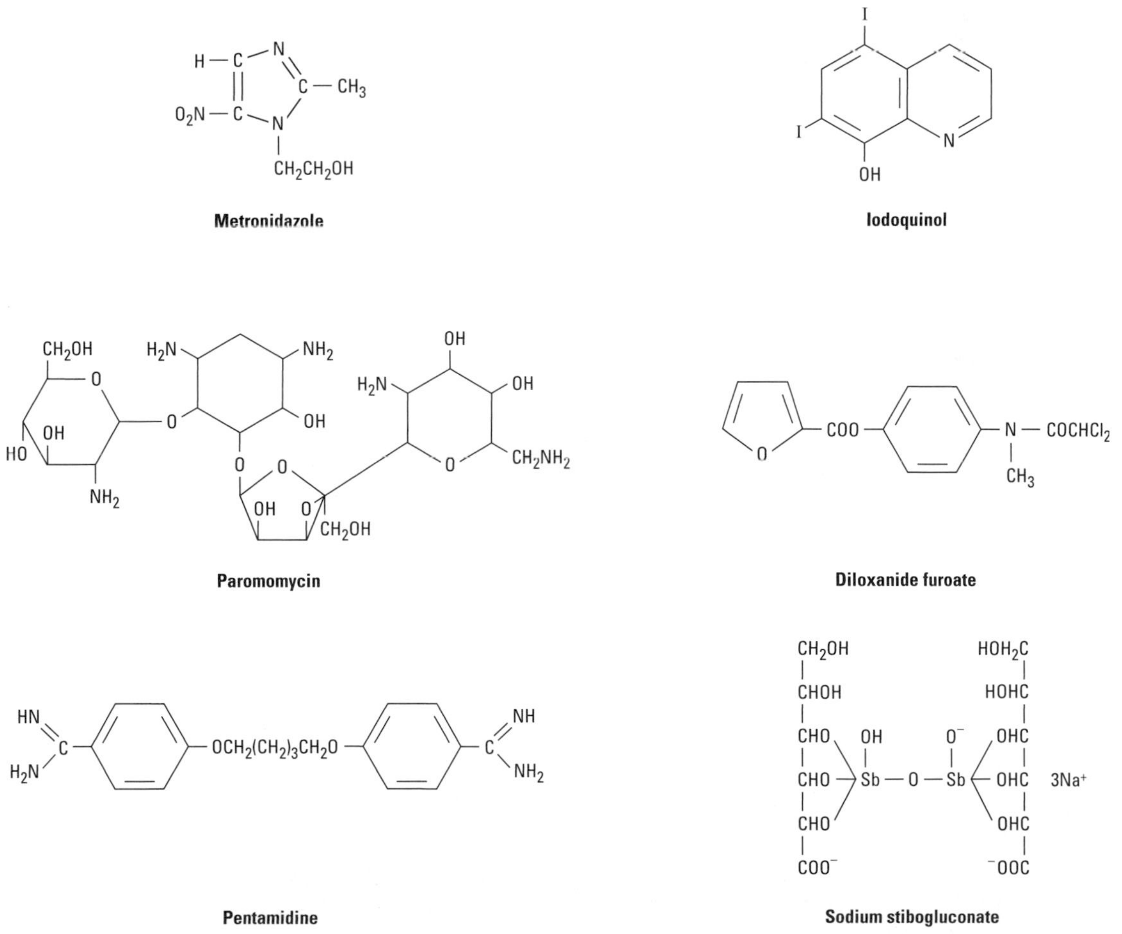

Figure 53–2. Structural formulas of other antiprotozoal drugs.

effective against luminal parasites and so must be used with a luminal amebicide to ensure eradication of the infection. Tinidazole, a related nitroimidazole, appears to have similar activity and a better toxicity profile than metronidazole, but it is not available in the USA.

B. GIARDIASIS

Metronidazole is the treatment of choice for giardiasis. The dosage for giardiasis is much lower—and the drug thus better tolerated—than that for amebiasis. Efficacy after a single treatment is about 90%. Tinidazole is equally effective.

C. TRICHOMONIASIS

Metronidazole is the treatment of choice. A single dose of 2 g is effective. Metronidazole-resistant organisms may lead to treatment failures. Tinidazole may be effective against some of these infections, but it is not available in the USA. Such cases may require repeat courses of metronidazole at higher doses than normally recommended—or topical therapy.

Adverse Effects & Cautions

Nausea, headache, dry mouth, or a metallic taste in the mouth occurs commonly. Infrequent adverse effects include vomiting, diarrhea, insomnia, weakness, dizziness, thrush, rash, dysuria, dark urine, vertigo, paresthesias, and neutropenia. Taking the drug with meals lessens gastrointestinal irritation. Pancreatitis and severe central nervous system toxicity (ataxia, encephalopathy, seizures) are rare. Metronidazole has a disulfiram-like effect, so that nausea and vomiting can occur if alcohol is ingested during therapy. The drug should be used with caution in patients with central nervous system disease. Intravenous infusions have rarely caused seizures or peripheral neuropathy. The dosage should be adjusted for patients with severe liver or renal disease.

Metronidazole has been reported to potentiate the anticoagulant effect of coumarin-type anticoagulants. Phenytoin and phenobarbital may accelerate elimination of the drug, while cimetidine may decrease plasma clearance. Lithium toxicity may occur when the drug is used with metronidazole.

Metronidazole and its metabolites are mutagenic in bacteria. Chronic administration of large doses led to tumorigenicity in mice. Data on teratogenicity are inconsistent. Metronidazole is thus best avoided in pregnant or nursing women, though congenital abnormalities have not clearly been associated with use in humans.

IODOQUINOL

Iodoquinol (diiodohydroxyquin) is a halogenated hydroxyquinoline. It is an effective luminal amebicide that is commonly used with metronidazole to treat amebic infections. Its pharmacokinetic properties are poorly understood. Ninety percent of the drug is retained in the intestine and excreted in the feces. The remainder enters the circulation, has a half-life of 11–14 hours, and is excreted in the urine as glucuronides.

The mechanism of action of iodoquinol against trophozoites is unknown. It is effective against organisms in the bowel lumen but not against trophozoites in the intestinal wall or extraintestinal tissues.

Infrequent adverse effects include diarrhea—which usually stops after several days—anorexia, nausea, vomiting, abdominal pain, headache, rash, and pruritus. The drug may increase protein-bound serum iodine, leading to a decrease in measured ^{131}I uptake that persists for months. Some halogenated hydroxyquinolines can produce severe neurotoxicity with prolonged use at greater than recommended doses. Iodoquinol is not known to produce these effects at its recommended dosage, and this dosage should never be exceeded.

Iodoquinol should be taken with meals to limit gastrointestinal toxicity. It should be used with caution in patients with optic neuropathy, renal or thyroid disease, or nonamebic hepatic disease. The drug should be discontinued if it produces persistent diarrhea or signs of iodine toxicity (dermatitis, urticaria, pruritus, fever). It is contraindicated in patients with intolerance to iodine.

DILOXANIDE FUROATE

Diloxanide furoate is a dichloroacetamide derivative. It is an effective luminal amebicide but is not active against tissue trophozoites. In the gut, diloxanide furoate is split into diloxanide and furoic acid; about 90% of the diloxanide is rapidly absorbed and then conjugated to form the glucuronide, which is promptly excreted in the urine. The unabsorbed diloxanide is the active antiamebic substance. The mechanism of action of diloxanide furoate is unknown.

Diloxanide furoate is considered by many the drug of choice for asymptomatic luminal infections, but it is no longer available in the USA. It is used with a tissue amebicide, usually metronidazole, to treat serious intestinal and extraintestinal infections. Diloxanide furoate does not produce serious adverse effects. Flatulence is common, but nausea and abdominal cramps are infrequent and rashes are rare. The drug is not recommended in pregnancy.

PAROMOMYCIN SULFATE

Paromomycin sulfate is an aminoglycoside antibiotic (see also Chapter 45) that is not significantly absorbed from the gastrointestinal tract. It is used only as a luminal amebicide and has no effect against extraintestinal amebic infections. The small amount absorbed is slowly excreted unchanged, mainly by glomerular filtration. However, the drug may accumulate with renal insufficiency and contribute to renal toxicity. Paromomycin is an effective luminal amebicide that appears to have similar efficacy and probably less toxicity than other agents; in a recent study, it was superior to diloxanide furoate in clearing asymptomatic infections. Adverse effects include occasional abdominal distress and diarrhea. Paromomycin should be avoided in patients with significant renal disease and used with caution in persons with gastrointestinal ulcerations. Parenteral paromomycin is under investigation for the treatment of visceral leishmaniasis.

EMETINE & DEHYDROEMETINE

Emetine, an alkaloid derived from ipecac, and dehydroemetine, a synthetic analog, are effective against tissue trophozoites of *E histolytica,* but because of major toxicity concerns they have been almost completely replaced by metronidazole. The drugs are administered parenterally because oral preparations are absorbed erratically. They accumulate in tissues and are eliminated slowly via the kidneys.

The use of emetine and dehydroemetine is limited to unusual circumstances in which severe amebiasis warrants effective therapy and metronidazole cannot be used. Dehydroemetine is preferred over emetine because of its somewhat better toxicity profile. The drugs should be used to treat amebic dysentery or amebic liver abscess for the minimum period needed to relieve severe symptoms (usually 3–5 days).

Emetine and dehydroemetine should be administered subcutaneously (preferred) or intramuscularly (but never intravenously) in a supervised setting. Adverse effects are generally mild when the drugs are used for 3–5 days but increase with prolonged use. They should not be used for more than 10 days. Pain and tenderness in the area of injection are frequent, and sterile abscesses may develop. Diarrhea is common. Other adverse effects are nausea, vomiting, muscle weakness and discomfort, and minor electrocardiographic changes. Serious toxicities include cardiac arrhythmias, heart failure, and hypotension. The drugs should not be used in patients with cardiac or renal disease, in young children, or in pregnancy unless absolutely necessary.

OTHER ANTIPROTOZOAL DRUGS

See Table 53–5 for a list of drugs used in the treatment of other protozoal infections. Important drugs that are not covered elsewhere in this or other chapters are discussed below.

PENTAMIDINE

Pentamidine has activity against trypanosomatid protozoans and against *P jiroveci,* but toxicity is significant.

Chemistry & Pharmacokinetics

Pentamidine is an aromatic diamidine (Figure 53–2) formulated as an isethionate salt. Pentamidine is only administered parenterally. The drug leaves the circulation rapidly, with an initial half-life of about 6 hours, but it is bound avidly by tissues. Pentamidine thus accumulates and is eliminated very slowly, with a terminal elimination half-life of about 12 days. The drug can be detected in urine 6 or more weeks after treatment. Only trace amounts of pentamidine appear in the central nervous system, so it is not effective against central nervous system African trypanosomiasis. Pentamidine can also be inhaled as a nebulized powder for the prevention of pneumocystosis. Absorption into the systemic circulation after inhalation appears to be minimal. The mechanism of action of pentamidine is unknown.

Clinical Uses

A. PNEUMOCYSTOSIS

Pentamidine is a well-established alternative therapy for pulmonary and extrapulmonary disease caused by *P jiroveci.* The drug has somewhat lower efficacy and greater toxicity than trimethoprim-sulfamethoxazole. The standard dosage is now 3 mg/kg/d intravenously for 21 days. Significant adverse reactions are common, and with multiple regimens now available to treat *P jiroveci* infection, pentamidine is best reserved for patients with severe disease who cannot tolerate or fail other drugs.

Pentamidine is also an alternative agent for primary or secondary prophylaxis against pneumocystosis in immunocompromised individuals, including patients with advanced AIDS. For this indication, pentamidine is administered as an inhaled aerosol (300 mg inhaled monthly). The drug is well-tolerated in this form. Its efficacy is very good but clearly less than that of daily trimethoprim-sulfamethoxazole. Because of its cost and ineffectiveness against nonpulmonary disease, it is best reserved for patients who cannot tolerate oral chemoprophylaxis with other drugs.

B. AFRICAN TRYPANOSOMIASIS (SLEEPING SICKNESS)

Pentamidine has been used since 1940 as an alternative to suramin for the early hemolymphatic stage of disease caused by *Trypanosoma brucei* (especially *T brucei gambiense*). The drug can also be used with suramin. Pentamidine should not be used to treat late trypanosomiasis with central nervous system involvement. A number of dosing regimens have been described, generally providing 2–4 mg/kg daily or on alternate days for a total of

Table 53–5. Treatment of other protozoal infections.

Organism or Clinical Setting	Drugs of Choice[1]	Alternative Drugs
Babesia species	Clindamycin, 600 mg 3 times daily for 7 days plus– Quinine, 650 mg for 7 days	Atovaquone *or* azithromycin
Balantidium coli	Tetracycline, 500 mg 4 times daily for 10 days	Metronidazole, 750 mg 3 times daily for 5 days
Cryptosporidium species	Paromomycin, 500–750 mg 3 or 4 times daily for 10 days	Azithromycin, 500 mg daily for 21 days[2]
Cyclospora cayetanensis	Trimethoprim-sulfamethoxazole, one double-strength tablet 4 times daily for 7–14 days	
Dientamoeba fragilis	Iodoquinol, 650 mg 3 times daily for 20 days	Tetracycline, 500 mg 4 times daily for 10 days or– Paromomycin, 500 mg 3 times daily for 7 days
Giardia lamblia	Metronidazole, 250 mg 3 times daily for 5 days or– Tinidazole,[3] 2 g once	Furazolidone, 100 mg 4 times daily for 7 days or– Albendazole, 400 mg daily for 5 days[2]
Isospora belli	Trimethoprim-sulfamethoxazole, one double-strength tablet 4 times daily for 10 days, then twice daily for 21 days	Pyrimethamine, 75 mg daily for 14 days plus– Folinic acid, 10 mg daily for 14 days
Microsporidia	Albendazole, 400 mg twice daily for 20–30 days	

Leishmaniasis
  Visceral
  (*L donovani,*
  L chagasi,
  L infantum)
  or mucosal
  (*L braziliensis*)
	Sodium stibogluconate,[4] 20 mg/kg/d IV or IM for 28 days	Meglumine antimonate[2]
		or–
		Pentamidine
		or–
		Amphotericin B
		or–
		Miltefosine[2]

Cutaneous
  (*L major,*
  L tropica,
  L mexicana,
  L braziliensis)
	Sodium stibogluconate,[4] 20 mg/kg/d IV or IM for 20 days	Meglumine antimonate[2]
		or–
		Ketoconazole
		or–
		Pentamidine
		or–
		Topical or intralesional therapies

Pneumocystis jiroveci, *P carinii* [5]	Trimethoprim-sulfamethoxazole, 15–20 mg trimethoprim component/kg/d IV, or two double-strength tablets every 8 hours for 21 days	Pentamidine or– Trimethoprim-dapsone or– Clindamycin *plus* primaquine or– Atovaquone
Toxoplasma gondii Acute, congenital, immunocom-promised	Pyrimethamine *plus* clindamycin *plus* folinic acid	Pyrimethamine *plus* sulfadiazine *plus* folinic acid
Pregnancy	Spiramycin, 3 g daily until delivery	

Table 53–5. Treatment of other protozoal infections (*continued*).

Organism or Clinical Setting	Drugs of Choice[1]	Alternative Drugs
Trichomonas vaginalis	Metronidazole, 2 g once or 250 mg 3 times daily for 7 days	Tinidazole[3]
Trypanosoma brucei Hemolymphatic	Suramin[4]	Pentamidine or– Eflornithine
Advanced CNS disease	Melarsoprol[4]	Eflornithine
Trypanosoma cruzi	Nifurtimox[4] or– Benznidizole[3]	

[1]Established, relatively simple dosing regimens are provided. Route is oral unless otherwise indicated. See text for additional information, toxicities, cautions, and discussions of dosing for the more rarely used drugs, many of which are highly toxic.

[2]Nitazoxanide is also available for pediatric use.

[3]Not available in the USA.

[4]Available in the USA only from the Drug Service, CDC, Atlanta (404-639-3670).

[5]*P jiroveci* (*carinii* in animals) has traditionally been considered a protozoan because of its morphology and drug sensitivity, but recent molecular analyses have shown it to be most closely related to fungi.

10–15 doses. Pentamidine has also been used for chemoprophylaxis against African trypanosomiasis, with dosing of 4 mg/kg every 3–6 months.

C. LEISHMANIASIS

Pentamidine is an alternative to sodium stibogluconate for the treatment of visceral leishmaniasis, although resistance has been reported. The drug has been successful in some cases that have failed therapy with antimonials. The dosage is 2–4 mg/kg intramuscularly daily or every other day for up to 15 doses, and a second course may be necessary. Pentamidine has also shown success against cutaneous leishmaniasis, but it is not routinely used for this purpose.

Adverse Effects & Cautions

Pentamidine is a highly toxic drug, with adverse effects noted in about 50% of patients receiving 4 mg/kg/d. Rapid intravenous administration can lead to severe hypotension, tachycardia, dizziness, and dyspnea, so the drug should be administered slowly (over 2 hours) and patients should be recumbent and monitored closely during treatment. With intramuscular administration, pain at the injection site is common and sterile abscesses may develop.

Pancreatic toxicity is common. Hypoglycemia due to inappropriate insulin release often appears 5–7 days after onset of treatment, can persist for days to several weeks, and may be followed by hyperglycemia. Reversible renal insufficiency is also common. Other adverse effects include rash, metallic taste, fever, gastrointestinal symptoms, abnormal liver function tests, acute pancreatitis, hypocalcemia, thrombocytopenia, hallucinations, and cardiac arrhythmias. Inhaled pentamidine is generally well-tolerated but may cause cough, dyspnea, and bronchospasm.

SODIUM STIBOGLUCONATE

Pentavalent antimonials, including sodium stibogluconate (pentostam; Figure 53–2) and meglumine antimonate, are generally considered first-line agents for cutaneous and visceral leishmaniasis. The drugs are rapidly absorbed after intravenous (preferred) or intramuscular administration and eliminated in two phases, with short (about 2 hour) and much longer (> 24 hour) half-lives. Treatment is given once daily at a dose of 20 mg/kg/d intravenously or intramuscularly for 20 days in cutaneous leishmaniasis and 28 days in visceral and mucocutaneous disease.

The mechanism of action of the antimonials is unknown. Their efficacy against different species may vary, possibly based on local drug resistance patterns.

Cure rates are generally quite good, but resistance to sodium stibogluconate is increasing in some endemic areas. Some authorities have advocated initial therapy with other agents (eg, amphotericin B) in areas (such as parts of India) where therapy with sodium stibogluconate is commonly ineffective.

Few adverse effects occur initially, but the toxicity of stibogluconate increases over the course of therapy. Most common are gastrointestinal symptoms, fever, headache, myalgias, arthralgias, and rash. Intramuscular injections can be very painful and lead to sterile abscesses. Electrocardiographic changes may occur, most commonly T wave changes and QT prolongation. These changes are generally reversible, but continued therapy may lead to dangerous arrhythmias. Thus, the electrocardiogram should be monitored during therapy. Hemolytic anemia and serious liver, renal, and cardiac effects are rare.

NITAZOXANIDE

Nitazoxanide is a nitrothiazolyl-salicylamide prodrug. Nitazoxanide was recently approved in the USA for use in children against *G lamblia* and *Cryptosporidium parvum*. The drug is converted to an active metabolite, tizoxanide, which inhibits the pyruvate:ferredoxin oxidoreductase pathway. It is rapidly absorbed and converted to tizoxanide and tizoxanide conjugates, which are subsequently excreted in both urine and feces. Nitazoxanide appears to have activity against metronidazole-resistant protozoal strains and is well tolerated. Unlike metronidazole, nitazoxanide and its metabolites appear to be free of mutagenic effects. Other organisms that may be susceptible to nitazoxanide include *E histolytica*, *Helicobacter pylori*, *A lumbricoides*, several tapeworms, and *Fasciola hepatica*.

The recommended dosage for children is 100–200 mg twice daily for 3 days. The adult dosage has not been established.

OTHER DRUGS FOR TRYPANOSOMIASIS & LEISHMANIASIS

Currently available therapies for all forms of trypanosomiasis are seriously deficient in both efficacy and safety. Availability of these therapies is also a concern, as they remain available mainly through donation or nonprofit production by pharmaceutical companies.

A. SURAMIN

Suramin is a sulfated naphthylamine that was introduced in the 1920s. It is the first-line therapy for early hemolymphatic African trypanosomiasis (especially *T brucei gambiense* infection), but because it does not enter the central nervous system, it is not effective against advanced disease. The drug's mechanism of action is unknown. It is administered intravenously and displays complex pharmacokinetics with very tight protein binding. It has a short initial half-life but a terminal elimination half-life of about 50 days. The drug is slowly cleared by renal excretion.

Suramin is administered after a 200-mg intravenous test dose. Regimens that have been used include 1 g on days 1, 3, 7, 14, and 21 or 1 g each week for 5 weeks. Combination therapy with pentamidine may improve efficacy. Suramin can also be used for chemoprophylaxis against African trypanosomiasis. Adverse effects are common. Immediate reactions can include fatigue, nausea, vomiting, and, more rarely, seizures, shock, and death. Later reactions include fever, rash, headache, paresthesias, neuropathies, renal abnormalities including proteinuria, chronic diarrhea, hemolytic anemia, and agranulocytosis.

B. MELARSOPROL

Melarsoprol is a trivalent arsenical that has been available since 1949 and is first-line therapy for advanced central nervous system African trypanosomiasis. After intravenous administration it is excreted rapidly, but clinically relevant concentrations accumulate in the central nervous system within 4 days. Melarsoprol is administered in propylene glycol by slow intravenous infusion at a dosage of 3.6 mg/kg/d for 3–4 days, with repeated courses at weekly intervals if needed. A new regimen of 2.2 mg/kg daily for 10 days had efficacy and toxicity similar to what was observed with three courses over 26 days. Melarsoprol is extremely toxic. The use of such a toxic drug is justified only by the severity of advanced trypanosomiasis and the lack of available alternatives. Immediate adverse effects include fever, vomiting, abdominal pain, and arthralgias. The most important toxicity is a reactive encephalopathy that generally appears within the first week of therapy (in 5–10% of patients) and is probably due to disruption of trypanosomes in the central nervous system. Common consequences of the encephalopathy include cerebral edema, seizures, coma, and death. Other serious toxicities include renal and cardiac disease and hypersensitivity reactions. Failure rates with melarsoprol appear to have increased recently in parts of Africa, suggesting the possibility of drug resistance.

C. EFLORNITHINE

Eflornithine (difluoromethylornithine), an inhibitor of ornithine decarboxylase, is the only new drug registered to treat African trypanosomiasis in the last half-century. It is a second therapy for advanced central nervous system African trypanosomiasis and is less toxic than melarsoprol but not as widely available. The drug had very limited availability until recently, when it was developed for use as a topical depilatory cream, leading to donation of the drug for the treatment of trypanosomiasis. Eflornithine is administered intravenously, and good central nervous system drug levels are achieved. Peak plasma levels are reached rapidly, and the elimination half-life is about 3 hours. The usual regimen is 100 mg/kg intravenously every 6 hours for 7–14 days (14 days was superior for a newly diagnosed infection). An oral formulation is also available and under clinical investigation. Eflornithine appears to be as effective as melarsoprol against advanced *T brucei gambiense* infection, but its efficacy against *T brucei rhodesiense* is limited by drug resistance. Toxicity from eflornithine is significant, but considerably less than that from melarsoprol. Adverse effects include diarrhea, vomiting, anemia, thrombocytopenia, leukopenia, and seizures. These effects are generally reversible. Increased experience with eflornithine and increased availability of the compound in endemic areas may lead to its replacement of suramin, pentamidine, and melarsoprol for the treatment of *T brucei gambiense* infection.

D. NIFURTIMOX

Nifurtimox, a nitrofuran, is the most commonly used drug for American trypanosomiasis (Chagas' disease). Nifurtimox is also under study for the treatment of African trypanosomiasis. Nifurtimox is well absorbed after oral administration and eliminated with a plasma half-life of about 3 hours. The drug is administered at a dose of 8–10 mg/kg/d (divided into 3–4 doses) orally for 3–4 months for the treatment of acute Chagas' disease. Nifurtimox decreases the severity of acute disease and usually eliminates detectable parasites, but it is often ineffective in fully eradicating infection. Thus, it often fails to prevent progression to the gastrointestinal and cardiac syndromes associated with chronic infection that are the most important clinical consequences of *Trypanosoma cruzi* infection. Efficacy may vary in different parts of South America, possibly related to drug resistance in some areas. Nifurtimox does not appear to be effective in the treatment of chronic Chagas' disease. Toxicity related to nifurtimox is common. Adverse effects include nausea, vomiting, abdominal pain, fever, rash, restlessness, insomnia, neuropathies, and seizures. These effects are generally reversible but often lead to cessation of therapy before completion of a standard course.

E. BENZNIDAZOLE

Benznidazole is an orally administered nitroimidazole that appears to have efficacy similar to that of nifurtimox for the treatment of acute Chagas' disease. Availability of the drug is currently limited. Important toxicities include peripheral neuropathy, rash, gastrointestinal symptoms, and myelosuppression.

F. AMPHOTERICIN

This important antifungal drug (see Chapter 48) is an alternative therapy for visceral leishmaniasis, especially in parts of India with high-level resistance to sodium stibogluconate, but its use is limited in developing countries by difficulty of administration, cost, and toxicity.

G. MILTEFOSINE

Miltefosine is an alkylphosphocholine analog that has recently shown efficacy for the treatment of visceral leishmaniasis. In a recent phase III study, the drug was administered orally with daily doses of 2.5 mg/kg for 28 days and provided excellent clinical results. A 100 mg daily dose is recommended in adults. Vomiting and diarrhea are common but generally short-lived toxicities. Transient elevations in liver enzymes are also seen. The drug should be avoided in pregnancy because of its teratogenic effects. Miltefosine is registered for the treatment of visceral leishmaniasis in India, and—considering the serious limitations of other drugs, including parenteral administration, toxicity, and resistance—it may become the treatment of choice for that disease.

PREPARATIONS AVAILABLE IN THE USA

Albendazole (Albenza)
  Oral: 200 mg tablets
Atovaquone (Mepron)
  Oral: 750 mg/5 mL suspension
Atovaquone-proguanil (Malarone)
  Oral: 250 mg atovaquone + 100 mg proguanil tablets; pediatric 62.5 mg atovaquone + 25 mg proguanil tablets
Chloroquine (generic, Aralen)
  Oral: 250, 500 mg tablets (equivalent to 150, 300 mg base, respectively)

  Parenteral: 50 mg/mL (equivalent to 40 mg/mL base) for injection
Clindamycin (generic, Cleocin)
  Oral: 75, 150, 300 mg capsules; 75 mg/5 mL suspension
  Parenteral: 150 mg/mL for injection
Doxycycline (generic, Vibramycin)
  Oral: 20, 50, 100 mg capsules; 50, 100 mg tablets; 25 mg/5 mL suspension; 50 mg/5 mL syrup
  Parenteral: 100, 200 mg for injection

Dehydroemetine*
Eflornithine (Ornidyl)
  Parenteral: 200 mg/mL for injection
Halofantrine (Halfan)
  Oral: 250 mg tablets
Iodoquinol (Yodoxin)
  Oral: 210, 650 mg tablets
Mefloquine (generic, Lariam)
  Oral: 250 mg tablets
Melarsoprol (Mel B)*
Metronidazole (generic, Flagyl)
  Oral: 250, 500 mg tablets; 375 mg capsules; extended-release 750 mg tablets
  Parenteral: 5 mg/mL
Nifurtimox*
Nitazoxanide (Alinia)
  Oral: powder for 100 mg/5 mL oral solution
Paromomycin (Humatin)
  Oral: 250 mg capsules

Pentamidine (Pentam 300, Pentacarinat, pentamidine isethionate)
  Parenteral: 300 mg powder for injection
  Aerosol (Nebupent): 300 mg powder
Primaquine (generic)
  Oral: 26.3 mg (equivalent to 15 mg base) tablet
Pyrimethamine (Daraprim)
  Oral: 25 mg tablets
Quinidine gluconate (generic)
  Parenteral: 80 mg/mL (equivalent to 50 mg/mL base) for injection
Quinine (generic)
  Oral: 260 mg tablets; 200, 260, 325 mg capsules
Sodium stibogluconate*
Sulfadoxine and pyrimethamine (Fansidar)
  Oral: 500 mg sulfadoxine plus 25 mg pyrimethamine tablets
Suramin*

* Available in the USA only from the Drug Service, CDC, Atlanta (404-639-3670).

REFERENCES

GENERAL

Drugs for parasitic infections. Med Lett Drugs Ther 2002;44:33. (Issue available at www.medicalletter.com/freedocs/parasitic.pdf.)

Rosenblatt JE: Antiparasitic agents. Mayo Clin Proc 1999;74:1161.

MALARIA

Adjuk M et al: Amodiaquine-artesunate versus amodiaquine for uncomplicated *Plasmodium falciparum* malaria in African children: a randomised, multicentre trial. Lancet 2002; 359:1365.

Baird JK, Hoffman SL: Prevention of malaria in travelers. Med Clin North Am 1999 83:923.

Bindschedler M et al: Comparison of the cardiac effects of the antimalarials coartemether and halofantrine in healthy participants. Am J Trop Med Hyg 2002;66:293.

Brockman A et al: *Plasmodium falciparum* antimalarial drug susceptibility on the north-western border of Thailand during five years of extensive use of artesunate-mefloquine. Trans R Soc Trop Med Hyg 2000;94:537.

Djimde A et al: A molecular marker for chloroquine-resistant falciparum malaria. N Engl J Med 2001;344:257.

Dorsey G et al: Sulfadoxine/pyrimethamine alone or with amodiaquine or artesunate for treatment of uncomplicated malaria: a longitudinal randomised trial. Lancet 2002;360:2031.

Ezzet F et al: Pharmacokinetics and pharmacodynamics of lumefantrine (benflumetol) in acute falciparum malaria. Antimicrob Agents Chemother 2000;44:697.

Fidock DA et al: Mutations in the *P. falciparum* digestive vacuole transmembrane protein PfCRT and evidence for their role in chloroquine resistance. Mol Cell 2000;6:861.

Foley M, Tilley L: Quinoline antimalarials: mechanisms of action and resistance and prospects for new agents. Pharmacol Ther 1998;79:55.

Guerin PJ et al: Malaria: current status of control, diagnosis, treatment, and a proposed agenda for research and development. Lancet Infect Dis 2002;2:564.

Ling J et al: Randomized, placebo-controlled trial of atovaquone/proguanil for the prevention of *Plasmodium falciparum* or *Plasmodium vivax* malaria among migrants to Papua, Indonesia. Clin Infect Dis 2002;35:825.

Lobel HO, Kozarsky PE: Update on prevention of malaria for travelers. JAMA 1997;278:1767.

Looareesuwan S et al: Malarone (atovaquone and proguanil hydrochloride): a review of its clinical development for treatment of malaria. Am J Trop Med Hyg 1999;60:533.

Looareesuwan S et al: Efficacy and safety of atovaquone/proguanil compared with mefloquine for treatment of acute *Plasmodium falciparum* malaria in Thailand. Am J Trop Med Hyg 1999;60:526.

Mutabingwa T et al: Chlorproguanil-dapsone for treatment of drug-resistant falciparum malaria in Tanzania. Lancet 2001; 358:1218.

Newton P, White NJ: Malaria: New developments in treatment and prevention. Annu Rev Med 1999;50:179.

Nosten F, Brasseur P: Combination therapy for malaria. Drugs 2002;62:1315.

Olliaro P: Mode of action and mechanisms of resistance for antimalarial drugs. Pharmacol Ther 2001;89:207.

Peragallo MS, Sabatinelli G, Sarnicola G: Compliance and tolerability of mefloquine and chloroquine plus proguanil for long-term malaria chemoprophylaxis in groups at particular risk (the military). Trans R Soc Trop Med Hyg 1999;93:73.

Price R et al: Adverse effects in patients with acute falciparum malaria treated with artemisinin derivatives. Am J Trop Med Hyg 1999;60:547.

Ridley RG: Medical need, scientific opportunity and the drive for antimalarial drugs. Nature 2002;415:686.

Rosenthal PJ (editor): *Antimalarial Chemotherapy: Mechanisms of Action, Resistance, and New Directions in Drug Discovery.* Humana Press, 2001.

Schlagenhauf P: Mefloquine for malaria chemoprophylaxis 1992–1998: a review. J Travel Med 1999;6:122.

Staedke SG et al: Amodiaquine, sulfadoxine/pyrimethamine, and combination therapy for treatment of uncomplicated falciparum malaria in Kampala, Uganda: a randomised trial. Lancet 2001;358:368.

Sukwa TY et al: A randomized, double-blind, placebo-controlled field trial to determine the efficacy and safety of Malarone (atovaquone/proguanil) for the prophylaxis of malaria in Zambia. Am J Trop Med Hyg 1999;60:521.

Sulo J et al: Chlorproguanil-dapsone versus sulfadoxine-pyrimethamine for sequential episodes of uncomplicated falciparum malaria in Kenya and Malawi: a randomised clinical trial. Lancet 2002;360:1136.

van Agtmael MA, Eggelte TA, van Boxtel CJ: Artemisinin drugs in the treatment of malaria: from medicinal herb to registered medication. Trends Pharmacol Sci 1999;20:199.

Van Vugt M et al: Artemether-lumefantrine for the treatment of multidrug-resistant falciparum malaria. Trans R Soc Trop Med Hyg 2000;94:545.

Winstanley P: Modern chemotherapeutic options for malaria. Lancet Infect Dis 2001;1:242.

AMEBIASIS

Blessmann J, Tannich E: Treatment of asymptomatic intestinal *Entamoeba histolytica* infection. N Engl J Med 2002; 347:1384.

Freeman CD, Klutman NE, Lamp KC: Metronidazole: a therapeutic review and update. Drugs 1997;54:679.

Petri WA, Singh U: Diagnosis and management of amebiasis. Clin Infect Dis 1999;29:1117.

OTHER PROTOZOAL INFECTIONS

Aronson NE et al: Safety and efficacy of intravenous sodium stibogluconate in the treatment of leishmaniasis: recent U.S. military experience. Clin Infect Dis 1998;27:1457.

Burri C et al: Efficacy of new, concise schedule for melarsoprol in treatment of sleeping sickness caused by *Trypanosoma brucei gambiense:* a randomised trial. Lancet 2000;355:1419.

Burchmore RJ et al: Chemotherapy of human African trypanosomiasis. Curr Pharm Des 2002;8:256.

Croft SL, Yardley V: Chemotherapy of leishmaniasis. Curr Pharm Des 2002;8:319.

Davidson RN: Practical guide for the treatment of leishmaniasis. Drugs 1998;56:1009.

Guerin PJ et al: Visceral leishmaniasis: current status of control, diagnosis, and treatment, and a proposed research and development agenda. Lancet Infect Dis 2002;2:494.

Hepburn NC: Management of cutaneous leishmaniasis. Curr Opin Infect Dis 2001;14:151.

Katz DE, Taylor DN: Parasitic infections of the gastrointestinal tract. Gastroenterol Clin North Am 2001;30:797.

Legros D et al: Treatment of human African trypanosomiasis—present situation and needs for research and development. Lancet Infect Dis 2002;2:437.

Nitazoxanide (Alinia)—a new antiprotozoal agent. Med Lett Drugs Ther 2003;45:29.

Okhuysen PC: Traveler's diarrhea due to intestinal protozoa. Clin Infect Dis 2001;33:110.

Pepin J et al: Short-course eflornithine in Gambian trypanosomiasis: a multicentre randomized controlled trial. Bull World Health Organ 2000;78:1283.

Sobel JD, Nyirjesy P, Brown W: Tinidazole therapy for metronidazole-resistant vaginal trichomoniasis. Clin Infect Dis 2001;33:1341.

Sundar S et al: Oral miltefosine for Indian visceral leishmaniasis. N Engl J Med 2002;347:1739.

Urbina JA: Specific treatment of Chagas disease: current status and new developments. Curr Opin Infect Dis 2001;14:717.

Clinical Pharmacology of the Anthelmintic Drugs

54

Philip J. Rosenthal, MD, & Robert S. Goldsmith, MD, DTM&H

CHEMOTHERAPY OF HELMINTHIC INFECTIONS

Table 54–1 lists the major helminthic infections and provides a guide to the drug of choice and alternative drugs for each infection. In the text that follows, these drugs are arranged alphabetically. In general, parasites should be identified before treatment is started.

ALBENDAZOLE

Albendazole, a broad-spectrum oral anthelmintic, is the drug of choice and is approved in the USA for treatment of hydatid disease and cysticercosis. It is also used for the treatment of pinworm and hookworm infections, ascariasis, trichuriasis, and strongyloidiasis, though it is not labeled for these conditions.

Chemistry & Pharmacokinetics

Albendazole is a benzimidazole carbamate. After oral administration, it is erratically absorbed (increased with a fatty meal) and then rapidly undergoes first-pass metabolism in the liver to the active metabolite albendazole sulfoxide. It reaches variable maximum plasma concentrations about 3 hours after a 400 mg oral dose, and its plasma half-life is 8–12 hours. The sulfoxide is mostly protein-bound, distributes well to tissues, and enters bile, cerebrospinal fluid, and hydatid cysts. Albendazole metabolites are excreted in the urine.

Albendazole

Anthelmintic Actions

Benzimidazoles are thought to act against nematodes by inhibiting microtubule synthesis. Albendazole also has larvicidal effects in hydatid disease, cysticercosis, ascariasis, and hookworm infection and ovicidal effects in ascariasis, ancylostomiasis, and trichuriasis.

Clinical Uses

Albendazole is administered on an empty stomach when used against intraluminal parasites but with a fatty meal when used against tissue parasites.

A. ASCARIASIS, TRICHURIASIS, AND HOOKWORM AND PINWORM INFECTIONS

For adults and children over 2 years of age, the treatment is a single dose of 400 mg orally (repeated for 2–3 days for heavy ascaris infections and in 2 weeks for pinworm infections). These treatments achieve high cure rates for these roundworm infections and marked reduction in egg counts in those not cured.

B. HYDATID DISEASE

Albendazole is the treatment of choice for medical therapy and is a useful adjunct to surgical removal or aspiration of cysts. It is more active against *E granulosus* than *E multilocularis*. Dosing is 400 mg twice daily with meals for 1 month or longer. Daily therapy for up to 6 months has been well tolerated. One reported therapeutic strategy is to treat with albendazole and praziquantel, to assess response after 1 month or more, and, depending on the response, to then manage the patient with continued chemotherapy or combined surgical and drug therapy.

C. NEUROCYSTICERCOSIS

Indications for medical therapy for neurocysticercosis are controversial, as anthelmintic therapy is not clearly superior to therapy with corticosteroids alone and may exacerbate neurologic disease. Therapy is probably most

Table 54–1. Drugs for the treatment of helminthic infections.

Infecting Organism	Drug of Choice	Alternative Drugs
Roundworms (nematodes)		
Ascaris lumbricoides (roundworm)	Albendazole[1] or pyrantel pamoate or mebendazole	Piperazine
Trichuris trichiura (whipworm)	Mebendazole or albendazole[1]	Oxantel/pyrantel pamoate[2]
Necator americanus (hookworm); *Ancylostoma duodenale* (hookworm)	Pyrantel pamoate[1] or mebendazole or albendazole[1]	
Strongyloides stercoralis (threadworm)	Ivermectin	Thiabendazole, albendazole[1]
Enterobius vermicularis (pinworm)	Mebendazole or pyrantel pamoate	Albendazole[1]
Trichinella spiralis (trichinosis)	Mebendazole;[1] add corticosteroids for severe infection	Albendazole;[1] add corticosteroids for severe infection
Trichostrongylus species	Pyrantel pamoate[1] or mebendazole[1]	Albendazole[1]
Cutaneous larva migrans (creeping eruption)	Albendazole[1] or ivermectin[1]	Thiabendazole (topical)
Visceral larva migrans	Albendazole[1]	Mebendazole[1]
Angiostrongylus cantonensis	Thiabendazole	Albendazole[1] or mebendazole[1]
Wuchereria bancrofti (filariasis); *Brugia malayi* (filariasis); tropical eosinophilia; *Loa loa* (loiasis)	Diethylcarbamazine[3]	Ivermectin[1]
Onchocerca volvulus (onchocerciasis)	Ivermectin	
Dracunculus medinensis (guinea worm)	Metronidazole[1]	Thiabendazole[1] or mebendazole[1]
Capillaria philippinensis (intestinal capillariasis)	Albendazole[1]	Mebendazole[1] or thiabendazole[1]
Flukes (trematodes)		
Schistosoma haematobium (bilharziasis)	Praziquantel	Metrifonate[2]
Schistosoma mansoni	Praziquantel	Oxamniquine
Schistosoma japonicum	Praziquantel	
Clonorchis sinensis (liver fluke); opisthorchis species	Praziquantel	Albendazole[1]
Paragonimus westermani (lung fluke)	Praziquantel[1]	Bithionol[3]
Fasciola hepatica (sheep liver fluke)	Bithionol[3] or triclabendazole[2]	
Fasciolopsis buski (large intestinal fluke)	Praziquantel[1] or niclosamide[2]	
Heterophyes heterophyes; *Metagonimus yokogawai* (small intestinal flukes)	Praziquantel[1] or niclosamide[2]	
Tapeworms (cestodes)		
Taenia saginata (beef tapeworm)	Praziquantel[1] or niclosamide[2]	Mebendazole[1,3]
Diphyllobothrium latum (fish tapeworm)	Praziquantel[1] or niclosamide[2]	

(continued)

Table 54–1. Drugs for the treatment of helminthic infections (*continued*).

Infecting Organism	Drug of Choice	Alternative Drugs
Tapeworms (cestodes)		
Taenia solium (pork tapeworm)	Praziquantel[1] or niclosamide[2]	
Cysticercosis (pork tapeworm larval stage)	Albendazole	Praziquantel[1]
Hymenolepis nana (dwarf tapeworm)	Praziquantel[1]	Niclosamide[2]
Echinococcus granulosus (hydatid disease); *Echinococcus multilocularis*	Albendazole	

[1]Available in the USA but not labeled for this indication.

[2]Not available in the USA but available in some other countries.

[3]Available in the USA only from the Parasitic Disease Drug Service, Parasitic Diseases Branch, Centers for Disease Control and Prevention, Atlanta 30333. Telephone 404-639-3670.

appropriate for symptomatic parenchymal or intraventricular cysts. Corticosteroids are usually given with the anthelmintic drug to decrease inflammation caused by dying organisms. Albendazole is now generally considered the drug of choice over praziquantel because of its shorter course, lower cost, improved penetration into the subarachnoid space, and increased drug levels (as opposed to decreased levels of praziquantel) when administered with corticosteroids. Albendazole is given in a dosage of 400 mg twice a day for up to 21 days.

D. OTHER INFECTIONS

Albendazole is the drug of choice in the treatment of **cutaneous larva migrans** (400 mg daily for 3 days), visceral larva migrans (400 mg twice daily for 5 days), **intestinal capillariasis** (400 mg daily for 10 days), microsporidial infections (400 mg twice daily for 2 weeks or longer), and **gnathostomiasis** (400 mg twice daily for 3 weeks). It also has activity against **trichinosis** (400 mg twice daily for 1–2 weeks) and **clonorchiasis** (400 mg twice daily for 1 week). There have been reports of some effectiveness in treatment of **opisthorchiasis, toxocariasis,** and **loiasis** and conflicting reports of effectiveness in **giardiasis** and **taeniasis.**

Adverse Reactions, Contraindications, & Cautions

When used for 1–3 days, albendazole is nearly free of significant adverse effects. Mild and transient epigastric distress, diarrhea, headache, nausea, dizziness, lassitude, and insomnia can occur. In long-term use for hydatid disease, albendazole is well tolerated, but it can cause abdominal distress, headaches, fever, fatigue, alopecia, increases in liver enzymes, and pancytopenia.

Blood counts and liver function studies should be followed during long-term therapy. The drug should not be given to patients with known hypersensitivity to other benzimidazole drugs or to those with cirrhosis. The safety of albendazole in pregnancy and in children under 2 years of age has not been established.

BITHIONOL

Bithionol is the drug of choice for the treatment of **fascioliasis (sheep liver fluke).** An alternative drug, triclabendazole, is not available in the USA.

Bithionol is also an alternative drug in the treatment of pulmonary paragonimiasis.

Pharmacokinetics

After ingestion, bithionol reaches peak blood levels in 4–8 hours. Excretion appears to be mainly via the kidney.

Clinical Uses

For treatment of paragonimiasis and fascioliasis, the dosage of bithionol is 30–50 mg/kg in two or three divided doses, given orally after meals on alternate days for 10–15 doses. For pulmonary paragonimiasis, cure rates are over 90%. For cerebral paragonimiasis, repeat courses of therapy may be necessary.

Adverse Reactions, Contraindications, & Cautions

Adverse effects, which occur in up to 40% of patients, are generally mild and transient, but occasionally their severity requires interruption of therapy. These problems include diarrhea, abdominal cramps, anorexia, nausea, vomiting, dizziness, and headache. Skin rashes may occur after a week or more of therapy, suggesting a reaction to antigens released from dying worms.

Bithionol should be used with caution in children under 8 years of age because there has been limited experience in this age group.

DIETHYLCARBAMAZINE CITRATE

Diethylcarbamazine is a drug of choice in the treatment of filariasis, loiasis, and tropical eosinophilia. It has been replaced by ivermectin for the treatment of onchocerciasis.

Chemistry & Pharmacokinetics

Diethylcarbamazine, a synthetic piperazine derivative, is marketed as a citrate salt. It is rapidly absorbed from the gastrointestinal tract; after a 0.5 mg/kg dose, peak plasma levels are reached within 1–2 hours. The plasma half-life is 2–3 hours in the presence of acidic urine but about 10 hours if the urine is alkaline. The drug rapidly equilibrates with all tissues except fat. It is excreted, principally in the urine, as unchanged drug and the N-oxide metabolite. Dosage may have to be reduced in patients with persistent urinary alkalosis or renal impairment.

Anthelmintic Actions

Diethylcarbamazine immobilizes microfilariae and alters their surface structure, displacing them from tissues and making them more susceptible to destruction by host defense mechanisms. The mode of action against adult worms is unknown.

Clinical Uses

The drug should be taken after meals.

A. *Wuchereria bancrofti, Brugia malayi, Brugia timori,* and *Loa loa*

Diethylcarbamazine is the drug of choice for treatment of infections with these parasites because of its efficacy and lack of serious toxicity. Microfilariae of all species are rapidly killed; adult parasites are killed more slowly, often requiring several courses of treatment. The drug is highly effective against adult *L loa*. The extent to which *W bancrofti* and *B malayi* adults are killed is not known, but after appropriate therapy microfilariae do not reappear in the majority of patients.

These infections are treated for 2 or (for *L loa*) 3 weeks, with initial low doses to reduce the incidence of allergic reactions to dying microfilariae. This regimen is 50 mg (1 mg/kg in children) on day 1, three 50 mg doses on day 2, three 100 mg doses (2 mg/kg in children) on day 3, and then 2 mg/kg three times per day to complete the 2–3 week course.

Antihistamines may be given for the first few days of therapy to limit allergic reactions, and corticosteroids should be started and doses of diethylcarbamazine lowered or interrupted if severe reactions occur. Cures may require several courses of treatment.

Diethylcarbamazine may also be used for chemoprophylaxis (300 mg weekly or 300 mg on 3 successive days each month for loiasis; 50 mg monthly for bancroftian and Malayan filariasis).

B. Other Uses

For tropical eosinophilia, diethylcarbamazine is given orally at a dosage of 2 mg/kg three times daily for 7 days. Diethylcarbamazine is effective in *Mansonella streptocerca* infections, since it kills both adults and microfilariae. Limited information suggests that the drug is not effective, however, against adult *Mansonella ozzardi* or *M perstans* and that it has limited activity against microfilariae of these parasites. An important application of diethylcarbamazine has been its use for mass treatment of *W bancrofti* infections to reduce transmission. Weekly or monthly administration regimens have been studied; and, most recently, yearly treatment (with or without ivermectin) markedly reduced reservoirs of infection in Papua New Guinea.

Adverse Reactions, Contraindications, & Cautions

Reactions to diethylcarbamazine, which are generally mild and transient, include headache, malaise, anorexia, weakness, nausea, vomiting, and dizziness. Adverse effects also occur as a result of the release of proteins from dying microfilariae or adult worms. Reactions are particularly severe with onchocerciasis, but diethylcarbamazine is generally no longer used for this infection, as ivermectin is equally efficacious and less toxic. Reactions to dying microfilariae are usually mild in *W bancrofti,* more intense in *B malayi,* and occasionally severe in *L loa* infections. Reactions include fever, malaise, papular rash, headache, gastrointestinal symptoms, cough, chest pain, and muscle or joint pain. Leukocytosis is common. Eosinophilia may increase with treatment. Proteinuria may also occur. Symptoms are most likely to occur in patients with heavy loads of microfilariae. Retinal hemorrhages and, rarely, encephalopathy have been described.

Between the third and twelfth days of treatment, local reactions may occur in the vicinity of dying adult or immature worms. These include lymphangitis with localized swellings in *W bancrofti* and *B malayi,* small wheals in the skin in *L loa,* and flat papules in *M strepto-*

cerca infections. Patients with attacks of lymphangitis due to *W bancrofti* or *B malayi* should be treated during a quiescent period between attacks.

Caution is advised when using diethylcarbamazine in patients with hypertension or renal disease.

IVERMECTIN

Ivermectin is the drug of choice in strongyloidiasis and onchocerciasis. It is also an alternative drug for a number of other helminthic infections.

Chemistry & Pharmacokinetics

Ivermectin, a semisynthetic macrocyclic lactone, is a mixture of avermectin B_{1a} and B_{1b}. It is derived from the soil actinomycete *Streptomyces avermitilis.*

Ivermectin is used only orally in humans. The drug is rapidly absorbed, reaching maximum plasma concentrations 4 hours after a 12 mg dose. The drug has a wide tissue distribution and a volume of distribution of about 50 L. Its half-life is about 16 hours. Excretion of the drug and its metabolites is almost exclusively in the feces.

Anthelmintic Actions

Ivermectin appears to paralyze nematodes and arthropods by intensifying GABA-mediated transmission of signals in peripheral nerves (see Chapter 52). In onchocerciasis, ivermectin is microfilaricidal. It does not effectively kill adult worms but blocks the release of microfilariae for some months after therapy. After a single standard dose, microfilariae in the skin diminish rapidly within 2–3 days, remain low for months, and then gradually increase; microfilariae in the anterior chamber of the eye decrease slowly over months, eventually clear, and then gradually return. With repeated doses of ivermectin, the drug does appear to have a low-level macrofilaricidal action and to permanently reduce microfilarial production.

Clinical Uses

A. ONCHOCERCIASIS

Treatment is with a single oral dose of 150 μg/kg with water on an empty stomach. Doses are repeated; regimens vary from monthly to less frequent (every 6–12 months) dosing schedules. After acute therapy, treatment is repeated at 12-month intervals until the adult worms die, which may take 10 years or longer. With the first treatment only, patients with microfilariae in the cornea or anterior chamber may be treated with corticosteroids to avoid inflammatory eye reactions.

Ivermectin also now plays a key role in onchocerciasis control. Annual mass treatments have led to major reductions in disease transmission.

B. STRONGYLOIDIASIS

Treatment consists of two daily doses of 200 μg/kg. In immunosuppressed patients with disseminated infection, repeated treatment is often needed, but cure may not be possible. In this case, suppressive therapy—ie, once monthly—may be helpful.

C. OTHER PARASITES

Ivermectin reduces microfilariae in *Brugia malayi* and *Mansonella ozzardi* infections but not in *M perstans* infections. It has been used with diethylcarbamazine for the control of *W bancrofti,* but it does not kill adult worms, and whether it offers added benefit is uncertain. In **loiasis,** although the drug reduces microfilaria concentrations, it can occasionally induce severe reactions. Ivermectin is also effective in controlling **scabies, lice,** and **cutaneous larva migrans** and in eliminating a large proportion of **ascarid worms.**

Adverse Reactions, Contraindications, & Cautions

In strongyloidiasis treatment, infrequent side effects include fatigue, dizziness, nausea, vomiting, abdominal pain, and rashes. In onchocerciasis treatment, the adverse effects are principally from the Mazotti reaction, due to killing of microfilariae. The reaction includes fever, headache, dizziness, somnolence, weakness, rash, increased pruritus, diarrhea, joint and muscle pains, hypotension, tachycardia, lymphadenitis, lymphangitis, and peripheral edema. This reaction starts on the first day and peaks on the second day after treatment. The Mazotti reaction occurs in 5–30% or persons and is generally mild, but it may be more frequent and more severe in individuals who are not long-term residents of onchocerciasis-endemic areas. A more intense Mazotti reaction occurs in 1–3% of persons and a severe reaction in 0.1%, including high fever, hypotension, and bronchospasm. Corticosteroids are indicated in these cases, at times for several days. The Mazotti reaction diminishes with repeated dosing. Swellings and abscesses occasionally occur at 1–3 weeks, presumably at sites of adult worms.

Some patients develop corneal opacities and other eye lesions several days after treatment. These are rarely severe and generally resolve without corticosteroid treatment.

It is best to avoid concomitant use of ivermectin and other drugs that enhance GABA activity, eg, barbiturates, benzodiazepines, and valproic acid. Ivermectin should not be used in pregnancy. Safety in children under 5 years has not been established.

MEBENDAZOLE

Mebendazole is a synthetic benzimidazole (compare with albendazole) that has a wide spectrum of anthelmintic activity and a low incidence of adverse effects.

Mebendazole

Chemistry & Pharmacokinetics

Less than 10% of orally administered mebendazole is absorbed. The absorbed drug is protein-bound (> 90%), rapidly converted to inactive metabolites (primarily during its first pass in the liver), and has a half-life of 2–6 hours. It is excreted mostly in the urine, principally as decarboxylated derivatives. In addition, a portion of absorbed drug and its derivatives are excreted in the bile. Absorption is increased if the drug is ingested with a fatty meal.

Anthelmintic Actions

Mebendazole probably acts by inhibiting microtubule synthesis; the parent drug appears to be the active form. Efficacy of the drug varies with gastrointestinal transit time, with intensity of infection, and perhaps with the strain of parasite. The drug kills hookworm, ascaris, and trichuris eggs.

Clinical Uses

In the USA, mebendazole has been approved for use in ascariasis, trichuriasis, and hookworm and pinworm infection. It can be taken before or after meals; the tablets should be chewed before swallowing. For pinworm infection, the dose is 100 mg once, repeated at 2 weeks. For ascariasis, trichuriasis, hookworm, and trichostrongylus infections, a dosage of 100 mg twice daily for 3 days is used for adults and for children over 2 years of age. Cure rates are 90–100% for pinworm infections, ascariasis, and trichuriasis. Cure rates are lower for hookworm infections, but a marked reduction in the worm burden occurs in those not cured. For intestinal capillariasis, mebendazole is used at a dosage of 400 mg/d in divided doses for 21 or more days. In trichinosis, limited reports suggest efficacy against adult worms in the intestinal tract and tissue larvae. Treatment is three times daily, with fatty foods, at 200–400 mg per dose for 3 days and then 400–500 mg per dose for 10 days. Corticosteroids should be coadministered for severe infections.

Adverse Reactions, Contraindications, & Cautions

Short-term mebendazole therapy for intestinal nematodes is nearly free of adverse effects. Mild nausea, vomiting, diarrhea, and abdominal pain have been reported infrequently. Rare side effects, usually with high-dose therapy, are hypersensitivity reactions (rash, urticaria), agranulocytosis, alopecia, and elevation of liver enzymes.

Mebendazole is teratogenic in animals and therefore contraindicated in pregnancy. It should be used with caution in children under 2 years of age because of limited experience and rare reports of convulsions in this age group. Plasma levels may be decreased by concomitant use of carbamazepine or phenytoin and increased by cimetidine. Mebendazole should be used with caution in those with cirrhosis.

METRIFONATE (TRICHLORFON)

Metrifonate is a safe, low-cost alternative drug for the treatment of *Schistosoma haematobium* infections. It is not active against *S mansoni* or *S japonicum*. It is not available in the USA.

Chemistry & Pharmacokinetics

Metrifonate, an organophosphate compound, is rapidly absorbed after oral administration. Following the standard oral dose, peak blood levels are reached in 1–2 hours; the half-life is about 1.5 hours. Clearance appears to be through nonenzymatic transformation to dichlorvos, its active metabolite. Metrifonate and dichlorvos are well distributed to the tissues and are completely eliminated in 24–48 hours.

Anthelmintic Actions

The mode of action is thought to be related to cholinesterase inhibition. This inhibition temporarily paralyzes the adult worms, resulting in their shift from the bladder venous plexus to small arterioles of the lungs, where they are trapped, encased by the immune system, and die. The drug is not effective against *S haematobium* eggs; live eggs continue to pass in the urine for several months after all adult worms have been killed.

Clinical Uses

In the treatment of *S haematobium*, a single oral dose of 7.5–10 mg/kg is given three times at 14-day intervals. Cure rates on this schedule are 44–93%, with marked reductions in egg counts in those not cured. Metrifonate was also effective as a prophylactic agent when given monthly to children in a highly endemic area, and it has been used in mass treatment programs. In mixed infections with *S haematobium* and *S mansoni*, metrifonate has been successfully combined with oxamniquine.

Adverse Reactions, Contraindications, & Cautions

Some studies note mild and transient cholinergic symptoms, including nausea and vomiting, diarrhea, abdominal pain, bronchospasm, headache, sweating, fatigue, weakness, dizziness, and vertigo. These symptoms may begin within 30 minutes and persist up to 12 hours.

Metrifonate should not be used after recent exposure to insecticides or drugs that might potentiate cholinesterase inhibition. Metrifonate is contraindicated in pregnancy.

NICLOSAMIDE

Niclosamide is a second-line drug for the treatment of most tapeworm infections, but it is not available in the United States.

Chemistry & Pharmacokinetics

Niclosamide is a salicylamide derivative. It appears to be minimally absorbed from the gastrointestinal tract—neither the drug nor its metabolites have been recovered from the blood or urine.

Niclosamide

Anthelmintic Actions

Adult worms (but not ova) are rapidly killed, presumably due to inhibition of oxidative phosphorylation or stimulation of ATPase activity.

Clinical Uses

The adult dose of niclosamide is 2 g once, given in the morning on an empty stomach. The tablets must be chewed thoroughly and are then swallowed with water.

A. *T SAGINATA* (BEEF TAPEWORM), *T SOLIUM* (PORK TAPEWORM), AND *DIPHYLLOBOTHRIUM LATUM* (FISH TAPEWORM)

A single 2 g dose of niclosamide results in cure rates of over 85% for *D latum* and about 95% for *T saginata*. It is

probably equally effective against *T solium*. Cysticercosis is theoretically possible after treatment of *T solium* infections, since viable ova are released into the gut lumen following digestion of segments. However, no such cases of cysticerosis following therapy have been reported.

B. OTHER TAPEWORMS

Praziquantel is superior for *Hymenolepis nana* (dwarf tapeworm) infection. Most patients treated for *Hymenolepis diminuta* and *Dipylidium caninum* infections are cured with a 7-day course of treatment; a few require a second course. Niclosamide is not effective against cysticerosis or hydatid disease.

C. INTESTINAL FLUKE INFECTIONS

Niclosamide can be used as an alternative drug for the treatment of *Fasciolopsis buski*, *Heterophyes heterophyes*, and *Metagonimus yokogawai* infections. The standard dose is given every other day for three doses.

Adverse Reactions, Contraindication, & Cautions

Infrequent, mild, and transitory adverse events include nausea, vomiting, diarrhea, and abdominal discomfort.

The consumption of alcohol should be avoided on the day of treatment and for 1 day afterward.

The safety of the drug has not been established in pregnancy or for children under 2 years of age.

OXAMNIQUINE

Oxamniquine is an alternative to praziquantel for the treatment of *S mansoni* infections. It has also been used extensively for mass treatment. It is not effective against *S haematobium* or *S japonicum*.

Pharmacokinetics

Oxamniquine, a semisynthetic tetrahydroquinoline, is readily absorbed orally. Its plasma half-life is about 2.5 hours. The drug is extensively metabolized to inactive metabolites and excreted in the urine—up to 75% in the first 24 hours. Intersubject variations in serum concentration have been noted, which may explain some treatment failures.

Anthelmintic Actions

Oxamniquine is active against both mature and immature stages of *S mansoni* but does not appear to be cercaricidal. The mechanism of action is unknown. Contraction and paralysis of the worms results in detachment from terminal venules in the mesentery and transit to the liver, where many die; surviving females return to the mesenteric vessels but cease to lay eggs.

Strains of *S mansoni* in different parts of the world vary in susceptibility. Oxamniquine has been effective in instances of praziquantel resistance.

Clinical Uses

Oxamniquine is safe and effective in all stages of *S mansoni* disease, including advanced hepatosplenomegaly. In the acute (Katayama) syndrome, treatment results in disappearance of acute symptoms and clearance of the infection. The drug is generally less effective in children, who require higher doses than adults. It is better-tolerated with food.

Optimal dosage schedules vary for different regions of the world. In the Western Hemisphere and western Africa, the adult oxamniquine dosage is 12–15 mg/kg given once. In northern and southern Africa, standard schedules are 15 mg/kg twice daily for 2 days. In eastern Africa and the Arabian peninsula, standard dosage is 15–20 mg/kg twice in 1 day. Cure rates are 70–95%, with marked reduction in egg excretion in those not cured.

In mixed schistosome infections, oxamniquine has been successfully used in combination with metrifonate.

Adverse Reactions, Contraindications, & Cautions

Mild symptoms, starting about 3 hours after a dose and lasting for several hours, occur in more than one third of patients. Central nervous system symptoms (dizziness, headache, drowsiness) are most common; nausea and vomiting, diarrhea, colic, pruritus, and urticaria also occur. Infrequent adverse effects are low-grade fever, an orange to red discoloration of the urine, proteinuria, microscopic hematuria, and a transient decrease in leukocytes. Seizures have been reported rarely.

Since the drug makes many patients dizzy or drowsy, it should be used with caution in patients whose work or activity requires mental alertness (eg, no driving for 24 hours). It should be used with caution in those with a history of epilepsy.

Oxamniquine is contraindicated in pregnancy.

PIPERAZINE

Piperazine is an alternative for the treatment of ascariasis, with cure rates over 90% when taken for 2 days, but it is not recommended for other helminth infections. Piperazine is available as the hexahydrate and as a variety of salts. It is readily absorbed, and maximum plasma levels are reached in 2–4 hours. Most of the drug is excreted unchanged in the urine in 2–6 hours, and excretion is complete within 24 hours.

Piperazine causes paralysis of ascaris by blocking acetylcholine at the myoneural junction; unable to maintain their position in the host, live worms are expelled by normal peristalsis.

For ascariasis, the dosage of piperazine (as the hexahydrate) is 75 mg/kg (maximum dose, 3.5 g) orally once daily for 2 days. For heavy infections, treatment should be continued for 3–4 days or repeated after 1 week.

Occasional mild adverse effects include nausea, vomiting, diarrhea, abdominal pain, dizziness, and headache. Neurotoxicity and allergic reactions are rare.

Piperazine compounds should not be given to women during pregnancy, to patients with impaired renal or hepatic function, or to those with a history of epilepsy or chronic neurologic disease.

PRAZIQUANTEL

Praziquantel is effective in the treatment of schistosome infections of all species and most other trematode and cestode infections, including cysticercosis. The drug's safety and effectiveness as a single oral dose have also made it useful in mass treatment of several infections.

Chemistry & Pharmacokinetics

Praziquantel is a synthetic isoquinoline-pyrazine derivative. It is rapidly absorbed, with a bioavailability of about 80% after oral administration. Peak serum concentrations are reached 1–3 hours after a therapeutic dose. Cerebrospinal fluid concentrations of praziquantel reach 14–20% of the drug's plasma concentration. About 80% of the drug is bound to plasma proteins. Most of the drug is rapidly metabolized to inactive mono- and polyhydroxylated products after a first pass in the liver. The half-life is 0.8–1.5 hours. Excretion is mainly via the kidneys (60–80%) and bile (15–35%). Plasma concentrations of praziquantel increase when the drug is taken with a high-carbohydrate meal or with cimetidine; bioavailability is markedly reduced with some antiepileptics (phenytoin, carbamazepine) or with corticosteroids.

Anthelmintic Actions

Praziquantel appears to increase the permeability of trematode and cestode cell membranes to calcium, resulting in paralysis, dislodgement, and death.

In schistosome infections of experimental animals, praziquantel is effective against adult worms and immature stages and it has a prophylactic effect against cercarial infection.

Clinical Uses

Praziquantel tablets are taken with liquid after a meal; they should be swallowed without chewing because their bitter taste can induce retching and vomiting.

A. Schistosomiasis

Praziquantel is the drug of choice for all forms of schistosomiasis. The dosage is 20 mg/kg for two (*S mansoni* and *S haematobium*) or three (*S japonicum* and *S mekongi*) doses at intervals of 4–6 hours. High cure rates (75–95%) are achieved when patients are evaluated at 3–6 months; there is marked reduction in egg counts in those not cured. The drug is effective in adults and children and is generally well tolerated by patients in the hepatosplenic stage of advanced disease. It is not clear, however, whether the drug can be safely or effectively used during the acute stage of the disease (Katayama fever) because release of antigens from dying immature worms may exacerbate symptoms. Increasing evidence indicates rare *S mansoni* drug resistance, which is treatable with oxamniquine. Effectiveness of the drug for chemoprophylaxis has not been established.

B. Clonorchiasis, Opisthorchiasis, and Paragonimiasis

The dosage of 25 mg/kg three times for 1 day results in nearly 100% cure rates for clonorchiasis and opisthorchiasis, and a 2 day's course provides 90–100% cure rates for pulmonary paragonimiasis.

C. Taeniasis and Diphyllobothriasis

A single dose of praziquantel, 5–10 mg/kg, results in nearly 100% cure rates for *T saginata*, *T solium*, and *D latum* infections. For *T solium*, since praziquantel does not kill eggs, it is theoretically possible that larvae released from eggs in the large bowel could penetrate the intestinal wall and give rise to cysticercosis, but this hazard is probably minimal.

D. Neurocysticercosis

Albendazole is now the preferred drug, but when it is not appropriate or available, praziquantel has similar efficacy. Indications are similar to those for albendazole. The praziquantel dosage is 50 mg/kg/d in three divided doses for 14 days or longer. Clinical responses to therapy vary from dramatic improvements of seizures and other neurologic findings to no response and even progression of the disease. Praziquantel—but not albendazole—has diminished bioavailability when taken concurrently with a corticosteroid. Recommendations on steroid use in neurocysticercosis vary.

E. *H nana*

Praziquantel is the drug of choice for *H nana* infections and the first drug to be highly effective. A single dose of 25 mg/kg is taken initially and repeated in 1 week.

F. Hydatid Disease

In hydatid disease, praziquantel kills protoscoleces but does not affect the germinal membrane. Praziquantel is being evaluated as an adjunct with albendazole pre- and postsurgery. In addition to its direct action, praziquantel enhances the plasma concentration of albendazole sulfoxide.

G. Other Parasites

Limited trials at a dosage of 25 mg/kg three times a day for 1–2 days indicate effectiveness of praziquantel against fasciolopsiasis, metagonimiasis, and other forms of heterophyiasis. Praziquantel was not effective for fascioliasis, however, even at dosages as high as 25 mg/kg three times daily for 3–7 days.

Adverse Reactions, Contraindications, & Cautions

Mild and transient adverse effects are common. They begin within several hours after ingestion and may persist for hours to 1 day. Most frequent are headache, dizziness, drowsiness, and lassitude; others include nausea, vomiting, abdominal pain, loose stools, pruritus, urticaria, arthralgia, myalgia, and low-grade fever. Mild and transient elevations of liver enzymes have been reported. Several days after starting praziquantel, low-grade fever, pruritus, and skin rashes (macular and urticarial), sometimes associated with worsened eosinophilia, may occur, probably due to the release of proteins from dying worms rather than direct drug toxicity. The intensity and frequency of adverse effects increase with dosage such that they occur in up to 50% of patients who receive 25 mg/kg three times in 1 day.

In neurocysticercosis, neurologic abnormalities may be exacerbated by inflammatory reactions around dying parasites. Common findings in patients who do not receive corticosteroids, usually presenting during or shortly after therapy, are headache, meningismus, nausea, vomiting, mental changes, and seizures (often accompanied by increased cerebrospinal fluid pleocytosis). More serious findings, including arachnoiditis, hyperthermia, and intracranial hypertension, may also occur. Corticosteroids are commonly used with praziquantel in the treatment of neurocysticercosis to decrease the inflammatory reaction, but this is controversial, and complicated by knowledge that corticosteroids decrease the plasma level of praziquantel up to 50%. Praziquantel is contraindicated in ocular cysticercosis, as parasite destruction in the eye may cause irreparable damage. Some workers also caution against use of the drug in spinal neurocysticercosis.

The safety of praziquantel in children under age 4 years is not established, but no specific problems in young children have been documented. Indeed, the drug appears to be better tolerated in children than in adults. Praziquantel increased abortion rates in rats and therefore should be avoided in pregnancy if possible. Because the drug induces dizziness and drowsiness, patients should not drive during therapy and should be warned regarding activities requiring particular physical coordination or alertness.

PYRANTEL PAMOATE

Pyrantel pamoate is a broad-spectrum anthelmintic highly effective for the treatment of pinworm, ascaris, and *Trichostrongylus orientalis* infections. It is moderately effective against both species of hookworm. It is not effective in trichuriasis or strongyloidiasis. Oxantel pamoate, an analog of pyrantel not available in the USA, has been used successfully in the treatment of trichuriasis; the two drugs have been combined for their broad-spectrum anthelmintic activity.

Chemistry & Pharmacokinetics

Pyrantel pamoate is a tetrahydropyrimidine derivative. It is poorly absorbed from the gastrointestinal tract and active mainly against luminal organisms. Peak plasma levels are reached in 1–3 hours. Over half of the administered dose is recovered unchanged in the feces.

Anthelmintic Actions

Pyrantel is effective against mature and immature forms of susceptible helminths within the intestinal tract but not against migratory stages in the tissues or against ova. The drug is a neuromuscular blocking agent that causes release of acetylcholine and inhibition of cholinesterase; this results in paralysis, which is followed by expulsion of worms.

Clinical Uses

The standard dose is 11 mg (base)/kg (maximum, 1 g), given orally once with or without food. For pinworm the dose is repeated in 2 weeks, and cure rates are greater than 95%. The drug is available in the USA without prescription for this indication.

For ascariasis, a single dose yields cure rates of 85–100%. Treatment should be repeated if eggs are found 2 weeks after treatment. For hookworm infections, a single dose is effective against light infections; but for heavy infections, especially with *N americanus,* a 3-day course is necessary to reach 90% cure rates. A course of treatment can be repeated in 2 weeks.

Adverse Reactions, Contraindications, & Cautions

Adverse effects are infrequent, mild, and transient. They include nausea, vomiting, diarrhea, abdominal cramps, dizziness, drowsiness, headache, insomnia, rash, fever, and weakness. Pyrantel should be used with caution in patients with liver dysfunction, since low, transient

aminotransferase elevations have been noted in a small number of patients. Experience with the drug in pregnant women and children under age 2 years is limited.

THIABENDAZOLE

Thiabendazole is an alternative to ivermectin for the treatment of strongyloidiasis and cutaneous larva migrans.

Chemistry & Pharmacokinetics

Thiabendazole is a benzimidazole compound. Although it is a chelating agent that forms stable complexes with a number of metals, including iron, it does not bind calcium.

Thiabendazole is rapidly absorbed after ingestion. With a standard dose, drug concentrations in plasma peak within 1–2 hours; the half-life is 1.2 hours. The drug is almost completely metabolized in the liver to the 5-hydroxy form; 90% is excreted in the urine in 48 hours, largely as the glucuronide or sulfonate conjugate. Thiabendazole can also be absorbed from the skin.

Anthelmintic Actions

The mechanism of action of thiabendazole is probably the same as that of other benzimidazoles (see above). The drug has ovicidal effects for some parasites.

Clinical Uses

The standard dosage, 25 mg/kg (maximum, 1.5 g) twice daily, should be given after meals. Tablets should be chewed. For strongyloides infection, treatment is for 2 days. Cure rates are reportedly 93%. A course can be repeated in 1 week if indicated. In patients with hyperinfection syndrome, the standard dose is continued twice daily for 5–7 days. For cutaneous larva migrans, thiabendazole cream can be applied topically or the oral drug can be given for 2 days (although albendazole is less toxic and therefore preferred).

Adverse Reactions, Contraindications, & Cautions

Thiabendazole is much more toxic than other benzimidazoles or ivermectin, so other agents are now preferred for most indications. Common adverse effects include dizziness, anorexia, nausea, and vomiting. Less frequent problems are epigastric pain, abdominal cramps, diarrhea, pruritus, headache, drowsiness, and neuropsychiatric symptoms. Irreversible liver failure and fatal Stevens-Johnson syndrome have been reported.

Experience with thiabendazole is limited in children weighing less than 15 kg. The drug should not be used in pregnancy or in the presence of hepatic or renal disease.

PREPARATIONS AVAILABLE

Albendazole (Albenza, Zentel)
Oral: 200 mg tablets; 100 mg/5 mL suspension
Note: Albendazole is approved in the USA for the treatment of cysticercosis and hydatid disease.

Bithionol (Bitin)
Oral: 200 mg tablets
Note: Bithionol is not marketed in the USA but is available from the Parasitic Disease Drug Service, Centers for Disease Control and Prevention, Atlanta; 404-639-3670.

Diethylcarbamazine (Hetrazan)
Oral: 50 mg tablets
Note: Diethylcarbamazine is no longer marketed in the USA but is available from the Parasitic Disease Drug Service, Centers for Disease Control and Prevention, Atlanta; 404-639-3670.

Ivermectin (Mectizan, Stromectol)
Oral: 3, 6 mg tablets
Note: Ivermectin is approved for use in the USA for the treatment of onchocerciasis and strongyloidiasis. See Chapter 66 for comment on the unlabeled use of drugs.

Levamisole (Decaris, Ethnor, Ketrax, Solaskil)
Oral: 50, 150 mg tablets and syrup

Mebendazole (generic, Vermox)
Oral: 100 mg chewable tablets; outside the USA, 100 mg/5 mL suspension

Metrifonate (trichlorfon, Bilarcil)
Oral: 100 mg tablets
Note: Metrifonate is not available in the USA.

Niclosamide (Niclocide)
Oral: 500 mg chewable tablets
Note: Niclosamide is not available in the USA.

Oxamniquine (Vansil, Mansil)
Oral: 250 mg capsules; outside the USA, 50 mg/mL syrup

Oxantel pamoate (Quantrel); oxantel/pyrantel pamoate (Telopar)
Oral: tablets containing 100 mg (base) of each drug; suspensions containing 20 or 50 mg (base) per mL
Note: Oxantel pamoate and oxantel/pyrantel pamoate are not available in the USA.

Piperazine (generic, Vermizine)
Oral: piperazine citrate tablets equivalent to 250 mg of the hexahydrate; piperazine citrate syrup equivalent to 500 mg of the hexahydrate per 5 mL

Praziquantel (Biltricide; others outside the USA)
Oral: 600 mg tablets (other strengths outside the USA)

Pyrantel pamoate (Antiminth, Combantrin, Pin-rid, Pin-X)
Oral: 50 mg (base)/mL suspension; 62.5 mg (base) capsules (available without prescription in the USA)

Suramin (Bayer 205, others)
Parenteral: ampules containing 0.5 or 1 g powder to be reconstituted as a 10% solution and used immediately
Note: Suramin is not marketed in the USA but can be obtained from the Parasitic Disease Drug Service, Centers for Disease Control, Atlanta, 404-639-3670.

Thiabendazole (Mintezol)
Oral: 500 mg chewable tablets; suspension, 500 mg/mL

REFERENCES

Ammann RW et al: Long-term mebendazole may be parasiticidal in alveolar echinococcosis. J Hepatol 1998;29:994.

Anadol D et al: Treatment of hydatid disease. Paediatr Drugs 2001;3:123.

Ayles HM et al: A combined medical and surgical approach to hydatid disease: 12 years' experience at the Hospital for Tropical Diseases, London. Ann R Coll Surg Engl 2002;84:100.

Bockarie MJ et al: Mass treatment to eliminate filariasis in Papua New Guinea. N Engl J Med 2002;347:1841.

Burnham G: Onchocerciasis. Lancet 1998;351:1341.

Carpio A: Neurocysticercosis: an update. Lancet Infect Dis 2002;2:751.

Caumes E: Treatment of cutaneous larva migrans. Clin Infect Dis 2000;30:811.

Cioli D: Chemotherapy of schistosomiasis: An update. Parasitology Today 1998;14:418.

Cobo F et al: Albendazole plus praziquantel versus albendazole alone as a preoperative treatment in intra-abdominal hydatidosis caused by *Echinococcus granulosus.* Trop Med Int Health 1998;3:462.

Cummings JF: Metrifonate: Overview of safety and efficacy. Pharmacotherapy 1998;18:43.

de Silva NR et al: Effect of mebendazole therapy during pregnancy on birth outcome. Lancet 1999;353:1145.

Drugs for parasitic infections. Med Lett Drugs Ther 2002;44:33. Issue available at http://www.medicalletter.com/freedocs/parasitic.pdf

Dunyo SK, Nkrumah FK, Simonsen PE: A randomized double-blind placebo-controlled field trial of ivermectin and albendazole alone and in combination for the treatment of lymphatic filariasis in Ghana. Trans R Soc Trop Med Hyg 2000;94:205.

Forrester JE et al: Randomized trial of albendazole and pyrantel in symptomless trichuriasis in children. Lancet 1998;352:1103.

Franchi C, Di Vico B, Teggi A: Long-term evaluation of patients with hydatidosis treated with benzimidazole carbamates. Clin Infect Dis 1999;29:304.

Garcia HH, Del Brutto OH: *Taenia solium* cysticercosis. Infect Dis Clin North Am 2000;14:97.

Gardon J et al: Effects of standard and high doses of ivermectin on adult worms of *Onchocerca volvulus*: a randomised controlled trial. Lancet 2002;360:203.

Georgiev VS: Parasitic infections. Treatment and developmental therapeutics 1. Necatoriasis. Curr Pharm Des 1999;5:545.

Haarbrink M et al: Adverse reactions following diethylcarbamazine (DEC) intake in "endemic normals," microfilaremics and elephantiasis patients. Trans R Soc Trop Med Hyg 1999;93:91.

Horton J: Albendazole: a review of anthelmintic efficacy and safety in humans. Parasitology 2000;121:S113.

Jackson TF et al: A comparison of mebendazole and albendazole in treating children with *Trichuris trichiura* infection in Durban, South Africa. S Afr Med J 1998;88:880.

Marti H et al: A comparative trial of single-dose ivermectin versus three days of albendazole for the treatment of strongyloidiasis stercoralis and other soil transmitted helminth infections in children. Am J Trop Med Hyg 1996;55:477.

Mataika JU et al: Efficacy of five annual single doses of diethylcarbamazine for treatment of lymphatic filariasis in Fiji. Bull World Health Organ 1998;76:575.

Proano JV et al: Medical treatment for neurocysticercosis characterized by giant subarachnoid cysts. N Engl J Med 2001;345:879

Rosenblatt JE: Antiparasitic agents. Mayo Clin Proc 1999;74:1161.

Sotelo J, Jung H: Pharmacokinetic optimization of the treatment of neurocysticercosis. Clin Pharmacokinet 1998;34:503.

Stelma FF et al: Oxamniquine cures *Schistosoma mansoni* infection in a focus in which cure rates with praziquantel are unusually low. J Infect Dis 1997;176:304.

Stephenson I, Wiselka M: Drug treatment of tropical parasitic infections: recent achievements and developments. Drugs 2000;60:985.

Venkatesan P: Albendazole. J Antimicrobial Chemotherapy 1998; 41:145.

Cancer Chemotherapy

Edward Chu, MD, & Alan C. Sartorelli, PhD

Cancer is basically a disease of cells characterized by a shift in the control mechanisms that govern cell proliferation and differentiation. Cells that have undergone neoplastic transformation usually express cell surface antigens that may be of normal fetal type, may display other signs of apparent immaturity, and may exhibit qualitative or quantitative chromosomal abnormalities, including various translocations and the appearance of amplified gene sequences. Such cells proliferate excessively and form local tumors that can compress or invade adjacent normal structures. A small subpopulation of cells within the tumor can be described as tumor stem cells. They retain the ability to undergo repeated cycles of proliferation as well as to migrate to distant sites in the body to colonize various organs in the process called metastasis. Such tumor stem cells thus can express clonogenic or colony-forming capability. Tumor stem cells often have chromosome abnormalities reflecting their genetic instability, which leads to progressive selection of subclones that can survive more readily in the multicellular environment of the host. Quantitative abnormalities in various metabolic pathways and cellular components accompany this neoplastic progression. The invasive and metastatic processes as well as a series of metabolic abnormalities resulting from the cancer cause illness and eventual death of the patient unless the neoplasm can be eradicated with treatment.

CAUSES OF CANCER

The incidence, geographic distribution, and behavior of specific types of cancer are related to multiple factors, including sex, age, race, genetic predisposition, and exposure to environmental carcinogens. Of these factors, environmental exposure is probably most important. Chemical carcinogens (particularly those in tobacco smoke) as well as azo dyes, aflatoxins, asbestos, and benzene have been clearly implicated in cancer induction in humans and animals. Identification of potential carcinogens in the environment has been greatly simplified by the widespread use of the Ames test for mutagenic agents. Ninety percent of carcinogens can be shown to be mutagenic with this assay. Ultimate

ACRONYMS	
ABVD	Doxorubicin (adriamycin), bleomycin, vinblastine, dacarbazine
CHOP	Cyclophosphamide, doxorubicin (hydroxydaunorubicin), vincristine (oncovin), prednisone
CMF	Cyclophosphamide, methotrexate, fluorouracil
COP	Cyclophosphamide, vincristine (oncovin), prednisone
FAC	Fluorouracil, doxorubicin (adriamycin), cyclophosphamide
FEC	Fluorouracil, epirubicin, cyclophosphamide
IFL	Irinotecan, fluorouracil, leucovorin
MP	Melphalan, prednisone
MOPP	Mechlorethamine, vincristine (oncovin), procarbazine, prednisone
PCV	Procarbazine, lomustine, vincristine
PEB	Cisplatin (platinum), etoposide, bleomycin
VAD	Vincristine, doxorubicin (adriamycin), dexamethasone

identification of potential human carcinogens, however, requires testing in at least two animal species.

Certain herpes and papilloma group DNA viruses and type C RNA viruses have also been implicated as causative agents in animal cancers and are responsible for some human cancers as well. Oncogenic RNA viruses all appear to contain a reverse transcriptase enzyme that permits translation of the RNA message of the tumor virus into the DNA code of the infected cell. Thus, the information governing transformation can become a stable part of the genome of the host cell. Expression of virus-induced neoplasia probably also depends on additional host and environmental factors that modulate the transformation process. A specific human retrovirus (HTLV-I) has been identified as being the causative agent for a specific type of human T cell leukemia. The virus that causes AIDS (HIV-1) is closely related. Cellular genes are known that are homologous to the transforming genes of the retroviruses, a family of RNA viruses, and induce oncogenic transformation. These mammalian cellular genes, known as oncogenes, have been shown to code for specific growth factors and their receptors and may be amplified (increased number of gene copies) or modified by a single nucleotide in malignant cells. The *bcl*-2 oncogene may be a generalized cell death suppressor gene that directly regulates apoptosis, a pathway of programmed cell death.

Another class of genes, tumor suppressor genes, may be deleted or damaged, with resulting neoplastic change. A single gene in this class, the *p53* gene, has been shown to have mutated from a tumor suppressor gene to an oncogene in a high percentage of cases of several human tumors, including liver, breast, colon, lung, cervix, bladder, prostate, and skin. The normal wild form of this gene appears to play an important role in suppressing neoplastic transformation; mutations in this gene place the cell at high risk.

CANCER THERAPEUTIC MODALITIES

Cancer is the second most common cause of death in the USA, after heart disease, causing over 500,000 fatalities annually. With present methods of treatment, one third of patients are cured with local modalities (surgery or radiation therapy), which are quite effective when the tumor has not metastasized by the time of treatment. Earlier diagnosis might lead to increased cure rates with such local treatment; however, in the remaining cases, early micrometastasis is a characteristic feature of the neoplasm, indicating that a systemic approach such as chemotherapy is required (often along with surgery or radiation) for effective cancer management. At present, about 50% of patients with cancer can be cured, with chemotherapy contributing to cure in 10–15% of patients.

Cancer chemotherapy, as currently employed, can be curative in certain disseminated neoplasms that have undergone either gross or microscopic spread by the time of diagnosis. These cancers include testicular cancer, non-Hodgkin's lymphoma, Hodgkin's disease, and choriocarcinoma as well as childhood cancers such as acute lymphoblastic leukemia, Burkitt's lymphoma, Wilms' tumor, and embryonal rhabdomyosarcoma. There are also growing numbers of cancers in which the use of chemotherapy combined with initial surgery can increase the cure rate in locally advanced early-stage breast cancer, esophageal cancer, rectal cancer, and osteogenic sarcoma.

For many other forms of disseminated cancer, chemotherapy provides palliative rather than curative therapy at present. Effective palliation results in temporary improvement of the symptoms and signs of cancer and enhancement in the overall quality of life. In the past decade, advances in cancer chemotherapy have also begun to provide evidence that chemical control of neoplasia may become a reality for many forms of cancer. This will probably be achieved through a combined-modality approach in which optimal combinations of surgery, radiotherapy, and chemotherapy are used to eradicate both the primary neoplasm and its occult micrometastases before gross spread can be detected on physical or x-ray examination. Use of hormonal agents to modulate tumor growth is playing an increasing role in hormone-responsive tumors thanks to the development of hormone antagonists and partial agonists. Several recombinant biologic agents have been identified as being active for cancer therapy, including interferon alfa and interleukin-2.

ANTICANCER DRUG DEVELOPMENT

A major effort to develop anticancer drugs through both empiric screening and rational design of new compounds has been under way for over 3 decades. Recent advances in this field have included the synthesis of peptides and proteins with recombinant DNA techniques and monoclonal antibodies. The drug development program has employed testing in a few well-characterized transplantable animal tumor systems. Simple in vitro assays for measuring drug sensitivity of a battery of human tumor cells augment and shorten the testing program and are used currently as the primary screening tests for new agents by the National Cancer Institute and many pharmaceutical firms. After new drugs with potential anticancer activity are identified, they are subjected to preclinical toxicologic and limited pharmacologic studies in animals as described in Chapter 5. Promising agents that do not have excessive toxicity are then advanced to phase I clinical trials, wherein their pharmacologic and toxic effects are usually tested in patients with advanced cancer. Other features of clinical testing are similar to the procedure for other drugs but may be accelerated.

Ideal anticancer drugs would eradicate cancer cells without harming normal tissues. Unfortunately, no currently available agents meet this criterion, and clinical use of these drugs involves a weighing of benefits against toxicity in a search for a favorable therapeutic index.

Classes of drugs that have recently entered clinical development include signal transduction inhibitors, focused on critical signaling pathways essential for cell growth and proliferation; microtubule inhibitors, directed against the mitotic spindle apparatus; differentiation agents, intended to force neoplastic cells past a maturation block to form end-stage cells with little or no proliferative potential; antimetastatic drugs, designed to perturb surface properties of malignant cells and thus alter their invasive and metastatic potential; antiangiogenic agents, designed to inhibit the formation of tumor vasculature; hypoxic tumor stem cell-specific agents, designed to exploit the greater capacity for reductive reactions in these often therapeutically resistant cells; tumor radiosensitizing and normal tissue radioprotecting drugs, aimed at increased therapeutic effectiveness of radiation therapy; cytoprotective agents, focused on protecting certain normal tissues against the toxic effects of chemotherapy; and biologic response modifiers, which alter tumor-host metabolic and immunologic relationships.

IMPORTANCE OF NEOPLASTIC CELL BURDEN

Patients with widespread cancer may have up to 10^{12} tumor cells throughout the body at the time of diagnosis (Figure 55–1). If tolerable dosing of an effective drug is capable of killing 99.99% of clonogenic tumor cells, treatment would induce a clinical remission of the neoplasm associated with symptomatic improvement. However, there would still be up to 8 logs of tumor cells (10^8) remaining in the body, including those that might be inherently resistant to the drug because of tumor heterogeneity. There may also be other tumor cells that reside in pharmacologic sanctuary sites (eg, the central nervous system, testes), where effective drug concentrations may be difficult to achieve. When cell cycle-specific drugs are used, the tumor stem cells must also be in the sensitive phase of the cell cycle (not in G_0). For this reason, scheduling of these agents is particularly important. In common bacterial infections, a three-log reduction in microorganisms might be curative because host resistance factors can eliminate residual bacteria through immunologic and microbicidal mechanisms; however, host mechanisms for eliminating even moderate numbers of cancer cells appear to be generally ineffective.

Combinations of agents with differing toxicities and mechanisms of action are often employed to overcome the limited log kill of individual anticancer drugs. If drugs display nonoverlapping toxicities, they can be used at almost full dosage, and at least additive cytotoxic effects can be achieved with combination chemotherapy; furthermore, subclones resistant to only one of the agents can potentially be eradicated. Some combinations of anticancer drugs also appear to exert true synergism, wherein the effect of the two drugs is greater than additive. The efficacy of combination chemotherapy has now been validated in many forms of human cancer, and the scientific rationale appears to be sound. As a

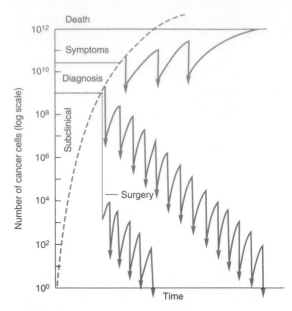

Figure 55–1. The log-kill hypothesis. Relationship of tumor cell number to time of diagnosis, symptoms, treatment, and survival. Three alternative approaches to drug treatment are shown for comparison with the course of tumor growth when no treatment is given *(dashed line)*. In the protocol diagrammed at top, treatment (indicated by the arrows) is given infrequently and the result is manifested as prolongation of survival but with recurrence of symptoms between courses of treatment and eventual death of the patient. The combination chemotherapy treatment diagrammed in the middle section is begun earlier and is more intensive. Tumor cell kill exceeds regrowth, drug resistance does not develop, and "cure" results. In this example, treatment has been continued long after all clinical evidence of cancer has disappeared (1–3 years). This approach has been established as effective in the treatment of childhood acute leukemia, testicular cancers, and Hodgkin's disease. In the treatment diagrammed near the bottom of the graph, early surgery has been employed to remove the primary tumor and intensive adjuvant chemotherapy has been administered long enough (up to 1 year) to eradicate the remaining tumor cells that comprise the occult micrometastases.

result, combination chemotherapy is now the standard approach to curative treatment of testicular cancer and lymphomas and to palliative treatment of many other tumor types. This important therapeutic approach was first formulated by Skipper and Schabel and described as the log-kill hypothesis (Figure 55–1).

Growth of acute leukemias and aggressive lymphomas closely follows exponential cell kinetics. In contrast, most human solid tumors do not grow in such a manner; instead, they follow a Gompertzian model of tumor growth and regression. Under Gompertzian kinetics, the growth fraction of the tumor is not constant and peaks when the tumor is about one third of its maximum size.

IMPORTANCE OF CELL CYCLE KINETICS

Information on cell and population kinetics of cancer cells explains, in part, the limited effectiveness of most available anticancer drugs. A schematic summary of cell cycle kinetics is presented in Figure 55–2. This information is relevant to the mode of action, indications, and scheduling of **cell cycle-specific (CCS)** and **cell cycle-nonspecific (CCNS)** drugs. Agents falling into these two major classes are summarized in Table 55–1.

In general, CCS drugs are most effective in hematologic malignancies and in solid tumors in which a relatively large proportion of the cells are proliferating or are in the growth fraction. CCNS drugs (many of which

Table 55–1. Cell cycle effects of major classes of anticancer drugs.

Cell Cycle-Specific (CCS) Agents	Cell Cycle-Nonspecific (CCNS) Agents
Antimetabolites	**Alkylating agents**
Capecitabine	Busulfan
Cladribine	Carmustine
Cytarabine	Cyclophosphamide
Fludarabine	Lomustine
Fluorouracil	Mechlorethamine
Gemcitabine	Melphalan
Mercaptopurine	Thiotepa
Methotrexate	**Anthracyclines**
Thioguanine	Daunorubicin
Antitumor antibiotic	Doxorubicin
Bleomycin	Epirubicin
Epipodophyllotoxins	Idarubicin
Etoposide	Mitoxantrone
Teniposide	**Antitumor antibiotics**
Taxanes	Dactinomycin
Docetaxel	Mitomycin
Paclitaxel	**Camptothecins**
Vinca alkaloids	Irinotecan
Vinblastine	Topotecan
Vincristine	**Platinum analogs**
Vinorelbine	Carboplatin
	Cisplatin
	Oxaliplatin

bind to cellular DNA and damage these macromolecules) are particularly useful in low growth fraction solid tumors as well as in high growth fraction tumors. In all instances, effective agents sterilize or inactivate tumor stem cells, which are often only a small fraction of the cells within a tumor. Non-stem cells (eg, those that have irreversibly differentiated) are considered sterile by definition and are not a significant component of the cancer problem.

Resistance to Cytotoxic Drugs

A major problem in cancer chemotherapy is drug resistance. Some tumor types, eg, malignant melanoma, renal cell cancer, and brain cancer, exhibit *primary* resistance, ie, absence of response on the first exposure, to currently available standard agents. The presence of inherent drug resistance is felt to be tightly associated with the genomic instability associated with the development of most cancers. *Acquired* resistance develops in a number of drug-sensitive tumor types. Experimentally, drug resistance can be highly specific to a single drug and usually is based on a change in the genetic apparatus of a given tumor cell with amplification or increased expression of one or more specific genes. In other instances, a multidrug-resistant

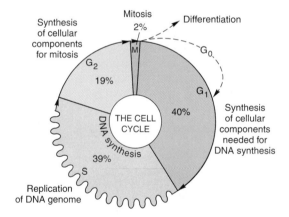

Figure 55–2. The cell cycle and cancer. A conceptual depiction of the cell cycle phases that all cells—normal and neoplastic—must traverse before and during cell division. The percentages given represent the approximate percentage of time spent in each phase by a typical malignant cell; the duration of G_1, however, can vary markedly. Many of the effective anticancer drugs exert their action on cells traversing the cell cycle and are called cell cycle-specific (CCS) drugs (Table 55–1). A second group of agents called cell cycle-nonspecific (CCNS) drugs can sterilize tumor cells whether they are cycling or resting in the G_0 compartment. CCNS drugs can kill both G_0 and cycling cells (although cycling cells are more sensitive).

phenotype occurs—resistance to a variety of natural product anticancer drugs of differing structures developing after exposure to a single agent. This form of multidrug resistance is often associated with increased expression of a normal gene (the *MDR1* gene) for a cell surface glycoprotein (P-glycoprotein) involved in drug efflux. This transport molecule requires ATP to expel a variety of foreign molecules (not limited to antitumor drugs) from the cell. It is expressed constitutively in normal tissues such as the epithelial cells of the kidney, large intestine, and adrenal gland as well as in a variety of tumors. Multidrug resistance can be reversed experimentally by calcium channel blockers, such as verapamil, and a variety of other drugs, which inhibit the transporter. Other mechanisms of multiple drug resistance involve overexpression of the multidrug resistance protein 1 (MRP1), a member of the ATP-binding cassette transmembrane transporter superfamily that now consists of nine members (MRP1-MRP9). MRP1, the most extensively studied, increases

resistance to natural product drugs such as anthracyclines, vinca alkaloids, taxanes, and epipodophyllotoxins by functioning as a drug export pump.

I. BASIC PHARMACOLOGY OF CANCER CHEMOTHERAPEUTIC DRUGS

POLYFUNCTIONAL ALKYLATING AGENTS

The major clinically useful alkylating agents (Figure 55–3) have a structure containing a bis-(chloroethyl)amine, ethyleneimine, or nitrosourea moiety. Among the bis(chloroethyl)amines, cyclophos-

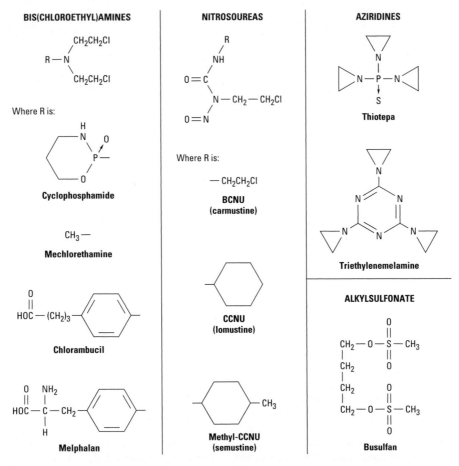

Figure 55–3. Structures of major classes of alkylating agents.

phamide, mechlorethamine, melphalan, and chlorambucil are the most useful. Ifosfamide is closely related to cyclophosphamide but has a somewhat different spectrum of activity and toxicity. Thiotepa and busulfan are used for specialized purposes for ovarian cancer and chronic myeloid leukemia, respectively. The major nitrosoureas are carmustine (BCNU), lomustine (CCNU), and semustine (methyl-CCNU). A variety of investigational alkylating agents have been synthesized that link various carrier molecules such as amino acids, nucleic acid bases, hormones, or sugar moieties to a group capable of alkylation; however, successful site-directed alkylation has not been achieved to date.

As a class, the alkylating agents exert cytotoxic effects via transfer of their alkyl groups to various cellular constituents. Alkylations of DNA within the nucleus probably represent the major interactions that lead to cell death. However, these drugs react chemically with sulfhydryl, amino, hydroxyl, carboxyl, and phosphate groups of other cellular nucleophiles as well. The general mechanism of action of these drugs involves intramolecular cyclization to form an ethyleneimonium ion that may directly or through formation of a carbonium ion transfer an alkyl group to a cellular constituent. In addition to alkylation, a secondary mechanism that occurs with nitrosoureas involves carbamoylation of lysine residues of proteins through formation of isocyanates.

The major site of alkylation within DNA is the N7 position of guanine (Figure 55–4); however, other bases are also alkylated to lesser degrees, including N1 and N3 of adenine, N3 of cytosine, and O6 of guanine, as well as phosphate atoms and proteins associated with DNA. These interactions can occur on a single strand or on both strands of DNA through cross-linking, as most major alkylating agents are bifunctional, with two reactive groups. Alkylation of guanine can result in miscoding through abnormal base pairing with thymine or in depurination by excision of guanine residues. The latter effect leads to DNA strand breakage through scission of the sugar-phosphate backbone of DNA. Cross-linking of DNA appears to be of major importance to the cytotoxic action of alkylating agents, and replicating cells are most susceptible to these drugs. Thus, although alkylating agents are not cell cycle-specific, cells are most susceptible to alkylation in late G_1 and S phases of the cell cycle and express block in G_2.

Drug Resistance

The mechanism of acquired resistance to alkylating agents may involve increased capability to repair DNA lesions, decreased permeability of the cell to the alkylating drug, and increased production of glutathione, which inactivates the alkylating agent through conjugation or through increased glutathione S-transferase activity, which catalyzes the conjugation.

Pharmacologic Effects

Active alkylating agents have direct vesicant effects and can damage tissues at the site of injection as well as produce

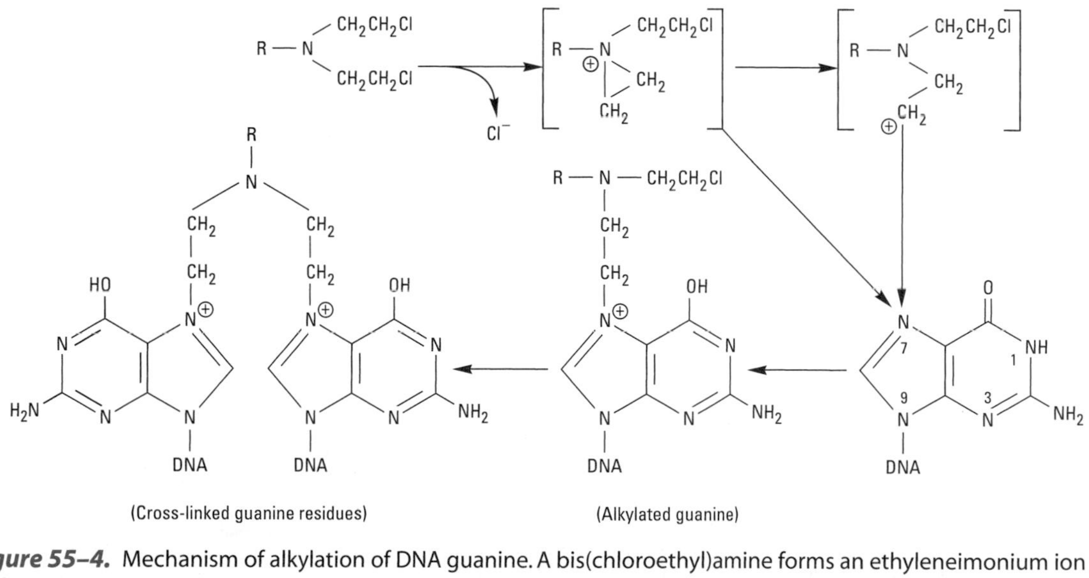

Figure 55–4. Mechanism of alkylation of DNA guanine. A bis(chloroethyl)amine forms an ethyleneimonium ion and a carbonium ion that react with a base such as N7 of guanine in DNA, producing an alkylated purine. Alkylation of a second guanine residue, through the illustrated mechanism, results in cross-linking of DNA strands.

systemic toxicity. Toxicities are generally dose-related and occur particularly in rapidly growing tissues such as bone marrow, the gastrointestinal tract, and the reproductive system. After intravenous injection, nausea and vomiting usually occur within 30–60 minutes with mechlorethamine, cyclophosphamide, or carmustine. The emetogenic effects are mediated by the central nervous system and can be reduced by pretreatment with 5-HT$_3$ (serotonin) receptor antagonists such as ondansetron or granisetron. Subcutaneous injection of mechlorethamine or carmustine leads to tissue necrosis and sloughing.

Cyclophosphamide in its parent form does not have direct cytotoxic effects, and it must be activated to cytotoxic forms by microsomal enzymes (Figure 55–5). The liver microsomal cytochrome P450 mixed-function oxidase system converts cyclophosphamide to 4-hydroxycyclophosphamide, which is in equilibrium with aldophosphamide. These active metabolites are believed to be delivered by the bloodstream to both tumor and normal tissue, where nonenzymatic cleavage of aldophosphamide to the cytotoxic forms—phosphoramide mustard and acrolein—occurs. The liver appears to be protected through the enzymatic formation of the inactive metabolites 4-ketocyclophosphamide and carboxyphosphamide.

The major toxicities of alkylating agents are set forth in Table 55–2 and discussed below.

Oral administration of alkylating agents has been of great value, and this approach has been developed using relatively less reactive alkylating drugs. Cyclophosphamide, melphalan, chlorambucil, busulfan, and, more recently, temozolomide are those most commonly given via the oral route, and their cytotoxic effects are similar to those observed with parenteral administration. In general, if a tumor is resistant to one alkylating agent, it will be relatively resistant to other agents of this class (though not necessarily to nitrosoureas); however, there are exceptions to this rule depending on the specific tumor. Cyclophosphamide is the most widely used alkylating agent. The oral drug busulfan has a major degree of specificity for the granulocyte series and is therefore of particular value in therapy of chronic myelogenous leukemia. With all oral alkylating agents, some degree of leukopenia is necessary to provide evidence that the drug has been absorbed adequately. Frequent monitoring of blood counts is essential during administration of these agents as the development of severe leukopenia or thrombocytopenia necessitates immediate interruption of therapy.

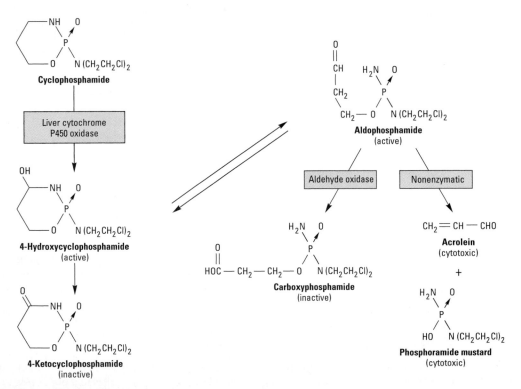

Figure 55–5. Cyclophosphamide metabolism.

Table 55–2. Alkylating agents: Dosages and toxicities.

Alkylating Agent	Single-Agent Dosage	Acute Toxicity	Delayed Toxicity
Mechlorethamine	0.4 mg/kg IV in single or divided doses	Nausea and vomiting, myelosuppression	Moderate depression of peripheral blood count; excessive doses produce severe bone marrow depression with leukopenia, thrombocytopenia, and bleeding; alopecia and hemorrhagic cystitis occasionally occur with cyclophosphamide; cystitis can be prevented with adequate hydration; busulfan is associated with skin pigmentation, pulmonary fibrosis, and adrenal insufficiency
Chlorambucil	0.1–0.2 mg/kg/d orally; 6–12 mg/d	Nausea and vomiting, myelosuppression	
Cyclophosphamide	3.5–5 mg/kg/d orally for 10 days; 1 g/m^2 IV as single dose	Nausea and vomiting, myelosuppression	
Melphalan	0.25 mg/kg/d orally for 4 days every 4–6 weeks	Nausea and vomiting, myelosuppression	
Thiotepa (triethylenethiophosphoramide)	0.2 mg/kg IV for 5 days	Nausea and vomiting, myelosuppression	
Busulfan	2–8 mg/d orally; 150–250 mg/course	Nausea and vomiting, myelosuppression	
Carmustine (BCNU)	200 mg/m^2 IV every 6 weeks	Nausea and vomiting	Leukopenia, thrombocytopenia, and rarely hepatitis
Lomustine (CCNU)	150 mg/m^2 orally every 6 weeks	Nausea and vomiting	
Altretamine	10 mg/kg/d for 21 days	Nausea and vomiting	Leukopenia, thrombocytopenia, and peripheral neuropathy
Procarbazine	50–200 mg/d orally	Nausea and vomiting, flu-like syndrome, drug interactions	Bone marrow depression, central nervous system depression, leukemogenic
Dacarbazine	300 mg/m^2 daily IV for 5 days	Nausea and vomiting	Bone marrow depression
Cisplatin	20 mg/m^2/d IV for 5 days or 50–70 mg/m^2 as single dose every 3 weeks	Nausea and vomiting, myelosuppression	Nephrotoxicity, peripheral sensory neuropathy, ototoxicity, nerve dysfunction.
Carboplatin	AUC 5–7 mgxmin/mL	Myelosuppression, nausea and vomiting	Rarely: peripheral neuropathy, renal toxicity, and hepatic dysfunction
Oxaliplatin	130 mg/m^2 IV every 3 weeks or 85 mg/m^2 IV every 2 weeks	Nausea and vomiting, laryngopharyngeal dysesthesias	Peripheral sensory neuropathy, diarrhea, myelosuppression, and renal toxicity

NITROSOUREAS

These drugs appear to be non-cross-resistant with other alkylating agents; all require biotransformation, which occurs by nonenzymatic decomposition, to metabolites with both alkylating and carbamoylating activities. The nitrosoureas are highly lipid-soluble and cross the blood-brain barrier, making them useful in the treatment of brain tumors. The nitrosoureas appear to function by cross-linking through alkylation of DNA. The drugs may be more effective against plateau phase cells than exponentially growing cells, though within a cycling cell population these agents appear to slow cell progression through the DNA synthetic phase. After oral administration of lomustine, peak plasma levels of metabolites appear within 1–4 hours; central nervous system concentrations reach 30–40% of the activity present in the plasma. While the initial plasma half-life is in the range of 6 hours, a second half-life is in the range of 1–2 days. Urinary excretion appears to be the major route of elimination from the body. One naturally occurring sugar-containing nitrosourea, streptozocin, is interesting because it has minimal bone marrow toxicity. This agent has activity in the treatment of insulin-secreting islet cell carcinoma of the pancreas.

RELATED DRUGS PROBABLY ACTING AS ALKYLATING AGENTS

A variety of other compounds have mechanisms of action that involve alkylation. These include procarbazine, dacarbazine, altretamine (hexamethylmelamine), cisplatin, and carboplatin. Dosages and major toxicities are listed in Table 55–2.

1. Procarbazine

The oral agent procarbazine is a methylhydrazine derivative, and it is commonly used in combination regimens for Hodgkin's disease, non-Hodgkin's lymphoma, and brain tumors. The drug is also leukemogenic and has teratogenic and mutagenic properties.

The mechanism of action of procarbazine is uncertain; however, the drug inhibits the synthesis of DNA, RNA, and protein; prolongs interphase; and produces chromosome breaks. Oxidative metabolism of this drug by microsomal enzymes generates azoprocarbazine and H_2O_2, which may be responsible for DNA strand scission. A variety of other metabolites of the drug are formed that may be cytotoxic. One metabolite is a weak monoamine oxidase (MAO) inhibitor, and adverse side effects can occur when procarbazine is given with other MAO inhibitors.

There is an increased risk of secondary cancers in the form of acute leukemia, and the carcinogenic potential of procarbazine is felt to be higher than that of most other alkylating agents.

2. Dacarbazine

Dacarbazine is a synthetic compound that functions as an alkylating agent following metabolic activation by liver microsomal enzymes by oxidative N-demethylation to the monomethyl derivative. This metabolite spontaneously decomposes to 5-aminoimidazole-4-carboxamide, which is excreted in the urine, and diazomethane. The diazomethane generates a methyl carbonium ion that is believed to be the likely cytotoxic species. Dacarbazine is administered parenterally and is not schedule-dependent. It produces marked nausea, vomiting, and myelosuppression. Its major applications are in melanoma, Hodgkin's disease, and soft tissue sarcomas.

3. Altretamine (Hexamethylmelamine)

Altretamine is structurally similar to triethylenemelamine. It is relatively insoluble and available only in oral form. It is rapidly biotransformed in the liver by demethylation to the pentamethylmelamine and tetramethylmelamine metabolites. This agent is approved for use in ovarian cancer patients who have progressed despite treatment with a regimen based on platinum or an alkylating agent (or both). The main dose-limiting toxicities include nausea, vomiting, and myelosuppression. Neurotoxicity in the form of somnolence, mood changes, and peripheral neuropathy is also observed.

4. Cisplatin, Carboplatin, & Oxaliplatin

Cisplatin (*cis*-diamminedichloroplatinum [II]) is an inorganic metal complex discovered through the serendipitous observation that neutral platinum complexes inhibited division and induced filamentous growth of *Escherichia coli*. Several platinum analogs have been subsequently synthesized. While the precise mechanism of action of cisplatin is still undefined, it is thought to act in somewhat the same way as alkylating agents. It kills cells in all stages of the cell cycle, inhibits DNA biosynthesis, and binds DNA through the formation of interstrand cross-links. The primary binding site is the N7 of guanine, but covalent interaction with adenine and cytosine also occurs. The platinum complexes appear to synergize with certain other anticancer drugs. Aggressive hydration with intravenous saline infusion alone or with saline and mannitol or other diuretics appears to significantly reduce the incidence of nephrotoxicity.

$$H_3N \diagdown \quad \diagup Cl$$
$$Pt$$
$$H_3N \diagup \quad \diagdown Cl$$

Cisplatin

Cisplatin has major antitumor activity in a broad range of solid tumors, including non-small cell and small cell lung cancer, esophageal and gastric cancer, head and neck cancer, and genitourinary cancers, particularly testicular, ovarian, and bladder cancer. When used in combination regimens with vinblastine and bleomycin or etoposide and bleomycin, cisplatin-based therapy has led to the cure of nonseminomatous testicular cancer.

Carboplatin is a second-generation platinum analog that exerts its cytotoxic effects exactly as cisplatin and has activity against the same spectrum of solid tumors. Its main dose-limiting toxicity is myelosuppression, and it has significantly less renal toxicity and gastrointestinal toxicity than cisplatin. Moreover, vigorous intravenously hydration is not required. As a result, carboplatin is now being used in place of cisplatin in combination chemotherapy.

Oxaliplatin is a third generation diaminocyclohexane platinum analog. Its mechanism of action is identical to that of cisplatin and carboplatin. However, it is not cross-resistant to cancer cells that are resistant to cisplatin or carboplatin on the basis of mismatch repair defects. This agent was recently approved for use as second-line therapy in metastatic colorectal cancer following treatment with the combination of fluorouracil-leucovorin and irinotecan, and it is now widely used as first-line therapy of this disease as well. Neurotoxicity is dose-limiting and characterized by a peripheral sensory neuropathy, often triggered or worsened upon exposure to cold. While this neurotoxicity is cumulative, it tends to be reversible—in contrast to cisplatin-induced neurotoxicity.

Clinical Uses of the Alkylating Agents

The alkylating agents are used in the treatment of a wide variety of hematologic and solid cancers, generally as part of a combination regimen. They are discussed along with various specific tumors (below).

ANTIMETABOLITES (STRUCTURAL ANALOGS)

The development of drugs with actions on intermediary metabolism of proliferating cells has been important both clinically and conceptually. While biochemical properties unique to all cancer cells have yet to be discovered, neoplastic cells do have a number of quantitative differences in metabolism from normal cells that render them more susceptible to a number of antimetabolites or structural analogs. Many of these agents have been rationally designed and synthesized based on knowledge of cellular processes, and a few have been discovered as antibiotics.

Mechanisms of Action

The biochemical pathways that have thus far proved to be most vulnerable to antimetabolites have been those relating to nucleotide and nucleic acid synthesis. In a number of instances, when an enzyme is known to have a major effect on pathways leading to cell replication, inhibitors of the reaction it catalyzes have proved to be useful anticancer drugs.

These drugs and their doses and toxicities are shown in Table 55–3. The principal drugs are discussed below.

METHOTREXATE

Methotrexate (MTX) is a folic acid antagonist that binds to the active catalytic site of dihydrofolate reductase (DHFR), interfering with the synthesis of the reduced form that accepts one-carbon units. Lack of this cofactor interrupts the synthesis of thymidylate, purine nucleotides, and the amino acids serine and methionine, thereby interfering with the formation of DNA, RNA, and proteins. The enzyme binds methotrexate with high affinity, and at pH 6.0, virtually no dissociation of the enzyme-inhibitor complex occurs (inhibition constant about 1 nmol/L). At physiologic pH, reversible competitive kinetics occur (inhibition constant about 1 μmol/L). Intracellular formation of polyglutamate derivatives appears to be important in the therapeutic action of methotrexate. The polyglutamates of methotrexate are selectively retained within cancer cells and have increased inhibitory effects on enzymes involved in folate metabolism, making them important determinants of the duration of action of methotrexate.

Folic acid

Methotrexate

Drug Resistance

Tumor cell resistance to methotrexate has been attributed to (1) decreased drug transport, (2) decreased polyglutamate formation, (3) synthesis of increased levels of DHFR through gene amplification, and (4) altered DHFR with reduced affinity for methotrexate. Recent studies have also suggested that decreased accumulation of drug through activation of the multidrug resistance P170 glycoprotein transporter may also result in drug resistance.

Dosage & Toxicity

Methotrexate is administered by the intravenous, intrathecal, or oral route. Up to 90% of an oral dose is

Table 55–3. Antimetabolites: Dosages and toxicities.

Chemotherapeutic Agent	Single-Agent Dosage	Delayed Toxicity[1]
Capecitabine	1250 mg/m^2/bid orally for 14 days followed by 1 week of rest. Repeat every 3 weeks.	Diarrhea, hand-and-foot syndrome,[2] myelosuppression, nausea and vomiting
Cladribine	0.09 mg/kg/d for 7 days by continuous IV infusion in sterile saline	Myelosuppression, nausea and vomiting, and immunosuppression
Cytarabine	100 mg/m^2/d for 5–10 days, either by continuous IV infusion or SC every 8 hours.	Nausea and vomiting, bone marrow depression, stomatitis, and cerebellar ataxia
Fludarabine	25 mg/m^2/d for 5 days every 28 days (administer IV over 30 minutes)	Myelosuppression, immunosuppression, fever, myalgias, and arthralgias
Fluorouracil	15 mg/kg/d IV for 5 days by 24-hour infusion; 15 mg/kg weekly IV	Nausea, mucositis, diarrhea, myelosuppression, hand and foot syndrome, and neurotoxicity
Gemcitabine	1000 mg/m^2 IV weekly for up to 7 weeks followed by 1 week of rest	Nausea, vomiting, diarrhea, myelosuppression
Mercaptopurine	2.5 mg/kg/d orally	Myelosuppression, immunosuppression, and hepatotoxicity
Methotrexate	2.5–5 mg/d orally (Rheumatrex); 10 mg intrathecally (Folex) once or twice weekly	Mucositis, diarrhea, bone marrow depression with leukopenia and thrombocytopenia
Thioguanine	2 mg/kg/d orally	Myelosuppression, immunosuppression, and hepatotoxicity

[1]These drugs do not cause acute toxicity.

[2]Hand and foot syndrome is a form of erythromelalgia manifested as tingling, numbness, pain, erythema, swelling, and increased pigmentation.

excreted in the urine within 12 hours. The drug is not subject to metabolism, and serum levels are therefore proportionate to dose as long as renal function and hydration status are adequate. Dosages and toxic effects are listed in Table 55–3. The effects of methotrexate can be reversed by administration of leucovorin (citrovorum factor). Leucovorin rescue has been used with accidental overdose or experimentally along with high-dose methotrexate therapy in a protocol intended to rescue normal cells while still leaving the tumor cells subject to its cytotoxic action.

Other Applications

Methotrexate is also used in the treatment of rheumatoid arthritis (Chapter 36) and psoriasis.

PURINE ANTAGONISTS

1. 6-Thiopurines

Mercaptopurine (6-MP) was the first of the thiopurine series found useful as an anticancer drug. Like other thiopurines, it must be metabolized by hypoxanthine-guanine phosphoribosyl transferase (HGPRT) to the nucleotide form (6-thioinosinic acid), which in turn inhibits a number of the enzymes of purine nucleotide interconversion. Significant amounts of thioguanylic acid and 6-methylmercaptopurine ribotide (MMPR) are also formed from 6-MP. These metabolites may also contribute to the action of the mercaptopurine. Mercaptopurine is used primarily in the treatment of childhood acute leukemia, and a closely related analog, azathioprine, is used as an immunosuppressive agent (see Chapter 56).

Thioguanine (6-TG) inhibits several enzymes in the purine nucleotide pathway. A variety of metabolic lesions are associated with the cytotoxic action of the purinethiols. These include inhibition of purine nucleotide interconversion; decrease in intracellular levels of guanine nucleotides, which leads to inhibition of glycoprotein synthesis; interference with the formation of DNA and RNA; and incorporation of thiopurine nucleotides into both DNA and RNA. 6-TG has a synergistic action when used together with cytarabine in the treatment of adult acute leukemia.

Drug Resistance

Resistance to both 6-MP and 6-TG occurs most commonly by decrease in HGPRT activity; an alternative mechanism in acute leukemia involves elevation of levels of alkaline phosphatase, which results in dephosphorylation of thiopurine nucleotide and cellular loss of the resulting ribonucleoside.

Dosage & Toxicity

Mercaptopurine and thioguanine are both given orally (Table 55–3) and excreted mainly in the urine. However, 6-MP is converted to an inactive metabolite (6-thiouric acid) by an oxidation catalyzed by xanthine oxidase, whereas 6-TG requires deamination before it is metabolized by this enzyme. This factor is important because the purine analog allopurinol, a potent xanthine oxidase inhibitor, is frequently used with chemotherapy in hematologic cancers to prevent hyperuricemia after tumor cell lysis. It does this by blocking purine oxidation, allowing excretion of cellular purines that are relatively more soluble than uric acid. Nephrotoxicity and acute gout produced by excessive uric acid are thereby prevented. Simultaneous therapy with allopurinol and 6-MP results in excessive toxicity unless the dose of mercaptopurine is reduced to 25% of the usual level. This effect does not occur with 6-TG, which can be used in full doses with allopurinol.

Hypoxanthine   **6-Mercaptopurine**   **Allopurinol**

Guanine   **6-Thioguanine**

2. Fludarabine Phosphate

Fludarabine phosphate (2-fluoro-arabinofuranosyladenine monophosphate) is rapidly dephosphorylated to 2-fluoro-arabinofuranosyladenine and then phosphorylated intracellularly by deoxycytidine kinase to the triphosphate. This metabolite interferes with DNA synthesis through inhibition of DNA polymerase-α and ribonucleotide reductase, and it also induces apoptosis. Fludarabine phosphate is used chiefly in the treatment of low-grade non-Hodgkin's lymphoma and chronic lymphocytic leukemia (CLL). Fludarabine phosphate is given parentally and is excreted primarily in the urine; its dose-limiting toxicity is myelosuppression.

3. Cladribine

Cladribine (2-chlorodeoxyadenosine) achieves high intracellular concentrations because of its resistance to adenosine deaminase; it is phosphorylated by deoxycytidine kinase and is incorporated into DNA. Cladribine causes DNA strand breaks (presumably through interference with DNA repair) and loss of NAD (through activation of poly[ADP-ribose]synthase). Cladribine is indicated for the treatment of hairy cell leukemia and is also used for CLL and low-grade non-Hodgkin's lymphoma. It is normally administered as a single continuous 7-day infusion; under these conditions, its toxicity usually consists of transient myelosuppression. In addition, it is an immunosuppressive agent, and a decrease in CD4 and CD8 cells, lasting for over 1 year, occurs in most patients.

PYRIMIDINE ANTAGONISTS

1. Fluorouracil

5-Fluorouracil (5-FU) is a prodrug and undergoes a complex series of biotransformation reactions to ribosyl and deoxyribosyl nucleotide metabolites. One of these metabolites, 5-fluoro-2'-deoxyuridine-5'-monophosphate (FdUMP), forms a covalently bound ternary complex with the enzyme thymidylate synthase and the reduced folate $N^{5,10}$-methylenetetrahydrofolate, a reaction critical for the synthesis of thymidylate. This results in inhibition of DNA synthesis through "thymineless death." 5-FU is converted to 5-fluorouridine-5'-triphosphate (FUTP), which is then incorporated into RNA, where it interferes with RNA processing and mRNA translation. In addition, 5-FU is converted to 5-fluorodeoxyuridine-5'-triphosphate (FdUTP), which can be incorporated into cellular DNA, resulting in inhibition of DNA synthesis and function. Thus, the cytotoxicity of fluorouracil is felt to be the result of effects on both DNA- and RNA-mediated events.

Uracil   **5-FU**

Fluorouracil is normally given intravenously (Table 55–3) and has a short metabolic half-life on the order of 15 minutes. It is not administered by the oral route because its bioavailability is erratic due to the high levels of the breakdown enzyme dihydropyrimidine dehydrogenase present in the gut mucosa. Floxuridine (5-fluoro-2′-deoxyuridine, FUDR) has an action similar to that of fluorouracil, and it is only used for hepatic artery infusions. A cream incorporating fluorouracil is used topically for treating basal cell cancers of the skin.

Fluorouracil is the most widely used agent for the treatment of colorectal cancer, both as adjuvant therapy as well as for advanced disease. In addition, it has activity against a wide variety of solid tumors, including cancers of the breast, stomach, pancreas, esophagus, liver, head and neck, and anus. Its major toxicities are listed in Table 55–3.

2. Capecitabine

Capecitabine is a fluoropyrimidine carbamate prodrug that has nearly 70–80% oral bioavailability. It undergoes extensive metabolism in the liver by the enzyme carboxylesterase to an intermediate, 5′-deoxy-5-fluorocytidine. This in turn is converted to 5′-deoxy-5-fluorouridine by the enzyme cytidine deaminase. The 5′-deoxy-5-fluorouridine metabolite is then hydrolyzed by thymidine phosphorylase to fluorouracil in the tumor. (The expression of thymidine phosphorylase is significantly higher in a broad range of solid tumors than in corresponding normal tissue.) Peak plasma levels are achieved in about 1.5 hours, and peak fluorouracil levels are reached at 2 hours after oral administration.

Capecitabine is used in the treatment of metastatic breast cancer as either a single agent or in combination with the taxane docetaxel. It has recently been approved for use in the treatment of metastatic colorectal cancer as monotherapy, and significant efforts are now directed at using this agent in combination with either irinotecan or oxaliplatin. The main toxicities of capecitabine are listed in Table 55–3. While myelosuppression, nausea and vomiting, and mucositis can be observed with this agent, the incidence is significantly less than that seen with intravenous fluorouracil.

3. Cytarabine

Cytarabine (cytosine arabinoside, ara-C) is an S phase-specific antimetabolite that is converted by deoxycytidine kinase to the 5′-mononucleotide (AraCMP). AraCMP is further metabolized to the triphosphate (AraCTP), which competitively inhibits DNA polymerase and results in blockade of DNA synthesis. Cytarabine is also incorporated into RNA and DNA. Incorporation into DNA leads to interference with chain elongation and defective ligation of fragments of newly synthesized DNA. The cel-

lular retention time for AraCTP appears to correlate with its lethality to malignant cells.

After intravenous administration (Table 55–3), the drug is cleared rapidly, with most being deaminated to an inactive form. The ratio of the anabolic enzyme deoxycytidine kinase to the inactivating catalyst cytidine deaminase is important in determining the cytotoxicity of cytarabine.

Cytosine deoxyriboside **Cytosine arabinoside (cytarabine)**

In view of cytarabine's S phase specificity, the drug is highly schedule-dependent and must be given either by continuous infusion or every 8–12 hours for 5–7 days. Its activity is limited almost entirely to treatment of acute myelogenous leukemia, for which it is a major drug. Adverse effects are listed in Table 55–3.

4. Gemcitabine

Gemcitabine is phosphorylated initially by the enzyme deoxycytidine kinase and then by other nucleoside kinases to the di- and triphosphate nucleotide forms, which then inhibit DNA synthesis. Inhibition is considered to result from two actions: inhibition of ribonucleotide reductase by gemcitabine diphosphate, which reduces the level of deoxyribonucleoside triphosphates required for the synthesis of DNA; and incorporation of gemcitabine triphosphate into DNA. Following incorporation of gemcitabine nucleotide, only one additional nucleotide can be added to the growing DNA strand, resulting in chain termination.

Gemcitabine

Gemcitabine was initially approved for use in pancreatic cancer but is now widely used in the treatment of non-small cell lung cancer and bladder cancer. Myelosuppression is the principal dose-limiting toxicity.

PLANT ALKALOIDS

VINBLASTINE

Vinblastine is an alkaloid derived from *Vinca rosea,* the periwinkle plant. Its mechanism of action involves depolymerization of microtubules, which are an important part of the cytoskeleton and the mitotic spindle. The drug binds specifically to the microtubule protein tubulin in dimeric form; the drug-tubulin complex adds to the forming end of the microtubules to terminate assembly, and depolymerization of the microtubules then occurs. This results in mitotic arrest at metaphase, dissolution of the mitotic spindle, and interference with chromosome segregation. Toxicity includes nausea and vomiting, bone marrow suppression, and alopecia. It has clinical activity in the treatment of Hodgkin's disease, non-Hodgkin's lymphomas, breast cancer, and germ cell cancer. See clinical section below and Table 55–4.

R: O=C—H **Vincristine**

R: CH₃ **Vinblastine**

VINCRISTINE

Vincristine is also an alkaloid derivative of *Vinca rosea* and is closely related in structure to vinblastine. Its mechanism of action is considered to be identical to that of vinblastine in that it functions as a mitotic spindle poison leading to arrest of cells in the M phase of the cell cycle. Despite these similarities to vinblastine, vincristine has a strikingly different spectrum of clinical activity and qualitatively different toxicities.

Vincristine has been effectively combined with prednisone for remission induction in acute lymphoblastic leukemia in children. It is also active in various hemato-logic malignancies such as Hodgkin's and non-Hodgkin's lymphoma and multiple myeloma and in several pediatric tumors including rhabdomyosarcoma, neuroblastoma, Ewing's sarcoma, and Wilms' tumor. The main dose-limiting toxicity is neurotoxicity, usually expressed as a peripheral sensory neuropathy, although autonomic nervous system dysfunction—with orthostatic hypotension, sphincter problems, and paralytic ileus—cranial nerve palsies, ataxia, seizures, and coma have been observed. While myelosuppression can occur, it is generally milder and much less significant than with vinblastine. The other potential side effect that can develop is the syndrome of inappropriate secretion of antidiuretic hormone (SIADH).

VINORELBINE

Vinorelbine is a semisynthetic vinca alkaloid whose mechanism of action is identical to that of vinblastine and vincristine, ie, inhibition of mitosis of cells in the M phase through inhibition of tubulin polymerization. Despite its similarities in mechanism of action, vinorelbine has activity in non-small cell lung cancer and in breast cancer. Myelosuppression with neutropenia is the dose-limiting toxicity, but nausea and vomiting, transient elevations in liver function tests, neurotoxicity, and SIADH are also reported.

EPIPODOPHYLLOTOXINS

Two compounds, **VP-16 (etoposide)** and a related drug, **VM-26 (teniposide)**, are semisynthetic derivatives of podophyllotoxin, which is extracted from the mayapple root *(Podophyllum peltatum)*. Both an intravenous and an oral formulation of etoposide are approved for clinical use in the USA.

Etoposide and teniposide are similar in chemical structure and in their effects—they block cell division in the late S-G₂ phase of the cell cycle. Their primary mode of action involves inhibition of topoisomerase II, which results in DNA damage through strand breakage induced by the formation of a ternary complex of drug, DNA, and enzyme. The drugs are water-insoluble and need to be formulated in a Cremophor vehicle for clinical use. These agents are administered via the intravenous route (Table 55–4) and are rapidly and widely distributed throughout the body except for the brain. Up to 90–95% of drug is protein-bound, mainly to albumin. Dose reduction is required in the setting of renal dysfunction. Etoposide has clinical activity in germ cell cancer, small cell and non-small cell lung cancer, Hodgkin's and non-Hodgkin's lymphomas, and gastric cancer and as high-dose therapy in the transplant setting for breast cancer and lymphomas. Teniposide's use is limited to acute lymphoblastic leukemia.

Table 55–4. Natural product cancer chemotherapy drugs: Dosages and toxicities.

Drug	Single-Agent Dosage	Acute Toxicity	Delayed Toxicity
Bleomycin	Up to 15 units/m² IV twice weekly to a total dose of 200–250 units	Allergic reactions, fever, hypotension	Skin toxicity, pulmonary fibrosis, mucositis, alopecia
Dactinomycin (actinomycin D)	0.04 mg/kg IV weekly	Nausea and vomiting	Stomatitis, gastrointestinal tract upset, alopecia, bone marrow depression
Daunorubicin (daunomycin)	30–60 mg/m² daily IV for 3 days, or 30–60 mg/m² IV weekly	Nausea, fever, red urine (not hematuria)	Cardiotoxicity (see text), alopecia, bone marrow depression
Docetaxel	100 mg/m² IV over 1 hour every 3 weeks	Hypersensitivity, rash	Neurotoxicity, fluid retention, neutropenia
Doxorubicin (Adriamycin)	60 mg/m² daily IV for 3 days, or 30–60 mg/m² IV weekly	Nausea, red urine (not hematuria)	Cardiotoxicity (see text), alopecia, bone marrow depression, stomatitis
Etoposide (VP-16)	50–100 mg/m² daily for 5 days	Nausea, vomiting, hypotension	Alopecia, bone marrow depression
Idarubicin	12 mg/m² IV daily for 3 days (with cytarabine)	Nausea and vomiting	Bone marrow depression, mucositis, cardiotoxicity
Irinotecan	125 mg/m² IV once weekly for 4 weeks; repeat every 6 weeks or 300–350 mg/m² IV every 3 weeks	Diarrhea, nausea, vomiting	Diarrhea, bone marrow depression, nausea and vomiting, liver function abnormalities
Mitomycin	20 mg/m² IV every 6 weeks	Nausea	Thrombocytopenia, anemia, leukopenia, mucositis
Paclitaxel	130–170 mg/m² IV over 3 or 24 hours every 3–4 weeks	Nausea, vomiting, hypotension, arrhythmias, hypersensitivity	Bone marrow depression, peripheral sensory neuropathy
Topotecan	1.5 mg/m² IV for 5 days, repeat every 21 days for 4 courses	Nausea and vomiting	Bone marrow depression, arthralgias
Vinblastine	0.1–0.2 mg/kg IV weekly	Nausea and vomiting	Alopecia, loss of reflexes, bone marrow depression
Vincristine	1.5 mg/m² IV (maximum: 2 mg weekly)	None	Areflexia, muscle weakness, peripheral neuritis, paralytic ileus, mild bone marrow depression, alopecia
Vinorelbine	30 mg/m² IV weekly	Nausea and vomiting	Bone marrow depression, fatigue, constipation, hyporeflexia, paresthesias

CAMPTOTHECINS

The camptothecins are natural products that are derived from the *Camptotheca acuminata* tree, and they inhibit the activity of topoisomerase I, the key enzyme responsible for cutting and religating single DNA strands. Inhibition of the enzyme results in DNA damage. **Topotecan** is indicated in the treatment of patients with advanced ovarian cancer who have failed platinum-based chemotherapy and is also approved as second-line therapy of small cell lung cancer. The main route of elimination is renal excretion, and for this reason caution must be exercised in patients with abnormal renal function, with dosage reduction being required.

Irinotecan is a prodrug that is converted mainly in the liver by the carboxylesterase enzyme to the SN-38 metabolite, which is a potent inhibitor of topoisomerase I. In contrast to topotecan, irinotecan and SN-38 are mainly eliminated in bile and feces, and dose reduction is required in the setting of liver dysfunction. Irinotecan is indicated as second-line monotherapy in patients with metastatic colorectal cancer who have failed fluorouracil-based therapy and as first-line therapy when used in combination with fluorouracil and leucovorin. Myelosuppression and diarrhea are the two most common adverse events. There are two forms of diarrhea: an early form that occurs within 24 hours after administration and is felt to be a cholinergic event effectively treated with atropine, and a late form which usually occurs 3–10 days after treatment. The late diarrhea can be severe, leading to significant electrolyte imbalance and dehydration in some cases.

TAXANES

Paclitaxel is an alkaloid ester derived from the Western yew *(Taxus brevifolia)* and the European yew *(Taxus baccata).* The drug functions as a mitotic spindle poison through high-affinity binding to microtubules with enhancement of tubulin polymerization. This promotion of microtubule assembly by paclitaxel occurs in the absence of microtubule-associated proteins and guanosine triphosphate and results in inhibition of mitosis and cell division.

Paclitaxel has significant activity in a wide variety of solid tumors, including ovarian, advanced breast, non-small cell and small cell lung, head and neck, esophageal, prostate, and bladder cancer and AIDS-related Kaposi's sarcoma. It is metabolized extensively by the liver P450 system, and nearly 80% of the drug is excreted in feces. For this reason, dose reduction is required in the setting of liver dysfunction. The primary dose-limiting toxicities are listed in Table 55–4. Hypersensitivity reactions may be observed in up to 5% of patients, but the incidence can be reduced by premedication with dexamethasone, diphenhydramine, and an H_2 blocker.

Docetaxel is a semisynthetic taxane derived from the European yew tree. Its mechanism of action, metabolism, and elimination are identical to those of paclitaxel. It is approved for use as second-line therapy in advanced breast cancer and non-small cell lung cancer, and it also has major activity in head and neck cancer, small cell lung cancer, gastric cancer, advanced platinum-refractory ovarian cancer, and bladder cancer. Its major toxicities are listed in Table 55–4.

ANTITUMOR ANTIBIOTICS

Screening of microbial products has led to the discovery of a number of growth inhibiting compounds that have proved to be clinically useful in cancer chemotherapy. Many of these antibiotics bind to DNA through intercalation between specific bases and block the synthesis of RNA, DNA, or both; cause DNA strand scission; and interfere with cell replication. All of the anticancer antibiotics now being used in clinical practice are products of various strains of the soil microbe *Streptomyces.* These include the anthracyclines, dactinomycin, bleomycin, and mitomycin.

ANTHRACYCLINES

The anthracycline antibiotics, isolated from *Streptomyces peucetius* var *caesius,* are among the most widely used cytotoxic anticancer drugs. Two congeners, **doxorubicin** and **daunorubicin,** are FDA-approved, and their structures are shown below. Several other anthracycline analogs have entered clinical practice, including idarubicin, epirubicin, and mitoxantrone. Daunorubicin was the first agent in this class to be isolated, and it is still used in the treatment of acute myeloid leukemia. Doxorubicin has a broad spectrum of clinical activity against hematologic malignancies as well as a wide range of solid tumors. The entire class of anthracyclines exert their cytotoxic action through four major mechanisms. These are (1) inhibition of topoisomerase II; (2) high-affinity binding to DNA through intercalation, with consequent blockade of the synthesis of DNA and RNA, and DNA strand scission; (3) binding to cellular membranes to alter fluidity and ion transport; and (4) generation of semiquinone free radicals and oxygen free radicals through an enzyme-mediated reductive process. This latter mechanism has now been established as being the cause of the drug's cardiac toxicity.

Daunorubicin   **Doxorubicin**

In the clinical setting, anthracyclines are administered via the intravenous route (Table 55–4). The anthracyclines are metabolized extensively in the liver, with reduction and hydrolysis of the ring substituents. The hydroxylated metabolite is an active species, whereas the aglycone is inactive. Up to 50% of drug is eliminated in the feces via biliary excretion, and for this reason dose reduction is required in the setting of liver dysfunction. Although anthracyclines are usually administered on an every-3-week schedule, alternative schedules of administration such as low-dose weekly or 72–96 hour continuous infusions have been shown to yield equivalent clinical efficacy with reduced overall toxicity.

Doxorubicin is one of the most important anticancer drugs, with major clinical activity in carcinomas of the breast, endometrium, ovary, testicle, thyroid, stomach, bladder, liver, and lung; in soft tissue sarcomas; and in several childhood cancers, including neuroblastoma, Ewing's sarcoma, osteosarcoma, and rhabdomyosarcoma. It is also widely used in hematologic malignancies, including acute lymphoblastic leukemia, multiple myeloma, and Hodgkin's and non-Hodgkin's lymphomas. It is generally used in combination with other anticancer agents (eg, cyclophosphamide, cisplatin, and fluorouracil), and responses and remission duration tend to be improved with combination regimens as opposed to single-agent therapy. Daunorubicin has a far narrower spectrum of activity than doxorubicin. Daunorubicin has been mainly used for the treatment of acute myeloid leukemia, although there has been a shift in clinical practice toward using idarubicin, an analog of daunorubicin. Its efficacy in solid tumors appears to be limited.

Idarubicin is a semisynthetic anthracycline glycoside analog of daunorubicin and is approved for use in combination with cytarabine for induction therapy of acute myeloid leukemia. When combined with cytarabine, idarubicin appears to be more active than daunorubicin in producing complete remissions and in improving survival in patients with acute myelogenous leukemia.

Epirubicin is a doxorubicin analog whose mechanism of action is identical to that of all other anthracyclines. It was initially approved for use as a component of adjuvant therapy of early-stage, node-positive breast cancer but is now also used for the treatment of metastatic breast cancer.

The main dose-limiting toxicity of all anthracyclines is myelosuppression, with neutropenia more commonly observed than thrombocytopenia. In some cases, mucositis is dose-limiting. Two forms of cardiotoxicity are observed. The acute form occurs within the first 2–3 days and presents as arrhythmias or conduction abnormalities, other electrocardiographic changes, pericarditis, and myocarditis. This form is usually transient and is asymptomatic in most cases. The chronic form results in

a dose-dependent, dilated cardiomyopathy associated with heart failure. The chronic cardiac toxicity appears to result from increased production of free radicals within the myocardium. This effect is rarely seen at total doxorubicin dosages below 500–550 mg/m². Use of lower weekly doses or continuous infusions of doxorubicin appear to reduce the incidence of cardiac toxicity. In addition, treatment with the iron-chelating agent dexrazoxane (ICRF-187) is currently approved to prevent or reduce anthracycline-induced cardiotoxicity in women with metastatic breast cancer who have received a total cumulative dose of doxorubicin of 300 mg/m². All anthracyclines can produce "radiation recall reaction," with erythema and desquamation of the skin observed at sites of prior radiation therapy.

MITOXANTRONE

Mitoxantrone (dihydroxyanthracenedione, DHAD) is an anthracene compound whose structure resembles the anthracycline ring. It binds to DNA to produce strand breakage and inhibits both DNA and RNA synthesis. It is currently used for treatment of advanced, hormone-refractory prostate cancer and low-grade non-Hodgkin's lymphoma. It is also indicated in breast cancer as well as in pediatric and adult acute myeloid leukemias. The plasma half-life of mitoxantrone in patients is approximately 75 hours, and it is predominantly excreted via the hepatobiliary route in feces. Myelosuppression with leukopenia is the dose-limiting toxicity, and mild nausea and vomiting, mucositis, and alopecia also occur. While the drug is felt to be less cardiotoxic than doxorubicin, both acute and chronic cardiac toxicity are reported. A blue discoloration of the fingernails, sclera, and urine can be observed up to 1–2 days after drug therapy.

DACTINOMYCIN

Dactinomycin is an antitumor antibiotic isolated from a *Streptomyces* organism. It binds tightly to double-stranded DNA through intercalation between adjacent guanine-cytosine base pairs and inhibits all forms of DNA-dependent RNA synthesis, with ribosomal RNA formation being most sensitive to drug action.

Dactinomycin is mainly used to treat pediatric tumors such as Wilms' tumor, rhabdomyosarcoma, and Ewing's sarcoma, but it has activity also against germ cell tumors and gestational trophoblastic disease. Dactinomycin can also induce a "radiation recall reaction." See Table 55–4 for other toxicities.

MITOMYCIN

Mitomycin (mitomycin C) is an antibiotic isolated from *Streptomyces caespitosus*. It is an alkylating agent that undergoes metabolic activation through an enzyme-mediated reduction to generate an alkylating agent that cross-links DNA. Hypoxic tumor stem cells of solid tumors exist in an environment conducive to reductive reactions and are more sensitive to the cytotoxic actions of mitomycin than normal cells and oxygenated tumor cells. It is thought to be a CCNS alkylating agent, and it is the best available drug for use in combination with radiation therapy to attack hypoxic tumor cells. Its main clinical use is in the treatment of squamous cell cancer of the anus along with fluorouracil and radiation therapy. In addition, it is used in combination chemotherapy for squamous cell carcinoma of the cervix and for adenocarcinomas of the stomach, pancreas, and lung. One special application of mitomycin has been in the intravesical treatment of superficial bladder cancer. Because virtually none of the agent is absorbed systemically, there is little or no systemic toxicity.

Mitomycin

See Table 55–4 for common toxicities. The hemolytic-uremic syndrome, manifested as microangiopathic hemolytic anemia, thrombocytopenia, and renal failure, as well as occasional instances of interstitial pneumonitis have been reported.

BLEOMYCIN

Bleomycin is a small peptide that contains a DNA-binding region and an iron-binding domain at opposite ends of the molecule. It acts by binding to DNA, which results in single-strand and double-strand breaks following free radical formation, and inhibition of DNA biosynthesis. The fragmentation of DNA is due to oxidation of a DNA-bleomycin-Fe(II) complex and leads to chromosomal aberrations. Bleomycin is a CCS drug that causes accumulation of cells in the G_2 phase of the cell cycle.

Bleomycin is indicated for the treatment of Hodgkin's and non-Hodgkin's lymphomas, germ cell tumor, head and neck cancer, and squamous cell cancer of the skin, cervix, and vulva. In addition, it can be used as a sclerosing agent for malignant pleural effusions and ascites. One advantage of this agent is that it can be given subcutaneously, intramuscularly, or intravenously

(Table 55–4). Peak blood levels of bleomycin after intramuscular injection appear within 30–60 minutes. Intravenous injection of similar dosages yields higher peak concentrations and a terminal half-life of about 2.5 hours. Elimination of bleomycin is mainly via renal excretion; for this reason, dose modification is recommended in the setting of renal dysfunction.

Pulmonary toxicity is dose-limiting for bleomycin and usually presents as pneumonitis with cough, dyspnea, dry inspiratory crackles on physical examination, and infiltrates on chest x-ray. The incidence of this adverse event is increased in patients older than 70 years of age and with cumulative doses greater than 400 units. In rare cases, pulmonary toxicity can be fatal. Other toxicities are listed in Table 55–4.

HORMONAL AGENTS

STEROID HORMONES & ANTISTEROID DRUGS

The relationship between hormones and hormone-dependent tumors was initially demonstrated in 1896 when Beatson showed that oophorectomy produced improvement in women with advanced breast cancer. Sex hormones and adrenocortical hormones are employed in the management of several other types of cancer. Since sex hormones are actively involved in the stimulation and control of proliferation and function of certain tissues, including the mammary and prostate glands, cancers arising from these tissues may be inhibited or stimulated by appropriate changes in hormonal balance. Cancer of the breast and cancer of the prostate can be effectively treated with sex hormone therapy or ablation of appropriate endocrine organs.

Corticosteroids have been useful in the treatment of acute leukemia, lymphoma, multiple myeloma, and other hematologic malignancies as well as in advanced breast cancer. In addition, they are effective as supportive therapy in the management of cancer-related hypercalcemia. The steroid hormones and related agents most useful in cancer therapy are listed in Table 55–5.

The mechanisms of action of steroid hormones on lymphoid, mammary, and prostatic cancer have been partially clarified. Specific cell surface receptors have been identified for estrogen, progesterone, corticosteroids, and androgens in neoplastic cells in these tissues. As in normal cells, steroid hormones also form an intracellular steroid-receptor complex that ultimately binds directly to nuclear proteins associated with DNA to activate transcription of a broad range of cellular genes involved in cell growth and proliferation (see Chapter 39).

Most steroid-sensitive cancers express specific cell

Table 55–5. Hormonally active agents: Dosages and toxicities.

Drug	Usual Adult Dosage	Acute Toxicity	Delayed Toxicity
Antiandrogen			
Flutamide	250 mg/tid orally	Mild nausea	Hot flushes, transient elevations in liver function tests
Antiestrogen			
Tamoxifen	20 mg/d orally	Transient flare of tumor symptoms	Menopausal symptoms, fluid retention and edema, thromboembolic events, increased incidence of endometrial hyperplasia and cancer
Progestins			
Megestrol acetate	40 mg orally 4 times daily	None	Fluid retention
Adrenocorticosteroids			
Hydrocortisone	40–200 mg/d orally	None	Fluid retention, hypertension, diabetes, increased susceptibility to infection, moon facies
Prednisone	20–100 mg/d orally	None	
Gonadotropin-releasing hormone agonists			
Goserelin acetate	3.6 mg SC monthly	Transient flare of tumor symptoms, pain at injection site	Hot flushes, impotence, gynecomastia
Leuprolide	7.5 mg SC monthly	Transient flare of tumor symptoms, pain at injection site	Hot flushes, impotence, gynecomastia
Aromatase inhibitors			
Aminoglutethimide	250 mg orally twice daily and hydrocortisone 20 mg twice daily	Fatigue, mild nausea	Skin rash, adrenal insufficiency, myelosuppression
Anastrozole	1 mg orally daily	Mild nausea, headache	Fatigue, hot flushes, arthralgias
Exemestane	25 mg orally daily	Mild nausea, headache	Fatigue, hot flushes
Letrozole	2.5 mg orally daily	Mild nausea, headache	Fatigue, hot flushes, arthralgias

surface receptors. Prednisone-sensitive lymphomas, estrogen-sensitive breast cancers, and prostatic cancers express specific receptors for corticosteroids, estrogens, and androgens, respectively. It is now possible to assay tumor specimens for steroid receptor content and to identify which individual patients are likely to benefit from hormonal therapy. Measurement of the estrogen receptor (ER) and progesterone receptor (PR) proteins in breast cancer tissue is now standard clinical practice. ER or PR positivity predicts response to hormonal therapy, whereas patients whose tumors are ER-negative generally fail to respond to such treatment.

The sex hormones are used in the treatment of cancers of the breast, prostate, and endometrium. With replacement doses, estrogen can stimulate the growth of breast and endometrial cancer. Surprisingly, high-dose estrogen is useful therapeutically in metastatic breast cancer but has been largely replaced by antiestrogen therapy. In prostate cancer, androgens stimulate growth while estrogen administration results in suppression of androgen production. Drugs that reduce androgen secretion or block the effect of androgens at the receptor level are also effective in prostate cancer.

The toxicities of adrenocortical hormones are presented in Chapter 39 and those of estrogens and androgens in Chapter 40.

ESTROGEN & ANDROGEN INHIBITORS

The antiestrogen **tamoxifen** has proved to be extremely useful for the treatment of both early-stage and metastatic breast cancer. It is now approved as a chemopreventive agent in women at high risk for breast cancer. In addition, this hormonal agent has activity in endometrial cancer. Tamoxifen functions as a competitive partial agonist-inhibitor of estrogen and binds to the estrogen receptors of estrogen-sensitive tumors. However, tamoxifen has a tenfold lower affinity for ER than does estradiol, indicating the importance of ablation of endogenous estrogen for optimal antiestrogen effect. In addition to its direct antiestrogen effects on tumor cells, tamoxifen also suppresses serum levels of insulin-like growth factor 1 and up regulates local production of transforming growth factor-beta (TGF-β).

Tamoxifen

Tamoxifen is given orally and is rapidly and completely absorbed. High plasma levels of tamoxifen are obtained within 4–6 hours after oral administration, and the agent has a much longer biologic half-life than estradiol—on the order of 7–14 days. It is extensively metabolized by the liver P450 system, and the main metabolites also possess antitumor activity similar to that of the parent drug. Tamoxifen is well tolerated, and its side effects are generally quite mild (Table 55–5). **Flutamide** and **bicalutamide** are nonsteroidal antiandrogen agents that bind to the androgen receptor and inhibit androgen effects. They are administered orally and are rapidly and completely absorbed by the gastrointestinal tract. At present they are used in combination with radiation therapy for the treatment of early-stage prostate cancer and in the setting of metastatic prostate cancer. Toxicities are listed in Table 55–5.

GONADOTROPIN-RELEASING HORMONE AGONISTS

Leuprolide and **goserelin** are synthetic peptide analogs of naturally occurring gonadotropin-releasing hormone (GnRH, LHRH). They are described in further detail in Chapters 37 and 40. These analogs are more potent than the natural hormone and function as LHRH ago-

nists. When given as depot preparations, these agents lead to a transient release of follicle-stimulating hormone (FSH) and luteinizing hormone (LH) followed by inhibition of the release of these gonadotropins. In men, this results in castration levels of testosterone after 2–4 weeks of therapy.

Leuprolide and goserelin are indicated in the treatment of advanced prostate cancer and more recently these agents have been incorporated as part of neoadjuvant therapy of early-stage prostate cancer. Leuprolide and goserelin are now formulated in long-acting depot forms, which allows for administration once every 3 months. The main side effects include hot flushes, impotence, and gynecomastia. Other toxicities are given in Table 55–5.

AROMATASE INHIBITORS

Aminoglutethimide is a nonsteroidal inhibitor of corticosteroid synthesis at the first step involving the conversion of cholesterol to pregnenolone; see Chapter 39). Aminoglutethimide also inhibits the extra-adrenal synthesis of estrone and estradiol. Aside from its direct effects on adrenal steroidogenesis, aminoglutethimide is an inhibitor of an aromatase enzyme that converts the adrenal androgen androstenedione to estrone (Figure 40–2). This aromatization of an androgenic precursor into an estrogen occurs in body fat. Since estrogens promote the growth of breast cancer, estrogen synthesis in adipose tissue can be important in breast cancer growth in postmenopausal women.

Aminoglutethimide is primarily used in the treatment of metastatic breast cancer in women whose tumors express significant levels of estrogen or progesterone receptors. It also has activity in advanced prostate cancer that is hormone-responsive. Aminoglutethimide is normally administered with hydrocortisone to prevent symptoms of adrenal insufficiency. Hydrocortisone is preferable to dexamethasone because the latter agent accelerates the rate of catabolism of aminoglutethimide. Adverse effects of aminoglutethimide are listed in Table 55–5.

Anastrozole is a selective nonsteroidal inhibitor of aromatase that has no inhibitory effect on adrenal glucocorticoid or mineralocorticoid synthesis. It is presently approved for first-line treatment of postmenopausal women with metastatic breast cancer that is ER-positive, for treatment of postmenopausal women with metastatic breast cancer that is ER-positive and has progressed while on tamoxifen therapy, and as adjuvant therapy of postmenopausal women with hormone-positive, early-stage breast cancer. **Letrozole** is a nonsteroidal competitive inhibitor of aromatase that is significantly more potent than aminoglutethimide and acts in the same way as anastrozole. It is also indicated for first-line treatment of postmenopausal women with hormone receptor-positive metastatic breast cancer and for second-line treatment of postmenopausal women with advanced breast cancer after progression on tamoxifen therapy. **Exemestane** is a steroidal hormonal agent that binds to and irreversibly inactivates aromatase. There appears to be a lack of cross-resistance between exemestane and nonsteroidal aromatase inhibitors. This agent is indicated for the treatment of advanced breast cancer in postmenopausal women whose disease has progressed on tamoxifen therapy. Each of these aromatase inhibitors exhibits a similar side effect profile (Table 55–5, see also Chapter 40).

MISCELLANEOUS ANTICANCER DRUGS (SEE TABLE 55–6.)

IMATINIB

Imatinib (STI571) is an inhibitor of the tyrosine kinase domain of the Bcr-Abl oncoprotein and prevents the phosphorylation of the kinase substrate by ATP. It is indicated for the treatment of chronic myelogenous leukemia (CML), a pluripotent hematopoietic stem cell disorder characterized by the t(9:22) Philadelphia chromosomal translocation. This translocation results in the Bcr-Abl fusion protein, the causative agent in CML, and is present in up to 95% of patients with this disease.

This agent inhibits other activated receptor tyrosine kinases for platelet-derived growth factor receptor (PDGFR), stem cell factor (SCF), and c-kit.

Imatinib is administered orally and is well absorbed; it is highly protein-bound in plasma. The drug is metabolized in the liver, and elimination of metabolites occurs mainly in feces via biliary excretion. This agent is approved for use as first-line therapy in chronic phase CML, in blast crisis, and as second-line therapy for chronic phase CML that has progressed on prior interferon-α therapy. Imatinib is effective also for treatment of gastrointestinal stromal tumors expressing the c-kit tyrosine kinase. Dosage and toxicities are listed in Table 55–6.

ASPARAGINASE

Asparaginase (L-asparagine amidohydrolase) is an enzyme that is isolated from various bacteria for clinical use. The drug is used to treat childhood acute lymphocytic leukemia. It hydrolyzes circulating L-asparagine to aspartic acid and ammonia. Because tumor cells lack asparagine synthetase, they require an exogenous source of L-asparagine. Thus, depletion of L-asparagine results in effective inhibition of protein synthesis. In contrast, normal cells can synthesize L-asparagine and thus are less susceptible to the cytotoxic action of asparaginase. The main side effect of this agent is a hypersensitivity reaction manifested by fever, chills, nausea and vomit-

Table 55–6. Miscellaneous anticancer drugs: Dosages and toxicities.

Drug	Usual Dosage	Acute Toxicity	Delayed Toxicity
Arsenic trioxide	0.15 mg/kg/d IV for 60 days as induction therapy; 0.15 mg/kg/d IV for 5 days per week for a total of 5 weeks as consolidation therapy	Headache and lightheadedness	Fatigue, cardiac dysrhythmias, fever, dyspnea, fluid retention and weight gain
Asparaginase	20,000 IU/m² daily IV for 5–10 days	Nausea, fever, and allergic reactions	Hepatotoxicity, mental depression, pancreatitis
Imatinib	400–600 mg/d orally	Nausea and vomiting	Fluid retention with ankle and periorbital edema, diarrhea, myalgias
Hydroxyurea	300 mg/m² orally for 5 days	Nausea and vomiting	Bone marrow depression
Mitotane	6–15 g/d orally	Nausea and vomiting	Diarrhea, lethargy, adrenal insufficiency, transient skin rash
Mitoxantrone	10–12 mg/m² IV every 3–4 weeks	Nausea	Bone marrow depression, occasional cardiac toxicity, mild alopecia
Trastuzumab[1]	4 mg/kg IV loading dose; 2 mg/kg/wk as maintenance	Nausea and vomiting, infusion-related hypersensitivity reaction	Cardiomyopathy, myelosuppression, pulmonary toxicity

[1]This monoclonal antibody is described in Chapter 56.

ing, skin rash, and urticaria. Severe cases can present with bronchospasm, respiratory failure, and hypotension. Other toxicities include an increased risk of both clotting and bleeding as a result of alterations in various clotting factors, pancreatitis, and neurologic toxicity with lethargy, confusion, hallucinations, and coma.

HYDROXYUREA

Hydroxyurea ($HONHCONH_2$) is an analog of urea whose mechanism of action involves the inhibition of DNA synthesis in the S phase by inhibiting the enzyme ribonucleotide reductase, resulting in depletion of deoxynucleoside triphosphate pools. The drug is administered orally and has nearly 100% oral bioavailability. It is mainly used in chronic myelogenous leukemia and treatment of the blast crisis of acute myeloid leukemia. However, it is also effective as an adjunct with radiation therapy for head and neck cancer and in treating essential thrombocytosis and polycythemia vera. Myelosuppression is the dose-limiting toxicity, but nausea and vomiting, mucositis and diarrhea, headache and increased lethargy, and a maculopapular skin rash with pruritus are also observed.

MITOTANE

This drug (Figure 39–5) is a dichloro analog of the insecticide DDT that was first found to be adrenolytic in dogs. Subsequently, it was found to be useful in the treatment of an adrenocortical carcinoma, and it is labeled for this clinical indication. The drug produces tumor regression and reduces the excessive adrenal steroid secretion that often occurs with this malignancy. Toxicities are listed in Table 55–6.

RETINOIC ACID DERIVATIVES

All-*trans*-Retinoic acid (**tretinoin**) produces remissions in patients with acute promyelocytic leukemia (APL) through the induction of terminal differentiation, in which the leukemic promyelocytes lose their ability to proliferate. APL is associated with a t(15;17) chromosomal translocation, which disrupts the gene for the nuclear receptor-α for retinoic acid and fuses it to a gene called *PML*. This chimeric gene, which expresses aberrant forms of the retinoic acid receptor-α, is present in virtually all patients with promyelocytic leukemia and appears to be responsible for sensitivity to all-*trans*-retinoic acid. This agent is approved for use in APL following progression or relapse with anthracycline-based chemotherapy and for patients in whom anthracycline-based chemotherapy is contraindicated. However, a number of serious adverse events have been observed, and they include vitamin A toxicity manifesting as headache, fever, dry skin and mucous membranes, skin rash, pruritus, and conjunctivitis; retinoic acid syndrome with fever, leukocytosis, dysp-

nea, weight gain, diffuse pulmonary infiltrates, and pleural or pericardial effusions; increased serum cholesterol and triglyceride levels; central nervous system toxicity in the form of dizziness, anxiety, depression, confusion, and agitation; abdominal pain and diarrhea; and transient elevations in liver function tests. Finally, this retinoid has been shown to be teratogenic.

13-*cis*-Retinoic acid (**isotretinoin**) is used for the treatment of severe cystic acne (Chapter 62). It also appears to have significant clinical activity as an adjuvant to prevent second primary tumors in patients with head and neck squamous cell carcinoma and may also have activity in the chemoprevention of non-small cell lung cancer. However, it remains an investigational agent for cancer chemotherapy in the USA, and further clinical studies are under way to confirm its true clinical benefit.

ARSENIC TRIOXIDE

Arsenic trioxide (AS_2O_3) is used for induction of remission in patients with acute promyelocytic leukemia with the t(15;17) chromosomal translocation refractory to or relapsed following first-line therapy with all-*trans*-retinoic acid- and anthracycline-based chemotherapy. It functions by inducing differentiation through degradation of the chimeric PML/RAR-alpha protein. In addition, it induces apoptosis through a mitochondrion-dependent process, resulting in subsequent release of cytochrome C with caspase activation. This drug is administered via the intravenous route and it is widely distributed in the body. The main toxicities are fatigue, electrocardiographic changes with QT prolongation, arrhythmias, and a syndrome characterized by fever, dyspnea, skin rash, fluid retention, and weight gain.

BONE MARROW GROWTH FACTORS

Use of bone marrow-stimulating factors with chemotherapy can reduce the frequency and severity of neutropenic sepsis and other complications. Two recombinant bone marrow growth factors that stimulate neutrophil growth are available: granulocyte colony-stimulating factor (G-CSF, filgrastim; and pegfilgrastim, long-acting filgrastim) and granulocyte-macrophage colony-stimulating factor (GM-CSF, sargramostim) (Chapter 33). Both sargramostim and filgrastim can reduce the incidence of neutropenia and prevent the onset of infection when used as an adjunct to chemotherapy and can also shorten hospitalization after bone marrow transplantation. There are currently two colony-stimulating growth factors for red blood cells: darbopoetin alfa and erythropoietin. They are indicated for chemotherapy-induced anemia in patients with nonmyeloid cancer, as well as for anemia associated with chronic renal failure.

AMIFOSTINE

Amifostine (WR-2721) is an organic thiophosphate analog designed to produce preferential cytoprotection of normal tissues from cytotoxic therapies. The preferential cytoprotection is due to the activation of amifostine by membrane-bound alkaline phosphatase to the free thiol, WR-1065, the active form. This activation occurs to a greater extent in normal tissue sites than in tumor cells. The free thiol acts as a potent scavenger of free radicals and superoxide anions to inactivate the reactive species of cisplatin and radiation therapy. At present, this agent is approved to reduce the incidence of nephrotoxicity in ovarian cancer and non-small cell lung cancer in conjunction with cisplatin-based chemotherapy and to reduce the incidence of xerostomia in patients undergoing radiation therapy for head and neck cancer. Amifostine does not appear to adversely affect the antitumor activity of cisplatin or radiation therapy. Recent studies suggest that amifostine can reduce the incidence of pneumonitis and esophagitis secondary to combined modality therapy for non-small cell lung cancer, and there is also evidence that it can stimulate bone marrow growth in patients with marrow disorders such as the myelodysplastic syndrome.

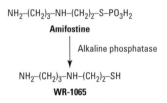

$$NH_2-(CH_2)_3-NH-(CH_2)_2-S-PO_3H_2$$

Amifostine

Alkaline phosphatase

$$NH_2-(CH_2)_3-NH-(CH_2)_2-SH$$

WR-1065

INVESTIGATIONAL AGENTS

Several of the drugs mentioned in the text remain investigational in the USA until their clinical efficacy and safety can be fully established. In specific instances where treatment with one of these agents seems warranted, it usually can be arranged through a compassionate use program either by contacting the pharmaceutical sponsor of the drug or by contacting the Division of Cancer Treatment of the National Cancer Institute and the Food and Drug Administration, which can provide further information and identify investigators who are authorized to administer these drugs. This status applies to gefitinib, a small molecule inhibitor of the tyrosine kinase domain of the epidermal growth factor (EGF) receptor; cetuximab, a chimeric monoclonal antibody directed specifically against the EGF receptor; pemetrexed, an inhibitor of thymidylate synthase, dihydrofolate reductase, and enzymes involved in de novo purine synthesis; suramin, an inhibitor of various

growth factors including basic fibroblast growth factor; and several others.

II. CLINICAL PHARMACOLOGY OF CANCER CHEMOTHERAPEUTIC DRUGS

A thorough knowledge of the kinetics of tumor cell proliferation along with an enhanced understanding of the pharmacology and mechanism of action of cancer chemotherapeutic agents is critically important in designing optimal regimens for patients with cancer (Table 55–7). The strategy for developing drug regimens requires a knowledge of the particular characteristics of specific tumors—eg, Is there a high growth fraction? Is there a high spontaneous cell death rate? Are most of the cells in G_0? Is a significant fraction of the tumor composed of hypoxic stem cells? Are their normal counterparts under hormonal control? Similarly, knowledge of the pharmacology of specific drugs is equally important—eg, Does the drug have a particular affinity for uptake by the tumor cells (streptozocin)? Are the tumor cells sensitive to the drug? Is the drug cell cycle-specific? Does the drug require activation in certain normal tissue such as the liver, or is it activated in the tumor tissue itself (capecitabine)? Similarly, for some tumor types, knowledge of receptor expression is important. For example, in patients with breast cancer, analysis of the tumor for expression of estrogen or progesterone receptors—or overexpression of HER-2 receptors—is important in guiding therapy. Knowledge of specific pathway abnormalities (eg, Ras pathway) for intracellular signaling may prove important for the next generation of anticancer drugs.

Drugs that affect cycling cells can often be used most effectively after treatment with a cell cycle-nonspecific agent (eg, alkylating agents); this principle has been tested in a few human tumors with increasing success. Similarly, recognition of true drug synergism (tumor cell kill by the drug combination greater than the additive effects of the individual drugs) or antagonism is important in the design of combination chemotherapeutic programs. The combination of cytarabine with an anthracycline in acute myelogenous leukemia and the use of vinblastine or etoposide along with cisplatin and bleomycin in testicular tumors are good examples of true drug synergism against cancer cells but not against normal tissues.

In general, it is preferable to use cytotoxic chemotherapeutic agents in intensive pulse courses every 3–4 weeks rather than to use continuous daily dosage schedules. This allows for maximum effects against neoplastic cell populations with complete hematologic and immunologic recovery between courses rather than leaving the patient continuously suppressed

Table 55–7. Malignancies responsive to chemotherapy.

Diagnosis	Current Treatment of Choice	Other Valuable Agents
Acute lymphocytic leukemia	Induction: vincristine plus prednisone. Remission maintenance: mercaptopurine, methotrexate, and cyclophosphamide in various combinations	Asparaginase, daunorubicin, carmustine, doxorubicin, cytarabine, allopurinol,[1] craniospinal radiotherapy
Acute myelocytic and myelomonocytic leukemia	Combination chemotherapy: cytarabine and mitoxantrone or daunorubicin or idarubicin	Methotrexate, thioguanine, mercaptopurine, allopurinol,[1] mitoxantrone, azacitidine,[2] amsacrine,[2] etoposide
Chronic lymphocytic leukemia	Chlorambucil and prednisone (if indicated), fludarabine	Allopurinol,[1] doxorubicin, cladribine
Chronic myelogenous leukemia	Imatinib, busulfan, or interferon, bone marrow transplantation (selected patients)	Vincristine, mercaptopurine, hydroxyurea, melphalan, interferon, allopurinol[1]
Hodgkin's disease (stages III and IV)	Combination chemotherapy: vinblastine, doxorubicin, dacarbazine, bleomycin	Lomustine, etoposide, ifosfamide, interferon, mechlorethamine, vincristine, procarbazine, prednisone
Non-Hodgkin's lymphoma	Combination chemotherapy: cyclophosphamide, doxorubicin, vincristine, prednisone	Bleomycin, lomustine, carmustine, etoposide, interferon, mitoxantrone, ifosfamide, rituximab
Multiple myeloma	Melphalan plus prednisone or multiagent combination chemotherapy	Cyclophosphamide, vincristine, carmustine, interferon, doxorubicin, epoetin alfa[1]
Macroglobulinemia	Chlorambucil or fludarabine	Prednisone
Polycythemia vera	Busulfan, chlorambucil, or cyclophosphamide	Radioactive phosphorus 32
Carcinoma of adrenal	Mitotane	Suramin[2]
Carcinoma of breast	(1) Adjuvant chemotherapy or tamoxifen after primary breast surgery (2) Combination chemotherapy or hormonal manipulation for late recurrence	Cyclophosphamide, doxorubicin, vincristine, methotrexate, fluorouracil, paclitaxel, mitoxantrone, prednisone,[1] megestrol, androgens,[1] aminoglutethimide, trastuzumab
Carcinoma of cervix	Radiation plus cisplatin (localized), cisplatin, carboplatin (metastatic)	Lomustine, cyclophosphamide, doxorubicin, methotrexate, mitomycin, bleomycin, vincristine, interferon, 13-*cis*-retinoic acid
Carcinoma of colon	Fluorouracil plus leucovorin plus irinotecan	Oxaliplatin
Carcinoma of endometrium	Progestins or tamoxifen	Doxorubicin, cisplatin, carboplatin
Carcinoma of lung	Cisplatin plus taxane	Methotrexate, vincristine, vinblastine, doxorubicin, mitomycin C
Carcinoma of ovary	Cisplatin or carboplatin plus paclitaxel	Cyclophosphamide, doxorubicin, melphalan, fluorouracil, vincristine, altretamine, bleomycin
Carcinoma of pancreas	Gemcitabine	Docetaxel, fluorouracil
Carcinoma of prostate	GnRH agonist plus androgen antagonist	Aminoglutethimide, doxorubicin, cisplatin, prednisone,[1] estramustine, fluorouracil, progestins, suramin[2]
Carcinoma of stomach	Fluorouracil plus cisplatin	Hydroxyurea, lomustine
Carcinoma of testis	Combination chemotherapy: cisplatin, bleomycin, and etoposide	Methotrexate, dactinomycin, plicamycin, vinblastine, doxorubicin, cyclophosphamide, etoposide, ifosfamide plus mesna[1]

(continued)

Table 55–7. Malignancies responsive to chemotherapy (*continued*).

Diagnosis	Current Treatment of Choice	Other Valuable Agents
Carcinoma of thyroid	Radioiodine (^{131}I), doxorubicin, cisplatin	Bleomycin, fluorouracil, melphalan
Carcinomas of head and neck	Fluorouracil plus cisplatin, cisplatin plus paclitaxel	Methotrexate, bleomycin, hydroxyurea, doxorubicin, vincristine, vinorelbine
Choriocarcinoma (trophoblastic neoplasms)	Methotrexate alone or etoposide and cisplatin	Vinblastine, mercaptopurine, chlorambucil, doxorubicin
Wilms' tumor	Vincristine plus dactinomycin after surgery and radiotherapy	Methotrexate, cyclophosphamide, doxorubicin
Neuroblastoma	Cyclophosphamide plus doxorubicin and vincristine	Dactinomycin, daunorubicin, cisplatin
Carcinoid	Doxorubicin plus cyclophosphamide, fluorouracil, octreotide	Interferon, dactinomycin, methysergide,[1] streptozocin
Insulinoma	Streptozocin, interferon	Doxorubicin, fluorouracil, mitomycin, streptozocin
Osteogenic sarcoma	Doxorubicin, or methotrexate with leucovorin rescue initiated after surgery	Cyclophosphamide, dacarbazine, interferon, ifosfamide plus mesna[1]
Miscellaneous sarcomas	Doxorubicin plus dacarbazine	Methotrexate, dactinomycin, ifosfamide plus mesna,[1] vincristine, vinblastine
Melanoma	Dacarbazine, cisplatin, temozolomide	Lomustine, hydroxyurea, mitomycin, dactinomycin, interferon, tamoxifen

[1]Supportive agent, not oncolytic.

[2]Investigational agent. Treatment available through qualified investigators and centers authorized by National Cancer Institute and Cooperative Oncology Groups.

with cytotoxic therapy. This approach reduces adverse effects but does not reduce therapeutic efficacy.

The application of these principles is well illustrated in the current approach to the treatment of acute leukemia, lymphomas, Wilms' tumor, and testicular neoplasms.

Adjuvant Chemotherapy

One of the most important roles for effective cancer chemotherapy is as an adjuvant to initial or primary field treatment with other methods such as surgery or radiation therapy. Failures with primary field therapy are due principally to occult micrometastases outside the primary field. With the currently available treatment modalities, this form of combined-modality therapy appears to offer the greatest chance of curing patients with solid tumors.

Distant micrometastases are usually present in patients with one or more positive lymph nodes at the time of surgery (eg, in breast cancer) and in patients with tumors having a known propensity for early hematogenous spread (eg, osteogenic sarcoma, Wilms' tumor). The risk of recurrent or metastatic disease in such patients is extremely high (80%). Only systemic therapy can adequately attack micrometastases. Chemotherapy regimens that are at least moderately effective against advanced cancer may have curative potential (at the right dosage and schedule) when combined with primary therapy such as surgery. Several studies show that adjuvant chemotherapy prolongs both disease-free and overall survival in patients with osteogenic sarcoma, rhabdomyosarcoma, or breast cancer. Similar comments apply to the use of three cycles of combination chemotherapy (eg, MOPP) prior to total nodal radiation in stage IIB Hodgkin's disease.

In breast cancer, premenopausal women with positive lymph nodes at the time of mastectomy have benefited from combination chemotherapy. It has been established that several programs of cytotoxic chemotherapy achieve prolonged disease-free and overall survival times; this method of treatment has increased the cure rate in high-risk primary breast cancer. In general, regimens with at least three active drugs have been useful. The results produced by combination chemotherapy are superior to those produced by single agents because combination chemotherapy copes better with tumor cell heterogeneity and produces a greater tumor cell log kill. Full protocol doses of cytotoxic agents are required to maximize the likelihood of efficacy. Clinical trials have proved tamoxifen to be an effective adjuvant in postmenopausal women with positive estrogen receptor tests on the primary tumor. Because it is cytostatic rather than cytocidal, adjuvant therapy with tamoxifen is usually administered for 5 years. A recent trial in women with node-negative disease showed no additional advantage with 10 years of tamoxifen therapy. Tamoxifen adjuvant chemotherapy is now standard in node-positive postmenopausal women with positive ER or PR tests on tumor specimens. Tamoxifen has also received regulatory approval for reducing the incidence of breast cancer in women who are at high risk for developing the disease.

Other applications of adjuvant chemotherapy include colorectal cancer, testicular cancer, head and neck cancer, and gynecologic neoplasms. In a recent large-scale trial in patients with primary melanoma at high risk of metastases, intensive administration of interferon alfa improved disease-free survival. Thus, adjuvant chemotherapy (with curative intent) should now be considered for patients who undergo primary surgical staging and therapy and are found to have a stage and histologic type of cancer with a high risk of micrometastasis. This policy is germane to those tumor types for which palliative chemotherapy has already been developed and has been shown to induce complete remissions in advanced stages of the disease. In each instance, the benefit:risk ratio must be closely examined.

Combined-modality therapy—radiation plus cisplatin—for localized carcinoma of the cervix has recently proved to achieve long-term survival rates superior to those reported with radiation alone.

Primary chemotherapy (prior to local surgery) is now extensively used in patients with osteogenic sarcoma and has facilitated limb-sparing procedures. Primary chemotherapy is also being evaluated in breast cancer to "downstage" patients prior to surgery.

THE LEUKEMIAS

1. *Acute Leukemia*

Childhood Leukemia

Acute lymphoblastic leukemia (ALL) is the predominant form of leukemia in childhood, and it is the most com-

mon form of cancer in children. Children with this disease have a relatively good prognosis. A subset of patients with neoplastic lymphocytes expressing surface antigenic features of T lymphocytes have a poor prognosis (see Chapter 56). A cytoplasmic enzyme expressed by normal thymocytes, terminal deoxycytidyl transferase (terminal transferase), is also expressed in many cases of ALL. T cell ALLs also express high levels of the enzyme adenosine deaminase (ADA). This led to interest in the use of the ADA inhibitor pentostatin (deoxycoformycin) for treatment of such T cell cases. Until 1948, the median length of survival in ALL was 3 months. With the advent of the folic acid antagonists, the length of survival was greatly increased. Subsequently, corticosteroids, mercaptopurine, cyclophosphamide, vincristine, daunorubicin, and asparaginase were all found to act against this disease. A combination of vincristine and prednisone plus other agents is currently used to induce remission. Over 90% of children enter complete remission with this therapy with only minimal toxicity. However, circulating leukemic cells often migrate to sanctuary sites located in the brain and testes. The value of prophylactic intrathecal methotrexate therapy for prevention of central nervous system leukemia (a major mechanism of relapse) has been clearly demonstrated. Intrathecal therapy with methotrexate should therefore be considered as a standard component of the induction regimen for children with ALL.

Adult Leukemia

Acute myelogenous leukemia (AML) is the most common leukemia seen in adults. The single most active agent for AML is cytarabine; however, it is best used in combination with an anthracycline, in which case complete remissions occur in about 70% of patients. Idarubicin has now replaced daunorubicin as the preferred anthracycline.

Patients often require intensive supportive care during the period of induction chemotherapy. Such care includes platelet transfusions to prevent bleeding, filgrastim to shorten periods of neutropenia, and antibiotics to combat infections. Younger patients (eg, < age 55) who are in complete remission and have an HLA-matched donor are candidates for allogeneic bone marrow transplantation. The transplant procedure is preceded by high-dose chemotherapy and total body irradiation followed by immunosuppression. This approach may cure up to 35–40% of eligible patients. Patients over age 60 respond less well to chemotherapy, primarily because their tolerance for aggressive therapy and their resistance to infection is lower.

Once remission of AML is achieved, consolidation chemotherapy is required to maintain a durable remission and to induce cure. The usual approach is to administer up to four courses of high-dose cytarabine.

2. Chronic Myelogenous Leukemia

Chronic myelogenous leukemia (CML) arises from a chromosomally abnormal hematopoietic stem cell in which a balanced translocation between the long arms of chromosomes 9 and 22, t(9:22), is observed in 90–95% of cases. This translocation results in expression of the Bcr-Abl fusion oncoprotein with a molecular weight of 210 kDa, which is constitutively expressed. The clinical symptoms and course are related to the white blood cell count and its rate of increase. Most patients with white cell counts over 50,000/μL should be treated. The goals of treatment are to reduce the granulocytes to normal levels, to raise the hemoglobin concentration to normal, and to relieve disease-related symptoms. There has been a significant change in the management of this disease. Recently, the signal transduction inhibitor imatinib was approved for use as first-line therapy in previously untreated patients with chronic phase CML. Imatinib is also recommended in patients with chronic phase disease who have failed prior interferon alfa therapy. Nearly all patients treated with imatinib exhibit a complete hematologic response, and up to 40–50% of patients will show a complete cytogenetic response. The usual dose for chronic phase disease is 400 mg/d, and an advantage of this drug is that it is given orally. As described previously, this drug is extremely well tolerated and is associated with relatively minor side effects. Other treatment options include interferon alfa, busulfan, other oral alkylating agents, and hydroxyurea.

3. Chronic Lymphocytic Leukemia

Patients with early-stage chronic lymphocytic leukemia (CLL) have a relatively good prognosis, and therapy has not changed the course of the disease. However, in the setting of high-risk disease or in the presence of disease-related symptoms, treatment is indicated.

The purine nucleoside analog fludarabine is rapidly becoming the treatment of choice in CLL. Fludarabine can be given alone or used in combination with cyclophosphamide and with mitoxantrone and dexamethasone. The most commonly used single chemotherapeutic agent has been the alkylating agent chlorambucil. The dosage is usually 0.1 mg/kg/d, with monitoring of blood counts at weekly intervals. Chlorambucil is frequently combined with prednisone, although there is no clear evidence that the combination yields better response rates or survival compared with chlorambucil alone. Alternatively, cyclophosphamide can be given, usually in dosages of 1–2 g/m² every 3–4 weeks. In most cases, cyclophosphamide is given in combination with vincristine and prednisone (COP protocol), or it can also be given with these same drugs along with doxorubicin (CHOP).

Monoclonal antibody-targeted therapies are being more widely used in CLL, especially in relapsed or refractory disease. Alemtuzumab is a chimeric monoclonal antibody directed against the CD52 antigen and is approved for use in CLL that is refractory to alkylating agent or fludarabine therapy. Response rates up to 30–35% are observed, with disease stabilization in another 30% of patients. Rituximab is an anti-CD20 antibody that also has clinical activity in this setting.

THE LYMPHOMAS

1. Hodgkin's Disease

The treatment of Hodgkin's disease has undergone dramatic evolution over the last 30 years. Hodgkin's disease is now recognized as a B cell neoplasm in which the malignant Reed-Sternberg cells have rearranged *VH* genes. In addition, the Epstein-Barr virus genome has been identified in up to 80% of tumor specimens.

Complete staging evaluation is required before a definitive treatment plan can be made. For patients with stage I and stage IIA disease, there has been a significant change in the treatment approach. Initially, these patients were treated with extended-field radiation therapy. However, given the late effects of radiation therapy, which include hypothyroidism and an increased risk of secondary cancers and coronary artery disease, combined-modality therapy with a brief course of combination chemotherapy and involved field radiation therapy is now the recommended approach. The main advance for patients with advanced stage III and IV Hodgkin's disease came with the development of MOPP (mechlorethamine, vincristine, procarbazine, and prednisone) chemotherapy in the 1960s. This regimen resulted initially in high complete response rates—on the order of 80–90%, with cures in up to 60% of patients. Over the past few years, the anthracycline-containing regimen ABVD (doxorubicin, bleomycin, vinblastine, and dacarbazine) has been shown to be more effective and less toxic than MOPP, especially with regard to the incidence of sterility and secondary malignancies. This regimen uses four cycles of ABVD. The Stanford group has developed an alternative regimen wherein a 12-week course of combination chemotherapy, termed Stanford V (doxorubicin, vinblastine, mechlorethamine, vincristine, bleomycin, etoposide, and prednisone) is followed by involved radiation therapy.

With all these regimens, over 80% of previously untreated patients with advanced Hodgkin's disease (stages III and IV) are expected to go into complete remission, with disappearance of all disease-related symptoms and objective evidence of disease. Approximately 50–60% of all patients with Hodgkin's disease are cured of their disease.

2. Non-Hodgkin's Lymphomas

Over the past 25 years, there has been a dramatic increase, by over 80%, in the incidence of non-Hodgkin's lymphoma. This is a heterogeneous disease, and the clinical characteristics of non-Hodgkin's lymphoma subsets are related to the underlying histopathologic features and the extent of disease involvement. In general, the nodular (or follicular) lymphomas have a far better prognosis, with a median survival up to 7 years, compared with the diffuse lymphomas, which have a median survival of about 1–2 years.

Combination chemotherapy is the treatment standard for patients with diffuse non-Hodgkin's lymphoma. The anthracycline-containing regimen CHOP (cyclophosphamide, doxorubicin, vincristine, and prednisone) has been considered the best treatment in terms of initial therapy. Recently, randomized phase III clinical studies have shown that the combination of CHOP with the anti-CD20 monoclonal antibody rituximab results in improved response rates, disease-free survival, and overall survival compared with CHOP chemotherapy alone.

The nodular follicular lymphomas are low-grade, indolent tumors that tend to present in an advanced stage and are usually confined to lymph nodes, bone marrow, and spleen. This form of non-Hodgkin's lymphomas, when presenting at an advanced stage, is considered incurable, and treatment is generally palliative. To date, there is no evidence that immediate treatment with combination chemotherapy offers clinical benefit over close observation and "watchful waiting" with initiation of chemotherapy at the time of disease symptoms.

MULTIPLE MYELOMA

This plasma cell malignancy is one of the models of neoplastic disease in humans because it arises from a single tumor stem cell, and the tumor cells produce a marker protein (myeloma immunoglobulin) that allows the total body burden of tumor cells to be quantified. Multiple myeloma principally involves the bone marrow and the surrounding bone, causing bone pain, lytic lesions, bone fractures, and anemia as well as an increased susceptibility to infection.

Most patients with multiple myeloma are symptomatic at the time of initial diagnosis and require treatment with cytotoxic chemotherapy. Treatment with the combination of the alkylating agent melphalan and prednisone (MP protocol) remains a standard regimen. About 40% of patients respond to the MP combination, and the median remission is on the order of 2–2.5 years. While a host of studies have investigated the efficacy of combination of multiple alkylating agents, none of these regimens have as yet been shown to be superior to MP.

Melphalan and other alkylating agents should be avoided in patients who are felt to be candidates for high-dose therapy with stem cell transplantation, as prior therapy will affect the success of stem cell harvesting. In this setting, the nonalkylator combination of vincristine, doxorubicin, and dexamethasone (VAD) has been used.

Thalidomide is now a well-established agent for treating refractory or relapsed disease, and about 30% of patients will achieve a response to this therapy. More recently, thalidomide has been used in combination with dexamethasone, and response rates on the order of 65% have been observed. Studies are now under way to directly compare VAD with the combination of thalidomide and dexamethasone. In some patients, especially those with poor performance status, single-agent pulse dexamethasone administered on a weekly basis can be effective in palliating symptoms.

Significant efforts are currently focused on developing novel agents for multiple myeloma. These include CC5013, a small molecule analog of thalidomide with immunomodulatory effects; the proteasome inhibitor PS341; and arsenic trioxide.

BREAST CANCER

1. Stage I & Stage II Disease

The management of primary breast cancer has undergone a remarkable evolution as a result of major efforts at early diagnosis (through encouragement of self-examination as well as through the use of cancer detection centers) and the implementation of combined modality approaches incorporating systemic chemotherapy as an adjuvant to surgery and radiation therapy. Women with stage I disease (small primaries and negative axillary lymph node dissections) are currently treated with surgery alone, and they have an 80% chance of cure.

Women with node-positive disease have a high risk of both local and systemic recurrence. Thus, lymph node status directly indicates the risk of occult distant micrometastasis. In this situation, postoperative use of systemic cytotoxic chemotherapy with six cycles of cyclophosphamide-methotrexate-fluorouracil (CMF protocol) or of fluorouracil, doxorubicin, and cyclophosphamide (FAC) has been shown to significantly reduce the relapse rate and prolong survival. Alternative regimens with equivalent clinical benefit include four cycles of doxorubicin and cyclophosphamide and six cycles of fluorouracil, epirubicin, and cyclophosphamide (FEC). Each of these chemotherapy regimens has benefited women with stage II breast cancer with one to three involved lymph nodes. Women with four or more involved nodes have had limited benefit thus far from adjuvant chemotherapy. High-dose chemotherapy with autologous stem cell rescue and growth factor support is presently being evaluated in women with ten or more involved nodes. Long-term analysis has clearly shown improved survival rates in node-positive premenopausal women who have been treated aggressively with multiagent combination chemotherapy.

Tamoxifen is beneficial in postmenopausal women when used alone or when combined with cytotoxic chemotherapy. The present recommendation is to administer tamoxifen for 5 years of continuous therapy after surgical resection. Longer durations of tamoxifen therapy do not appear to add additional clinical benefit. Results from several randomized trials for breast cancer have established that adjuvant chemotherapy for premenopausal women and adjuvant tamoxifen for postmenopausal women are of benefit to women with stage I (node-negative) breast cancer. While this group of patients has the lowest overall risk of recurrence after surgery alone (about 35–50% over 15 years), this risk can be further reduced with adjuvant therapy.

2. Stage III & Stage IV Disease

The approach to women with advanced breast cancer remains a major problem, as current treatment options are only palliative. Combination chemotherapy, endocrine therapy, or a combination of both results in overall response rates of 40–50%, with only a 10–20% complete response rate. Breast cancers expressing estrogen receptors (ER) or progesterone receptors (PR), retain the intrinsic hormonal sensitivities of the normal breast—including the growth-stimulatory response to ovarian, adrenal, and pituitary hormones. Patients who show improvement with hormonal ablative procedures also respond to the addition of tamoxifen. The aromatase inhibitors anastrozole and letrozole have recently been approved as first-line therapy in women with advanced breast cancer whose tumors are hormone-receptor positive. In addition, these agents and exemestane are approved as second-line therapy following treatment with tamoxifen.

Patients with significant visceral involvement of the lung, liver, or brain and those with rapidly progressive disease rarely benefit from hormonal maneuvers, and initial systemic chemotherapy is indicated in such cases. For the 25–30% of breast cancer patients whose tumors express the HER-2/*neu* cell surface receptor, a humanized monoclonal anti-HER-2/*neu* antibody, trastuzumab, is available for therapeutic use alone or in combination chemotherapy.

Systemic Chemotherapy

About 50–60% of patients with metastatic disease respond to initial chemotherapy. A broad range of anti-

cancer agents have activity in this disease, including the anthracyclines (doxorubicin, mitoxantrone, and epirubicin), the taxanes (docetaxel and paclitaxel), navelbine, capecitabine, gemcitabine, cyclophosphamide, methotrexate, and cisplatin. Doxorubicin and the taxanes are the most active cytotoxic drugs. Combination chemotherapy has been found to induce higher and more durable remissions in up to 50–80% of patients. Anthracycline-containing regimens including fluorouracil, doxorubicin, and cyclophosphamide or epirubicin, cyclophosphamide, and fluorouracil are now considered standard first-line regimens. With most combination regimens, partial remissions have a median duration of about 10 months and complete remissions have a duration of about 15 months. Unfortunately, only 10–20% of patients achieve complete remissions with any of these regimens, and as noted, complete remissions are usually not long-lasting. The addition of tamoxifen to combination chemotherapy yields only modest additional improvement.

PROSTATE CANCER

Prostate cancer was the second type of cancer shown to be responsive to hormonal manipulation. The treatment of choice for patients with advanced prostate cancer is elimination of testosterone production by the testes either through surgical or chemical castration. Bilateral orchiectomy or estrogen therapy in the form of diethylstilbestrol were previously used as first-line therapy. However, at present, the use of LHRH agonists—including leuprolide and goserelin agonists, alone or in combination with an antiandrogen (eg, flutamide, bicalutamide, or nilutamide)—has become the preferred approach. There appears to be no survival advantage of total androgen blockade using a combination of LHRH agonist and antiandrogen agent compared with single-agent therapy. Hormonal treatment reduces symptoms—especially bone pain—in 70–80% of patients and may cause a significant reduction in the PSA level, which is now widely accepted as a surrogate marker for response to treatment in prostate cancer. Although initial hormonal manipulation is able to control symptoms for up to 2 years, patients usually present with progressive disease. Second-line hormonal therapies include aminoglutethimide plus hydrocortisone, the antifungal agent ketoconazole plus hydrocortisone, or hydrocortisone alone.

Unfortunately, nearly all patients with advanced prostate cancer eventually become refractory to hormone therapy. A regimen of mitoxantrone and prednisone is approved in patients with hormone-refractory prostate cancer since it provides effective palliation in those who experience significant bone pain. Estramustine is an antimicrotubule agent that produces an almost 20% response rate as a single agent. However, when used in combination with either etoposide or a taxane such as docetaxel or paclitaxel, response rates are more than doubled to 40–50%. To date, no combination regimen has resulted in improved survival benefit. For this reason, intense efforts are focused on identifying novel agents and treatment regimens for patients with hormone-refractory prostate cancer.

GASTROINTESTINAL CANCERS

Colorectal adenocarcinoma is the most common type of gastrointestinal malignancy. There are approximately 145,000 new cases diagnosed each year in the USA; worldwide, there are nearly one million cases diagnosed each year. At the time of initial presentation, only about 40–45% of cases are potentially curable with surgery. Patients presenting with high-risk stage II disease and stage III disease with involvement of regional lymph nodes are candidates for adjuvant chemotherapy with fluorouracil plus leucovorin and are generally treated for up to 6–8 months following surgical resection. Treatment with this combination regimen reduces the recurrence rate after surgery by 35% in these patients and clearly improves overall patient survival compared with surgery alone. For patients with rectal carcinoma, surgical adjuvant therapy with protracted intravenous infusion of fluorouracil along with pelvic irradiation provides a modest albeit significant improvement in both relapse-free and overall survival.

As a single agent, the topoisomerase I inhibitor irinotecan is approved as second-line therapy in patients who are no longer responding to fluorouracil. The combination of irinotecan, fluorouracil, and leucovorin (IFL protocol) when given either in a weekly bolus fashion or via a biweekly infusion schedule has now been shown to provide significant clinical benefit in terms of overall response rates, time to disease progression, and survival when compared with treatment with the combination of fluorouracil and leucovorin. Oxaliplatin has recently received approval in the USA for use in combination with a biweekly infusion schedule of fluorouracil and leucovorin as second-line therapy in patients who have failed the IFL regimen.

The incidence of gastric cancer, esophageal cancer, and pancreatic cancer is much lower than for colorectal cancer, but these malignancies are more aggressive. In most cases, they cannot be completely resected surgically, as most patients present with either locally advanced or metastatic disease at the time of their initial diagnosis. Fluorouracil-based chemotherapy has been the usual approach for gastroesophageal cancers. Recently, there has been a shift toward incorporating cisplatin-based regimens in combination with either the topoisomerase I inhibitor irinotecan or with one of the taxanes, paclitaxel or docetaxel, and response rates in the range of 40–50% are now being reported. In addition, neoadjuvant approaches with combination chemotherapy and radiation therapy prior to surgery appear to have some promise in selected patients. Although gemcitabine is approved for use as a single-agent in metastatic pancreas cancer, the overall response rate is less than 10%, with no complete responses. Intense efforts are now being placed on incorporating gemcitabine into various combination regimens and on identifying novel agents that target signal transduction pathways felt to be critical for the growth of pancreatic cancer.

LUNG CANCER

Lung cancer can be divided into two main histopathologic subtypes, non-small cell and small cell. Non-small cell lung cancer (NSCLC) makes up about 75–80% of all cases of lung cancer, and this group includes adenocarcinoma, squamous cell cancer, and large cell cancer, while small cell lung cancer (SCLC) makes up the remaining 20–25%. When NSCLC is diagnosed in an advanced stage with metastatic disease, the prognosis is extremely poor, with a median survival of about 8 months. It is clear that prevention (primarily through avoidance of cigarette smoking) and early detection remain the most important means of control. When diagnosed at an early stage, surgical resection can result in patient cure. However, in most cases, distant metastases have occurred at the time of diagnosis. In certain instances, radiation therapy can be offered for palliation of pain, airway obstruction, or bleeding and to treat patients whose performance status would not allow for more aggressive treatments.

Patients with small cell lung cancer (the most aggressive type) show the best responses to platinum-based combination regimens, including cisplatin and etoposide or cisplatin and irinotecan. The topoisomerase I inhibitor topotecan is used as second-line monotherapy in patients who have failed a platinum-based regimen.

OVARIAN CANCER

In the majority of patients, this cancer remains occult and becomes symptomatic after it has already metastasized to the peritoneal cavity. At this stage, it usually presents with malignant ascites. It is important to accurately stage this cancer with laparoscopy, ultrasound, and CT scanning. Patients with stage I disease appear to benefit from whole-abdomen radiotherapy and may receive additional benefit from combination chemotherapy with cisplatin and cyclophosphamide.

Combination chemotherapy is the standard approach to stage III and stage IV disease. Randomized clinical studies have shown that the combination of paclitaxel and cisplatin provides survival benefit compared with the previous standard combination of cisplatin plus cyclophosphamide. More recently, several studies have shown that carboplatin and paclitaxel yields clinical results similar to what is achieved with the cisplatin plus paclitaxel combination; however, because of reduced toxicity and greater ease of administration, carboplatin plus paclitaxel has now become the treatment of choice. In patients who present with recurrent disease, the topoisomerase I inhibitor topotecan, the alkylating agent altretamine, and liposomal doxorubicin are used as single agent monotherapy.

TESTICULAR CANCER

The introduction of platinum-based combination chemotherapy has made an impressive change in the treatment of patients with advanced testicular cancer. At present, chemotherapy is recommended for patients with stage IIC or stage III seminomas and nonseminomatous disease. Over 90% of patients respond to chemotherapy, and, depending upon the extent and severity of disease, complete remissions up to 70–80% are observed. Over 50% of patients achieving complete remission are cured with chemotherapy. In patients with good-risk features, three cycles of cisplatin, etoposide, and bleomycin (PEB protocol) or four cycles of cisplatin and etoposide give virtually identical results. In patients with high-risk disease, the combination of cisplatin, etoposide, and ifosfamide can be used as well as etoposide and bleomycin with high-dose cisplatin. Clinical studies are ongoing to determine the role of high-dose therapy and bone marrow transplantation in this setting.

MALIGNANT MELANOMA

Malignant melanoma is one of the most difficult neoplasms to treat because it is relatively resistant to drugs. Dacarbazine, temozolomide, and cisplatin are the most active cytotoxic agents for this disease. Biologic agents, including interferon alfa and interleukin-2 (IL-2), may have greater activity than traditional anticancer agents, and treatment with high-dose IL-2 has led to cures in a small subset of patients. Several clinical studies are actively investigating the combination of biologic therapy with combination chemotherapy in what has been labeled biochemotherapy regimens. Thus far, overall response rates as well as complete response rates appear to be much higher with biochemotherapy regimens compared with chemotherapy alone. Unfortunately, treatment toxicity also seems to be increased. This approach remains investigational, and further studies are required to determine whether this approach can lead to improved patient survival.

BRAIN CANCER

Chemotherapy has only limited efficacy in the treatment of malignant gliomas. In general, the nitrosoureas, because of their ability to cross the blood-brain barrier, are the most active agents in this disease. Carmustine (BCNU) can be used a single agent, or lomustine (CCNU) can be used in combination with procarbazine and vincristine. In addition, the nonclassic alkylating agent temozolomide has activity in the setting of recurrent disease, and it is approved for this indication. The histopathologic subtype oligodendroglioma has now been shown to be especially chemosensitive, and the combination of procarbazine, lomustine, and vincristine (PCV protocol) is the treatment of choice for this disease.

CHORIOCARCINOMA

This rare tumor arises from fetal trophoblastic tissue and was the first metastatic cancer cured with chemotherapy. Single-agent methotrexate produced complete regression of metastatic lesions, resulting in a high percentage of cures. At present, treatment with single-agent methotrexate or dactinomycin is recommended for low-risk disease, while intense combination regimens including methotrexate and leucovorin rescue, etoposide, dactinomycin, vincristine, and cyclophosphamide are recommended for intermediate or high-risk disease.

EVALUATION OF CLINICAL RESPONSE

Since cancer chemotherapy can induce clinical improvement, significant toxicity, or both, it is critically important to carefully assess the effects of treatment. The goal of therapy in most cancers is to palliate symptoms and to improve the overall quality of life.

Shrinkage in tumor size is a useful measure of clinical response, and this effect can be demonstrated by physical examination, chest film or other x-ray, or special scanning procedures such as bone scanning (breast, prostate cancer), CT scan, magnetic resonance imaging (MRI), or ultrasonography.

Another sign of therapeutic response is a significant decrease in the quantity of a tumor product or marker substance that reflects the amount of tumor in the body.

Normalization of organ function is another useful indicator of drug effectiveness. Examples of such improvement include the normalization of liver function (eg, increased serum albumin) in patients known to have liver metastases and improvement in neurologic findings in patients with cerebral metastases.

Finally, a valuable sign of clinical improvement is the general well-being of the patient. Although this finding is a combination of subjective and objective factors and may be subject to placebo effects, it nonetheless serves as an obvious and useful sign of clinical improvement and can be used to reassess some of the objective observations listed above. Factors to be considered in determining general well-being include improved appetite, weight gain, and improved performance status (eg, ambulatory versus bedridden).

SECONDARY MALIGNANCIES & CANCER CHEMOTHERAPY

The development of secondary malignancies is a late complication of some types of cancer chemotherapy. The most frequent secondary malignancy is acute myelogenous leukemia (AML). The alkylating agents, procarbazine, etoposide, and ionizing radiation are all considered to be leukemogenic. AML has been observed in up to 15% of patients with Hodgkin's disease who have received radiotherapy plus MOPP chemotherapy and in patients with multiple myeloma, ovarian carcinoma, or breast carcinoma treated with melphalan. The risk of AML is observed as early as 2–4 years after the initiation of chemotherapy and peaks at 5 and 9 years. With improvements in the clinical efficacy of various combination chemotherapy regimens resulting in prolonged survival and in some cases actual cure of cancer, the issue of how second cancers may affect long-term survival assumes greater importance. There is already evidence that certain alkylating agents (eg, cyclophosphamide) may be less carcinogenic than others (eg, melphalan). Systematic testing of the carcinogenicity of anticancer drugs in several animal models should allow less toxic agents to be identified and substituted for other more carcinogenic ones in chemotherapy regimens.

PREPARATIONS AVAILABLE

The reader is referred to the manufacturers' literature for the most recent information.

REFERENCES

Books & Monographs

Abbruzzesse JL et al: *Gastrointestinal Oncology.* Oxford Univ Press, 2003.

Abraham J, Allegra CJ: *Bethesda Handbook of Clinical Oncology.* Lippincott Williams & Wilkins, 2000.

Armitage JO, Antman KH: *High-Dose Cancer Therapy,* 3rd ed. Lippincott Williams & Wilkins, 1999.

Chabner BA, Longo DL: *Cancer Chemotherapy and Biotherapy: Principles and Practice,* 3rd ed. Lippincott Williams & Wilkins, 2001.

Chao KSC, Perry CA, Brady LW: *Radiation Oncology: Management Decisions,* 2nd ed. Lippincott Williams & Wilkins, 2001.

Chu E, DeVita VT Jr: *Cancer Chemotherapy Drug Manual 2003,* 3rd ed. Jones & Bartlett, 2002.

DeVita VT Jr, Hellman S, Rosenberg SA: *Cancer: Principles and Practice of Oncology,* 6th ed. Lippincott Williams & Wilkins, 2001.

Fischer DE: *Tumor Suppressor Genes in Human Cancer.* Humana Press, 2000.

Frank DA: *Signal Transduction in Cancer.* Kluwer Academic, 2002

Harris JR et al: *Diseases of the Breast,* 2nd ed. Lippincott Williams & Wilkins, 1999.

Harrison LB et al: *Head and Neck Cancer: A Multidisciplinary Approach.* Lippincott Williams & Wilkins, 1998.

Holland JF et al: *Cancer Medicine,* 4th ed. BC Decker, 2000.

Hoskins WJ, Perez CA, Young RC: *Principles and Practice of Gynecologic Oncology,* 3rd ed. Lippincott Williams & Wilkins, 2000.

Kantoff PW et al: *Prostate Cancer: Principles and Practice.* Lippincott Williams & Wilkins, 2001.

Kelsen DP et al: *Gastrointestinal Oncology: Principles and Practices.* Lippincott Williams & Wilkins, 2001.

Pass HI et al: *Lung Cancer: Principles and Practice,* 2nd ed. Lippincott Williams & Wilkins, 2000.

Pazdur R et al (editors): *Cancer Management: A Multidisciplinary Approach,* 5th ed. PRR, 2001.

Perez CA, Brady LW: *Principles and Practice of Radiation Oncology,* 4th ed. Lippincott Williams & Wilkins, 2003.

Perry MC: *The Chemotherapy Source Book,* 3rd ed. Lippincott Williams & Wilkins, 2001.

Pizzo PA, Poplack AG: *Principles and Practice of Pediatric Oncology,* 4th ed. Lippincott Williams & Wilkins, 2001.

Rosenberg SA: *Principles and Practice of the Biologic Therapy of Cancer,* 3rd ed. Lippincott Williams & Wilkins. 2000.

Articles & Reviews

Abal M, Andreu JM, Barasoain I: Taxanes: microtubule and centrosome targets, and cell cycle dependent mechanisms of action. Curr Cancer Drug Targets 2003;3:193.

Bonadonna GS et al: Adjuvant cyclophosphamide, methotrexate, and fluorouracil in node-positive breast cancer: The results of 20 years of follow-up. N Engl J Med 1995;333:596.

Dombret H et al: A controlled study of recombinant human granulocyte colony-stimulating factor in elderly patients after treatment for acute myelogenous leukemia. N Engl J Med 1995;332:1678.

Gianni AM et al: High dose chemotherapy and autologous bone marrow transplantation compared with MACOP-B in aggressive B-cell lymphoma. N Engl J Med 1997;336:1290.

Khalil MY, Grandis JR, Shin DM: Targeting epidermal growth factor receptor: novel therapeutics in the management of cancer. Expert Rev Anticancer Ther 2003;3:367.

Kuwano M et al: Multidrug resistance-associated protein subfamily transporters and drug resistance. Anticancer Drug Des 1999;14:123.

McGuire WE, Hoskins WJ, Brady WF: Cyclophosphamide and cisplatin compared with paclitaxel and cisplatin in patients with stage III and stage IV ovarian cancer. N Engl J Med 1996;334:1.

Rozman C, Montserrat E: Chronic lymphocytic leukemia. N Engl J Med 1995;333:1052.

Seymour JF et al: Long-term follow-up of a prospective study of combined modality therapy for stage I-II indolent non-Hodgkin's lymphoma. J Clin Oncol 2003;21:2115.

Skipper HE et al: Implications of biochemical, pharmacologic, and toxicologic relationships in the design of optimal therapy. Cancer Chemother Rep 1970;54:431.

Smith IE, Dowsett M: Aromatase inhibitors in breast cancer. N Engl J Med 2003;348:2431.

Ueda K, Yoshida A, Amachi T: Recent progress in p-glycoprotein research. Anticancer Drug Des 1999;14:115.

Wu K, Brown P: Is low-dose tamoxifen useful for the treatment and prevention of breast cancer? J Natl Cancer Inst 2003;95:766.

Immunopharmacology

*Douglas F. Lake, PhD, Adrienne D. Briggs, MD,
& Emmanuel T. Akporiaye, PhD*

Agents that suppress the immune system play an important role in the retention of organ or tissue grafts and in the treatment of certain diseases that arise from dysregulation of the immune response. While the details of the mechanisms of action of a number of these agents are still obscure, a knowledge of the elements of the immune system is useful in understanding their effects. Agents that augment the immune response or selectively alter the balance of various components of the immune system are also becoming important in the management of certain diseases such as cancer, AIDS, and autoimmune or inflammatory diseases. A growing number of other diseases (infections, cardiovascular diseases) may also be candidates for immune manipulation.

I. ELEMENTS OF THE IMMUNE SYSTEM

NORMAL IMMUNE RESPONSES

The immune system is designed to protect the host from invading pathogens and to eliminate disease. At its functioning best, the immune system is exquisitely responsive to invading pathogens while retaining the capacity to recognize "self" antigens to which it is tolerant. Protection from infection and disease is provided by the innate and the adaptive immune systems.

The Innate Immune System

The innate immune system is the first line of defense against an antigenic insult and includes physical (eg, skin), biochemical (eg, complement, lysozyme, interferons), and cellular components (neutrophils, monocytes, macrophages). An intact skin or mucosa is the first barrier to infection. When this barrier is breached, bacterial destruction is accomplished by lysozyme, which breaks the peptidoglycan cell wall, and by the split products arising from complement activation. These complement components (Figure 56–1) enhance macrophage and

ACROYNMS	
ADA	Adenosine deaminase
ALG	Antilymphocyte globulin
APC	Antigen-presenting cell
ATG	Antithymocyte globulin
CD	Cluster of differentiation
CSF	Colony-stimulating factor
CTL	Cytotoxic T lymphocyte
DC	Dendritic cell
DTH	Delayed-type hypersensitivity
FKBP	FK-binding protein
HAMA	Human antimouse antibody
IFN	Interferon
IL	Interleukin
IGIV	Immunoglobulin intravenous
LAK cell	Lymphokine-activated killer cell
LFA	Lymphocyte functional antigen
MAb	Monoclonal antibody
MHC	Major histocompatibility complex
MCP-1	Macrophage chemotactic protein-1
MIP-1	Macrophage inflammatory protein-1
NK cell	Natural killer cell
PAF	Platelet-activating factor
RA	Rheumatoid arthritis
SCID	Severe combined immunodeficiency disease
SLE	Systemic lupus erythematosus
TCR	T cell receptor
TGF-β	Transforming growth factor-β
TH1, TH2	T helper cell types 1 and 2
TNF	Tumor necrosis factor

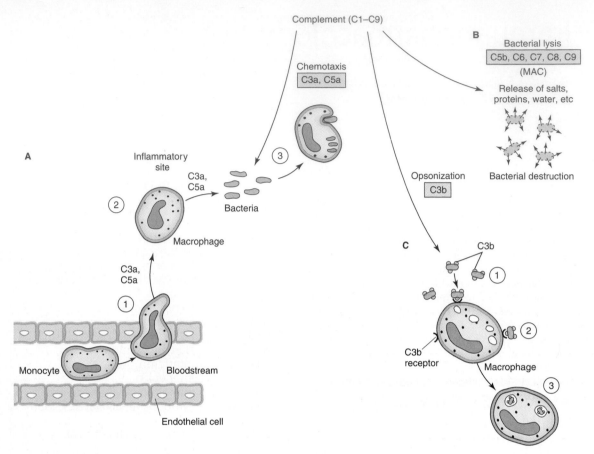

Figure 56–1. Role of complement in innate immunity. Complement is made up of nine proteins (C1–C9), which are split into fragments during activation. **A:** Complement components (C3a, C5a) attract phagocytes (1) to inflammatory sites (2), where they ingest and degrade pathogens (3). **B:** Complement components C5b, C6, C7, C8, and C9 associate to form a membrane attack complex (MAC) that lyses bacteria, causing their destruction. **C:** Complement component C3b is an opsonin that coats bacteria (1) and facilitates their ingestion (2) and digestion (3) by phagocytes.

neutrophil phagocytosis by acting as opsonins (C3b), attracting immunocytes to inflammatory sites (C3a, C5a), and causing bacterial lysis via the generation of a membrane attack complex. During the inflammatory response triggered by infection, neutrophils and monocytes enter the tissue sites from the peripheral circulation. This influx is mediated by the release of chemokines (IL-8, MIP-1, MCP-1) from activated endothelial cells and immune cells (mostly macrophages) at the inflammatory site and is triggered by the adhesion of immune cells to ligands on the activated endothelial cell surface. If these mechanisms are successful, the invading pathogen is ingested, degraded, and eliminated, and disease is either prevented or is of short duration.

The Adaptive Immune System

When the innate immune response is inadequate to cope with infection, the adaptive immune system is mobilized by cues from the innate response. The adaptive immune system has a number of characteristics that contribute to its success in eliminating pathogens. These include the ability (1) to respond to a variety of antigens, each in a specific manner; (2) to discriminate between foreign ("nonself") antigens and self antigens of the host; and (3) to respond to a previously encountered antigen in a learned way by initiating a vigorous memory response. This adaptive response culminates in the production of **antibodies,** which are the effectors of **humoral immunity;** and the activation of **T lympho-**

cytes, which are the effectors of **cell-mediated immunity.**

The induction of specific immunity requires the participation of antigen-presenting cells (APCs), which include macrophages, dendritic cells, Langerhans cells, and B lymphocytes. These cells play pivotal roles in the immune response by enzymatically digesting protein antigens and presenting the derived peptides in association with class I and class II major histocompatibility complex (MHC) proteins to the T cell receptor (TCR) expressed on CD4 and CD8 T lymphocytes, respectively. At least two signals are necessary for the activation of CD4 and CD8 T cells. The first signal is delivered following engagement of the TCR with peptide-bound MHC molecules (see Figure 56–3 inset). In the absence of a second signal, the T cells become unresponsive (anergic) or undergo apoptosis. A second signal that involves ligation of costimulatory molecules (CD40, CD80, CD86) on the antigen-presenting cell to their respective ligands (CD40L for CD40, CD28 for CD80 and CD86) is required for T cell activation (see Figure 56–3 inset). Binding of CD80 or CD86 to CTLA-4 on activated T cells provides a negative feedback loop for regulating the immune response.

T lymphocytes develop and learn to recognize self and nonself in the thymus; those T cells that bind with high affinity to self antigens in the thymus undergo apoptosis (negative selection), while those that are capable of recognizing foreign antigens in the context of self MHC are retained and expanded (positive selection) (Figure 56–2) for export to the periphery (lymph nodes, spleen, mucosa-associated lymphoid tissue, peripheral blood), where they become activated after encountering MHC-presented peptides (Figure 56–3).

Studies using T cell clones have demonstrated the presence of two subsets of T helper lymphocytes (TH1 and TH2) based on the cytokines they secrete after activation. The TH1 subset characteristically produces interferon-γ (IFN-γ), interleukin-2 (IL-2), and tumor necrosis factor-β (TNF-β) and induces cell-mediated immunity by activation of macrophages, cytotoxic T cells (CTLs), and natural killer cells (NKs). The TH2 subset produces IL-4, IL-5, IL-6, and IL-10, which induce B cell proliferation and differentiation into antibody-secreting plasma cells. IL-10 produced by TH2 cells inhibits cytokine production by TH1 via the downregulation of MHC expression by APCs. Conversely, IFN-γ produced by TH1 cells inhibits the proliferation of TH2 cells (Figure 56–3). Although these subsets have been well described in vitro, the nature of the antigenic challenge that elicits a TH1 or TH2 phenotype is less clear. Extracellular bacteria typically cause the elaboration of TH2 cytokines, culminating in the production of neutralizing or opsonic antibodies. In contrast, intracellular organisms (eg, mycobacterium species) elicit the production of TH1 cytokines, which lead to the activation of effector cells such as macrophages. A less well defined T cell subset (TH3) has been described that produces transforming growth factor-β (TGF-β), whose numerous functions include down-regulation of proliferation and differentiation of T lymphocytes.

Cytotoxic T lymphocytes (CTLs) recognize endogenously processed peptides presented by virus-infected cells or tumor cells. These peptides are usually nonapeptide (nine amino acid) fragments derived from virus or protein tumor antigens in the cytoplasm and are loaded onto MHC class I molecules (Figure 56–3, inset) in the endoplasmic reticulum. In contrast, MHC class II molecules present peptides (11–22 amino acids) that have been internalized from the extracellular environment and enzymatically digested foreign antigens to CD4 T helper cells. Upon activation, CTLs induce target cell death via lytic granule enzymes ("granzymes"), perforin, and the Fas-Fas ligand (Fas-FasL) apoptosis pathways. Nitric oxide may also be released, which inhibits cellular enzyme functions.

Natural killer (NK) cells are large granular lymphocyte-like cells that play an important role in innate immunity. Studies with monoclonal antisera originally suggested that NK cells may be of T cell or monocytic origin. More recent studies have shown that they may be derived from CD34 stem cells in the bone marrow that give rise to precursors of the NK cell lineage. NK cells are able to recognize and destroy tumor cells and pathogen-infected normal cells in vitro without prior stimulation. This activity is regulated by so-called "killer cell immunoglobulin-like receptors" (KIRs) on the NK cell surface that are specific for MHC class I molecules. When NK cells bind self MHC proteins (expressed on all nucleated cells), these receptors deliver inhibitory signals, preventing them from killing normal host cells. Tumor cells or virus-infected cells that have down-regulated MHC expression in order to avoid T cell destruction do not engage these KIRs. This results in activation of NK cells and subsequent destruction of the NK target cell. NK cells are also the main precursors of lymphokine-activated killer (LAK) cells. LAK cells are stimulated by high concentrations of IL-2 and are termed "promiscuous killers" because they can kill across MHC barriers and can also kill target cells that do not express MHC. As with CTL-mediated killing, NK cell killing involves the release of cytotoxic granules that induce programmed cell death of the target cell.

Natural killer T (NKT) cells are T cells that express T cell receptors as well as the NK1.1 receptors commonly found on NK cells. NKT cells recognize microbial lipid antigens presented by a unique class of MHC-like molecules known as CD1. They have been implicated in host defense against microbial agents, autoimmune diseases, and tumors.

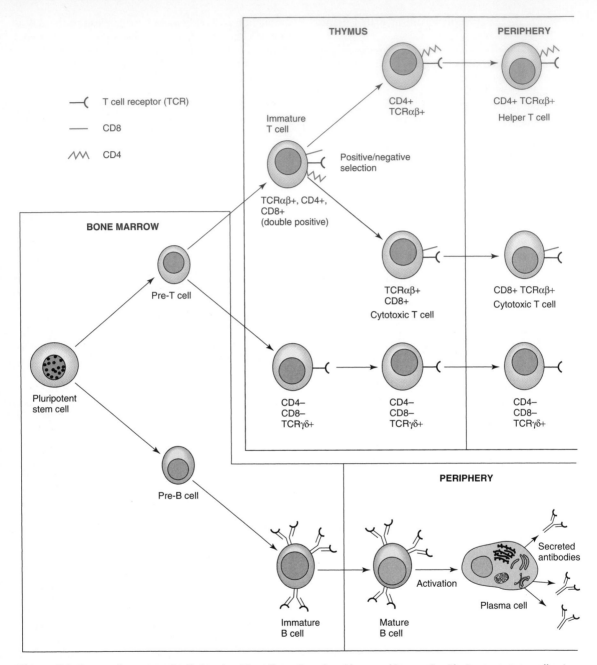

Figure 56–2. Development of cells involved in cell-mediated and humoral immunity. Pluripotent stem cells give rise to pre-T and pre-B lymphocytes in the bone marrow. Under the influence of thymic hormones, pre-T cells migrate to the fetal thymus, where they acquire the T cell receptor and undergo selection to become mature helper CD4 or cytotoxic CD8 T cells that are exported to the periphery. B lymphocytes develop in the bone marrow and differentiate into antibody-secreting plasma cells following encounter with specific antigens.

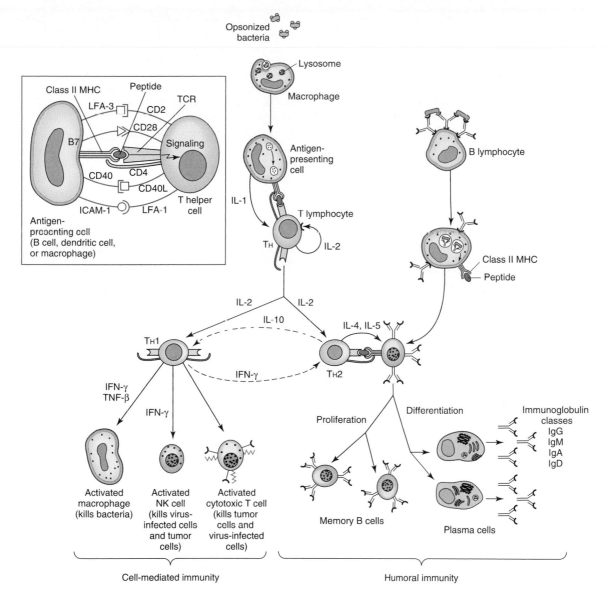

Figure 56–3. Scheme of cellular interactions during the generation of cell-mediated and humoral immune responses (see text). The cell-mediated arm of the immune response involves the ingestion and digestion of antigen by APCs such as macrophages. The resulting processed peptides bound to class II MHC surface proteins are presented to T helper cells. TH cell activation is optimally achieved when costimulatory molecules (B7) and adhesion molecules (ICAM-1, LFA-3) and CD40-CD40 ligand on the APC are bound to their appropriate ligands on the T cell (see inset). Activated TH cells secrete IL-2, which causes proliferation and activation of CTLs, and TH1 and TH2 cell subsets. TH1 cells also produce IFN-γ and TNF-β, which can directly activate macrophages and NK cells. The humoral response is triggered when B lymphocytes bind antigen via their surface immunoglobulin. They are then induced by TH2-derived IL-4 and IL-5 to proliferate and differentiate into memory cells and antibody-secreting plasma cells. Regulatory cytokines such as IFN-γ and IL-10 down-regulate TH2 and TH1 responses, respectively.

B lymphocytes undergo selection in the bone marrow, during which self-reactive B lymphocytes are clonally deleted while B cell clones specific for foreign antigens are retained and expanded. The repertoire of antigen specificities by T cells is genetically determined and arises from T cell *receptor* gene rearrangement while the specificities of B cells arise from *immunoglobulin* gene rearrangement; for both types of cells, these determinations occur prior to encounters with antigen. Upon an encounter with antigen, a mature B cell binds the antigen, internalizes and processes it, and presents its peptide in the MHC class II to CD4 helper cells, which in turn secrete IL-4 and IL-5. These interleukins stimulate B cell proliferation and differentiation into memory B cells and antibody-secreting plasma cells. The primary antibody response consists mostly of IgM-class immunoglobulins. Subsequent antigenic stimulation results in a vigorous "booster" response accompanied by class (isotype) switching to produce IgG, IgA, and IgE antibodies with diverse effector functions. These antibodies also undergo affinity maturation, which allows the antibody to bind more efficiently to the antigen. With the passage of time, this results in accelerated elimination of microorganisms in subsequent infections. Antibodies mediate their functions by acting as opsonins to enhance phagocytosis and cellular cytotoxicity and by activating complement to elicit an inflammatory response and induce bacterial lysis (Figure 56–4).

ABNORMAL IMMUNE RESPONSES

Whereas the normally functioning immune response can successfully neutralize toxins, inactivate viruses, destroy transformed cells, and eliminate pathogens, inappropriate responses can lead to extensive tissue damage (hypersensitivity) or reactivity against self antigens (autoimmunity); conversely, impaired reactivity to appropriate targets (immunodeficiency) may occur.

Hypersensitivity

Hypersensitivity can be classified as immediate or delayed depending on the time required for clinical symptoms to become manifest following exposure of the host to the sensitizing antigen.

A. IMMEDIATE HYPERSENSITIVITY

Immediate hypersensitivity is antibody-mediated, with symptoms usually occurring within minutes or a few hours following the patient's encounter with antigen. Three categories of immediate hypersensitivity are recognized.

1. Type I—Type I hypersensitivity results from cross-linking of membrane-bound IgE on blood basophils or tissue mast cells by antigen. This cross-linking causes cells to degranulate, releasing substances such as histamine, leukotrienes, and eosinophil chemotactic factor that induce asthma, hay fever, or urticaria (hives) in affected individuals (Figure 56–5). A severe type I hypersensitivity reaction such as systemic anaphylaxis (eg, from insect envenomation, ingestion of certain foods, or drug hypersensitivity) requires immediate medical intervention.

2. Type II—Type II hypersensitivity results from the formation of antigen-antibody complexes between foreign antigen and IgM or IgG immunoglobulins. One example of this type of hypersensitivity is a blood transfusion reaction that can occur if blood is not cross-matched properly. Preformed antibodies bind to red blood cell membrane antigens that activate the complement cascade, generating a membrane attack complex that destroys the transfused red blood cells. In hemolytic disease of the newborn, anti-Rh IgG antibodies produced by an Rh-negative mother cross the placenta, bind to red blood cells of an Rh-positive fetus, and damage them. The disease can be prevented by the administration of anti-Rh antibodies to the mother 24–48 hours after delivery (see below). Type II hypersensitivity can also be drug-induced and occurs during the administration of penicillin to allergic patients. In these patients, penicillin binds to red blood cells or other host tissue to form a neoantigen that evokes production of antibodies capable of inducing complement-mediated red cell lysis. In some circumstances, subsequent administration of the drug can lead to systemic anaphylaxis (type I hypersensitivity).

3. Type III—Type III hypersensitivity is due to the presence of elevated levels of antigen-antibody complexes that cause tissue damage. The formation of these complexes, followed by deposition on basement membranes, activates complement to produce components with anaphylatoxic and chemotactic activities (C5a, C3a, C4a) that increase vascular permeability and recruit neutrophils to the site of complex deposition. Complex deposition and the action of lytic enzymes released by neutrophils can cause skin rashes, glomerulonephritis, and arthritis in these individuals.

B. TYPE IV: DELAYED TYPE HYPERSENSITIVITY

Unlike immediate hypersensitivity, delayed-type hypersensitivity (DTH) is cell-mediated, and responses occur 2–3 days after exposure to the sensitizing antigen. Delayed-type hypersensitivity induces a local inflammatory response and causes tissue damage characterized by the influx of antigen-nonspecific inflammatory cells, especially macrophages and neutrophils. These cells are recruited under the influence of TH1-produced cytokines (Figure 56–6), which collectively induce extravasation and chemotaxis of circulating monocytes

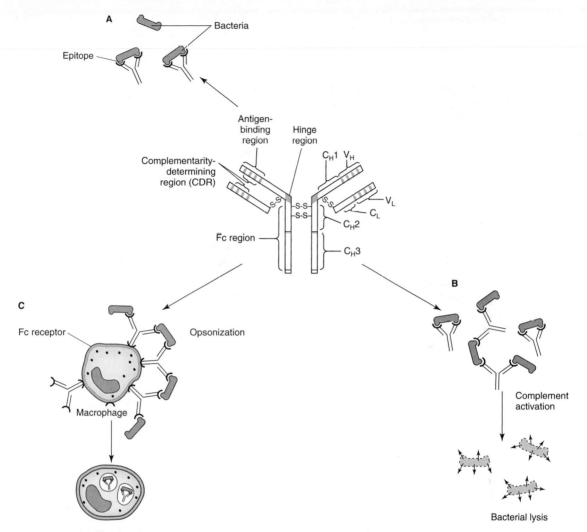

Figure 56–4. Antibody has multiple functions. The prototypical antibody consists of two heavy (H) and two light (L) chains, each subdivided into constant (C_L, C_H) and variable (V_L, V_H) domains. The structure is held together by intra- and interchain disulfide bridges. **A:** The complementarity-determining region (CDR) of the antigen-binding portion of the antibody engages the antigenic determinant (epitope) in a lock and key fashion. **B:** Antigen-antibody complexes activate complement to produce split complement components that cause bacterial lysis. **C:** The Fc portion of antibodies binds to Fc receptors on phagocytes (eg, macrophages, neutrophils) and facilitates uptake of bacteria (opsonization).

and neutrophils, induce myelopoiesis, and activate macrophages. The activated macrophages display increased phagocytic, microbicidal, and antigen-presenting functions and release copious amounts of digestive enzymes that contribute to the tissue damage associated with delayed-type hypersensitivity. Although widely considered to be deleterious, delayed-type hypersensitivity responses are very effective in eliminating infections caused by intracellular pathogens such as *M*

tuberculosis and leishmania species. Tuberculosis exposure is determined using a DTH skin test.

Autoimmunity

Autoimmune disease arises when the body mounts an immune response against itself as a result of failure to distinguish self tissues and cells from foreign (nonself) antigens. This phenomenon derives from the activation of

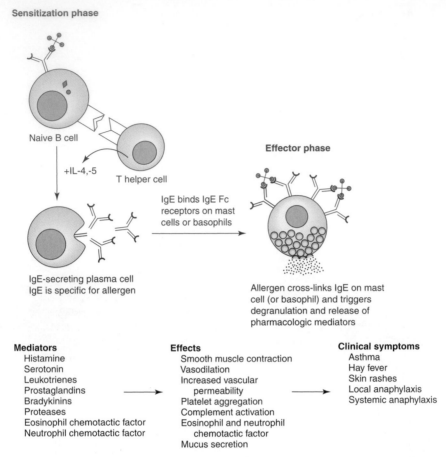

Sensitization phase

Naive B cell

+IL-4,-5

T helper cell

IgE-secreting plasma cell
IgE is specific for allergen

Effector phase

IgE binds IgE Fc
receptors on mast
cells or basophils

Allergen cross-links IgE on mast
cell (or basophil) and triggers
degranulation and release of
pharmacologic mediators

Mediators	Effects	Clinical symptoms
Histamine	Smooth muscle contraction	Asthma
Serotonin	Vasodilation	Hay fever
Leukotrienes	Increased vascular	Skin rashes
Prostaglandins	permeability	Local anaphylaxis
Bradykinins	Platelet aggregation	Systemic anaphylaxis
Proteases	Complement activation	
Eosinophil chemotactic factor	Eosinophil and neutrophil	
Neutrophil chemotactic factor	chemotactic factor	
	Mucus secretion	

Figure 56–5. Mechanism of type I hypersensitivity. Initial exposure to allergen leads to production of IgE by plasma cells differentiated from allergen-specific B cells (not shown). The secreted IgE binds cognate IgE-specific receptors on blood basophils and tissue mast cells. Reexposure to allergen leads to cross-linking of membrane-bound IgE. This union causes degranulation of cytoplasmic granules and release of mediators that induce vasodilation, smooth muscle contraction, and increased vascular permeability. These effects lead to the clinical symptoms characteristic of type I hypersensitivity.

self-reactive T and B lymphocytes that generate cell-mediated or humoral immune responses directed against self antigens. The pathologic consequences of this reactivity constitute different types of autoimmune diseases. Autoimmune diseases are highly complex due to MHC genetics, environmental conditions, infectious entities, and dysfunctional immune regulation. Examples of autoimmune diseases include rheumatoid arthritis, systemic lupus erythematosus, multiple sclerosis, and type 1 diabetes mellitus. In rheumatoid arthritis, IgM antibodies (rheumatoid factors) are produced that react with the Fc portion of IgG and may form immune complexes that activate the complement cascade, causing inflammation of the joints and kidneys. In systemic lupus erythe-

matosus, antibodies are made against DNA, histones, red blood cells, platelets, and other cellular components. In multiple sclerosis and type 1 diabetes, cell-mediated autoimmune attack destroys myelin surrounding nerve cells and insulin-producing B cells of the pancreas, respectively. In type 1 diabetes, activated CD4 T_{DTH} cells that infiltrate the islets of Langerhans and recognize self islet B cell peptides are thought to produce cytokines which stimulate macrophages to produce lytic enzymes that destroy islet B cells. Autoantibodies directed against the islet B cell antigens are produced but probably do not contribute significantly to disease.

A number of mechanisms have been proposed to explain autoimmunity:

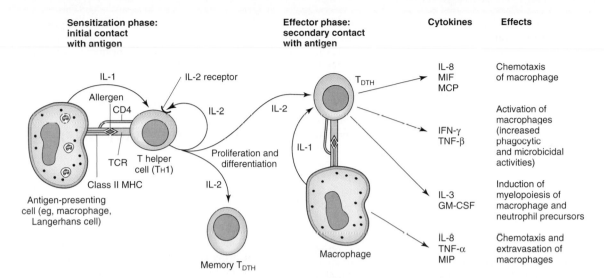

Sensitization phase:
initial contact
with antigen

Effector phase:
secondary contact
with antigen

Cytokines

Effects

IL-8
MIF
MCP

Chemotaxis
of macrophage

IFN-γ
TNF-β

Activation of
macrophages
(increased
phagocytic
and microbicidal
activities)

IL-3
GM-CSF

Induction of
myelopoiesis of
macrophage and
neutrophil precursors

IL-8
TNF-α
MIP

Chemotaxis and
extravasation of
macrophages

Figure 56–6. Mechanism of delayed type IV hypersensitivity (DTH). In the **sensitization phase,** the processed allergen (eg, from poison oak) is presented to CD4 TH1 cells by antigen-presenting cells (APC) in association with class II MHC. T cells are induced to express IL-2 receptors and are stimulated to proliferate and differentiate into memory T$_{DTH}$ cells. Secondary contact with antigen triggers the **effector phase,** in which memory T$_{DTH}$ cells release cytokines that attract and activate nonspecific inflammatory macrophages and neutrophils. These cells display increased phagocytic and microbicidal activities and release large quantities of lytic enzymes that cause extensive tissue damage.

(1) Exposure of self-reactive T lymphocytes to antigens previously sequestered from the immune system (eg, lens protein, myelin basic protein).

(2) Molecular mimicry by invading pathogens, in which immune responses are directed at antigenic determinants on pathogens that share identical or similar epitopes with normal host tissue. This phenomenon occurs in rheumatic fever following *Streptococcus pyogenes* infection, in which heart damage is thought to arise from an immune response directed against streptococcal antigens shared with heart muscle. The suggested viral cause of autoimmune diseases has been ascribed to immune responses (both cell-mediated and humoral) directed against virus epitopes that mimic sequestered self antigens.

(3) Inappropriate expression of class II MHC molecules on the membranes of cells that normally do not express class II MHC (eg, islet B cells). Increased expression of MHC II may increase presentation of self peptides to T helper cells, which in turn induce CTL, T$_{DTH}$, and B lymphocyte cells that react against self antigens.

Immunodeficiency Diseases

Immunodeficiency diseases result from abnormalities in the immune system; the consequences of these abnormalities include increased susceptibility to infections

and prolonged duration and severity of disease. Immunodeficiency diseases are either congenitally acquired or arise from extrinsic factors such as bacterial or viral infections or drug treatment. Affected individuals frequently succumb to infections caused by opportunistic organisms that have low pathogenicity for immunocompetent hosts. Examples of congenitally acquired immunodeficiency disease include X-linked agammaglobulinemia, DiGeorge's syndrome, and severe combined immunodeficiency disease (SCID) due to adenosine deaminase (ADA) deficiency. X-linked agammaglobulinemia is a disease affecting males that is characterized by a failure of immature B lymphocytes to mature into antibody-producing plasma cells. These individuals are susceptible to recurrent bacterial infections, though the cell-mediated responses directed against viruses and fungi are preserved. DiGeorge's syndrome is due to failure of the thymus to develop, resulting in diminished T cell responses (T$_{DTH}$, CTL). The ADA enzyme normally prevents the accumulation of toxic deoxy-ATP in cells. Deoxy-ATP is particularly toxic to lymphocytes and leads to death of T and B cells. Absence of the enzyme therefore results in SCID. Infusion of the purified enzyme (**pegademase**, from bovine sources) and transfer of ADA gene-modified lymphocytes have both been used successfully to treat this disease.

AIDS represents the classic example of immunodeficiency disease caused by extrinsic factors, in this instance the human immunodeficiency virus (HIV). This virus exhibits a strong tropism for CD4 helper T cells; these become depleted, giving rise to increased frequency of opportunistic infections and malignancies in infected individuals. This results from the failure of T helper cells to maintain the cytotoxic lymphocyte response. AIDS is also characterized by an imbalance in TH1 and TH2 cells, and the ratios of cells and their functions are skewed toward TH2. This results in a loss of cytotoxic lymphocyte activity and delayed hypersensitivity, with concurrent hypergammaglobulinemia.

The clinical conditions that arise when the immune system goes awry demonstrate the importance of immune regulation in ensuring the induction of a successful immune response specific for an invading pathogen without being injurious to the host.

Immunosuppressive agents have proved very useful in minimizing the occurrence or impact of deleterious effects of exaggerated or inappropriate immune responses. Unfortunately, these agents also have the potential to cause disease and to increase the risk of infection and malignancies.

TESTS OF IMMUNOCOMPETENCE

A wide variety of techniques have been used to test immunologic competence and drug-induced immune dysfunction. The simplest tests that can be used to detect the effects of immunosuppressive or immunostimulating agents include the following:

(1) Delayed-type hypersensitivity testing with skin test antigens to detect the ability to respond to recall antigens, including antigens derived from common microbial pathogens such as candida. The Merieux skin test device is an effective approach to skin testing.

(2) Measurement of serum immunoglobulins, serum complement, and specific antibodies to various natural and acquired antigens.

(3) Serial measurements of antibody response after primary immunization or a secondary booster injection.

(4) Total circulating lymphocyte count.

(5) Measurement of the percentages of B cells, T cells, and subsets such as CD4, CD8, CD11a, and CD56 (eg, with monoclonal antibodies) that comprise the circulating blood lymphocyte count.

(6) In vitro lymphocyte proliferative responses to mitogens such as phytohemagglutinin, concanavalin A, and pokeweed mitogen or to specific antigens of interest. The response may be measured by tritiated thymidine incorporation or by cytokine production (IFN-γ, IL-2, TNF, and others).

(7) Mixed lymphocyte reaction, in which the lymphocytes of one individual are mixed with and proliferate in response to allogeneic lymphocytes of another individual.

Many of these tests are available through the pathology departments of major medical centers.

IMMUNOSUPPRESSIVE AGENTS

GLUCOCORTICOIDS

Glucocorticoids were the first hormonal agents recognized as having lympholytic properties. Administration of a glucocorticoid (eg, prednisone, dexamethasone) reduces the size and lymphoid content of the lymph nodes and spleen, though it has essentially no toxic effect on proliferating myeloid or erythroid stem cells in the bone marrow. Glucocorticoids are thought to interfere with the cell cycle of activated lymphoid cells (Figure 56–7). The mechanism of their action is described in Chapter 39. Glucocorticoids are quite cytotoxic to certain subsets of T cells, but their immunologic effects are probably due to their ability to modify cellular functions rather than to direct cytotoxicity. Glucocorticoids inhibit the production of inflammatory mediators, including PAF, leukotrienes, prostaglandins, histamine, and bradykinin. In monocytes and neutrophils, glucocorticoids cause diminished chemotaxis and impaired bactericidal and fungicidal activities but do not alter their phagocytic ability. Leukocyte distribution is also

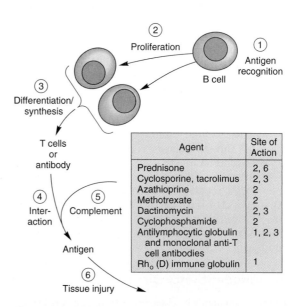

Figure 56–7. The sites of action of immunosuppressive agents on the immune response.

changed by glucocorticoids, which can cause lymphopenia (probably due to lymphoid tissue sequestration) and neutrophilia (due to demargination and impaired extravasation of neutrophils). By inhibiting IL-1 production by monocytes, glucocorticoids also cause a decrease in IL-2 and IFN-γ production. Although cellular immunity is affected more than humoral immunity, the primary antibody response can be diminished—and, with continued use, previously established antibody responses are also decreased. Additionally, continuous administration of prednisone increases the fractional catabolic rate of IgG, the major class of antibody immunoglobulins, thus lowering the effective concentration of specific antibodies. Cutaneous delayed hypersensitivity is usually abrogated by glucocorticoid therapy.

Glucocorticoids are used in a wide variety of conditions. It is thought that the immunosuppressive and anti-inflammatory properties of steroids account for their beneficial effects in diseases like idiopathic thrombocytopenic purpura and rheumatoid arthritis. Glucocorticoids modulate allergic reactions and are useful in the treatment of bronchial asthma or as premedication for other agents (eg, blood products, chemotherapy) that might cause undesirable immune responses. Steroids are first-line immunosuppressive therapy for both solid organ and hematopoietic stem cell transplant recipients. High doses, eg, 4 mg/kg/d of prednisone, can be used to treat organ rejection or graft-versus-host disease without fear of marrow toxicity.

The toxicity of high-dose, long-term glucocorticoid therapy can be severe and is discussed in Chapter 39.

CYCLOSPORINE

Cyclosporine is an immunosuppressive agent with efficacy in human organ transplantation, in the treatment of graft-versus-host disease after hematopoietic stem cell transplantation, and in the treatment of selected autoimmune disorders. Patients in whom it is used as the only immunosuppressant or in combination with prednisone have similar graft survival rates and a lower incidence of rejection and infectious complications than patients treated with combinations of drugs such as azathioprine, prednisone, and antilymphocyte antibodies. The drug is a fat-soluble peptide antibiotic that appears to act at an early stage in the antigen receptor-induced differentiation of T cells and blocks their activation. Cyclosporine binds to cyclophilin, a member of a class of intracellular proteins called immunophilins. Cyclosporine and cyclophilin form a complex that inhibits a cytoplasmic phosphatase, calcineurin, that is necessary for the activation of a T cell-specific transcription factor. This transcription factor, NF-AT, is involved in the synthesis of interleukins (eg, IL-2) by activated T cells. In vitro studies have indicated that cyclosporine inhibits the gene transcription of IL-2, IL-3, IFN-γ, and other factors produced by antigen-stimulated T cells, but it does not block the effect of such factors on primed T cells nor does it block interaction with antigen.

Cyclosporine may be given orally or intravenously. Cyclosporine is slowly and incompletely absorbed (20–50%) after oral administration. It has an elimination half-life of 24 hours. The absorbed drug is almost totally metabolized and excreted in the bile. The dosage is based on a predetermined therapeutic blood level, measured as the trough level in steady state. Cyclosporine is metabolized primarily by P450 isoforms, and there is a potential for many drug interactions.

Toxicities are numerous and frequently include nephrotoxicity, hypertension, hyperglycemia, liver dysfunction, and hirsutism. A significant increase in the incidence of cholelithiasis has been observed in children treated with cyclosporine after heart transplantation. Cyclosporine causes very little bone marrow toxicity. While an increased incidence of lymphoma and other cancers (Kaposi's sarcoma, skin cancer) has been documented in transplant recipients receiving cyclosporine, other immunosuppressive agents may also predispose recipients to cancer. Some evidence suggests that tumors may arise after cyclosporine treatment because it induces TGF-β, which promotes tumor invasion and metastasis.

Cyclosporine may be effective without the simultaneous use of other immunosuppressive drugs in some patients, but in other patients it must be combined with them. It has been used successfully as the sole immunosuppressant for cadaveric transplants of the kidney, pancreas, and liver, and it has proved extremely useful in cardiac transplants as well. Low-dosage cyclosporine (7.5 mg/kg/d or less) has also proved useful in a variety of autoimmune disorders, including uveitis and rheumatoid arthritis. Cyclosporine may also have potential utility in the clinical management of other conditions, including psoriasis and asthma. In asthma it has been able to significantly improve the pulmonary function of some patients suffering from the disease and long-term glucocorticoid toxicity.

Cyclosporine is a major step in the direction of a more specific and selective agent that is effective against a subpopulation of lymphocytes. Its adverse effects are still considerable, though perhaps less severe than those of glucocorticoids and other cytotoxic agents used for immunosuppression. Its combination with newer agents is showing considerable efficacy in clinical and experimental settings where effective and less toxic immunosuppression is needed.

TACROLIMUS (FK506)

Tacrolimus is an immunosuppressant macrolide antibiotic produced by *Streptomyces tsukubaensis*. It is not chemically related to cyclosporine, but their mechanisms of action are similar. Both drugs bind to cytoplasmic peptidyl-prolyl isomerases that are abundant in all tissues. While cyclosporine binds to cyclophilin, tacrolimus binds to the immunophilin FK-binding protein (FKBP). Both complexes inhibit calcineurin, which is necessary for the activation of the T cell-specific transcription factor NF-AT.

On a weight basis, tacrolimus is 10–100 times more potent than cyclosporine in inhibiting immune responses. Tacrolimus is utilized for the same indications as cyclosporine, particularly in organ transplantation. Multicenter studies in the United States and in Europe indicate that both graft and patient survival are similar for the two drugs. Tacrolimus has been proved to be effective therapy for preventing rejection in solid-organ transplant patients even after failure of standard rejection therapy, including anti-T cell antibodies.

Tacrolimus can be administered orally or intravenously. After oral administration, peak concentrations are reached after 1–4 hours. The half-life of the intravenous form is approximately 9–12 hours. Like cyclosporine, tacrolimus is metabolized primarily by P450 enzymes in the liver, and there is a potential for drug interactions. The dosage is determined by trough blood level at steady state. Its toxic effects are similar to those of cyclosporine and include nephrotoxicity, neurotoxicity, hyperglycemia, hypertension, hyperkalemia, and gastrointestinal complaints.

Because of the effectiveness of systemic tacrolimus in some dermatologic diseases, a topical preparation is now available. Tacrolimus ointment is currently used in the therapy of atopic dermatitis and psoriasis.

SIROLIMUS

Sirolimus (rapamycin) is a newer agent, derived from *Streptomyces hygroscopicus,* that binds immunophilins and inhibits calcineurin, as do cyclosporine and tacrolimus. However, sirolimus does not block interleukin production by activated T cells but instead blocks the response of T cells to cytokines. In vitro, it antagonizes tacrolimus-induced T cell responses but seems to be synergistic with cyclosporine. Furthermore, it is a potent inhibitor of B cell proliferation and immunoglobulin production. Sirolimus also inhibits the mononuclear cell proliferative response to colony-stimulating factors and suppresses hematopoietic recovery after myelotoxic treatment in mice. Sirolimus has been used effectively alone or in combination with other immunosuppressants (cyclosporine, tacrolimus, and mycophenolate mofetil) in the preservation of solid organ allografts. Sirolimus is being investigated as therapy for steroid-refractory acute and chronic graft-versus-host disease in hematopoietic stem cell transplant recipients. Topical sirolimus is also used in some dermatologic disorders and, in combination with cyclosporine, in the management of uveoretinitis.

Toxicities of sirolimus can include profound myelosuppression (especially thrombocytopenia), hepatotoxicity, diarrhea, hypertriglyceridemia, and headache.

INTERFERONS

The interferons (IFNs) are proteins that are currently grouped into three families: **IFN-α, IFN-β,** and **IFN-γ.** The IFN-α and IFN-β families comprise type I IFNs, ie, acid-stable proteins that act on the same receptor on target cells. Type I IFNs are usually induced by virus infections, with leukocytes producing IFN-α. Fibroblasts and epithelial cells produce IFN-β. IFN-γ, a type II IFN, is acid-labile and acts on a separate receptor on target cells. IFN-γ is usually the product of activated T lymphocytes.

IFNs interact with cell receptors to produce a wide variety of effects that depend on the cell and IFN types. IFNs, particularly IFN-γ, display immune enhancing properties, which include increased antigen presentation and macrophage, natural killer cell, and cytotoxic T lymphocyte activation. IFNs also inhibit cell proliferation. In this respect, IFN-α and IFN-β are more potent than IFN-γ. Another striking IFN action is increased expression of MHC molecules on cell surfaces. While all three types of IFN induce MHC class I molecules, only IFN-γ induces class II expression. In glial cells, IFN-β antagonizes this effect and may, in fact, decrease antigen presentation within the nervous system.

In clinical practice, IFNs have been used mainly as therapeutic agents in cancers such as melanoma, renal cell carcinoma, and chronic myelogenous leukemia. Interferon-α, in combination with the antiviral drug ribavirin, is efficacious in the therapy of hepatitis C. Clinical trials of IFN-β in patients with multiple sclerosis have shown a favorable effect of this cytokine in relapsing-remitting multiple sclerosis. Patients treated with this cytokine had a reduced rate of exacerbations and less severe disease; they also showed fewer abnormalities on magnetic resonance imaging. Furthermore, these beneficial effects were accompanied by minimal side effects. IFN-β has therefore been approved for use in relapsing multiple sclerosis. The mechanism of cytokine action in multiple sclerosis still needs to be elucidated, and it remains to be determined whether the drug will benefit all patients with progressive disease.

Toxicities of interferons include fever, chills, malaise, myalgias, myelosuppression, headache, and depression.

Mycophenolate Mofetil

Mycophenolate mofetil is a semisynthetic derivative of mycophenolic acid, isolated from the mold *Penicillium glaucum.* In vitro, it inhibits a series of T and B lymphocyte responses, including mitogen and mixed lymphocyte responses. Its action involves inhibition of de novo synthesis of purines. Mycophenolate mofetil is hydrolyzed to mycophenolic acid, the active immunosuppressive moiety; it is synthesized and administered as mycophenolate mofetil to enhance bioavailability. Mycophenolate mofetil is used in solid organ transplant patients for refractory rejections and, in combination with prednisone, as an alternative to cyclosporine or tacrolimus in patients who do not tolerate those drugs. In a placebo-controlled multicenter study, its administration (at 2–3 g/d), along with tacrolimus and glucocorticoids, to recipients of cadaveric renal allografts significantly reduced acute rejection episodes. Mycophenolate mofetil is used to treat steroid-refractory graft-versus-host disease in hematopoietic stem cell transplant patients. It is in clinical trial in combination with tacrolimus as the primary immunosuppressant therapy after stem cell transplant. Newer immunosuppressant applications for mycophenolate mofetil include lupus nephritis, rheumatoid arthritis, and some dermatologic disorders. Mycophenolate mofetil is available in both oral and intravenous forms. The standard dose is one gram twice a day. Drug concentrations are measured in some centers, although the therapeutic range is not well established. Toxicities of mycophenolate mofetil include gastrointestinal disturbances (nausea and vomiting, diarrhea, abdominal pain) and myelosuppression (primarily neutropenia).

Thalidomide

Thalidomide is a sedative drug that was withdrawn from the market in the 1960s because of its disastrous teratogenic effects when used during pregnancy. Nevertheless, it has significant immunomodulatory actions and is currently in active use or in clinical trials for over 40 different conditions. Thalidomide inhibits angiogenesis and is anti-inflammatory and immunomodulatory. It inhibits TNF-α, reduces phagocytosis by neutrophils, increases production of IL-10, alters adhesion molecule expression, and enhances cell-mediated immunity via interactions with T cells. The complex actions of thalidomide continue to be studied as its clinical use evolves.

Thalidomide is currently used for the treatment of multiple myeloma, at initial diagnosis and for relapsed-refractory disease. Patients generally show signs of response within 2–3 months of starting the drug, and reported response rates range from 20% to 70% depending on the conditions and disease state. When combined with dexamethasone, the response rates in myeloma are 80% or more in some studies. Many patients have durable responses—up to 12–18 months.

The success of thalidomide in myeloma has lead to numerous clinical trials in other diseases such as myelodysplastic syndrome, acute myelogenous leukemia, and graft-versus-host disease, as well as in solid tumors like colon cancer, renal cell carcinoma, melanoma, and prostate cancer. The efficacy of thalidomide in these diseases is not yet known. Thalidomide has been used for many years in the treatment of some manifestations of leprosy and was recently reintroduced in the USA for erythema nodosum leprosum; it is also useful in management of the skin manifestations of lupus erythematosus.

The side effect profile of thalidomide is extensive. The most important toxicity is teratogenesis. Because of this effect, thalidomide use is closely regulated by the manufacturer. The regulatory program involves mandatory pregnancy testing and contraceptive measures that are acknowledged in writing by the patient and the prescribing physician. Pharmacists may dispense the drug in amounts sufficient for only 1 month of therapy and only with appropriate patient registries and consents.

Other adverse effects of thalidomide include peripheral neuropathy, constipation, rash, fatigue, hypothyroidism, and increased risk of deep vein thrombosis. Thrombosis is sufficiently frequent, particularly in the myeloma population, that most patients are placed on warfarin when thalidomide treatment is initiated.

Owing to thalidomide's serious toxicity profile, considerable effort has been expended in the development of analogs. Immunomodulatory derivatives of thalidomide are termed IMiDs. Some IMiDs are much more potent than thalidomide in regulating cytokines and affecting T cell proliferation. CC-5013 (Revimid) is an IMiD that in in vitro and animal studies has been shown to be similar to thalidomide in action but without the sedative effects or teratogenicity. CC-5013 is currently in phase I and II clinical trials for the treatment of myeloma, some myelodysplastic syndromes, and melanoma. Preliminary results show efficacy with decreased toxicity compared with thalidomide.

Another group of thalidomide analogs are called selective cytokine inhibitory drugs (SelCIDs). These agents are phosphodiesterase type 4 inhibitors with potent anti-TNF-α activity but no T cell costimulatory activity. Several SelCIDs are currently under investigation for clinical use.

CYTOTOXIC AGENTS

Azathioprine

Azathioprine is a derivative of mercaptopurine and, like the parent drug, functions as a structural analog or antimetabolite (Chapter 55). Although its action is presumably mediated by conversion to mercaptopurine, it has been more widely used than mercaptopurine for immunosuppression in humans. These agents represent prototypes of the antimetabolite group of cytotoxic immunosuppressive drugs, and many other agents that kill proliferative cells appear to work at a similar level in the immune response.

Azathioprine is well absorbed from the gastrointestinal tract and is metabolized primarily to mercaptopurine. Xanthine oxidase splits much of the active material to 6-thiouric acid prior to excretion in the urine. After administration of azathioprine, small amounts of unchanged drug and mercaptopurine are also excreted by the kidney, and as much as a twofold increase in toxicity may occur in anephric or anuric patients. Since much of the drug's inactivation depends on xanthine oxidase, patients who are also receiving allopurinol (see Chapters 36 and 55) for control of hyperuricemia should have the dose of azathioprine reduced to one-fourth to one-third the usual amount to prevent excessive toxicity.

Azathioprine and mercaptopurine appear to produce immunosuppression by interfering with purine nucleic acid metabolism at steps that are required for the wave of lymphoid cell proliferation that follows antigenic stimulation. The purine analogs are thus cytotoxic agents that destroy stimulated lymphoid cells. Although continued messenger RNA synthesis is necessary for sustained antibody synthesis by plasma cells, these analogs appear to have less effect on this process than on nucleic acid synthesis in proliferating cells. Cellular immunity as well as primary and secondary serum antibody responses can be blocked by these cytotoxic agents.

Azathioprine

Azathioprine and mercaptopurine appear to be of definite benefit in maintaining renal allografts and may be of value in transplantation of other tissues. These antimetabolites have been used with some success in the management of acute glomerulonephritis and in the renal component of systemic lupus erythematosus. They have also proved useful in some cases of rheumatoid arthritis, Crohn's disease, and multiple sclerosis. The drugs have been of occasional use in prednisone-resistant antibody-mediated idiopathic thrombocytopenic purpura and autoimmune hemolytic anemias.

The chief toxic effect of azathioprine and mercaptopurine is bone marrow suppression, usually manifested as leukopenia, although anemia and thrombocytopenia may occur. Skin rashes, fever, nausea and vomiting, and sometimes diarrhea occur, with the gastrointestinal symptoms seen mainly at higher dosages. Hepatic dysfunction, manifested by very high serum alkaline phosphatase levels and mild jaundice, occurs occasionally, particularly in patients with preexisting hepatic dysfunction.

Leflunomide

Leflunomide is a prodrug of an inhibitor of pyrimidine synthesis rather than purine synthesis. It is orally active, and the active metabolite has a long half-life of several weeks. Thus, the drug should be started with a loading dose, but it can be taken once daily after reaching steady state. It is approved only for rheumatoid arthritis at present, though studies are under way combining leflunomide with mycophenolate mofetil for a variety of autoimmune and inflammatory skin disorders.

Toxicities include elevation of liver enzymes with some risk of liver damage, renal impairment, and teratogenic effects. A low frequency of cardiovascular effects (angina, tachycardia) was reported in clinical trials of leflunomide.

Cyclophosphamide

The alkylating agent cyclophosphamide is one of the most efficacious immunosuppressive drugs available. Cyclophosphamide destroys proliferating lymphoid cells (see Chapter 55) but also appears to alkylate some resting cells. It has been observed that very large doses (eg, > 120 mg/kg intravenously over several days) may induce an apparent specific tolerance to a new antigen if the drug is administered simultaneously with—or shortly after—the antigen. In smaller doses, it has been very effective against autoimmune disorders (including systemic lupus erythematosus and multiple sclerosis) and in patients with autoimmune hemolytic anemia, antibody-induced pure red cell aplasia, and Wegener's granulomatosis.

Treatment with large doses of cyclophosphamide carries considerable risk of pancytopenia and hemorrhagic cystitis and therefore is generally combined with stem cell rescue (transplant) procedures. Although cyclophosphamide appears to induce tolerance for marrow or immune cell grafting, its use does not prevent the subsequent graft-versus-host disease syndrome, which may be serious or lethal if the donor is a poor histocompatibility match (despite the severe immunosuppression induced by high doses of cyclophosphamide). Other adverse effects of cyclophosphamide include nausea, vomiting, cardiac toxicity, and electrolyte disturbances.

Other Cytotoxic Agents

Other cytotoxic agents, including vincristine, methotrexate, and cytarabine (see Chapter 55), also have immunosuppressive properties. Methotrexate has been used extensively in rheumatoid arthritis (see Chapter 36) and in the treatment of graft-versus-host disease. Although the other agents can be used for immunosuppression, they have not received as widespread use as the purine antagonists, and their indications for immunosuppression are less certain. The use of methotrexate (which can be given orally) appears reasonable in patients with idiosyncratic reactions to purine antagonists. The antibiotic dactinomycin has also been used with some success at the time of impending renal transplant rejection. Vincristine appears to be quite useful in idiopathic thrombocytopenic purpura refractory to prednisone. The related vinca alkaloid vinblastine has been shown to prevent mast cell degranulation in vitro by binding to microtubule units within the cell and to prevent release of histamine and other vasoactive compounds.

ANTIBODIES AS IMMUNOSUPPRESSIVE AGENTS

The development of hybridoma technology by Milstein and Kohler in 1975 revolutionized the antibody field and radically increased the purity and specificity of antibodies used in the clinic and for diagnostic tests in the laboratory. Hybridomas consist of antibody-forming cells fused to immortal plasmacytoma cells. Hybrid cells that are stable and produce the required antibody can be cloned for mass culture for antibody production. Large-scale fermentation facilities are now used for this purpose in the pharmaceutical industry.

More recently, molecular biology has been used to develop monoclonal antibodies that are specific for a single molecule. Combinatorial libraries of cDNAs encoding immunoglobulin heavy and light chains expressed on bacteriophage surfaces are screened against purified antigens. The result is an antibody fragment with specificity and high affinity for the antigen of interest. This technique has been used to develop antibodies specific for viruses (eg, HIV), bacterial proteins, and even tumor antigens. Several antibodies developed in this manner are in clinical trials.

Another genetic engineering technique involves "humanization" of murine monoclonal antibodies in order to increase the half-life of the antibody. Murine antibodies administered to human patients evoke production of antimouse antibodies (HAMAs), which clear the original murine protein very rapidly. Humanization involves replacing the murine Fc portion with a human Fc region while keeping the specificity intact. The procedure has been successful in reducing or preventing HAMA production for several drugs, including infliximab and etanercept, discussed below.

Antilymphocyte & Antithymocyte Antibodies

Antisera directed against lymphocytes have been prepared sporadically for over 100 years. With the advent of human organ transplantation as a therapeutic option, heterologous antilymphocyte globulin (ALG) took on new importance. ALG and antithymocyte globulin (ATG) are now in clinical use in many medical centers, especially in transplantation programs. The antiserum is usually obtained by immunization of large animals such as horses or sheep with human lymphoid cells.

Antilymphocyte antibody acts primarily on the small, long-lived peripheral lymphocytes that circulate between the blood and the lymph. With continued administration, "thymus-dependent" lymphocytes from the cuffs of lymphoid follicles are also depleted, as they normally participate in the recirculating pool. As a result of destruction or inactivation of the T cells, an impairment of delayed hypersensitivity and cellular immunity occurs while humoral antibody formation remains relatively intact. ALG and ATG are useful for suppressing certain major compartments (eg, T cells) of the immune system and play a definite role in the management of organ and bone marrow transplantation.

Monoclonal antibodies directed against specific antigens such as CD3, CD4, CD40, IL-2 receptor, and TNF (discussed below) much more selectively influence T cell subset function. The high specificity of these antibodies improves selectivity, reduces the toxicity of therapy, and alters the disease course in several different autoimmune disorders.

In the management of transplants, ALG and monoclonal antibodies can be used in the induction of immunosuppression, in the treatment of initial rejections, and in the treatment of steroid-resistant rejections. There has been some success in the use of ALG and ATG plus cyclosporine for recipient preparation for bone marrow transplantation. In this procedure, the recipient is treated with ALG or ATG in large doses for 7–10 days prior to transplantation of bone marrow cells from the donor. Residual ALG appears to destroy the T cells in the donor marrow graft, and the probability of severe graft-versus-host disease is reduced.

The adverse effects of ALG are mostly those associated with injection of a foreign protein obtained from heterologous serum. Local pain and erythema often occur at the injection site. Since the humoral antibody mechanism remains active, skin-reactive and precipitating antibodies may be formed against the foreign IgG. Similar reactions occur with monoclonal antibodies of murine origin, and reactions thought to be caused by the release of cytokines by T cells and monocytes have also been described.

Anaphylactic and serum sickness reactions to ALG and murine monoclonal antibodies have been observed and usually require cessation of therapy. Complexes of host antibodies with horse ALG may precipitate and localize in the glomeruli of the kidneys. Even more disturbing has been the development of histiocytic lymphomas in the buttock at the site of ALG injection. The incidence of lymphoma as well as other forms of cancer is increased in kidney transplant patients. It appears likely that part of the increased risk of cancer is related to the suppression of a normally potent defense system against oncogenic viruses or transformed cells. The preponderance of lymphoma in these cancer cases is thought to be related to the concurrence of chronic immune suppression with chronic low-level lymphocyte proliferation.

Monoclonal antibodies against T cell surface proteins are increasingly being used in the clinic for autoimmune disorders and in transplantation settings. Clinical studies have shown that the murine monoclonal antibody muromonab-CD3 (OKT3) directed against the CD3 molecule on the surface of human thymocytes and mature T cells can also be useful in the treatment of renal transplant rejection. In vitro, muromonab-CD3 blocks both killing by cytotoxic human T cells and several other T cell functions. In a prospective randomized multicenter trial with cadaveric renal transplants, use of muromonab-CD3 (along with lower doses of steroids or other immunosuppressive drugs) proved more effective at reversing acute rejection than did conventional steroid treatment. Muromonab-CD3 is now marketed for the treatment of renal allograft rejection crises. Several other monoclonal antibodies directed against surface markers on lymphocytes are approved for certain indications (see monoclonal antibody section below), while others are in various stages of development and clinical trials.

Immune Globulin Intravenous (IGIV)

A quite different approach to immunomodulation is the intravenous use of polyclonal human immunoglobulin. This immunoglobulin preparation is prepared from pools of thousands of healthy donors, and no specific antigen is the target of the therapeutic antibody. Rather, one expects that the pool of different antibodies will have a "normalizing" effect upon the patient's immune network.

IGIV in high doses (2 g/kg) has proved effective in a variety of different conditions ranging from asthma to autoimmune disorders. In patients with Kawasaki's disease, it has been shown to be safe and effective, reducing systemic inflammation and preventing coronary artery aneurysms. It has also brought about good clinical responses in subacute lupus erythematosus and refractory idiopathic thrombocytopenic purpura. Possible mechanisms of action of intravenous immunoglobulin include a reduction of helper T cells, increase of suppressor T cells, and a decrease in spontaneous immunoglobulin production and idiotypic-anti-idiotypic interactions with "pathologic antibodies." Though its precise mechanism of action is still controversial, IGIV brings undeniable clinical benefit to many patients with a variety of immune syndromes.

$Rh_o(D)$ Immune Globulin Micro-Dose

One of the major advances in immunopharmacology was the development of a technique for preventing Rh hemolytic disease of the newborn. The technique is based on the observation that a *primary* antibody response to a foreign antigen can be blocked if specific antibody to that antigen is administered passively at the time of exposure to antigen. $Rh_o(D)$ immune globulin is a concentrated (15%) solution of human IgG containing a higher titer of antibodies against the $Rh_o(D)$ antigen of the red cell.

Sensitization of Rh-negative mothers to the D antigen usually occurs at the time of birth of an $Rh_o(D)$-positive or D^u-positive infant, when fetal red cells may leak into the mother's bloodstream. Sensitization might also occur occasionally with miscarriages or ectopic pregnancies. In subsequent pregnancies, maternal antibody against Rh-positive cells is transferred to the fetus during the third trimester, leading to the development of erythroblastosis fetalis (hemolytic disease of the newborn).

If an injection of $Rh_o(D)$ antibody is administered to the mother within 24–72 hours after the birth of an Rh-positive baby, the mother's own antibody response to the foreign $Rh_o(D)$-positive cells is suppressed because the baby's red cells are cleared from circulation before the mother can generate a B cell response against $Rh_o(D)$. Therefore, she has no memory B cells that can activate upon subsequent pregnancies with an $Rh_o(D)$-positive fetus.

When the mother has been treated in this fashion, Rh hemolytic disease of the newborn has not been observed in subsequent pregnancies. For this prophylactic treatment to be successful, the mother must be $Rh_o(D)$-negative and D^u-negative and must not already be immunized to the Rh$_o$(D) factor. Treatment is also often advised for Rh-negative mothers who have had miscarriages, ectopic pregnancies, or abortions when the blood type of the fetus is unknown. ***Note:*** *Rh$_o$(D) immune globulin is administered to the mother and must not be given to the infant.*

The usual dose of Rh$_o$(D) immune globulin is 2 mL intramuscularly, containing approximately 300 μg anti-Rh$_o$(D) IgG. Adverse reactions are infrequent and consist of local discomfort at the injection site or, rarely, a slight temperature elevation.

Hyperimmune Immunoglobulins

Hyperimmune immunoglobulin preparations are IGIV preparations made from pools of selected human or animal donors with high-titer antibodies against particular agents of interest such as viruses or toxins (see also Appendix I). Various hyperimmune IGIVs are available for treatment of infections with respiratory syncytial virus, cytomegalovirus, varicella-zoster virus, human herpes virus 3, and hepatitis B virus and for patients with rabies, tetanus, and digoxin overdose. Intravenous administration of the hyperimmune globulins is a passive transfer of high-titer antibodies that either reduces risk or reduces the severity of infection. Rabies hyperimmune globulin is injected around the wound and given intravenously. Tetanus hyperimmune globulin is administered intravenously when indicated for prophylaxis. Rattlesnake and coral snake hyperimmune globulins (antivenins) are effective for North and South American rattlesnakes and some coral snakes (but not Arizona coral snake). Equine and ovine antivenins are available for rattlesnake envenomations, but only equine antivenin is available for coral snake bite.

MONOCLONAL ANTIBODIES

Recent advances in the ability to manipulate the genes of immunoglobulins have resulted in development of a wide array of humanized and chimeric monoclonal antibodies directed against therapeutic targets. The only murine elements of humanized monoclonal antibodies are the complementarity-determining regions (CDRs) in the variable domains of immunoglobulin heavy and light chains. CDR loops are primarily responsible for the antigen-binding capacity of antibodies. Chimeric antibodies typically contain the antigen-binding murine variable regions and human constant regions. The following are brief descriptions of the engineered antibodies that have been approved by the FDA.

Trastuzumab is a recombinant DNA-derived, humanized monoclonal antibody that binds to the extracellular domain of the human epidermal growth factor receptor HER-2/*neu*. This antibody blocks the natural ligand from binding and down-regulates the receptor. Trastuzumab is approved for the treatment of metastatic breast cancer in patients whose tumors over-express HER-2/*neu*. As a single agent it induces remission in about 15–20% of patients; in combination with chemotherapy, it increases response rate and duration as well as 1-year survival. Trastuzumab is under investigation for other tumors that express HER-2.

Rituximab is a murine-human monoclonal IgG1 (human Fc) that binds to the CD20 molecule on normal and malignant B lymphocytes and is approved for the therapy of patients with relapsed or refractory low-grade or follicular B cell non-Hodgkin's lymphoma. The mechanism of action includes complement-mediated lysis, antibody-dependent cellular cytotoxicity, and induction of apoptosis in the malignant lymphoma cells. This drug appears to be synergistic with chemotherapy for lymphoma. **Ibritumomab tiuxetan** is an anti-CD20 murine monoclonal antibody labeled with either Yttrium-90 or Indium-111 approved for use in patients with relapsed or refractory low-grade, follicular, or B cell non-Hodgkin's lymphoma (NHL), including patients with rituximab-refractory follicular NHL. It is used in conjunction with rituximab in a two step therapeutic regimen.

Daclizumab is a humanized IgG1 that binds to CD25 (alpha subunit of IL-2 receptor). It functions as an IL-2 antagonist, blocking IL-2 from binding to activated lymphocytes, and is therefore immunosuppressive. It is indicated for prophylaxis of acute organ rejection in renal transplant patients and is usually used as part of an immunosuppressive regimen that also includes glucocorticoids and cyclosporine. Daclizumab is administered in doses of 1 mg/kg, the first 24 hours prior to transplant followed by four separate doses at 14-day intervals.

Basiliximab also binds to the IL-2 receptor alpha chain on activated lymphocytes but is a chimeric human-mouse IgG1. Its indication is identical to that of daclizumab; however, basiliximab is given in two bolus or intravenous infusions, the first administered no more than 2 hours prior to transplant and the second 4 days after the transplant procedure.

Abciximab is a Fab fragment of a murine-human monoclonal antibody that binds to the integrin GPIIb/IIIa receptor on activated platelets, inhibiting fibrinogen, Von Willebrand factor, and other adhesive molecules from binding to activated platelets and preventing their aggregation. See Chapter 34 for additional details.

Palivizumab is a monoclonal antibody that binds to the fusion protein of respiratory syncytial virus, preventing infection in susceptible cells in the airways. Its use in neonates at risk for respiratory syncytial virus infection reduces the frequency of infection and hospitalization by about 50% (see Chapter 49).

Infliximab, etanercept, and **adalimumab** are new biologic agents that bind TNF-α, a proinflammatory cytokine. Blocking TNF-α from binding to TNF receptors on inflammatory cell surfaces results in suppression of downstream inflammatory cytokines such as IL-1 and IL-6 and adhesion molecules involved in leukocyte activation and migration. Infliximab is a human-mouse chimeric IgG1 monoclonal antibody possessing human constant (Fc) regions and murine variable regions. In clinical trials in Crohn's disease, Infliximab reduced symptoms in 25% of patients who were refractory to all other agents. In clinical trials in rheumatoid arthritis, 52% of patients showed improvement of arthritic symptoms. Infliximab is currently approved for use in Crohn's disease of the colon and in rheumatoid arthritis. Toxicities of all three drugs include an increased incidence of lymphoma.

Etanercept is a dimeric fusion protein composed of human IgG1 constant regions (C_H2, C_H3, and hinge, not C_H1) fused to the TNF *receptor.* Etanercept binds to both TNF-α and TNF-β and appears to have effects similar to that of infliximab, ie, inhibition of TNF-α-mediated inflammation, but its half-life is shorter due to its physical form (fusion protein) and the route of injection (subcutaneously, twice weekly). Etanercept is approved for adult rheumatoid arthritis, polyarticular course juvenile rheumatoid arthritis, and psoriatic arthritis. It may be used in combination with methotrexate.

Adalimumab is a completely human IgG1 that was generated using antibody-phage display technology. It is approved for use in rheumatoid arthritis. Like the other anti-TNF-α biologicals, adalimumab blocks the interaction of TNF-α with TNF receptors on cell surfaces; it does not bind TNF-β. Pharmacodynamic studies showed that administration of adalimumab reduced levels of C-reactive protein, erythrocyte sedimentation rate, serum IL-6, and matrix metalloproteinases MMP-1 and MMP-3. In vitro, adalimumab lyses cells expressing TNF-α in the presence of complement. Patients may self-administer single doses (40 mg/0.8 mL) of the antibody subcutaneously every other week. Adalimumab has a serum half-life of 2 weeks, which can be increased by 29–44% in patients who are also taking methotrexate.

Alefacept is an engineered protein consisting of the CD2-binding portion of LFA-3 fused to a human IgG1 Fc region (hinge, C_H1, and C_H2), approved for the treatment of plaque psoriasis. It inhibits activation of T cells by binding to cell surface CD2, inhibiting the normal CD2/LFA-3 interaction. Treatment of patients with alefacept also results in a dose-dependent reduction of circulating T cells overall and also in those that predominate in psoriatic plaques. Therefore, T cell numbers of patients receiving alefacept must be monitored and the drug discontinued if CD4 lymphocyte levels fall below 250 cells/μL. Dosing of 7.5 mg is once per week for 12 weeks as a bolus intravenous or intramuscular injection.

Alemtuzumab is a humanized IgG1 with a kappa chain that binds to CD52 found on normal and malignant B and T lymphocytes, NK cells, monocytes, macrophages, and a small population of granulocytes. Currently, alemtuzumab is approved for the treatment of B cell chronic lymphocytic leukemia in patients who have been treated with alkylating agents and have failed fludarabine therapy. Alemtuzumab appears to deplete leukemic and normal cells by direct antibody-dependent lysis. Patients receiving this antibody become lymphopenic and may also become neutropenic, anemic, and thrombocytopenic. As a result, patients should be closely monitored for opportunistic infections and hematologic toxicity. Partial response rates in clinical trials were between 21 and 31%.

CLINICAL USES OF IMMUNOSUPPRESSIVE DRUGS

Immunosuppressive agents are commonly used in two clinical circumstances: transplantation and autoimmune disorders. The agents used differ somewhat for the specific disorders treated (see specific agents and Table 56–1), as do administration schedules. Because autoimmune disorders are very complex, optimal treatment schedules have yet to be established in many clinical situations.

Solid Organ & Bone Marrow Transplantation

In organ transplantation, tissue typing—based on donor and recipient histocompatibility matching with the human leukocyte antigen (HLA) haplotype system—is required. Close histocompatibility matching reduces the likelihood of graft rejection and may also reduce the requirements for intensive immunosuppressive therapy. Prior to transplant, patients may receive an immunosuppressive regimen including antithymocyte globulin, muromonab-CD3, daclizumab, or basiliximab. Four types of rejection can occur in a solid organ transplant recipient: hyperacute, accelerated, acute, and chronic. Hyperacute rejection is due to preformed antibodies against the donor organ, such as anti-blood group antibodies. Hyperacute rejection occurs within hours after the transplant procedure and cannot be stopped with immunosuppressive drugs. It results in rapid necrosis and failure of the transplanted organ. Accelerated rejection is mediated by both antibodies and T cells, but it also cannot be stopped by immuno-

Table 56–1. Clinical uses of immunosuppressive agents.

	Immunosuppressive Agents Used	Response
Autoimmune diseases		
Idiopathic thrombocytopenic purpura	Prednisone,[1] vincristine, occasionally cyclophosphamide, mercaptopurine, or azathioprine; commonly high-dose gamma globulin, plasma immunoadsorption or plasma exchange	Usually good
Autoimmune hemolytic anemia	Prednisone,[1] cyclophosphamide, chlorambucil, mercaptopurine, azathioprine, high-dose gamma globulin	Usually good
Acute glomerulonephritis	Prednisone,[1] mercaptopurine, cyclophosphamide	Usually good
Acquired factor XIII antibodies	Cyclophosphamide plus factor XIII	Usually good
Autoreactive tissue disorders (autoimmune diseases)[2]	Prednisone, cyclophosphamide, methotrexate, interferon alfa and interferon beta, azathioprine, cyclosporine, infliximab, etanercept, adalimumab	Often good, variable
Isoimmune disease		
Hemolytic disease of the newborn	Rh_o(D) immune globulin	Excellent
Organ transplantation		
Renal	Cyclosporine, azathioprine, prednisone, ALG, OKT3,	Very good
Heart	tacrolimus, basiliximab,[3] daclizumab[3]	Good
Liver	Cyclosporine, prednisone, azathioprine, tacrolimus	Fair
Bone marrow	Cyclosporine, cyclophosphamide, prednisone, methotrexate, ALG	Good

[1]Drug of choice.

[2]Including systemic lupus erythematosus, rheumatoid arthritis, scleroderma, dermatomyositis, mixed tissue disorder, multiple sclerosis, Wegener's granulomatosis, chronic active hepatitis, lipoid nephrosis, inflammatory bowel disease.

[3]Basiliximab and daclizumab are approved for renal transplant only.

suppressive drugs. Acute rejection of an organ occurs within days to months and involves mainly cellular immunity. Reversal of acute rejection is usually possible with general immunosuppressive drugs such as azathioprine, mycophenolate mofetil, cyclosporine, tacrolimus, glucocorticoids, cyclophosphamide, methotrexate, or rapamycin. Recently, biologicals such as anti-CD3 monoclonal antibody have been used to combat acute rejection. Chronic rejection usually occurs months or even years after transplantation. It is characterized by thickening and fibrosis of the vasculature of the transplanted organ, involving both cellular and humoral immunity. Chronic rejection is treated with the same drugs as those used for acute rejection.

Allogeneic hematopoietic stem cell transplantation is a well-established treatment for many malignant and nonmalignant diseases. An HLA-matched donor, usually a family member, is located; patients are conditioned with high-dose chemotherapy or radiation therapy (or both); and donor stem cells are then infused. The conditioning regimen is used not only to kill cancer cells in the case of malignant disease but also to totally

suppress the immune system so that the patient does not reject the donor stem cells. As patients' blood counts recover (after reduction by the conditioning regimen), they develop a new immune system that is created from the donor stem cells. Rejection of donor stem cells is uncommon and can only be treated by infusion of more stem cells from the donor. Graft-versus-host disease, however, is very common, occurring in the majority of patients who receive an allogeneic transplant. Graft-versus-host disease occurs as donor T cells fail to recognize the patient's skin, liver, and gut (usually) as self and attack those tissues. Patients are immunosuppressed (cyclosporine, methotrexate, and others) early in their transplant course to help prevent graft-versus-host disease, but it usually occurs despite these medications. Acute graft-versus-host disease occurs within the first 100 days and is usually manifested as a skin rash, severe diarrhea, or hepatotoxicity. Additional medications are added, invariably starting with high-dose steroids and moving to additional drugs such as mycophenolate mofetil, rapamune, tacrolimus, daclizumab, and others, with variable success rates. Patients generally progress to chronic graft-versus-host disease (after 100 days) and require therapy for variable periods thereafter. Unlike solid organ transplantation, however, stem cell transplant patients generally are able to discontinue immunosuppressive drugs as the graft-versus-host disease resolves (generally 1–2 years after the transplant procedure).

Autoimmune Disorders

The effectiveness of immunosuppressive drugs in autoimmune disorders varies widely. Nonetheless, with immunosuppressive therapy, remissions can be obtained in many instances of autoimmune hemolytic anemia, idiopathic thrombocytopenic purpura, type 1 diabetes mellitus, Hashimoto's thyroiditis, and temporal arteritis. Apparent improvement is also often seen in patients with systemic lupus erythematosus, acute glomerulonephritis, acquired factor VIII inhibitors (antibodies), rheumatoid arthritis, inflammatory myopathy, scleroderma, and certain other autoimmune states.

Some cases of idiopathic aplastic anemia also appear to have an autoimmune basis. A recent series of aplastic anemia patients showed significant clinical improvement and prolonged survival when treated with ATG alone. Some prior cases treated with bone marrow transplantation after conditioning with cyclophosphamide, cyclosporine, or ALG have also shown prolonged improvement in blood counts even though there was evidence of graft rejection and recovery of recipient marrow function—again supporting an autoimmune basis for some cases of aplastic anemia. Another novel approach to control this condition is plasma immunoabsorption using protein A columns. This presumably removes the immunoreactive antibody, particularly in the form of immune complexes.

Immunosuppressive therapy is currently an option in chronic severe asthma, where cyclosporine seems to be an effective drug and rapamycin promises to be another alternative. Tacrolimus is currently under clinical investigation for the management of autoimmune chronic active hepatitis and of multiple sclerosis, where IFN-β has a definitive role.

IMMUNOMODULATING AGENTS

The development of agents that modulate the immune response rather than suppress it has become an important area of pharmacology. The rationale underlying this research is that such drugs may increase the immune responsiveness of patients who have either selective or generalized immunodeficiency. The major potential uses are in immunodeficiency disorders, chronic infectious diseases, and cancer. At present, all but two of the immunostimulating or immunomodulating agents (BCG and levamisole) are classed as investigational drugs for this purpose. The AIDS epidemic has greatly increased interest in developing more effective immunomodulating drugs.

Cytokines

The cytokines are a large and heterogeneous group of proteins with diverse functions. Some are immunoregulatory proteins synthesized within lymphoreticular cells and play numerous interacting roles in the function of the immune system and in the control of hematopoiesis. The cytokines that have been clearly identified are summarized in Table 56–2. In most instances, cytokines mediate their effects via receptors on or in relevant target cells and appear to act in a manner similar to the mechanism of action of hormones. In other instances, cytokines may have antiproliferative, antimicrobial, and antitumor effects.

The first group of cytokines discovered, the interferons, were followed by the colony-stimulating factors (CSFs, also discussed in Chapter 33). The latter regulate the proliferation and differentiation of bone marrow progenitor cells. Most of the more recently discovered cytokines have been classified as interleukins and numbered in the order of their discovery. The identification of most interleukins and the production of highly purified cytokines of all types have been greatly facilitated by the development and pharmaceutical application of gene cloning techniques.

IFN-α is approved for the treatment of several neoplasms, including hairy cell leukemia, chronic myelogenous leukemia, malignant melanoma, and Kaposi's sarcoma, and for use in hepatitis B and C infections. It has also shown activity as an anticancer agent in renal cell carcinoma, carcinoid syndrome, and T cell leukemia. IFN-β is approved for use in relapsing-type multiple sclerosis. IFN-γ is approved for the treatment of chronic granulomatous disease and IL-2 for metastatic renal cell carcinoma and malignant melanoma. Numerous clinical investigations of the other cytokines, including IL-1, IL-3, IL-4, IL-6, IL-11, and IL-12, are now in progress. TNF-α has been extensively tested in the therapy of various malignancies, but results have been disappointing. One exception is the use of intra-arterial high-dose TNF-α for malignant melanoma and soft tissue sarcoma of the extremities. In these settings, response rates greater than 80% have been noted.

Cytokines as adjuvants to vaccines have also been under clinical investigation. Interferons and IL-2 have shown some positive effects in the response of human subjects to hepatitis B vaccine. IL-12 and GM-CSF (sargramostim) have also shown adjuvant effects with vaccines. GM-CSF is of particular interest because it promotes recruitment of professional antigen-presenting

Table 56–2. The cytokines.

Cytokine	Properties
Interferon α (IFN-α)	Antiviral, oncostatic, activates NK cells
Interferon-β (IFN-β)	Antiviral, oncostatic, activates NK cells
Interferon-γ (IFN-γ)	Antiviral, oncostatic, secreted by and activates or upregulates TH1 cells, NK cells, CTLs, and macrophages
Interleukin-1 (IL-1)	T cell activation, B cell proliferation and differentiation, HCF[1]
Interleukin-2 (IL-2)	T cell proliferation, TH1, NK, and LAK cell activation
Interleukin-3 (IL-3)	Hematopoietic precursor proliferation and differentiation
Interleukin-4 (IL-4)	TH2 and CTL activation, B cell proliferation
Interleukin-5 (IL-5)	Eosinophil proliferation, B cell proliferation and differentiation
Interleukin-6 (IL-6)	HCF, TH2, CTL, and B cell proliferation
Interleukin-7 (IL-7)	CTL, NK, LAK, and B cell proliferation, thymic precursor stimulation
Interleukin-8 (IL-8)	Neutrophil chemotaxis, proinflammatory
Interleukin-9 (IL-9)	T cell proliferation
Interleukin-10 (IL-10)	TH1 suppression, CTL activation, B cell proliferation
Interleukin-11 (IL-11)	Megakaryocyte proliferation, B cell differentiation
Interleukin-12 (IL-12)	TH1 and CTL proliferation and activation
Interleukin-13 (IL-13)	Macrophage function modulation, B cell proliferation
Interleukin-14 (IL-14)	B cell proliferation and differentiation
Interleukin-15 (IL-15)	TH1, CTL, and NK/LAK activation, expansion of T cell memory pools
Interleukin-16 (IL-16)	T lymphocyte chemotaxis, suppresses HIV replication
Interleukin-17 (IL-17)	Stromal cell cytokine production
Interleukin-18 (IL-I8)	Induces TH1 responses
Interleukin-19 (IL-19)	Proinflammatory
Interleukin-20 (IL-20)	Promotes skin differentiation
Interleukin-21 (IL-21)	Proliferation of activated T cells, maturation of NK cells
Interleukin-22 (IL-22)	Regulator of TH2 cells
Interleukin-23 (IL-23)	Proliferation of TH1 memory cells
Interleukin-24 (IL-24)	Induces tumor apoptosis, induces TH1 responses
Tumor necrosis factor-α (TNF-α)	Oncostatic, macrophage activation, proinflammatory
Tumor necrosis factor-β (TNF-β)	Oncostatic, proinflammatory, chemotactic
Granulocyte colony stimulating factor	Granulocyte production
Granulocyte-macrophage colony stimulating factor	Granulocyte, monocyte, eosinophil production
Macrophage colony stimulating factor	Monocyte production, activation
Erythropoietin (EPO)	Red blood cell production
Thymopoietin (TPO)	Platelet production

[1]Hematopoietic cofactor (HCF): Plays some role, but not the central role, in growth and differentiation of bone marrow derived cells.

cells such as dendritic cells required for priming naive antigen-specific T lymphocyte responses. There are some claims that GM-CSF can itself stimulate an anti-tumor immune response, resulting in tumor regression in melanoma and prostate cancer. However, recombinant cytokines are expensive drugs and may never reach wide use as vaccine adjuvants.

It is important to emphasize that cytokine interactions with target cells often result in the release of a cascade of different endogenous cytokines, which exert their effects sequentially or simultaneously. For example, IFN-γ exposure increases the number of cell surface receptors on target cells for TNF-α. Therapy with IL-2 induces the production of TNF-α, while therapy with IL-12 induces the production of IFN-γ.

Most cytokines (including TNF-α, IFN-γ, IL-2, G-CSF (filgrastim), and GM-CSF) have very short serum half-lives (minutes). The usual subcutaneous route of administration provides slower release into the circulation. Each cytokine has its own unique toxicity, but some toxicities are shared. Thus, IFN-α, IFN-β, IFN-γ, IL-2, and TNF-α all induce fever, flu-like symptoms, anorexia, fatigue, and malaise.

A more recent approach to immunomodulation involves the use of cytokine inhibitors for the treatment of inflammatory diseases and septic shock, conditions where cytokines such as IL-1 and TNF-α are involved in the pathogenesis. Now under investigation are anticytokine monoclonal antibodies, soluble cytokine receptors (both soluble IL-1 receptors and soluble TNF-α receptors occur naturally in humans), and the IL-1 receptor antagonist IL-1Ra (also a naturally occurring molecule that binds to IL-1 receptors but does not induce biologic responses). These molecules have shown efficacy in animal models of septic shock, experimental arthritis, immune complex-mediated colitis, and diabetes. Phase I clinical studies have demonstrated the safety of monoclonal anti-TNF-α and anti-IL-1Ra antibodies in human volunteers. Preliminary data from phase III studies with monoclonal anti-TNF-α antibodies suggest that these antibodies may be effective in the treatment of septic shock when bacteremia is present. Furthermore, results from a phase III study of IL-1Ra indicated that among high-risk patients, treatment with IL-1Ra improved survival significantly. Other clinical trials using IL-1Ra for the treatment of ulcerative colitis, rheumatoid arthritis, and myelogenous leukemia are also underway.

LEVAMISOLE

Levamisole was first synthesized for the treatment of parasitic infections. Later studies suggested that it increases the magnitude of delayed hypersensitivity or T cell-mediated immunity in humans. In immunodeficiency associ-

ated with Hodgkin's disease, levamisole has been noted to increase the number of T cells in vitro and to enhance skin test reactivity. Levamisole has also been widely tested in rheumatoid arthritis and found to have some efficacy. However, it has induced severe agranulocytosis (mainly in HLA-B27-positive patients), which required discontinuation of its use. The drug may also potentiate the action of fluorouracil (5-FU) in adjuvant therapy of colorectal cancer, and this combination has been approved for clinical use in the treatment of Dukes class C colorectal cancer after surgery. Its use in these cases reduces recurrences, and the mechanism probably relates to macrophage activation and the killing of residual tumor cells by activated macrophages. However, based on recent results from several randomized clinical trials, the 5-FU-levamisole regimen is being replaced by 5-FU-leucovorin since the latter was more effective at increasing disease-free survival and decreasing overall mortality.

BCG (Bacille Calmette-Guérin) & Other Adjuvants

BCG is a viable strain of *Mycobacterium bovis* that has been used for immunization against tuberculosis. It has also been employed as a nonspecific adjuvant or immunostimulant in cancer therapy but has been successful only in intravesical therapy for superficial bladder cancer. BCG appears to act at least in part via activation of macrophages to make them more effective killer cells in concert with lymphoid cells in the cellular efferent limb of the immune response. Lipid extracts of BCG as well as nonviable preparations of *Corynebacterium parvum* may have similar nonspecific immunostimulant properties. A chemically defined derivative of the BCG cell wall, [Lys^{18}]-muramyl dipeptide, has been licensed in Japan to enhance bone marrow recovery after cancer chemotherapy.

A variety of microbial products, including whole organisms and extracts, have been used in Japan as immunomodulators in standard cancer treatments. These have included **picibanil** (OK432), **lentinan,** and **pachymaran.** Clinical trials, usually historically controlled, showed a prolongation of remission and survival. These agents stimulate macrophages to release various cytokines, including IL-1, colony-stimulating factors, and TNF-α. TNF-α is released into the serum of BCG-treated animals after endotoxin challenge. TNF-α is also considered an important mediator of the hypotensive reaction observed in patients with endotoxic shock associated with gram-negative bacteremia.

Other Immunomodulators

Inosiplex (isoprinosine) has immunomodulating activities in various experimental and clinical settings. This agent increased natural killer cell cytotoxicity as well as T cell and monocyte functional activities. Inosiplex is approved in several European countries for the treatment of diverse immunodeficiency diseases but is not approved in the USA. Other synthetic drugs, including cyanoaziridine compounds (**azimexon, ciamexon,** and **imexon**) and **methylinosine monophosphate**, have been under investigation for the treatment of AIDS and neoplasia. Several sulfur-containing compounds have also been under investigation as immunomodulators. **Diethyl dithiocarbamate (DTC)** was found to reduce infections and slow progression in some patients with advanced HIV infection. The drug was not active in earlier stages of HIV infection and is not currently approved.

Thymosin consists of a group of protein hormones synthesized by the epithelioid component of the thymus. These proteins have been isolated and purified from bovine and human thymus glands. Thymosin, which has a molecular weight of approximately 10,000, appears to convey T cell specificity to uncommitted lymphoid stem cells. Smaller peptides and recombinant molecules such as thymosin-α1, thymic humoral factor, and thymopentin, may have similar activity. Thymosin levels are high through normal childhood and early adulthood, begin to fall in the third to fourth decades, and are low in elderly people. Serum levels are also low in DiGeorge's syndrome of T cell deficiency. In vitro treatment of lymphocytes with thymosin increases the number of cells that manifest T cell surface markers and function. Mechanistically, thymosin is considered to induce the maturation of pre-T cells. The effects of fetal thymus transplantation in DiGeorge's syndrome are probably attributable to the action of thymosin.

While thymic hormones are licensed in Europe and Asia, their use has not been approved in the USA. Recent clinical trials have demonstrated some effectiveness of thymosin-α1 plus IFN-α in treating hepatitis B and C.

II. IMMUNOLOGIC REACTIONS TO DRUGS & DRUG ALLERGY

The basic immune mechanism and the ways in which it can be suppressed or stimulated by drugs have been discussed in foregoing sections of this chapter. Drugs also activate the immune system in undesirable ways manifested as adverse drug reactions. These reactions are generally lumped in a broad classification as "drug allergy." Indeed, many drug reactions such as those to penicillin, iodides, phenytoin, and sulfonamides are allergic in nature. These drug reactions are manifested as skin eruptions, edema, anaphylactoid reactions, glomerulonephritis, fever, and eosinophilia. The underlying mechanism of the allergic sensitization to drugs is IgE-mediated and occurs by sensitization and effector phases (see Figure 56–5).

Drug reactions mediated by immune responses may have different mechanisms. Thus, any of the four major types of hypersensitivity can be associated with allergic drug reactions:

Type I: IgE-mediated acute allergic reactions to stings, pollens, and drugs, including anaphylaxis, urticaria, and angioedema. IgE is fixed to tissue mast cells and blood basophils, and after interaction with antigen the cells release potent mediators.

Type II: Drugs often modify host proteins, thereby eliciting antibody responses to the modified protein. These allergic responses involve IgG or IgM in which the antibody becomes fixed to a host cell, which is then subject to complement-dependent lysis or to antibody-dependent cellular cytotoxicity (ADCC).

Type III: Drugs may cause serum sickness, which involves immune complexes containing IgG and is a multisystem complement-dependent vasculitis that may result in urticaria.

Type IV: Cell-mediated allergy is the mechanism involved in allergic contact dermatitis from topically applied drugs or induration of the skin at the site of an antigen injected intradermally.

In a number of drug reactions, several of these hypersensitivity reactions may present simultaneously. Some adverse reactions to drugs may be mistakenly classified as allergic or immune when they are actually genetic deficiency states or are idiosyncratic and not mediated by immune mechanisms (eg, hemolysis due to primaquine in glucose-6-phosphate dehydrogenase deficiency, or aplastic anemia due to chloramphenicol).

IMMEDIATE (TYPE I) DRUG ALLERGY

Type I (immediate) allergy to certain drugs occurs when the drug, not capable of inducing an immune response by itself, covalently links to a host carrier protein (hapten). When this happens, the immune system detects the drug-hapten conjugate as "modified self" and responds by generating IgE antibodies specific for the drug-hapten. It is not known why some people mount an IgE response to a drug while others mount IgG responses. Under the influence of IL-4, IL-5, and IL-13 secreted by TH2 cells, B cells specific for the drug secrete IgE antibody. The mechanism for IgE-mediated immediate hypersensitivity is diagrammed in Figure 56–5.

Fixation of the IgE antibody to high-affinity Fc receptors (Fc$_\varepsilon$R) on blood basophils or their tissue equivalent (mast cells) sets the stage for an acute allergic reaction. The most important sites for mast cell distribution are skin, nasal epithelium, lung, and gastrointestinal tract. When the offending drug is reintroduced into the body, it binds and cross-links basophil and mast cell-surface IgE to signal release of the mediators (eg, histamine, leukotrienes; see Chapters 16 and 18) from granules. Mediator release is associated with a fall in intracellular cAMP within the mast cell. Many of the drugs that block mediator release appear to act through the cAMP mechanism (eg, catecholamines, glucocorticoids, theophylline), others block histamine release, and still others block histamine receptors. Other vasoactive substances such as kinins may also be generated during histamine release. These mediators initiate immediate vascular smooth muscle relaxation and increased vascular permeability, resulting in hypotension as well as bronchoconstriction.

Drug Treatment of Immediate Allergy

One can test an individual for possible sensitivity to a drug by a simple scratch test, ie, by applying an extremely dilute solution of the drug to the skin and making a scratch with the tip of a needle. If allergy is present, an immediate wheal (edema) and flare (increased blood flow) will often occur. However, skin tests may be negative in spite of marked hypersensitivity to a hapten or to a metabolic product of the drug, especially if the patient is taking steroids or antihistamines.

Drugs that modify allergic responses act at several links in this chain of events. Prednisone, which is often used in severe allergic reactions, is immunosuppressive and blocks proliferation of the IgE-producing clones and inhibits IL-4 production by helper T cells in the IgE response, since glucocorticoids are generally toxic to lymphocytes. In the efferent limb of the allergic response, isoproterenol, epinephrine, and theophylline reduce the release of mediators from mast cells and basophils and produce bronchodilation. Epinephrine causes both relaxation of bronchiolar smooth muscle and contraction of vascular muscle, relieving both bronchospasm and hypotension. The antihistamines competitively inhibit histamine, which would otherwise produce bronchoconstriction and increased capillary permeability in the end organ. Glucocorticoids may also act to reduce tissue injury and edema in the inflamed tissue as well as facilitating the actions of catecholamines in cells that may have become refractory to epinephrine or isoproterenol. Several agents directed toward the inhibition of leukotriene synthesis may be useful in acute allergic and inflammatory disorders (see Chapter 20).

Desensitization to Drugs

When reasonable alternatives are not available, certain drugs (eg, penicillin, insulin) must be used for life-threatening illnesses even in the presence of known allergic sensitivity. In such cases, desensitization can sometimes be accomplished by starting with very small doses of the drug and gradually increasing the dose over a period of hours or days to the full therapeutic range. This practice is hazardous and must be performed under direct medical supervision, as anaphylaxis may occur before desensitization has been achieved. It is thought that slow and progressive administration of the drug gradually binds all available IgE on mast cells, triggering a gradual release of granules. Once all of the IgE on the mast cell surfaces has been bound and the cells have been degranulated, the therapeutic doses of the offending drug may be given with minimal further immune reaction. Therefore, a patient is only "desensitized" during administration of the drug.

AUTOIMMUNE (TYPE II) REACTIONS TO DRUGS

Certain autoimmune syndromes can be induced by drugs. Examples of this phenomenon include systemic lupus erythematosus following hydralazine or procainamide therapy, "lupoid hepatitis" due to cathartic sensitivity, autoimmune hemolytic anemia resulting from methyldopa administration, thrombocytopenic purpura due to quinidine, and agranulocytosis due to a variety of drugs. As indicated in other chapters of this book, a number of drugs are associated with type I and type II reactions. In these drug-induced autoimmune states, IgG antibodies to tissue constituents or to the drug can be demonstrated. Immune mechanisms also appear to be involved in many additional cases of so-called idiopathic thrombocytopenic purpura, but it is more difficult to demonstrate the presence of specific antibodies. Blood platelets or granulocytes are sometimes innocent bystanders in an immunologic reaction to a drug but manage to be damaged or activated by antigen-antibody complexes or destroyed by the reticuloendothelial system, leading to the development of "idiopathic" thrombocytopenic purpura or agranulocytosis.

Fortunately, autoimmune reactions to drugs usually subside within several months after the offending drug is withdrawn. Immunosuppressive therapy is warranted only when the autoimmune response is unusually severe.

SERUM SICKNESS & VASCULITIC (TYPE III) REACTIONS

Immunologic reactions to drugs resulting in serum sickness are more common than immediate anaphylactic responses, but type II and type III hypersensitivities often overlap. The clinical features of serum sickness include urticarial and erythematous skin eruptions, arthralgia or arthritis, lymphadenopathy, peripheral edema, and fever. The reactions generally last 6–12 days and usually subside once the offending drug is eliminated. Antibodies of the IgM or IgG class are usually involved. The mechanism of tissue injury is immune complex formation and deposition on basement membranes (eg, lung, kidney), followed by complement activation and infiltration of leukocytes, causing tissue destruction. Glucocorticoids are useful in attenuating severe serum sickness reactions to drugs. In severe cases, plasmapheresis also removes the offending drug from circulation.

Immune vasculitis can also be induced by drugs. The sulfonamides, penicillin, thiouracil, anticonvulsants, and iodides have all been implicated in the initiation of hypersensitivity angiitis. Erythema multiforme is a relatively mild vasculitic skin disorder that may be secondary to drug hypersensitivity. Stevens-Johnson syndrome is probably a more severe form of this hypersensitivity reaction and consists of erythema multiforme, arthritis, nephritis, central nervous system abnormalities, and myocarditis. It has frequently been associated with sulfonamide therapy. Administration of nonhuman monoclonal or polyclonal antibodies such as rattlesnake antivenin may cause serum sickness.

PREPARATIONS AVAILABLE*

Abciximab (ReoPro)
Parenteral: 2 mg/mL solution for IV injection
Adalimumab (Humira)
Parenteral: 40 mg/vial for IV injection
Alefacept (Amivive)
Parenteral: 7.5, 15 mg for IV injection
Alemtuzumab (Campath)
Parenteral: 30 mg/3 mL vial for IV injection
Anti-Thymocyte Globulin (Thymoglobulin)
Parenteral: 25 mg/vial for IV injection
Azathioprine (generic, Imuran)
Oral: 50 mg tablets
Parenteral: 100 mg/vial for IV injection
Basiliximab (Simulect)
Parenteral: 20 mg powder for IV injection
BCG (Bacillus Calmette-Guérin) (Tice BCG)
Parenteral: 30 mg, 1×10^8 organism/vial for percutaneous vaccination
Cyclophosphamide (Cytoxan, Neosar)
Oral: 25, 50 mg tablets
Parenteral: 100 mg/mL for injection
Cyclosporine (Sandimmune, Neoral, SangCya)
Oral: 25, 50, 100 mg capsules; 100 mg/mL solution
Parenteral: 50 mg/mL for IV administration
Daclizumab (Zenapax)
Parenteral: 25 mg/5 mL vial for IV infusion
Etanercept (Enbrel)
Parenteral: 25 mg lyophilized powder for subcutaneous injection
Gemtuzumab (Mylotarg)
Parenteral: 5 mg powder for injection
Glatiramer (Copaxone)
Parenteral: 20 mg for SC injection

Ibritumomab tiuxetan (Cevalin)
Parenteral: 3.2 mg/2 mL for injection
Immune Globulin Intravenous (IGIV) (Gamimune, Gammagard, Iveegam, Polygam, others)
Parenteral: 5, 10% solutions; 2.5, 5, 6, 10, 12 g powder for injection
Infliximab (Remicade)
Parenteral: 100 mg lyophilized powder for IV injection
Interferon alfa-2a (Roferon-A)
Parenteral: 3–36 million units in vials or prefilled single-use syringes
Interferon alfa-2b (Intron-A)
Parenteral: 3–50 million units in vials or multidose pens
Interferon beta-1a (Avonex, Rebif)
Parenteral: 22, 33, 44 μg powder for IV injection
Interferon beta-1b (Betaseron)
Parenteral: 0.3 mg powder for SC injection
Interferon gamma-1b (Actimmune)
Parenteral: 100 μg vials
Interleukin-2, IL-2, aldesleukin (Proleukin)
Parenteral: 22 million unit vials
Leflunomide (Arava)
Oral: 10, 20, 100 mg tablets
Levamisole (Ergamisol)
Oral: 50 mg tablets
Lymphocyte immune globulin (Atgam)
Parenteral: 50 mg/mL for injection (in 5 mL ampules)
Methylprednisolone sodium succinate (Solu-Medrol, others)
Parenteral: 40, 125, 500, 1000, 2000 mg powder for injection
Muromonab-CD3 [OKT3] (Orthoclone OKT3)
Parenteral: 5 mg/5 mL ampule for injection

---

* Several drugs discussed in this chapter are available as orphan drugs but are not listed here. Other drugs not listed here will be found in other chapters (see Index).

Mycophenolate mofetil (CellCept)
Oral: 250 mg capsules; 500 mg tablets; 200 mg powder for suspension
Parenteral: 500 mg powder for injection
Pegademase Bovine (Adagen)
Parenteral: 250 units/mL for IM injection
Note: Pegademase is bovine adenosine deaminase
Peginterferon alfa-2a (Pegasys)
Parenteral: 180 µg/mL
Peginterferon alfa-2b (PEG-Intron)
Parenteral: 50, 80, 120, 150 µg/0.5 mL
Prednisone (generic)
Oral: 1, 2.5, 10, 20, 50 mg tablets; 1, 5 mg/mL solution
Rh$_o$(D) Immune Globulin Micro-dose (BayRho-D, BayRho-D Mini-Dose, MICRhoGAM, RhoGam, Win-Rho)
Parenteral: in single-dose and micro-dose vials

Rituximab (Rituxan)
Parenteral: 10 mg/mL for IV infusion
Sirolimus (Rapamune)
Oral: 1 mg tablets; 1 mg/mL solution
Tacrolimus [FK506] (Prograf)
Oral: 0.5, 1, 5 mg capsules
Parenteral: 5 mg/mL
Topical (Protopic): 0.03%, 0.1% ointment
Thalidomide (Thalomid)
Oral: 50 mg capsules
Note: Thalidomide is labeled for use only in erythema nodosum leprosum in the USA.
Trastuzumab (Herceptin)
Parenteral: 440 mg powder for IV infusion

REFERENCES

GENERAL IMMUNOLOGY

Diefenbach A, DH Raulet: Strategies for target cell recognition by natural killer cells. Immunol Rev 2001;181:170.

Goldsby RA et al: *Immunology 3,* 5th ed. Freeman, 2003.

Janeway C et al: *Immunobiology: The Immune System in Health and Disease,* 5th ed. Current Biology Publications, 2001.

INFLAMMATION

Fearon DT, Locksley RM: The instructive role of innate immunity in the acquired immune response. Science 1996;272:50.

Gallin JI, Goldstein IM, Snyderman R: *Inflammation—Basic Principles and Clinical Correlates,* 3rd ed. Raven Press, 1999.

T HELPER CELLS: T$_H$1 & T$_H$2

Grewe M et al: A role for T$_H$1 and T$_H$2 cells in the immunopathogenesis of atopic dermatitis. Immunol Today 1998;19:359.

Ramachandra L et al: Phagocytic antigen processing and effects of microbial products on antigen processing and T cell responses. Immunol Rev 1999;168:217.

HYPERSENSITIVITY

Curotto de Lafaille MA, Lafaille JJ: CD4(+) regulatory T cells in autoimmunity and allergy. Curr Opin Immunol 2002;14:771.

Girolomoni G et al: T cell subpopulations in the development of atopic and contact allergy. Curr Opin Immunol 2001;13:733

von Bubnoff D et al: The central role of FcεRI in allergy. Clin Exp Dermatol 2003;28:184.

AUTOIMMUNITY

Brand SJ et al: Pharmacological treatment of chronic diabetes by stimulating pancreatic beta-cell regeneration with systemic co-administration of EGF and gastrin. Pharmacol Toxicol 2002;91:414.

Czaja AJ: Treatment strategies in autoimmune hepatitis. Clin Liver Dis 2002;6:511.

Housman TS et al: Low-dose thalidomide therapy for refractory cutaneous lesions of lupus erythematosus. Arch Dermatol 2003;139:50.

Kalman B, Albert RH, Leist TP: Genetics of multiple sclerosis: determinants of autoimmunity and neurodegeneration. Autoimmunity 2002;35:225.

Kato H, Yamakawa M, Ogino T: Complement mediated vascular endothelial injury in rheumatoid nodules: a histopathological and immunohistochemical study. J Rheumatol 2000;27:1839.

Morahan G, Morel L: Genetics of autoimmune diseases in humans and in animal models. Curr Opin Immunol 2002;14:803.

Shlomchik MJ, Craft JE, Mamula MJ: From T to B and back again: positive feedback in systemic autoimmune disease. Nat Rev Immunol 2001;1:147.

Umetsu DT et al: Asthma: an epidemic of dysregulated immunity. Nat Immunol 2002;3:715.

Zhang J, Hutton G, Zang Y: A comparison of the mechanisms of action of interferon beta and glatiramer acetate in the treatment of multiple sclerosis. Clin Ther 2002;24:1998.

IMMUNODEFICIENCY DISEASES

Ballow M: Primary immunodeficiency disorders: antibody deficiency. J Allergy Clin Immunol 2002;109:581.

Cavazzana-Calvo M et al: Gene therapy of severe combined immunodeficiencies. J Gene Med 2001;3:201.

Cham B, Bonilla MA, Winkelstein J: Neutropenia associated with primary immunodeficiency syndromes. Semin Hematol 2002;39:107.

Markert ML et al: Thymic transplantation in complete DiGeorge syndrome: immunologic safety evaluations in twelve patients. Blood 2003;102:1121.

IMMUNOSUPPRESSIVE AGENTS

Barlogie B et al: Thalidomide in the management of multiple myeloma. Semin Hem 2001;38:250.

Benito AI et al: Sirolimus (rapamycin) for the treatment of steroid-refractory acute graft-versus-disease. Transplantation 2001; 72:1924.

Davidson RJ, Marley SB, Gordon MY: Rapamycin for GVHD prophylaxis—potential for severe myelotoxicity. Bone Marrow Transplant 2001;27:115.

Dredge K et al: Novel thalidomide analogues display anti-angiogenic activity independently of immunomodulatory effects. Br J Cancer 2002;87:1166.

Gerards AH et al: Cyclosporine A monotherapy versus cyclosporine A and methotrexate combination therapy in patients with early rheumatoid arthritis: a double blind randomised placebo controlled trial. Ann Rheum Dis 2003;62:291.

MacDonald AS: Rapamycin in combination with cyclosporine or tacrolimus in liver pancreas, and kidney transplantation. Transplant Proc 2003;35(3 Suppl):S201.

Matthews SJ, McCoy C: Thalidomide: a review of approved and investigational uses. Clin Ther 2003;25:342.

McHutchison JG, Fried MW: Current therapy for hepatitis C: pegylated interferon and ribavirin. Clin Liver Dis 2003;7:149.

McMurray RW, Harisdangkul V: Mycophenolate mofetil: selective T cell inhibition. Am J Med Sci 2002;323:194.

Moder KG: Mycophenolate mofetil: new applications for this immunosuppressant. Ann Allergy Asthma Immunol 2003; 90:15.

Radovancevic B, Vrtovec B: Sirolimus therapy in cardiac transplantation. Transplant Proc 2003;35(3 Suppl):S171.

Richardson PG et al: Immunomodulatory drug CC-5013 overcomes drug resistance and is well tolerated in patients with relapsed multiple myeloma. Blood 2002:100:3063.

ANTILYMPHOCYTE GLOBULIN & MONOCLONAL ANTIBODIES

Bashey A: Immunosuppression with limited toxicity: the characteristics of nucleoside analogs and anti-lymphocyte antibodies used in non-myeloablative hematopoietic cell transplantation. Cancer Treat Res 2002;110:39.

Illei GG, Lipsky PE: Novel, non-antigen-specific therapeutic approaches to autoimmune/inflammatory diseases. Curr Opin Immunol 2000;12:712.

Kazatchkine MD, Kaveri SV: Immunomodulation of autoimmune and inflammatory diseases with intravenous immune globulin. N Engl J Med 2001;345:747.

Reichert JM: Therapeutic monoclonal antibodies: trends in development and approval in the US. Curr Opin Mol Ther 2002;4:110.

Thompson J: Haemolytic disease of the newborn: the new NICE guidelines. J Fam Health Care 2002;12:133.

Tutuncu Z, Morgan GJ Jr, Kavanaugh A: Anti-TNF therapy for other inflammatory conditions. Clin Exp Rheumatol 2002;20(6 Suppl 28):S146.

Wall WJ: Use of antilymphocyte induction therapy in liver transplantation. Liver Transpl Surg 1999;5(4 Suppl 1):S64.

CYTOKINES & CHEMOKINES

Auron PE: The interleukin 1 receptor: ligand interactions and signal transduction. Cytokine Growth Factor Rev 1998;9:221.

Baggiolini M: Chemokines and leukocyte traffic. Nature 1998; 392:565.

Cortes JE et al: A pilot study of interleukin-2 for adult patients with acute myelogenous leukemia in first complete remission. Cancer 1999;85:1506.

Ducreux M, Boige V: Adjuvant chemotherapy of colon cancer. Best Practice & Res Clin Gastroenterol 2002;16:283.

Ferrari R: The role of TNF in cardiovascular disease. Pharmacol Res 1999;40:97.

Harris DT et al: Immunologic approaches to the treatment of prostate cancer. Semin Oncol 1999;26:439.

Hasko G, Szabo C: IL-12 as a therapeutic target for pharmacological modulation in immune-mediated and inflammatory diseases: regulation of T helper 1/T helper 2 responses. Br J Pharmacol 1999;127:1295.

Kollias G et al: On the role of tumor necrosis factor and receptors in models of multiorgan failure, rheumatoid arthritis, multiple sclerosis and inflammatory bowel disease. Immunol Rev 1999;169:175.

Mellstedt H et al: Augmentation of the immune response with granulocyte-macrophage colony-stimulating factor and other hematopoietic growth factors. Curr Opin Hematol 1999; 6:169.

Morse MA, Lyerly K: Clinical applications of dendritic cell vaccines. Curr Opinion Mol Ther 2000;2:20.

Orme IM: Beyond BCG: the potential for a more effective TB vaccine. Mol Med Today 1999;5:487.

Rosenberg SA. Progress in the development of immunotherapy for the treatment of patients with cancer. J Int Med 2001; 250:462.

Sinkovics JG, Horvath JC: Vaccination against human cancers. Int J Oncol 2000;16:81.

Tompkins WA: Immunomodulation and therapeutic effects of the oral use of interferon-alpha: mechanism of action. J Interferon Cytokine Res 1999;19:817.

DRUG ALLERGY

Ju C, Uetrecht JP: Mechanism of idiosyncratic drug reactions: reactive metabolite formation, protein binding and the regulation of the immune system. Curr Drug Metab 2002;3:367.

Naisbitt DJ et al: Reactive metabolites and their role in drug reactions. Curr Opin Allergy Clin Immunol 2001;1:317.

Brogan BL, Olsen NJ: Drug-induced rheumatic syndromes. Curr Opin Rheumatol 2003;15:76.

Shipley D, Ormerod AD: Drug-induced urticaria. Recognition and treatment. Am J Clin Dermatol 2001;2:151.

SECTION IX
Toxicology

Introduction to Toxicology: Occupational & Environmental

Gabriel L. Plaa, PhD

Humans live in a chemical environment and inhale, ingest, or absorb from the skin many of these chemicals. Toxicology is concerned with the deleterious effects of these chemical agents on all living systems. In the biomedical area, however, the toxicologist is primarily concerned with adverse effects in humans resulting from exposure to drugs and other chemicals as well as the demonstration of safety or hazard associated with their use.

Occupational Toxicology

Occupational toxicology deals with the chemicals found in the workplace. The major emphasis of occupational toxicology is to identify the agents of concern, define the conditions leading to their safe use, and prevent absorption of harmful amounts. Guidelines have been elaborated to establish safe ambient air concentrations for many chemicals found in the workplace. The American Conference of Governmental Industrial Hygienists periodically prepares lists of recommended **threshold limit values** (**TLVs**) for about 600 such chemicals (Doull, 2001). These guidelines are reevaluated as new information becomes available.

Environmental Toxicology

Environmental toxicology deals with the potentially deleterious impact of chemicals, present as pollutants of the environment, to living organisms. The term **envi-**

ronment includes all the surroundings of an individual organism, but particularly the air, soil, and water. While humans are considered a target species of particular interest, other terrestrial and aquatic species are of considerable importance as potential biologic targets.

Air pollution is a product of industrialization, technologic development, and increased urbanization. Humans may also be exposed to chemicals used in the agricultural environment as pesticides or in food processing that may persist as residues or ingredients in food products. The Food and Agriculture Organization and the World Health Organization (FAO/WHO) Joint Expert Commission on Food Additives adopted the term **acceptable daily intake** (**ADI**) to denote the daily intake of a chemical which, during an entire lifetime, appears to be without appreciable risk. These guidelines are reevaluated as new information becomes available.

Ecotoxicology

Ecotoxicology is concerned with the toxic effects of chemical and physical agents on populations and communities of living organisms within defined ecosystems; it includes the transfer pathways of those agents and their interactions with the environment. Traditional toxicology is concerned with toxic effects on individual organisms; ecotoxicology is concerned with the impact on populations of living organisms or on ecosystems. It is possible that an environmental event, while exerting severe effects on *individual* organisms, may have no important impact on populations or on an ecosystem. Thus, the terms "environmental toxicology" and "eco-toxicology" are not interchangeable.

TOXICOLOGIC TERMS & DEFINITIONS

Hazard & Risk

Hazard is *the ability of a chemical agent to cause injury in a given situation or setting;* the conditions of use and exposure are primary considerations. To assess hazard, one needs to have knowledge about both the inherent toxicity of the substance and the amounts to which individuals are liable to be exposed. Humans can safely use potentially toxic substances when the necessary conditions minimizing absorption are established and respected.

Risk is defined as *the expected frequency of the occurrence of an undesirable effect* arising from exposure to a chemical or physical agent. Estimation of risk makes use of dose-response data and extrapolation from the observed relationships to the expected responses at doses occurring in actual exposure situations. The quality and suitability of the biologic data used in such estimates are major limiting factors.

Routes of Exposure

The route of entry for chemicals into the body differs in different exposure situations. In the industrial setting, inhalation is the major route of entry. The transdermal route is also quite important, but oral ingestion is a relatively minor route. Consequently, preventive measures are largely designed to eliminate absorption by inhalation or by topical contact. Atmospheric pollutants gain entry by inhalation, whereas for pollutants of water and soil, oral ingestion is the principal route of exposure for humans.

Duration of Exposure

Toxic reactions may differ qualitatively depending on the duration of the exposure. A single exposure—or multiple exposures occurring over 1 or 2 days—represents **acute exposure.** Multiple exposures continuing over a longer period of time represent a **chronic exposure.** In the occupational setting, both acute (eg, accidental discharge) and chronic (eg, repetitive handling of a chemical) exposures may occur, whereas with chemicals found in the environment (eg, pollutants in ground water), chronic exposure is more likely.

ENVIRONMENTAL CONSIDERATIONS

Certain chemical and physical characteristics are known to be important for estimating the potential hazard involved for environmental toxicants. In addition to information regarding effects on different organisms, knowledge about the following properties is essential to predict the environmental impact: The **degradability** of the substance; its **mobility** through air, water, and soil; whether or not **bioaccumulation** occurs; and its transport and **biomagnification** through food chains. (See Box, Bioaccumulation & Biomagnification.) Chemicals that are poorly degraded (by abiotic or biotic pathways) exhibit *environmental persistence* and thus can accumulate. Lipophilic substances tend to bioaccumulate in body fat, resulting in tissue residues. When the toxicant is incorporated into the food chain, biomagnification occurs as one species feeds upon others and concentrates the chemical. The pollutants that have the widest environmental impact are poorly degradable; are relatively mobile in air, water, and soil; exhibit bioaccumulation; and also exhibit biomagnification.

SPECIFIC CHEMICALS

AIR POLLUTANTS

Five major substances account for about 98% of air pollution: carbon monoxide (about 52%), sulfur oxides (about 14%), hydrocarbons (about 14%), nitrogen oxides (about 14%), and particulate matter (about 4%). The sources of these chemicals include transportation, industry, generation of electric power, space heating, and refuse disposal. Sulfur dioxide and smoke resulting from incomplete combustion of coal have been associated with acute adverse effects, particularly among the elderly and individuals with preexisting cardiac or respiratory disease. Ambient air pollution has been implicated as a contributing factor in bronchitis, obstructive ventilatory disease, pulmonary emphysema, bronchial asthma, and lung cancer.

1. Carbon Monoxide

Carbon monoxide (CO) is a colorless, tasteless, odorless, and nonirritating gas, a byproduct of incomplete combustion. The average concentration of CO in the atmosphere is about 0.1 ppm; in heavy traffic, the concentration may exceed 100 ppm. The recommended 1999–2000 threshold limit values (TLV-TWA and TLV-STEL) are shown in Table 57–1.

Mechanism of Action

CO combines reversibly with the oxygen-binding sites of hemoglobin and has an affinity for hemoglobin that is about 220 times that of oxygen. The product formed,

BIOACCUMULATION & BIOMAGNIFICATION

If the intake of a long-lasting contaminant by an organism exceeds the latter's ability to metabolize or excrete the substance, the chemical accumulates within the tissues of the organism. This is called **bioaccumulation.**

Although the concentration of a contaminant may be virtually undetectable in water, it may be magnified hundreds or thousands of time as the contaminant passes up the food chain. This is called **biomagnification.**

The biomagnification of PCBs in the Great Lakes of North America is illustrated by the following residue values available from *Environment Canada,* a report published by the Canadian government, and other sources.

Thus, the biomagnification for this substance in the food chain, beginning with phytoplankton and ending with the herring gull, is nearly 50,000-fold. Domesticated animals and humans may eat fish from the Great Lakes, resulting in PCB residues in these species as well.

Source	PCB Concentration (ppm)[1]	Concentration Relative to Phytoplankton
Phytoplankton	0.0025	1
Zooplankton	0.123	49.2
Rainbow smelt	1.04	416
Lake trout	4.83	1,932
Herring gull	124	49,600

[1]Sources: *Environment Canada, The State of Canada's Environment,* 1991. Government of Canada, Ottawa, and other publications.

Table 57–1. Threshold limit values (TLV) of some common air pollutants and solvents. (NA = none assigned.)

Compound	TLV (ppm)	
	TWA[1]	STEL[2]
Benzene	0.5	2.5
Carbon monoxide	25	NA
Carbon tetrachloride	5	10
Chloroform	10	NA
Nitrogen dioxide	3	5
Ozone	0.05	NA
Sulfur dioxide	2	5
Tetrachloroethylene	25	100
Toluene	50	NA
1,1,1-Trichloroethane	350	450
Trichloroethylene	50	100

[1]TLV-TWA is the concentration for a normal 8-hour workday or 40-hour workweek to which workers may be repeatedly exposed without adverse effects.

[2]TLV-STEL is the maximum concentration that should not be exceeded at any time during a 15-minute exposure period.

carboxyhemoglobin, cannot transport oxygen. Furthermore, the presence of carboxyhemoglobin interferes with the dissociation of oxygen from the remaining oxyhemoglobin, thus reducing the transfer of oxygen to tissues. The brain and the heart are the organs most affected. Normal nonsmoking adults have carboxyhemoglobin levels of less than 1% saturation (1% of total hemoglobin is in the form of carboxyhemoglobin); this level has been attributed to the endogenous formation of CO from heme catabolism. Smokers may exhibit 5–10% saturation, depending on their smoking habits. An individual breathing air containing 0.1% CO (1000 ppm) would have a carboxyhemoglobin level of about 50%.

Clinical Effects

The principal signs of CO intoxication are those of hypoxia and progress in the following sequence: (1) psychomotor impairment; (2) headache and tightness in the temporal area; (3) confusion and loss of visual acuity; (4) tachycardia, tachypnea, syncope, and coma; and (5) deep coma, convulsions, shock, and respiratory failure. There is great variability in individual responses to a given carboxyhemoglobin concentration. Carboxyhemoglobin levels below 15% rarely produce symptoms; collapse and syncope may appear around 40%; above 60%, death may ensue. Prolonged hypoxia and posthypoxic unconsciousness can result in irreversible damage to the brain and the myocardium. The clinical effects may be aggravated by heavy labor, high altitudes, and high ambient temperatures. The presence of cardiovascular disease is considered to increase the risks associated with CO exposure. Delayed neuropsychiatric impairment can occur after poisoning, and the resolution of behavioral consequences can be slow. While CO intoxication is usually thought of as a form of acute toxicity, there is some evidence that chronic exposure to low levels may lead to undesirable effects, including the development of atherosclerotic coronary disease in cigarette smokers. However, convincing experimental evidence is lacking. The fetus may be quite susceptible to the effects of CO exposure.

Treatment

In cases of acute intoxication, removal of the individual from the exposure source and maintenance of respiration is essential, followed by administration of oxygen—the specific antagonist to CO—within the limits of oxygen toxicity. With room air at 1 atm, the elimination half-time of CO is about 320 minutes; with 100% oxygen, the half-time is about 80 minutes; and with hyperbaric oxygen (2–3 atm), the half-time can be reduced to about 20 minutes.

2. Sulfur Dioxide

Sulfur dioxide (SO_2) is a colorless, irritant gas generated primarily by the combustion of sulfur-containing fossil fuels. The 1999–2000 threshold limit values are given in Table 57–1.

Mechanism of Action

On contact with moist membranes, SO_2 forms sulfurous acid, which is responsible for its severe irritant effects on the eyes, mucous membranes, and skin. It is estimated that approximately 90% of inhaled SO_2 is absorbed in the upper respiratory tract, the site of its principal effect. The inhalation of SO_2 causes bronchial constriction; altered smooth muscle tone and parasympathetic reflexes appear to be involved in this reaction. Exposure to 5 ppm for 10 minutes leads to increased resistance to airflow in most humans. Exposures to 5–10 ppm are reported to cause severe bronchospasm; 10–20% of the healthy young adult population is estimated to be reactive to even lower concentrations. The phenomenon of adaptation to irritating concentrations is a recognized occurrence in workers. Asthmatic individuals are especially sensitive to SO_2.

Clinical Effects & Treatment

The signs and symptoms of intoxication include irritation of the eyes, nose, and throat and reflex bronchoconstriction. If severe exposure has occurred, delayed onset pulmonary edema may be observed. Cumulative effects from chronic low-level exposure to SO_2 are not striking, particularly in humans. Chronic exposure, however, has been associated with aggravation of chronic cardiopulmonary disease. Treatment is not specific for SO_2 but depends on therapeutic maneuvers utilized in the treatment of irritation of the respiratory tract.

3. Nitrogen Oxides

Nitrogen dioxide (NO_2) is a brownish irritant gas sometimes associated with fires. It is formed also from fresh silage; exposure of farmers to NO_2 in the confines of a silo can lead to silo-filler's disease. The 1999–2000 threshold limit values are shown in Table 57–1.

Mechanism of Action

NO_2 is a deep lung irritant capable of producing pulmonary edema. The type I cells of the alveoli appear to be the cells chiefly affected on acute exposure. Exposure to 25 ppm is irritating to some individuals; 50 ppm is moderately irritating to the eyes and nose. Exposure for 1 hour to 50 ppm can cause pulmonary edema and perhaps subacute or chronic pulmonary lesions; 100 ppm can cause pulmonary edema and death.

Clinical Effects & Treatment

The signs and symptoms of acute exposure to NO_2 include irritation of the eyes and nose, cough, mucoid or frothy sputum production, dyspnea, and chest pain. Pulmonary edema may appear within 1–2 hours. In some individuals, the clinical signs may subside in about 2 weeks; the patient may then pass into a second stage of abruptly increasing severity, including recurring pulmonary edema and fibrotic destruction of terminal bronchioles (bronchiolitis obliterans). Chronic exposure of laboratory animals to 10–25 ppm NO_2 has resulted in emphysematous changes; thus, chronic effects in humans are of concern. There is no specific treatment for acute intoxication by NO_2; therapeutic measures for the management of deep lung irritation and noncardiogenic pulmonary edema are employed. These measures include maintenance of gas exchange with adequate oxygenation and alveolar ventilation. Drug therapy may include bronchodilators, sedatives, and antibiotics.

4. Ozone

Ozone (O_3) is a bluish irritant gas that occurs normally in the earth's atmosphere, where it is an important absorbent of ultraviolet light. In the workplace, it can occur around high-voltage electrical equipment and around ozone-producing devices used for air and water purification. It is also an important oxidant found in polluted urban air. The effect of low ambient levels of ozone on admission to Ontario, Canada, hospitals for respiratory problems revealed a near-linear gradient between exposure (1-hour level, 20–100 ppb) and response. See Table 57–1 for 1999–2000 threshold limit values.

Clinical Effects & Treatment

O_3 is an irritant of mucous membranes. Mild exposure produces upper respiratory tract irritation. Severe exposure can cause deep lung irritation, with pulmonary edema when inhaled at sufficient concentrations. Ozone penetration in the lung depends on tidal volume; consequently, exercise can increase the amount of ozone reaching the distal lung. Some of the effects of O_3 resemble those seen with radiation, suggesting that O_3 toxicity may result from the formation of reactive free radicals. The gas causes shallow, rapid breathing and a decrease in pulmonary compliance. Enhanced sensitivity of the lung to bronchoconstrictors is also observed. Exposure around 0.1 ppm for 10–30 minutes causes irritation and dryness of the throat; above 0.1 ppm, one finds changes in visual acuity, substernal pain, and dyspnea. Pulmonary function is impaired at concentrations exceeding 0.8 ppm. Airway hyperresponsiveness and airway inflammation have been observed in humans.

Animal studies indicate that the response of the lung to O_3 is a dynamic one. The morphologic and biochemical changes are the result of both direct injury and secondary responses to the initial damage. Long-term exposure in animals results in morphologic and functional pulmonary changes. Chronic bronchitis, bronchiolitis, fibrosis, and emphysematous changes have been reported in a variety of species exposed to concentrations above 1 ppm. There is no specific treatment for acute O_3 intoxication. Management depends on therapeutic measures utilized for deep lung irritation and noncardiogenic pulmonary edema (see Nitrogen Oxides, above.)

SOLVENTS

1. Halogenated Aliphatic Hydrocarbons

These agents find wide use as industrial solvents, degreasing agents, and cleaning agents. The substances include carbon tetrachloride, chloroform, trichloroethylene, tetrachloroethylene (perchloroethylene), and 1,1,1-trichloroethane (methyl chloroform). See Table 57–1 for recommended threshold limit values.

Mechanism of Action & Clinical Effects

In laboratory animals, the halogenated hydrocarbons cause central nervous system depression, liver injury, kidney injury, and some degree of cardiotoxicity. These substances are depressants of the central nervous system in humans, though their relative potencies vary considerably; chloroform is the most potent and was widely used as an anesthetic agent. Chronic exposure to tetrachloroethylene can cause impaired memory and peripheral neuropathy. In 1994, evidence was presented suggesting that 1,1,1-trichloroethane used in some degreasing operations may be associated with peripheral neuropathy. This proposed association requires confirmation because of the widespread use of this agent. Hepatotoxicity is also a common toxic effect that can occur in humans after acute or chronic exposures, the severity of the lesion being dependent on the amount absorbed. Carbon tetrachloride is the most potent of the series in this regard. Nephrotoxicity can occur in humans exposed to carbon tetrachloride, chloroform, and trichloroethylene. With chloroform, carbon tetrachloride, trichloroethylene, and tetrachloroethylene, carcinogenicity has been observed in lifetime exposure studies performed in rats or mice. The potential effects of low-level, long-term exposures in humans, however, are yet to be determined. Data indicate that the margin of safety for humans is very large with respect to the potential carcinogenic effect of household exposure to chloroform or environmentally relevant concentrations of trichloroethylene.

Treatment

There is no specific treatment for acute intoxication resulting from exposure to halogenated hydrocarbons. Management depends upon the organ system involved.

2. Aromatic Hydrocarbons

Benzene is widely used for its solvent properties and as an intermediate in the synthesis of other chemicals. The 1999–2000 recommended threshold limit values are given in Table 57–1. The acute toxic effect of benzene is depression of the central nervous system. Exposure to 7500 ppm for 30 minutes can be fatal. Exposure to concentrations larger than 3000 ppm may cause euphoria, nausea, locomotor problems, and coma; vertigo, drowsiness, headache, and nausea may occur at concentrations ranging from 250 to 500 ppm. No specific treatment exists for the acute toxic effect of benzene.

Chronic exposure to benzene can result in very serious toxic effects, the most significant being an insidious and unpredictable injury to the bone marrow; aplastic anemia, leukopenia, pancytopenia, or thrombocytopenia may occur. Bone marrow cells in early stages of development appear to be most sensitive to benzene. The early symptoms of chronic benzene intoxication may be rather vague (headache, fatigue, and loss of appetite). Epidemiologic data suggest an association between chronic benzene exposure and an increased incidence of leukemia in workers.

Toluene (methylbenzene) does not possess the myelotoxic properties of benzene, nor has it been associated with leukemia. It is, however, a central nervous system depressant. See Table 57–1 for the threshold limit values. Exposure to 800 ppm can lead to severe fatigue and ataxia; 10,000 ppm can produce rapid loss of consciousness. Chronic effects of long-term toluene exposure are unclear because human studies indicating behavioral effects usually concern exposures to several solvents, not toluene alone. In limited occupational studies, however, metabolic interactions and modification of toluene's effects have not been observed in workers also exposed to other solvents.

INSECTICIDES

1. Chlorinated Hydrocarbon Insecticides

These agents are usually classified in four groups: DDT (chlorophenothane) and its analogs, benzene hexachlorides, cyclodienes, and toxaphenes (Table 57–2). They are aryl, carbocyclic, or heterocyclic compounds containing chlorine substituents. The individual compounds differ widely in their biotransformation and capacity for storage in tissues; toxicity and storage are not always correlated. They can be absorbed through the skin as well as by inhalation or oral ingestion. There are, however, important quantitative differences between the various derivatives; DDT in solution is poorly absorbed through the skin, whereas dieldrin absorption from the skin is very efficient.

Human Toxicology

The acute toxic properties of the chlorinated hydrocarbon insecticides in humans are qualitatively similar. These agents interfere with inactivation of the sodium channel in excitable membranes and cause rapid repetitive firing in most neurons. Calcium ion transport is also inhibited. These events affect repolarization and enhance the excitability of neurons. The major effect is central nervous stimulation. With DDT, tremor may be the first manifestation, possibly continuing on to convulsions, whereas with the other compounds convulsions often appear as the first sign of intoxication. There is no specific treatment for the acute intoxicated state, management being symptomatic.

Chronic administration of some of these agents to laboratory animals over long periods has resulted in enhanced tumorigenicity; there is no agreement regarding the potential carcinogenic properties of these substances, and extrapolation of these observations to humans is controversial. Evidence of carcinogenic effects in humans has not been established. In a large epidemiologic study, no relationship was observed between the risk of breast cancer and serum levels of DDE, the major metabolite of DDT. A case-control study conducted to investigate the relation between DDE and DDT breast adipose tissue levels and breast cancer risk yielded results that did not support a positive association.

Environmental Toxicology

The chlorinated hydrocarbon insecticides are considered persistent chemicals (Jorgenson, 2001). Degrada-

Table 57–2. Chlorinated hydrocarbon insecticides.

Chemical Class	Compounds	Toxicity Rating[1]	ADI[2]
DDT and analogs	Dichlorodiphenyltrichloroethane (DDT)	4	0.005
	Methoxychlor	3	0.1
	Tetrachlorodiphenylethane (TDE)	3	—
Benzene hexachlorides	Benzene hexachloride (BHC; hexachlorocyclohexane)	4	0.008
	Lindane	4	0.008
Cyclodienes	Aldrin	5	0.0001
	Chlordane	4	0.0005
	Dieldrin	5	0.0001
	Heptachlor	4	0.0001
Toxaphenes	Toxaphene (camphechlor)	4	—

[1]Toxicity rating: Probable human oral lethal dosage for class 3 = 500–5000 mg/kg, class 4 = 50–500 mg/kg, and class 5 = 5–50 mg/kg. (See Gosselin et al, 1984.)

[2]ADI = acceptable daily intake (mg/kg/d).

tion is quite slow when compared to other insecticides, and bioaccumulation, particularly in aquatic ecosystems, is well documented. Their mobility in soil depends on the composition of the soil; the presence of organic matter favors the adsorption of these chemicals onto the soil, whereas adsorption is poor in sandy soils. Once adsorbed, they do not readily desorb.

Because of their environmental impact, use of the chlorinated hydrocarbon insecticides has been largely curtailed in North America and Europe. Some of them are still used, however, in equatorial countries.

2. Organophosphorus Insecticides

These agents, some of which are listed in Table 57–3, are utilized to combat a large variety of pests. They are useful pesticides when in direct contact with insects or when used as **plant systemics,** where the agent is translocated within the plant and exerts its effects on insects that feed on the plant. Some of these agents are used in human and veterinary medicine as local or systemic antiparasitics (Chapter 54). The compounds are absorbed by the skin as well as by the respiratory and gastrointestinal tracts. Biotransformation is rapid, particularly when compared with the rates observed with the chlorinated hydrocarbon insecticides. Current and suggested human inhalation occupational exposure lim-

Table 57–3. Organophosphorus insecticides.

Compound	Toxicity Rating[1]	ADI[2]
Azinphos-methyl	5	0.005
Chlorfenvinphos	—	0.002
Diazinon	4	0.002
Dichlorvos	—	0.004
Dimethoate	4	0.01
Fenitrothion	—	0.005
Leptophos	—	—
Malathion	4	0.02
Parathion	6	0.005
Parathion-methyl	5	0.02
Trichlorfon	4	0.01

[1]Toxicity rating: Probable human oral lethal dosage for class 4 = 50–500 mg/kg, class 5 = 5–50 mg/kg, and class 6 = ≤ 5 mg/kg. (See Gosselin et al, 1984.)
[2]ADI = acceptable daily intake (mg/kg/d).

its for 30 organophosphate pesticides have been reviewed (Storm et al, 2000).

Human Toxicology

In mammals as well as insects, the major effect of these agents is inhibition of acetylcholinesterase through phosphorylation of the esteratic site. The signs and symptoms that characterize acute intoxication are due to inhibition of this enzyme and accumulation of acetylcholine; some of the agents also possess direct cholinergic activity. These effects and their treatment are described in Chapters 7 and 8 in this book and in Steenland et al, 1994. Altered neurologic and cognitive function, as well as psychological symptoms of variable duration, have been associated with exposure to high concentrations of these insecticides (Ecobichon, 1994). Furthermore, there is some indication of an association of low arylesterase activity with neurologic symptom complexes in Gulf War veterans (Haley et al, 1999).

In addition to—and independently of—inhibition of acetylcholinesterase, some of these agents are capable of phosphorylating another enzyme present in neural tissue, the so-called **neuropathy target esterase.** This results in development of a delayed neurotoxicity characterized by polyneuropathy, associated with paralysis and axonal degeneration (organophosphorus ester–induced delayed polyneuropathy; OPIDP); hens are particularly sensitive to these properties and have proved very useful for studying the pathogenesis of the lesion and for identifying potentially neurotoxic organophosphorus derivatives. In humans, neurotoxicity has been observed with **triorthocresyl phosphate** (TOCP), a noninsecticidal organophosphorus compound, and is thought to occur with the insecticides dichlorvos, trichlorfon, leptophos, methamidophos, mipafox, and trichloronat. The polyneuropathy usually begins with burning and tingling sensations, particularly in the feet, with motor weakness following a few days later. Sensory and motor difficulties may extend to the legs and hands. Gait is affected, and ataxia may be present. There is no specific treatment for this form of delayed neurotoxicity.

Environmental Toxicology

Organophosphorus insecticides are not considered to be persistent pesticides because they are relatively unstable and break down in the environment. As a class they are considered to have a small impact on the environment in spite of their acute effects on organisms.

3. Carbamate Insecticides

These compounds (Table 57–4) inhibit acetylcholinesterase by carbamoylation of the esteratic site.

Table 57–4. Carbamate insecticides.

Compound	Toxicity Rating[1]	ADI[2]
Aldicarb	6	0.005
Aminocarb	5	—
Carbaryl	4	0.01
Carbofuran	5	0.01
Dimetan	4	—
Dimetilan	4	—
Isolan	5	—
Methomyl	5	—
Propoxur	4	0.02
Pyramat	4	—
Pyrolan	5	—
Zectran	5	—

[1]Toxicity rating: Probable human oral lethal dosage for class 4 = 50–500 mg/kg, class 5 = 5–50 mg/kg, and class 6 = ≤ 5 mg/kg. (See Gosselin et al, 1984.)

[2]ADI = acceptable daily intake (mg/kg/d).

Thus, they possess the toxic properties associated with inhibition of this enzyme as described for the organophosphorus insecticides. The effects and treatment are described in Chapters 7 and 8. The clinical effects due to carbamates are of shorter duration than those observed with organophosphorus compounds. The range between the doses that cause minor intoxication and those which result in lethality is larger with carbamates than that observed with the organophosphorus agents. Spontaneous reactivation of cholinesterase is more rapid after inhibition by the carbamates. While the clinical approach to carbamate poisoning is similar to that for organophosphates, the use of pralidoxime is not recommended.

The carbamate insecticides are considered to be nonpersistent pesticides and are thought to exert only a small impact on the environment.

4. Botanical Insecticides

Insecticides derived from natural sources include **nicotine, rotenone,** and **pyrethrum.** Nicotine is obtained from the dried leaves of *Nicotiana tabacum* and *Nicotiana rustica.* It is rapidly absorbed from mucosal surfaces; the free alkaloid, but not the salt, is readily absorbed from the skin. Nicotine reacts with the acetylcholine receptor of the postsynaptic membrane (sympathetic and parasympathetic ganglia, neuromuscular junction), resulting in depolarization of the membrane. Toxic doses cause stimulation rapidly followed by blockade of transmission. These actions are described in Chapter 7. Treatment is directed toward maintenance of vital signs and suppression of convulsions.

Rotenone (Figure 57–1) is obtained from *Derris elliptica, Derris mallaccensis, Lonchocarpus utilis,* and *Lonchocarpus urucu.* The oral ingestion of rotenone produces gastrointestinal irritation. Conjunctivitis, dermatitis, pharyngitis, and rhinitis can also occur. Treatment is symptomatic.

Pyrethrum consists of six known insecticidal esters: pyrethrin I (Figure 57–1), pyrethrin II, cinerin I, cinerin II, jasmolin I, and jasmolin II. Synthetic pyrethroids account for about 30% of worldwide insecticide usage. Pyrethrum may be absorbed after inhalation or ingestion; absorption from the skin is not significant. The esters are extensively biotransformed. Pyrethrum insecticides are not highly toxic to mammals. When absorbed in sufficient quantities, the major site of toxic action is the central nervous system; excitation, convulsions, and tetanic paralysis can occur. Voltage-sensitive sodium, calcium, and chloride channels are considered targets, as well as peripheral-type benzodiazepine receptors. Treatment is with anticonvulsants. The most frequent injury reported in humans results from the allergenic properties of the substance, especially contact dermatitis. Cutaneous paresthesias have been observed in workers spraying synthetic pyrethroids. Severe occupational exposures to synthetic pyrethroids in China resulted in marked effects on the central nervous system, including convulsions.

HERBICIDES

1. Chlorophenoxy Herbicides

2,4-Dichlorophenoxyacetic acid (2,4-D), 2,4,5-trichlorophenoxyacetic acid (2,4,5-T), and their salts and esters are the major compounds of interest as herbicides used for the destruction of weeds (Figure 57–1). They have been assigned toxicity ratings of 4 or 3, respectively, which place the probable human lethal dosages at 50–500 or 500–5000 mg/kg, respectively (Gosselin et al, 1984).

In humans, 2,4-D in large doses can cause coma and generalized muscle hypotonia. Rarely, muscle weakness and marked myotonia may persist for several weeks. With 2,4,5-T, coma may occur, but the muscular dysfunction is less evident. In laboratory animals, signs of liver and kidney dysfunction have also been reported. There is limited evidence that occupational exposure to phenoxy herbicides is associated with an increased risk of non-Hodgkin's lymphoma; the evidence for soft-tissue sarcoma, however, is considered equivocal.

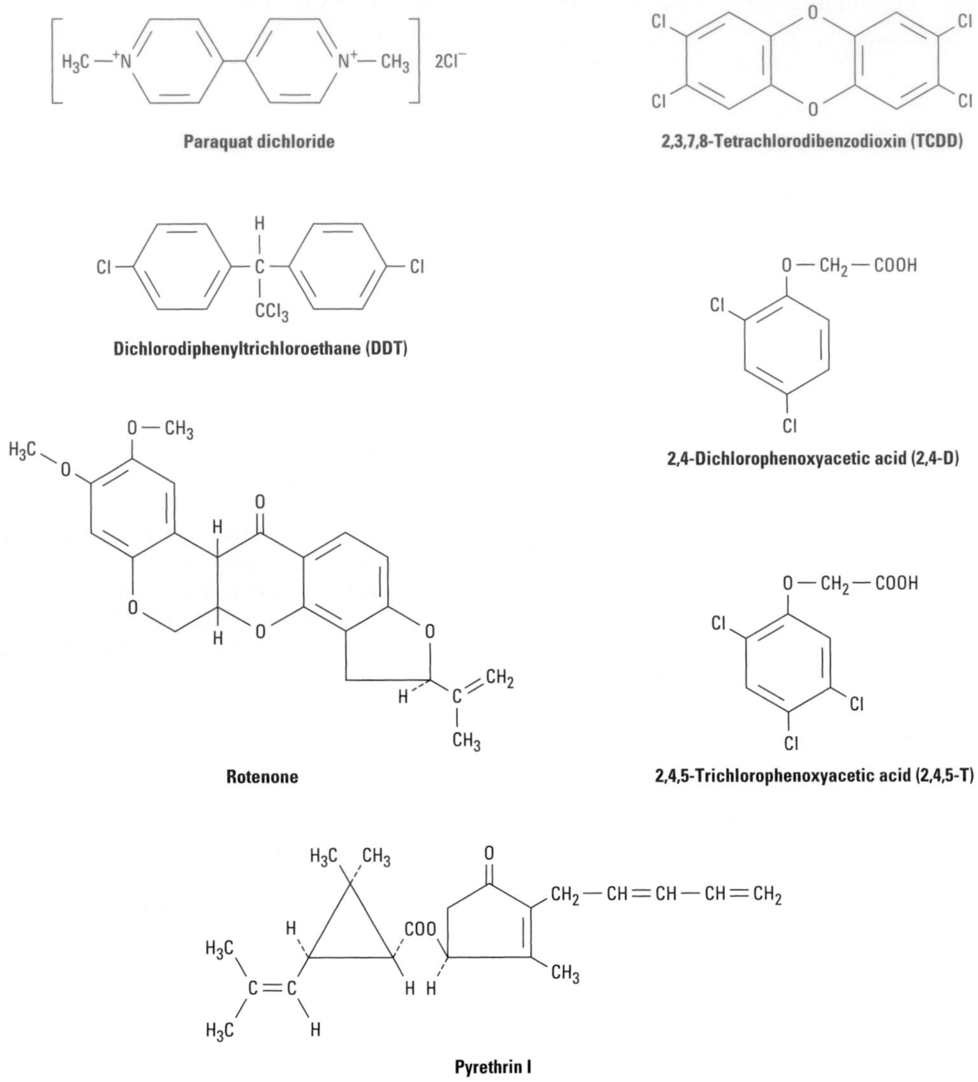

Figure 57–1. Chemical structures of selected herbicides and pesticides.

The toxicologic profile for these agents, particularly that of 2,4,5-T, has been confusing because of the presence of chemical contaminants (**dioxins**) produced during the manufacturing process (see below). 2,3,7,8-Tetrachlorodibenzo-*p*-dioxin (TCDD) is the most important of these contaminants.

2. Bipyridyl Herbicides

Paraquat is the most important agent of this class (Figure 57–1). Its mechanism of action is said to be similar in plants and animals and involves single-electron

reduction of the herbicide to free radical species. It has been given a toxicity rating of 4, which places the probable human lethal dosage at 50–500 mg/kg. A number of lethal human intoxications (accidental or suicidal) have been reported. Paraquat accumulates slowly in the lung by an active process and causes lung edema, alveolitis, and progressive fibrosis.

In humans, the first signs and symptoms after oral exposure are attributable to gastrointestinal irritation (hematemesis and bloody stools). Within a few days, however, delayed toxicity occurs, with respiratory distress and the development of congestive hemorrhagic pulmonary edema accompanied by widespread cellular proliferation. Hepatic, renal, or myocardial involvement may also be evident. The interval between ingestion and death may be several weeks. Because of the delayed pulmonary toxicity, prompt removal of paraquat from the digestive tract is important. Gastric lavage, the use of cathartics, and the use of adsorbents to prevent further absorption have all been advocated; after absorption, treatment is successful in fewer than 50% of cases. Oxygen should be used cautiously to combat dyspnea or cyanosis, as it may aggravate the pulmonary lesions. Patients require prolonged observation, because the proliferative phase begins 1–2 weeks after ingestion.

ENVIRONMENTAL POLLUTANTS

1. Polychlorinated Biphenyls

The **polychlorinated biphenyls (PCBs, coplanar biphenyls)** have been used in a large variety of applications as dielectric and heat transfer fluids, plasticizers, wax extenders, and flame retardants. Their industrial use and manufacture in the USA was terminated by 1977. Unfortunately, they persist in the environment. The products used commercially were actually mixtures of PCB isomers and homologs containing 12–68% chlorine. These chemicals are highly stable and highly lipophilic, poorly metabolized, and very resistant to environmental degradation; they bioaccumulate in food chains. Food is the major source of PCB residues in humans.

A serious exposure to PCBs—lasting several months—occurred in Japan in 1968 as a result of cooking oil contamination with PCB-containing transfer medium (Yusho disease). Possible effects on the fetus and on the development of the offspring of poisoned women were reported. It is now known that the contaminated cooking oil contained not only PCBs but also polychlorinated dibenzofurans (PCDFs) and polychlorinated quaterphenyls (PCQs). Consequently, the effects that were initially attributed to the presence of PCBs are now thought to have been largely caused by the other contaminants. Workers occupationally exposed to PCBs have exhibited the following clinical signs: dermatologic problems (chloracne, folliculitis, erythema, dryness, rash, hyperkeratosis, hyperpigmentation), some hepatic involvement, and elevated plasma triglycerides.

The effects of PCBs alone on reproduction and development, as well as their carcinogenic effects, have yet to be established in humans—whether workers or the general population—even though some subjects have been exposed to very high levels of PCBs. Some adverse behavioral effects in infants are reported to have been observed in two studies involving subjects from the general population, but the adverse effects observed in the two studies were dissimilar; furthermore, there are a number of uncertainties about the exposure assessments in both studies (Kimbrough, 1995). An association between prenatal exposure to PCBs and deficits in childhood intellectual function was described for children born to mothers who had eaten large quantities of contaminated fish (Jacobson & Jacobson, 2002). The bulk of the evidence from human studies indicates that PCBs pose little hazard to human health except in situations where food is contaminated with high concentrations of these congeners.

The **polychlorinated dibenzo-*p*-dioxins (PCDDs), or dioxins,** have been mentioned above as a group of congeners of which the most important is **2,3,7,8-tetrachlorodibenzo-*p*-dioxin (TCDD).** In addition, there is a larger group of dioxin-like compounds, including certain **polychlorinated dibenzofurans (PCDFs)** and **coplanar biphenyls.** While PCBs were used commercially, PCDDs and PCDFs are unwanted by-products that appear in the environment as contaminants because of improperly controlled combustion processes. PCDD and PCDF contamination of the global environment is considered to represent a contemporary problem produced by human activities. Like PCBs, these chemicals are very stable and highly lipophilic. They are poorly metabolized and very resistant to environmental degradation.

In laboratory animals, TCDD administered in suitable doses has produced a wide variety of toxic effects, including a wasting syndrome (severe weight loss accompanied by reduction of muscle mass and adipose tissue), thymic atrophy, epidermal changes, hepatotoxicity, immunotoxicity, effects on reproduction and development, teratogenicity, and carcinogenicity. Fortunately, most of these actions have not been observed in humans. The effects observed in workers involved in the manufacture of 2,4,5-T (and therefore presumably exposed to TCDD) consisted primarily of contact dermatitis and chloracne. In severely TCDD-intoxicated patients, only discrete chloracne may be present.

The presence of TCDD in 2,4,5-T is believed to be largely responsible also for other human toxicities associated with the herbicide. There is some epidemiologic evidence indicating an association between occupational exposure to the phenoxy herbicides and an excess incidence of non-Hodgkin's lymphoma. The evidence of an association of increased soft tissue sarcomas with herbicides themselves, however, is considered equivocal. On the other hand, the TCDD contaminant in these herbicides may play a role in soft tissue sarcomas.

2. "Endocrine Disruptors"

The potential hazardous effects of some chemicals found in the environment are receiving considerable attention because of their estrogen-like or antiandrogenic properties. These so-called endocrine disruptors that mimic, enhance, or inhibit a hormonal action include a number of plant constituents (phytoestrogens) and some mycoestrogens as well as industrial chemicals, particularly persistent organochlorine agents like DDT and PCBs. In vitro assays alone are unreliable for regulatory purposes, and animal studies are considered indispensable. Modified endocrine responses in some reptiles and marine invertebrates have been observed. In humans, however, a causal relationship between exposure to a specific environmental agent and an adverse health effect due to endocrine modulation has not been established. At present, the evidence is not considered compelling.

REFERENCES

AIR POLLUTION

Burnett RT et al: Effects of low ambient levels of ozone and sulfates on the frequency of respiratory admissions to Ontario hospitals. Environ Res 1994;65:172.

Costa DL: Air Pollution. In: Klaassen CD (editor). *Casarett and Doull's Toxicology,* 6th ed. McGraw-Hill, 2001.

Folinsbee LJ: Human health effects of air pollution. Environ Health Perspect 1993;100:45.

Penney DG, Howley JW: Is there a connection between carbon monoxide exposure and hypertension? Environ Health Perspect 1991;95:191.

Raub JA et al: Carbon monoxide poisoning—a public health perspective. Toxicology 2000;145:1.

Samet JM, Utell MJ: The environment and the lung. JAMA 1991;266:670.

Wright ES, Dziedzic D, Wheeler CS: Cellular, biochemical, and functional effects of ozone: New research and perspectives on ozone health effects. Toxicol Lett 1990;51:125.

OCCUPATIONAL TOXICOLOGY

Cullen MR, Cherniak MG, Rosenstock L: Occupational medicine. (Two parts.) N Engl J Med 1990;322:594, 675.

Doull J: Recommended Limits for Occupational Exposure to Chemicals. In: Klaassen CD (editor). *Casarett and Doull's Toxicology,* 6th ed. McGraw-Hill, 2001.

Faustman EM, Omenn GS: Risk Assessment. In: Klaassen CD (editor). *Casarett and Doull's Toxicology,* 6th ed. McGraw-Hill, 2001.

House RA, Liss GM, Wills MC: Peripheral sensory neuropathy associated with 1,1,1-trichlorethane. Arch Environ Health 1994;51:196.

Proctor NH, Hughes JP: *Chemical Hazards of the Workplace,* 3rd ed. Lippincott, 1991.

Ukai H et al: Occupational exposure to solvent mixtures: Effects on health and metabolism. Occup Environ Health 1994;51:523.

ENVIRONMENTAL TOXICOLOGY & ECOTOXICOLOGY

Crisp TM et al: Environmental endocrine disruption: an effects assessment and analysis. Environ Health Persp 1998; 106(Suppl 1):11.

Degen GH, Bolt HM: Endocrine disruptors: update on xenoestrogens. Int Arch Occup Environ Health 2000;73:433.

Geusau A et al: Severe 2,3,7,8-tetrachlorodibenzo-*p*-dioxin (TCDD) intoxication: clinical and laboratory effects. Environ Health Persp 2001;109:865.

Jacobson JL, Jacobson SW: Association of prenatal exposure to an environmental contaminant with intellectual function in childhood. J Toxicol Clin Toxicol 2002;40:467.

Kimbrough RD: Polychlorinated biphenyls (PCBs) and human health: An update. CRC Crit Rev Toxicol 1995;25:133.

Lavin AL, Jacobson OF, DeSesso JM: An assessment of the carcinogenic potential of trichloroethylene in humans. Human Ecol Risk Assess 2000;6:575.

Lévesque B et al: Cancer risk associated with household exposure to chloroform. J Toxicol Environ Health A 2002;65:489.

Safe SH: Endocrine disruptors and human health—is there a problem? An update. Environ Health Persp 2000;108:487.

Schecter A: *Dioxins and Health.* Plenum, 1994.

Silberhorn EM, Glauert HP, Robertson LW: Carcinogenicity of polyhalogenated biphenyls: PCBs and PBBs. CRC Crit Rev Toxicol 1990;20:440.

PESTICIDES & HERBICIDES

Ecobichon DJ: Organophosphorus ester insecticides. In: Ecobichon DJ, Joy RM (editors). *Pesticides and Neurological Diseases,* 2nd ed. CRC, 1994.

Ecobichon DJ: Our changing perspectives on benefits and risks of pesticides: a historical overview. Neurotoxicology 2000;21:211.

Ecobichon DJ: Toxic effects of pesticides. In: Klaassen CD (editor). *Casarett and Doull's Toxicology,* 6th ed. McGraw-Hill, 2001.

Haley RW et al: Association of low PON1 type Q (type A) arylesterase activity with neurologic symptom complexes in Gulf War veterans. Toxicol Appl Pharmacol 1999;157:227.

Jorgenson JL: Aldrin and dieldrin: a review of research on their production, environmental deposition and fate, bioaccumulation, toxicology, and epidemiology in the United States. Environ Health Perspect 2001;109(Suppl 1):113.

Krieger N et al: Breast cancer and serum organochlorines: A prospective study among white, black and Asian women. J Natl Cancer Inst 1994;86:589.

Lotti M: The pathogenesis of organophosphate polyneuropathy. CRC Crit Rev Toxicol 1992;213:465.

Machemer LD, Pickel M: Carbamate insecticides. Toxicology 1994;91:29.

MacMahon B: Pesticide residues and breast cancer? J Natl Cancer Inst 1994;86:572.

Morrison HI et al: Herbicides and cancer. J Natl Cancer Inst 1992;84:1866.

Sabapathy NN: Quaternary ammonium compounds. Toxicology 1994;91:93.

Soderlund DM et al: Mechanisms of pyrethroid neurotoxicity: implications for cumulative risk assessment. Toxicology 2002;171:3.

Steenland K et al: Chronic neurological sequelae to organophosphate pesticide poisoning. Am J Public Health 1994;84:731.

Storm JE, Rozman KK, Doull J: Occupational exposure limits for 30 organophosphate pesticides based on inhibition of red blood cell acetylcholinesterase. Toxicology 2000;150:1.

Zheng T et al: DDE and DDT in breast adipose tissue and risk of female breast cancer. Am J Epidemiol 1999;150:453.

CLINICAL TOXICOLOGY

Ellenhorn MJ: *Ellenhorn's Medical Toxicology,* 2nd ed. Lippincott Williams & Wilkins, 1997.

Gosselin RE, Smith RP, Hodge HC: *Clinical Toxicology of Commercial Products,* 5th ed. Williams & Wilkins, 1984.

Heavy Metal Intoxication & Chelators

58

Michael J. Kosnett, MD, MPH

Some metals such as iron are essential for life, while others such as lead are present in all organisms but serve no useful biologic purpose. Some of the oldest diseases of humans can be traced to heavy metal poisoning associated with metal mining, refining, and use. Even with the present recognition of the hazards of heavy metals, the incidence of intoxication remains significant and the need for preventive strategies and effective therapy remains high. When intoxication occurs, chelator molecules (from *chela* "claw") may be used to bind the metal and facilitate its excretion from the body. Chelator drugs are discussed in the second part of this chapter.

TOXICOLOGY OF HEAVY METALS

LEAD

Lead poisoning is one of the oldest occupational and environmental diseases in the world. Despite its recognized hazards, lead continues to have widespread commercial application. Environmental lead exposure, ubiquitous by virtue of the anthropogenic distribution of lead to air, water, and food, has declined considerably in the past 2 decades as a result of diminished use of lead in gasoline and other applications. While these public health measures, together with improved workplace conditions, have decreased the incidence of serious overt lead poisoning, there remains considerable concern over the effects of low-level lead exposure. Extensive evidence indicates that lead may have subtle subclinical adverse effects on neurocognitive function and on blood pressure at blood lead concentrations once considered "normal" or "safe." Lead serves no useful purpose in the human body. In key target organs such as the developing central nervous system, no safe threshold of lead exposure has been established.

Pharmacokinetics

Inorganic lead is slowly but consistently absorbed via the respiratory and gastrointestinal tracts. Inorganic lead is poorly absorbed through the skin, but organic lead compounds, eg, leaded antiknock gasoline, are well absorbed by this route. Absorption of lead dust via the respiratory tract is the most common cause of industrial poisoning. The intestinal tract is the primary route of entry in nonindustrial exposure (Table 58–1). Absorption via the gastrointestinal tract varies with the nature of the lead compound, but in general, adults absorb about 10% of the ingested amount while young children absorb up to 50%. Low dietary calcium, iron deficiency, and ingestion on an empty stomach have all been associated with increased lead absorption.

Once absorbed from the respiratory or gastrointestinal tract, lead is bound to erythrocytes and widely distributed initially to soft tissues such as the bone marrow, brain, kidney, liver, muscle, and gonads; then to the subperiosteal surface of bone; and later to bone matrix. Lead also crosses the placenta and poses a potential hazard to the fetus. The kinetics of lead clearance from the body follows a multi-compartment model, composed predominantly of the blood and soft tissues, with a half-life of 1–2 months; and the skeleton, with a half-life of years to decades. Approximately 70% of the lead that is eliminated appears in the urine, with lesser amounts excreted through the bile, skin, hair, nails, sweat, and breast milk. The fraction not undergoing prompt excretion, approximately half of the absorbed lead, may be incorporated into the skeleton, the repository of more than 90% of the body lead burden in most adults. In patients with high bone lead burdens, slow release from the skeleton may elevate blood lead concentrations for years after exposure ceases; and pathologic high bone turnover states such as hyperthyroidism or prolonged immobilization may result in frank lead intoxication. The lead burden in bone has been quantitated using noninvasive x-ray fluorescence, a technique that may provide the best measure of long-term, cumulative lead absorption.

Pharmacodynamics

Lead exerts multisystemic toxic effects through at least three mechanisms: by inhibiting enzyme activity, some-

Table 58–1. Toxicology of selected arsenic, lead, and mercury compounds.

	Form Entering Body	Major Route of Absorption	Distribution	Major Clinical Effects	Key Aspects of Mechanism	Metabolism and Elimination
Arsenic	Inorganic arsenic salts	Gastrointestinal, respiratory (all mucosal surfaces), skin	Predominantly soft tissues (highest in liver, kidney). Avidly bound in skin, hair, nails	Cardiovascular: shock, arrhythmias. CNS: encephalopathy, peripheral neuropathy. Gastroenteritis; pancytopenia; cancer (many sites)	Inhibits enzymes via sulfhydryl binding; interferes with oxidative phosphorylation	Methylation. Renal (major); sweat and feces (minor)
Lead	Inorganic lead oxides and salts	Gastrointestinal, respiratory	Soft tissues; redistributed to skeleton (> 90% of adult body burden)	CNS deficits, peripheral neuropathy; anemia; nephropathy; hypertension (?)	Inhibits enzymes; interferes with essential cations; alters membrane structure	Renal (major); breast milk (minor)
	Organic (tetraethyl lead)	Skin, gastrointestinal, respiratory	Soft tissues, especially liver, CNS	Encephalopathy	Hepatic dealkylation (fast) → trialkymetabolites (slow) → dissociation to lead	Urine and feces (major); sweat (minor)
Mercury	Elemental mercury	Respiratory tract	Soft tissues, especially kidney, CNS	CNS: behavioral (erethism); gingivostomatitis; peripheral neuropathy; acrodynia; pneumonitis (high-dose)	Inhibits enzymes; alters membranes	Elemental Hg converted to Hg^{2+}. Urine (major); feces (minor)
	Inorganic: Hg^+ (less toxic); Hg^{2+} (more toxic)	Gastrointestinal, skin (minor)	Soft tissues, especially kidney	Acute tubular necrosis; gastroenteritis; CNS effects (rare)	Inhibits enzymes; alters membranes	Urine
	Organic: alkyl, aryl	Gastrointestinal, skin, respiratory (minor)	Soft tissues	CNS effects, birth defects	Inhibits enzymes; alters neuronal structure	Deacylation. Fecal (alkyl, major); urine (Hg^{2+} after deacylation, minor)

times as a consequence of binding to sulfhydryl groups; by interfering with the action of essential cations, particularly calcium, iron, and zinc; and by altering the structure of cell membranes and receptors.

A. Nervous System

The developing central nervous system of the fetus and young child is the most sensitive target organ for lead's toxic effect. Epidemiologic studies suggest that blood lead concentrations less than 5 μg/dL may result in sub-

clinical deficits in neurocognitive function in lead-exposed young children, with no demonstrable threshold for a "no effect" level (Canfield et al, 2003). Hearing acuity may also be diminished. Adults are less sensitive to the CNS effects of lead, but at blood lead concentrations in excess of 30 μg/dL, behavioral, constitutional, and neurocognitive effects may gradually emerge, producing signs and symptoms such as irritability, fatigue, decreased libido, anorexia, sleep disturbance, impaired visual-motor coordination, and slowed reaction time.

Headache, arthralgias, and myalgias are also frequent complaints. Tremor occurs but is less common. Lead encephalopathy, usually occurring at blood lead concentrations in excess of 100 μg/dL, is typically accompanied by increased intracranial pressure and may produce ataxia, stupor, coma, convulsions, and death. There is wide interindividual variation in the magnitude of lead exposure required to cause overt lead-related signs and symptoms.

Peripheral neuropathy may appear after chronic high-dose lead exposure, usually following months to years of blood lead concentrations in excess of 100 μg/dL. Predominantly motor in character, the neuropathy may present clinically with painless weakness of the extensors, particularly in the upper extremity, resulting in classic wrist-drop. Preclinical signs of lead-induced peripheral nerve dysfunction may be detectable by electrodiagnostic testing.

B. BLOOD

Lead can induce an anemia that may be either normocytic or microcytic and hypochromic. Lead interferes with heme synthesis by blocking the incorporation of iron into protoporphyrin IX and by inhibiting the function of enzymes in the heme synthesis pathway, including aminolevulinic acid dehydratase and ferrochelatase. Within 2–8 weeks after an elevation in blood lead concentration (generally to 30–50 μg/dL or greater), increases in heme precursors, notably free erythrocyte protoporphyrin or its zinc chelate, zinc protoporphyrin, may be detectable in whole blood. Lead also contributes to anemia by increasing erythrocyte membrane fragility and decreasing red cell survival time. Frank hemolysis may occur with high exposure. The presence of basophilic stippling on the peripheral blood smear, thought to be a consequence of lead inhibition of the enzyme 3',5'-pyrimidine nucleotidase, is sometimes a suggestive—albeit insensitive and nonspecific—diagnostic clue to the presence of lead intoxication.

C. KIDNEYS

Chronic high-dose lead exposure, usually associated with months to years of blood lead concentrations in excess of 80 μg/dL, may result in renal interstitial fibrosis and nephrosclerosis. Lead nephropathy may have a latency period of years. Lead may alter uric acid excretion by the kidney, resulting in recurrent bouts of gouty arthritis ("saturnine gout"). Acute high-dose lead exposure sometimes produces transient azotemia, possibly as a consequence of intrarenal vasoconstriction.

D. REPRODUCTIVE ORGANS

High-dose lead exposure is a recognized risk factor for stillbirth or spontaneous abortion. Epidemiologic studies of the impact of low-level lead exposure on reproductive outcome such as low birth weight, preterm delivery, or spontaneous abortion have yielded mixed results. However, a well-designed nested case-control study recently detected an odds ratio for spontaneous abortion of 1.8 (95% CI 1.1–3.1) for every 5 μg/dL increase in maternal blood lead across an approximate range of 5–20 μg/dL (Borja-Aburto et al, 1999). In males, blood lead concentrations in excess of 40 μg/dL have been associated with diminished or aberrant sperm production.

E. GASTROINTESTINAL TRACT

Moderate lead poisoning may cause loss of appetite, constipation, and, less commonly, diarrhea. At high dosage, intermittent bouts of severe colicky abdominal pain ("lead colic") may occur. The mechanism of lead colic is unclear but is believed to involve spasmodic contraction of the smooth muscles of the intestinal wall. In heavily exposed individuals with poor dental hygiene, the reaction of circulating lead with sulfur ions released by microbial action may produce dark deposits of lead sulfide at the gingival margin ("gingival lead lines"). Although frequently mentioned as a diagnostic clue, this is a far from universal sign of lead exposure.

F. CARDIOVASCULAR SYSTEM

Epidemiologic, experimental, and in vitro mechanistic data indicate that lead exposure elevates blood pressure in susceptible individuals. In populations with environmental or occupational lead exposure, blood lead concentration is linked with increases in systolic and diastolic blood pressure. Studies of middle-aged and elderly men and women have identified cumulative lead exposure to be an independent risk factor for hypertension (Korrick et al, 1999). Lead can also elevate blood pressure in experimental animals, an effect that may be caused by interaction with calcium-mediated constriction of vascular smooth muscle.

Major Forms of Lead Intoxication

A. INORGANIC LEAD POISONING (TABLE 58–1)

1. Acute—Acute inorganic lead poisoning is uncommon today. It usually results from industrial inhalation of large quantities of lead oxide fumes or, in small children, from ingestion of a large oral dose of lead in lead-based paints or contaminated food or drink. The onset of severe symptoms usually requires several days or weeks of recurrent exposure and presents with signs and symptoms of encephalopathy or colic. Evidence of hemolytic anemia (or anemia with basophilic stippling if exposure has been subacute) and elevated hepatic aminotransferases may be present. The diagnosis of acute inorganic lead poisoning may be difficult, and depending on the presenting symptoms, the condition has sometimes been mistaken for appendicitis, peptic ulcer, pancreatitis, or infectious meningitis. Subacute presentation, featuring headache, fatigue, intermittent abdominal cramps, myalgias, and arthralgias, has often been mistaken for a flu-like viral illness and may not come to medical attention. When there has been recent ingestion of lead-containing paint chips, glazes, or weights, radiopacities may be visible on abdominal radiographs.

2. Chronic—The patient with chronic lead intoxication usually presents with multisystemic findings, including constitutional complaints of anorexia, fatigue, and malaise; neurologic complaints, including headache, difficulty in concentrating, irritability or depressed mood; weakness, arthralgias or myalgias; and gastrointestinal symptoms. Lead poisoning should be strongly suspected in any patient presenting with headache, abdominal pain, and anemia; and less commonly with motor neuropathy, gout, and renal insufficiency. Chronic lead intoxication should be considered in any child with neurocognitive deficits, growth retardation, or developmental delay.

The diagnosis is best confirmed by measuring lead in whole blood. Although this test reflects lead currently circulating in blood and soft tissues and is not a reliable marker of either recent or cumulative lead exposure, most patients with lead-related disease will have blood lead concentrations above the normal range. Average background blood lead concentrations in North America and Europe have declined considerably in recent decades, and the geometric mean blood lead concentration in the United States in 1999–2000 was estimated to be 1.66 μg/dL (CDC, 2003). Although predominantly a research tool, the concentration of lead in bone assessed by noninvasive K x-ray fluorescence measurement of lead in bone has been correlated with long-term cumulative lead exposure, and its relationship to numerous lead-related disorders is a subject of ongoing investigation. Measurement of lead excretion in the urine following a single dose of a chelating agent (sometimes called a "chelation challenge test") primarily reflects the lead content of soft tissues and may not be a reliable marker of long-term lead exposure, remote past exposure, or skeletal lead burden.

B. Organolead Poisoning

Poisoning from organolead compounds is now very rare, in large part due to the worldwide phase-out of tetraethyl and tetramethyl lead as antiknock additives in gasoline. However, organolead compounds such as lead stearate or lead naphthenate are still used in certain commercial processes. Because of their volatility or lipid solubility, organolead compounds tend to be well absorbed through either the respiratory tract or the skin.

Organolead compounds predominantly target the central nervous system, producing dose-dependent effects that may include neurocognitive deficits, insomnia, delirium, hallucinations, tremor, convulsions, and death.

Treatment

A. Inorganic Lead Poisoning

Treatment of inorganic lead poisoning involves immediate termination of exposure, supportive care, and the judicious use of chelation therapy. (Chelation is discussed further later in this chapter.) Lead encephalopathy is a medical emergency that requires intensive supportive care. Cerebral edema may improve with corticosteroids and mannitol, and anticonvulsants may be required to treat seizures. Radiopacities on abdominal radiographs may suggest the presence of retained lead objects requiring gastrointestinal decontamination. Adequate urine flow should be maintained, but overhydration should be avoided. Intravenous edetate calcium disodium ($CaNa_2EDTA$) is administered at a dosage of 1000–1500 mg/m²/d (approximately 30–50 mg/kg/d) by continuous infusion for up to 5 days. Some clinicians advocate that chelation treatment for lead encephalopathy be initiated with an intramuscular injection of dimercaprol, followed in 4 hours by concurrent administration of dimercaprol and EDTA. Parenteral chelation is limited to 5 or fewer days, at which time oral treatment with another chelator, succimer, may be instituted. In symptomatic lead intoxication without encephalopathy, treatment may sometimes be initiated with succimer. The end point for chelation is usually resolution of symptoms or return of the blood lead concentration to the premorbid range. In patients with chronic exposure, cessation of chelation may be followed by an upward rebound in blood lead concentration as the lead reequilibrates from bone lead stores.

While most clinicians support chelation for symptomatic patients with elevated blood lead concentrations, the decision to chelate asymptomatic subjects is more controversial. Since 1991, the CDC has recommended chelation for all children with blood lead concentrations of 45 μg/dL or greater. However, a recent randomized, double-blind, placebo-controlled clinical trial of succimer in children with blood lead concentrations between 25 μg/dL and 44 μg/dL found no benefit on neurocognitive function or long-term blood lead reduction (Rogan et al, 2001). Prophylactic use of chelating agents in the workplace should never be a substitute for reduction or prevention of excessive exposure.

B. Organic Lead Poisoning

Initial treatment consists of decontaminating the skin and preventing further exposure. Treatment of seizures requires appropriate use of anticonvulsants. Empiric chelation may be attempted if high blood lead concentrations are present.

ARSENIC

Arsenic is a naturally occurring element in the earth's crust with a long history of use as a constituent of commercial and industrial products, as a component in pharmaceuticals, and as an agent of deliberate poisoning. Recent commercial applications of arsenic include its use in the manufacture of semiconductors, wood preservatives, herbicides, cotton desiccants, nonferrous alloys, glass, insecticides, and veterinary pharmaceuticals. In some regions of the world, groundwater may contain high levels of arsenic that has leached from natural mineral deposits. Arsenic in drinking water in the Ganges delta of India and Bangladesh is now recognized as one of the world's most pressing environmental health problems. Arsine, a hydride gas with potent hemolytic effects, is manufactured predominantly for use in the semiconductor industry but may also be generated accidentally when arsenic-containing ores come in contact with acidic solutions.

It is of historical interest that Fowler's solution, which contains 1% potassium arsenite, was widely used as a medicine for many conditions from the eighteenth century through the mid twentieth century. Organic arsenicals were the first pharmaceutical antibiotics* and were widely used for the first half of the twentieth century until supplanted by penicillin and other more effective and less toxic agents.

Other organoarsenicals, most notably lewisite (dichloro[2-chlorovinyl]arsine), were developed in the early twentieth century as chemical warfare agents. Arsenic trioxide was reintroduced into the United States Pharmacopeia in 2000 as an orphan drug for the treatment of relapsed acute promyelocytic leukemia (Chapter 55).

Pharmacokinetics

Soluble arsenic compounds are well absorbed through the respiratory and gastrointestinal tracts (Table 58–1). Percutaneous absorption is limited but may be clinically significant after heavy exposure to concentrated arsenic reagents. Most of the absorbed inorganic arsenic undergoes methylation, mainly in the liver, to monomethylarsonic acid and dimethylarsinic acid, which are excreted, along with residual inorganic arsenic, in the urine. When chronic daily absorption is less than 1000 μg of soluble inorganic arsenic, approximately two thirds of

the absorbed dose is excreted in the urine. After massive ingestions, the elimination half-life is prolonged. Inhalation of arsenic compounds of low solubility may result in prolonged retention in the lung and may not be reflected by urinary arsenic excretion. Arsenic binds to sulfhydryl groups present in keratinized tissue, and following cessation of exposure, hair, nails, and skin may contain elevated levels after urine values have returned to normal. However, arsenic present in hair and nails as a result of external deposition may be indistinguishable from that incorporated after internal absorption.

Pharmacodynamics

Arsenic compounds are believed to exert their toxic effects by several modes of action. Interference with enzymatic function may result from sulfhydryl group binding by trivalent arsenic or by substitution for phosphate. Inorganic arsenic or its metabolites may induce oxidative stress, alter gene expression, and interfere with cell signal transduction. Although on a molar basis trivalent arsenic (As^{3+}, arsenite) is generally two to ten times more acutely toxic than pentavalent arsenic (As^{5+}, arsenate), in vivo interconversion is known to occur, and the full spectrum of arsenic toxicity has occurred after sufficient exposure to either form. Arsine gas is oxidized in vivo and exerts a potent hemolytic effect associated with alteration of ion flux across the erythrocyte membrane; however, it also disrupts cellular respiration in other tissues. Arsenic is a recognized human carcinogen and has been associated with cancer of the lung, skin, and bladder (National Research Council, 2001). Marine organisms may contain large amounts of a well-absorbed trimethylated organoarsenic, arsenobetaine, as well as a variety of arsenosugars. Arsenobetaine exerts no known toxic effects when ingested by mammals and is excreted in the urine unchanged; arsenosugars are partially metabolized to dimethylarsinic acid.

Major Forms of Arsenic Intoxication

A. ACUTE INORGANIC ARSENIC POISONING

Within minutes to hours after exposure to high doses (tens to hundreds of milligrams) of soluble inorganic arsenic compounds, many systems are affected. Initial gastrointestinal signs and symptoms include nausea, vomiting, diarrhea, and abdominal pain. Diffuse capillary leak, combined with gastrointestinal fluid loss, may result in hypotension, shock, and death. Cardiopulmonary toxicity, including congestive cardiomyopathy, cardiogenic or noncardiogenic pulmonary edema, and ventricular arrhythmias, may occur promptly or after a delay of several days. Pancytopenia usually develops within a week, and basophilic stippling of erythrocytes may be present soon after. Central nervous system

---

* Paul Ehrlich's "magic bullet" for syphilis (arsphenamine; Salvarsan) was an arsenical.

effects, including delirium, encephalopathy, and coma, may occur within the first few days of intoxication. An ascending sensorimotor peripheral neuropathy may begin to develop after a delay of 2–6 weeks. This neuropathy may ultimately involve the proximal musculature and result in neuromuscular respiratory failure. Months after an episode of acute poisoning, transverse white striae (Aldrich-Mees lines) may be visible in the nails.

Acute inorganic arsenic poisoning should be considered in an individual presenting with abrupt onset of gastroenteritis in combination with hypotension and metabolic acidosis. The diagnosis may be confirmed by demonstration of elevated amounts of inorganic arsenic and its metabolites in the urine (typically in the range of several thousand micrograms in the first 2–3 days following acute symptomatic poisoning). Arsenic disappears rapidly from the blood, and except in anuric patients, blood arsenic levels should not be used for diagnostic purposes. Treatment is based on appropriate gut decontamination, intensive supportive care, and prompt chelation with unithiol, 3–5 mg/kg intravenously every 4–6 hours, or dimercaprol, 3–5 mg/kg intramuscularly every 4–6 hours. In animal studies, the efficacy of chelation has been highest when it is administered within minutes to hours after arsenic exposure; therefore, if diagnostic suspicion is high, treatment should not be withheld for the several days to weeks often required to obtain laboratory confirmation. Succimer has also been effective in animal models and has a higher therapeutic index than dimercaprol. However, because it is available in the United States only for oral administration, its use may not be advisable in the initial treatment of acute arsenic poisoning, when severe gastroenteritis and splanchnic edema may limit absorption by this route.

B. Chronic Inorganic Arsenic Poisoning

Chronic inorganic arsenic poisoning also results in multisystemic signs and symptoms. Overt noncarcinogenic effects may be evident after chronic absorption of more than 500–1000 µg/d. The time to appearance of symptoms will vary with dose and interindividual tolerances. Constitutional symptoms of fatigue, weight loss, and weakness may be present, along with anemia, nonspecific gastrointestinal complaints, and a sensorimotor peripheral neuropathy, particularly featuring a stocking-glove pattern of dysesthesia. Skin changes—among the most characteristic effects—typically develop after years of exposure and include a "raindrop" pattern of hyperpigmentation, and hyperkeratoses involving the palms and soles. Peripheral vascular disease and noncirrhotic portal hypertension may also occur. Epidemiologic studies suggest a possible link to hypertension and diabetes. Cancer of the lung, skin, bladder, and possibly other sites, may appear years after exposure to doses of arsenic that are not high enough to elicit other acute or chronic effects.

The diagnosis of chronic arsenic poisoning involves integration of the clinical findings with confirmation of exposure. Urinary levels of total arsenic, usually less than 50 µg/24 h, may return to normal within days to weeks after exposure ceases. Because it may contain large amounts of nontoxic organoarsenic, all seafood should be avoided for at least 3 days prior to submission of a urine sample for diagnostic purposes. The arsenic content of hair and nails (normally less than 1 ppm) may sometimes reveal past elevated exposure, but results should be interpreted cautiously in view of the potential for external contamination.

C. Arsine Gas Poisoning

Arsine gas poisoning produces a distinctive pattern of intoxication dominated by profound hemolytic effects. After a latent period that may range from 2 hours to 24 hours postinhalation (depending on the magnitude of exposure), massive intravascular hemolysis may occur. Initial symptoms may include malaise, headache, dyspnea, weakness, nausea, vomiting, abdominal pain, jaundice, and hemoglobinuria. Oliguric renal failure, a consequence of hemoglobin deposition in the renal tubules, often appears within 1–3 days. In massive exposures, lethal effects on cellular respiration may occur before renal failure develops. Urinary arsenic levels are elevated but will seldom be available to confirm the diagnosis during the critical period of illness. Intensive supportive care—including exchange transfusion, vigorous hydration, and, in the case of acute renal failure, hemodialysis—is the mainstay of therapy. Currently available chelating agents have not been demonstrated to be of clinical value in arsine poisoning.

MERCURY

Metallic mercury as "quicksilver"—the only metal that is liquid under ordinary conditions—has attracted scholarly and scientific interest from antiquity. In early times it was recognized that the mining of mercury was hazardous to health. As industrial use of mercury became common during the past 200 years, new forms of toxicity were recognized that were found to be associated with various transformations of the metal. In the early 1950s, a mysterious epidemic of birth defects and neurologic disease occurred in the Japanese fishing village of Minamata. The causative agent was determined to be methylmercury in contaminated seafood, traced to industrial discharges into the bay from a nearby factory. In addition to elemental mercury and alkylmercury (including methylmercury), other key mercurials include inorganic mercury salts and aryl mercury compounds, each of which exerts a relatively unique pattern of clinical toxicity.

Mercury is mined predominantly as HgS in cinnabar ore and is then converted commercially to a variety of chemical forms. Key industrial and commercial applications of mercury are found in the electrolytic production of chlorine and caustic soda; the manufacture of electrical equipment, thermometers, and other instruments; paint and pigment production; dental amalgam; and gold refining. Use in pharmaceuticals and in biocides has declined substantially in recent years, but occasional use in antiseptics and folk medicines is still encountered. Environmental exposure to mercury from the burning of fossil fuels—or the bioaccumulation of methylmercury in fish—remains a concern in some regions of the world. Low-level exposure to mercury released from dental amalgam fillings occurs, but no evidence of toxicity from this source has been demonstrated.

Pharmacokinetics

The absorption of mercury varies considerably depending on the chemical form of the metal. Elemental mercury is quite volatile and can be absorbed from the lungs (Table 58–1). It is poorly absorbed from the intact gastrointestinal tract. Inhaled mercury is the primary source of occupational exposure. Organic short-chain alkylmercury compounds are volatile and potentially harmful by inhalation as well as by ingestion. Percutaneous absorption of all types of mercurials is limited but may be of clinical concern when there is heavy exposure. After absorption, mercury is distributed to the tissues within a few hours, with the highest concentration occurring in the kidney. Inorganic mercury is excreted through the urine and the feces. Excretion of inorganic mercury follows a multicomponent model: most is excreted within days to weeks, but a fraction may be retained in the kidneys and brain for years. Methylmercury undergoes biliary excretion and enterohepatic circulation, with 90% eventually excreted in the feces. Mercury binds to sulfhydryl groups in keratinized tissue, and, as with lead and arsenic, traces appear in the hair and nails.

Major Forms of Mercury Intoxication

Mercury interacts with sulfhydryl groups in vivo, inhibiting enzymes and altering cell membranes. The pattern of clinical intoxication from mercury depends to a great extent on the chemical form of the metal and the route and severity of exposure.

A. ACUTE

Acute inhalation of elemental mercury vapors may cause chemical pneumonitis and noncardiogenic pulmonary edema. Acute gingivostomatitis may occur, and neurologic sequelae (see below) may also ensue. Acute ingestion of inorganic mercury salts, such as mercuric chloride, can result in a corrosive, potentially life-threatening hemorrhagic gastroenteritis followed within hours to days by acute tubular necrosis and oliguric renal failure.

B. CHRONIC

Chronic poisoning from inhalation of mercury vapor results in a classic triad of tremor, neuropsychiatric disturbance, and gingivostomatitis. The tremor usually begins as a fine intention tremor of the hands, but the face may also be involved, and progression to choreiform movements of the limbs may occur. Neuropsychiatric manifestations, including memory loss, fatigue, insomnia, and anorexia, are common. There may be an insidious change in mood to shyness, withdrawal, and depression along with explosive anger or blushing (a behavioral pattern referred to as **erethism**). Recent studies suggest that low-dose exposure may produce subclinical neurologic effects. Gingivostomatitis, sometimes accompanied by loosening of the teeth, may be reported after high-dose exposure. Evidence of peripheral nerve damage may be detected on electrodiagnostic testing, but overt peripheral neuropathy is rare. Acrodynia is an uncommon idiosyncratic reaction to subacute or chronic mercury exposure and occurs mainly in children. It is characterized by painful erythema of the extremities and may be associated with hypertension, diaphoresis, anorexia, insomnia, irritability or apathy, and a miliarial rash.

Methylmercury intoxication affects mainly the central nervous system and results in paresthesias, ataxia, hearing impairment, dysarthria, and progressive constriction of the visual fields. Signs and symptoms may first appear several weeks or months after exposure begins. Methylmercury is a reproductive toxin. High-dose prenatal exposure to methylmercury may produce mental retardation and a cerebral palsy-like syndrome in the offspring. Low-level prenatal exposures have been associated with a risk of subclinical neurodevelopmental deficits (National Research Council, 2000). Dimethylmercury is a rarely encountered but extremely neurotoxic form of organomercury that may be lethal in small quantities.

The diagnosis of mercury intoxication involves integration of the history and physical findings with confirmatory laboratory testing or other evidence of exposure. In the absence of occupational exposure, the urine mercury concentration is usually less than 5 μg/L, and whole blood mercury is less than 5 μg/L (CDC, 2003). In 1990, the Biological Exposure Index (BEI) Committee of the American Conference of Governmental Industrial Hygienists (ACGIH) recommended that workplace exposures should result in urinary mercury concentrations less than 35 µg per gram of creatinine and end-of-workweek whole blood mercury concentrations less than 15 µg/L.

Treatment

A. Acute Exposure

In addition to intensive supportive care, prompt chelation with oral or intravenous unithiol, intramuscular dimercaprol, or oral succimer may be of value in diminishing nephrotoxicity after acute exposure to inorganic mercury salts. Vigorous hydration may help to maintain urine output, but if acute renal failure ensues, days to weeks of hemodialysis may be necessary. Because the efficacy of chelation declines with time since exposure, treatment should not be delayed until the onset of oliguria or other major systemic effects.

B. Chronic Exposure

Unithiol and succimer increase urine mercury excretion following acute or chronic elemental mercury inhalation, but the impact of such treatment on clinical outcome is unknown. Dimercaprol has been shown to redistribute mercury to the central nervous system from other tissue sites, and since the brain is a key target organ, dimercaprol should not be used in treatment of exposure to elemental or organic mercury. Limited data suggest that succimer, unithiol, and N-acetyl-L-cysteine (NAC) may enhance body clearance of methylmercury.

PHARMACOLOGY OF CHELATORS

Chelating agents are drugs used to prevent or reverse the toxic effects of a heavy metal on an enzyme or other cellular target, or to accelerate the elimination of the metal from the body. Chelating agents are usually flexible molecules with two or more electronegative groups that form stable coordinate-covalent bonds with a cationic metal atom. In some cases, eg, succimer, the parent compound may require in vivo biotransformation to become an active complexing agent. The chelator-metal complexes formed are excreted by the body. Edetate (ethylenediaminetetraacetate, Figure 58–1) is an important example.

The efficiency of the chelator is partly determined by the number of ligands available for metal binding. The greater the number of these ligands, the more stable the metal-chelator complex. Depending on the number of metal-ligand bonds, the complex may be referred to as mono-, bi-, or polydentate. The chelating ligands include functional groups such as –OH, –SH, and –NH, which can donate electrons for coordination with the metal. Such bonding effectively prevents interaction of the metal with similar functional groups of enzymes

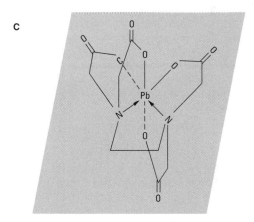

Figure 58–1. Salt and chelate formation with edetate (ethylenediaminetetraacetate; EDTA). **A:** In a solution of the disodium salt of EDTA, the sodium and hydrogen ions are chemically and biologically available. **B:** In solutions of calcium disodium edetate, calcium is bound by coordinate-covalent bonds with nitrogens as well as by the usual ionic bonds. Calcium ions are effectively removed from solution. **C:** In the lead-edetate chelate, lead is incorporated into five heterocyclic rings. (Modified and reproduced, with permission, from Meyers FH, Jawetz E, Goldfien A: *Review of Medical Pharmacology*, 7th ed. Originally published by Lange Medical Publications. McGraw-Hill, 1980.)

or other proteins, coenzymes, cellular nucleophiles, and membranes.

In addition to removing the target metal that is exerting toxic effects on the body, some chelating agents (such as calcium EDTA used for lead intoxication) may enhance the excretion of essential cations such as zinc or copper. However, this side effect is seldom of clinical significance during the limited time frame that characterizes most courses of therapeutic chelation.

In some cases, the metal-mobilizing effect of a therapeutic chelating agent may not only enhance that metal's excretion—a desired effect—but may also redistribute some of the metal to other vital organs. This has been demonstrated for dimercaprol, which redistributes mercury and arsenic to brain while also enhancing urinary mercury and arsenic excretion. Although several chelating agents have the capacity to mobilize cadmium, their tendency to redistribute cadmium to the kidney and increase nephrotoxicity has negated their therapeutic value in cadmium intoxication.

In most cases, the capacity of chelating agents to prevent or reduce the adverse effects of toxic metals appears to be greatest when they are administered very soon after an acute metal exposure. Use of chelating agents days to weeks after an acute metal exposure ends—or their use in the treatment of chronic metal intoxication—may still be associated with increased metal excretion. However, at that point, the capacity of such enhanced excretion to mitigate the pathologic effect of the metal exposure may be reduced.

The most important chelating agents currently in use in the United States are described below.

DIMERCAPROL (2,3-DIMERCAPTOPROPANOL, BAL)

Dimercaprol (Figure 58–2), an oily, colorless liquid with a strong mercaptan-like odor, was developed in Great Britain during World War II as a therapeutic antidote against poisoning by the arsenic-containing warfare agent lewisite. It thus became known as British anti-Lewisite, or BAL. Because aqueous solutions of dimercaprol are unstable and oxidize readily, it is dispensed in 10% solution in peanut oil and must be administered by intramuscular injection, which is often painful.

In animal models, dimercaprol prevents and reverses arsenic-induced inhibition of sulfhydryl-containing enzymes and, if given soon after exposure, may protect against the lethal effects of inorganic and organic arsenicals. Human data indicate that it can increase the rate of excretion of arsenic and lead and may offer therapeutic benefit in the treatment of acute intoxication by arsenic, lead, and mercury.

Indications & Toxicity

Dimercaprol is FDA-approved as single-agent treatment of acute poisoning by arsenic and inorganic or elemental mercury and for the treatment of severe lead poisoning

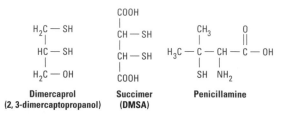

Figure 58–2. Chemical structures of several chelators. Ferroxamine (ferrioxamine) without the chelated iron is deferoxamine. It is represented here to show the functional groups; the iron is actually held in a caged system. The structures of the in vivo metal-chelator complexes for dimercaprol, succimer, penicillamine, and unithiol (not shown), are not known and may involve the formation of mixed disulfides with amino acids. (Modified and reproduced, with permission, from Meyers FH, Jawetz E, Goldfien A: *Review of Medical Pharmacology*, 7th ed. McGraw-Hill, 1980.)

when used in conjunction with edetate calcium disodium (EDTA; see below). Although studies of its metabolism in humans are limited, intramuscularly administered dimercaprol appears to be readily absorbed, metabolized, and excreted by the kidney within 4–8 hours. Animal models indicate that it may also undergo biliary excretion, but the role of this excretory route in humans and other details of its biotransformation are uncertain.

When used in therapeutic doses, dimercaprol is associated with a high incidence of adverse effects, including hypertension, tachycardia, nausea, vomiting, lacrimation, salivation, fever (particularly in children), and pain at the injection site. Its use has also been associated with thrombocytopenia and increased prothrombin time—factors that may limit intramuscular injection because of the risk of hematoma formation at the injection site. Despite its protective effects in acutely intoxicated animals, dimercaprol may redistribute arsenic and mercury to the central nervous system, and it is not advocated for treatment of chronic poisoning. Water-soluble analogs of dimer-caprol—unithiol and succimer—have higher therapeutic indices and have replaced dimercaprol in many settings.

SUCCIMER (DIMERCAPTOSUCCINIC ACID, DMSA)

Succimer is a water-soluble analog of dimercaprol, and like that agent it has been shown in animal studies to prevent and reverse metal-induced inhibition of sulfhydryl-containing enzymes and to protect against the acute lethal effects of arsenic. In humans, treatment with succimer is associated with an increase in urinary lead excretion and a decrease in blood lead concentration. It may also decrease the mercury content of the kidney, a key target organ of inorganic mercury salts. In the United States, succimer is formulated exclusively for oral use, but intravenous formulations have been used successfully elsewhere. It is absorbed rapidly but somewhat variably after oral administration. Peak blood levels occur at approximately 3 hours. The drug binds in vivo to the amino acid cysteine to form 1:1 and 1:2 mixed disulfides, possibly in the kidney, and it may be these complexes that are the active chelating moieties. The elimination half-time of transformed succimer is approximately 2–4 hours.

Indications & Toxicity

Succimer is currently FDA-approved for the treatment of children with blood lead concentrations greater than 45 μg/dL, but it is also commonly used in adults. The usual dosage is 10 mg/kg orally three times a day. Oral administration of succimer is comparable to parenteral EDTA in reducing blood lead concentration and has supplanted EDTA in outpatient treatment of patients capable of absorbing the oral drug. However, despite the demonstrated capacity of both succimer and EDTA to enhance lead elimination, their value in reversing established lead toxicity or in otherwise improving therapeutic outcome has yet to be established by a placebo-controlled clinical trial. Based on its protective effects against arsenic in animals and its ability to mobilize mercury from the kidney, succimer has also been used in the treatment of arsenic and mercury poisoning. Succimer has been well tolerated in limited clinical trials. It has a negligible impact on body stores of calcium, iron, and magnesium. It induces a mild increase in urinary excretion of zinc that is of minor or no clinical significance. Gastrointestinal disturbances, including anorexia, nausea, vomiting, and diarrhea, are the most common side effects, occurring in less than 10% of patients. Rashes, sometimes requiring discontinuation of the medication, have been reported in less than 5% of patients. Mild, reversible increases in liver aminotransferases have been noted in 6–10% of

patients, and isolated cases of mild to moderate neutropenia have been reported.

EDETATE CALCIUM DISODIUM (ETHYLENEDIAMINETETRAACETIC ACID [EDTA])

Ethylenediaminetetraacetic acid (Figure 58–1) is an efficient chelator of many divalent and trivalent metals in vitro. The drug is administered as a calcium disodium salt to prevent potentially life-threatening depletion of calcium.

EDTA penetrates cell membranes relatively poorly and therefore chelates extracellular metal ions much more effectively than intracellular ions.

The highly polar ionic character of EDTA limits its oral absorption. Moreover, oral administration may increase lead absorption from the gut. Consequently, EDTA should be administered by intravenous infusion. In patients with normal renal function, EDTA is rapidly excreted by glomerular filtration, with 50% of an injected dose appearing in the urine within 1 hour. EDTA mobilizes lead from soft tissues, causing a marked increase in urinary lead excretion and a corresponding decline in blood lead concentration. In patients with renal insufficiency, excretion of the drug—and its metal-mobilizing effects—may be delayed.

Indications & Toxicity

Edetate calcium disodium is indicated chiefly for the chelation of lead, but it may also have utility in poisoning by zinc, manganese, and certain heavy radionuclides. In spite of repeated claims in the alternative medicine literature, EDTA has no demonstrated utility in the treatment of atherosclerotic cardiovascular disease.

Because the drug and the mobilized metals are excreted via the urine, the drug is contraindicated in anuric patients. Nephrotoxicity from EDTA has been reported, but in most cases this can be prevented by maintenance of adequate urine flow, avoidance of excessive doses, and limitation of a treatment course to 5 or fewer consecutive days. EDTA may result in temporary zinc depletion that is of uncertain clinical significance. An experimental analog of EDTA, calcium disodium diethylenetriaminepentaacetic acid (DTPA), has been used for removal ("decorporation") of uranium, plutonium, and other heavy radioisotopes from the body.

UNITHIOL (DIMERCAPTOPROPANESULFONIC ACID, DMPS)

Unithiol, a dimercapto chelating agent that is a water-soluble analog of dimercaprol, has been available in the official formularies of Russia and other former Soviet countries since 1958 and in Germany since 1976. It has been legally available from compounding pharmacists in the United States since 1999. Unithiol can be administered orally and intravenously. Bioavailability by the oral route is approximately 50%, with peak blood levels occurring in approximately 3.7 hours. Over 80% of an intravenous dose is excreted in the urine, mainly as cyclic DMPS sulfides. The elimination half-time for total unithiol (parent drug and its transformation products) is approximately 20 hours. Unithiol exhibits protective effects against the toxic action of mercury and arsenic in animal models, and it increases the excretion of mercury, arsenic, and lead in humans.

Indications & Toxicity

Unithiol has no FDA-approved indications, but experimental studies and its pharmacologic and pharmacodynamic profile suggest that intravenous unithiol offers advantages over intramuscular dimercaprol or oral succimer in the initial treatment of severe acute poisoning by inorganic mercury or arsenic. Aqueous preparations of unithiol (usually 50 mg/mL in sterile water) can be administered at a dose of 3–5 mg/kg every 4 hours by slow intravenous infusion over 20 minutes. If a few days of treatment are accompanied by stabilization of the patient's cardiovascular and gastrointestinal status, it may be possible to change to oral administration at a dose of 4–8 mg/kg every 6–8 hours. Oral unithiol may also be considered as an alternative to oral succimer in the treatment of lead intoxication.

Unithiol has been reported to have a low overall incidence of adverse effects (< 4%). Self-limited dermatologic reactions (drug exanthems or urticaria) are the most commonly reported adverse effects, though isolated cases of major allergic reactions, including erythema multiforme and Stevens-Johnson syndrome, have been reported. Because rapid intravenous infusion may cause vasodilation and hypotension, unithiol should be infused slowly over an interval of 15–20 minutes.

PENICILLAMINE (D-DIMETHYLCYSTEINE)

Penicillamine (Figure 58–2) is a white crystalline, water-soluble derivative of penicillin. D-Penicillamine is less toxic than the L isomer and consequently is the preferred therapeutic form. Penicillamine is readily absorbed from the gut and is resistant to metabolic degradation.

Indications & Toxicity

Penicillamine is used chiefly for treatment of poisoning with copper or to prevent copper accumulation, as in Wilson's disease (hepatolenticular degeneration). It is also used occasionally in the treatment of severe rheumatoid arthritis (Chapter 36). Its ability to increase urinary excretion of lead and mercury had occasioned its use as outpatient treatment for intoxication with these metals, but succimer, with its stronger metal-mobilizing capacity and lower side effect profile, has generally replaced penicillamine for these purposes.

Adverse effects have been seen in up to one third of patients receiving penicillamine. Hypersensitivity reactions include rash, pruritus, and drug fever, and the drug should be used with extreme caution, if at all, in patients with a history of penicillin allergy. Nephrotoxicity with proteinuria has also been reported, and protracted use of the drug may result in renal insufficiency. Pancytopenia has been associated with prolonged drug intake. Pyridoxine deficiency is a frequent toxic effect of other forms of the drug but is rarely seen with the D form. An acetylated derivative, N-acetylpenicillamine, has been used experimentally in mercury poisoning and may have superior metal-mobilizing capacity, but it is not commercially available.

DEFEROXAMINE

Deferoxamine is isolated from *Streptomyces pilosus*. It binds iron avidly but essential trace metals poorly. Furthermore, while competing for loosely bound iron in iron-carrying proteins (hemosiderin and ferritin), it fails to compete for biologically chelated iron, as in microsomal and mitochondrial cytochromes and hemoproteins. Consequently, it is the chelator of choice for iron poisoning (Chapters 33 and 59). Deferoxamine plus hemodialysis may also be useful in the treatment of aluminum toxicity in renal failure. Deferoxamine is poorly absorbed when administered orally and may increase iron absorption when given by this route. It should therefore be administered intramuscularly or, preferably, intravenously. It is believed to be metabolized, but the pathways are unknown. The iron-chelator complex is excreted in the urine, often turning the urine an orange-red color.

Rapid intravenous administration may result in hypotension. Adverse idiosyncratic responses such as flushing, abdominal discomfort, and rash have also been observed. Pulmonary complications (eg, acute respiratory distress syndrome) have been reported in some patients undergoing deferoxamine infusions lasting longer than 24 hours, and neurotoxicity and increased susceptibility to certain infections (eg, with *Yersinia enterocolitica*) have been described after long-term therapy of iron overload conditions (eg, thalassemia major).

PREPARATIONS AVAILABLE

Deferoxamine (Desferal)
  Parenteral: Powder to reconstitute, 500 mg/vial
Dimercaprol (BAL in Oil)
  Parenteral: 100 mg/mL for IM injection
Edetate calcium [calcium EDTA] (Calcium Dis
  odium Versenate)
  Parenteral: 200 mg/mL for injection

Penicillamine (Cuprimine, Depen)
  Oral: 125, 250 mg capsules; 250 mg tablets
Succimer (Chemet)
  Oral: 100 mg capsules
Unithiol (Dimaval)
  Bulk powder available for compounding as oral
  capsules, or for infusion (50 mg/mL).

REFERENCES

LEAD

Borja-Aburto VH et al: Blood lead levels measured prospectively and risk of spontaneous abortion. Am J Epidemiol 1999; 150:590.

Canfield RL et al: Intellectual impairment in children with blood lead concentrations below 10 μg per deciliter. N Engl J Med 2003;348:1517.

Korrick SA et al: Lead and hypertension in a sample of middle-aged women. Am J Public Health 1999;89:330.

Lanphear BP et al: Cognitive deficits associated with blood lead concentrations < 10 μg/dL in US children and adolescents. Publ Health Rep 2000;115:521.

Rogan WJ et al: The effect of chelation therapy with succimer on neuropsychological development in children exposed to lead. N Engl J Med 2001;344:1421.

Second National Report on Exposure to Environmental Chemicals. Lead. CDC, 2003. [http://www.cdc.gov/exposurereport/metals/ pdf/lead.pdf]

ARSENIC

National Research Council. *Arsenic in Drinking Water: 2001 Update.* National Academy Press, 2001. [http://search.nap. edu/books/0309076293/html/]

Petrick JS et al: Monomethylarsonous acid (MMA[III]) and arsenite: LD50 in hamsters and in vitro inhibition of pyruvate dehydrogenase. Chem Res Toxicol 2001;14:651.

Unnikrishnan D et al: Torsades de pointes in 3 patients with leukemia treated with arsenic trioxide. Blood 2001;97:1514.

MERCURY

Clarkson TW: The three modern faces of mercury. Environ Health Perspect 2002;110(Suppl 1).11.

National Research Council. Toxicological Effects of Methylmercury. National Academy Press, 2000. [http://www.nap.edu/books/ 0309071402/html/]

Nierenberg DW et al: Delayed cerebellar disease and death after accidental exposure to dimethylmercury. N Engl J Med 1998;338:1672.

Second National Report on Exposure to Environmental Chemicals. Mercury. CDC, 2003. [www.cdc.gov/exposurereport/metals/pdf/mercury.pdf]

CHELATING AGENTS

Cremin JD Jr et al: Efficacy of succimer chelation for reducing brain lead in a primate model of human lead exposure. Toxicol Appl Pharmacol 1999;161:283.

Cremin JD et al: Oral succimer decreases the gastrointestinal absorption of lead in juvenile monkeys. Environ Health Perspect 2001;109:613.

Lin JL et al: Environmental lead exposure and progression of chronic renal diseases in patients without diabetes. N Engl J Med 2003;348:277.

Nakamura H et al: Acute encephalopathy due to aluminum toxicity successfully treated by combined intravenous deferoxamine and hemodialysis. J Clin Pharmacol 2000;40:296.

Management of the Poisoned Patient

Kent R. Olson, MD

Over a million cases of acute poisoning occur in the USA each year, although only a small fraction are fatal. Most deaths are due to intentional suicidal overdose by an adolescent or adult. Childhood deaths due to accidental ingestion of a drug or toxic household product have been markedly reduced in the past 30 years as a result of safety packaging and effective poisoning prevention education.

Even with a serious exposure, poisoning is rarely fatal if the victim receives prompt medical attention and good supportive care. Careful management of respiratory failure, hypotension, seizures, and thermoregulatory disturbances has resulted in improved survival of patients who reach the hospital alive.

This chapter reviews the basic principles of poisoning, initial management and specialized treatment of poisoning including methods of increasing the elimination of drugs and toxins.

TOXICOKINETICS & TOXICODYNAMICS

The term "toxicokinetics" denotes the absorption, distribution, excretion, and metabolism of toxins, toxic doses of therapeutic agents, and their metabolites. The term "toxicodynamics" is used to denote the injurious effects of these substances on vital function. Although there are many similarities between the pharmacokinetics and toxicokinetics of most substances, there are also important differences. The same caution applies to pharmacodynamics and toxicodynamics.

SPECIAL ASPECTS OF TOXICOKINETICS

Volume of Distribution

The volume of distribution (V_d) is defined as the apparent volume into which a substance is distributed (see Chapter 3). A large V_d implies that the drug is not readily accessible to measures aimed at purifying the blood, such as hemodialysis. Examples of drugs with large volumes of distribution (> 5 L/kg) include antidepressants, antipsychotics, antimalarials, narcotics, propranolol, and verapamil. Drugs with relatively small volumes of distribution (< 1 L/kg) include salicylate, phenobarbital, lithium, valproic acid, warfarin, and phenytoin (see Table 3–1).

Clearance

Clearance is a measure of the volume of plasma that is cleared of drug per unit time (see Chapter 3). For most drugs the total clearance is the sum of clearances by excretion by the kidneys and metabolism by the liver. In planning detoxification strategy, it is important to know the contribution of each organ to total clearance. For example, if a drug is 95% cleared by liver metabolism and only 5% cleared by renal excretion, even a dramatic increase in urinary concentration of the poison will have little effect on overall elimination.

Overdosage of a drug can alter the usual pharmacokinetic processes, and this must be considered when applying kinetics to poisoned patients. For example, dissolution of tablets or gastric emptying time may be slowed so that absorption and peak toxic effects are delayed. Drugs may injure the epithelial barrier of the gastrointestinal tract and thereby increase absorption. If the capacity of the liver to metabolize a drug is exceeded, more drug will be delivered to the circulation. With a dramatic increase in the concentration of drug in the blood, protein-binding capacity may be exceeded, resulting in an increased fraction of free drug and greater toxic effect. At normal dosage, most drugs are eliminated at a rate proportionate to the plasma concentration (first-order kinetics). If the plasma concentration is very high and normal metabolism is saturated, the rate of elimination may become fixed (zero-order kinetics). This change in kinetics may markedly prolong the apparent serum half-life and increase toxicity.

SPECIAL ASPECTS OF TOXICODYNAMICS

The general dose-response principles described in Chapter 2 are relevant when estimating the potential severity of an intoxication. When considering quantal dose-response data, both the therapeutic index and the overlap of therapeutic and toxic response curves must be considered. For instance, two drugs may have the same therapeutic index but unequal safe dosing ranges if the slopes of their dose-response curves are not the same. For some drugs, eg, sedative-hypnotics, the major toxic effect is a direct extension of the therapeutic action, as shown by their graded dose-response curve (see Figure 22–1). In the case of a drug with a linear dose-response curve (drug A), lethal effects may occur at ten times the normal therapeutic dose. In contrast, a drug with a curve that reaches a plateau (drug B) may not be lethal at 100 times the normal dose.

For many drugs, at least part of the toxic effect may be quite different from the therapeutic action. For example, intoxication with drugs that have atropine-like effects (eg, tricyclic antidepressants) will reduce sweating, making it more difficult to dissipate heat. In tricyclic antidepressant intoxication, there may also be increased muscular activity or seizures; the body's production of heat is thus enhanced, and lethal hyperpyrexia may result. Overdoses of drugs that depress the cardiovascular system, eg, β-blockers or calcium channel blockers, can profoundly alter not only cardiac function but all functions that are dependent on blood flow. These include renal and hepatic elimination of the toxin and any other drugs that may be given.

APPROACH TO THE POISONED PATIENT

HOW DOES THE POISONED PATIENT DIE?

An understanding of common mechanisms of death due to poisoning can help prepare the physician to treat patients effectively. Many toxins depress the central nervous system (CNS), resulting in obtundation or coma. Comatose patients frequently lose their airway protective reflexes and their respiratory drive. Thus, they may die as a result of airway obstruction by the flaccid tongue, aspiration of gastric contents into the tracheobronchial tree, or respiratory arrest. These are the most common causes of death due to overdoses of narcotics, barbiturates, alcohol, and other sedative-hypnotic drugs.

Cardiovascular toxicity is also frequently encountered in poisoning. Hypotension may be due to depression of cardiac contractility; hypovolemia resulting from vomiting, diarrhea, or fluid sequestration; peripheral vascular collapse due to blockade of α-adrenoceptor-mediated vascular tone; or cardiac arrhythmias. Hypothermia or hyperthermia due to exposure as well as the temperature-dysregulating effects of many drugs can also produce hypotension. Lethal arrhythmias such as ventricular tachycardia and fibrillation can occur with overdoses of many cardioactive drugs such as ephedrine, amphetamines, cocaine, tricyclic antidepressants, digitalis, and theophylline.

Cellular hypoxia may occur in spite of adequate ventilation and oxygen administration when poisoning is due to cyanide, hydrogen sulfide, carbon monoxide, and other poisons that interfere with transport or utilization of oxygen. In such patients, cellular hypoxia is evident by the development of tachycardia, hypotension, severe lactic acidosis, and signs of ischemia on the ECG.

Seizures, muscular hyperactivity, and rigidity may result in death. Seizures may cause pulmonary aspiration, hypoxia, and brain damage. Hyperthermia may result from sustained muscular hyperactivity and can lead to muscle breakdown and myoglobinuria, renal failure, lactic acidosis, and hyperkalemia. Drugs and poisons that often cause seizures include antidepressants, theophylline, isoniazid (INH), diphenhydramine, antipsychotics, cocaine, and amphetamines.

Other organ system damage may occur after poisoning, and is sometimes delayed in onset. Paraquat attacks lung tissue, resulting in pulmonary fibrosis, beginning several days after ingestion. Massive hepatic necrosis due to poisoning by acetaminophen or certain mushrooms results in hepatic encephalopathy and death 48–72 hours or longer after ingestion.

Finally, some patients may die before hospitalization because the behavioral effects of the ingested drug may result in traumatic injury. Intoxication with alcohol and other sedative-hypnotic drugs is a frequent contributing factor to motor vehicle accidents. Patients under the influence of hallucinogens such as phencyclidine (PCP) or LSD may die in fights or falls from high places.

INITIAL MANAGEMENT OF THE POISONED PATIENT

The initial management of a patient with coma, seizures, or otherwise altered mental status should follow the same approach regardless of the poison involved. Attempting to make a specific toxicologic diagnosis only delays the application of supportive measures that form the basis ("ABCDs") of poisoning treatment.

First, the **airway** should be cleared of vomitus or any other obstruction and an oral airway or endotracheal tube inserted if needed. For many patients, simple positioning in the lateral decubitus position is sufficient to move the flaccid tongue out of the airway. **Breathing** should be assessed by observation and oximetry and, if in doubt, by measuring arterial blood gases. Patients with respiratory insufficiency should be intubated and mechanically ventilated. The **circulation** should be assessed by continuous monitoring of pulse rate, blood pressure, urinary output, and evaluation of peripheral perfusion. An intravenous line should be placed and blood drawn for serum glucose and other routine determinations.

At this point, every patient with altered mental status should receive a challenge with concentrated **dextrose,** unless a rapid bedside blood sugar test demonstrates that the patient is not hypoglycemic. Adults are given 25 g (50 mL of 50% dextrose solution) intravenously, children 0.5 g/kg (2 mL/kg of 25% dextrose). Hypoglycemic patients may appear to be intoxicated, and there is no rapid and reliable way to distinguish them from poisoned patients. Alcoholic or malnourished patients should also receive 100 mg of thiamine intramuscularly or in the intravenous infusion solution at this time to prevent Wernicke's syndrome.

The opioid antagonist naloxone may be given in a dose of 0.4–2 mg intravenously. Naloxone will reverse respiratory and CNS depression due to all varieties of opioid drugs (see Chapter 31). It is useful to remember that these drugs cause death primarily by respiratory depression; therefore, if airway and breathing assistance have already been instituted, naloxone may not be necessary. Larger doses of naloxone may be needed for patients with overdose involving propoxyphene, codeine, and some other opioids. The benzodiazepine antagonist flumazenil (see Chapter 22) may be of value in patients with suspected benzodiazepine overdose, but it should not be used if there is a history of tricyclic antidepressant overdose or a seizure disorder, as it can induce convulsions in such patients.

History & Physical Examination

Once the essential initial "ABCD" interventions have been instituted, one can begin a more detailed evaluation to make a specific diagnosis. This includes gathering any available history and performing a toxicologically oriented physical examination. Other causes of coma or seizures such as head trauma, meningitis, or metabolic abnormalities should be looked for and treated. Some common toxic syndromes are described beginning on page 988.

A. HISTORY

Oral statements about the amount and even the type of drug ingested in toxic emergencies may be unreliable. Even so, family members, police, and fire department or paramedical personnel should be asked to describe the environment in which the toxic emergency occurred and should bring to the emergency department any syringes, empty bottles, household products, or over-the-counter medications in the immediate vicinity of the possibly poisoned patient.

B. PHYSICAL EXAMINATION

A brief examination should be performed, emphasizing those areas most likely to give clues to the toxicologic diagnosis. These include vital signs, eyes and mouth, skin, abdomen, and nervous system.

1. Vital signs—Careful evaluation of vital signs (blood pressure, pulse, respirations, and temperature) is essential in all toxicologic emergencies. Hypertension and tachycardia are typical with amphetamines, cocaine, and antimuscarinic (anticholinergic) drugs. Hypotension and bradycardia are characteristic features of overdose with calcium channel blockers, β-blockers, clonidine, and sedative-hypnotics. Hypotension with tachycardia is common with tricyclic antidepressants, phenothiazines, vasodilators, and theophylline. Rapid respirations are typical of salicylates, carbon monoxide, and other toxins that produce metabolic acidosis or cellular asphyxia. Hyperthermia may be associated with sympathomimetics, anticholinergics, salicylates, and drugs producing seizures or muscular rigidity. Hypothermia can be caused by any CNS-depressant drug, especially when accompanied by exposure to a cold environment.

2. Eyes—The eyes are a valuable source of toxicologic information. Constriction of the pupils (miosis) is typical of opioids, clonidine, phenothiazines, and cholinesterase inhibitors (eg, organophosphate insecticides), and deep coma due to sedative drugs. Dilation of the pupils (mydriasis) is common with amphetamines, cocaine, LSD, and atropine and other anticholinergic drugs. Horizontal nystagmus is characteristic of intoxication with phenytoin, alcohol, barbiturates, and other sedative drugs. The presence of both vertical and horizontal nystagmus is strongly suggestive of phencyclidine poisoning. Ptosis and ophthalmoplegia are characteristic features of botulism.

3. Mouth—The mouth may show signs of burns due to corrosive substances, or soot from smoke inhalation. Typical odors of alcohol, hydrocarbon solvents, or ammonia may be noted. Poisoning due to cyanide can be recognized by some examiners as an odor like bitter almonds.

4. Skin—The skin often appears flushed, hot, and dry in poisoning with atropine and other antimuscarinics.

Excessive sweating occurs with organophosphates, nicotine, and sympathomimetic drugs. Cyanosis may be caused by hypoxemia or by methemoglobinemia. Icterus may suggest hepatic necrosis due to acetaminophen or *Amanita phalloides* mushroom poisoning.

5. Abdomen—Abdominal examination may reveal ileus, which is typical of poisoning with antimuscarinic, opioid, and sedative drugs. Hyperactive bowel sounds, abdominal cramping, and diarrhea are common in poisoning with organophosphates, iron, arsenic, theophylline, and *A phalloides.*

6. Nervous system—A careful neurologic examination is essential. Focal seizures or motor deficits suggest a structural lesion (such as intracranial hemorrhage due to trauma) rather than toxic or metabolic encephalopathy. Nystagmus, dysarthria, and ataxia are typical of phenytoin, carbamazepine, alcohol, and other sedative intoxication. Twitching and muscular hyperactivity are common with atropine and other anticholinergic agents, and cocaine and other sympathomimetic drugs. Muscular rigidity can be caused by haloperidol and other antipsychotic agents and by strychnine. Seizures are often caused by overdose with antidepressants (especially tricyclic antidepressants and bupropion), cocaine, amphetamines, theophylline, isoniazid, and diphenhydramine. Flaccid coma with absent reflexes and even an isoelectric EEG may be seen with deep coma due to opioid or sedative-hypnotic intoxication and may be mistaken for brain death.

Laboratory & Imaging Procedures

A. ARTERIAL BLOOD GASES

Hypoventilation will result in an elevated PCO_2 (hypercapnia) and a low PO_2 (hypoxia). The PO_2 may also be low with aspiration pneumonia or drug-induced pulmonary edema. Poor tissue oxygenation due to hypoxia, hypotension, or cyanide poisoning will result in metabolic acidosis. The PO_2 measures only oxygen dissolved in the plasma and not total blood oxygen content or oxyhemoglobin saturation, and may appear normal in patients with severe carbon monoxide poisoning. Pulse oximetry may also give falsely normal results in carbon monoxide intoxication.

B. ELECTROLYTES

Sodium, potassium, chloride, and bicarbonate should be measured. The anion gap is then calculated by subtracting the measured anions from cations:

$$\text{Anion gap} = (Na^+ + K^+) - (HCO_3^- + Cl^-)$$

It is normally no greater than 12–16 meq/L. A larger-than-expected anion gap is caused by the presence of

Table 59–1. Examples of drug-induced anion gap acidosis.

Type of Elevation of the Anion Gap	Agents
Organic acid metabolites	Methanol, ethylene glycol, diethylene glycol
Lactic acidosis	Cyanide, carbon monoxide, ibuprofen, isoniazid, metformin, salicylates, valproic acid; any drug-induced seizures, hypoxia, or hypotension

Note: The normal anion gap calculated from $(Na^+ + K^+) - (HCO_3^- + Cl^-)$ is 12–16 meq/L; calculated from $(Na^+) - (HCO_3^- + Cl^-)$, it is 8–12 meq/L.

unmeasured anions accompanying metabolic acidosis. This may occur with numerous conditions, such as diabetic ketoacidosis, renal failure, or shock-induced lactic acidosis. Drugs that may induce an elevated anion gap metabolic acidosis (Table 59–1) include aspirin, metformin, methanol, ethylene glycol, isoniazid, and iron.

Alterations in the serum potassium level are hazardous because they may result in cardiac arrhythmias. Drugs that may cause hyperkalemia despite normal renal function include potassium itself, β-blockers, digitalis glycosides, potassium-sparing diuretics, and fluoride. Drugs associated with hypokalemia include barium, β-agonists, caffeine, theophylline, and thiazide and loop diuretics.

C. RENAL FUNCTION TESTS

Some toxins have direct nephrotoxic effects; in other cases, renal failure is due to shock or myoglobinuria. Blood urea nitrogen and creatinine levels should be measured and urinalysis performed. Elevated serum creatine kinase (CK) and myoglobin in the urine suggest muscle necrosis due to seizures or muscular rigidity. Oxalate crystals in the urine suggest ethylene glycol poisoning.

D. SERUM OSMOLALITY

The calculated serum osmolality is dependent mainly on the serum sodium and glucose and the blood urea nitrogen and can be estimated from the following formula:

$$2 \times Na^+ (meq/L) + \frac{\text{Glucose (mg/dL)}}{18} + \frac{\text{BUN (mg/dL)}}{3}$$

This calculated value is normally 280–290 mosm/L. Ethanol and other alcohols may contribute significantly to the measured serum osmolality but, since they are not included in the calculation, cause an osmolar gap:

$$\frac{\text{Osmolar}}{\text{gap}} = \frac{\text{Measured}}{\text{osmolality}} - \frac{\text{Calculated}}{\text{osmolality}}$$

Table 59–2 lists the concentration and expected contribution to the serum osmolality in ethanol, methanol, ethylene glycol, and isopropanol poisonings.

E. ELECTROCARDIOGRAM

Widening of the QRS complex duration to greater than 100 milliseconds is typical of tricyclic antidepressant and quinidine overdoses (Figure 59–1). The QT_c interval may be prolonged to more than 440 milliseconds in many poisonings, including quinidine, tricyclic antidepressants, several newer antidepressants and antipsychotics, lithium, and arsenic (see also http://www.torsades.org/). Variable atrioventricular (AV) block and a variety of atrial and ventricular arrhythmias are common with poisoning by digoxin and other cardiac glycosides. Hypoxemia due to carbon monoxide poisoning may result in ischemic changes on the ECG.

F. IMAGING FINDINGS

A plain film of the abdomen may be useful because some tablets, particularly iron and potassium, may be radiopaque. Chest x-ray may reveal aspiration pneumonia, hydrocarbon pneumonia, or pulmonary edema. When head trauma is suspected, a CT scan is recommended.

Table 59–2. Some substances that cause an osmolar gap.

Substance[1]	Serum Level (mg/dL)	Corresponding Osmolar Gap (mosm/kg)
Ethanol	350	75
Methanol	80	25
Ethylene glycol	200	35
Isopropanol	350	60

[1] Other substances that can increase the osmolar gap include acetone, mannitol, and magnesium.

Note: Most laboratories use the freezing point method of determining osmolality. However, if the vaporization point method is used, the alcohols may be driven off and their contribution to osmolality will be lost.

Toxicology Screening Tests

It is a common misconception that a broad toxicology "screen" is the best way to diagnose and manage an acute poisoning. However, comprehensive toxicology screening is time-consuming, expensive, and often unreliable. Moreover, many highly toxic drugs such as calcium channel blockers, β-blockers, and isoniazid are not included in the screening process. The clinical examina-

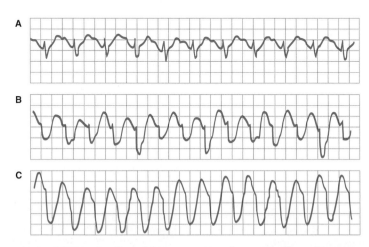

Figure 59–1. Changes in the ECG in tricyclic antidepressant overdosage. **A:** Slowed intraventricular conduction results in prolonged QRS interval (0.18 s; normal, 0.08 s). **B:** and **C:** Supraventricular tachycardia with progressive widening of QRS complexes mimics ventricular tachycardia. (Reproduced, with permission, from Benowitz NL, Goldschlager N: Cardiac disturbances in the toxicologic patient. In: Haddad LM, Winchester JF [editors]. *Clinical Management of Poisoning and Drug Overdose.* WB Saunders, 1983.)

tion of the patient and selected routine laboratory tests are usually sufficient to generate a tentative diagnosis and an appropriate treatment plan. While screening tests may be helpful in confirming a suspected intoxication or for ruling out intoxication as a cause of apparent brain death, they should not delay needed treatment.

When a specific antidote or other treatment is under consideration, quantitative laboratory testing may be indicated. For example, determination of the acetaminophen serum level is useful in assessing the need for antidotal therapy with acetylcysteine. Serum levels of theophylline, carbamazepine, lithium, salicylates, valproic acid, and other drugs may indicate the need for hemodialysis (Table 59–3).

Table 59–3. Indications for hemodialysis (HD) and hemoperfusion (HP) in drug poisoning.

Intoxicating Drug	Intervention
Intervention may be indicated depending on degree of intoxication or blood concentration	
Carbamazepine	HP
Ethchlorvynol	HP
Ethylene glycol	HD
Lithium	HD
Methanol	HD
Meprobamate	HP
Metformin	HD
Phenobarbital	HP
Procainamide	HD or HP
Salicylate	HD
Theophylline	HP or HD
Valproic acid	HD
Intervention not indicated (ineffective)	
Amphetamines	
Antidepressants	
Antipsychotics	
Benzodiazepines	
Calcium channel blockers	
Digoxin	
Metoprolol	
Opioids	
Propanolol	
Quinidine	
Many other drugs and poisons	

Decontamination

Decontamination procedures should be undertaken simultaneously with initial stabilization, diagnostic assessment, and laboratory evaluation. Decontamination involves removing toxins from the skin or gastrointestinal tract.

A. Skin

Contaminated clothing should be completely removed and double-bagged to prevent illness in health care providers and for possible laboratory analysis. Wash contaminated skin with soap and water.

B. Gastrointestinal Tract

There remains controversy regarding the efficacy of gut emptying by emesis or gastric lavage, especially when treatment is initiated more than 1 hour after ingestion. For most ingestions, clinical toxicologists recommend simple administration of activated charcoal to bind ingested poisons in the gut before they can be absorbed. In unusual circumstances, induced emesis or gastric lavage may also be used.

1. Emesis—Emesis can be induced with ipecac *syrup* (never *extract* of ipecac), and this method is sometimes used to treat childhood ingestions at home under telephone supervision of a physician or poison control center personnel. Ipecac should not be used if the suspected intoxicant is a corrosive agent, a petroleum distillate, or a rapidly acting convulsant. Previously popular methods of inducing emesis such as fingertip stimulation of the pharynx, salt water, and apomorphine are ineffective or dangerous and should not be used.

2. Gastric lavage—If the patient is awake or if the airway is protected by an endotracheal tube, gastric lavage may be performed using an orogastric or nasogastric tube. As large a tube as possible should be used. Lavage solutions (usually 0.9% saline) should be at body temperature to prevent hypothermia.

3. Activated charcoal—Owing to its large surface area, activated charcoal can adsorb many drugs and poisons. It is most effective if given in a ratio of at least 10:1 of charcoal to estimated dose of toxin by weight. Charcoal does not bind iron, lithium, or potassium, and it binds alcohols and cyanide only poorly. It does not appear to be useful in poisoning due to corrosive mineral acids and alkali. Recent studies suggest that oral activated charcoal given alone may be just as effective as gut emptying followed by charcoal. Also, other studies have shown that repeated doses of oral activated charcoal may enhance systemic elimination of some drugs (including carbamazepine, dapsone, and theophylline) by a mechanism referred to as "gut dialysis."

4. Cathartics—Administration of a cathartic (laxative) agent may hasten removal of toxins from the gastrointestinal tract and reduce absorption, although no controlled studies have been done. Whole bowel irrigation with a balanced polyethylene glycol-electrolyte solution (GoLYTELY, CoLyte) can enhance gut decontamination after ingestion of iron tablets, enteric-coated medicines, illicit drug-filled packets, and foreign bodies. The solution is administered at 1–2 L/h (500 mL/h in children) for several hours until the rectal effluent is clear.

Specific Antidotes

There is a popular misconception that there is an antidote for every poison. Actually, selective antidotes are available for only a few classes of toxins. The major antidotes and their characteristics are listed in Table 59–4.

Methods of Enhancing Elimination of Toxins

After appropriate diagnostic and decontamination procedures and administration of antidotes, it is important to consider whether measures for enhancing elimination, such as hemodialysis or urinary alkalinization, can improve clinical outcome. Table 59–3 lists intoxications requiring immediate dialysis, those in which it is used only if supportive measures fail, and those for which dialysis is not indicated.

A. Dialysis Procedures (Table 59–3)

1. Peritoneal dialysis—This is a relatively simple and available technique but is inefficient in removing most drugs.

2. Hemodialysis—Hemodialysis is more efficient than peritoneal dialysis and has been well studied. It assists in correction of fluid and electrolyte imbalance and may also enhance removal of toxic metabolites (eg, formate in methanol poisoning, oxalate and glycolate in ethylene glycol poisoning). The efficiency of both peritoneal dialysis and hemodialysis is a function of the molecular weight, water solubility, protein binding, endogenous clearance, and distribution in the body of the specific toxin. Hemodialysis is especially useful in overdose cases in which fluid and electrolyte imbalances are present (eg, salicylate intoxication).

3. Hemoperfusion—Blood is pumped from the patient via a venous catheter through a column of adsorbent material and then recirculated to the patient. Hemoperfusion does not improve fluid and electrolyte balance. However, it does remove many high-molecular-weight toxins that have poor water solubility because the perfusion cartridge has a large surface area for adsorption that is directly perfused with the blood and is not impeded by a membrane. The rate-limiting factors in removal of toxins by hemoperfusion are the affinity of the charcoal or adsorbent resin for the drug, the rate of blood flow through the cartridge, and the rate of equilibration of the drug from the peripheral tissues to the blood. Hemoperfusion may enhance whole body clearance of salicylate, phenytoin, etchlorvynol, phenobarbital, theophylline, and carbamazepine.

B. Forced Diuresis and Urinary pH Manipulation

Previously popular but of unproved value, forced diuresis may cause volume overload and electrolyte abnormalities and is not recommended. Renal elimination of a few toxins can be enhanced by alteration of urinary pH. For example, urinary alkalinization is useful in cases of salicylate overdose. Acidification may increase the urine concentration of drugs such as phencyclidine and amphetamines but is not advised because it may worsen renal complications from rhabdomyolysis, which often accompanies the intoxication.

COMMON TOXIC SYNDROMES

ACETAMINOPHEN

Acetaminophen is one of the drugs most commonly involved in suicide attempts and accidental poisonings, both as the sole agent and in combination with other drugs. Acute ingestion of more than 150–200 mg/kg (children) or 7 g total (adults) is considered potentially toxic. A highly toxic metabolite is produced in the liver (see Figure 4–4).

Initially, the patient is asymptomatic or has mild gastrointestinal upset (nausea, vomiting). After 24–36 hours, evidence of liver injury appears, with elevated aminotransferase levels and hypoprothrombinemia. In severe cases, fulminant liver failure occurs, leading to hepatic encephalopathy and death. Renal failure may also occur.

The severity of poisoning is estimated from a serum acetaminophen concentration measurement. If the level is greater than 150–200 mg/L approximately 4 hours after ingestion, the patient is at risk for liver injury. (Chronic alcoholics or patients taking drugs that enhance P450 production of toxic metabolites are at risk with lower levels, perhaps as low as 100 mg/L at 4 hours.) The antidote acetylcysteine acts as a glutathione substitute, binding the toxic metabolite as it is being produced. It is most effective when given early and should be started within 8–10 hours if possible. A liver transplant may be required for patients with fulminant hepatic failure.

Table 59–4. Examples of specific antidotes.

Antidote	Poison(s)	Comments
Acetylcysteine (Mucomyst)	Acetaminophen	Best results if given within 8–10 hours of overdose. Follow liver function tests and acetaminophen blood levels. Acetylcysteine is given orally in the USA. Intravenous acetylcysteine has been used successfully in Europe and is under trial in the USA.
Atropine	Anticholinesterases: organophosphates, carbamates	A test dose of 1–2 mg (for children, 0.05 mg/kg) is given IV and repeated until symptoms of atropinism appear (tachycardia, dilated pupils, ileus). Dose may be repeated every 10–15 minutes, with decrease of secretions as therapeutic end point.
Bicarbonate, sodium	Membrane-depressant cardiotoxic drugs (tricyclic antidepressants, quinidine, etc)	1–2 mEq/kg IV bolus usually reverses cardiotoxic effects (wide QRS, hypotension). Give cautiously in heart failure (avoid sodium overload).
Calcium	Fluoride; calcium channel blockers	Large doses may be needed in severe calcium channel blocker overdose. Start with 15 mg/kg IV.
Deferoxamine	Iron salts	If poisoning is severe, give 15 mg/kg/h IV. Urine may become pink. 100 mg of deferoxamine binds 8.5 mg of iron.
Digoxin antibodies	Digoxin and related cardiac glycosides	One vial binds 0.5 mg digoxin; indications include serious arrhythmias, hyperkalemia.
Esmolol	Theophylline, caffeine, metaproterenol	Short-acting β-blocker reverses β_1-induced tachycardia and (possibly) β_2-induced vasodilation. Infuse 25–50 µg/kg/min IV.
Ethanol	Methanol, ethylene glycol	Ethanol therapy can be started before laboratory diagnosis is confirmed. A loading dose is calculated so as to give a blood level of at least 100 mg/dL (42 g/70 kg in adults).
Flumazenil	Benzodiazepines	Adult dose is 0.2 mg IV, repeated as necessary to a maximum of 3 mg. *Do not give to patients with seizures, benzodiazepine dependence, or tricyclic overdose.*
Fomepizole	Methanol, ethylene glycol	More convenient and easier to use than ethanol. Loading dose 15 mg/kg; repeat every 12 hours.
Glucagon	β-blockers	5–10 mg IV bolus may reverse hypotension and bradycardia that was resistant to β-agonist drugs. May cause vomiting.
Naloxone	Narcotic drugs, other opioid derivatives	A specific antagonist of opioids; 1–2 mg initially by IV, IM, or subcutaneous injection. Larger doses may be needed to reverse the effects of overdose with propoxyphene, codeine, or fentanyl derivatives. Duration of action (2–3 hours) may be significantly shorter than that of the opioid being antagonized.
Oxygen	Carbon monoxide	Give 100% by high-flow nonrebreathing mask; use of hyperbaric chamber is controversial.
Physostigmine	Suggested for antimuscarinic anticholinergic agents; not for tricyclic antidepressants	Adult dose is 0.5–1 mg IV slowly. The effects are transient (30–60 minutes), and the lowest effective dose may be repeated when symptoms return. May cause bradycardia, increased bronchial secretions, seizures. Have atropine ready to reverse excess effects. *Do not use for tricyclic antidepressant overdose.*
Pralidoxime (2-PAM)	Organophosphate cholinesterase inhibitors	Adult dose is 1 g IV, which should be repeated every 3–4 hours as needed or preferably as a constant infusion of 250–400 mg/h. Pediatric dose is approximately 250 mg. No proved benefit in carbamate poisoning.

AMPHETAMINES & OTHER STIMULANTS

Stimulant drugs commonly abused in the USA include methamphetamine ("crank," "crystal"), methylene-dioxymethamphetamine (MDMA, "ecstasy"), and cocaine ("crack") as well as legal substances such as pseudoephedrine (Sudafed) and ephedrine (as such and in the herbal agent *Ma-huang*) (see Chapter 32). Caffeine is often added to dietary supplements sold as "metabolic enhancers" or "fat-burners" and is also found combined with pseudoephedrine or ephedrine in pills sold as amphetamine substitutes.

At the doses usually used by stimulant abusers, euphoria and wakefulness are accompanied by a sense of power and well-being. At higher doses, restlessness, agitation, and acute psychosis may occur, accompanied by hypertension and tachycardia. Prolonged muscular hyperactivity can cause dehydration and eventually, hypotension. Seizures and muscle activity may contribute to hyperthermia and rhabdomyolysis. Body temperatures as high as 42°C have been recorded. Hyperthermia can cause brain damage, hypotension, coagulopathy, and renal failure.

Treatment includes general supportive measures as outlined earlier. There is no specific antidote. Seizures and hyperthermia are the most dangerous manifestations and must be treated aggressively. Seizures are usually managed with intravenous benzodiazepines (eg, lorazepam). Temperature is reduced by removing clothing, spraying with tepid water, and encouraging evaporative cooling with fanning. For very high body temperatures (eg, > 40–41°C), neuromuscular paralysis is used to abolish muscle activity quickly.

ANTICHOLINERGIC AGENTS

A large number of prescription and nonprescription drugs, as well as a variety of plants and mushrooms, can inhibit the effects of acetylcholine. Many drugs used for other purposes (eg, antihistamines) also have anticholinergic effects. Many of them have other potentially toxic actions as well—eg, antihistamines such as diphenhydramine can cause seizures; tricyclic antidepressants, which have anticholinergic, quinidine-like, and α-blocking effects, can cause severe cardiovascular toxicity.

The classic anticholinergic syndrome is remembered as "red as a beet" (skin flushed), "hot as a hare" (hyperthermia), "dry as a bone" (dry mucous membranes, no sweating), "blind as a bat" (blurred vision), and "mad as a hatter" (confusion, delirium). Patients usually have sinus tachycardia, and the pupils are usually dilated (see Chapter 8). There may be agitated delirium or coma. Muscle twitching is common, but seizures are unusual unless the patient has ingested an antihistamine or a tricyclic antidepressant. Urinary retention is common, especially in older men.

Treatment is largely supportive. Agitated patients may require sedation with a benzodiazepine or an antipsychotic agent (eg, haloperidol). The specific antidote for peripheral and central anticholinergic syndrome is physostigmine, which has a prompt and dramatic effect and is especially useful for patients who are very agitated. It is given in small intravenous doses (0.5–1 mg), with careful monitoring, because it can cause bradycardia and seizures if given too rapidly. Physostigmine should not be given to a patient with suspected tricyclic antidepressant overdose because it can aggravate cardiotoxicity, resulting in heart block or asystole. Catheterization may be needed to prevent excessive distention of the bladder.

ANTIDEPRESSANTS

Tricyclic antidepressants (eg, amitriptyline, desipramine, doxepin, many others; see Chapter 30) are among the most common prescription drugs involved in life-threatening drug overdose. Ingestion of more than 1 g of a tricyclic (or about 15–20 mg/kg) is considered potentially lethal.

Tricyclic antidepressants are competitive antagonists at muscarinic cholinergic receptors, and anticholinergic findings (tachycardia, dilated pupils, dry mouth) are common even at moderate doses. The tricyclics are also strong α-blockers, which can lead to vasodilation. Centrally mediated agitation and seizures may be followed by depression and hypotension. Most importantly, the tricyclics have quinidine-like depressant effects that cause slowed conduction with a wide QRS interval and depressed cardiac contractility. This cardiac toxicity may result in serious arrhythmias (Figure 59–1), including ventricular conduction block and ventricular tachycardia.

Treatment of tricyclic antidepressant overdose includes general supportive care as outlined earlier. Endotracheal intubation should be carried out and ventilation assisted as needed. Intravenous fluids are given for hypotension, and dopamine or norepinephrine is added if needed. Because of blockade of catecholamine reuptake, nerve endings may be depleted of norepinephrine, and dopamine may be relatively ineffective; therefore, many toxicologists recommend norepinephrine as the initial drug of choice for tricyclic-induced hypotension. The antidote for quinidine-like cardiac toxicity (manifested by a wide QRS complex) is sodium bicarbonate: a bolus of 50–100 meq (or 1–2 meq/kg) provides a rapid increase in extracellular sodium that helps overcome sodium channel blockade. *Do not use physostigmine!* Although this agent does effectively reverse anticholinergic symptoms, it can aggravate depression of cardiac conduction and can cause seizures.

Monoamine oxidase inhibitors (eg, tranylcypromine, phenelzine) are a group of older antidepressants that are occasionally used for resistant depression. They can cause severe hypertensive reactions when interacting foods or drugs are taken (see Chapter 9); and they can interact with the selective serotonin reuptake inhibitors (SSRIs).

Newer antidepressants (eg, fluoxetine, paroxetine, citalopram, venlafaxine) are mostly selective serotonin reuptake inhibitors and are generally safer than the tricyclic antidepressants and monoamine oxidase inhibitors, although they can can cause seizures. Bupropion (not an SSRI) has caused seizures even in therapeutic doses. Some antidepressants have been associated with QT prolongation and torsade de pointes arrhythmia. The SSRIs may interact with each other or especially with monoamine oxidase inhibitors to cause the **serotonin syndrome,** characterized by agitation, muscle hyperactivity, and hyperthermia.

ANTIPSYCHOTICS

Antipsychotic drugs include the older phenothiazines and butyrophenones, as well as newer atypical drugs. All of these can cause CNS depression, seizures, and hypotension. Some can cause QT prolongation. The potent dopamine D_2 blockers are also associated with parkinsonian-like movement disorders (dystonic reactions) and in rare cases with the neuroleptic malignant syndrome, characterized by "lead-pipe" rigidity, hyperthermia, and autonomic instability (see Chapter 29).

ASPIRIN (SALICYLATE)

Salicylate poisoning (see Chapter 36) is a much less common cause of childhood poisoning deaths since the introduction of child-resistant containers and the reduced use of children's aspirin. It still accounts for numerous suicidal and accidental poisonings. Acute ingestion of more than 200 mg/kg is likely to produce intoxication. Poisoning can also result from chronic overmedication; this occurs most commonly in elderly patients using salicylates for chronic pain who become confused about their dosing. Poisoning causes uncoupling of oxidative phosphorylation and disruption of normal cellular metabolism.

The first sign of salicylate toxicity is often hyperventilation and respiratory alkalosis due to medullary stimulation (see Figure 36–4). Metabolic acidosis follows, and an increased anion gap results from accumulation of lactate as well as excretion of bicarbonate by the kidney to compensate for respiratory alkalosis. Arterial blood gas testing often reveals this mixed respiratory alkalosis and metabolic acidosis. Body temperature may be elevated due to uncoupling of oxidative phosphorylation.

Severe hyperthermia may occur in serious cases. Vomiting and hyperpnea as well as hyperthermia contribute to fluid loss and dehydration. With very severe poisoning, profound metabolic acidosis, seizures, coma, pulmonary edema, and cardiovascular collapse may occur. Absorption of salicylate and signs of toxicity may be delayed after very large overdoses or ingestion of enteric-coated tablets.

General supportive care as described earlier is essential. After massive aspirin ingestions (eg, more than 100 tablets), aggressive gut decontamination is advisable, including gastric lavage, repeated doses of activated charcoal, and consideration of whole bowel irrigation. Intravenous fluids are used to replace fluid losses caused by tachypnea, vomiting, and fever. For moderate intoxications, intravenous sodium bicarbonate is given to alkalinize the urine and promote salicylate excretion by trapping the salicylate in its ionized, polar form. For severe poisoning (eg, patients with severe acidosis, coma, and serum salicylate level > 100 mg/dL), emergency hemodialysis is performed to remove the salicylate more quickly and restore acid-base balance and fluid status.

BETA BLOCKERS

In overdose, these drugs block both β_1- and β_2-adrenoceptors—ie, selectivity, if any, is lost at high dosage. The most toxic β-blocker is propranolol. As little as two to three times the therapeutic dose can cause serious toxicity. This may be because propranolol has additional properties: At high doses it may cause sodium channel blocking effects similar to those seen with quinidine-like drugs, and it is lipophilic, allowing it to enter the CNS (see Chapter 10).

Bradycardia and hypotension are the most common manifestations of toxicity. Agents with partial agonist activity (eg, pindolol) can cause tachycardia and hypertension. Seizures and cardiac conduction block (wide QRS complex) may be seen with propranolol overdose.

General supportive care should be provided as outlined earlier. The usual measures used to raise the blood pressure and heart rate, such as intravenous fluids, β-agonist drugs, and atropine, are generally ineffective. Glucagon is a useful antidote that—like β-agonists—acts on cardiac cells to raise intracellular cAMP but does so through stimulation of glucagon receptors rather than β-adrenoceptors. It can improve heart rate and blood pressure when given in high doses (5–20 mg intravenously).

CALCIUM CHANNEL BLOCKERS

Calcium antagonists can cause serious toxicity or death with relatively small overdoses. These channel blockers depress sinus node automaticity and slow AV node conduction (see Chapter 12). They also reduce cardiac output and blood pressure. Serious hypotension is mainly seen with nifedipine and related dihydropyridines, but in severe overdose all of the listed cardiovascular effects can occur with any of the calcium channel blockers.

Treatment requires general supportive care as outlined earlier. Since most ingested calcium antagonists are in a sustained-release form, it may be possible to expel them before they are completely absorbed; initiate whole bowel irrigation and oral activated charcoal as soon as possible, before calcium antagonist-induced ileus intervenes. Calcium, given intravenously in doses of 2–10 g, is a useful antidote for depressed cardiac contractility but less effective for nodal block or peripheral vascular collapse.

CARBON MONOXIDE & OTHER TOXIC GASES

Carbon monoxide (CO) is a colorless, odorless gas that is ubiquitous because it is created whenever carbon-containing materials are burned (see Table 57–1). Carbon monoxide poisoning is the leading cause of death due to poisoning in the USA. Most cases occur in victims of fires, but accidental and suicidal exposures are also common. Diagnosis and treatment of carbon monoxide poisoning are described in Chapter 57. Many other toxic gases are produced in fires or released in industrial accidents (Table 59–5).

CHOLINESTERASE INHIBITORS

Organophosphate and carbamate cholinesterase inhibitors (see Chapter 7) are widely used to kill insects and other pests. Most cases of serious organophosphate or carbamate poisoning result from intentional ingestion by a suicidal person, but poisoning has also occurred at work (pesticide application or packaging) or, rarely, as a result of food contamination or terrorist attack (eg, release of the chemical warfare nerve agent sarin in the Tokyo subway system in 1995).

Stimulation of muscarinic receptors causes abdominal cramps, diarrhea, excessive salivation, sweating, urinary frequency, and increased bronchial secretions (see Chapters 6 and 7). Stimulation of nicotinic receptors causes generalized ganglionic activation, which can lead to hypertension and either tachycardia or bradycardia. Muscle twitching and fasciculations may progress to weakness and respiratory muscle paralysis. CNS effects include agitation, confusion, and seizures. The mnemonic DUMBELS (diarrhea, urination, miosis and muscle weakness, bronchospasm, excitation, lacrimation, and seizures, sweating, and salivation) helps recall the common findings. Blood testing may be used to document depressed activity of red blood cell (acetylcholinesterase) and plasma (butyrylcholinesterase) enzymes, which provide an indirect estimate of synaptic cholinesterase activity.

General supportive care should be provided as outlined above. Extra precautions should be taken to ensure that rescuers and health care providers are not poisoned

Table 59–5. Characteristics of poisoning with some gases.

Gas	Mechanism of Toxicity	Clinical Features and Treatment
Irritant gases (eg, chlorine, ammonia, sulfur dioxide, nitrogen oxides)	Corrosive effect on upper and lower airways	Cough, stridor, wheezing, pneumonia **Treatment:** Humidified oxygen, bronchodilators
Carbon monoxide	Binds to hemoglobin, reducing oxygen delivery to tissues	Headache, dizziness, nausea, vomiting, seizures, coma **Treatment:** 100% oxygen
Cyanide	Binds to cytochrome, blocks cellular oxygen use	Headache, nausea, vomiting, syncope, seizures, coma **Treatment:** CN antidote kit consists of nitrites to induce methemoglobinemia (which binds CN) and thiosulfate (which hastens conversion of CN to less toxic thiocyanate)
Hydrogen sulfide	Similar to cyanide	Similar to cyanide. Smell of rotten eggs **Treatment:** No specific antidote
Oxidizing agents (eg, nitrogen oxides)	Can cause methemoglobinemia	Dyspnea, cyanosis (due to brown color of methemoglobin), syncope, seizures, coma **Treatment:** Methylene blue (which hastens conversion back to normal hemoglobin)

by exposure to contaminated clothing or skin. This is especially critical for the most potent substances such as parathion or nerve gas agents. Antidotal treatment consists of atropine and pralidoxime (see Chapter 8). Atropine is an effective competitive inhibitor at muscarinic sites but has no effect at nicotinic sites. Pralidoxime given early enough is capable of restoring the cholinesterase activity and is active at both muscarinic and nicotinic sites.

DIGOXIN

Digitalis and other cardiac glycosides are found in many plants (see Chapter 13) and in the skin of some toads. Toxicity may occur as a result of acute overdose or from accumulation of digoxin in a patient with renal insufficiency or one taking a drug that interferes with digoxin elimination. Patients receiving long-term digoxin treatment are often also taking diuretics, which can lead to electrolyte depletion (especially potassium).

Vomiting is common in patients with digitalis overdose. Hyperkalemia may be caused by acute digitalis overdose or severe poisoning, while hypokalemia may be present in patients as a result of long-term diuretic treatment. (Digitalis does not cause hypokalemia.) A variety of cardiac rhythm disturbances may occur, including sinus bradycardia, AV block, atrial tachycardia with block, accelerated junctional rhythm, premature ventricular beats, bidirectional ventricular tachycardia, and other ventricular arrhythmias.

General supportive care should be provided as outlined earlier. Atropine is often effective for bradycardia or AV block. Lidocaine is sometimes effective for arrhythmias. *Administration of calcium should be avoided because it may precipitate lethal arrhythmias.* Cardioversion should be used only for ventricular fibrillation. The use of digoxin antibodies (see Chapter 13) has revolutionized the treatment of digoxin toxicity; they should be administered intravenously in the dosage indicated in the package insert. Symptoms usually improve within 30–60 minutes after antibody administration. Digoxin antibodies may also be tried in cases of poisoning by other cardiac glycosides (eg, digitoxin, oleander), although larger doses may be needed due to incomplete cross-reactivity.

ETHANOL & SEDATIVE-HYPNOTIC DRUGS

Overdosage with ethanol and sedative-hypnotic drugs (eg, benzodiazepines, barbiturates, γ-hydroxybutyrate [GHB], carisoprodol [Soma]; see Chapters 22 and 23) occurs frequently because of their common availability and use.

Patients with ethanol or sedative-hypnotic overdose may be euphoric and rowdy ("drunk") or in a state of stupor or coma ("dead drunk"). Comatose patients often have depressed respiratory drive. Depression of protective airway reflexes may result in aspiration of gastric contents. Hypothermia may be present because of environmental exposure and depressed shivering. Ethanol blood levels greater than 300 mg/dL usually cause deep coma, but regular users are often tolerant to the effects of ethanol and may be ambulatory despite even higher levels. Patients with GHB overdose are often deeply comatose for 3–4 hours and then awaken fully in a matter of minutes.

General supportive care should be provided. With careful attention to protecting the airway (including endotracheal intubation) and assisting ventilation, most patients will recover as the drug effects wear off. Hypotension usually responds to body warming (if cold), intravenous fluids and, if needed, dopamine. Patients with isolated benzodiazepine overdose may awaken after intravenous flumazenil, a benzodiazepine antagonist. However, this drug is not widely used as empiric therapy for drug overdose because it may precipitate seizures in patients who are addicted to benzodiazepines or who have ingested a convulsant drug (eg, a tricyclic antidepressant). There are no antidotes for ethanol, barbiturates, or most other sedative-hypnotics. Hemoperfusion is occasionally used for very severe phenobarbital poisoning.

ETHYLENE GLYCOL & METHANOL

These alcohols are important toxins because of their metabolism to highly toxic organic acids (see Chapter 23). They are capable of causing CNS depression and a drunken state similar to ethanol overdose. However, their products of metabolism—formic acid (from methanol) or hippuric, oxalic, and glycolic acids (from ethylene glycol)—cause a severe metabolic acidosis and can lead to coma and blindness (in the case of formic acid) or renal failure (from oxalic acid and glycolic acid). Initially, the patient appears drunk, but after a delay of up to several hours, a severe anion gap metabolic acidosis becomes apparent, accompanied by hyperventilation and altered mental status. Patients with methanol poisoning may complain of severe visual disturbances, eg, "like being in a snowstorm."

Metabolism of ethylene glycol and methanol to their toxic products can be blocked by inhibiting the enzyme alcohol dehydrogenase with a competing drug. Ethanol is metabolized preferentially by alcohol dehydrogenase, so ethanol can be given orally or intravenously (5% pharmaceutical grade) to a level of approximately 100 mg/dL. Alternatively, the antidote fomepizole—an effective blocker of alcohol dehydrogenase that does not induce ethanol intoxication—can be used.

IRON & OTHER METALS

Iron is widely used in over-the-counter vitamin preparations and is a leading cause of childhood poisoning deaths. As few as 10–12 prenatal multivitamins with iron may cause serious illness in a small child. Poisoning with other metals (lead, mercury, arsenic) is also important, especially in industry. See Chapters 33 and 58 for detailed discussions of poisoning by iron and other metals.

OPIOIDS

Opioids (opium, morphine, heroin, meperidine, methadone, etc) are common drugs of abuse (see Chapters 31 and 32), and overdose is a frequent result of using the poorly standardized preparations sold on the street. See Chapter 31 for a detailed discussion of opioid overdose and its treatment.

RATTLESNAKE ENVENOMATION

In the USA, rattlesnakes are the most common venomous reptiles. Bites are rarely fatal, and 20% do not involve envenomation. However, about 60% of bites cause significant morbidity due to the destructive digestive enzymes found in the venom. Evidence of rattlesnake envenomation includes severe pain, swelling, bruising, hemorrhagic bleb formation, and obvious fang marks. Systemic effects include nausea, vomiting, muscle fasciculations, tingling and metallic taste in the mouth, shock, and systemic coagulopathy with prolonged clotting time and reduced platelet count.

Studies have shown that emergency field remedies such as incision and suction, tourniquets, and ice packs are far more damaging than useful. Avoidance of unnecessary motion, on the other hand, does help to limit the spread of the venom. Definitive therapy relies on intravenous antivenin and should be started as soon as possible.

THEOPHYLLINE

Although it has been largely replaced by inhaled β-agonists, theophylline continues to be used for the treatment of bronchospasm by some patients with asthma and bronchitis (see Chapter 20). A dose of 20–30 tablets can cause serious or fatal poisoning. Chronic or subacute theophylline poisoning can also occur as a result of accidental overmedication or use of a drug that interferes with theophylline metabolism (eg, cimetidine, ciprofloxacin, erythromycin; see Chapter 4).

In addition to sinus tachycardia and tremor, vomiting is common after overdose. Hypotension, tachycardia, hypokalemia, and hyperglycemia may occur, probably due to β_2-adrenergic activation. The cause of this activation is not fully understood, but the effects can be ameliorated by the use of β-blockers (see below). Cardiac arrhythmias include atrial tachycardias, premature ventricular contractions, and ventricular tachycardia. In severe poisoning (eg, acute overdose with serum level > 100 mg/L), seizures often occur and are usually resistant to common anticonvulsants. Toxicity may be delayed in onset for many hours after ingestion of sustained-release tablet formulations.

General supportive care should be provided. Aggressive gut decontamination should be carried out using repeated doses of activated charcoal and whole bowel irrigation. Propranolol or other β-blockers (eg, esmolol) are useful antidotes for β-mediated hypotension and tachycardia. Phenobarbital is preferred over phenytoin for convulsions; most anticonvulsants are ineffective. Hemodialysis is indicated for serum concentrations > 100 mg/L and for intractable seizures in patients with lower levels.

REFERENCES

Dart RD (editor): *The 5 Minute Toxicology Consult.* Lippincott Williams & Wilkins, 2000.

Ford M et al (editors): *Clinical Toxicology.* Saunders, 2000.

Goldfrank LR et al (editors): *Goldfrank's Toxicologic Emergencies,* 7th ed. Copyright © 2002 The McGraw-Hill Companies.

Haddad LM, Shannon MW, Winchester JF (editors): *Clinical Management of Poisoning and Drug Overdose,* 3rd ed. Saunders, 1998.

Klaassen CD, Amdur MO, Doull J (editors): *Casarett and Doull's Toxicology: The Basic Science of Poisons,* 5th ed. Macmillan, 1995.

Olson KR et al (editors): *Poisoning & Drug Overdose,* 4th ed. Copyright © 2004 The McGraw-Hill Companies.

POISINDEX. (Revised Quarterly.) Thompson/Micromedex.

SECTION X
Special Topics

Special Aspects of Perinatal & Pediatric Pharmacology*

Gideon Koren, MD

The effects of drugs on the fetus and newborn infant are based on the general principles set forth in Chapters 1–4 of this book. However, the physiologic contexts in which these pharmacologic laws operate are different in pregnant women and in rapidly maturing infants. At present, the special pharmacokinetic factors operative in these patients are beginning to be understood, whereas information regarding pharmacodynamic differences (eg, receptor characteristics and responses) is still incomplete. This chapter presents basic principles of pharmacology in the special context of perinatal and pediatric therapeutics.

DRUG THERAPY IN PREGNANCY

Pharmacokinetics

Most drugs taken by pregnant women can cross the placenta and expose the developing embryo and fetus to their pharmacologic and teratogenic effects. Critical factors affecting placental drug transfer and drug effects on the fetus include the following: (1) the physicochemical properties of the drug; (2) the rate at which the drug crosses the placenta and the amount of drug reaching the fetus; (3) the duration of exposure to the drug; (4) distribution characteristics in different fetal tissues; (5)

the stage of placental and fetal development at the time of exposure to the drug; (6) the effects of drugs used in combination.

A. LIPID SOLUBILITY

As is true also of other biologic membranes, drug passage across the placenta is dependent on lipid solubility and the degree of drug ionization. Lipophilic drugs tend to diffuse readily across the placenta and enter the fetal circulation. For example, thiopental, a drug commonly used for cesarean sections, crosses the placenta almost immediately and can produce sedation or apnea in the newborn infant. Highly ionized drugs such as succinylcholine and tubocurarine, also used for cesarean sections, cross the placenta slowly and achieve very low concentrations in the fetus. Impermeability of the placenta to polar compounds is relative rather than absolute. If high enough maternal-fetal concentration gradients are achieved, polar compounds cross the placenta in measurable amounts. Salicylate, which is almost completely ionized at physiologic pH, crosses the placenta rapidly. This occurs because the small amount of salicylate that is not ionized is highly lipid-soluble.

B. MOLECULAR SIZE

The molecular weight of the drug also influences the rate of transfer and the amount of drug transferred across the placenta. Drugs with molecular weights of 250–500 can cross the placenta easily, depending upon their lipid solubility and degree of ionization; those with

* Supported by a grant from The Canadian Institutes for Health Research.

molecular weights of 500–1000 cross the placenta with more difficulty; and those with molecular weights greater than 1000 cross very poorly. An important clinical application of this property is the choice of heparin as an anticoagulant in pregnant women. Because it is a very large (and polar) molecule, heparin is unable to cross the placenta. Unlike warfarin, which is teratogenic and should be avoided during the first trimester and even beyond (as the brain continues to develop), heparin may be safely given to pregnant women who need anticoagulation. Yet the placenta contains drug transporters, which can carry to the fetus larger molecules. For example, a variety of maternal antibodies cross the placenta and may cause fetal morbidity, as in Rh incompatibility.

C. Placental Transporters

During the last decade, increasing numbers of drug transporters have been identified in the placenta, with substantial effects of drug transfer to the fetus. For example, the P-glycoprotein transporter encoded by the *MDR1* gene pumps back into the maternal circulation a variety of drugs, including cancer drugs (eg, vinblastine, doxorubicin) and other agents (eg, digoxin). Inhibition of this transporter may cause drug accumulation in the fetus.

D. Protein Binding

The degree to which a drug is bound to plasma proteins (particularly albumin) may also affect the rate of transfer and the amount transferred. However, if a compound is very lipid-soluble (eg, some anesthetic gases), it will not be affected greatly by protein binding. Transfer of these more lipid-soluble drugs and their overall rates of equilibration are more dependent on (and proportionate to) placental blood flow. This is because very lipid-soluble drugs diffuse across placental membranes so rapidly that their overall rates of equilibration do not depend on the free drug concentrations becoming equal on both sides. If a drug is poorly lipid-soluble and is ionized, its transfer is slow and will probably be impeded by its binding to maternal plasma proteins. Differential protein binding is also important since some drugs exhibit greater protein binding in maternal plasma than in fetal plasma because of a lower binding affinity of fetal proteins. This has been shown for sulfonamides, barbiturates, phenytoin, and local anesthetic agents.

E. Placental and Fetal Drug Metabolism

Two mechanisms help protect the fetus from drugs in the maternal circulation: (1) The placenta itself plays a role both as a semipermeable barrier and as a site of metabolism of some drugs passing through it. Several different types of aromatic oxidation reactions (eg, hydroxylation, N-dealkylation, demethylation) have been shown to occur in placental tissue. Pentobarbital is

oxidized in this way. Conversely, it is possible that the metabolic capacity of the placenta may lead to creation of toxic metabolites, and the placenta may therefore augment toxicity (eg, ethanol, benzpyrenes). (2) Drugs that have crossed the placenta enter the fetal circulation via the umbilical vein. About 40–60% of umbilical venous blood flow enters the fetal liver; the remainder bypasses the liver and enters the general fetal circulation. A drug that enters the liver may be partially metabolized there before it enters the fetal circulation. In addition, a large proportion of drug present in the umbilical artery (returning to the placenta) may be shunted through the placenta back to the umbilical vein and into the liver again. It should be noted that metabolites of some drugs may be more active than the parent compound and may affect the fetus adversely.

Pharmacodynamics

A. Maternal Drug Actions

The effects of drugs on the reproductive tissues (breast, uterus, etc) of the pregnant woman are sometimes altered by the endocrine environment appropriate for the stage of pregnancy. Drug effects on other maternal tissues (heart, lungs, kidneys, central nervous system, etc) are not changed significantly by pregnancy, though the physiologic context (cardiac output, renal blood flow, etc) may be altered and may require the use of drugs that are not needed by the same woman when she is not pregnant. For example, cardiac glycosides and diuretics may be needed for heart failure precipitated by the increased cardiac workload of pregnancy, or insulin may be required for control of blood glucose in pregnancy-induced diabetes.

B. Therapeutic Drug Actions in the Fetus

Fetal therapeutics is an emerging area in perinatal pharmacology. This involves drug administration to the pregnant woman with the fetus as the target of the drug. At present, corticosteroids are used to stimulate fetal lung maturation when preterm birth is expected. Phenobarbital, when given to pregnant women near term, can induce fetal hepatic enzymes responsible for the glucuronidation of bilirubin, and the incidence of jaundice is lower in newborns when mothers are given phenobarbital than when phenobarbital is not used. Before phototherapy became the preferred mode of therapy for neonatal indirect hyperbilirubinemia, phenobarbital was used for this indication. Administration of phenobarbital to the mother was suggested recently as a means of decreasing the risk of intracranial bleeding in preterm infants. However, large randomized studies failed to confirm this effect. Antiarrhythmic drugs have also been given to mothers for treatment of fetal cardiac arrhythmias. Although their efficacy has not yet been established by controlled studies, digoxin, flecainide, procainamide, verapamil, and other antiarrhythmic agents have been shown to be effective in case series. During the last decade it has been shown that maternal use of zidovudine decreases by two thirds transmission of HIV from the mother to the fetus, and use of combinations of three antiretroviral agents can eliminate fetal infection almost entirely (Chapter 49).

C. PREDICTABLE TOXIC DRUG ACTIONS IN THE FETUS

Chronic use of opioids by the mother may produce dependence in the fetus and newborn. This dependence may be manifested after delivery as a neonatal withdrawal syndrome. A less well understood fetal drug toxicity is caused by the use of angiotensin-converting enzyme inhibitors during pregnancy. These drugs can result in significant and irreversible renal damage in the fetus and are therefore contraindicated in pregnant women. Adverse effects may also be delayed, as in the case of female fetuses exposed to diethylstilbestrol, who may be at increased risk for adenocarcinoma of the vagina after puberty.

D. TERATOGENIC DRUG ACTIONS

A single intrauterine exposure to a drug can affect the fetal structures undergoing rapid development at the time of exposure. Thalidomide is an example of a drug that may profoundly affect the development of the limbs after only brief exposure. This exposure, however, must be at a critical time in the development of the limbs. The thalidomide phocomelia risk occurs during the fourth through the seventh weeks of gestation because it is during this time that the arms and legs develop (Figure 60–1).

1. Teratogenic mechanisms—The mechanisms by which different drugs produce teratogenic effects are poorly understood and are probably multifactorial. For example, drugs may have a direct effect on maternal tissues with secondary or indirect effects on fetal tissues. Drugs may interfere with the passage of oxygen or nutrients through the placenta and therefore have effects on the most rapidly metabolizing tissues of the fetus. Finally, drugs may have important direct actions on the processes of differentiation in developing tissues. For example, vitamin A (retinol) has been shown to have important differentiation-directing actions in normal tissues. Several vitamin A analogs (isotretinoin, etretinate) are powerful teratogens, suggesting that they alter the normal processes of differentiation. Finally, deficiency of a critical substance appears to play a role in some types of abnormalities. For example, folic acid supplementation during pregnancy appears to reduce the incidence of neural tube defects (eg, spina bifida).

Continued exposure to a teratogen may produce cumulative effects or may affect several organs going through varying stages of development. Chronic consumption of high doses of ethanol during pregnancy, particularly during the first and second trimesters, may result in the fetal alcohol syndrome (Chapter 23). In this syndrome, the central nervous system, growth, and facial development may be affected.

2. Defining a teratogen—To be considered teratogenic, a candidate substance or process should (1) result in a characteristic set of malformations, indicating selectivity for certain target organs; (2) exert its effects at a particular stage of fetal development, ie, during the limited time period of organogenesis of the target organs (Figure 60–1); and (3) show a dose-dependent incidence. Some drugs with known teratogenic or other adverse effects in pregnancy are listed in Table 60–1.

3. Counseling women about teratogenic risk—Since the thalidomide disaster, medicine has been practiced as if every drug were a potential human teratogen when, in fact, fewer than 30 such drugs have been identified, with hundreds of agents proved safe for the unborn. Owing to high levels of anxiety among pregnant women—and because half of the pregnancies in North America are unplanned—every year many thousands of women need counseling about fetal exposure to drugs, chemicals, and radiation. In the Motherisk program in Toronto, thousands of women are counseled every month, and the ability of appropriate counseling to prevent unnecessary abortions has been documented. Clinicians who wish to provide such counsel to pregnant women must ensure that their information is up to date and evidence-based and that the woman understands that the baseline teratogenic risk in pregnancy (ie, the risk of a neonatal abnormality in the absence of any known teratogenic exposure) is about 3%. It is also critical to address the maternal-fetal risks of the untreated condition. Recent studies show serious morbidity in women who discontinued SSRI therapy for depression in pregnancy.

DRUG THERAPY IN INFANTS & CHILDREN

Physiologic processes that influence pharmacokinetic variables in the infant change significantly in the first year of life, particularly during the first few months. Therefore, special attention must be paid to pharmacokinetics in this age group. Pharmacodynamic differences between pediatric and other patients have not been explored in great detail and are probably small except for those specific target tissues that mature at birth or immediately thereafter (eg, the ductus arteriosus).

Drug Absorption

Drug absorption in infants and children follows the same general principles as in adults. Unique factors that

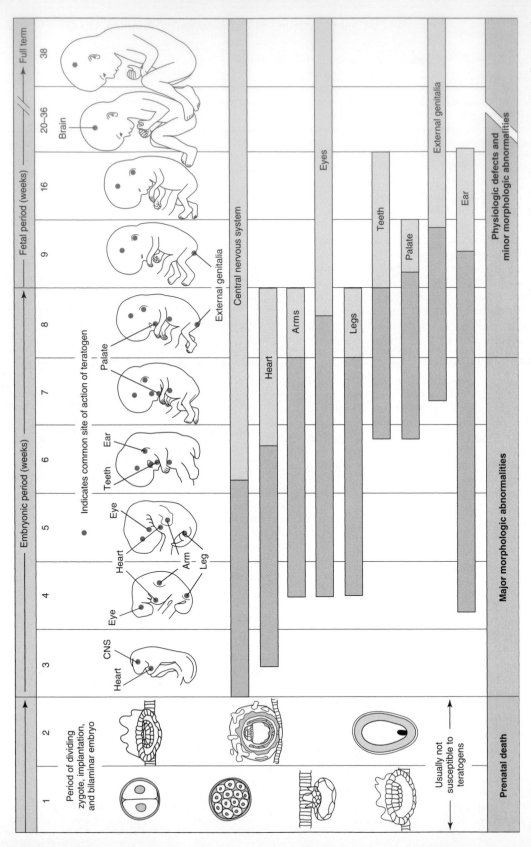

Figure 60–1. Schematic diagram of critical periods of human development. (Reproduced, with permission, from Moore KL: *The Developing Human: Clinically Oriented Embryology*, 4th ed. Saunders, 1988.)

Table 60–1. Drugs with significant adverse effects on the fetus.

Drug	Trimester	Effect
ACE inhibitors	All, especially second and third	Renal damage
Aminopterin	First	Multiple gross anomalies
Amphetamines	All	Suspected abnormal developmental patterns, decreased school performance
Androgens	Second and third	Masculinization of female fetus
Antidepressants, tricyclic	Third	Neonatal withdrawal symptoms have been reported in a few cases with clomipramine, desipramine, and imipramine
Barbiturates	All	Chronic use can lead to neonatal dependence. Cognitive loss has been described.
Busulfan	All	Various congenital malformations; low birth weight
Carbamazepine	First	Neural tube defects
Chlorpropamide	All	Prolonged symptomatic neonatal hypoglycemia
Clomipramine	Third	Neonatal lethargy, hypotonia, cyanosis, hypothermia
Cocaine	All	Increased risk of spontaneous abortion, abruptio placentae, and premature labor; neonatal cerebral infarction, abnormal development, and decreased school performance
Cyclophosphamide	First	Various congenital malformations
Cytarabine	First, second	Various congenital malformations
Diazepam	All	Chronic use may lead to neonatal dependence and increase risk for oral cleft
Diethylstilbestrol	All	Vaginal adenosis, clear cell vaginal adenocarcinoma
Ethanol	All	Risk of fetal alcohol syndrome and alcohol-related neurodevelopmental defects
Etretinate	All	High risk of multiple congenital malformations
Heroin	All	Chronic use leads to neonatal dependence
Iodide	All	Congenital goiter, hypothyroidism
Isotretinoin	All	Extremely high risk of CNS, face, ear, and other malformations
Lithium	First	Ebstein's anomaly
Methadone	All	Chronic use leads to neonatal dependence
Methotrexate	First	Multiple congenital malformations
Methylthiouracil	All	Hypothyroidism
Metronidazole	First	May be mutagenic (from animal studies; there is no evidence for mutagenic or teratogenic effects in humans)
Organic solvents	First	Multiple malformations and effects on brain development
Misoprostol	First	Möbius sequence
Penicillamine	First	Cutis laxa, other congenital malformations
Phencyclidine	All	Abnormal neurologic examination, poor suck reflex and feeding
Phenytoin	All	Fetal hydantoin syndrome
Propylthiouracil	All	Congenital goiter
Streptomycin	All	Eighth nerve toxicity described in a few cases
Smoking (constituents of tobacco smoke)	All	Intrauterine growth retardation; prematurity; sudden infant death syndrome; perinatal complications

(continued)

Table 60–1. Drugs with significant adverse effects on the fetus (*continued*).

Drug	Trimester	Effect
Tamoxifen	All	Increased risk of spontaneous abortion or fetal damage
Tetracycline	All	Discoloration and defects of teeth
Thalidomide	First	Phocomelia (shortened or absent long bones of the limbs) and many internal malformations
Trimethadione	All	Multiple congenital anomalies
Valproic acid	All	Neural tube defects
Warfarin	First	Hypoplastic nasal bridge, chondrodysplasia
	Second	CNS malformations
	Third	Risk of bleeding. Discontinue use 1 month before delivery.

influence drug absorption include blood flow at the site of administration, as determined by the physiologic status of the infant or child; and, for orally administered drugs, gastrointestinal function, which changes rapidly during the first few days after birth. Age after birth also influences the regulation of drug absorption.

A. Blood Flow at the Site of Administration

Absorption after intramuscular or subcutaneous injection depends mainly, in neonates as in adults, on the rate of blood flow to the muscle or subcutaneous area injected. Physiologic conditions that might reduce blood flow to these areas are cardiovascular shock, vasoconstriction due to sympathomimetic agents, and heart failure. However, sick preterm infants requiring intramuscular injections may have very little muscle mass. This is further complicated by diminished peripheral perfusion to these areas. In such cases, absorption becomes irregular and difficult to predict, because the drug may remain in the muscle and be absorbed more slowly than expected. If perfusion suddenly improves, there can be a sudden and unpredictable increase in the amount of drug entering the circulation, resulting in high and potentially toxic concentrations of drug. Examples of drugs especially hazardous in such situations are cardiac glycosides, aminoglycoside antibiotics, and anticonvulsants.

B. Gastrointestinal Function

Significant biochemical and physiologic changes occur in the neonatal gastrointestinal tract shortly after birth. In full-term infants, gastric acid secretion begins soon after birth and increases gradually over several hours. In preterm infants, the secretion of gastric acid occurs more slowly, with the highest concentrations appearing on the fourth day of life. Therefore, drugs that are partially or totally inactivated by the low pH of gastric contents should not be administered orally.

Gastric emptying time is prolonged (up to 6 or 8 hours) in the first day or so after delivery. Therefore, drugs that are absorbed primarily in the stomach may be absorbed more completely than anticipated. In the case of drugs absorbed in the small intestine, therapeutic effect may be delayed. Peristalsis in the neonate is irregular and may be slow. The amount of drug absorbed in the small intestine may therefore be unpredictable; more than the usual amount of drug may be absorbed if peristalsis is slowed, and this could result in potential toxicity from an otherwise standard dose. Table 60–2 summarizes data on oral bioavailability of various drugs in neonates as opposed to older children and adults. An increase in peristalsis, as in diarrheal conditions, tends to decrease the extent of absorption, since contact time with the large absorptive surface of the intestine is decreased.

Gastrointestinal enzyme activities tend to be lower in the newborn than in the adult. Activities of α-amylase and other pancreatic enzymes in the duodenum are low in infants up to 4 months of age. Neonates also have low concentrations of bile acids and lipase, which may decrease the absorption of lipid-soluble drugs.

Drug Distribution

As body composition changes with development, the distribution volumes of drugs are also changed. The neonate has a higher percentage of its body weight in the form of water (70–75%) than does the adult (50–60%). Differences can also be observed between the full-term neonate (70% of body weight as water) and the small preterm neonate (85% of body weight as water). Similarly, extracellular water is 40% of body weight in the neonate, compared with 20% in the adult. Most neonates will experience diuresis in the first 24–48 hours of life. Since many drugs are distributed through-

Table 60–2. Oral drug absorption (bioavailability) of various drugs in the neonate compared with older children and adults.

Drug	Oral Absorption
Acetaminophen	Decreased
Ampicillin	Increased
Diazepam	Normal
Digoxin	Normal
Penicillin G	Increased
Phenobarbital	Decreased
Phenytoin	Decreased
Sulfonamides	Normal

out the extracellular water space, the size (volume) of the extracellular water compartment may be important in determining the concentration of drug at receptor sites. This is especially important for water-soluble drugs (such as aminoglycosides) and less crucial for lipid-soluble agents.

Preterm infants have much less fat than full-term infants. Total body fat in preterm infants is about 1% of total body weight, compared with 15% in full-term neonates. Therefore, organs that generally accumulate high concentrations of lipid-soluble drugs in adults and older children may accumulate smaller amounts of these agents in less mature infants.

Another major factor determining drug distribution is drug binding to plasma proteins. Albumin is the plasma protein with the greatest binding capacity. In general, protein binding of drugs is reduced in the neonate. This has been seen with local anesthetic drugs, diazepam, phenytoin, ampicillin, and phenobarbital. Therefore, the concentration of free (unbound) drug in plasma is increased initially. Because the free drug exerts the pharmacologic effect, this can result in greater drug effect or toxicity despite a normal or even low plasma concentration of total drug (bound plus unbound). Consider a therapeutic dose of a drug (eg, diazepam) given to a patient. The concentration of total drug in the plasma is 300 µg/L. If the drug is 98% protein-bound in an older child or adult, then 6 µg/L is the concentration of free drug. Assume that this concentration of free drug produces the desired effect in the patient without producing toxicity. However, if this drug is given to a preterm infant in a dosage adjusted for body weight and it produces a total drug concentration of 300 µg/L—and protein binding is only 90%—then the free drug concentration will be 30 µg/L, or five times

higher. Although the higher free concentration may result in faster elimination (Chapter 3), this concentration may be quite toxic initially.

Some drugs compete with serum bilirubin for binding to albumin. Drugs given to a neonate with jaundice can displace bilirubin from albumin. Because of the greater permeability of the neonatal blood-brain barrier, substantial amounts of bilirubin may enter the brain and cause kernicterus. This was in fact observed when sulfonamide antibiotics were given to preterm neonates as prophylaxis against sepsis. Conversely, as the serum bilirubin rises for physiologic reasons or because of a blood group incompatibility, bilirubin can displace a drug from albumin and substantially raise the free drug concentration. This may occur without altering the total drug concentration and would result in greater therapeutic effect or toxicity at normal concentrations. This has been shown to happen with phenytoin.

Drug Metabolism

The metabolism of most drugs occurs in the liver (Chapter 4). The drug-metabolizing activities of the cytochrome P450-dependent mixed-function oxidases and the conjugating enzymes are substantially lower (50–70% of adult values) in early neonatal life than later. The point in development at which enzymatic activity is maximal depends upon the specific enzyme system in question. Glucuronide formation reaches adult values (per kilogram body weight) between the third and fourth years of life. Because of the neonate's decreased ability to metabolize drugs, many drugs have slow clearance rates and prolonged elimination half-lives. If drug doses and dosing schedules are not altered appropriately, this immaturity predisposes the neonate to adverse effects from drugs that are metabolized by the liver. Table 60–3 demonstrates how neonatal and adult drug elimination half-lives can differ and how the half-lives of phenobarbital and phenytoin decrease as the neonate grows older. The process of maturation must be considered when administering drugs to this age group, especially in the case of drugs administered over long periods.

Another consideration for the neonate is whether or not the mother was receiving drugs (such as phenobarbital) that can induce early maturation of fetal hepatic enzymes. In this case, the ability of the neonate to metabolize certain drugs will be greater than expected, and one may see less therapeutic effect and lower plasma drug concentrations when the usual neonatal dose is given.

Drug Excretion

The glomerular filtration rate is much lower in newborns than in older infants, children, or adults, and this

Table 60–3. Approximate elimination half-lives of various drugs in neonates and adults.

Drug	Neonatal Age	Neonates $t_{1/2}$ (hours)	Adults $t_{1/2}$ (hours)
Acetamino-phen		2.25	0.9–2.2
Diazepam		25–100	40–50
Digoxin		60–70	30–60
Phenobar-bital	0–5 days 5–15 days 1–30 months	200 100 50	64–140
Phenytoin	0–2 days 3–14 days 14–50 days	80 18 6	12–18
Salicylate		4.5–11	10–15
Theophylline	Neonate Child	13–26 3–4	10–15

limitation persists during the first few days of life. Calculated on the basis of surface area, glomerular filtration in the neonate is only 30–40% of the adult value. The glomerular filtration rate is even lower in neonates born before 34 weeks of gestation. Function improves substantially during the first week of life. At the end of the first week, the glomerular filtration rate and renal plasma flow have increased 50% from the first day. By the end of the third week, glomerular filtration is 50–60% of the adult value; by 6–12 months, it reaches adult values (per unit surface area). Therefore, drugs that depend on renal function for elimination are cleared from the body very slowly in the first weeks of life.

Penicillins, for example, are cleared by preterm infants at 17% of the adult rate based on comparable surface area and 34% of the adult rate when adjusted for body weight. The dosage of ampicillin for a neonate less than 7 days old is 50–100 mg/kg/d in two doses at 12-hour intervals. The dosage for a neonate over 7 days old is 100–200 mg/kg/d in three doses at 8-hour intervals. A decreased rate of renal elimination in the neonate has also been observed with aminoglycoside antibiotics (kanamycin, gentamicin, neomycin, and streptomycin). The dosage of gentamicin for a neonate less than 7 days old is 5 mg/kg/d in two doses at 12-hour intervals. The dosage for a neonate over 7 days old is 7.5 mg/kg/d in three doses at 8-hour intervals. Total body clearance of digoxin is directly dependent upon adequate renal function, and accumulation of digoxin can occur when glomerular filtration is decreased. Since renal function

in a sick infant may not improve at the predicted rate during the first weeks and months of life, appropriate adjustments in dosage and dosing schedules may be very difficult. In this situation, adjustments are best made on the basis of plasma drug concentrations determined at intervals throughout the course of therapy.

While great focus is naturally concentrated on the neonate, it is important to remember that toddlers may have shorter elimination half-lives of drugs than older children and adults, due probably to increased renal elimination and metabolism. For example, the dose per kilogram of digoxin is much higher in toddlers than in adults. The mechanisms for these developmental changes are still poorly understood.

Special Pharmacodynamic Features in the Neonate

The appropriate use of drugs has made possible the survival of neonates with severe abnormalities who would otherwise die within days or weeks after birth. For example, administration of indomethacin (Chapter 35) causes the rapid closure of a patent ductus arteriosus, which would otherwise require surgical closure in an infant with a normal heart. Infusion of prostaglandin E_1, on the other hand, causes the ductus to remain open, which can be life-saving in an infant with transposition of the great vessels or tetralogy of Fallot (Chapter 18). An unexpected effect of such PGE_1 infusion has recently been described. The drug caused antral hyperplasia with gastric outlet obstruction as a clinical manifestation in 6 of 74 infants who received it. This phenomenon appears to be dose-dependent.

PEDIATRIC DOSAGE FORMS & COMPLIANCE

The form in which a drug is manufactured and the way in which the parent dispenses the drug to the child determine the actual dose administered. Many drugs prepared for children are in the form of elixirs or suspensions. **Elixirs** are alcoholic solutions in which the drug molecules are dissolved and evenly distributed. No shaking is required, and unless some of the vehicle has evaporated, the first dose from the bottle and the last dose should contain equivalent amounts of drug. **Suspensions** contain undissolved particles of drug that must be distributed throughout the vehicle by shaking. If shaking is not thorough each time a dose is given, the first doses from the bottle may contain less drug than the last doses, with the result that less than the expected plasma concentration or effect of the drug may be achieved early in the course of therapy. Conversely, toxicity may occur late in the course of therapy, when it is not expected. This uneven distribution is a potential cause of inefficacy or toxicity in children taking phenytoin suspensions. It is thus essential that the prescriber know the form in which the drug will be dispensed and provide proper instructions to the pharmacist and patient or parent.

Compliance may be more difficult to achieve in pediatric practice than otherwise, since it involves not only the parent's conscientious effort to follow directions but also such practical matters as measuring errors, spilling, and spitting out. For example, the measured volume of "teaspoons" ranges from 2.5 to 7.8 mL. The parents should obtain a calibrated medicine spoon or syringe from the pharmacy. These devices improve the accuracy of dose measurements and simplify administration of drugs to children.

When evaluating compliance, it is often helpful to ask if an attempt has been made to give a further dose after the child has spilled half of what was offered. The parents may not always be able to say with confidence how much of a dose the child actually received. The parents must be told whether or not to wake the baby for its every-6-hour dose day or night. These matters should be discussed and made clear, and no assumptions should be made about what the parents may or may not do. Noncompliance frequently occurs when antibiotics are prescribed to treat otitis media or urinary tract infections and the child feels well after 4 or 5 days of therapy. The parents may not feel there is any reason to continue giving the medicine even though it was prescribed for 10 or 14 days. This common situation should be anticipated so the parents can be told why it is important to continue giving the medicine for the prescribed period even if the child seems to be "cured."

Practical and convenient dosage forms and dosing schedules should be chosen to the extent possible. The easier it is to administer and take the medicine and the easier the dosing schedule is to follow, the more likely it is that compliance will be achieved.

Consistent with their ability to comprehend and cooperate, children should also be given some responsibility for their own health care and for taking medications. This should be discussed in appropriate terms both with the child and with the parents. Possible adverse effects and drug interactions with over-the-counter medicines or foods should also be discussed. Whenever a drug does not achieve its therapeutic effect, the possibility of noncompliance should be considered. There is ample evidence that in such cases parents' or children's reports may be grossly inaccurate. Random pill counts and measurement of serum concentrations may help disclose noncompliance. The use of computerized pill containers, which record each lid opening, has been shown to be very effective in measuring compliance.

Because many pediatric doses are calculated—eg, using body weight—rather than simply read from a list, major dosing errors may result from incorrect calculations. Typically, tenfold errors due to incorrect placement of the decimal point have been described. In the case of digoxin, for example, an intended dose of 0.1 mL containing 5 µg of drug, when replaced by 1.0 mL—which is still a small volume—can result in fatal overdosage. A good rule for avoiding such "decimal point" errors is to use a leading "0" plus decimal point when dealing with doses less than "1" and to avoid using a zero after a decimal point (see Chapter 66).

DRUG USE DURING LACTATION

Despite the fact that most drugs are excreted into breast milk in amounts too small to adversely affect neonatal health, thousands of women taking medications do not breast-feed because of misperception of risk. Unfortunately, physicians contribute heavily to this bias. It is important to remember that formula feeding is associated with higher morbidity and mortality in all socioeconomic groups.

Most drugs administered to lactating women are detectable in breast milk. Fortunately, the concentration of drugs achieved in breast milk is usually low (Table 60–4). Therefore, the total amount the infant would receive in a day is substantially less than what would be considered a "therapeutic dose." If the nursing mother must take medications and the drug is a relatively safe one, she should optimally take it 30–60 minutes after nursing and 3–4 hours before the next feeding. This allows time for many drugs to be cleared from the mother's blood, and the concentrations in breast milk will be relatively low. Drugs for which no data are available on safety during lactation should be avoided or breast-feeding discontinued while they are being given.

Most antibiotics taken by nursing mothers can be detected in breast milk. Tetracycline concentrations in breast milk are approximately 70% of maternal serum concentrations and present a risk of permanent tooth staining in the infant. Isoniazid rapidly reaches equilibrium between breast milk and maternal blood. The concentrations achieved in breast milk are high enough so that signs of pyridoxine deficiency may occur in the infant if the mother is not given pyridoxine supplements.

Most sedatives and hypnotics achieve concentrations in breast milk sufficient to produce a pharmacologic effect in some infants. Barbiturates taken in hypnotic doses by the mother can produce lethargy, sedation, and poor suck reflexes in the infant. Chloral hydrate can produce sedation if the infant is fed at peak milk concentrations. Diazepam can have a sedative effect on the nursing infant, but, most importantly, its long half-life can result in significant drug accumulation.

Table 60–4. Drugs often used during lactation and possible effects on the nursing infant.

Drug	Effect on Infant	Comments
Ampicillin	Minimal	No significant adverse effects; possible occurrence of diarrhea or allergic sensitization.
Aspirin	Minimal	Occasional doses probably safe; high doses may produce significant concentration in breast milk, but infant dose is nevertheless low.
Caffeine	Minimal	Caffeine intake in moderation is safe; concentration in breast milk is about 1% of that in maternal blood.
Chloral hydrate	Significant	May cause drowsiness if infant is fed at peak concentration in milk.
Chloramphenicol	Significant	Concentrations too low to cause gray baby syndrome; possibility of bone marrow suppression does exist; recommend not taking chloramphenicol while breast-feeding.
Chlorothiazide	Minimal	No adverse effects reported.
Chlorpromazine	Minimal	Appears insignificant.
Codeine	Minimal	No adverse effects reported.
Diazepam	Significant	May cause sedation in breast-fed infants; clinical monitoring recommended.
Dicumarol	Minimal	No adverse side effects reported; may wish to follow infant's prothrombin time.
Digoxin	Minimal	Insignificant quantities enter breast milk.
Ethanol	Moderate	Large amounts consumed by mother can produce alcohol effects in infant. Calculate "time to zero" concentration to schedule consumption or breast-feeding (see Chapter 23).
Heroin	Significant	Enters breast milk and can prolong neonatal narcotic dependence.
Iodine (radioactive)	Significant	Enters milk in quantities sufficient to cause thyroid suppression in infant.
Isoniazid (INH)	Minimal	Milk concentrations equal maternal plasma concentrations. Possibility of pyridoxine deficiency developing in the infant.
Kanamycin	Minimal	No adverse effects reported.
Lithium	Significant	Breast-feeding with caution; levels can be measured in milk.
Methadone	Significant	(See heroin.) Under close physician supervision, breast-feeding can be continued. Signs of opioid withdrawal in the infant may occur if mother stops taking methadone or stops breast feeding abruptly.
Oral contraceptives	Minimal	May suppress lactation in high doses.
Penicillin	Minimal	Very low concentrations in breast milk.
Phenobarbital	Moderate	Hypnotic doses can cause sedation in the infant. Close monitoring of infant.
Phenytoin	Moderate	Amounts entering breast milk are not sufficient to cause adverse effects in infant.
Prednisone	Moderate	Low maternal doses (5 mg/d) probably safe. Doses two or more times physiologic amounts (> 15 mg/d) should probably be avoided.
Propranolol	Minimal	Very small amounts enter breast milk.
Propylthiouracil	Significant	May suppress thyroid function in infant.
Spironolactone	Minimal	Very small amounts enter breast milk.
Tetracycline	Moderate	Possibility of permanent staining of developing teeth in the infant. Should be avoided during lactation.

(continued)

Table 60–4. Drugs often used during lactation and possible effects on the nursing infant (*continued*).

Drug	Effect on Infant	Comments
Theophylline	Moderate	Can enter breast milk in moderate quantities but not likely to produce significant effects.
Thyroxine	Minimal	No adverse effects in therapeutic doses.
Tolbutamide	Minimal	Low concentrations in breast milk.
Warfarin	Minimal	Very small quantities found in breast milk.

Opioids such as heroin, methadone, and morphine enter breast milk in quantities potentially sufficient to prolong the state of neonatal narcotic dependence if the drug was taken chronically by the mother during pregnancy. If conditions are well controlled and there is a good relationship between the mother and the physician, an infant could be breast-fed while the mother is taking methadone. She should not, however, stop taking the drug abruptly; the infant can be tapered off the methadone as the mother's dose is tapered. The infant should be watched for signs of narcotic withdrawal.

Minimal use of alcohol by the mother has not been reported to harm nursing infants. Excessive amounts of alcohol, however, can produce alcohol effects in the infant. Nicotine concentrations in the breast milk of smoking mothers are low and do not produce effects in the infant. Very small amounts of caffeine are excreted in the breast milk of coffee-drinking mothers.

Lithium enters breast milk in concentrations equal to those in maternal serum. Clearance of this drug is almost completely dependent upon renal elimination, and women who are receiving lithium may expose the baby to relatively large amounts of the drug.

Radioactive substances such as iodinated ^{125}I albumin and radioiodine can cause thyroid suppression in infants and may increase the risk of subsequent thyroid cancer as much as tenfold. Breast-feeding is contraindicated after large doses and should be withheld for days to weeks after small doses. Similarly, breast-feeding should be avoided in mothers receiving cancer chemotherapy or being treated with cytotoxic or immune-modulating agents for collagen diseases such as lupus erythematosus or after an organ transplant.

PEDIATRIC DRUG DOSAGE

Because of differences in pharmacokinetics in infants and children, simple proportionate reduction in the adult dose may not be adequate to determine a safe and effective pediatric dose. The most reliable pediatric dose information is usually that provided by the manufacturer in the package insert. However, such information is not available for the majority of products even when studies have been published in the medical literature—reflecting the reluctance of manufacturers to label their products for children. Recently, the Food & Drug Administration has moved toward more explicit expectations that manufacturers test their new products in infants and children. In the absence of explicit pediatric dose recommendations, an approximation can be made by any of several methods based on age, weight, or surface area. These rules are not precise and should not be used if the manufacturer provides a pediatric dose. Most drugs approved for use in children have recommended pediatric doses, generally stated as milligrams per kilogram or per pound. However, most drugs in the common formularies, eg, *Physicians' Desk Reference,* are still not specifically approved for children. This is due to lack of interest by manufacturers because the pediatric market for drugs is relatively small. When pediatric doses are calculated (either from one of the methods set forth below or from a manufacturer's dose), the pediatric dose should never exceed the adult dose.

Surface Area

Calculations of dosage based on age or weight (see below) are conservative and tend to underestimate the required dose. Doses based on surface area (Table 60–5) are more likely to be adequate.

Age (Young's rule):

$$\text{Dose} = \text{Adult dose} \times \frac{\text{Age (years)}}{\text{Age} + 12}$$

Weight (somewhat more precise is Clark's rule):

$$\text{Dose} = \text{Adult dose} \times \frac{\text{Weight (kg)}}{70}$$

or

$$\text{Dose} = \text{Adult dose} \times \frac{\text{Weight (lb)}}{150}$$

Table 60–5. Determination of drug dosage from surface area.[1]

Weight (kg)	(lb)	Approximate Age	Surface Area (m²)	Percent of Adult Dose
3	6.6	Newborn	0.2	12
6	13.2	3 months	0.3	18
10	22	1 year	0.45	28
20	44	5.5 years	0.8	48
30	66	9 years	1	60
40	88	12 years	1.3	78
50	110	14 years	1.5	90
60	132	Adult	1.7	102
70	154	Adult	1.76	103

Reproduced, with permission, from Silver HK, Kempe CH, Bruyn HB: *Handbook of Pediatrics,* 14th ed. Originally published by Lange Medical Publications. Copyright © 1983 by the McGraw-Hill Companies, Inc.

[1] For example, if adult dose is 1 mg/kg, dose for 3-month-old infant would be 2 mg/kg (18% of 70 mg/6 kg).

In spite of these approximations, only by conducting studies in children can safe and effective doses for a given age group and condition be determined.

REFERENCES

American Academy of Pediatrics, Committee on Drugs: Emergency drug doses for infants and children. Pediatrics 1988;81:462.

Benitz WE, Tatro DS: *The Pediatric Drug Handbook,* 3rd ed. Year Book, 1995.

Bennett PN: *Drugs and Human Lactation,* 2nd ed. Elsevier, 1996.

Berlin CM Jr: Advances in pediatric pharmacology and toxicology. Adv Pediatr 1997;44:545.

Besunder JB, Reed MD, Blumer JL: Principles of drug biodisposition in the neonate: A critical evaluation of the pharmacokinetic-pharmacodynamic interface. (Two parts.) Clin Pharmacokinet 1988;14:189, 261.

Briggs GG, Freeman RK, Yaffe SJ: *Drugs in Pregnancy and Lactation. A Reference Guide to Fetal and Neonatal Risk,* 6th ed. Williams & Wilkins, 2002.

Gavin PJ, Yogev R: The role of protease inhibitor therapy in children with HIV infection. Paediatr Drugs 2002;4:581.

Gilman JT: Therapeutic drug monitoring in the neonate and paediatric age group: Problems and clinical pharmacokinetic implications. Clin Pharmacokinet 1990;19:1.

Hansten PD, Horn JR: *Drug Interactions, Analysis and Management.* Facts & Comparisons. [Quarterly.]

Hendrick V et al: Birth outcomes after prenatal exposure to antidepressant medication. Am J Obstet Gynecol 2003;188:812.

Iqbal MM, Sohhan T, Mahmud SZ: The effects of lithium, valproic acid, and carbamazepine during pregnancy and lactation. J Toxicol Clin Toxicol 2001;39:381.

Ito S, Koren G: Fetal drug therapy. Perinat Clin North Am 1994;21:1.

Koren G: *Maternal-Fetal Toxicology; A Clinician's Guide,* 3rd ed. Dekker, 2001.

Koren G, Klinger G, Ohlsson A: Fetal pharmacotherapy. Drugs 2002;62:757.

Koren G, Pastuszak A: Prevention of unnecessary pregnancy terminations by counseling women on drug, chemical, and radiation exposure during the first trimester. Teratology 1990; 41:657.

Koren G, Pastuszak A, Ito E: Drugs in pregnancy. N Engl J Med 1998;338:1128.

Koren G, Prober C, Gold R: *Antimicrobial Therapy in Infants and Children.* Dekker, 1987.

Loebstein R, Koren G: Clinical pharmacology and therapeutic drug monitoring in neonates and children. Pediatr Rev 1998; 19:423.

Nau H: Clinical pharmacokinetics in pregnancy and perinatology: 2. Penicillins. Dev Pharmacol Ther 1987;10:174.

Neubert D: Reproductive toxicology: the science today. Teratog Carcinog Mutagen 2002;22:159.

Nottarianni LJ: Plasma protein binding of drugs in pregnancy and in neonates. Clin Pharmacokinet 1990;18:20.

Paap CM, Nahata MC: Clinical pharmacokinetics of antibacterial drugs in neonates. Clin Pharmacokinet 1990;19:280.

Peled N et al: Gastric-outlet obstruction induced by prostaglandin therapy in neonates. N Engl J Med 1992;327:505.

Rousseaux CG, Blakely PM: Fetus. In: Haschek WM, Rousseaux CG (editors). *Handbook of Toxicologic Pathology.* Academic Press, 1991.

Safety of antimicrobial drugs in pregnancy. Med Lett Drugs Ther 1987;29:61.

Stewart CF, Hampton EM: Effect of maturation on drug disposition in pediatric patients. Clin Pharm 1987;6:548.

Valdes-Dapena M: Iatrogenic disease in the perinatal period. Pediatr Clin North Am 1989;36:67.

van Lingen RA et al: The effects of analgesia in the vulnerable infant during the perinatal period. Clin Perinatol 2002;29:511.

Special Aspects of Geriatric Pharmacology

Bertram G. Katzung, MD, PhD

61

Society often classifies everyone over 65 as "elderly," but most authorities consider the field of geriatrics to apply to persons over 75—even though this too is an arbitrary definition. Furthermore, chronologic age is only one determinant of the changes pertinent to drug therapy that occur in older people. Important changes in responses to some drugs occur with increasing age in many individuals. For other drugs, age-related changes are minimal, especially in the "healthy old." Drug usage patterns also change as a result of the increasing incidence of disease with age and the tendency to prescribe heavily for patients in nursing homes. General changes in the lives of older people have significant effects on the way drugs are used. Among these changes are the increased incidence with advancing age of multiple diseases, nutritional problems, reduced financial resources, and—in some patients—decreased dosing compliance for a variety of reasons. The health practitioner thus should be aware of the changes in pharmacologic responses that may occur in older people and how to deal with these changes.

PHARMACOLOGIC CHANGES ASSOCIATED WITH AGING

In the general population, measurements of functional capacity of most of the major organ systems show a decline beginning in young adulthood and continuing throughout life. As shown in Figure 61–1, there is no "middle-age plateau" but rather a linear decrease beginning no later than age 45. However, these data reflect the mean and do not apply to every person above a certain age; approximately one third of healthy subjects have no age-related decrease in, for example, creatinine clearance up to the age of 75. Thus, the elderly do not lose specific functions at an accelerated rate compared with young and middle-aged adults but rather accumulate more deficiencies with the passage of time. Some of these changes result in altered pharmacokinetics. For the pharmacologist and the clinician, the most important of these is the decrease in renal function. Other changes

and concurrent diseases may alter the pharmacodynamic characteristics of particular drugs in certain patients.

Pharmacokinetic Changes

A. ABSORPTION

There is little evidence that there is any major alteration in drug absorption with age. However, conditions associated with age may alter the rate at which some drugs are absorbed. Such conditions include altered nutritional habits, greater consumption of nonprescription drugs (eg, antacids, laxatives), and changes in gastric emptying, which is often slower in older persons.

B. DISTRIBUTION

Compared to young adults, the elderly have reduced lean body mass, reduced total and percentage body water, and an increase in fat as a percentage of body mass. Some of these changes are shown in Table 61–1. There is usually a decrease in serum albumin, which binds many drugs, especially weak acids. There may be a concurrent *increase* in serum orosomucoid (α-acid glycoprotein), a protein that binds many basic drugs. Thus, the ratio of bound to free drug may be significantly altered. As explained in Chapter 3, these changes may alter the appropriate loading dose of a drug. However, since both the clearance and the effects of drugs are related to the free concentration, the steady state effects of a maintenance dosage regimen should not be altered by these factors alone. For example, the loading dose of digoxin in an elderly patient with heart failure should be reduced (if used at all) because of the decreased apparent volume of distribution. The maintenance dose may have to be reduced because of reduced clearance of the drug.

C. METABOLISM

The capacity of the liver to metabolize drugs does not appear to decline consistently with age for all drugs. Animal studies and some clinical studies have suggested that certain drugs are metabolized more slowly; some of

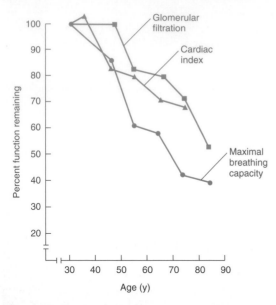

Figure 61–1. Effect of age on some physiologic functions. (Modified and reproduced, with permission, from Kohn RR: *Principles of Mammalian Aging.* Prentice-Hall, 1978.)

Table 61–2. Effects of age on hepatic clearance of some drugs.

Age-Related Decrease in Hepatic Clearance Found	No Age-Related Difference Found
Alprazolam	Ethanol
Barbiturates	Isoniazid
Carbenoxolone	Lidocaine
Chlordiazepoxide	Lorazepam
Chlormethiazole	Nitrazepam
Clobazam	Oxazepam
Desmethyldiazepam	Prazosin
Diazepam	Salicylate
Flurazepam	Warfarin
Imipramine	
Meperidine	
Nortriptyline	
Phenylbutazone	
Propranolol	
Quinidine, quinine	
Theophylline	
Tolbutamide	

these drugs are listed in Table 61–2. The greatest changes are in phase I reactions, ie, those carried out by the microsomal mixed-function oxidase system; there are much smaller changes in the ability of the liver to carry out conjugation (phase II) reactions (see Chapter

4). Some of these changes may be caused by decreased liver blood flow (Table 61–1), an important variable in the clearance of drugs that have a high hepatic extraction ratio. In addition, there is a decline with age of the liver's ability to recover from injury, eg, that caused by alcohol or viral hepatitis. Therefore, a history of recent liver disease in an older person should lead to caution in dosing with drugs that are cleared primarily by the liver, even after apparently complete recovery from the hepatic insult. Finally, malnutrition and diseases that affect hepatic function—eg, heart failure—are more common in the elderly. Heart failure may dramatically alter the ability of the liver to metabolize drugs and may also reduce hepatic blood flow. Similarly, severe nutritional deficiencies, which occur more often in old age, may impair hepatic function.

Table 61–1. Some changes related to aging that affect pharmacokinetics of drugs.

Variable	Young Adults (20–30 years)	Older Adults (60–80 years)
Body water (% of body weight)	61	53
Lean body mass (% of body weight)	19	12
Body fat (% of body weight)	26–33 (women) 18–20 (men)	38–45 36–38
Serum albumin (g/dL)	4.7	3.8
Kidney weight (% of young adult)	(100)	80
Hepatic blood flow (% of young adult)	(100)	55–60

D. Elimination

Because the kidney is the major organ for clearance of drugs from the body, the age-related decline of renal functional capacity referred to above is very important. The decline in creatinine clearance occurs in about two thirds of the population. It is important to note that this decline is not reflected in an equivalent rise in serum creatinine because the production of creatinine is also reduced as muscle mass declines with age. The practical result of this change is marked prolongation of the half-life of many drugs and the possibility of accumulation to toxic levels if dosage is not reduced in size or frequency. Dosing recommendations for the elderly often include an allowance for reduced renal clearance. If only the young adult dosage is known for a drug that requires renal clearance, a rough correction can be made by using the Cockcroft-Gault formula (Cockcroft et al, 1976), which is applicable to patients from age 40 through age 80:

$$\text{Creatinine clearance (mL/min)} = \frac{(140 - \text{Age}) \times (\text{Weight in kg})}{72 \times \text{Serum creatinine in mg/dL}}$$

For women, the result should be multiplied by 0.85. It must be emphasized that this estimate is, at best, a *population* estimate and may not apply to a particular patient (Goldberg et al, 1987). If the patient has normal renal function (up to one third of patients), a dose corrected on the basis of this estimate will be too low—but a low dose is initially desirable if one is uncertain of the renal function in any patient. If a precise measure is needed, a standard 12- or 24-hour creatinine clearance determination should be done. As indicated above, nutritional changes alter pharmacokinetic parameters. A patient who is severely dehydrated (not uncommon in patients with stroke or other motor impairment) may have an additional marked reduction in renal drug clearance that is completely reversible by rehydration.

The lungs are important for the excretion of volatile drugs. As a result of reduced respiratory capacity (Figure 61–1) and the increased incidence of active pulmonary disease in the elderly, the use of inhalation anesthesia is less common and parenteral agents more common in this age group. (See Chapter 25.)

Pharmacodynamic Changes

It was long believed that geriatric patients were much more "sensitive" to the action of many drugs, implying a change in the pharmacodynamic interaction of the drugs with their receptors. It is now recognized that many—perhaps most—of these apparent changes result from altered pharmacokinetics or diminished homeostatic responses. Clinical studies have supported the idea that the elderly are more sensitive to *some* sedative-hypnotics and analgesics. In addition, there are some data from animal studies that suggest actual changes with age in the characteristics or numbers of a few receptors. The most extensive studies show a decrease in responsiveness to β-adrenoceptor stimulants. Other examples are discussed below.

Certain homeostatic control mechanisms appear to be blunted in the elderly. Since homeostatic responses are often important components of the total response to a drug, these physiologic alterations may change the pattern or intensity of drug response. In the cardiovascular system, the cardiac output increment required by mild or moderate exercise is successfully provided to at

least age 75 (in individuals without obvious cardiac disease), but the increase is the result primarily of increased stroke volume in the elderly and not tachycardia, as in young adults. Average blood pressure goes up with age (in most Western countries), but the incidence of symptomatic orthostatic hypotension also increases markedly. It is thus particularly important to check for orthostatic hypotension on every visit. Similarly, the average 2-hour postprandial blood sugar increases by about 1 mg/dL for each year of age above 50. Temperature regulation is also impaired, and hypothermia is poorly tolerated in the elderly.

Behavioral & Lifestyle Changes

Major changes in the conditions of daily life accompany the aging process and impact health. Some of these (eg, forgetting to take one's pills) are the result of cognitive changes associated with vascular or other pathology. Others relate to economic stresses associated with greatly reduced income and possibly, increased expenses due to illness. One of the most important changes is the loss of a spouse.

MAJOR DRUG GROUPS

CENTRAL NERVOUS SYSTEM DRUGS

Sedative-Hypnotics

The half-lives of many benzodiazepines and barbiturates increase 50–150% between age 30 and age 70. Much of this change occurs during the decade from 60 to 70. For many of the benzodiazepines, both the parent molecule and its metabolites (produced in the liver) are pharmacologically active (see Chapter 22). The age-related decline in renal function and liver disease, if present, both contribute to the reduction in elimination of these compounds. In addition, an increased volume of distribution has been reported for some of these drugs. Lorazepam and oxazepam may be less affected by these changes than the other benzodiazepines. In addition to these pharmacokinetic factors, it is generally believed that the elderly vary more in their sensitivity to the sedative-hypnotic drugs on a pharmacodynamic basis as well. Among the toxicities of these drugs, ataxia and other aspects of motor impairment should be particularly watched for in order to avoid accidents.

Analgesics

The opioid analgesics show variable changes in pharmacokinetics with age. However, the elderly are often markedly more sensitive to the respiratory effects of these agents because of age-related changes in respiratory function. Therefore, this group of drugs should be used with caution until the sensitivity of the particular patient has been evaluated, and the patient should then be dosed appropriately for full effect. Unfortunately, studies show that opioids are consistently *underutilized* in patients who require strong analgesics for chronic painful conditions such as cancer. There is no justification for underutilization of these drugs, especially in the care of the elderly, and good pain management plans are readily available (Ashburn et al, 1993; Schug et al, 1992).

Antipsychotic & Antidepressant Drugs

The antipsychotic agents (phenothiazines and haloperidol) have been very heavily used (and probably misused) in the management of a variety of psychiatric diseases in the elderly. There is no doubt that they are useful in the management of schizophrenia in old age, and they are probably useful also in the treatment of some symptoms associated with delirium, dementia, agitation, combativeness, and a paranoid syndrome that appears in some geriatric patients. However, they are not fully satisfactory in these geriatric conditions, and dosage should not be increased on the assumption that full control is possible. There is no evidence that these drugs have any beneficial effects in Alzheimer's dementia, and on theoretical grounds the antimuscarinic effects of the phenothiazines might be expected to worsen memory impairment and intellectual dysfunction (see below). Much of the apparent improvement in agitated and combative patients may simply reflect the sedative effects of the drugs. When a sedative antipsychotic is desired, a phenothiazine such as thioridazine is appropriate. If sedation is to be avoided, haloperidol is more appropriate. The latter drug has increased extrapyramidal toxicity, however, and should be avoided in patients with preexisting extrapyramidal disease. The phenothiazines, especially older drugs such as chlorpromazine, often induce orthostatic hypotension in young adults because of their α-adrenoceptor-blocking effects. They are even more prone to do so in the elderly.

Because of increased responsiveness to all these drugs, dosage should usually be started at a fraction of that used in young adults. The half-lives of some phenothiazines are increased in the geriatric population. Thioridazine's half-life, for example, is more than doubled. Plasma protein binding of fluphenazine is reduced, which results in an increase of the free drug:total drug ratio.

Lithium is often used in the treatment of mania in the aged. Because it is cleared by the kidneys, dosages must be adjusted appropriately. Concurrent use of thiazide diuretics reduces the clearance of lithium and should be accompanied by further reduction in dosage and more frequent measurement of lithium blood levels.

Psychiatric depression is thought to be underdiagnosed and undertreated in the elderly. The suicide rate in the over-65 age group (twice the national average) supports this view. Unfortunately, the apathy, flat affect, and social withdrawal of major depression may be mistaken for senile dementia. Clinical evidence suggests that the elderly are as responsive to the antidepressants (of all types) as younger patients but are more likely to experience toxic effects. This factor along with the reduced clearance of some of these drugs underlines the importance of careful dosing and strict attention to the appearance of toxic effects. If a tricyclic antidepressant is to be used, a drug with reduced antimuscarinic effects should be selected, eg, nortriptyline or desipramine (see Table 30–3). To minimize autonomic effects, a selective serotonin reuptake inhibitor may be chosen.

Drugs Used in Alzheimer's Disease

Alzheimer's disease is characterized by progressive impairment of memory and cognitive functions and may lead to a completely vegetative state and early death. The biochemical defects responsible for these changes have not been identified, but in addition to evidence for abnormalities of neuronal lipoprotein processing, there is much evidence for a marked decrease in choline acetyltransferase and other markers of cholinergic neuron activity and for changes in brain glutamate, dopamine, norepinephrine, serotonin, and somatostatin activity. Eventually, cholinergic and perhaps other neurons die or are destroyed. Patients with Alzheimer's disease are often exquisitely sensitive to the central nervous system toxicities of drugs with antimuscarinic effects.

Many methods of treatment of Alzheimer's disease have been explored. Most attention has been focused on the cholinomimetic drugs because of the evidence for loss of cholinergic neurons noted above. MAO type B inhibition with selegiline (L-deprenyl) has been suggested to have some beneficial effects. "Ampakines," substances that facilitate synaptic activity at glutamate AMPA* receptors and nerve growth factors, are also under intense study. So-called cerebral vasodilators are ineffective.

Tacrine (tetrahydroaminoacridine, THA), a long-acting cholinesterase inhibitor and muscarinic modulator, has been extensively studied. Tacrine is orally active, enters the central nervous system readily, and has a duration of effect of 6–8 hours. Tacrine blocks both acetylcholinesterase and butyrylcholinesterase and has

---

* See Chapter 21.

complex inhibitory effects on M_1 and M_2 cholinoceptors. It is also a weak nicotinic blocker. The drug apparently increases the release of acetylcholine from cholinergic nerve endings as well. Finally, tacrine may inhibit MAO, decrease the release of GABA, and increase the release of norepinephrine, dopamine, and serotonin from nerve endings. Tacrine causes cholinomimetic adverse effects, including nausea and vomiting, and significant hepatic toxicity. The latter is manifested by a reversible increase in serum AST or ALT levels of sufficient magnitude to require dose reduction or withdrawal in 40–50% of patients. Hepatocellular necrosis with jaundice has been reported.

Donepezil, rivastigmine, and **galantamine** are newer cholinesterase inhibitors with adequate penetration into the CNS and a spectrum of action more limited to indirect cholinomimetic effects than tacrine's. The cholinesterase inhibitors should be used with caution in patients receiving other drugs that inhibit cytochrome P450 enzymes (eg, ketoconazole, quinidine; see Chapter 4).

According to several double-blind trials, these drugs can improve cognitive measures in some patients with Alzheimer's disease. Very tentative evidence suggests that they may even reduce morbidity from other diseases and prolong life slightly. Preparations available are listed in Chapter 7. More effective and less toxic drugs are urgently needed for the treatment of Alzheimer's disease.

CARDIOVASCULAR DRUGS

Antihypertensive Drugs

As noted previously, blood pressure, especially systolic pressure, increases with age in Western countries and in most cultures in which salt intake is high. In women, the increase is especially marked after age 50. The high frequency and sometimes benign course of this form of late-onset systolic hypertension encouraged a conservative approach to its treatment in the past. It is now clear, however, that uncontrolled hypertension leads to the same sequelae in the elderly as in younger individuals. Most clinicians believe that hypertension should be treated vigorously in the elderly.

The basic principles of therapy are not different in the geriatric age group from those described in Chapter 11, but the usual cautions regarding altered pharmacokinetics and sensitivity apply. Because of its safety, nondrug therapy (weight reduction in the obese and salt restriction) should be encouraged. Thiazides are a reasonable first step in drug therapy. The hypokalemia, hyperglycemia, and hyperuricemia caused by of these agents are more relevant in the elderly because of the higher incidence in these patients of arrhythmias, type 2 diabetes, and gout. Thus, use of low antihypertensive doses—rather than maximum diuretic doses—is important. Calcium channel blockers are effective and safe if titrated to the appropriate response. They are especially useful if the patient also has atherosclerotic angina (Chapter 12). Beta blockers are potentially hazardous in patients with obstructive airway disease and are considered less useful than calcium channel blockers in the older patient unless heart failure is present. ACE inhibitors are also considered less useful in the elderly unless heart failure or diabetes is present. The most powerful drugs, such as guanethidine and minoxidil, are rarely needed. Every patient receiving antihypertensive drugs should be checked regularly for orthostatic hypotension because of the danger of cerebral ischemia and falls.

Positive Inotropic Agents

Heart failure is a common and particularly lethal disease in the elderly. Fear of this condition may be one reason why physicians overuse cardiac glycosides in this age group. The toxic effects of this drug group are particularly dangerous in the geriatric population, since the elderly are more susceptible to arrhythmias. The clearance of digoxin is usually decreased in the older age group, and while the volume of distribution is often decreased as well, the half-life of this drug may be increased by 50% or more. Because the drug is cleared mostly by the kidneys, renal function must be considered in designing a dosage regimen. There is no evidence that there is any increase in pharmacodynamic sensitivity to the therapeutic effects of the cardiac glycosides; in fact, animal studies suggest a possible decrease in therapeutic sensitivity. On the other hand, as noted above, there is probably an increase in sensitivity to the toxic arrhythmogenic actions. Hypokalemia, hypomagnesemia, hypoxemia (from pulmonary disease), and coronary atherosclerosis all contribute to the high incidence of digitalis-induced arrhythmias in geriatric patients. The less common toxicities of digitalis such as delirium, visual changes, and endocrine abnormalities (see Chapter 13) also occur more often in the elderly than in younger patients.

Antiarrhythmic Agents

The treatment of arrhythmias in the elderly is particularly challenging because of the lack of good hemodynamic reserve, the frequency of electrolyte disturbances, and the high incidence of severe coronary disease. The clearances of quinidine and procainamide decrease and their half-lives increase with age. Disopyramide should probably be avoided in the geriatric population because its major toxicities—antimuscarinic action, leading to voiding problems in men; and negative inotropic cardiac effects, leading to heart failure—are particularly undesirable in these patients. The clearance of lidocaine appears to be little changed, but the half-life is increased in the elderly. Although this observation implies an increase in the volume of distribution, it has been recommended that the loading dose of this drug be reduced in geriatric patients because of their greater sensitivity to its toxic effects.

Recent evidence indicates that many patients with atrial fibrillation—a very common arrhythmia in the elderly—do as well with simple control of ventricular rate as with conversion to normal sinus rhythm. Of course, measures should be taken to reduce the risk of thromboembolism in chronic atrial fibrillation (aspirin or anticoagulant drugs).

ANTIMICROBIAL DRUGS

Several age-related changes contribute to the high incidence of infections in geriatric patients. There appears to be a reduction in host defenses in the elderly; this is manifested in the increase in both serious infections and cancer. This may reflect an alteration in T lymphocyte function. In the lungs, a major age- and tobacco-dependent decrease in mucociliary clearance significantly increases susceptibility to infection. In the urinary tract, the incidence of serious infection is greatly increased by urinary retention and catheterization in men.

Since 1940, the antimicrobial drugs have contributed more to the prolongation of life than any other drug group because they can compensate to some extent for this deterioration in natural defenses. The basic principles of therapy of the elderly with these agents are no different from those applicable in younger patients and have been presented in Chapter 51. The major pharmacokinetic changes relate to decreased renal function; because most of the β-lactam, aminoglycoside, and fluoroquinolone antibiotics are excreted by this route, important changes in half-life may be expected. This is particularly important in the case of the aminoglycosides, because they cause concentration- and time-dependent toxicity in the kidney and in other organs. For gentamicin, kanamycin, and netilmicin, the half-lives are more than doubled. According to one study, the increase may not be so marked for tobramycin.

ANTI-INFLAMMATORY DRUGS

Osteoarthritis is a very common disease of the elderly. Rheumatoid arthritis is less exclusively a geriatric problem, but the same drug therapy is usually applicable. The basic principles laid down in Chapter 36 and the properties of the anti-inflammatory drugs described there apply fully here.

The nonsteroidal anti-inflammatory agents must be used with special care in the geriatric patient because they cause toxicities to which the elderly are very susceptible. In the case of aspirin, the most important of these is gastrointestinal irritation and bleeding. In the case of the newer NSAIDs, the most important is renal damage, which may be irreversible. Because they are cleared primarily by the kidneys, these drugs will accumulate more rapidly in the geriatric patient and especially in the patient whose renal function is already compromised beyond the average range for his or her age. A vicious circle is easily set up in which cumulation of the NSAID causes more renal damage, which causes more cumulation. There is no evidence that the COX-2-selective NSAIDs are safer with regard to renal function. Elderly patients receiving high doses of any NSAID should be carefully monitored for changes in renal function.

Corticosteroids are extremely useful in elderly patients who cannot tolerate full doses of NSAIDs. However, they consistently cause a dose- and duration-related osteoporosis, an especially hazardous toxic effect in the elderly. It is not certain whether this drug-induced effect can be reduced by increased calcium and vitamin D intake, but it would seem prudent to consider these agents (and bisphosphonates if osteoporosis is already present) and to encourage frequent exercise in any patient taking corticosteroids.

ADVERSE DRUG REACTIONS IN THE ELDERLY

The positive relationship between number of drugs taken and the incidence of adverse reactions to them has been well documented. In long-term care facilities, which have a high population of the elderly, the average number of prescriptions per patient varies between 6 and 8. Studies have shown that the percentage of patients with adverse reactions increases from about 10% when a single drug is being taken to nearly 100% when ten drugs are taken. Thus, it may be expected that about half of patients in long-term care facilities will have recognized or unrecognized reactions at some time. The overall incidence of drug reactions in geriatric patients is estimated to be at least twice that in the younger population. Reasons for this high incidence undoubtedly include errors in prescribing on the part of the practitioner and errors in drug usage by the patient.

Practitioner errors sometimes occur because the physician does not appreciate the importance of changes in pharmacokinetics with age and age-related diseases. Some errors occur because the practitioner is unaware of incompatible drugs prescribed by other practitioners for the same patient. For example, cimetidine, a drug heavily prescribed to the elderly, causes a much higher incidence of untoward effects (eg, confusion, slurred speech) in the geriatric population than in younger patients. It also inhibits the hepatic metabolism of many drugs, including phenytoin, warfarin, β blockers, and other agents. A patient who has been taking one of the latter agents without untoward effect may develop markedly elevated blood levels and severe toxicity if cimetidine is added to the regimen without adjustment of dosage of the other drugs. Additional examples of drugs that inhibit liver microsomal enzymes and lead to adverse reactions are described in Chapter 4 and Appendix II.

Patient errors may result from noncompliance for reasons described below. In addition, they often result from use of nonprescription drugs taken without the knowledge of the physician. As noted in Chapters 64 and 65, many OTC agents and herbal medications contain "hidden ingredients" with potent pharmacologic effects. For example, many antihistamines have significant sedative effects and are inherently more hazardous in patients with impaired cognitive function. Similarly, their antimuscarinic action may precipitate urinary retention in the geriatric male or glaucoma in a patient with a narrow anterior chamber angle. If the patient is also taking a metabolism inhibitor such as cimetidine, the probability of an adverse reaction is greatly increased. A patient taking a herbal medication containing gingko is more likely to experience bleeding while taking low doses of aspirin.

PRACTICAL ASPECTS OF GERIATRIC PHARMACOLOGY

The quality of life in elderly patients can be greatly improved and life span can be prolonged by the intelligent use of drugs. However, there are several practical obstacles to compliance that the prescriber must recognize.

The expense of drugs can be a major disincentive in patients receiving marginal retirement incomes who are not covered or inadequately covered by health insurance. The prescriber must be aware of the cost of the prescription and of cheaper alternative therapies. For example, the monthly cost of arthritis therapy with newer NSAIDs may exceed $100, while that for generic aspirin is about $5 and for ibuprofen, an older NSAID, about $20.

Noncompliance may result from forgetfulness or confusion, especially if the patient has several prescriptions and different dosing intervals. A survey carried out in 1986 showed that the population over 65 years of age accounted for 32% of drugs prescribed in the USA though these patients represented only 11–12% of the population at that time. Since the prescriptions are often written by several different practitioners, there is usually no attempt to design "integrated" regimens that use drugs with similar dosing intervals for the conditions being treated. Patients may forget instructions regarding the need to complete a fixed duration of therapy when a course of anti-infective drug is being given. The disappearance of symptoms is often regarded as the best reason to halt drug taking, especially if the prescription was expensive.

Noncompliance may also be deliberate. A decision not to take a drug may be based on prior experience with it. There may be excellent reasons for such "intelligent" noncompliance, and the practitioner should try to elicit them. Such efforts may also improve compliance with alternative drugs, because enlisting the patient as a participant in therapeutic decisions tends to increase the motivation to succeed.

Some errors in drug taking are caused by physical disabilities. Arthritis, tremor, and visual problems may all contribute. Liquid medications that are to be measured out "by the spoonful" are especially inappropriate for patients with any type of tremor or motor disability. The use of a pediatric dosing syringe may be helpful in such cases. Because of decreased production of saliva, older patients often have difficulty swallowing large tablets. "Childproof" containers are often "patient-proof" if the patient has arthritis. Cataracts and macular degeneration occur in a large number of patients over 70; therefore, labels on prescription bottles should be large enough for the patient with diminished vision to read, or color-coded if the patient can see but can no longer read.

Drug therapy has considerable potential for both helpful and harmful effects in the geriatric patient. The balance may be tipped in the right direction by adherence to a few principles:

(1) Take a careful drug history. The disease to be treated may be drug-induced, or drugs being taken may lead to interactions with drugs to be prescribed.

(2) Prescribe only for a specific and rational indication. Do not prescribe omeprazole for "dyspepsia."

(3) Define the goal of drug therapy. Then start with small doses and titrate to the response desired. Wait at least three half-lives (adjusted for age) before increasing the dose. If the expected response does not occur at the normal adult dosage, check blood levels. If the expected response does not occur at the appropriate blood level, switch to a different drug.

(4) Maintain a high index of suspicion regarding drug reactions and interactions. Know what other drugs the patient is taking.

(5) Simplify the regimen as much as possible. When multiple drugs are prescribed, try to use drugs that can be taken at the same time of day. Whenever possible, reduce the number of drugs being taken.

REFERENCES

Abrams WB: Cardiovascular drugs in the elderly. Chest 1990; 98:980.

Ashburn MA, Lipman AG: Management of pain in the cancer patient. Anesth Analg 1993;76:402.

Birnbaum LS: Pharmacokinetic basis of age-related changes in sensitivity to toxicants. Annu Rev Pharmacol Toxicol 1991; 31:101.

Chatap G, Giraud K, Vincent JP: Atrial fibrillation in the elderly: facts and management. Drugs Aging 2002;19:819.

Cockcroft DW, Gault MH: Prediction of creatinine clearance from serum creatinine. Nephron 1976;16:31.

Cody RJ: Physiologic changes due to age: Implications for drug therapy of congestive heart failure. Drugs Aging 1993;3:320.

Dergal JM et al: Potential interactions between herbal medicines and conventional drug therapies used by older adults attending a memory clinic. Drugs Aging 2002;19:879.

Dhondt T et al: Depressogenic medication as an aetiological factor in major depression: An analysis in a clinical population of depressed elderly people. Int J Geriatr Psychiatry 1999; 14:875.

Docherty JR: Age-related changes in adrenergic neuroeffector transmission. Auton Neurosci 2002;96:8.

Ferrari AU: Modifications of the cardiovascular system with aging. Am J Geriatr Cardiol 2002;11:30.

Flynn BL, Theeson KA: Pharmacologic management of Alzheimer disease part III: Nonsteroidal antiinflammatory drugs—emerging protective evidence? Ann Pharmacother 1999; 33:840.

Goldberg TH, Finkelstein MS: Difficulties in estimating glomerular filtration rate in the elderly. Arch Intern Med 1987;147:1430.

Hayflick L: Theories of biological aging. Exp Gerontol 1985; 20:145.

Karlsson I: Drugs that induce delirium. Dement Geriatr Cogn Disord 1999;10:412.

Knapp MJ et al: A 30-week randomized controlled trial of high-dose tacrine in patients with Alzheimer's disease. JAMA 1994;271:985.

Lamy PP: The role of cholinesterase inhibitors in Alzheimer's disease. CNS Drugs 1994;1:145.

Lindeman RD, Tobin J, Shock NW: Longitudinal studies on the rate of decline in renal function with age. J Am Geriatr Soc 1985;33:278.

Materson BJ et al: Treatment of hypertension in the elderly: I. Blood pressure and clinical changes. Results of a Department of Veterans Affairs Cooperative Study. Hypertension 1990;15:348.

Moore AR, O'Keefe ST: Drug-induced cognitive impairment in the elderly. Drugs Aging 1999;15:15.

Muhlberg W, Platt D: Age-dependent changes of the kidneys: pharmacological implications. Gerontology 1999;45:243.

Nicolle LE: Quinolones in the aged. Drugs 1999;58(Suppl 2):49.

Ouslander JG, Schnelle JF: Incontinence in the nursing home. Ann Intern Med 1995;122:438.

Ott BR, Lapane KL: Tacrine therapy is associated with reduced mortality in nursing home residents with dementia. J Am Geriatr Soc 2002;50:35.

Pilotto A et al: Long-term outcome of elderly patients with reflux esophagitis: a six-month to three-year follow-up study. Am J Ther 2002;9:295.

Poirer J, Minnich A, Davignon J: Apolipoprotein E, synaptic plasticity and Alzheimer's disease. Ann Med 1995;27:663.

Portenoy RK et al: Pain in ambulatory patients with lung or colon cancer: Prevalence, characteristics and impact. Cancer 1992;70:1616.

Preskorn SH: Recent advances in antidepressant therapy for the elderly. Am J Med 1993;95(Suppl 5):2S.

Prinz PN et al: Geriatrics: Sleep disorders and aging. N Engl J Med 1990;323:520.

Ray WA: Psychotropic drugs and injuries among the elderly: A review. J Clin Psychopharmacol 1992;12:386.

Ray WA, Daugherty JR, Griffin MR: Lipid-lowering agents and the risk of hip fracture in a Medicaid population. Injury Prevention 2002;8:276.

Richards SS, Hendrie HC: Diagnosis, management, and treatment of Alzheimer disease: A guide for the internist. Arch Intern Med 1999;159:789.

Rodriguez EG et al: use of lipid-lowering drugs in older adults with and without dementia: A community-based epidemiological study. J Am Geriatr Soc 2002;50:1852.

Schug SA, Dunlap R, Zech D: Pharmacologic management of cancer pain. Drugs 1992;43:44.

Sival RC et al: Sodium valproate in the treatment of aggressive behavior in patients with dementia—a randomized placebo-controlled clinical trial. Int J Geriatr Psychiatry 2002;17:579.

Sproule BA et al: The use of non-prescription sleep products in the elderly. Int J Geriatr Psychiatry 1999;14:851.

Thompson TL II et al: Lack of efficacy of Hydergine in patients with Alzheimer's disease. N Engl J Med 1990;323:445.

Tonkin A, Wing L: Aging and susceptibility to drug-induced orthostatic hypotension. Clin Pharmacol Ther 1992;52:277.

Tumer N, Scarpace PJ, Lowenthal DT: Geriatric pharmacology: Basic and clinical considerations. Annu Rev Pharmacol Toxicol 1992;32:271.

Veehof LJ et al: Adverse drug reactions and polypharmacy in the elderly in general practice. Eur J Clin Pharmacol 1999; 55:533.

Wade PR: Aging and neural control of the GI tract. I. Age-related changes in the enteric nervous system. Am J Physiol Gastrointest Liver Physiol 2002;283:G489.

Wagg A, Cohen M: Medical therapy for the overactive bladder in the elderly. Age Aging 2002;31:241.

Watkins PB et al: Hepatotoxic effects of tacrine administration in patients with Alzheimer's disease. JAMA 1994;271:992.

Dermatologic Pharmacology

62

Dirk B. Robertson, MD, & Howard I. Maibach, MD

The skin offers a number of special opportunities to the therapist. For example, the topical route of administration is especially appropriate for diseases of the skin, though some dermatologic diseases respond as well or better to drugs administered systemically.

The general pharmacokinetic principles governing the use of drugs applied to the skin are the same as those involved in other routes of drug administration (Chapters 1 and 3). However, human skin, though often depicted as a simple three-layered structure, is a complex series of diffusion barriers. Quantitation of the flux of drugs and drug vehicles through these barriers is the basis of pharmacokinetic analysis of dermatologic therapy; techniques for making such measurements are rapidly increasing in number and sensitivity.

Major variables that determine pharmacologic response to drugs applied to the skin include the following:

(1) Regional variation in drug penetration: For example, the scrotum, face, axilla, and scalp are far more permeable than the forearm and may require less drug for equivalent effect.

(2) Concentration gradient: Increasing the concentration gradient increases the mass of drug transferred per unit time, just as in the case of diffusion across other barriers (Chapter 1). Thus, resistance to topical corticosteroids can sometimes be overcome by use of higher concentrations of drug.

(3) Dosing schedule: Because of its physical properties, the skin acts as a reservoir for many drugs. As a result, the "local half-life" may be long enough to permit once-daily application of drugs with short systemic half-lives. For example, once-daily application of corticosteroids appears to be just as effective as multiple applications in many conditions.

(4) Vehicles and occlusion: An appropriate vehicle maximizes the ability of the drug to penetrate the outer layers of the skin. In addition, through their physical properties (moistening or drying effects), vehicles may themselves have important therapeutic effects. Occlusion (application of a plastic wrap to hold the drug and its vehicle in close contact with the skin) is extremely effective in maximizing efficacy.

DERMATOLOGIC VEHICLES

Topical medications usually consist of active ingredients incorporated in a vehicle that facilitates cutaneous application. Important considerations in selection of a vehicle include the solubility of the active agent in the vehicle; the rate of release of the agent from the vehicle; the ability of the vehicle to hydrate the stratum corneum, thus enhancing penetration; the stability of the therapeutic agent in the vehicle; and interactions, chemical and physical, of the vehicle, stratum corneum, and active agent.

Depending upon the vehicle, dermatologic formulations may be classified as tinctures, wet dressings, lotions, gels, aerosols, powders, pastes, creams, and ointments. The ability of the vehicle to retard evaporation from the surface of the skin increases in this series, being least in tinctures and wet dressings and greatest in ointments. In general, acute inflammation with oozing, vesiculation, and crusting is best treated with drying preparations such as tinctures, wet dressings, and lotions, while chronic inflammation with xerosis, scaling, and lichenification is best treated with more lubricating preparations such as creams and ointments. Tinctures, lotions, gels, and aerosols are convenient for application to the scalp and hairy areas. Emulsified vanishing type creams may be used in intertriginous areas without causing maceration.

Emulsifying agents are used to provide homogeneous, stable preparations when mixtures of immiscible liquids such as oil-in-water creams are compounded. Some patients develop irritation from these agents. Substituting a preparation that does not contain them or using one containing a lower concentration may resolve the problem.

ANTIBACTERIAL AGENTS

TOPICAL ANTIBACTERIAL PREPARATIONS

Topical antibacterial agents may be useful in preventing infections in clean wounds, in the early treatment of infected dermatoses and wounds, in reducing colonization of the nares by staphylococci, in axillary deodorization, and in the management of acne vulgaris. The efficacy of antibiotics in these topical applications is not uniform. The general pharmacology of the antimicrobial drugs is discussed in Chapters 43–51.

Numerous topical anti-infectives contain corticosteroids in addition to antibiotics. There is no convincing evidence that topical corticosteroids inhibit the antibacterial effect of antibiotics when the two are incorporated in the same preparation. In the treatment of secondarily infected dermatoses, which are usually colonized with streptococci, staphylococci, or both, combination therapy may prove superior to corticosteroid therapy alone. Antibiotic-corticosteroid combinations may be useful in treating diaper dermatitis, otitis externa, and impetiginized eczema.

The selection of a particular antibiotic depends of course upon the diagnosis and, when appropriate, in vitro culture and sensitivity studies of clinical samples. The pathogens isolated from most infected dermatoses are group A beta-hemolytic streptococci, *Staphylococcus aureus*, or both. The pathogens present in surgical wounds will be those resident in the environment. Information about regional patterns of drug resistance is therefore important in selecting a therapeutic agent. Prepackaged topical antibacterial preparations that contain multiple antibiotics are available in fixed dosages well above the therapeutic threshold. These formulations offer the advantages of efficacy in mixed infections, broader coverage for infections due to undetermined pathogens, and delayed microbial resistance to any single component antibiotic.

1. Bacitracin & Gramicidin

Bacitracin and gramicidin are peptide antibiotics, active against gram-positive organisms such as streptococci, pneumococci, and staphylococci. In addition, most anaerobic cocci, neisseriae, tetanus bacilli, and diphtheria bacilli are sensitive. Bacitracin is compounded in an ointment base alone or in combination with neomycin, polymyxin B, or both. The use of bacitracin in the anterior nares may temporarily decrease colonization by pathogenic staphylococci. Microbial resistance may develop following prolonged use. Bacitracin-induced

contact urticaria syndrome, including anaphylaxis, occurs rarely. Allergic contact dermatitis occurs frequently. Bacitracin is poorly absorbed through the skin, so systemic toxicity is rare.

Gramicidin is available only for topical use, in combination with other antibiotics such as neomycin, polymyxin, bacitracin, and nystatin. Systemic toxicity limits this drug to topical use. The incidence of sensitization following topical application is exceedingly low in therapeutic concentrations.

2. Mupirocin

Mupirocin (pseudomonic acid A) is structurally unrelated to other currently available topical antibacterial agents. Most gram-positive aerobic bacteria, including methicillin-resistant *S aureus,* are sensitive to mupirocin. It is effective in the treatment of impetigo caused by *S aureus* and group A beta-hemolytic streptococci.

Intranasal (Bactroban Nasal ointment) use for eliminating nasal carriage of *S aureus* may be associated with irritation of mucous membranes caused by the polyethylene glycol vehicle. Mupirocin is not appreciably absorbed systemically after topical application to intact skin.

3. Polymyxin B Sulfate

Polymyxin B is a peptide antibiotic effective against gram-negative organisms, including *Pseudomonas aeruginosa, Escherichia coli,* enterobacter, and klebsiella. Most strains of proteus and serratia are resistant, as are all gram-positive organisms. Topical preparations may be compounded in either a solution or ointment base. Numerous prepackaged antibiotic combinations containing polymyxin B are available. Detectable serum concentrations are difficult to achieve from topical application, but the total daily dose applied to denuded skin or open wounds should not exceed 200 mg in order to reduce the likelihood of neurotoxicity and nephrotoxicity. Hypersensitivity to topically applied polymyxin B sulfate is uncommon.

4. Neomycin & Gentamicin

Neomycin and gentamicin are aminoglycoside antibiotics active against gram-negative organisms, including *E coli,* proteus, klebsiella, and enterobacter. Gentamicin generally shows greater activity against *P aeruginosa* than neomycin. Gentamicin is also more active against staphylococci and group A beta-hemolytic streptococci. Widespread topical use of gentamicin, especially in a hospital environment, should be avoided to slow the appearance of gentamicin-resistant organisms.

Neomycin is available in numerous topical formulations, both alone and in combination with polymyxin, bacitracin, and other antibiotics. It is also available as a sterile powder for topical use. Gentamicin is available as an ointment or cream.

Topical application of neomycin rarely results in detectable serum concentrations. However, in the case of gentamicin, serum concentrations of 1–18 μg/mL are possible if the drug is applied in a water-miscible preparation to large areas of denuded skin, as in burned patients. Both drugs are water-soluble and are excreted primarily in the urine. Renal failure may permit the accumulation of these antibiotics, with possible nephrotoxicity, neurotoxicity, and ototoxicity.

Neomycin frequently causes sensitization, particularly if applied to eczematous dermatoses or if compounded in an ointment vehicle. When sensitization occurs, cross-sensitivity to streptomycin, kanamycin, paromomycin, and gentamicin is possible.

5. Topical Antibiotics in Acne

Several systemic antibiotics that have traditionally been used in the treatment of acne vulgaris have been shown to be effective when applied topically. Currently, four antibiotics are so utilized: clindamycin phosphate, erythromycin base, metronidazole, and sulfacetamide. The effectiveness of topical therapy is less than that achieved by systemic administration of the same antibiotic. Therefore, topical therapy is generally suitable in mild to moderate cases of inflammatory acne.

Clindamycin

Clindamycin has in vitro activity against *Propionibacterium acnes;* this has been postulated as the mechanism of its beneficial effect in acne therapy. Approximately 10% of an applied dose is absorbed, and rare cases of bloody diarrhea and pseudomembranous colitis have been reported following topical application. The hydroalcoholic vehicle may cause drying and irritation of the skin, with complaints of burning and stinging. The water-based gel and lotion formulations are well tolerated and less likely to cause irritation. Allergic contact dermatitis is uncommon. Clindamycin is also available in a fixed-combination topical gel with benzoyl peroxide (BenzaClin).

Erythromycin

In topical preparations, the base of erythromycin rather than a salt is used to facilitate penetration. Although the mechanism of action of topical erythromycin in inflammatory acne vulgaris is unknown, it is presumed to be due to its inhibitory effects on *P acnes*. One of the possible complications of topical therapy is the development of antibiotic-resistant strains of organisms, including staphylococci. If this occurs in association with a clinical infection, topical erythromycin should be discontinued and appropriate systemic antibiotic therapy started. Adverse local reactions to erythromycin solution may include a burning sensation at the time of application and drying and irritation of the skin. The topical water-based gel is less drying and may be better-tolerated. Allergic hypersensitivity appears to be uncommon. Erythromycin is also available in a fixed combination preparation with benzoyl peroxide (Benzamycin) for topical treatment of acne vulgaris.

Metronidazole

Topical metronidazole is effective in the treatment of acne rosacea. The mechanism of action is unknown, but it may relate to the inhibitory effects of metronidazole on *Demodex brevis* or as an anti-inflammatory agent by direct effect on neutrophil cellular function. Oral metronidazole had been shown to be a carcinogen in susceptible rodent species, and topical use during pregnancy and by nursing mothers and children is therefore not recommended.*

Adverse local effects of the water-based gel formulation (MetroGel) include dryness, burning, and stinging. Less drying formulations may be better-tolerated (MetroCream, MetroLotion, and Noritate cream). Caution should be exercised when applying metronidazole near the eyes to avoid excessive tearing.

Sodium Sulfacetamide

Topical sulfacetamide is available alone as a 10% lotion (Klaron) and as a 10% wash (Ovace), and in several preparations in combination with sulfur for the treatment of acne vulgaris and acne rosacea. The mechanism of action is thought to be due to inhibition of *P acnes* by competitive inhibition of *p*-aminobenzoic acid utilization. Approximately 4% of topically applied sulfacetamide is absorbed percutaneously, and its use is therefore contraindicated in patients having a known hypersensitivity to sulfonamides.

ANTIFUNGAL AGENTS

The treatment of superficial fungal infections caused by dermatophytic fungi may be accomplished (1) with topical antifungal agents, eg, clotrimazole, miconazole, econazole, ketoconazole, oxiconazole, sulconazole,

---

* See Chapter 53 for a more detailed discussion.

ciclopirox olamine, naftifine, terbinafine, and tolnaftate; or (2) with orally administered agents, ie, griseofulvin, terbinafine, ketoconazole, fluconazole, and itraconazole. Superficial infections caused by candida species may be treated with topical applications of clotrimazole, miconazole, econazole, ketoconazole, oxiconazole, ciclopirox olamine, nystatin, or amphotericin B. Chronic generalized mucocutaneous candidiasis is responsive to long-term therapy with oral ketoconazole.

TOPICAL ANTIFUNGAL PREPARATIONS

1. Topical Azole Derivatives

The imidazoles, which currently include clotrimazole, econazole, ketoconazole, miconazole, oxiconazole, and sulconazole, have a wide range of activity against dermatophytes (epidermophyton, microsporum, and trichophyton) and yeasts, including *Candida albicans* and *Pityrosporum orbiculare,* the cause of tinea versicolor.

Miconazole (Monistat, Micatin) is available for topical application as a cream or lotion and as vaginal cream or suppositories for use in vulvovaginal candidiasis. Clotrimazole (Lotrimin, Mycelex) is available for topical application to the skin as a cream or lotion and as vaginal cream and tablets for use in vulvovaginal candidiasis. Econazole (Spectazole) is available as a cream for topical application. Oxiconazole (Oxistat) is available as a cream and lotion for topical use. Ketoconazole (Nizoral) is available as a cream for topical treatment of dermatophytosis and candidiasis and as a shampoo for the treatment of seborrheic dermatitis. Sulconazole (Exelderm) is available as a cream or solution. Topical antifungal-corticosteroid fixed combinations have recently been introduced on the basis of providing more rapid symptomatic improvement than an antifungal agent alone. Clotrimazole-betamethasone dipropionate cream (Lotrisone) is one such example.

Once- or twice-daily application to the affected area will generally result in clearing of superficial dermatophyte infections in 2–3 weeks, although the medication should be continued until eradication of the organism is confirmed. Paronychial and intertriginous candidiasis can be treated effectively by any of these agents when applied three or four times daily. Seborrheic dermatitis should be treated with twice-daily applications of ketoconazole until clinical clearing is obtained.

Adverse local reactions to the imidazoles may include stinging, pruritus, erythema, and local irritation. Allergic contact dermatitis appears to be uncommon.

2. Ciclopirox Olamine

Ciclopirox olamine is a synthetic broad-spectrum antimycotic agent with inhibitory activity against dermatophytes, candida species, and *P orbiculare.* This agent appears to inhibit the uptake of precursors of macromolecular synthesis; the site of action is probably the cell membrane.

Pharmacokinetic studies indicate that 1–2% of the dose is absorbed when applied as a solution on the back under an occlusive dressing. Ciclopirox olamine is available as a 1% cream and lotion (Loprox) for the topical treatment of dermatomycosis, candidiasis, and tinea versicolor. The incidence of adverse reactions has been low. Pruritus and worsening of clinical disease have been reported. The potential for delayed allergic contact hypersensitivity appears small.

Topical 8% ciclopirox olamine (Penlac nail lacquer) has been approved for the treatment of mild to moderate onychomycosis of fingernails and toenails. Although well tolerated with minimal side effects, the overall cure rates in clinical trials are less than 12%.

3. Naftifine

Naftifine hydrochloride is an allylamine that is highly active against dermatophytes but less active against yeasts. The antifungal activity derives from selective inhibition of squalene epoxidase, a key enzyme for the synthesis of ergosterol.

Naftifine (Naftin) is available as a 1% cream and gel for the topical treatment of dermatophytosis, to be applied on a twice-daily dosing schedule. Adverse reactions include local irritation, burning sensation, and erythema. Contact with mucous membranes should be avoided.

4. Terbinafine

Terbinafine (Lamisil) is an allylamine with activity similar to that of naftifine hydrochloride. It is available as a 1% cream and solution for the topical treatment of dermatophyte infections. Treatment should be for a minimum of 1 week and should not exceed 4 weeks. Clinical improvement may continue for 2–4 weeks following cessation of therapy. Reported adverse reactions include local irritation with erythema, dryness, and stinging. Contact with eyes and mucous membranes should be avoided.

5. Butenafine

Butenafine hydrochloride (Mentax) is a benzylamine that is structurally related to the allylamines. As with the allylamines, butenafine inhibits the epoxidation of squalene, thus blocking the synthesis of ergosterol, an essential component of the fungal cell membranes. Butenafine is available as a 1% cream to be applied once daily for the treatment of superficial dermatophytosis.

6. Tolnaftate

Tolnaftate is a synthetic antifungal compound that is effective topically against dermatophyte infections caused by epidermophyton, microsporum, and trichophyton. It is also active against *P orbiculare* but not against candida.

Tolnaftate (Aftate, Tinactin) is available as a cream, solution, powder, or powder aerosol for application twice daily to infected areas. Recurrences following cessation of therapy are common, and infections of the palms, soles, and nails are usually unresponsive to tolnaftate alone. The powder or powder aerosol may be used chronically following initial treatment in patients susceptible to tinea infections. Tolnaftate is generally well tolerated and rarely causes irritation or allergic contact sensitization.

7. Nystatin & Amphotericin B

Nystatin and amphotericin B are useful in the topical therapy of *C albicans* infections but ineffective against dermatophytes. Nystatin is limited to topical treatment of cutaneous and mucosal candida infections because of its narrow spectrum and negligible absorption from the gastrointestinal tract following oral administration. Amphotericin B has a broader antifungal spectrum and is used intravenously in the treatment of many systemic mycoses (Chapter 48) and to a lesser extent in the treatment of cutaneous candida infections.

The recommended dosage for topical preparations of nystatin in treating paronychial and intertriginous candidiasis is application two or three times a day. Oral candidiasis (thrush) is treated by holding 5 mL (infants, 2 mL) of nystatin oral suspension in the mouth for several minutes four times daily before swallowing. An alternative therapy for thrush is to retain a vaginal tablet in the mouth until dissolved four times daily. Recurrent or recalcitrant perianal, vaginal, vulvar, and diaper area candidiasis may respond to oral nystatin, 0.5–1 million units in adults (100,000 units in children) four times daily in addition to local therapy. Vulvovaginal candidiasis may be treated by insertion of 1 vaginal tablet twice daily for 14 days, then nightly for an additional 14–21 days.

Amphotericin B (Fungizone) is available for topical use in cream and lotion form. The recommended dosage in the treatment of paronychial and intertriginous candidiasis is application two to four times daily to the affected area.

Adverse effects associated with oral administration of nystatin include mild nausea, diarrhea, and occasional vomiting. Topical application is nonirritating, and allergic contact hypersensitivity is exceedingly uncommon. Topical amphotericin B is well tolerated and only occasionally locally irritating. Hypersensitivity is very rare. The drug may cause a temporary yellow staining of the skin, especially when the cream vehicle is used.

ORAL ANTIFUNGAL AGENTS

1. Griseofulvin

Griseofulvin is effective orally against dermatophyte infections caused by epidermophyton, microsporum, and trichophyton. It is ineffective against candida and *P orbiculare*.

Griseofulvin's antifungal activity has been attributed to inhibition of hyphal cell wall synthesis, effects on nucleic acid synthesis, and inhibition of mitosis. Griseofulvin interferes with microtubules of the mitotic spindle and with cytoplasmic microtubules. The destruction of cytoplasmic microtubules may result in impaired processing of newly synthesized cell wall constituents at the growing tips of hyphae. Griseofulvin is active only against growing cells.

Following the oral administration of 1 g of micronized griseofulvin, peak serum levels of 1.5–2 μg/mL are obtained in 4–8 hours. The drug can be detected in the stratum corneum 4–8 hours following oral administration, with the highest concentration in the outermost layers and the lowest in the base. Reducing the particle size of the medication greatly increases absorption of the drug. Formulations that contain the smallest particle size are labeled "ultramicronized." Ultramicronized griseofulvin achieves bioequivalent plasma levels with half the dose of micronized drug. In addition, solubilizing griseofulvin in polyethylene glycol enhances absorption even further. Micronized griseofulvin is available as 250 mg and 500 mg tablets, and ultramicronized drug is available as 125 mg, 165 mg, 250 mg, and 330 mg tablets and as 250 mg capsules.

The usual adult dosage of the micronized ("microsize") form of the drug is 500 mg daily in single or divided doses with meals; occasionally, 1 g/d is indicated in the treatment of recalcitrant infections. The pediatric dosage is 10 mg/kg of body weight daily in single or divided doses with meals. An oral suspension is available for use in children.

Griseofulvin is most effective in treating tinea infections of the scalp and glabrous (nonhairy) skin. In general, infections of the scalp respond to treatment in 4–6 weeks, and infections of glabrous skin will respond in 3–4 weeks. Dermatophyte infections of the nails respond only to prolonged administration of griseofulvin. Fingernails may respond to 6 months of therapy, whereas toenails are quite recalcitrant to treatment and may require 8–18 months of therapy; relapse almost invariably occurs.

Adverse effects seen with griseofulvin therapy

include headaches, nausea, vomiting, diarrhea, photosensitivity, peripheral neuritis, and occasionally mental confusion. Griseofulvin is derived from a penicillium mold, and cross-sensitivity with penicillin may occur. It is contraindicated in patients with porphyria or hepatic failure or those who have had hypersensitivity reactions to it in the past. Its safety in pregnant patients has not been established. Leukopenia and proteinuria have occasionally been reported. Therefore, in patients undergoing prolonged therapy, routine evaluation of the hepatic, renal, and hematopoietic systems is advisable. Coumarin anticoagulant activity may be altered by griseofulvin, and anticoagulant dosage may require adjustment.

2. Oral Azole Derivatives

Azole derivatives currently available for oral treatment of systemic mycosis include fluconazole (Diflucan), itraconazole (Sporonax), and ketoconazole (Nizoral). As discussed in Chapter 48, imidazole derivatives act by affecting the permeability of the cell membrane of sensitive cells through alterations of the biosynthesis of lipids, especially sterols, in the fungal cell.

Ketoconazole was the first imidazole derivative used for oral treatment of systemic mycoses. Patients with chronic mucocutaneous candidiasis respond well to a once-daily dose of 200 mg of ketoconazole, with a median clearing time of 16 weeks. Most patients require long-term maintenance therapy. Variable results have been reported in treatment of chromomycosis.

Ketoconazole has been shown to be quite effective in the therapy of cutaneous infections caused by epidermophyton, microsporum, and trichophyton species. Infections of the glabrous skin often respond within 2–3 weeks to a once-daily oral dose of 200 mg. Palmar-plantar skin is slower to respond, often taking 4–6 weeks at a dosage of 200 mg twice daily. Infections of the hair and nails may take even longer before resolving with low cure rates noted for tinea capitis. Tinea versicolor is very responsive to short courses of a once-daily dose of 200 mg.

Nausea or pruritus has been noted in approximately 3% of patients taking ketoconazole. More significant side effects include gynecomastia, elevations of hepatic enzyme levels, and hepatitis. Caution is advised when using ketoconazole in patients with a history of hepatitis. Routine evaluation of hepatic function is advisable for patients on prolonged therapy.

The newer azole derivatives for oral therapy include fluconazole and itraconazole. Fluconazole is well absorbed following oral administration, with a plasma half-life of 30 hours. In view of this long half-life, daily doses of 100 mg are sufficient to treat mucocutaneous candidiasis; alternate-day doses are sufficient for der-

matophyte infections. The plasma half-life of itraconazole is similar to fluconazole, with detectable therapeutic concentrations remaining in the stratum corneum for up to 28 days following termination of therapy. Itraconazole has been demonstrated to be effective for the treatment of onychomycosis in a dosage of 200 mg daily taken with food to ensure maximum absorption for 3 consecutive months. Recent reports of heart failure in patients receiving itraconazole for onychomycosis have resulted in recommendations that it not be given for treatment of onychomycosis in patients with ventricular dysfunction. Additionally, routine evaluation of hepatic function is recommended for patients receiving itraconazole for onychomycosis.

Administration of oral azoles with midazolam or triazolam has resulted in elevated plasma concentrations and may potentiate and prolong hypnotic and sedative effects of these agents. Administration with HMG-CoA reductase inhibitors has been shown to cause a significant risk of rhabdomyolysis. *Therefore, administration of the oral azoles with midazolam, triazolam, or HMG-CoA inhibitors is contraindicated.*

3. Terbinafine

Terbinafine (Lamisil) is an allylamine antifungal agent that has been shown to be quite effective for the treatment of onychomycosis. Recommended oral dosing consists of 250 mg daily for 6 weeks for fingernail infections and 12 weeks for toenail infections. Recent reports of serious hepatic toxicity, including liver failure and death, have led to recommendations that patients receiving terbinafine for onychomycosis be monitored closely with periodic laboratory evaluations for possible hepatic dysfunction.

TOPICAL ANTIVIRAL AGENTS

ACYCLOVIR, VALACYCLOVIR, PENCICLOVIR, & FAMCICLOVIR

Acyclovir, valacyclovir, penciclovir, and famciclovir are synthetic guanine analogs with inhibitory activity against members of the herpesvirus family, including herpes simplex types 1 and 2. As explained in Chapter 49, these guanine derivatives are phosphorylated preferentially by herpes simplex virus-coded thymidine kinase, and, following further phosphorylation, the resultant triphosphate interferes with herpesvirus DNA polymerase and viral DNA replication. Indications and usage of oral and parenteral acyclovir, valacyclovir, and famciclovir in the treatment of cutaneous infections are discussed in Chapter 49.

Topical acyclovir (Zovirax) is available as a 5% ointment for application to primary cutaneous herpes simplex infections and to limited mucocutaneous herpes simplex virus infections in immunocompromised patients. In primary infections, the use of topical acyclovir shortens the duration of viral shedding and may decrease healing time. In localized, limited mucocutaneous infections in immunocompromised patients, its use may be associated with a decrease in the duration of viral shedding.

Topical penciclovir (Denavir) is available as a 1% cream for the treatment of recurrent orolabial herpes simplex virus infection in immunocompetent adults. Application of penciclovir within 1 hour after appearance of the first sign or symptom of a recurrence and repeat application every 2 hours while awake for 4 days shortens viral shedding and reduces time to healing by approximately 1 day. Adverse local reactions to acyclovir and penciclovir may include pruritus and mild pain with transient stinging or burning.

IMMUNOMODULATORS

IMIQUIMOD

Imiquimod (Aldara) is an immunomodulator approved for the treatment of external genital and perianal warts in adults. The precise mechanism of its action is not fully understood but is thought to be related to imiquimod's ability to stimulate peripheral mononuclear cells to release interferon-α and to stimulate macrophages to produce interleukins-1, -6, -8, and tumor necrosis factor-α. Imiquimod should be applied to the wart tissue 3 times per week and left on the skin for 6–10 hours prior to washing off with mild soap and water. Treatment should be continued until eradication of the warts is accomplished, but not for more than a total of 16 weeks. Percutaneous absorption is minimal, with less than 0.9% absorbed following a single-dose application. Adverse side effects consist of local inflammatory reactions, including pruritus, erythema, and superficial erosion.

TACROLIMUS & PIMECROLIMUS

Tacrolimus (Protopic) and pimecrolimus (Elidel) are macrolide immunosuppressants that have been shown to be of significant benefit in the treatment of atopic dermatitis. Both agents inhibit T lymphocyte activation and prevent the release of inflammatory cytokines and mediators from mast cells in vitro after stimulation by antigen-IgE complexes. Tacrolimus is available as 0.03% and 0.1% ointments, and pimecrolimus is available as a 1% cream. Both are indicated for short-term and intermittent long-term therapy for mild to moderate atopic dermatitis. Tacrolimus 0.03% ointment and pimecrolimus 1% cream are approved for use in children over 2 years of age, while all strengths are approved for adult use. Recommended dosing of both agents is twice-daily application to affected skin until clearing is noted. Neither medication should be used with occlusive dressings. The most common side effect of both drugs is a burning sensation in the applied area that improves with continued use.

ECTOPARASITICIDES

LINDANE (HEXACHLOROCYCLOHEXANE)

The gamma isomer of hexachlorocyclohexane was commonly called gamma benzene hexachloride, which was a misnomer, since no benzene ring is present in this compound. Lindane is an effective pediculicide and scabicide.

Percutaneous absorption studies using a solution of lindane in acetone have shown that almost 10% of a dose applied to the forearm is absorbed, to be subsequently excreted in the urine over a 5-day period. Serum levels following the application of a commercial lindane lotion reach maximum at 6 hours and decline thereafter with a half-life of 24 hours. After absorption, lindane is concentrated in fatty tissues, including the brain.

Lindane (Kwell, etc) is available as a shampoo or lotion. For pediculosis capitis or pubis, one application of 30 mL of shampoo is worked into a lather and left on the scalp or genital area for 5 minutes and then rinsed off. No additional application is indicated unless living lice are present 1 week after treatment. Then reapplication may be required. Recent concerns about the toxicity of lindane have altered treatment guidelines for its use in scabies; the current recommendation calls for a single application to the entire body from the neck down, left on for 8–12 hours, and then washed off. Patients should be retreated only if active mites can be demonstrated, and never within 1 week of initial treatment.

Much controversy exists about the possible systemic toxicities of topically applied lindane used for medical purposes. Concerns about neurotoxicity and hematotoxicity have resulted in warnings that lindane should be used with caution in infants, children, and pregnant women. The current USA package insert recommends that it not be used as a scabicide in premature infants and in patients with known seizure disorders. The risk of adverse systemic reactions to lindane appears to be minimal when it is used properly and according to directions in adult patients. However, local irritation may occur, and contact with the eyes and mucous membranes should be avoided.

CROTAMITON

Crotamiton, *N*-ethyl-*o*-crotonotoluidide, is a scabicide with some antipruritic properties. Its mechanism of action is not known, and studies on percutaneous absorption have not been published.

Crotamiton (Eurax) is available as a cream or lotion. Suggested guidelines for scabies treatment call for two applications to the entire body from the chin down at 24-hour intervals, with a cleansing bath 48 hours after the last application. Crotamiton is an effective agent that can be used as an alternative to lindane. Allergic contact hypersensitivity and primary irritation may occur, necessitating discontinuance of therapy. Application to acutely inflamed skin or to the eyes or mucous membranes should be avoided.

SULFUR

Sulfur has a long history of use as a scabicide. Although it is nonirritating, it has an unpleasant odor, is staining, and is thus disagreeable to use. It has been replaced by more aesthetic and effective scabicides in recent years, but it remains a possible alternative drug for use in infants and pregnant women. The usual formulation is 5% precipitated sulfur in petrolatum.

PERMETHRIN

Permethrin is neurotoxic to *Pediculus humanus, Pthirus pubis,* and *Sarcoptes scabiei.* Less than 2% of an applied dose is absorbed percutaneously. Residual drug persists up to 10 days following application.

It is recommended that permethrin 1% cream rinse (Nix) be applied undiluted to affected areas of pediculosis for 10 minutes and then rinsed off with warm water. For the treatment of scabies, a single application of 5% cream (Elimite) is applied to the body from the neck down, left on for 8–14 hours, and then washed off. Adverse reactions to permethrin include transient burning, stinging, and pruritus. Cross-sensitization to pyrethrins or chrysanthemums may occur.

MALATHION

Malathion is an organophosphate cholinesterase inhibitor that is hydrolyzed by plasma carboxylesterases much faster in humans than in insects, thereby providing a therapeutic advantage in treating pediculosis (Chapter 7). Malathion is available as a 0.5% lotion (Ovide) that should be applied to the hair when dry and

the hair then combed to remove nits and lice after 4–6 hours.

AGENTS AFFECTING PIGMENTATION

HYDROQUINONE & MONOBENZONE

Hydroquinone and monobenzone (Benoquin), the monobenzyl ether of hydroquinone, are used to reduce hyperpigmentation of the skin. Topical hydroquinone usually results in temporary lightening, whereas monobenzone causes irreversible depigmentation.

The mechanism of action of these compounds appears to involve inhibition of the enzyme tyrosinase, thus interfering with the biosynthesis of melanin. In addition, monobenzone may be toxic to melanocytes, resulting in permanent depigmentation. Some percutaneous absorption of these compounds takes place, because monobenzone may cause hypopigmentation at sites distant from the area of application. Both hydroquinone and monobenzone may cause local irritation. Allergic sensitization to these compounds does occur, and a prescription combination of hydroquinone, fluocinolone acetonide, and retinoic acid (Tri-Luma) is more effective than hydroquinone alone.

TRIOXSALEN & METHOXSALEN

Trioxsalen and methoxsalen are psoralens used for the *repigmentation* of depigmented macules of vitiligo. With the recent development of high-intensity long-wave ultraviolet fluorescent lamps, photo-chemotherapy with oral methoxsalen for psoriasis and with oral trioxsalen for vitiligo has been under intensive investigation.

Psoralens must be photoactivated by long-wavelength ultraviolet light in the range of 320–400 nm (UVA) to produce a beneficial effect. Psoralens intercalate with DNA and, with subsequent UVA irradiation, cyclobutane adducts are formed with pyrimidine bases. Both monofunctional and bifunctional adducts may be formed, the latter causing interstrand cross-links. These DNA photoproducts may inhibit DNA synthesis. The major long-term risks of psoralen photochemotherapy are cataracts and skin cancer.

SUNSCREENS

Topical medications useful in protecting against sunlight contain either chemical compounds that absorb ultraviolet light, called sunscreens; or opaque materials such as titanium dioxide that reflect light, called sunshades. The three classes of chemical compounds most commonly used in sunscreens are *p*-aminobenzoic acid (PABA) and its esters, the benzophenones, and the dibenzoylmethanes.

Most sunscreen preparations are designed to absorb ultraviolet light in B ultraviolet wavelength range from 280 to 320 nm, which is the range responsible for most of the erythema and tanning associated with sun exposure. Chronic exposure to light in this range induces aging of the skin and photocarcinogenesis. Para-aminobenzoic acid and its esters are the most effective available absorbers in the B region.

The benzophenones include oxybenzone, dioxybenzone, and sulisobenzone. These compounds provide a broader spectrum of absorption from 250 to 360 nm, but their effectiveness in the UVB erythema range is less than that of *p*-aminobenzoic acid. The dibenzoylmethanes include Parasol and Eusolex. These compounds absorb wavelengths throughout the longer ultraviolet A range, 320 nm to 400 nm, with maximum absorption at 360 nm. Patients particularly sensitive to ultraviolet A wavelengths include individuals with polymorphous light eruption, cutaneous lupus erythematosus, and drug-induced photosensitivity. In these patients, dibenzoylmethane-containing sunscreen may provide superior photoprotection.

The protection factor (PF) of a given sunscreen is a measure of its effectiveness in absorbing erythrogenic ultraviolet light. It is determined by measuring the minimal erythema dose (MED) with and without the sunscreen in a group of normal people. The ratio of the minimal erythema dose with sunscreen to the minimal erythema dose without sunscreen is the protection factor. Fair-skinned individuals who sunburn easily are advised to use a product with a protection factor of 15 or greater.

ACNE PREPARATIONS

RETINOIC ACID & DERIVATIVES

Retinoic acid, also known as tretinoin or *all-trans*-retinoic acid, is the acid form of vitamin A. It is an effective topical treatment for acne vulgaris. Several analogs of vitamin A, eg, 13-*cis*-retinoic acid (isotretinoin), have been shown to be effective in various dermatologic diseases when given *orally*. Vitamin A alcohol is the physiologic form of vitamin A. The topical therapeutic agent, retinoic acid, is formed by the oxidation of the alcohol group, with all four double bonds in the side chain in the *trans* configuration as shown.

Retinoic acid

Retinoic acid is insoluble in water but soluble in many organic solvents. It is susceptible to oxidation and ester formation, particularly when exposed to light. Topically applied retinoic acid remains chiefly in the epidermis, with less than 10% absorption into the circulation. The small quantities of retinoic acid absorbed following topical application are metabolized by the liver and excreted in bile and urine.

Retinoic acid has several effects on epithelial tissues. It stabilizes lysosomes, increases ribonucleic acid polymerase activity, increases prostaglandin E_2, cAMP, and cGMP levels, and increases the incorporation of thymidine into DNA. Its action in acne has been attributed to decreased cohesion between epidermal cells and increased epidermal cell turnover. This is thought to result in the expulsion of open comedones and the transformation of closed comedones into open ones.

Topical retinoic acid is applied initially in a concentration sufficient to induce slight erythema with mild peeling. The concentration or frequency of application may be decreased if too much irritation is produced. Topical retinoic acid should be applied to dry skin only, and care should be taken to avoid contact with the corners of the nose, eyes, mouth, and mucous membranes. During the first 4–6 weeks of therapy, comedones not previously evident may appear and give the impression that the acne has been aggravated by the retinoic acid. However, with continued therapy, the lesions will clear, and in 8–12 weeks optimal clinical improvement should occur. A timed-release formulation of tretinin containing microspheres (Retin-A Micro) delivers the medication over time and may be less irritating for sensitive patients.

The effects of tretinoin on keratinization and desquamation offer benefits for patients with photodamaged skin. Prolonged use of tretinoin promotes dermal collagen synthesis, new blood vessel formation, and thickening of the epidermis, which helps diminish fine lines and wrinkles. A specially formulated moisturizing 0.05% cream (Renova) is marketed for this purpose.

The most common adverse effects of topical retinoic acid are erythema and dryness that occur in the first few weeks of use, but these can be expected to resolve with continued therapy. Animal studies suggest that this drug may increase the tumorigenic potential of ultraviolet radiation. In light of this, patients using retinoic acid should be advised to avoid or minimize sun exposure and use a protective sunscreen. Allergic contact dermatitis to topical retinoic acid is rare.

Adapalene (Differin) is a derivative of naphthoic acid that resembles retinoic acid in structure and effects. It is applied as a 0.1% gel once daily. Unlike tretinoin, adapalene is photochemically stable and shows little decrease in efficacy when used in combination with benzoyl peroxide. Adapalene is less irritating than tretinoin and is most effective in patients with mild to moderate acne vulgaris.

Tazarotene (Tazorac) is an acetylenic retinoid that is available as a 0.1% gel and cream for the treatment of mild to moderately severe facial acne. Topical tazarotene should be used by women of childbearing age only after contraceptive counseling. It is recommended that tazarotene should not be used by pregnant women.

ISOTRETINOIN

Isotretinoin (Accutane) is a synthetic retinoid currently restricted to the treatment of severe cystic acne that is recalcitrant to standard therapies. The precise mechanism of action of isotretinoin in cystic acne is not known, although it appears to act by inhibiting sebaceous gland size and function. The drug is well absorbed, extensively bound to plasma albumin, and has an elimination half-life of 10–20 hours.

Most cystic acne patients respond to 1–2 mg/kg, given orally in two divided doses daily for 4–5 months. If severe cystic acne persists following this initial treatment, after a period of 2 months, a second course of therapy may be initiated. Common adverse effects resemble hypervitaminosis A and include dryness and itching of the skin and mucous membranes. Less common side effects are headache, corneal opacities, pseudotumor cerebri, inflammatory bowel disease, anorexia, alopecia, and muscle and joint pains. These effects are all reversible on discontinuance of therapy. Skeletal hyperostosis has been observed in patients receiving isotretinoin with premature closure of epiphyses noted in children treated with this medication. Lipid abnormalities (triglycerides, HDL) are frequent; their clinical relevance is unknown at present.

Teratogenicity is a significant risk in patients taking isotretinoin; therefore, women of childbearing potential *must* use an effective form of contraception for at least 1 month before, throughout isotretinoin therapy, and for one or more menstrual cycles following discontinuance of treatment. A serum pregnancy test *must* be obtained within 2 weeks before starting therapy in these patients, and therapy should be initiated only on the second or third day of the next normal menstrual period.

BENZOYL PEROXIDE

Benzoyl peroxide is an effective topical agent in the treatment of acne vulgaris. It penetrates the stratum corneum or follicular openings unchanged and is converted metabolically to benzoic acid within the epidermis and dermis. Less than 5% of an applied dose is absorbed from the skin in an 8-hour period.

It has been postulated that the mechanism of action of benzoyl peroxide in acne is related to its antimicrobial activity against *P acnes* and to its peeling and comedolytic effects.

To decrease the likelihood of irritation, application should be limited to a low concentration (2.5%) once daily for the first week of therapy and increased in frequency and strength if the preparation is well tolerated. Fixed-combination formulations of 5% benzoyl peroxide with 3% erythromycin base (Benzamycin) or 1% clindamycin (BenzaClin) appear to be more effective than individual agents alone.

Benzoyl peroxide is a potent contact sensitizer in experimental studies, and this adverse effect may occur in up to 1% of acne patients. Care should be taken to avoid contact with the eyes and mucous membranes. Benzoyl peroxide is an oxidant and may rarely cause bleaching of the hair or colored fabrics.

AZELAIC ACID

Azelaic acid (Azelex) is a straight-chain saturated dicarboxylic acid that has been demonstrated to be effective in the treatment of acne vulgaris. Its mechanism of action has not been fully determined, but preliminary studies demonstrate antimicrobial activity against *P acnes* as well as an in vitro inhibitory effect on the conversion of testosterone to dihydrotestosterone. Initial therapy is begun with once-daily applications of the 20% cream to the affected areas for 1 week and twice daily thereafter. Most patients will experience mild irritation with redness and dryness of the skin during the first week of treatment. Clinical improvement is noted in 6–8 weeks of continuous therapy.

DRUGS FOR PSORIASIS

ACITRETIN

Acitretin (Soriatane), a metabolite of the aromatic retinoid etretinate, is quite effective in the treatment of psoriasis, especially pustular forms. It is given orally at a dosage of 25–50 mg/d. Adverse effects attributable to acitretin therapy are similar to those seen with isotretinoin and resemble hypervitaminosis A. Elevations in cholesterol and triglycerides may be noted with acitretin, and hepatotoxicity with liver enzyme elevations has been reported. Acitretin is more teratogenic than isotretinoin in the animal species studied to date, which is of special concern in view of the drug's prolonged elimination time of over 3 months after chronic administration. In cases where etretinate is formed by concomitant administration of acitretin and ethanol, etretinate may be found in plasma and subcutaneous fat for many years.

Acitretin must not be used by women who are pregnant or may become pregnant while undergoing treatment or at any time for at least 3 years after treatment is discontinued. Ethanol must be strictly avoided during treatment with acitretin and for 2 months after discontinuing therapy. Patients must not donate blood during treatment and for 3 years after acitretin is stopped.

TAZAROTENE

Tazarotene (Tazorac) is an acetylenic retinoid prodrug that is hydrolyzed to its active form by an esterase. The active metabolite, tazarotenic acid, binds to retinoic acid receptors, resulting in modified gene expression. The precise mechanism of action in psoriasis is unknown but may relate to both anti-inflammatory and antiproliferative actions. Tazarotene is absorbed percutaneously, and teratogenic systemic concentrations may be achieved if applied to more than 20% of total body surface area. Women of childbearing potential must therefore be advised of the risk prior to initiating therapy, and adequate birth control measures must be utilized while on therapy.

Treatment of psoriasis should be limited to once-daily application not to exceed 20% of total body surface area. Adverse local effects include a burning or stinging sensation (sensory irritation) and peeling, erythema, and localized edema of the skin (irritant dermatitis). Potentiation of photosensitizing medication may occur, and patients should be cautioned to minimize sunlight exposure and to use sunscreens and protective clothing.

CALCIPOTRIENE

Calcipotriene (Dovonex) is a synthetic vitamin D_3 derivative that has been shown to be effective in the treatment of plaque type psoriasis vulgaris of moderate severity. Approximately 6% of the topically applied 0.005% ointment is absorbed through psoriatic plaques, resulting in a transient elevation of serum calcium in fewer than 1% of subjects treated in clinical trials. Improvement of psoriasis was generally noted following 2 weeks of therapy, with continued improvement for up to 8 weeks of treatment. Fewer than 10% of patients demonstrate total clearing while on calcipotriene as single-agent therapy. Adverse effects include burning, itching, and mild irritation, with dryness and erythema of the treatment area. Care should be taken to avoid facial contact, which may cause ocular irritation.

ANTI-INFLAMMATORY AGENTS

TOPICAL CORTICOSTEROIDS

The remarkable efficacy of topical corticosteroids in the treatment of inflammatory dermatoses was noted soon after the introduction of hydrocortisone in 1952. Subsequently, numerous analogs have been developed that offer extensive choices of potencies, concentrations, and vehicles. The therapeutic effectiveness of topical corticosteroids is based primarily on their anti-inflammatory activity. Definitive explanations of the effects of corticosteroids on endogenous mediators of inflammation such as histamine, kinins, lysosomal enzymes, prostaglandins, and leukotrienes await further experimental clarification. The antimitotic effects of corticosteroids on human epidermis may account for an additional mechanism of action in psoriasis and other dermatologic diseases associated with increased cell turnover. The general pharmacology of these endocrine agents is discussed in Chapter 39.

Chemistry & Pharmacokinetics

The original topical glucocorticosteroid was hydrocortisone, the natural glucocorticosteroid of the adrenal cortex. The 9α-fluoro derivative of hydrocortisone was active topically, but its salt-retaining properties made it undesirable even for topical use. Prednisolone and methylprednisolone are as active topically as hydrocortisone. The 9α-fluorinated steroids dexamethasone and betamethasone subsequently developed did not have any advantage over hydrocortisone. However, triamcinolone and fluocinolone, the acetonide derivatives of the fluorinated steroids, have a distinct advantage in topical therapy. Similarly, betamethasone is not very active topically, but attaching a 5-carbon valerate chain to the 17-hydroxyl position results in a compound over 300 times as active as hydrocortisone for topical use. Fluocinonide is the 21-acetate derivative of fluocinolone acetonide; the addition of the 21-acetate enhances the topical activity about fivefold. Fluorination of the steroid is not required for high potency; hydrocortisone valerate and butyrate have activity similar to that of triamcinolone acetonide.

Corticosteroids are only minimally absorbed following application to normal skin; for example, approximately 1% of a dose of hydrocortisone solution applied to the ventral forearm is absorbed. Long-term occlusion with an impermeable film such as plastic wrap is an effective method of enhancing penetration, yielding a tenfold increase in absorption. There is a marked regional anatomic variation in corticosteroid penetration. Compared with the absorption from the forearm, hydrocortisone is absorbed 0.14 times as well through the plantar foot arch, 0.83 times as well through the palm, 3.5 times as well through the scalp, 6 times as well through the forehead, 9 times as well through vulvar skin, and 42 times as well through scrotal skin. Penetration is increased severalfold in the inflamed skin of atopic dermatitis; and in severe exfoliative diseases, such as erythrodermic psoriasis, there appears to be little barrier to penetration.

Experimental studies on the percutaneous absorption of hydrocortisone fail to reveal a significant increase in absorption when applied on a repetitive basis compared to a single dose, and a single daily application may be effective in most conditions. Ointment bases tend to give better activity to the corticosteroid than do cream or lotion vehicles. Increasing the concentration of a corticosteroid increases the penetration but not to the same degree. For example, approximately 1% of a 0.25% hydrocortisone solution is absorbed from the forearm. A tenfold increase in concentration causes only a fourfold increase in absorption. Solubility of the corticosteroid in the vehicle is a significant determinant of the percutaneous absorption of a topical steroid. Marked increases in efficacy are noted when optimized vehicles are used, as demonstrated by newer formulations of betamethasone dipropionate and diflorasone diacetate.

Table 62–1 groups topical corticosteroid formulations according to approximate relative efficacy. Table 62–2 lists major dermatologic diseases in order of their responsiveness to these drugs. In the first group of diseases, low- to medium-efficacy corticosteroid preparations often produce clinical remission. In the second group, it is often necessary to use high-efficacy preparations, occlusion therapy, or both. Once a remission has been achieved, every effort should be made to maintain the patient with a low-efficacy corticosteroid.

The limited penetration of topical corticosteroids can be overcome in certain clinical circumstances by the intralesional injection of relatively insoluble corticosteroids, eg, triamcinolone acetonide, triamcinolone diacetate, triamcinolone hexacetonide, and betamethasone acetate-phosphate. When these agents are injected into the lesion, measurable amounts remain in place and are gradually released for 3–4 weeks. This form of therapy is often effective for the lesions listed in Table 62–2 that are generally unresponsive to topical corticosteroids. The dosage of the triamcinolone salts should be limited to 1 mg per treatment site, ie, 0.1 mL of 10 mg/mL suspension, to decrease the incidence of local atrophy (see below).

Adverse Effects

All absorbable topical corticosteroids possess the potential to suppress the pituitary-adrenal axis (Chapter 39). Although most patients with pituitary-adrenal axis suppression demonstrate only a laboratory test abnormality, cases of severely impaired stress response can occur. Iatrogenic Cushing's syndrome may occur as a result of protracted use of topical corticosteroids in large quantities. Applying potent corticosteroids to extensive areas of the body for prolonged periods, with or without occlusion, increases the likelihood of systemic side effects. Fewer of these factors are required to produce adverse systemic effects in children, and growth retardation is of particular concern in the pediatric age group.

Adverse local effects of topical corticosteroids include the following: atrophy, which may present as depressed, shiny, often wrinkled "cigarette paper"-appearing skin with prominent telangiectases and a tendency to develop purpura and ecchymosis; steroid rosacea, with persistent erythema, telangiectatic vessels, pustules, and papules in central facial distribution; perioral dermatitis, steroid acne, alterations of cutaneous infections, hypopigmentation, hypertrichosis, and increased intraocular pressure; and allergic contact dermatitis. The latter may be confirmed by patch testing with high concentrations of corticosteroids, ie, 1% in petrolatum, because topical corticosteroids are not irritating. Screening for allergic contact dermatitis potential is performed with tixocortol pivalate, budesonide, and hydrocortisone valerate or butyrate. Topical corticosteroids are contraindicated in individuals who demonstrate hypersensitivity to them. Some sensitized subjects develop a generalized flare when dosed with ACTH or oral prednisone.

ALEFACEPT

Alefacept (Amevive) is an immunosuppressive dimeric fusion protein that consists of the extracellular CD2-binding portion of the human leukocyte function antigen-3 linked to the Fc portion of human IgG1. Alefacept interferes with lymphocyte activation, which plays a role in the pathophysiology of psoriasis, resulting in a reduction in subsets of CD2 T lymphocytes and circulating total CD4 and CD8 T lymphocyte counts. Alefacept is indicated for the treatment of adult patients with moderate to severe chronic plaque psoriasis. The recommended dosage is 7.5 mg given once weekly as an intravenous bolus or 15 mg once weekly as an intramuscular injection for a 12-week course of treatment. Patients should have CD4 lymphocyte counts monitored weekly while on alefacept, and dosing should be withheld if CD4 counts are below 250 cells/μL. The drug should be discontinued if the counts remain below

Table 62–1. Relative efficacy of some topical corticosteroids in various formulations.

Lowest efficacy	
0.25–2.5%	Hydrocortisone
0.25%	Methylprednisolone acetate (Medrol)
0.1%	Dexamethasone[1] (Decaderm)
1.0%	Methylprednisolone acetate (Medrol)
0.5%	Prednisolone (MetiDerm)
0.2%	Betamethasone[1] (Celestone)
Low efficacy	
0.01%	Fluocinolone acetonide[1] (Fluonid, Synalar)
0.01%	Betamethasone valerate[1] (Valisone)
0.025%	Fluorometholone[1] (Oxylone)
0.05%	Alclometasone dipropionate (Aclovate)
0.025%	Triamcinolone acetonide[1] (Aristocort, Kenalog, Triacet)
0.1%	Clocortolone pivalate[1] (Cloderm)
0.03%	Flumethasone pivalate[1] (Locorten)
Intermediate efficacy	
0.2%	Hydrocortisone valerate (Westcort)
0.1%	Mometasone furoate (Elocon)
0.1%	Hydrocortisone butyrate (Locoid)
0.1%	Hydrocortisone probutate (Pandel)
0.025%	Betamethasone benzoate[1] (Uticort)
0.025%	Flurandrenolide[1] (Cordran)
0.1%	Betamethasone valerate[1] (Valisone)
0.1%	Prednicarbate (Dermatop)

Intermediate efficacy (continued)	
0.05%	Fluticasone propionate (Cutivate)
0.05%	Desonide (Desowen)
0.025%	Halcinonide[1] (Halog)
0.05%	Desoximetasone[1] (Topicort L.P.)
0.05%	Flurandrenolide[1] (Cordran)
0.1%	Triamcinolone acetonide[1]
0.025%	Fluocinolone acetonide[1]
High efficacy	
0.05%	Fluocinonide[1] (Lidex)
0.05%	Betamethasone dipropionate[1] (Diprosone, Maxivate)
0.1%	Amcinonide[1] (Cyclocort)
0.25%	Desoximetasone[1] (Topicort)
0.5%	Triamcinolone acetonide[1]
0.2%	Fluocinolone acetonide[1] (Synalar-HP)
0.05%	Diflorasone diacetate[1] (Florone, Maxiflor)
0.1%	Halcinonide[1] (Halog)
Highest efficacy	
0.05%	Betamethasone dipropionate in optimized vehicle (Diprolene)[1]
0.05%	Diflorasone diacetate[1] in optimized vehicle (Psorcon)
0.05%	Halobetasol propionate[1] (Ultravate)
0.05%	Clobetasol propionate[1] (Temovate)

[1]Fluorinated steroids.

250 cells/μL for 1 month. Alefacept is an immunosuppressive agent and should not be administered to patients with clinically significant infection. Because of the possibility of an increased risk of malignancy, it should not be administered to patients with a history of systemic malignancy.

TAR COMPOUNDS

Tar preparations are used mainly in the treatment of psoriasis, dermatitis, and lichen simplex chronicus. The phenolic constituents endow these compounds with antipruritic properties, making them particularly valu-able in the treatment of chronic lichenified dermatitis. Acute dermatitis with vesiculation and oozing may be irritated by even weak tar preparations, which should be avoided. However, in the subacute and chronic stages of dermatitis and psoriasis, these preparations are quite useful and offer an alternative to the use of topical corticosteroids.

The most common adverse reaction to coal tar compounds is an irritant folliculitis, necessitating discontinuance of therapy to the affected areas for a period of 3–5 days. Phototoxicity and allergic contact dermatitis may also occur. Tar preparations should be avoided in patients who have previously exhibited sensitivity to them.

Table 62–2. Dermatologic disorders responsive to topical corticosteroids ranked in order of sensitivity.

Very responsive
  Atopic dermatitis
  Seborrheic dermatitis
  Lichen simplex chronicus
  Pruritus ani
  Later phase of allergic contact dermatitis
  Later phase of irritant dermatitis
  Nummular eczematous dermatitis
  Stasis dermatitis
  Psoriasis, especially of genitalia and face

Less responsive
  Discold lupus erythematosus
  Psoriasis of palms and soles
  Necrobiosis lipoidica diabeticorum
  Sarcoidosis
  Lichen striatus
  Pemphigus
  Familial benign pemphigus
  Vitiligo
  Granuloma annulare

Least responsive: intralesional injection required
  Keloids
  Hypertrophic scars
  Hypertrophic lichen planus
  Alopecia areata
  Acne cysts
  Prurigo nodularis
  Chondrodermatitis nodularis chronica helicis

KERATOLYTIC & DESTRUCTIVE AGENTS

SALICYLIC ACID

Salicylic acid was chemically synthesized in 1860 and has been extensively used in dermatologic therapy as a keratolytic agent. It is a white powder quite soluble in alcohol but only slightly soluble in water.

Salicylic acid

The mechanism by which salicylic acid produces its keratolytic and other therapeutic effects is poorly understood. The drug may solubilize cell surface proteins that keep the stratum corneum intact, thereby resulting in desquamation of keratotic debris. Salicylic acid is keratolytic in concentrations of 3–6%. In concentrations greater than 6%, it can be destructive to tissues.

Salicylism and death have occurred following topical application. In an adult, 1 g of a topically applied 6% salicylic acid preparation will raise the serum salicylate level not more than 0.5 mg/dL of plasma; the threshold for toxicity is 30–50 mg/dL. Higher serum levels are possible in children, who are therefore at a greater risk to develop salicylism. In cases of severe intoxication, hemodialysis is the treatment of choice (see Chapter 59). It is advisable to limit both the total amount of salicylic acid applied and the frequency of application. Urticarial, anaphylactic, and erythema multiforme reactions may occur in patients allergic to salicylates. Topical use may be associated with local irritation, acute inflammation, and even ulceration with the use of high concentrations of salicylic acid. Particular care must be exercised when using the drug on the extremities of diabetics or patients with peripheral vascular disease.

PROPYLENE GLYCOL

Propylene glycol is extensively used in topical preparations because it is an excellent vehicle for organic compounds. Propylene glycol has recently been used alone as a keratolytic agent in 40–70% concentrations, with plastic occlusion, or in gel with 6% salicylic acid.

Only minimal amounts of a topically applied dose are absorbed through normal stratum corneum. Percutaneously absorbed propylene glycol is oxidized by the liver to lactic acid and pyruvic acid, with subsequent utilization in general body metabolism. Approximately 12–45% of the absorbed agent is excreted unchanged in the urine.

Propylene glycol is an effective keratolytic agent for the removal of hyperkeratotic debris. Propylene glycol is also an effective humectant and increases the water content of the stratum corneum. The hygroscopic characteristics of the agent may help it to develop an osmotic gradient through the stratum corneum, thereby increasing hydration of the outermost layers by drawing water out from the inner layers of the skin.

Propylene glycol is used under polyethylene occlusion or with 6% salicylic acid for the treatment of ichthyosis, palmar and plantar keratodermas, psoriasis, pityriasis rubra pilaris, keratosis pilaris, and hypertrophic lichen planus.

In concentrations greater than 10%, propylene glycol may act as an irritant in some patients; those with eczematous dermatitis may be more sensitive. Allergic contact dermatitis occurs with propylene glycol, and a 4% aqueous propylene glycol solution is recommended for the purpose of patch testing.

UREA

Urea in a compatible cream vehicle or ointment base has a softening and moisturizing effect on the stratum corneum. It has the ability to make creams and lotions feel less greasy, and this has been utilized in dermatologic preparations to decrease the oily feel of a preparation that otherwise might feel unpleasant. It is a white crystalline powder with a slight ammonia odor when moist.

Urea is absorbed percutaneously, although the precise amount absorbed is not well documented. It is distributed predominantly in the extracellular space and excreted in urine. Urea is a natural product of metabolism, and systemic toxicities with topical application do not occur.

Urea allegedly increases the water content of the stratum corneum, presumably as a result of the hygroscopic characteristics of this naturally occurring molecule. Urea is also keratolytic. The mechanism of action appears to involve alterations in prekeratin and keratin, leading to increased solubilization. In addition, urea may break hydrogen bonds that keep the stratum corneum intact.

As a humectant, urea is used in concentrations of 2–20% in creams and lotions. As a keratolytic agent, it is used in 20% concentration in diseases such as ichthyosis vulgaris, hyperkeratosis of palms and soles, xerosis, and keratosis pilaris. Concentrations of 30–50% applied to the nail plate have been useful in softening the nail prior to avulsion.

PODOPHYLLUM RESIN & PODOFILOX

Podophyllum resin, an alcoholic extract of *Podophyllum peltatum,* commonly known as mandrake root or May apple, is used in the treatment of condyloma acuminatum and other verrucae. It is a mixture of podophyllotoxin, alpha and beta peltatin, desoxypodophyllotoxin, dehydropodophyllotoxin, and other compounds. It is soluble in alcohol, ether, chloroform, and compound tincture of benzoin.

Percutaneous absorption of podophyllum resin occurs, particularly in intertriginous areas and from applications to large moist condylomas. It is soluble in lipids and therefore is distributed widely throughout the body, including the central nervous system.

The major use of podophyllum resin is in the treatment of condyloma acuminatum. Podophyllotoxin and its derivatives are active cytotoxic agents with specific affinity for the microtubule protein of the mitotic spindle. Normal assembly of the spindle is prevented, and epidermal mitoses are arrested in metaphase. A 25%

concentration of podophyllum resin in compound tincture of benzoin is recommended for the treatment of condyloma acuminatum. Application should be restricted to wart tissue only, to limit the total amount of medication used and to prevent severe erosive changes in adjacent tissue. In treating cases of large condylomas, it is advisable to limit application to sections of the affected area to minimize systemic absorption. The patient is instructed to wash off the preparation 2–3 hours after the initial application, since the irritant reaction is variable. Depending on the individual patient's reaction, this period can be extended to 6–8 hours on subsequent applications. If three to five applications have not resulted in significant resolution, other methods of treatment should be considered.

Toxic symptoms associated with excessively large applications include nausea, vomiting, alterations in sensorium, muscle weakness, neuropathy with diminished tendon reflexes, coma, and even death. Local irritation is common, and inadvertent contact with the eye may cause severe conjunctivitis. Use during pregnancy is contraindicated in view of possible cytotoxic effects on the fetus.

Pure podophyllotoxin (podofilox) is approved for use as a 0.5% podophyllotoxin preparation (Condylox) for application by the patient in the treatment of genital condylomas. The low concentration of podofilox significantly reduces the potential for systemic toxicity. Most men with penile warts may be treated with less than 70 µL per application. At this dose, podofilox is not routinely detected in the serum. Treatment is self administered in treatment cycles of twice-daily application for 3 consecutive days followed by a 4-day drug-free period. Local adverse effects include inflammation, erosions, burning pain, and itching.

FLUOROURACIL

Fluorouracil is a fluorinated pyrimidine antimetabolite that resembles uracil, with a fluorine atom substituted for the 5-methyl group. Its systemic pharmacology is described in Chapter 55. Fluorouracil is used topically for the treatment of multiple actinic keratoses..

Approximately 6% of a topically applied dose is absorbed—an amount insufficient to produce adverse systemic effects. Most of the absorbed drug is metabolized and excreted as carbon dioxide, urea, and α-fluoro-β-alanine. A small percentage is eliminated unchanged in the urine. Fluorouracil inhibits thymidylate synthetase activity, interfering with the synthesis of deoxyribonucleic acid and to a lesser extent ribonucleic acid. These effects are most marked in atypical, rapidly proliferating cells.

The response to treatment begins with erythema and progresses through vesiculation, erosion, superficial ulceration, necrosis, and finally reepithelialization. Fluorouracil should be continued until the inflammatory reaction reaches the ulceration and necrosis stage, usually in 3–4 weeks, at which time treatment should be terminated. The healing process may continue for 1–2 months after therapy is discontinued. Local adverse reactions may include pain, pruritus, a burning sensation, tenderness, and residual postinflammatory hyperpigmentation. Excessive exposure to sunlight during treatment may increase the intensity of the reaction and should be avoided. Allergic contact dermatitis to fluorouracil has been reported, and its use is contraindicated in patients with known hypersensitivity.

Trials demonstrated similar effectiveness of 10% masoprocol cream (Actinex), but usage has been limited because of frequency of allergic contact dermatitis.

AMINOLEVULINIC ACID

Aminolevulinic acid (ALA) is an endogenous precursor of photosensitizing porphyrin metabolites. When exogenous ALA is provided to the cell through topical applications, protoporphyrin IX (PpIX) accumulates in the cell. When exposed to light of appropriate wavelength and energy, the accumulated PpIX produces a photodynamic reaction resulting in the formation of cytotoxic superoxide and hydroxyl radicals. Photosensitization of actinic keratoses using ALA (Levulan Kerastick) and illumination with a blue light photodynamic therapy illuminator (BLU-U) is the basis for ALA photodynamic therapy.

Treatment consists of applying ALA 20% topical solution to individual actinic keratoses followed by blue light photodynamic illumination 14–18 hours later. Transient stinging or burning at the treatment site occurs during the period of light exposure. Patients *must* avoid exposure to sunlight or bright indoor lights for at least 40 hours after ALA application. Redness, swelling, and crusting of the actinic keratoses will occur and gradually resolve over a 3- to 4-week time course.

ANTIPRURITIC AGENTS

DOXEPIN

Topical doxepin hydrochloride 5% cream (Zonalon) may provide significant antipruritic activity when utilized in the treatment of pruritus associated with atopic dermatitis or lichen simplex chronicus. The precise mechanism of action is unknown but may relate to the potent H_1 and H_2-receptor antagonist properties of dibenzoxepin tricyclic compounds. Percutaneous absorption is variable and may result in significant

drowsiness in some patients. In view of the anticholinergic effect of doxepin, topical use is contraindicated in patients with untreated narrow-angle glaucoma or a tendency to urinary retention.

Plasma levels of doxepin similar to those achieved during oral therapy may be obtained with topical application; the usual drug interactions associated with tricyclic antidepressants may occur. Therefore, MAO inhibitors must be discontinued at least 2 weeks prior to the initiation of doxepin cream. Topical application of the cream should be performed four times daily for up to 8 days of therapy. The safety and efficacy of chronic dosing has not been established. Adverse local effects include marked burning and stinging of the treatment site which may necessitate discontinuation of the cream in some patients. Allergic contact dermatitis appears to be frequent, and patients should be monitored for symptoms of hypersensitivity.

PRAMOXINE

Pramoxine hydrochloride is a topical anesthetic that can provide temporary relief from pruritus associated with mild eczematous dermatoses. Pramoxine is available as a 1% cream, lotion, or gel and in combination with hydrocortisone acetate. Application to the affected area two to four times daily may provide short-term relief of pruritus. Local adverse effects include transient burning and stinging. Care should be exercised to avoid contact with the eyes.

TRICHOGENIC & ANTITRICHOGENIC AGENTS

MINOXIDIL

Topical minoxidil (Rogaine) is effective in reversing the progressive miniaturization of terminal scalp hairs associated with androgenic alopecia. Vertex balding is more responsive to therapy than frontal balding. The mechanism of action of minoxidil on hair follicles is unknown. Chronic dosing studies have demonstrated that the effect of minoxidil is not permanent, and cessation of treatment will lead to hair loss in 4–6 months. Percutaneous absorption of minoxidil in normal scalp is minimal, but possible systemic effects on blood pressure (Chapter 11) should be monitored in patients with cardiac disease.

FINASTERIDE

Finasteride (Propecia) is a 5α-reductase inhibitor that blocks the conversion of testosterone to dihydrotestosterone, the androgen responsible for androgenic alopecia in genetically predisposed men. Oral finasteride, 1 mg/d, promotes hair growth and prevents further hair loss in a significant proportion of men with androgenic alopecia. Treatment for at least 3–6 months is necessary to see increased hair growth or prevent further hair loss. Continued treatment with finasteride is necessary to sustain benefit. Reported side effects include decreased libido, ejaculation disorders, and erectile dysfunction, which resolve in most men who remain on therapy and in all men who discontinue finasteride.

There are no data to support the use of finasteride in women with androgenic alopecia. Pregnant women should not be exposed to finasteride either by use or by handling crushed tablets because of the risk of hypospadias developing in a male fetus.

EFLORNITHINE

Eflornithine (Vaniqa) is an irreversible inhibitor of ornithine decarboxylase that catalyzes the rate-limiting step in the biosynthesis of polyamines. Polyamines are required for cell division and differentiation, and inhibition of ornithine decarboxylase affects the rate of hair growth. Eflornithine has been shown to be effective in reducing facial hair growth in approximately 30% of women when applied twice daily for 6 months of ther-

Table 62–3. Antiseborrhea agents.

Betamethasone valerate foam (Luxiq)
Chloroxine shampoo (Capitrol)
Coal tar shampoo (Ionil-T, Pentrax, Theraplex-T, T-Gel)
Fluocinolone acetonide shampoo (FS Shampoo)
Ketoconazole shampoo (Nizoral)
Selenium sulfide shampoo (Selsun, Exsel)
Zinc pyrithione shampoo (DHS-Zinc, Theraplex-Z)

apy. Hair growth was observed to return to pretreatment levels 8 weeks after discontinuation. Local adverse effects include stinging, burning, and folliculitis.

ANTINEOPLASTIC AGENTS

Alitretinoin (Panretin) is a topical formulation of 9-*cis*-retinoic acid which is approved for the treatment of cutaneous lesions in patients with AIDS-related Kaposi's sarcoma. Localized reactions may include intense erythema, edema, and vesiculation necessitating discontinuation of therapy. Patients who are applying alitretinoin

Table 62–4. Miscellaneous medications and the dermatologic conditions in which they are used.

Drug or Group	Conditions	Comment
Alitretinoin	AIDS-related Kaposi's sarcoma	See also Chapter 49.
Antihistamines	Pruritus (any cause), urticaria	See also Chapter 16.
Antimalarials	Lupus erythematosus, photosensitization	See also Chapter 36.
Antimetabolites	Psoriasis, pemphigus, pemphigoid	See also Chapter 55.
Becaplermin	Diabetic neuropathic ulcers	See also Chapter 41.
Bexarotene	Cutaneous T cell lymphoma	See also Chapter 55.
Corticosteroids	Pemphigus, pemphigoid, lupus erythematosus, allergic contact dermatoses, and certain other dermatoses	See also Chapter 39.
Cyclosporine	Psoriasis	See also Chapter 56.
Dapsone	Dermatitis herpetiformis, erythema elevatum diutinum, pemphigus, pemphigoid, bullous lupus erythematosus	See also Chapter 47.
Denileukin diftitox	Cutaneous T cell lymphoma	See also Chapter 56.
Etanercept	Psoriatic arthritis	See also Chapters 36 and 56.
Interferon	Melanoma, viral warts	See also Chapter 56.
Mycophenolate mofetil	Bullous disease	See also Chapter 56.
Thalidomide	Erythema nodosum leprosum	See also Chapters 47 and 56.

should not concurrently use products containing deet, a common component of insect repellant products.

Bexarotene (Targretin) is a member of a subclass of retinoids that selectively binds and activates retinoid X receptor subtypes. It is available both in an oral formulation and as a topical gel for the treatment of cutaneous T cell lymphoma. Teratogenicity is a significant risk for both systemic and topical treatment with bexarotene, and women of childbearing potential must avoid becoming pregnant throughout therapy and for at least 1 month following discontinuation of the drug.

ANTISEBORRHEA AGENTS

Table 62–3 lists topical formulations for the treatment of seborrheic dermatitis. These are of variable efficacy and may necessitate concomitant treatment with topical corticosteroids for severe cases.

MISCELLANEOUS MEDICATIONS

A number of drugs used primarily for other conditions also find use as oral therapeutic agents for dermatologic conditions. A few such preparations are listed in Table 62–4.

REFERENCES

GENERAL

Baran R, Maibach HI: *Cosmetic Dermatology,* 2nd ed. Martin Dunitz, 1998.

Bronaugh R, Maibach HI: *Percutaneous Penetration: Principles and Practices,* 3rd ed. Marcel Dekker, 1999.

Lorette G, Vaillant L: Pruritus: Current concepts in pathogenesis and treatment. Drugs 1990;39:218.

Orkin M, Maibach HI, Dahl MV (editors): *Dermatology.* Appleton & Lange, 1992.

Reeves J, Maibach HI: *Clinical Dermatology, Illustrated.* Lippincott Williams & Wilkins, 1997.

Phillips TJ, Dover JS: Recent advances in dermatology. N Engl J Med 1992;326:167.

Steigleder G, Maibach HI: *Pocket Atlas of Dermatology.* Thieme, 1994.

Wakelin S, Maibach HI: *Systemic Drugs in Dermatology.* Decker, 2003.

ANTIBACTERIAL DRUGS

Aly R, Beutner K, Maibach HI: *Cutaneous Microbiology.* Marcel Dekker, 1996.

Aly R, Maibach I: *Atlas of Cutaneous Microbiology.* Saunders, 1999.

Leyden JJ: Therapy for acne vulgaris. N Engl J Med 1997; 336:1156.

Milstone EM, McDonald AJ, Scholhamer CF: Pseudomembranous colitis after topical application of clindamycin. Arch Dermatol 1981;117:154.

Wachs GN, Maibach HI: Cooperative double blind trial of an antibiotic corticoid combination in impetiginized atopic dermatitis. Br J Dermatol 1976;95:323.

ANTIFUNGAL DRUGS

Graybill JR et al: Ketoconazole treatment of chronic mucocutaneous candidiasis. Arch Dermatol 1980;116:1137.

Knight AG: The activity of various griseofulvin preparations and the appearance of oral griseofulvin in the stratum corneum. Br J Dermatol 1974;91:49.

McClellan KJ et al: Terbinafine. An update of its use in superficial mycoses. Drugs 1999;58:179.

Sheehan DS et al: Current and emerging azole antifungal agents. Clin Microbiol Rev 1999;12:40.

Urcuyo FG, Zaias N: The successful treatment of pityriasis versicolor by systemic ketoconazole. J Am Acad Dermatol 1982;6:24.

ANTIVIRAL AGENTS

Diaz-Mitoma F et al: Oral famciclovir for the suppression of recurrent genital herpes: a randomized controlled trial. JAMA 1998;280:887.

Douglas JM et al: A double-blind study of oral acyclovir for suppression of recurrences of genital herpes simplex virus infection. N Engl J Med 1984;310:1551.

Spruance SL et al: Treatment of recurrent herpes simplex labialis with oral acyclovir. J Infect Dis 1990;161:185.

ECTOPARASITICIDES

Elgart ML: A risk-benefit assessment of agents used in the treatment of scabies. Drug Saf 1996;14:386.

Franz TJ et al: Comparative percutaneous absorption of lindane and permethrin. Arch Dermatol 1996;132:901.

Konstantinou D, Stanoeva L, Yawalkar SJ: Crotamiton cream and lotion in the treatment of infants and young children with scabies. J Int Med Res 1979;7:443.

Orkin M et al (editors): *Scabies and Pediculosis.* CRC Press, 1990.

Schacter B: Treatment of scabies and pediculosis with lindane preparation: An evaluation. J Am Acad Dermatol 1981;5:517.

Taplin D et al: Malathion for treatment of *Pediculus humanus* var *capitis* infestation. JAMA 1982;247:3103.

AGENTS AFFECTING PIGMENTATION

Engasser PG, Maibach HI: Cosmetics and dermatology: Bleaching creams. J Am Acad Dermatol 1981;5:143.

Mosher DB, Parrish JA, Fitzpatrick TB: Monobenzylether of hydroquinone: A retrospective study of treatment of 18 vitiligo patients and a review of the literature. Br J Dermatol 1977;97:669.

Pathak MA, Kramer DM, Fitzpatrick TB: Photobiology and photochemistry of furocoumarins (psoralens). In: *Sunlight and*

Man: Normal and Abnormal Photobiologic Responses. Tokyo Univ Press, 1974.

Stolk LML, Siddiqui AH: Biopharmaceutics, pharmacokinetics, and pharmacology of psoralens. Gen Pharmacol 1988;19:649.

Thompson SC et al: Reduction of solar keratoses by regular sunscreen use. N Engl J Med 1993;329:1147.

RETINOIDS & OTHER ACNE PREPARATIONS

Ehmann CW, Voorhees JJ: International studies of the efficacy of etretinate in the treatment of psoriasis. J Am Acad Dermatol 1982;6:692.

Ellis CN et al: Etretinate therapy reduces inpatient treatment of psoriasis. J Am Acad Dermatol 1987;17:787.

Lammer EJ et al: Retinoic acid embryopathy. N Engl J Med 1985;313:837.

Larsen FG et al: Pharmacokinetics and therapeutic efficacy of retinoids in skin diseases. Clin Pharmacokinetic 1992;23:42.

Leyden JJ: Topical treatment of acne vulgaris: retinoids and cutaneous irritation. J Am Acad Dermatol 1998;38:S1.

Nacht S et al: Benzoyl peroxide: Percutaneous penetration and metabolic disposition. J Am Acad Dermatol 1981;4:31.

Orfanos CE, Ehlert R, Gollnick H: The retinoids: A review of their clinical pharmacology and therapeutic use. Drugs 1987;34:459.

Shalita AR et al: Tazarotene gel is safe and effective in the treatment of acne vulgaris. a multicenter, double-blind, vehicle-controlled study. Cutis 1999;63:349.

Weinstein GD et al: Topical tretinoin for treatment of photodamaged skin. Arch Dermatol 1991;127:659.

Weiss JS et al: Topical tretinoin improves photoaged skin: A double-blind vehicle-controlled study. JAMA 1988;259:527.

ANTI-INFLAMMATORY AGENTS

Grupper C: The chemistry, pharmacology and use of tar in the treatment of psoriasis. In: *Psoriasis: Proceedings of the International Symposium,* Stanford University. Farber E, Cos AJ (editors). Stanford Univ Press, 1971.

Jackson DB et al: Bioequivalence (bioavailability) of generic topical corticosteroids. J Am Acad Dermatol 1989;20:791.

Korting HC, Maibach HI: *Topical Glucocorticoids.* Karger, 1993.

Maibach HI, Stoughton RB: Topical corticosteroids. In: Arzanoff DL (editor). *Steroid Therapy.* Saunders, 1975.

Miller JA, Munro DD: Topical corticosteroids: Clinical pharmacology and therapeutic use. Drugs 1980;19:119.

Robertson DB, Maibach HI: Topical corticosteroids: A review. Int J Dermatol 1982;21:59.

Surber C, Maibach HI: *Topical Corticosteroids.* Karger, 1994.

KERATOLYTIC & DESTRUCTIVE AGENTS

Ashton H, Frenk E, Stevenson CJ: Urea as a topical agent. Br J Dermatol 1971;84:194.

Chamberlain MJ, Reynolds AL, Yeoman WB: Toxic effects of podophyllum applications in pregnancy. Br Med J 1972;3:391.

Fine JD, Arndt KA: *Propylene Glycol: A Review.* Excerpta Medica, 1980.

Roenigk H, Maibach HI (editors): *Psoriasis,* 3rd ed. Marcel Dekker, 1998.

Taylor JR, Halprin KM: Percutaneous absorption of salicylic acid. Arch Dermatol 1975;111:740.

ANTIPRURITIC AGENTS

Drake LA, Millikan LE: The antipruritic effect of 5% doxepin cream in patients with eczematous dermatitis. Doxepin Study Group. Arch Dermatol 1995;131:1403.

Drugs Used in the Treatment of Gastrointestinal Diseases

Kenneth R. McQuaid, MD

Many of the drug groups discussed elsewhere in this book have important applications in the treatment of diseases of the gastrointestinal tract and other organs. Other groups are used almost exclusively for their effects on the gut; these are discussed below according to their therapeutic uses.

I. DRUGS USED IN ACID-PEPTIC DISEASES

Acid-peptic diseases include gastroesophageal reflux, peptic ulcer (gastric and duodenal), and stress-related mucosal injury. In all these conditions, mucosal erosions or ulceration arise when the caustic effects of aggressive factors (acid, pepsin, bile) overwhelm the defensive factors of the gastrointestinal mucosa (mucus and bicarbonate secretion, prostaglandins, blood flow, and the processes of restitution and regeneration after cellular injury). Over 99% of peptic ulcers are caused by infection with the bacterium *Helicobacter pylori* or by use of nonsteroidal anti-inflammatory drugs (NSAIDs). Drugs used in the treatment of acid-peptic disorders may be divided into two classes: agents that reduce intragastric acidity and agents that promote mucosal defense.

AGENTS THAT REDUCE INTRAGASTRIC ACIDITY

PHYSIOLOGY OF ACID SECRETION

The parietal cell contains receptors for gastrin, histamine (H_2), and acetylcholine (muscarinic, M_3) (Figure 63–1). When acetylcholine or gastrin bind to the parietal cell receptors, they cause an increase in cytosolic calcium, which in turn stimulates protein kinases that stimulate acid secretion from a H^+/K^+ ATPase (the proton pump) on the canalicular surface.

In close proximity to the parietal cells are gut endocrine cells called enterochromaffin-like (ECL) cells. ECL cells have receptors for gastrin and acetylcholine and are the major source for histamine release. Histamine binds to the H_2 receptor on the parietal cell, resulting in activation of adenylyl cyclase, which increases intracellular cyclic adenosine monophosphate (cAMP). cAMP activates protein kinases that stimulate acid secretion by the H^+/K^+ ATPase. In humans, it is believed that the major effect of gastrin upon acid secretion is mediated indirectly through the release of histamine from ECL cells rather than through direct parietal cell stimulation.

ANTACIDS

Antacids have been used for centuries in the treatment of patients with dyspepsia and acid-peptic disorders. They were the mainstay of treatment for acid-peptic disorders until the advent of H_2-receptor antagonists and proton pump inhibitors. They continue to be used commonly by patients as nonprescription remedies for the intermittent treatment of heartburn and dyspepsia.

Antacids are weak bases that react with gastric hydrochloric acid to form a salt and water. Although their principle mechanism of action is reduction of intragastric acidity, they may also promote mucosal defense mechanisms through stimulation of mucosal prostaglandin production. After a meal, approximately 45 meq/h of hydrochloric acid is secreted. A single dose of 156 meq of antacid given 1 hour after a meal effectively neutralizes gastric acid for up to 2 hours. However, the acid-neutralization capacity among different proprietary formulations of antacids is highly variable, depending on their rate of dissolution (tablet versus liquid), water solubility, rate of reaction with acid, and rate of gastric emptying.

Sodium bicarbonate (eg, baking soda, Alka Seltzer) reacts rapidly with HCl to produce carbon dioxide and NaCl. Formation of carbon dioxide results in gastric distention and belching. Unreacted alkali is readily absorbed, potentially causing metabolic alkalosis when

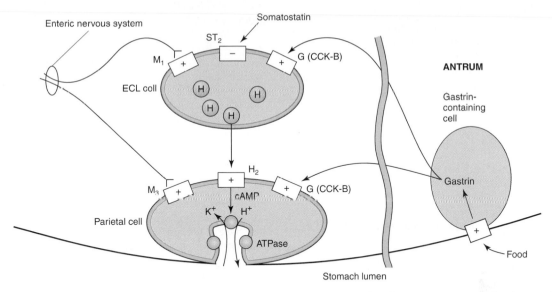

Figure 63–1. Schematic diagram of one model of the physiologic control of hydrogen ion secretion by the gastric parietal cell. ECL cell, enterochromaffin-like cell; G(CCK-B), gastrin-cholecystokinin-B receptor; H, histamine; H_2, histamine H_2 receptor; M_1, M_3, muscarinic receptors; ST_2, somatostatin$_2$ receptor; ATPase, K^+/H^+ ATPase proton pump. Some investigators place histamine receptors—and possibly cholinoceptors—on nearby tissue cells rather than on the parietal cell itself. (Modified and redrawn from Sachs G, Prinz C: Gastric enterochromaffin-like cells and the regulation of acid secretion. News Physiol Sci 1996;11:57, and other sources.)

given in high doses or to patients with renal insufficiency. Sodium chloride absorption may exacerbate fluid retention in patients with heart failure, hypertension, and renal insufficiency.

Calcium carbonate (eg, Tums, Os-Cal) is less soluble and reacts more slowly than sodium bicarbonate with HCl to form carbon dioxide and $CaCl_2$. Like sodium bicarbonate, calcium carbonate may cause belching or metabolic alkalosis. Calcium carbonate is used for a number of other indications apart from its antacid properties (see Chapter 42). Excessive doses of either sodium bicarbonate or calcium carbonate with calcium-containing dairy products can lead to hypercalcemia, renal insufficiency, and metabolic alkalosis (milk-alkali syndrome).

Formulations containing **magnesium hydroxide** or **aluminum hydroxide** react slowly with HCl to form magnesium chloride or aluminum chloride and water. Because no gas is generated, belching does not occur. Metabolic alkalosis is also uncommon because of the efficiency of the neutralization reaction. Because unabsorbed magnesium salts may cause an osmotic diarrhea and aluminum salts may cause constipation, these agents are commonly administered together in propri-

etary formulations (eg, Gelusil, Maalox, Mylanta) to minimize the impact upon bowel function. Both magnesium and aluminum are absorbed and excreted by the kidneys. Hence, patients with renal insufficiency should not take these agents long-term.

All antacids may affect the absorption of other medications by binding the drug (reducing its absorption) or by increasing intragastric pH that affects the drug's dissolution or solubility (especially weakly basic or acidic drugs). Hence, antacids should not be given within 2 hours of doses of tetracyclines, fluoroquinolones, itraconazole, and iron.

H_2-RECEPTOR ANTAGONISTS

From their introduction in the 1970s until the early 1990s, H_2-receptor antagonists (commonly referred to as H_2-blockers) were the most commonly prescribed drugs in the world (see Clinical Uses). With the recognition of the role of *H pylori* in ulcer disease (which may be treated with appropriate antibacterial therapy) and the advent of proton pump inhibitors, the use of prescription H_2-blockers has declined markedly.

Chemistry & Pharmacokinetics

Four H_2 antagonists are in clinical use: **cimetidine, ranitidine, famotidine,** and **nizatidine** (Figure 63–2). All four agents are rapidly absorbed from the intestine. Cimetidine, ranitidine, and famotidine undergo first-pass hepatic metabolism resulting in a bioavailability of approximately 50%. Nizatidine has little first-pass metabolism and a bioavailability of almost 100%. The serum half-lives of the four agents range from 1.1–4 hours; however, duration of action depends on the dose given (Table 63–1). H_2 antagonists are cleared by a combination of hepatic metabolism, glomerular filtration, and renal tubular secretion. Dose reduction is required in patients with moderate to severe renal (and possibly severe hepatic) insufficiency. In the elderly, there is a decline of up to 50% in drug clearance as well as a significant reduction in volume of distribution.

Pharmacodynamics

The H_2 antagonists exhibit competitive inhibition at the parietal cell H_2 receptor, and suppress basal and meal-stimulated acid secretion in a linear, dose-dependent manner. They are highly selective and do not affect H_1 or H_3 receptors. The volume of gastric secretion and concentration of pepsin are also reduced (Figure 63–3).

H_2 antagonists reduce acid secretion stimulated by histamine as well as by gastrin and cholinomimetic agents through two mechanisms. First, histamine released from ECL cells by gastrin or vagal stimulation is blocked from binding to the parietal cell H_2 receptor. Second, direct stimulation of the parietal cell by gastrin or acetylcholine results in diminished acid secretion in the presence of H_2 receptor blockade. It appears that reduced parietal cell cAMP levels attenuate the intracellular activation of protein kinases by gastrin or acetylcholine.

The potencies of the four H_2-receptor antagonists vary over a 50-fold range (Table 63–1). When given in usual prescription doses however, all of the H_2 antagonists inhibit 60–70% of total 24-hour acid secretion. H_2 antagonists are especially effective at inhibiting nocturnal acid secretion (which depends largely on histamine) but have a modest impact on meal-stimulated acid secretion (which is stimulated by gastrin and acetylcholine as well as histamine). Thus, they block more than 90% of nocturnal acid but only 60–80% of daytime acid secretion. Therefore, nocturnal and fasting intragastric pH is raised to 4–5 but the impact upon the daytime, meal-stimulated pH profile is less. Recommended prescription doses maintain greater than 50% acid inhibition for 10 hours; hence, these drugs are commonly given twice daily. At doses available in over-

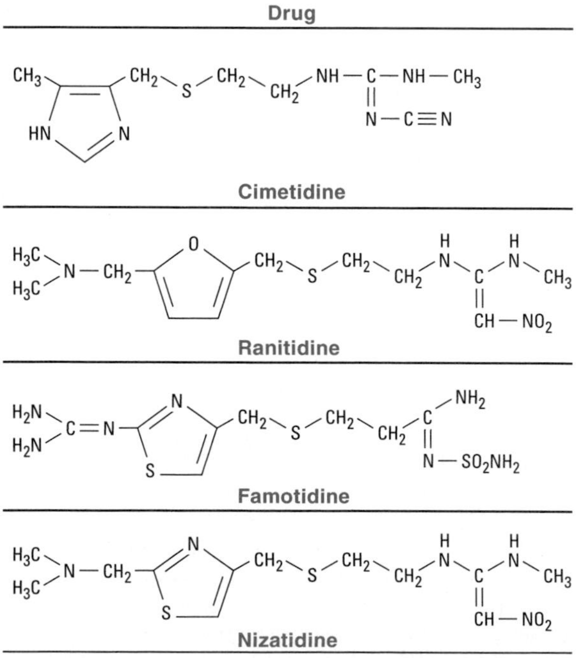

Figure 63–2. H_2 receptor-blocking drugs.

Table 63–1. Clinical comparisons of H_2 receptor blockers.

Drug	Relative Potency	Dose to Achieve > 50% Acid Inhibition for 10 Hours	Usual Dose for Acute Duodenal or Gastric Ulcer	Usual Dose for Gastroesophageal Reflux Disease	Usual Dose for Prevention of Stress-Related Bleeding
Cimetidine	1	400–800 mg	800 mg HS or 400 mg bid	800 mg bid	50 mg/h continuous infusion
Ranitidine	4–10×	150 mg	300 mg HS or 150 mg bid	150 mg bid	6.25 mg/h continuous infusion or 50 mg IV every 6–8 h
Nizatidine	4–10×	150 mg	300 mg HS or 150 mg bid	150 mg bid	Not available
Famotidine	20–50×	20 mg	40 mg HS or 20 mg bid	20 mg bid	20 mg IV every 12 h

the-counter formulations, the duration of acid inhibition is less than 6 hours.

Clinical Uses

H_2-receptor antagonists continue to be prescribed commonly. However, due to their superior acid inhibition and safety profile, proton pump inhibitors (see below) are steadily replacing H_2 antagonists for most clinical indications.

A. GASTROESOPHAGEAL REFLUX DISEASE (GERD)

Patients with infrequent heartburn or dyspepsia (fewer than 3 times per week) may take either antacids or intermittent H_2 antagonists. Because antacids provide rapid acid neutralization, they afford faster symptom relief than H_2 antagonists. However, the effect of antacids is short-lived (1–2 hours) compared with H_2 antagonists (6–10 hours). H_2 antagonists may be taken prophylactically before meals in an effort to reduce the likelihood of

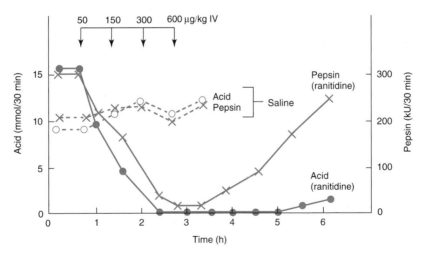

Figure 63–3. Effects of ranitidine on hypersecretion of pepsin and acid secretion in a patient. Gastric contents were collected by gastric tube for two 6-hour periods. Pepsin is quantitated as thousands of units and acid as millimoles per 30 minutes. During the first period, intravenous saline (placebo) injections were made at 40-minute intervals. During the second period, increasing intravenous ranitidine doses were given at 40-minute intervals as shown by the arrows. Ranitidine had a marked and long-lasting effect on acid secretion and a shorter but significant effect on pepsin production. (Modified and reproduced, with permission, from Danilewith M et al: Ranitidine suppression of gastric hypersecretion resistant to cimetidine. N Engl J Med 1982;306:20.)

heartburn. Frequent heartburn is better treated with twice daily H_2 antagonists; this regimen provides effective symptom control in 50–75% of people (Table 63–1). In patients with erosive esophagitis (approximately half of patients with GERD), H_2 antagonists afford healing in less than 50% of patients. Although higher doses of H_2 antagonists increase healing rates, proton pump inhibitors are preferred.

B. PEPTIC ULCER DISEASE

Proton pump inhibitors have largely replaced H_2 antagonists in the treatment of peptic ulcer disease. Nocturnal acid suppression affords effective ulcer healing in the majority of patients with uncomplicated gastric and duodenal ulcers. Hence, all the agents may be administered once daily at bedtime for acute, uncomplicated ulcers, resulting in ulcer healing rates greater than 80–90% after 6–8 weeks of therapy. For patients with acute peptic ulcers caused by *H pylori*, H_2 antagonists no longer play a significant therapeutic role. For the minority of patients in whom *H pylori* cannot be successfully eradicated, H_2 antagonists may be given daily at bedtime in half of the usual ulcer therapeutic dose in order to prevent ulcer recurrence (eg, ranitidine 150 mg, famotidine 20 mg). For patients with ulcers caused by aspirin or other NSAIDs, H_2 antagonists provide rapid ulcer healing so long as the NSAID is discontinued. If the NSAID must be continued for clinical reasons despite active ulceration, a proton pump inhibitor should be given to promote ulcer healing.

C. NONULCER DYSPEPSIA

H_2 antagonists are commonly used as over-the-counter agents and prescription agents for treatment of intermittent dyspepsia not caused by peptic ulcer. However, benefit compared with placebo has never been convincingly demonstrated.

D. PREVENTION OF BLEEDING FROM STRESS-RELATED GASTRITIS

H_2-receptor antagonists significantly reduce the incidence of bleeding from stress-related gastritis in seriously ill patients in the intensive care unit. H_2 antagonists are given intravenously, either as intermittent injections or continuous infusions. For maximal efficacy, the pH of gastric aspirates should be measured and the doses titrated to achieve a gastric pH $\geq$ 4.

Adverse Effects

H_2 antagonists are extremely safe drugs. Side effects occur in fewer than 3% of patients and include diarrhea, headache, fatigue, myalgias, and constipation.

A. CENTRAL NERVOUS SYSTEM

Mental status changes (confusion, hallucinations, agitation) may occur with administration of intravenous H_2 antagonists, especially in patients in the intensive care unit who are elderly or who have renal or hepatic dysfunction. These events may be more common with cimetidine. Mental status changes rarely occur in ambulatory patients.

B. ENDOCRINE EFFECTS

Cimetidine inhibits binding of dihydrotestosterone to androgen receptors, inhibits metabolism of estradiol, and increases serum prolactin levels. When used long-term or in high doses, it may cause gynecomastia or impotence in men and galactorrhea in women. These effects are specific to cimetidine and do not occur with the other H_2 antagonists.

C. PREGNANCY AND NURSING MOTHERS

Although there are no known harmful effects on the fetus, these agents cross the placenta. Therefore, they should not be administered to pregnant women unless absolutely necessary. The H_2 antagonists are secreted into breast milk and may therefore affect nursing infants.

D. OTHER EFFECTS

H_2 antagonists may rarely cause blood dyscrasias. Blockade of cardiac H_2 receptors may cause bradycardia but this is rarely of clinical significance. Rapid intravenous infusion may cause bradycardia and hypotension through blockade of cardiac H_2 receptors; therefore, intravenous injection should be given over 30 minutes. H_2 antagonists rarely cause reversible abnormalities in liver chemistry.

Drug Interactions

Cimetidine interferes with several important hepatic cytochrome P450 drug metabolism pathways, including those catalyzed by CYP1A2, CYP2C9, CYP2D6, and CYP3A4 (see Chapter 4). Hence, the half-lives of drugs metabolized by these pathways may be prolonged. These drugs include warfarin, theophylline, phenytoin, lidocaine, quinidine, propranolol, labetalol, metoprolol, tricyclic antidepressants, several benzodiazepines, calcium channel blockers, sulfonylureas, metronidazole, and ethanol. It is best to avoid cimetidine in patients using these drugs. Ranitidine binds 4–10 times less avidly than cimetidine to cytochrome P450. Negligible interaction occurs with nizatidine and famotidine.

H_2 antagonists compete with certain drugs (such as procainamide) for renal tubular secretion. All of these agents except famotidine inhibit gastric first-pass metabolism of ethanol (especially in women). Although the importance of this is debated, increased bioavailability of ethanol could lead to increased blood ethanol levels.

PROTON PUMP INHIBITORS (PPI)

Since their introduction in the late 1980s, these efficacious acid inhibitory agents have rapidly assumed the major role for the treatment of acid-peptic disorders. They are now among the most widely selling drugs worldwide due to their outstanding efficacy and safety.

Chemistry & Pharmacokinetics

Five proton pump inhibitors are available for clinical use: **omeprazole, lansoprazole, rabeprazole, pantoprazole,** and **esomeprazole.** All are substituted benzimidazoles that resemble H_2 antagonists in structure (Figure 63–4) but have a completely different mechanism of action. Omeprazole is a racemic mixture of R- and S-isomers. Esomeprazole is the S-isomer of omeprazole. All agents are available in oral formulations. Pantoprazole is also available in an intravenous formulation.

Proton pump inhibitors are administered as inactive prodrugs. To protect the acid-labile prodrug from rapid destruction within the gastric lumen, they are formulated as acid-resistant enteric-coated formulations. For patients with dysphagia or enteral feeding tubes, capsules may be opened and the microgranules mixed with apple juice or applesauce. After passing through the stomach into the alkaline intestinal lumen, the enteric coatings dissolve and the prodrug is absorbed. These prodrugs are lipophilic weak bases (pK_a 4–5) and therefore diffuse readily across lipid membranes into acidified compartments (such as the parietal cell canaliculus). Within the acidified compartment the prodrug rapidly becomes protonated and is concentrated > 1000-fold within the parietal cell canaliculus. There, it rapidly undergoes a molecular conversion to the active, reactive thiophilic sulfonamide cation. The sulfonamide reacts with the H^+/K^+ ATPase, forms a covalent disulfide linkage, and irreversibly inactivates the enzyme.

The pharmacokinetics of available proton pump inhibitors are shown in Table 63–2. Their bioavailability is decreased approximately 50% by food; hence, the drugs should be administered on an empty stomach. In a fasting state, only 10% of proton pumps are actively secreting acid and susceptible to inhibition. Proton pump inhibitors should be administered approximately 1 hour before a meal (usually breakfast or dinner), so that the peak serum concentration coincides with the maximal activity of proton pump secretion. The drugs have a short serum half-life of about 1.5 hours; however, the duration of acid inhibition lasts up to 24 hours due to the irreversible inactivation of the proton pump. At least 18 hours are required for synthesis of new H^+/K^+ ATPase pump molecules. Because not all proton pumps are inactivated with the first dose of medication, up to 3–4 days of daily medication are required before the full acid-inhibiting potential is reached. Similarly, after stopping the drug, it takes 3–4 days for full acid secretion to return.

Proton pump inhibitors undergo rapid first-pass and systemic hepatic metabolism and have negligible

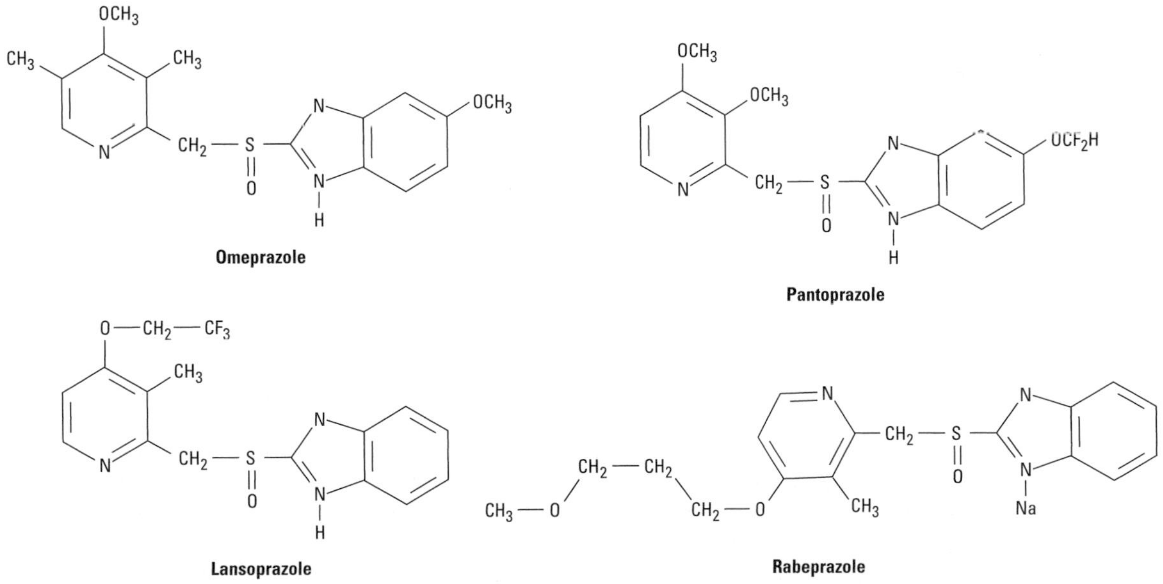

Figure 63–4. Molecular structure of the proton pump inhibitors: omeprazole, lansoprazole, pantoprazole, and the sodium salt of rabeprazole. Omeprazole and esomeprazole have the same chemical structure (see text).

Table 63–2. Pharmacokinetics of proton pump inhibitors.

Drug	Bioavailability	Half-Life (h)	T$_{max}$ (h)[1]	AUC (mg × h/L)[1]
Omeprazole	40–65%	0.5–1	1–3.5	0.2–1.2
Esomeprazole	50–89%	1.2	1..5	4.2 (20 mg dose) 12.6 (40 mg dose)
Lansoprazole	80–90%	1.5	1–1.7	1.7–5
Pantoprazole	77%	1.9	2.0–4.0	2–5
Rabeprazole	52%	0.7–2.0	2.0–5.0	0.8

[1]T$_{max}$, time of maximum concentration; AUC, area under the curve.

renal clearance. Dose reduction is not needed for patients with renal insufficiency or mild to moderate liver disease but should be considered in patients with severe liver impairment (Table 63–3). Although other proton pumps exist in the body, the H$^+$/K$^+$ ATPase appears to exist only in the parietal cell and is distinct structurally and functionally from other H$^+$ transporting enzymes.

The intravenous formulation of pantoprazole has similar characteristics to the oral drugs. When given to a fasting patient, intravenous pantoprazole inactivates acid pumps that are actively secreting but has no effect on pumps in quiescent, nonsecreting vesicles. Because the half-life of a single injection of the intravenous formulation is short, acid secretion returns several hours later as pumps move from the tubulo-vesicles to the canalicular surface. Thus, in order to provide maximal inhibition, intravenous pantoprazole must be given over 24–48 hours as a continuous infusion or as repeated bolus injections. The optimal dosing of intravenous pantoprazole to achieve maximal blockade is not yet established.

Table 63–3. Clinical comparisons of proton pump inhibitors.

Agent	Usual Dosage for Peptic Ulcer or GERD[1]	Maintenance Therapy
Esomeprazole	20–40 mg qd	20 mg qd
Lansoprazole	30 mg qd	15 mg qd
Omeprazole	20 mg qd	20 mg qd
Pantoprazole	40 mg qd	40 mg qd
Rabeprazole	20 mg qd	20 mg qd

[1]GERD, gastroesophageal reflux disease.

Pharmacodynamics

From a pharmacokinetic perspective, proton pump inhibitors are ideal drugs: they have a short serum half-life, they are concentrated and activated near their site of action, and they have a long duration of action. In contrast to H$_2$ antagonists, proton pump inhibitors inhibit both fasting and meal-stimulated secretion because they block the final common pathway of acid secretion, the proton pump. In standard doses, proton pump inhibitors inhibit 90–98% of 24-hour acid secretion. In patients receiving long-term therapy with proton pump inhibitors, the median 24-hour intragastric pH varies from 3.6 to 4.9 (esomeprazole 40 mg); the mean number of hours the pH is higher than 4 varies from 10.5 hours to 16.8.

Clinical Uses

A. GASTROESOPHAGEAL REFLUX DISEASE (GERD)

Proton pump inhibitors are the most effective agents for the treatment of nonerosive and erosive reflux disease, esophageal complications of reflux disease (peptic stricture or Barrett's esophagus), and extraesophageal manifestations of reflux disease. Once-daily dosing provides effective symptom relief and tissue healing in 85–90% of patients; up to 15% of patients require twice daily dosing.

Symptoms of erosive esophagitis recur in over 80% of patients within 6 months after discontinuation of a proton pump inhibitor. For this reason, long-term daily maintenance therapy with a full-dose or half-dose proton pump inhibitor often is needed, particularly for patients with erosive esophagitis or esophageal complications.

In current clinical practice, many patients with symptomatic gastroesophageal reflux are treated empirically with medications without prior endoscopy, ie, without knowledge of whether the patient has erosive or nonerosive reflux disease. Empiric treatment with proton pump inhibitors provides sustained symptomatic relief in 70–80% of patients, compared with 50–60% with H_2 antagonists. Due to recent cost reductions, proton pump inhibitors are increasingly being used as first-line therapy for patients with symptomatic GERD.

Sustained acid suppression with twice-daily proton pump inhibitors for at least 3 months is used to treat extraesophageal complications of reflux disease (asthma, chronic cough, laryngitis, and noncardiac chest pain).

B. Peptic Ulcer Disease

Compared with H_2 antagonists, proton pump inhibitors afford more rapid symptom relief and faster ulcer healing for duodenal ulcers and, to a lesser extent, gastric ulcers. All of the pump inhibitors heal more than 90% of duodenal ulcers within 4 weeks and a similar percentage of gastric ulcers within 6–8 weeks.

1. H pylori–associated ulcers—For *H pylori*–associated ulcers, there are two therapeutic goals: heal the ulcer and eradicate the organism. The most effective regimens for *H pylori* eradication are combinations of two antibiotics and a proton pump inhibitor. Proton pump inhibitors promote eradication of *H pylori* through several mechanisms: direct antimicrobial properties (minor) and—by raising intragastric pH—lowering the minimal inhibitory concentrations of antibiotics against *H pylori*. The best treatment regimen consists of a 10–14 day regimen of "triple therapy": a proton pump inhibitor twice daily, clarithromycin 500 mg twice daily, and amoxicillin 1 g twice daily. For patients who are allergic to penicillin, metronidazole 500 mg twice daily should be substituted for amoxicillin. After completion of triple therapy, the proton pump inhibitor should be continued once daily for a total of 4–6 weeks to ensure complete ulcer healing.

2. NSAID-associated ulcers—For patients with ulcers caused by aspirin or other NSAIDs, either H_2 antagonists or proton pump inhibitors provide rapid ulcer healing so long as the NSAID is discontinued; continued use of the NSAID impairs ulcer healing. Treatment with a once daily proton pump inhibitor promotes ulcer healing despite continued NSAID therapy.

Proton pump inhibitors are also given to prevent ulcer complications from NSAIDs. Asymptomatic peptic ulceration develops in 10–20% of people taking frequent NSAIDs, and ulcer-related complications (bleeding, perforation) develop in 1–2% of persons per year. Proton pump inhibitors taken once daily are effective in reducing the incidence of ulcers and ulcer complications in patients taking aspirin or other NSAIDs.

3. Prevention of rebleeding from peptic ulcers—In patients with acute gastrointestinal bleeding due to peptic ulcers, the risk of rebleeding from ulcers that have a visible vessel or adherent clot is increased. Ulcer rebleeding is reduced significantly with use of proton pump inhibitors administered for 3–5 days either as high-dose oral therapy (eg, omeprazole 40 mg orally twice daily) or as a continuous intravenous infusion. The optimal dosing for intravenous pantoprazole is under investigation.

C. Nonulcer Dyspepsia

Proton pump inhibitors have modest efficacy for treatment of nonulcer dyspepsia, benefiting 10–20% more patients than placebo. Despite their increasing use for this indication, superiority to H_2 antagonists (or even placebo) has not been conclusively demonstrated.

D. Prevention of Stress Gastritis

Intravenous proton pump inhibitors increasingly are being used in critically ill patients to reduce the incidence of stress-related mucosal bleeding despite a lack of any controlled trials demonstrating their efficacy. In the absence of trials that establish efficacy and optimal dosing for proton pump inhibitors, intravenous H_2 antagonists remain the preferred drugs for this indication.

E. Gastrinoma and Other Hypersecretory Conditions

Patients with isolated gastrinomas are best treated with surgical resection. In patients with metastatic or unresectable gastrinomas, massive acid hypersecretion results in peptic ulceration, erosive esophagitis, and malabsorption. Previously, these patients required vagotomy and extraordinarily high doses of H_2 antagonists, which resulted in suboptimal acid suppression. With proton pump inhibitors, excellent acid suppression can be achieved in all patients. Dosage is titrated to reduce basal acid output to less than 5–10 meq/h. Typical doses of omeprazole are 60–120 mg/d.

Adverse Effects

A. General

Proton pump inhibitors are extremely safe. Diarrhea, headache, and abdominal pain are reported in 1–5% of patients, although the frequency of these events is only slightly increased compared with placebo. Proton pump inhibitors do not have teratogenicity in animal models; however, safety during pregnancy has not been established.

B. Nutrition

Acid is important in releasing vitamin B_{12} from food. A minor reduction in oral cyanocobalamin absorption occurs during proton pump inhibition, potentially leading to subnormal B_{12} levels with prolonged therapy. Acid also promotes absorption of food-bound minerals (iron, calcium, zinc); however, no mineral deficiencies have been reported with proton pump inhibitor therapy.

C. ENTERIC INFECTIONS

Gastric acid is an important barrier to colonization and infection of the stomach and intestine from ingested bacteria. Hypochlorhydria from any cause increases the risk for enteric infections (eg, salmonella, shigella). A small increased risk of enteric infections may exist in patients taking proton pump inhibitors, especially when traveling in underdeveloped countries.

D. POTENTIAL PROBLEMS DUE TO INCREASED SERUM GASTRIN

Gastrin levels are regulated by a feedback loop. During meals, intraluminal food proteins stimulate gastrin release from antral G-cells. The rise in serum gastrin stimulates parietal cell acid secretion. Increased intragastric acidity stimulates antral D-cells to release somatostatin, which binds to receptors on adjacent antral G-cells, turning off further gastrin release. Acid suppression alters this feedback inhibition so that gastrin levels rise two- to four-fold in patients taking proton pump inhibitors. In approximately 3%, gastrin levels exceed 500 pg/mL (normal < 100 pg/mL). Upon stopping the drug, the levels normalize.

The rise in serum gastrin levels in patients receiving long-term therapy with proton pump inhibitors has raised two theoretical concerns. First, gastrin is a trophic hormone that stimulates hyperplasia of ECL cells. Hypergastrinemia due to gastrinoma (Zollinger-Ellison syndrome) or atrophic gastritis is associated with the development of gastric carcinoids in up to 3% of patients. In female rats given proton pump inhibitors for prolonged periods, gastric carcinoid tumors developed in areas of ECL hyperplasia. Although humans who take proton pump inhibitors for a long time may exhibit ECL hyperplasia in response to hypergastrinemia, carcinoid tumor formation has not been documented. Second, hypergastrinemia increases the proliferative rate of colonic mucosa, potentially promoting carcinogenesis. In humans, hypergastrinemia caused by vagotomy, atrophic gastritis, or Zollinger-Ellison syndrome has not been associated with increased colon cancer risk. At present, routine monitoring of serum gastrin levels is not recommended in patients receiving prolonged proton pump inhibitor therapy.

E. POTENTIAL PROBLEMS DUE TO DECREASED GASTRIC ACIDITY

As noted above, gastric acid serves as an important barrier to bacterial colonization of the stomach and small intestine. Increases in gastric bacterial concentrations are detected in patients taking proton pump inhibitors.

An increase in nitrate-reductase positive strains could theoretically increase carcinogenic nitrites and N-nitrosamines. However, most studies do not demonstrate this.

Among patients infected with *H pylori*, long-term acid suppression leads to increased chronic inflammation in the gastric body and decreased inflammation in the antrum. Concerns have been raised that increased gastric inflammation may accelerate gastric gland atrophy (atrophic gastritis) and intestinal metaplasia—known risk factors for gastric adenocarcinoma. A special US Food and Drug Administration Gastrointestinal Advisory Committee concluded that there is no evidence that prolonged proton pump inhibitor therapy produces the kind of atrophic gastritis (multifocal atrophic gastritis) or intestinal metaplasia that is associated with increased risk of adenocarcinoma. Routine testing for *H pylori* is no longer recommended in patients who require long-term proton pump inhibitor therapy.

Drug Interactions

Decreased gastric acidity may alter absorption of drugs for which intragastric acidity affects drug bioavailability, eg, ketoconazole and digoxin. All proton pump inhibitors are metabolized by hepatic P450 cytochromes, including CYP2C19 and CYP3A4. Omeprazole may inhibit the metabolism of coumadin, diazepam, and phenytoin. Esomeprazole also may decrease metabolism of diazepam. Lansoprazole may enhance clearance of theophylline. However, clinically significant interactions with these drugs are rare. Rabeprazole and pantoprazole have no significant drug interactions.

MUCOSAL PROTECTIVE AGENTS

The gastroduodenal mucosa has evolved a number of defense mechanisms to protect itself against the noxious effects of acid and pepsin. Both mucus and epithelial cell-cell tight junctions restrict back diffusion of acid and pepsin. Epithelial bicarbonate secretion establishes a pH gradient within the mucous layer in which the pH ranges from 7 at the mucosal surface to 1–2 in the gastric lumen. Blood flow carries bicarbonate and vital nutrients to surface cells. Areas of injured epithelium are quickly repaired by restitution, a process in which migration of cells from gland neck cells seals small erosions to reestablish intact epithelium. Mucosal prostaglandins appear to be important in stimulating mucus and bicarbonate secretion and mucosal blood flow. A number of agents that potentiate these mucosal defensive mechanisms are available for the prevention and treatment of acid-peptic disorders.

SUCRALFATE

Chemistry & Pharmacokinetics

Sucralfate is a salt of sucrose complexed to sulfated aluminum hydroxide. In water or acidic solutions it forms a viscous, tenacious paste that binds selectively to ulcers or erosions for up to 6 hours. Sucralfate has limited solubility, breaking down into sucrose sulfate (strongly negatively charged) and an aluminum salt. Less than 3% of intact drug and 0.01% of aluminum is absorbed from the intestinal tract; the remainder is excreted in the feces.

Pharmacodynamics

A variety of beneficial effects have been attributed to sucralfate, but the precise mechanism of action is unclear. It is believed that the negatively charged sucrose sulfate binds to positively charged proteins in the base of ulcers or erosion, forming a physical barrier that restricts further caustic damage and stimulates mucosal prostaglandin and bicarbonate secretion. It may also bind epithelial growth factor and fibroblast growth factor, enhancing mucosal repair.

Clinical Uses

Sucralfate is administered in a dosage of 1 g four times daily on an empty stomach (at least 1 hour before meals). At present, its clinical uses are limited. It has been shown to be effective for the healing of duodenal ulcers, but with the advent of more effective agents (proton pump inhibitors), it is seldom used for this indication. In critically ill patients hospitalized in the intensive care unit, sucralfate is effective for the prevention of bleeding from stress-related gastritis. It is still unclear which is the preferred agent for this indication: sucralfate (administered as a slurry through a nasogastric tube), intravenous H_2 antagonists, or intravenous proton pump inhibitors. Some clinicians administer sucralfate to patients taking NSAIDs who are experiencing dyspepsia. It is not an effective agent in preventing or healing NSAID-induced ulcers.

Adverse Effects

Because it is not absorbed, sucralfate is virtually devoid of systemic side effects. Constipation occurs in 2% due to the aluminum salt. Because a small amount of aluminum is absorbed, it should not be used for prolonged periods in patients with renal insufficiency.

Drug Interactions

Sucralfate may bind to other medications, impairing their absorption.

PROSTAGLANDIN ANALOGS

Chemistry & Pharmacokinetics

The human gastrointestinal mucosa synthesizes a number of prostaglandins (see Chapter 18), however the primary ones are prostaglandins E and F. **Misoprostol**, a methyl analog of PGE_1, has been approved for gastrointestinal conditions. Following oral administration, it is rapidly absorbed and metabolized to a metabolically active free acid. The serum half-life is less than 30 minutes; hence, it must be administered 3–4 times daily. It is excreted in the urine, however dose reduction is not needed in patients with renal insufficiency.

Pharmacodynamics

Misoprostol has both acid inhibitory and mucosal protective properties. It is believed to stimulate mucus and bicarbonate secretion and enhance mucosal blood flow. In addition, it binds to a prostaglandin receptor on parietal cells, reducing histamine-stimulated cAMP production and causing modest acid inhibition. Prostaglandins have a variety of other actions, including stimulation of intestinal electrolyte and fluid secretion, intestinal motility and uterine contractions.

Clinical Uses

Peptic ulcers develop in approximately 10–20% of patients who receive long-term NSAID therapy (see Proton Pump Inhibitors, above). Misoprostol reduces the incidence of NSAID-induced ulcers to less than 3% and the incidence of ulcer complications by 50%. It is approved for prevention of NSAID-induced ulcers in high-risk patients; however, it has never achieved widespread use due to its high side effect profile and need for multiple daily dosing. As discussed, proton pump inhibitors may be as effective and better tolerated than misoprostol for this indication. Cyclooxygenase-2-selective NSAIDs, which may have less gastrointestinal toxicity (see Chapter 36), offer another option for patients at high-risk for NSAID-induced complications.

Adverse Effects & Drug Interactions

Diarrhea and cramping abdominal pain occurs in 10–20% of patients. Because misoprostol stimulates uterine contractions (see Chapter 18), it should not be used during pregnancy or in women of childbearing potential unless they have a negative serum pregnancy test and are compliant with effective contraceptive measures. No significant drug interactions are reported.

COLLOIDAL BISMUTH COMPOUNDS

Chemistry & Pharmacokinetics

The only bismuth compound available in the USA is **bismuth subsalicylate,** a nonprescription formulation containing bismuth and salicylate. In other countries, **bismuth subcitrate** and **bismuth dinitrate** are also available. Bismuth subsalicylate undergoes rapid dissociation within the stomach, allowing absorption of salicylate. Over 99% of the bismuth appears in the stool. Although minimal (< 1%) bismuth is absorbed, it is stored in many tissues and has slow renal excretion. Salicylate (like aspirin) is readily absorbed and excreted in the urine.

Pharmacodynamics

Like sucralfate, bismuth probably coats ulcers and erosions, creating a protective layer against acid and pepsin. It may also stimulate prostaglandin, mucus, and bicarbonate secretion. Bismuth subsalicylate reduces stool frequency and liquidity in acute infectious diarrhea, due to salicylate inhibition of intestinal prostaglandin and chloride secretion. Bismuth has direct antimicrobial effects and binds enterotoxins, accounting for its benefit in preventing and treating traveler's diarrhea. Bismuth compounds have direct antimicrobial activity against *H pylori*.

Clinical Uses

In spite of the lack of comparative trials, nonprescription bismuth compounds are widely used by patients for the nonspecific treatment of dyspepsia and acute diarrhea. Bismuth subsalicylate also is used for the prevention of traveler's diarrhea (30 mL or 2 tablets four times daily)

Bismuth compounds have been used in multidrug regimens for the eradication of *H pylori* infection. In the USA, a "triple therapy" regimen has been used, consisting of bismuth subsalicylate (2 tablets; 262 mg each), tetracycline (500 mg), and metronidazole (250 mg), each taken four times daily for 14 days. Because of the need for four-times daily dosing and the high side effect profile, this regimen is no longer used as first-line therapy for *H pylori* eradication (see Proton Pump Inhibitors above). For patients with resistant infections, "quadruple therapy" consisting of a proton pump inhibitor twice daily in addition to the three-drug bismuth-based regimen four times daily for 14 days is highly effective. In Europe, bismuth subcitrate is used instead of bismuth subsalicylate, and treatment for 7–10 days may be sufficient.

Adverse Effects

All bismuth formulations have an excellent safety profile. Bismuth causes blackening of the stool, which may be confused with gastrointestinal bleeding. Liquid formulations may cause harmless darkening of the tongue. Bismuth agents should be used for only short periods and should be avoided in patients with renal insufficiency. Prolonged usage of some bismuth compounds may rarely lead to bismuth toxicity resulting in encephalopathy (ataxia, headaches, confusion, seizures). However, such toxicity is not reported with bismuth subsalicylate or bismuth citrate. High dosages of bismuth subsalicylate may lead to salicylate toxicity.

II. DRUGS STIMULATING GASTROINTESTINAL MOTILITY

Drugs that can selectively stimulate gut motor function (**prokinetic** agents) have significant potential clinical usefulness. Agents that increase lower esophageal sphincter pressures may be useful for GERD. Drugs that improve gastric emptying may be helpful for gastroparesis and postsurgical gastric emptying delay. Agents that stimulate the small intestine may be beneficial for postoperative ileus or chronic intestinal pseudo-obstruction. Finally, agents that enhance colonic transit may be useful in the treatment of constipation. Unfortunately, only a limited number of agents are available for clinical use at this time.

PHYSIOLOGY OF THE ENTERIC NERVOUS SYSTEM

The enteric nervous system (see Chapter 6) is composed of interconnected networks of ganglion cells and nerve fibers mainly located in the submucosa (submucosal plexus) and between the circular and longitudinal muscle layers (myenteric plexus). These networks give rise to nerve fibers that connect with the mucosa and deep muscle. Although extrinsic sympathetic and parasympathetic nerves project onto the submucosal and myenteric plexuses, the enteric nervous system can independently regulate gastrointestinal motility and secretion. Afferent fibers present in the mucosa and muscularis connect to cell bodies in the plexuses that mediate local reflexes.

Myenteric plexus interneurons containing **calcitonin gene related peptide** (CGRP) may be important in controlling the peristaltic reflex, promoting release of excitatory mediators proximally and inhibitory mediators distally. Excitatory muscle activity (contraction) is promoted by enteric interneurons and motor neurons that release **acetylcholine, serotonin,** and **substance P.** Inhibition of muscle activity and relaxation is promoted by enteric motor neurons that release **vasoactive intesti-**

nal peptide, nitric oxide, and ATP. **Motilin** may stimulate excitatory neurons or muscle cells directly. **Dopamine** acts as an inhibitory neurotransmitter in the gastrointestinal tract, decreasing the intensity of esophageal and gastric contractions.

Although there are at least 14 serotonin (5-HT) receptor subtypes, drug development for gastrointestinal applications to date has focused on **5-HT$_3$ receptor antagonists** and **5-HT$_4$ receptor agonists**. These agents—which have effects upon gastrointestinal motility and visceral afferent sensation—are discussed under Drugs Used for the Treatment of Irritable Bowel Syndrome and Antiemetics. Other drugs acting on 5-HT receptors are discussed in Chapters 16, 29, and 30.

CHOLINOMIMETIC AGENTS

Cholinomimetic agonists such as **bethanechol** stimulate muscarinic M$_3$ receptors on muscle cells and at myenteric plexus synapses (see Chapter 7). Bethanechol was used in the past for the treatment of GERD and gastroparesis. Due to multiple cholinergic side effects and the advent of newer agents, it is now seldom used. The acetylcholinesterase inhibitor **neostigmine** can enhance gastric, small intestine, and colonic emptying. Intravenous neostigmine (2 mg) has enjoyed a resurgence in clinical usage for the treatment of hospitalized patients with acute large bowel distention (known as acute colonic pseudo-obstruction or Ogilvie's syndrome), resulting in prompt colonic evacuation of flatus and feces in the majority of patients. Cholinergic side effects include excessive salivation, nausea, vomiting, diarrhea, and bradycardia.

METOCLOPRAMIDE, DOMPERIDONE, & CISAPRIDE

Metoclopramide and **cisapride** are substituted benzamides and **domperidone** is a butyrophenone. The primary prokinetic mechanism of action of all three agents is mediated through cholinergic stimulation. In addition to agonist activity at 5-HT$_4$ receptors on enteric neurons, which promotes release of acetylcholine, cisapride exhibits some antagonist activity at 5-HT$_3$ receptors. Metoclopramide and domperidone (but not cisapride) are dopamine D$_2$ receptor antagonists. Within the gastrointestinal tract dopamine receptor antagonism may potentiate cholinergic smooth muscle stimulation. Metoclopramide and domperidone also block dopamine D$_2$ receptors in the chemoreceptor trigger zone of the medulla (area postrema), resulting in potent antinausea and antiemetic action.

These agents increase esophageal peristaltic amplitude, increase lower esophageal sphincter (LES) pressure, and enhance gastric emptying. Cisapride also enhances small bowel and colonic motility.

Clinical Uses

A. GASTROESOPHAGEAL REFLUX DISEASE (GERD)

Metoclopramide is available for clinical use in the USA; domperidone is available in many other countries. Cisapride was removed from the United States market by the manufacturer due to cardiac arrhythmias and is now available only for compassionate use. All three agents are used for the treatment of symptomatic GERD but none are effective for treatment of erosive esophagitis. Due to the superior efficacy and safety of antisecretory agents for treatment of heartburn, prokinetic agents are used mainly in combination with antisecretory agents for treatment of regurgitation or refractory heartburn.

B. IMPAIRED GASTRIC EMPTYING

All three agents have been widely used for the treatment of patients with delayed gastric emptying due to postsurgical disorders (vagotomy, antrectomy) and diabetic gastroparesis. Metoclopramide is sometimes administered in hospitalized patients to promote advancement of nasoenteric feeding tubes from the stomach into the duodenum.

C. NONULCER DYSPEPSIA

These agents lead to symptomatic improvement in a small number of patients with chronic dyspepsia.

D. PREVENTION OF VOMITING

Due to their potent antiemetic action, metoclopramide and domperidone are used for the prevention and treatment of emesis (see page 1051).

E. POSTPARTUM LACTATION STIMULATION

Domperidone is sometimes recommended to promote postpartum lactation (see also Adverse Effects).

Adverse Effects

The most common adverse effects of **metoclopramide** involve the central nervous system. Restlessness, drowsiness, insomnia, anxiety, and agitation occur in 10–20% of patients, especially the elderly. Extrapyramidal effects (dystonias, akathisia, parkinsonian features) due to central dopamine receptor blockade occur acutely in 25% of patients given high doses and in 5% of patients receiving long-term therapy. Tardive dyskinesia, sometime irreversible, has developed in patients treated for a prolonged period with metoclopramide. For this reason, long-term use should be avoided unless absolutely necessary, especially in the elderly. Elevated prolactin levels (caused by both metoclopramide and domperidone) can cause galactorrhea, gynecomastia, impotence, and menstrual disorders.

Domperidone is extremely well tolerated. Because it does not cross the blood-brain barrier to a significant degree, neuropsychiatric and extrapyramidal side effects are rare.

Due to prokinetic effects in the colon, abdominal cramps and diarrhea occur in up to 15% of patients taking **cisapride**; however significant problems are unusual. In addition, cisapride is metabolized by the hepatic cytochrome P450 CYP3A4 enzyme. When coadministered with drugs that inhibit this enzyme (such as ketoconazole, fluconazole, macrolide antibiotics, and HIV protease inhibitors), significant increases in serum levels of cisapride may occur that rarely lead to QT prolongation on the ECG and serious cardiac arrhythmias. For this reason, cisapride was removed from the market by the manufacturer.

MACROLIDES

Macrolide antibiotics such as erythromycin directly stimulate motilin receptors on gastrointestinal smooth muscle and promote the onset of a migrating motor complex. Intravenous erythromycin (3 mg/kg) is beneficial in some patients with gastroparesis; however, tolerance rapidly develops. Specific motilin agonists are under investigation.

III. LAXATIVES

The overwhelming majority of people do not need laxatives, yet they are self-prescribed by a large portion of the population. For most people, intermittent constipation is best prevented with a high fiber diet, adequate fluid intake, regular exercise, and the heeding of nature's call. Patients not responding to dietary changes or fiber supplements should undergo medical evaluation prior to the initiation of long-term laxative treatment. Laxatives may be classified by their major mechanism of action, but many work through more than one mechanism.

BULK-FORMING LAXATIVES

Bulk-forming laxatives are indigestible, hydrophilic colloids that absorb water, forming a bulky, emollient gel that distends the colon and promotes peristalsis. Common preparations include natural plant products (**psyllium, methylcellulose**) and synthetic fibers (**polycarbophil**). Bacterial digestion of plant fibers within the colon may lead to increased bloating and flatus.

STOOL SURFACTANT AGENTS (SOFTENERS)

These agents soften stool material, permitting water and lipids to penetrate. They may be administered orally or rectally. Common agents include **docusate** (oral or enema) or **glycerin suppository.** In hospitalized patients, docusate is commonly prescribed to prevent constipation and minimize straining. **Mineral oil** is a clear, viscous oil that lubricates fecal material, retarding water absorption from the stool. It is used to prevent and treat fecal impaction in young children and debilitated adults. It is not palatable but may be mixed with juices. Aspiration can result in a severe lipid pneumonitis. Long-term use can impair absorption of fat-soluble vitamins (A, D, E, K).

OSMOTIC LAXATIVES

The colon can neither concentrate nor dilute fecal fluid: fecal water is isotonic throughout the colon. Osmotic laxatives are soluble but nonabsorbable compounds that result in increased stool liquidity due to an obligate increase in fecal fluid.

Nonabsorbable Sugars or Salts

These agents may be used for the treatment of acute constipation or the prevention of chronic constipation. **Magnesium oxide (milk of magnesia)** is a commonly used osmotic laxative. It should not be used for prolonged periods in patients with renal insufficiency due to risk of hypermagnesemia. **Sorbitol** and **lactulose** are nonabsorbable sugars that can be used to prevent or treat chronic constipation. These sugars are metabolized by colonic bacteria, producing severe flatus and cramps.

High doses of osmotically active agents produce prompt bowel evacuation (purgation) within 1–3 hours. The rapid movement of water into the distal small bowel and colon leads to a high volume of liquid stool followed by rapid relief of constipation. The most commonly used **purgatives** are **magnesium citrate** and **sodium phosphate.** These hyperosmolar agents may lead to intravascular volume depletion and electrolyte fluctuations; hence they should not be used in patients who are frail, elderly, have renal insufficiency, or have significant cardiac disease.

Balanced Polyethylene Glycol

Lavage solutions containing **polyethylene glycol (PEG)** are used for complete colonic cleansing prior to gastrointestinal endoscopic procedures. These balanced, isotonic solutions contain an inert, nonabsorbable, osmotically active sugar (PEG) with sodium sulfate, sodium chloride, sodium bicarbonate, and potassium chloride. The solution is designed so that no significant intravascular fluid or electrolyte shifts occur. Therefore, they are safe for all patients. The solution should be ingested rapidly (4 L over 2 hours) to promote bowel cleansing. For treatment or prevention of chronic constipation, smaller doses of PEG powder may be mixed with water or juices (17 g/8 oz) and ingested daily. In contrast to sorbitol or lactulose, PEG does not produce significant cramps or flatus.

STIMULANT LAXATIVES

Stimulant laxatives (cathartics) induce bowel movements through a number of poorly understood mechanisms. These include direct stimulation of the enteric nervous system and colonic electrolyte and fluid secretion. There has been concern that long-term use of cathartics could lead to dependency and destruction of the myenteric plexus, resulting in colonic atony and dilation. More recent research suggests that long-term use of these agents probably is safe in most patients. Cathartics may be required on a long-term basis, especially in patients who are neurologically impaired and in bed-bound patients in long-term care facilities.

Anthraquinone Derivatives

Aloe, senna, and cascara occur naturally in plants. These laxatives are poorly absorbed and after hydrolysis in the colon, produce a bowel movement in 6–12 hours when given orally and within 2 hours when given rectally. Chronic use leads to a characteristic brown pigmentation of the colon known as "melanosis coli." There has been some concern that these agents may be carcinogenic, but epidemiologic studies do not suggest a relationship to colorectal cancer.

Diphenylmethane Derivatives

Due to concerns about possible cardiac toxicity, these agents (eg, phenolphthalein) were recently removed from the market.

Castor Oil

This oil is a potent stimulant laxative. It is hydrolyzed in the upper small intestine to ricinoleic acid, a local irritant that stimulates intestinal motility. Formerly used as a purgative to clean the colon before procedures, it is now seldom used.

IV. ANTIDIARRHEAL AGENTS

Antidiarrheal agents may be used safely in patients with mild to moderate acute diarrhea. However, they should not be used in patients with bloody diarrhea, high fever, or systemic toxicity because of the risk of worsening the underlying condition. They should be discontinued in patients whose diarrhea is worsening despite therapy. Antidiarrheals are also used to control chronic diarrhea caused by such conditions as irritable bowel syndrome (IBS) or inflammatory bowel disease (IBD).

OPIOID AGONISTS

Opioids have significant constipating effects (see Chapter 31). They increase colonic phasic segmenting activity through inhibition of presynaptic cholinergic nerves in the submucosal and myenteric plexuses and lead to increased colonic transit time and fecal water absorption. They also decrease mass colonic movements and the gastrocolic reflex. Although all opioids have antidiarrheal effects, central nervous system effects and potential for addiction limit the usefulness of most. **Loperamide** is a nonprescription opioid agonist that does not cross the blood-brain barrier and has no analgesic properties or potential for addiction. Tolerance to long-term use has not been reported. It is typically administered in doses of 2 mg taken one to four times daily. **Diphenoxylate** is another opioid agonist that has no analgesic properties in standard doses; however, higher doses have central nervous system effects and prolonged use can lead to opioid dependence. Commercial preparations commonly contain small amounts of atropine to discourage overdosage (2.5 mg diphenoxylate with 0.025 mg atropine). The anticholinergic properties of atropine may contribute to the antidiarrheal action.

COLLOIDAL BISMUTH COMPOUNDS

See the section under Mucosal Protective Agents on page 1044.

KAOLIN & PECTIN

Kaolin is a naturally occurring hydrated magnesium aluminum silicate (attapulgite), and pectin is an indigestible carbohydrate derived from apples. Both appear to act as absorbents of bacteria, toxins, and fluid, thereby decreasing stool liquidity and number. They may be useful in acute diarrhea but are seldom used on a chronic basis. A common commercial preparation is Kaopectate. The usual dose is 1.2–1.5 g after each loose bowel movement (maximum: 9 g/d). Kaolin-pectin formulations are not absorbed and have no significant side effects except constipation. They should not be taken within 2 hours of other medications (to which they may bind).

BILE SALT BINDING RESINS

Conjugated bile salts are normally absorbed in the terminal ileum. Disease of the terminal ileum (eg, Crohn's disease) or surgical resection leads to malabsorption of bile salts, which may cause colonic secretory diarrhea. The bile salt binding resins **cholestyramine** or **colestipol** may decrease diarrhea caused by excess fecal bile acids (see Chapter 35). The usual dose is 4–5 g one to three times daily before meals. Side effects include bloating, flatulence, constipation, and fecal impaction. In patients with diminished circulating bile acid pools, further removal of bile acids may lead to an exacerbation of fat malabsorption. These agents bind a number of drugs and reduce their absorption; hence, they should not be given within 2 hours of other drugs.

OCTREOTIDE

Somatostatin is a 14 amino acid peptide that is released in the gastrointestinal tract and pancreas from paracrine cells, D-cells, and enteric nerves as well as from the hypothalamus (see Chapter 37). It is a key regulatory peptide that has myriad physiologic effects:

1. It inhibits the secretion of numerous hormones, including gastrin, cholecystokinin, glucagon, growth hormone, insulin, secretin, pancreatic polypeptide, vasoactive intestinal peptide, and 5-HT$_3$.
2. It reduces intestinal fluid secretion and pancreatic secretion.
3. It slows gastrointestinal motility and inhibits gallbladder contraction.
4. It induces direct contraction of vascular smooth muscle, leading to a reduction of portal and splanchnic blood flow.
5. It inhibits secretion of some anterior pituitary hormones.

The clinical usefulness of somatostatin is limited by its short half-life in the circulation (3 minutes) when it is administered by intravenous injection. **Octreotide** is a synthetic octapeptide with actions similar to somatostatin. When administered intravenously, it has a serum half-life of 1.5 hours. It also may be administered by subcutaneous injection, resulting in a 6- to 12-hour duration of action. A longer-acting formulation is available for once-monthly depot intramuscular injection.

Clinical Uses

A. INHIBITION OF ENDOCRINE TUMOR EFFECTS

Two gastrointestinal neuroendocrine tumors (carcinoid, VIPoma) cause secretory diarrhea and systemic symptoms such as flushing and wheezing. For patients with advanced symptomatic tumors that cannot be completely removed by surgery, octreotide decreases secretory diarrhea and systemic symptoms through inhibition of hormonal secretion and may slow tumor progression.

B. OTHER CAUSES OF DIARRHEA

Octreotide inhibits intestinal secretion and has dose-related affects on bowel motility. In low doses (50 μg subcutaneously) it stimulates motility, whereas at higher doses (eg, 100–250 μg subcutaneously), it inhibits motility. Octreotide is effective in higher doses for the treatment of diarrhea due to vagotomy or dumping syndrome as well as for diarrhea caused by short bowel syndrome or AIDS. Octreotide has been used in low doses (50 μg subcutaneously) to stimulate small bowel motility in patients with small bowel bacterial overgrowth or intestinal pseudo-obstruction secondary to scleroderma.

C. OTHER USES

Because it inhibits pancreatic secretion, octreotide may be of value in patients with pancreatic fistula. The role of octreotide in the treatment of pituitary tumors (eg, acromegaly) is discussed in Chapter 37. Octreotide is sometimes used in gastrointestinal bleeding (see below).

Adverse Effects

Impaired pancreatic secretion may cause steatorrhea, which can lead to fat-soluble vitamin deficiency. Alterations in gastrointestinal motility cause nausea, abdominal pain, flatulence, and diarrhea. Due to inhibition of gallbladder contractility and alterations in fat absorption, long-term use can cause formation of sludge or gallstones in over half of patients, which rarely results in the development of acute cholecystitis. Because octreotide alters the balance between insulin, glucagon, and growth hormone, hyperglycemia or, less frequently, hypoglycemia (usually mild) can occur. Prolonged treatment with octreotide may result in hypothyroidism. Octreotide also can cause bradycardia.

V. DRUGS USED FOR THE TREATMENT OF IRRITABLE BOWEL SYNDROME (IBS)

Irritable bowel syndrome is an idiopathic chronic, relapsing disorder characterized by abdominal discomfort (pain, bloating, distention, or cramps) in association with alterations in bowel habits (diarrhea, constipation, or both). With episodes of abdominal pain or discomfort, patients note a change in the frequency or consistency of their bowel movements.

Pharmacologic therapies for irritable bowel syndrome are directed at relieving abdominal pain and discomfort and improving bowel function. For patients with predominant diarrhea, antidiarrheal agents, especially loperamide, are helpful in reducing stool frequency and fecal urgency. For patients with predominant constipation, fiber supplements may lead to softening of stools and reduced straining; however, increased gas production may exacerbate bloating and abdominal discomfort. Consequently, osmotic laxatives, especially milk of magnesia, are commonly used to soften stools and promote increased stool frequency.

For the treatment of chronic abdominal pain, low doses of tricyclic antidepressants (eg, amitriptyline or desipramine 10–25 mg/d) appear to be helpful (see Chapter 30). At these doses, these agents have no effect on mood but may alter central processing of visceral afferent information. The anticholinergic properties of these agents also may have effects on gastrointestinal motility and secretion, reducing stool frequency and liquidity of stools. Finally, tricyclic antidepressants may alter receptors for enteric neurotransmitters such as serotonin, affecting visceral afferent sensation.

Several other agents are available that are specifically intended for the treatment of irritable bowel syndrome.

ANTISPASMODICS (ANTICHOLINERGICS)

Some agents are promoted as providing relief of abdominal pain or discomfort through "antispasmodic" actions. However, small or large bowel spasm has not been found to an important factor in symptom causation in patients with irritable bowel syndrome. These agents work primarily through anticholinergic activities. Commonly used medications in this class include **dicyclomine** (Bentyl) and **hyoscyamine** (Levsin). These drugs inhibit muscarinic cholinergic receptors in the enteric plexus and on smooth muscle. Efficacy of these agents for relief of abdominal symptoms has never been convincingly demonstrated. At low doses, they have minimal autonomic effects. However, at higher doses they exhibit significant anticholinergic side effects including dry mouth, visual disturbances, urinary retention, and constipation. For these reasons, these drugs are infrequently used.

SEROTONIN 5-HT$_3$ RECEPTOR ANTAGONISTS

Inhibition of 5-HT$_3$ receptors in the gastrointestinal tract results in modulation of visceral afferent pain sensation and intestinal motility. **Alosetron** is a 5-HT$_3$ antagonist that has been approved for the treatment of patients with severe irritable bowel syndrome with diarrhea (Figure 63–5). Three other 5-HT$_3$ antagonists (ondansetron, granisetron, dolasetron) have been approved for the prevention and treatment of nausea and vomiting (see Antiemetics); however, their efficacy in the treatment of irritable bowel syndrome has not

been determined. The relative differences between these 5-HT$_3$ antagonists that determine their pharmacodynamic effects have not been well studied.

Pharmacokinetics & Pharmacodynamics

Alosetron is a highly potent and specific antagonist of the 5-HT$_3$ receptor. It is rapidly absorbed from the gastrointestinal tract with a bioavailability of 50–60% and has a plasma half-life of 1.5 hours but a much longer duration of effect. It undergoes extensive hepatic cytochrome P450 metabolism with renal excretion of most metabolites.

Alosetron blocks 5-HT$_3$ receptors on enteric afferent neurons, inhibiting distention-induced sensory and motor reflex activation. Blockade of central 5-HT$_3$ receptors also reduces central response to visceral stimulation. 5-HT$_3$ receptor blockade on enteric cholinergic neurons inhibits colonic motility, especially in the left colon, increasing total colonic transit time. Alosetron binds with higher affinity and dissociates more slowly from 5-HT$_3$ receptors than other 5-HT$_3$ antagonists, which may account for its long duration of action.

Clinical Uses

Alosetron currently is approved for the treatment of women with severe irritable bowel syndrome in whom diarrhea is the predominant symptom ("diarrhea-predominant IBS"). Efficacy in men has not been established. In a dosage of 1 mg once or twice daily, it reduces IBS-related lower abdominal pain, cramps, urgency, and diarrhea. Approximately 50–60% of patients report adequate relief of pain and discomfort compared with 30–40% of patients treated with placebo. It also leads to a reduction in the mean number of bowel movements per day and improvement in stool consistency. This agent has not been evaluated for the treatment of other causes of diarrhea.

Adverse Events

In contrast to the excellent safety profile of other 5-HT$_3$ receptor antagonists, alosetron is associated with rare but serious gastrointestinal toxicity. Constipation occurs in up to 30% of patients with diarrhea-predominant IBS, requiring discontinuation of the drug in 10%. Serious complications of constipation requiring hospitalization or surgery have occurred in 1 of every 1000 patients. Episodes of ischemic colitis—some fatal—have been reported in up to 3 of every 1000 patients. Given the seriousness of these adverse events, alosetron is restricted to women with severe diarrhea-predominant IBS who have not responded to conventional therapies and who have been educated about the relative risks and benefits.

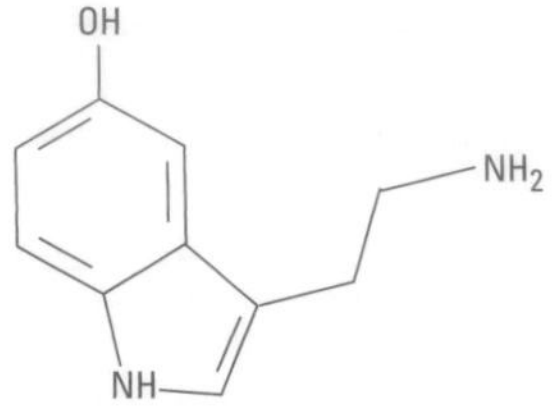

Serotonin

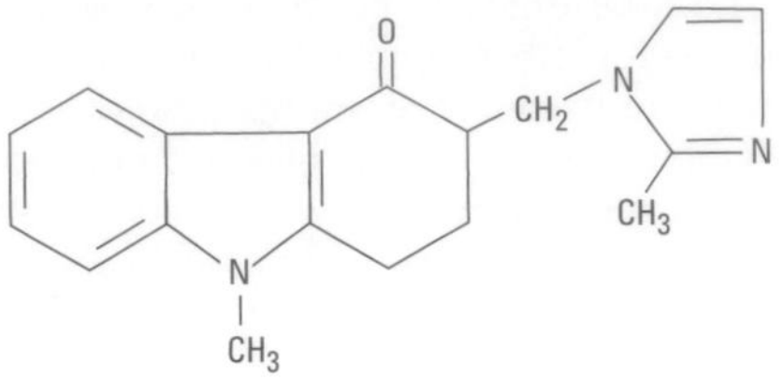

Ondansetron

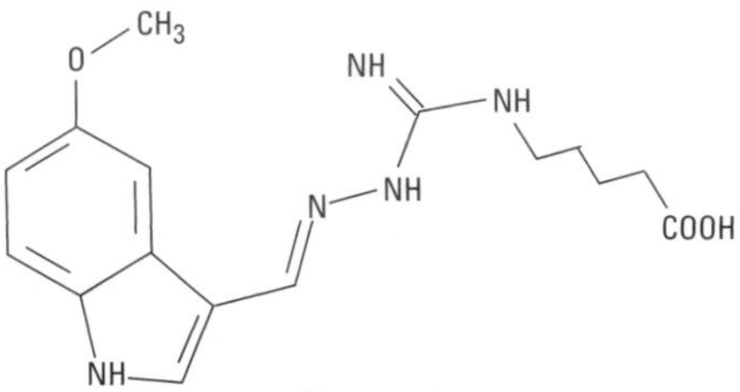

Tegaserod

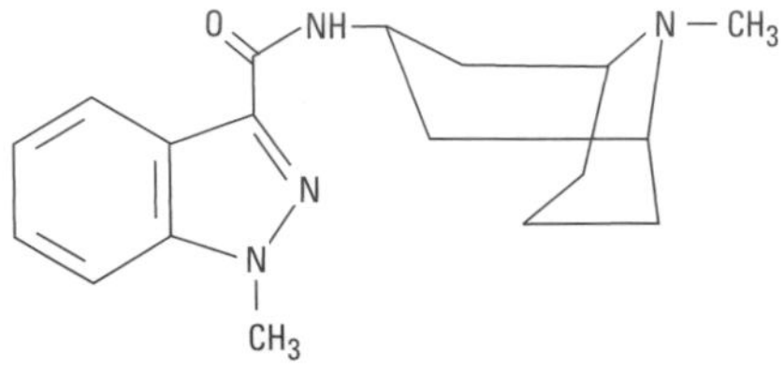

Granisetron

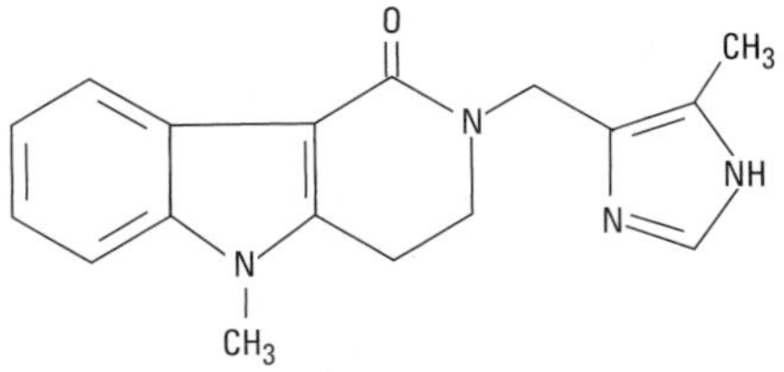

Alosetron

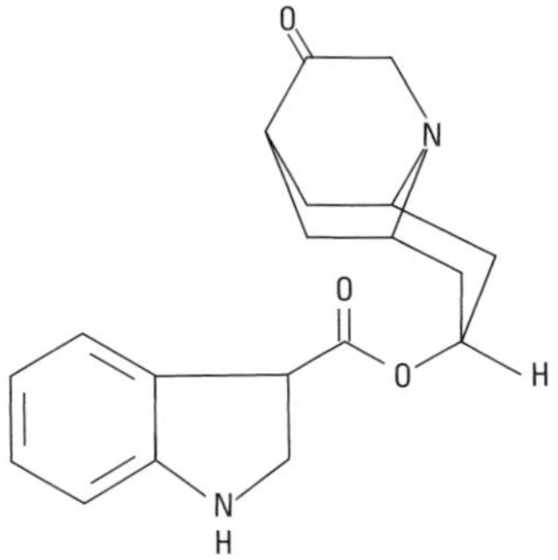

Dolasetron

Figure 63–5. Chemical structure of serotonin, the $5HT_3$-antagonists ondansetron, granisetron, dolasetron, and alosetron and the 5-HT_4 partial agonist tegaserod.

Drug Interactions

Despite being metabolized by a number of CYP enzymes, alosetron does not appear to have clinically significant interactions with other drugs.

SEROTONIN 5-HT_4 RECEPTOR AGONIST

Pharmacokinetics & Pharmacodynamics

Tegaserod is a partial serotonin 5-HT_4 agonist that resembles serotonin in structure. Although it binds with high affinity to 5-HT_4 receptors, it has no appreciable binding to 5-HT_3 (unlike cisapride) or dopamine receptors (unlike metoclopramide or domperidone). Tegaserod has a bioavailability of only 10%. It should be taken before meals because food further reduces bioavailability by 50%. The drug is metabolized both by gastric acid-catalyzed hydrolysis and hepatic glucuronidation. Approximately 66% of drug is excreted unchanged in the feces and 33% as a metabolite in the urine. It should not be given to patients with severe hepatic or renal impairment.

Research with tegaserod suggests that stimulation of 5-HT_4 receptors on mucosal afferent nerve fibers triggers the release of neurotransmitters from the submucosal and myenteric plexuses, including calcitonin gene-related peptide, that stimulate the peristaltic reflex. These neurotransmitters stimulate proximal bowel contraction (via acetylcholine and substance P) and distal bowel relaxation (via nitric oxide and vasoactive intestinal peptide). Thus, tegaserod binding to mucosal 5-HT_4 receptors promotes gastric emptying and enhances small and large bowel transit. Stimulation of 5-HT$_4$ receptors activates cAMP-dependent chloride secretion from the colon, leading to increased stool liquidity. In animal models, stimulation of 5-HT$_4$ receptors appears to modulate visceral afferent sensation of bloating and distention.

Clinical Uses

Tegaserod was recently approved for the treatment of patients with irritable bowel syndrome with predominant constipation. Controlled studies have demonstrated a modest improvement in patient global satisfaction and a reduction in severity of pain and bloating in patients treated with tegaserod 6 mg twice daily compared with placebo. Tegaserod also increases the number of bowel movements per week and reduces the hardness of stools. The role of tegaserod in the treatment of other gastrointestinal motility disorders such as nonulcer dyspepsia, gastroparesis, and chronic constipation is under investigation.

Adverse Effects

Tegaserod appears to be an extremely safe agent. Diarrhea occurs in 9% of patients within the first few days of treatment, but resolves in the majority of patients. Less than 2% of patients discontinue the drug because of diarrhea. Although it is stated that the drug does not cross the blood-brain barrier (and does not affect central serotonin receptors), headache may occur.

Drug Interactions

Tegaserod has no known effects on cytochrome P450 enzymes and no known drug interactions. Unlike cisapride, tegaserod does not inhibit cardiac repolarization and does not prolong the QT interval.

VI. ANTIEMETIC AGENTS

Nausea and vomiting may be manifestations of a wide variety of conditions, including adverse effects from medications; systemic disorders or infections; pregnancy; vestibular dysfunction; central nervous system infection or increased pressure; peritonitis; hepatobiliary disorders; radiation or chemotherapy; and gastrointestinal obstruction, dysmotility, or infections.

PATHOPHYSIOLOGY

The brainstem vomiting center is located in the lateral medullary reticular formation and coordinates the complex act of vomiting through interactions with cranial nerves VIII and X and neural networks in the nucleus tractus solitarius that control respiratory, salivatory, and vasomotor centers. High concentrations of muscarinic, histamine H$_1$, and serotonin 5-HT$_3$ receptors have been identified in the vomiting center.

There are five sources of afferent input to the vomiting center:

1. The chemoreceptor trigger zone is located in the fourth ventricle in the area postrema. This is outside the blood-brain barrier and is accessible to emetogenic stimuli in the blood or cerebrospinal fluid. The chemoreceptor trigger zone is rich in dopamine D$_2$ receptors, serotonin 5-HT$_3$ receptors, and opioid receptors.

2. The vestibular system is important in motion sickness via cranial nerve VIII. It is rich in muscarinic and histamine H$_1$ receptors.

3. Irritation of the pharynx, innervated by the vagus nerve, provokes a prominent gag and retch response.

4. Vagal and enteric afferents in the mucosa of the gastrointestinal tract are rich in 5-HT$_3$ receptors. Irritation of the gastrointestinal mucosa by chemotherapy, radiation therapy, distention, or acute infectious gastroenteritis leads to release of mucosal serotonin and activation of these receptors, which stimulate vagal afferent input to the vomiting center and chemoreceptor trigger zone.

5. The central nervous system plays a role in vomiting due to psychiatric disorders, stress, and anticipatory vomiting prior to chemotherapy.

Identification of the different neurotransmitters involved with emesis has allowed development of a diverse group of antiemetic agents that have affinity for various receptors. Combinations of antiemetic agents with different mechanisms of action are often used, especially in patients with vomiting due to chemotherapeutic agents.

SEROTONIN 5-HT$_3$ ANTAGONISTS

Pharmacokinetics & Pharmacodynamics

Selective 5-HT$_3$ receptor antagonists have potent antiemetic properties that are mediated mainly through peripheral 5-HT$_3$ receptor blockade on intestinal vagal afferents. In addition, central 5-HT$_3$ receptor blockade in the vomiting center and chemoreceptor trigger zone probably plays an important role. The antiemetic action of these agents is restricted to emesis attributable to vagal stimulation; other emetic stimuli such as motion sickness are poorly controlled.

Three agents are available: **ondansetron, granisetron, and dolasetron.** The drugs have a long serum half-life of

4–9 hours and may be administered once or twice daily by oral or intravenous routes. The drugs undergo extensive hepatic metabolism and are eliminated by renal and hepatic excretion. However, dose reduction is not required in geriatric patients or patients with renal insufficiency. For patients with hepatic insufficiency, dose reduction may be required with ondansetron.

These agents do not exhibit dopamine receptor or muscarinic receptor antagonism. They do not have effects on esophageal or gastric motility but may slow colonic transit.

Clinical Uses

A. Chemotherapy-Induced Nausea and Vomiting

5-HT$_3$ receptor antagonists are the primary agents for the prevention and treatment of chemotherapy induced nausea and emesis. The drugs are most effective when given by intravenous injection 30 minutes prior to administration of chemotherapy in the following doses: ondansetron 32 mg, granisetron 10 μg/kg, and dolasetron 1.8 mg/kg. These doses may be repeated every 24 hours. For less emetogenic regimens, oral administration may be effective in the following regimens: ondansetron 8 mg every 8–12 hours, granisetron 2 mg/d, and dolasetron 100 mg/d. Clinical studies suggest that the efficacy of 5-HT$_3$ receptor antagonists is enhanced by administration of dexamethasone 6–10 mg every 6 hours for two to four doses. Other antiemetics may also be used in combination with 5-HT$_3$ receptor antagonists to prevent emesis or to treat delayed emesis; these include phenothiazines or metoclopramide (for dopaminergic blockade), and benzodiazepines.

B. Postoperative and Post-Radiation Nausea and Vomiting

5-HT$_3$ receptor antagonists are used to prevent or treat postoperative nausea and vomiting. Due to side effects and increased restrictions on use of other antiemetic agents, 5-HT$_3$ receptor antagonists are increasingly used for this indication. They are also effective in the prevention and treatment of nausea and vomiting in patients undergoing radiation therapy to the whole body or abdomen.

C. Other Indications

The efficacy of 5-HT$_3$ receptor antagonists for the treatment of nausea and vomiting due to acute or chronic medical illness or acute gastroenteritis has not been evaluated.

Adverse Effects

These 5-HT$_3$ receptor antagonists are well-tolerated agents with excellent safety profiles. The most com-

monly reported side effects are headache, dizziness, and constipation. All three agents cause a small but statistically significant prolongation of the QT interval, but this is most pronounced with dolasetron. Although cardiac arrhythmias have not been linked to use of dolasetron, it should not be administered to patients with prolonged QT or in conjunction with other medications that may prolong the QT interval.

Drug Interactions

No significant drug interactions have been reported. All three agents undergo some metabolism by the hepatic cytochrome P450 system but they do not appear to affect the metabolism of other drugs metabolized by these enzyme systems. However, other drugs may reduce hepatic clearance of the 5-HT$_3$ receptor antagonists, altering their half-life.

PHENOTHIAZINES & BUTYROPHENONES

Phenothiazines are antipsychotic agents that can be used for their potent antiemetic and sedative properties (see Chapter 29). The antiemetic properties of phenothiazines are mediated through inhibition of dopamine and muscarinic receptors. Sedative properties are due to their antihistamine activity. The agents most commonly used as antiemetics are **prochlorperazine, promethazine,** and **thiethylperazine.**

Antipsychotic butyrophenones also possess antiemetic properties due to their central dopaminergic blockade (see Chapter 29). The main agent used is **droperidol,** which can be given by intramuscular or intravenous injection. In antiemetic doses, droperidol is extremely sedating. Until recently, it was used extensively for postoperative nausea and vomiting, in conjunction with opiates and benzodiazepines for sedation for surgical and endoscopic procedures, for neuroleptanalgesia, and for induction and maintenance of general anesthesia. Extrapyramidal side effects and hypotension may occur. Droperidol may prolong the QT interval, rarely resulting in fatal episodes of ventricular tachycardia including torsade de pointes. Therefore, droperidol should not be used in patients with QT prolongation and should only be used in patients who have not responded adequately to alternative agents.

SUBSTITUTED BENZAMIDES

Substituted benzamides include **metoclopramide** and **trimethobenzamide.** Their primary mechanism of antiemetic action is believed to be dopamine-receptor blockade. Trimethobenzamide also has weak antihistaminic activity. For prevention and treatment of nausea and vomiting, metoclopramide may be given in the relatively high dosage of 10–20 mg orally or intravenously every 6 hours. The usual dose of trimethobenzamide is 250 mg orally, 200 mg rectally, or 200 mg by intramuscular injection. As discussed previously, the principal side effects of these central dopamine antagonists are extrapyramidal: restlessness, dystonias, and parkinsonian symptoms.

H₁ ANTIHISTAMINES & ANTICHOLINERGICS

The pharmacology of anticholinergic agents is discussed in Chapter 8 and of H₁ antihistaminic agents in Chapter 16. As single agents, these drugs have weak antiemetic activity, although they are particularly useful for the prevention or treatment of motion sickness. Their use may be limited by sedation, dizziness, sedation, confusion, dry mouth, cycloplegia, and urinary retention. **Diphenhydramine** and one of its salts, **dimenhydrinate**, are first-generation histamine H₁ antagonists that have significant anticholinergic properties. Because of its sedating properties, diphenhydramine is commonly used in conjunction with other antiemetics for treatment of emesis due to chemotherapy. **Meclizine** is an H₁ antihistaminic agent with minimal anticholinergic properties that also has less sedation. It is used for the prevention of motion sickness and treatment of vertigo due to labyrinth dysfunction.

Hyoscine (scopolamine), a prototypic muscarinic receptor antagonist, is one of the best agents for the prevention of motion sickness. However, it has a very high incidence of anticholinergic effects when given orally or parenterally. It is better tolerated as a transdermal patch. Superiority to dimenhydrinate has not been proved.

BENZODIAZEPINES

Benzodiazepines such as lorazepam or diazepam are used prior to the initiation of chemotherapy to reduce anticipatory vomiting or vomiting caused by anxiety. The pharmacology of these agents is presented in Chapter 22.

CANNABINOIDS

Dronabinol is Δ^9-tetrahydrocannabinol, the major psychoactive chemical in marijuana (see Chapter 32). After oral ingestion, the drug is almost completely absorbed but undergoes significant first-pass hepatic metabolism. It undergoes hepatic metabolism and its metabolites are excreted slowly over days to weeks in the feces and urine. Like crude marijuana, dronabinol is a psychoactive agent that is used medically as an appetite stimulant and as an antiemetic, but the mechanisms for these effects are not understood. For the prevention of chemotherapy-induced nausea and vomiting, it is usually administered in conjunction with other antiemetic agents. Combination therapy with phenothiazines provides synergistic antiemetic action and appears to attenuate the adverse effects of both agents. Dronabinol is usually administered in a dosage of 5 mg/m² prior to chemotherapy and every 2–4 hours as needed. Adverse effects include euphoria, dysphoria, sedation, hallucinations, dry mouth, and increased appetite. It has some autonomic effects that may result in tachycardia, conjunctival injection, and orthostatic hypotension. Dronabinol has no significant drug-drug interactions but may potentiate the clinical effects of other psychoactive agents.

CORTICOSTEROIDS

Corticosteroids (dexamethasone, methylprednisolone) have antiemetic properties, but the basis for these effects is unknown. These agents are commonly used in combination with other agents in the treatment of chemotherapy-induced vomiting. The pharmacology of this class of drugs is discussed in Chapter 39.

VII. DRUGS USED TO TREAT INFLAMMATORY BOWEL DISEASE (IBD)

Inflammatory bowel disease comprises two distinct disorders: ulcerative colitis and Crohn's disease. The etiology and pathogenesis of these disorders remains unknown. For this reason, pharmacologic treatment of inflammatory bowel disorders often involves drugs that belong to different therapeutic classes and have different but nonspecific mechanisms of anti-inflammatory action.

AMINOSALICYLATES

Chemistry & Formulations

Drugs that contain **5-aminosalicylic acid (5-ASA)** have been used successfully for decades in the treatment of inflammatory bowel diseases. 5-ASA differs from salicylic acid only by the addition of an amino group at the 5 (meta) position. Aminosalicylates are believed to work topically (not systemically) in areas of diseased gastrointestinal mucosa. Up to 80% of unformulated, aqueous 5-ASA is absorbed from the small intestine and does not reach the distal small bowel or colon in appreciable quantities. To overcome the rapid absorption of 5-ASA from the proximal small intestine, a number of formulations have been designed to deliver 5-ASA to various distal segments of the small bowel or the colon. These include **sulfasalazine, olsalazine, balsalazide**, and various forms of **mesalamine**.

A. AZO COMPOUNDS

Sulfasalazine, balsalazide, and olsalazine contain 5-ASA bound by an azo (N=N) bond to an inert compound or to another 5-ASA molecule (Figure 63–6). In sulfasalazine, 5-ASA is bound to sulfapyridine; in balsalazide, 5-ASA is bound to 4-aminobenzoyl-B-alanine; and in olsalazine, two 5-ASA molecules are bound together. The azo structure markedly reduces absorption of the parent drug from the small intestine. In the terminal ileum and colon, resident bacteria cleave the azo bond by means of an azoreductase enzyme, releasing the active 5-ASA. Consequently, high concentrations of active drug are made available in the terminal ileum or colon.

B. MESALAMINE COMPOUNDS

A number of proprietary formulations have been designed that package 5-ASA in various ways in order to deliver it to different segments of the small or large bowel. These 5-ASA formulations are known generically as **mesalamine**. **Pentasa** is a mesalamine formulation that contains time-release microgranules that release 5-ASA throughout the small intestine. **Asacol** has 5-ASA coated in a pH-sensitive resin that dissolves at pH 7 (the pH of the distal ileum and proximal colon). 5-ASA also may be delivered in high concentrations to the rectum and sigmoid colon by means of enema formulations (**Rowasa**) or suppositories (**Canasa**).

Pharmacokinetics & Pharmacodynamics

Although unformulated 5-ASA is readily absorbed from the small intestine, absorption of 5-ASA from the colon is extremely low. In contrast, approximately 20–30% of 5-ASA from oral mesalamine formulations is systemically absorbed in the small intestine. Absorbed 5-ASA undergoes N-acetylation in the gut epithelium and liver to a metabolite that does not possess significant antiinflammatory activity. The acetylated metabolite is excreted by the kidneys.

Of the azo compounds, 10% of sulfasalazine and less than 1% of balsalazide are absorbed as native compounds. After azoreductase breakdown of sulfasalazine, over 85% of the carrier molecule sulfapyridine is systemically absorbed from the colon. Sulfapyridine undergoes hepatic metabolism (including acetylation) followed by renal excretion. By contrast, after azoreductase breakdown of balsalazide, over 70% of the carrier peptide is recovered intact in the feces and only a small amount of systemic absorption occurs.

The mechanism of action of 5-ASA is not certain. The primary action of salicylate and other NSAIDs is due to blockade of prostaglandin synthesis by inhibition of cyclooxygenase. However, the aminosalicylates have variable effects on prostaglandin production. It is believed that 5-ASA modulates inflammatory mediators derived from both the cyclooxygenase and lipoxygenase pathways. Other potential mechanisms of action of the 5-ASA drugs relate to their ability to interfere with the production of inflammatory cytokines. 5-ASA inhibits the activity of nuclear factor-κB (NF-κB), an important transcription factor for proinflammatory cytokines. 5-ASA may also inhibit cellular functions of natural killer

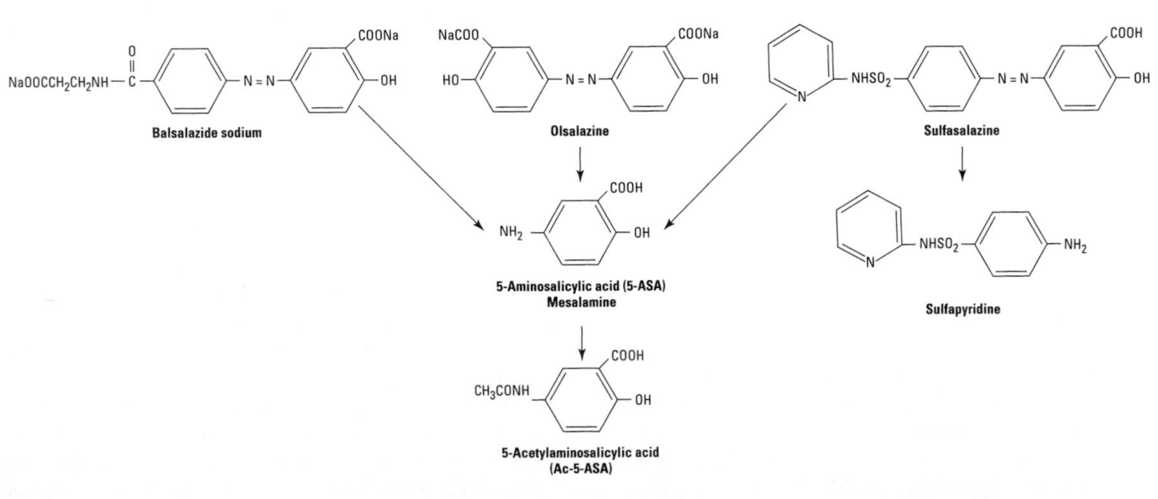

Figure 63–6. Chemical structures of aminosalicylates. Azo compounds (balsalazide, olsalazine, sulfasalazine) are converted by bacterial azoreductase to 5-aminosalicylic acid (mesalamine), the active therapeutic moiety.

cells, mucosal lymphocytes, and macrophages, and it may scavenge reactive oxygen metabolites.

Clinical Uses

5-ASA drugs induce and maintain remission in ulcerative colitis and are considered to be the first-line agents for treatment of mild to moderate active ulcerative colitis. Their efficacy in Crohn's disease is not as well established, although many clinicians use 5-ASA agents as first-line therapy for mild to moderate disease involving the colon or distal ileum.

The effectiveness of 5-ASA therapy depends in part on achieving high drug concentration at the site of active disease. Thus, 5-ASA suppositories or enemas are useful in patients with ulcerative colitis or Crohn's disease confined to the rectum (proctitis) or distal colon (proctosigmoiditis). In patients with ulcerative colitis or Crohn's colitis that extends to the proximal colon, both the azo compounds and mesalamine formulations are useful. For the treatment of Crohn's disease involving the small bowel, mesalamine compounds, which release 5-ASA in the small intestine, have a theoretic advantage over the azo compounds.

Adverse Effects

Sulfasalazine has a high incidence of adverse effects, most of which are attributable to systemic effects of the sulfapyridine molecule. Slow acetylators of sulfapyridine have more frequent and more severe adverse effects than fast acetylators. Up to 40% of patients cannot tolerate therapeutic doses of sulfasalazine. The most common problems are dose-related and include nausea, gastrointestinal upset, headaches, arthralgias, myalgias, bone marrow suppression, and malaise. Hypersensitivity to sulfapyridine (or, rarely, 5-ASA) results in fever, exfoliative dermatitis, pancreatitis, pneumonitis, hemolytic anemia, pericarditis, or hepatitis. Sulfasalazine has also been associated with oligospermia, which reverses upon discontinuation of the drug. Sulfasalazine impairs folate absorption and processing; hence, dietary supplementation with 1 mg/d folic acid is recommended.

In contrast to sulfasalazine, other aminosalicylate formulations are well tolerated. In most clinical trials, the frequency of drug adverse events is similar to patients treated with placebo. For unclear reasons, olsalazine may stimulate a secretory diarrhea—which should not be confused with active inflammatory bowel disease—in 10% of patients. Rare hypersensitivity reactions may occur with all aminosalicylates but are much less common than with sulfasalazine. Careful studies have documented subtle changes indicative of renal tubular damage in patients receiving high doses of aminosalicylates. Rare cases of interstitial nephritis are reported, particu-

larly in association with high doses of mesalamine formulations; this may be attributable to the higher serum 5-ASA levels attained with these drugs. Sulfasalazine and other aminosalicylates rarely cause worsening of colitis, which may be misinterpreted as refractory colitis.

GLUCOCORTICOIDS

Pharmacokinetics & Pharmacodynamics

In gastrointestinal practice, prednisone and prednisolone are the most commonly used oral glucocorticoids. These drugs have an intermediate duration of biologic activity allowing once daily dosing.

Hydrocortisone enemas, foam, or suppositories are used to maximize colonic tissue effects and minimize systemic absorption via topical treatment of active inflammatory bowel disease in the rectum and sigmoid colon. Absorption of hydrocortisone is reduced with rectal administration, although 15–30% of the administered dosage is absorbed.

Budesonide is a potent synthetic analog of prednisolone that has high affinity for the glucocorticoid receptor but is subject to rapid first-pass hepatic metabolism (in part by CYP3A4) resulting in low oral bioavailability. A controlled-release oral formulation of budesonide (Entocort) is now available that releases the drug in the distal ileum and colon where it is absorbed. The bioavailability of controlled-release budesonide capsules is approximately 10%.

As in other tissues, glucocorticoids inhibit production of inflammatory cytokines (TNF-α, IL-1) and chemokines(IL-8); reduce expression of inflammatory cell adhesion molecules; and inhibit gene transcription of nitric oxide synthase, phospholipase A_2, cyclooxygenase-2, and NF-κB.

Clinical Uses

Glucocorticoids are commonly used in the treatment of patients with moderate to severe active inflammatory bowel disease. Active disease is commonly treated with an initial oral dosage of 40–60 mg/d of prednisone or prednisolone. Higher doses have not been shown to be more efficacious but have significantly greater adverse effects. Once a patient responds to initial therapy (usually within 1–2 weeks), the dosage is tapered to minimize development of adverse effects. In severely ill patients, the drugs are usually administered intravenously.

For the treatment of inflammatory bowel disease involving the rectum or sigmoid colon, rectally administered glucocorticoids are preferred because of their lower systemic absorption.

Oral controlled-release budesonide (9 mg/d) is increasingly used in the treatment of active mild to moderate Crohn's disease involving the ileum and proximal colon. It appears to be slightly less effective than prednisolone in achieving clinical remission, but has significantly less adverse systemic effects.

Corticosteroids are not useful to maintain disease remission. Other medications such as aminosalicylates or immunosuppressive agents should be used for this purpose.

Adverse Effects

Side effects of glucocorticoids are reviewed in Chapter 39.

PURINE ANALOGS: AZATHIOPRINE & 6-MERCAPTOPURINE

Pharmacokinetics & Pharmacodynamics

Azathioprine and 6-mercaptopurine are purine antimetabolites that have immunosuppressive properties (see Chapters 55 and 56).

Azathioprine and 6-mercaptopurine have a serum half-life of less than 2 hours; however, the active metabolites, 6-thioguanine nucleotides, are concentrated in cells resulting in a prolonged half-life of days. The prolonged kinetics of 6-thioguanine nucleotide results in a median delay of 17 weeks before onset of therapeutic benefit from oral azathioprine or 6-mercaptopurine is observed in patients with inflammatory bowel disease.

The molecular basis for the therapeutic effects of the purine analogs is unknown. Intracellular 6-thioguanine causes inhibition of purine nucleotide metabolism and DNA synthesis and repair, resulting in inhibition of cell division and proliferation.

Clinical Uses

Azathioprine and 6-mercaptopurine are important agents in the induction and maintenance of remission of ulcerative colitis and Crohn's disease. After 3–6 months of treatment, 50–60% of patients with active disease achieve remission. These agents help maintain remission in up to 80% of patients. Among patients who depend on long-term glucocorticoid therapy to control active disease, purine analogs allow dose reduction or elimination of steroids in the majority.

Adverse Effects

Dose-related toxicities of azathioprine or 6-mercaptopurine include nausea, vomiting, bone marrow depression (leading to leukopenia, macrocytosis, anemia, or thrombocytopenia), and hepatic toxicity. Routine laboratory monitoring with complete blood count and liver function tests is required. Leukopenia or elevations in liver chemistries usually respond to medication dose reduction. Severe leukopenia may predispose to opportunistic infections; leukopenia may respond to therapy with granulocyte stimulating factor. Hypersensitivity reactions to azathioprine or 6-mercaptopurine occur in 5% of patients. These include fever, rash, pancreatitis, diarrhea, and hepatitis.

Although there appears to be an increased risk of lymphoma in transplant recipients receiving long-term 6-mercaptopurine or azathioprine therapy, it is unclear whether the risk is increased among patients with inflammatory bowel disease. These drugs cross the placenta; however, there are many reports of successful pregnancies in women taking these agents, and the risk of teratogenicity appears to be small.

Drug Interactions

Allopurinol markedly reduces metabolism of the purine analogs, potentially leading to severe leukopenia. The dose of 6-mercaptopurine or azathioprine should be reduced by at least half in patients taking allopurinol.

METHOTREXATE

Pharmacokinetics & Pharmacodynamics

Methotrexate is another antimetabolite that has beneficial effects in a number of chronic inflammatory diseases, including Crohn's disease and rheumatoid arthritis (see Chapter 36), and in cancer (see Chapter 55). Methotrexate may be given orally, subcutaneously, and intramuscularly. Reported oral bioavailability is 50–90% at doses used in chronic inflammatory diseases. Intramuscular and subcutaneous methotrexate exhibit nearly complete bioavailability.

The principal mechanism of action is inhibition of dihydrofolate reductase, an enzyme important in the production of thymidine and purines. At the high doses used for chemotherapy, methotrexate inhibits cellular proliferation. However, at the low doses used in the treatment of inflammatory bowel disease (12–25 mg/wk), the antiproliferative effects may not be evident. Methotrexate shares structural homology with interleukin-1 and may interfere with its inflammatory actions. It may also stimulate increased release of adenosine, an endogenous anti-inflammatory autacoid. Methotrexate may also stimulate apoptosis and death of activated T lymphocytes.

Clinical Uses

Methotrexate is used to induce and maintain remission in patients with Crohn's disease. Its efficacy in ulcerative colitis is uncertain. To induce remission, patients are treated with 15–25 mg of methotrexate once weekly by subcutaneous injection. If a satisfactory response is achieved within 8–12 weeks, the dose is reduced to 15 mg/wk.

Adverse Effects

At higher dosage, methotrexate may cause bone marrow depression, megaloblastic anemia, alopecia, and mucositis. At the doses used in the treatment of inflammatory bowel disease, these events are uncommon but warrant dose reduction if they do occur. Folate supplementation reduces the risk of these events without impairing the anti-inflammatory action.

In patients with psoriasis treated with methotrexate, hepatic damage is common; however, among patients with inflammatory bowel disease and rheumatoid arthritis, the risk is significantly lower. Renal insufficiency may increase risk of hepatic accumulation and toxicity.

ANTI-TNF-ALPHA THERAPY

Pharmacokinetics & Pharmacodynamics

A dysregulation of the TH1 T cell response is present in inflammatory bowel disease, especially Crohn's disease. One of the key proinflammatory cytokines in the TH1 response is TNF-α. **Infliximab** is a chimeric mouse-human monoclonal antibody to human TNF-α. It consists of human IgG1 constant regions, human κ light chains and transplanted monoclonal murine variable regions that have a high affinity for TNF-α. The molecule is 25% murine and 75% human.

Infliximab is administered as an intravenous infusion. The plasma concentration is linearly proportionate to dose and its elimination follows first-order kinetics. At therapeutic doses of 5–10 mg/kg, the half-life of infliximab is approximately 8–10 days, resulting in plasma disappearance of antibodies over 8–12 weeks.

The biologic activity of TNF-α is mediated by binding of soluble or membrane-bound TNF-α trimers to cell-surface TNF-α receptors. Infliximab binds to soluble TNF-α trimers with high affinity, preventing the cytokine from binding to its receptors. Serum TNF-α concentrations may actually increase because binding to infliximab slows TNF-α clearance. Infliximab also binds to membrane-bound TNF-α and neutralizes its activity. Furthermore, the Fc portion of human IgG1 region of infliximab promotes complement activation and antibody-mediated cellular cytotoxicity of inflammatory cells.

Clinical Uses

Infliximab leads to symptomatic improvement in two thirds and disease remission in one third of patients with moderately severe or fistulizing Crohn's disease, including patients who have been dependent on glucocorticoids or who have not responded to 6-mercaptopurine

or methotrexate. The median time to clinical response is 2 weeks. Infliximab induction therapy is generally given in a dosage of 5 mg/kg at 0, 2, and 6 weeks. Patients who respond may be treated with repeat infusions every 6–12 weeks to maintain remission with or without other therapies.

Adverse Effects

The most important adverse effect of infliximab therapy is infection due to suppression of the TH1 inflammatory response. Reactivation of latent tuberculosis, with dissemination, has occurred. Before administering infliximab, all patients must undergo purified protein derivative (PPD) testing; prophylactic therapy for tuberculosis is warranted for patients with positive test results. Other infections include pneumonia, sepsis, pneumocystosis, and listeriosis.

Infliximab infusions result in acute adverse infusion reactions in > 10% of patients, but discontinuation of the infusion is required in only 1%. Early reactions include fever, chills, pruritus, urticaria, or cardiopulmonary symptoms that include chest pain, dyspnea, or hemodynamic instability. Infusion reactions are more common with the second or subsequent infusions than with the first. Reactions may be reduced with prophylactic administration of acetaminophen and diphenhydramine.

An antibody directed at the murine epitope of infliximab may develop in patients. A delayed infusion reaction, which occurs 1–2 weeks after infusion, develops in approximately 5% patients who are re-treated with infliximab. Delayed infusion reaction is more common in patients with circulating anti-infliximab antibodies (20–30% of those getting multiple infusions) than in those without the antibodies. These reactions consist of myalgia; arthralgia; fever; rash; urticaria; and facial, hand, and lip edema. Delayed reactions respond to symptomatic treatment with antihistamines or corticosteroids. Positive antinuclear antibodies (ANA) and anti-dsDNA develop in a small number of patients. Development of a lupus-like syndrome has been reported that resolved after discontinuation of the drug.

Several malignancies have developed in patients who were treated with infliximab. However, the observed rates may be similar to those expected in patients with inflammatory bowel disease.

VIII. PANCREATIC ENZYME SUPPLEMENTS

Exocrine pancreatic insufficiency is most commonly caused by cystic fibrosis, chronic pancreatitis, or pancreatic resection. When secretion of pancreatic enzymes falls below 10% of normal, fat and protein maldigestion occur which can lead to steatorrhea, azotorrhea, vitamin malabsorption, and weight loss. Pancreatic enzyme supplements, which contain a mixture of amylase, lipase, and proteases, are the mainstay of treatment for pancreatic enzyme insufficiency. Two major types of preparations in use are **pancreatin** and **pancrelipase**. Pancreatin is an alcohol-derived extract of hog pancreas with relatively low concentrations of lipase and proteolytic enzymes, whereas pancrelipase is an enriched preparation. On a per weight basis, pancrelipase has approximately 12 times the lipolytic activity and more than 4 times the proteolytic activity of pancreatin. Consequently, pancreatin is no longer in common clinical use. Only pancrelipase will be discussed here.

Pancrelipase is available in both nonenteric-coated and enteric-coated preparations. Pancrelipase enzymes are rapidly and permanently inactivated by gastric acids. Therefore, nonenteric-coated preparations (eg, Cotazym, Viokase) should be given concomitantly with acid suppression therapy (proton pump inhibitor or H_2 antagonist) in order to reduce acid-mediated destruction within the stomach. Encapsulated formulations contain acid-resistant microspheres (Creon) or microtablets (Pancrease, Ultrase). Enteric-coated formulations are more commonly used because they do not require concomitant acid suppression therapy.

Pancrelipase preparations are administered with each meal and snack. Formulations are available in sizes containing varying amounts of lipase, amylase, and protease. However, manufacturers' listings of enzyme content do not always reflect true enzymatic activity. Dosing should be individualized according to the age and weight of the patient, the degree of pancreatic insufficiency, and the amount of dietary fat intake. Therapy is initiated at a dose that provides 30,000 units of lipase activity in the prandial and postprandial period—a level that is sufficient to reduce steatorrhea to a clinically insignificant level in most cases. Suboptimal response to enteric-coated formulations may be due to poor mixing of granules with food and/or slow dissolution and release of enzymes. Gradual increase of dose, change to a different formulation, or addition of acid suppression therapy may improve response.

Pancreatic enzyme supplements are well-tolerated. The capsules should be swallowed, not chewed, as pancreatic enzymes may cause oropharyngeal mucositis. Excessive doses may cause diarrhea and abdominal pain. The high purine content of pancreas extracts may lead to hyperuricosuria and renal stones. Several cases of colonic strictures were reported in patients with cystic fibrosis receiving high doses of pancrelipase with high lipase activity. These high dose formulations have since been removed from the market.

IX. BILE ACID THERAPY FOR GALLSTONES

Ursodiol (ursodeoxycholic acid) is a naturally occurring bile acid that makes up less than 5% of the circulating bile salt pool in humans and a much higher percentage in bears. After oral administration, it is absorbed, conjugated in the liver with glycine or taurine, and excreted in the bile. Conjugated ursodiol undergoes extensive enterohepatic recirculation. The serum half-life is approximately 100 hours. With long-term daily administration, ursodiol constitutes 30–50% of the circulating bile acid pool. A small amount of unabsorbed conjugated or unconjugated ursodiol passes into the colon where it is either excreted or undergoes dehydroxylation by colonic bacteria to lithocholic acid, a substance with potential hepatic toxicity.

Pharmacodynamics

Ursodiol is used for the dissolution of cholesterol gallstones. The solubility of cholesterol in bile is determined by the relative proportions of bile acids, lecithin, and cholesterol. Although prolonged ursodiol therapy expands the bile acid pool, this does not appear to be the principal mechanism of action for dissolution of gallstones. Ursodiol decreases the cholesterol content of bile by reducing hepatic cholesterol secretion. Ursodiol also appears to stabilize hepatocyte canalicular membranes, possibly through a reduction in the concentration of other endogenous bile acids or through inhibition of immune-mediated hepatocyte destruction.

Clinical Use

Ursodiol is used for dissolution of small cholesterol gallstones in patients with symptomatic gallbladder disease who refuse cholecystectomy or who are poor surgical candidates. At a dosage of 10 mg/kg/d for 12–24 months, dissolution occurs in up to half of patients with small (< 5–10 mm) noncalcified gallstones. It is also effective for the prevention of gallstones in obese patients undergoing rapid weight loss therapy. Several trials demonstrate that ursodiol 13–15 mg/kg/d is helpful for patients with early-stage primary biliary cirrhosis, reducing liver function abnormalities and improving liver histology.

Adverse Effects

Ursodiol is practically free of serious adverse effects. Bile salt-induced diarrhea is uncommon. Unlike its predecessor, chenodeoxycholate, ursodiol has not been associated with hepatotoxicity.

X. DRUGS USED TO TREAT VARICEAL HEMORRHAGE

Portal hypertension most commonly occurs as a consequence of chronic liver disease. Portal hypertension is caused by increased blood flow within the portal venous system and increased resistance to portal flow within the liver. Splanchnic blood flow is increased in patients with cirrhosis due to low arteriolar resistance that is mediated by increased circulating vasodilators and decreased vascular sensitivity to vasoconstrictors. Intrahepatic resistance to blood flow is increased in cirrhosis due to fixed fibrosis within the spaces of Disse and hepatic veins as well as reversible vasoconstriction of hepatic sinusoids and venules. Among the consequence of portal hypertension are ascites, hepatic encephalopathy, and the development of portosystemic collaterals—especially gastric or esophageal varices. Varices can rupture, leading to massive upper gastrointestinal bleeding.

Several drugs are available that reduce portal pressures. These may be used in the short term for the treatment of active variceal hemorrhage or long term to reduce the risk of hemorrhage.

SOMATOSTATIN & OCTREOTIDE

The pharmacology of octreotide is discussed above. In patients with cirrhosis and portal hypertension, intravenous somatostatin (250 µg/h) or octreotide (50 µg/h) reduces portal blood flow and variceal pressures; however, the mechanism by which they do so is poorly understood. They do not appear to induce direct contraction of vascular smooth muscle. Their activity may be mediated through inhibition of release of glucagon and other gut neuropeptides that alter mesenteric blood flow. Although data from clinical trials are conflicting, these agents are probably effective in promoting initial hemostasis from bleeding esophageal varices. They are generally administered for 3–5 days.

VASOPRESSIN & TERLIPRESSIN

Vasopressin (antidiuretic hormone) is a polypeptide hormone secreted by the hypothalamus and stored in the posterior pituitary. Its pharmacology is discussed in Chapters 17 and 37. Although its primary physiologic role is to maintain serum osmolality, it is also a potent arterial vasoconstrictor. When administered intra-venously by continuous infusion, it causes splanchnic arterial vasoconstriction that leads to reduced splanchnic perfusion and lowered portal venous pressures. Prior to the advent of octreotide, vasopressin was commonly used to treat acute variceal hemorrhage. However, because of its high side effect profile, it is no longer used for this purpose. However, for patients with acute gastrointestinal bleeding from small bowel or large bowel vascular ectasias or diverticulosis, vasopressin may be infused into one of the branches of the superior or inferior mesenteric artery through an angiographically placed catheter to promote vasospasm. Side effects with systemic vasopressin are common. Systemic and peripheral vasoconstriction can lead to hypertension, myocardial ischemia or infarction, or mesenteric infarction. These may be reduced by coadministration of nitroglycerin, which may further reduce portal venous pressures (by reducing portohepatic vascular resistance) and may also reduce the coronary and peripheral vascular vasospasm caused by vasopressin. Other common adverse effects are nausea, abdominal cramps and diarrhea (due to intestinal hyperactivity). Furthermore, the antidiuretic effects of vasopressin promote retention of free fluid which can lead to hyponatremia, fluid retention, and pulmonary edema.

Terlipressin is a vasopressin analog that appears to have similar efficacy to vasopressin with fewer adverse effects. This agent is undergoing clinical testing in the USA.

BETA-RECEPTOR BLOCKING DRUGS

The pharmacology of these agents is discussed in Chapter 10. Beta-receptor antagonists reduce portal venous pressures via a decrease in portal venous inflow. This decrease is due to a decrease in cardiac output (β_1 blockade) and to splanchnic vasoconstriction (β_2 blockade) caused by the unopposed effect of systemic catecholamines on α receptors. Thus, nonselective β blockers such as propranolol and nadolol are more effective than selective β_1 blockers in reducing portal pressures. Among patients with cirrhosis and esophageal varices who have not previously had an episode of variceal hemorrhage, the incidence of bleeding among patient treated with nonselective β blockers is 15% compared with 25% in control groups. Among patients with a history of variceal hemorrhage, the likelihood of recurrent hemorrhage is 80% within 2 years. Nonselective β blockers significantly reduce the rate of recurrent bleeding, although a reduction in mortality is unproved.

PREPARATIONS AVAILABLE

ANTACIDS
Aluminum hydroxide gel* (Amphojel, ALternaGEL, others)
Oral: 300, 500, 600 mg tablets; 400, 500 mg capsules; 320, 450, 675 mg/5 mL suspension
Calcium carbonate* (Tums, others)
Oral: 350, 420, 500, 600, 650, 750, 1000, 1250 mg chewable tablets; 1250 mg/5 mL suspension
Combination aluminum hydroxide and magnesium hydroxide preparations* (Maalox, Mylanta, Gaviscon, Gelusil, others)
Oral: 400 to 800 mg combined hydroxides per tablet, capsule, or 5 mL suspension

H₂ HISTAMINE RECEPTOR BLOCKERS
Cimetidine (generic, Tagamet, Tagamet HB*)
Oral: 100*, 200, 300, 400, 800 mg tablets; 300 mg/5 mL liquid
Parenteral: 300 mg/2 mL, 300 mg/50 mL for injection
Famotidine (generic, Pepcid, Pepcid AC*)
Oral: 10 mg tablets*, gelcaps*; 20, 40 mg tablets; powder to reconstitute for 40 mg/5 mL suspension
Parenteral: 10 mg/mL for injection
Nizatidine (Axid, Axid AR*)
Oral: 75 mg tablets*; 150, 300 mg capsules
Ranitidine (generic, Zantac, Zantac 75*)
Oral: 75*, 150, 300 mg tablets; 150 mg effervescent tablets; 150, 300 mg capsules; 15 mg/mL syrup
Parenteral: 1.0, 25 mg/mL for injection

SELECTED ANTICHOLINERGIC DRUGS
Atropine (generic)
Oral: 0.4 mg tablets
Parenteral: 0.05, 0.1, 0.3, 0.4, 0.5, 0.8, 1 mg/mL for injection
Belladonna alkaloids tincture (generic)
Oral: 0.27–0.33 mg/mL liquid
Dicyclomine (generic, Bentyl, others)
Oral: 10, 20 mg capsules; 20 mg tablets; 10 mg/5 mL syrup
Parenteral: 10 mg/mL for injection
Glycopyrrolate (generic, Robinul)
Oral: 1, 2 mg tablets
Parenteral: 0.2 mg/mL for injection
l-Hyoscyamine (Anaspaz, others)
Oral: 0.125, 0.15 mg tablets; 0.375 mg timed-release capsules; 0.125 mg/5 mL oral elixir and solution
Parenteral: 0.5 mg/mL for injection
Methscopolamine (Pamine)
Oral: 2.5 mg tablets

Propantheline (generic, Pro-Banthine)
Oral: 7.5, 15 mg tablets
Scopolamine (generic)
Oral: 0.4 mg tablets
Parenteral: 0.3, 0.4, 0.86, 1 mg/mL for injection
Tridihexethyl (Pathilon)
Oral: 25 mg tablets

PROTON PUMP INHIBITORS
Esomeprazole (Nexium)
Oral: 20, 40 mg delayed-release capsules
Omeprazole (Prilosec)
Oral: 10, 20, 40 mg delayed-release capsules
Lansoprazole (Prevacid)
Oral: 15, 30 mg delayed-release capsules; 15, 30 mg enteric-coated granules for oral suspension
Pantoprazole (Protonix)
Oral: 20, 40 mg delayed release tablets
Parenteral: 40 mg/vial powder for IV injection
Rabeprazole (Aciphex)
Oral: 20 mg delayed-release tablets

MUCOSAL PROTECTIVE AGENTS
Misoprostol (Cytotec)
Oral: 100, 200 μg tablets
Sucralfate (generic, Carafate)
Oral: 1 g tablets; 1 g/10 mL suspension

DIGESTIVE ENZYMES
Pancrelipase (Cotazym, Pancrease, Viokase, others)
Oral: Capsules, tablets, or powder containing lipase, protease, and amylase activity. See manufacturers' literature for details.

DRUGS FOR MOTILITY DISORDERS
& SELECTED ANTIEMETICS
Alosetron (Lotronex)
Oral: 1 mg tablets
Cisapride (Propulsid)
Available in the USA only from the manufacturer, 877-795-4247
Dolasetron (Anzemet)
Oral: 50, 100 mg tablets
Parenteral: 20 mg/mL for injection
Dronabinol (Marinol)
Oral: 2.5, 5, 10 mg capsules
Granisetron (Kytril)
Oral: 1 mg tablets
Parenteral: 1 mg/mL for injection
Metoclopramide (generic, Reglan, others)
Oral: 5, 10 mg tablets; 5 mg/5 mL syrup, 10 mg/mL concentrated solution
Parenteral: 5 mg/mL for injection

Ondansetron (Zofran)
Oral: 4, 8, 24 mg tablets; 4 mg/5 mL solution
Parenteral: 2 mg/mL for IV injection
Prochlorperazine (Compazine)
Oral: 5, 10, 25 mg tablets; 10, 15, 30 mg capsules;
1 mg/mL solution
Rectal: 2.5, 5, 25 mg suppositories
Parenteral: 5 mg/mL for injection
Tegaserod (Zelnorm)
Oral: 2, 6 mg tablets

Selected Anti-Inflammatory Drugs Used in Gastrointestinal Disease

Balsalazide (Colazal)
Oral: 750 mg capsules
Budesonide (Entocort)
Oral: 3 mg capsules
Hydrocortisone (Cortenema, Cortifoam)
Rectal: 100 mg/60 mL unit retention enema; 90
mg/applicatorful intrarectal foam
Mesalamine (5-ASA)
Oral: Asacol: 400 mg delayed-release tablets; Pentasa: 250 mg controlled-release capsules
Rectal: Rowasa: 4 g/60 mL suspension; 500 mg
suppositories
Methylprednisolone (Medrol Enpack)
Rectal: 40 mg/bottle retention enema
Olsalazine (Dipentum)
Oral: 250 mg capsules
Sulfasalazine (generic, Azulfidine, others)
Oral: 500 mg tablets and enteric-coated tablets
Infliximab (Remicade)
Parenteral: 100 mg powder for injection

Selected Antidiarrheal Drugs

Bismuth subsalicylate* (Pepto-Bismol, others)
Oral: 262 mg caplets, chewable tablets; 130, 262,
524 mg/15 mL suspension
Difenoxin (Motofen)
Oral: 1 mg (with 0.025 mg atropine sulfate) tablets
Diphenoxylate (generic, Lomotil, others)
Oral: 2.5 mg (with 0.025 mg atropine sulfate)
tablets and liquid
Kaolin/pectin* (generic, Kaopectate, others)
Oral (typical): 5.85 g kaolin and 260 mg pectin per
30 mL suspension

Loperamide* (generic, Imodium, others)
Oral: 2 mg tablets, capsules; 1 mg/5 mL liquid

Selected Laxative Drugs*

Bisacodyl (generic, Dulcolax, others)
Oral: 5 mg enteric-coated tablets
Rectal: 10 mg suppositories
Cascara sagrada (generic)
Oral: 325 mg tablets; 5 mL per dose fluid extract
(approximately 18% alcohol)
Castor oil (generic, others)
Oral: liquid or liquid emulsion
Docusate (generic, Colace, others)
Oral: 50, 100, 250 mg capsules; 100 mg tablets; 20,
50, 60, 150 mg/15 mL syrup
Glycerin liquid (Fleet Babylax)
Rectal liquid: 4 mL per applicator
Glycerin suppository (generic, Sani-Supp)
Lactulose (Chronulac, Cephulac)
Oral: 10 g/15 mL syrup
**Magnesium hydroxide [milk of magnesia,
Epsom Salt]** (generic)
Oral: 400, 800 mg/5 mL aqueous suspension
Methylcellulose
Oral: bulk powder
Mineral oil (generic, others)
Oral: liquid or emulsion
Polycarbophil (Equalactin, Mitrolan, FiberCon,
Fiber-Lax)
Oral: 500, 625 mg tablets; 500 mg chewable
tablets
Polyethylene glycol electrolyte solution (CoLyte,
GoLYTELY, others)
Oral: Powder for oral solution, makes one gallon
(approximately 4 L)
Psyllium (generic, Serutan, Metamucil, others)
Oral: 3.3, 3.4, 3.5, 4.03, 6 g psyllium granules or
powder per packet
Senna (Senokot, Ex•Lax, others)
Oral: 8.6, 15, 17, 25 mg tablets; 8.8, 15 mg/mL
liquid

Drugs that Dissolve Gallstones

Monoctanoin (Moctanin)
Parenteral: 120 mL bottle for bile duct perfusion
Ursodiol (Actigall)
Oral: 300 mg (Actigall) capsules

---

*Over-the-counter formulations.

REFERENCES

ACID-PEPTIC DISEASES

Chan FK, Leung WK: Peptic-ulcer disease. Lancet 2002;360:933.

Davies NM, Longstreth J, Jamali F: Misoprostol therapeutics revisited. Pharmacotherapy 2001;21:60.

Feldman M, Burton ME: Histamine2-receptor antagonists. Standard therapy for acid-peptic disorders. 1. N Engl J Med 1990;323:1672.

Gisbert J et al: Proton pump inhibitors versus H2-antagonists: a meta-analysis of their efficacy in treating bleeding peptic ulcer. Aliment Pharmacol Ther 2001;15:917.

Laine L et al: Potential gastrointestinal effects of long-term acid suppression with proton pump inhibitors. Aliment Pharmacol Ther 2000;14:651.

Laine L: Approaches to nonsteroidal anti-inflammatory drug use in the high-risk patient. Gastroenterology 2001;120:594.

Scott LJ et al: Esomeprazole: a review of its use in the management of acid-related disorders. Drugs 2002;62:1503.

Stedman CA, Barclay ML: Comparison of the pharmacokinetics, acid suppression and efficacy of proton pump inhibitors. Aliment Pharmacol Ther 2000;14:963.

Suerbaum S, Michetti P: Helicobacter pylori infection. N Engl J Med 2002;347:1175.

Wolfe WM, Sachs G: Acid suppression: optimizing therapy for gastroduodenal ulcer healing, gastroesophageal reflux disease, and stress-related erosive syndrome. Gastroenterology 2000; 118(2 Suppl 1):S9.

MOTILITY DISORDERS

Booth CM, Heyland DK, Paterson WG: Gastrointestinal promotility drugs in the critical care setting: a systemic review of the evidence. Crit Care Med 2002;30:1429.

Bytzer P: H(2) receptor antagonists and prokinetics in dyspepsia: a critical review. Gut 2002;50(Suppl 4):58.

Curry JI, Lander TD, Stringer MD: Erythromycin as a prokinetic agent in infants and children. Aliment Pharmacol Ther 2001;15:595.

De Giorgio R et al: The pharmacological treatment of acute colonic pseudo-obstruction. Aliment Pharmacol Ther 2001;15:1717.

Holte K, Kehlet H: Postoperative ileus: progress towards effective management. Drugs 2002;62:2603.

Quigley EM: Pharmacotherapy of gastroparesis. Expert Opin Pharmacother 2000;1:881.

LAXATIVES

Toledo TK, DiPalma JA: Colon cleansing preparation for gastrointestinal procedures. Aliment Pharmacol Ther 2001;15:605.

Schiller LR: The therapy of constipation. Aliment Pharmacol Ther 2001;15:749.

Van Gorkom BA et al: Anthranoid laxatives and their potential carcinogenic effects. Aliment Pharmacol Ther 1999;13:443.

Xing JH, Soffer EE: Adverse effects of laxatives. Dis Colon Rectum 2001;44:1201.

ANTIDIARRHEAL AGENTS

Farthing MG: Novel targets for the control of secretory diarrhea. Gut 2002;50(Suppl 3):III15.

Ramzan NN: Traveler's diarrhea. Gastroenterol Clin North Am 2001;30:665.

Ung KA et al: Role of bile acids and bile acid binding agents in patients with collagenous colitis. Gut 2000;46:170.

Wingate D et al: Guidelines for adults on self-medication for the treatment of acute diarrhoea. Aliment Pharmacol Ther 2001;15:773.

DRUGS USED FOR IRRITABLE BOWEL SYNDROME

American College of Gastroenterology Functional Gastrointestinal Task Force: An evidence-based position statement on the management of irritable bowel syndrome in North America. Am J Gastroenterol 2002;97:S1.

Camilleri M: Tegaserod. Aliment Pharmacol Ther 2001;15:277.

Drossman DA et al: AGA technical review on irritable bowel syndrome. Gastroenterology 2002;123:2108.

Gunput MD: Clinical pharmacology of alosetron. Aliment Pharmacol Ther 1999;13(Suppl 2):70.

Kamm MA: The complexity of drug development for irritable bowel syndrome. Aliment Pharmacol Ther 2002;16:343.

ANTIEMETIC AGENTS

Goodin S, Cunningham R: 5-HT$_3$-receptor antagonists for the treatment of nausea and vomiting: a reappraisal of their side-effect profile. Oncologist 2002;7:424.

Gralla RJ: New agents, new treatment, and antiemetic therapy. Semin Oncol 2002;29(Suppl 4):119.

Hesketh PJ: Comparative review of 5-HT$_3$ receptor antagonists in the treatment of acute chemotherapy-induced nausea and vomiting. Cancer Invest 2000;18:163.

Magee LA, Mazzotta P, Koren G: Evidence-based view of safety and effectiveness of pharmacologic therapy for nausea and vomiting of pregnancy (NVP). Am J Obstet Gynecol 2002; 185(Suppl):S256.

Tramer MR et al: Cannabinoids for control of chemotherapy-induced nausea and vomiting: quantitative systematic review. BMJ 2001;323:16.

Tramer MR: A rational approach to the control of postoperative nausea and vomiting: evidence from systematic reviews. Part I. Efficacy and harm of antiemetic interventions, and methodological issues. Acta Anaesthesiol Scand 2001;45:4.

Tramer MR: A rational approach to the control of postoperative nausea and vomiting: evidence from systematic reviews. Part II. Recommendations for prevention and treatment, and research agenda. Acta Anaesthesiol Scand 2001;45:14.

DRUGS USED FOR INFLAMMATORY BOWEL DISEASE

Blam ME, Stein RB, Lichtenstein GR: Integrating anti-tumor necrosis factor therapy in inflammatory bowel disease: current and future perspectives. Am J Gastroenterol 2001;96:1977.

De Vos M: Clinical pharmacokinetics of slow release mesalazine. Clin Pharmacokinet 2000;39:85.

Gionchetti P et al: Treatment of mild to moderate ulcerative colitis and pouchitis. Aliment Pharmacol Ther 2002;16(Suppl 4):13.

Kane SV et al: The effectiveness of budesonide therapy for Crohn's disease. Aliment Pharmacol Ther 2002;16:1509.

Klotz U: The role of aminosalicylates at the beginning of the new millennium in the treatment of chronic inflammatory bowel disease. Eur J Clin Pharmacol 2000;56:353.

Muijsers RB, Goa KL: Balsalazide: a review of its therapeutic use in mild-to-moderate ulcerative colitis. Drugs 2002;62:1689.

Nielsen OH, Vainer B, Rask-Madsen J: The treatment of inflammatory bowel disease with 6-mercaptopurine or azathioprine. Aliment Pharmacol Ther 2001;15:1699.

Plevy SE: Corticosteroid-sparing treatments in patients with Crohn's disease. Am J Gastroenterol 2002;97:1607.

Schwab M, Klotz U: Pharmacokinetic considerations in the treatment of inflammatory bowel disease. Clin Pharmacokinet 2001;40:723.

Vandell AG, DiPiro JT: Low-dosage methotrexate for treatment and maintenance of remission in patients with inflammatory bowel disease. Pharmacotherapy 2002;22:613.

PANCREATIC ENZYME SUPPLEMENTS

Greenberger NJ: Enzymatic therapy in patients with chronic pancreatitis. Gastroenterol Clin North Am 1999;28:687.

Stern RC et al: A comparison of the efficacy and tolerance of pancrelipase and placebo in the treatment of steatorrhea in cystic fibrosis patients with clinical exocrine pancreatic insufficiency. Am J Gastroenterol 2000;95:1932.

BILE ACIDS FOR GALLSTONE THERAPY

Crosignani A et al: Clinical pharmacokinetics of therapeutic bile acids. Clin Pharmacokinet 1996;30:333.

Gluud C, Christensen E: Ursodeoxycholic acid for primary biliary cirrhosis. Cochrane Database Syst Rev 2002;(1):CD000551.

Krowdley KV: Ursodeoxycholic acid therapy in hepatobiliary disease. Am J Med 2000;108:481.

Paumgartner G, Beuers U: Ursodeoxycholic acid in cholestatic liver disease: mechanisms of action and therapeutic use revisited. Hepatology 2002;36:525.

DRUGS FOR PORTAL HYPERTENSION

Corley D et al: Octreotide for acute esophageal variceal bleeding: a meta-analysis. Gastroenterology 2001;120:946.

D'Amico G, Pagliaro L, Bosch J: Pharmacological treatment of portal hypertension: an evidence-based approach. Semin Liver Dis 1999;19:475.

Garcia-Tsao G: Current management of the complications of cirrhosis and portal hypertension: variceal hemorrhage, ascites, and spontaneous bacterial peritonitis. Gastroenterology 2001;120:726.

Gotzsche PC: Somatostatin analogues for acute bleeding esophageal varices. Cochrane Database Syst Rev 2002;(1):CD000193.

Ioannou G, Doust J, Rockey DC: Terlipressin for acute esophageal variceal hemorrhage. Cochrane Database Syst Rev 2001;(1):CD002147.

Lebrec D: Drug therapy for portal hypertension. Gut 2001;49:441.

Lui HG et al: Primary prophylaxis of variceal hemorrhage: a randomized controlled trial comparing band ligation, propranolol, and isosorbide mononitrate. Gastroenterology 2002; 123:735.

Therapeutic & Toxic Potential of Over-the-Counter Agents

64

Robin L. Corelli, PharmD

In the USA, drugs are divided by law into two classes: those restricted to sale by prescription only and those for which directions for safe use by the public can be written. The latter category constitutes the nonprescription or over-the-counter (OTC) drugs. In 2001, the American public spent approximately $18 billion on over 125,000 OTC products to medicate themselves for ailments ranging from acne to warts. These products contain approximately 1000 active ingredients in various forms and combinations.

It is apparent that many OTC drugs are no more than "me too" products advertised to the public in ways that suggest that there are significant differences between them. For example, there are over 100 different systemic analgesic products, almost all of which contain aspirin, acetaminophen, nonsteroidal antiinflammatory drugs (NSAIDs) such as ibuprofen, or a combination of these agents as primary ingredients. They are made different from one another by the addition of questionable ingredients such as caffeine or antihistamines; by brand names chosen to suggest a specific use or strength ("women's," "migraine," "arthritis," "maximum"); or by special dosage formulations (enteric-coated tablets, geltabs, liquids, sustained-release products, powders, seltzers). There is a price attached to all of these features, and in most cases a less expensive generic product can be equally effective. It is probably safe to assume that the public is generally overwhelmed and confused by the wide array of products presented and will probably use those that are most heavily advertised.

Since 1972, the Food and Drug Administration (FDA) has been engaged in a methodical review of OTC ingredients for both safety and efficacy. There have been two major outcomes of this review: (1) Ingredients designated as ineffective or unsafe for their claimed therapeutic use are being eliminated from OTC product formulations (eg, antimuscarinic agents have been eliminated from OTC sleep aids); and (2) Agents previously available by prescription only have been made available for OTC use because they were judged by the review panel to be generally safe and effective for consumer use without medical supervision (Table 64–1). Since the appointment of the Nonprescription Drugs Advisory Committee in 1993, the rate of switches from prescription to OTC status has accelerated. Indeed, more than 700 OTC products contain ingredients and dosages that were available only by prescription less than 30 years ago. Some agents such as docosanol and the nicotine polacrilex lozenge have bypassed the prescription route altogether and have been released directly to the OTC market. Other OTC ingredients previously available in low doses only are now available in higher-strength formulations. Examples of other prescription drugs currently under consideration for OTC reclassification include cyclobenzaprine, sucralfate, nonsedating antihistamines (cetirizine, fexofenadine), and topical penciclovir. The prescription to OTC reclassification process is very rigorous, and many agents have not been approved for OTC use. For example, the cholesterol-lowering agents cholestyramine, lovastatin, and pravastatin were denied OTC status on the basis that these agents could not be used safely and effectively in an OTC setting. The advisory committee believed that diagnosis and ongoing management by a health care provider was necessary for the management of hyperlipidemia, a chronic, asymptomatic condition with potentially life-threatening consequences. In a similar recommendation, oral acyclovir for OTC use in the treatment of recurrent genital herpes was not approved because of concerns about misdiagnosis and inappropriate use leading to increased viral resistance.

There are three reasons why it is essential for clinicians to be familiar with this class of products. First, many OTC medications are effective in treating common ailments, and it is important to be able to help the patient select a safe, effective product. Because managed care practices encourage clinicians to limit the cost of drugs they prescribe, many will begin to recommend effective OTC treatments to their patients, since these drugs are rarely paid for by the insurance plan. (See Table 64–2.) Second, many of the active ingredients contained in OTC

Table 64–1. Selected agents switched from prescription to OTC status by the Food and Drug Administration.

Ingredient	Indication	Year Ingredient First Switched	Single-Ingredient Product Examples
Systemic agents			
Brompheniramine	Antihistamine	1976	Dimetapp[1]
Chlorpheniramine	Antihistamine	1976	Chlor-Trimeton
Cimetidine	Acid reducer	1995	Tagamet HB
Clemastine	Antihistamine	1992	Tavist Allergy
Dexbrompheniramine	Antihistamine	1982	Drixoral Cold & Allergy[2]
Diphenhydramine	Antihistamine, sleep aid	1981	Benadryl Allergy, Sominex, Nytol
Doxylamine	Sleep aid, antihistamine	1978	Unisom
Famotidine	Acid reducer	1995	Pepcid AC
Ibuprofen	Analgesic, antipyretic	1984	Advil, Motrin IB, Nuprin
Ketoprofen	Analgesic, antipyretic	1995	Orudis KT
Loperamide	Antidiarrheal	1988	Imodium A-D
Loratadine	Antihistamine	2002	Claritin, Alavert
Naproxen sodium	Analgesic, antipyretic	1994	Aleve
Nicotine polacrilex (gum)	Smoking cessation	1996	Nicorette
Nicotine transdermal system	Smoking cessation	1996	Nicotrol, Nicoderm CQ
Nizatidine	Acid reducer	1996	Axid AR
Omeprazole	Acid reducer	2003	Prilosec OTC
Phenylpropanolamine	Nasal decongestant	1981	Not applicable[3]
Pseudoephedrine	Nasal decongestant	1976	Sudafed
Pyrantel pamoate	Anthelmintic (pinworm)	1986	Pin-X, Antiminth
Ranitidine	Acid reducer	1995	Zantac 75
Triprolidine	Antihistamine	1982	Actifed[4]
Topical agents			
Butenafine	Antifungal (topical)	2001	Lotrimin Ultra
Butoconazole	Antifungal (vaginal)	1995	Femstat-3, Mycelex-3
Clotrimazole	Antifungal (topical)	1989	Lotrimin AF, Mycelex
Clotrimazole	Antifungal (vaginal)	1990	Gyne-Lotrimin, Mycelex-7, Gyne-Lotrimin-3
Cromolyn	Nasal antiallergy	1997	Nasalcrom
Hydrocortisone	Antipruritic	1979	Cortaid, Cortizone
Ketoconazole	Dandruff shampoo	1997	Nizoral AD

Table 64–1. Selected agents switched from prescription to OTC status by the Food and Drug Administration *(continued).*

Ingredient	Indication	Year Ingredient First Switched	Single-Ingredient Product Examples
Topical agents *(cont'd)*			
Miconazole	Antifungal (topical)	1982	Micatin
Miconazole	Antifungal (vaginal)	1991	Monistat-7, Monistat-3
Minoxidil	Hair growth stimulant	1996	Rogaine Regular and Extra Strength For Men, Rogaine For Women
Naphazoline/antazoline	Ophthalmic decongestant-antihistamine	1994	Vasocon A
Naphazoline/pheniramine	Ophthalmic decongestant-antihistamine	1994	Naphcon A, Opcon A, Ocuhist
Oxymetazoline	Nasal decongestant	1976	Neo-Synephrine 12 Hour, Afrin 12 Hour
Permethrin	Pediculicide (head lice)	1990	Nix
Terbinafine	Antifungal (topical)	1999	Lamisil AT
Tioconazole	Antifungal (vaginal)	1997	Vagistat-1
Xylometazoline	Nasal decongestant	1976	Otrivin

[1] No single ingredient product available (brompheniramine/pseudoephedrine combination).

[2] No single ingredient product available (dexbrompheniramine/pseudoephedrine combination).

[3] Products containing phenylpropanolamine were withdrawn from the US market in 2000 based on reports of an increased risk of hemorrhagic stroke in patients using this agent.

[4] No single ingredient product available (triprolidine/pseudoephedrine combination).

drugs may worsen existing medical conditions or interact with prescription medications. (See Appendix II, Drug Interactions.) Finally, the misuse or abuse of OTC products may actually produce significant medical complications. Phenylpropanolamine, for example, a sympathomimetic previously found in many cold, allergy, and weight control products, was withdrawn from the United States market by the FDA in 2000 based on reports that the drug increased the risk of hemorrhagic stroke. A general awareness of these products and their formulations will enable clinicians to more fully appreciate the potential for OTC drug-related problems in their patients.

Table 64–2 lists examples of OTC products that may be used effectively to treat common medical problems. The selection of one ingredient over another may be important in patients with certain medical conditions or in patients taking other medications. These are discussed in detail in other chapters. The recommendations listed in Table 64–2 are based upon the efficacy of the ingredients and on the principles set forth in the following paragraphs.

(1) Select the product that is simplest in formulation with regard to ingredients and dosage form. In general, single-ingredient products are preferred. Although some combination products contain effective doses of all ingredients, others contain therapeutic doses of some ingredients and subtherapeutic doses of others. Furthermore, there may be differing durations of action among the ingredients, and there is always a possibility that the clinician or patient will be unaware of the presence of certain active ingredients in the product. Acetaminophen, for example, is present in many cough and cold preparations; a patient unaware of this may take separate doses of analgesic in addition to that contained in the cold preparation, potentially leading to toxicity.

(2) Select a product that contains a therapeutically effective dose.

(3) Carefully read the product labeling to determine which ingredients are appropriate based on the patient's symptoms and underlying health conditions and whatever is known about the medications the patient is already taking. (Text continues on page 1072.)

Table 64–2. Ingredients of known efficacy for selected over-the-counter (OTC) classes.

OTC Category	Ingredient and Usual Adult Dosage	Product Examples	Comments
Acid reducers, H$_2$ antagonists	Cimetidine, 200 mg once or twice daily	Tagamet HB	These products have been approved at lower than prescription doses for the relief of "heartburn, acid indigestion, and sour stomach." They should not be taken for longer than 2 weeks and are not recommended for children under 12 years of age.
	Famotidine, 10 mg once or twice daily	Pepcid AC	
	Nizatidine, 75 mg once or twice daily	Axid AR	
	Ranitidine, 75 mg once or twice daily	Zantac 75	
Acid reducers, Proton pump inhibitors	Omeprazole magnesium, 20.6 mg once daily for 14 days	Prilosec OTC	Omeprazole is the first proton pump inhibitor approved for the treatment of frequent heartburn in adults with symptoms of heartburn 2 or more days per week. The product should not be taken for more than 14 days or more often than every 4 months unless directed by a physician. Omeprazole magnesium 20.6 mg is equivalent to 20 mg of omeprazole (prescription strength).
Acne preparations	Benzoyl peroxide, 2.5%, 5%, 10%	Clearasil, Fostex, Oxy-5, Oxy-10, various generic	One of the most effective acne preparations. Apply sparingly once or twice daily. Decrease dose if excessive skin irritation occurs.
Allergy and "cold" preparations	Chlorpheniramine, 4 mg every 4–6 hours; 8–12 mg (extended release) every 8–12 hours	Chlor-Trimeton Allergy 4 Hour, Chlor-Trimeton Allergy 12 Hour, various generic	Antihistamines alone relieve most symptoms associated with allergic rhinitis or hay fever. Chlorpheniramine, brompheniramine, and clemastine cause less drowsiness than diphenhydramine and doxylamine. Loratadine, a second-generation antihistamine, was recently approved for OTC use; therapeutically comparable to first-generation agents but with a much lower incidence of sedation. Occasionally, symptoms unrelieved by the antihistamine respond to the addition of a sympathomimetic.
	Brompheniramine, 4 mg every 4–6 hours; 12 mg (extended release) every 12 hours	Dimetane Extentabs, Dimetapp Allergy, various generic	
	Clemastine 1.34 mg every 12 hours	Tavist Allergy	
	Diphenhydramine, 25–50 mg every 6–8 hours	Benadryl Allergy, various generic	
	Loratadine (10 mg) every 24 hours	Alavert, Claritin	
	Chlorpheniramine (2–4 mg) with pseudoephedrine (30–60 mg) every 4–6 hours	Allerest Maximum Strength, Sudafed Cold & Allergy, various generic	
	Diphenhydramine (25 mg) with pseudoephedrin (60 mg) every 4–6 hours	Benadryl Allergy/Sinus, various generic	
	Loratadine (10 mg with pseudoephedrine (240 mg) every 24 hours	Claritin-D 24 Hour	
	Triprolidine (2.5 mg) with pseudoephedrine (60 mg) every 4–6 hours	Actifed, various generic	

(continued)

Table 64–2. Ingredients of known efficacy for selected over-the-counter (OTC) classes *(continued)*.

OTC Category	Ingredient and Usual Adult Dosage	Product Examples	Comments
Analgesics and antipyretics	Acetaminophen, 325–650 mg every 4–6 hours	Panadol, Tylenol, various generic	There are numerous product modifications, including the addition of antacids and caffeine; enteric-coated tablets and seltzers; long-acting or extra-strength formulations; and various mixtures of analgesics. None have any substantial advantage over a single-ingredient product. Acetaminophen lacks anti-inflammatory activity but is available as a liquid; this dosage form is used primarily for infants and children who cannot chew or swallow tablets. Do not exceed a total daily acetaminophen dose of 4 grams (2 grams/day in regular alcohol users. Aspirin should be used cautiously in certain individuals (see text). Use of OTC products containing aspirin, other salicylates, acetaminophen, ibuprofen, naproxen, or ketoprofen may increase the risk of hepatotoxicity and gastrointestinal hemorrhage in individuals who consume three or more alcoholic drinks daily.
	Aspirin, 325–650 mg every 4–6 hours	Bayer Aspirin, Ecotrin, Bufferin, various generic	
	Ibuprofen, 200–400 mg every 4–6 hours (not to exceed 1200 mg daily)	Advil, Motrin IB, Nuprin, various generic	
	Ketoprofen, 12.5 mg every 4–6 hours	Orudis KT	
	Naproxen sodium, 220 mg every 8–12 hours	Aleve	
Antacids	Magnesium hydroxide and aluminum hydroxide alone or in combination; calcium carbonate, dosage varies; consult product labeling	Amphojel, Maalox, Milk of Magnesia, Mylanta, Tums, various generic	Combinations of magnesium and aluminum hydroxide are less likely to cause constipation or diarrhea and offer high neutralizing capacity. Some preparations include simethicone, an antiflatulent to relieve symptoms of bloating and pressure.
Anthelmintics (pinworm infection)	Pyrantel pamoate, 11 mg/kg (maximum: 1 g)	Antiminth, Pin-X, Reese's Pinworm	Treat all members of the household. Consult physician for children under age 2 years or under 25 lb. Undergarments, pajamas and linens should be washed daily until the infection is resolved.
Antidiarrheal agents	Attapulgite, 1200 mg after each loose bowel movement up to 7 doses daily	Donnagel, Kaopectate, Parepectolin, various generic	Antidiarrheals should not be used if diarrhea is accompanied by fever > 101°F or if blood or mucus is present in stool.
	Bismuth subsalicylate, 524 mg every 30–60 minutes as needed up to 8 doses daily	Pepto-Bismol, various generic	Bismuth salts can cause dark discoloration of the tongue and stools. Salicylates are absorbed and can cause tinnitus if coadministered with aspirin.
	Loperamide, 4 mg initially, then 2 mg after each loose stool, not to exceed 8 mg daily	Imodium A-D	A synthetic opioid that acts on intestinal smooth muscle to decrease motility allowing for absorption of water and electrolytes. Poorly penetrates the CNS and has a lower risk of side effects compared to diphenoxylate or opiates. Not considered a controlled substance.
Antifungal topical preparations	Butenafine, 1% (cream) apply to affected areas once daily	Lotrimin Ultra	Effective for the treatment of tinea pedis (athlete's foot), tinea cruris (jock itch), and tinea corporis (ringworm). Clotrimazole and miconazole also effective against *Candida albicans*.

Table 64–2. Ingredients of known efficacy for selected over-the-counter (OTC) classes *(continued)*.

OTC Category	Ingredient and Usual Adult Dosage	Product Examples	Comments
Antifungal topical preparations *(continued)*	Clotrimazole, 1% (cream, lotion, solution), apply to affected areas twice daily	Lotrimin AF Cream/Lotion/Solution, Mycelex OTC	
	Miconazole, 2% (cream, powder, solution), apply to affected areas twice daily	Lotrimin AF Powder/Spray, Micatin, Zeasorb-AF	
	Terbinafine, 1% (cream), apply to affected areas once or twice daily	Lamisil AT	
	Tolnaftate, 1% (cream, powder, solution), apply to affected areas twice daily	Aftate, Tinactin, Ting, various generic	
	Undecylenic acid, 10–25% (powder, spray powder, cream, liquid) apply to affected areas twice daily	Cruex, Desenex, various generic	
Antifungal vaginal preparations	Butoconazole, 2% cream, one applicatorful intravaginally at bedtime for 3 consecutive days	Femstat-3, Mycelex-3	Topical vaginal antifungals should only be used for treatment of recurrent vulvovaginal candidiasis previously diagnosed by a clinician in otherwise healthy, nonpregnant women.
	Clotrimazole (1%, 2% vaginal cream, 100 mg, 200 mg tablet); see comments for dosage	Gyne-Lotrimin, Mycelex-7, Gyne-Lotrimin-3, various generic	Insert one applicatorful (1%) or one tablet (100 mg) intravaginally at bedtime for 7 consecutive days. Alternatively: Insert one applicatorful (2%) or one tablet (200 mg), intravaginally at bedtime for 3 consecutive days.
	Miconazole (2%, 4% vaginal cream; 100 mg, 200 mg vaginal suppositories); see comments for dosage	Monistat-7, Monistat-3	Insert one applicatorful intravaginally at bedtime for 7 consecutive days (2%) or 3 consecutive days (4%). Alternatively: insert one suppository intravaginally at bedtime for 7 consecutive days (100 mg) or 3 consecutive days (200 mg).
	Tioconazole, 6.5% vaginal ointment, one applicatorful intravaginally at bedtime (single-dose)	Monistat-1, Vagistat-1	
Anti-inflammatory topical preparations	Hydrocortisone, 0.5% (cream, ointment, lotion), 1% (cream ointment, lotion, spray)	Anusol HC, Cortaid, Cortizone-5, Cortizone-10, various generic	Used to temporarily relieve itching and inflammation associated with minor rashes due to contact or allergic dermatitides, insect bites, and hemorrhoids. Apply sparingly to affected areas two to four times daily.

(continued)

Table 64–2. Ingredients of known efficacy for selected over-the-counter (OTC) classes *(continued)*.

OTC Category	Ingredient and Usual Adult Dosage	Product Examples	Comments
Antiseborrheal agents	Coal tar, 0.5-15% shampoo, dosage varies; consult product labeling	Denorex, Ionil T Plus, Tegrin, Zetar, various generic	Tar derivatives inhibit epidermal proliferation and may possess antipruritic and antimicrobial activity.
	Ketoconazole, 1% shampoo, apply every 3–4 days	Nizoral A-D	Synthetic azole antifungal agent with activity versus *Pityrosporum ovale,* a fungus that may cause seborrhea and dandruff. Massage over entire scalp for 3 minutes. Rinse thoroughly and repeat application.
	Pyrithione zinc, 1–2% shampoo, apply once or twice weekly	Denorex, Head & Shoulders, Sebulon, various generic	Both selenium sulfide and zinc pyrithione are cytostatic agents that decrease epidermal turnover rates. Massage into wet scalp for 2–3 minutes. Rinse thoroughly and repeat application. Selenium sulfide can be irritating to the eyes and skin.
	Selenium sulfide, 1% shampoo, apply once or twice weekly	Head & Shoulders Intensive Treatment, Selsun Blue, various generic	
Antitussives	Codeine, 10–20 mg every 4–6 hours (with guaifenesin)	Robitussin A-C, Guiatuss AC, various generic	Acts centrally to increase the cough threshold. In doses required for cough suppression, the addictive liability associated with codeine is low. Many codeine-containing antitussive combinations are schedule V narcotics, and OTC sale is restricted in some states.
	Dextromethorphan, 10–20 mg every 4 hours or 30 mg every 6–8 hours	Benylin Adult Formula Cough, Hold DM, Vicks 44 Cough Relief, various generic	Dextromethorphan is a nonopioid congener of levorphanol without analgesic or addictive properties. Often is used with antihistamines, decongestants, and expectorants in combination products.
Decongestants, topical	Oxymetazoline, 0.05% nasal solution, 2–3 sprays per nostril every 10–12 hours	Afrin, Dristan 12 Hour Nasal, Neo-Synephrine 12 Hour, various generic	Topical sympathomimetics are effective for the temporary acute management of rhinorrhea associated with common colds and allergies. Long-acting agents (oxymetazoline and xylometazoline) are generally preferred, though phenylephrine is equally effective. Topical decongestants should not be used for longer than 3 days to prevent rebound nasal congestion.
	Phenylephrine (0.125%, 0.25%, 0.5%, 1%), nasal solution, 2–3 sprays/drops per nostril every 3–4 hours	Neo-Synephrine, various generic	
	Xylometazoline (0.05%, 0.1%), nasal solution, 2–3 sprays/drops per nostril every 8–10 hours	Otrivin	

Table 64–2. Ingredients of known efficacy for selected over-the-counter (OTC) classes *(continued).*

OTC Category	Ingredient and Usual Adult Dosage	Product Examples	Comments
Decongestants, systemic	Phenylephrine, 10 mg every 4 hours	Novahistine Elixir, various generic combination products	Oral decongestants have a prolonged duration of action but may cause more systemic effects, including nervousness, excitability, restlessness, and insomnia. Also available in antihistamine, antitussive, expectorant, and analgesic combination products. Phenylephrine is unpredictably absorbed from the gastrointestinal tract.
	Pseudoephedrine, 60 mg every 4–6 hours or 120 mg (extended release) every 12 hours	Sudafed, various generic	
Expectorants	Guaifenesin, 100–400 mg every 4 hours	Robitussin, various generic	The only OTC expectorant recognized as safe and effective by the FDA. Often used with antihistamines, decongestants, and antitussives in combination products.
Hair growth stimulants	Minoxidil, 2%, 5% solution, apply 1 mL to affected areas of scalp twice daily.	Rogaine for Men, Rogaine for Women, Rogaine Extra Strength for Men	Minoxidil appears to directly stimulate hair follicles resulting in increased hair thickness and reduced hair loss. Treatment for four months or longer may be necessary to achieve visible results. If new hair growth is observed, continued treatment is necessary as hair density returns to pretreatment levels within months following drug discontinuation.
Laxatives	Bulk formers: Polycarbophil, psyllium and methylcellulose preparations. Dosage varies; consult product labeling	Citrucel, Equalactin, Konsyl, Metamucil, Perdiem, various generic	The safest laxatives for chronic use include the bulk formers and stool softeners. Saline laxatives and stimulants may be used acutely but not chronically (see text). Bulk formers hold water and expand in stool, promoting peristalsis.
	Stool softeners: Docusate sodium, 50–500 mg daily Docusate calcium, 240 mg daily	Colace, Surfak, various generic	Soften fecal material via detergent action that allows water to penetrate stool.
	Stimulant laxatives: Bisacodyl, 5–15 mg daily. Senna: dosage varies, consult product labeling	Correctol, Dulcolax, Ex-Lax, Senokot, various generic	Stimulant laxative actions include direct irritation of intestinal mucosa or stimulation of the myenteric plexus, resulting in peristalsis. These agents may also cause alteration of fluid and electrolyte absorption, resulting in luminal fluid accumulation and bowel evacuation.
Pediculicides (head lice)	Permethrin 1%	Nix	Instructions for use varies; consult product labeling. Avoid contact with eyes. Comb out nits. Linens, pajamas, combs, and brushes should be washed daily until the infestation is eliminated. Repeat application 7 days later if live nits are still visible.
	Pyrethrins (0.3%) combined with piperonyl butoxide (3–4%)	A-200, RID	

(continued)

Table 64–2. Ingredients of known efficacy for selected over-the-counter (OTC) classes *(continued)*.

OTC Category	Ingredient and Usual Adult Dosage	Product Examples	Comments
Sleep aids	Diphenhydramine, 25–50 mg at bedtime	Compoz, Nytol, Sominex, various generic	Diphenhydramine and doxylamine are antihistamines with well-documented CNS depressant effects. Because insomnia may be indicative of a serious underlying condition requiring medical attention, patients should consult a physician if insomnia persists continuously for longer than 2 weeks.
	Doxylamine, 25 mg at bedtime	Unisom, various generic	
Smoking cessation aids	Nicotine (transdermal patch), dosage varies; consult product labeling	Nicoderm CQ, Nicotrol, various generic	Nicotine replacement products in combination with behavioral support approximately double abstinence rates compared to placebo. Review directions for use carefully, since product strengths vary and self-titration and tapering may be necessary.
	Nicotine polacrilex gum or lozenge; dosage varies; consult product labeling	Nicorette, Commit, various generic	

(4) Recommend a generic product if one is available.

(5) Be wary of "gimmicks" or advertising claims of specific superiority over similar products.

(6) For children, the dose, dosage form, and palatability of the product will be prime considerations.

Certain ingredients in OTC products should be avoided or used with caution in selected patients because they may exacerbate existing medical problems or interact with other medications the patient is taking. Many of the more potent OTC ingredients are hidden in products where their presence would not ordinarily be expected (Table 64–3). While most OTC medications are clearly labeled with the specific ingredients contained in the product, many products do not presently conform to the new FDA-mandated standardized OTC medication labeling requirements that are being phased in through 2005. Lack of awareness of the ingredients present in OTC products and the belief by many physicians that OTC products are ineffective and harmless may cause diagnostic confusion and perhaps interfere with therapy. For example, innumerable OTC products, including analgesics and allergy, cough, and cold preparations, contain sympathomimetics. These agents should be avoided or used cautiously by type 1 diabetics and patients with hypertension, angina, or hyperthyroidism. Aspirin should not be used in children and adolescents for viral infections (with or without fever) because of an increased risk of Reye's syndrome. Aspirin and other NSAIDs should be avoided by individuals with active peptic ulcer disease, certain platelet disorders, and patients taking oral anticoagulants.

Cimetidine, an H_2-receptor antagonist, is a well-known inhibitor of hepatic drug metabolism and can increase the blood levels and toxicity of drugs such as phenytoin, theophylline, and warfarin.

Overuse or misuse of OTC products may induce significant medical problems. A prime example is rebound congestion from the regular use of decongestant nasal sprays for more than 3 days. The improper and chronic use of some antacids (eg, aluminum hydroxide) may cause constipation and even impaction in elderly people, as well as hypophosphatemia. Laxative abuse can result in abdominal cramping and fluid and electrolyte disturbances. Insomnia, nervousness, and restlessness can result from the use of sympathomimetics or caffeine hidden in many OTC products (Table 64–3). The chronic systemic use of some analgesics containing large amounts of caffeine may produce rebound headaches, and long-term use of analgesics has been associated with interstitial nephritis. Recent evidence suggests that use of OTC products containing aspirin, other salicylates, acetaminophen, ibuprofen, naproxen, or ketoprofen may increase the risk of hepatotoxicity and gastrointestinal hemorrhage in individuals who consume three or more alcoholic drinks daily. Furthermore, acute ingestion of large amounts of aspirin or acetaminophen by adults or children can cause serious toxicity. Antihistamines may cause sedation or drowsiness, especially when taken concurrently with sedative-hypnotics, tranquilizers, alcohol, or other central nervous system depressants. Finally, antihistamines, local anesthetics, antimicrobial agents, counterirritants, *p*-aminobenzoic acid (PABA) and preservatives contained in a myriad of OTC topical and vaginal products may induce allergic reactions.

Table 64–3. Hidden ingredients in over-the-counter (OTC) products.

Hidden Drug or Drug Class	OTC Class Containing Drug	Product Examples
Alcohol (percent ethanol)	Cough syrups, cold preparations	Cheracol Plus (5%) Comtrex Multi-Symptom Cold & Cough Relief (10%) Vicks 44M (10%) Vicks NyQuil Liquid (10%)
	Mouthwashes	Cepacol Mouthwash (14%) Listerine (27%) Scope (15%)
Antihistamines	Analgesics	Aspirin Free Anacin PM Aspirin Free Excedrin PM Extra Strength Bayer PM Percogesic Extra Strength Tylenol PM Tylenol Severe Allergy
	Menstrual products	Midol PM Maximum Strength Midol Menstrual Maximum Strength Midol PMS Maximum Strength Multi-Symptom Pamprin Menstrual Relief Premsyn PMS
	Sleep aids	Compoz Nytol Sominex Twilite Caplets Unisom
Aspirin and other salicylates	Antidiarrheals	Pepto-Bismol (bismuth subsalicylate)
	Cold/allergy preparations	Alka-Seltzer Plus Cold & Cough Liqui-Gels BC Allergy Sinus Cold Powder
Caffeine	Analgesics	Alka-Seltzer Morning Relief Anacin Cope Excedrin Extra Strength Excedrin Migraine Goody's Extra Strength Fast Relief Goody's Extra Strength Headache Powder Vanquish
	Menstrual products	Maximum Strength Midol Menstrual
	Stimulants	Lucidex NoDoz Vivarin

(continued)

Table 64–3. Hidden ingredients in over-the-counter (OTC) products *(continued).*

Hidden Drug or Drug Class	OTC Class Containing Drug	Product Examples
Local anesthetics (usually benzocaine)	Antitussives/Lozenges	Cepacol Maxium Strength Lozenges Spec T Sore Throat/Cough Suppressant Vicks Chloraseptic Lozenges
	Dermatologic preparations	Americaine Bactine Dermoplast Lanacane Solarcaine
	Hemorrhoidal products	Americaine Anusol Ointment Medicone Tronolane
	Toothache, cold sore, and teething products	(Many) Anbesol Baby Orajel Kank-A Orabase B Zilactin-B
Sodium (mg/tablet or mg/5 mL or as stated)	Analgesics	Alka-Seltzer Original Effervescent Tablet (568) Alka-Seltzer Extra Strength Effervescent Tablet (588) Bromo-Seltzer Granules (959/pre-measured packet)
	Antacids	Alka-Seltzer Original Effervescent Tablet (568) Alka-Seltzer Extra Strength Effervescent Tablet (588) Alka-Seltzer Gold (299) Alka-Seltzer Heartburn Relief (569) Bromo-Seltzer Granules (959/pre-measured packet) Citrocarbonate Effervescent Granules (780/ teaspoon)
	Laxatives	Fleets Enema (4,439 mg, of which 275–400 mg/enema is absorbed) Fleet Phospho-Soda (554/teaspoon)
Sympathomimetics	Analgesics	Motrin Sinus Headache Sinarest No Drowsiness Sine-Aid Sinus Headache Tablets Sinutab Tylenol Flu Day Non-Drowsy Tylenol Sinus Day Non-Drowsy
	Asthma products	Bronkaid Dual Action Primatene
	Cold/allergy preparations	(Many) Advil Cold and Sinus Alka-Seltzer Plus Comtrex Maximum Strength Day and Night Flu Contac Severe Cold and Flu Dimetapp Cold & Allergy PediaCare Cold & Allergy Motrin Cold & Flu Sudafed

Table 64–3. Hidden ingredients in over-the-counter (OTC) products *(continued).*

Hidden Drug or Drug Class	OTC Class Containing Drug	Product Examples
Sympathomimetics *(continued)*	Cold/allergy preparations *(continued)*	TheraFlu Severe Cold & Congestion Triaminic Chest Congestion Vicks 44M Vicks DayQuil Vicks NyQuil
	Cough preparations	(Many) PediaCare Long Lasting Cough Plus Cold Robitussin PM Cold & Cough Robitussin Maximum Strength Cough & Cold Triaminic Cough Vicks 44D
	Hemorrhoidal products	Hem-Prep Pazo Hemorrhoid Ointment Preparation H
	Sore throat products	Spec-T Sore Throat/Decongestant

There are three major drug information sources for OTC products. *Handbook of Nonprescription Drugs* is the most comprehensive resource for OTC medications; it evaluates ingredients contained in major OTC drug classes and lists the ingredients included in many OTC products. *Nonprescription Drug Therapy* is a loose-leaf reference, updated quarterly, that provides detailed OTC product information and patient counseling instructions. *Physicians' Desk Reference for Nonprescription Drugs,* a compendium of manufacturers' information regarding OTC products, is published annually but is somewhat incomplete with regard to the number of products included and the consistency of information provided. Any health care provider who seeks more specific information regarding OTC products may find useful the references listed below.

REFERENCES

Brass EP: Changing the status of drugs from prescription to over-the-counter availability. N Engl J Med 2001;345:810.

Consumer Healthcare Products Association Web Page: http://www.chpa-info.org/

U.S. Food and Drug Administration. Center for Drug Evaluation and Research. Over-the-Counter (OTC) Drugs Web Page: http://www.fda.gov/cder/offices/otc/default.htm

U.S. Food and Drug Administration. Center for Drug Evaluation and Research. Phenylpropanolamine (PPA) Information Web Page: http://www.fda.gov/cder/drug/infopage/ppa/default.htm

Handbook of Nonprescription Drugs, 14th ed. American Pharmaceutical Association, 2004.

Newton GD et al: New OTC drugs and devices 2001: a selective review. J Am Pharm Assoc (Wash) 2003;43:249.

Nonprescription Drug Therapy: Guiding Patient Self-Care, Facts and Comparisons, 2003.

Physicians' Desk Reference for Nonprescription Drugs and Dietary Supplements, 25rd ed. Medical Economics, 2004.

Botanicals ("Herbal Medications") & Nutritional Supplements

Cathi E. Dennehy, PharmD, & Candy Tsourounis, PharmD

65

The medical use of botanicals in their natural and unprocessed form undoubtedly began when the first intelligent animals noticed that certain food plants altered particular body functions. Much information exists about the historical use and effectiveness of botanical products. Unfortunately, the quality of this information is extremely variable. One of the most complete compendiums of clinical recommendations regarding the use of botanicals is the *Report of the German Commission E* (a committee that sets standards for herbal medications in that country; Blumenthal, 2000). Interest in the endocrine effects and possible nutritional benefits of certain purified chemicals such as dehydroepiandrosterone, melatonin, high-dose vitamins, and minerals has led to a parallel development of consumer demand for such substances. These substances, together with the botanicals, constitute a substantial source of profits for those who exploit the concept of "alternative medicine."

The alternative medicinal substances are distinguished from similar botanical substances used in traditional medicine (morphine, digitalis, atropine, etc) by virtue of being available without a prescription and, unlike over-the-counter medications, being legally considered dietary supplements rather than drugs (thus avoiding conventional FDA oversight). Among the purified chemicals, dehydroepiandrosterone and melatonin are of significant pharmacologic interest.

This chapter provides an evidence-based approach to the pharmacology and clinical efficacy of several of the commonly used and commercially available botanicals and dietary supplements. Ephedrine, the active principle in Ma-huang, is discussed in Chapter 9.

REGULATORY FACTORS

Dietary supplements (which include vitamins, minerals, cofactors, herbal medications, and amino acids) are not considered over-the-counter drugs in the USA but rather food supplements. In 1994, the United States Congress, influenced by growing "consumerism" as well as strong manufacturer lobbying efforts, passed the Dietary Supplement and Health Education Act (DSHEA). This landmark act prevented adequate FDA oversight of these substances. Thus, DSHEA has allowed a variety of substances with pharmacologic activity—if classified as dietary supplements—to be sold without a prescription or any FDA review of efficacy or safety prior to product marketing. Dietary supplements are governed under Current Good Manufacturing Practice in Manufacturing, Packaging or Holding Human Food (CGMP) regulations. Although administered by the FDA, CGMP regulations are often inadequate to ensure product purity, potency, and other variables such as accurate product identification and appropriate botanical harvesting. Therefore, much of the criticism regarding the dietary supplement industry involves a lack of product purity and variations in potency.

In 1999, the FDA announced labeling recommendations for dietary supplements marketed in the USA. These recommendations were not mandated; some manufacturers, however, have adopted them in an effort to increase sales. According to these recommendations, the term "dietary supplement" should be included in the product label name. A "Supplement Facts Panel" similar to the "Nutrition Facts Panels" found on processed foods was also recommended. According to these new labeling recommendations, up to 14 "inactive" ingredients can be listed.

CLINICAL ASPECTS OF THE USE OF BOTANICALS

Many United States consumers have embraced the use of botanicals and other supplements as a "natural" approach to their health care. Unfortunately, misconceptions regarding safety and efficacy of the agents are common, and the fact that a substance can be called "natural" of course does not guarantee its safety. In fact, these products can be adulterated, misbranded, or contaminated either intentionally or unintentionally in a variety of ways. Furthermore, the doses recommended for active botanical substances may be much higher than those considered clinically safe. For example, the doses recommended for several Ma-huang preparations contain three to five times the medically recommended daily dose of the active ingredient, ephedrine—doses that impose significant risks for patients with cardiovascular disease.

Adverse effects have been documented for a variety of botanical medications. Unfortunately, chemical analysis is rarely performed on the products involved. This leads to uncertainty about whether the primary herb or an adulterant caused the adverse effect. In some cases, the chemical constituents of the herb can clearly lead to toxicity. Some of the herbs that should be used cautiously or not at all, based on the severity of their reported effects, are listed in Table 65–1.

Table 65–1. Botanical supplements and some associated risks.

Commercial Name, Scientific Name, Plant Parts	Intended Use	Toxic Agents, Effects	Comments
Comfrey *Symphytum species* Leaves and roots	Internal digestive aid, topical for wound healing	Pyrrolizidine alkaloids, hepatotoxicity	Avoid internal ingestion: topical use should be limited to 4–6 weeks
Coltsfoot *Tussilago farfara* Leaves, flower	Upper respiratory tract infections	Pyrrolizidine alkaloids, hepatotoxicity	Avoid ingestion of any parts of plant; leaves may be used topically for anti-inflammatory effects for up to 4–6 weeks
Germander *Teucrium chamaedrys* Leaves, tops	Diet aid	Hepatotoxicity	Avoid
Borage *Borago officinalis* Tops, leaves	Anti-inflammatory, diuretic	Pyrrolizidine alkaloids, hepatotoxicity	Avoid
Chaparral *Larrea tridentata* Twigs, leaves	Anti-infective, antioxidant, anticancer	Hepatotoxicity	Avoid
Sassafras *Sassafras albidum* Root bark	Blood thinner	Safrole oil, hepatocarcinogen in animals	Avoid
Aconite *Aconitum species*	Analgesic	Alkaloid, cardiac and central nervous system effects	Avoid
Pennyroyal *Mentha pulegium* or *Hedeoma pulegioides* Extract	Digestive aid, induction of menstrual flow, abortifacient	Pulegone and pulegone metabolite, liver failure, renal failure	Avoid
Poke root *Phytolacca americana*	Antirheumatic	Hemorrhagic gastritis	Avoid
Jin Bu Huan	Analgesic; sedative	Hepatotoxicity	Avoid
Ephedra, Ma huang *Ephedra species*	Diet aid; stimulant; bronchodilator	Central nervous system toxicity, cardiac toxicity	Avoid in patients at risk for stroke, myocardial infarction, uncontrolled blood pressure, seizures, general anxiety disorder
Royal jelly *Apis mellifera* (honeybee)	Tonic	Bronchospasm, anaphylaxis	Avoid in patients with chronic allergies or respiratory diseases; asthma, chronic obstructive pulmonary disease, emphysema, atopy

BOTANICAL SUBSTANCES

ECHINACEA (*ECHINACEA PURPUREA*)

Chemistry

The three most widely used species of Echinacea are *Echinacea purpurea, E pallida,* and *E angustifolia.* The chemical constituents include flavonoids, lipophilic constituents (eg, alkamides, polyacetylenes), water-soluble polysaccharides, and water-soluble caffeoyl conjugates (eg, echinacoside, chicoric acid, caffeic acid). Within any marketed Echinacea formulation, the relative amounts of these components are dependent upon the species used, the method of manufacture, and the plant parts used. The German Commission E has approved two formulations for clinical use: the fresh pressed juice of aerial parts of *E purpurea* and the alcoholic root extract of *E pallida.* While the active constituents of Echinacea are not completely known, chicoric acid, alkamide, and polysaccharides are most often noted as having immune-modulating properties. Commercial formulations, however, are not standardized for any particular constituent.

Pharmacologic Effects

A. IMMUNE MODULATION

The effect of Echinacea on the immune system is controversial. Human studies using commercially marketed formulations of Echinacea have shown increased phagocytosis but not immunostimulation. In vitro, however, *E purpurea* juice increased production of interleukin-1, -6, -10, and tumor necrosis factor-α by human phagocytes. Enhanced natural killer cell activity and antibody-dependent cellular toxicity was also observed with *E purpurea* extract in cell lines from both healthy and immunocompromised patients. Studies using the isolated purified polysaccharides from Echinacea have also shown cytokine activation. The latter compounds, however, are unlikely to accurately reproduce the activity of the entire extract.

B. ANTI-INFLAMMATORY EFFECTS

Certain Echinacea constituents have demonstrated anti-inflammatory properties in vitro. Inhibition of cyclooxygenase and 5-lipoxygenase may be involved. In animals, application of Echinacea prior to application of a topical irritant reduced both paw and ear edema. There are too few clinical trials in humans to warrant the use of Echinacea in wound healing.

C. ANTIBACTERIAL, ANTIFUNGAL, ANTIVIRAL, AND ANTIOXIDANT EFFECTS

Some in vitro studies have reported weak antibacterial, antifungal, antiviral, and antioxidant activity with Echinacea constituents. The applicability of these findings to clinical trials is discussed below.

Clinical Trials

Echinacea is most often used to enhance immune function in individuals who have colds and other respiratory tract infections. Systematic reviews and cold treatment trials generally report favorable results for Echinacea in reducing symptoms or time to recovery if the agent was administered within the first 24 hours of a cold. To date, however, most of these trials have contained multiple variables (eg, formulation, dose, duration) that make it difficult to make a clear therapeutic recommendation or ensure reproducible outcomes. At best, symptoms and duration may be reduced by about 25–30%. Echinacea has also been evaluated as a prophylactic agent in the prevention of upper respiratory tract infection. These trials have generally been less favorable and have reported no effect.

Echinacea has been used investigationally to enhance hematologic recovery following chemotherapy. It has also been used as an adjunct in the treatment of urinary tract and vaginal fungal infections. These indications require further research before they can be accepted in clinical practice. Echinacea is ineffective in treating recurrent genital herpes.

Adverse Effects

Flu-like symptoms (eg, fever, shivering, headache, vomiting) have been reported following the intravenous use of Echinacea extracts. Adverse effects with oral commercial formulations are minimal and most often include unpleasant taste, gastrointestinal upset, or central nervous system effects (eg, headache, dizziness). Allergic reactions such as rash, acute asthma, and anaphylaxis have been infrequently reported.

Drug Interactions & Precautions

Until the role of Echinacea in immune modulation is better defined, this agent should be avoided in patients with immune deficiency disorders (eg, AIDS, cancer), autoimmune disorders (eg, multiple sclerosis, rheumatoid arthritis), patients with tuberculosis, and patients using immunosuppressant medications (eg, organ transplant recipients). The German Commission E recommends limiting the chronic use of Echinacea to no more than 8 weeks. While there are no reported drug interactions for Echinacea, some preparations have a high alcohol content and should not be used with medications known to cause a disulfiram-like reaction.

Dosage

Dried *Echinacea pallida* root extract (1:5 tincture, 50% ethanol) is given at a dosage of 900 mg/d. *E purpurea* freshly pressed juice is given at a dosage of 6–9 mL/d in divided doses two to five times daily. Echinacea is generally taken at the first sign of a cold.

FEVERFEW (*TANACETUM PARTHENIUM*)

Chemistry

Feverfew contains flavonoid glycosides, monoterpenes (eg, camphor, other pinene derivatives), and sesquiterpene lactones. The most prevalent sesquiterpene is parthenolide, which is primarily found in the seeds and leaves of the plant, with concentrations ranging from 1% to 3%.

Feverfew products should be standardized to contain no less than 0.2% parthenolide since this agent is considered to be one of the primary active constituents. It is likely, however, that other constituents also contribute to the overall biologic activity. Parthenolide content in commercially marketed formulations can vary depending on growing conditions, manufacturing process, and duration of storage. Some commercial dried leaf formulations contain no parthenolide, due to polymerization with prolonged storage.

Pharmacologic Effects

A. MIGRAINE HEADACHE

Feverfew is most often used as a prophylactic remedy for migraine headache. This action has been related to the serotonin hypothesis for migraine causation (see also Chapter 16). In vitro, feverfew and parthenolide inhibit platelet aggregation and serotonin release from platelets.

B. ANTI-INFLAMMATORY EFFECTS

Feverfew has been used as an anti-inflammatory agent to treat rheumatoid arthritis. In vitro inhibition of prostaglandin, thromboxane, and leukotriene B_4 synthesis as well as cytokine (TNF-α and IL-1) expression have been reported.

C. OTHER ACTIONS

Additional in vitro effects of feverfew include inhibition of histamine release from mast cells and granular components from leukocytes; inhibition of smooth muscle contraction; cytotoxic effects on human tumor cell lines; and antimicrobial effects against gram-positive bacteria, yeasts, and filamentous fungi.

Clinical Trials

A. MIGRAINE

The use of feverfew as a prophylactic remedy for migraine headache is extensively described in the anecdotal literature. Unfortunately, most of the reported formal trials used small samples and had variable outcomes.

In a recent systematic review, three of four randomized, double-blind, placebo-controlled trials reported a positive effect. In these studies, the feverfew group generally had significant reductions in headache frequency, severity, and nausea compared with placebo. Feverfew products were standardized to contain 0.2–0.66% parthenolide, dosing ranged from 50 mg/d to 143 mg/d, and study durations from 1 month to 6 months. In contrast to studies reporting beneficial effects, which used freeze-dried or air-dried whole feverfew leaves, trials using an ethanol extract of feverfew leaves (standardized to 0.35% parthenolide) and a special extract showed no prophylactic benefit. Since one of these formulations contained 0.35% parthenolide, this may indicate that other chemical constituents necessary for biologic activity were absent from the ethanol formulation.

Overall, the benefits of feverfew in the prevention of migraine headache are weakly substantiated. Additional research is required to establish its place in therapy.

B. ARTHRITIS

The use of feverfew in rheumatoid arthritis has been poorly studied. A double blind, placebo-controlled trial in 41 patients failed to find a significant benefit of feverfew over placebo at 6 weeks. Until further clinical trials are conducted, feverfew should not be recommended as a treatment for rheumatoid arthritis.

Adverse Effects

Mouth ulcers and gastrointestinal upset are the most common side effects associated with the use of feverfew. In a survey of 300 feverfew users, 11.3% reported mouth ulcers. External contact dermatitis may also occur. A rebound syndrome, consisting of nervousness, tension headache, insomnia, and joint stiffness has been reported in some patients who abruptly discontinued using feverfew.

Drug Interactions, Precautions, & Dosing

Patients taking anticoagulant and antiplatelet drugs should use feverfew cautiously, because the herb may inhibit platelet aggregation.

Recommended dosing of feverfew is two or three fresh leaves daily or up to 125 mg/d of the dried leaf formulation. Long-term effects of feverfew are unknown, as clinical studies typically lasted only 4–6 months or less.

GARLIC (*ALLIUM SATIVUM*)

Chemistry

The pharmacologic activity of garlic involves a variety of organosulfur compounds. The most notable of these is allicin, which is responsible for the characteristic garlic odor.

Pharmacologic Effects

A. CARDIOVASCULAR EFFECTS

In vitro, allicin and related compounds inhibit HMG-CoA reductase, which is involved in cholesterol biosynthesis (see Chapter 35). Several clinical trials have investigated the lipid-lowering potential of garlic. Some have shown significant reductions in cholesterol and others no effect. The most recent meta-analysis suggested a minor (5%) reduction of total cholesterol that was insignificant when dietary controls were in place.

Clinical trials report antiplatelet effects following garlic ingestion and mixed effects on fibrinolytic activity. These effects in combination with antioxidant effects and reductions in total cholesterol may be beneficial in patients with atherosclerosis. In preliminary trials involving atherosclerotic patients, significant reductions in plaque volume were observed for patients taking garlic versus placebo.

Garlic constituents may affect blood vessel elasticity and blood pressure. Proposed mechanisms include opening of potassium channels in vascular smooth muscle, stimulation of nitric oxide synthesis, and inhibition of angiotensin-converting enzyme. Epidemiologic studies suggest that individuals chronically consuming low doses of garlic (averaging 460 mg/d) may have reductions in aortic stiffness. A meta-analysis of garlic's antihypertensive properties revealed a mild effect with a 7.7 mm Hg decrease in systolic pressure and a 5 mm Hg decrease in diastolic pressure.

B. ENDOCRINE EFFECTS

The effect of garlic on glucose homeostasis is controversial. Certain organosulfur constituents in garlic have demonstrated hypoglycemic effects in nondiabetic animal models. There has been no effect, however, in animal models or humans with diabetes.

C. ANTIMICROBIAL EFFECTS

In vitro, allicin has demonstrated activity against gram-positive and gram-negative bacteria as well as fungi (*Candida albicans*), protozoa (*Entamoeba histolytica*), and certain viruses. The primary mechanism involves the inhibition of thiol-containing enzymes needed by these microbes. The antimicrobial effect of garlic has not been extensively studied in clinical trials. Given the availability of effective prescription antimicrobials, the usefulness of garlic in this area appears limited.

D. ANTINEOPLASTIC EFFECTS

In vitro, garlic inhibits procarcinogens for colon, esophageal, lung, breast, and stomach cancer, probably by detoxification of carcinogens and reduced carcinogen activation. The evidence for anticarcinogenic properties in vivo is largely epidemiologic. For example, certain populations with high dietary garlic consumption appear to have a reduced incidence of stomach cancer.

Adverse Effects

Following oral ingestion, adverse effects may include nausea (6%), hypotension (1.3%), allergy (1.1%), and bleeding (rare). Breath odor has been reported with an incidence of 20–40% at recommended doses using enteric-coated formulations. Contact dermatitis may occur with the handling of raw garlic.

Drug Interactions & Precautions

Because of reported antiplatelet effects, patients using anticlotting medications (eg, warfarin, aspirin, ibuprofen) should use garlic cautiously. Additional monitoring of blood pressure and signs and symptoms of bleeding is warranted. Garlic may reduce the bioavailability of saquinavir, an antiviral protease inhibitor, but it does not appear to affect the bioavailability of ritonavir.

Dosage

Products should be standardized to contain 1.3% alliin (the allicin precursor) or have an allicin-generating potential of 0.6%. Enteric-coated formulations are recommended to minimize degradation of the active substances. A daily dose of 600–900 mg/d of powdered garlic is most common. This is equivalent to one clove of raw garlic (2–4 g) per day.

GINKGO (*GINKGO BILOBA*)

Chemistry

Ginkgo biloba extract is prepared from the leaves of the ginkgo tree. The most common formulation is prepared by concentrating 50 parts of the crude leaf to prepare one part of extract. The active constituents in ginkgo are flavone glycosides and terpenoids (ie, ginkgolides A, B, C, J, and bilobalide).

Pharmacologic Effects

A. CARDIOVASCULAR EFFECTS

In animal models and some human studies, ginkgo has been shown to increase blood flow and reduce blood viscosity. Enhancement of endogenous nitric oxide (Chapter 19) may be involved. A meta-analysis suggested that ginkgo was more effective than placebo and possibly comparable to pentoxifylline (Chapter 20) in relieving symptoms of intermittent claudication.

B. METABOLIC EFFECTS

Antioxidant and radical-scavenging properties have been observed for the flavonoid fraction of ginkgo as well as some of the terpene constituents. In vitro, ginkgo has demonstrated superoxide dismutase-like activity and superoxide anion and hydroxyl radical-scavenging properties. It has also demonstrated a protective effect in limiting free radical formation in animal models of ischemic injury and in reducing markers of oxidative stress in patients undergoing coronary artery bypass surgery.

C. CENTRAL NERVOUS SYSTEM EFFECTS

In aged animal models, chronic administration of ginkgo for 3–4 weeks led to modifications in central nervous system receptors and neurotransmitters. Receptor densities increased for muscarinic, α_2, and 5-HT$_{1a}$ receptors and decreased for β-adrenoceptors. Increased serum levels of acetylcholine and norepinephrine and enhanced synaptosomal reuptake of serotonin have also been reported. Additional mechanisms that may be involved include reversible inhibition of MAO-A and MAO-B, reduced corticosterone synthesis, inhibition of amyloid-beta fibril formation, and enhanced GABA levels.

Ginkgo is frequently used to treat "cerebral insufficiency" and dementia of the Alzheimer type. The term "cerebral insufficiency," however, includes a variety of manifestations ranging from poor concentration and confusion to anxiety and depression as well as physical complaints such as hearing loss and headache. For this reason, studies evaluating "cerebral insufficiency" tend to be more inclusive and difficult to assess than trials evaluating dementia. A systematic review and meta-analysis agree that ginkgo is significantly better than placebo at improving symptoms of dementia, but the clinical relevance of these improvements is questionable and amounts to an improvement of approximately 3% in cognition. The duration of the largest of these studies was 1 year. Recent studies on the effects of ginkgo for memory enhancement in healthy nondemented elderly adults did not show a benefit with 6 weeks of use. Ginkgo is currently under investigation as a prophylactic agent for dementia of the Alzheimer type.

D. MISCELLANEOUS EFFECTS

Various ginkgolides, particularly ginkgolide B, have platelet-activating factor (PAF) antagonist properties. This action could explain some antiplatelet and anti-inflammatory effects of these substances.

Ginkgo has also been studied for its effects in allergic and asthmatic bronchoconstriction, erectile dysfunction, tinnitus and hearing loss, short-term memory loss in healthy nonelderly adults, and macular degeneration. A systematic review of randomized controlled trials for chronic tinnitus suggests an improvement with up to 3 months of use. In all of these miscellaneous conditions, with the exception of tinnitus, the evidence is insufficient to warrant clinical use at this time.

Adverse Effects

Adverse effects have been reported with a frequency comparable to that of placebo. These include nausea, headache, stomach upset, diarrhea, allergy, anxiety, and insomnia. A few case reports noted bleeding complications in patients using ginkgo. In two of these cases, the patients were also using either aspirin or warfarin.

Drug Interactions & Precautions

Ginkgo may have antiplatelet properties and should not be used in combination with other antiplatelet or anticoagulant medications. A case report of an enhanced sedative effect was reported when ginkgo was combined with trazodone. Seizures have been reported as a toxic effect of ginkgo, most likely related to seed contamination in the leaf formulations. Ginkgo seeds are epileptogenic. Ginkgo formulations should be avoided in individuals with preexisting seizure disorders.

Dosage

Ginkgo biloba dried leaf extract should be standardized to contain 24% flavone glycosides and 6% terpene lactones. Products should be concentrated to a 50:1 ratio. The daily dose ranges from 120–240 mg of the dried extract in two or three divided doses. Onset of effect may require 2–4 weeks.

GINSENG

Chemistry

Ginseng botanical preparations may be derived from any of several species of the genus Panax. Of these, crude preparations or extracts of *Panax ginseng*, the Chinese or Korean variety, and *Panax quinquefolium*, the American variety, are most often available to consumers in the United States. The active principles appear to be a dozen or more triterpenoid saponin glycosides called ginsenosides or panaxosides. It is recommended that commercial Panax ginseng formulations be standardized to contain 7% ginsenosides.

Other plant materials are commonly sold under the name ginseng but are not from Panax species. These include Siberian ginseng (*Eleutherococcus senticosus*) and Brazilian ginseng (*Pfaffia paniculata*). Of these, Siberian ginseng is more widely available in the United States. Siberian ginseng contains eleutherosides but no ginsenosides. Currently, there is no recommended standardization for eleutheroside content in Siberian ginseng products.

Pharmacology

An extensive literature exists on the potential pharmacologic effects of ginsenosides. Unfortunately, the studies differ widely in the species of Panax used, the ginsenosides studied, the degree of purification applied to the extracts, the animal species studied, and the measurements used to evaluate the responses. Some of the more commonly reported beneficial pharmacologic effects include modulation of immune function, ergogenic ("energizing") activity, nootropic ("mind-enhancing") activity, vasoregulatory effects, anti-inflammatory effects, antistress activity, analgesia, antiplatelet activity, improved glucose homeostasis, and anticancer properties.

Clinical Trials

Ginseng is most often used to help improve physical and mental performance. Unfortunately, the clinical trials are of small sample size and report either an improvement in mental function and physical performance or no effect. Some randomized controlled trials evaluating "quality of life" and enhancement of immune function have claimed significant benefits with *P ginseng*. American ginseng appears to lower postprandial glucose indices in subjects with and without diabetes. Some epidemiologic trials suggest a reduction in several types of cancer with *P ginseng*. Systematic reviews, however, have generally failed to find conclusive evidence for the use of *P ginseng* for any particular condition. Until better clinical studies are published, no recommendation can be made regarding the use of ginseng.

Adverse Effects

A variety of adverse effects have been reported. Weak estrogenic properties may cause the vaginal bleeding and mastalgia reported by some patients. Central nervous system stimulation (eg, insomnia, nervousness) and hypertension have been reported in patients using high doses (more than 3 g/d) of Panax ginseng. Methylxanthines found in the ginseng plant may contribute to this effect. The German Commission E lists high blood pressure as a contraindication to the use of Siberian ginseng but not Panax ginseng.

Drug Interactions & Precautions

Irritability, sleeplessness, and manic behavior have been reported in psychiatric patients using ginseng in combination with other medications (phenelzine, lithium, neuroleptics). Ginseng should be used cautiously in patients taking any psychiatric, estrogenic, or hypoglycemic medications. Ginseng has antiplatelet properties and should not be used in combination with warfarin. Similar to echinacea, cytokine stimulation has been observed for both *P ginseng* and *P quinquefolium*, necessitating cautious use in individuals who are immunocompromised, are taking immune stimulants or suppressants, or have autoimmune disorders.

Dosing

The German Commission E recommends 1–2 g/d of crude *P ginseng* root or its equivalent. Two hundred milligrams of ginseng extract is equivalent to 1 g of the crude root. Ginsana has been used as a standardized extract in some clinical trials and is available in the United States. Dosing for Siberian ginseng is 2–3 g/d of the crude root.

KAVA (*PIPER METHYSTICUM*)

Kava is an extract derived from the root of the pepper plant, *Piper methysticum* Forster. Kava has been used as a ceremonial drink for many centuries in Polynesia, Melanesia, and Micronesia. In many parts of the world, kava is used for its relaxing properties in the same way as alcohol is used in Western societies.

Chemistry

Extracts of the kava root contain both lipophilic and hydrophilic components. The active constituents of kava are referred to as kavalactones or kavapyrones. The active enolides and dienolides are thought to be kawain (kavain), methysticin, and yangonin.

Pharmacologic Effects

A. CENTRAL NERVOUS SYSTEM EFFECTS

The mechanism of action of kava on the central nervous system is not known. Since kava shares similar central nervous system effects with the benzodiazepines, GABA receptors were thought to be involved. In vitro, kavalactones have been shown to bind readily to $GABA_A$ receptors located in the hypothalamus and amygdala, areas thought to be largely responsible for emotion and memory rather than cognition and movement. However, kavalactones do not compete with flunitrazepam or diazepam for benzodiazepine binding sites. Kava may also increase the number of GABA-binding sites.

Other suggested mechanisms include reduced excitatory neurotransmission by decreasing the release of glutamate, inhibition of norepinephrine uptake, reversible MAO-B inhibition, or dopamine antagonism.

Kava has also been shown to have mild anticonvulsant properties in animals, possibly involving voltage-dependent sodium channels.

Research is needed to assess reported analgesic effects in humans. Animal data suggest that opioid receptors are not involved in the actions of kava.

B. ANTIPLATELET EFFECTS

One of the kavalactones, kavain, has in vitro cyclooxygenase-inhibiting activity. The potential for antiplatelet and anti-inflammatory effects needs further study.

Clinical Trials

A. ANXIETY

Kava is most often used as a sedative-hypnotic to treat anxiety. The substance has been evaluated in Europe and in the USA for the treatment of anxiety in several placebo-controlled studies. Most of these trials have shown significant improvements in anxiety symptoms in patients with moderate to severe anxiety within 8 weeks after starting treatment. In one study, kava was compared with oxazepam, a benzodiazepine. Similar reductions in anxiolytic effects and fewer adverse effects were reported for the kava group. Kava appears to have a slow onset of action for the treatment of anxiety symptoms, most patients responding only after 4–8 weeks. Kava should not be used to treat acute symptoms of anxiety or panic attacks.

Adverse Effects

In most patients, kava's adverse effects are mild at recommended doses. These effects include tingling in the mouth and gastrointestinal upset. Kava does not seem to impair memory or cognitive function to the same degree as benzodiazepines.

Kava can cause central nervous system effects such as sedation, euphoria, and visual and auditory changes. Ataxia, muscle weakness, paresthesias, and even ascending paralysis have also been reported with excessive kava doses. Clinical evidence suggests that kava does not induce physiologic dependence, though it may lead to psychologic dependence. Reactions resembling dopaminergic antagonism have been reported. All patients were using kava at recommended doses and experienced dystonic extrapyramidal reactions.

Kava has been shown to alter uterine tone in vitro and should be avoided during pregnancy. Kavalactones are soluble and excreted into breast milk. Women who are nursing should avoid kava.

An ichthyosiform skin rash has been seen when kava is taken at very high doses chronically. It is associated with facial swelling and photosensitivity. Exfoliation on the palms of the hands and soles of the feet, forearms, back, and shins has also been described. Sebaceous gland skin eruptions have been reported, with lymphocytic infiltrates on biopsy. Kava dermopathy is reversible on cessation of consumption.

Since 1999, eleven cases of kava-induced hepatitis have been reported in the USA, Germany, and Switzerland. Various kava products were used at varying doses (60–240 mg/d). Liver biopsies revealed hepatic necrosis requiring liver transplants. As a result, kava products have been removed from the market in Canada, Germany, Switzerland, and Australia.

Drug Interactions

Kava predictably potentiates the effects of other central nervous system depressants such as alcohol and possibly barbiturates. Combining kava with alcohol may result in additive or greater impairment of cognitive performance. Impaired motor function can also occur when kava is combined with central nervous system depressants. One case has been reported of a patient who combined alprazolam with kava and presented in a semicomatose state. Kavalactones inhibit cytochrome P450 isozymes, particularly 3A4, 2C9, 2C19, 2D6, and 1A2. Alprazolam is primarily metabolized by CYP3A4. A decrease in levodopa effectiveness was reported in one patient with Parkinson's disease. The use of kava with dopamine agonists or antagonists should be avoided.

Dosage

Fifty to 70 milligrams of purified kavalactones three times daily appears to be the optimal antianxiety dosage. This is equivalent to 100–250 mg of dried kava root extract three times daily. As a hypnotic, 180–210 mg of kavalactones may be taken 30 minutes to 1 hour before bedtime. Until more is known about the risk of kava-induced hepatotoxicity and drug interactions, kava is not recommended for use. If patients insist on using kava, use should be limited to 3 months or less to minimize the potential for dependence and hepatotoxicity.

MILK THISTLE (*SILYBUM MARIANUM*)

Chemistry

The fruit and seeds of the milk thistle plant contain a lipophilic mixture of flavonolignans known as silymarin. Silymarin comprises 2–3% of the dried herb and is composed of three primary isomers, silybin (also known as silybinin or silibinin), silychristin (silichristin), and silydianin (silidianin). Silybin is the most prevalent and potent of the three isomers and accounts for about 50% of the silymarin complex. Products should be standardized to contain 70–80% silymarin.

Pharmacologic Effects

A. LIVER DISEASE

In animal models, milk thistle limits hepatic injury associated with a variety of toxins, including Amanita mushrooms, galactosamine, carbon tetrachloride, acetaminophen, radiation, cold ischemia, and ethanol. In vitro studies and some in vivo studies demonstrate that silymarin reduces lipid peroxidation, scavenges free radicals, and enhances glutathione and superoxide dismutase levels. This may contribute to membrane stabilization and reduce toxin entry.

Milk thistle may have anti-inflammatory properties. In vitro, silybin strongly and noncompetitively inhibits lipoxygenase and leukotriene formation. On the other hand, concentrations required to inhibit thromboxane and prostaglandin formation in vivo probably exceed dosing capabilities. Inhibition of leukocyte migration has also been observed in vivo and may be a factor when acute inflammation is present.

One of the most unusual mechanisms claimed for milk thistle involves an increase in RNA polymerase I activity in nonmalignant hepatocytes but not in hepatoma or other malignant cell lines. By increasing this enzyme's activity, enhanced protein synthesis and cellular regeneration may occur in diseased but not malignant cells. Milk thistle may have a role in hepatic fibrosis. In an animal model of cirrhosis, it reduced collagen accumulation, and in an in vitro model it reduced expression of the profibrogenic cytokine TGF-β.

It has been suggested that milk thistle may be beneficial in the management of hypercholesterolemia and gallstones. A small trial in humans showed a reduction in bile saturation index and biliary cholesterol concentration. The latter may reflect a reduction in liver cholesterol synthesis. To date, however, there is insufficient evidence to warrant the use of milk thistle for either of these disorders.

B. CHEMOTHERAPEUTIC EFFECTS

Preliminary in vitro and mouse studies have been carried out with skin, breast, and prostate cancer cell lines. In murine models of skin cancer, milk thistle reduced tumor initiation and promotion. It also inhibited cell growth and proliferation by inducing a G_1 cell cycle arrest in cultured human breast and prostate cancer cell lines. However, the use of milk thistle in the treatment of cancer has not yet been adequately studied and should not be recommended to patients.

Clinical Trials

Milk thistle has been used to treat acute and chronic viral hepatitis, alcoholic liver disease, and toxin-induced liver injury in human patients. Milk thistle has most often been studied in the treatment of alcoholic hepatitis and cirrhosis. In both of these disorders, outcomes have been mixed and reports include significant reductions in markers of liver dysfunction and in mortality, as well as no effect. In acute viral hepatitis, studies have generally involved small sample sizes and have shown mixed outcomes of improved liver function (eg, aminotransferase values, bilirubin, prothrombin time) or no effect. Studies in chronic viral hepatitis and toxin-induced injury have also been of small size but have reported mostly favorable results. Parenteral silybin is marketed and used in Europe as an antidote in *Amanita phalloides* mushroom poisoning, based on favorable outcomes reported in case-control studies.

Overall, milk thistle may be effective in improving survival and liver function in a variety of conditions, but additional well-designed clinical trials are needed to confirm these findings.

Adverse Effects

Milk thistle has rarely been reported to cause adverse effects. Loose stools associated with increased bile secretion may occur at high doses.

Drug Interactions, Precautions, & Dosing

There are no reported drug-drug interactions or precautions for milk thistle. Recommended dosage is 200–400 mg/d, calculated as silybin, in three divided doses.

ST. JOHN'S WORT (*HYPERICUM PERFORATUM*)

Chemistry

St. John's wort, also known as hypericum, contains a variety of constituents that may contribute to its pharmacologic activity. Hypericin, a marker of standardization for currently marketed products, was thought to be the primary antidepressant constituent. Recent attention has focused on hyperforin, but a combination of several compounds is probably involved. Commercial formulations are usually prepared by soaking the dried chopped flowers in methanol to create a hydroalcoholic extract that is then dried.

Pharmacologic Effects

A. ANTI-DEPRESSANT ACTION

The hypericin fraction was initially reported to have MAO-A and -B inhibitor properties. Later studies found that the concentration required for this inhibition was higher than that which could be achieved with recommended dosages. In vitro studies using the commercially formulated hydroalcoholic extract have shown inhibition of serotonin, norepinephrine, and dopamine reuptake. While the hypericin constituent did not show reuptake inhibition for any of these systems, a concentrated hyperforin extract did. Chronic administration of the commercial extract has also been shown to significantly down-regulate the expression of cortical β-adrenoceptors and up-regulate the expression of serotonin receptors in a rodent model.

Other effects observed in vitro include opioid sigma receptor binding using the hypericin fraction and GABA receptor binding using the commercial extract. Interleukin-6 production is also reduced in the presence of the extract.

A number of clinical trials have shown St. John's wort to be more efficacious than placebo and just as efficacious as some prescription antidepressants for mild to moderate depression. It does not appear to be effective, however, for more severe depression. Most trials used doses of St. John's wort ranging from 300 mg/d to 1000 mg/d and lasted 4–8 weeks.

B. ANTIVIRAL AND ANTICARCINOGENIC EFFECTS

The hypericin constituent of St. John's wort is photolabile and can be activated by exposure to certain wavelengths of visible or UVA light. Parenteral formulations of hypericin (photoactivated just before administration) have been used investigationally to treat HIV infection (given intravenously) and basal and squamous cell carcinoma (given by intralesional injection). In vitro, photoactivated hypericin inhibits a variety of enveloped and nonenveloped viruses as well as the growth of cells in some neoplastic tissues. Inhibition of protein kinase C and of singlet oxygen radical generation have been proposed as possible mechanisms. The latter could inhibit cell growth or cause cell apoptosis. These studies were carried out using the isolated hypericin constituent of St. John's wort; the usual hydroalcoholic extract of St. John's wort has not been studied for these indications and should not be recommended for patients with viral illness or cancer.

Adverse Effects

Photosensitization has been reported, and patients should be instructed to wear sunscreen while using this product. Hypomania, mania, and autonomic arousal have also been reported in patients using St. John's wort.

Drug Interactions & Precautions

Inhibition of reuptake of various amine transmitters has been highlighted as a potential mechanism of action for St. John's wort. Drugs with similar mechanisms (ie, antidepressants, stimulants) should be used cautiously or avoided in patients using St. John's wort due to the risk of serotonin syndrome or MAO crisis (see Chapters 30 and 59). This herb may induce hepatic CYP enzymes and the P-glycoprotein drug transporter. This has led to case reports of subtherapeutic levels of digoxin, birth control drugs (and subsequent pregnancy), cyclosporine, HIV protease and nonnucleoside reverse transcriptase inhibitors, warfarin, irinotecan, theophylline, and anticonvulsants.

Dosage

The most common commercial formulation of St. John's wort is the dried hydroalcoholic extract. Products are currently standardized to contain 0.3% hypericin. This may change to reflect the new results implicating hyperforin, which should be 2–5%. The recommended dosing for mild to moderate depression is 900 mg of the dried extract per day in three divided doses. Onset of effect may take 2–4 weeks. Long-term benefits beyond 8 weeks have not been sufficiently studied.

SAW PALMETTO (SERENOA REPENS or SABAL SERRULATA)

Chemistry

The active constituents in saw palmetto berries are not well defined. Phytosterols (eg, β-sitosterol), aliphatic alcohols, polyprenic compounds, and flavonoids are all present. Marketed preparations are lipophilic extracts that contain 85–95% fatty acids and sterols.

Pharmacologic Effects

Saw palmetto is most often used in the treatment of benign prostatic hyperplasia. Enzymatic conversion of testosterone to dihydrotestosterone (DHT) by 5α-reductase is inhibited by saw palmetto in vitro. This effect is similar to that of finasteride, which is also used to treat the disorder (Chapter 40). In vitro, saw palmetto also inhibits the binding of DHT to androgen receptors. Additional effects that have been observed in vitro include inhibition of prostatic growth factors, blockade of α_1-adrenoceptors, and inhibition of inflammatory mediators produced by the 5-lipoxygenase pathway.

The clinical pharmacology of saw palmetto is not well defined. One week of treatment in healthy volunteers failed to influence 5α-reductase activity, DHT concentration, or testosterone concentration. Six months of treatment in patients with benign prostatic hyperplasia also failed to affect prostate-specific antigen (PSA) levels, a marker that is typically reduced by enzymatic inhibition of 5α-reductase. In contrast, other researchers have reported a reduction in epidermal growth factor, DHT levels, and estrogen expression after three months of treatment in patients with benign prostatic hyperplasia. The largest clinical trial to date compared saw palmetto, 320 mg/d, with finasteride, 5 mg/d, in 1098 patients. At 6 months, overall symptom score, quality of life, and peak urinary flow were significantly improved for both groups. Finasteride was significantly better at reducing prostate volume (18% versus 6%, respectively). Adverse effects were comparable in both groups except for a significantly greater degree of sexual dysfunction in patients receiving finasteride versus saw palmetto. Shortcomings in the latter trial included lack of placebo control and failure to extend the study duration beyond 6 months.

In a systematic review of seven double-blind placebo-controlled trials, saw palmetto was found to be significantly more effective than placebo in reducing nocturnal urinary frequency (33–74% versus 13–39%, respectively), in reducing daytime urinary frequency (11–43% versus 1–29%, respectively), and in increasing peak urinary flow (26–50% versus 2–35%, respectively). A recent meta-analysis of randomized controlled trials also indicated a therapeutic advantage of saw palmetto over placebo in improving urologic symptoms and flow measures.

Small comparative trials of saw palmetto versus α-blockers showed greater symptomatic improvement with α-blockers.

Adverse Effects

In the largest clinical trial conducted to date, adverse events reported with an incidence of 1–3% included hypertension, decreased libido, abdominal pain, impotence, back pain, urinary retention, and headache. In another large-scale trial, gastrointestinal upset was the most common side effect.

Drug Interactions, Precautions, & Dosing

No drug-drug interactions have been reported for saw palmetto. Patients should be instructed that it may take 4–6 weeks for onset of clinical effects. Recommended dosing of a standardized dried extract (containing 85–95% fatty acids and sterols) is 160 mg orally twice daily. The efficacy of saw palmetto in benign prostatic hyperplasia beyond 6 months has not been established.

PURIFIED NUTRITIONAL SUPPLEMENTS

DEHYDROEPIANDROSTERONE

Dehydroepiandrosterone (DHEA) is a precursor hormone secreted by the adrenal cortex and to a lesser extent by the central nervous system (Chapter 40). It is readily converted to androstenedione, testosterone, and androsterone. In peripheral tissues, aromatase converts DHEA to estradiol. In the plasma, DHEA is converted to DHEA sulfate (DHEAS).

Although no specific physiologic function has been attributed to DHEA or DHEAS, the relationships between their endogenous levels and various diseases have been widely studied. Exogenous DHEA supplementation has been advocated for a variety of indications, including relief of age-related disorders, promotion of weight loss, reduction of heart disease risk, prevention of a variety of cancers, and strengthening of the immune system.

Clinical Uses

A. WEIGHT LOSS

Only a few poorly designed studies have assessed the effects of DHEA supplements in facilitating weight loss. Each of these studies employed a very small sample size and varying measures of weight loss. The effects of DHEA on weight loss are therefore uncertain. Until more is known, DHEA should not be recommended as a weight loss agent.

B. CARDIOVASCULAR DISEASE

DHEA may affect the synthesis of cholesterol and other lipids involved in atherogenesis. Many studies have assessed the relationship between endogenous DHEA levels and the risk for developing cardiovascular disease. Both high and low DHEA levels have been associated with increased risk of cardiovascular morbidity in men. In postmenopausal women, cardiovascular morbidity was greater in women with high DHEAS levels.

C. HYPERCHOLESTEROLEMIA

The effects on cholesterol values in the few studies reported to date have been modest and variable. Thus, the role of DHEA in hypercholesterolemia in men and women has not been determined. According to existing information, endogenous levels of DHEA do not correlate with cholesterol regulation or synthesis. DHEA supplementation might have a role in decreasing HDL cholesterol in postmenopausal women since DHEA is converted to estradiol and to a lesser extent testosterone. These proposed effects need to be assessed using adequate study design.

D. Aging

Because DHEA and DHEAS levels decline with age, DHEA has been advocated as replacement therapy to prevent age-associated changes (especially in sexual function in men) and diseases. DHEA has demonstrated some antioxidant effects. The extent to which DHEA may decrease free radical formation, however, requires further study.

A low DHEA dose is adequate to increase DHEAS levels to those of a 20- or 30-year-old individual, and some evidence suggests that DHEA replacement dosing increases mean free testosterone levels in elderly men (by 5–10% after DHEA initiation, remaining slightly elevated for 2–3 months). The clinical significance of this effect is not known.

There is insufficient evidence at present to recommend DHEA in preventing any age-associated diseases.

E. Alzheimer's Disease

The role of DHEA supplementation in Alzheimer's disease remains controversial. Some research suggests that low endogenous DHEA and DHEAS levels correlate with dementia, while other reports are negative. Research is continuing to assess the effects of DHEA supplementation on dementia and Alzheimer's disease.

F. Treatment of HIV Infection and AIDS

Early studies in mice demonstrated that DHEA supplementation afforded protection against certain virus infections. Furthermore, DHEA affected T lymphocytes by increasing IL-2 production and decreasing IL-4, IL-5, and IL-6 release. The effect of DHEA supplementation on HIV disease progression has therefore been assessed in both men and women. Women reported improvements in energy, cognitive and physical functioning, emotional well-being, and health perception. Modest increases in body weight and CD4 cell counts were seen in women receiving DHEA. No patients displayed a statistically significant decline in viral load. Although male subjects reported improvements in well being, changes in CD4 cell counts were not observed.

G. Systemic Lupus Erythematosus (SLE)

SLE is associated with low levels of endogenous DHEA and DHEAS in women. In one study, patients receiving DHEA for 6 months had fewer lupus flares and improved global assessment scores of disease activity as measured by retrospective medical record review. Adverse effects included acne, hirsutism, menstrual alterations, emotional changes, and weight gain. In another study, statistically significant improvements were observed in the SLE disease activity index during the first 3 months of therapy. However, nearly 60% of patients discontinued DHEA supplementation prior to the 1-year study completion. Reasons for discontinuation included lack of efficacy (30%) and androgenic side effects (14%).

H. Diabetes

Early evidence suggested that DHEA might be used to ameliorate insulin resistance in patients with diabetes. DHEA and DHEAS levels appear to decline in a variety of disease states characterized by insulin resistance or states associated with hyperinsulinism such as hypertension, obesity, and type 2 diabetes mellitus. These relationships have prompted the promotion of DHEA as a regulator of blood glucose levels. However, a role for DHEA in regulating blood glucose and the management of diabetes has not been adequately demonstrated. Until more information is available, patients with diabetes should not rely on DHEA to help control blood glucose.

Adverse Effects & Risks of DHEA & DHEAS Use

A. Benign Prostatic Hyperplasia and Prostate Cancer

The effects of DHEA on the prostate are still unknown. However, since DHEA supplementation can increase mean testosterone levels, it might contribute to increased prostate cell growth, and worsening of prostate cancer must be considered. Because the ultimate effects are unknown, patients with benign prostatic hyperplasia should avoid using DHEA. If a patient uses DHEA therapy, he should be closely monitored for signs and symptoms of prostate disease.

B. Other Cancers

DHEA supplementation can increase production of gonadal hormones. Therefore, DHEA should be avoided by patients with any type of hormone-dependent cancer.

C. Endocrine Effects

Endocrine adverse effects depend on gender and DHEA dose. DHEA is a precursor of gonadal hormones, and it appears to be preferentially converted to the hormone present in lowest quantities. In premenopausal women, DHEA is converted mainly to testosterone and minimally to estrogen. In men, conversion favors increased production of estrogen and to a lesser extent testosterone. Women therefore may complain of masculinizing effects such as hirsutism, acne, and deepening of the voice. Men may experience gynecomastia and breast tenderness.

Reports of euphoria or an increased sense of well-being are also common and may be related to increased release of corticosteroid congeners. DHEA has also been reported to cause mania and cardiac arrhythmias. Although these reports are rare, patients at risk for these effects should avoid taking DHEA.

Drug Interactions

Drug-drug interactions have not been systematically studied for DHEA. It is unknown whether DHEA interacts with over-the-counter medicine or prescription drugs.

Dosage

Replacement dosage sufficient to maintain DHEA levels at young adult values varies with gender and the individual. Approximately 25–50 mg daily is adequate for women, whereas 25–100 mg may be required for men. Adverse effects appear to be uncommon at these doses. Doses greater than 100 mg daily have been used to increase androgens and other hormones. Doses of 1600 mg daily have resulted in significant adverse effects, often requiring drug discontinuation.

MELATONIN

Melatonin, a serotonin derivative produced by the pineal gland and some other tissues (see also Chapter 16), is believed to be responsible for regulating sleep-wake cycles. Melatonin release coincides with darkness; it typically begins around 9 PM and lasts until about 4 AM. Melatonin release is suppressed by daylight. Melatonin has also been studied for a number of other functions, including contraception, protection against endogenous oxidants, prevention of aging, and treatment of depression, HIV infection, and a variety of cancers. Currently, melatonin is most often administered to induce sleep and to prevent jet lag.

Pharmacologic Effects & Clinical Uses

A. JET LAG

Jet lag, a disturbance of the sleep-wake cycle, occurs when there is a disparity between the external time and the traveler's endogenous circadian clock (internal time). The internal time regulates not only daily sleep rhythms but also body temperature and many metabolic systems. The synchronization of the circadian clock relies on light as the most potent "zeitgeber" (time giver).

Jet lag is especially common among frequent travelers and airplane cabin crews. Typical symptoms of jet lag may include daytime drowsiness, insomnia, frequent awakenings, and gastrointestinal upset. Clinical studies with administration of melatonin have reported subjective reduction in daytime fatigue, improved mood, and a quicker recovery time (return to normal sleep patterns, energy, and alertness). Unfortunately, many of these studies were characterized by inconsistencies in dosing, duration of therapy, and time of drug administration. In addition to melatonin, maximizing exposure to daylight on arrival at the new destination can aid in resetting the internal clock.

B. INSOMNIA

Melatonin has been studied in the treatment of various sleep disorders, including insomnia and delayed sleep-phase syndrome. Melatonin has been shown to improve sleep onset, duration, and quality when administered to healthy volunteers, suggesting a pharmacologic hypnotic effect. Melatonin has also been shown to increase rapid-eye-movement (REM) sleep.

Clinical studies in patients with sleep disorders have shown that oral melatonin supplementation may alter sleep architecture. Subjective improvements in sleep quality and improvements in sleep onset and sleep duration have been reported. However, the significance of these findings is impaired by many study limitations.

Patients over 65 years of age tend to suffer from sleep maintenance insomnia; melatonin serum levels have been reported to be low in these patients. Elderly patients with sleep maintenance insomnia who received immediate-release and sustained-release melatonin had improved sleep onset time. They did not, however, experience an improvement in sleep maintenance or total sleep time.

C. FEMALE REPRODUCTIVE FUNCTION

Melatonin receptors have been identified in granulosa cell membranes, and significant amounts of melatonin have been detected in ovarian follicular fluid. Melatonin has been associated with midcycle suppression of luteinizing hormone surge and secretion. This may result in partial inhibition of ovulation. Nightly doses of melatonin (75–300 mg) given with a progestin through days 1–21 of the menstrual cycle resulted in lower mean LH levels. Therefore, melatonin should not be used by women who are pregnant or attempting to conceive. Furthermore, melatonin supplementation may decrease prolactin release in women and therefore should be used cautiously or not at all while nursing.

D. MALE REPRODUCTIVE FUNCTION

In healthy men, chronic melatonin administration (≥ 6 months) decreased sperm quality, possibly by aromatase inhibition in the testes. Until more is known, melatonin should not be used by couples who are actively trying to conceive.

Adverse Effects

Melatonin appears to be well tolerated and is often used in preference to over-the-counter "sleep-aid" drugs. Although melatonin is associated with few adverse effects, some next-day drowsiness has been reported as well as tachycardia, depression, vivid dreams, and headache. Sporadic case reports of movement disorders and psychoses have also appeared.

Drug Interactions

Melatonin drug interactions have not been formally studied. Various studies, however, suggest that melatonin concentrations are altered by a variety of drugs, including NSAIDs, antidepressants, β-adrenoceptor agonists and antagonists, scopolamine, and sodium valproate. The relevance of these effects is unknown.

Dosage

A. JET LAG

The optimal timing and dose of melatonin have not been established. Current information suggests 5–8 mg of the immediate-release formulation given on the evening of departure and for 1–3 nights after arrival at the new destination. Exposure to daylight at the new time zone is also important to regulate the sleep-wake cycle.

B. INSOMNIA

Doses of 0.3–10 mg of the immediate-release formulation orally given once nightly have been tried. The lowest effective dose should be used first and may be repeated in 30 minutes up to a maximum of 10–20 mg. Sustained-release formulations may be used but currently do not offer any notable advantages over the immediate-release formulations. Sustained-release formulations are also more costly.

REFERENCES

GENERAL

Blumenthal M et al: *Herbal medicine: expanded commission E monograph.* American Botanical Council. Integrative Medicine Communications, 2000.

Dietary Supplement Health and Education Act of 1994. 103rd Congress, 2nd Session, Report 103-410, January 25, 1994.

DeSmet PAGM: Herbal remedies. N Engl J Med 2002;347:2046.

Jellin JM et al: *Pharmacist's Letter/Prescriber's Letter Natural Medicines Comprehensive Database.* 4th edition. Therapeutic Research Faculty, 2002.

ECHINACEA

Barrett BP et al: Treatment of the common cold with unrefined echinacea. Ann Intern Med 2002;137:939.

Grimm W et al: A randomized controlled trial of the effect of fluid extract of *Echinacea purpurea* on the incidence and severity of colds and respiratory infections. Am J Med 1999;106:138.

Hoheisel O et al: Echinagard treatment shortens the course of the common cold: A double-blind, placebo-controlled trial. Eur J Clin Res 1997;9:261.

Melchart D et al: Echinacea for preventing and treating the common cold (Cochrane Review). In: The Cochrane Library Issue 4, 2002. Oxford: Update Software.

Turner RB et al: Ineffectiveness of echinacea for prevention of experimental rhinovirus colds. Antimicrob Agents Chemother 2000;44:1708.

FEVERFEW

Paltevich D et al: Feverfew (*Tanacetum parthenium*) as a prophylactic treatment for migraine: A double-blind placebo controlled study. Phytother Res 1997;11:508.

Pfaffenrath V et al: The efficacy and safety of *Tanacetum parthenium* (feverfew) in migraine prophylaxis: a double-blind, multicentre, randomized, placebo-controlled dose-response study. Cephalalgia 2002;22:523.

GARLIC

Ackermann RT et al: Garlic shows promise for improving some cardiovascular risk factors. Arch Intern Med 2001;161:813.

Ankri S, Mirelman D: Antimicrobial properties of allicin from garlic. Microbes Infect 1999;1:125.

Fleischauer AT et al: Garlic consumption and cancer prevention: meta-analyses of colorectal and stomach cancers. Am J Clin Nutr 2000;72:1047.

GINKGO

Ernst E et al: *Ginkgo biloba* for dementia—A systematic review of double-blind, placebo-controlled trials. Clin Drug Invest 1999;17:301.

Maclennan KM et al: The CNS effects of *Ginkgo biloba* extracts and ginkgolide B. Progress Neurobiol 2002;67:235.

Pittler MH et al: *Ginkgo biloba* extract for the treatment of intermittent claudication: a meta-analysis of randomized trials. Am J Med 2000;108:276.

Solomon PR et al: Ginkgo for memory enhancement—A randomized controlled trial. JAMA 2002;288:835.

GINSENG

Assinewe VA et al: Extractable polysaccharides of *Panax quinquefolius* L. (North American ginseng) root stimulate TNF alpha production by alveolar macrophages. Phytomedicine 2002;9:398.

Bahrke MS et al: Evaluation of the ergogenic properties of ginseng. Sports Med 2000;29:113.

Engels HJ, Wirth JC: No ergogenic effects of ginseng (*Panax ginseng* C.A. Meyer) during graded maximal aerobic exercise. J Am Diet Assoc 1997;97:1110.

Shin HR et al: The cancer preventive potential of *Panax ginseng:* a review of human and experimental evidence. Cancer Causes Control 2000;11:565.

Sorenson H, Sonne J: A double-masked study of the effects of ginseng on cognitive functions. Curr Ther Res 1996;57:959.

Thompson Coon J et al: *Panax ginseng*—A systematic review of adverse effects and drug interactions Drug Saf 2002;25:323.

Vogler BK et al: The efficacy of ginseng—A systematic review of randomised clinical trials. Eur J Clin Pharmacol 1999;55:567.

KAVA

Almeida JC et al: Coma from the health food store: Interaction between kava and alprazolam. Ann Intern Med 1996;125:940.

Foo H, Lemon J: Acute effects of kava, alone or in combination with alcohol, on subjective measures of impairment and intoxication and on cognitive performance. Drug Alcohol Rev 1997;16:147.

Singh YN: Kava: An overview. J Ethnopharmacol 1992;37:13.

Strahl S et al: Necrotizing hepatitis after taking herbal remedies. Dtsch Med Wochenschr 1998;123:1410.

MILK THISTLE

Buzelli G et al: A pilot study on the liver protective effect of silybin-phosphatidylcholine complex (IdB1016) in chronic active hepatitis. Int J Clin Pharmacol Ther Toxicol 1993;31:456.

Hruby C: Silibinin in the treatment of deathcap fungus poisoning. Forum 1984;6:23.

Jacobs BP et al: Milk thistle for the treatment of liver disease: a systematic review and meta-analysis. Am J Med 2002;113:506.

Pares A et al: Effects of silymarin in alcoholic patients with cirrhosis of the liver: Results of a controlled, double-blind, randomized and multicenter trial. J Hepatol 1998;28:615.

Valenzuela A, Garrido A: Biochemical bases of the pharmacological action of the flavonoid silymarin and of its structural isomer silibinin. Biol Res 1994;27:105.

ST. JOHN'S WORT

Bennett DA et al: Neuropharmacology of St. John's wort (*Hypericum*). Ann Pharmacother 1998;32:1201.

Gulick RM et al: Phase I studies of hypericin, the active compound in St. John's wort, as an antiretroviral agent in HIV-infected adults. Ann Intern Med 1999;130:510.

Henderson L et al: St John's wort (*Hypericum perforatum*): drug interactions and clinical outcomes. Br J Clin Pharmacol 2002;54:349.

Hypericum Depression Trial Study Group:Effect of *Hypericum perforatum* (St John's wort) in major depressive disorder. JAMA 2002;287:1807.

Muller WE et al: Hyperforin—Antidepressant activity by a novel mechanism of action. Pharmacopsychiatry 2001;34:S98.

Muller WE et al: Hyperforin represents the neurotransmitter reuptake inhibiting constituent of hypericum extract. Pharmacopsychiatry 1998;31(Suppl 1):16.

Nahrstedt A, Butterweck A: Biologically active and other chemical constituents of the herb of *Hypericum perforatum* L. Pharmacopsychiatry 1997;30(Suppl 2):129.

SAW PALMETTO

Boyle P et al: Meta-analysis of clinical trials of Permixon in the treatment of symptomatic prostatic hyperplasia. Urology 2000;55:533.

Plosker GL, Brogden RN: *Serenoa repens* (Permixon): A review of its pharmacology and therapeutic efficacy in benign prostatic hyperplasia. Drugs Aging 1996;9:379.

Wilt T et al: Saw palmetto extracts for treatment of benign prostatic hyperplasia. JAMA 1998;280:1604.

DEHYDROEPIANDROSTERONE

Chang DM et al: Dehydroepiandrosterone treatment of women with mild to moderate systemic lupus erythematosus: A multicenter randomized, double-blind placebo-controlled trial. Arthritis Rheum 2002;46:2924.

Flynn MA et al: Dehydroepiandrosterone replacement in aging humans. J Clin Endocrinol Metab 1999;84:1527.

Piketty C et al: Double-blind placebo-controlled trial of oral dehydroepiandrosterone in patients with advanced HIV disease. Clin Endocrinol 2001;55:325.

Wellman M et al: The role of dehydroepiandrosterone in diabetes mellitus. Pharmacotherapy 1999;19:582.

MELATONIN

Brzezinski A: Melatonin in humans. N Engl J Med 1997;336:186.

Haimov I et al: Melatonin replacement therapy of elderly insomniacs. Sleep 1995;18:598.

Hughes RJ et al: The role of melatonin and circadian phase in age-related sleep-maintenance insomnia: Assessment in a clinical trial of melatonin replacement. Sleep 1998;21:52.

Petrie K et al: A double-blind trial of melatonin as a treatment for jet lag in international cabin crew. Biol Psychiatry 1993;33:526.

Rational Prescribing & Prescription Writing

Paul W. Lofholm, PharmD, & Bertram G. Katzung, MD, PhD

Once a patient with a clinical problem has been evaluated and a diagnosis has been reached, the practitioner can often select from a variety of therapeutic approaches. Medication, surgery, psychiatric treatment, radiation, physical therapy, health education, counseling, further consultation, and no therapy are some of the options available. Of these options, drug therapy is by far the one most commonly chosen. In most cases, this requires the writing of a prescription. A prescription is the prescriber's order to prepare or dispense a specific treatment—usually medication—for a specific patient. When a patient comes for an office visit, the physician or other authorized health professional will prescribe medications 67% of the time, and an average of one prescription per office visit is written because more than one prescription may be written at a single visit.

In this chapter, a plan for prescribing is presented. The physical form of the prescription, common prescribing errors, and legal requirements that govern various features of the prescribing process are then discussed. Finally, some of the social and economic factors involved in prescribing and drug use are described.

RATIONAL PRESCRIBING

Like any other process in medicine, writing a prescription should be based on a series of rational steps.

(1) **Make a specific diagnosis:** Prescriptions based merely on a desire to satisfy the patient's psychological need for some type of therapy are often unsatisfactory and may result in adverse effects. A specific diagnosis, even if it is tentative, is required to move to the next step. In a 35-year-old woman with symmetric joint stiffness, pain, and inflammation that are worse in the morning and not associated with a history of infection, a diagnosis of rheumatoid arthritis would be considered. This diagnosis and the reasoning underlying it should be shared with the patient.

(2) **Consider the pathophysiologic implications of the diagnosis:** If the disorder is well understood, the prescriber is in a much better position to offer effective therapy. For example, increasing knowledge about the mediators of inflammation makes possible more effective use of NSAIDs and other agents used in rheumatoid arthritis. The patient should be provided with the appropriate level and amount of information about the pathophysiology. Many disease-oriented public and private agencies (eg, American Heart Association, American Cancer Society, Arthritis Foundation) provide information sheets suitable for patients.

(3) **Select a specific therapeutic objective:** A therapeutic objective should be chosen for each of the pathophysiologic processes defined in the preceding step. In a patient with rheumatoid arthritis, relief of pain by reduction of the inflammatory process is one of the major therapeutic goals that identifies the drug groups which will be considered. Arresting the course of the disease process in rheumatoid arthritis is a different therapeutic goal that might lead to consideration of other drug groups and prescriptions.

(4) **Select a drug of choice:** One or more drug groups will be suggested by each of the therapeutic goals specified in the preceding step. Selection of a drug of choice from among these groups will follow from a consideration of the specific characteristics of the patient and the clinical presentation. For certain drugs, characteristics such as age, other diseases, and other drugs being taken are extremely important in determining the most suitable drug for management of the present complaint. In the example of the patient with probable rheumatoid arthritis, it would be important to know whether she has a history of aspirin intolerance or ulcer disease, whether the cost of medication is an especially important factor, and whether there is a need for once-daily dosing. Based on this information, a drug would probably be selected from the nonsteroidal anti-inflammatory group. If the patient is intolerant of aspirin and does not have ulcer disease but does have a need for low-cost treatment, ibuprofen would be a rational choice.

(5) **Determine the appropriate dosing regimen:** The dosing regimen is determined primarily by the pharmacokinetics of the drug in that patient. If the patient is known to have disease of the organs required for elimination of the drug selected, adjustment of the "average" regimen will be needed. For a drug such as ibuprofen, which is eliminated mainly by the kidneys, renal function should be assessed. If renal function is normal, the half-life of ibuprofen (about 2 hours) requires administration three or four times daily. The dose suggested in drug handbooks and the manufacturer's literature is 400–800 mg four times daily.

(6) **Devise a plan for monitoring the drug's action and determine an end point for therapy:** The prescriber should be able to describe to the patient the kinds of drug effects that will be monitored and in what way, including laboratory tests (if necessary) and signs and symptoms that the patient should report. For conditions that call for a limited course of therapy (eg, most infections), the duration of therapy should be made clear so that the patient will not stop taking the drug prematurely and will understand why the prescription probably need not be renewed. For the patient with rheumatoid arthritis, the need for prolonged—perhaps indefinite—therapy should be explained. The prescriber should also specify any changes in the patient's condition that would call for changes in therapy. For example, in the patient with rheumatoid arthritis, development of gastrointestinal bleeding would require an immediate change in drug therapy and a prompt workup of the bleeding. Major toxicities that require immediate attention should be explained clearly to the patient.

(7) **Plan a program of patient education:** The prescriber and other members of the health team should be prepared to repeat, extend, and reinforce the information transmitted to the patient as often as necessary. The more toxic the drug prescribed, the greater the importance of this educational program. The importance of informing and involving the patient in each of the above steps must be recognized, as shown by experience with teratogenic drugs (see Chapter 60; Shulman, 1989).

THE PRESCRIPTION

While a prescription can be written on any piece of paper (as long as all of the legal elements are present), it usually takes a specific form. A typical printed prescription form for outpatients is shown in Figure 66–1.

In the hospital setting, drugs are prescribed on a particular page of the patient's hospital chart called the **physician's order sheet** (POS) or **chart order.** The contents of that prescription are specified in the medical staff rules by the hospital's Pharmacy and Therapeutics Committee. The patient's name is typed or written on the

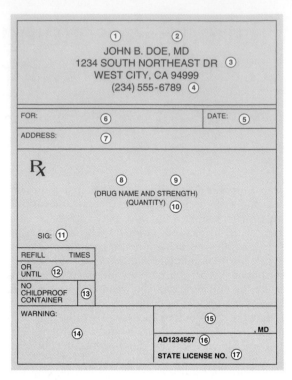

Figure 66–1. Common form of outpatient prescription. Circled numbers are explained in the text.

form; therefore, the orders consist of the name and strength of the medication, the dose, the route and frequency of administration, the date, other pertinent information, and the signature of the prescriber. The duration of therapy or the number of doses is often not specified; therefore, medications are continued until the prescriber discontinues the order or until it is terminated as a matter of policy routine, eg, a stop order policy.

A typical chart order might be as follows:

11/13/03
10:30 a.m.

  (1) **Ampicillin 500 mg IV q6h × 5 days**
  (2) **Aspirin 0.6 g per rectum q6h prn temp over 101**

  [Signed] **Janet B. Doe, MD**

Thus, the elements of the hospital chart order are equivalent to the central elements (5, 8–11, 15) of the outpatient prescription.

Elements of the Prescription

The first four elements (see circled numerals in Figure 66–1) of the outpatient prescription establish the identity of the prescriber: name, license classification (ie, professional degree), address, and office telephone number. Before dispensing a prescription, the pharmacist must establish the prescriber's bona fides and should be able to contact the prescriber by telephone if any questions arise. Element [5] is the date the prescription was written. It should be near the top of the prescription form or at the beginning (left margin) of the chart order. Since the order has legal significance and usually has some temporal relationship to the date of the patient-prescriber interview, a pharmacist should refuse to fill a prescription without verification by telephone if too much time has elapsed since its writing.

Elements [6] and [7] identify the patient by name and address. The patient's name and full address should be clearly spelled out.

The body of the prescription contains the elements [8] to [11] that specify the medication, the strength and quantity to be dispensed, the dosage, and complete directions for use. When writing the drug name (element [8]), either the brand name (proprietary name) or generic name (nonproprietary name) may be used. Reasons for using one or the other are discussed below. The strength of the medication (element [9]) should be written in metric units. However, the prescriber should be familiar with both systems now in use: apothecary and metric. For practical purposes, the following approximate conversions are useful:

1 grain (gr) = 0.065 grams (g), **often rounded to 60 milligrams (mg)**

15 gr = 1 g

1 ounce (oz) by volume = 30 milliliters (mL)

1 teaspoonful (tsp) = 5 mL

1 tablespoonful (tbsp) = 15 mL

1 quart (qt) = 1000 mL

1 minim = 1 drop (gtt)

20 drops = 1 mL

2.2 pounds (lb) = 1 kilogram (kg)

The strength of a solution is usually expressed as the quantity of solute in sufficient solvent to make 100 mL; for instance, 20% potassium chloride solution is 20 grams of KCl per deciliter (g/dL). Both the concentration and the volume should be explicitly written out.

The quantity of medication prescribed should reflect the anticipated duration of therapy, the cost, the need for continued contact with the clinic or physician, the potential for abuse, and the potential for toxicity or overdose. Consideration should be given also to the standard sizes in which the product is available and whether this is the initial prescription of the drug or a repeat prescription or refill. If 10 days of therapy are required to effectively cure a streptococcal infection, an

appropriate quantity for the full course should be prescribed. Birth control pills are often prescribed for 1 year or until the next examination is due; however, some patients may not be able to afford a year's supply at one time; therefore, a 3-month supply might be ordered, with refill instructions to renew three times or for 1 year (element [12]). Finally, when first prescribing medications that are to be used for the treatment of a chronic disease, the initial quantity should be small, with refills for larger quantities. The purpose of beginning treatment with a small quantity of drug is to reduce the cost if the patient cannot tolerate it. Once it is determined that intolerance is not a problem, a larger quantity purchased less frequently is sometimes less expensive.

The directions for use (element [11]) must be both drug-specific and patient-specific. The simpler the directions, the better; and the fewer the number of doses (and drugs) per day, the better. Patient noncompliance (failure to adhere to the drug regimen) is a major cause of treatment failure. To help patients remember to take their medications, prescribers often give an instruction that medications be taken at or around mealtimes and at bedtime. However, it is important to inquire about the patient's eating habits and other lifestyle patterns, since many patients do not eat three regularly spaced meals a day—especially if they are sick or dieting.

The instructions on how and when to take medications, the duration of therapy, and the purpose of the medication must be explained to each patient by the physician and by the pharmacist. (Neither should assume that the other will do it.) Furthermore, the drug name, the purpose for which it is given, and the duration of therapy should be written on each label so that the drug may be identified easily in case of overdose. An instruction to "take as directed" may save the time it takes to write the orders out but often leads to noncompliance, patient confusion, and medication error. The directions for use must be clear and concise to avoid toxicity and to obtain the greatest benefits from therapy.

Although directions for use are no longer written in Latin, many Latin apothecary abbreviations (and some others included below) are still in use. Knowledge of these abbreviations is essential for the dispensing pharmacist and often useful for the prescriber. Some of the abbreviations still used are listed in Table 66–1.

Elements [12] to [14] of the prescription include refill information, waiver of the requirement for childproof containers, and additional labeling instructions (eg, warnings such as "may cause drowsiness," "do not drink alcohol"). Pharmacists put the name of the medication on the label unless directed otherwise by the prescriber, and some medications have the name of the drug stamped or imprinted on the tablet or capsule. Pharmacists must place the expiration date for the drug on the label. If the patient or prescriber does not request

Table 66–1. Abbreviations used in prescriptions and chart orders. **Note:** It is always safer to write out the direction without abbreviating.

ABBREVIATION	EXPLANATION	ABBREVIATION	EXPLANATION
ā	before	pr n	when needed
ac	before meals	q	every
agit	shake, stir	qam, om	every morning
Aq	water	qd	every day
Aq dest	distilled water	qh, q1h	every hour
bid	twice a day	q2h, q3h, etc	every 2 hours, every 3
c̄	with		hours, etc
cap	capsule	qhs	every night at bed-
D5W, D_5W	dextrose 5% in water		time
dil	dissolve, dilute	qid	four times a day
disp, dis	dispense	qod	every other day
elix	elixir	qs	sufficient quantity
ext	extract	rept, repet	may be repeated
g	gram	Rx	take
gr	grain	s̄	without
gtt	drops	SC, SQ	subcutaneous
h	hour	Sig, S	label
hs	at bedtime	sos	if needed
IA	intra-arterial	s̄s̄, ss	one-half
IM	intramuscular	stat	at once
IV	intravenous	sup, supp	suppository
IVPB	IV piggyback	susp	suspension
kg	kilogram	tab	tablet
mEq, meq	milliequivalent	tbsp, T (do not use)	tablespoon (always
mg	milligram		write out "15 mL")
mcg, μg (do not use)	microgram (always	tid	three times a day
	write out "microgram")	tr, tinct	tincture
no	number	tsp (do not use)	teaspoon (always
non rep	do not repeat		write out "5 mL")
OD	right eye	U (do not use)	units (always write out
OS, OL	left eye		"units")
OTC	over-the-counter	vag	vaginal
OU	both eyes	i, ii, iii, iv, etc	one, two, three, four, etc
p̄	after	ʒ (do not use)	dram (in fluid measure,
pc	after meals		3.7 mL)
PO	by mouth	℥ (do not use)	ounce (in fluid measure,
PR	per rectum		29.6 mL)

waiver of childproof containers, the pharmacist or dispenser must place the medication in such a container. Pharmacists may not refill a prescription medication without authorization from the prescriber. Prescribers may grant authorization to renew prescriptions at the time of writing the prescription or over the telephone. Elements [15] to [17] are the prescriber's signature and other identification data.

PRESCRIBING ERRORS

All prescription orders should be legible, unambiguous, dated (and timed in the case of a chart order), and signed clearly for optimal communication between prescriber, pharmacist, and nurse. Furthermore, a good prescription or chart order should contain sufficient information to permit the pharmacist or nurse to discover possible errors before the drug is dispensed or administered.

Several types of prescribing errors are particularly common. These include errors involving omission of needed information; poor writing perhaps leading to errors of drug dose or timing; and prescription of drugs that are inappropriate for the specific situation.

Omission of Information

Errors of omission are common in hospital orders and may include instructions to "resume pre-op meds," which assumes that a full and accurate record of the "pre-op meds" is available; "continue present IV fluids," which fails to state exactly what fluids are to be given, in what volume, and over what time period; or "continue eye drops," which omits mention of which eye is to be treated as well as the drug, concentration, and frequency of administration. Chart orders may also fail to discontinue a prior medication when a new one is begun; may fail to state whether a regular or long-acting form is to be used; may fail to specify a strength or notation for long-acting forms; or may authorize "as-needed" (prn) use that fails to state what conditions will justify the need.

Poor Prescription Writing

Poor prescription writing is traditionally exemplified by illegible handwriting. However, other types of poor writing are common and often more dangerous. One of the most important is the misplaced or ambiguous decimal point. Thus ".1" is easily misread as "1," a tenfold overdose, if the decimal point is not unmistakably clear. This danger is easily avoided by always preceding the decimal point with a zero. On the other hand, appending an unnecessary zero after a decimal point increases the risk of a tenfold overdose, because "1.0 mg" is easily misread as "10 mg," whereas "1 mg" is not. The slash or virgule ("/") was traditionally used as a substitute for a decimal point. This should be abandoned because it is too easily misread as the numeral "1." Similarly, the abbreviation "U" for units should never be used because "10U" is easily misread as "100"; the word "units" should *always* be written out. Doses in micrograms should *always* have this unit written out because the abbreviated form ("μg") is very easily misread as "mg," a 1000-fold overdose! Orders for drugs specifying only the number of dosage units and not the total dose required should not be filled if more than one size dosage unit exists for that drug. For example, ordering "one ampule of furosemide" is unacceptable because furosemide is available in ampules that contain 20, 40, or 100 mg of the drug. The abbreviation "OD" should be used (if at all) only to mean "the right eye"; it has been used for "every day" and has caused inappropriate administration of drugs into the eye. Similarly, "Q.D." or "QD" should not be used because it is often read as "QID," resulting in four daily doses instead of one. Acronyms such as "ASA" (aspirin), "5-ASA" (5-aminosalicylic acid), "6MP" (6-mercaptopurine), etc, should not be used; drug names should be written out. Unclear handwriting can be lethal when drugs with similar names but very different effects are available, eg, acetazolamide and acetohexamide, methotrexate and metolazone. In this situation, errors are best avoided by noting the indication for the drug in the body of the prescription, eg, "acetazolamide, for glaucoma."

Inappropriate Drug Prescriptions

Prescribing an inappropriate drug for a particular patient results from failure to recognize contraindications imposed by other diseases the patient may have, failure to obtain information about other drugs the patient is taking (including over-the-counter drugs), or failure to recognize possible physicochemical incompatibilities between drugs that may react with each other. Contraindications to drugs in the presence of other diseases or pharmacokinetic characteristics are listed in the discussions of the drugs described in this book. The manufacturer's package insert usually contains similar information. Some of the important drug interactions are listed in Appendix II of this book as well as in package inserts.

Physicochemical incompatibilities are of particular concern when parenteral administration is planned. For example, when calcium and phosphate ion concentrations are excessively high in a total parenteral nutrition (TPN) solution, precipitation will occur. Similarly, the simultaneous administration of antacids or products high in metal content may compromise the absorption of many drugs in the intestine, eg, tetracyclines. The package insert and the *Handbook on Injectable Drugs* (Trissel 2003) are good sources for this information.

COMPLIANCE

Compliance (sometimes called "adherence") is the extent to which patients follow treatment instructions. There are four types of noncompliance leading to medication errors.

(1) The patient fails to obtain the medication. Some studies suggest that one third of patients never have

their prescriptions filled. Some patients leave the hospital without obtaining their discharge medications, while others leave the hospital without having their prehospitalization medications resumed. Some patients cannot afford the medications prescribed.

(2) The patient fails to take the medication as prescribed. Examples include wrong dosage, wrong frequency of administration, improper timing or sequencing of administration, wrong route or technique of administration, or taking medication for the wrong purpose. This usually results from inadequate communication between the patient and the prescriber and the pharmacist.

(3) The patient prematurely discontinues the medication. This can occur, for instance, if the patient incorrectly assumes that the medication is no longer needed because the bottle is empty or symptomatic improvement has occurred.

(4) The patient (or another person) takes medication inappropriately. For example, the patient may share a medication with others for any of several reasons.

Several factors encourage noncompliance. Some diseases cause no symptoms (eg, hypertension); patients with these diseases therefore have no symptoms to remind them to take their medications. Patients with very painful conditions, such as arthritis, may continually change medications in hope of finding a better one. Characteristics of the therapy itself can limit the degree of compliance; patients taking a drug once a day are much more likely to be compliant than those taking a drug four times a day. Various patient factors also play a role in compliance. Patients living alone are much less likely to be compliant than married patients of the same age. Packaging may also be a deterrent to compliance—elderly arthritic patients often have difficulty opening their medication containers. Lack of transportation as well as various social or personal beliefs about the use of medications are likewise barriers to compliance.

Strategies for improving compliance include enhanced communication between the patient and health care team members; assessment of personal, social, and economic conditions (often reflected in the patient's lifestyle); development of a routine for taking medications (eg, at mealtimes if the patient has regular meals); and provision of systems to assist taking medications (ie, containers that separate drug doses by day of the week, or medication alarm clocks that remind patients to take their medications); and mailing of refill reminders by the pharmacist to patients taking drugs chronically. The patient who is likely to discontinue a medication because of a perceived drug-related problem should receive instruction and education about how to monitor and understand the effects of the medication.

Compliance can often be improved by enlisting the patient's active participation in the treatment.

LEGAL FACTORS (USA)

The United States government recognizes two classes of drugs: (1) over-the-counter (OTC) drugs and (2) those that require a prescription from a licensed prescriber (Rx Only). OTC drugs are those that can be safely self-administered by the layman for self-limiting conditions and for which appropriate labels can be written for lay comprehension. Half of all drug doses consumed by the American public are OTC drugs.

Physicians, dentists, podiatrists, and veterinarians—and, in some states, specialized pharmacists, nurses, physician's assistants, and optometrists—are granted authority to prescribe dangerous drugs (those bearing the federal legend statement, "Rx Only") on the basis of their training in diagnosis and treatment (see Box, Who May Prescribe?). Pharmacists are authorized to dispense prescriptions pursuant to a prescriber's order provided that the medication order is appropriate and rational for the patient. Nurses are authorized to administer medications to patients subject to a prescriber's order.

Prescription drugs are controlled by the United States Food and Drug Administration as described in Chapter 5. The federal legend statement as well as the package insert are part of the packaging requirements for all prescription drugs. The package insert is the official brochure setting forth the indications, contraindications, warnings, and dosing for the drug.

The prescriber, by writing and signing a prescription order, controls who may obtain prescription drugs. The pharmacist may purchase these drugs, but they may be dispensed only on the order of a legally qualified prescriber. Thus, a "prescription" is actually three things: the physician's order in the patient's chart, the written order to which the pharmacist refers when dispensing, and the patient's medication container with a label affixed.

While the federal government controls the drugs and their labeling and distribution, the state legislatures control who may prescribe drugs through their licensing boards, eg, the Board of Medical Examiners. Prescribers must pass examinations, pay fees, and—in the case of some states and some professions—meet other requirements for relicensure such as continuing education. If these requirements are met, the prescriber is licensed to order dispensing of drugs.

The federal government and the states further impose special restrictions on drugs according to their perceived potential for abuse (Table 66–3). Such drugs include opioids, hallucinogens, stimulants, depressants, and anabolic steroids (see Chapter 32). Special requirements must be met when these drugs are to be prescribed. The Controlled Drug Act requires prescribers

---

WHO MAY PRESCRIBE?*

The right to prescribe drugs and much of the legal responsibility for any harm that derives from the prescription were largely limited to just two groups in the past: physicians and osteopaths. In recent years, this power has diffused and now includes—in a number of states and in varying degrees—pharmacists, nurse practitioners, physician's assistants, and optometrists (see Table 66–2). This development began with the growth of a sense of independence within different health professions and was actively promoted by their professional societies. The more recent development of large health maintenance organizations has greatly strengthened the movement because it offers these extremely powerful economic bodies a way to reduce their expenses.

For example, under a plan of pharmacist care, a patient diagnosed as asthmatic by a physician might be referred to a pharmacist for coordination and follow-up of therapy. The pharmacist would be responsible for generating a problem list, prescribing and dispensing the appropriate drugs after consultation with the physician, educating the patient with regard to his or her disease and medications, and then following the patient's responses to the medications by means of appropriate tests (peak airflow metering, etc).

The primary organizations controlling the privilege of prescribing in the USA are the state boards, under the powers delegated to them by the state legislatures. As indicated in Table 66–2, many state boards have attempted to reserve some measure of the primary responsibility for prescribing to physicians by requiring that the ancillary professional work with or under a physician according to a specific "protocol." In the state of California, this protocol must include a statement of the training, supervision, and documentation requirements of the arrangement and must specify referral requirements, limitations to the list of drugs that may be prescribed (ie, a formulary), and a method of evaluation by the supervising physician. The protocol must be in writing and must be periodically updated (An Explanation of the Scope of RN Practice, 1994).

---

* This section prepared with the assistance of Ronda Malone, PharmD.

---

and dispensers to register with the Drug Enforcement Agency (DEA), pay a fee, receive a personal registration number, and keep records of all controlled drugs prescribed or dispensed. Every time a controlled drug is prescribed, a valid DEA number must appear on the prescription blank.

Prescriptions for substances with a high potential for abuse (schedule II) cannot be refilled. Prescriptions for schedule III, IV, and V drugs can be refilled, but there is a five-refill maximum, and in no case may the prescription be refilled after 6 months from the date of writing. Schedule II drug prescriptions may not be transmitted over the telephone, and some states require a special state-issued prescription blank. These restrictive prescribing laws are intended to limit the amount of drugs of abuse that are made available to the public.

Unfortunately, the inconvenience occasioned by these laws—and an unwarranted fear by medical professionals themselves regarding the risk of patient tolerance and addiction—continues to hamper adequate treatment of patients with terminal conditions. This has been shown to be particularly true in children and elderly patients with cancer. *There is no excuse for inadequate treatment of pain in a terminal patient; not only is addiction irrelevant in such a patient, it is actually uncommon in patients who are being treated for pain* (see Chapter 31). Some states have recognized the underutiliza-tion of pain medications in the treatment of pain associated with chronic and terminal conditions. California, for example, has enacted an "intractable pain treatment" act that reduces the difficulty of renewing prescriptions for opioids. Under the provisions of this act, upon receipt of a copy of the order from the prescriber, eg, by fax, a pharmacist may write a "triplicate" prescription* for a Schedule II substance for a patient under hospice care or living in a skilled nursing facility or in cases where the patient is expected to live less than 6 months; the word "exemption" with regulatory code number is written on a typical prescription, thus providing easier access for the terminally ill.

Labeled & Unlabeled Uses of Drugs

In the USA, the FDA approves a drug only for the specific uses proposed and documented by the manufacturer in its New Drug Application (NDA; see Chapter 5). These approved (labeled) uses or indications are set forth in the package insert that accompanies the drug. For a variety of reasons, these labeled indications may not include all the conditions in which the drug might be useful. Therefore, a

---

* The "triplicate" is the special California prescription form required for Schedule II substances.

Table 66–2. Prescribing authority of certain allied health professionals in selected states.

State	Pharmacists	Nurse Practitioners	Physician's Assistants	Optometrists
California	Yes, under protocol;[1] must be trained in clinical practice	Yes[2]	Yes, under protocol[1]	Yes; limited to certain drug classes
Florida	Yes, according to state formulary; protocol not required	Yes[2]	Yes[2]	Yes; limited to certain drug classes
Michigan	Yes, under protocol; must be specially qualified by education, training, or experience	Yes; do not need physician supervision	Yes[2]	Yes; limited to certain drug classes
Mississippi	Yes, under protocol in an institutional setting	Yes,[2] under narrowly specified conditions	No	Yes; limited to certain certain drug classes
Nevada	Yes, under protocol, within a licensed medical facility	Yes[2]	Yes[2]	Yes; limited to certain drug classes
New Mexico	Yes, under protocol, must be "pharmacist clinician"	Yes; do not need physician supervision	Yes[2]	Yes; limited to certain drug classes
North Dakota	Yes, under protocol in an institutional setting	Yes; do not need physician supervision	Yes	Yes; limited to certain drug classes
Oregon	Yes, under guidelines set by the state board	Yes; do not need physician supervision	Yes[2]	Yes; limited to certain drug classes
Texas	Yes, under protocol set for a particular patient in an institutional setting	Yes; do not need physician supervision	Yes	Yes; limited to certain drug classes
Washington	Yes, under guidelines set by the state board	Yes; do not need physician supervision	Yes[2]	Yes; limited to certain drug classes

[1]Under protocol: see box: Who May Prescribe.
[2]In collaboration with or under the supervision of a physician.

clinician may wish to prescribe the agent for some other, unapproved (unlabeled) clinical condition, often on the basis of adequate or even compelling scientific evidence. Federal laws governing FDA regulations and drug use place no restrictions on such unapproved use.[†]

[†]"Once a product has been approved for marketing, a physician may prescribe it for uses or in treatment regimens or patient populations that are not included in the approved labeling. Such 'unapproved' or, more precisely, 'unlabeled' uses may be appropriate and rational in certain circumstances, and may, in fact, reflect approaches to drug therapy that have been extensively reported in medical literature."—FDA Drug Bull 1982;12:4.

Even if the patient suffers injury from the drug, its use for an unlabeled purpose does not in itself constitute "malpractice." However, the courts may consider the package insert labeling as a complete listing of the indications for which the drug is considered safe unless the clinician can show that other use is considered safe by competent expert testimony.

SOCIOECONOMIC FACTORS

Generic Prescribing

Prescribing by generic name offers the pharmacist flexibility in selecting the particular drug product to fill the

Table 66–3. Classification of controlled substances. (See Inside Front Cover for examples.)

Schedule	Potential for Abuse	Other Comments
I	High	No accepted medical use; lack of accepted safety as drug.
II	High	Current accepted medical use. Abuse may lead to psychologic or physical dependence.
III	Less than I or II	Current accepted medical use. Moderate or low potential for physical dependence and high potential for psychologic dependence.
IV	Less than III	Current accepted medical use. Limited potential for dependence.
V	Less than IV	Current accepted medical use. Limited dependence possible.

order and the patient a potential savings if there is price competition. The brand name of a popular sedative is, for example, Valium by Roche. The generic (public nonproprietary) name of the same chemical substance adopted by United States Adopted Names (USAN) and approved by the Food and Drug Administration (FDA) is diazepam. All diazepam drug products in the USA meet the pharmaceutical standards expressed in *United States Pharmacopeia (USP)*. However, there are several manufacturers, and prices vary greatly. For some drugs in common use, the difference in cost between the trade-named product and generic products varies from less than twofold to more than 100-fold.

In most states and in many hospitals, pharmacists have the option of supplying a generically equivalent drug product even if a proprietary name has been specified in the order. If the physician wants a particular brand of drug product dispensed, handwritten instruction to "dispense as written" or words of similar meaning are required. Some government-subsidized health care programs and many third-party insurance payers require that pharmacists dispense the cheapest generically equivalent product in the inventory. However, the principles of drug product selection by private pharmacists do not permit substituting one therapeutic agent for another (therapeutic substitution)—ie, dispensing trichlormethiazide for hydrochlorothiazide would not be permitted without the prescriber's permission even though these two diuretics may be considered pharmacodynamically equivalent. Pharmacists within managed care organizations may follow different policies; see below.

It should not be assumed that every generic drug product is as satisfactory as the trade-named product, though most generics are satisfactory. Bioavailability— the effective absorption of the drug product—varies between manufacturers and sometimes between different lots of a drug produced by the same manufacturer.

In the case of a very small number of drugs, which usually have a low therapeutic index, poor solubility, or a high ratio of inert ingredients to active drug content, a specific manufacturer's product may give more consistent results. In the case of life-threatening diseases, the advantages of generic substitution are probably outweighed by the clinical urgency so that the prescription should be filled as written.

In an effort to codify bioequivalence information, the FDA publishes *Approved Drug Products With Therapeutic Equivalence Evaluations,* with monthly supplements, commonly called "the Orange Book." The book contains listings of multisource products in one of two categories: Products coded "A" are considered bioequivalent to all other versions of that product with a similar "A" coding. Products not considered bioequivalent are coded "B." Of the approximately 8000 products listed, 90% are coded "A."

Mandatory drug product selection on the basis of price is common practice in the USA as third-party payers (insurance companies, health maintenance organizations, etc) enforce money-saving regulations. If outside a managed care organization, the prescriber can sometimes override these controls by writing "dispense as written" on a prescription that calls for a brand-named product. However, in such cases, the patient may have to pay the difference between the dispensed product and the cheaper one.

Within most managed care organizations, formulary controls have been put in place that force the selection of less expensive medications whenever they are available. In a managed care environment, the prescriber often selects the drug group rather than a specific agent, and the pharmacist dispenses the formulary drug from that group. For example, if a prescriber in such an organization decides that a patient needs a thiazide diuretic, the pharmacist will automatically dispense the single thiazide diuretic carried on the organization's formulary.

THE COST OF PRESCRIPTIONS

The cost of prescriptions has risen dramatically in the last several decades. The average price for a single prescription in the USA in 2003 was more than $50.00. This rise is occasioned by new technology, marketing costs, and stockholder expectations. The pharmaceutical industry typically posts double-digit profits annually while the retail business sector shows a 3% profit. The cost to the patient for many new drugs like "statins" exceeds $1000 per year. Pharmaceuticals are the highest out-of-pocket health-related cost for the health sector because many other health care services are covered by health insurance whereas prescriptions are often not.

These high drug costs have caused payers and consumers alike to seek alternative sources or to ask the government to subsidize personal pharmaceutical needs. Because the Canadian government has done a better job in controlling drug prices, their prices are less than those in the United States. This fact has caused a number of United States citizens to purchase their drugs "off-shore" for "personal use" in quantities up to a 3-month supply—at substantial savings. However, there is no assurance that these drugs are what they are purported to be or that they will be delivered in a timely manner—or that there is a traditional doctor-pharmacist-patient relationship and the safeguards that such a relationship offers. Pharmacists and physicians are asking the question: Why can't we purchase drugs at "off-shore" prices and thus lower the overall cost to the patients? The Veterans Administration system for controlling costs through bulk purchases of drugs and serious negotiation of prices with manufacturers shows that it is possible.

Other Cost Factors

The private pharmacy bases its charges on the cost of the drug plus a fee for providing a professional service. Each time a prescription is dispensed, there is a fee. The prescriber controls the frequency of filling prescriptions by authorizing refills and specifying the quantity to be dispensed. Thus, the prescriber can save the patient money by prescribing standard sizes (so that drugs do not have to be repackaged) and, when chronic treatment is involved, by ordering the largest quantity consistent with safety, expense, and third-party plan. Optimal prescribing for cost savings often involves consultation between the prescriber and the pharmacist. Because of continuing increases in the wholesale prices of drugs in the USA, prescription costs have risen dramatically over the past 3 decades (see Box, The Cost of Prescriptions).

REFERENCES

An explanation of the scope of RN practice including standardization procedures. Board of Registered Nursing, State of California, August 1994.

Bloom BS, Wierz DJ, Pauly MV: Cost and price of comparable branded and generic pharmaceuticals. JAMA 1986;256:2523.

California Business and Professions Code, Chapter 9, Division 2, Pharmacy Law. Department of Consumer Affairs, Sacramento, California, 2003.

Do we pay too much for prescriptions? Consumer Reports 1993;58:668.

Final Report: *Task Force on Prescription Drugs.* Department of Health, Education, and Welfare, 1969.

Frazier LM et al: Can physician education lower the cost of prescription drugs? Ann Intern Med 1991;115:116.

Friedman D et al: Physician attitudes toward and knowledge about generic drug substitution. N Y State J Med 1987;87:539.

Gennaro AR (editor): *Remington's Pharmaceutical Sciences,* 18th ed. Mack, 1990.

Huseby JS, Anderson P: Confusion about drug names. (Letter.) N Engl J Med 1991;325:588.

Jerome JB, Sagan P: The USAN nomenclature system. JAMA 1975;232:294.

Krawelski JE, Pitt L, Dowd B: The effects of competition on prescription-drug product substitution. N Engl J Med 1983;309:213.

Kuehm SL, Doyle MJ: Medication errors: 1977 to 1988. Experience in medical malpractice claims. N J Med 1990;87:27.

Lesar TS, Briceland L, Stein DS: Factors related to errors in medication prescribing. JAMA 1997;277:312.

Lindley CM et al: Inappropriate medication is a major cause of adverse drug reactions in elderly patients. Age Aging 1992;21:294.

Shulman SR: The broader message of Accutane. Am J Public Health 1989;79:1565.

Strom BL: Generic drug substitution revisited. N Engl J Med 1987;316:1456.

Trissel LA: *Handbook on Injectable Drugs,* 12th ed. American Society of Hospital Pharmacists, 2003. (With supplements.)

Use of approved drugs for unlabeled indications. FDA Drug Bull 1982;12:4.

WHO Drug Action Committee: *Model Guide to Good Prescribing.* WHO, 1994.

Wu AW et al: Do house officers learn from their mistakes? JAMA 1991;265:2089.

Appendix I: Vaccines, Immune Globulins, & Other Complex Biologic Products

Harry W. Lampiris, MD, & Daniel S. Maddix, PharmD

Vaccines and related biologic products constitute an important group of agents that bridge the disciplines of microbiology, infectious diseases, immunology, and immunopharmacology. A listing of the most important preparations is provided here. The reader who requires more complete information is referred to the sources listed at the end of this appendix.

ACTIVE IMMUNIZATION

Active immunization consists of the administration of antigen to the host to induce formation of antibodies and cell-mediated immunity. Immunization is practiced to induce protection against many infectious agents and may utilize either inactivated (killed) materials or live attenuated agents (Table I–1). Desirable features of the ideal immunogen include complete prevention of disease, prevention of the carrier state, production of prolonged immunity with a minimum of immunizations, absence of toxicity, and suitability for mass immunization (eg, cheap and easy to administer). Active immunization is generally preferable to passive immunization—in most cases because higher antibody levels are sustained for longer periods of time, requiring less frequent immunization, and in some cases because of the development of concurrent cell-mediated immunity. However, active immunization requires time to develop and is therefore generally inactive at the time of a specific exposure (eg, for parenteral exposure to hepatitis B, concurrent hepatitis B IgG [passive antibodies] and active immunization are given to prevent illness).

Current recommendations for routine active immunization of children are given in Table I–2.

PASSIVE IMMUNIZATION

Passive immunization consists of transfer of immunity to a host using preformed immunologic products. From a practical standpoint, only immunoglobulins have been utilized for passive immunization, since passive administration of cellular components of the immune system has been technically difficult and associated with graft-versus-host reactions. Products of the cellular immune system (eg, interferons) have also been used in the therapy of a wide variety of hematologic and infectious diseases (Chapter 56).

Passive immunization with antibodies may be accomplished with either animal or human immunoglobulins in varying degrees of purity. These may contain relatively high titers of antibodies directed against a specific antigen or, as is true for pooled immune globulin, may simply contain antibodies found in most of the population. Passive immunization is useful for (1) individuals unable to form antibodies (eg, congenital agammaglobulinemia); (2) prevention of disease when time does not permit active immunization (eg, postexposure); (3) for treatment of certain diseases normally prevented by immunization (eg, tetanus); and (4) for treatment of conditions for which active immunization is unavailable or impractical (eg, snakebite).

Complications from administration of *human* immunoglobulins are rare. The injections may be moderately painful and rarely a sterile abscess may occur at the injection site. Transient hypotension and pruritus occasionally occur with the administration of IGIV products, but generally are mild. Individuals with certain immunoglobulin deficiency states (IgA deficiency,

(continued on page 1105)

Table I–1. Materials commonly used for active immunization in the United States.[1]

Vaccine	Type of Agent	Route of Administration	Primary Immunization	Booster[2]	Indications
Diphtheria-tetanus-acellular pertussis (DTaP)	Toxoids and inactivated bacterial components	Intramuscular	See Table I–2		For all children
Haemophilus influenzae type b conjugate (Hib)	Bacterial polysaccharide conjugated to protein	Intramuscular	One dose (see Table I–2 for childhood schedule)	Not recommended	1. For all children 2. Asplenia and other at-risk conditions
Hepatitis A	Inactivated virus	Intramuscular	One dose (administer at least 2–4 weeks before travel to endemic areas)	At 6–12 months for long-term immunity	1. Travelers to hepatitis A endemic areas 2. Homosexual and bisexual men 3. Illicit drug users 4. Chronic liver disease or clotting factor disorders 5. Persons with occupational risk for infection 6. Persons living in, or relocating to, endemic areas 7. Household and sexual contacts of individuals with acute hepatitis A
Hepatitis B	Inactive viral antigen, recombinant	Intramuscular (subcutaneous injection is acceptable in individuals with bleeding disorders)	Three doses at 0, 1, and 6 months (see Table I–2 for childhood schedule)	Not routinely recommended	1. For all infants 2. Preadolescents, adolescents, and young adults 3. Persons with occupational, lifestyle, or environmental risk 4. Hemophiliacs 5. Hemodialysis patients 6. Postexposure prophylaxis
Influenza	Inactivated virus or viral components	Intramuscular	One dose (children ≤ 12 years of age should receive split virus vaccine only; children < 9 who are receiving influenza vaccine for the first time should receive two doses administered at least 1 month apart)	Yearly with current vaccine	1. Adults ≥ 50 years of age 2. Persons with high risk conditions (eg, asthma) 3. Health care workers and others in contact with high-risk groups 4. Residents of nursing homes and other residential chronic care facilities

Vaccine	Type	Route	Primary Schedule	Booster	Indications
Measles	Live virus	Subcutaneous	Two doses at least 1 month apart	None	1. Adults and adolescents born after 1956 without a history of measles or live virus vaccination on or after their first birthday 2. Postexposure prophylaxis in unimmunized persons
Measles-mumps-rubella (MMR)	Live virus	Subcutaneous	See Table I–2	None	For all children
Menningococcal vaccine	Bacterial polysaccharides of serotypes A/C/Y/W-135	Subcutaneous	One dose	Every 3 to 5 years if there is continuing high risk of exposure	1. Military recruits 2. Travelers to areas with epidemic meningococcal disease 3. Individuals with asplenia, complement deficiency, or properdin deficiency 4. Control of outbreaks in closed or semi-closed populations 5. College freshmen who live in dormitories
Mumps	Live virus	Subcutaneous	One dose	None	Adults born after 1956 without a history of mumps or live virus vaccination on or after their first birthday
Pneumococcal vaccine	Bacterial polysaccharides of 23 serotypes	Intramuscular or subcutaneous	One dose	Repeat after 5 years in patients at high risk	1. Adults ≥ 65 years of age 2. Persons at increased risk for pneumococcal disease or its complications
Poliovirus vaccine, inactivated (IPV)	Inactivated viruses of all three serotypes	Subcutaneous	See Table I–2 for childhood schedule. Adults: Two doses 4 to 8 weeks apart, and a third dose 6 to 12 months after the second	One-time booster dose for adults at increased risk of exposure	1. For all children 2. Previously unvaccinated adults at increased risk for occupational or travel exposure to polioviruses
Rabies	Inactivated virus	Intramuscular (IM) or intradermal (ID)	**Preexposure:** Three doses (IM or ID) at days 0, 7, and 21 or 28 **Postexposure:** Five-doses (IM only) at days 0, 3, 7, 14, and 28	Serologic testing every 6 months to 2 years in persons at high risk	1. **Preexposure** prophylaxis in persons at risk for contact with rabies virus 2. **Postexposure** prophylaxis (administer with rabies immune globulin)

(continued)

Table I–1. Materials commonly used for active immunization in the United States[1] (continued).

Vaccine	Type of Agent	Route of Administration	Primary Immunization	Booster[2]	Indications
Rubella	Live virus	Subcutaneous	One or two doses (at least 28 days apart)	None	Adults born after 1956 without a history of rubella or live virus vaccination on or after their first birthday
Tetanus-diphtheria (Td or DT)[3]	Toxoids	Intramuscular	Two doses 4–8 weeks apart, and a third dose 6–12 months after the second	Every 10 years	1. All adults who have not been immunized as children 2. Postexposure prophylaxis if > 5 years has passed since last dose
Typhoid, Ty21a oral	Live bacteria	Oral	Four doses administered every other day	Four doses every 5 years	Risk of exposure to typhoid fever
Typhoid, Vi capsular polysaccharide	Bacterial polysaccharide	Intramuscular	One dose	Every 2 years	Risk of exposure to typhoid fever
Varicella	Live virus	Subcutaneous	Two doses 4–8 weeks apart in persons past their 13th birthday (see Table I–2 for childhood schedule)	Unknown	1. For all children 2. Persons (at high risk for exposure) past their 13th birthday without a history of varicella infection or immunization 3. Postexposure prophylaxis in susceptible persons
Yellow Fever	Live virus	Subcutaneous	One dose 10 days to 10 years before travel	Every 10 years	1. Laboratory personnel who may be exposed to yellow fever virus 2. Travelers to areas where yellow fever occurs

[1] Dosages for the specific product, including variations for age, are best obtained from the manufacturer's package insert. Does not include all combination products.

[2] One dose unless otherwise indicated.

[3] Td = Tetanus and diphtheria toxoids for use in persons ≥ 7 years of age (contains less diphtheria toxoid than DPT and DT). DT = Tetanus and diphtheria toxoids for use in persons < 7 years of age (contains the same amount of diphtheria toxoid as DPT).

Table I–2. Recommended routine childhood immunization schedule.[1]

Age	Immunization	Comments
Birth to 2 months	Hepatitis B vaccine (HBV)	**Infants born to seronegative mothers:** Administration should begin at birth, with the second dose administered at least 4 weeks after the first dose. **Infants born to seropositive mothers:** Should receive the first dose within 12 hours after birth (with hepatitis B immune globulin), the second dose at 1–2 months of age, and the third dose at 6 months of age.
2 months	Diphtheria and tetanus toxoids and acellular pertussis vaccine (DTaP), inactivated poliovirus vaccine (IPV), *Haemophilus influenzae* type b conjugate vaccine (Hib)[2] pneumococcal conjugate vaccine (PCV)	
1–4 months	HBV	The second dose should be given at least 4 weeks after the first dose.
4 months	DTaP, Hib[2], IPV, PCV	
6 months	DTaP, Hib[2], PCV	
6–18 months	HBV, IPV	The third dose of HBV should be given at least 16 weeks after the first dose and at least 8 weeks after the second dose, but not before age 6 months.
6–23 months	Influenza, split virus vaccine	Two doses ≥ 1 month apart are recommended for children ≤ 9 years who are receiving influenza vaccine for the first time.
12–15 months	Measles-mumps-rubella vaccine (MMR), Hib[2], PCV	
12–18 months	DTaP at 15–18 months, varicella vaccine	DTaP may be given as early as age 12 months. Varicella vaccine is recommended at any visit after the first birthday for susceptible children. Susceptible children ≥ 13 years of age should receive two doses given at least 4 weeks apart.
4–6 years	DTaP IPV, MMR	The second dose of MMR should be routinely administered at 4–6 years of age but may be given during any visit if at least 4 weeks have elapsed since administration of the first dose. The second dose should be given no later than age 11–12 years.
11–12 years	Diphtheria and tetanus toxoids (Td)	Vaccination is recommended if at least 5 years has elapsed since administration of the last dose of DTaP. Routine booster doses of Td should be given every 10 years thereafter.

[1]Adapted from MMWR Morb Mortal Wkly Rep 2002;31:31.

[2]Three Hib conjugate vaccines are available for use: (a) oligosaccharide conjugate Hib vaccine (HbOC), (b) polyribosylribitol phosphate-tetanus toxoid conjugate (PRP-T), and (c) *Haemophilus influenzae* type b conjugate vaccine (meningococcal protein conjugate) (PRP-OMP). Children immunized with PRP-OMP at 2 and 4 months of age do not require a dose at 6 months of age.

etc) may occasionally develop hypersensitivity reactions to immune globulin that may limit therapy. Conventional immune globulin contains aggregates of IgG; it will cause severe reactions if given intravenously. However, if the passively administered antibodies are derived from *animal* sera, hypersensitivity reactions ranging from anaphylaxis to serum sickness may occur. Highly purified immunoglobulins, especially from rodents or lagomorphs are the least likely to cause reactions. To avoid anaphylactic reactions, tests for hypersensitivity to the animal serum must be performed. If an alternative preparation is not available and administration of the specific antibody is deemed essential, desensitization can be carried out.

Antibodies derived from human serum not only avoid the risk of hypersensitivity reactions but also have a much longer half-life in humans (about 23 days for IgG antibodies) than those from animal sources (5–7 days or less). Consequently, much smaller doses of human antibody can be administered to provide therapeutic concentrations for several weeks. These advantages point to the desirability of using human antibodies for passive protection whenever possible. Materials available for passive immunization are summarized in Table I–3.

LEGAL LIABILITY FOR UNTOWARD REACTIONS

It is the physician's responsibility to inform the patient of the risk of immunization and to employ vaccines and antisera in an appropriate manner. This may require skin testing to assess the risk of an untoward reaction. Some of the risks described above are, however, currently unavoidable; on the balance, the patient and society are clearly better off accepting the risks for routinely administered immunogens (eg, influenza and tetanus vaccines).

Manufacturers should be held legally accountable for failure to adhere to existing standards for production of biologicals. However, in the present litigious atmosphere of the United States, the filing of large liability claims by the statistically inevitable victims of good public health practice has caused many manufacturers to abandon efforts to develop and produce low-profit but medically valuable therapeutic agents such as vaccines. Since the use and sale of these products are subject to careful review and approval by government bodies such as the Surgeon General's Advisory Committee on Immunization Practices and the Food and Drug Administration, "strict product liability" (liability without fault) may be an inappropriate legal standard to apply when rare reactions to biologicals, produced and administered according to government guidelines, are involved.

RECOMMENDED IMMUNIZATION OF ADULTS FOR TRAVEL

Every adult, whether traveling or not, should be immunized with tetanus toxoid and should also be fully immunized against poliomyelitis, measles (for those born after 1956), and diphtheria. In addition, every traveler must fulfill the immunization requirements of the health authorities of the countries to be visited. These are listed in *Health Information for International Travel,* available from the Superintendent of Documents, United States Government Printing Office, Washington, DC 20402. A useful website is www.cdc.gov/travel/vaccinat.htm. *The Medical Letter on Drugs and Therapeutics* also offers periodically updated recommendations for international travelers (see issue of April 15, 2002). Immunizations received in preparation for travel should be recorded on the International Certificate of Immunization. *Note:* Smallpox vaccination is not recommended or required for travel in any country.

Table I–3. Materials available for passive immunization.[1]

Indication	Product	Dosage	Comments
Black widow spider bite	Antivenin (*Latrodectus mactans*), equine	One vial (6000 units) IV or IM.	For persons with hypertensive cardiovascular disease or age < 16 or > 60 years.
Bone marrow transplantation	Immune globulin (intravenous)[2]	500 mg/kg IV on days 7 and 2 prior to transplantation and then once weekly through day 90 after transplantation.	Prophylaxis to decrease the risk of infection, interstitial pneumonia, and acute graft-versus-host disease in adults undergoing bone marrow transplantation.
Botulism	Botulism antitoxin (trivalent, types A, B, and E), equine	Consult the CDC.[3]	Treatment and prophylaxis of botulism. Available from the CDC.[3] Ten to 20 percent incidence of serum reactions.
Chronic lymphocytic leukemia (CLL)	Immune globulin (intravenous)[3]	Initial dose of 400 mg/kg IV every 3–4 weeks. Dosage should be adjusted upward if bacterial infections occur.	CLL patients with hypogammaglobulinemia and a history of at least one serious bacterial infection.
Cytomegalovirus (CMV)	Cytomegalovirus immune globulin (intravenous)	Consult the manufacturer's dosing recommendations.	Prophylaxis of CMV infection in bone marrow, kidney, liver, lung, pancreas, heart transplant recipients.
Diphtheria	Diphtheria antitoxin, equine	20,000–120,000 units IV or IM depending on the severity and duration of illness.	Early treatment of respiratory diphtheria. Available from the CDC.[3] Anaphylactic reactions in ≥ 7% of adults and serum reactions in ≥ 5–10% of adults.
Hepatitis A	Immune globulin (intramuscular)	**Preexposure prophylaxis:** 0.02 mL/kg IM for anticipated risk of ≤ 3 months, 0.06 mL/kg for anticipated risk of > 3 months, repeated every 4–6 months for continued exposure. **Postexposure:** 0.02 mL/kg IM as soon as possible after exposure up to 2 weeks.	Preexposure and postexposure hepatitis A prophylaxis. The availability of hepatitis A vaccine has greatly reduced the need for preexposure prophylaxis.
Hepatitis B	Hepatitis B immune globulin (HBIG)	0.06 mL/kg IM as soon as possible after exposure up to 1 week for percutaneous exposure or 2 weeks for sexual exposure. 0.5 mL IM within 12 hours after birth for perinatal exposure.	Postexposure prophylaxis in nonimmune persons following percutaneous, mucosal, sexual, or perinatal exposure. Hepatitis B vaccine should also be administered.
HIV-infected children	Immune globulin (intravenous)[2]	400 mg/kg IV every 28 days.	HIV-infected children with recurrent serious bacterial infections or hypogammaglobulinemia.
Kawasaki disease	Immune globulin (intravenous)[2]	400 mg/kg IV daily for 4 consecutive days within 4 days after the onset of illness. A single dose of 2 g/kg IV over 10 hours is also effective.	Effective in the prevention of coronary aneurysms. For use in patients who meet strict criteria for Kawasaki disease.

(continued)

Table I–3. Materials available for passive immunization *(continued)*.

Indication	Product	Dosage	Comments
Measles	Immune globulin (intramuscular)	**Normal hosts:** 0.25 mL/kg IM. **Immunocompromised hosts:** 0.5 mL/kg IM (maximum 15 mL for all patients).	Postexposure prophylaxis (within 6 days after exposure) in nonimmune contacts of acute cases.
Idiopathic thrombocyto-penic purpura (ITP)	Immune globulin (intravenous)[2]	Consult the manufacturer's dosing recommendations for the specific product being used.	Response in children with ITP is greater than in adults. Corticosteroids are the treatment of choice in adults, except for severe pregnancy-associated ITP.
Primary immuno-deficiency disorders	Immune globulin (intravenous)[2]	Consult the manufacturer's dosing recommendations for the specific product being used.	Primary immunodeficiency disorders include specific antibody deficiencies (eg, X-linked agammaglobulinemia) and combined deficiencies (eg, severe combined immunodeficiencies).
Rabies	Rabies immune globulin	20 IU/kg. The full dose should be infiltrated around the wound and any remaining volume should be given IM at an anatomic site distant from vaccine administration.	Postexposure rabies prophylaxis in persons not previously immunized with rabies vaccine. Must be combined with rabies vaccine.
Respiratory syncytial virus (RSV)	Palivizumab	15 mg/kg IM once prior to the beginning of the RSV season and once monthly until the end of the season.	For use in infants and children younger than 24 months with chronic lung disease or a history of premature birth (≤ 35 weeks' gestation).
	RSV immune globulin	750 mg/kg IV once prior to the beginning of the RSV season and once monthly until the end of the season.	As for palivizumab. Palivizumab is preferred for selected high-risk children, but RSV-IGIV may be pre-ferred for selected high-risk children.
Rubella	Immune globulin (intramuscular)	0.55 mL/kg IM.	Nonimmune pregnant women exposed to rubella who will not consider therapeutic abortion. Administration does not prevent rubella in the fetus of an exposed mother.
Snake bite (coral snake)	Antivenin *(Micrurus fulvius)*, equine	At least 3–5 vials (30–50 mL) IV initially within 4 hours after the bite. Additional doses may be required.	Neutralizes venom of eastern coral snake and Texas coral snake. Serum sickness occurs in almost all patients who receive > 7 vials.
Snake bite (pit vipers)	Antivenin (Crotalidae) polyvalent, equine	The entire dose should be given within 4 hours after the bite by the IV or IM route (1 vial = 10 mL): Minimal envenomation: 2–4 vials Moderate envenomation: 5–9 vials Severe envenomation: 10–15 vials Additional doses may be required.	Neutralizes the venom of rattlesnakes, copperheads, cottonmouths, water moccasins, and tropical and Asiatic crotalids. Serum sickness occurs in almost all patients who receive > 7 vials.

Table I–3. Materials available for passive immunization *(continued)*.

Indication	Product	Dosage	Comments
Tetanus	Tetanus immune globulin	**Postexposure prophylaxis:** 250 units IM. For severe wounds or when there has been a delay in administration, 500 units is recommended. **Treatment:** 3000–6000 units IM.	Treatment of tetanus and postexposure prophylaxis of nonclean, nonminor wounds in inadequately immunized persons (less than two doses of tetanus toxoid or less than three doses if wound is more than 24 hours old).
Vaccinia	Vaccinia immune globulin	Consult the CDC.[3]	Treatment of severe reactions to vaccinia vaccination, including eczema vaccinatum, vaccinia necrosum, and ocular vaccinia. Available from the CDC.[3]
Varicella	Varicella-zoster immune globulin	**Weight (kg) Dose (units)** ≤ 10 125 IM 10.1–20 250 IM 20.1–30 375 IM 30.1–40 500 IM > 40 625 IM	**Postexposure prophylaxis** (preferably within 48 hours but no later than within 96 hours after exposure) in susceptible immunocompromised hosts, selected pregnant women, and perinatally exposed newborns.

[1]Passive immunotherapy or immunoprophylaxis should always be administered as soon as possible after exposure. Prior to the administration of animal sera, patients should be questioned and tested for hypersensitivity.

[2]See the following references for an analysis of additional uses of intravenously administered immune globulin: Ratko TA et al: Recommendations for off-label use of intravenously administered immunoglobulin preparations. JAMA 1995;273:1865; and Dalakas MC: Intravenous immune globulin therapy for neurologic diseases. Ann Intern Med 1997;126:721.

[3]Centers for Disease Control and Prevention, 404-639-3670 during weekday business hours; 404-639-2888 during nights, weekends, and holidays (emergency requests only).

REFERENCES

Ada G: Vaccines and vaccination. N Engl J Med 2001;345:1042.

Advice for travelers. Med Lett Drugs Ther 2002;44:33.

Avery RK: Immunizations in adult immunocompromised patients: which to use and which to avoid. Cleve Clin J Med 2001;68:337.

CDC Website: www.cdc.gov/travel/vaccinat.htm.

Combination vaccines for childhood immunization. MMWR Morb Mortal Wkly Rep 1999;48(RR-5):1.

Dennehy PH: Active immunization in the United States: developments over the past decade. Clin Micro Rev 2001;14:872.

Gardner P, Peter G: Vaccine recommendations: challenges and controversies. Infect Dis Clin North Am 2001;15:1.

Gardner P et al: Guidelines for quality standards for immunization. Clin Infect Dis 2002;35:503.

General recommendations on immunization. Recommendations of the Advisory Committee on Immunization Practices (ACIP) and the American Academy of Family Physicians (AAFP). MMWR Morb Mortal Wkly Rep 2002;51(RR-2):1.

Keller MA, Stiehm ER: Passive immunity in prevention and treatment of infectious diseases. Clin Microbiol Rev 2000;13:602.

Lutwick LI: New vaccines and new vaccine technology. Infect Dis Clin North Am 1999;13:1.

Recommended adult immunization schedule—United States, 2002-2003. MMWR Morb Mortal Wkly Rep 2002;51:904.

Recommended childhood immunization schedule—United States, 2002. MMWR Morb Mortal Wkly Rep 2002;51:31.

Vaccine-preventable diseases: Improving vaccination coverage in children, adolescents, and adults. A report on recommendations from the Task Force on Community Preventive Services. MMWR Morb Mortal Wkly Rep 1999;48(RR-8):1.

Appendix II: Important Drug Interactions & Their Mechanisms

Philip D. Hansten, PharmD

One of the factors that can alter the response to drugs is the concurrent administration of other drugs. There are several mechanisms by which drugs may interact, but most can be categorized as pharmacokinetic (absorption, distribution, metabolism, excretion), pharmacodynamic, or combined interactions. Knowledge of the mechanism by which a given drug interaction occurs is often clinically useful, since the mechanism may influence both the time course and the methods of circumventing the interaction. Some important drug interactions occur as a result of two or more mechanisms.

Pharmacokinetic Mechanisms

The gastrointestinal absorption of drugs may be affected by concurrent use of other agents that (1) have a large surface area upon which the drug can be adsorbed, (2) bind or chelate, (3) alter gastric pH, (4) alter gastrointestinal motility, or (5) affect transport proteins such as P-glycoprotein. One must distinguish between effects on adsorption rate and effects on extent of absorption. A reduction in only the absorption rate of a drug is seldom clinically important, whereas a reduction in the extent of absorption will be clinically important if it results in subtherapeutic serum levels.

The mechanisms by which drug interactions alter drug distribution include (1) competition for plasma protein binding, (2) displacement from tissue binding sites, and (3) alterations in local tissue barriers, eg, P-glycoprotein inhibition in the blood-brain barrier. Although competition for plasma protein binding can increase the free concentration (and thus the effect) of the displaced drug in plasma, the increase will be transient owing to a compensatory increase in drug disposition. The clinical importance of protein binding displacement has been overemphasized; current evidence suggests that such interactions are unlikely to result in adverse effects. Displacement from tissue binding sites would tend to transiently increase the blood concentration of the displaced drug.

The metabolism of drugs can be stimulated or inhibited by concurrent therapy. Induction (stimulation) of cytochrome P450 isozymes in the liver and small intestine can be caused by drugs such as barbiturates, carbamazepine, efavirenz, glutethimide, nevirapine, phenytoin, primidone, rifampin, and rifabutin. Enzyme inducers can also increase the activity of phase II metabolism such as glucuronidation. Enzyme induction does not take place quickly; maximal effects usually occur after 7–10 days and require an equal or longer time to dissipate after the enzyme inducer is stopped. Rifampin, however, may produce enzyme induction after only a few doses. Inhibition of metabolism generally takes place more quickly than enzyme induction and may begin as soon as sufficient tissue concentration of the inhibitor is achieved. However, if the half-life of the affected drug is long, it may take a week or more to reach a new steady-state serum level. Drugs that may inhibit cytochrome P450 metabolism of other drugs include allopurinol, amiodarone, androgens, chloramphenicol, cimetidine, ciprofloxacin, clarithromycin, cyclosporine, delavirdine, diltiazem, disulfiram, enoxacin, erythromycin, fluconazole, fluoxetine, fluvoxamine, grapefruit juice, indinavir, isoniazid, itraconazole, ketoconazole, metronidazole, mexiletine, miconazole, nefazodone, omeprazole, paroxetine, phenylbutazone, propoxyphene, quinidine, ritonavir, sulfonamides, verapamil, zafirlukast, and zileuton.

The renal excretion of active drug can also be affected by concurrent drug therapy. The renal excretion of certain drugs that are weak acids or weak bases may be influenced by other drugs that affect urinary pH. This is due to changes in ionization of the drug, as described in Chapter 1 under Ionization of Weak Acids and Weak Bases; the Henderson-Hasselbalch Equation. For some drugs, active secretion into the renal tubules is an important elimination pathway. The ABC transporter P-glycoprotein is involved in active tubular secretion of some drugs, and inhibition of this transporter can inhibit renal elimination with attendant increase in serum drug concentrations.

Pharmacodynamic Mechanisms

When drugs with similar pharmacologic effects are administered concurrently, an additive or synergistic response is usually seen. The two drugs may or may not act on the same receptor to produce such effects. Conversely, drugs with opposing pharmacologic effects may reduce the response to one or both drugs. Pharmacodynamic drug interactions are relatively common in clinical practice, but adverse effects can usually be minimized if one understands the pharmacology of the drugs involved. In this way, the interactions can be anticipated and appropriate countermeasures taken.

Combined Toxicity

The combined use of two or more drugs, each of which has toxic effects on the same organ, can greatly increase the likelihood of organ damage. For example, concurrent administration of two nephrotoxic drugs can produce kidney damage even though the dose of either drug alone may have been insufficient to produce toxicity. Furthermore, some drugs can enhance the organ toxicity of another drug even though the enhancing drug has no intrinsic toxic effect on that organ.

PREDICTABILITY OF DRUG INTERACTIONS

The designations listed in Table II–1 will be used here to *estimate* the predictability of the drug interactions. These estimates are intended to indicate simply whether or not the interaction will occur and do not always mean that the interaction is likely to produce an adverse effect. Whether the interaction occurs and produces an adverse effect or not depends upon (1) the presence or absence of factors that predispose to the adverse effects of the drug interaction (diseases, organ function, dose of drugs, etc) and (2) awareness on the part of the prescriber, so that appropriate monitoring can be ordered or preventive measures taken.

Table II–1. Important drug interactions.

HP = Highly predictable. Interaction occurs in almost all patients receiving the interacting combination.	
P = Predictable. Interaction occurs in most patients receiving the combination.	
NP = Not predictable. Interaction occurs only in some patients receiving the combination.	
NE = Not established. Insufficient data available on which to base estimate of predictability.	

Drug or Drug Group	Properties Promoting Drug Interaction	Clinically Documented Interactions

Alcohol	Chronic alcoholism results in enzyme induction. Acute alcoholic intoxication tends to inhibit drug metabolism (whether person is alcoholic or not). Severe alcohol-induced hepatic dysfunction may inhibit ability to metabolize drugs. Disulfiram-like reaction in the presence of certain drugs. Additive central nervous system depression with other central nervous system depressants.	**Acetaminophen:** [NE] Increased formation of hepatotoxic acetaminophen metabolites (in chronic alcoholics).
		Acitretin: [P] Increased conversion of acitretin to etretinate (teratogenic).
		Anticoagulants, oral: [NE] Increased hypoprothrombinemic effect with acute alcohol intoxication.
		Central nervous system depressants: [HP] Additive or synergistic central nervous system depression.
		Insulin: [NE] Acute alcohol intake may increase hypoglycemic effect of insulin (especially in fasting patients).
		Drugs that may produce a disulfiram-like reaction:
		    Cephalosporins: [NP] Disulfiram-like reactions noted with cefamandole, cefoperazone, cefotetan, and moxalactam.
		    Chloral hydrate: [NP] Mechanism not established.
		    Disulfiram: [HP] Inhibits aldehyde dehydrogenase.
		    Metronidazole: [NP] Mechanism not established.
		    Sulfonylureas: [NE] Chlorpropamide is most likely to produce a disulfiram-like reaction; acute alcohol intake may increase hypoglycemic effect (especially in fasting patients).

Allopurinol	Inhibits hepatic drug-metabolizing enzymes.	**Anticoagulants, oral:** [NP] Increased hypoprothrombinemic effect. **Azathioprine:** [P] Decreased azathioprine detoxification resulting in increased azathioprine toxicity. **Mercaptopurine:** [P] Decreased mercaptopurine metabolism resulting in increased mercaptopurine toxicity.
Antacids	Antacids may adsorb drugs in gastrointestinal tract, thus reducing absorption. Antacids tend to speed gastric emptying, thus delivering drugs to absorbing sites in the intestine more quickly. Some antacids (eg, magnesium hydroxide with aluminum hydroxide) alkalinize the urine somewhat, thus altering excretion of drugs sensitive to urinary pH.	**Digoxin:** [NP] Decreased gastrointestinal absorption of digoxin. **Iron:** [P] Decreased gastrointestinal absorption of iron with calcium-containing antacids. **Itraconazole:** [P] Reduced gastrointestinal absorption of itraconazole due to increased pH (itraconazole requires acid for absorption). **Ketoconazole:** [P] Reduced gastrointestinal absorption of ketoconazole due to increased pH (ketoconazole requires acid for absorption). **Quinolones:** [HP] Decreased gastrointestinal absorption of ciprofloxacin, norfloxacin, enoxacin (and probably other quinolones). **Salicylates:** [P] Increased renal clearance of salicylates due to increased urine pH; occurs only with large doses of salicylates. **Sodium polystyrene sulfonate:** [NE] Binds antacid cation in gut, resulting in metabolic alkalosis. **Tetracyclines:** [HP] Decreased gastrointestinal absorption of tetracyclines. **Thyroxine:** [NP] Reduced gastrointestinal absorption of thyroxine.

Table II–1. Important drug interactions *(continued).*

HP = Highly predictable. Interaction occurs in almost all patients receiving the interacting combination.	
P = Predictable. Interaction occurs in most patients receiving the combination.	
NP = Not predictable. Interaction occurs only in some patients receiving the combination.	
NE = Not established. Insufficient data available on which to base estimate of predictability.	

Drug or Drug Group	Properties Promoting Drug Interaction	Clinically Documented Interactions
Anticoagulants, oral	Metabolism inducible. Susceptible to inhibition of metabolism by CYP2C9. Highly bound to plasma proteins. Anticoagulation response altered by drugs that affect clotting factor synthesis or catabolism.	*Drugs that may increase anticoagulant effect:* **Amiodarone:** [P] Inhibits anticoagulant metabolism. **Anabolic steroids:** [P] Alter clotting factor disposition? **Chloramphenicol:** [NE] Decreased dicumarol metabolism (probably also warfarin). **Cimetidine:** [HP] Decreased warfarin metabolism. **Ciprofloxacin.** [NP] Decreased anticoagulant metabolism? **Clofibrate:** [P] Mechanism not established. **Danazol:** [NE] Impaired synthesis of clotting factors? **Dextrothyroxine:** [P] Enhances clotting factor catabolism? **Disulfiram:** [P] Decreased warfarin metabolism. **Erythromycin:** [NP] Probably inhibits anticoagulant metabolism. **Fluconazole:** [P] Decreased warfarin metabolism. **Gemfibrozil:** [NE] Mechanism not established. **Lovastatin:** [NE] Probably decreased anticoagulant metabolism. **Metronidazole:** [P] Decreased warfarin metabolism. **Miconazole:** [NE] Decreased warfarin metabolism. **Nonsteroidal anti-inflammatory drugs:** [P] Inhibition of platelet function, gastric erosions; some agents increase hypoprothrombinemic response (unlikely with diclofenac, ibuprofen, or naproxen). **Propafenone:** [NE] Probably decreased anticoagulant metabolism. **Quinidine:** [NP] Additive hypoprothrombinemia. **Salicylates:** [HP] Platelet inhibition with aspirin but not with other salicylates; [P] large doses have hypoprothrombinemic effect. **Sulfinpyrazone:** [NE] Inhibits warfarin metabolism. **Sulfonamides:** [NE] Inhibit warfarin metabolism; displace protein binding. **Thyroid hormones:** [P] Enhance clotting factor catabolism. **Trimethoprim-sulfamethoxazole:** [P] Inhibits warfarin metabolism; displaces from protein binding. *See also* Alcohol; Allopurinol. *Drugs that may decrease anticoagulant effect:* **Aminoglutethimide:** [P] Enzyme induction. **Barbiturates:** [P] Enzyme induction. **Carbamazepine:** [P] Enzyme induction. **Cholestyramine:** [P] Reduces absorption of anticoagulant. **Glutethimide:** [P] Enzyme induction. **Nafcillin:** [NE] Enzyme induction. **Phenytoin:** [NE] Enzyme induction; anticoagulant effect may increase transiently at start of phenytoin therapy due to protein-binding displacement. **Primidone:** [P] Enzyme induction.

(continued)

Table II–1. Important drug interactions *(continued).*

HP = Highly predictable. Interaction occurs in almost all patients receiving the interacting combination.
P = Predictable. Interaction occurs in most patients receiving the combination.
NP = Not predictable. Interaction occurs only in some patients receiving the combination.
NE = Not established. Insufficient data available on which to base estimate of predictability.

Drug or Drug Group	Properties Promoting Drug Interaction	Clinically Documented Interactions
Anticoagulants, oral *(continued)*	(See preceding page.)	**Rifabutin:** [P] Enzyme induction. **Rifampin:** [P] Enzyme induction. **St. John's wort:** [NE] Enzyme induction. *Effects of anticoagulants on other drugs:* 　**Hypoglycemics, oral:** [P] Dicumarol inhibits hepatic metabolism of tolbutamide and chlorpropamide. 　**Phenytoin:** [P] Dicumarol inhibits metabolism of phenytoin.
Antidepressants, tricyclic and heterocyclic	Inhibition of amine uptake into postganglionic adrenergic neuron. Antimuscarinic effects may be additive with other antimuscarinic drugs. Metabolism inducible. Susceptible to inhibition of metabolism by CYP2D6 and other CYP450 enzymes.	**Barbiturates:** [P] Increased antidepressant metabolism. **Carbamazepine:** [NE] Enhanced metabolism of antidepressants. **Cimetidine:** [P] Decreased antidepressant metabolism. **Clonidine:** [P] Decreased clonidine antihypertensive effect. **Guanadrel:** [P] Decreased uptake of guanadrel into sites of action. **Guanethidine:** [P] Decreased uptake of guanethidine into sites of action. **Monoamine oxidase inhibitors:** [NP] Some cases of excitation, hyperpyrexia, mania, and convulsions, especially with serotonergic antidepressants such as clomipramine and imipramine, but many patients have received combination without ill effects. **Quinidine:** [NE] Decreased antidepressant metabolism. **Rifampin:** [P] Increased antidepressant metabolism. **Selective serotonin reuptake inhibitors (SSRIs):** [P] Fluoxetine and paroxetine inhibit CYP2D6 and decrease metabolism of antidepressants metabolized by this enzyme (eg, desipramine). Citalopram, sertraline, and fluvoxamine are only weak inhibitors of CYP2D6, but fluvoxamine inhibits CYP1A2 and CYP3A4 and thus can inhibit the metabolism of antidepressants metabolized by these enzymes. **Sympathomimetics:** [P] Increased pressor response to norepinephrine, epinephrine, and phenylephrine.
Azole antifungals	Inhibition of CYP3A4 (itraconazole = ketoconazole > voriconazole > fluconazole). Inhibition of CYP2C9 (fluconazole, voriconazole). Susceptible to enzyme inducers (itraconazole, ketoconazole, voriconazole). Gastrointestinal absorption pH-dependent (itraconazole, ketoconazole). Inhibition of P-glycoprotein (itraconazole, ketoconazole).	**Barbiturates:** [P] Increased metabolism of itraconazole, ketoconazole, voriconazole. **Calcium channel blockers:** [P] Decreased calcium channel blocker metabolism. **Carbamazepine:** [P] Decreased carbamazepine metabolism. **H₂-receptor antagonists:** [NE] Decreased absorption of itraconazole and ketoconazole. **Cisapride:** [NP] Decreased metabolism of cisapride; possible ventricular arrhythmias. **Cyclosporine:** [P] Decreased metabolism of cyclosporine. **Digoxin:** [NE] Increased gastrointestinal absorption and decreased renal excretion of digoxin with itraconazole and ketoconazole.

Table II–1. Important drug interactions *(continued).*

HP = Highly predictable. Interaction occurs in almost all patients receiving the interacting combination.		
P = Predictable. Interaction occurs in most patients receiving the combination.		
NP = Not predictable. Interaction occurs only in some patients receiving the combination.		
NE = Not established. Insufficient data available on which to base estimate of predictability.		

Drug or Drug Group	Properties Promoting Drug Interaction	Clinically Documented Interactions
Azole antifungals *(continued)*	(See preceding page.)	**HMG CoA reductase inhibitors:** Decreased metabolism of lovastatin, simvastatin, and, to a lesser extent, atorvastatin. **Phenytoin:** [P] Decreased metabolism of phenytoin with fluconazole and probably voriconazole. **Pimozide:** [NE] Decreased pimozide metabolism. **Proton pump inhibitors:** [P] Decreased absorption of itraconazole and ketoconazole. **Rifampin:** [P] Increased metabolism of itraconazole, ketoconazole, and voriconazole. *See also* Antacids; Anticoagulants, oral.
Barbiturates	Induction of hepatic microsomal drug-metabolizing enzymes. Additive central nervous system depression with other central nervous system depressants.	**Beta-adrenoceptor blockers:** [P] Increased β-blocker metabolism. **Calcium channel blockers:** [P] Increased calcium channel blocker metabolism. **Central nervous system depressants:** [HP] Additive central nervous system depression. **Corticosteroids:** [P] Increased corticosteroid metabolism. **Cyclosporine:** [NE] Increased cyclosporine metabolism. **Delavirdine:** [P] Increased delavirdine metabolism. **Doxycycline:** [P] Increased doxycycline metabolism. **Estrogens:** [P] Increased estrogen metabolism. **Methadone:** [NE] Increased methadone metabolism. **Phenothiazine:** [P] Increased phenothiazine metabolism. **Protease inhibitors:** [NE] Increased protease inhibitor metabolism. **Quinidine:** [P] Increased quinidine metabolism. **Sirolimus:** [NE] Increased sirolimus metabolism. **Tacrolimus:** [NE] Increased tacrolimus metabolism. **Theophylline:** [NE] Increased theophylline metabolism; reduced theophylline effect. **Valproic acid:** [P] Decreased phenobarbital metabolism. *See also* Anticoagulants, oral; Antidepressants, tricyclic.
Beta-adrenoceptor blockers	Beta-blockade (especially with nonselective agents such as propranolol) alters response to sympathomimetics with β-agonist activity (eg, epinephrine). Beta-blockers that undergo extensive first-pass metabolism may be affected by drugs capable of altering this process. Beta-blockers may reduce hepatic blood flow.	*Drugs that may increase β-blocker effect:* **Cimetidine:** [P] Decreased metabolism of β-blockers that are cleared primarily by the liver, eg, propranolol. Less effect (if any) on those cleared by the kidneys, eg, atenolol, nadolol. *Drugs that may decrease β-blocker effect:* **Enzyme inducers:** [P] Barbiturates, phenytoin, and rifampin may enhance β-blockers metabolism; other enzyme inducers may produce similar effects. **Nonsteroidal anti-inflammatory drugs:** [P] Indomethacin reduces antihypertensive response; other prostaglandin inhibitors probably also interact. *Effects of β-blockers on other drugs:* **Clonidine:** [NE] Hypertensive reaction if clonidine is withdrawn while patient is taking propranolol.

(continued)

Table II–1. Important drug interactions *(continued).*

HP = Highly predictable. Interaction occurs in almost all patients receiving the interacting combination.		
P = Predictable. Interaction occurs in most patients receiving the combination.		
NP = Not predictable. Interaction occurs only in some patients receiving the combination.		
NE = Not established. Insufficient data available on which to base estimate of predictability.		

Drug or Drug Group	Properties Promoting Drug Interaction	Clinically Documented Interactions
Beta-adrenoceptor blockers *(continued)*	(See preceding page.)	**Insulin:** [P] Inhibition of glucose recovery from hypoglycemia; inhibition of symptoms of hypoglycemia (except sweating); increased blood pressure during hypoglycemia. **Lidocaine:** [NE] Decreased clearance of intravenous lidocaine; increased plasma lidocaine levels. **Prazosin:** [P] Increased hypotensive response to first dose of prazosin. **Sympathomimetics:** [P] Increased pressor response to epinephrine (and possibly other sympathomimetics); this is more likely to occur with nonspecific β-blockers.
Bile acid-binding resins	Resins may bind with orally administered drugs in gastrointestinal tract. Resins may bind in gastrointestinal tract with drugs that undergo enterohepatic circulation, even if the latter are given parenterally.	**Acetaminophen:** [NE] Decreased gastrointestinal absorption of acetaminophen. **Digitalis glycosides:** [NE] Decreased gastrointestinal absorption of digitoxin (possibly also digoxin). **Furosemide:** [P] Decreased gastrointestinal absorption of furosemide. **Methotrexate:** [NE] Reduced gastrointestinal absorption of methotrexate. **Mycophenolate:** [P] Reduced gastrointestinal absorption of mycophenolate. **Thiazide diuretics:** [P] Reduced gastrointestinal absorption of thiazides. **Thyroid hormones:** [P] Reduced thyroid absorption. *See also* Anticoagulants, oral.
Calcium channel blockers	Verapamil, diltiazem, and perhaps nicardipine (but not nifedipine) inhibit hepatic drug-metabolizing enzymes. Metabolism of diltiazem, nifedipine, verapamil, and probably other calcium channel blockers subject to induction and inhibition.	**Carbamazepine:** [P] Decreased carbamazepine metabolism with diltiazem and verapamil; possible increase in calcium channel blocker metabolism. **Cimetidine:** [NP] Decreased metabolism of calcium channel blockers. **Cyclosporine:** [P] Decreased cyclosporine metabolism with diltiazem, nicardipine, verapamil. **Phenytoin:** [NE] Increased metabolism of calcium channel blockers. **Rifampin:** [P] Increased metabolism of calcium channel blockers. *See also* Azole antifungals, Barbiturates, Theophylline.
Carbamazepine	Induction of hepatic microsomal drug-metabolizing enzymes. Susceptible to inhibition of metabolism, primarily by CYP3A4.	**Cimetidine:** [P] Decreased carbamazepine metabolism. **Clarithromycin:** [P] Decreased carbamazepine metabolism. **Corticosteroids:** [P] Increased corticosteroid metabolism. **Cyclosporine:** [P] Increased cyclosporine metabolism. **Danazol:** [P] Decreased carbamazepine metabolism. **Diltiazem:** [P] Decreased carbamazepine metabolism. **Doxycycline:** [P] Increased doxycycline metabolism. **Erythromycin:** [NE] Decreased carbamazepine metabolism.

Table II–1. Important drug interactions (continued).

HP = Highly predictable. Interaction occurs in almost all patients receiving the interacting combination.	
P = Predictable. Interaction occurs in most patients receiving the combination.	
NP = Not predictable. Interaction occurs only in some patients receiving the combination.	
NE = Not established. Insufficient data available on which to base estimate of predictability.	

Drug or Drug Group	Properties Promoting Drug Interaction	Clinically Documented Interactions
Carbamazepine (*continued*)	(See preceding page.)	**Fluvoxamine:** [NE] Decreased carbamazepine metabolism. **Estrogens:** [P] Increased estrogen metabolism. **Haloperidol:** [P] Increased haloperidol metabolism. **Isoniazid:** [P] Decreased carbamazepine metabolism. **Nefazodone:** [NE] Decreased carbamazepine metabolism. **Propoxyphene:** [HP] Decreased carbamazepine metabolism. **Selective serotonin reuptake inhibitors (SSRIs):** [NE] Fluoxetine and fluvoxamine decrease carbamazepine metabolism. **Tacrolimus:** [P] Increased tacrolimus metabolism. **Theophylline:** [NE] Increased theophylline metabolism. **Troleandomycin:** [P] Decreased carbamazepine metabolism. **Verapamil:** [P] Decreased carbamazepine metabolism. *See also* Anticoagulants, oral; Antidepressants, tricyclic; Azole antifungals; Calcium channel blockers.
Chloramphenicol	Inhibits hepatic drug-metabolizing enzymes.	**Phenytoin:** [P] Decreased phenytoin metabolism. **Sulfonylurea hypoglycemics:** [P] Decreased sulfonylurea metabolism. *See also* Anticoagulants, oral.
Cimetidine	Inhibits hepatic microsomal drug-metabolizing enzymes. (Ranitidine, famotidine, and nizatidine do not appear to do so.) May inhibit the renal tubular secretion of weak bases. Purportedly reduces hepatic blood flow, thus reducing first-pass metabolism of highly extracted drugs. (However, the ability of cimetidine to affect hepatic blood flow has been disputed.)	**Benzodiazepines:** [P] Decreased metabolism of alprazolam, chlordiazepoxide, diazepam, halazepam, prazepam, and clorazepate but not oxazepam, lorazepam, or temazepam. **Carmustine:** [NE] Increased bone marrow suppression. **Ketoconazole:** [NE] Decreased gastrointestinal absorption of ketoconazole due to increased pH in gut; other H_2 blockers and proton pump inhibitors would be expected to have the same effect. **Itraconazole:** [NE] Decreased gastrointestinal absorption of itraconazole due to increased pH in gut; other H_2-receptor antagonists and proton pump inhibitors would be expected to have the same effect. **Lidocaine:** [P] Decreased metabolism of lidocaine; increased serum lidocaine. **Phenytoin:** [NE] Decreased phenytoin metabolism; increased serum phenytoin. **Procainamide:** [P] Decreased renal excretion of procainamide; increased serum procainamide levels. Similar effect with ranitidine but smaller. **Quinidine:** [P] Decreased metabolism of quinidine; increased serum quinidine levels. **Theophylline:** [P] Decreased theophylline metabolism; increased plasma theophylline. *See also* Anticoagulants, oral; Antidepressants, tricyclic; Beta-adrenoceptor blockers; Calcium channel blockers, Carbamazepine.

(continued)

Table II–1. Important drug interactions *(continued).*

HP = Highly predictable. Interaction occurs in almost all patients receiving the interacting combination.	
P = Predictable. Interaction occurs in most patients receiving the combination.	
NP = Not predictable. Interaction occurs only in some patients receiving the combination.	
NE = Not established. Insufficient data available on which to base estimate of predictability.	

Drug or Drug Group	Properties Promoting Drug Interaction	Clinically Documented Interactions
Cisapride	Susceptible to inhibition of metabolism by CYP3A4 inhibitors. High cisapride serum concentrations can result in ventricular arrhythmias.	**Clarithromycin:** [NP] Decreased metabolism of cisapride; possible ventricular arrhythmia. **Cyclosporine:** [NE] Decreased metabolism of cisapride; possible ventricular arrhythmia. **Erythromycin:** [NP] Decreased metabolism of cisapride; possible ventricular arrhythmia. **Fluconazole:** [NE] Decreased metabolism of cisapride; possible ventricular arrhythmia. **Itraconazole:** [NP] Decreased metabolism of cisapride; possible ventricular arrhythmia. **Ketoconazole:** [NP] Decreased metabolism of cisapride; possible ventricular arrhythmia. **Nefazodone:** [NP] Possible decreased metabolism of cisapride by CYP3A4; possible ventricular arrhythmia. **Ritonavir:** [NE] Decreased metabolism of cisapride; possible ventricular arrhythmia. **Selective serotonin reuptake inhibitors (SSRIs):** [NP] Fluvoxamine inhibits CYP3A4 and probably decreases cisapride metabolism; possible ventricular arrhythmia.
Cyclosporine	Metabolism inducible. Susceptible to inhibition of metabolism by CYP3A4. (Tacrolimus and sirolimus appear to have similar interactions.)	**Aminoglycosides:** [NE] Possible additive nephrotoxicity. **Amphotericin B:** [NE] Possible additive nephrotoxicity. **Androgens:** [NE] Increased serum cyclosporine. **Barbiturates:** [P] Increased cyclosporine metabolism. **Carbamazepine:** [P] Increased cyclosporine metabolism. **Clarithromycin:** [P] Decreased cyclosporine metabolism. **Diltiazem:** [NE] Decreased cyclosporine metabolism. **Erythromycin:** [NE] Decreased cyclosporine metabolism. **Lovastatin:** [NE] Myopathy and rhabdomyolysis noted in patients taking lovastatin and cyclosporine. **Nefazodone:** [P] Decreased cyclosporine metabolism. **Phenytoin:** [NE] Increased cyclosporine metabolism. **Pimozide:** [NE] Decreased pimozide metabolism. **Rifampin:** [P] Increased cyclosporine metabolism. **Ritonavir:** [P] Decreased cyclosporine metabolism. **St. John's wort:** [NE] Increased cyclosporine metabolism. **Verapamil:** [NE] Decreased cyclosporine metabolism. *See also* Azole antifungals, Barbiturates; Calcium channel blockers.
Digitalis glycosides	Digoxin susceptible to inhibition of gastrointestinal absorption. Digitalis toxicity may be increased by drug-induced electrolyte imbalance (eg, hypokalemia). Digitoxin metabolism inducible. Renal excretion of digoxin susceptible to inhibition.	*Drugs that may increase digitalis effect:* **Amiodarone:** [P] Reduced renal digoxin excretion leads to increased plasma digoxin concentrations. **Clarithromycin:** [NE] Reduced renal excretion of digoxin. **Diltiazem:** [P] Increased plasma digoxin (usually 20–30%) due to reduced renal and nonrenal clearance. **Erythromycin:** [NE] Reduced renal excretion of digoxin. **Itraconazole:** [NE] Reduced renal excretion of digoxin. **Potassium-depleting drugs:** [P] Increased likelihood of digitalis toxicity.

Table II–1. Important drug interactions *(continued)*.

HP = Highly predictable. Interaction occurs in almost all patients receiving the interacting combination.	
P = Predictable. Interaction occurs in most patients receiving the combination.	
NP = Not predictable. Interaction occurs only in some patients receiving the combination.	
NE = Not established. Insufficient data available on which to base estimate of predictability.	

Drug or Drug Group	Properties Promoting Drug Interaction	Clinically Documented Interactions
Digitalis glycosides *(continued)*	(See preceding page.)	**Propafenone:** [P] Increased plasma digoxin levels. **Quinidine:** [HP] Reduced digoxin excretion; displacement of digoxin from tissue binding sites; digitoxin may also be affected. **Spironolactone:** [NE] Decreased renal digoxin excretion and interference with some serum digoxin assays. **Verapamil:** [P] Increased plasma digoxin levels *Drugs that may decrease digitalis effect:* **Kaolin-pectin:** [P] Decreased gastrointestinal digoxin absorption. **Penicillamine:** [NE] Decreased plasma digoxin. **Rifampin:** [NE] Increased metabolism of digitoxin and possibly digoxin. **Sulfasalazine:** [NE] Decreased gastrointestinal digoxin absorption. *See also* Antacids; Azole antifungals; Bile acid-binding resins.
Disulfiram	Inhibits hepatic microsomal drug-metabolizing enzymes. Inhibits aldehyde dehydrogenase.	**Benzodiazepines:** [P] Decreased metabolism of chlordiazepoxide and diazepam but not lorazepam and oxazepam. **Metronidazole:** [NE] Confusion and psychoses reported in patients receiving this combination; mechanisms unknown. **Phenytoin:** [P] Decreased phenytoin metabolism. *See also* Alcohol; Anticoagulants, oral.
Estrogens	Metabolism inducible. Enterohepatic circulation of estrogen may be interrupted by alteration in bowel flora (eg, due to antibiotics).	**Ampicillin:** [NP] Interruption of enterohepatic circulation of estrogen; possible reduction in oral contraceptive efficacy. Some other oral antibiotics may have a similar effect. **Corticosteroids:** [P] Decreased metabolism of corticosteroids leading to increased corticosteroid effect. **Diazepam:** [NE] Decreased diazepam metabolism. **Griseofulvin:** [NE] Possible inhibition of oral contraceptive efficacy; mechanism unknown. **Phenytoin:** [NP] Increased estrogen metabolism; possible reduction in oral contraceptive efficacy. **Primidone:** [NP] Increased estrogen metabolism; possible reduction in oral contraceptive efficacy. **Rifabutin:** [NP] Increased estrogen metabolism; possible reduction in oral contraceptive efficacy. **Rifampin:** [NP] Increased estrogen metabolism; possible reduction in oral contraceptive efficacy. **St. John's wort:** [NE] Increased estrogen metabolism; possible reduction in oral contraceptive efficacy. *See also* Barbiturates; Carbamazepine.
HMG-CoA reductase inhibitors	Lovastatin, simvastatin, and, to a lesser extent, atorvastatin are susceptible to CYP3A4	**Clarithromycin:** [P] Decreased statin metabolism. **Clofibrate:** [NP] Increased risk of myopathy. **Diltiazem:** [NE] Decreased statin metabolism.

(continued)

Table II–1. Important drug interactions *(continued)*.

HP = Highly predictable. Interaction occurs in almost all patients receiving the interacting combination.
P = Predictable. Interaction occurs in most patients receiving the combination.
NP = Not predictable. Interaction occurs only in some patients receiving the combination.
NE = Not established. Insufficient data available on which to base estimate of predictability.

Drug or Drug Group	Properties Promoting Drug Interaction	Clinically Documented Interactions
HMG-CoA reductase inhibitors *(continued)*	inhibitors; lovastatin, simvastatin, and, to a lesser extent, atorvastatin are susceptible to CYP3A4 inducers; increased risk of additive myopathy risk with other drugs that can cause myopathy.	**Cyclosporine:** [P] Decreased statin metabolism. **Erythromycin:** [P] Decreased statin metabolism. **Gemfibrozil:** [NP] Increased plasma lovastatin and simvastatin. **Nefazodone:** [NE] Decreased statin metabolism. **Ritonavir:** [NE] Decreased statin metabolism. **Verapamil:** [NE] Decreased statin metabolism. *See also* Azole antifungals.
Iron	Binds with drugs in gastrointestinal tract, reducing absorption.	**Methyldopa:** [NE] Decreased methyldopa absorption. **Quinolones:** [P] Decreased absorption of ciprofloxacin. **Tetracyclines:** [P] Decreased absorption of tetracyclines; decreased efficacy of iron. **Thyroid hormones:** [P] Decreased thyroxine absorption. *See also* Antacids.
Levodopa	Levodopa degraded in gut prior to reaching sites of absorption. Agents that alter gastrointestinal motility may alter degree of intraluminal degradation. Antiparkinsonism effect of levodopa susceptible to inhibition by other drugs.	**Clonidine:** [NE] Inhibits antiparkinsonism effect. **Monoamine oxidase inhibitors:** [P] Hypertensive reaction (carbidopa prevents the interaction). **Papaverine:** [NE] Inhibits antiparkinsonism effect. **Phenothiazines:** [P] Inhibits antiparkinsonism effect. **Phenytoin:** [NE] Inhibits antiparkinsonism effect. **Pyridoxine:** [P] Inhibits antiparkinsonism effect (carbidopa prevents the interaction). *See also* Antimuscarinics.
Lithium	Renal lithium excretion sensitive to changes in sodium balance. (Sodium depletion tends to cause lithium retention.) Susceptible to drugs enhancing central nervous system lithium toxicity.	**ACE inhibitors:** [NE] Probable reduced renal clearance of lithium; increased lithium effect. **Angiotensin II receptor blockers:** [NE] Probable reduced renal clearance of lithium; increased lithium effect. **Diuretics (especially thiazides):** [P] Decreased excretion of lithium; furosemide may be less likely to produce this effect than thiazide diuretics. **Haloperidol:** [NP] Occasional cases of neurotoxicity in manic patients, especially with large doses of one or both drugs. **Methyldopa:** [NE] Increased likelihood of central nervous system lithium toxicity. **Nonsteroidal anti-inflammatory drugs:** [NE] Reduced renal lithium excretion (except sulindac and salicylates). **Theophylline:** [P] Increased renal excretion of lithium; reduced lithium effect.
Monoamine oxidase inhibitors (MAOIs)	Increased norepinephrine stored in adrenergic neuron. Displacement of these stores by other drugs may produce acute hypertensive response. MAOIs have intrinsic hypoglycemic activity.	**Anorexiants:** [P] Hypertensive episodes due to release of stored norepinephrine (benzphetamine, diethylpropion, mazindol, phendimetrazine, phentermine). **Antidiabetic agents:** [P] Additive hypoglycemic effect. **Buspirone:** [NE] Possible serotonin syndrome; avoid concurrent use. **Dextromethorphan:** [NE] Severe reactions (hyperpyrexia, coma, death) have been reported.

Table II–1. Important drug interactions *(continued).*

| HP = Highly predictable. Interaction occurs in almost all patients receiving the interacting combination. |
| P = Predictable. Interaction occurs in most patients receiving the combination. |
| NP = Not predictable. Interaction occurs only in some patients receiving the combination. |
| NE = Not established. Insufficient data available on which to base estimate of predictability. |

Drug or Drug Group	Properties Promoting Drug Interaction	Clinically Documented Interactions
Monoamine oxidase inhibitors (MAOIs) *(continued)*	(See preceding page.)	**Guanethidine:** [P] Reversal of the hypotensive action of guanethidine. **Mirtazapine:** [NE] Possible serotonin syndrome; avoid concurrent use. **Narcotic analgesics:** [NP] Some patients develop hypertension, rigidity, excitation; meperidine may be more likely to interact than morphine. **Nefazodone:** [NE] Possible serotonin syndrome; avoid concurrent use. **Phenylephrine:** [P] Hypertensive episode, since phenylephrine is metabolized by monoamine oxidase. **Selective serotonin reuptake inhibitors (SSRIs):** [P] Fatalities have occurred due to serotonin syndrome; SSRIs are contraindicated in patients taking MAOIs. **Sibutramine:** [NE] Possible serotonin syndrome; avoid concurrent use. **Sympathomimetics (indirect-acting):** [HP] Hypertensive episode due to release of stored norepinephrine (amphetamines, ephedrine, isometheptene, phenylpropanolamine, pseudoephedrine). **Tramadol:** [NE] Possible serotonin syndrome; avoid concurrent use. **Venlafaxine:** [NE] Possible serotonin syndrome; avoid concurrent use. *See also* Antidepressants, tricyclic and heterocyclic; Levodopa.
Nonsteroidal anti-inflammatory drugs	Prostaglandin inhibition may result in reduced renal sodium excretion, impaired resistance to hypertensive stimuli, and reduced renal lithium excretion. Most NSAIDs inhibit platelet function; may increase likelihood of bleeding due to other drugs that impair hemostasis. Most NSAIDs are highly bound to plasma proteins. Phenylbutazone may inhibit hepatic microsomal drug metabolism (also seems to act as enzyme inducer in some cases). Phenylbutazone may alter renal excretion of some drugs.	**ACE inhibitors:** [P] Decreased antihypertensive response. **Furosemide:** [P] Decreased diuretic, natriuretic, and antihypertensive response to furosemide. **Hydralazine:** [NE] Decreased antihypertensive response to hydralazine. **Methotrexate:** [NE] Possible increase in methotrexate toxicity (especially with anticancer doses of methotrexate). **Phenytoin:** [P] Decreased hepatic phenytoin metabolism. **Triamterene:** [NE] Decreased renal function noted with triamterene plus indomethacin in both healthy subjects and patients. *See also* Anticoagulants, oral; Beta-adrenoceptor blockers; Lithium.

(continued)

Table II–1. Important drug interactions *(continued).*

HP = Highly predictable. Interaction occurs in almost all patients receiving the interacting combination.		
P = Predictable. Interaction occurs in most patients receiving the combination.		
NP = Not predictable. Interaction occurs only in some patients receiving the combination.		
NE = Not established. Insufficient data available on which to base estimate of predictability.		

Drug or Drug Group	Properties Promoting Drug Interaction	Clinically Documented Interactions
Phenytoin	Induces hepatic microsomal drug metabolism. Susceptible to inhibition of metabolism by CYP2C9 and, to a lesser extent, CYP2C19.	*Drugs whose metabolism is stimulated by phenytoin:* **Corticosteroids:** [P] Decreased serum corticosteroid levels. **Doxycycline:** [P] Decreased serum doxycycline levels. **Methadone:** [P] Decreased serum methadone levels; withdrawal symptoms. **Mexiletine:** [NE] Decreased serum mexiletine levels. **Quinidine:** [P] Decreased serum quinidine levels. **Theophylline:** [NE] Decreased serum theophylline levels. **Verapamil:** [NE] Decreased serum verapamil levels. *See also* Calcium channel blockers, Cyclosporine, Estrogens. *Drugs that inhibit phenytoin metabolism:* **Amiodarone:** [P] Increased serum phenytoin; possible reduction in serum amiodarone. **Capecitabine:** [NE] Increased serum phenytoin. **Chloramphenicol:** [P] Increased serum phenytoin. **Felbamate:** [P] Increased serum phenytoin. **Fluorouracil:** [NE] Increased serum phenytoin. **Fluvoxamine:** [NE] Increased serum phenytoin. **Isoniazid:** [NP] Increased serum phenytoin; problem primarily with slow acetylators of isoniazid. **Miconazole:** [P] Increased serum phenytoin. **Ticlopidine:** [NP] Increased serum phenytoin. *See also* Cimetidine; Disulfiram; Phenylbutazone. *Drugs that enhance phenytoin metabolism:* **Rifampin:** [P] Decreased serum phenytoin levels.
Pimozide	Susceptible to CYP3A4 inhibitors; may exhibit additive effects with other agents that prolong QT$_c$ interval.	**Clarithromycin:** [NE] Decreased pimozide metabolism. **Erythromycin:** [NE] Decreased pimozide metabolism **Nefazodone:** [NE] Decreased pimozide metabolism. *See also* Azole antifungals, Cyclosporine.
Potassium-sparing diuretics (amiloride, spironolactone, triamterene)	Additive effects with other agents increasing serum potassium concentration. May alter renal excretion of substances other than potassium (eg, digoxin, hydrogen ions).	**ACE inhibitors:** [NE] Additive hyperkalemic effect. **Potassium supplements:** [P] Additive hyperkalemic effect; especially a problem in presence of renal impairment. *See also* Digitalis glycosides; Nonsteroidal anti-inflammatory drugs.
Probenecid	Interference with renal excretion of drugs that undergo active tubular secretion, especially weak	**Clofibrate:** [P] Reduced glucuronide conjugation of clofibric acid. **Methotrexate:** [P] Decreased renal methotrexate excretion; possible methotrexate toxicity.

Table II–1. Important drug interactions *(continued).*

Drug or Drug Group	Properties Promoting Drug Interaction	Clinically Documented Interactions
Probenecid *(continued)*	acids. Inhibition of glucuronide conjugation of other drugs.	**Penicillin:** [P] Decreased renal penicillin excretion. **Salicylates:** [P] Decreased uricosuric effect of probenecid (interaction unlikely with less than 1.5 g of salicylate daily).
Quinidine	Metabolism inducible. Inhibits CYP2D6. Renal excretion susceptible to changes in urine pH. Additive effects with other agents that prolong the QT_c interval.	**Acetazolamide:** [P] Decreased renal quinidine excretion due to increased urinary pH; elevated serum quinidine. **Amiodarone:** [NF] Increased serum quinidine levels; mechanism not established. **Kaolin-pectin:** [NE] Decreased gastrointestinal absorption of quinidine. **Rifampin:** [P] Increased hepatic quinidine metabolism. **Thioridazine:** [NE] Decreased thioridazine metabolism; additive prolongation of QT_c interval. *See also* Anticoagulants, oral; Antidepressants, tricyclic; Barbiturates; Cimetidine; Digitalis glycosides; Phenytoin.
Quinolone antibiotics	Susceptible to inhibition of gastrointestinal absorption. Some quinolones inhibit CYP1A2.	**Caffeine:** [P] Ciprofloxacin, enoxacin, pipedemic acid, and to a lesser extent, norfloxacin, inhibit caffeine metabolism. **Sucralfate:** [HP] Reduced gastrointestinal absorption of ciprofloxacin, norfloxacin, and probably other quinolones. **Theophylline:** [P] Ciprofloxacin, enoxacin, and, to a lesser extent, norfloxacin inhibit theophylline metabolism; gatifloxacin, levofloxacin, lomefloxacin, ofloxacin, and sparfloxacin appear to have little effect. *See also* Antacids; Anticoagulants, oral.
Rifampin	Induction of hepatic microsomal drug-metabolizing enzymes.	**Corticosteroids:** [P] Increased corticosteroid hepatic metabolism; reduced corticosteroid effect. **Mexiletine:** [NE] Increased mexiletine metabolism; reduced mexiletine effect. **Sulfonylurea hypoglycemics:** [P] Increased hepatic metabolism of tolbutamide and probably other sulfonylureas metabolized by the liver (including chlorpropamide). **Theophylline:** [P] Increased theophylline metabolism; reduced theophylline effect. *See also* Anticoagulants, oral; Azole antifungals; Beta-adrenoceptor blockers; Calcium channel blockers; Cyclosporine; Digitalis glycosides; Estrogens.
Salicylates	Interference with renal excretion of drugs that undergo active tubular secretion. Salicylate renal excretion dependent on urinary pH when large doses of	**Carbonic anhydrase inhibitors:** [NE] Increased acetazolamide serum concentrations; increased salicylate toxicity due to decreased blood pH. **Corticosteroids:** [P] Increased salicylate elimination; possible additive toxic effect on gastric mucosa.

(continued)

Table II–1. Important drug interactions *(continued).*

> **HP** = Highly predictable. Interaction occurs in almost all patients receiving the interacting combination.
> **P** = Predictable. Interaction occurs in most patients receiving the combination.
> **NP** = Not predictable. Interaction occurs only in some patients receiving the combination.
> **NE** = Not established. Insufficient data available on which to base estimate of predictability.

Drug or Drug Group	Properties Promoting Drug Interaction	Clinically Documented Interactions
Salicylates *(continued)*	salicylate used. Aspirin (but not other salicylates) interferes with platelet function. Large doses of salicylates have intrinsic hypoglycemic activity. Salicylates may displace drugs from plasma protein binding sites.	**Heparin:** [NE] Increased bleeding tendency with aspirin, but probably not with other salicylates. **Methotrexate:** [P] Decreased renal methotrexate clearance; increased methotrexate toxicity (primarily at anticancer doses). **Sulfinpyrazone:** [HP] Decreased uricosuric effect of sulfinpyrazone (interaction unlikely with less than 1.5 g of salicylate daily). *See also* Antacids; Anticoagulants, oral; Probenecid.
Theophylline	Susceptible to inhibition of hepatic metabolism by CYP1A2. Metabolism inducible.	**Benzodiazepines:** [NE] Inhibition of benzodiazepine sedation. **Diltiazem:** [P] Decreased theophylline metabolism by CYP1A3. **Clarithromycin:** [NE] Decreased theophylline metabolism. **Erythromycin:** [P] Decreased theophylline metabolism. **Fluvoxamine:** [P] Decreased theophylline metabolism. **Smoking:** [HP] Increased theophylline metabolism. **Tacrine:** [P] Decreased theophylline metabolism. **Ticlopidine:** [NE] Decreased theophylline metabolism. **Troleandomycin:** [P] Decreased theophylline metabolism. **Verapamil:** [P] Decreased theophylline metabolism. **Zileuton:** [P] Decreased theophylline metabolism. *See also* Barbiturates; Carbamazepine; Cimetidine; Lithium; Phenytoin; Quinolones; Rifampin.

REFERENCES

Abebe W: Herbal medication: potential for adverse interactions with analgesic drugs. J Clin Pharm Ther 2002;27:391.

Asberg A: Interactions between cyclosporin and lipid-lowering drugs: implications for organ transplant recipients. Drugs. 2003;63:367.

Bergendal L, Fribert A, Schaffrath A: Potential drug-drug interactions in 5125 mostly elderly out-patients in Gothenburg, Sweden. Pharm World Sci 1995;17:152.

Bertz RJ, Granneman GR: Use of in vitro and in vivo data to estimate the likelihood of metabolic pharmacokinetic interactions. Clin Pharmacokinet 1997;32:210.

deMaat MM et al: Drug interactions between antiretroviral drugs and comedicated agents. Clin Pharmacokinet 2003;42:223.

Doucet J et al: Drug-drug interactions related to hospital admissions in older adults: A prospective study of 1000 patients. J Am Geriatr Soc 1996;44:944.

Hansten PD: Understanding drug interactions. Science & Medicine 1998;5:16.

Hansten PD, Horn JR: *Drug Interactions, Analysis and Management.* Facts & Comparisons. [Quarterly.]

Hansten PD, Horn JR: *The Top 100 Drug Interactions. A Guide to Patient Management.* H&H Publications, 2003.

Juurlink DN et al: Drug-drug interactions among elderly patients hospitalized for drug toxicity. JAMA 2003;289:1652.

Kim RB (editor): *The Medical Letter Handbook of Adverse Interactions.* Medical Letter, 2003.

Levy RH et al (editors): *Metabolic Drug Interactions.* Lippincott Williams & Wilkins, 2000.

Lin JH, Yamazaki M: Role of P-glycoprotein in pharmacokinetics: clinical implications. Clin Pharmacokinet 2003;42:59.

Quinn DI, Day RO: Drug interactions of clinical importance: An updated guide. Drug Saf 1995;12:393.

Riesenman C: Antidepressant drug interactions and the cytochrome P450 system: A critical appraisal. Pharmacotherapy 1995;15:84S.

Tatro DS (editor): *Drug Interaction Facts.* Facts & Comparisons. [Quarterly.]

Index

Note: Page numbers in boldface type indicate major discussions. A *t* following a page number indicates tabular material and an *i* following a page number indicates an illustration. Most drugs are listed under their generic names. Insofar as possible, when a drug trade name is listed, page numbers are for preparations available. For further detail, refer to the generic name provided.